KT-363-387

Davidson's
Principles and Practice of
Medicine

21st Edition

The Editors

Nicki R. Colledge BSc FRCP(Ed)
Consultant Geriatrician, Liberton Hospital, Edinburgh,
and Royal Infirmary of Edinburgh;
Honorary Senior Lecturer in Geriatric Medicine,
University of Edinburgh

Brian R. Walker BSc MD FRCP(Ed)
Professor of Endocrinology, University of Edinburgh;
Honorary Consultant Physician, Royal Infirmary of Edinburgh

Stuart H. Ralston MD FRCP FMedSci FRSE
ARC Professor of Rheumatology, University of Edinburgh;
Honorary Consultant Rheumatologist, Western General Hospital, Edinburgh

Illustrated by *Robert Britton*

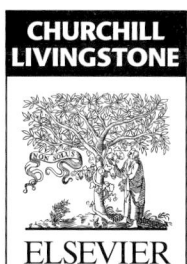

CHURCHILL
LIVINGSTONE

ELSEVIER

Edinburgh   London   New York   Oxford   Philadelphia   St Louis   Sydney   Toronto   2010

CHURCHILL
LIVINGSTONE
ELSEVIER

An imprint of Elsevier Limited
© 2010, Elsevier Limited. All rights reserved.

No part of this publication may be reproduced or transmitted in any form or by any means, electronic or mechanical, including photocopying, recording, or any information storage and retrieval system, without permission in writing from the publisher. Permissions may be sought directly from Elsevier's Rights Department: phone: (+1) 215 239 3804 (US) or (+44) 1865 843830 (UK); fax: (+44) 1865 853333; e-mail: healthpermissions@elsevier.com. You may also complete your request online via the Elsevier website at http://www.elsevier.com/permissions.

First edition 1952
Second edition 1954
Third edition 1956
Fourth edition 1958
Fifth edition 1960
Sixth edition 1962
Seventh edition 1964
Eighth edition 1966
Ninth edition 1968
Tenth edition 1971
Eleventh edition 1974

Twelfth edition 1977
Thirteenth edition 1981
Fourteenth edition 1984
Fifteenth edition 1987
Sixteenth edition 1991
Seventeenth edition 1995
Eighteenth edition 1999
Nineteenth edition 2002
Twentieth edition 2006
Twenty-first edition 2010

Main Edition
ISBN-13: 978-0-7020-3085-7
   Reprinted 2011
International Edition
ISBN-13: 978-0-7020-3084-0
   Reprinted 2010

British Library Cataloguing in Publication Data
A catalogue record for this book is available from the British Library

Library of Congress Cataloging in Publication Data
A catalog record for this book is available from the Library of Congress

Notice
Knowledge and best practice in this field are constantly changing. As new research and experience broaden our knowledge, changes in practice, treatment and drug therapy may become necessary or appropriate. Readers are advised to check the most current information provided (i) on procedures featured or (ii) by the manufacturer of each product to be administered, to verify the recommended dose or formula, the method and duration of administration, and contraindications. It is the responsibility of the practitioner, relying on their own experience and knowledge of the patient, to make diagnoses, to determine dosages and the best treatment for each individual patient, and to take all appropriate safety precautions. To the fullest extent of the law, neither the Publisher nor the Editors assume any liability for any injury and/or damage to persons or property arising out of or related to any use of the material contained in this book.

The Publisher

ELSEVIER your source for books,
journals and multimedia
in the health sciences
www.elsevierhealth.com

Working together to grow
libraries in developing countries

www.elsevier.com | www.bookaid.org | www.sabre.org

ELSEVIER   BOOK AID International   Sabre Foundation

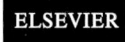

The
Publisher's
policy is to use
**paper manufactured
from sustainable forests**

Printed in China

Contents

Preface

Since *Davidson's Principles and Practice of Medicine* was first published in 1952, over two million copies have been sold and the book has acquired a large following of medical students, doctors and other health professionals all over the world. It has been translated into many languages, most recently Russian and Polish, and has won numerous prizes, the last edition receiving an award from the Society of Authors and the Royal Society of Medicine. *Davidson's* has endured because with each new edition it has evolved to provide comprehensive updated information in a format suitable for its contemporary readership, and yet it has remained concise and easy to read. This 21st Edition has been extensively updated and revised, but has not increased in length or size.

Since its beginnings, *Davidson's* has sought to explain the basis for medical practice. The integration of 'preclinical' science with clinical practice is now a feature of many undergraduate medical curricula, and many students use *Davidson's* from the outset of their medical course. In recognition of this, the first part of the book, 'Principles of Medicine', highlights the mechanisms of health and disease, along with the professional and ethical principles underlying medical practice. Many examples of clinical problems are included to bring the medical sciences to life for the new student and to rejuvenate the interest of the experienced clinician. The second part of the book, 'Practice of Medicine', covers the major medical specialties. Every chapter has been rewritten for this edition to ensure that it reflects the 'cutting edge' of medical knowledge and practice, pitched at a level of detail to meet the needs of candidates preparing for examination for Membership of the Royal College of Physicians or its equivalent.

Many of the innovations introduced in recent editions have been warmly received. We have retained the ever-popular 'Clinical Examination' overview pages and the patient-orientated approach in the 'Presenting Problems' sections, while enhancing the book's practical content with a new series of 'Emergency' and 'Practice Point' boxes. Embedding horizontal themes within the book—for example, with the 'In Old Age' boxes—has been applauded, and we have extended this approach by adding 'In Pregnancy' boxes in relevant chapters. The inclusion of both SI and non-SI units in the last edition proved popular and has been maintained.

We are proud of *Davidson's* international heritage. As well as recruiting authors from around the globe, particularly for topics such as Infectious Diseases and Envenoming, we have welcomed new members on to our International Advisory Board. These leading experts provide detailed comments that, along with the feedback received from our global readership, are crucial to our planning of every chapter in each new edition. In 2006, we had the privilege of visiting several medical schools on the Indian subcontinent and were delighted with the enthusiasm of the students and teachers that we met, and the very useful criticisms and feedback they provided. We have tried to address as many of these as possible in this edition.

Education is achieved by assimilating information from many sources and we are delighted that readers of this book can enhance their learning experience using complementary resources. The StudentConsult platform continues to provide online access to the text and illustrations of the main edition. *Davidson's* has had a long-standing association with its sister books, *Macleod's Clinical Examination* (now in its 12th Edition) and *Principles and Practice of Surgery* (now in its 5th Edition). The *Davidson's* 'family' has now expanded with the publication of *Essential Davidson's*, a long-requested pocket-size version of the main text; *Davidson's Foundations of Clinical Practice*, an indispensable guide to starting work as a junior doctor; and *Davidson's Clinical Cases*, which contains over 90 cases based on the 'Presenting Problems' in the main text. We congratulate the editors and authors of these books for continuing the tradition of concise, easily read and beautifully illustrated text.

The regular introduction of new authors and editors to *Davidson's* is important to maintain the freshness of each new edition. On this occasion, Professor Stuart Ralston has joined the editorial team and 14 new authors have contributed material. We all take immense pride in producing an outstanding book for the next generation of doctors, and in continuing the great tradition first established by Sir Stanley Davidson and passed on by all the previous editors and authors, for what remains one of the world's leading textbooks of medicine.

NRC, BRW, SHR
Edinburgh 2010

The *Davidson* family of textbooks

Medical learning is a life-long process that is facilitated by many different tools. *Davidson's Principles and Practice of Medicine* has stood the test of time because it provides an overview that is both comprehensive and concise. Its long-standing partner textbooks, *Macleod's Clinical Examination* and *Principles and Practice of Surgery*, share a similar ethos. To add value for readers of *Davidson's*, its highly successful style has now been employed in a 'family' of new companion books. These complement the main textbook, both by presenting its material in different formats to enhance learning, and by including supplementary material that could not be accommodated in the main edition.

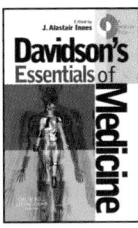

Davidson's Essentials of Medicine is a 'handbook' version of *Davidson's Principles and Practice of Medicine*, helping those who need portable information to study while on the move—whether commuting between training sites, or during remote attachments and electives. It also serves as a condensed revision aid. Every effort has been made to maximise readability and avoid dry and unmemorable lists. The text presents the essential elements in a structured format, key *Davidson's* illustrations are adapted and retained, and several new 'added value' sections have been included: Major Investigations describes key diagnostic tests; Therapeutics describes the clinical use of common drugs; and typical OSCE scenarios are included to help the reader to prepare for this examination format.

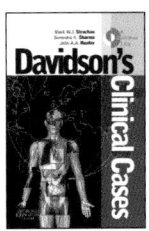

In the real world, patients do not present with a specific disease; instead they come with problems that might involve many systems, and the primary pathology may not be at all clear. In recognition of this, *Davidson's Clinical Cases* has been written by an impressive international group of physicians with wide clinical experience. This book guides the reader step by step to find the correct path in the maze between a patient's presenting complaint and the final diagnosis. The selection of cases is closely based on the 'Presenting Problems' of *Davidson's Principles and Practice of Medicine* and includes illnesses that reflect an international outlook.

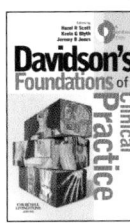

For those just qualified and starting out on their initial years of hospital training, *Davidson's Foundations of Clinical Practice* provides key guidance on how to manage the practicalities of working life. The emphasis is on acute rather than chronic symptom presentation and management in a wide range of disci-

plines. It also provides an invaluable step-by-step guide to undertaking a range of core clinical procedures, along with an insight into the non-clinical aspects of managing a medical career. Much of the text is written by junior doctors, and so provides a real view of what it is like to work as a trainee hospital doctor today.

Davidson's is also closely linked to its two sister titles, *Macleod's Clinical Examination* and *Principles and Practice of Surgery*.

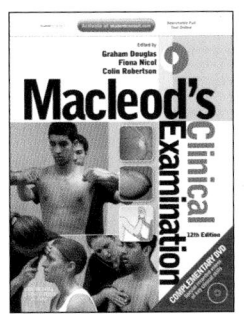
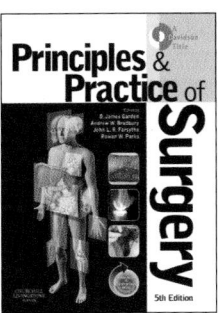

Also available on StudentCONSULT

Davidson's 500 'Best of Five' self-testing questions

Single best answer questions are now widely used for examination purposes as a reliable and discriminatory test of the factual knowledge necessary for good medical practice. To help to consolidate this knowledge, 500 questions based on the content of this edition of *Davidson's* are available at:

www.studentconsult.com/Gopaperless/ davidsonsquestionbank.cfm

The questions concentrate on those topics which are of greatest importance in passing examinations, especially evidence-based medicine. The detailed answers help clarify why a particular answer is right or wrong and are linked to selected portions of the main textbook for in-depth exploration of a specific topic. The questions are suitable for all levels, and range in difficulty from core knowledge to more advanced topics.

Contributors

Albiruni Ryan Abdul Razak
MRCPI
Clinical Research Associate and Honorary Specialist
Registrar, Northern Centre for Cancer Care, Freeman
Hospital, Newcastle upon Tyne, UK

Chris Allen
MA MD FRCP
Consultant Neurologist, Addenbrooke's Hospital,
Cambridge; Associate Lecturer, School of Clinical
Medicine, University of Cambridge, UK

Brian J. Angus
BSc DTM&H FRCP MD FFTM(Glas)
Reader in Infectious Diseases, Nuffield Department
of Medicine, University of Oxford; Director, Oxford
Centre for Tropical Medicine, UK

Jeffrey K. Aronson
MA DPhil MBChB FRCP FBPharmacolS FFPM (Hon)
Reader in Clinical Pharmacology and Consultant
Physician, University of Oxford, UK

Andrew W. Bradbury
BSc MBChB (Hons) MBA MD FRCSEd
Sampson Gamgee Professor of Vascular Surgery and
Director of Quality Assurance and Enhancement,
College of Medical and Dental Sciences, University of
Birmingham; Consultant Vascular and Endovascular
Surgeon, Heart of England NHS Foundation Trust,
Birmingham, UK

Leslie Burnett
MB BS PhD DBA FRCPA MAACB FHGSA
Clinical Professor in Pathology, Sydney Medical
School, University of Sydney; Director and Chief
Executive, Pathology North, Royal North Shore
Hospital, Sydney, Australia

Mark Byers
MSc MRCGP MCEM MFSEM
Senior Medical Officer, Army Medical
Directorate, Camberley, UK

Nicki Colledge
BSc FRCP(Ed)
Consultant Geriatrician, Liberton Hospital, Edinburgh
and Royal Infirmary of Edinburgh; Honorary
Senior Lecturer in Geriatric Medicine, University of
Edinburgh, UK

Jane D. Collier
MD FRCP
Consultant Hepatologist, John Radcliffe Hospital,
Oxford; Honorary Senior Lecturer in Hepatology,
University of Oxford, UK

Jenny I.O. Craig
MD FRCP(Ed) FRCPath
Consultant Haematologist, Addenbrooke's Hospital,
Cambridge, UK

Allan D. Cumming
BSc MBChB MD FRCP(Ed) FRCP(Lond)
Consultant Nephrologist, Royal Infirmary of
Edinburgh; Professor of Medical Education,
University of Edinburgh, UK

Graham G. Dark
MBBS FRCP FHEA
Senior Lecturer in Medical Oncology and Cancer
Education, Newcastle University, Northern Centre
for Cancer Care, Freeman Hospital, Newcastle upon
Tyne, UK

Martin Dennis
MD FRCP(Ed)
Professor of Stroke Medicine, University of
Edinburgh, UK

David H. Dockrell
MD FRCPI FRCP FACP
Professor of Infectious Diseases, University of
Sheffield, UK

Michael Doherty
MA MD FRCP
Professor of Rheumatology, University of
Nottingham, UK

Michael John Field
MD BS BSc FRACP
Professor of Medicine, University of Sydney;
Associate Dean and Head, Northern Clinical School,
Royal North Shore Hospital, Sydney, Australia

Miles Fisher
MD FRCP(Glas) FRCP(Ed)
Consultant Physician, Glasgow Royal Infirmary;
Honorary Professor, University of
Glasgow, UK

David R. FitzPatrick
MD FRCP(Ed)
Professor and Consultant in Clinical Genetics, MRC
Human Genetics Unit, Edinburgh, UK

Brian M. Frier
BSc(Hons) MD FRCP(Ed) FRCP(Glas)
Consultant Physician, Royal Infirmary of Edinburgh;
Honorary Professor of Diabetes, University of
Edinburgh, UK

Jane Goddard
PhD FRCP(Ed)
Consultant Nephrologist, Royal Infirmary of
Edinburgh; Senior Lecturer, University of
Edinburgh, UK

Ian S. Grant
FRCP(Ed) FFARCSI
Consultant in Intensive Care Medicine and
Anaesthesia,Western General Hospital,
Edinburgh, UK

Neil Robert Grubb
MD MRCP
Consultant Cardiologist, Royal Infirmary of
Edinburgh; Honorary Senior Lecturer, University of
Edinburgh, UK

Phil Hanlon
BSc MD MRCGP FRCP FFPH MPH
Professor of Public Health, University of Glasgow, UK

Richard P. Hobson
PhD MRCP(UK) FRCPath
Senior Lecturer, University of Leeds; Honorary
Consultant Microbiologist, Leeds Teaching Hospitals
NHS Trust, UK

J. Alastair Innes
PhD FRCP(Ed)
Consultant Physician and Honorary Reader in
Respiratory Medicine, Western General Hospital,
Edinburgh, UK

Stephen M. Lawrie
MD(Hons) FRCPsych HonFRCP(Ed)
Professor of Psychiatry and Neuro-Imaging,
University of Edinburgh; Honorary Consultant
Psychiatrist, Royal Edinburgh Hospital,
Edinburgh, UK

Christian J. Lueck
PhD FRCP FRACP
Senior Staff Neurologist, The Canberra Hospital,
Canberra; Associate Professor, Australian National
University Medical School, Canberra, Australia

D.B.L. McClelland
PhD (Leiden) FRCP FRCPath
Former Strategy Director, Scottish National
Blood Transfusion Service, Edinburgh, UK

Helen Macdonald
BSc PhD
Senior Lecturer in Nutrition and Translational
Musculoskeletal Science, University of Aberdeen, UK

Sara E. Marshall
FRCP(Ed) FRCPath PhD
Professor of Clinical Immunology, University of
Dundee, UK

David E. Newby
DM PhD DSc FRCP FRSE
BHF Professor of Cardiology, University of
Edinburgh, UK

Graham R. Nimmo
MD FRCP FFARCSI
Consultant Physician in Intensive Care Medicine
and Clinical Education, Western General Hospital,
Edinburgh, UK

Simon I.R. Noble
MBBS FRCP Dip Pall MEd PGCE
Clinical Senior Lecturer in Palliative Medicine,
Cardiff University; Honorary Consultant in Palliative
Medicine, Royal Gwent Hospital, Newport, UK

David R. Oxenham
MRCP FAChPM
Consultant in Palliative Care, Marie Curie Hospice,
Edinburgh, UK

Kelvin R. Palmer
MD FRCP(Ed) FRCP(Lond) FRCSE
Consultant Gastroenterologist, Western General
Hospital, Edinburgh, UK

Ian D. Penman
BSc MD FRCP(Ed)
Consultant Gastroenterologist, Western General
Hospital, Edinburgh, UK

Stuart H. Ralston
MD FRCP FMedSci FRSE
ARC Professor of Rheumatology, University of
Edinburgh; Honorary Consultant Rheumatologist,
Western General Hospital, Edinburgh, UK

Jonathan L. Rees
BMedSci FRCP FRCPE FMedSci
Grant Chair of Dermatology, University of
Edinburgh, UK

Peter T. Reid
MD FRCP(Ed)
Consultant Physician and Honorary Senior Lecturer,
Western General Hospital, Edinburgh, UK

Olivia M.V. Schofield
FRCP(Ed)
Consultant Dermatologist, Royal Infirmary of
Edinburgh, UK

x

Gordon R. Scott
BSc FRCP
Consultant in Genitourinary Medicine, Royal
Infirmary of Edinburgh, UK

Jonathan R. Seckl
FRCP(Ed) FMedSci FRSE
Moncrieff-Arnott Professor of Molecular Medicine
and Director of Research, College of Medicine and
Veterinary Medicine, University of Edinburgh, UK

Michael C. Sharpe
MA MD FRCP FRCP(Ed) FRCPsych
Professor of Psychological Medicine, Psychological
Medicine Research, University of Edinburgh, UK

Laurence H. Stewart
MD FRCS(Ed) FRCS(Urol)
Consultant Urological Surgeon, Western General
Hospital, Edinburgh, UK

Peter Stewart
FRACP FRCPA
Director of Pathology, Sydney South West Area Health
Service, Sydney; Associate Professor, University of
Sydney, Australia

Mark W.J. Strachan
BSc(Hons) MD FRCP(Ed)
Consultant Physician, Western General Hospital,
Edinburgh; Part-Time Senior Lecturer, University of
Edinburgh, UK

David R. Sullivan
MBBS FRACP FRCPA
Clinical Associate Professor, University of Sydney,
Australia

Shyam Sundar
MD FRCP FNA
Professor of Medicine, Institute of Medical Sciences,
Banaras Hindu University, Varanasi, India

Simon H.L. Thomas
BSc MD FRCP
Professor of Clinical Pharmacology and Therapeutics,
Newcastle University; Consultant Physician,
Newcastle Hospitals NHS Foundation Trust, UK

Neil Turner
PhD FRCP
Professor of Nephrology, University of Edinburgh;
Honorary Consultant Nephrologist, Royal Infirmary
of Edinburgh, UK

Brian R. Walker
BSc MD FRCP(Ed)
Professor of Endocrinology, University of Edinburgh;
Honorary Consultant Physician, Royal Infirmary of
Edinburgh, UK

Simon R. Walker
MA DM FRCPath
Senior Lecturer and Honorary Consultant in Clinical
Biochemistry, University of Edinburgh, UK

Henry G. Watson
MD FRCP FRCPath
Consultant Haematologist, Aberdeen Royal
Infirmary, UK

George Webster
BSc MD FRCP
Consultant Gastroenterologist/Hepatologist,
University College London Hospitals, UK

Julian White
MBBS MD FACTM
Consultant Clinical Toxinologist and Head of
Toxinology, Women's and Children's Hospital,
Adelaide; Associate Professor, Department of
Paediatrics, University of Adelaide, Australia

Ed Wilkins
FRCP FRCPath
Consultant Physician in Infectious Diseases,
North Manchester General Hospital, UK

International Advisory Board

xii

Professor Tofayel Ahmed
Chairman, Governing Body Ibrahim Medical College, Dhaka; Professor of Medicine, Pioneer Dental College, Dhaka, Bangladesh

Dr Samar Banerjee
Professor, Department of Medicine, Vivekananda Institute of Medical Sciences and Ramkrishna Mission Seva Pratisthan, Kolkata, India

Professor Jan D. Bos
Professor and Chairman, Department of Dermatology, Academic Medical Centre, University of Amsterdam, Netherlands

Professor M.A. Brown
Professor of Immunogenetics, Diamantina Institute of Cancer, Immunology and Metabolic Medicine, Princess Alexandra Hospital, University of Queensland, Brisbane, Australia

Professor Y.-C. Chee
Assistant Chief Executive Officer (Clinical), National Healthcare Group, and Senior Physician, Department of General Medicine, Tan Tock Seng Hospital, Singapore

Dr M.K. Daga
Professor of Medicine and In-charge ICU, Maulana Azad Medical College, New Delhi, India

Dr D. Dalus
Professor of Internal Medicine, Medical College and Hospital, Trivandrum, India

Dr Tapas Das
Professor and Head, Department of Medicine, Institute of Post-graduate Medical Education and Research, and SSKM Hospital, Kolkata, India

Professor Md. Abul Faiz
Professor of Medicine, Sir Salimullah Medical College, Mitford, Dhaka, Bangladesh

Professor A.G. Frauman
Professor of Clinical Pharmacology & Therapeutics, University of Melbourne and Medical Director, Austin Centre for Clinical Studies, Austin Health, Heidelberg, Victoria, Australia

Professor H.A. Goubran
Professor of Medicine and Haematology, Faculty of Medicine, Cairo University, Egypt

Professor Saman B. Gunatilake
Professor of Medicine, Faculty of Medical Sciences, University of Sri Jayawardenepura, Sri Lanka

Dr R. Gupta
Associate Professor of Medicine, All India Institute of Medical Sciences, New Delhi, India

Dr S.M. Wasim Jafri
Alticharan Professor of Medicine, Associate Dean, Aga Khan University, Karachi, Pakistan

Dr A.L. Kakrani
Professor and Head of Department of Medicine, Dr D.Y. Patil Medical College and Hospital, Pimpri, Pune, India

Dr V. Kamath
Professor and Head, Department of Medicine, Victoria Hospital, Bangalore Medical College and Research Institute, India

Professor Piotr Kuna
Professor of Medicine, Department of Internal Medicine, Asthma and Allergy, Medical University of Lodz, Poland

Professor Gary Maartens
Division of Clinical Pharmacology, Department of Medicine, University of Cape Town, South Africa

Professor W.F. Mollentze
Head of Internal Medicine, University of the Free State, Bloemfontein, South Africa

Professor Ammar F. Mubaidin
Associate Professor of Neurology, King Hussein Medical Center, Amman, Jordan

Dr Milind Nadkar
Professor of Medicine (Emergency Medicine) and Chief, Rheumatology Services, Seth G S Medical College and KEM Hospital, Mumbai, India

Dr Prem Pais
Dean and Professor of Medicine, St John's Medical College, Bangalore, India

Professor A. Ramachandran
President, India Research Foundation and Chairman, Dr A. Ramachandran's Diabetes Hospitals, Chennai, India

Dr Medha Y. Rao
Professor and Head of Department, Department of Medicine, MS Ramaiah Medical College, Bangalore, India

Dr (Mrs) H.R. Salkar
Professor and Head of Medicine, NKP Salve Institute of Medical Science, Nagpur, India

Dr K.R. Sethuraman
Deputy VC (Academics) and Faculty Dean of Medicine, AIMST University, Malaysia

Dr Surendra K. Sharma
Chief, Division of Pulmonary and Critical Care Medicine; Professor and Head, Department of Medicine, All India Institute of Medical Sciences, New Delhi, India

Professor Ibrahim Sherif
Professor of Medicine and Programs Director, The Libyan Board for Medical Specialties, Tripoli, Libya

Professor Ian J Simpson
Emeritus Professor of Medicine, Faculty of Medical and Health Sciences, University of Auckland and Nephrologist, Auckland City Hospital, Auckland, New Zealand

Professor Dato' Tahir Azhar
Dean, Faculty of Medicine, International Islamic University Malaysia, Malaysia

Professor C.F. Van der Merwe
Professor and Head of Department of Gastroenterology, University of Limpopo, South Africa

Dr S. Varma
Professor and Head of Department of Internal Medicine, Postgraduate Institute of Medical Education and Research, Chandigarh, India

Dr G.A. Wittert
Professor of Medicine and Head, School of Medicine, University of Adelaide; Senior Consultant Endocrinologist, Royal Adelaide Hospital, Australia

Dr M.E. Yeolekar
Director-Professor, University Department of Tribal Health, Maharashtra University of Health Sciences, Regional Centre, GMC Campus, Nagpur, India

Introduction

The first section of the book, 'Principles of Medicine', describes the basis on which medicine is practised and the fundamental mechanisms determining health and disease which are relevant to all medical specialties. The second section, 'Practice of Medicine', is devoted to individual medical specialties. Each chapter has been written by experts in the field to provide the level of detail expected of young trainees in their discipline. However, to maintain the book's virtue of being concise, care has been taken to avoid unnecessary duplication between chapters.

The system-based chapters follow a standard format, beginning with an overview of relevant clinical examination, followed by an account of functional anatomy, physiology and investigations, then the common presentations of disease, and finishing with details of the individual diseases and treatments of that system. Where appropriate, the chapters in the first section follow a similar format; the introduction of a problem-based approach in chapters which describe the immunological, cellular and molecular basis of disease brings the close links between modern medical science and clinical practice into sharp focus.

The methods used to present information throughout the book are described below.

Clinical examination overviews

The value of good clinical skills is highlighted by a two-page overview of the important elements of the clinical examination at the beginning of most chapters. The left-hand page of these sections includes a manikin to illustrate the key steps in the examination of the relevant system, beginning with simple observations and progressing in a logical sequence around the body. The right-hand page expands on selected themes and includes tips on examination technique and the interpretation of physical signs. These overviews are intended to act as an aide-mémoire and not as a replacement for a detailed text on clinical examination, as provided in our sister title, *Macleod's Clinical Examination*.

Presenting problems

Medical students and junior doctors must not only learn a great many facts about various disorders, but also develop an analytical approach to formulating a differential diagnosis and a plan of investigation for patients who present with particular symptoms or signs. In *Davidson's* this is addressed by incorporating a 'Presenting Problems' section into all system-based chapters. Over 200 presentations are included, which represent the most common reasons for referral to each medical specialty. The same approach has been used in several of the chapters in the 'Principles of Medicine' section, to reinforce the close connection between clinical problems and fundamental mechanisms of disease. Many patients present with symptoms such as weight loss, dizziness or breathlessness, which are not specific to a particular system; these are described in the most relevant chapter and cross-referenced elsewhere. An index of presenting problems may be found on the inside back cover.

Boxes and tables

Boxes and tables are a popular way of presenting information and are particularly useful for revision. They are classified by the type of information they contain using the following symbols:

 Causes

 Clinical Features

 Investigations

 Treatment

 In Old Age

EBM Evidence-based Medicine

 In Pregnancy

 Practice Point

 Emergency

 Other Information

In Old Age

In most developed countries, older people comprise 20% of the population and are the chief users of health care. While they contract the same diseases as those who are younger, there are often important differences in the way they present and how they are best managed.

Chapter 7, 'Ageing and Disease', concentrates on the principles of managing the frailest group who suffer from multiple pathology and disability, and who tend to present with non-specific problems such as falls or delirium. However, many older people suffer from specific single-organ pathology. 'In Old Age' boxes are thus included in each chapter, and describe common presentations, implications of physiological changes of ageing, effects of age on investigations, problems of treatment in old age, and the benefits and risks of intervention in older people.

Evidence-based Medicine

Clinicians must base their practice on the best available evidence, which needs to be up to date, relevant, authoritative and easily accessible. Over 150 evidence-based medicine (EBM) boxes are included in this edition. They contain recommendations that are supported by evidence obtained from meta-analysis of several randomised controlled trials (RCTs) or one (or more) high-quality RCT, as described in Chapter 2 (p. 22). Recommendations conform to 'Grade A' criteria, as described in Chapter 1 (pp. 7–8).

In Pregnancy

Many conditions, both acute and chronic, are different in the context of pregnancy, while some arise only during or shortly after pregnancy. Particular care must be taken with investigations (to avoid, for example, radiation exposure to the fetus) and treatment (to avoid the use of drugs which harm the fetus). These issues are highlighted in new 'In Pregnancy' boxes distributed throughout the book.

Practice Point

There are many practical skills that students must learn in order to become effective junior doctors. These vary from inserting a nasogastric tube to reading an ECG or X-ray, or interpreting investigations such as arterial blood gases or thyroid function tests. 'Practice Point' boxes have been introduced in this edition to provide straightforward guidance on how these and many other skills can be acquired and applied.

Emergency

New in the 21st edition, these boxes describe management of many of the most common emergencies in medicine.

Terminology

Recommended International Non-proprietary Names (rINNs) are used for all drugs, with the exception of adrenaline and noradrenaline. However, British spellings have been retained for drug classes and groups (e.g. amphetamines not amfetamines).

Units of measurement

The International System of Units (SI units) is the recommended means of presentation for laboratory data and has been used throughout *Davidson's*. However, we recognise that many laboratories around the world continue to provide data in non-SI units, so these have been included in the text for the commonly measured analytes. Both SI and non-SI units are also given in Chapter 28, which describes the reference ranges used in Edinburgh's laboratories. It should be appreciated that these reference ranges may vary from those used in other laboratories.

Finding what you are looking for

A detailed contents list is given on the opening page of each chapter. In addition, the book contains numerous cross-references to help readers find their way around, along with an extensive index of over 10 000 subject entries. The online text available on StudentConsult (www.studentconsult.com) allows for detailed searches of the content by keyword. A list of up-to-date reviews and useful websites with links to management guidelines appears at the end of each chapter.

Acknowledgements

Following the publication of the 20th Edition of *Davidson's Principles and Practice of Medicine*, Dr Nick Boon and Professor John Hunter retired as Editors. We would like to express our gratitude for the immense contribution they made. We are also indebted to former authors who have stepped down from this edition. They include Dr P. Bloomfield, Dr D.A. Cameron, Dr R.W. Chapman, Professor P.C. Hayes, Dr G.C.W. Howard, Professor G. John, Dr A.L. Jones, Dr L. Karalliedde, Dr P. Lanyon, Dr D.N.J. Lockwood, Professor C.A. Ludlam, Dr S. Paterson-Brown, Dr S.G. Potts, Dr R. Sandford, Dr C. Summerton, Dr W.T.A. Todd and Dr D.F. Treacher.

We are grateful to members of the International Advisory Board, all of whom provided detailed suggestions which have improved the book. Several members have stepped down and we are grateful for their support during the preparation of previous editions. They include Dr S. Aaron, Dr S.K. Agarwal, Professor V. Diehl, Professor K.V. Johny, Professor J.A. Ker, Professor C.-L. Lai, Professor S.K. Rajan and Dr P.S. Shankar.

Detailed chapter reviews were commissioned to help plan this new edition and we are grateful to all those who assisted, including Dr Alison Avenell, Professor Pradeep Bamberry, Dr Richard Davenport, Dr David Eedy, Dr John English, Professor John Iredale, Professor Alan Jardine, Dr Dilip Nathwani, Dr Marianne Nicholson, Dr Denis O'Reilly, Professor John Pettifor, Dr John Saunders, Professor Tom Strachan and Dr Andrew Ustianowski.

As part of the publishers' review, students from several medical schools supplied many innovative ideas on how to enhance the book. We are indebted to the following for their enthusiastic support: Jonathan Beavers, Sarah Edwards, Gulnaz Gill, Akhil D. Goel, Reiyal Goveas, Amanda Jewison, Rohit Kumar, Richard McGregor, Chris McLure, Puja Mehta, David Miller, Aparajita Mitra, Eliza Mohammed, Talha Patel, Jason Reynolds, Kar Teoh, Michael Wilson and Danny Wong.

The authors of Chapter 21 would like to acknowledge Professor Paul Dodson, Dr Robert Lindsay and Dr Ewan Pearson for their specialist advice.

We would like to extend our thanks to the many readers who have used the email feedback address to contact us with suggestions for improvements. Their input has been invaluable and is much appreciated; they are unfortunately too numerous to mention individually.

We are grateful to colleagues who have generously provided many of the illustrations that appear in this edition. They are acknowledged on pages 1299–1300.

We are especially grateful to all those working for Churchill Livingstone, in particular Laurence Hunter, Wendy Lee and Robert Britton, for their endless support and expertise in the shaping, collation and illustration of this edition. We would also like to thank Susan Boobis for her labours in compiling the extensive index and Ruth Noble for expert proofreading.

NRC, BRW, SHR
Edinburgh 2010

A.D. Cumming
S.I.R. Noble

Good medical practice

1

1

1

Since the time of Hippocrates, the role of the doctor has extended beyond the narrow remit of curing patients of their ailments. Good medical practice, or the art of medicine, hinges on recognising and respecting the breadth of physical, cultural, spiritual, experiential and psychosocial characteristics of each patient, and understanding their impact on the patient's beliefs, attitudes and expectations. Doctors must deliver appropriate care which considers the technical complexities of modern treatment, and at the same time deals with the communication and interpersonal needs of the patient, at a time when he or she may feel most vulnerable. In addition to the diagnosis and treatment of illness, the scope of medicine has expanded to preventing disease through measures such as screening, vaccination and health promotion. Doctors are centrally involved in tackling lifestyle-related issues of the modern world such as obesity, alcohol excess, cigarette smoking and sexual health.

Medical professionalism has been described by a Royal College of Physicians working party (2005) as 'a set of values, behaviours and relationships that underpin the trust the public has in doctors'. They stated that, in their day-to-day practice, doctors should be committed to integrity, compassion, altruism, continuous improvement, excellence, and working in partnership with members of the wider health-care team. They perceived that medical professionalism was relevant to leadership, education, career pathways, appraisal and research.

This chapter outlines how doctors must provide patients and their families with relevant but complex information, discuss management options, and reach appropriate clinical decisions that are commensurate with the available resources. It also describes pathways and processes to develop, maintain and assure medical professionalism.

MEDICAL PRACTICE

The doctor–patient relationship

The contents of this book are not all based on indisputable contemporary evidence; many reflect wisdom and understanding distilled over hundreds of years and passed from generation to generation of doctors. This perceived wisdom lies at the heart of the way that doctors and patients interact; it demands respect, and if the doctor also displays compassion, sets the scene for the development of trust.

Due to the complexities of many chronic diseases and treatments, and the multifaceted impact of illness on a patient, there is an increasing role for health care to be delivered by a multidisciplinary team (Box 1.1). This model of care recognises the different skills of each allied health professional and focuses patient care beyond surgical procedures or pharmacological manipulation. The doctor usually takes the lead in determining the overall direction of care but must also:

- guide the patient through the unfamiliar landscape, language and customs of clinical care
- interpret, synthesise and convey complex information
- help patients and families to participate fully in thinking about their care and in the decision-making process.

ℹ️ **1.1 Members and roles of a multidisciplinary team**	
Professional	**Roles**
Doctor	Diagnosis and treatment Overall coordination of care
Specialist nurse	Patient and family support Information-giving
Physiotherapist	Improving physical function Physical rehabilitation
Occupational therapist	Maximising skills and abilities Complex re-enablement
Speech and language therapist	Optimising communication Swallowing assessment
Dietitian	Nutritional advice Parenteral feeding support
Pharmacist	Safe prescribing Complex medicines delivery
Social worker	Coordination of home care Financial advice
Clinical psychologist	Cognitive interventions Psychological support
Pastoral care	Psychological support Spiritual support

ℹ️ 1.2 The duties of a doctor registered with the UK General Medical Council

Patients must be able to trust doctors with their lives and health. To justify that trust you must show respect for human life and you must:

- Make the care of your patient your first concern
- Protect and promote the health of patients and the public
- Provide a good standard of practice and care
    - Keep your professional knowledge and skills up to date
    - Recognise and work within the limits of your competence
    - Work with colleagues in the ways that best serve patients' interests
- Treat patients as individuals and respect their dignity
    - Treat patients politely and considerately
    - Respect patients' right to confidentiality
- Work in partnership with patients
    - Listen to patients and respond to their concerns and preferences
    - Give patients the information they want or need in a way they can understand
    - Respect patients' right to reach decisions with you about their treatment and care
    - Support patients in caring for themselves to improve and maintain their health
- Be honest and open, and act with integrity
    - Act without delay if you have good reason to believe that you or a colleague may be putting patients at risk
    - Never discriminate unfairly against patients or colleagues
    - Never abuse your patients' trust in you or the public's trust in the profession.

You are personally accountable for your professional practice and must always be prepared to justify your decisions and actions.

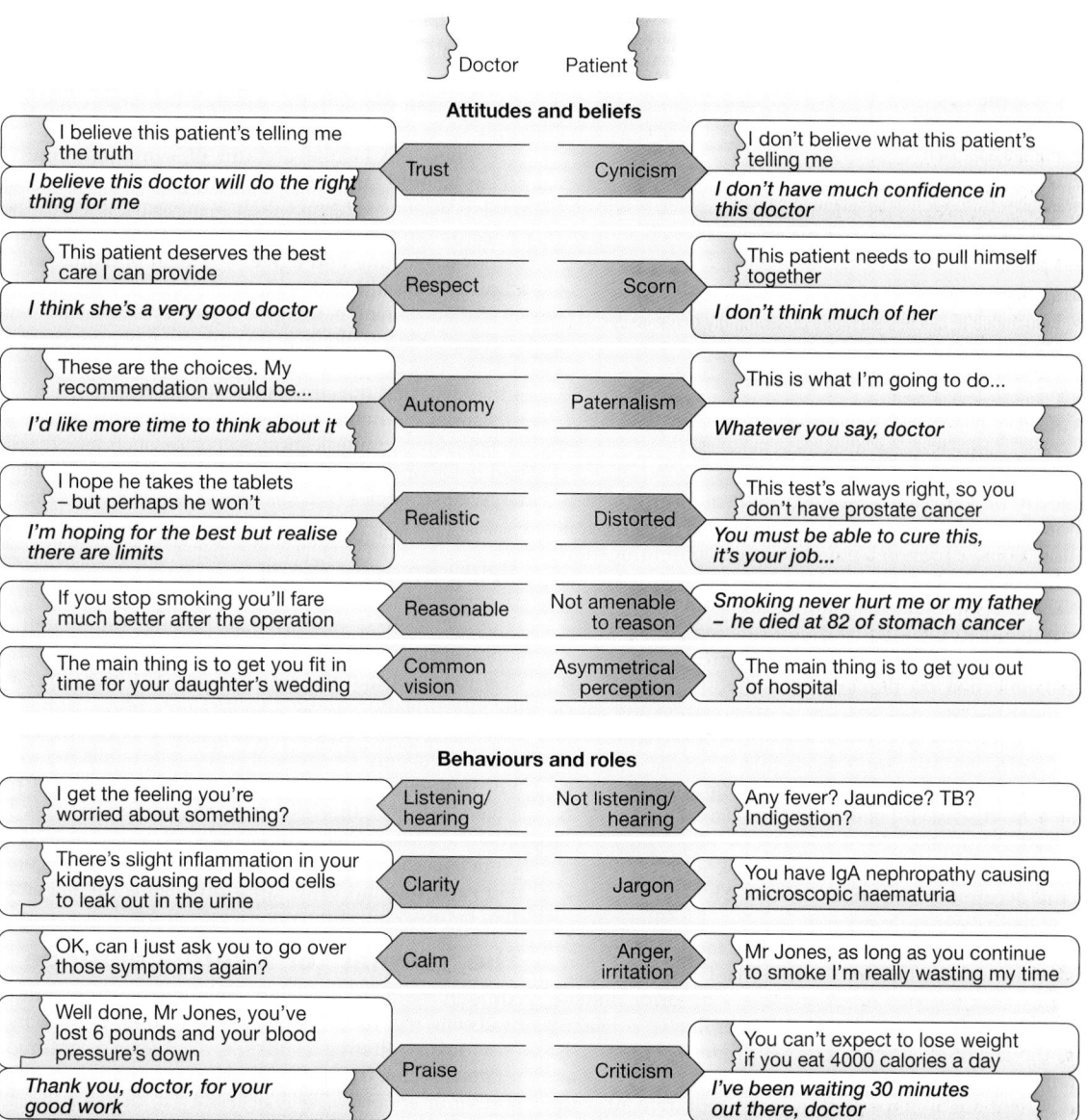

Fig. 1.1 Some aspects of the doctor–patient relationship.

In many clinical disciplines, doctors from several specialties form a multidisciplinary team in order to formulate a treatment plan. In oncology, for example, this ensures that various modalities of treatment (surgical, oncological and palliative) are considered.

The doctor–patient relationship is in itself therapeutic; a successful consultation with a trusted and respected practitioner will therefore have beneficial effects irrespective of any other therapy given. The doctor–patient relationship is also multilayered, dynamic and bilateral. Figure 1.1 illustrates how it may be influenced by differences in attitudes or beliefs, and behaviours or roles.

Regulatory bodies such as the UK General Medical Council seek to define the medical side of the doctor–patient relationship in terms of the duties of a doctor (Box 1.2). It is common for medical schools to require undergraduate students to sign an ethical code of conduct based on statements like this.

Clinical and communication skills

Communication lies at the heart of good medical practice. The most technically capable clinician will fail in the duty of care if he or she is unable to communicate effectively with patients or relatives, since this is essential for accurate history-taking, information-giving and decision-making. Likewise, the delivery of holistic care requires effective communication with other doctors and members of the multidisciplinary team, failure of which may lead to clinical errors. Clear and appropriately detailed clinical note-keeping is essential, as are timely and accurate written communications between professionals.

Failures in communication may also lead to poor health outcomes, strained working relations, widespread dissatisfaction among patients, their families and health professionals, anger and litigation. The

1

1.3 Some barriers to good communication in health care

The clinician

- Authoritarian or dismissive attitude
- Hurried approach
- Use of jargon
- Inability to speak first language of patient
- No experience of patient's cultural background

The patient

- Anxiety
- Reluctance to discuss sensitive or seemingly trivial issues
- Misconceptions
- Conflicting sources of information
- Cognitive impairment
- Hearing/speech/visual impediment

majority of complaints received by health-care professionals could have been avoided by effective communication. Some common barriers to good communication are listed in Box 1.3.

The development of communication skills to facilitate accurate history-taking and information-giving takes many years and requires frequent opportunities for personal reflection on previous consultations. A detailed account of history-taking, clinical examination and communication skills is beyond the scope of this chapter but is provided in Davidson's sister title, *MacLeod's Clinical Examination*. However, some basic communication principles are discussed below and these can be applied to most consultations.

The main aim of a medical interview is to establish a factual account of the patient's illness. The clinician must allow the patient to describe the problems without overbearing questioning, but should try to facilitate the process with appropriate questions (Box 1.4). Techniques such as an unhurried approach, checking prior understanding, making it clear that the interviewer is listening, the use of silence when appropriate, recapping on what has been said, and reflection of key points back to the patient are all important. A major requirement is to express complex information and concepts in language

1.4 Communication skills in the medical interview

- **Open questions** allow patients to express their own thoughts and feelings, e.g. 'How have you been since we last saw you?', 'Is there anything else that you want to mention?'
- **Closed questions** are requests for factual information, e.g. 'When did this pain start?'
- **Leading questions** invite specific responses and suggest options, e.g. 'You'll be glad when this treatment is over, won't you?'
- **Reflecting questions** help to develop or expand topics, e.g. 'Can you tell me more about your family?'
- **Active listening** encourages further dialogue, e.g. 'Go on,' 'I see,' 'Hmm' etc.
- **Requesting clarification** encourages further detail, e.g. 'How do mean?', 'In what way?' etc.
- **Summarising** ensures accurate understanding, e.g. 'Tell me if I've got this right.'

with which the patient can readily engage. Non-verbal communication is equally important. The patient's facial expressions and body language may betray hidden fears. The clinician can help the patient to talk more freely by smiling or nodding appropriately.

Beyond the factual account of symptoms, the clinician should also explore patients' feelings, determine how they interpret their symptoms, unearth their concerns and fears, and explore their expectations before suggesting and agreeing a plan of management. Clinicians should demonstrate understanding, sensitivity and empathy (i.e. imagine themselves in the patient's position). Most patients have more than one concern and will be reluctant to discuss potentially important issues if they feel that the clinician is not interested or is likely to dismiss their complaints as irrational or trivial.

Specific communication scenarios such as breaking bad news or dealing with aggression require additional targeted strategies (see *MacLeod's Clinical Examination*).

Using investigations

Modern medical practice has become dominated by sophisticated and often expensive investigations. It is easy to forget that the judicious use of these tools, and the interpretation of the data that they provide, are crucially dependent on good basic clinical skills. Indeed, a test should only be ordered if it is clear that the result will influence the patient's management and the perceived value of the resulting information exceeds the anticipated discomfort, risk and cost of the procedure. Clinicians should therefore analyse their patient's condition carefully and draw up a provisional management plan before requesting any investigations.

The 'normal' (or reference) range

Although some tests provide qualitative results (present or absent, e.g. faecal occult blood testing, p. 856), most provide quantitative results (i.e. a value on a continuous numeric scale). In order to classify quantitative results as normal or abnormal, it is necessary to define a 'normal range'. Many quantitative measurements in populations exhibit a bell-shaped, or Gaussian, frequency distribution (Fig. 1.2); this is called a 'normal distribution' and is characteristic of biological variables determined by a complex mixture of genetic and environmental factors (e.g. height) and of test results (e.g. plasma sodium concentration). A normal distribution can be described by the mean value (which places the centre of the bell-shaped curve on the x axis) and the standard deviation (SD, which describes the width of the bell-shaped curve). Within each SD away from the mean there is a fixed percentage of the population. By convention, the 'normal range' is usually defined as those values which encompass 95% of the population, i.e. the values within 2 SDs above and below the mean. If this convention is used, however, 2.5% of the normal population will have values above, and 2.5% will have values below, the normal range; for this reason, it is more precise to describe 'reference' rather than 'normal' ranges.

'Abnormal' results, i.e. those lying beyond 2 SDs from the mean, may occur either because the person is one of the 2.5% of the normal population whose test result is outside the reference range, or because he or she has

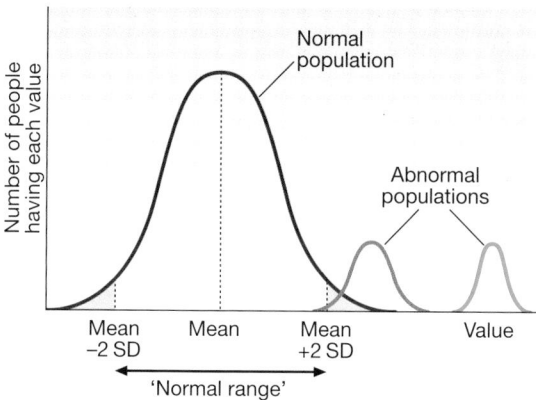

Fig. 1.2 Normal distribution and 'normal' (reference) range. For many tests, the frequency distribution of results in the normal healthy population (red line) is a symmetrical bell-shaped curve. The mean ± 2 standard deviations (SD) encompasses 95% of the normal population and usually defines the 'normal range' (or 'reference range'); 2.5% of the normal population have values above, and 2.5% below, the reference range (shaded areas). For some diseases (blue line), test results overlap with the normal population or even with the reference range. For other diseases (green line), tests may be more reliable because there is no overlap between the normal and abnormal population.

a disease characterised by a different result from the test. Test results in 'abnormal' populations also have a bell-shaped distribution with a different mean and SD (see Fig. 1.2). In some diseases, there is typically no overlap between results from the normal and abnormal population (e.g. elevated serum creatinine in renal failure, p. 465). In many diseases, however, there is overlap, sometimes extending into the reference range (e.g. elevated serum thyroxine in toxic multinodular goitre, p. 750). In these circumstances, the greater the difference between the test result and the limits of the reference range, the higher the chance that the person has a disease, but there is a risk that results within the reference range may be 'false negatives' and results outside the reference range may be 'false positives'.

Each time a test is performed in a member of the normal population there is a 5% (1 in 20) chance that the result will be outside the reference range. If two tests are performed, the chance that one of them will be 'abnormal' is 10% (2 in 20), and so on; the chance of detecting an 'abnormal' result increases as more tests are performed, so multiple indiscriminate testing should be avoided.

In practice, reference ranges are usually established by performing the test in a number of healthy volunteers who are assumed to be a random sample of the normal population. Not all populations are the same, however, and while it is common to have different reference ranges for tests in men and women, or in children and adults, clinicians need to be aware that reference ranges defined either by test manufacturers or even within the local laboratory may have been established in small numbers of healthy young people who are not necessarily representative of their patient population. This is another reason to recognise that reference ranges do not discriminate perfectly between health and disease.

For some tests, the clinical decision does not depend on whether or not the patient is a member of the normal population. This commonly applies to quantitative risk factors for future disease. For example, higher plasma total cholesterol levels are associated with a higher risk

of future myocardial infarction (p. 579) within the normal population. Although a reference range for cholesterol can be calculated, cholesterol-lowering therapy is commonly recommended for people with values within the reference range; the 'cutoff' value at which therapy is recommended depends upon the presence of other risk factors for cardiovascular disease. The reference range for plasma cholesterol is therefore redundant and the phrase 'normal plasma cholesterol level' is unhelpful. Similar arguments apply for interpretation of values of blood pressure (p. 579), blood glucose (p. 805), bone mineral density (p. 1118) and so on.

Some quantitative test results are not normally distributed, usually because a substantial proportion of the normal population will have an unrecordably low result (e.g. serum prostate-specific antigen, p. 513, and serum troponin, p. 531), and the distribution cannot be described by mean and SDs. Alternative statistical procedures can be used to calculate 95th centiles, but it is common in these circumstances to use information from normal and abnormal people to identify 'cutoff' values which are associated with a certain risk of disease, as described below.

Sensitivity and specificity

Many tests are potentially hazardous and none is completely reliable. All diagnostic tests can produce false positives (an abnormal result in the absence of disease) and false negatives (a normal result in a patient with disease). The diagnostic accuracy of a test can be expressed in terms of its sensitivity and its specificity (Box 1.5).

Sensitivity is defined as the percentage of the test population who are affected by the index condition and test positive for it. In contrast, specificity is defined as the percentage of the test population who are healthy and test negative. A very sensitive test will detect most disease but may generate abnormal findings in healthy people. A negative result will therefore reliably exclude disease but a positive test is likely to require further evaluation. On the other hand, a very specific test may miss significant pathology but is likely to establish the diagnosis, beyond doubt, when the result is positive.

In choosing how a test is used to guide decision-making there is an inevitable trade-off between emphasising sensitivity as opposed to specificity. For example, defining an exercise electrocardiogram (p. 530) as abnormal if there is ≥ 0.5 mm ST depression will ensure that very few cases of coronary artery disease are missed but will generate a lot of false positive tests (high sensitivity, low specificity).

1.5 The accuracy of diagnostic tests

	Affected	Unaffected
Positive test	True +ve (a)	False +ve (b)
Negative test	False −ve (c)	True −ve (d)

Sensitivity (%) = [a/(a + c)] × 100
Specificity (%) = [d/(b + d)] × 100

Positive predictive value = a/(a + b)
Negative predictive value = d/(c + d)

Likelihood ratio: positive test = sensitivity/(1 − specificity)
negative test = (1 − sensitivity)/specificity

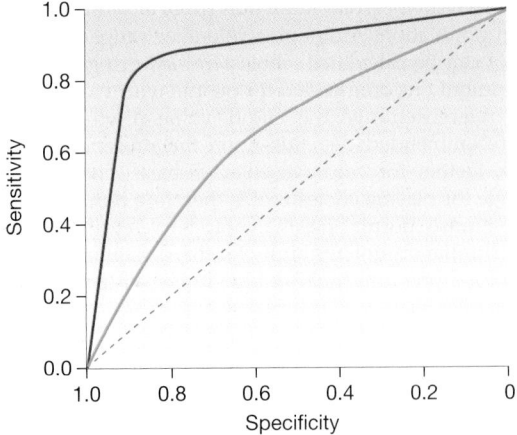

Fig. 1.3 Receiver operating characteristic graphs illustrating the trade-off between sensitivity and specificity for a given test. The curve is generated by 'adjusting' the cutoff values defining normal and abnormal results, calculating the effect on sensitivity and specificity, then plotting these against each other. The closer the curve lies to the top left-hand corner, the more useful the test. The red line illustrates a test with useful discriminant value and the green line illustrates a less useful poorly discriminant test.

On the other hand, using a cutoff point of $\geq 2.0\,\text{mm}$ ST depression will detect most cases of important coronary disease with far fewer false positive results. This trade-off can be illustrated by the receiver operating characteristic curve of the test (Fig. 1.3).

Predictive value

The predictive value of a test is determined by its sensitivity and specificity, and can be expressed in several ways. The positive predictive value is the probability that a patient with a positive test has the index condition, whilst the negative predictive value is the probability that a patient with a negative test does not have the condition (see Box 1.5). The likelihood ratio expresses the odds that a given finding would occur in a patient with, as opposed to a patient without, the index condition (see Box 1.5) (as the odds rise above 1 the probability that disease is present rises).

The interpretation, and therefore the utility, of a test are critically dependent on the circumstances in which it is used. Bayes' theorem dictates that the value of a diagnostic test is determined by the prevalence of the condition in the test population. The probability that a subject has a particular condition (the post-test probability) can be calculated if the pre-test probability and the sensitivity and specificity of the test are known (Box 1.6). Thus, a test is most valuable when there is an intermediate pre-test probability of disease. Clinicians seldom have access to such precise information but must appreciate the importance of integrating clinical and laboratory data.

Screening

Many health-care systems run screening programmes to detect important (and treatable) disease in apparently healthy but at-risk individuals. These initiatives may be directed towards a single pathology (e.g. mammography for breast cancer, p. 274) or may comprise a battery of tests for a wide range of conditions. Screening inevitably generates a number of false-positive results that

1.6 Bayes' theorem: post-test likelihood of disease

Positive test

$$\text{Post-test probability of disease} = \frac{\text{pre} \times \text{sens}}{(\text{pre} \times \text{sens}) + ((1-\text{sens}) \times (1-\text{spec}))}$$

Negative test

$$\text{Post-test probability of disease} = \frac{\text{pre} \times (1-\text{sens})}{(\text{pre} \times (1-\text{sens})) + ((1-\text{pre}) \times \text{spec})}$$

(pre = pre-test probability of disease; sens = sensitivity; spec = specificity)

Example

Assume: Exercise tolerance testing for the diagnosis of coronary artery disease (CAD) (using cutoff of 2 mm ST depression) has 70% sensitivity (0.7) and 90% specificity (0.9) The pre-test odds of significant CAD in a 65-yr-old woman with atypical angina on effort are 50% (0.5)

Post-test odds of significant CAD will be:

Positive test $\dfrac{0.5 \times 0.7}{(0.5 \times 0.7) + (0.3 \times 0.1)} = 92\%$

Negative test $\dfrac{0.5 \times 0.3}{(0.5 \times 0.3) + (0.5 \times 0.9)} = 25\%$

In contrast, the pre-test probability of significant coronary disease in a 45-yr-old man with typical angina on effort would be 90%, with post-test odds of 95% in the event of a positive exercise test and 75% in the event of a negative test.

1.7 Factors that influence the cost-effectiveness of health screening

- The prevalence of the index condition in the target population
- The cost of the screening test
- The sensitivity and specificity of the screening test
- The availability and effectiveness of treatment for the index condition
- The cost of not detecting and treating the condition

require further, potentially expensive and sometimes risky, investigation. This may engender a good deal of anxiety for the patient and create dilemmas for the clinician; for example, it may be difficult to determine how to evaluate minor abnormalities of the liver function tests in an otherwise healthy person (p. 930).

Some of the criteria that must be considered before deciding if the wider costs of a screening programme can be justified are listed in Box 1.7.

Estimating and communicating risk

Medical management decisions are usually made by weighing up the anticipated benefits of a particular procedure or treatment against the potential risks. To allow patients to contribute to the decision-making process, health professionals must be able to explain risk in an accurate and understandable way.

Providing the relevant biomedical facts is seldom sufficient to guide decision-making because a patient's perception of risk is often coloured by emotional, and sometimes irrational, factors. Most patients will have access to information from a wide variety of sometimes conflicting sources, including the Internet, books, magazines, self-help groups, other health-care professionals, friends and family. The clinician must be aware of and sensitive to the way in which these resources influence the individual, while building trust with the patient, clarifying the problem and conveying the key facts.

Research evidence provides statistics and probabilities, but these can be confusing and can be presented in many ways (Box 1.8). Relative risk describes the proportional increase in risk; it is a useful measure of the size of an effect. In contrast, absolute risk describes the actual chance of an event and is what matters to most patients.

 1.8 Explaining the risks and benefits of therapy

Would you take a drug once a day for a year to prevent stroke if:
- it reduced your risk of having a stroke by 47%?
- it reduced your chance of suffering a stroke from 0.26% to 0.14%?
- there was one chance in 850 that it would prevent you having a stroke?
- 849 out of 850 patients derived no benefit from the treatment?
- there was a 99.7% chance that you would not have a stroke anyway?

All these statements are derived from the same data and describe an equivalent effect*

*MRC trial of treatment of mild hypertension (bendroflumethiazide vs placebo). BMJ 1985; 291:97–104.

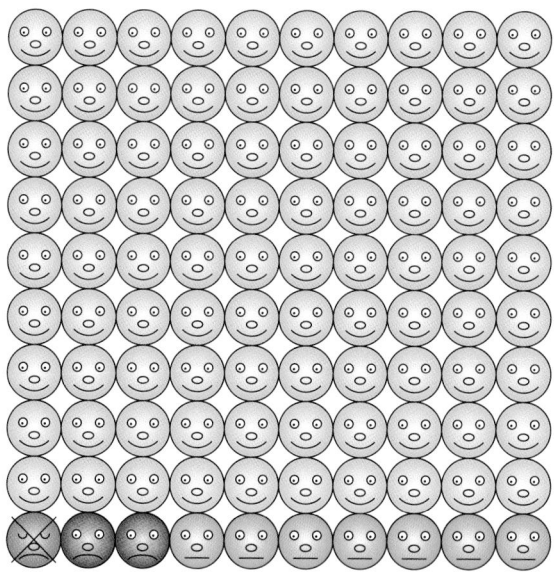

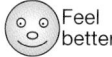 Feel better   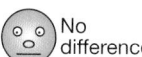 No difference   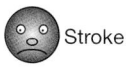 Stroke   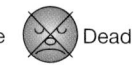 Dead

Fig. 1.4 Visual portrayal of benefit and risks. The image refers to an operation that is expected to relieve symptoms in 90% of patients, but cause stroke in 2% and death in 1%.

Terms such as 'common', 'rare', 'probable' and 'unlikely' are elastic. Whenever possible, the clinician should quote numerical information using consistent denominators (e.g. '90 of every 100 patients who have this operation feel much better, 1 will die during the operation and 2 will suffer a stroke'). Positive framing ('There is a 99% chance of survival') and negative framing ('There is a 1% chance of death') may both be appropriate. A variety of visual aids can be used to present complex statistical information in a digestible way (Fig. 1.4).

Finally, it is essential to allow the patient to place his or her own weighting on the potential benefits and adverse effects of each course of action. Thus, some patients may choose to sacrifice a good chance of pain relief because they are not prepared to run even a small risk of paralysis, whilst others may opt to proceed with very high-risk spinal surgery because they find their current circumstances intolerable.

Clinical decision-making

Assimilating symptoms, signs and results of investigations into a diagnosis and then planning treatment are highly complex tasks that require not only factual knowledge but also a highly developed set of skills in decision-making. Diagnostic decision-making is guided by Ockham's razor, originally expressed by the 14th-century Englishman William of Ockham as 'plurality should not be posited without necessity.' In short, all things being equal, the simplest explanation is the best. In practice, clinicians formulate hypotheses about the underlying diagnosis (or shortlist of diagnoses, the 'differential' diagnosis) during the consultation with the patient and refine this hypothesis both by collecting selected additional information and by choosing to ignore other information which they regard as irrelevant, in order to reach the most parsimonious diagnosis.

Decision-making in health care often operates under conditions of uncertainty, where it is uncertain what is wrong with the patient or which treatment is most appropriate. This can lead to variations in how clinicians make decisions, and subsequently variations in the care that patients receive. Clinicians often employ a process of 'ad hoc' decision-making, where they use some form of global judgement about what might be the best course of action for an individual patient. These ad hoc decisions may be based on a number of factors, including what a clinician has been taught, his or her clinical experience of other patients with that particular disease, or what is common practice within a particular institution. However, such decisions may be governed by heuristics or bias, which may lead to errors. Heuristics are cognitive processes or 'rules of thumb' used unconsciously when making decisions (Box 1.9). Such processes may lead to mistakes, most commonly when there is a lack of evidence to inform practice. Whenever possible, clinical decision-making should be guided by evidence-based medicine.

Evidence-based medicine

Patient treatment should be based on the integration of best research evidence alongside clinical expertise and patient values. The discipline of evidence-based medicine (EBM) came into being in order to introduce a more

1.9 Heuristics in clinical decision-making

Availability

- The probability of an event is estimated based on how easily an individual can recall a similar event from his or her memory
- E.g. a doctor judges that a patient has a particular disease because the case reminds him or her of a similar case seen recently
- This can lead to errors, as individuals often recall recent or vivid events more easily, rather than considering the actual likelihood of an event in the wider population

Representativeness

- The probability of an event is estimated based on how similar (or representative) it is of a wider category of events
- E.g. a doctor judges that a patient has a particular disease because the patient's signs and symptoms are 'representative' of that disease
- This can lead to errors such as neglecting to take into account the prevalence of the disease in a specific patient population

Anchoring and adjustment

- The probability of an event is estimated by taking an initial reference point (anchor) and then adjusting this to reach a final judgement about likelihood
- E.g. a doctor judges that the likelihood of a patient having a particular disease is 60%. The doctor collects information (perhaps from diagnostic tests) and reassesses his or her estimation on the basis of these results to reach a final diagnosis
- This can lead to errors, as final estimations of likelihood are linked to the original anchor, so if this is incorrect, the final judgement is also likely to be inaccurate

1.10 Categories in evidence-based medicine (EBM)*

Levels of evidence (in descending order of strength)

Ia	Evidence obtained from meta-analysis of randomised clinical trials
Ib	Evidence obtained from at least one randomised controlled trial
IIa	Evidence obtained from at least one well-designed controlled study without randomisation
IIb	Evidence obtained from at least one other type of well-designed quasi-experimental study
III	Evidence obtained from well-designed non-experimental descriptive studies, such as comparative studies, correlation studies and case studies
IV	Evidence obtained from expert committee reports or opinions and/or clinical experiences of respected authorities

Grades of recommendation

A	Directly based on level I studies
B	Directly based on level II studies *or* extrapolations from level I studies
C	Directly based on level III studies *or* extrapolations from level I or II studies
D	Directly based on level IV studies *or* extrapolations from level I, II or III studies

*From the Scottish Intercollegiate Guidelines Network (SIGN; see www.sign. ac.uk). This scheme is widely used, although other modified schemes exist.

systematic approach to the use of evidence in making clinical decisions. This was made possible by:

- the development of statistical methods to analyse data systematically
- recognition of the importance of analysing all data, both published and unpublished
- the development of databases of relevant information and systems by which to access such information.

The principles of EBM are based on the tenet that well-formulated questions about medical management can be answered by:

- conducting high-quality randomised controlled trials
- tracing all the available evidence
- critically appraising the evidence
- applying the evidence to the management of the individual patient.

EBM categorises different types of clinical evidence and ranks them according to their freedom from the various biases that beset medical research. It therefore places greater emphasis on evidence from a meta-analysis of randomised controlled trials than on a series of case reports or expert opinion (Box 1.10).

Guidelines and protocols

The terms 'clinical guidelines' and 'protocols' are often used together, yet they are inherently different.

Guidelines

Clinical guidelines aim to guide clinicians on how to manage specific clinical scenarios using the best available evidence. They have been in existence throughout the history of medicine, although many were based on tradition or authority. A large number of local, national and international bodies have produced guidelines, following a range of different methodologies (see www.library.nhs.uk/guidelinesfinder). Some are based on systematic reviews of the medical literature and others on consensus of expert opinion. When considering guidelines, it is important for clinicians to be aware of the strength of the evidence on which the recommendations are based (see Box 1.10).

Properly developed guidelines recognise that medicine is an art as well as a science and that the evidence on which the guidelines are based is, strictly speaking, only applicable to the study population in the trial(s). Clinicians must therefore use their judgement to ascertain whether the recommendations are applicable to the patient in front of them and follow the guidance accordingly.

Some guidelines are formulated not only from evidence-based best practice but also from cost effectiveness (see below). An example in the UK is guidance produced by the government-commissioned body, the National Institute for Health and Clinical Excellence (NICE; see www.nice.org.uk). These guidelines recognise that health services have limited resources, and that treatments should be funded which offer the greatest improvement in health for the largest number of people per unit of resource.

Protocols

Whilst guidelines recognise the individuality of the patient and help clinicians decide on which action is best, protocols are far more directive and are written to be followed exactly. Protocols usually apply in situations where the clinical decision has already been made and the treatment or intervention is then being instigated. Protocols aim to ensure that treatment will be identical irrespective of where and by whom it is given. For example, a guideline may help a multidisciplinary team decide which modality of treatment is best for someone with lung cancer; it will allow the team to evaluate the best evidence alongside the individual psychosocial needs of the patient. However, once a decision has been made in favour of a certain treatment, e.g. chemotherapy, the clinician will be expected to follow a strict protocol outlining dosages, routes of administration, monitoring and so on to ensure parity of treatment wherever the chemotherapy is given.

Cost-effectiveness

The best available health care can be expensive. No country can now afford to provide unlimited state-of-the-art medicine for all its citizens. Health-care systems must therefore take account of the cost-effectiveness of the treatments they provide. This can create difficult dilemmas for clinicians who may be asked to withhold expensive but effective therapies (e.g. implantable defibrillators) from individual patients on the basis that the money will do more good for more patients if it is spent elsewhere (e.g. offering angioplasty to all acute myocardial infarction patients). Assessing the cost-effectiveness of interventions and allocating resources accordingly follows ethical principles such as justice, which are covered in greater detail below. One way to assess the cost-effectiveness of an intervention is to calculate the number of quality-adjusted life years that an intervention will provide for a patient.

Quality-adjusted life years

Outcomes from health care can be measured in terms of changes in the quality and quantity of life. Life expectancy is easily defined but quality of life is difficult to measure. Nevertheless, it is possible to construct a continuum between perfect health (score 1), survival with no quality of life (score 0) and states that are perceived to be worse than death (minus score). Quality and quantity of life can then be combined in a measure known as the quality-adjusted life year (QALY). For example, an intervention that results in a patient living an additional 4 years with an average quality of life rated as 0.6 on the continuum would yield 2.4 QALYs (4 × 0.6). Thus a cost per QALY can be calculated and compared with other interventions. This sort of approach has many failings but, for the time being at least, offers the best means of comparing the cost-effectiveness of a wide range of treatments.

Practising medicine in low-resource settings

The problems associated with medical care in low-resource areas cluster in four domains:

- *Prevention versus cure*. Prevention is easier, cheaper and more effective than cure for many diseases. On the other hand, curative medicine is immediate, highly visible and glamorous. This tension is most evident when a disease is common and the benefits of prevention have yet to be realised. The allocation of adequate resources for long-term prevention needs both political will and social acceptance.
- *Acute versus chronic care*. Acute medical care produces immediate and often gratifying results whilst treating chronic illness can be time-consuming and less rewarding. Facilities for chronic care are therefore accorded a low priority in many health-care systems. Unfortunately, this often results in patients who require long-term care being denied treatment altogether or being managed inappropriately (at high cost) in the acute sector.
- *The ideal versus the possible*. Most medical management guidelines are derived from studies that were conducted in well-resourced health-care systems. In trying to apply this knowledge to the developing world, there are tensions between best practice and what is possible. For example, anticoagulant therapy (p. 1014) may pose risks that were not evident in the studies that underpin guidelines if it is prescribed in areas where reliable laboratories are not available and medications that interact with warfarin are commonly purchased 'over the counter'.
- *Channels of health-care provision*. In developing countries health care may be delivered through government-run public clinics (usually free or subsidised services) or non-governmental organisations (sometimes subsidised but usually privately funded services). Many of the available services are too costly for the average patient, so for the benefit of the community as a whole there is a need for constructive cooperation between all of the health-care sectors.

The best possible practice is that which can be delivered within the available resources in a specific setting. Compassionate care given with empathy, understanding and good communication is always within the physician's reach, even when physical resources are inadequate.

MEDICAL ETHICS

Ethics is the 'science' of morality. Medical ethics is concerned both with the standards of conduct and competence expected of members of the medical profession, and with the study of ethical problems raised by the practice of medicine. Recent advances in biomedical science and their application to clinical care have thrown up many difficult ethical problems. These include human cloning, predictive genetic testing, eugenics, women's health, new reproductive technologies, antenatal screening, abortion, priority-setting, global medicine, underserved populations, brain death, organ transplantation, end-of-life issues, assisted suicide and advance directives. Detailed discussion of these is beyond the scope of this chapter but a framework for the application of ethics to medical practice will be described.

In general, ethical problems relate to the intentions or motives of those involved, their actions, the consequences of their actions, and the context in which their

1

actions take place. Ethical problems can be analysed in a variety of ways, and different analytical approaches may lead to different conclusions. To find the best solution, it may be necessary to apply several different analytical approaches and attempt to reconcile the conclusions. In modern medical practice there is not always time to do this systematically. However, the process of applying an ethical framework to a given situation is a key element in clinical decision-making and helps to ensure that a decision is both morally acceptable and legally defensible.

- *Virtue ethics* is concerned with the character of the persons involved and with their actions. Are my intentions (what my actions aim at) and my motives (what moves me to act) good or bad, wise or unwise, sensible or unrealistic, patient-centred or self-centred, and so on? Is the course of action I propose to take one which would be considered appropriate by a prudent doctor—or by a prudent patient? The focus here is on the characteristics of a virtuous person. Right action flows from the nature of that person.
- *Deontological ethics* is concerned with whether a proposed action or course of action, in itself and regardless of its consequences, is right or wrong. Is it ever right or always wrong to kill, to tell a lie, to break a promise? Deontological (from the Greek for 'duty') considerations include rights as well as duties, and omissions as well as acts. An action is right if it is in accordance with an established moral rule or principle.
- *Teleological ethics* (or consequentialism) is concerned with the consequences of a proposed action or course of action. Are they likely to be good or bad, in the short term and long term, for the patient, doctor, family and society? What will promote a net balance of good over harm for the individual as well as 'the greatest good for the greatest number'? Who decides (or can predict) what is the 'best' outcome?

An ethical problem can therefore be addressed by trying to decide what a virtuous person would do, whether an action or course of action is right or wrong in itself, or what its consequences might be. Yet the circumstances in which any decision is made will vary, and what may be right in one context may be wrong in another. *Situation ethics* recognises this, emphasising the need to consider carefully the context (or situation) in which a course of action is chosen.

Ethics are applied to the practice of medicine in three broad areas:

- *Clinical ethics* deal with the relationship between clinicians and individual patients, as described below.
- *Public health ethics* deal with the health issues of groups of people—the community. Examples include the banning of smoking in public places, where the autonomy of the individual may be coerced for the greater good of the community.
- *Research ethics* deal with issues related to clinical research. This is to ensure not only that research is conducted safely but also that the rights of the participants are paramount. No research can be undertaken unless it has undergone ethical scrutiny.

Key principles of clinical ethics

In clinical ethics, four key principles are frequently used to underpin the analysis of a problem, and are often abbreviated to 'autonomy, beneficence, non-maleficence and justice'.

Respect for persons and their autonomy

This respect is a significant aspect of the relationship between patient and doctor. The patient seeks out a doctor based on a desire to attain freedom from a disability or disease which limits his or her ability to exercise autonomy (the power or right of self-determination). Unless the patient is a child, is unconscious or is mentally incapacitated, it is the patient's choice to seek advice. The physician must therefore respect the patient's autonomy. This includes the patient's right to refuse therapy. The doctor must also actively seek to empower the patient with adequate information.

Respect for persons and their autonomy has important implications for truth-telling, informed consent and confidentiality.

Truth-telling

Telling the truth is essential to generating and maintaining trust between the doctor and the patient. This includes providing information about the nature of the illness, expected outcome and therapeutic alternatives, and answering questions honestly. The facts should not be given 'brutally' but with due sensitivity to appropriate timing and to the patient's capacity to cope with bad news. However, the clinical uncertainties described earlier in the chapter must also be acknowledged. There are two rare situations where the truth may, at least for a time, be withheld:

- If it will cause real harm to the patient (e.g. a depressed patient likely to commit suicide who has to be told that he or she has cancer). This is sometimes called 'therapeutic privilege', since it should be exercised only in the patient's vital interests and for very serious clinical reasons.
- If the patient makes it clear that he or she does not want to hear the bad news (but always bearing in mind that this may be a stage in the patient's adjustment to the condition).

In no case should false information be given, and the physician should always be prepared to justify any decision to withhold relevant information.

Informed consent

This term describes the participation of patients in decisions about their health care. In order to facilitate this, the clinician must provide the patient with an adequate explanation of the nature of the decision, and details of the relevant risks, benefits and uncertainties of each possible course of action. The amount of information to provide will vary, depending on the patient's condition and the complexity of the treatment, and on the physician's assessment of the patient's understanding of the situation. Not all options need be explained, but those that a 'prudent patient' would consider significant should be explored—for example, by open questioning (see Box 1.4, p. 4).

From both a legal and an ethical perspective the patient retains the right to decide what is in his or her best interests. All adults have decision-making capacity if they can understand the relevant information (which may have to be explained in simple terms), consider the implications of the relevant options, and make a communicable decision. If a patient makes choices that seem irrational or are at variance with professional advice, it does not mean that they lack capacity.

When the patient does lack decision-making capacity, the clinician should always act in the best interests of the patient. In an emergency, consent may be presumed, but only for treatment immediately necessary to preserve the patient's life and health, and if there is no clear evidence that this would be against the previous settled wishes of the patient when competent (for example, blood transfusion in the case of an adult Jehovah's Witness). If the patient has a legally entitled surrogate decision-maker, the consent of the latter should be sought wherever possible. It is also good practice to involve close relatives in decision-making but the hierarchy of surrogate decision-makers will depend on local laws and culture.

Confidentiality

Confidentiality in relation to the appropriate management of patient-specific information is important in generating and maintaining trust in the doctor–patient relationship. Health-care teams must take precautions to prevent unauthorised access to patient records, and may disclose patient-identifying information only when the patient has given consent or when required by law. Where such information is shared with other health-care professionals in order to optimise individual patient care, this should be done on a strictly 'need-to-know' basis.

Beneficence

This is the principle of doing good, or acting in another person's best interests. In clinical ethics, the term refers to the good of the individual patient. It means considering the patient's view of his or her own best interests as well as his or her medical best interests. Situations may arise where there is a conflict between what is good for the individual and what is best for society, but the traditional medical approach is that stated in the Declaration of Geneva (World Medical Association): 'The health of my patient will be my first consideration.'

Non-maleficence

This is the principle of doing no harm: in medicine, the traditional 'primum non nocere'. In balancing beneficence and non-maleficence (benefit versus risk), the clinician must share the relevant information with the patient, who can then be helped to make an informed decision.

Justice

In the context of clinical ethics, justice relates primarily to the distribution of medical care and the allocation of resources. In order to distribute health resources justly, the concept of utility—'greatest good for the greatest number'—must be considered. In the case of individual patients, however, justice is also equated with being 'fair' and 'even-handed'. The concept of fair delivery of health care can be viewed from three perspectives:

- Respect for the *needs* of the individual. Health care is delivered first to those who need it most. This perspective is particularly relevant when need must be assessed by some kind of triage.
- Respect for the *rights* of a person. Everyone who needs health care is entitled to a fair share of the resources available. This perspective is particularly relevant when local or global economic, social, educational or other inequalities prevent or reduce equitable access to health care.
- Respect for *merit*. Health care is delivered on the basis of value judgements, according to financial, political, social or other factors relating to the value of the individual to society. For example, the President of the USA is cared for by an in-house personal physician and the White House Medical Unit. The relevance of this perspective to health care is widely disputed, not least because such value judgements are difficult to make in practice and to defend ethically.

Types of ethical problem

When faced with an ethical problem, it is often helpful to characterise it in terms of certain patterns which can be recognised (Fig. 1.5).

A gap or block

The ideal goal is clearly seen but there are major obstacles to achieving it. The obstacles may be economic or social, or in the belief system of the patient. The obvious answer—to bridge the gap or remove the block—may not be possible within the available time frame and resources. A young boy from a poor family in a developing country,

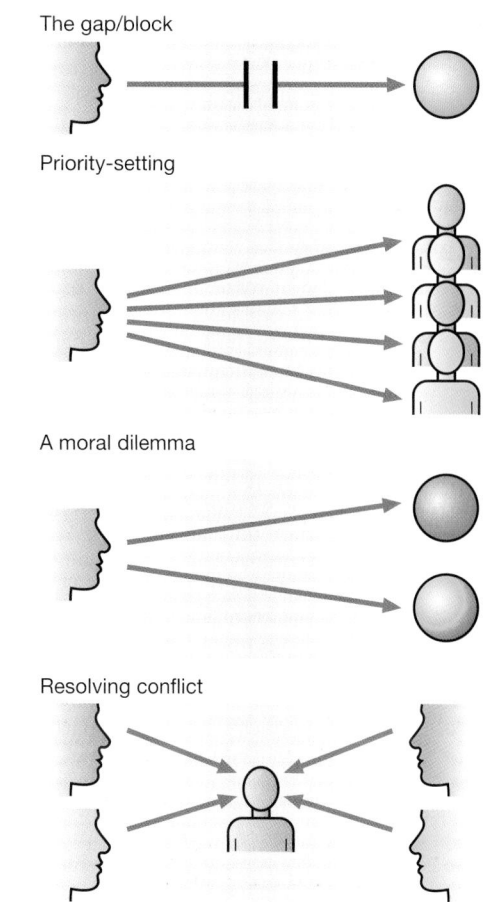

The gap/block

Priority-setting

A moral dilemma

Resolving conflict

Fig. 1.5 A classification of ethical problems.

who has Wilson's disease and needs a liver transplant, is an example of an economic block. Some problems of this kind cannot be resolved satisfactorily in the clinical context until or unless they are resolved in the economic or political context.

Priority-setting

The right course of action is clear but prioritisation is necessary and the principles to guide that process have to be defined. A decision to allot the last bed in intensive care to either an 80-year-old patient with pneumonia or a 20-year-old with advanced lymphoma is an example. While it is not possible to cover all eventualities, guidelines agreed in advance with relevant stakeholders are often helpful.

A moral dilemma

Acting in accordance with one ethical principle may conflict with another ethical principle. This can create a moral dilemma—a choice between two alternatives, neither of which is ethically satisfactory. For example, a physician may decide that a particular mode of therapy is best (principle of beneficence) while the patient makes a different choice (principle of respect for autonomy). In theory, the dilemma can be resolved only if one of the ethical principles is given priority; ethical analysis (see below) can help to achieve resolution. True moral dilemmas are less common in practice than in theory; apparent dilemmas can often be resolved by good doctor–patient communication.

Resolving conflict

A conflict of opinion may arise between members of the team responsible for care of the patient. Differing views should normally be resolved through discussion, but if this does not work, decision-making authority allocated in advance may have to be invoked. The challenge then is to ensure consistent and accurate implementation of the decision.

Ethical analysis

Ethical analysis (or moral reasoning) is the process of thinking through ethical problems and reaching a conclusion. It helps the decision-maker to grow personally and professionally, allows communication of the process by which a decision is made, and permits the process to be constructively criticised. It can be used systematically: for example, in retrospective review of difficult cases. When, in everyday practice, time for reflection is limited, knowledge of methods of moral reasoning provides a useful background and aid for decision-making, and is often employed in ways analogous to those of 'the novice–expert shift' (see Box 1.13, p. 14). Some approaches that can be applied are as follows:

- *A principles approach*. This involves analysing an ethical problem in terms of the principles of respect for autonomy, beneficence, non-maleficence and justice. If all of these principles support a particular course of action, then that course of action is probably correct and there may in fact no longer be an ethical problem. If, however, different principles suggest different courses of action, this approach has no intrinsic mechanism for deciding which principle has priority. On the other hand, analysing the problem in terms of these principles can help

to clarify the nature of the ethical problem and the issues which need to be addressed if the problem is to be resolved.
- *A casuistry (cases) approach*. This uses precedent as a guide to what to do. A case is recalled or imagined which is similar to that under discussion but where the right choice of action/behaviour was obvious. Then the features which make the present case different, if any, are analysed and considered to see if and why they lead to a different conclusion. A variation on this approach, related to virtue ethics, is to imagine what a physician who was particularly skilled or experienced in this type of situation would do, or how a previous patient might have viewed the problem.
- *A perspectives (or narrative) approach*. A perspectives approach involves considering the views of all the stakeholders: the patient, the family or carers, the health-care team, the health service and society. The greater the degree of concordance of these views on a particular outcome, the more likely it is that the decision leading to that outcome is right. A narrative approach is similar to this but involves listening attentively to the different 'stories' told by the stakeholders about the problem and how they perceive it in their own experience. Where these stories differ can provide clues to a more nuanced understanding of the problem and how, if possible, it might be resolved.
- *A counter-argument approach*. A particular course of action is chosen and the best ethical arguments against it are then marshalled and evaluated. This may or may not cause the decision to be reconsidered.
- *Application of rules*. In certain common and clearly defined situations, externally imposed rules (including the law) may require, or guide towards, a specific course of action. This does not obviate the need for ethical analysis. Moreover, any such rules must be reviewed regularly.

While all of these approaches may be useful, it is important to remember that none of them removes the need on the one hand for the exercise of judgement, and on the other for good communication and consensus decision-making. No less important is the requirement for all of this to be based on sound and shared information about the clinical and human facts of the case. In this respect a useful, integrated way of addressing ethical problems is provided by what has been called:

- *An onion-peel approach*. This uses a layered framework to analyse the problem systematically (Box 1.11).

Discussion with colleagues and others is crucial in reaching ethical decisions. Many hospitals have a clinical ethics committee to review difficult decisions. Up-to-date, accurate, valid and reliable data should inform the decision-making progress. Local legal issues must be considered. Once a conclusion has been reached, a strategy to complete the action must be implemented. Post-hoc evaluation of decisions is important, and again is best carried out collectively by an ethics committee or some other means of retrospective review.

A clinical ethics scenario

A 70-year-old man who has chronic obstructive pulmonary disease, hypertension and diabetes mellitus is admitted to hospital with pneumonia. His memory

1.11 Ethical analysis: an 'onion-peel' approach

Patient preferences: data gathered from patient and relatives/carers

- What is the quality of life expected after therapy—from the patient's perspective?
- If the patient is competent, has he or she been offered options and made choices?
- If the patient is not competent, who will make the decisions?

Medical goals: data gathered from literature, guidelines, expert opinion

- What are the prospects of a successful outcome?
- What are the best therapeutic options available based on evidence?
- Has the therapy been optimised and matched to this individual patient?

Regional issues: data gathered from local sources

- What decisions are most consistent with local laws and with social and cultural values?

Basic ethical principles, type of ethical problem, ethical analysis (see text)

- Consider the basic principles of medical ethics
- Consider the type of ethical problem
- Choose the ethical analytical approach(es) to use and apply it/them to the problem

has been deteriorating for 3 years with a rapid decline in cognition over the last 3 months and he now needs help to carry out his activities of daily living. A neurologist has evaluated him and has excluded reversible causes of dementia. The patient deteriorates and needs mechanical ventilation. His wife states that he told her (when he was well) that he did not want to be put on 'life support machines' and is therefore opposed to mechanical ventilation. Two of his children fail to confirm this and request active treatment. What care should be given?

On the one hand, considered mainly in teleological terms:

The patient is incapable of making an autonomous decision. The closest surrogate indicates that he would have preferred to forego life-sustaining therapy at this stage. (Respect for autonomy might support this.) The consequences of ventilation would probably be to prolong the process of dying (which non-maleficence could argue against) rather than increase his chances of recovery to a good quality of life. Beneficence requires that he receive general care and symptom relief immediately. An appropriate action therefore is not to ventilate the patient but to continue basic medical (fluids, oxygen and antibiotics) and nursing care in a general ward setting in order to optimise patient comfort.

On the other hand, considered in deontological as well as teleological terms:

The present illness is due to a potentially reversible infection. The patient's real preference is uncertain and his family, who have difficulty in looking after him, have expressed differing views. In terms of the duty of a doctor to make the patient's health the first consideration, and of the patient's right to appropriate health care regardless of his age or mental condition, it would

therefore be appropriate to institute all possible care, including ventilation on an intensive care unit.

In practice:

The physician responsible for the patient's care should consider the different courses of action suggested, but not determined, by these ethical analyses, explain the reasons for and against each course of action to the patient's family and, if one of them is the patient's legal surrogate, help that person come to a decision. Where there is no legal surrogate, the physician will have to reach a judgement about what is in the patient's best interests, recognising that, while judgement is always fallible, whatever decision is made must be defensible if challenged on legal or ethical grounds. Decisions that are reached on the basis of ethical and moral reasoning will be relatively easy to defend.

In this case, further discussion of the relevant issues with the relatives and other members of the health-care team led to concordance. The patient was treated by artificial ventilation in the intensive care unit for 3 days. He made a good recovery and appeared grateful for the care he had received.

Some basic concepts related to end-of-life care are discussed in Chapter 12.

PERSONAL AND PROFESSIONAL DEVELOPMENT

Good doctors never stop learning, and continue to develop their knowledge, skills and attributes throughout their working lives, to the benefit of their patients and themselves. This has become an essential component of clinical governance, which is a mechanism for ensuring high standards of clinical care (Box 1.12). Personal and professional development (PPD) requires a reflective and self-directed approach to the study and practice of medicine (Fig. 1.6), and will maximise both lifelong effectiveness and personal satisfaction. Linked to this is the concept of the novice–expert shift (Box 1.13).

PPD begins in the first days at medical school and continues through postgraduate training and subsequent professional practice. Maintaining competence and expertise requires continuous professional development (CPD). In the UK this is formally regulated by professional bodies such as the Royal Colleges, and is linked to processes of appraisal (Box 1.14) and re-accreditation for established practitioners.

To support this process, outcomes and competences for PPD are being defined at all levels of medical training, including undergraduate and postgraduate study. These sit alongside and complement curricula that focus on discipline-based knowledge and skills. As adult learners, doctors are expected to reflect on their own practice and identify their own particular learning or

1.12 Key components in clinical governance

- Continuing education
- Clinical audit
- Clinical effectiveness
- Risk management
- Research and development
- Openness

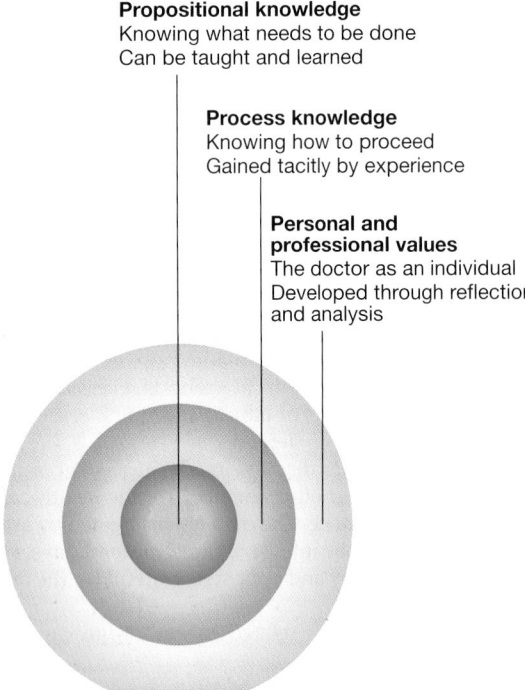

Propositional knowledge
Knowing what needs to be done
Can be taught and learned

Process knowledge
Knowing how to proceed
Gained tacitly by experience

Personal and professional values
The doctor as an individual
Developed through reflection and analysis

Fig. 1.6 The personal and professional development of a doctor.

1.13 The novice–expert shift

- **Novices** use pre-determined methods which they learn
- **Advanced beginners** recognise that these methods are not effective in all circumstances and can adapt them according to context
- **Competent professionals** are able to make conscious, independent choices and can manage and regulate their own practice
- **Proficient professionals** make use of intuition based on experience, and integrate multiple aspects of practice into a holistic model
- **Experts** function largely through 'unconscious competence' and are inseparable from the tasks they undertake

1.14 Some techniques used in the appraisal process

- Formal, structured assessment (e.g. postgraduate examinations)
- 360° assessment (surveying colleagues from medicine and other disciplines who work alongside the practitioner)
- Educational supervision and mentoring (a specific colleague has nominated responsibility to guide, and also assess, the practitioner)
- Logbooks (records of work undertaken and outcomes)
- Portfolio-based assessment (the practitioner accumulates a record of educational and clinical experiences together with evidence of reflective practice)

developmental needs. This recognises that doctors will have different learning needs throughout their career which will be affected by their current clinical practice, their future career plans and any areas of educational need that have become apparent through the appraisal process.

Whilst the individual learning needs of doctors are important, each doctor has a duty to ensure that his or her clinical knowledge and skills are up-to-date and comparable with his or her peers. Clinical audit is one method of assessing practice in this context.

Clinical audit

Clinical audit is the process by which the clinical practice of a doctor or medical team and the outcomes of that practice are evaluated against an agreed standard. Where practice fails to meet the standard, changes to practice are implemented; after a period, practice can be re-evaluated to identify any improvement. The continuing evaluation, implementation of change and re-evaluation process is known as the audit loop or cycle (Fig. 1.7). The standard against which practice is measured is usually an externally agreed one, rather than a local one. It is important to know that clinical care is comparable to that delivered elsewhere. For this reason, national standards are the norm in most countries, often set alongside national guidelines which signpost the practice necessary to achieve them. Clinical audit may be conducted by the doctor or team themselves, or by an external body. Outcome measures may include success rates or complication rates of clinical procedures such as surgical operations; process variables such as waiting times for clinical care; or the perspective of patients and relatives. In the UK, all practising clinicians are now expected to participate in audit, and it is an integral part of appraisal procedures and proposals for revalidation and relicensing of doctors.

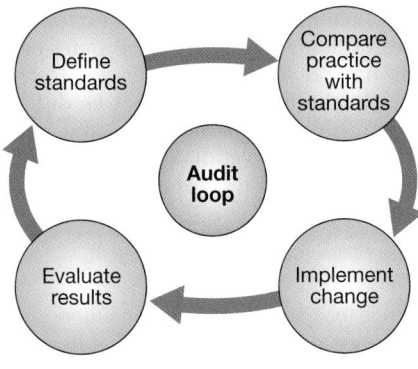

Fig. 1.7 The clinical audit loop.

COMPLEMENTARY AND ALTERNATIVE MEDICINE

Complementary and alternative medicine (CAM) refers to a group of medical and health-care systems, practices and products that are not considered to be part of conventional medicine. It covers an enormous and ever-changing range of activities, from well-established physical therapies such as osteopathy to spiritual measures such as prayer specifically for health. Proponents suggest that CAM focuses on the whole person: his or her lifestyle, environment, diet, and mental, emotional and spiritual health, as well as physical complaints.

'Complementary medicine' is the term used to describe the use of these treatments in conjunction with conventional medicine (e.g. acupuncture to reduce pain after surgery). 'Alternative medicine' describes their use in place of conventional medicine (e.g. reflexology instead of anti-inflammatory drugs for arthritis). Clearly, most forms of treatment can be used in either way, so the term CAM is often used generically. 'Integrative medicine' describes the use of conventional therapy in combination with one or more complementary therapies for which there is evidence of efficacy and safety.

A variety of different taxonomies are used for CAM therapies. The National Center for Complementary and Alternative Medicine in the USA uses the following classification:

- *Alternative medical systems.* These have their own constructs of theory and practice, often based on ancient historical beliefs. Examples are homeopathy, naturopathy, traditional Chinese medicine and Ayurveda.
- *Mind–body interactions.* These rely on the mind's capacity to influence physical function. Examples are meditation, prayer, mental healing, music therapy and dance.
- *Biologically based therapies.* These involve the use or regulation of an extraneous agent or preparation. Examples include herbal medicine, dietary supplementation and nutritional medicine.
- *Manipulative and body-based methods.* These are based on manipulation or movement of parts of the body. They include osteopathy, chiropractic, reflexology and massage (which is often combined with aromatherapy).
- *Energy therapies.* These involve use of energy fields. Examples include gi gong, reiki and therapeutic touch.

Some forms of CAM are embedded in the cultural norms of particular social and ethnic groups, e.g. traditional Chinese medicine. In Western society, the use of CAM is extensive and growing. For example, in 2002 in the USA, at any one time 36% of the population were using some form of CAM. If prayer for health reasons was included, this figure rose to 62%. The most common medical conditions involved were back, neck, head or joint pain, upper respiratory tract infections, anxiety or depression, gastrointestinal symptoms and sleep disturbance.

The popularity of CAM may reflect a lack of confidence in conventional medicine, particularly a belief that it will not help the condition or may cause harm. CAM is particularly popular with cancer patients who have disease which is unresponsive to conventional medicines. In addition, it may reflect the increasing ease of access to information and therapies via the Internet, although such information is not formally regulated. CAM is often perceived to be completely safe; patients may therefore be willing to experiment with it as a 'no-lose' measure. Moreover, many forms of CAM are, regardless of any therapeutic benefit, inherently pleasurable.

Safety

Not all CAM therapies are entirely safe; some are toxic in their own right (e.g. dietary supplements containing ephedrine alkaloids, now banned in the USA) and others are harmful if used in combination with conventional treatment (e.g. garlic supplements that interfere with the action of anti-HIV chemotherapy). Others have been reported to be associated with rare but serious side-effects, which can be life-threatening (e.g. bowel perforation from coffee enemas, hyponatraemia from noni juice).

There is also a potential for harm when alternative medicine is used to treat serious or life-threatening medical conditions if the resultant delay in seeking conventional treatment compromises clinical outcome, in a way that patients would not have chosen had they been fully informed at the outset.

On balance, however, the relative safety of most CAM therapies is a positive feature; homeopathy is an obvious example.

Evidence

In an era where EBM is the norm, practitioners and advocates of CAM are increasingly challenged to justify these treatments through independent, well-conducted, randomised controlled clinical trials. In some cases this may be difficult (e.g. the placebo arm of a double-blind trial of acupuncture). In addition, it can be argued that different types and standards of evidence, focusing on patient satisfaction and subjective benefit rather than measurable clinical outcomes, are more appropriate for CAM. The literature in this area is growing rapidly but, at present, only a minority of CAM therapies are supported by evidence that would be acceptable for conventional medicine. These are primarily the 'big five' CAM therapies: homeopathy, osteopathy, chiropractic, acupuncture and herbal medicine. Moreover, where evidence does exist, it is often limited to a small subset of the clinical conditions for which the treatment is used.

Regulation

Many CAM therapies have professional regulatory frameworks in place, and others are following suit. Nevertheless, for many CAM therapies, there is still no established structure of training, certification and accreditation, and practice is effectively open to all. Set against the demanding training and life-long continuous professional development that pertain to conventional medicine, this constitutes an important barrier to integrative medicine.

Integrated health care

There is a considerable popular and political impetus behind moves to integrate CAM with conventional medicine and health care at the level of resource allocation, service design, clinical practice, education and research. Almost 50% of general practices in the UK now offer some form of access to CAM and this is an increasing trend in hospitals. Historically, patients using both types of therapy have often experienced conflicting advice and value judgements, poor or absent communication between practitioners, and even hostility or ridicule. They often revert to secrecy, an inherently undesirable and potentially dangerous outcome. Integrated health care aims to understand and remove the barriers that create such dilemmas for patients. It aims to let them exercise their choice of treatment in an open environment characterised by good communication, respect, and due consideration of autonomy, efficacy and risk.

1

Further information

www.dh.gov.uk *UK Department of Health guidance and policy on confidentiality and consent.*

www.gmc-uk.org *UK General Medical Council. Includes access to guidance on professional conduct (Duties of a Doctor, Good Medical Practice) and guidance on medical education, such as Tomorrow's Doctors.*

www.library.nhs.uk/guidelinesfinder *A UK National Health Service resource providing a searchable library of clinical guidelines from all sources.*

www.nice.org.uk *National Institute for Health and Clinical Excellence. Includes recommendations for evidence-based treatments.*

www.rcplondon.ac.uk *Royal College of Physicians. Includes access to a working party report: Doctors in Society: Medical Professionalism in a Changing World.*

www.sign.ac.uk *Scottish Intercollegiate Guidelines Network. Includes evidence-based guidelines for clinical practice.*

www.who.int *World Health Organization.*

J.K. Aronson

Therapeutics and good prescribing

2

2

WHAT MAKES A GOOD PRESCRIBER?

The purpose of drug therapy is to cure or ameliorate disease or to alleviate symptoms. However, all drugs have adverse effects and before a drug is prescribed clinicians need to weigh the potential benefit of therapy against the potential for doing harm. A good prescriber:

- prescribes only when necessary, having carefully assessed the balance of benefit and harm
- chooses medicines that are appropriate for the disease and the patient
- chooses a dosage regimen that is appropriate to the disease and the patient
- continues therapy for an appropriate time and alters doses when necessary.

BASIC PRINCIPLES OF PHARMACOLOGY RELEVANT TO PRESCRIBING

The essence of good prescribing is to pick the most appropriate drug for the disease in question, taking pathophysiology into account. For example, rheumatoid arthritis and osteoarthritis both cause joint pain. Although some aspects of management are similar (such as the use of analgesics), other aspects differ (such as the use of immunosuppressives in rheumatoid arthritis) because the pathophysiology is different. Similar comments apply to the treatment of haemorrhagic as compared with embolic stroke.

Mechanisms of action of drugs

Drugs act on a wide variety of targets, as discussed below.

Drugs that act on receptors

Many drugs act by binding to receptors, which are proteins that affect cellular function by modulating intracellular signalling pathways (p. 46). Although most receptors are located on the cell surface, some—such as steroid hormone receptors—are located intracellularly. There are four subtypes of drugs that interact with receptors:

- *Agonists* cause activation of receptors and their downstream intracellular signalling pathways.
- *Pure antagonists* prevent agonists from binding and inhibit receptors and their downstream intracellular signalling pathways.
- *Partial agonists* activate receptors to an extent, but not to the same degree as a full agonist; depending on the milieu, they can act as agonists or antagonists.
- *Inverse agonists* bind to receptors and block the effects of endogenous ligands, but also stimulate the receptor, causing effects opposite to those of agonists.

Drugs that act on transport processes

Many drugs act on ion channels, which are responsible for transporting cations (such as sodium, potassium and calcium) and other substances (such as organic acids in the kidneys and neurotransmitters in the nervous system) across cell membranes. Drugs that act on transport proteins can exert their effects in several ways:

- by blocking transport of an endogenous substance
- by increasing release of an endogenous ligand
- by inhibiting reuptake of an endogenous ligand.

Drugs that act on enzymes

Several drugs act on enzymes and work by modulating synthesis of a second messenger or a substance involved in the pathophysiology of disease.

Drug action by other miscellaneous effects

- *Chelating agents* bind metal ions and are used to treat, for example, iron and copper overload syndromes.
- *Osmotic agents* are used as diuretics and in the treatment of cerebral oedema.
- *General anaesthetics* do not have a specific molecular target but act on the lipid matrix of biological membranes, changing its biophysical properties.
- *Enzymes* are used as replacement therapy in patients with deficiency or to activate specific pathways.

Stereoisomerism and drug action

If a carbon atom has four different substituents it is called asymmetric; the conformation of the four other atoms or molecules around it can vary. Sometimes other atoms (such as phosphorus) are asymmetric in an analogous way. This leads to forms with different optical activities, rotating polarised light to the left or right. By convention, a substance that rotates polarised light to the right is called dextrorotatory (d), while a substance that rotates polarised light to the left is called laevorotatory (l). If the actual spatial arrangement of the molecules is known, the right- and left-handedness of the configuration about an asymmetric atom is designated by 'R' and 'S' (Latin, *rectus* and *sinister*), or 'D' and 'L'. Stereoisomers are of two types, enantiomers and diastereomers (or 'epimers').

- In *enantiomers*, asymmetry occurs at all the centres of potential asymmetry (chiral centres). Enantiomers can be considered as 'mirror images' of one another (Fig. 2.1) and tend to have similar physicochemical properties.
- In *diastereomers*, asymmetry occurs at only one chiral centre, even though the molecule may have more than one; in such cases the isomers are not mirror images of each other. Diastereomers do not usually share similar physicochemical properties.

About 40% per cent of the drugs used in routine clinical practice are chiral, and about 90% of these are marketed in the racemic form (as an equal mixture of the two stereoisomers). Examples of drugs that are marketed as single stereoisomers include naproxen, levodopa (L-dopa), levothyroxine (L-thyroxine) and dextrose (D-glucose). Often there are important pharmacological differences between stereoisomers, as the following examples show:

- S-warfarin is about five times more potent than R-warfarin; the two isomers are differently metabolised and are subject to different drug interactions.
- L-sotalol is a beta-adrenoceptor antagonist while D-sotalol is a class III anti-arrhythmic drug.
- R-thalidomide is a hypnotic, while S-thalidomide is immunomodulatory and teratogenic.

Although it is theoretically desirable to take advantage of these differences by using individual isomers,

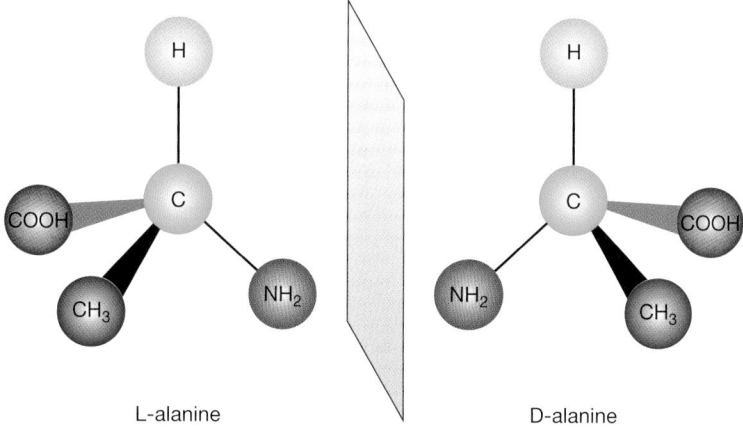

L-alanine   D-alanine

Fig. 2.1 An example of stereoisomerism. The central carbon atom in amino acids is asymmetrical, i.e. it is attached to four different moieties; two configurations are possible, mirror images of each other and not superimposable. These are L-alanine and D-alanine. Levodopa (L-dihydroxyphenylalanine) has a similar structure to L-alanine, but the CH_3 group is replaced by $C_6H_3(OH)_2CH_2$.

it is generally too difficult to prepare them in practice, and in any case administration of a single isomer often results in back-conversion to the racemic form in vivo. In a few cases drug companies have extended the patent lives of some of their drugs by marketing them as isomers; examples include esomeprazole and escitalopram. These drugs generally have few or no advantages over the corresponding racemic mixtures.

Pharmacokinetics

Following administration, disposition of drugs in the body is determined by drug absorption, distribution, metabolism and excretion. Taken together, these processes define the pharmacokinetics of a drug. A few simple pharmacokinetic principles are worth knowing in relation to practical prescribing.

Drug absorption and systemic availability

After oral administration drugs are mainly absorbed in the small bowel. The *speed* of absorption is affected by the rate of gastric emptying and the formulation. The absolute *amount* of absorption is generally unaffected by these factors. Some drugs are inactivated in the gut and need to be given parenterally, whereas others are removed by metabolism during absorption, or by enzymes in the gut and liver. This is called first-pass metabolism. The systemic availability of a drug (bioavailability) depends on the extent to which it is absorbed and metabolised. Drug interactions that involve inhibition of gut or liver metabolism reduce bioavailability. Impaired liver function reduces first-pass metabolism and increases bioavailability.

Drug distribution

Drugs are distributed by binding to plasma and tissue proteins. In the plasma, acidic drugs, such as warfarin and phenytoin, are bound to albumin, whereas basic drugs, such as propranolol, are bound to alpha$_1$ acid glycoproteins (such as C-reactive protein). Changes in the concentrations of these proteins can alter the disposition of drugs markedly. Furthermore, the affinity of albumin for drugs changes in chronic renal failure, probably because of dialysable endogenous inhibitors of binding.

Drug metabolism

Most drug metabolism occurs in the liver. The main routes are through:
- oxidation by the family of enzymes known as cytochrome P450 (CYP)
- conjugation to glucuronides, sulphates and other derivatives (acetyl, methyl) by various enzymes
- direct enzymatic breakdown.

The CYP family plays a key role in drug metabolism, and the various subtypes are designated by a combination of letters and numbers (e.g. CYP3A4, CYP2D6). Each metabolises a range of drugs, and they can also be inhibited by drugs. Many clinically important drug interactions occur through inhibition of CYP activity.

Drug excretion

The main route of drug excretion is by the kidney, where drugs are filtered at the glomerulus and reabsorbed or secreted by the renal tubules. Drug excretion is reduced in renal insufficiency, and this can result in toxicity unless the dosage is adjusted. For some drugs, excretion also occurs through the gut as the result of secretion by enterocytes, with subsequent reabsorption. The secretory process is active, mediated by P glycoprotein, and is potentially susceptible to inhibition by other drugs. After overdose, reabsorption after enteric secretion can be prevented by repeated administration of activated charcoal, increasing the rate of clearance. This can be used to treat overdose with some drugs such as carbamazepine, theophylline and cardiac glycosides.

THE BALANCE OF BENEFIT AND HARM IN DRUG THERAPY

The balance of benefit and harm in drug therapy depends on various factors (Box 2.1). Generally, it will be favourable if the disease is life-threatening, the drug highly effective and the only one available, and the risk of serious adverse effects negligible. For example, acetylcysteine is highly effective in preventing liver damage after paracetamol overdose (p. 211), its adverse effects are

2.1 Factors that determine the balance of benefit and harm in drug therapy

Factor	Balance of benefit and harm	
	Favourable	Unfavourable
Seriousness of the disease	Life-threatening	Trivial
Efficacy of the drug	High	Low
Seriousness of adverse effects	Trivial	Serious
Frequency of adverse effects	Rare	Frequent
Efficacy of alternative drugs	Poor	Good
Safety of alternative drugs	Poor	Good

2.2 Some drugs with a low therapeutic index

- Aminoglycoside antibiotics
- Anticoagulants
- Anticonvulsants
- Antihypertensive drugs
- Cardiac glycosides
- Cytotoxic and immunosuppressant drugs
- Drugs that act on the central nervous system
- Oral contraceptives

uncommon and usually mild, and no other agent is as effective. The balance of benefit and harm is unfavourable when the disease is trivial, the drug poorly effective with more effective and safer competitors, and the risk of serious adverse effects high. For example, aminophenazone, used in some countries to treat headache, can cause severe bone marrow depression, and there are much safer and equally effective alternatives. Most cases lie somewhere between these two extremes.

When assessing the balance of benefit and harm, remember that some drugs can cause adverse effects when given in dosages that are within or only a little above the usual therapeutic range; these drugs are said to have a low therapeutic index (Box 2.2). Assessment of the balance of benefit and harm is best made by using evidence-based medicine.

EVIDENCE-BASED MEDICINE IN DRUG THERAPY

For many years doctors have based decisions about the use of drugs or other therapeutic measures on the available evidence, but until recently this was done in a haphazard fashion. For example, treatment strategies would often be formulated using selected pieces of evidence that experts in the field judged to be the most valuable or relevant. Inevitably, bias occurred. The discipline of evidence-based medicine (EBM) introduced a more systematic approach. The tenets of EBM are shown in Box 2.3.

The most important but most difficult task is to apply EBM to management of the individual patient. This is because evidence from large-scale clinical trials is often derived from populations that may not have included

2.3 Principles of evidence-based medicine

- Carrying out high-quality, randomised, controlled clinical trials
- Tracing all the available evidence (published and unpublished)
- Analysing the evidence systematically
- Determining how valid and useful the evidence is
- Developing computerised databases of relevant information
- Applying that evidence to the management of the individual patient

patients like those the prescriber wants to treat. For example, trials that are undertaken by pharmaceutical companies to gain marketing authorisation often have strict inclusion and exclusion criteria and may not be representative of 'real-life' patients. Methods for dealing with this are available, but are not as well developed or easily applied as the methods for obtaining the evidence. In addition, there are many therapeutic problems for which evidence from high-quality randomised trials is not available, and in such cases the prescriber has to use clinical judgement and whatever evidence is available. The evidence-based medicine movement has tended to devalue forms of evidence that are not based on randomised trials, but this view needs to be corrected; observational studies and sometimes even anecdotal reports can contribute usefully in different circumstances and should be used when necessary.

Beneficial effects and the number needed to treat for benefit (NNT$_B$)

Benefit in drug therapy is often expressed as the so-called number needed to treat (NNT or NNT$_B$), which is the number of patients who need to be treated in order to produce benefit. A simple example illustrates how this is calculated. Of 239 patients with the acute pain of third molar extraction, 122 were given placebo, of whom 9 (7.4%) had at least 50% pain relief by 6 hours, compared with 65 (55.6%) of the 117 patients who were given ibuprofen; the difference was therefore 55.6−7.4 = 48.2%, or an effect size of 0.482. This is known as the absolute risk reduction, and the NNT$_B$ is the inverse of this: 1/0.482 = 2.1. In other words 1 out of every 2 people who take a single dose of ibuprofen will have better than 50% pain relief in the 6 hours after the dose. The 95% confidence interval of this estimate (the calculation of which is more complicated) was 1.7–2.6; in other words, the mean estimate of the NNT$_B$ was 2.1 and there was a 95% chance that the true value lay between 1.7 and 2.6.

When a drug is given repeatedly, rather than as a single dose, the duration of therapy also has to be considered. For example, in a systematic analysis of the use of warfarin to prevent strokes in patients with atrial fibrillation there were 53 strokes in 1450 patients who took warfarin (3.66%) and 133 in 1450 patients who took placebo (9.17%). The effect size was thus 9.17−3.66 = 5.51% (0.0551) and the NNT$_B$ was 18 (1/0.0551). The confidence interval was 14–27. So, on the basis of these results, if 18 patients were treated with warfarin for 1 year, one stroke would be prevented. It is not valid to extrapolate effects to durations of treatment that were not studied in the original trial; in other words, we cannot conclude that if 18 patients were treated for 2 years, two strokes would be prevented; a longer trial would be needed to investigate this.

For a further perspective on NNT_B, consider oral contraception. On average a woman who has unprotected sex for 1 year has a 40% chance of becoming pregnant, while a woman who takes some form of oral contraception has a 3% chance; this 37% difference translates into an NNT_B of 2.7 (1/0.37). Now because oral contraception is so effective it might be expected that the NNT_B would be very close to 1 but that is not so, since the NNT_B takes into account the rate that occurs without treatment. In other words, if 100 women are treated for a year with an oral contraceptive only 37 (100/2.7) pregnancies that would otherwise have occurred will be prevented, because the other 63 women would not have become pregnant anyway. However with the passage of time, the NNT_B for oral contraceptives falls and approaches 1.0, as unprotected sexually active women will mostly become pregnant eventually.

Adverse effects and the number needed to treat for harm (NNT_H)

The other side of the coin, the number needed to treat for harm to occur (NNT_H), can be similarly calculated from data on adverse effects of drugs. For example, in a meta-analysis of 13 trials of the effect of thiazide diuretics in essential hypertension, 205 out of 3275 patients taking a thiazide had erectile impotence (6.26%), compared with 67 out of 5295 patients taking placebo (1.27%); the difference is 5% and so the NNT_H for this effect is 20 (Box 2.4).

The balance of benefit and harm assessed from the NNT_B and NNT_H

Although one might expect to be able to express the balance of benefit to harm as the simple ratio of the NNT_B to the NNT_H, the comparison is not straightforward, since the quality of the benefit and the severity and seriousness of the harm need to be weighed against each other.

Consider tamoxifen, which prolongs survival in breast cancer (by an anti-oestrogenic effect on the tumour) and reduces the risk of myocardial infarction, but causes endometrial cancer and venous thromboembolism (by oestrogenic effects on lipids, the endometrium and clotting factors):

- NNT_B to prevent one death = 17
- NNT_B to prevent one myocardial infarction = 29
- NNT_H for one case of endometrial cancer = 143
- NNT_H for one venous thromboembolism = 130.

These figures suggest that treating 1000 women with breast cancer for 2–5 years with tamoxifen will prevent about 60 deaths and 34 myocardial infarctions, at the cost of 7 cases of endometrial cancer and 7 cases of venous thromboembolism, clearly a favourable benefit to harm balance. However, calculations of this sort yield probabilities that relate to the patients that have been studied in clinical trials. They do not necessarily apply to the whole population and do not predict what the outcome will be in the individual patient.

There are other ways of expressing results of this kind. For example, it is possible to calculate the risk ratio (RR) or odds ratio (OR), each with its confidence interval (see Box 2.4). The larger the effect, the higher the odds ratio is relative to the risk ratio; at incidences of up to about 15% the risk ratio and odds ratio are very similar, but at higher incidences the odds ratio starts to overestimate the risk ratio considerably. Note that two treatments can have exactly the same risk ratio but different values of NNT_H. For example, a treatment that increases the risk

---

i 2.4 Calculation of NNT_H, risk ratio and odds ratio

(A) A THEORETICAL CASE

Group	Number with the adverse event	Number without the adverse event	Total
Active treatment	a	b	a+b
Placebo	c	d	c+d
Total	a+c	b+d	a+b+c+d

1. Calculation of number needed to treat for harm (NNT_H)
Rate of event in treated group = a/(a+b)
Rate of event in placebo group = c/(c+d)
Difference (absolute harm increase) = a/(a+b) − c/(c+d) = A

$NNT_H = 1/A$

2. Calculation of risk ratio (RR)
Rate of event in treated group = a/(a+b)
Rate of event in placebo group = c/(c+d)
Relative risk = [a/(a+b)]/[c/(c+d)]

3. Calculation of odds ratio (OR)
Odds of event in treated group = a/b
Odds of event in placebo group = c/d
Odds ratio = (a/b)/(c/d)

(B) A REAL CASE*

Group	Number with the adverse event	Number without the adverse event	Total
Drug	205	3070	3275
Placebo	67	5228	5295
Total	272	8298	8570

1. Calculation of number needed to treat for harm (NNT_H)
Rate of event in treated group = 205/3275
Rate of event in placebo group = 67/5295
Difference (absolute harm increase) = 205/3275 − 67/5295 = 0.0499

$NNT_H = \dfrac{1}{0.0499} = 20$

2. Calculation of risk ratio (RR)
Rate of event in treated group = 205/3275
Rate of event in placebo group = 67/5295
Relative risk = [205/3275]/[67/5295] = 5.0 (i.e. a five-fold risk)

3. Calculation of odds ratio (OR)
Odds of event in treated group = 205/3070
Odds of event in placebo group = 67/5228
Odds ratio = [205/3070]/[67/5228] = 5.2 (i.e. relative odds of about 5 to 1 on)

*Erectile impotence with thiazide diuretics in hypertension over a mean of 4 years, a meta-analysis of 13 RCTs (Hypertension 1999; 34:710).

of an adverse event from 1% to 2% would have a risk ratio of 2 but an NNT_H of 100 (1/0.01), while a treatment that increased the risk of an adverse event from 25% to 50% would also have a risk ratio of 2 but an NNT_H of 4 (1/0.25), a much more important effect. When it was reported that third-generation progestogens approximately doubled the risk of deep venous thrombosis compared with older progestogens, the announcement caused some women to panic; they did not appreciate that the baseline risk was very low and the NNT_H therefore very high.

Obtaining the best evidence

Randomised trials are highly desirable as sources of evidence that treatments are effective. However, randomised trials are not perfect. They may be underpowered and give results that are contradictory or implausible. Conversely, non-randomised evidence is sometimes sufficient to make a clear case for the effectiveness of an intervention. Some ways of obtaining evidence are listed in Box 2.5. Depending on the quality of the design and conduct, the evidence that any of these forms of study provides can be

2.5 Some methods of obtaining evidence in drug therapy

- Systematic review (meta-analysis)
- Systematic review (other types of analysis)
- Prospective, randomised, double-blind, placebo-controlled trial
- Prospective, randomised, double-blind, comparative trial (drug vs. drug)
- Cohort study
- Case-control study
- Point prevalence study
- Subgroup analysis of a large trial (generates hypotheses for further trials)
- N-of-one trial
- Other trials (e.g. non-randomised, non-controlled, historical controls, retrospective analysis)
- Case series and case reports
- Non-systematic review

of value in clinical decision-making. Accordingly, there is no absolute index of the usefulness of evidence, because in different circumstances one form of evidence may be better than another.

Any form of evidence of causation can be assessed, using guidelines to help decide whether an association is causative or an intervention effective (Box 2.6). The guidelines, adapted from ones originally devised by Sir Austin Bradford Hill, can be organised into three categories:

1. direct evidence from studies (randomised or non-randomised) that a probabilistic association between intervention and outcome is causal and not spurious
2. mechanistic evidence for the alleged causal process that connects the intervention and the outcome
3. parallel evidence that supports the causal hypothesis suggested in a study, by noting that related studies have consistent results.

DRUG DISCOVERY AND DEVELOPMENT

Most drug discovery nowadays is carried out by pharmaceutical companies. However, they rely heavily on research in academic institutions, and governments in developed countries spend about twice as much on drug research as pharmaceutical companies. Current estimates of the costs to a company of developing a new drug range from $250 million to $1000 million.

Drug discovery

There are several ways in which drugs are discovered:
- *from herbal remedies*: for example, morphine from the opium poppy (*Papaver somniferum*) and digoxin from foxgloves (*Digitalis lanata*)
- *from studies of endogenous agents in animals*: for example, the anticoagulant hirudin from the medicinal leech (*Hirudo medicinalis*)
- *serendipity*: for example, penicillins from Alexander Fleming's chance observation of the effect of *Penicillium* mould on bacterial growth

2.6 Guidelines for assessing the strength of evidence for a cause and effect relationship of interventions*

Type of evidence	Guideline	Comment
Direct	Size of effect not attributable to plausible confounding	The larger the effect and the fewer the identifiable confounding factors, the stronger the evidence in favour of an association
	Appropriate temporal and/or spatial proximity	The cause/intervention should precede the effect and the effect should occur after a plausible interval; the effect should occur at the same site as the intervention
	Dose-responsiveness and reversibility	The presence of dose-responsiveness and reversibility provides strong evidence in favour of an association; its absence is unhelpful
Mechanistic	Evidence for a mechanism of action	The absence of biological, chemical or mechanical plausibility provides evidence against an association
	Coherence	Absence of consistency with the current scientific paradigm provides strong evidence against an association
Parallel	Replicability	Replicability in different settings and at different times provides strong evidence in favour of an association
	Similarity	If similar effects are produced by analogous interventions, this provides strong evidence in favour of an association

*Adapted from Howick J, et al. J R Soc Med 2009; 102:186–194.

- *metabolites of existing drugs*: for example, mesalazine (the active metabolite of sulfasalazine)
- *applied pharmacology and empirical chemistry*: for example, the development of β-adrenoceptor antagonists (β-blockers) based on the structure of isoprenaline
- *rational drug design based on knowledge of pathophysiology*: for example, the development of tumour necrosis factor alpha (TNF-α) blocking agents for the treatment of rheumatoid arthritis, based on the finding of increased TNF-α concentrations in the joints of affected patients
- *rational design based on the human genome*: for example, the development of cathepsin K inhibitors as bone resorption inhibitors, based on the observation that mutations of cathepsin K result in increased bone mass with reduced bone resorption.

The current issue of the *British National Formulary (BNF)* contains about 1200 compounds. About 75% of these have human targets; the rest are either antimicrobial drugs or have no specific pharmacological targets (e.g. vitamins, plasma substitutes). About 150 pharmacological targets are known. A comparison of this figure with the number of genes in the human genome (about 25 000) shows how much therapeutic potential there is still to be realised. Of these targets, about 25% are G protein-coupled receptors, 25% enzymes, 20% other types of receptor (ionotropic, kinase-linked and nuclear receptors), 10% ion channels and transporters, and 10% a variety of proteins (including TNF-α, VEGF, HER-2, interferons, cell surface antigens such as CD20, CD25 and CD52, and various tumour-associated antigens).

Targets can be discovered by understanding the pathophysiology of the disease, by analysing the mechanisms of action of existing drugs, or by analysing the human genome. Examples of targets that have been discovered in these respective ways are angiotensin-converting enzyme in the management of hypertension, cyclo-oxygenase in the development of non-steroidal anti-inflammatory drugs (NSAID), and *Abl* kinase in the development of anticancer drugs.

Drug development

When a new drug has been discovered it goes through a defined development process, after which it is licensed for use and marketed.

Preclinical pharmacology and toxicology

Preclinical studies include extensive pharmacological testing in vitro and in animals, including short- and long-term toxicity testing.

Clinical testing (volunteer studies)

Next the pharmacokinetics of the drug are studied after single and multiple doses. If it has measurable effects in healthy people, its pharmacology is studied and clinical, biochemical and haematological adverse effects are assessed. In some cases (for example, drugs for AIDS or cancer), healthy volunteer studies are not possible and the drug is tried immediately in patients.

Phase 0 studies

Phase 0 studies are first-in-human studies that involve the administration of tiny doses (microdoses) of the drug in a few subjects, in order to collect preliminary pharmacokinetic and pharmacodynamic information. They do not cover safety or efficacy.

Phase I studies

Phase I studies in patients or healthy volunteers concentrate on the clinical pharmacology of the drug, short-term safety, efficacy, pharmacological effects and pharmacokinetics. These early studies also provide information about the likely dose range to be used in phase II studies.

Phase II studies

In phase II studies further evidence of safety and efficacy is obtained in larger numbers of patients, often with a surrogate clinical endpoint, with further attention to dose-ranging and adverse effects.

Phase III studies

Phase III studies are full-scale clinical trials, in which the effects of the drug are studied in relation to an important clinical endpoint. These may be placebo-controlled studies or comparisons with other active compounds. In comparative studies the intention is usually to demonstrate superiority or, at the very least, non-inferiority. So-called 'real-life' trials involve a comparison of the new agent with standard therapy; such trials often include a pharmacoeconomic assessment of the added value that a new treatment brings in relation to its cost.

Phase IV studies

Phase IV studies are carried out after a drug has been marketed. They are designed to obtain information on the effects of the drug in populations who have not been studied before marketing and to detect adverse drug reactions or interactions. The latter are sometimes called phase V studies.

Marketing and post-marketing surveillance

If the regulatory authorities are convinced about quality, safety and efficacy, the drug will be formulated as a medicinal product, and will receive marketing authorisation and a product licence. Marketing authorisations are issued by different regulatory authorities in different countries (e.g. the Medicines and Healthcare products Regulatory Agency in the UK and the Food and Drug Administration in the USA) or by a supranational organisation, such as the European Medicines Evaluation Agency (EMEA).

Surveillance of the effects of a new drug continues after marketing, both formally and informally. There is a post-marketing event monitoring (PEM) scheme in the UK, for research into adverse drug reactions after marketing, and doctors are also encouraged to report suspected adverse effects informally to regulatory agencies (for example, the yellow card scheme in the UK and Medwatch in the USA). If new serious adverse effects are noted, the drug may be withdrawn or its licensed indications may be changed. Examples in the UK include:

- *aspirin*, which is now restricted to those over 16 years of age, because of the risk of Reye's syndrome
- *clozapine*, for which a blood monitoring scheme is mandatory to detect neutropenia, should it occur
- *rofecoxib*, which was voluntarily withdrawn from the market by the manufacturers in 2004 because of an increased risk of cardiovascular disease.

23

2

PRACTICAL PRESCRIBING

When to prescribe a drug

Drug therapy is not always necessary. For example, a mild tremor in Parkinson's disease may not be unduly troublesome and drug treatment to alleviate it may cause harm, outweighing the benefit. Do not be tempted to prescribe a drug simply to end a consultation. If a patient expects drug therapy, discuss the pros and cons. Try to estimate the balance of benefit and harm and prescribe only if it seems favourable.

How to choose a drug to prescribe

After deciding to prescribe a drug, first choose the therapeutic class. The choice may be restricted or wide, as a few examples illustrate (Box 2.7).

Having chosen the class of drug, choose a therapeutic subgroup (Box 2.8). For example, the choice of an anticoagulant depends partly on whether short-term or long-term treatment is indicated. Drug interactions can also affect treatment choice, as in the case of antibiotics (Box 2.9).

2.7 Examples of choosing a therapeutic class of drug

Indication	Therapeutic class
Infection	Antibiotic
Depression	Antidepressant
Acute attack of asthma	Bronchodilators
Diabetes mellitus	Insulin Oral or parenteral (non-insulin) hypoglycaemic drugs
Congestive cardiac failure	Diuretics ACE inhibitors Vasodilators
Hypertension	Diuretics ACE inhibitors β-adrenoceptor antagonists Calcium channel blockers

2.8 Examples of choosing a group of drugs from within a class

Therapeutic class	Therapeutic group
Anticoagulants	Coumarin anticoagulants Heparins Anticoagulant factor inhibitors (e.g. direct thrombin inhibitors)
Diuretics	Thiazides Loop diuretics Potassium-sparing diuretics
Antibiotics	Penicillins Cephalosporins Tetracyclines Aminoglycosides Macrolides Quinolones

2.9 Examples of drug interactions with antibiotics

Antibiotic	Interacting drug	Mechanism	Effect
Gentamicin	Furosemide	Additive	Ototoxicity
Metronidazole	Alcohol	Inhibition of aldehyde dehydrogenase	'Disulfiram reaction'
Metronidazole	Warfarin	Inhibition of metabolism	Potentiation of anticoagulation
Rifampicin	Oestrogens (oral contraceptives)	Induction of metabolism	Reduced contraceptive effect
Rifampicin	Warfarin	Induction of metabolism	Reduced effect of warfarin
Tetracycline	Antacids	Chelation	Reduced effect of tetracycline
Tetracycline	Warfarin	Altered clotting factor activity	Potentiation of anticoagulation

Finally, choose a specific drug from within the class. In doing so, take account of the characteristics of the drugs that are available. For example, in a patient with cardiac failure, when the gut is congested with fluid, bumetanide may be preferable to furosemide because it is better absorbed from the gut. Similarly, the choice of β-blocker will depend upon whether selectivity is required for a receptor subtype, on whether vasodilatory actions are desirable and on other properties (Box 2.10). In other cases the choice may be unimportant; for example, all thiazide diuretics have equal efficacy and similar adverse effects, and there is little to choose between them.

How to make a rational choice

Many factors dictate the choice of a particular drug:

- *Absorption*. It is generally advisable to choose drugs that are well absorbed from the gut.
- *Distribution*. The distribution of a drug to a particular tissue sometimes dictates choice; for example, tetracyclines and rifampicin are

2.10 Examples of choosing a particular drug from within a group

Drug	Distinguishing features
Atenolol	Moderately β_1-selective; water-soluble (poor brain penetration); poor vasodilator
Bisoprolol	Highly β_1-selective; good vasodilator
Carvedilol	Non-selective and also an α-blocker; excellent vasodilator
Metoprolol	Moderately β_1-selective; short-acting; good vasodilator
Propranolol	Non-selective; lipid-soluble; poor vasodilator
Sotalol	Non-selective; poor vasodilator; double action (β-blockade + class III anti-arrhythmic action)

concentrated in the bile, and lincomycin and clindamycin in bones.

- *Metabolism.* In severe liver disease try to avoid drugs that are extensively metabolised (for example, opiate analgesics). Genetic factors can influence the extent of metabolism of a drug, and many examples of genetically determined variations in response have been described. These factors do not make a large impact on drug prescribing but there are some important exceptions (Box 2.11).
- *Excretion.* In renal insufficiency try to avoid drugs that are excreted by the kidney; for example, avoid the aminoglycoside antibiotics if alternatives are suitable.

i **2.11 Some examples of genetic factors that cause variability in drug response**

Genetic factor	Example of drug affected	Clinical outcome
Pharmacokinetic		
Acetylation	Isoniazid	Better response and increased risk of some adverse effects (e.g. peripheral neuropathy) in slow acetylators
Oxidation (CYP2D6)	Nortriptyline	Increased risk of toxicity in poor metabolisers
Oxidation (CYP2C18)	Proguanil (active metabolite cycloguanil)	Reduced efficacy in poor metabolisers
Oxidation (CYP2C9)	Warfarin	Polymorphisms partly determine dosages
Sulphoxidation	Penicillamine	Increased risk of toxicity in poor metabolisers
Pseudocholinesterase	Suxamethonium (succinylcholine)	Prolonged duration of effect in pseudocholinesterase deficiency
Pharmacodynamic		
Glucose-6-phosphate dehydrogenase (G6PD)	Many antimalarial drugs	Risk of haemolysis in G6PD deficiency
Porphyria	Enzyme-inducing drugs	Increased risk of an acute attack
SLCO1B1 polymorphism	Statins	Increased risk of rhabdomyolysis
HLA-B*5701 polymorphism	Abacavir	Increased risk of skin hypersensitivity reactions
HLA-B*5801 polymorphism	Allopurinol	Increased risk of skin rashes in Han Chinese
HLA-B*1502 polymorphism	Carbamazepine	Increased risk of skin hypersensitivity reactions in Han Chinese

- *Efficacy.* It is best to choose drugs with the greatest efficacy, although this is not always necessary if the less efficacious drug works adequately and is easier or safer to use. For example, insulin is more efficacious at lowering the blood sugar than the oral hypoglycaemic drugs but type 2 diabetes can usually be adequately controlled without the need for insulin.
- *Features of the disease.* Choose an antibiotic to match the known or suspected sensitivity of the infective organism: for example, amoxicillin + erythromycin for a patient with a community-acquired bronchopneumonia (p. 680), since the likeliest organisms will be *Streptococcus pneumoniae* or *Legionella pneumophila*.
- *Severity of disease.* Choose a drug appropriate to the severity of the disease. For example, mild pain will generally respond well to paracetamol, whereas more severe pain may require more potent analgesics, such as opiates.
- *Coexisting diseases.* In hypertension coexisting left ventricular failure would prompt the use of a diuretic combined with an ACE inhibitor, whereas coexisting angina pectoris would prompt the use of a β-blocker.
- *Avoiding adverse effects.* Make sure that the treatment chosen does not worsen an associated condition. For example, β-blockers should be avoided as treatment for hypertension in patients with asthma.
- *Avoiding adverse drug interactions.* Try to avoid giving combinations of drugs that might interact, either directly or indirectly. For example, avoid NSAIDs in patients taking warfarin, since they increase the risk of bleeding, both by inhibiting platelet aggregation and by causing gastric ulceration; their effects on warfarin protein binding are probably not important.
- *Patient adherence to therapy.* Try to choose drugs with a simple dosing schedule. For example, when using an ACE inhibitor it is better to choose an agent that can be given once daily (e.g. enalapril) as opposed to one that needs to be given several times a day (e.g. captopril).
- *Cost.* Choose the cheaper drug if two drugs are of equal efficacy and safety. However, the true costs of drug therapy cannot always be calculated simply on the basis of the relative costs of the medication. For example, a more expensive drug that is better tolerated might be better value than a cheaper drug because of the difference in adherence to therapy.

Choosing the route of administration

There are several reasons for choosing a particular route of administration, as some examples illustrate (Box 2.12).

Choosing a formulation

Drugs come in various different formulations. The formulation can essentially be considered as a sort of packaging that influences the mode of administration and the frequency with which the drug needs to be taken. Oral formulations include tablets, capsules, granules, elixirs and suspensions. Drugs for injection come as lyophilised

2.12 Reasons for choosing a particular route of administration

Reason	Example
Only one route possible	Dopamine (intravenous) Glibenclamide (oral)
Patient adherence	Phenothiazines and thioxanthenes (intramuscular depot injections in schizophrenia)
Poor absorption	Furosemide (intravenous, in severe heart failure)
Vomiting	Phenothiazines (rectal or buccal) Sumatriptan (nasal spray)
Avoiding first-pass metabolism	Glyceryl trinitrate (sublingual)
Rapid action	Glyceryl trinitrate (sublingual) Insulin (intravenous, in diabetic ketoacidosis)
Direct access to the site of action	Bronchodilators (inhalation, in asthma) Corticosteroids (rectal, in ulcerative colitis) Local application to skin, eyes, etc.
Ease of access	Benzodiazepines (rectal diazepam if intravenous access is difficult in status epilepticus) Subcutaneous fluids (hypodermoclysis)
Controlled release	Insulin (subcutaneous)

powders for reconstitution before injection or as solutions ready for injection; solutions come in single-dose ampoules, single-dose or multiple-dose vials, and half-litre or litre bottles for infusion. Some examples show how the choice of formulation can be important.

Lithium salts and theophylline come in several different ordinary and modified-release formulations, each with different absorption characteristics. A formulation that produces adequate serum lithium or theophylline concentrations in one patient may not be suitable for another, and it is sometimes worth changing the formulation if serum concentrations are suboptimal. These are examples of drugs that should be prescribed by specific brand name rather than the International Non-proprietary Name (INN), which is otherwise recommended.

Iron salts are available as tablets for twice- or thrice-daily administration or as modified-release formulations for once-daily administration. Adverse effects are fewer with the modified-release formulations, but the iron is more erratically absorbed. It is usual to start with an ordinary formulation of iron and change to a modified-release formulation if adverse effects occur.

Choosing a dosage regimen

The dose of the drug and the frequency and timing of its administration constitute the dosage regimen. Each prescription should be treated as an experiment to try to find the regimen that produces the best therapeutic effect with minimal adverse effects, according to some simple principles:

- Generally, start with a dose at the lower end of the recommended range. There are some exceptions to this rule; glucocorticoids and carbimazole are initially given at high doses and then the dose is reduced to a maintenance level. Drugs such as digoxin, warfarin and amiodarone are also given using a 'loading dose' followed by a maintenance dose.
- Increase the dose slowly, monitoring the therapeutic effect at regular intervals and looking for adverse effects.
- If adverse effects occur, reduce the dose or try another drug; in some cases lower doses may be possible by combining drugs (for example, the immunosuppressant azathioprine reduces glucocorticoid requirements in patients with inflammatory disease).
- Think of drug interactions and avoid potentially dangerous combinations.
- Remember that pharmacokinetic and pharmacodynamic variability can alter dosage requirements, as discussed below.
- Take particular care with drugs that have a low therapeutic index (see Box 2.2, p. 20).

Pharmacokinetic variability

Because absorption, distribution and elimination of drugs vary from patient to patient, flexibility in dosages is necessary. The examples in Box 2.13 show how to respond to differences or changes in pharmacokinetics.

Pharmacodynamic variability

Pharmacological responses are usually governed by the dose-response curve, an example of which is shown in Figure 2.2: the effects of the loop diuretics bumetanide and furosemide on urinary sodium excretion. The two diuretics have different *potencies* (reflected by the fact that the curve for bumetanide lies to the left of the curve for furosemide), which can be dealt with by using different doses; however, they both have the same *efficacy* (reflected by the maximum height that the dose-response curve reaches), so that comparable doses produce the same diuretic effect.

2.13 Therapeutic approaches to pharmacokinetic problems

Pharmacokinetic problem	Therapeutic approach
Poor absorption	Increase the dose Choose another route of administration Use another drug
Altered tissue distribution	One-off doses may have to be altered Usually does not affect chronic therapy, unless distribution to the target tissue is altered; may have to choose a different drug
Altered protein binding	Usually does not affect long-term therapy (but does alter steady-state total plasma drug concentration of low-clearance drugs*)
Reduced renal elimination	Reduce dosage (use creatinine clearance or eGFR as a guide)
Reduced hepatic elimination	Low-clearance drugs*: reduce oral and intravenous doses High-clearance drugs*: reduce oral (but not intravenous) doses

*See Box 2.16

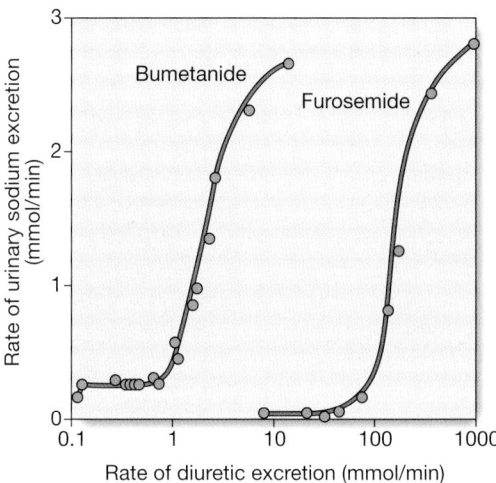

Fig. 2.2 Dose-response curves for bumetanide and furosemide.
The two drugs have different potencies (the doses required to produce the same effect differ) but the same efficacy (the maximal effect is the same).

Variability in dose-responsiveness dictates flexibility in prescribing. If a therapeutic effect does not occur with the first dosage chosen, an effect may be achieved by making small increases within the therapeutic dosage range. Of course, increasing the dosage will also increase the risk of adverse effects. Certain diseases can alter a dose-response curve (for example, there is resistance to digoxin in hyperthyroidism) and the pharmacodynamics of one drug can be affected by another drug.

Choosing the frequency of drug administration

Patient adherence to therapy is probably inversely related to the number of doses that are required per day. In general, therefore, try to choose drugs that can be given no more than twice daily. A modified-release formulation can be useful in this respect. In some special cases the frequency of drug administration is an important consideration in therapy (Box 2.14).

Choosing the time of drug administration

For many drugs the time of administration is unimportant. However, there are occasionally pharmacokinetic or therapeutic reasons for giving drugs at particular times (see Box 2.14). Meal times do not usually affect drug administration, since although food may reduce the speed of absorption of a drug, it generally does not reduce the extent of absorption; notable exceptions are bisphosphonates and tetracyclines, since their absorption is greatly reduced by divalent and trivalent cations, and they should not be taken with food or antacids. Food sometimes helps to reduce adverse gastrointestinal effects; for instance, the effects of aspirin on the stomach are partly reduced by taking it with food.

Prescribing in special circumstances

Prescribing in renal insufficiency

If a drug or its active metabolites are eliminated by the kidneys, the maintenance dose must be altered in

Drug	Recommended frequency or timing	Reasons
2.14 Some special examples of frequency and timing of drug administration		
Furosemide	Once in the morning	Kidney refractory to a second dose within 6 hrs; night-time diuresis undesirable
Glucocorticoids	Once in the morning	Minimises inhibitory effects on adrenal function
Salmeterol	Once at night	Prevents early morning symptoms
Antidepressants	Once at night	Allows adverse effects to occur during sleep
Digoxin	Once at night	So that when blood samples for plasma concentration measurement are taken it is at least 6 hrs (preferably 11 hrs) after the last dose
Glyceryl trinitrate (sublingual)	When required	Relief of acute symptoms
Glyceryl trinitrate patches or long-acting nitrates	Staggered doses (see *British National Formulary*)	To avoid tolerance
Tetracyclines	2 hours before or after food or antacids	Divalent and trivalent cations chelate tetracyclines, preventing absorption
Opiates	In anticipation of pain	Better relief in chronic pain
Levodopa	Several times a day	Dictated by the duration of action (often wears off quickly during long-term therapy)
Statins	Once at night	Inhibition of HMG CoA reductase is greater at night

renal insufficiency, although it is not usually necessary to alter a one-off dose. Creatinine clearance can be used as a guide to reducing maintenance dosages. Nowadays this is usually estimated (eGFR) by measurement of serum creatinine, taking age, sex and ethnic group into account. Many laboratories now report eGFR along with the serum creatinine concentration. In some cases dosages should be reduced because the pharmacological effects interact with renal impairment (for example, ACE inhibitors worsen potassium retention). Some drugs should be avoided entirely in renal insufficiency, for either pharmacokinetic or pharmacodynamic reasons (Box 2.15).

Diuretics are relatively ineffective in severe renal insufficiency because they cannot gain access to their site of action, the luminal epithelium. Potassium-sparing diuretics should not be used because of the increased risk of hyperkalaemia.

2.15 Some drugs whose dosages are affected by renal insufficiency

Mild renal insufficiency (GFR 20–50 mL/min or serum creatinine 150–300 μmol/L)

- ACE inhibitors (monitor carefully; increase dosages if renal function does not worsen with low doses)
- Aminoglycosides
- Chlorpropamide
- Digoxin
- Fibrates
- Lithium
- Zidovudine

Moderate renal insufficiency (GFR 10–20 mL/min or serum creatinine 300–700 μmol/L)

- Some β-blockers (e.g. atenolol, sotalol)
- Opioid analgesics

Severe renal insufficiency (GFR < 10 mL/min or serum creatinine > 700 μmol/L; many of these patients receive renal replacement therapy, which can affect drug pharmacokinetics)

- Azathioprine
- Cephalosporins
- Cimetidine
- Isoniazid
- Penicillins
- Sulphonylurea hypoglycaemic drugs (gliclazide, glipizide, gliquidone)

Drugs to avoid in renal insufficiency

Any degree of renal insufficiency
- Mesalazine
- Metformin
- NSAIDs
- Tetracyclines (except doxycycline and minocycline)

Moderate or severe renal insufficiency
- Lithium
- Methotrexate

Severe renal insufficiency
- Sulphonylurea hypoglycaemic drugs (chlorpropamide, glibenclamide)
- Chloramphenicol
- Chloroquine
- Fibrates

(GFR = glomerular filtration rate)

2.16 Some drugs of low and high hepatic clearance rates

Low

- Aspirin
- Codeine
- Diazepam
- Isoniazid
- Nortriptyline
- Paracetamol
- Phenobarbital
- Phenytoin
- Procainamide
- Quinidine
- Theophylline
- Warfarin

High

- Clomethiazole
- Glyceryl trinitrate
- Labetalol
- Lidocaine
- Morphine
- Pethidine
- Propranolol
- Simvastatin

2.17 Some drugs whose actions are increased in liver disease

Drug	Adverse effect
Oral anticoagulants	Increased anticoagulation (reduced clotting factor synthesis)
Metformin	Lactic acidosis
Chloramphenicol	Bone-marrow suppression
NSAIDs	Gastrointestinal bleeding
Sulphonylureas	Hypoglycaemia

Prescribing in hepatic failure

The liver has a large capacity for drug metabolism and hepatic insufficiency has to be considerable before drug dosages need to be modified. In patients with chronic liver disease who have jaundice, ascites, hypoalbuminaemia, malnutrition or encephalopathy, clinically important impairment of drug metabolism is likely. Hepatic drug clearance may also be reduced in acute hepatitis, in hepatic congestion due to cardiac failure, and if there is intrahepatic arteriovenous shunting (for example, in hepatic cirrhosis).

There is no easy way of calculating dosage changes in patients with impaired hepatic function, since there are no good tests of hepatic drug-metabolising capacity or of biliary excretion. Doses of drugs that are metabolised by the liver should therefore be altered according to the therapeutic response, with careful monitoring for adverse effects.

If a drug has a high rate of hepatic clearance (Box 2.16) it will be mostly cleared during its first passage through the liver (so-called 'first-pass' metabolism). In such cases, hepatic impairment increases the amount of drug that escapes metabolism in the liver after oral administration, reducing oral dosage requirements but not altering intravenous dosage requirements. For example, clomethiazole is extensively metabolised by the liver, and metabolism is reduced by chronic liver disease. It is therefore important to ensure that overdose does not occur when using oral clomethiazole in a patient with liver disease. The pharmacological effects of several drugs are altered in liver disease, with increased risks of adverse effects (Box 2.17).

Prescribing for older people

The handling of, and response to, drugs change as people age, and responses to drugs are much more variable in older people. Great care must be exercised when prescribing in old age and the broad principles are outlined in Box 2.18. The dosage regimens of many drugs need to be adjusted and toxicity is more likely for several reasons (Box 2.19).

Inappropriate polypharmacy is common in old people and the scope for drug interactions is large (p. 173); in patients over 60 years of age the error rate in taking drugs is about 60% and the rate of errors increases markedly if more than three drugs are prescribed. However,

2.18 How to prescribe in old age

- Use as few drugs as possible
- Start with low doses, and increase carefully only if required
- Choose oral drugs with easily swallowed formulations
- Keep therapy as simple as possible
- Take great care in frail old people

2.19 Mechanisms of drug toxicity in old age

- **Reduced renal function**: impaired urinary excretion.
- **Smaller liver**: reduced hepatic metabolism.
- **Impaired homeostatic mechanisms**: exaggerated response.
- **Swallowing difficulty**: medication sticks in oesophagus.
- **Polypharmacy and cognitive impairment**: wrong medication taken or medication missed.
- **Increased proportion of body fat**: accumulation of lipid-soluble drugs.

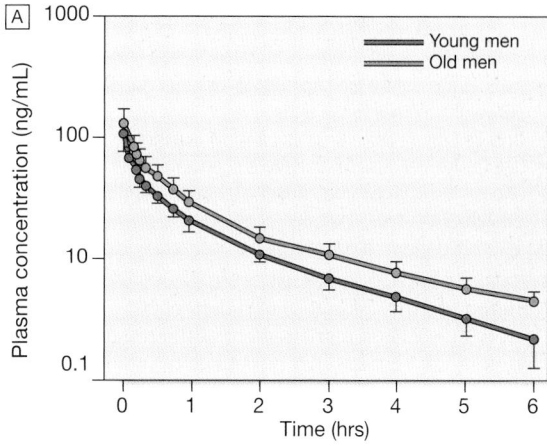

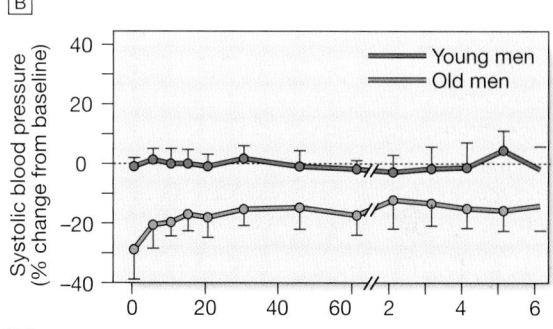

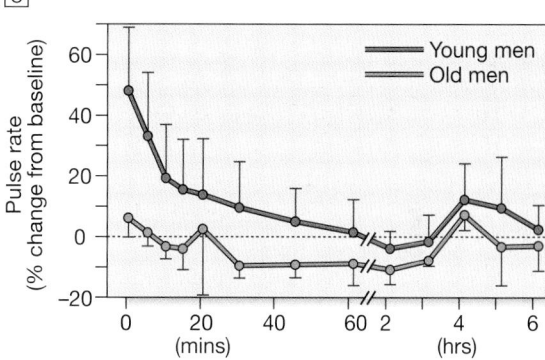

Fig. 2.3 Differences between young men and old men given an intravenous dose of nifedipine. [A] Old men have higher plasma concentrations than young men. [B] and [C] Old men have a greater fall in blood pressure and a smaller rise in heart rate than young men.

polypharmacy may be appropriate and justified in some elderly people.

Many old people find it difficult to swallow tablets. Some tablets and capsules can adhere to the oesophageal mucosa and drugs should be taken with at least 60 mL of water to avoid this. Elixirs may be preferable but not all drugs are available in this form. Drug distribution may be altered in old people and dosages should be adjusted for body weight, particularly for drugs with a low therapeutic index. Some of these principles are illustrated in Figure 2.3, which shows the difference in nifedipine pharmacokinetics and pharmacodynamic responses between young and old men. After an intravenous dose of nifedipine (2.5 mg) the old men had higher plasma nifedipine concentrations and a fall in blood pressure; the difference in blood pressure response was partly due to the difference in plasma concentration, but was mostly due to a difference in baroreceptor reflexes, as shown by the difference in heart rate responses.

Examples of drugs for which special care is required in older people are shown in Box 2.20.

2.20 Drugs whose actions are frequently altered in old age

Drug	Mechanism	Consequence
Digoxin	Increased sensitivity of Na/K pump Renal impairment Hypokalaemia due to diuretics	Increased risk of toxicity
Antihypertensive drugs	Reduced baroreceptor function	Increased risk of postural hypotension
Antidepressants Hypnotics Sedatives Tranquillisers	Increased brain sensitivity; reduced metabolism	Increased risk of toxicity
Warfarin	Increased sensitivity to inhibition of clotting factor synthesis	Increased risk of bleeding
Clomethiazole Lidocaine Nifedipine Phenobarbital Propranolol Theophylline	Metabolism reduced	Increased risk of toxicity

Prescribing in pregnancy

Drug therapy in relation to pregnancy may be required either for a pre-existing problem (e.g epilepsy, asthma, hyperthyroidism, hypertension) or for a problem that arises or threatens to arise as a result of pregnancy (e.g. morning sickness, anaemia, prevention of neural tube defects, hypertension).

About 35% of women take drug therapy at least once during pregnancy and 6% take drug therapy during the first trimester (excluding iron, folic acid and vitamins). The most commonly used drugs are simple analgesics, antibacterial drugs and antacids. The principles of prescribing in pregnancy are summarised in Box 2.21. Problems can arise under several headings:

2

- Avoid drugs unless the benefit to the mother greatly outweighs the risk to the fetus
- Only use drugs when there is previous experience
- Use the lowest dose for the shortest time possible
- Choose the least harmful drug if a range of alternatives is available

- altered pharmacokinetics in pregnancy
- teratogenesis and management of the pregnant woman who has taken a possible teratogen
- adverse effects of drugs on the fetus during the later stages of pregnancy
- therapeutic intervention on behalf of the fetus
- termination of pregnancy and the management of preterm labour and of labour (beyond the scope of this text)
- breastfeeding.

Altered pharmacokinetics

Vomiting can affect drug absorption. Plasma albumin concentration falls during pregnancy and the albumin-bound fraction of drugs may be altered; for example, the unbound fraction of phenytoin increases during pregnancy and total plasma phenytoin concentrations fall because of increased clearance, but the concentration of *unbound* phenytoin does not fall to the same extent. This means that care must be taken in adjusting dosages and in interpreting plasma concentrations. The glomerular filtration rate increases by about 70% during pregnancy and drugs that are mainly eliminated by renal excretion are cleared more quickly.

Teratogenesis

Teratogenesis is the induction of a developmental abnormality in a fetus by a drug taken during the early stages of pregnancy; the period from 2 to 8 weeks of gestation is the most critical. Information about teratogenic risks in humans is scarce but well-known examples include thalidomide, retinoids (e.g. isotretinoin) and cytotoxic drugs. The *BNF* contains a list of drugs that should be avoided or used with care. If a woman takes a potentially teratogenic drug, identify the exact time of exposure and the likely time of conception; investigations may be necessary to determine whether fetal abnormalities are present and specialist advice should be sought about the question of termination. Some conditions such as epilepsy are difficult to manage during pregnancy because of the risk of teratogenesis.

Later stages of pregnancy

Some drugs adversely affect the fetus at any time during pregnancy. Tetracyclines adversely affect growing teeth and bones; sulphonamides displace fetal bilirubin from plasma proteins and the unbound bilirubin enters the brain, potentially causing kernicterus; sulphonylureas can cause fetal and neonatal hypoglycaemia. Anticoagulation in pregnancy is highly problematic because of the teratogenic effects of warfarin in the first trimester. Heparin is usually used as an alternative, but it has potential adverse effects on the fetus and mother around term, and potential adverse effects such as osteoporosis in the mother.

Therapeutic intervention on behalf of the fetus

Examples include the administration of anti-D immunoglobulin to a mother to prevent rhesus disease of the newborn and the use of anti-arrhythmic drugs in the treatment of fetal arrhythmias.

Breastfeeding

Drugs that are excreted in breast milk can cause adverse effects in the baby if they are present in large enough amounts or if they cause hypersusceptibility reactions in small amounts (e.g. penicillin hypersensitivity; haemolysis in G6PD deficiency). The *BNF* contains a list of drugs that should be avoided or used with care.

When to stop drug treatment

The duration of drug treatment is straightforward for conditions that require one-off therapy (e.g. post-operative analgesia) and those that require life-long treatment (e.g. thyroxine for hypothyroidism). However, the optimal duration of drug treatment has not been established for many diseases, partly because the clinical trials that form the basis of marketing authorisation for many drugs often have short durations. For example, it is still not clear for how long treatment with warfarin should be continued in the treatment of deep venous thrombosis and pulmonary embolism (p. 1015). When a drug treatment is started, it is wise to plan the likely duration of therapy. It is also important to review long-term treatment at regular intervals to assess whether continued treatment is required. A hospital admission is often an opportunity for revising drug therapy, and it is not uncommon for drugs to be withdrawn temporarily, or even permanently, following an acute severe illness.

Prescribing in constrained circumstances

Prescribing in a developing country may have economic constraints, limiting the list of drugs available. The World Health Organization (WHO) has published a so-called Model Formulary, including a list of essential medicines and helpful advice about how to use them.

However, economic constraints can also affect developed countries, since health budgets are limited. Also, new drugs are more expensive than long-established treatments, since pharmaceutical companies need to recoup the costs of development to make a profit and to support further research and development. In some countries expenditure is controlled by limiting prescribing to drugs that are considered to be cost-effective. In the UK the National Institute for Health and Clinical Excellence (NICE) and the Scottish Medicines Consortium (SMC) issue advice about the cost-effectiveness of medicines after they have been approved for therapy by the regulatory authorities. This is based on the incremental cost-effectiveness ratio (ICER), which is the cost of the drug per quality-adjusted life year (QALY) gained. If the ICER for the use of an intervention in a particular condition is greater than £20 000, the intervention is generally considered not to be cost-effective and its use is not recommended, although the restrictions may be relaxed for end-of-life treatments. The calculations involved are based on complicated economic models. Individual National Health Service trust hospitals often restrict the use of drugs to those contained in a local formulary, the contents of which are based on similar considerations.

Even for interventions that are considered to be cost-effective, prescribing may be limited to certain individuals. For a junior doctor (e.g. a doctor in the Foundation Years in the UK) the ability to prescribe will be constrained by limited knowledge and experience. A suggested formulary of drugs with which medical students should familiarise themselves as a first step in learning the art of prescribing is listed on the Davidson website (www.studentconsult.com). Similar considerations apply to some other prescribers; for example, a UK nurse prescriber in a coronary care unit, although theoretically empowered to prescribe any drug in the *British National Formulary*, will prescribe only drugs that are relevant to the work of the unit. Some drugs are limited to specialist use, such as those that are used to treat cancer.

ADVERSE DRUG REACTIONS

Adverse drug reactions are classified mechanistically and clinically. This can be done using two complementary classification systems: EIDOS and DoTS (Fig. 2.4). Understanding adverse reactions in this way contributes to areas such as drug development and regulation, pharmacovigilance, monitoring therapy, and the prevention, diagnosis and treatment of adverse drug reactions.

Mechanistic classification of adverse drug reactions—EIDOS

The EIDOS mechanistic classification of adverse drug effects considers five elements:

- the **E**xtrinsic species that initiates the effect
- the **I**ntrinsic species that it affects
- the **D**istribution of these species in the body
- the (physiological or pathological) **O**utcome
- the **S**equela, which is the adverse effect.

Extrinsic species

This can be the parent compound, an excipient, a contaminant or adulterant, a degradation product, or a derivative of any of these (e.g. a metabolite).

Intrinsic species

This is usually the endogenous molecule with which the extrinsic species interacts. This can be a nucleic acid, an enzyme, a receptor, an ion channel or transporter, or some other protein.

Distribution

A drug will not produce an adverse effect if it is not distributed to the same site as the target protein that mediates the adverse effect. Thus, the pharmacokinetics of the extrinsic species can affect the occurrence of adverse effects.

Outcome

Interactions between extrinsic and intrinsic species in the production of an adverse effect can result in physiological or pathological changes. Physiological changes can involve either increased actions (e.g. clotting due to tranexamic acid) or decreased actions (e.g. bradycardia due to β-blockers). Pathological changes can involve cellular adaptations (atrophy, hypertrophy, hyperplasia, metaplasia and neoplasia), altered cell function (e.g. mast cell degranulation in IgE-mediated anaphylactic reactions) or cell damage (e.g. cell lysis, necrosis or apoptosis).

Sequela

The sequela of the changes induced by a drug describes the clinically recognisable adverse drug reaction, of which there may be more than one. Sequelae can be classified using the DoTS system.

Clinical classification of adverse drug reactions—DoTS

The DoTS clinical classification of adverse drug reactions takes into account three aspects of the interaction between the patient and the drug that produces an adverse effect (see Fig. 2.4):

- the relation of the adverse effect to the **Do**se of the drug
- the **T**ime course of the effect
- the **S**usceptibility of the patient.

Dose-responsiveness of adverse drug reactions

There are three types of adverse drug effect:

- A *toxic effect* is one that occurs as an exaggeration of the desired therapeutic effect and occurs at doses at or near the top of the dose-response curve. For example, syncope due to a β-blocker is a toxic effect; it occurs by the same mechanism as the therapeutic effect (lowering of the blood pressure).
- *Collateral effects* occur at doses in the middle of the usual dose-response curve but in a tissue other than

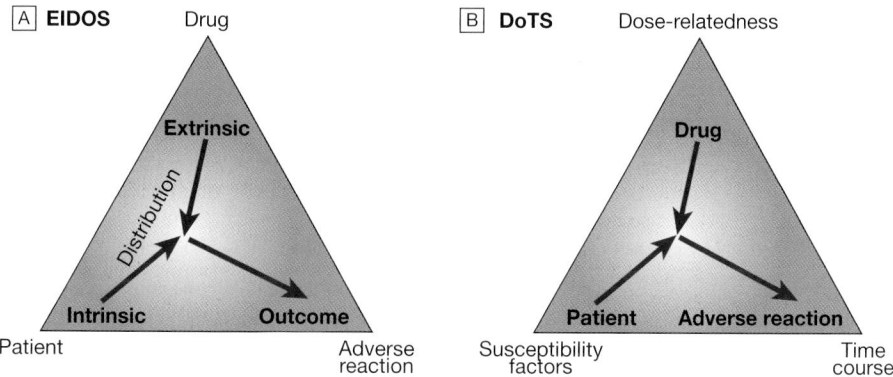

Fig. 2.4 Two complementary forms of classification of adverse drug reactions. **A** The EIDOS mechanistic classification describes how the combination of drug and patient causes the adverse reaction. **B** The DoTS clinical classification defines the important aspects of the drug (dose-relatedness), the patient (susceptibility factors) and the reaction (its time course).

that in which the therapeutic action is sought. They can occur:

— through the same pharmacological effect as that whereby the therapeutic action is produced (for example, colour vision disturbance from sildenafil)

— through a distinct pharmacological effect (for example, a dry mouth due to an anticholinergic effect of a tricyclic antidepressant).

• *Hypersusceptibility effects* occur at subtherapeutic doses in susceptible patients. Penicillin allergy is a hypersusceptibility effect.

Toxic effects can be avoided by using dosages at the lower end of the recommended range and increasing cautiously, monitoring carefully for therapeutic and adverse effects. Collateral adverse effects may not be avoidable; if they occur despite careful dosage adjustment, it may be necessary to use a different drug. Hypersusceptibility effects can be avoided by identify-ing the susceptibility factors that contribute to them; for example, a history of penicillin allergy is a contraindication to the use of any penicillin.

Time courses of adverse effects

The different patterns of time course of adverse reactions are listed in Box 2.22, with illustrative examples.

Susceptibility to adverse drug reactions

The sources of the various factors that can increase the susceptibility of an individual to an adverse effect of a drug are listed in Box 2.23.

DRUG INTERACTIONS

A drug interaction occurs when the effects of one drug (the object drug) are altered (increased or decreased) by the effects of another drug (the precipitant drug).

2.22 Time-related classification of adverse drug reactions

Type of reaction	Examples	Implications
Time-independent		
Due to a change in dose or concentration (*pharmaceutical effects*)	Toxicity due to increased systemic availability	Beware of changing formulations of some drugs (e.g. modified-release formulations of lithium)
Due to a change in dose or concentration (*pharmacokinetic effects*)	Digitalis toxicity due to renal insufficiency	Forewarn the patient; monitor carefully throughout treatment; alter dosage when pharmacokinetics change (e.g. renal insufficiency); avoid interacting drugs
Occuring without a change in dose (*pharmacodynamic effects*)	Digitalis toxicity due to hypokalaemia	Forewarn the patient; monitor carefully throughout treatment; avoid precipitating (pharmacodynamic) factors; avoid interacting drugs
Time-dependent		
Rapid (due to rapid administration)	Red man syndrome (vancomycin) Hypertension (digitalis) Hypotension (adipiodone)	Administer slowly
First dose (of a course)	Hypotension (α_1-adrenoceptor antagonists and ACE inhibitors) Type I hypersensitivity reactions	Take special precautions for the first dose Careful history taking; if a reaction occurs, avoid re-exposure; counsel the patient
Early tolerant (abates with repeated exposure)	Adverse reactions that involve tolerance (e.g. nitrate-induced headache)	Monitor during the early stages; give appropriate reassurance; expect adverse effects if strategies to avoid tolerance are adopted
Early permanent (occurs early and does not abate)	Some adverse effects of corticosteroids	Monitor during the early stages; withdraw or use preventive measures
Intermediate (risk increases at first, then diminishes)	Venous thromboembolism (antipsychotic drugs) Hypersensitivity reactions types II, III and IV	Monitoring not needed after the high-risk period unless susceptibility changes; withdraw drug if a reaction develops
Late (risk increases with time)	Osteoporosis (glucocorticoids) Tardive dyskinesia (dopamine receptor antagonists) Retinopathy (chloroquine) Tissue phospholipid deposition (amiodarone)	Assess baseline function; forewarn the patient; monitor periodically during prolonged treatment
Late (effects occur after withdrawal)	Withdrawal syndromes: opiates, benzodiazepines, hypertension (clonidine and methyldopa), myocardial infarction (β-blockers)	Withdraw slowly; forewarn the patient; replace with a longer-acting drug if withdrawal is not possible
Delayed	Carcinogenesis (ciclosporin, diethylstilbestrol) Teratogenesis (thalidomide)	Avoid or screen; counsel or forewarn the patient

2.23 Sources of altered susceptibility to adverse drug reactions

Source of susceptibility	Examples	Implications
Genetic (see also Box 2.11, p. 25)	Porphyria Suxamethonium (succinylcholine) sensitivity Malignant hyperthermia CYP isozyme polymorphisms HLA polymorphisms	Screen for abnormalities; avoid specific drugs
Age	Neonates (chloramphenicol) Elderly people (hypnotics)	Adjust doses according to age
Sex	Alcohol intoxication Mefloquine, neuropsychiatric effects ACE inhibitors, cough Lupus-like syndrome (e.g. hydralazine)	Use different doses in men and women
Physiology altered	Phenytoin in pregnancy	Alter dose or avoid
Exogenous factors	Drug interactions Interactions with food (e.g. grapefruit juice with drugs cleared by CYP3A4)	Alter dose or avoid co-administration
Disease	Renal insufficiency (e.g. lithium) Hepatic cirrhosis (e.g. morphine)	Screen for abnormalities; avoid specific drugs; use reduced doses

2.24 Classification of drug interactions by mechanism

Mechanism	Example		
	Object drug	Precipitant drug	Result
Pharmaceutical	Sodium bicarbonate	Calcium gluconate	Precipitation of insoluble calcium carbonate
Pharmacokinetic			
Reduced absorption	Tetracyclines	Calcium, aluminium, magnesium salts	Reduced tetracycline absorption
Reduced protein binding	Phenytoin	Aspirin	Reduced phenytoin plasma concentration with same therapeutic effect
Reduced metabolism (CYP3A4)	Terfenadine	Grapefruit juice	Cardiac arrhythmias (prolonged QT interval, p. 529)
Reduced metabolism (CYP2C19)	Phenytoin	Ticlopidine	Phenytoin toxicity
Reduced metabolism (CYP2D6)	Clozapine	Paroxetine	Clozapine toxicity
Reduced metabolism (other enzymes)	Azathioprine (xanthine oxidase) Catecholamines (monoamine oxidase)	Allopurinol Monoamine oxidase inhibitors	Azathioprine toxicity Hypertensive crisis due to monoamine toxicity
Increased metabolism (induction)	Ciclosporin	St John's wort	Loss of immunosuppression
Reduced renal elimination	Lithium	Diuretics	Lithium toxicity
Pharmacodynamic Direct antagonism	Opiates	Naloxone	Reversal of opiate effects
Direct potentiation	Alcohol	Antidepressants	Increased sedation
Indirect potentiation	Anti-arrhythmic drugs	Diuretics	Cardiac arrhythmias (hypokalaemia)

Although a drug interaction usually results in an adverse effect, in some cases it can prove beneficial. An example is pharmacodynamic synergy between diuretics and ACE inhibitors in the treatment of hypertension. The classification of drug interactions by mechanism is shown in Box 2.24.

Pharmaceutical interactions

Pharmaceutical interactions are physicochemical interactions, either of a drug with an intravenous infusion solution or of two drugs in the same solution, resulting in the loss of activity of the drugs involved. Pharmaceutical interactions are too numerous to remember in detail, but they can be simply avoided:

- by giving intravenous drugs via bolus injection or an infusion burette or syringe pump
- by using only dextrose or saline for drug infusion
- by not mixing drugs in the same infusion solution, unless the mixture is known to be safe (e.g. potassium chloride with insulin).

Pharmacokinetic interactions

Pharmacokinetic interactions occur when the absorption, distribution or elimination (metabolism or excretion) of one drug is altered by another drug.

Absorption interactions

Absorption interactions are seldom important. Exceptions include impaired absorption of tetracyclines, bisphosphonates and fluoroquinolones by chelation with divalent and trivalent cations. Parenteral metoclopramide increases the rate of gastric emptying and this hastens the absorption of analgesics in the treatment of an acute attack of migraine, a beneficial interaction.

Distribution interactions: protein-binding displacement

Protein-binding displacement causes an increase in the circulating concentration of unbound drug. However, this is only important if the object drug is highly protein-bound (greater than 90%) and is not widely distributed to body tissues. In practice, important interactions of this type occur with warfarin and phenytoin. When these drugs are displaced, their clearance rate increases in proportion to the degree of displacement, and so at steady state the total concentration of drug in the plasma falls to a new equilibrium value and the unbound *concentration* is the same as it was before the precipitant drug was introduced, in spite of an increase in the unbound *fraction*. This means that the interaction may not have significant clinical consequences, provided the patient can 'weather' the increase in unbound concentration of the object drug until a new steady state is reached.

Metabolism interactions

Drug interactions involving metabolism are important. They occur when the metabolism of one drug is either inhibited or increased by another drug. There are two phases of hepatic drug metabolism. Phase I metabolic reactions (for example, dealkylation, deamination, hydroxylation, sulphoxidation) are carried out by isoenzymes of the mixed-function oxidase (cytochrome p450 or CYP) system and are subject to interactions. Phase II reactions are conjugations (for example, acetylation, methylation, glucuronidation, sulphatation); they are not affected by interactions. Some drugs are metabolised by specific enzymes and may be the subject of interactions.

- *Induction of drug metabolism.* Induction of the metabolism of a drug reduces the amount of drug in the body and therefore reduces its effects. An important example is unwanted pregnancy when an enzyme-inducing drug such as carbamazepine, phenytoin or rifampicin is taken along with an oral contraceptive.
- *Inhibition of drug metabolism.* Drug metabolism can be reduced by inhibition of either CYP isoenzymes

or other metabolic pathways. Examples of the former include inhibition of warfarin metabolism by chloramphenicol, cimetidine, erythromycin, ketoconazole, metronidazole and quinolones, inhibition of phenytoin metabolism by isoniazid, and inhibition of theophylline metabolism by quinolone and macrolide antibiotics (for example, erythromycin). Examples of the latter include inhibition by allopurinol of xanthine oxidase, inhibiting the metabolism of azathioprine and 6-mercaptopurine, and inhibition of the metabolism of dietary amines by monoamine oxidase inhibitors.

Excretion interactions

Competition for renal tubular secretion reduces drug excretion. For example, probenecid inhibits the tubular secretion of penicillin, increasing the blood concentration of penicillin and prolonging its therapeutic effects: a beneficial interaction. Amiodarone, quinidine and verapamil inhibit the tubular secretion of digoxin by inhibiting the transport protein P glycoprotein, increasing plasma digoxin concentrations and potentially causing toxicity.

Pharmacodynamic interactions

In pharmacodynamic interactions the effect of a drug is altered at its site of action. Such interactions are either direct or indirect.

Direct pharmacodynamic interactions

Direct pharmacodynamic interactions occur when two drugs either act at the same site (antagonism or synergism) or act at two different sites with a similar end result. For example, naloxone reverses the effects of opiates and vitamin K reverses the effects of warfarin. The anticoagulant effects of warfarin are increased in direct synergistic interactions with anabolic steroids and tetracyclines. Any drug that has a depressant action on central nervous function can potentiate the effect of another such drug, whether or not the two drugs have effects on the same receptors; for example, alcohol potentiates the action of any other centrally acting drug.

Indirect pharmacodynamic interactions

Indirect pharmacodynamic interactions occur when one drug affects the pharmacological, therapeutic or toxic effect of another drug, but the two effects are independent. For example, the effects of anticoagulants can be increased by three indirect effects:

- reduced platelet aggregation (due for example to salicylates, dipyridamole, clopidogrel and NSAID)
- gastrointestinal ulceration (due, for example, to NSAID)
- increased fibrinolysis (due, for example, to metformin).

Diuretic-induced alterations in fluid and electrolyte balance (especially potassium) increase the effects of cardiac glycosides and class I anti-arrhythmic drugs (for example, lidocaine, quinidine, flecainide and phenytoin).

Avoiding adverse drug interactions

The simple way of avoiding adverse drug interactions is to avoid combinations that are known to be dangerous. If that is not possible, the dosage of the object drug should be reduced in advance of starting the precipitant drug and the precipitant drug should be introduced slowly. When a theoretical interaction is anticipated on the basis of the known properties of two drugs, even if it has not been previously described, careful monitoring may help recognise adverse effects early.

WRITING A DRUG PRESCRIPTION

A prescription should be a precise, accurate, clear, readable set of instructions, sufficient for a nurse to administer a drug accurately in hospital, or for a pharmacist to provide a patient with both the correct drug and the instructions on how to take it. The information that should be written on a prescription is given in Box 2.25.

Writing drug doses

- Quantities of 1 gram or more should be written in grams. For example, write 2 g.
- Quantities less than 1 gram but more than 1 milligram should be written in milligrams. For example, write 100 mg, not 0.1 g.
- Quantities less than 1 milligram should be written in micrograms or nanograms as appropriate. Do not abbreviate micrograms or nanograms. For example, write 100 micrograms, not 0.1 mg, 100 µg, 100 mcg or 100 ug.
- If a decimal point cannot be avoided for values less than 1, write a zero before it. For example, write 0.5 mL, not .5 mL.
- For liquid medicines given orally the dose should be stated as the number of milligrams in either 5 mL or 10 mL of solution.

Prescribing controlled drugs

Because of the problems of drug addiction and misuse of drugs, in the UK drugs likely to be abused are the subject of the *Misuse of Drugs Act* (1971), the *Misuse of Drugs (Notification of and Supply to Addicts) Regulations* (1973) and the *Misuse of Drugs Regulations* (1985). The requirements for prescription of controlled drugs in the UK are listed in Box 2.26. Doctors in other countries should make themselves familiar with local regulations.

Abbreviations

Some abbreviations that are used in prescribing are listed in Box 2.27. Other abbreviations should be avoided and instructions should be written in plain English whenever possible.

2.25 Information to be given on a UK prescription outside hospital

- The date
- The patient's name, initials and address
- The age of a child under 12
- The name of the drug, preferably in capitals (use generic names when possible)
- The formulation to be prescribed
- The strength of the formulation
- The dose
- The frequency of administration
- The route of administration
- The doctor's name, address and signature

2.26 How to write a prescription for a controlled drug

- Complete the prescription in handwriting in ink
- Sign and date it
- Include your address
- Include the name and address of the patient
- State the form and strength (if appropriate) of the drug
- State the total quantity of the drug or the number of dose units to be dispensed in both words and figures
- State the exact size of each dose in both words and figures

2.27 Acceptable abbreviations in prescriptions

Abbreviation	Latin meaning	English meaning
b.d. or b.i.d.	Bis in die	Twice a day
gutt.	Guttae	Drops
i.m.	–	Intramuscular(ly)
i.v.	–	Intravenous(ly)
o.d.	Omni die	(Once) every day
o.m.	Omni mane[1]	(Once) every morning
o.n.	Omni nocte[1]	(Once) every night
p.o.	Per os	By mouth
PR	Per rectum	By the anal route
p.r.n.	Pro re nata	Whenever required
PV	Per vaginam	By the vaginal route
q.d.s.	Quater die sumendum[2]	Four times a day
s.c.	–	Subcutaneous(ly)
stat.	Statim	Immediately
t.d.s.	Ter die sumendum[2]	Three times a day

[1]Sometimes written simply as 'mane' or 'nocte'.
[2]The abbreviation t.i.d. or q.i.d. (ter or quater in die) is sometimes used instead; do not use q.d. to mean once a day.

DRUG NOMENCLATURE

Drugs have different kinds of name:

- The chemical name, whose form generally follows the rules issued by the International Union of Pure and Applied Chemistry (IUPAC).
- The approved (official or generic) name. This is usually the International Non-proprietary Name (INN), either recommended (rINN) or proposed (pINN) by the WHO, but it may be some locally approved name (for example, the British Approved Name (BAN) or United States Adopted Name, (USAN)).
- The proprietary name (brand name or trade name), given to it by the manufacturer.
  For example:
- chemical name: (R)-1-(3,4-dihydroxyphenyl) -2-methylaminoethanol
- INN: epinephrine; BAN: adrenaline
- proprietary names: Epipen® for intramuscular injection and Eppy® or Simplene® eyedrops.

Since the chemical name is generally unsuitable for routine prescribing, either the approved name or proprietary name is used. Which should one choose? For some drugs the question is trivial, since only one proprietary formulation exists; for example, trastuzumab is currently available in the UK only as Herceptin®.

However, several proprietary formulations of the same chemical entity usually become available when the patent expires on a drug with a previously unique proprietary name. For instance, amoxicillin was first marketed as Amoxil®. When the patent expired the number of proprietary brands multiplied. This can cause prescribing and dispensing problems. For example, in the UK, whether the prescriber writes 'trastuzumab BP' or 'Herceptin' the patient will receive Herceptin®. However, if the prescriber writes 'amoxicillin BP' the pharmacist may dispense any proprietary formulation, provided that it conforms to the description laid out in the *British Pharmacopoeia* (BP), and will generally dispense the cheapest available.

By writing the proprietary name the prescriber can ensure that a particular formulation of a drug is prescribed. However, in some UK hospitals the pharmacy may stock only one formulation, and even if the hospital doctor writes 'Amoxil' on a prescription chart, the pharmacist may dispense some other approved formulation for which the hospital will have negotiated an economic deal with the supplier.

There are advantages and disadvantages to the prescribing of drugs by their generic (non-proprietary) as opposed to their proprietary names. The advantages include:

- *Awareness of the prescription*. The name of the compound often indicates to what class it belongs, usually by virtue of its suffix; e.g. -vastatin (HMGCoA reductase inhibitors), -olol (β-blockers, although beware stanozolol), -floxacin (quinolone antibiotics).
- *Drug stocks*. If, say, 'Amoram' rather than 'amoxicillin' is prescribed and a pharmacy stocks only Amoxil, the pharmacist cannot legally dispense

the prescription without first consulting the doctor; clearly, this can cause inconvenience to all concerned and can result in delayed treatment.
- *Expense*. It is generally cheaper to prescribe by the approved name, since the pharmacist will dispense the cheapest variant held in stock.

The disadvantages of prescribing by non-proprietary name include:

- *Remembering names*. Proprietary names are chosen by pharmaceutical companies because they are catchy, usually easier to remember than the corresponding generic name, and shorter and easier to spell (compare, for example, 'Serc' with 'betahistine'). Furthermore, a single proprietary name will do when the formulation contains two or more drugs (compare, for example, 'Fefol' with 'ferrous sulphate plus folic acid'). In a few cases, to counteract this problem, BANs have been coined for common combinations of drugs; for example, the combination of dihydrocodeine with paracetamol (acetaminophen) is known as co-dydramol.
- *Quality of product*. For a few drugs a change in tablet excipients has large effects on the absorption of the drug from the formulation. Important examples include lithium salts, nifedipine and theophylline, which should always be prescribed by brand name.
- *Continuity of treatment*. Patients not infrequently become confused if the drug they are being given changes its form with every prescription. Continuity can be achieved by prescribing the same proprietary formulation every time.

2.28 Usual therapeutic and toxic plasma concentrations of commonly measured drugs

Drug	Optimal sampling time	Concentration below which a therapeutic effect is unlikely		Concentration above which a toxic effect is more likely	
		Mass units	Molar units	Mass units	Molar units
Carbamazepine	Just before next dose	4 mg/L	17 µmol/L	10 mg/L	42 µmol/L
Cardiac glycosides					
Digitoxin	Just before next dose	15 µg/L	20 nmol/L	30 µg/L	39 nmol/L
Digoxin	11 hrs after last dose	0.8 µg/L	1.0 nmol/L	2 µg/L	2.6 nmol/L
Ciclosporin*	Just before next dose	125 µg/L	104 nmol/L	200 µg/L	166 nmol/L
Lithium	12 hrs after last dose	–	0.4 mmol/L	–	1.0 mmol/L
Phenytoin	Just before next dose	10 mg/L	40 µmol/L	20 mg/L	80 µmol/L
Theophylline	Just before next dose	10 mg/L	55 µmol/L	20 mg/L	110 µmol/L

*Measured in whole blood by specific radioimmunoassay or high-performance liquid chromatography (hplc).

Notes

1. Care should be taken in comparing results between different laboratories (particularly with ciclosporin).
2. The concentration below which a therapeutic effect is unlikely and the concentration above which a toxic effect is more likely together constitute a target range within which satisfactory therapy is likely to be achieved; however, dosages should be adjusted according to the clinical response, not the concentration, which should only be used as a guide.
3. Note the units used when interpreting results. Laboratories may report in SI mass units (e.g. mg/L) or SI molar units (e.g. µmol/L), or both. The volume term should ideally be the litre, but for mass units some laboratories use millilitres instead: µg/L = ng/mL; mg/L = µg/mL.
4. Remember that pharmacokinetics differ from individual to individual. For within-patient comparisons always use the same time after the last dose. For lithium the sample must be taken at 12 hours after the previous dose.
5. Remember that pharmacodynamics differ from individual to individual and that different individuals respond differently to the same concentration of drug. Other factors that can alter the individual response should be considered.
6. For paracetamol, see Figure 9.2 (p. 211).
7. For aminoglycosides, consult your laboratory.

In hospital it is usually better to prescribe by approved name, since the pharmacy will dispense whatever formulation is held in stock. The proprietary name can be used when a combination product is prescribed for which no single approved name exists (for example, 'Fefol'). In general practice it is also usually best to prescribe by approved name. Doctors who make the effort to prescribe by approved name when possible will generally find it just as easy as prescribing by proprietary name.

Countries in the European Community are required to use INNs, except for adrenaline and noradrenaline (BANs that are permitted instead of the rINNs epinephrine and norepinephrine, primarily for reasons of safety).

MONITORING DRUG THERAPY

There is no space here for a detailed discussion of how to monitor drug therapy, which should be done using (in order of preference) clinical, pharmacodynamic or pharmacokinetic methods. For some drugs whose effects can be monitored by measuring plasma concentrations, target concentrations are given in Box 2.28.

Further information

Books and journal articles

British National Formulary. London: British Medical Association and the Pharmaceutical Society of Great Britain; new edition every 6 months. *Guide to currently available formulations, with notes on dosages, uses, adverse effects and interactions; chapters on prescribing, especially in renal failure, in liver disease, in pregnancy and during breastfeeding, and appendices on drug interactions and intravenous additives. The British National Formulary for Children (BNFC) is specifically designed for paediatric prescribing.*

Glasziou P, Irwig L, Aronson JK, eds. Evidence-based Medical Monitoring: From Principles to Practice. Oxford: Wiley–Blackwell, 2008. *An introduction to monitoring drug therapy.*

Grahame-Smith DG, Aronson JK. Oxford Textbook of Clinical Pharmacology and Drug Therapy. 3rd edn. Oxford: Oxford University Press; 2002. *Contains a more detailed account of the principles outlined here.*

Rang HP (ed.). Drug Discovery and Development. Edinburgh: Churchill Livingstone, 2006. *A comprehensive but highly accessible account.*

Rawlins M. De testimonio: on the evidence for decisions about the use of therapeutic interventions. Lancet 2008; 372:2152–2161. *A discussion of the use of different types of evidence.*

Richards D, Aronson JK. Oxford Handbook of Practical Drug Therapy. Oxford: Oxford University Press; 2005. *Contains practical guidance.*

WHO Model Formulary. World Health Organization; 2004. *The equivalent of the British National Formulary for developing countries.*

Websites

http://mednet3.who.int/medicine/organization/par/edl/eml.shtml *The WHO limited list and formulary.*

www.bnf.org *British National Formulary.*

www.clinicalevidence.org *A compendium of best evidence, published by the British Medical Journal.*

www.cochrane.co.uk *The Cochrane Collaboration.*

2

D.R. FitzPatrick
J.R. Seckl

Molecular and genetic factors in disease

3

3

Almost all diseases have a genetic component, and many disorders that cause long-term morbidity and mortality in children and young adults are genetically determined. The past decade has witnessed an exponential increase in identification of the genes that are mutated in genetic diseases and in our understanding of the abnormalities in cell function responsible for the clinical presentation. There is also an increasing appreciation that a combination of common genetic variants can contribute to the aetiology of common diseases like inflammatory bowel disease, rheumatoid arthritis and osteoporosis. In this chapter, we review key principles of cell biology, cellular signalling and molecular genetics, with a specific emphasis on the diagnosis and assessment of patients with genetic diseases.

FUNCTIONAL ANATOMY AND PHYSIOLOGY

Cell and molecular biology

All human cells are derived from the zygote (the fertilised ovum), a single totipotent stem cell capable of producing all cell types. During development, organs and tissues are formed by the integration of four closely regulated cellular processes: cell division, migration, differentiation and programmed cell death. These processes continue in adult life by small populations of stem cells capable of self-renewal. These cells can also differentiate to maintain and repair the tissues in which they are found. Cell biology is the study of these processes and of intracellular compartments, called organelles, which maintain cellular homeostasis. Dysfunction of any of these processes may lead to disease.

DNA, chromosomes and chromatin

The nucleus is a membrane-bound compartment found in all cells, with the exception of erythrocytes and platelets. In humans, the nucleus contains 46 chromosomes, each of which comprises a single linear molecule of deoxyribonucleic acid (DNA), which is intimately complexed with proteins in the form of chromatin. The basic unit of chromatin is the nucleosome, which is a structure of approximately 147 base pairs (bp) of DNA bound round a complex of four different histone proteins.

The vast majority of chromosomal DNA is double-stranded, with exception of the ends of chromosomes where 'knotted' domains of single-stranded DNA, called telomeres, are found. Telomeres prevent degradation and accidental fusion of chromosomal DNA.

The human genome comprises approximately 3.1 billion bp of DNA. Each nucleus contains two copies of the genome and thus humans are diploid organisms. The diploid status is present as 22 identical chromosomal pairs—the autosomes—named 1–22 in descending size order (see Fig. 3.9, p. 54), and two sex chromosomes (XX in females and XY in males). Each DNA strand consists of a linear sequence of four bases—guanine (G), cytosine (C), adenine (A) and thymine (T)—covalently linked by phosphate bonds. The sequence of one strand of double-stranded DNA determines the sequence of the opposite strand because the helix is held together by hydrogen bonds between adenine and thymine or guanine and cytosine.

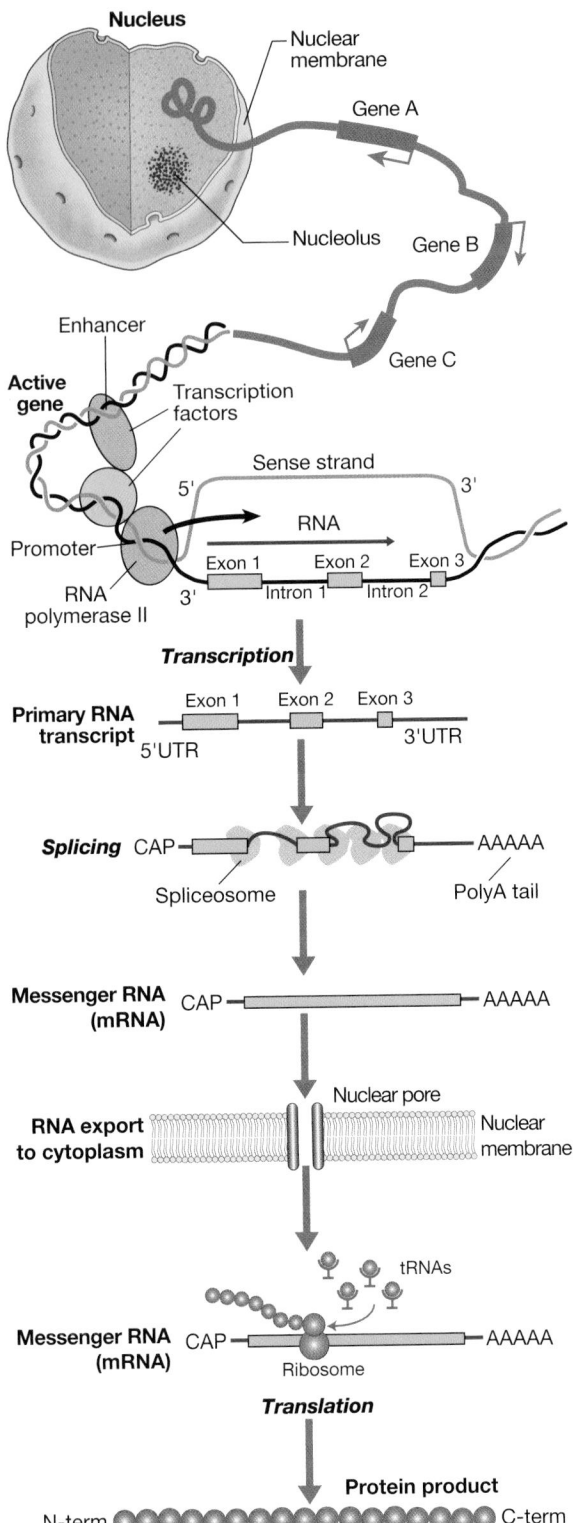

Fig. 3.1 RNA synthesis and its translation into protein. Gene transcription involves binding of RNA polymerase II to the promoter of genes being transcribed with other proteins (transcription factors) that regulate the transcription rate. The primary RNA transcript is a copy of the whole gene and includes both introns and exons, but the introns are removed within the nucleus by splicing and the exons are joined to form the messenger RNA (mRNA). Prior to export from the nucleus, a methylated guanosine nucleotide is added to the 5′ end of the RNA ('cap') and a string of adenine nucleotides are added to the 3′ ('poly A tail'). This protects the RNA from degradation and facilitates transport into the cytoplasm. In the cytoplasm the mRNA binds to ribosomes and forms a template for protein production.

Genes and transcription

Genes are functional units of the chromosome that result in a flow of information from the DNA template via the production of messenger ribonucleic acid (mRNA) to the production of proteins. The human genome contains an estimated 21 500 different genes. Genes may be silent or active; genes that are active undergo transcription which requires binding of an enzyme called RNA polymerase II to a segment of DNA at the start of the gene termed the promoter. Once bound, RNA polymerase II proceeds along one strand of DNA, producing an RNA molecule which is complementary to the DNA template. A DNA sequence close to the end of the gene, called the polyadenylation signal, acts as a signal for termination of the RNA transcript (Fig. 3.1). The activity of RNA polymerase II is regulated by transcription factors. These proteins bind to specific DNA sequences at the promoter or to enhancer elements that may be many thousands of base pairs away from the promoter. The enhancer region forms a loop, enabling the transcription factors to interact directly with other proteins bound to the promoter.

There are over 1200 different transcription factors in humans and mutations in many of these can cause genetic diseases (Fig. 3.2). Alterations of the DNA sequence within promoters and enhancers also cause disease. For example, the blood disorder alpha-thalassaemia can result from loss of an enhancer located more than 100 000 bp from the alpha-globin gene promoter, leading to greatly reduced transcription. Similarly, variation in the promoter of the gene encoding intestinal lactase determines whether or not this is 'shut off' in adulthood, producing lactose intolerance (p. 886).

The availability of the gene promoter to bind RNA polymerase II is regulated by the configuration of chromatin. Chromosomal regions that are transcriptionally active are maintained in a state in which the chromatin is in an open configuration. Conversely, the chromatin is

3

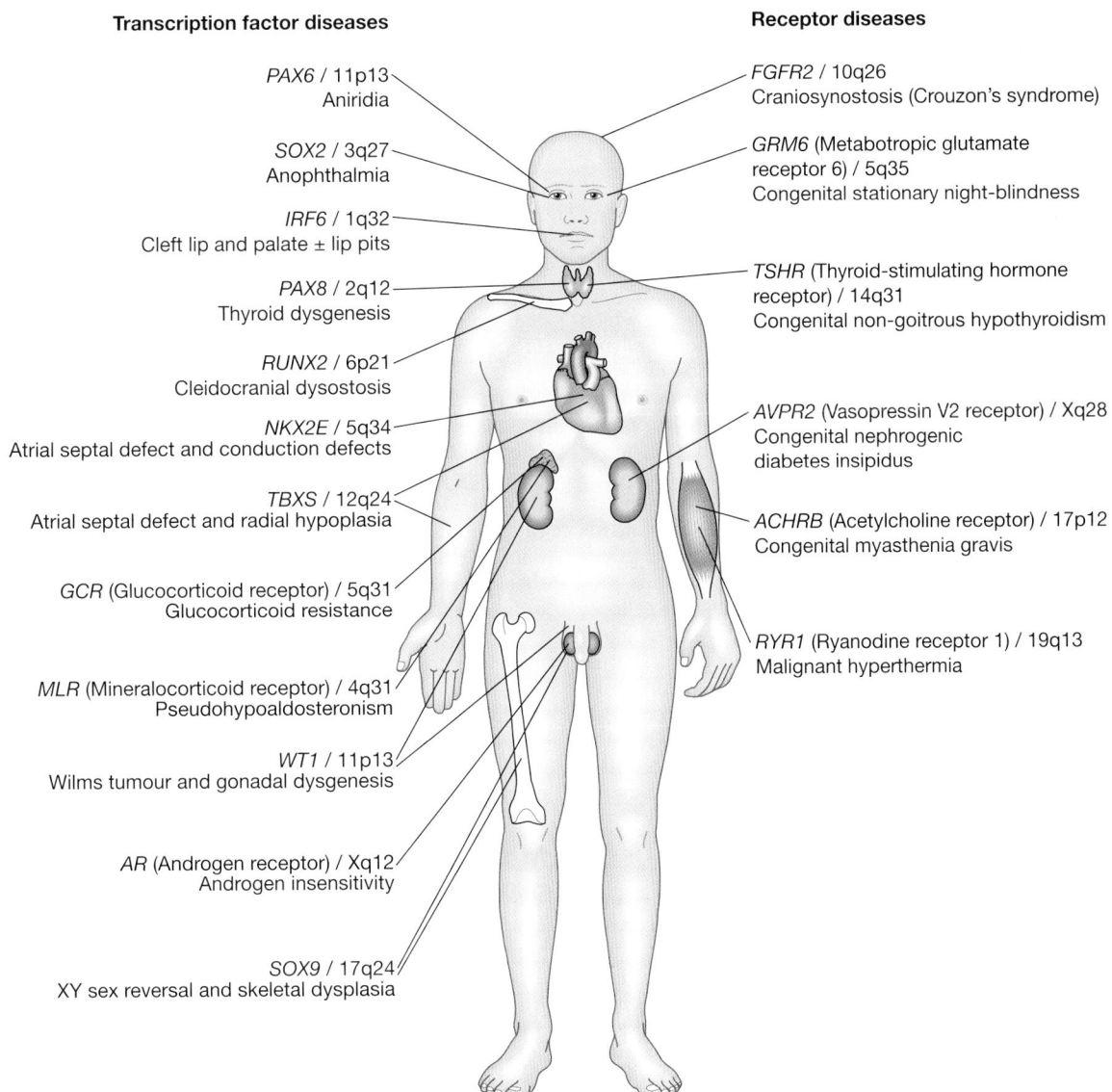

Transcription factor diseases

PAX6 / 11p13
Aniridia

SOX2 / 3q27
Anophthalmia

IRF6 / 1q32
Cleft lip and palate ± lip pits

PAX8 / 2q12
Thyroid dysgenesis

RUNX2 / 6p21
Cleidocranial dysostosis

NKX2E / 5q34
Atrial septal defect and conduction defects

TBXS / 12q24
Atrial septal defect and radial hypoplasia

GCR (Glucocorticoid receptor) / 5q31
Glucocorticoid resistance

MLR (Mineralocorticoid receptor) / 4q31
Pseudohypoaldosteronism

WT1 / 11p13
Wilms tumour and gonadal dysgenesis

AR (Androgen receptor) / Xq12
Androgen insensitivity

SOX9 / 17q24
XY sex reversal and skeletal dysplasia

Receptor diseases

FGFR2 / 10q26
Craniosynostosis (Crouzon's syndrome)

GRM6 (Metabotropic glutamate receptor 6) / 5q35
Congenital stationary night-blindness

TSHR (Thyroid-stimulating hormone receptor) / 14q31
Congenital non-goitrous hypothyroidism

AVPR2 (Vasopressin V2 receptor) / Xq28
Congenital nephrogenic diabetes insipidus

ACHRB (Acetylcholine receptor) / 17p12
Congenital myasthenia gravis

RYR1 (Ryanodine receptor 1) / 19q13
Malignant hyperthermia

Fig. 3.2 Examples of genetic diseases caused by mutations in genes encoding either transcription factors or receptors.

3

very densely packed into heterochromatin in regions of the genome which are not being transcribed. The DNA and histone proteins associated with heterochromatin are chemically distinct from those of open chromatin. A proportion of the cytosine molecules are enzymatically modified by addition of a methyl group (methylation). This silences transcription, since methyl cytosines are usually not available for transcription factor binding or RNA transcription. The histone proteins associated with chromatin can also be methylated, phosphorylated or acetylated at specific amino acid residues in a pattern that reflects the functional state of the chromatin; this is called the histone code. Such modifications are termed epigenetic, as they do not alter the primary sequence of the DNA code but do have biological significance in chromosomal function. Abnormal epigenetic changes are increasingly recognised as important events in the progression of cancer, allowing re-expression of genes which are normally silenced during development to support cancer cell dedifferentiation (see Fig. 3.7 and Box 3.3, pp. 49 and 51).

RNA splicing, editing and degradation

Transcription produces an RNA molecule that is a copy of the whole gene, termed the primary or nascent transcript. RNA differs from DNA in three main ways:

- RNA is single-stranded.
- The sugar residue within the nucleotide is ribose, rather than deoxyribose.
- Uracil (U) is used in place of thymine (T).

The nascent RNA molecule then undergoes a process called splicing, to generate an mRNA molecule which provides the template for protein production. Splicing involves the removal of regions of the RNA molecule which are not required to make protein (introns) from those which are retained in the mRNA to make protein (exons). Splicing is a highly regulated process which is carried out by a multimeric protein complex called the spliceosome. Following splicing, the mRNA molecule is exported from the nucleus and used as a template for protein synthesis. It should be noted that many genes produce more than one form of mRNA (and thus protein) by a process termed alternative splicing. This allows production of different proteins from the same gene, which can have entirely distinct functions. For example, the calcitonin gene expressed in thyroid C cells produces mRNA molecules with one complement of exons encoding the osteoclast inhibitor calcitonin (p. 736), but the same gene is differently spliced in neurons to produce an alternative mRNA encoding the neurotransmitter calcitonin-gene-related peptide.

Most mRNA molecules contain a segment called the open reading frame (ORF), which contains the code that directs synthesis of a protein product. This code comprises a contiguous series of three sequential bases (codon), which specifies that a particular amino acid should be incorporated into the protein. There are 64 different codons; 61 of these specify incorporation of one of the 20 amino acids, whereas the remaining three codons—UAA, UAG and UGA (stop codons)—cause termination of the growing polypeptide chain. ORFs in humans most commonly start with the amino acid methionine. All mRNA molecules have domains before and after the ORF called the 5′ untranslated region (5′UTR) and 3′ untranslated region (3′UTR), respectively. The start of the 5′UTR contains a cap structure that protects mRNA from enzymatic degradation, and other elements within the 5′UTR are required for efficient translation. The 3′UTR also contains elements that regulate efficiency of translation and mRNA stability, including a stretch of adenine bases known as a polyA tail.

There are approximately 4500 genes in humans in which the transcribed RNA molecules do not code for proteins. There are various categories of non-coding RNA (ncRNA), including transfer RNA (tRNA), ribosomal RNA (rRNA), ribozymes and microRNA (miRNA). There is increasing evidence to suggest that miRNAs play a role in normal development, cancer and common degenerative disorders by regulating the stability of other RNA molecules.

Translation and protein production

Following splicing and export from the nucleus, mRNAs associate with ribosomes, which are the sites of protein production (see Fig. 3.1). Each ribosome consists of two subunits (40S and 60S), which comprise non-coding rRNA molecules complexed with proteins. During translation, tRNA binds to the ribosome. The tRNAs deliver amino acids to the ribosome so that the newly synthesised protein can be assembled in a step-wise fashion. Individual tRNA molecules bind a specific amino acid and 'read' the mRNA ORF via an 'anticodon' of three nucleotides that is complementary to the codon in mRNA. Some ribosomes are bound to the membrane of the endoplasmic reticulum (ER), a complex tubular structure that surrounds the nucleus. Proteins synthesised on these ribosomes are translocated into the lumen of the ER, where they undergo folding and processing. From here the protein may be transferred to the Golgi apparatus, where it undergoes post-translational modifications, such as glycosylation (covalent attachment of sugar moieties), to form the mature protein that can be exported into the cytoplasm or packaged into vesicles for secretion. The clinical importance of post-translational modification of proteins is shown by the severe developmental, neurological, haemostatic and soft tissue abnormalities that are associated with the dozen or so congenital disorders of glycosylation, rare deficiencies of the enzymes that catalyse the addition of chains of sugar moieties to proteins (e.g. phosphomannose isomerase deficiency). Post-translational modifications can also be disrupted by the synthesis of proteins with abnormal amino acid sequences. For example, the most common mutation in cystic fibrosis (ΔF508) results in an abnormal protein that cannot be exported from the ER and Golgi.

Mitochondria and energy production

The mitochondrion has both an inner and outer membrane, and is the main site of energy production within the cell. Mitochondria arose via the symbiotic association with an intracellular bacterium at some point during evolution. Energy, in the form of adenosine triphosphate (ATP) production, is mostly derived from the metabolism of glucose and fat (Fig. 3.3). Glucose cannot enter mitochondria directly but is first metabolised to pyruvate via glycolysis. Pyruvate is then imported into the mito-

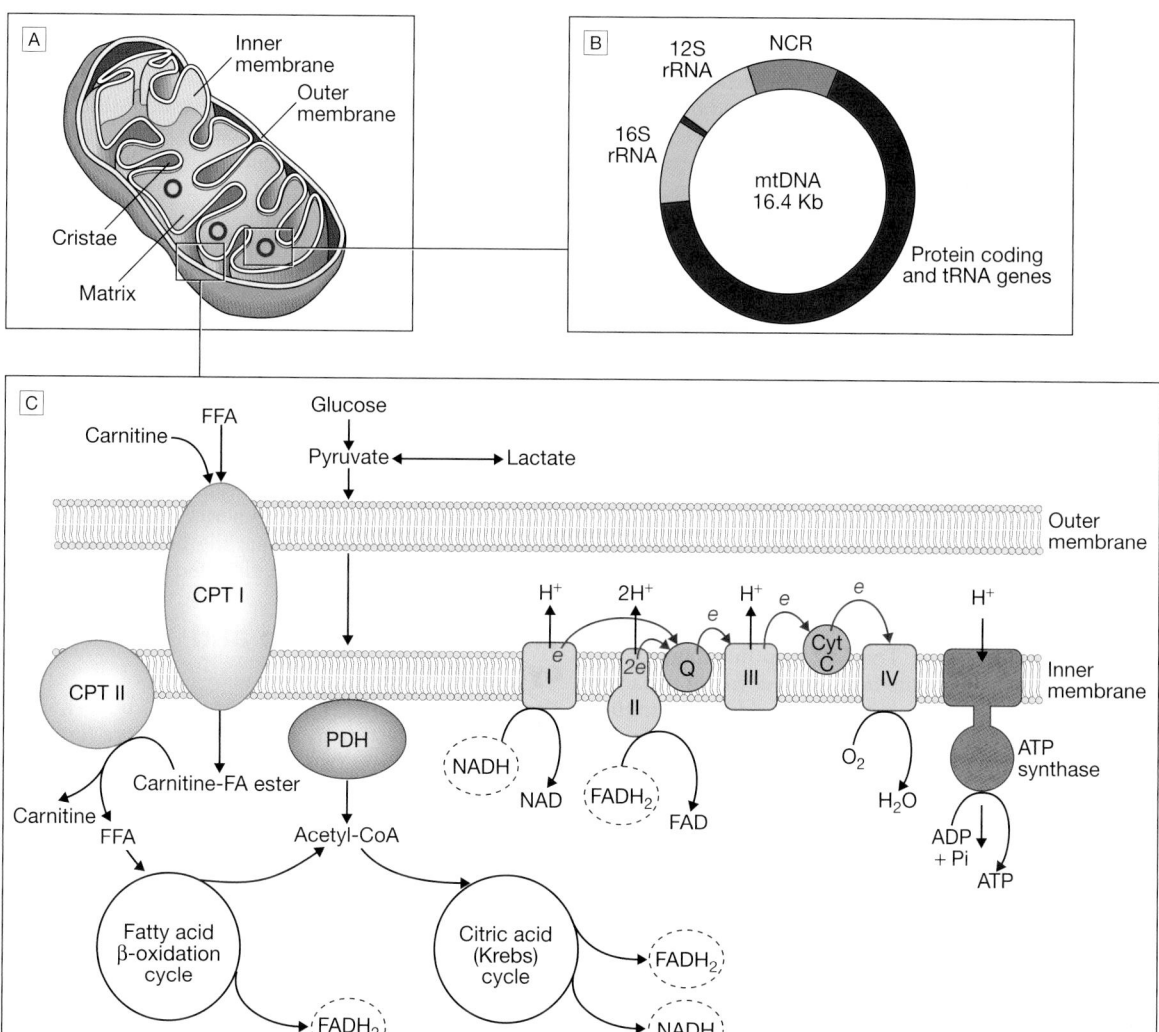

Fig. 3.3 Mitochondria. **A** Mitochondrial structure. There is a smooth outer membrane surrounding a convoluted inner membrane which has inward projections called cristae. The membranes create two compartments: the inter-membrane compartment, which plays a crucial role in the electron transport chain, and the inner compartment (or matrix), which contains mitochondrial DNA and the enzymes responsible for the citric acid (Krebs) cycle and the fatty acid β-oxidation cycle. **B** Mitochondrial DNA. The mitochondrion contains several copies of a circular double-stranded DNA molecule which has a non-coding region (NCR), and a coding region which encodes the genes responsible for energy production, mitochondrial tRNA molecules and mitochondrial rRNA molecules. **C** Mitochondrial energy production. Fatty acids enter the mitochondrion conjugated to carnitine by carnitine-palmityl transferase type 1 (CPT I) and, once inside the matrix, are unconjugated by CPT II to release free fatty acids (FFA). These are broken down by the β-oxidation cycle to produce acetyl-CoA. Pyruvate can enter the mitochondrion directly and is metabolised by pyruvate dehydrogenase (PDH) to produce acetyl-CoA. The acetyl-CoA enters the Krebs cycle, leading to the production of NADH and FADH$_2$ which are used by proteins in the electron transport chain to generate a hydrogen ion gradient across the inter-membrane compartment. Reduction of NADH and FADH$_2$ by proteins I and II respectively releases electrons (e), and the energy released is used to pump protons into the inter-membrane compartment. As these electrons are exchanged between proteins in the chain, more protons are pumped across the membrane, until the electrons reach complex IV (cytochrome oxidase) which uses the energy to reduce oxygen to water. The hydrogen ion gradient is used to produce ATP by the enzyme ATP synthase which consists of a proton channel and catalytic sites for the synthesis of ATP from ADP. When the channel opens, hydrogen ions enter the matrix down the concentration gradient and energy is released which is used to make ATP.

chondrion and metabolised to acetyl-CoA. Fatty acids are transported into the mitochondria following conjugation with carnitine and are sequentially catabolised by a process called β-oxidation to produce acetyl-CoA. The acetyl-CoA from both pyruvate and fatty acid oxidation is used in the citric acid (Krebs) cycle—a series of enzymatic reactions that produces CO$_2$, NADH and FADH$_2$. Both NADH and FADH$_2$ then donate electrons to the respiratory chain, which transfers the electrons in a complex series of reactions which results in the pro-

duction of a proton gradient across the inner mitochondrial membrane. The proton gradient is then used by the inner mitochondrial membrane protein, ATP synthase, to produce ATP. ATP is then transported to other parts of the cell, where it can be dephosphorylated to produce the energy required for most reactions within the cell.

Each mitochondrion contains 2–10 copies of a 16 kilobase (kB) double-stranded circular DNA molecule (mtRNA). mtDNA contains 13 protein-coding genes, all involved in the respiratory chain, and the ncRNA genes required for protein synthesis within the mitochondria (see Fig. 3.3). The mutational rate of mtDNA is relatively high due to the lack of protection by chromatin. Several mtDNA diseases characterised by defects in ATP production have been described. mtDNA diseases are inherited exclusively down the maternal line (see Fig. 3.6, p. 48), since all mtDNA is derived from the mother, as sperm contribute no mitochondria to the zygote. Mitochondria are most numerous in cells with high metabolic demands, such as muscle, retina and the basal ganglia, and these tissues tend to be the ones most severely affected in mitochondrial diseases (Box 3.1). There are many other mitochondrial diseases that are caused by mutations in nuclear genes, which encode proteins that are then imported into the mitochondrion and are critical for energy production.

Protein degradation

The cell has developed three organelles, the lysosome, the peroxisome and the 26S proteasome, for the degradation of proteins and other molecules that are damaged, are potentially toxic or have simply served their purpose. The proteasome is the main site of protein degradation within the cell. The first step in proteasomal degradation is ubiquitination—the covalent attachment of a protein called ubiquitin as a side chain to the target protein. Ubiquitination is carried out by a large group of enzymes called E3 ligases, whose function is to recognise specific proteins that should be targeted for degradation by the proteasome. The E3 ligases ubiquitinate their target protein, which is then transported to a large multiprotein complex called the 26S proteasome, where it is degraded. There is mounting evidence that defects in the proteasome are responsible for many diseases; a severe genetic disease termed Angelman's syndrome is due to a mutation in a specific E3 ligase.

Proteins with complex post-translational modifications are degraded in membrane-bound structures called lysosomes, which have an acidic pH and contain proteolytic enzymes that degrade proteins. There are many inherited defects in lysosomal enzymes which result in failure to degrade intracellular toxic substances.

For instance, in Gaucher's disease, mutations of the gene encoding lysosomal (acid) beta-glucosidase lead to undigested lipid accumulating in macrophages, producing hepatosplenomegaly and, if severe, deposition in the brain leading to mental retardation.

Peroxisomes are small single membrane-bound cytoplasmic organelles containing many different oxidative enzymes such as catalase. Peroxisomes are involved in the degradation of hydrogen peroxide, bile acids and amino acids. However, the beta-oxidation of very long-chain fatty acids appears to be their most important function since mutations in the peroxisomal beta-oxidation enzymes (or the proteins that import these enzymes into the peroxisome) result in the same severe congenital disorder as mutations that cause complete failure of peroxisomal biogenesis. This group of disorders is called Zellweger's syndrome (cerebrohepatorenal syndrome) and is characterised by severe developmental delay, seizures, hepatomegaly and renal cysts; the biochemical diagnosis is made on the basis of elevated plasma levels of very long-chain fatty acids.

The cell membrane and cytoskeleton

The cell membrane is a phospholipid bilayer, with hydrophilic surfaces and a hydrophobic core (Fig. 3.4). The cell membrane is, however, much more than a simple wall. Cholesterol-rich 'rafts' float within the membrane, with proteins anchored to them via the post-translational addition of complex lipid moieties. The membrane also hosts a series of transmembrane proteins that function as receptors, pores, ion channels, pumps and associated energy suppliers. These proteins allow the cell to monitor the extracellular milieu, import crucial molecules for function, and exclude or exchange unwanted substances. Many proteins within the cell membrane are highly dynamic and associate and disassociate to subserve their functions.

The cell membrane is permeable to hydrophobic substances such as anaesthetic gases. Water is able to pass through the membrane via a pore formed by aquaporin

3.1 The structure of the respiratory chain complexes and the diseases associated with their dysfunction

Complex	Enzyme	nDNA subunits[1]	mtDNA subunits[2]	Diseases
I	NADH dehydrogenase	38	7	MELAS, bilateral striatal necrosis, LHON, myopathy and exercise intolerance, Parkinsonism, Leigh's disease, exercise myoglobinuria, leukodystrophy/myoclonic epilepsy
II	Succinate dehydrogenase	4	0	Phaeochromocytoma
III	Cytochrome bc$_1$ complex	10	1	Parkinsonism/MELAS, cardiomyopathy, myopathy, exercise myoglobinuria
IV	Cytochrome c oxidase	10	3	Sideroblastic anaemia, myoclonic ataxia, deafness, myopathy, MELAS, mitochondrial encephalomyopathy, motor neuron disease-like, exercise myoglobinuria
V	ATP synthase	14	2	Leigh's disease, NARP, bilateral striatal necrosis

[1]nDNA subunits (nDNA = nuclear DNA)
[2]mtDNA subunits = number of different protein subunits in each complex that are encoded in the nDNA and mtDNA respectively.
(LHON = Leber hereditary optic neuropathy; MERRF = myoclonic epilepsy and ragged-red fibres; MELAS = myopathy, encephalopathy, lactic acidosis and stroke-like episodes; mtDNA = mitochondrial DNA; NARP = neuropathy, ataxia and retinitis pigmentosa.

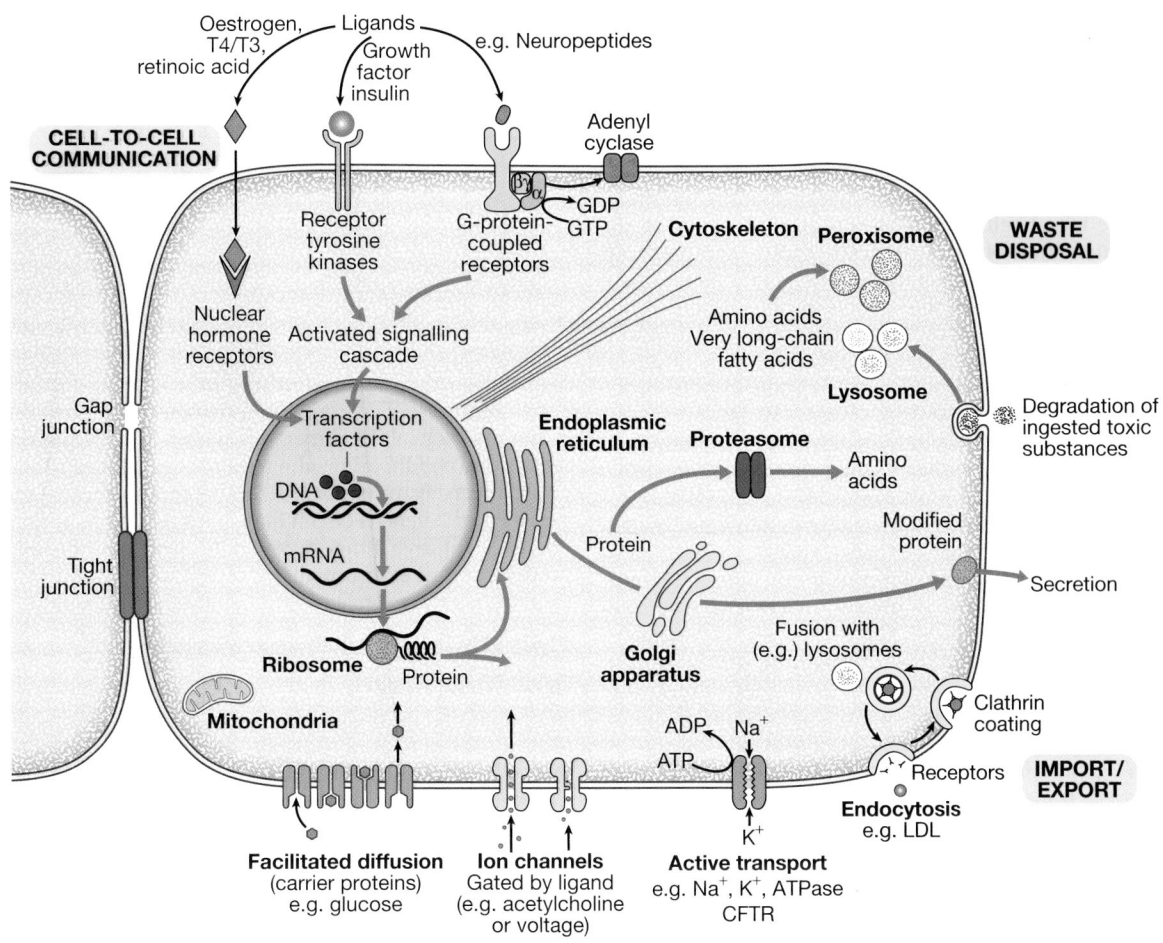

Fig. 3.4 An archetypal human cell. The basic cell components required for function within a tissue: (1) cell-to-cell communication taking place via gap junctions and the various types of receptor that receive signals from the extracellular environment and transduce these into intracellular messengers; (2) the nucleus containing the chromosomal DNA; (3) intracellular organelles including the mechanisms for proteins and lipid catabolism; (4) the cellular mechanisms for import and export of molecules across the cell membrane. (ABC = ATP-binding cassette transporters; ATP = adenosine triphosphate; cAMP = cyclic adenosine monophosphate; CFTR = cystic fibrosis transmembrane regulator; CREB = cAMP response element-binding protein; GDP/GTP = guanine diphosphate/triphosphate; LDL = low-density lipoproteins)

proteins; mutations of an aquaporin gene cause congenital nephrogenic diabetes insipidus (p. 792). Other molecules, including ions, glucose and other fuels, amino acids and peptides, must be actively transported using either channels or pumps. Channels are responsible for the transport of ions and other small molecules across the cell membrane. They open and close in a highly regulated manner. The cystic fibrosis transmembrane conductance regulator (CFTR) is an example of an ion channel which is responsible for transport of chloride ions across epithelial cell membranes. Mutation of the CFTR chloride channel, highly expressed in the lung and gut, leads to defective chloride transport, producing cystic fibrosis. Pumps are highly specific for their substrate and often use energy (ATP) to drive transport against a concentration gradient.

Endocytosis is a cellular process that allows internalisation of larger complexes and molecules via an invaginated fold of plasma membrane. Such engulfing is typically mediated by specific binding of the particle to surface receptors. This can involve phagocytosis of large particles and whole cells. An example of endocy-

tosis of smaller structures is the uptake of low-density lipoprotein (LDL) cholesterol, which binds to cell membranes via a specialised region of the membrane called a clathrin pit LDL receptor. In familial hypercholesterol-aemia (p. 451), mutation of the receptor leads to failure to bind LDL cholesterol. Intriguingly, in some families, mutations in a specific tyrosine in the intracellular tail of the receptor, which normally attaches the protein to clathrin, prevents receptors concentrating in clathrin-coated pits and hence impairs uptake of LDL, even though the receptors are present elsewhere in the cell membrane.

The shape and structure of the cell are maintained by the cytoskeleton, which consists of a series of proteins which form microfilaments (actin), microtubules (tubulins) and intermediate filaments (keratins, desmin, vimentin, laminins) that facilitate cellular movement and provide pathways for intracellular transport. Dysfunction of the cytoskeleton may result in a variety of human disorders. For instance, some keratin genes encode intermediate filaments in epithelia. In epidermolysis bullosa simplex (p. 1249), mutations in keratin

45

genes (*KRT5, KRT14*) lead to cell fragility, producing the characteristic blistering on mild trauma.

Cellular signalling

Cells communicate with one another directly through gap junctions, and indirectly by release of hormones, cytokines and growth factors which bind to receptors on the target cell. Gap junctions are pores formed by the interaction of 'hemichannels' in the membrane of adjacent cells. This interaction results in a direct communication between the cytoplasm of adjacent cells. Many diseases are due to mutations in gap junction proteins, including the most common form of autosomal recessive hearing loss (GJB2) and the X-linked form of Charcot–Marie–Tooth disease (GJB1).

As organisms have become larger and more complex, mechanisms have evolved which enable communication between cells that operates over greater distances. Cell signalling is a very important mechanism in medicine. In a typical signalling pathway, a ligand will bind to a receptor that will then directly or indirectly activate gene expression to produce a cellular response (see Fig. 3.4).

There are several different signalling pathways; for example, in nuclear steroid hormone signalling, the ligands (steroid hormones or thyroid hormone) bind to their cognate receptor in the cytoplasm and the receptor/ligand complex then enters the nucleus, where it acts as a transcription factor to regulate the expression of target genes (Box 3.2). However, the most diverse and abundant types of receptor are located at the cell surface, and these usually activate gene expression and cellular responses indirectly. When a cell surface receptor is activated by its ligand, a series of events ensue, usually involving the phosphorylation and activation of a cascade of enzymes called kinases. This, in turn, typically culminates in phosphorylation and activation of transcription factors which bind DNA and modulate gene expression. Some membrane receptors, like the insulin receptor, contain a kinase domain which is activated by ligand binding. Others, like the tumour necrosis factor (TNF) receptor, do not have intrinsic kinase activity but recruit other effector proteins. Transmembrane receptors can be grouped into:

- ion channel-linked receptors (e.g. glutamate and the nicotinic acetylcholine receptor)
- G protein-coupled receptors (e.g. rhodopsin, olfactory receptors, parathyroid hormone receptor)
- receptors with intrinsic enzyme activity (e.g. insulin receptor, growth factor receptors)
- receptors which do not have intrinsic enzymatic activity, but which recruit other proteins with kinase activity to their intracellular domain when activated by ligand (TNF receptor, interleukin (IL)-1 receptor) (see Box 3.2).

Many receptors need to form dimers for full activity, and in some cases, active receptors form trimers. Mutations which interfere with receptor dimerisation can result in disease. For example, mutations of the insulin receptor which inhibit dimerisation have been described that lead to childhood insulin resistance and growth failure. Conversely, mutations in the fibroblast growth factor receptor 2 gene (*FGFR2*) have been described which cause constitutive dimerisation in the absence of ligand, producing bone overgrowth and an autosomal dominant form of craniosynostosis called Crouzon's syndrome.

Cell division, differentiation and migration

In normal tissues, molecules such as hormones, growth factors and cytokines provide the signal to activate the cell cycle, a controlled programme of biochemical events that culminates in cell division. During the first phase, G1, synthesis of the cellular components necessary to complete cell division occurs. In S phase, the cell produces an identical copy of each chromosome—which carries the cell's genetic information—via a process called DNA replication. The cell then enters G2, when any errors in the replicated DNA are repaired before proceeding to mitosis, in which identical copies of all chromosomes are segregated to the daughter cells. The progression from one phase to the next is tightly controlled by cell cycle checkpoints. For example, the checkpoint between G2 and mitosis ensures that all damaged DNA is repaired prior to segregation of the chromosomes. Failure of these control processes is a crucial factor in the pathogenesis of cancer, as discussed in Chapter 11 (p. 258).

3.2 Examples of molecules involved in specific signalling cascades

Ligand	Receptor (type)	Signal transduction	Effector/target genes	Medical significance
TNF-α	TNFR1 (TNFR)	TRADD, FADD IKK, NFκB	Caspase 8 → apoptosis Inflammatory cytokines	TNF-α is an important cytokine that results in apoptosis, but binding of the same receptor also activates inflammation by the NFκB pathway
Insulin	Insulin receptor (RTK)	IRS1, PI3K, PIP3, AKT/PKB, PDK1, mTORC2, GSK3	Glycogen synthase	Insulin has many roles; activation of this cascade stimulates conversion of blood glucose to muscle glycogen
Thyroid hormones	THRA or THRB (NHR)	Ligand/receptor complex	*GH, SERCA2A, PEPCK* etc.	Thyroid hormone signalling has many roles in embryogenesis and adult life. The different receptors seem to have subtly different roles
Gonadotrophin-releasing hormone (GnRH)	GnRHR (GPCR)	Gq/G(11), PLCbetal, PLA(2), PLD, PKC, MAPK	Gonadotrophin subunits, GnRHR	This cascade produces a pulsatile cascade that is important in control of fertility

(GPCR = G protein-coupled receptor; NHR = nuclear hormone receptor; RTK = receptor tyrosine kinase receptor; TNFR = tumour necrosis superfamily of receptors)

During development or tissue repair, cells must progressively replace their stem cell identity with the morphological and biochemical configuration of an individual tissue. This process is called differentiation and requires the programmed gain and loss of specific functions in individual cells. This is achieved by activation or repression of genes which are functional elements coded within the chromosomal DNA. It is the ability to switch genes on and off that allows cells containing the same genetic material to become very different in shape and function. The programme of differentiation is often deranged or partially reversed in cancer cells.

Another process that is of particular importance during development and tissue repair is cell migration. This requires the activation of a set of genes which give the cell polarity and enable the leading edge of the cell to interact with the extracellular environment to control the speed and direction of travel. Again, this process can be reactivated in cancer cells and is thought to facilitate tumour metastasis.

Cell death, apoptosis and senescence

With the exception of stem cells, human cells have only a limited capacity for cell division. The Hayflick limit is the number of divisions a cell population can go through in culture before division stops (senescence). The molecular nature of this 'biological clock' is of great interest in the study of the normal ageing process, and the study of rare human diseases associated with premature ageing has been very helpful in identifying the importance of DNA repair mechanisms in senescence (pp. 46 and 166).

A very different mechanism of cell death is seen in apoptosis, or programmed cell death. Apoptosis is an active process that occurs in normal tissues and plays an important role in development, tissue remodelling and the immune response. The signal that triggers apoptosis is specific to each tissue or cell type. This signal activates enzymes, called caspases, which actively destroy cellular components, including chromosomal DNA. This degradation results in cell death, but the cellular corpse contains characteristic vesicles called apoptotic bodies. The corpse is then recognised and removed by phagocytic cells of the immune system, such as macrophages, in a manner that does not provoke an inflammatory response.

A third mechanism of cell death is necrosis. This is a pathological process in which the cellular environment loses one or more of the components necessary for cell viability. Hypoxia is probably the most common cause of necrosis.

GENETIC DISEASE AND INHERITANCE

Meiosis

Meiosis is a special form of cell division that only occurs in the postpubertal testis and the fetal and adult ovary (Fig. 3.5). Meiosis differs from mitosis in two main ways. Firstly, there is extensive swapping of genetic material between homologous chromosomes, a process known as recombination, before the first of the two meiotic cell

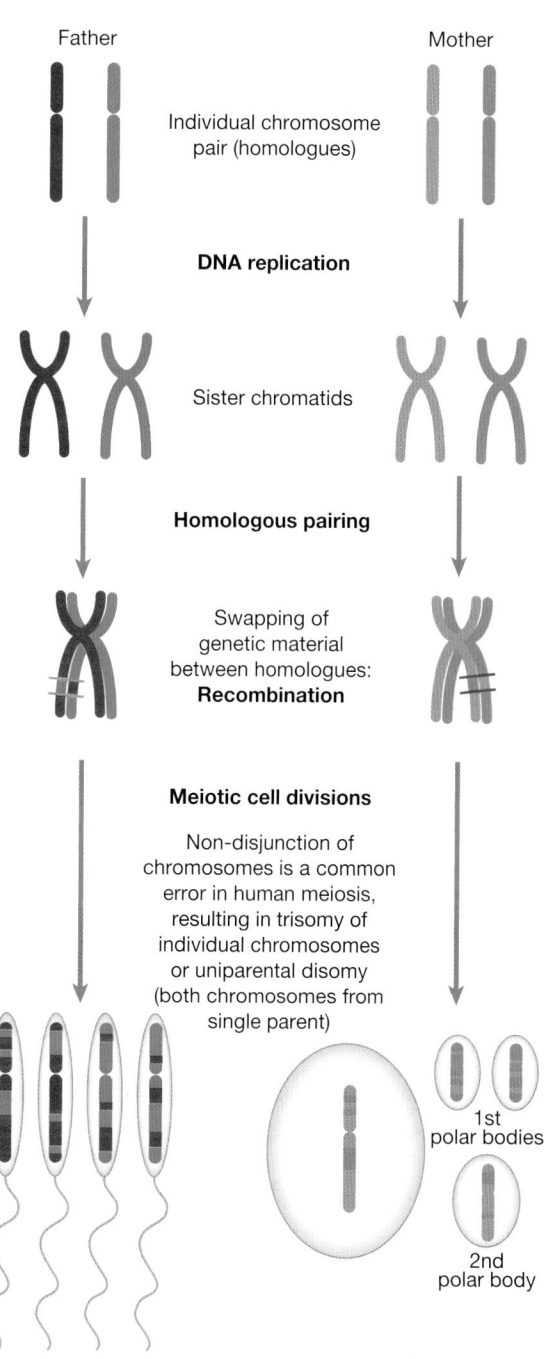

Fig. 3.5 Meiosis and gametogenesis. The main chromosomal stages of meiosis in both males and female. A single homologous pair of chromosomes is represented in different colours. The final step is the production of haploid germ cells. Each round of meiosis in the male results in four sperm cells; in the female, however, only one egg cell is produced, as the other divisions are sequestered on the periphery of the mature egg as peripheral polar bodies.

divisions. As a result of recombination, each chromosome that a parent passes to his or her offspring is a mix of the chromosomes which the parent inherited from his or her own mother and father. Secondly, the cells that are produced as the result of meiosis (sperm and egg cells) are haploid, in that they each have only 23 chromosomes: one of each homologous pair of autosomes and

3

a sex chromosome. The requirement for this reductive process is obvious; when a sperm cell fertilises the egg, the resulting zygote will have a diploid chromosome complement of 46 chromosomes. The sperm thus determines the sex of the offspring, since 50% of sperm will carry an X chromosome and 50% a Y chromosome, with each egg cell carrying an X chromosome.

The individual steps in meiotic cell division are similar in males and females. However, the timing of the cell divisions is very different (see Fig. 3.5). In females, meiosis begins in fetal life but does not complete until after ovulation. A single meiotic cell division can thus take more than 40 years to complete. In males, meiotic division does not begin until puberty and continues throughout life. In the testes, both meiotic divisions are completed in a matter of days.

Patterns of disease inheritance

Five modes of genetic disease inheritance are discussed below and illustrated in Figures 3.6 and 3.7.

Autosomal dominant inheritance

Autosomal dominant disorders are caused by inheritance of a genetic abnormality in only one of the two copies (alleles) of a single gene. The risk of an affected individual transmitting an autosomal disease to his or her offspring is 50% for each pregnancy, since half the affected individual gametes (sperm or egg cells) will contain the affected chromosome and half will contain the normal chromosome. However, even within a family, individuals with the same mutation rarely have identical patterns of disease due to variable penetrance and/or expressivity. Penetrance is defined as the proportion of individuals bearing a mutated allele who develop the disease phenotype. The mutation is said to be fully penetrant if all individuals who inherit a mutation develop the disease. Expression of a disease describes the degree to which the severity of various aspects of the disease phenotype may vary. Neurofibromatosis type 1 (*NF1*, neurofibromin, 17q11.2) is an example of a disease that is fully (100%) penetrant but which shows extremely variable expressivity. The factors that alter penetrance and expressivity are not clearly understood. It is very likely that other genes act as modifiers of the mutated gene's function, along with environmental factors. A good example of an environmental influence which can profoundly influence expression of autosomal dominant disease is seen in the triggering of malignant hyperpyrexia by anaesthetic agents in the presence of *RYR1*

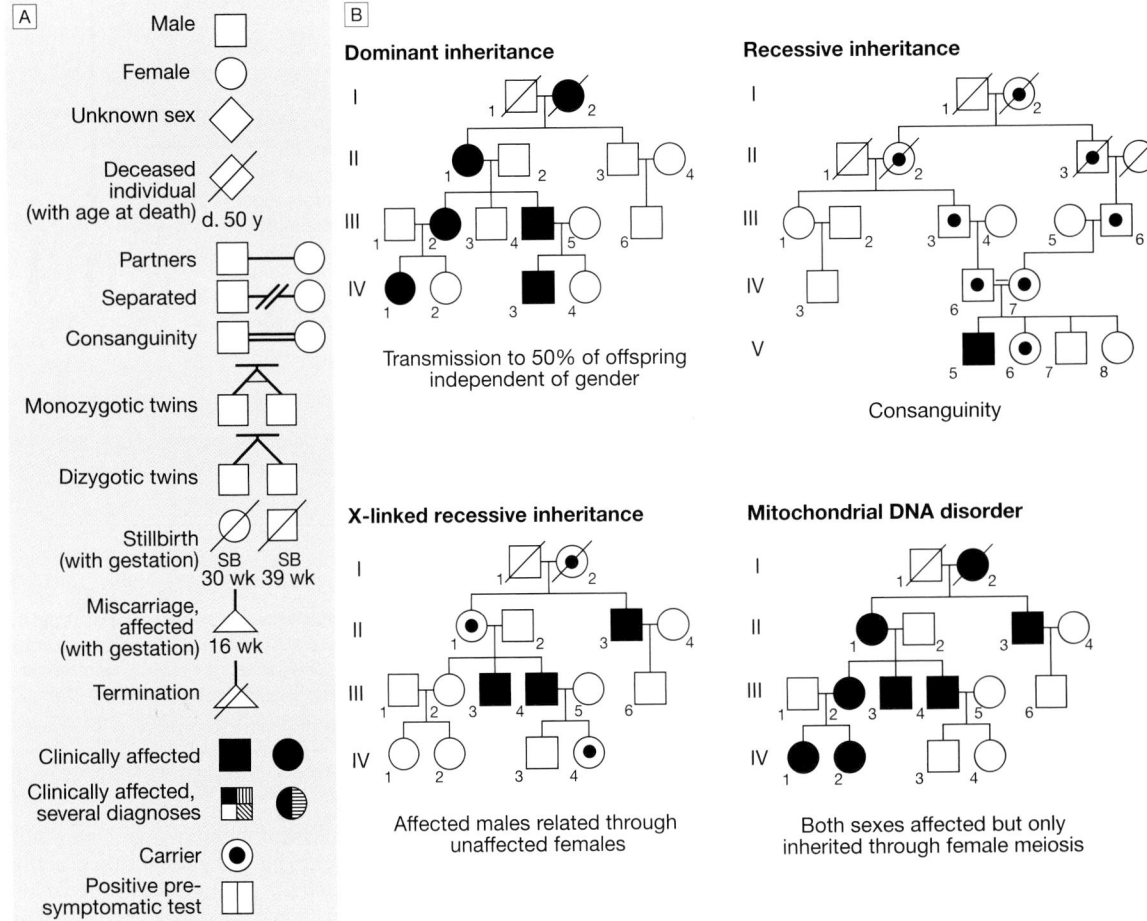

Fig. 3.6 Drawing a pedigree and patterns of inheritance. A The main symbols used to represent pedigrees in diagrammatic form. B The main modes of disease inheritance, as discussed in the text.

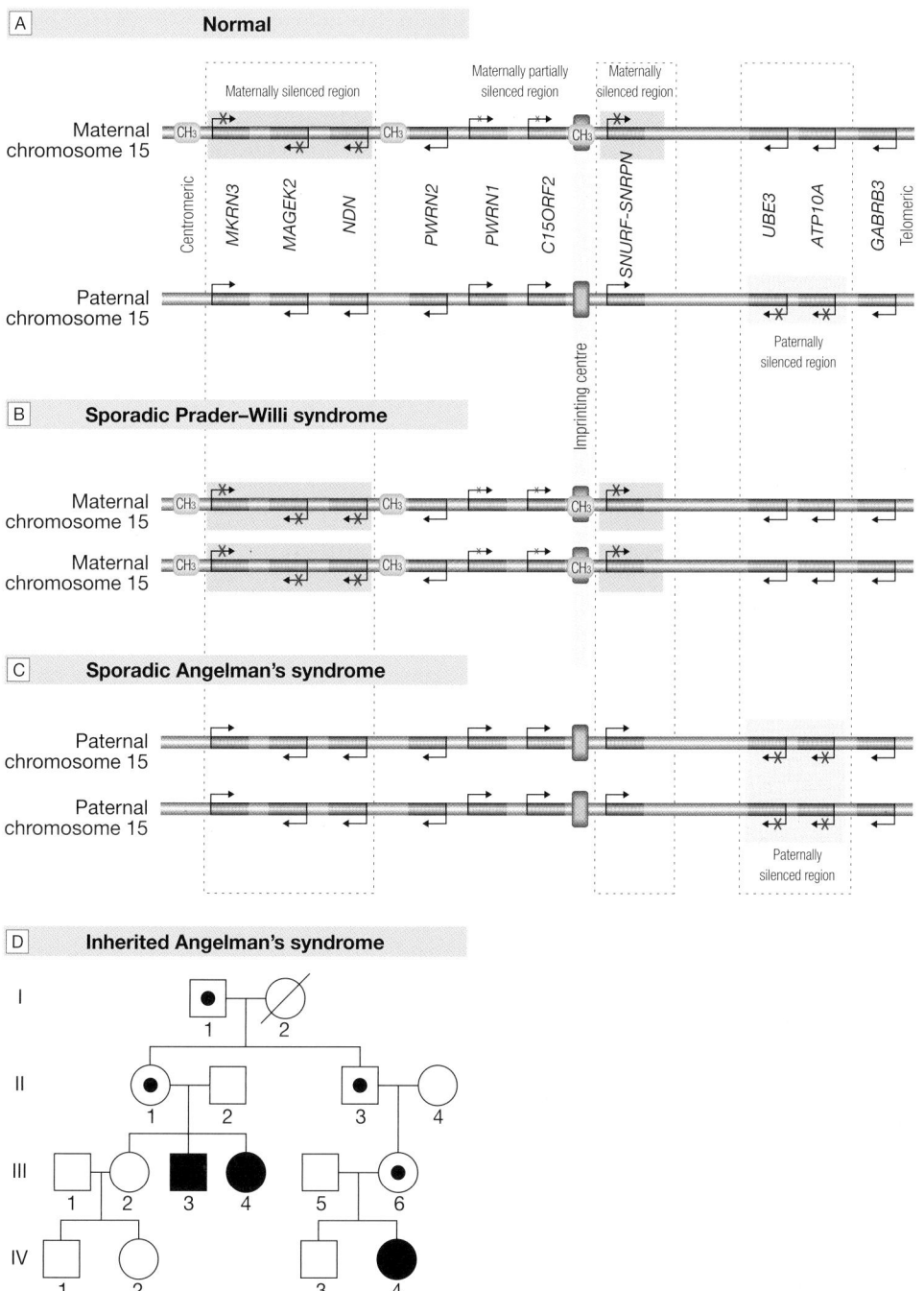

3

Fig. 3.7 Genomic imprinting and associated diseases. Several regions of the genome exhibit the phenomenon of imprinting whereby expression of one or a group of genes is influenced by whether the chromosome is derived from the mother or the father; one such region lies on chromosome 15.
A Normal imprinting. Under normal circumstances expression of several genes is suppressed (silenced) on the maternal chromosome (red), whereas these are expressed normally by the paternal chromosome (blue). However, two genes in the paternal chromosome (*UBE3* and *ATP10A*) are silenced.
B In sporadic Prader–Willi syndrome (PWS) there is a non-disjunction defect on chromosome 15, and both copies of the chromosomal region are derived from the mother (maternal uniparental disomy). In this case Prader–Willi syndrome occurs because there is loss of function of several paternally expressed genes, including *MKRN3*, *MAGEK2*, *NDN*, *PWRN2*, *C15ORF2* and *SNURF-SNRNP*. **C** In sporadic Angelman's syndrome, both chromosomal regions are derived from the father (paternal uniparental disomy) due to non-disjunction during paternal meiosis. As a result, both copies of the *UBE3* gene are silenced and this causes Angelman's syndrome. Note that the syndrome can also be caused by deletion of this region on the maternal chromosome or a loss of function mutation on the maternal copy of *UBE3*, causing an inherited form of Angelman's as illustrated in panel D. **D** Pedigree of a family with inherited Angelman's syndrome due to a loss of function mutation in *UBE3*. Inheriting this mutation from a father causes no disease (because the gene is normally silenced in the paternal chromosome) (see individuals I-1, II-1, II-3, III-6), but the same mutation inherited from the mother causes the syndrome (individuals III-3, III-4, IV-4), as this is the only copy expressed and the *UBE3* gene is mutated.

mutations. Other examples of autosomal dominant disorders (with the affected gene, the name of the protein encoded by the gene and the locus) include adult polycystic kidney disease type 1 (*PKD1*, polycystin I, 16p13.1) and hereditary motor and sensory neuropathy type 1 (*PMP22*, peripheral myelin protein 22, 17p11.2). Autosomal dominant disorders can occur as a result of either loss or gain of function of the affected gene.

Autosomal recessive inheritance

In autosomal recessive disorders, both alleles of a gene must be mutated before the disease is manifest in an individual, and an affected individual must inherit one mutant allele from each parent. The distinguishing feature of recessive diseases is that carrying one mutant allele does not produce a phenotype. Autosomal recessive disorders are rare in most populations. For example, the most common serious autosomal recessive disorder in the UK is cystic fibrosis, which has a birth incidence of 1:2500. The frequency of autosomal recessive disorders increases with the degree of inbreeding of a population because the risk of inheriting the same mutant allele from both parents (homozygosity) is increased. Genetic risk calculation for a fully penetrant autosomal recessive disorder is straightforward. Each subsequent pregnancy of a couple who have had a previous child affected by an autosomal recessive disorder will have a 25% (1:4) risk of being affected; a healthy individual who has a sibling with an autosomal recessive disorder will have 2/3 chance of being a carrier. The risk of an affected individual having children with the same condition is usually low but is dependent on the carrier rate of mutant allele of the gene in the population.

X-linked inheritance

Genetic diseases caused by mutations on the X chromosome have specific characteristics. X-linked diseases are mostly recessive and restricted to males who carry the mutant allele. This is because males have only one X chromosome, whereas females have two. Thus females who carry a single mutant allele are generally unaffected. Occasionally, female carriers may exhibit signs of an X-linked disease due to a phenomenon called skewed X-inactivation. All females will inactivate one of their two X chromosomes in each cell at a point during development. This process is random in each cell but if, by chance, there is a disproportionate inactivation of normal X chromosomes carrying the normal allele, then an affected female carrier will be more likely. X-linked recessive disorders have a recognisable pattern of inheritance, with transmission of the disease from carrier females to affected males and absence of father-to-son transmission. The risk of a female carrier having an affected child is 25% (1:4; half her male offspring). If the carrier status of a woman is unclear, then the risk may be altered by conditional information, as discussed in the autosomal dominant disease section above. Bayes' theorem is commonly used to calculate such modified risks and this is discussed in more detail later in this chapter (p. 64).

Mitochondrial inheritance

The inheritance of mtDNA disorders is characterised by transmission from females, but males and females are generally equally affected. Unlike all the other inheritance patterns mentioned above, mitochondrial inheritance has nothing to do with meiosis but reflects the fact that mitochondrial DNA is transmitted by oöcytes. Mitochondrial disorders tend to be very variable in penetrance and expressivity within families, and this is mostly accounted for by the fact that only a proportion of mtDNA molecules within mitochondria contain the causal mutation (the degree of mtDNA heteroplasmy).

Epigenetic inheritance (including imprinting)

Several loci have been identified where gene repression is inherited in a parent of origin-specific manner; these are called imprinted loci. Within these loci the paternal alleles of a gene may be active while the maternal one may be silenced, or vice versa (see Fig. 3.7). Mutations within imprinted loci lead to a very unusual pattern of inheritance where the phenotype is only manifest if inherited from the parent who contributes the transcriptionally active allele (see Fig. 3.7). Examples of these disorders are listed in Box 3.3.

Classes of genetic variant

There are many different classes of variation in the human genome (Fig. 3.8). Rare genetic variations which result in a disease are generally referred to as mutations, whereas common variations and those which do not cause disease are referred to as polymorphisms. These different types of variation are further categorised by the size of the DNA segment involved and/or by the mechanism giving rise to the variation.

Nucleotide substitutions

The substitution of one nucleotide for another is the most common type of variation in the human genome. Depending on their frequency and functional consequences, these changes are known as a point mutation or a single nucleotide polymorphism (SNP). They occur by misincorporation of a nucleotide during DNA synthesis or by the action of a chemical mutagen. When these substitutions occur within ORFs of a protein-coding gene, they are further classified into:

- *synonymous* (resulting in a change in the codon but no change in the amino acid and thus no phenotype)
- *missense* (altering a codon, resulting in an amino acid change in the protein)
- *nonsense* (introducing a premature stop codon, resulting in truncation of the protein).

Single-base changes can also affect splicing of a gene if they occur at the junction of an intron or an exon, and those which adversely affect splicing are called splice site mutations.

Insertions and deletions

One or more nucleotides may be inserted or lost in a DNA sequence, resulting in an insertion/deletion (indel) polymorphism or mutation (see Fig. 3.8). If an indel change affects one or two nucleotides within the ORF of a protein-coding gene, this can have serious consequences because the triple nucleotide sequence of the codons is disrupted, resulting in a frameshift mutation. The effect upon the gene is typically severe because the amino acid sequence is totally disrupted.

3.3 Epigenetic disease

Disease	Locus and genes	Notes
Imprinting disorders		
Beckwith–Wiedemann syndrome	11p15 $p57^{KIP2}$ HASH2, INS2, IGF2, H19	General 'over-growth', advanced bone age and increased childhood tumours. Some cases due to mutations in $p57^{KIP2}$
Prader–Willi syndrome	15q11–q13 SNRPN, Necdin and others	Obesity, hypogonadism and learning disability. Lack of paternal contribution (due to deletion of paternal 15q11–q13, or inheritance of both chromosome 15q11–q13 regions from the mother)
Angelman's syndrome (AS)	15q11–q13 UBE3A	Severe mental retardation, ataxia, epilepsy and inappropriate laughing bouts. Due to loss-of-function mutations in the maternal UBE3A gene. The neurological phenotype results because most tissues express both maternal and paternal alleles of UBE3A, whereas the brain expresses predominantly the maternal allele
X-inactivation disorders		
Duchenne muscular dystrophy (DMD) in females	Xp22, DMD	If, by chance, a sufficient number of the X chromosomes containing the normal dystrophin gene are inactivated in muscle, heterozygous females may rarely develop full-blown DMD. Conversely, if a higher proportion of the disease gene-carrying chromosome is inactivated, a carrier female may test negative on biochemical screening for elevated creatine kinase levels
Epigenetic silencing (oncogenesis)		
Colon cancer	3p21 MLH1	Hypermethylation of the promoter results in silencing of MLH1, which encodes a DNA repair gene

Simple tandem repeat mutation

Variations in the length of simple tandem repeats of DNA are thought to arise as the result of slippage of DNA during meiosis and are termed microsatellite (small) or minisatellite (larger) repeats. These repeats are unstable and can expand or contract in different generations. This instability is related to the size of the original repeat, in that longer repeats tend to be more unstable. Many microsatellites and minisatellites occur in introns or in chromosomal regions between genes and have no obvious adverse effects. However, some genetic diseases, including Huntington disease and myotonic dystrophy, are caused by microsatellite repeats which result in duplication of amino acids within the affected gene product or affect gene expression (Box 3.4).

Copy number variations

Variation in the number of copies of an individual segment of the genome from the usual diploid (two copies) content can be categorised by the size of the segment involved. Rarely, individuals may gain or lose a whole chromosome. Such numerical chromosome anomalies most commonly occur by a process known as meiotic non-dysjunction (Box 3.5). This is the most common cause of Down's syndrome, known as trisomy (three copies) of chromosome 21.

Large insertions or deletions of chromosomal DNA also occur and are usually associated with learning disability and/or malformations. Such structural chromosomal anomalies arise as the result of two different processes:

- non-homologous end-joining
- non-allelic homologous recombination.

Random double-stranded breaks in DNA are a necessary process in meiotic recombination and also occur during mitosis at a predictable rate. The rate of these breaks is dramatically increased by exposure to ionising radiation. When such breaks occur, they are usually repaired accurately by DNA repair mechanisms within the cell. However, a proportion of breaks will undergo non-homologous end-joining, which results in the joining of two segments of DNA that are not normally contiguous. If the joined fragments are from different chromosomes, this results in a translocation. If they are from the same chromosome, this will result in either an inversion or a deletion (Fig. 3.9). Large insertions and deletions may be cytogenetically visible as chromosomal deletions or duplications. If the anomalies are too small to be detected by microscopy, they are termed microdeletions and microduplications. Many microdeletion syndromes have been described and most stem from non-allelic homologous recombination between locus-specific repeat of highly similar DNA sequences, which results in identical chromosome anomalies—and clinical syndromes—occurring in unrelated individuals (see Fig. 3.9 and Box 3.5).

Polymorphic copy number variants (CNVs)

It has recently been appreciated that, in addition to the disease-causing structural chromosomal anomalies mentioned above, there are also a considerable number of CNVs that exist as common genetic polymorphisms in humans. These involve duplication of large segments of the genome, often containing multiple genes and regulatory elements. These duplications usually result from non-allelic homologous recombination via misalignment of tandem repeated DNA elements in the chromosome during recombination (see Fig. 3.9). The consequences of CNV for genetic disease have not been fully explored, although recent studies have shown a strong association between an increased copy number of the gene FCGR3B and the risk of systemic lupus erythematosus.

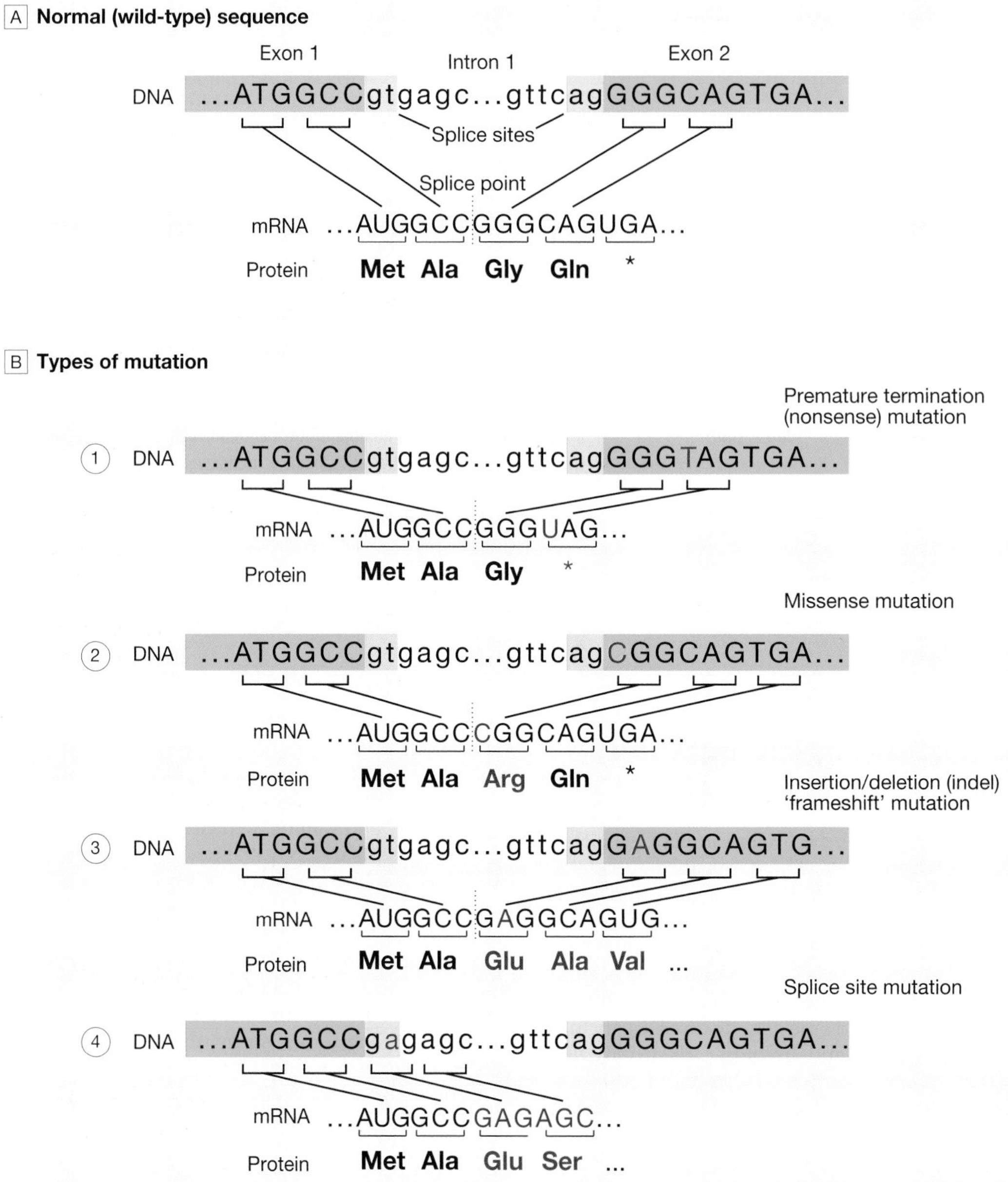

A **Normal (wild-type) sequence**

B **Types of mutation**

Fig. 3.8 Categories of mutation and summary of mutation types. A Normal genomic DNA spanning two exons and an intervening intron. Note that the 'coding strand' DNA sequence is shown; RNA is actually read from the complementary strand and, following splicing, the intron is removed, giving rise to the mRNA and protein sequence as shown (see also Fig. 3.1, p. 40). B Various examples of mutation are illustrated.

1. A nonsense mutation results in change from the normal sequence (CAG), encoding glutamine to a stop codon (TAG) which causes premature termination of the polypeptide chain; this would be expected to result in loss of protein function.
2. A missense mutation in exon 2 results in a change from the normal sequence encoding glycine (GGG) to (CGG) which encodes arginine. The change from a neutral amino acid to a charged residue would be expected to alter protein function.
3. An insertion of a single 'A' nucleotide in exon 2 causes a 'frameshift' mutation, resulting in disruption of the normal triple nucleotide sequence. The amino acids downstream of the insertion are completely different from those of the normal protein. This usually results in a loss of function mutation.
4. A splice site mutation which changes the second nucleotide of intron 1 from a 't' to an 'a' residue disrupts the normal 'gt' splice site donor motif, causing the RNA to 'read' through the intron and producing an abnormal protein. Splice site mutations often result in the production of mRNA molecules with a premature termination codon downstream of the mutation.

Consequences of genetic variation

Genetic variants can generally be classed into three groups:

- those with no detectable (neutral variants)
- those which cause loss of function
- those which cause a gain of function of the gene product.

The consequence of an individual mutation depends on many factors, including the mutation type, the nature of the gene product and the position of the variant in the protein. Mutations can have profound effects or subtle effects on gene and cell function (Box 3.6). Variations which have profound effects are responsible for 'classical' genetic diseases, whereas those with subtle effects

3.4 Diseases associated with triplet and other repeat sequences

		No. of repeats				
	Repeat	Normal	Mutant	Gene	Gene location	Inheritance
Coding repeat expansion						
Huntington disease	[CAG]	6–34	> 35	*Huntingtin*	4p16	AD
Spinocerebellar ataxia (type 1)	[CAG]	6–39	> 40	*Ataxin*	6p22–23	AD
Spinocerebellar ataxia (types 2, 3, 6, 7)	[CAG]	Various	Various	Various	Various	AD
Dentatorubral-pallidoluysian atrophy	[CAG]	7–25	> 49	*Atrophin*	12p12–13	AD
Machado–Joseph disease	[CAG]	12–40	> 67	*MJD*	14q32	AD
Spinobulbar muscular atrophy	[CAG]	11–34	> 40	Androgen receptor	Xq11–12	XL recessive
Non-coding repeat expansion						
Myotonic dystrophy	[CTG]	5–37	> 50	*DMPK-3′UTR*	19q13	AD
Friedreich's ataxia	[GAA]	7–22	> 200	*Frataxin-intronic*	9q13	AR
Progressive myoclonic epilepsy	[CCCCGCCCCGCG]$_{4-6}$	2–3	> 25	*Cystatin B-5′UTR*	21q	AR
Fragile X mental retardation	[CGG]	5–52	> 200	*FMR1-5′UTR*	Xq27	XL dominant
Fragile site mental retardation 2 (FRAXE)	[GCC]	6–35	> 200	*FMR2*	Xq28	XL, probably recessive

Note The triplet repeat diseases fall into two major groups: those with disease resulting from expansion of [CAG]$_n$ repeats in coding DNA, resulting in multiple adjacent glutamine residues (polyglutamine tracts), and those with non-coding repeats. The latter tend to be longer. Unaffected parents usually display 'pre-mutation' allele lengths that are just above the normal range.
(AD = autosomal dominant; AR = autosomal recessive; UTR = untranslated region; XL = X-linked)

3.5 Chromosome and contiguous gene disorders

Disease	Locus	Incidence	Clinical features
Numerical chromosomal abnormalities			
Down's syndrome (trisomy 21)	47,XY,+21 or 47,XX+21	1:800	Characteristic facies, IQ usually < 50, congenital heart disease, reduced life expectancy
Edwards' syndrome (trisomy 18)	47,XY,+18 or 47, XX,+18	1:6000	Early lethality, characteristic skull and facies, frequent malformations of heart, kidney and other organs
Patau's syndrome (trisomy 13)	47,XY, +13 or 47, XX,+13	1:15 000	Early lethality, cleft lip and palate, polydactyly, small head, frequent congenital heart disease
Klinefelter's syndrome	47,XXY	1:1000	Phenotypic male, infertility, gynaecomastia, small testes—p. 763
XYY	47,XYY	1:1000	Usually asymptomatic, some impulse control problems
Triple X syndrome	47,XXX	1:1000	Usually asymptomatic, may have reduced IQ
Turner's syndrome	45,X	1:5000	Phenotypic female, short stature, webbed neck, coarctation of the aorta, primary amenorrhoea—p. 761
Recurrent deletions, microdeletions and contiguous gene defects			
Di George/velocardiofacial syndrome	22q11.2	1 in 4000	Cardiac outflow tract defects, distinctive facial appearance, thymic hypoplasia, cleft palate and hypocalcaemia. Major gene seems to be *TBX1* (cardiac defects and cleft palate)
Prader–Willi syndrome	15q11–q13	1:15 000	Distinctive facial appearance, hyperphagia, small hands and feet, distinct behavioural phenotype. Imprinted region, deletions on paternal allele in 70% of cases
Angelman's syndrome	15q11–q13	1:15 000	Distinctive facial appearance, absent speech, EEG abnormality, characteristic gait. Imprinted region, deletions on maternal allele in *UBE3A*
Williams' syndrome	7q11.23	1:10 000	Distinctive facial appearance, supravalvular aortic stenosis, learning disability and infantile hypercalcaemia. Major gene for supravalvular aortic stenosis is *elastin*
Smith–Magenis syndrome	17p11.2	1 in 25 000	Distinctive facial appearance and behavioural phenotype, self-injury and rapid eye movement (REM) sleep abnormalities. Major gene seems to be *RAI1*

3

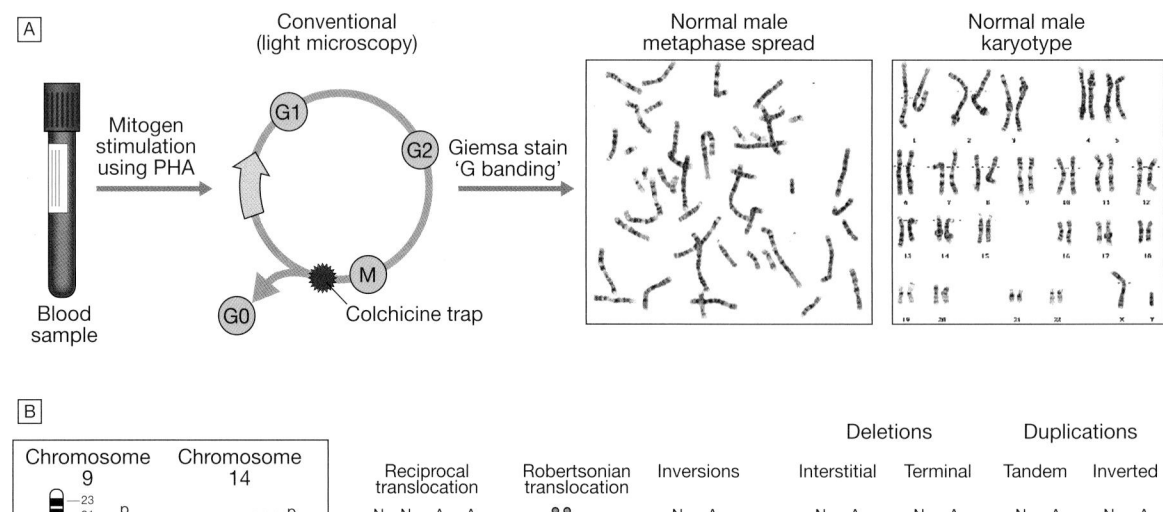

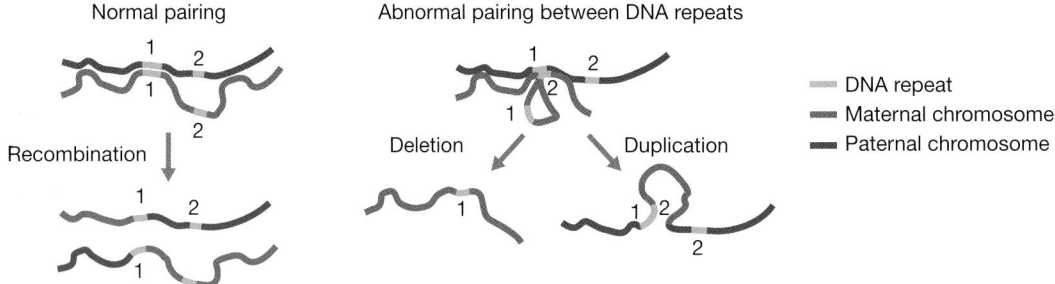

Fig. 3.9 Chromosomal analysis and structural chromosomal disorders. **A** How chromosome analysis is carried out. Starting with a blood sample, the white cells are stimulated to divide by adding the mitogen phytohaemagglutinin (PHA) and colchicine is used to trap the cells in metaphase, which allows the chromosomes to be seen using light microscopy following staining with Giemsa, resulting in a banding pattern. **B** How structural chromosomal anomalies are described. Human chromosomes can be classed as metacentric if the centromere is near the middle, or acrocentric if the centromere is at the end. The bands of each chromosome are given a number starting at the centromere and working out along the short (p) arm and long (q) arm. Translocations and inversions are balanced structural chromosome anomalies where no genetic material is missing but it is in the wrong order. Translocations can be divided into reciprocal (direct swap of chromosomal material between non-homologous chromosomes) and Robertsonian (fusion of acrocentric chromosomes). Deletions and duplications can also occur due to non-allelic homologous recombination (illustrated in panel C). Deletions are classified as interstitial if they lie within a chromosome and terminal if the terminal region of the chromosome is affected. Duplications can either be in tandem (where the duplicated fragment is orientated in the correct direction) or inverted (where the duplicated fragment is in the wrong direction). (N = normal; A = abnormal) **C** A common error of meiotic recombination, know as non-allelic homologous recombination, can occur (right panel) resulting in a deletion on one chromosome and a duplication in the homologous chromosome. The error is induced by tandem repeats in the DNA sequences (green) which can misalign and bind to each other, thereby 'fooling' the DNA into thinking the pairing prior to recombination is correct.

may contribute to the pathogenesis of complex diseases with a genetic component.

Loss-of-function (LOF) mutations

These mutations cause the normal function of a protein to be reduced or lost. Deletion of the whole gene is the most obvious example but the same phenotype is likely to be seen with a nonsense or frameshift mutation early in the ORF. Missense mutations that alter a critical domain within the protein can also result in LOF. In autosomal recessive diseases, mutations that result in no protein function whatsoever are known as null mutations. If LOF mutations result in an autosomal dominant disease,

the genetic mechanism is known as haplo-insufficiency and indicates that both functional copies of the gene are required for normal cellular function. Mutations in *PKD1* or *PKD2* which cause autosomal dominant adult polycystic kidney disease are mostly LOF.

Gain-of-function mutations

These are usually the result of missense mutations or, occasionally, triplet repeat expansion mutations. In this type of mutation the protein function is altered in a manner that results in a change in the original function of the gene. For example, heterozygous mutations (mutations on one allele in the presence of a wild-type allele) in *FBN1* cause Marfan's syndrome by the production of a protein with an abnormal amino acid sequence that disrupts the normal assembly of microfibrils. In comparison, complete loss of function of one allele of *FBN1* is usually completely benign. This is an example of how some missense mutations can be worse than 'null' mutations; this is called a 'dominant negative' effect. Constitutive activation of fibroblast growth factor receptors by missense mutation, which causes achondroplasia, is another example of such a mutation.

Polymorphisms

A polymorphism is defined as one that exists with a population frequency of > 1%. Most common polymorphisms are neutral (see below), but some cause subtle changes in gene expression or in protein structure and function (see Box 3.17, p. 65). It is thought that these polymorphisms lead to variations in phenotype within the general population, including variations in susceptibility to common diseases. An example is polymorphism in the gene *SLC2A9* that not only explains a significant proportion of the normal population variation in serum urate concentration but also predisposes 'high-risk' allele carriers to the development of gout. Other examples are listed in Box 3.6.

Neutral variants

The vast majority of variations within the human genome have no discernible effect on the cell or organism. This may be because the variation lies within an intron of a gene or a region of the genome which does not code for a gene or a regulatory element. Also, some variations within the coding regions of a gene do not change the amino acid, typically when the third base of a codon is affected. Some variations that do change the amino acid result in a conservative substitution, which does not change protein function appreciably.

Evolutionary selection

Genetic variants play an important role in evolutionary selection. Some variants can be advantageous to an organism, in which case they will be under positive selection through evolution via improved reproductive fitness. Conversely, other variations that decrease reproductive fitness become less common and are excluded through evolution. Given this simple paradigm, it would be tempting to assume that common mutations are all advantageous and all rare mutations

are pathogenic. Unfortunately, it is often difficult to classify any common mutation as either advantageous or deleterious—or indeed neutral. Mutations that are advantageous in early life and thus enhance reproductive fitness may be deleterious in later life. There may be mutations that are advantageous for survival in particular conditions (for example, famine or pandemic), which may be disadvantageous in more benign circumstances by resulting in a predisposition to obesity or autoimmune disorders. This complexity of balancing selection through evolution is likely to be an important feature of the genetics of common disease.

Constitutional genetic disease

All familial genetic disease is caused by constitutional mutations, which are inherited through the germ line. However, different mutations in the same gene can lead to different consequences, depending on the genetic mechanism underlying that disease. About 1% of the human population carries constitutional mutations that cause disease.

Allelic heterogeneity

Allelic heterogeneity is the term given to the phenomenon whereby several different mutations cause the same phenotype. In familial adenomatous polyposis coli, whole gene deletions, nonsense mutations, frameshift mutations and some missense mutations result in exactly the same phenotype because they all cause loss of function in the *FAP* gene on chromosome 5q. Many other Mendelian disorders show this phenomenon with loss-of-function mutations, including adult polycystic kidney disease (*PKD1*, 16p13; *PKD2*, 4q21). Allelic heterogeneity can also be seen in gain-of-function mutations. In connective tissue disorders, gain-of-function mutations are almost always missense mutations or in-frame deletions or insertions, since the protein has to be made for the disease to manifest. In other diseases, particularly those caused by gain-of-function mutations, allelic heterogeneity is severely restricted. A good example of this is achondroplasia, in which the mutations in *FGFR3* are restricted to a few specific codons which cause constitutive activation of the receptor that is required to cause the disease.

3.6 Examples of recessive diseases caused by common polymorphisms*

Disease	Inheritance	Gene	Genetic variant	Population frequency
Haemochromatosis	AR	*HFE*	p.Cys282Tyr (p.C282Y; nucleotide c.845G>A)	3%
			p.His63Asp (p.H63D; nucleotide c.187C>G)	5%
α₁-antitrypsin deficiency	AR	*SERPINA1*	p.Glu342Lys (p.E342K, c.1197G>A)	3%
Spinal muscular atrophy	AR	*SMN1*	Gene deletion by non-allelic homologous recombination	2–3%
Cystic fibrosis	AR	*CFTR*	p.Phe508del (p.F508del aka ΔF508, c.1521_1523delCTT)	4%

*The genetic variants shown are common in the general population but heterozygotes do not exhibit any evidence of disease. In the homozygous form, however, these variants cause recessive disease due to loss of function of the affected gene.

3

Locus heterogeneity

Locus heterogeneity is the term given to the phenomenon whereby a similar phenotype results from mutations in several different genes. One of the best examples is retinitis pigmentosa, which can occur as the result of mutations in more than 75 genes, each of which has a different chromosomal location.

De novo mutations

Although the vast majority of constitutional mutations are inherited, each gamete will contain mutations that have occurred as a result of meiosis; these are called de novo mutations. A certain number of de novo mutations in each generation are presumably required for evolution to occur. Such mutations also cause human disease. The best-known examples of de novo mutations cause severe congenital disorders such as thanatophoric dysplasia (*FGFR3* gain-of-function mutation), bilateral anophthalmia (*SOX2* haplo-insufficiency), campomelic dysplasia (*SOX9* loss of function) (see Fig. 3.2, p. 41) and the severe form of osteogenesis imperfecta (dominant negative mutations in *COL1A1* or *COL1A2*).

Somatic genetic disease

Somatic mutations are not inherited but instead occur following meiosis during development or adult life. An example of this phenomenon is polyostotic fibrous dysplasia, in which a somatic mutation in the G_s alpha protein causes constitutive activation of GPCR signalling, resulting in focal lesions in the skeleton and endocrine dysfunction (McCune–Albright syndrome, p. 768).

The most important example of human disease caused by somatic mutations is cancer. Here, mutations occur within genes that are involved in regulating cell division or apoptosis, resulting in abnormal cell growth and tumour formation. Two general types of cancer-causing mutation are recognised: gain-of-function mutations in growth-promoting genes (oncogenes) and loss-of-function mutations in growth-suppressing genes (tumour suppressor genes). Whatever the mechanism, most tumours seem to require an initiating mutation in a single cell that can then escape from normal growth controls. This cell replicates more frequently or fails to undergo programmed death and therefore forms a clone. As the clone of mutated cells expands, one or more cells may be subject to additional mutations which confer further growth advantage, leading to proliferation of these subclones, and ultimately to aggressive metastatic cancer. The cell's complex self-regulating machinery means that more than one mutation is usually required to produce a malignant tumour (see Fig. 11.2, p. 259). For example, if a cell mutates to produce a growth factor for which it already expresses the receptor (autocrine stimulation), that cell will replicate more frequently but will still be subject to cell cycle checkpoints to promote DNA integrity in its progeny. If an additional mutation occurs which overrides a cell cycle checkpoint, that cell and its progeny may go on to accumulate further mutations, some of which may allow it to replicate an unlimited number of times, or to separate from its matrix and cellular attachments without undergoing apoptosis. As deregulated growth continues, cancer cells become increasingly unable to differentiate, fail to respond to the normal local signals in their tissue of origin, and cease

to ensure appropriate chromosomal segregation pre-division, generating the classical malignant pathological appearances of disorganised growth, variable levels of differentiation, and gain of additional chromosomes (aneuploidy). Somatic mutations occur more frequently in response to external mutagens, such as those contained in cigarette smoke, or if the cell has defects in DNA repair systems. Cancer is thus a disease that affects the fundamental processes of molecular and cell biology.

In many familial cancer syndromes, somatic mutations interact with inherited mutations to cause a familial increase in the risk of specific cancer. A proportion of familial cancer syndromes are due to loss-of-function mutations in DNA repair enzymes. This increases the rate at which they accumulate somatic mutations, which predisposes to cancer. Autosomal recessive disorders that result in complete loss of specific DNA repair enzymes usually cause a severe multifaceted degenerative disorder with cancer susceptibility as a significant component (e.g. xeroderma pigmentosum, p. 63). Autosomal dominant mutations in genes encoding components of specific DNA repair systems are more common and cause some forms of familial colon cancer and breast cancer (e.g. *BRCA1*).

Other cancer syndromes are caused by loss-of-function mutations in tumour suppressor genes. At the cellular level, loss of one functional copy of a tumour suppressor gene does not have any immediate consequences, since the cell is protected by the remaining normal copy. However, there is a high chance of a somatic mutation developing in the normal allele at some point during life, which leads to tumour development due to complete loss of tumour suppressor activity in the affected cell. This is the so-called Knudsen two-hit hypothesis, which clinically explains why tumours may not develop for many years (or ever) in some members of these cancer-prone families. Yet another group of cancer syndromes are the result of gain-of-function mutations in tumour promoter genes (proto-oncogenes) (see Box 3.13, p. 63).

INVESTIGATION OF GENETIC DISEASE

General principles of diagnosis

Many genetic diseases can be diagnosed by a careful clinical history and examination and an awareness and knowledge of rare disease entities. Although DNA-based diagnostic tools are now widely used, it is important to be aware that not all diagnostic genetic tests involve analysis of DNA. For example, an electrocardiogram (ECG) can establish the diagnosis in long QT syndrome or a renal ultrasound can detect adult polycystic kidney disease. By definition, all genetic testing (whether it is DNA-based or not) has implications both for the patient and for other members of the family. These should be considered before genetic testing is undertaken and systems should be in place to deliver medical information and support to family members and to organise any relevant downstream investigations.

Constructing a family tree

The family tree—or pedigree—is fundamental to the diagnosis of genetic diseases. The basic symbols and nomenclature used in drawing a pedigree are shown in Figure 3.6 (p. 48). A three-generation family history taken in a routine medical clerking may reveal important genetic information of relevance to the presenting complaint, particularly relating to cancer.

A pedigree must include details from both sides of the family, any history of pregnancy loss or infant death, consanguinity, and details of all medical conditions in family members. Other significant information includes dates of birth and age at death.

It is important to be aware that a diagnosis given by a family member, or even obtained from a death certificate, may be wrong. This is often true in cases of cancer where 'stomach' may mean any part of the bowel, and 'brain' may refer to secondary deposits or be used where the primary site has not been identified.

Polymerase chain reaction (PCR) and DNA sequencing

PCR is a very widely used laboratory technique that amplifies targeted sections of the human genome for analysis. It is the most important technique in DNA diagnostic analysis. Almost any tissue can be used to extract DNA for PCR analysis, but most commonly, a sample of peripheral blood is used. The ability to determine the exact sequence of a fragment of DNA amplified by PCR is also of critical importance in DNA diagnostics. The most widely used DNA sequencing technique is illustrated in Figure 3.10. There are many other laboratory approaches for detecting individual mutations and polymorphisms but they almost all involve PCR at some stage.

Assessing DNA copy number

Visible microscopy of standard metaphase chromosome preparations has been the mainstay of clinical cytogenetic analysis for decades and is very useful for detecting the gain or loss of whole chromosomes or large chromosomal segments (> 4 million bp). Many clinically recognisable syndromes are the result of microdeletions. The specific phenotype associated with individual microdeletion syndromes is the result of loss of one copy of several adjacent genes—a contiguous gene syndrome (see Box 3.5, p. 53). Detection of submicroscopic chromosome anomalies requires special techniques for identification (see Box 3.5). Fluorescent in situ hybridisation (FISH, Fig. 3.11A) and multiplex ligation-dependent probe amplification (MLPA) are two of the most widely used techniques to identify such syndromes. However, the availability of whole-genome microarrays has revolutionised chromosome analysis, as it allows the rapid detection of gain or loss of any segment of DNA throughout the genome (see Box 3.5). These microarrays consist of millions of short sequences of DNA (probes) that are complementary to known sequences in the genome (Fig. 3.11B). Each probe is fixed at a known position on the array (often printed on to a specially coated glass slide). The patient's sample is hybridised to the array, and positive and negative results for each probe are read using a laser scanner that detects fluorescent 'labels' inserted in the DNA. This allows a map of the patient's DNA to be constructed from just one test and missing sequences to be identified.

Non-DNA-based methods of assessment

Although DNA-based diagnostic tools are used in the vast majority of patients with suspected genetic disease, it may sometimes be more economical or convenient to measure enzyme activity rather than sequencing the coding region of the genes involved. An example of this is the investigation of myopathy thought to be due to defects in mitochondrial complex 1 proteins (Box 3.7). Complex 1 is made up of at least 36 nuclear-encoded and 7 mitochondrial DNA-encoded subunits, and mutations in any of these subunits can cause the disorder, which makes sequence analysis impractical as a first-line clinical test. Conversely, the biochemical measurement of respiratory chain complex I proteins can easily be analysed in muscle biopsies, and this can be diagnostic of a specific mitochondrial cytopathy (see Fig. 3.3, p. 43, and Box 3.1, p. 44).

Genetic testing in pregnancy

Genetic testing may be performed during pregnancy. Invasive tests, such as amniocentesis and chorionic villus sampling, are most often performed to diagnose conditions that result in early infant death or severe disability. Such tests are only offered after careful explanation of the risks involved. Many couples will use the result of such tests to decide about termination of pregnancy. Some indications for testing are listed in Box 3.8; the methods used are summarised in Boxes 3.9 and 3.10. Non-invasive ultrasound scanning is usually offered to all pregnant couples and is particularly important if there is a previous history of serious developmental abnormalities. As the range of tests for genetic diseases increases, demand for prenatal testing is likely to rise. A considerable ethical debate is taking place about the types of disease for which prenatal testing is appropriate.

Genetic testing in children

Ethical issues often arise with regard to genetic testing of children. In childhood-onset conditions for which proven treatments are available or screening is appropriate, it is clearly important to test a child: for example, neonatal testing for cystic fibrosis, when early therapy reduces disease progression (p. 678), or testing a child at risk of developing multiple endocrine neoplasia type 2B (MEN2B), when early thyroidectomy prevents medullary thyroid carcinoma (p. 793). However, testing a healthy child for an adult-onset disorder where no benefit from early intervention exists should be avoided. Instead, the child should be left to make his or her own informed decision as an adult.

Identifying a disease gene in families

For diseases which have a significant genetic contribution but are of unknown cause, the process of attributing an inherited disease to a specific gene typically begins with investigation of the affected family or families. DNA polymorphisms identified in normal populations (p. 51) can be used to track or 'map' disease genes by a technique called genome-wide linkage analysis. There are now techniques that allow > 500 000 SNPs to be typed in a single experiment, and comparison of the segregation of patterns of contiguous SNPs (called haplotypes) in affected and unaffected individuals allows identification

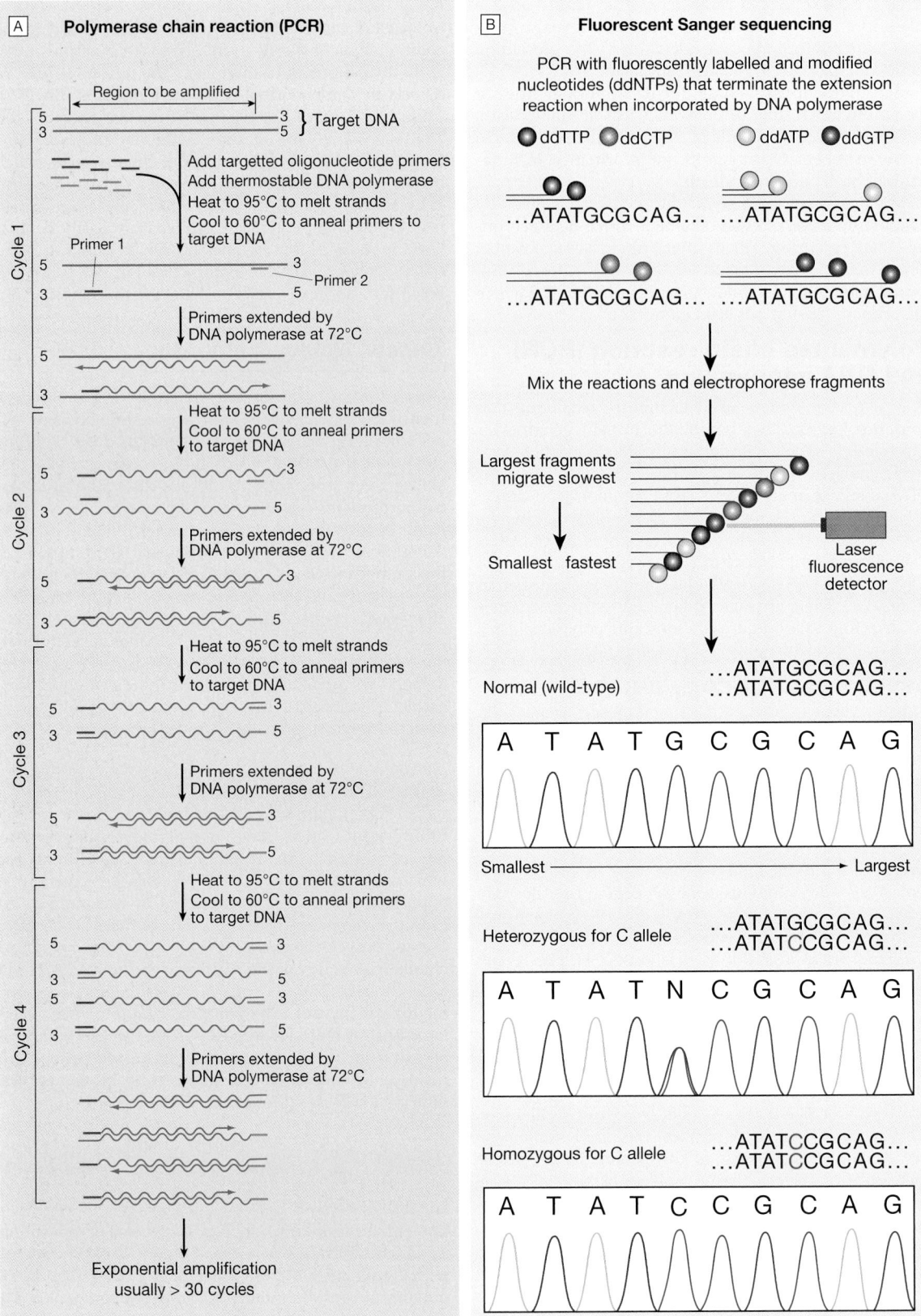

Fig. 3.10 The polymerase chain reaction (PCR) and sequencing. **A** A summary of the steps involved in PCR, which amplifies targeted segments of DNA. **B** Sanger sequencing of DNA, very widely used—together with PCR—in DNA diagnostics.

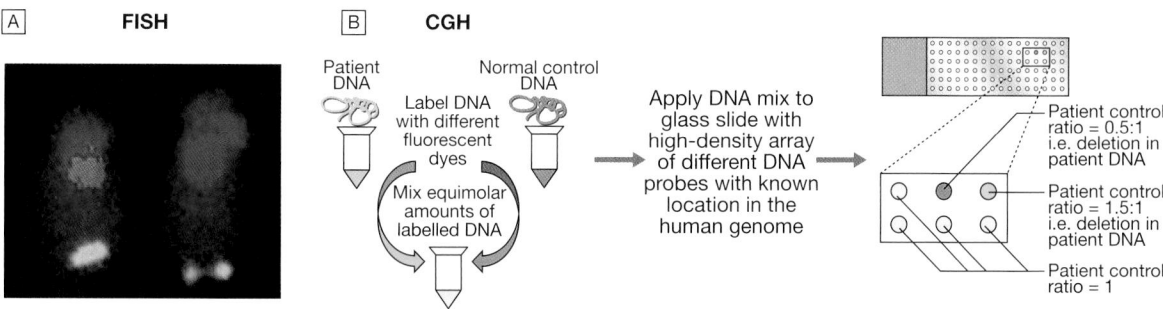

| A | FISH | B | CGH |

Fig. 3.11 Detection of chromosomal abnormalities by FISH and CGH. [A] An example of FISH analysis showing a pair of homologous metaphase chromosome 22 stained with a blue fluorescent dye. The green spots represent a telomeric probe that has hybridised to both sister chromatids (there are two spots on the right-hand chromosome, whereas on the left the two spots are overlapping). The pink spot shows hybridisation of a probe mapping to band 22q11.2. The left chromosome has a normal signal that is absent on the right. This represents the microdeletion associated with velo-cardio-facial syndrome on the chromosome on the right. [B] Overview of comparative genomic hybridisation (CGH). Deletions and duplications are detected by looking for deviation from the 1:1 ratio of patient and control DNA in a microarray. Ratios in excess of 1 indicate duplications, whereas ratios below 1 indicate deletions.

3

3.7 Examples of non-DNA-based investigations for common genetic diseases

Disease	Investigation	Page reference
Haemoglobinopathy e.g. sickle-cell disease	Haemoglobin electrophoresis	1027
Coagulation disorders e.g. haemophilia	Clotting factor levels	1046
Immune deficiencies e.g. hypogammaglobulinaemia	Ig levels, complement levels	76
Inborn errors of metabolism e.g. phenylketonuria	Enzyme assays, amino acid levels	447
Endocrine disease e.g. congenital adrenal hyperplasia	Hormone levels, enzyme assays	780
Renal disease e.g. autosomal dominant polycystic kidney disease	Radiology, renal biopsy	506
Myopathy e.g. mitochondrial myopathy	Muscle biopsy, enzyme assay	1234
Skeletal dysplasias e.g. osteogenesis imperfecta	Radiology	1126

3.8 Some indications for prenatal testing

- Advanced maternal age and a high-risk serum screening result
- A previous child with a detectable chromosome abnormality or a parent with a chromosome abnormality such as a balanced translocation
- A parent or child with a genetic disease for which testing is available
- Abnormal antenatal scan

3.9 Methods used in prenatal testing

Test	Gestation	Comments
Ultrasound	1st trimester onwards	Increased nuchal translucency (an oedematous flap of skin at the base of the neck) for trisomies and Turner's; all major abnormalities such as NTD, congenital heart disease
Chorionic villus biopsy	From 11 weeks	2% risk of miscarriage; used for early chromosomal, DNA and biochemical analysis; a specialised test
Amniocentesis	From 14 weeks	< 1% risk of miscarriage; used for chromosomal and some biochemical analysis, e.g. α-fetoprotein for NTD
Cordocentesis	From 19 weeks	2–3% risk of miscarriage; a highly specialised test; used for chromosomal and DNA analysis

(NTD = neural tube defect)

of the 'locus' of DNA where the responsible gene resides. The confidence of association ('linkage') with the disease in question is influenced by the number of subjects studied, the strength of the effect of the gene on the disease, and the closeness of the SNP to the gene in question. The confidence can be expressed as a LoD (logarithm of the odds) score, which is $-\log_{10}$ of the probability (p value) of linkage; by convention a LoD score of > 3 (p < 0.001) is taken to be statistically significant. Once a locus has been identified, more detailed mapping within the locus can be undertaken and the relevant mutation confirmed by sequencing the relevant gene.

EBM 3.10 **Screening for Down's syndrome**

'Antenatal screening in the first and second trimesters identifies fetuses at risk of Down's syndrome. Tests which currently have sensitivity > 60% and specificity > 95% include:
- *First trimester* (11–14 weeks): nuchal translucency; or nuchal translucency, human chorionic gonadotrophin (hCG) and pregnancy-associated plasma protein-A (PAPP-A)
- *Second trimester* (13–20 weeks): triple test (hCG, α-fetoprotein, unconjugated oestriol, uE3)
- Other combinations are available for use from 11–20 weeks.'

For further information: www.nice.org.uk

Genetic investigation in populations

Genetic screening may be applied to whole populations. The criteria for the use of population screening are well established; they depend on the incidence of specific conditions in individual populations and on whether an intervention is available to ameliorate the effects of the disease. In the UK, examples include screening for phenylketonuria and cystic fibrosis in the newborn, and prenatal screening for neural tube defects and Down's syndrome in pregnant women (see Box 3.10). Screening for carriers of haemoglobinopathies and Tay–Sachs disease is also carried out in some countries where the incidence of these conditions may be high enough to merit screening the entire population (p. 1027).

Predictive genetic testing

In the absence of symptoms or signs of disease in an individual at risk, a genetic test can be used to determine whether that individual carries the disease-causing mutation. This is known as presymptomatic or predictive genetic testing. Predictive tests are usually carried out for adult-onset disorders such as familial cancer syndromes (see Box 3.13) and neurodegenerative disorders such as Huntington's disease (Box 3.11), or when a positive result in children will affect screening and management, such as in familial polyposis coli (pp. 63 and 908). However, many complicated ethical issues arise with testing of children and such tests should only be carried out by clinicians experienced in their use.

Whilst a negative predictive test is clearly a favourable outcome for the individual concerned, a positive test may

3.11 Predictive testing for Huntington disease

- Currently, no medical benefit can be derived from knowing presymptomatic genetic status. In this situation, predictive testing is not offered to children but is available to capable adults
- Individuals have several reasonably spaced appointments with a genetic counsellor (or medical geneticist or specialist psychiatrist) prior to testing to ensure the implications of testing are fully understood
- Fully informed patient consent is required prior to testing and individuals must be free to withdraw from testing at any time
- Follow-up support must be available and the result must not be disclosed to any other person without written consent of the tested individual

have significant negative consequences. These should have been explained fully in the counselling process (see below), and include employment discrimination and psychological effects. Providing this is done, current evidence suggests that serious psychological sequelae are uncommon.

PRESENTING PROBLEMS IN GENETIC DISEASE

There are many thousands of known single-gene diseases. Individually, these are rare, but collectively they are relatively common. This diversity makes clinical genetics a fascinating clinical specialty (Box 3.12) but it does mean

i 3.12 **Common monogenic disorders affecting major organ systems**

System	Disease	Inheritance
Multisystem	Neurofibromatosis	AD
	Tuberous sclerosis	AD
Respiratory	α₁-antitrypsin deficiency	AR
	Cystic fibrosis	AR
Cardiovascular	Hypertrophic cardiomyopathy	AD
	Long QT syndromes	AD and AR
Renal	Polycystic kidney disease	AD
	Alport's syndrome	XLR
Gastrointestinal	Hereditary pancreatitis	AD
	Familial adenomatous polyposis coli	AD
Hepatic	Gilbert's disease	AD
	Haemochromatosis	AR
	Wilson's disease	AR
Metabolic	Phenylketonuria	AR
	Familial hypercholesterolaemia	AD
	Hypophosphataemic rickets	XLD, AD
Endocrine	Congenital adrenal hyperplasia	AR
	Multiple endocrine neoplasia	AD
	Kallmann's syndrome	XLR or AD
Haematological	Sickle-cell disease	AR
	Alpha- and beta-thalassaemia	AR
	Haemophilia A and B	XLR
Neuromuscular	Duchenne muscular dystrophy	XLR
	Myotonic dystrophy	AD
	Spinal muscular atrophy	AR
CNS	Huntington's disease	AD
	Familial Alzheimer's disease	AD
	Friedreich's ataxia	AR
Musculoskeletal	Ehlers–Danlos syndrome	AD
	Marfan's syndrome	AD
	Osteogenesis imperfecta	AD and AR
Skin	Albinism	AR
	Neurofibromatosis	AD
	Xeroderma pigmentosum	AR
Eye	Retinitis pigmentosa	AR, AD, XLR
	Ocular albinism	XLR

(AD = autosomal dominant; AR = autosomal recessive; XLD = X-linked dominant; XLR = X-linked recessive)

that it is difficult, if not impossible, for any individual clinician to memorise the features associated with all these disorders. It is therefore important to have an awareness of the existence of genetic diseases and some general rules or 'triggers' in mind. Although single-gene disorders can present at any age (see Box 13.15) and affect any tissue or organ system, they share some general characteristics:

- positive family history
- early age of onset
- multisystem involvement
- no obvious non-genetic explanation.

It is important to recognise any unusual clinical presentation and to consider genetic disease in the context of the clinical findings and the family history. Publicly accessible online catalogues of Mendelian diseases can be useful sources of potential diagnoses.

MAJOR CATEGORIES OF GENETIC DISEASE

It would clearly be impossible to discuss all genetic diseases in this chapter. However, the major categories of genetic disease that are commonly encountered by clinical geneticists in adult practice are discussed below.

Inborn errors of metabolism

Inborn errors of metabolism (IEM) are caused by mutations that disrupt the normal function of a biochemical pathway. Most IEM are due to autosomal or X-linked recessive loss-of-function mutations in genes encoding specific enzymes or enzymatic co-factors. Knowledge of the biochemical pathway involved means that specific blocks have predictable consequences, including deficiency of the end product and build-up of intermediary compounds. Many hundreds of different IEM have been identified and these disorders have contributed a great deal to our understanding of human biochemistry. Most IEM are very rare and some are restricted to paediatric practice; however, a growing number may now present during adult life and some of these are discussed below.

Intoxicating IEM

A subgroup of IEM, termed 'intoxicating IEM', can present as a sudden deterioration in a previously well individual. Such deteriorations are usually precipitated by some form of stress, such as infection, pregnancy, exercise or changes in diet. The intoxication is due to the build-up of intermediary, water-soluble compounds, which will vary according to the pathway involved. For example, in urea cycle disorders ammonia is the toxic substance, but in maple syrup urine disease it is branch-chain amino acids. The intoxication is often associated with derangement of the acid–base balance and, if not recognised and treated, will often proceed to multi-organ failure, coma and death. The diagnosis of these disorders requires specialist biochemical analysis of blood and/or urine. Treatment relies on removal of the toxic substance using haemodialysis or chemical conjugation, and prevention of further accumulation by restricting intake of the precursors: total protein restriction in urea cycle disorders and branch-chain amino acid intake in maple syrup urine disease.

Mitochondrial disorders

Disorders of energy production are the most common type of IEM presenting in adult life and some of these disorders have been mentioned in the section on mitochondrial function (see Fig. 3.3, p. 43, and Box 3.1, p. 44). The tissues that are most commonly affected in this group of disorders are those with the highest metabolic energy requirements, such as muscle, heart, retina and brain. Therapy in this group of disorders is based on giving antioxidants and co-factors such as vitamin C and ubiquinone that can improve the function of the respiratory chain.

Storage disorders

Storage disorders are most commonly caused by loss-of-function mutations affecting enzymes involved in lysosomal degradation pathways. The clinical consequences depend on the specific enzyme involved. For example, Fabry disease, an X-linked recessive deficiency of alpha-galactosidase A, results in abdominal pain, episodic diarrhoea, renal failure and angiokeratoma. Niemann–Pick disease type C is caused by autosomal recessive loss-of-function mutations in either the *NPC1* or *NPC2* gene. This results in hepatosplenomegaly, dysphagia, loss of speech, very early dementia, spasticity and dystonia. An increasing number of storage disorders are treatable with enzyme replacement therapy, making awareness and diagnosis more important.

Neurological disorders

Progressive neurological deterioration is one of the most common presentations of adult genetic disease. These diseases are mostly autosomal dominant and can be grouped into specific neurological syndromes and early-onset forms of well-known non-Mendelian clinical entities. In the latter group the best examples would be early-onset familial forms of dementia, Parkinson's disease and motor neuron disease. The triplet repeat disorders cause an interesting group of syndromes and have specific features that are dealt with below.

Huntington disease

Huntington disease (HD) is the paradigm of triplet repeat disorders. This condition can present with a movement disorder, weight loss or psychiatric symptoms (depression, addiction, psychosis, dementia), or with a combination of all three. The disease is the result of a [CAG]$_n$ triplet repeat expansion mutation in the *HD* gene on chromosome 4. Since CAG is a codon for glutamine and this mutation is positioned in the ORF, this results in an expansion of a polyglutamine tract in the protein. The mutation probably leads to gain of function, as deletions of the gene do not cause HD. The function of the protein encoded by the *HD* gene is not fully understood, but expansion of the repeat to above the normal range of 3–35 results in neurological disease. In general, the severity of disease and age at onset are related to the repeat length. In HD, atrophy of the caudate nuclei and the putamen is obvious on magnetic resonance imaging (MRI) of the brain, and in later stages cerebral atrophy is also apparent. There is currently no therapy that will alter the progression of the disease, which will often be the cause of the patient's death. Within families there is a tendency for disease severity to increase and age at onset to fall due to further expansion of the repeat, a phenomenon known as anticipation. The mutation is more likely to expand through the male germ line than through female meiosis.

Other triplet repeat disorders

Other progressive neurological disorders caused by triplet repeat expansion mutations in different genes include several forms of autosomal dominant spinocerebellar ataxias, dentatorubral-pallidoluysian atrophy (DRPLA), Machado–Joseph disease, Kennedy disease and myotonic dystrophy. One common feature of the neuropathology of the polyglutamine disorder is the presence of intracellular inclusions in affected cells. It is thought that this accumulation may, in itself, be deleterious and is the result of defective protein degradation.

Connective tissue disorders

Mutations in different types of collagen, fibrillin and elastin make up the majority of connective tissue disorders. The clinical features of these disorders vary, depending on the structural function and tissue distribution of the protein which is mutated. For example, autosomal dominant loss-of-function mutations in the gene encoding elastin cause either supravalvular aortic stenosis, cutis laxa or a combination of both conditions. The most commonly involved systems are:

- *skin* (increased or decreased elasticity, poor wound healing)
- *eyes* (myopia, lens dislocation)
- *blood* vessels (vascular fragility)
- *bones* (osteoporosis, skeletal dysplasia)
- *joints* (hypermobility, dislocation, arthropathy).

Learning disability, dysmorphism and malformations

Congenital global cognitive impairment (also called mental handicap or learning disability) affects about 3% of the population. It is commonly divided into broad categories of mild to moderate (IQ 50–70), moderate to severe (IQ 20–50) and severe to profound (IQ < 20). There are important 'environmental' causes of global cognitive impairment, including:

- *teratogen exposure* during pregnancy (alcohol, anticonvulsants)
- *congenital infections* (cytomegalovirus, rubella, toxoplasmosis, syphilis)
- *the sequelae of prematurity* (intraventricular haemorrhage)
- *birth injury* (hypoxic ischaemic encephalopathy).

However, genetic disorders contribute very significantly to the aetiology of global cognitive impairment. Given the complexity of brain development, it is not surprising that global cognitive impairment shows extreme locus heterogeneity. The three most important groups of disorder are reviewed below.

Chromosome disorders

Any significant gain or loss of autosomal chromosomal material (known as aneuploidy) usually results in learning disability and other phenotypic abnormalities (see Fig. 3.9, p. 54). Down's syndrome is the most frequently found and best known of these disorders, and is caused by an increased dosage of genes on chromosome 21. Most cases of Down's syndrome are due to a numerical chromosome abnormality with trisomy of chromosome 21, e.g. 47,XX,+21 or 47,XY,+21. The clinical features are:

- globally delayed development
- short stature
- a significant risk of specific malformations (atrioventricular septal defect, duodenal atresia)
- a predisposition to several late-onset disorders, including hypothyroidism, acute leukaemias and Alzheimer's disease.

Recent surveys have shown that DNA microarray analysis can identify causative structural chromosome abnormalities in 10–25% of cases of significant learning disability. These deletions and duplications are mostly de novo and unique. An interest group of recurrent deletions and duplication due to non-allelic homologous recombination events has been mentioned above. These result in specific microdeletion or microduplication syndromes, such as:

- *velocardiofacial syndrome* due to deletion of 22q11.2 (learning disability, malformations of the cardiac outflow tract, cleft palate, distinctive facial appearance and immune disorders)
- *Williams' syndrome* due to deletion of 7q11.23 (learning disability, supravalvular aortic stenosis and mild cutis laxa as a result of deletion of the *elastin* gene, distinctive facial appearance and over-friendly, chatty personality).

Dysmorphic syndromes

There are several thousand different dysmorphic syndromes; all are rare but they are characterised by the occurrence of cognitive impairment, malformations and a distinctive facial appearance—or 'gestalt'—associated with various other clinical features. Making the correct diagnosis is important, as it has profound implications on immediate patient management, detection of future complications and assessment of recurrence risks in the family. Clinical examination remains the mainstay of diagnosis and the patient often needs to be evaluated by a clinician who specialises in the diagnosis of these syndromes. The differential diagnosis in dysmorphic syndromes is often very wide and this has resulted in computer-aided diagnosis becoming an established clinical tool. Dysmorphology databases have been established that are curated catalogues of the many thousands of known syndrome entities which can be searched to identify possible explanations of unusual combinations of clinical features. The clinical diagnosis may then be confirmed by specific genetic investigations, as the genetic basis of a wide range of dysmorphic syndromes has been identified.

X-linked mental handicap

X-linked mental handicap (XLMH) accounts for approximately 10% of cases of moderate to severe learning disability. There are over one hundred genes on the X chromosome that can cause learning disability but the most common disorder is fragile X syndrome, characterised by a distinctive facial appearance, attention deficit, joint hypermobility, macro-orchism (increased testicular size) and a non-staining gap on the X chromosome on chromosome analysis. Fragile X is caused by a triplet repeat expansion mutation but of a different type from the polyglutamine repeat disorders mentioned above. The repeat in fragile X syndrome is not in the coding region and is a $[CGG]_n$ expansion (see Box 3.4, p. 53). Methylation of the expanded repeat results in silencing of a specific gene called *FMR1*, which encodes an RNA-binding protein.

Familial cancer syndromes

Most cancers are not inherited but occur as the result of an accumulation of somatic mutations, as discussed previously in this chapter. However, it has been recognised for many decades that some families are prone to one or more specific types of cancer (Box 3.13). Affected individuals tend to present with tumours at an early age and are more likely to have multiple primary foci of carcinogenesis.

Retinoblastoma

Patients with autosomal dominant familial retinoblastoma have an inherited mutation in one copy of the *RB* gene, which is a tumour suppressor. This strongly predisposes individuals to the formation of retinoblastoma in one or both eyes. It is possible for more than one primary tumour to form in the same eye and for retinoblastoma to occur in the pineal gland. From a clinical perspective, it is important to screen the eyes and pineal gland of such individuals regularly so that tumours can be treated early and sight preserved. This gene is widely expressed and it is not clear why the retina is the main site of oncogenesis in this syndrome. It is clear that the bone is also sensitive, as there is an increased incidence of osteogenic sarcoma in affected individuals.

Familial adenomatous polyposis coli

Familial adenomatous polyposis coli (FAP) is an autosomal dominant condition due to inactivation mutations in the *FAP* tumour suppressor gene on 5q. The gene product is thought to modulate a specific signalling cascade (Wnt signalling) that regulates cell proliferation.

Mutation carriers usually develop many thousands of intestinal polyps in their second and third decades and have a very high risk of malignant change in the colon. Prophylactic colectomy in the third decade is necessary in most cases. Regular screening for polyps in the upper gastrointestinal tract is also recommended.

Li–Fraumeni syndrome

Heterozygous loss-of-function mutations in the gene encoding p53 cause Li–Fraumeni syndrome. Families with this condition have a very significant increased predisposition to early-onset leukaemias, sarcomas, and breast and brain malignancies. Screening for pre-symptomatic tumours in this condition is very difficult and of unproven benefit, as almost any tissue can be affected.

Hereditary non-polyposis colorectal cancer

Hereditary non-polyposis colorectal cancer (HNPCC) is an autosomal dominant disorder that presents with early-onset familial colon cancer, particularly affecting the proximal colon. Other cancers, such as endometrial cancer, are often observed in affected families. This disorder shows marked locus heterogeneity, as mutations can occur in several different genes encoding proteins involved in DNA mismatch repair.

Familial breast cancer

Familial breast cancer is an autosomal dominant disorder that is most often due to mutations in genes encoding either *BRCA1* or *BRCA2*. Both these proteins are involved in DNA repair. Individuals who carry a *BRCA1* or *BRCA2* mutation are at high risk of early-onset breast and ovarian tumours, and require regular screening for both these conditions. Many affected women will opt for prophylactic bilateral mastectomy and oophorectomy.

Xeroderma pigmentosum

Xeroderma pigmentosum (XP) is the name given to a group of rare disorders in which there are autosomal recessive defects in DNA repair genes which deal primarily with the effects of non-ionising radiation. The skin is particularly involved, and affected patients develop skin cancers with increased frequency.

3.13 Examples of familial cancer syndromes

Disease	Inheritance	Gene	Tumour(s)	Page reference
Retinoblastoma	AD	*RB1*	Retinoblastoma, osteosarcoma	–
Familial breast/ovarian cancer	AD	*BRCA1* and *BRCA2*	Breast, ovary	Ch. 11
Hereditary non-polyposis colorectal cancer (HNPCC)	AD	*hMSH2, hMLH1, hPMS1, hPMS2*	Colorectal, endometrial, stomach, breast, urinary tract	910
Von Hippel–Lindau disease	AD	*VHL*	CNS haemangioblastoma, renal, pancreas, phaeochromocytoma	1219
Peutz–Jeghers syndrome	AD	*STK11*	Gastrointestinal, endometrial, breast, ovary	909
Li–Fraumeni syndrome	AD	*p53*	Sarcoma, brain, breast, leukaemia, adrenal	–

3

Werner's syndrome

Werner's syndrome is a form of premature ageing (progeria), caused by mutation of one of a series of DNA repair enzymes; it presents with premature skin ageing, degenerative disorders and cancer.

GENETIC COUNSELLING

Genetic counselling is the process of providing information about the medical and family implications of a specific disease in a clear and non-directive manner. Such counselling aims to help individuals make informed decisions about planning a family, taking part in screening programmes and accepting prophylactic therapies. Genetic counselling may be provided by a medical geneticist, a specialist nurse, or a clinician with particular skills in this area, such as an obstetrician or paediatrician (Box 3.14). Perception of genetic risks clearly depends on perceived hazard. For example, a 5% (or 1:20) risk of genetic disease may be perceived as low if the disease is treatable, but unacceptably high if not.

Specific problems encountered in genetic counselling include:

- accurate assessment of genetic risk
- identification of children at risk of genetic disorders
- the increase in genetic risks associated with consanguinity
- non-paternity as an incidental finding in DNA diagnostic tests.

3.14 Clinical genetics services

Component	Role
Medical geneticist	Diagnosis and management of genetic disease, assessment of genetic risk, managing screening programmes, interpretation of genetic test results. Subspecialties include prenatal genetics, dysmorphology (syndrome identification), cancer genetics
Genetic counsellor	Assessing genetic risk, provision of genetic counselling (providing accurate risk information in a comprehensible format), predictive testing for genetic disease and provision of information and support
DNA diagnostic laboratory	Identifying and reporting disease-causing mutations in validated disease genes. Some laboratories also provide linkage analysis to track diseases in families. Laboratories often work in a consortium, as so many different disease genes have now been identified
Cytogenetics laboratory	Identifying pathogenic numerical and structural chromosome anomalies in prenatal, postnatal and oncology samples
Biochemical genetics laboratory	Metabolite and enzymatic-based diagnosis of IEM. Metabolite-based monitoring of treatment of IEM
Newborn screening laboratory	Provision of population-based newborn screening, e.g. PKU, cystic fibrosis, etc.

(IEM = inborn errors of metabolism; PKU = phenylketonuria)

3.15 Genetic disease and counselling in old age

- **Genetic disease**: may present for the first time in elderly patients, e.g. Huntington's disease.
- **Family investigation**: remains essential in the management of genetic disease presenting in old age and referral to clinical genetics services should be considered.

Genetic tests are increasingly used for the diagnosis and prediction of Mendelian disease in a medical context, and such skills will become increasingly important for many clinicians.

Genetic risk is often calculated using Bayes' theorem, which takes prior risk into account to calculate future risk. A simple Bayesian calculation is illustrated here. Consider a woman who is at risk of being a carrier of an X-linked recessive disease. Her grandfather and brother are affected, which makes her mother an obligate gene carrier. Her risk of being a carrier is therefore 50%. However, she has two unaffected sons. This information can be used to modify her risk. The prior probability that she is a carrier is 1/2 and that she is not a carrier also 1/2. The conditional probability that she would have two normal sons if she were a carrier is 1/2 × 1/2 = 1/4. If she were not a carrier, the probability of having normal sons is 1. From this, the joint probability for each outcome can be calculated (the prior risk × the conditional risk). This is 1/2 × 1/4 = 1/8 for being a carrier and 1/2 × 1 = 1/2 for not being a carrier. The final risk, or relative probability, for each outcome can then be obtained by dividing the joint probability for that outcome by the sum of the joint probabilities. Therefore, in this instance, probability that she is a carrier is 1/8/(1/8 + 1/2) = 1/5 (20%).

GENETICS OF COMMON DISEASES

Many common disorders, such as diabetes, atherosclerosis, hypertension, cancer, osteoarthritis, inflammatory bowel disease and osteoporosis, have an important genetic component but are not caused by a single mutation. Techniques are now available both to measure the contribution and to identify genes with significant effects. This means that the result of genetic testing is beginning to have an impact on diagnosis, prognosis and therapy for common diseases, and this trend is likely to expand significantly in the years to come. Some of the most useful approaches to clinical interpretation of the genetic aspects of common disorders are outlined below.

Measuring the genetic contribution to complex disease

Genetic contributions to complex disease can be detected and quantified by twin studies and/or by analysing familial clustering. Twin studies use the difference in disease concordance between monozygotic (MZ) and dizygotic (DZ) twins to calculate genetic contribution. MZ twins are genetically identical, whereas DZ twins, like all siblings, are identical for only about 50% of their genetic variation. However, both MZ and DZ twins

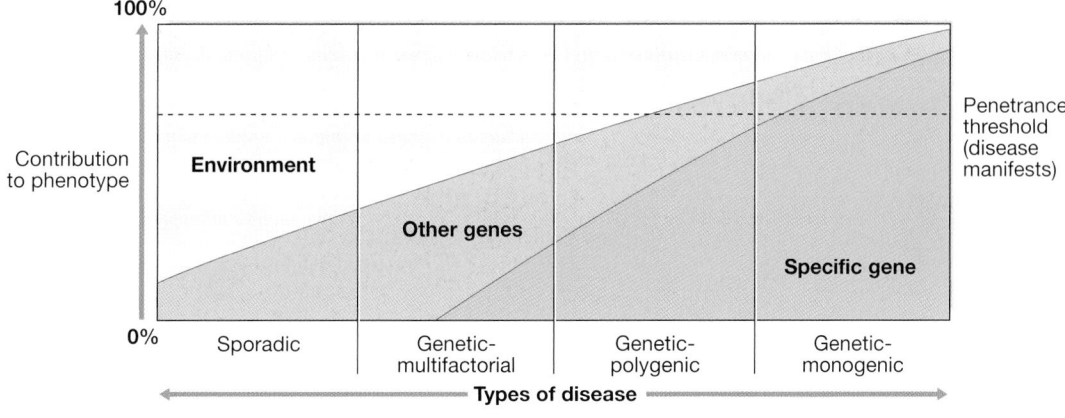

Fig. 3.12 The spectrum of genetic disease: how the genotype influences the phenotype. A particular characteristic or disease in an individual may be due to a specific genetic abnormality (monogenic disease), or may reflect several predisposing genes (polygenic disease). In each case, environmental factors may further influence the phenotype; in their absence, genetic factors alone may be insufficient to allow the disease to develop, resulting in non-penetrance (see text).

share a similar intrauterine environment and similar postnatal environment. Thus, any evidence of a higher concordance of the disease in MZ compared to DZ twins is assumed to be evidence of genetic contribution. Many common diseases and quantitative traits, such as height, weight, blood pressure and bone mineral density, show higher concordance rates in MZ twins compared to DZ twins. Genetic contributions to common diseases can also be assessed by studying the incidence of the disease in first-degree relatives of affected individuals as compared with the general population (Fig. 3.12). The difference in incidence is used to calculate a disease risk, which is measured by the λ_s value (Box 3.16).

Genetic testing in complex disease

Most common diseases are determined by interactions between a number of genes and the environment. In this situation, the genetic contribution to disease is termed polygenic. Until recently, very little progress had been made in identifying the genetic variants that predispose to common diseases, but this has been changed by the advent of genome-wide association studies (GWAS). A GWAS typically involves genotyping between 300 000 and 500 000 genetic markers spread across the genome in a large group of individuals with the disease and controls. By comparing the genotypes in cases and controls, it is possible to identify regions of the genome and candidate genes which contribute to the disease under study. Some of the candidate genes for common diseases identified by this approach are listed in Box 3.17.

Pharmacogenomics

Pharmacogenomics is the science of dissecting the genetic determinants of drug kinetics and effects using information from the human genome. For more than 50 years, it has been appreciated that polymorphic mutations within genes can affect individual responses to some drugs, such as loss-of-function mutations in

3.16 Risk to siblings of affected patients for common polygenic diseases

Disease	λ_s
Type 1 diabetes mellitus	15
Systemic lupus erythematosus	10–20
Multiple sclerosis	20–40
Schizophrenia	10
Ischaemic heart disease	4–12

3.17 Examples of disease-associated polymorphisms

Disease	Inheritance	Gene	Mutation	Population frequency
Breast cancer	Complex	FGFR2 (intron 2)	rs1219648	39%
Colorectal cancer	Complex	11q23	rs3802842	24%
Gout	Complex	SLC2A9 (intron 3)	rs1014290	23%
Inflammatory bowel disease	Complex	IL23R	rs11465804	93%

CYP2D6 causing hypersensitivity to debrisoquine, an adrenergic-blocking medication formerly used for the treatment of hypertension in 3% of the population. This gene is part of a large family of highly polymorphic genes encoding cytochrome P450 proteins, mostly expressed in the liver, which determine the metabolism of a host of specific drugs. Polymorphisms in the CYP2D6 gene also determine codeine activation, while those in the CYP2C9 gene affect warfarin inactivation. Polymorphisms in these and other drug metabolic genes determine the persistence of drugs and, therefore, should provide information about dosages and toxicity. At the present time, genetic testing for assessment of drug response is seldom used routinely, but in the future

3

STEM CELL THERAPY

Properties of stem cells

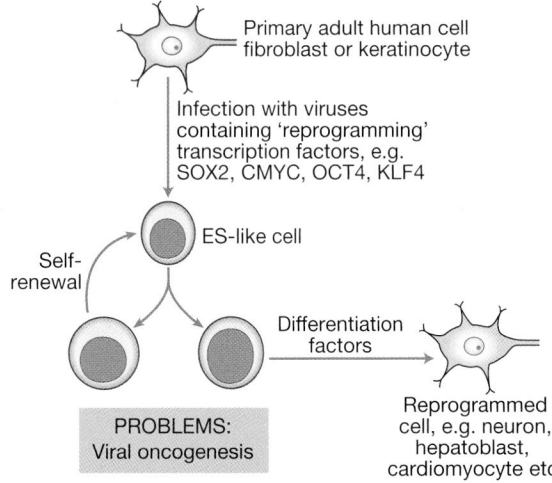

Stem cell — Self-renewal

↓ Differentiation factors

Mature cell, e.g. neuron

Human (ES) cells

Embryo biopsy following IVF

↓

Culture ES cells using growth factor cocktail

↓ In vitro differentiation

Inject into e.g. CNS, myocardium

PROBLEMS:
Ethical issues
Technically difficult

Isolation and culture of adult stem cells

e.g. bone marrow transplantation

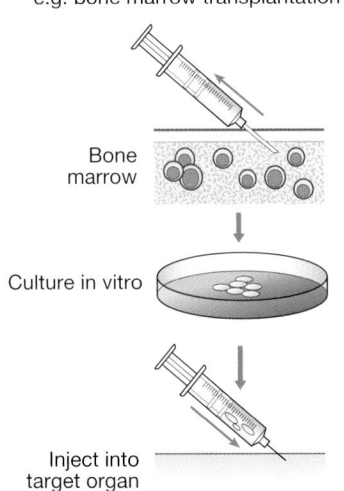

Bone marrow

↓

Culture in vitro

↓

Inject into target organ

PROBLEMS:
Stem cells are often inaccessible or difficult to culture
Immune response

Reprogramming adult human cells

Primary adult human cell fibroblast or keratinocyte

↓ Infection with viruses containing 'reprogramming' transcription factors, e.g. SOX2, CMYC, OCT4, KLF4

ES-like cell

Self-renewal

↓ Differentiation factors → Reprogrammed cell, e.g. neuron, hepatoblast, cardiomyocyte etc.

PROBLEMS:
Viral oncogenesis

GENE THERAPY

In vivo gene therapy

Replacement of deficient gene using either:
retrovirus (inserts into host genome)
or
DNA virus (directly expressed gene)

Inject into target tissue (muscle, bone marrow)

PROBLEMS:
Viral oncogenesis
Immune response

Ex vivo gene therapy

Bone marrow

↓

Culture in vitro

Retrovirus containing gene of interest

↓ Infection

↓

Inject into target organ

Fig. 3.13 Experimental gene and cell therapies. The general approaches to novel gene and stem cell therapies, with their potential or real problems and current limitations. (ES cells = embryonal stem cells)

it may be possible to predict the best specific drugs and dosages for individual patients based on genetic profiling: so-called 'personalised medicine'.

RESEARCH FRONTIERS IN MOLECULAR MEDICINE

Gene therapy

Attempts to replace or repair mutated genes (gene therapy) in humans have met with very limited success so far. Most notable has been replacement of the defective gene in the treatment of severe combined immune deficiency syndrome using retroviral vectors (p. 79). Bone marrow that has been genetically engineered ex vivo to express the normal gene product can be returned to the patient. There have been two major problems with the clinical trials of virally delivered gene therapy conducted to date:

- First, the random integration of the retroviral DNA (which contains the replacement gene) into the genome has caused leukaemia in some treated children via activation of proto-oncogenes.
- Second, a severe immune response to the viral vector may be induced. It has not yet been possible to use non-viral means to introduce sufficient numbers of copies of replacement genes to produce significant biological effects.

Other potentially exciting genetic therapies do not involve gene replacement. Several recently identified compounds, including PTC124, can 'force' cells to read through a mutation that results in a premature termination codon in an ORF with the aim of producing a near-normal protein product. The advantage of this type of therapeutic approach is that it can be applied to a subset of patients with any genetic disease where the genetic mechanism is loss of function.

Stem cell therapy and regenerative medicine

The identification of adult stem cells and the ability to purify and maintain such cells in vitro offer very exciting therapeutic potential (Fig. 3.13). Indeed, adult stem cell therapy has been in wide use for decades in the form of bone marrow transplantation. The recent discovery that adult fibroblasts can be transdifferentiated to form cells with almost all the characteristics of embryonal stem cells derived from the early blastocyst has negated much of the controversy surrounding this approach to therapy. In mammalian model species, such cells can be taken and used to regenerate differentiated tissue cells, such as in heart and brain. They have the ability to produce any cell in the body and proliferate rapidly in culture, and so could be used to refashion damaged organs. Such experiments are still in their infancy but are progressing fast.

Pathway medicine

The ability to manipulate pathways that have been altered in genetic disease has tremendous therapeutic potential for Mendelian disease, but a firm understanding of both disease pathogenesis and drug action at a biochemical level is required. An exciting example of this has been the discovery that the vascular pathology associated with Marfan's syndrome is due to the defective fibrillin molecules causing up-regulation of transforming growth factor (TGF)-β signalling in the vessel wall. Losartan is an antihypertensive drug that is marketed as an angiotensin II receptor antagonist. However, it also acts as a partial antagonist of TGF-β signalling and is effective in preventing aortic dilatation in a mouse model of Marfan's syndrome, showing promising effects in early human clinical trials.

Further information

Books and journal articles

Alberts B. Molecular biology of the cell. 4th edn. New York: Garland Science; 2002.

Strachan T, Read A. Human molecular genetics. 3rd edn. Wilmington, Delaware: Wiley–Liss; 2003.

Young ID. Introduction to risk calculation in genetic counselling. 2nd edn. Oxford: Oxford University Press; 1999.

Websites

www.bshg.org.uk *British Society for Human Genetics; has report on genetic testing of children.*

www.ensembl.org *Annotated genome databases from multiple organisms.*

www.ncbi.nlm.nih.gov/ *Extensive collection of genome databases.*

www.ncbi.nlm.nih.gov/Omim *Online Mendelian Inheritance in Man (OMIM).*

www.nhgri.nih.gov *Human Genome Project.*

3

Immunological factors in disease

S.E. Marshall

4

4

The immune system has evolved to protect the host from pathogens while minimising damage to self tissue. Despite the ancient observation that recovery from a disease frequently results in protection against that condition, the existence of the immune system as a functional entity was not recognised until the end of the 19th century. More recently, it has become clear that the immune system not only protects against infection, but also governs the responses that can lead to autoimmune diseases. Dysfunction or deficiency of the immune response leads to a wide variety of diseases, involving every organ system in the body.

The aim of this chapter is to provide a general understanding of immunology and how it contributes to human disease. A review of the key components of the immune response is followed by five sections that illustrate the clinical presentation of the most common forms of immune dysfunction. Clinical immunologists are usually involved in managing patients with allergy and immune deficiency. More detailed discussion of individual conditions can be found in the relevant organ-specific chapters of this book.

FUNCTIONAL ANATOMY AND PHYSIOLOGY OF THE IMMUNE SYSTEM

The immune system consists of an intricately linked network of cells, proteins and lymphoid organs which are strategically placed to ensure maximal protection against infection. Immune defences are normally categorised into the innate immune response, which provides immediate protection against an invading pathogen, and the adaptive or acquired immune response, which takes more time to develop but confers exquisite specificity and long-lasting protection.

The innate immune system

Innate defences against infection include anatomical barriers, phagocytic cells, soluble molecules such as complement and acute phase proteins, and natural killer cells. The innate immune system recognises generic microbial structures present on non-mammalian tissue and can be mobilised within minutes. A specific stimulus will elicit essentially identical responses in different individuals (in contrast with antibody and T-cell responses, which vary greatly between individuals).

Constitutive barriers to infection

The tightly packed, highly keratinised cells of the skin constantly undergo renewal and replacement, which physically limits colonisation by microorganisms. Microbial growth is inhibited by physiological factors such as low pH and low oxygen tension, and sebaceous glands secrete hydrophobic oils that further repel water and microorganisms. Sweat also contains lysozyme, an enzyme that destroys the structural integrity of bacterial cell walls; ammonia, which has antibacterial properties; and several antimicrobial peptides such as defensins. Similarly, the mucous membranes of the respiratory, gastrointestinal and genitourinary tract provide a constitutive barrier to infection. Secreted mucus acts as a physical barrier to trap invading pathogens, and secretory immunoglobulin A (IgA) prevents bacteria and viruses attaching to and penetrating epithelial cells. As in the skin, lysozyme and antimicrobial peptides within mucosal membranes can directly kill invading pathogens, and additionally lactoferrin acts to starve invading bacteria of iron. Within the respiratory tract, cilia directly trap pathogens and contribute to removal of mucus, assisted by physical manœuvres such as sneezing and coughing. In the gastrointestinal tract, hydrochloric acid and salivary amylase chemically destroy bacteria, while normal peristalsis and induced vomiting or diarrhoea assist clearance of invading organisms.

Endogenous commensal bacteria provide an additional constitutive defence against infection. Approximately 100 trillion (10^{14}) bacteria normally reside at epithelial surfaces in symbiosis with the human host (p. 134). They compete with pathogenic microorganisms for scarce resources, including space and nutrients. In addition, they produce fatty acids and bactericidins that inhibit the growth of many pathogens. Eradication of the normal flora with broad-spectrum antibiotics commonly results in opportunistic infection by organisms which rapidly colonise an undefended ecological niche.

These constitutive barriers are highly effective, but if external defences are breached by a wound or pathogenic organism, the specific soluble proteins and cells of the innate immune system are activated.

Phagocytes

Phagocytes ('eating cells') are specialised cells which ingest and kill microorganisms, scavenge cellular and infectious debris, and produce inflammatory molecules which regulate other components of the immune system. They include neutrophils, monocytes and macrophages, and are particularly important for defence against bacterial and fungal infections.

Phagocytes express a wide range of surface receptors that allow them to identify microorganisms. These pattern recognition receptors include the Toll-like receptors, NOD (nucleotide-oligomerisation domain protein)-like receptors and mannose receptors. They recognise generic molecular motifs not present on mammalian cells, including bacterial cell wall components, bacterial DNA and viral double-stranded RNA. While phagocytes can recognise microorganisms through pattern recognition receptors alone, engulfment of microorganisms is greatly enhanced by opsonisation. Opsonins include acute phase proteins such as C-reactive protein (CRP), antibodies and complement. They bind both to the pathogen and to phagocyte receptors, acting as a bridge between the two to facilitate phagocytosis (Fig. 4.1).

Neutrophils

Neutrophils, also known as polymorphonuclear leucocytes, are derived from the bone marrow and circulate freely in the blood (Fig. 4.2). They are short-lived cells with a half-life of 6 hours, and are produced at the rate of 10^{11} cells daily. Their functions are to kill microorganisms directly, facilitate the rapid transit of cells through tissues, and non-specifically amplify the immune response. This is mediated by enzymes contained in granules which also provide an intracellular milieu for the killing and degradation of microorganisms.

Two main types of granule are recognised: primary or azurophil granules, and the more numerous secondary or

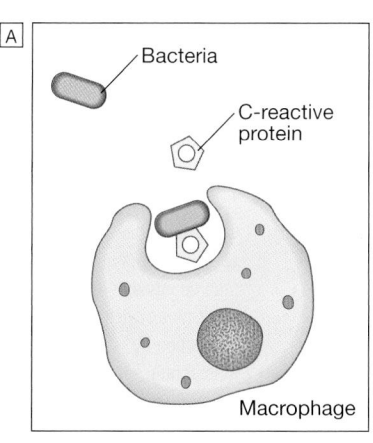
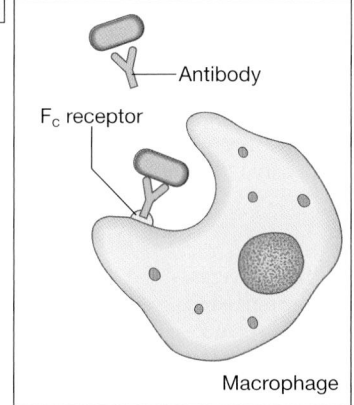

Fig. 4.1 Opsonisation. Phagocytosis of microbial products may be augmented by several opsonins. **A** C-reactive protein. **B** Antibody. **C** Complement fragments.

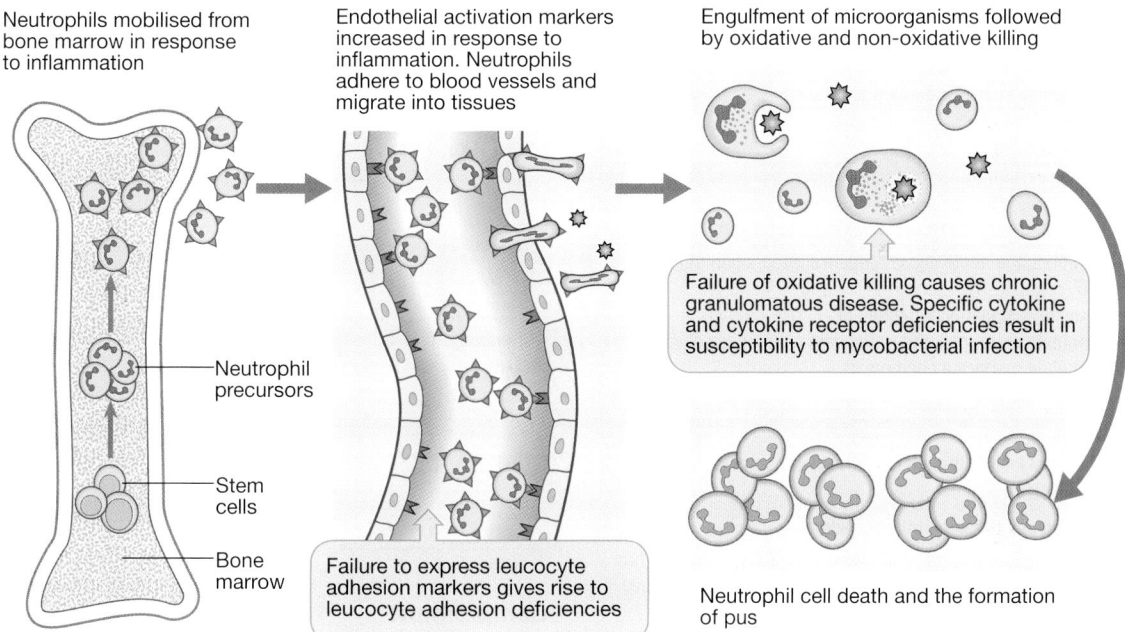

Fig. 4.2 Neutrophil function and dysfunction (green boxes).

specific granules. Primary granules contain myeloperoxidase and other enzymes important for killing ingested microbes and digesting their remains. Secondary granules are smaller and contain other enzymes including lysozyme, collagenase and lactoferrin. These can be released into the extracellular space, while the contents of primary granules are released into phagocytic vesicles. Granule staining becomes more intense in response to infection and is termed 'toxic granulation'.

Changes in damaged or infected cells trigger the local production of inflammatory molecules and cytokines. These stimulate the production and maturation of neutrophils in the bone marrow. The neutrophils are recruited to the site by chemotactic agents and by activation of local endothelium. The transit of neutrophils through the blood stream is responsible for the rise in leucocyte count that occurs in early infection. Once within infected tissue, activated neutrophils

seek out and engulf invading microorganisms. These are initially enclosed within membrane-bound vesicles which fuse with cytoplasmic granules to form the phagolysosome. Within this protected compartment, killing of the organism occurs through a combination of oxidative and non-oxidative killing. Oxidative killing, also known as the respiratory burst, is mediated by the NADPH oxidase enzyme complex, which converts oxygen into reactive oxygen species such as hydrogen peroxide and superoxide that are lethal to microorganisms. When combined with myeloperoxidase, hypochlorous ions (HOCl⁻, analogous to bleach) are produced, which are highly effective oxidants and antimicrobial agents. Non-oxidative (oxygen-independent) killing occurs through the release of bactericidal enzymes into the phagolysosome. Each enzyme has a distinct antimicrobial spectrum, providing broad coverage against bacteria and fungi.

The process of phagocytosis depletes neutrophil glycogen reserves and is followed by neutrophil cell death. As the cells die, their contents are released and lysosomal enzymes degrade collagen and other components of the interstitium, causing liquefaction of closely adjacent tissue. The accumulation of dead and dying neutrophils results in the formation of pus which, if extensive, may result in abscess formation.

Monocytes and macrophages

Monocytes are the precursors of tissue macrophages. They are produced in the bone marrow and exported to the circulation, where they constitute about 5% of leucocytes. From the blood stream, they migrate to peripheral tissues where they differentiate into tissue macrophages and reside for long periods. Specialised populations of tissue macrophages include Kupffer cells in the liver, alveolar macrophages in the lung, mesangial cells in the kidney, and microglial cells in the brain. Macrophages, like neutrophils, are capable of phagocytosis and killing of microorganisms but also play an important role in the amplification and regulation of the inflammatory response (Box 4.1). Unlike neutrophils, macrophages do not die after killing pathogens.

4.1 Functions of macrophages

Initiation and amplification of the inflammatory response

- Stimulate the acute phase response (production of IL-1, TNF-α and IL-6)
- Activate vascular endothelium (IL-1, TNF-α)
- Stimulate neutrophil maturation and chemotaxis (IL-1, IL-8)
- Stimulate monocyte chemotaxis

Killing of microorganisms

- Phagocytosis
- Microbial killing through oxidative and non-oxidative mechanisms

Resolution and repair of inflammation

- Scavenging of necrotic and apoptotic cells and other debris
- Tissue remodelling (elastase, collagenase, matrix proteins)
- Down-regulation of inflammatory cytokines
- Scar formation (IL-1, platelet-derived growth factor, fibroblast growth factor)

Link between innate and adaptive immune system

- Activate T cells by presenting antigen in a recognisable form
- T cell-derived cytokines increase phagocytosis and microbicidal activity of macrophages in a positive feedback loop

(IL = interleukin; TNF = tumour necrosis factor)

Cytokines

Cytokines are small soluble proteins that act as multipurpose chemical messengers. They are produced by cells involved in innate and adaptive immune responses and by stromal tissue. More than 100 cytokines have been described, with overlapping, complex roles in modifying the immune microenvironment. Subtle differences in cytokine composition, particularly at the initiation of an immune response, may have a major effect on outcome. The most important cytokines are listed in Box 4.2.

4.2 Important cytokines in regulation of the immune response

Cytokine	Source	Actions
Interferon-alpha (IFN-α)	T cells and macrophages	Antiviral activity Activates NK cells, CD8+ T cells and macrophages
Interferon-gamma (IFN-γ)	T cells and NK cells	Increases antimicrobial and antitumour activity of macrophages Determines cytokine production by T cells and macrophages
Tumour necrosis factor alpha (TNF-α)	Macrophages and NK cells	Pro-inflammatory Increases apoptosis and expression of cytokines and adhesion molecules Directly cytotoxic
Interleukin-1 (IL-1)	Macrophages and neutrophils	Acute phase reactant Stimulates neutrophil recruitment, fever, T-cell and macrophage activation, immunoglobulin production
Interleukin-2 (IL-2)	CD4+ T cells	Stimulates proliferation and differentiation of antigen-specific T lymphocytes
Interleukin-4 (IL-4)	CD4+ T cells and mast cells	Stimulates maturation of B and T cells, and production of IgE antibody
Interleukin-6 (IL-6)	Monocytes and macrophages	Acute phase reactant Stimulates maturation of B cells into plasma cells
Interleukin-12 (IL-12)	Monocytes and macrophages	Stimulates IFN-γ and TNF-α release by T cells, activates NK cells

(NK = natural killer)

Complement

The complement system is a group of more than 20 tightly regulated, functionally linked proteins that act to promote inflammation and eliminate invading pathogens. Complement proteins are produced in the liver and are present in the circulation as inactive molecules. When triggered, they enzymatically activate other proteins in a rapidly amplified biological cascade analogous to the coagulation cascade (p. 993).

There are three mechanisms by which the complement cascade may be triggered (Fig. 4.3):

- *The alternative pathway* is triggered directly by binding of C3 to bacterial cell wall components such as lipopolysaccharide of Gram-negative bacteria and teichoic acid of Gram-positive bacteria.
- *The classical pathway* is initiated when two or more IgM or IgG antibody molecules bind to antigen. The associated conformational change exposes binding sites on the antibodies for the first protein in the classical pathway, C1. C1 is a multi-headed molecule which can bind up to six antibody molecules. Once two or more 'heads' of a C1 molecule are bound to antibody, the classical cascade is triggered.

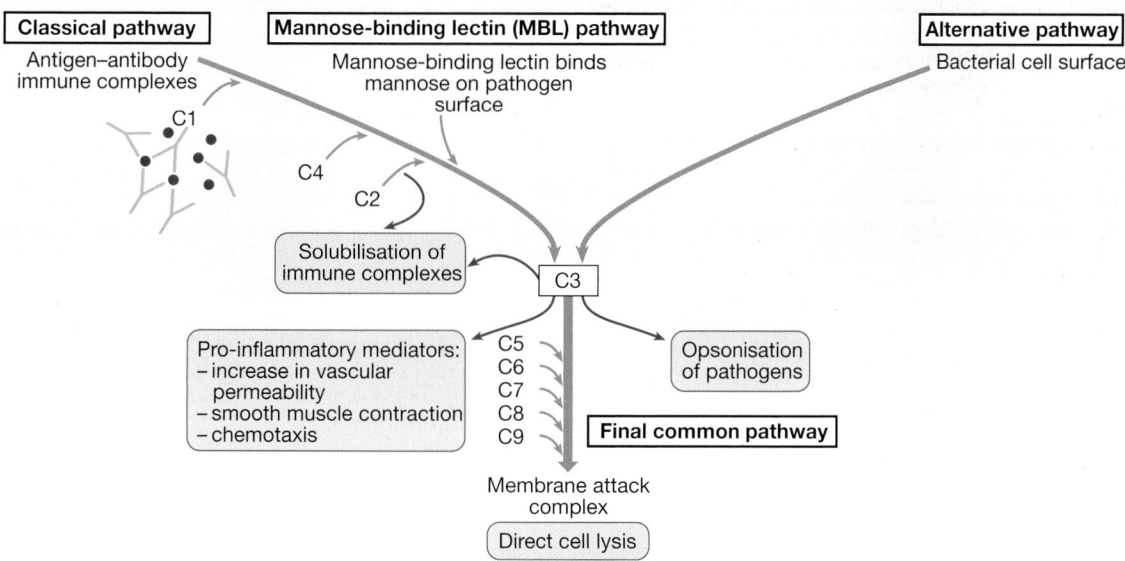

Fig. 4.3 The complement pathway. The activation of C3 is central to complement activation.

- *The lectin pathway* is activated by the direct binding of mannose-binding lectin to microbial cell surface carbohydrates. This mimics the binding of C1 to immune complexes and directly stimulates the classical pathway, bypassing the need for immune complex formation.

Activation of complement by any of these pathways results in activation of C3. This in turn activates the final common pathway, in which the complement proteins C5–C9 assemble together to form the membrane attack complex. This can insert into and puncture target cell walls, leading to osmotic cell lysis. This step is particularly important in the defence against encapsulated bacteria such as *Neisseria* spp. and *Haemophilus influenzae*. Complement fragments generated by activation of the cascade can also act as opsonins, rendering microorganisms more susceptible to phagocytosis by macrophages and neutrophils (see Fig. 4.1). In addition, they are chemotactic agents, promoting leucocyte trafficking to sites of inflammation. Some fragments act as anaphylotoxins, binding to complement receptors on mast cells and triggering release of histamine, which increases vascular permeability. The products of complement activation also help to target immune complexes to antigen-presenting cells, providing a link between the innate and the acquired immune systems. Finally, activated complement products dissolve the immune complexes that triggered the cascade, minimising bystander damage to surrounding tissues.

Mast cells and basophils

Mast cells and basophils are bone marrow-derived cells which play a central role in allergic disorders. Mast cells reside predominantly in tissues exposed to the external environment, such as the skin and gut, while basophils are located in the circulation and are recruited into tissues in response to inflammation. Both contain large cytoplasmic granules which enclose preformed vasoactive substances such as histamine (see Fig. 4.9, p. 87). Mast cells and basophils express IgE receptors on their cell surface. These bind IgE antibody via the antibody constant region (see Fig. 4.5). On encounter with specific antigen, the cell is triggered to release preformed mediators and synthesise additional mediators, including leukotrienes, prostaglandins and cytokines. An inflammatory cascade is initiated which increases local blood flow and vascular permeability, stimulates smooth muscle contraction, and increases secretion at mucosal surfaces.

Natural killer cells

Natural killer (NK) cells are large granular lymphocytes which play a major role in defence against tumours and viruses. They exhibit features of both the adaptive and innate immune systems: they are morphologically similar to lymphocytes and recognise similar ligands, but they are not antigen-specific and cannot generate immunological memory.

NK cells express a variety of cell surface receptors. Some recognise stress signals, while others recognise the absence of human leucocyte antigen (HLA) molecules on cell surfaces (down-regulation of HLA molecules by viruses and tumour cells is an important mechanism by which they evade the T-lymphocyte response). NK cells can also be activated by the binding of antigen–antibody complexes to surface receptors. This physically links the NK cell to its target in a manner analogous to opsonisation and is known as antibody-dependent cellular cytotoxicity (ADCC).

Activated NK cells can kill their targets in various ways. Pore-forming proteins such as perforin induce direct cell lysis, while granzymes are proteolytic enzymes which stimulate apoptosis. In addition, NK cells produce a variety of cytokines such as tumour necrosis factor (TNF)-α and interferon-γ (IFN-γ) which have direct antiviral and antitumour effects.

Dendritic cells

Dendritic cells are present in tissues and sample the environment for foreign particles. They carry microbial

73

4

antigens to regional lymph nodes, where they prime adaptive immune responses including B-cell production of antibody and T-cell responses to diverse pathogens.

The adaptive immune system

If the innate immune system fails to provide effective protection against an invading pathogen, the adaptive immune system (Fig. 4.4) is mobilised. This has three key characteristics:

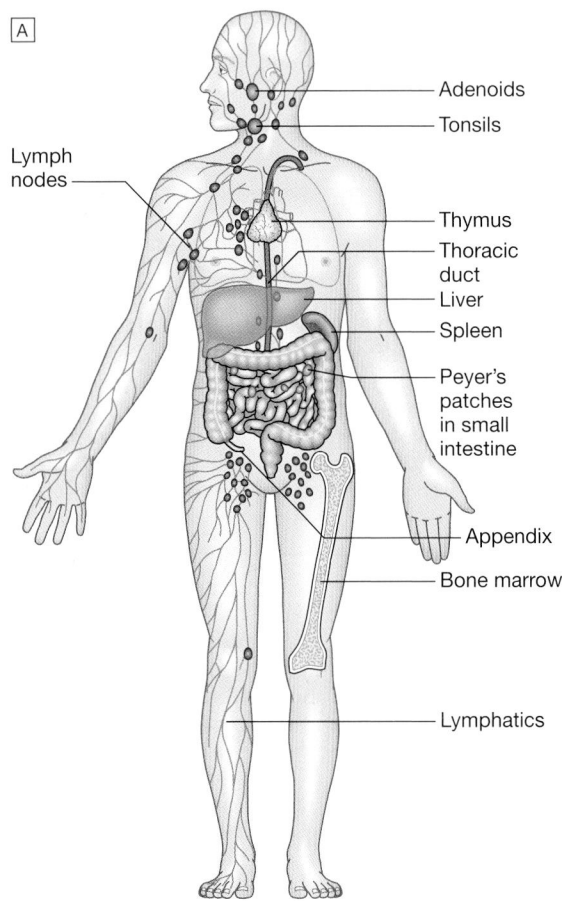

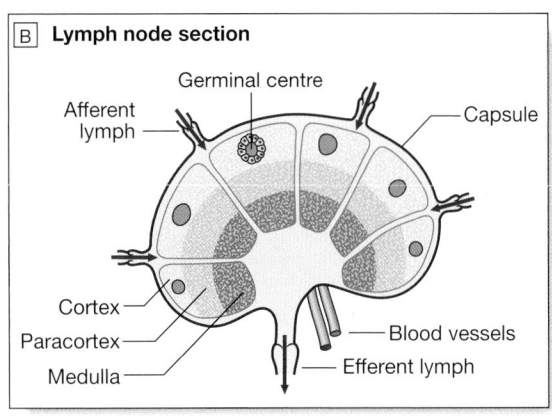

B **Lymph node section**

Fig. 4.4 Anatomy of the adaptive immune system. **A** Macroanatomy. **B** Anatomy of a lymph node.

- It has exquisite specificity and is able to discriminate between very small differences in molecular structure.
- It is highly adaptive and can respond to an unlimited number of molecules.
- It possesses immunological memory, being able to recall previous encounter with an antigen and respond more effectively than on the first occasion.

There are two major arms of the adaptive immune response. Humoral immunity involves antibodies that are produced by B lymphocytes; cellular immunity is mediated by T lymphocytes, which synthesise and release cytokines that affect other cells. These interact closely with each other and with the components of the innate immune system, to maximise the effectiveness of the immune response.

Lymphoid organs

- *Primary lymphoid organs.* The primary lymphoid organs are involved in lymphocyte development. They include the bone marrow, where both T and B lymphocytes are derived from haematopoietic stem cells (p. 989) and where B lymphocytes also mature, and the thymus, which is the site of T-cell maturation.
- *Secondary lymphoid organs.* After maturation, lymphocytes migrate to the secondary lymphoid organs. These include the spleen, lymph nodes and mucosa-associated lymphoid tissue. These organs trap and concentrate foreign substances, and are the major sites of interaction between naïve lymphocytes and microorganisms.

The thymus

The thymus is a bilobed structure organised into cortical and medullary areas. The cortex is densely populated with immature T cells, which migrate to the medulla to undergo selection and maturation. The thymus is most active in the fetal and neonatal period, and involutes after puberty. Absence of thymic development is associated with profound T-cell immune deficiency (p. 78), but surgical removal of the thymus in childhood (usually in the context of major cardiac surgery) is not associated with significant immune dysfunction.

The spleen

The spleen is the largest of the secondary lymphoid organs. It is highly effective at filtering blood and is an important site of phagocytosis of senescent erythrocytes, bacteria, immune complexes and other debris. It is also a major site of antibody synthesis. It is particularly important for defence against encapsulated bacteria, and asplenic individuals are at risk of overwhelming *Streptococcus pneumoniae* and *H. influenzae* infection (Box 24.41, p. 1024).

Lymph nodes

Lymph nodes are positioned to maximise exposure to lymph draining from sites of external contact. Their structure is highly organised, as shown in Fig. 4.4B:

- The *cortex* contains primary lymphoid follicles which are the site of B-lymphocyte interactions. When B cells encounter antigen they undergo intense proliferation, forming germinal centres within the cortex.

- The *paracortex* is rich in T lymphocytes and dendritic cells.
- The *medulla* is the major site of antibody-secreting plasma cells.
- Within the medulla there are many *sinuses*, which contain large numbers of macrophages.

Mucosa-associated lymphoid tissue

These tissues have similar structure and function to lymph nodes. They include Peyer's patches in the small intestine, submucosal lymphoid follicles in the appendix, and tonsils in the pharynx.

Lymphatics

The lymphoid tissue is physically connected by lymphatics, which have three major functions: they provide access to lymph nodes, return interstitial fluid to the venous system, and transport fat from the small intestine to the blood stream (see Fig. 16.14, p. 450). The lymphatics begin as blind-ending capillaries, which come together to form lymphatic ducts. These enter and then leave regional lymph nodes as afferent and efferent ducts respectively. They eventually coalesce and drain into the thoracic duct and thence into the left subclavian vein. Lymphatics may be either deep or superficial, and in general follow the distribution of major blood vessels.

Humoral immunity

B lymphocytes

These specialised cells arise from bone marrow stem cells, and their major functions are to produce antibody and interact with T cells. Mature B lymphocytes can be found in the bone marrow, lymphoid tissue, spleen and, to a lesser extent, the blood stream. They express a unique immunoglobulin receptor on their cell surface (the B-cell receptor), which binds to soluble antigen. Encounters with antigen usually occur within the lymph nodes, where, if provided with appropriate signals from nearby T lympho-

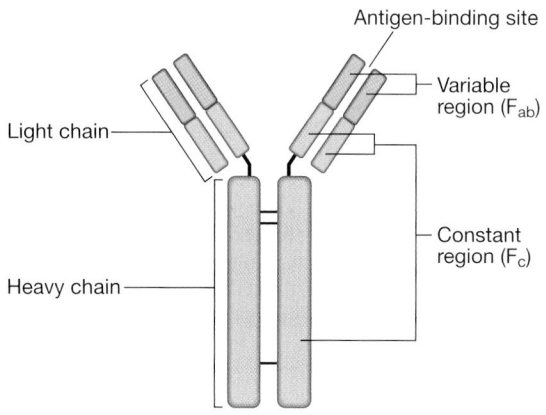

Fig. 4.5 The structure of an immunoglobulin (antibody) molecule.

cytes, stimulated antigen-specific B cells respond by rapidly proliferating in a process known as clonal expansion. This is accompanied by a highly complex series of genetic rearrangements which generates B-cell populations that express receptors with greater affinity for antigen than the original. These cells differentiate into either long-lived memory cells, which reside in the lymph nodes, or plasma cells, which produce antibody.

Immunoglobulins

Immunoglobulins (Ig) are soluble proteins made up of two heavy and two light chains (Fig. 4.5). The heavy chain determines the antibody class or isotype, i.e. IgG, IgA, IgM, IgE or IgD. Subclasses of IgG and IgA also occur. The antigen is recognised by the antigen-binding regions (F_{ab}) of both heavy and light chains, while the consequences of antibody-binding are determined by the constant region of the heavy chain (F_c) (Box 4.3).

Antibodies can initiate a number of different actions. They facilitate phagocytosis by acting as opsonins (see Fig. 4.1, p. 71). A similar bridging mechanism facilitates

4.3 Classes and properties of antibody

Antibody	Concentration in adult serum	Complement activation*	Opsonisation	Presence in external secretions	Other properties
IgG	8.0–16.0 g/L	IgG1 +++ IgG2 + IgG3 +++	IgG1 ++ IgG3 ++	++	4 subclasses: IgG1, IgG2, IgG3, IgG4 Distributed equally between blood and extracellular fluid, and transported across placenta IgG2 is particularly important in making antibodies against polysaccharides
IgA	1.5–4.0 g/L	–	–	++++	2 subclasses: IgA1, IgA2 Highly effective at neutralising toxins Particularly important at mucosal surfaces
IgM	0.5–2.0 g/L	++++	–	+	Highly effective at agglutinating pathogens
IgE	0.003–0.04 g/L	–	–	–	Majority of IgE is bound to mast cells, basophils and eosinophils Important in allergic disease and defence against parasite infection
IgD	Not detected	–	–	–	Function unknown

*I.e. activation of the classical pathway, also called 'complement fixation'.

cell killing by cytotoxic cells, particularly NK cells (ADCC, p. 73). Binding of antibodies to antigen can trigger activation of the classical complement pathway (see Fig. 4.3). In addition, antibodies may act directly to neutralise the biological activity of their antigen target. This is a particularly important feature of IgA antibodies, which act predominantly at mucosal surfaces.

The humoral immune response is characterised by immunological memory; that is, the antibody response to successive exposures to antigen is qualitatively and quantitatively different from that on first exposure. When a previously unstimulated (naïve) B lymphocyte is activated by antigen, the first antibody to be produced is IgM, which appears in the serum after 5–10 days. Depending on additional stimuli provided by T lymphocytes, other antibody classes (IgG, IgA and IgE) are produced 3–7 days later. If, some time later, a memory B cell is re-exposed to antigen, the lag time between antigen exposure and the production of antibody is decreased (to 2–3 days). In addition, the titre of antibodies produced is greatly increased and the response is dominated by IgG antibodies of high affinity. Furthermore, in contrast to the initial antibody response, secondary antibody responses do not require input from T lymphocytes. This allows the rapid generation of highly specific responses on pathogen re-exposure.

Cellular immunity

T lymphocytes mediate cellular immunity and are important for defence against viruses, fungi and intracellular bacteria. They also play an important immunoregulatory role, orchestrating and regulating the responses of other components of the immune system. T-lymphocyte precursors arise in bone marrow and are exported to the thymus while still immature (see Fig. 4.6). Within the thymus, each cell expresses a T-cell receptor with a unique specificity. These cells undergo a process of stringent selection to ensure that autoreactive T cells are deleted. Mature T lymphocytes leave the thymus and expand to populate other organs of the immune system. It has been estimated that an individual possesses 10^7–10^9 T-cell clones, each with a unique T-cell receptor, ensuring at least partial coverage for any antigen encountered.

T cells respond to protein antigens, but they cannot recognise these in their native form. Instead, intact protein must be processed into component peptides which can bind to a structural framework on the cell surface known as HLA (human leucocyte antigen). This process is known as antigen processing and presentation, and it is the peptide/HLA complex which is recognised by individual T cells. While all nucleated cells have the capacity to process and present antigens, specialised antigen-presenting cells include dendritic cells, macrophages and B lymphocytes. HLA molecules exhibit extreme polymorphism; for example, more than 500 different HLA-B alleles have been identified. As each HLA molecule presents a subtly different peptide repertoire to T lymphocytes, this ensures enormous diversity in recognition of antigens within the population.

T lymphocytes can be segregated into two subgroups on the basis of function, recognition of HLA molecules and expression of cell surface proteins. Leucocyte cell surface molecules are named systematically by assigning them a 'cluster of differentiation' (CD) antigen number.

CD8+ ('cytotoxic') T lymphocytes

These cells recognise antigenic peptides in association with HLA class I molecules (HLA-A, HLA-B, HLA-C). They kill infected cells directly through the production of pore-forming molecules such as perforin, or by triggering apoptosis of the target cell.

CD4+ ('helper') T lymphocytes

These cells recognise peptides presented on HLA class II molecules (HLA-DR, HLA-DP and HLA-DQ) and have mainly immunoregulatory functions. They produce cytokines and provide co-stimulatory signals that support the activation of CD8+ T lymphocytes and assist the production of mature antibody by B cells. In addition, their close interaction with phagocytes determines cytokine production by both cell types.

CD4+ lymphocytes can be further subdivided into subsets on the basis of the cytokines they produce:

- Typically, Th1 cells produce IL-2, IFN-γ and TNF-α, and support the development of delayed type hypersensitivity responses (p. 86).
- Th2 cells typically secrete IL-4, IL-5 and IL-10, and promote allergic responses (p. 86).
- A further subset of specialised CD4+ lymphocytes known as regulatory cells are important in the regulation of other CD4+ cells and the prevention of autoimmune disease.

IMMUNE DEFICIENCY

The consequences of deficiencies of the immune system include recurrent infections, autoimmunity and susceptibility to malignancy. Immune deficiency may arise through intrinsic defects in immune function, but is much more commonly due to secondary causes including infection, drug therapy, malignancy and ageing. This chapter gives an overview of the rare primary immune deficiencies. More than a hundred such deficiencies have been described, most of which are genetically determined and usually present in childhood or adolescence. The clinical manifestations are dictated by the component of the immune system involved (Box 4.4). However, there is considerable overlap and redundancy in the immune network, and some diseases do not fall easily into this classification.

Presenting problems in immune deficiency

Recurrent infections

Many patients with an immune deficiency present with recurrent infections. While there is no accepted definition of 'too many' infections, features that may indicate immune deficiency are shown in Box 4.5. Frequent, severe infections or infections caused by unusual organisms or at unusual sites are the most useful indicator.

Baseline investigations include full blood count and white cell differential, acute phase reactants (CRP, see below), renal and liver function tests, urine dipstick and serum immunoglobulins with protein electrophoresis.

4.4 Immune deficiencies and common patterns of infection

	Phagocyte deficiency	Complement deficiency	T-lymphocyte deficiency	Antibody deficiency
Bacteria	Staphylococcus aureus Pseudomonas aeruginosa Serratia marcescens Burkholderia cenocepacia Mycobacterium tuberculosis Atypical mycobacteria	Neisseria meningitidis Neisseria gonorrhoeae Haemophilus influenzae Streptococcus pneumoniae	Mycobacterium tuberculosis Atypical mycobacteria	Haemophilus influenzae Streptococcus pneumoniae Staphylococcus aureus
Fungi	Candida spp. Aspergillus spp.		Candida spp. Aspergillus spp.	
Viruses			Cytomegalovirus (CMV) Enteroviruses Epstein–Barr virus (EBV) Herpes zoster	
Protozoa			Pneumocystis jirovecii Toxoplasma gondii Cryptosporidia	Giardia lamblia

4.5 Warning signs of immune deficiency

- ≥ 8 ear infections within 1 year
- ≥ 2 serious sinus infections within 1 year
- ≥ 2 months on antibiotics with little effect
- ≥ 2 pneumonias within 1 year
- Failure of an infant to gain weight or grow normally
- Recurrent deep skin or organ abscesses
- Persistent thrush in mouth or elsewhere on skin after infancy
- Need for intravenous antibiotics to clear infections
- ≥ 2 deep-seated infections such as sepsis, meningitis or cellulitis
- A family history of primary immune deficiency

Additional microbiological, virological and radiological tests may be appropriate. At this stage it may be clear which category of immune deficiency is being considered, and specific investigation can be undertaken as described below.

If an immune deficiency is suspected but has not yet been formally characterised, patients should not receive live vaccines because of the risk of vaccine-induced disease. Discussion with specialists will help determine whether additional preventative measures, such as prophylactic antibiotics, are indicated.

Primary phagocyte deficiencies

Primary phagocyte deficiencies (see Fig. 4.2, p. 71) usually present with recurrent bacterial and fungal infections which may affect unusual sites. The majority present in childhood but milder forms may present in adults. Affected patients require aggressive management of existing infections, including intravenous antibiotics and surgical drainage of abscesses, and long-term prophylaxis with antifungal agents and trimethoprim-sulfamethoxazole. Specific treatment depends upon the nature of the defect; bone marrow transplantation may be considered (p. 1013).

Leucocyte adhesion deficiencies

These are disorders of phagocyte migration, when failure to express adhesion molecules on vascular endothelium results in the inability of phagocytes to exit the blood stream. They are characterised by recurrent bacterial infections but sites of infection lack pus or neutrophil infiltration. Peripheral blood neutrophil counts may be very high during acute infection because of the failure of mobilised neutrophils to exit blood vessels. Specialised tests show reduced or absent expression of adhesion molecules on neutrophils.

Chronic granulomatous disease

This is caused by mutations in the genes encoding the NADPH oxidase enzymes, which results in failure of oxidative killing. This can be demonstrated with the nitroblue tetrazolium reduction test (NBT). The defect leads to susceptibility to catalase-positive organisms such as Staphylococcus aureus, Burkholderia cenocepacia and aspergillus. Intracellular killing of mycobacteria in macrophages is also impaired. Infections most commonly involve the lungs, lymph nodes, soft tissues, bone, skin and urinary tract, and are characterised histologically by granuloma formation.

Defects in cytokines and cytokine receptors

Defects of cytokines such as IFN-γ, IL-12 or their receptors also result in failure of intracellular killing, and individuals are particularly susceptible to mycobacterial infections. Detailed assessment of cytokine deficiencies is currently only performed in specialised laboratories.

Complement pathway deficiencies

Genetic deficiencies of almost all the complement pathway proteins (see Fig. 4.3, p. 73) have been described. Many can present with recurrent infection with encapsulated bacteria, particularly Neisseria species. This reflects the importance of the membrane attack complex in defence against these bacteria. In addition, genetic deficiencies of the classical complement pathway (C1, C2 and C4) are associated with a high prevalence of autoimmune disease, particularly systemic lupus erythematosus (SLE, p. 1107).

In contrast to other complement deficiencies, mannose-binding lectin deficiency is very common (5% of the population). Individuals with complete mannose-binding lectin deficiency have an increased incidence of bacterial infections if subjected to an additional cause of immune compromise, such as premature birth or chemotherapy. However, the importance of this deficiency in otherwise healthy individuals remains uncertain.

Deficiency of the regulatory protein C1 esterase inhibitor is not associated with recurrent infections but causes recurrent angioedema. This is discussed on page 91.

Investigations and management

Complement C3 and C4 are the only complement components that are routinely measured. Screening for complement deficiencies is performed using more specialised functional tests. The CH50 (classical haemolytic pathway 50, also known as total haemolytic complement (THC)) involves adding the patient's serum to sheep red blood cells (SRBC) which have been coated with anti-SRBC antibody. If the cells lyse, the serum contains all the components of the classical and membrane attack pathways. Absence of lysis indicates a complement deficiency and should be followed by measurement of individual components. However, complement proteins degrade rapidly at room temperature, and the most common cause of an absent CH50 is delay in transportation of the sample to the laboratory. A similar assay is also available for specific measurement of alternative pathway function (AP50).

There is no definitive treatment for complement deficiencies. Patients should be vaccinated with meningococcal, pneumococcal and *H. influenzae* B vaccines in order to boost their adaptive immune responses. Lifelong prophylactic penicillin to prevent meningococcal infection is also recommended. At-risk family members should be screened for complement deficiencies with functional complement assays.

Primary deficiencies of the adaptive immune system

Primary T-lymphocyte deficiencies

These are characterised by recurrent viral, protozoal and fungal infections (see Box 4.4). In addition, many T-cell deficiencies are associated with defective antibody production because of the importance of T cells in providing help for B cells. These disorders generally present in childhood and are illustrated in Figure 4.6.

DiGeorge syndrome

This results from failure of development of the 3rd/4th pharyngeal pouch, usually caused by a deletion of 22q11. It is associated with abnormalities of the aortic arch, hypocalcaemia, tracheo-oesophageal fistulae, cleft lip and palate, and absent thymic development. It is characterised by very low numbers of mature T cells despite normal development in the bone marrow.

Bare lymphocyte syndromes

These are caused by absent expression of HLA molecules within the thymus. If HLA class I molecules are affected, CD8+ lymphocytes fail to develop, while absent expression of HLA class II molecules affects CD4+ lymphocyte maturation. In addition to recurrent

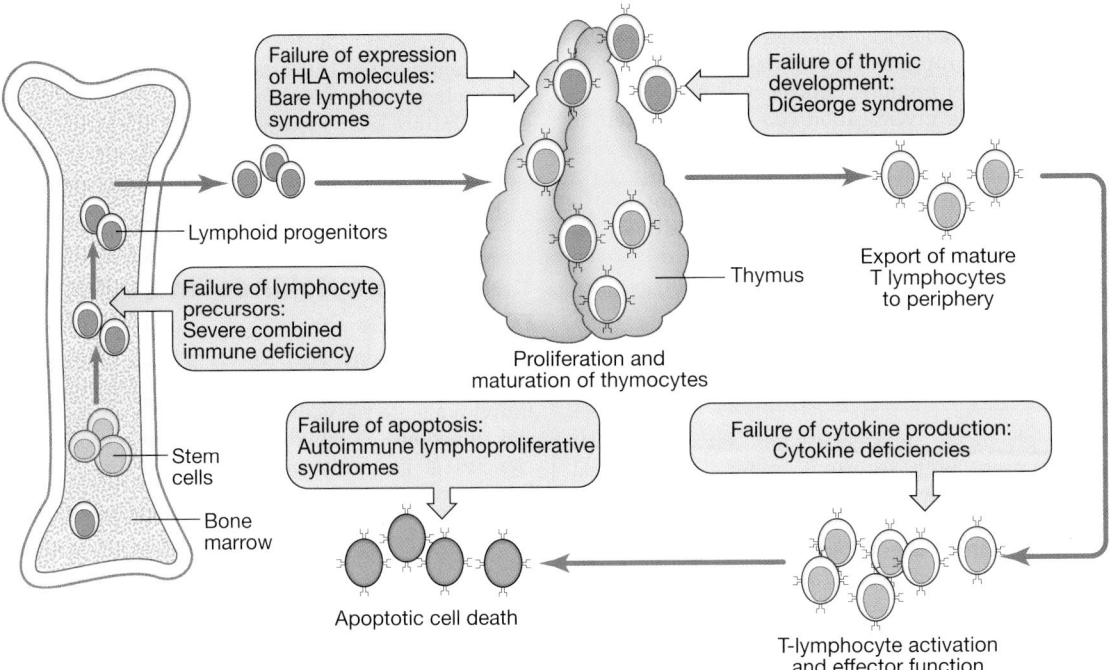

Fig. 4.6 T-lymphocyte function and dysfunction (green boxes).

infections, failure to express HLA class I is associated with systemic vasculitis caused by uncontrolled activation of natural killer cells.

Autoimmune lymphoproliferative syndrome

This is caused by failure of apoptosis of lymphocytes (p. 47). It is characterised by accumulation of autoreactive cells causing lymphadenopathy, splenomegaly and a variety of autoimmune diseases.

Investigations and management

The principal tests for T-lymphocyte deficiencies are a total lymphocyte count and quantitation of lymphocyte subpopulations by flow cytometry. Serum immunoglobulins should also be quantified. Functional tests of T-cell activation and proliferation may be indicated. Patients in whom T-lymphocyte deficiencies are suspected should be tested for HIV infection (p. 385).

Patients should receive anti-*Pneumocystis* and antifungal prophylaxis, and require aggressive management of specific infections. Immunoglobulin replacement may be indicated if disease is associated with defective antibody production. Stem cell transplantation (p. 1013) may be appropriate in bare lymphocyte syndromes, and thymic transplantation has been used for DiGeorge syndrome.

Combined B- and T-lymphocyte immune deficiencies

Severe combined immune deficiency (SCID) is caused by defects in lymphoid precursors and results in the combined failure of B- and T-cell maturation. The absence of an effective adaptive immune response causes recurrent bacterial, fungal and viral infections soon after birth. Bone marrow transplantation (p. 1013) is the only current treatment option, although specific gene therapy is under investigation.

Primary antibody deficiencies

Primary antibody deficiencies (Fig. 4.7) are characterised by recurrent bacterial infections, particularly of the respiratory and gastrointestinal tract. The most common causative organisms are bacteria such as *Strep. pneumoniae* and *H. influenzae*. These disorders may present in infancy, when the protective benefit of transferred maternal immunoglobulin has waned. However, three forms of primary antibody deficiency can also present in adulthood:

- *Selective IgA deficiency* is the most common primary immune deficiency, affecting 1:600 northern Europeans. In most patients, low (< 0.05 g/L) or undetectable IgA is an incidental finding with no clinical sequelae. However, 30% of individuals experience recurrent mild respiratory and gastrointestinal infections. In some patients, there is a compensatory increase in serum IgG levels.
- *Common variable immune deficiency (CVID)* is a heterogeneous adult-onset primary immune deficiency of unknown cause. It is characterised by low serum IgG levels and failure to make antibody responses to exogenous pathogens. Paradoxically, antibody-mediated autoimmune diseases such as idiopathic thrombocytopenic purpura and autoimmune haemolytic anaemia are common. CVID is also associated with an increased risk of malignancy, particularly lymphoproliferative disease.
- *Specific antibody deficiency or functional IgG antibody deficiency* is a poorly characterised condition which causes defective antibody responses to polysaccharide antigens. Some patients are deficient in the antibody subclasses IgG2 and IgG4, and this condition was previously called IgG subclass deficiency.

There is overlap between specific antibody deficiency, IgA deficiency and CVID, and some patients may progress to a more global antibody deficiency over time.

Investigations

Serum immunoglobulins (Box 4.6) should be measured in conjunction with protein and urine electrophoresis

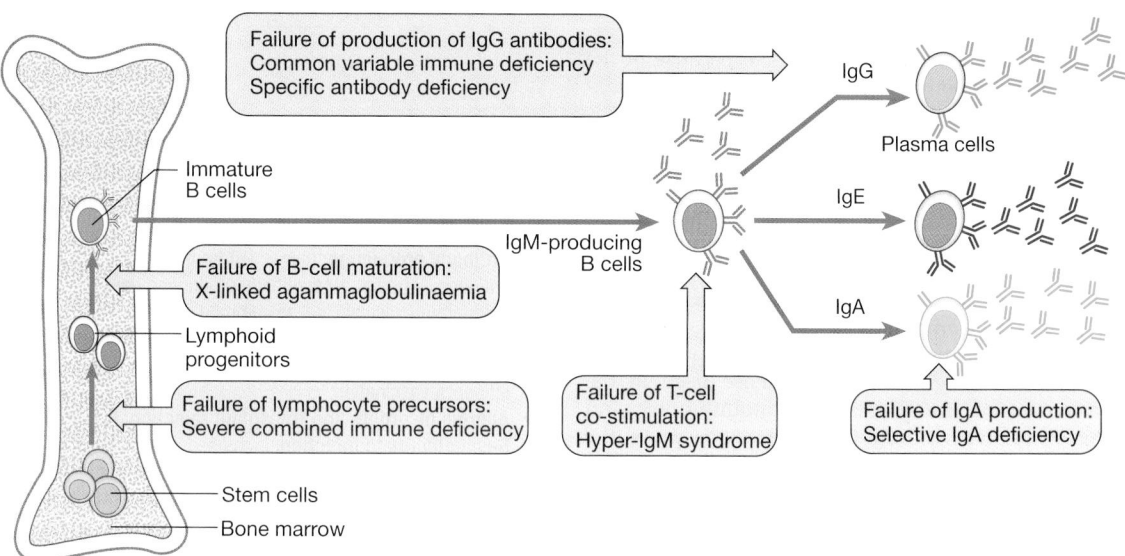

Fig. 4.7 B-lymphocyte function and primary antibody deficiencies (green boxes).

4.6 Investigation of primary antibody deficiencies

	Serum immunoglobulin concentrations				Circulating lymphocyte numbers		Test immunisation
	IgM	IgG	IgA	IgE	B cells	T cells	
Selective IgA deficiency	Normal	Often elevated	Absent	Normal	Normal	Normal	
Common variable immune deficiency	Normal or low	Low	Low or absent	Low or absent	Variable	Variable	No antibody response
Specific antibody deficiency	Normal	Normal	Normal	Normal	Normal	Normal	No antibody response to polysaccharide antigens

to exclude secondary causes of hypogammaglobulin-aemia. In addition, specific antibody responses to known pathogens should be assessed by measuring IgG antibodies against tetanus, *H. influenzae* and *Strep. pneumoniae* (most patients will have been exposed to some of these antigens through either infection or immunisation). If specific antibody levels are low, immunisation with the appropriate killed vaccine should be followed by repeat antibody measurement 6–8 weeks later; failure to mount a response indicates a significant defect in antibody production. These functional tests have generally superseded IgG subclass quantitation. Quantitation of B and T lymphocytes by flow cytometry is also useful.

Management

All patients with antibody deficiencies require aggressive treatment of infections and prophylactic antibiotics may be indicated. The mainstay of treatment is immunoglobulin replacement (intravenous immunoglobulin, IVIgG), which is derived from pooled plasma (p. 1007) and contains IgG antibodies to a wide variety of common organisms. IVIgG is usually administered every 3–4 weeks with the aim of maintaining trough IgG levels within the normal adult range. Treatment may be self-administered and is life-long.

With the exception of selective IgA deficiency, immunisation is generally not effective because of the defect in IgG antibody production. As with all primary immune deficiencies, live vaccines should be avoided.

Secondary immune deficiencies

Secondary immune deficiencies are much more common than primary immune deficiencies and occur if the immune system is compromised by external factors (Box 4.7). Common causes include infections, such as HIV and measles, and cytotoxic and immunosuppressive drugs, particularly those used in the management of transplantation, autoimmunity and cancer. Physiological immune deficiency occurs at the extremes of life; the decline of the immune response in the elderly is known as immune senescence (Box 4.8). Management of secondary immune deficiency is described in the relevant chapters on infectious diseases (Ch. 13), HIV (Ch. 14), oncology (Ch. 11) and haematological disorders (Ch. 24).

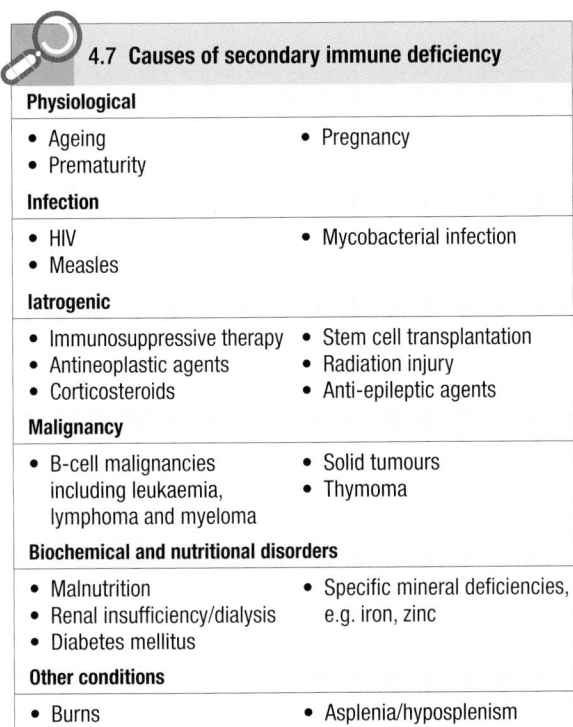

4.7 Causes of secondary immune deficiency

Physiological
- Ageing
- Prematurity
- Pregnancy

Infection
- HIV
- Measles
- Mycobacterial infection

Iatrogenic
- Immunosuppressive therapy
- Antineoplastic agents
- Corticosteroids
- Stem cell transplantation
- Radiation injury
- Anti-epileptic agents

Malignancy
- B-cell malignancies including leukaemia, lymphoma and myeloma
- Solid tumours
- Thymoma

Biochemical and nutritional disorders
- Malnutrition
- Renal insufficiency/dialysis
- Diabetes mellitus
- Specific mineral deficiencies, e.g. iron, zinc

Other conditions
- Burns
- Asplenia/hyposplenism

4.8 Immune senescence

- **T-cell responses:** decline, with reduced delayed type hypersensitivity responses.
- **Antibody production:** decreased for many exogenous antigens. Although autoantibody production rises, autoimmune disease is less common.
- **Response to vaccination:** reduced, e.g. 30% of healthy older people may not develop protective immunity after influenza vaccination.
- **Allergic disorders and transplant rejection:** less common.
- **Susceptibility to infection:** increased, e.g. community-acquired pneumonia by threefold and urinary tract infection by 20-fold. Latent infections including tuberculosis and herpes zoster, may be reactivated.
- **Manifestations of inflammation:** may be absent, e.g. lack of pyrexia or leucocytosis.

THE INFLAMMATORY RESPONSE

Inflammation is the response of tissues to injury or infection, and is necessary for normal repair and healing. This section focuses on the generic inflammatory response and its multisystem manifestations. The role of inflammation in specific diseases is illustrated in many other chapters of this book.

Physiology and pathology of inflammation

Acute inflammation

Acute inflammation is the result of rapid and complex interplay between the cells and soluble molecules of the innate immune system. The classical external signs include heat, redness, pain and swelling (calor, rubor, dolor and oedema, Fig. 4.8).

The inflammatory process is initiated by local tissue injury or infection. Damaged epithelial cells produce cytokines and antimicrobial peptides, causing early infiltration of phagocytic cells. As a result, there

is production of leukotrienes, prostaglandins, histamine, kinins, anaphylotoxins and inducible nitric oxide synthase within inflamed tissue. The effect is vasodilatation and increased local vascular permeability, which increases flow of fluid and cells to the affected tissue. In addition, pro-inflammatory cytokines produced at the site of injury have profound systemic effects. IL-1, TNF-α and IL-6 act on the hypothalamus to raise the temperature set-point, causing fever, and also stimulate the production of acute phase proteins by the liver.

Acute phase proteins

Acute phase proteins are produced by the liver in response to inflammatory stimuli and have a wide range of activities. C-reactive protein (CRP) and serum amyloid A may be increased 1000-fold, contributing to host defence and stimulating repair and regeneration. Fibrinogen plays an essential role in wound healing, and α₁-antitrypsin and α₁-antichymotrypsin control the pro-inflammatory cascade by neutralising the enzymes produced by activated neutrophils, preventing widespread tissue destruction. In addition, antioxidants such as haptoglobin and manganese superoxide dismutase scavenge for oxygen free radicals, while increased levels

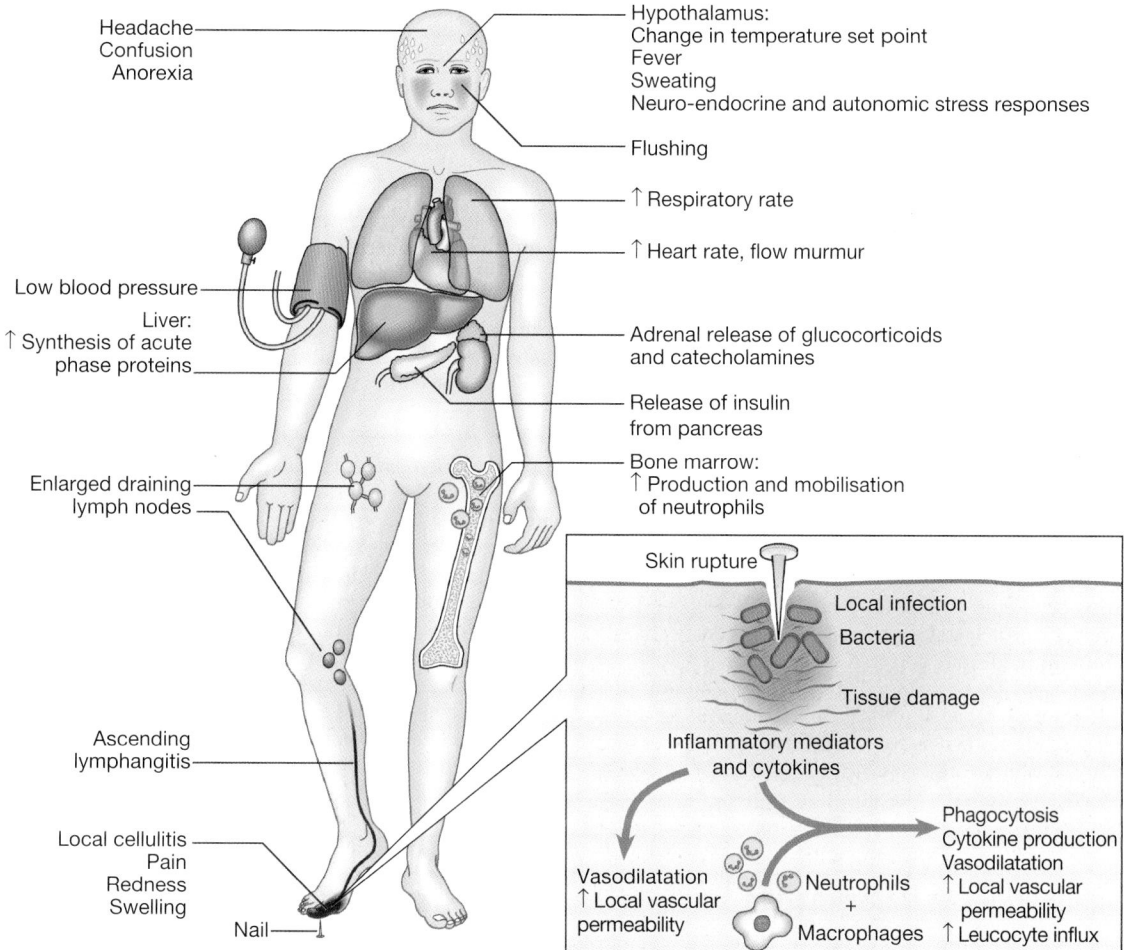

Fig. 4.8 Clinical features of acute inflammation. In this example, the response is to a penetrating injury and infection of the foot.

of iron-binding proteins such as transferrin, ferritin and lactoferrin decrease the iron available for uptake by bacteria. Immunoglobulins are not acute phase proteins but are often increased in chronic inflammation.

Resolution of inflammation

Resolution of an inflammatory response is crucial for normal healing. This involves active down-modulation of inflammatory stimuli and repair of bystander damage to local tissues. Extravasated neutrophils undergo apoptosis and are phagocytosed by macrophages, along with the remains of microorganisms. Macrophages also synthesise collagenase and elastase, which break down local connective tissue and aid in the removal of debris. Macrophage-derived cytokines, including transforming growth factor (TGF)-β and platelet-derived growth factor, attract fibroblasts and promote the synthesis of new collagen, while angiogenic factors stimulate new vessel formation.

Sepsis and septic shock

Septic shock is the clinical manifestation of overwhelming inflammation (p. 186). Failure of normal inhibitory mechanisms results in excessive production of pro-inflammatory cytokines by macrophages, causing hypotension, hypovolaemia, decreased perfusion and tissue oedema. In addition, uncontrolled neutrophil activation causes release of proteases and oxygen free radicals within blood vessels, damaging the vascular endothelium and further increasing capillary permeability. Direct activation of the coagulation pathway combines with endothelial cell disruption to form clots within the damaged vessels. The clinical consequences include cardiovascular collapse, acute respiratory distress syndrome, disseminated intravascular coagulation, multi-organ failure and often death. Septic shock most frequently results from infection with Gram-negative bacteria, because lipopolysaccharide is particularly effective at activating the inflammatory cascade.

Chronic inflammation

In most instances, the development of an active immune response results in either clearance or control of the inflammatory stimulus with minimal local damage. Failure of elimination may result in chronic inflammation. Persisting microorganisms stimulate the ongoing accumulation of neutrophils, macrophages and activated T lymphocytes. If this is associated with local deposition of fibrous connective tissue, a granuloma may form. Granulomas are characteristic of infections such as tuberculosis and leprosy, in which the microorganism is protected by a robust cell wall which shields it from killing, despite phagocytosis.

Inappropriately vigorous or prolonged immune responses may cause significant bystander tissue damage. These are known as hypersensitivity responses and may involve either antibody- or cell-mediated responses. The Gell and Coombs classification of hypersensitivity responses is discussed on page 86.

Investigations in inflammation

The changes associated with inflammation are reflected in many laboratory investigations. Leucocytosis is common, and reflects the transit of activated neutrophils and monocytes to the site of infection. The platelet count may also be increased. Chronic inflammation is frequently associated with a normocytic normochromic anaemia of chronic disease (p. 1019). The CRP (see below) is the most widely used clinical measure of acute inflammation, but increased levels of fibrinogen, ferritin and complement components are also associated with the acute phase response, while albumin levels are reduced.

C-reactive protein

C-reactive protein is an acute phase reactant synthesised by the liver, which opsonises invading pathogens. Levels of CRP increase within 6 hours of an inflammatory stimulus and may rise up to 1000-fold. Measurement of CRP provides a direct index of acute inflammation and, because the plasma half-life of CRP is 19 hours, levels fall promptly once the stimulus is removed. Sequential measurement is useful in monitoring disease activity (Box 4.9). For reasons which remain unclear, some diseases are associated with only minor elevations of CRP concentration despite unequivocal evidence of active inflammation. These include SLE, systemic sclerosis, ulcerative colitis and leukaemia. An important practical point is that intercurrent infection does provoke a significant CRP response in these conditions.

Erythrocyte sedimentation rate (ESR)

In contrast to the CRP, the ESR is an indirect measure of the acute phase response. It measures the rate of fall of erythrocytes through plasma, and a major determinant of this is aggregation of red cells. Normally, erythrocytes do not clump together because of their repellent negative charge. Plasma proteins are positively charged and act to neutralise the surface charge of erythrocytes; therefore an increase in plasma proteins, particularly fibrinogen, overcomes the repulsive forces of erythrocytes, causing them to stack together like tyres, or rouleaux. Rouleaux have a higher mass/surface area ratio than single red cells, and therefore sediment faster. Thus the ESR is a composite measure of erythrocyte morphology and of plasma protein composition and concentration.

The most common cause of an increased ESR is an acute phase response, which causes an increase in plasma protein concentration. This is accompanied by a corresponding increase in circulating CRP levels. However, other conditions that do not affect acute phase proteins may alter plasma protein composition and concentration (see Box 4.9). For example, immunoglobulins comprise a significant proportion of plasma proteins, but do not participate in the acute phase response. Thus any condition that causes a monoclonal or polyclonal increase in serum immunoglobulins will increase the ESR without a corresponding increase in CRP. In addition, changes in erythrocyte surface area and density influence sedimentation, and abnormal red cell morphology can make rouleaux formation impossible. For these reasons, an inappropriately low ESR occurs in spherocytosis and sickle cell anaemia.

As CRP is a simpler and more sensitive early indicator of the acute phase response, it is increasingly used in preference to the ESR. If both ESR and CRP are used, any discrepancy should be resolved by assessing the individual determinants of the ESR, i.e. full blood count and film, serum immunoglobulins (IgG, IgA and IgM) and protein

4.9 Conditions commonly associated with abnormal CRP and/or ESR

Condition	Consequence	Effect on CRP[1]	Effect on ESR[2]
Acute bacterial, fungal or viral infection	Stimulates acute phase response	Increased (range 50–150 mg/L; in severe infections may be > 300 mg/L)	Increased
Necrotising bacterial infection	Stimulates profound acute inflammatory response	Increased +++ (may be > 300 mg/L)	Increased
Chronic bacterial or fungal infection, e.g. localised abscess, bacterial endocarditis or tuberculosis	Stimulates acute and chronic inflammatory response with polyclonal increase in immunoglobulins as well as increased acute phase proteins	Increased (range 50–150 mg/L)	Increase disproportionate to CRP
Acute inflammatory diseases, e.g. Crohn's disease, polymyalgia rheumatica	Stimulates acute phase response	Increased (range 50–150 mg/L)	Increased
SLE, Sjögren's syndrome	Chronic inflammatory response	Normal (paradoxically)	Increased
Multiple myeloma	Monoclonal increase in serum immunoglobulin without acute inflammation	Normal	Increased
Pregnancy, old age, end-stage renal disease	Increased fibrinogen	Normal	Moderately increased

[1]Normal range < 10 mg/L.
[2]Normal range: adult males < 10 mm/hr, adult females < 20 mm/hr.

4

electrophoresis. The IgE concentration in plasma is very low and does not contribute significantly to the ESR.

Plasma viscosity

Plasma viscosity is another surrogate measure of plasma protein concentration. Like the ESR, it is affected by the concentration of large plasma proteins, including fibrinogen and immunoglobulins, especially IgM. However, it is not affected by haematocrit variations or by delay in analysis, and is generally considered to be more reliable than the ESR.

Presenting problems in inflammation

In most patients presenting with the manifestations of acute inflammation shown in Figure 4.8, it is possible to identify the source of the problem quickly and to assess the consequences, as discussed in other chapters. Systemic manifestations of inflammation include fever (p. 292), leucocytosis (p. 1000) and shock (p. 186).

Unexplained raised ESR

The ESR should not be used to screen asymptomatic patients for the presence of disease. However, in the era of frequent routine laboratory testing, an unexplained raised ESR is a common problem.

Clinical assessment

A comprehensive history and examination are crucial. Extreme elevations in the ESR (> 100 mm/hr) rarely occur in the absence of significant disease (see Box 4.9).

Investigations

Assessing the CRP, serum immunoglobulins and urine electrophoresis will help determine whether the eleva-

tion in ESR is due to an acute inflammatory process (see Box 4.9).

A full blood count and film may show a normocytic, normochromic anaemia, which occurs in many chronic diseases. Leucocytosis may reflect infection, inflammatory disease or tissue necrosis. Neutrophilia suggests infection or acute inflammation. Atypical lymphocytes may occur in some chronic infections, such as CMV and EBV.

Abnormalities in liver function suggest either a local infective process (hepatitis, hepatic abscess or biliary sepsis) or systemic disease, including malignancy.

Blood and urine cultures should be performed.

Imaging

A chest X-ray and abdominal CT scan may identify a source of unknown infection or malignancy. An abdominal and pelvic ultrasound may identify hepatic lesions, abdominal nodes and local intra-abdominal or pelvic abscesses. An MRI scan is more appropriate for the diagnosis of soft tissue or bone/joint infections. Echocardiography is used to look for vegetations and assess valve function in suspected bacterial endocarditis. White cell scans are rarely indicated but may occasionally be useful in identification of the site of pyogenic infection. An isotope scan may identify evidence of malignancy or focal bone infection.

Periodic fever syndromes

These rare disorders are characterised by recurrent episodes of fever and organ inflammation associated with an elevated acute phase response.

Familial Mediterranean fever (FMF)

This is the most common of the familial periodic fevers, predominantly affecting Mediterranean people, including Arabs, Turks, Sephardic Jews and Armenians. It results from mutations of the *MEFV* gene, which encodes a protein called pyrin. Pyrin regulates neutrophil-mediated inflammation by indirectly suppressing the production of IL-1. FMF is characterised by painful attacks of fever associated with peritonitis, pleuritis and arthritis, and lasts from a few hours to 4 days. During acute episodes, CRP levels are markedly increased. The majority of individuals have their first attack before the age of 20. The major complication of FMF is AA amyloidosis (see below). Colchicine significantly reduces the number of febrile episodes in 90% of patients but is ineffective during acute attacks.

Hyper-IgD syndrome (HIDS)

HIDS is an autosomal recessive disorder that causes recurrent attacks of fever, abdominal pain, diarrhoea, lymphadenopathy, arthralgia, skin lesions and aphthous ulceration. Most patients are from Western Europe, particularly the Netherlands and northern France. The defect is a mutation in the gene for mevalonate kinase, which is involved in the metabolism of cholesterol, but why this causes an inflammatory periodic fever remains unknown. Serum IgD levels are persistently elevated, and CRP levels are increased during acute attacks. No specific treatment is available, although trials of HMG CoA reductase inhibitors are ongoing.

TNF receptor-associated periodic syndrome (TRAPS)

TRAPS, also known as Hibernian fever, is an autosomal dominant syndrome causing recurrent periodic fever, arthralgia, myalgia, serositis and rashes. Attacks may be prolonged (> 1 week). During a typical attack, laboratory findings include neutrophilia, increased CRP and elevated IgA levels. The diagnosis can be confirmed by low serum levels of the soluble type 1 TNF receptor and by analysis of the *TNFRSF1A* gene. As in FMF, the major complication is amyloidosis, and regular screening for proteinuria is advised. TRAPS responds to systemic corticosteroids, and soluble TNF receptor therapy may be effective (p. 1080).

Amyloidosis

The amyloidoses are a group of acquired and hereditary disorders characterised by the extracellular deposition of insoluble proteins. These complex deposits consist of fibrils of the specific protein involved linked to glycosaminoglycans, proteoglycans and serum amyloid P (SAP). Protein accumulation may be localised or systemic, and the clinical manifestations depend upon the organ(s) affected. The diagnosis of amyloidosis should be considered in all cases of unexplained nephrotic syndrome (p. 481), cardiomyopathy (p. 635) and peripheral neuropathy (p. 1225).

Amyloid diseases are classified by aetiology and type of protein deposited (Box 4.10).

4.10 Amyloid disorders

Disorder	Pathological basis	Predisposing conditions	Other features
Acquired systemic amyloidosis			
Reactive (AA) amyloidosis	Increased production of serum amyloid A as part of prolonged or recurrent acute inflammatory response	Chronic infection (TB, bronchiectasis, chronic abscess, osteomyelitis) Chronic inflammatory diseases (rheumatoid arthritis, FMF)	90% of patients present with non-selective proteinuria or nephrotic syndrome
Light chain amyloidosis (AL)	Increased production of monoclonal light chain	Monoclonal gammopathies, including myeloma, benign gammopathies and plasmacytoma	Restrictive cardiomyopathy, peripheral and autonomic neuropathy, carpal tunnel syndrome, proteinuria, spontaneous purpura, amyloid nodules and plaques. Macroglossia occurs rarely but is pathognomonic. Prognosis is poor
Dialysis-associated (Aβ2M) amyloidosis	Accumulation of circulating β_2-microglobulin due to failure of renal catabolism in kidney failure	Renal dialysis	Carpal tunnel syndrome, chronic arthropathy and pathological fractures secondary to amyloid bone cyst formation. Manifestations occur 5–10 years after the start of dialysis
Senile systemic amyloidosis	Normal transthyretin protein deposited in tissues	Age > 70 yrs	Feature of normal ageing (affects > 90% of 90 year olds). Usually asymptomatic
Hereditary systemic amyloidosis			
> 20 forms of hereditary systemic amyloidosis	Production of protein with an abnormal structure that predisposes to amyloid fibril formation. Most commonly due to mutations in *transthyretin* gene	Autosomal dominant inheritance	Peripheral and autonomic neuropathy, cardiomyopathy Renal involvement unusual 10% of gene carriers are asymptomatic throughout life

Diagnosis

The diagnosis is established by biopsy, which may be of an affected organ, rectum or subcutaneous fat. The pathognomonic histological feature is apple-green bi-refringence of amyloid deposits when stained with Congo red dye and viewed under polarised light. Immunohistochemical staining can identify the type of amyloid fibril present. Quantitative scintigraphy with radiolabelled serum amyloid P is a valuable tool in determining the overall load and distribution of amyloid deposits.

Management

The aims of treatment are to support the function of affected organs and, in acquired amyloidosis, to prevent further amyloid deposition through treatment of the primary cause. When the latter is possible, regression of existing amyloid deposits may occur. Liver transplantation may provide definitive treatment in selected patients with hereditary transthyretin amyloidosis.

AUTOIMMUNE DISEASE

Autoimmunity can be defined as the presence of immune responses against self tissue, and is to some extent ubiquitous. It is often a harmless phenomenon, identified only by the presence of low titre autoantibodies or autoreactive T cells. However, autoimmune diseases occur if these responses cause significant organ damage. These are a major cause of chronic morbidity and disability, affecting up to 1 in 30 adults at some time (Box 4.11).

4.11 The spectrum of autoimmune disease

Type	Disease	Page no.
Organ-specific		
Immune response directed against localised antigens	Graves' disease	745
	Hashimoto's thyroiditis	748
	Addison's disease	775
	Pernicious anaemia	1021
	Type 1 diabetes	800
	Sympathetic ophthalmoplegia	1162
	Goodpasture's syndrome	502
	Pemphigus vulgaris	1275
	Bullous pemphigoid	1275
	Idiopathic thrombocytopenic purpura	1045
	Autoimmune haemolytic anaemia	1025
	Myasthenia gravis	1231
	Primary antiphospholipid syndrome	1050
	Rheumatoid arthritis	1088
	Dermatomyositis	1111
	Primary biliary cirrhosis	963
	Autoimmune hepatitis	962
	Sjögren's syndrome	1111
Multisystem		
Immune response directed to widespread target antigens	Systemic sclerosis	1109
	Mixed connective tissue disease	1111
	SLE	1107

Physiology and pathology of autoimmunity

Immunological tolerance

This is the process by which the immune system distinguishes self from foreign tissue, failure of which may result in autoimmune disease.

Central tolerance occurs during lymphocyte development and operates in the thymus and bone marrow. Here, T and B lymphocytes that recognise self antigens are eliminated before they develop into fully immunocompetent cells. This process is most active in fetal life, but continues throughout life as immature lymphocytes are generated.

Some autoreactive cells inevitably evade deletion and escape into the peripheral circulation. These cells are controlled through peripheral tolerance mechanisms. These include the suppression of autoreactive cells by regulatory T cells, and the generation of hyporesponsiveness ('anergy') in lymphocytes which encounter antigen in the absence of the co-stimulatory signals that accompany inflammation. Some tissues such as the eye are not normally patrolled by lymphocytes. Antigens within these 'immunologically privileged' sites are inaccessible to autoreactive cells.

Factors predisposing to autoimmune disease

Both genetic and environmental factors contribute. Autoimmune diseases are much more common in women than in men, for reasons which remain unclear. The most important genetic determinants of autoimmune susceptibility are the HLA genes, reflecting their importance in shaping lymphocyte responses (Box 4.12). Other susceptibility genes include those determining cytokine activity, co-stimulation and cell death.

Several environmental factors can trigger autoimmunity in genetically predisposed individuals. The most widely studied of these is infection, as occurs in acute rheumatic fever following streptococcal infection or reactive arthritis following bacterial infection. A number of mechanisms have been postulated, such as cross-reactivity between the infectious pathogen and self determinants (molecular mimicry), and release of sequestered antigens, which are not usually visible to the immune system, from damaged tissue. Alternatively, infection may result in the production of inflammatory cytokines which overwhelm the normal control mechanisms that prevent bystander damage. Occasionally, the development of autoimmune disease is a side-effect of drug treatment. For example, the metabolic products of

4.12 HLA associations in autoimmune disease

Disease	HLA association	Relative risk
Ankylosing spondylitis	B27	~90:1
Type 1 diabetes	DR3/DR4	~20:1
Rheumatoid arthritis	DR4	~5:1
Graves' disease	DR3	~5:1
Myasthenia gravis	DR3	~3:1

i **4.13 Gell and Coombs classification of hypersensitivity diseases**

Type	Mechanism	Example of disease in response to exogenous agent	Example of autoimmune disease
Type I Immediate hypersensitivity	IgE-mediated mast cell degranulation	Allergic disease	None described
Type II Antibody-mediated	Binding of cytotoxic IgG or IgM antibodies to antigens on cell surface causes cell killing	ABO blood transfusion reaction Hyperacute transplant rejection	Autoimmune haemolytic anaemia Idiopathic thrombocytopenic purpura Goodpasture's disease
Type III Immune complex-mediated	IgG or IgM antibodies bind soluble antigen to form immune complexes which trigger classical complement pathway activation	Serum sickness Farmer's lung	SLE
Type IV Delayed type	Activated T cells, phagocytes and NK cells	Acute cellular transplant rejection Nickel hypersensitivity	Type 1 diabetes Hashimoto's thyroiditis

the anaesthetic agent halothane bind to liver enzymes, resulting in a structurally novel protein. This is recognised as a new (foreign) antigen by the immune system, and the autoantibodies and activated T cells directed against it may cause hepatic necrosis.

Classification of autoimmune diseases

The spectrum of autoimmune diseases is broad. These diseases be classified as organ-specific or multisystem (see Box 4.11), or by the predominant mechanism responsible for tissue damage. The Gell and Coombs classification of hypersensitivity is the most widely used, and distinguishes four types of immune response which result in bystander tissue damage (Box 4.13).

- *Type I hypersensitivity* is relevant in allergy but is not associated with autoimmune disease.
- In *type II hypersensitivity*, injury is localised to a single tissue or organ.
- *Type III hypersensitivity* is a generalised reaction resulting from immune complex deposition in blood vessel walls, skin, joints and glomeruli, where they cause a chronic inflammatory response. This triggers the classical complement cascade as well as recruitment and activation of phagocytes and CD4+ lymphocytes. The site of immune complex deposition is determined by the relative amount of antibody, size of the immune complexes, nature of the antigen and local haemodynamics. Generalised deposition of immune complexes gives rise to systemic diseases such as SLE.
- In *type IV hypersensitivity*, activated T cells and macrophages mediate phagocytosis and NK cell recruitment. Autoantibodies may occur but these are not primarily responsible for the tissue damage.

Investigations in autoimmunity

Autoantibodies

An increasing number of autoantibodies can be identified in the laboratory and are useful in disease diagnosis and monitoring, as discussed elsewhere in this book (e.g. p. 1063). Antibody is quantified either by titre (the

minimal dilution at which the antibody can be detected) or by concentration in standardised units.

Cryoglobulins

Cryoglobulins are antibodies directed against other immunoglobulins that form immune complexes which precipitate in the cold. They are classified into three types on the basis of the properties of the immunoglobulin involved (Box 4.14). Testing for cryoglobulins requires the transport of a serum specimen to the laboratory at 37°C. Cryoglobulins should not be confused with cold agglutinins; the latter are autoantibodies specifically directed against the I/i antigen on the surface of red cells, which can cause intravascular haemolysis in the cold (p. 1026).

Measures of complement activation

Quantitation of complement components may be useful in the evaluation of immune complex-mediated diseases. Classical complement pathway activation leads to a decrease in circulating (unactivated) C4, and is often also associated with decreased C3 levels. Serial measurement of C3 and C4 is a useful surrogate measure of immune complex formation.

ALLERGY

Allergic diseases are a common and increasing cause of illness, affecting between 15% and 20% of the population at some time. They comprise a range of disorders from mild to life-threatening, and affect many organs. Atopy is the tendency to produce an exaggerated IgE immune response to otherwise harmless environmental substances, and an allergic disease may be defined as the clinical manifestation of this inappropriate IgE immune response.

Pathology of allergy

Normally, the immune system does not make detectable responses to the many environmental substances to which it is exposed on a daily basis. However, in an allergic reaction, initial exposure to an otherwise harmless

4.14 Classification of cryoglobulins

	Type I	Type II	Type III
Immunoglobulin isotype and specificity	Monoclonal IgM paraprotein with no particular specificity	Monoclonal IgM paraprotein directed towards constant region of IgG	Polyclonal IgM or IgG directed towards constant region of IgG
Prevalence	25%	25%	50%
Disease association	Lymphoproliferative disease, especially Waldenström's macroglobulinaemia (p. 1041)	Infection, particularly hepatitis B and hepatitis C; lymphoproliferative disease	Infection, particularly hepatitis B and C; autoimmune disease, including rheumatoid arthritis and SLE

Symptoms	Hyperviscosity:
	  Raynaud's phenomenon
	  Acrocyanosis
	  Retinal vessel occlusion
	  Arterial and venous thrombosis
		Small-vessel vasculitis:
		  Purpuric rash
		  Arthralgia
		  Cutaneous ulceration
		  Hepatosplenomegaly
		  Glomerulonephritis
		  Raynaud's phenomenon
			Small-vessel vasculitis:
			  Purpuric rash
			  Arthralgia
			  Cutaneous ulceration
			  Hepatosplenomegaly
			  Glomerulonephritis
			  Raynaud's phenomenon

Protein electrophoresis	Monoclonal IgM paraprotein	Monoclonal IgM paraprotein	No monoclonal paraprotein
Rheumatoid factor	Negative	Strongly positive	Strongly positive
Complement	Normal	Decreased C4	Decreased C4
Serum viscosity	Raised	Normal	Normal

4

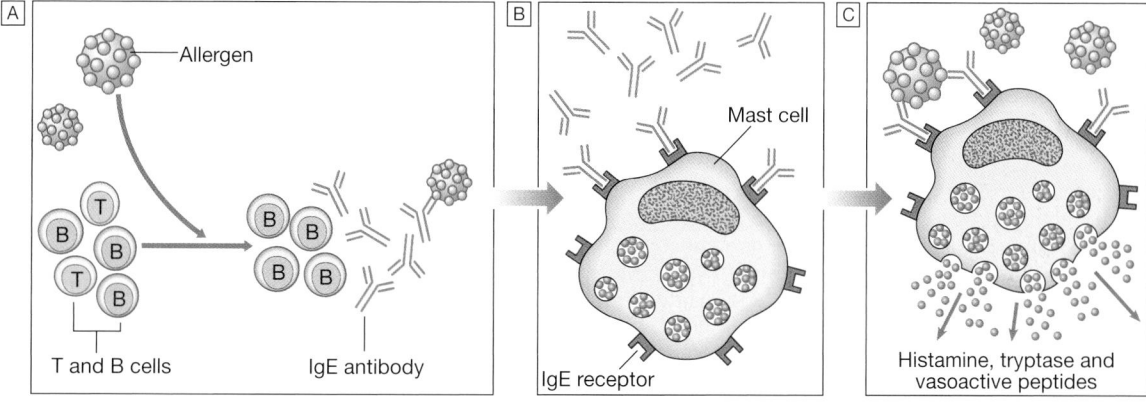

Fig. 4.9 Type I (immediate) hypersensitivity response. [A] After an encounter with allergen, B cells produce IgE antibody against the allergen. [B] Specific IgE antibodies bind to circulating mast cells via high-affinity IgE cell surface receptors. [C] On re-encounter with allergen, the allergen binds to the IgE antibody-coated mast cells. This triggers mast cell activation with release of vasoactive mediators (see Box 4.15).

exogenous substance (known as an allergen) triggers the production of specific IgE antibodies by activated B cells (Fig. 4.9 and Box 4.15). These IgE antibodies bind to the surface of mast cells via high-affinity IgE receptors, a step that is not immediately associated with clinical sequelae. However, upon re-exposure, the allergen binds to membrane-bound IgE which activates the mast cells, releasing a variety of vasoactive mediators (the early phase response) and causing a type I hypersensitivity reaction and the symptoms of allergy. The latter range from sneezing and rhinorrhoea to anaphylaxis (Box 4.16).

Persistent activation of mast cells may result in the recruitment of other cells, and in some patients the early phase response is followed 4–8 hours later by persistent swelling and local inflammation. This is known as the late phase reaction and is mediated by basophils, eosin-ophils and macrophages. Long-standing or recurrent allergic inflammation may give rise to a chronic inflammatory response characterised by a complex infiltrate of macrophages, eosinophils and T lymphocytes, in addition to mast cells and basophils. Once this has been established, inhibition of mast cell mediators with antihistamines is clinically ineffective.

Mast cell activation may also be non-specifically triggered through a variety of other signals such as neuropeptides, anaphylotoxins and bacterial peptides.

Factors influencing susceptibility to allergic diseases

The incidence of allergic diseases is increasing in both industrialised and non-industrialised countries. This trend is largely unexplained but one widely held theory

i 4.15 Products of mast cell degranulation

Mediator	Biological effects
Preformed and stored within granules	
Histamine	Vasodilatation, chemotaxis, bronchoconstriction and mucus secretion. Increases capillary permeability
Tryptase	Activates complement C3
Eosinophil chemotactic factor	Eosinophil chemotaxis
Neutrophil chemotactic factor	Neutrophil chemotaxis
Synthesised on activation of mast cells	
Leukotrienes	Increase vascular permeability, chemotaxis, mucus secretion and smooth muscle contraction
Prostaglandins	Bronchoconstriction, platelet aggregation and vasodilatation
Thromboxanes	Bronchoconstriction
Platelet-activating factor	Bronchoconstriction, chemotaxis of eosinophils and neutrophils

i 4.16 Common allergic diseases

- Urticaria — p. 1248
- Angioedema — p. 91
- Atopic dermatitis — p. 1257
- Allergic conjunctivitis — pp. 1094, 1096
- Allergic rhinitis (hayfever) — p. 721
- Allergic asthma — p. 662
- Food allergy — p. 886
- Drug allergy — p. 1286
- Allergy to insect venom — p. 91
- Anaphylaxis — p. 89

is the 'hygiene hypothesis'. This proposes that infections in early life bias the immune system against the development of allergies, and that allergy is the penalty for the decreased incidence of infection that has resulted from improvements in sanitation and health care.

A number of other factors contribute to the development of allergic diseases, the strongest of which is a family history. A wide array of genetic determinants of disease susceptibility have been identified, including genes controlling cytokine production, IgE levels and the ability of the epithelial barrier to protect against environmental agents. The expression of a genetic predisposition is governed by environmental factors such as pollutants and cigarette smoke, and the incidence of bacterial and viral infection.

Presenting problems in allergy

A general approach to the allergic patient

Common presentations of allergic disease are shown in Box 4.16. This chapter describes the general principles of the approach to the allergic patient and some of the more severe manifestations of allergy.

Clinical assessment

When assessing possible allergic disease, it is important to identify what the patient means by allergy, as up to 20% of the UK population describe themselves as having a food allergy, although < 1% have an IgE-mediated hypersensitivity reaction confirmed on double blind challenge. The nature of symptoms should be established and specific triggers identified, along with the predictability of a reaction, and the time lag between exposure to a potential allergen and onset of symptoms. An allergic reaction usually occurs within minutes of exposure and provokes predictable symptoms (angioedema, urticaria, wheezing

and so on). Specific enquiry should be made about other allergic symptoms, past and present, and about family history of allergic disease. Potential allergens in the home and workplace should be identified, and a detailed drug history should always be taken, including compliance, side-effects and the use of complementary therapies.

Investigations

Skin prick tests

Skin prick testing is the 'gold standard' of allergy testing. A droplet of diluted standardised allergen solution is placed on the forearm and the skin is superficially punctured through the droplet with a sterile lancet. After 15 minutes, a positive response is indicated by a local weal and flare response ≥ 2 mm larger than the negative control. A major advantage of skin prick testing is that patients can clearly see the results, which may be useful in gaining compliance with avoidance measures. Disadvantages include the remote risk of a severe allergic reaction, so resuscitation facilities should be available. Results are unreliable in patients with extensive skin disease. Antihistamines inhibit the magnitude of the response and should be discontinued for at least 4 days before testing; corticosteroids do not influence test results.

Specific IgE tests

An alternative to skin prick testing is the quantitation of IgE directed against the putative allergen. The sensitivity and specificity of specific IgE tests (previously known as radioallergosorbent tests, RAST) are lower than skin prick tests. However, IgE tests may be very useful if skin testing is inappropriate: for example, in patients taking antihistamines or those who have severe skin disease or dermatographism. They can also be used to test for cross-reactivity with multiple insect venoms, and post mortem to identify allergens responsible for lethal anaphylaxis.

There is no indication for routine testing of specific IgG antibodies in the investigation of allergic diseases.

Supervised exposure to allergen (challenge test)

Allergen challenges are usually performed in specialist centres, and include bronchial provocation testing, nasal challenge and food challenge. These may be particularly useful in the investigation of occupational asthma or food allergy.

Mast cell tryptase

After a systemic allergic reaction, the circulating level of mast cell mediators increases dramatically. Tryptase is the most stable of these and serum levels peak at 1–2 hours, remaining elevated for 24 hours. Measurement of serum mast cell tryptase is extremely useful in investigating a possible anaphylactic event. Ideally, measurements should be made at the time of the reaction, and 3 hours and 24 hours later.

Non-specific markers of atopic disease: total serum IgE and eosinophilia

Peripheral blood eosinophilia is common in atopic individuals. However, eosinophilia > 20% or an absolute eosinophil count > 1.5×10^9/L should initiate a search for a non-atopic cause (p. 307).

Atopy is the most common cause of elevated total IgE in developed countries. However, there are many other causes of raised total IgE, including parasite and helminth infections (pp. 364 and 376), lymphoma (p. 1037), drug reactions and Churg–Strauss vasculitis (p. 1114). Moreover, significant allergic disease can occur despite a normal total IgE level. Thus total IgE quantitation is not indicated in the routine investigation of allergic disease.

Management

- *Avoidance of the allergen* should be rigorously attempted, and the advice of specialist dietitians and occupational physicians may be required.
- *Antihistamines* block histamine H₁ tissue receptors, thereby inhibiting the effects of histamine release. Long-acting, non-sedating preparations are particularly useful for prophylaxis against frequent attacks.
- *Corticosteroids* down-regulate pro-inflammatory cytokine production. They are highly effective in allergic disease, and if used topically their adverse effects may be minimised.
- *Sodium cromoglicate* stabilises the mast cell membrane, inhibiting release of vasoactive mediators. It is effective as a prophylactic agent in asthma and allergic rhinitis, but has no role in management of acute attacks. It is poorly absorbed and therefore ineffective in the management of food allergies.
- *Antigen-specific immunotherapy* involves the sequential administration of escalating amounts of dilute allergen over a prolonged period of time. Its mechanism of action is unknown, but it is highly effective in the prevention of insect venom anaphylaxis, and allergic rhinitis secondary to grass pollen (Box 4.17). The traditional route of administration is via subcutaneous injections, which carry a risk of anaphylaxis and should only be performed in specialised centres. More recently, sublingual immunotherapy has been shown to be effective in the management of moderate grass pollen allergy.
- *Omalizumab*, a monoclonal antibody against IgE, inhibits the binding of IgE to mast cells and basophils. It is effective in moderate and severe allergic asthma and rhinitis.
- *Preloaded self-injectable adrenaline (epinephrine)* may be life-saving in the acute management of anaphylaxis.

EBM 4.17 **Immunotherapy for allergy**

'Immunotherapy is effective for treatment of allergic rhinitis, allergic asthma and stinging insect hypersensitivity. Clinical studies to date do not support the use of allergen immunotherapy for food hypersensitivity, chronic urticaria and/or angioedema.'

- Joint Task Force on Practice Parameters. Ann Allergy Asthma Immunol 2003; 90:1–40.

For further information: www.cochrane.org

4

Anaphylaxis

Anaphylaxis is a potentially life-threatening, systemic allergic reaction caused by the release of histamine and other vasoactive mediators from mast cells. The risk of death is increased in patients with pre-existing asthma, particularly if this is poorly controlled, and in individuals in whom treatment with adrenaline (epinephrine) is delayed.

Clinical assessment

The clinical features are shown in Figure 4.10. The severity of a reaction should be assessed; the time between allergen exposure and onset of symptoms provides a guide. Enquiry should be made about potential triggers; if these are not immediately obvious, a detailed history of the previous 24 hours may be helpful. The most common allergens are foods, latex, insect venom and drugs (Box 4.18). A history of previous local allergic responses to the offending agent is common. The route of allergen exposure may influence the principal clinical features of a reaction; for example, if an allergen is inhaled,

4.18 Common causes of immediate generalised reactions

Anaphylaxis: IgE-mediated mast cell degranulation

Foods
- Peanuts
- Tree nuts
- Fish and shellfish
- Milk
- Eggs
- Soy products

Insect stings
- Bee venom
- Wasp venom

Chemicals, drugs and other foreign proteins
- Intravenous anaesthetic agents, e.g. suxamethonium, propofol
- Penicillin and other antibiotics
- Latex

Anaphylactoid: non-IgE-mediated mast cell degranulation

Drugs
- Aspirin and non-steroidal anti-inflammatory drugs (NSAIDs)
- Opiates
- Radiocontrast media

Physical
- Exercise
- Cold

Idiopathic
- No cause is identified in 20% of patients with anaphylaxis

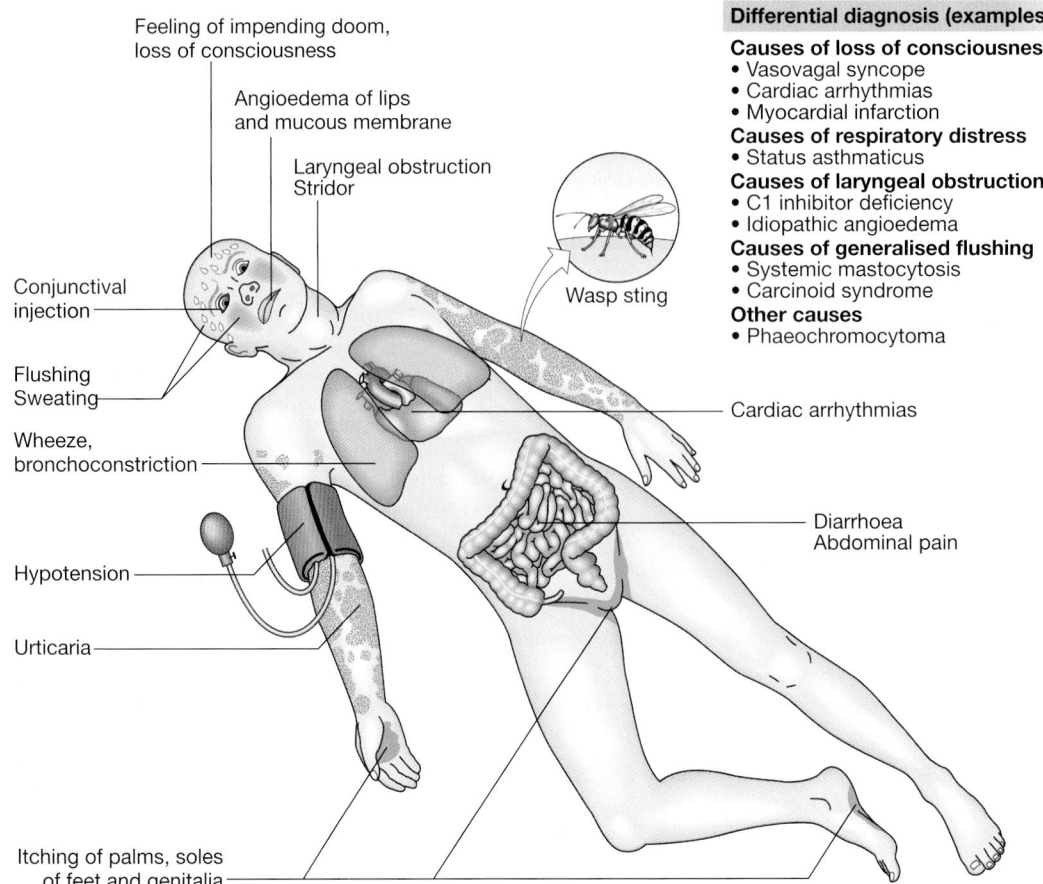

Fig. 4.10 Clinical manifestations of anaphylaxis. In this example, the response is to an insect sting containing venom to which the patient is allergic.

the major symptom is frequently wheezing. Features of anaphylaxis may overlap with the direct toxic effects of drugs and venoms (Ch. 9). Potentiating factors such as exercise or alcohol can lower the threshold for an anaphylactic event.

A number of conditions may mimic anaphylaxis (see Fig. 4.10). Anaphylactoid reactions result from the non-specific degranulation of mast cells by drugs, chemicals or other triggers (see Box 4.18), and do not involve IgE antibodies. The clinical presentations are indistinguishable, and in the acute situation discriminating between them is unnecessary. However, this may be important in identifying precipitating factors and appropriate avoidance measures.

Investigations

Measurement of acute and convalescent serum mast cell tryptase concentrations is useful to confirm the diagnosis. Specific IgE tests may be preferable to skin prick tests when investigating patients with a history of anaphylaxis.

Management

Anaphylaxis is an acute medical emergency (Box 4.19).

Individuals who have recovered from an anaphylactic event should be referred for specialist assessment. The aim is to identify the trigger factor, to educate the patient

---

4.19 Emergency management of anaphylaxis

Prevent further contact with allergen
- e.g. Removal of bee sting

Ensure airway patency

Administer *intramuscular* adrenaline (epinephrine) promptly
- Adult dose: 0.3–1.0 mL 1:1000 solution
- Acts within minutes
- Repeat at 5–10 min intervals if initial response is inadequate

Administer antihistamines
- e.g. Chlorphenamine 10 mg i.m. or slow i.v. injection
- Directly opposes effects of mast cell activation

Administer corticosteroids
- e.g. Hydrocortisone 200 mg i.v.
- Prevents rebound symptoms in severely affected patients

Provide supportive treatments
- e.g. Nebulised β_2-agonists to decrease bronchoconstriction
- I.v. fluids to restore or maintain blood pressure
- Oxygen

4.20 Prescribing self-injectable adrenaline (epinephrine)

Prescription of an adrenaline auto-injector is usually initiated by a specialist (e.g. immunologist or allergist)

Indications

- Anaphylaxis to allergens which are not easy to avoid, e.g. venom and foods
- Idiopathic anaphylactic reactions
- History of localised reactions with high risk of future anaphylaxis, e.g. reaction to trace allergen or likely repeated exposure to allergen
- History of localised reactions with high risk of adverse outcome, should anaphylaxis occur, e.g. poorly controlled asthma, lack of access to emergency care

Relative contraindications

Risk of arrhythmia or acute coronary syndrome
- Ischaemic heart disease, uncontrolled hypertension
- Tricyclic antidepressants, monoamine oxidase inhibitors, cocaine

Risk of hypertension

Key practice points

Patient and family education
- Know when and how to use the device
- Carry the device at all times
- Seek medical assistance immediately after use
- Wear an alert bracelet or necklace
- Include the school in education for young patients (www.allergyinschools.org.uk)

Prescriptions
- Specify the brand of auto-injector (Epipen® or Anapen®), as they have different triggering mechanisms
- Always prescribe two syringes
- Avoid β-blockers, as they may increase the severity of an anaphylactic reaction and reduce the response to adrenaline

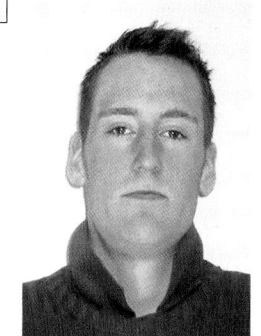 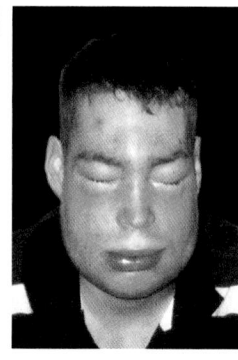

Fig. 4.11 Angioedema. This young man has hereditary angioedema. **A** Normal appearance. **B** During an acute attack.

regarding avoidance and management of subsequent episodes, and to identify whether specific treatment such as immunotherapy is indicated. If the trigger factor cannot be identified or cannot be avoided, recurrence is common. Patients who have previously experienced an anaphylactic event should be prescribed self-injectable adrenaline and they and their families or carers should be instructed on its use (Box 4.20). The use of a MedicAlert (or similar) bracelet will increase the likelihood that adrenaline (epinephrine) will be administered in an emergency.

Angioedema

Angioedema is the episodic, localised, non-pitting swelling of submucous or subcutaneous tissues. This most frequently affects the face (Fig. 4.11), extremities and genitalia. Involvement of the larynx or tongue may cause life-threatening respiratory tract obstruction, and oedema of the intestine may cause abdominal pain and distension.

In most cases, the underlying mechanism is degranulation of mast cells. However, angioedema may occasionally be mediated by increased local bradykinin concentration (Box 4.21). Differentiating the mechanism of angioedema is important in determining appropriate investigations and treatment.

Specific allergies

Insect venom allergy

Local non-IgE-mediated reactions to insect stings are common and may cause extensive swelling around the site lasting as long as 7 days. These usually do not require specific treatment. Toxic reactions to venom after multiple (50–100) simultaneous stings may mimic anaphylaxis. In addition, exposure to large amounts of insect venom frequently stimulates the production of IgE antibodies, and thus may be followed by allergic reactions to single stings. Allergic IgE-mediated reactions vary from mild to life-threatening. Antigen-specific immunotherapy with bee or wasp venom reduces the incidence of recurrent anaphylaxis from 50–60% to 10% after 2 years of treatment (see Box 4.17).

Peanut allergy

Peanut allergy is the most common food-related allergy. More than 50% of patients present before the age of 3 years and some individuals react to their first known exposure to peanuts, possibly because of sensitisation by topical creams. Peanuts are ubiquitous in the Western diet, and every year up to 25% of peanut-allergic individuals will experience a reaction as a result of inadvertent exposure. Peanut allergy only occasionally resolves and life-long avoidance is recommended.

Birch oral allergy syndrome

This syndrome is characterised by birch pollen hayfever, and local angioedema after contact with fresh fruit (especially apples), vegetables and nuts. Cooked fruits and vegetables are tolerated without difficulty. It is due to shared or cross-reactive allergens which are destroyed by cooking or digestion, and can be confirmed by skin prick testing using fresh fruit. Severe allergic reactions are unusual.

C1 inhibitor deficiency

Hereditary angioedema (HAE)

HAE, also known as inherited C1 esterase inhibitor deficiency, is an autosomal dominant disorder caused by

i 4.21 Types of angioedema

	Allergic reaction to specific trigger	Idiopathic angioedema	Hereditary angioedema	ACE-inhibitor associated angioedema
Pathogenesis	IgE-mediated degranulation of mast cells	Non-IgE-mediated degranulation of mast cells	C1 inhibitor deficiency, with resulting increased local bradykinin concentration	Inhibition of breakdown of bradykinin
Key mediator	Histamine	Histamine	Bradykinin	Bradykinin
Prevalence	Common	Common	Rare autosomal dominant disorder	0.1–0.2% of patients treated with ACE inhibitors
Clinical features	Usually associated with urticaria History of other allergies common Follows exposure, e.g. to food, animal dander or insect venom	Usually associated with urticaria May be triggered by physical stimuli such as heat, pressure or exercise Dermatographism common Occasionally associated with underlying infection or thyroid disease	Not associated with urticaria or other features of allergy Does not cause anaphylaxis May cause life-threatening respiratory tract obstruction Can cause severe abdominal pain	Not associated with urticaria Does not cause anaphylaxis Usually affects the head and neck, and may cause life-threatening respiratory tract obstruction Can occur years after the start of treatment
Investigations	Specific IgE tests or skin prick tests	Specific IgE tests and skin prick tests often negative Exclude hypothyroidism	Complement C4 (invariably low in acute attacks) C1 inhibitor levels	No specific investigations
Treatment	Allergen avoidance Antihistamines	Antihistamines are mainstay of treatment and prophylaxis	Unresponsive to antihistamines Attenuated androgens C1 inhibitor concentrate for acute attacks	Discontinue ACE inhibitor Avoid angiotensin II receptor blockers
Associated drug reactions	Specific drug allergies, e.g. penicillin	NSAIDs Opioids Radiocontrast		ACE inhibitors Angiotensin II receptor antagonists

decreased production or activity of C1 inhibitor protein. This complement regulatory protein inhibits spontaneous activation of the classical complement pathway (see Fig. 4.3, p. 73). C1 inhibitor is also a regulatory protein for the kinin cascade, activation of which increases local bradykinin levels and gives rise to local pain and swelling.

In HAE, angioedema may be spontaneous or triggered by local trauma or infection. Multiple parts of the body may be involved, especially the face, extremities, upper airway and gastrointestinal tract. Oedema of the intestinal wall causes severe abdominal pain and many patients with undiagnosed HAE undergo exploratory laparotomy. The most important complication is laryngeal obstruction, often associated with minor dental procedures, which can be fatal. Episodes of angioedema are self-limiting and usually resolve within 48 hours. Patients with HAE generally present in adolescence, but may go undiagnosed for many years. A family history can be identified in 80% of cases. HAE is not associated with allergic diseases and is specifically not associated with urticaria.

Acute episodes are always accompanied by low C4 levels and the diagnosis can be confirmed by C1 inhibitor measurement. Prevention is with modified androgens (e.g. danazol), which increase endogenous production of complement proteins. Severe acute attacks should be treated with infusion of purified C1 inhibitor or fresh frozen plasma.

4.22 Immunological diseases in pregnancy

Allergic disease
- **Maternal dietary restrictions during pregnancy or lactation:** current evidence does not support these for prevention of allergic disease.
- **Breastfeeding for at least 4 months:** prevents or delays the occurrence of atopic dermatitis, cow's milk allergy and wheezing in early childhood, as compared with feeding formula milk containing intact cow's milk protein.

Autoimmune disease
- **Suppressed T cell-mediated immune responses in pregnancy:** may suddenly reactivate post-partum. Autoimmune diseases often improve during pregnancy but flare immediately after delivery. However, an exception is SLE, which is prone to exacerbation in pregnancy.
- **Passive transfer of maternal antibodies:** can mediate autoimmune disease in the fetus and newborn, including SLE, Graves' disease and myasthenia gravis.
- **Antiphospholipid syndrome (p. 1050):** an important cause of fetal loss, intrauterine growth restriction and pre-eclampsia.

Acquired C1 inhibitor deficiency

This rare disorder is clinically indistinguishable from HAE but presents in late adulthood. It is associated with autoimmune and lymphoproliferative diseases. Treatment of the underlying disorder may induce remission of angioedema.

TRANSPLANTATION AND GRAFT REJECTION

Transplantation provides the opportunity for definitive treatment of end-stage organ disease (Box 4.23). The major complications are graft rejection, drug toxicity and infection consequent on immunosuppression. Transplant survival has significantly improved over the last 20 years, as a result of less toxic immunosuppressive agents and increased understanding of the process of transplant rejection.

Bone marrow stem cell transplantation and its complications are discussed on pages 1013–1014.

4.23 Number of solid organ transplants in UK per year, 2007–8[1]		
Organ	Number transplanted	Number waiting[2]
Kidney	2282	6790
Liver	660	259
Heart	127	91
Heart and lung	7	18
Lung	116	268
Kidney and pancreas	188	178

[1]From www.uktransplant.org.uk.
[2]Patients actively waiting for a transplant on 31 March 2008.

Transplant rejection

Solid organ transplantation inevitably stimulates an aggressive immune response by the recipient, unless the transplant is between monozygotic twins. The type and severity of the rejection response is determined by the genetic disparity between the donor and recipient, the immune status of the host and the nature of the tissue transplanted (Box 4.24). The most important genetic determinant is the difference between donor and recipient HLA proteins (p. 73). The extensive polymorphism of these proteins means that donor HLA antigens are almost invariably recognised as foreign by the recipient immune system, unless an active attempt has been made to minimise incompatibility.

- *Acute cellular rejection* is the most common form of graft rejection. It is mediated by activated T lymphocytes and results in deterioration in graft function. If allowed to progress, it may cause fever, pain and tenderness over the graft. It is usually amenable to increased immunosuppressive therapy.
- *Hyperacute rejection* results in rapid and irreversible destruction of the graft. It is mediated by pre-existing recipient antibodies against donor HLA antigens, which arise as a result of previous exposure through transplantation, blood transfusion or pregnancy. It is very rarely seen in clinical practice as the use of screening for anti-HLA antibodies and pre-transplant cross-matching ensures the prior identification of recipients with antibodies against a potential donor.
- *Acute vascular rejection* is mediated by antibody formed de novo after transplantation. It is more curtailed than the hyperacute response because of the use of intercurrent immunosuppression, but it is also associated with reduced graft survival. Aggressive immunosuppressive therapy is indicated, and physical removal of antibody through plasmapheresis may be effective. Not all post-transplant anti-donor antibodies cause graft damage; their consequences are determined by specificity and ability to trigger other immune components such as the complement cascade.
- *Chronic allograft failure*, also known as chronic rejection, is a major cause of graft loss. It is associated with proliferation of transplant vascular smooth muscle, interstitial fibrosis and scarring. The pathogenesis is poorly understood but contributing factors include immunological damage caused by subacute rejection, hypertension, hyperlipidaemia and chronic drug toxicity.

Investigations

Pre-transplantation testing

HLA typing determines an individual's HLA polymorphisms and facilitates donor–recipient matching.

4.24 Classification of transplant rejection				
Type	Time	Pathological findings	Mechanism	Treatment
Hyperacute rejection	Minutes to hours	Thrombosis, necrosis	Preformed antibody and complement activation (type II hypersensitivity)	None—irreversible graft loss
Acute vascular rejection	5–30 days	Vasculitis	Antibody and complement activation	Increase immunosuppression
Acute cellular rejection	5–30 days	Cellular infiltration	CD4+ and CD8+ T cells (type IV hypersensitivity)	Increase immunosuppression
Chronic allograft failure	> 30 days	Fibrosis, scarring	Immune and non-immune mechanisms	Minimise drug toxicity, control hypertension and hyperlipidaemia

4.25 Immunosuppressive drugs used in transplantation

Drug	Mechanism of action	Major adverse effects
Anti-proliferative agents e.g. azathioprine, mycophenolate mofetil	Inhibit lymphocyte proliferation by blocking DNA synthesis. May be directly cytotoxic at high doses	Increased susceptibility to infection Leucopenia Hepatotoxicity
Calcineurin inhibitors e.g. ciclosporin, tacrolimus	Inhibit T-cell signalling; prevent lymphocyte activation and block cytokine transcription	Increased susceptibility to infection Hypertension Nephrotoxicity Diabetogenic (especially tacrolimus) Gingival hypertrophy, hirsutism (ciclosporin)
Corticosteroids	Decrease phagocytosis and release of proteolytic enzymes; decrease lymphocyte activation and proliferation; decrease cytokine production; decrease antibody production	Increased susceptibility to infection Other complications (p. 774)
Anti-T-cell induction agents e.g. anti-thymocyte globulin (ATG), anti-CD3 monoclonal antibody	Depletion or blockade of T cells by antibodies to cell surface proteins	Profound non-specific immunosuppression Increased susceptibility to infection

Potential transplant recipients are screened for the presence of anti-HLA antibodies using either recombinant HLA proteins or a pool of lymphocytes from individuals with broadly representative HLA types. If antibodies are detected, their specificity is further characterised and the recipient is excluded from receiving a transplant which carries these alleles.

Donor–recipient cross-matching is a functional assay that directly tests whether serum from a recipient (which potentially contains anti-donor antibodies) is able to bind and/or kill donor lymphocytes. It is specific to a prospective donor–recipient pair and is done immediately prior to transplantation. A positive cross-match is a contraindication to transplantation because of the risk of hyperacute rejection.

C4d staining

C4d is a fragment of the complement protein C4 (see Fig. 4.3, p. 73). Deposition of C4d in graft capillaries indicates local activation of the classical complement pathway and provides evidence for antibody-mediated damage. This is useful in the early diagnosis of vascular rejection.

Complications of transplant immunosuppression

The prevention of transplant rejection requires indefinite treatment with immunosuppressive agents. In general, two or more immunosuppressive drugs are used in synergistic combinations in order to minimise drug side-effects (Box 4.25). The major complications of long-term immunosuppression are infection and malignancy.

The risk of some opportunistic infections may be minimised through the use of prophylactic medication (e.g. ganciclovir for CMV prophylaxis and trimethoprim-sulfamethoxazole for *Pneumocystis* prophylaxis). Immunisation with killed vaccines is appropriate, although the immune response may be curtailed. Live vaccines should not be given.

The increased risk of malignancy arises because T-cell suppression results in failure to control viral infections.

Virus-associated tumours include lymphoma (associated with EBV), Kaposi's sarcoma (associated with human herpesvirus 8) and skin tumours (associated with human papillomavirus). Immunosuppression is also associated with a small increase in the incidence of common cancers not associated with viral infection (such as lung, breast and colon cancer), reflecting the importance of T cells in anti-cancer surveillance.

Organ donation

The major problem in transplantation is the shortage of organ donors (see Box 4.23). Cadaveric organ donors are usually previously healthy individuals who experience brain stem death (p. 1158), frequently as a result of road traffic accidents or cerebrovascular events. However, even if organs were obtained from all potential cadaveric donors, their numbers would be insufficient to meet current needs. An alternative is the use of living donors. Altruistic living donation, usually from close relatives, is widely used in renal transplantation. Living organ donation is inevitably associated with some risk to the donor, and it is highly regulated to ensure appropriate appreciation of the risks involved. Because of concerns about coercion and exploitation, non-altruistic organ donation (the sale of organs) is illegal in most countries.

Further information

www.allergy.org.au *An Australasian site providing information on allergy, asthma and immune diseases.*

www.anaphylaxis.org.uk *Provides information and support for patients with severe allergies.*

www.immunopaedia.org *A South African site designed for healthcare providers requiring a general understanding of immunology, providing clinical case studies, articles, links and news, with a particular focus on HIV immunology.*

www.ukpin.org.uk *Provides practical guidelines on primary immune deficiency.*

P. Hanlon
M. Byers
B.R. Walker
H.M. Macdonald

Environmental and nutritional factors in disease

5

5

PRINCIPLES AND INVESTIGATION OF ENVIRONMENTAL FACTORS IN DISEASE

Environmental effects on health

Health emerges from a highly complex interaction between factors intrinsic to the patient and his or her environment. Many factors within the environment influence health, including aspects of the physical environment, biological environment (bacteria, viruses), built environment and social environment, but also encompass more distant influences such as the global ecosystem (Fig. 5.1). Environmental changes affect many physiological systems and do not respect boundaries between medical specialties. The specialty of 'public health' in the UK is concerned with the investigation and management of health in communities and populations, but the principles apply in all specialties.

Exposure to infectious agents is a major environmental determinant of health and is described in Chapter 6. This chapter describes the approach to other common environmental factors that influence health.

The hierarchy of systems—from molecules to ecologies

When assessing a patient, a clinician subconsciously considers many levels at which problems may be occurring, including molecular, cellular, tissue, organ and body systems. When the environment's influence on health is being considered, this 'hierarchy of systems' extends beyond the individual to include the family, community, population and ecology. Box 5.1 shows an example of the utility of this concept in describing determinants of coronary heart disease operating at each level of a hierarchy.

5.1 'Hierarchy of systems' applied to ischaemic heart disease

Level in the hierarchy	Example of effect
Molecular	ApoB mutation causing hypercholesterolaemia
Cellular	Foam cells accumulate in vessel wall
Tissue	Atheroma and thrombosis of coronary artery
Organ	Ischaemia and infarction of myocardium
System	Cardiac failure
Person	Limited exercise capacity, impact on employment
Family	Passive smoking, diet
Community	Shops and leisure opportunities
Population	Prevalence of obesity
Society	Policies on smoking, screening for risk factors
Ecology	Agriculture influencing fat content in diet

Interactions between people and their environment

The hierarchy of systems demonstrates that the clinician should not focus too quickly on the disease process without considering the context. Health is an emergent quality of a complex interaction between many determinants, including genetic inheritance, the physical circumstances in which people live (e.g. housing, air quality, working environment), the social environment (e.g. levels of friendship, support and trust), personal behaviour (smoking, diet, exercise), and access to money and the other resources that give people control over their lives. Health care is not the only determinant—and usually not the major determinant—of health status in the population.

These systems do not operate in isolation in separate communities. When one group responds to ill health by manipulating its environment, the consequences may be global. For example, an Afghan farmer who starts growing opium in order to feed his children influences the environment of a teenager in Europe; in turn, drug misuse in Europe has fostered higher prevalence of blood-borne infectious diseases such as human immunodeficiency virus/acquired immunodeficiency syndrome (HIV/AIDS); in turn, these have spilled out into sexually transmitted disease. This process contributes to the tragedy of the epidemic of HIV/AIDS.

The life course

The determinants of health operate over the whole lifespan. Values and behaviours acquired during childhood and adolescence have a profound influence on educational outcomes, job prospects and risk of disease. Attributes such as the ability to form empathetic relationships or assess risk have a strong influence on whether a young person takes up damaging behaviour like smoking, risky sexual behaviours and drug misuse. Influences on health can even operate before birth.

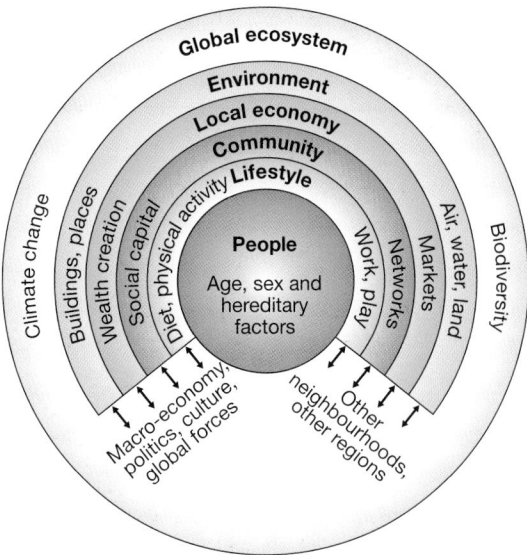

Fig. 5.1 Hierarchy of systems that influence population health.

Individuals with low birth weight have been shown to have higher prevalence of conditions such as hypertension and type 2 diabetes as young adults and of cardiovascular disease in middle age. It has been suggested that under-nutrition during middle to late gestation permanently 'programmes' cardiovascular and metabolic responses.

This 'life course' perspective highlights the cumulative effect on health of exposures to episodes of illness, adverse environmental conditions and behaviours that damage health. In this way biological and social risk factors at each stage of life link to form pathways to disease and health.

Investigations in environmental health

Incidence and prevalence

The first task is to establish how common a problem is within the population. This is expressed in two ways (Box 5.2).

- If the problem is a continuing condition (e.g. enlarged spleen due to malaria), then prevalence is the appropriate measurement and is calculated by dividing the number of people with the condition at a specified time by the number of people in the population at risk at that time. Prevalence tends to be higher if the problem is common (many new cases) and/or if it is of longer duration.
- If the problem is an event that occurs at a clear point in time (e.g. fever due to malaria), then incidence is used. Incidence is a measure of the rate at which new cases occur (e.g. confirmed pyrexia with malaria parasites on a blood film) in the population at risk during a defined period of time.

Variability by time, person and place

The next task is to establish how the problem varies in terms of time, person and place. The incidence may fluctuate throughout the year; for example, malaria occurs in the wet season but not the dry. Observation over longer

periods establishes whether a problem is becoming more or less common: malaria may re-emerge due to drug resistance. The next question is, who are the victims? Are males or females more commonly affected? What is the age pattern? What are the occupations and social positions of those affected? In this example, symptomatic malaria is more common in poorer, rural-dwelling children. Finally, there is the question of variability by place: the prevalence of malaria is dictated by the distribution of anopheles mosquitoes.

Measuring risk

Epidemiology is also concerned with the numerical estimation of risk. This is best illustrated by a simple example. In a rural African town with a population of 5000, disease 'd' is under investigation. The majority of the cases of disease 'd' (300 out of 360) occurred among women and children who use the river, which recently had its flow of water reduced because of a new irrigation scheme. A formal experiment is established to measure risk. The 1000 women and children who use the river are followed up for 1 year and compared to a cohort with a similar age and sex distribution who use stand pipes as their source of water.

The incidence (new cases) of disease 'd' in the 1000 exposed to risk 'r' (river water) was 300. The incidence (new cases) of disease 'd' in 1000 not exposed to risk 'r' was 60. The relative risk is the incidence in the exposed population (300 per 1000 per year) divided by the incidence in the non-exposed population (60 per 1000 per year). $300/60 = 5$, meaning that those exposed to the river water are 5 times more likely to contract the disease—their relative risk is 5. The attributable risk of exposure 'r' for disease 'd' is the incidence in the exposed population (300) minus the incidence in the non-exposed population (60), which is 240 per 1000 per year. The fraction, or proportion, of the disease in the exposed population which can be attributed to risk (r) is called the attributable fraction, in this case $(300-60)/300 = 0.8$. This means that 80% of the disease can be attributed to exposure to river water.

Establishing cause and effect

Associations between a risk factor and a disease do not prove that the risk factor causes the disease. In the northern hemisphere, both multiple sclerosis and blue eyes are more common but it is implausible that having blue eyes is the cause of multiple sclerosis. Cause and effect can only be proven by more detailed investigation. In the above example, further investigation of the river water for infectious agents will be needed, using the criteria for causation defined in Koch's postulates (p. 132).

Preventive medicine

There are many examples of epidemiological associations defining causative factors in disease, e.g. the association between cigarette smoking and lung cancer (p. 698). However, as illustrated above, the complexity of the interactions between physical, social and economic determinants of health means that successful prevention is often difficult. Moreover, the life course perspective illustrates that it may be necessary to intervene early in life or even before birth, to prevent important disease in

---

5.2 Calculation of risk using descriptive epidemiology

Prevalence

- The ratio of the number of people with longer-term disease or condition at a specified time, to the number of people in the population who are at risk

Incidence

- The number of events (new cases or episodes) occurring in the population at risk during a defined period of time

Attributable risk

- The difference between the risk (or incidence) of disease in exposed and non-exposed populations

Attributable fraction

- The ratio of the attributable risk to the incidence

Relative risk

- The ratio of the risk (or incidence) in the exposed population to the risk (or incidence) in the non-exposed population

later life. Successful prevention is likely to require many interventions across the life course and at several levels in the hierarchy of systems. The examples below illustrate this principle.

ENVIRONMENTAL DISEASES

The term 'homeostasis' describes the capacity to maintain the internal milieu by adapting to increases or decreases in a given environmental factor. However, there are limits to the coping abilities of any system, at which 'too much' or 'too little' of a given environmental factor will result in ill health. Too many calories lead to obesity while too few lead to malnutrition. Either involuntarily or deliberately, we expose ourselves to many poisons and hazards. Examples discussed elsewhere include industrial/occupational hazards, such as asbestos (p. 712) and other carcinogens (p. 261). 'Social' poisons, such as tobacco, alcohol and drugs of misuse, also need to be considered (p. 237).

Alcohol

Rates of alcohol-related harm have been rising dramatically in the UK, with Scotland (Fig. 5.2) showing the highest rates. Why did Scotland experience a dramatic increase in alcohol deaths from the early 1990s onwards? The most likely explanation is that the environment changed. The price of alcohol fell in real terms and availability increased (more supermarkets sold alcohol and opening times of pubs were extended). Also, the culture changed in a way that fostered higher levels of consumption and more binge drinking. These changes have caused a trebling of male and a doubling of female deaths due to alcohol. Public, professional and governmental concern has now led to increased tax on alcohol, tightening of licensing regulations and curtailment of some promotional activity (e.g. two for one offers in bars). Many experts judge that even more aggressive public health measures will be needed to reverse the levels of harm in the community. The approach for individual patients

suffering adverse effects of alcohol is described on pages 237 and 246.

Smoking

Smoking tobacco dramatically increases the risk of developing many diseases. It is responsible for a substantial majority of cases of lung cancer and chronic obstructive pulmonary disease, and most smokers die either from these respiratory diseases or from ischaemic heart disease. Smoking also causes cancers of the upper respiratory and gastrointestinal tracts, pancreas, bladder and kidney, and increases risks of peripheral vascular disease, stroke and peptic ulceration. Maternal smoking is an important cause of fetal growth retardation. Moreover, there is increasing evidence that passive (or 'secondhand') smoking has adverse effects on cardiovascular and respiratory health.

When the ill-health effects of smoking were first discovered, doctors imagined that warning people about the dangers of smoking would result in them giving up. However, it also took increased taxation of tobacco, banning of advertising and support for smoking cessation to maintain a decline in smoking rates. In several European countries (including the UK), this has culminated in a complete ban on smoking in all public places—legislation that only became possible as the public became convinced of the dangers of secondhand smoke. However, smoking rates remain high in many poorer areas and are increasing amongst young women. In many developing countries tobacco companies have found new markets and rates are rising. World-wide, there are ~1 billion smokers, and 3 million die prematurely each year as a result of their habit.

In reality, there is a complex hierarchy of systems that interact to cause smokers to initiate and maintain their habit. At the molecular and cellular levels, nicotine acts on the nervous system to create dependence, so that smokers experience unpleasant effects when they attempt to quit. So, even if they know it is harmful, the role of addiction in maintaining the habit is important. Influences at the personal and social level are just as important. Many individuals bolster their denial of the harmful effects of smoking by focusing on someone they knew personally who smoked until he or she was very old and died peacefully in bed. Such strong counter-examples help smokers to maintain internal beliefs that comfort them when presented with statistical evidence. Young female smokers are often motivated more by the desire to 'stay thin' or 'look cool' than to avoid an illness in middle life.

Even if a smoker decides to quit, there are a variety of influences in the wider environment that reduce the chances of sustained success, including peer pressure, cigarette advertising, and finding oneself in circumstances where one previously smoked. The tobacco industry works very hard to maintain and expand the smoking habit, and its advertising budget is much greater than that available to health promoters.

Strategies to help individuals quit smoking are outlined in Boxes 5.3 and 5.4. Although the success rates are modest, these interventions are cost-effective and form an important part of the overall anti-tobacco strategy.

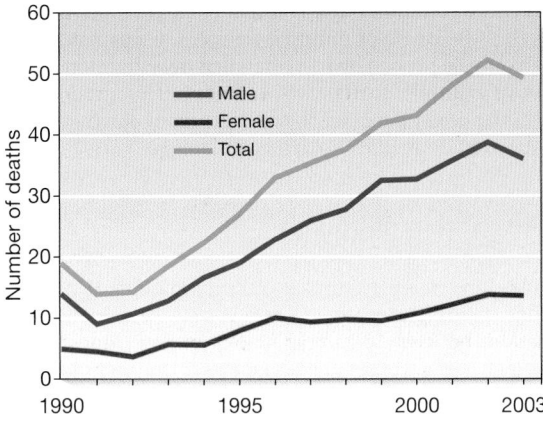

Fig. 5.2 Alcohol-related deaths in Scotland by year and sex (1990–2003). Principal ('underlying') and secondary ('contributing') causes of death. (Source: General Register Office (Scotland))

5.3 Methods for smoking cessation

Smokers who are not motivated to try to stop smoking

- Record smoking status at regular intervals
- Anti-smoking advice
- Encourage change in attitude towards smoking to improve motivation

Motivated light smokers (< 10/day)

- Anti-smoking advice
- Anti-smoking support programme

Motivated heavy smokers (10–15/day)

- As above plus nicotine replacement therapy (NRT) (minimum 8 weeks)

Motivated heavy smokers (> 15/day)

- As above plus bupropion if NRT and behavioural support are unsuccessful and patient remains motivated

---

EBM 5.4 Smoking cessation

'Placebo or will-power alone has a ~2% chance of abstinence for ≥ 6 months. This can be increased by the percentage shown by:
- written self-help materials: 1%
- opportunistic advice from doctor: 2%
- face-to-face behavioural support from specialist: 4–7%
- proactive telephone counselling: 2%
- NRT with limited or intensive behavioural support: 5–12%
- bupropion with intensive behavioural support: 9%.'

- Health Education Board for Scotland, Edinburgh; 2000.

5.5 Examples of effects of financial resources on health

Poverty

- Respiratory disease exacerbated or caused by air pollution
- Exposure to unnecessary hazards in the workplace or living environment
- Poor hygiene causing diarrhoeal diseases and debilitating intestinal parasitic infections
- Malnutrition
- Cardiovascular disease

Affluence

- Physical inactivity
- Alcohol and drug consumption
- High rates of suicide, depression, anxiety and stress
- Sexually transmitted infection
- Obesity

5.6 Environmental factors in disease in old age

- **Quality of life**: the major goal of public health policy in the young is to prolong lifespan; in old age, quality of life may be more important than its duration.
- **Life course**: the environmental factors that determine life expectancy operate throughout the lifespan and begin before birth.
- **Susceptibility to risk**: decline in many physiological functions increases risks from, for example, extremes of temperature, poverty, pollution and accidents in the home.
- **Reliance on support**: in many societies, financial, family and community support for older people is declining, with increasing risks of social isolation, poverty, malnutrition and neglect.

Poverty and affluence

The adverse health and social consequences of poverty are well documented: high birth rates, high death rates and short life expectancy (Box 5.5). Typically, with industrialisation the pattern changes: low birth rates, low death rates and longer life expectancy. Instead of infections, chronic conditions such as heart disease dominate in an older population. Adverse health consequences of excessive affluence are also becoming apparent. Despite experiencing sustained economic growth for the last 50 years, people in many industrialised countries are not growing any happier and the litany of socioeconomic problems—crime, congestion, inequality—persists. Living in societies that give pride of place to economic growth means that there is constant pressure to contribute by performing ever harder at work and by consuming as much as—or more than—we can afford. As a result, people become stressed and may adopt unhealthy strategies to mitigate their discomfort; they overeat, overshop, or use sex or drugs (legal and illegal) as 'pain-killers'. These behaviours often lead to the problems listed in Box 5.5.

Many countries are now experiencing a 'double burden'. They have large populations still living in poverty who are suffering from problems such as diarrhoea and malnutrition, alongside affluent populations (often in cities) who suffer from chronic illness such as diabetes and heart disease. Recent research suggests that uneven distribution of wealth is a more important determinant of health than the absolute level of wealth; countries with a more even distribution of wealth enjoy longer life expectancies than countries with similar or higher gross domestic products (GDPs) but wider distributions of wealth.

Atmospheric pollution

Emissions from industry, power plants and motor vehicles of sulphur oxides, nitrogen oxides, respirable particles and metals are severely polluting cities and towns in Asia, Africa, Latin America and Eastern Europe. Increased deaths from respiratory and cardiovascular disease occur in vulnerable adults, such as those with established respiratory disease and the elderly, while children experience an increase in bronchitic symptoms. In nations like the UK that have reduced their primary emissions, the new issue of greenhouse gases has emerged. Developing countries also suffer high rates of respiratory disease as a result of indoor pollution caused mainly by heating and cooking combustion.

Carbon dioxide and global warming

Climate change is arguably the world's most important environmental health issue. A combination of increased production of carbon dioxide and habitat destruction, both caused primarily by human activity, seems to be the main cause. The temperature of the globe is rising, climate is being affected, and if the trend continues, sea levels will rise and rainfall patterns will be altered so that both droughts and floods will become more common. These have already claimed millions of lives during the past 20 years and have adversely affected the lives of many more. The economic costs of property damage and the impact on agriculture, food supplies and prosperity have also been substantial. The health impacts of global warming will also include changes in the geographical range of some vector-borne infectious diseases.

Currently, politicians cannot agree on an effective framework of actions to tackle the problem. Meanwhile, the industrialised world continues with lifestyles and waste that are beyond the planet's limits to sustain. Rapidly growing economies in the world's two most populous states, India and China, are going to be a vital part of the unfolding problem or solution.

Radiation exposure

Radiation includes ionising (Box 5.7) and non-ionising radiations (ultraviolet (UV), visible light, laser, infrared and microwave). Whilst global industrialisation and the generation of fluorocarbons have raised concerns about loss of the ozone layer, leading to an increased exposure to UV rays, and disasters such as the Chernobyl nuclear power station explosion have demonstrated the harm of ionising radiation, it can be harnessed for medical benefit. Ionising radiation is used in X-rays, computed tomography (CT), radionucleotide scans and radiotherapy, and non-ionising UV for therapy in skin diseases and laser therapy for diabetic retinopathy.

Types of ionising radiation

These include charged subatomic alpha and beta particles, uncharged neutrons or high-energy electromagnetic radiations such as X-rays and gamma rays. When they interact with atoms, energy is released and the resulting ionisation can lead to molecular damage. The clinical effects of different forms of radiation depend upon their range in air and tissue penetration (see Box 5.7).

Dosage and exposure

The dose of radiation is based upon the energy absorbed by a unit mass of tissue and is measured in grays (Gy), with 1 Gy representing 1 J/kg. To take account of different types of radiation and variations in the sensitivity of various tissues, weighting factors are used to produce a unit of effective dose, measured in sieverts (Sv). This value reflects the absorbed dose weighted for the damaging effects of a particular form of radiation and is most valuable in evaluating the long-term effects of exposure.

i | **5.7 Properties of ionising radiations**

	Range in air	Range in tissue	Protection
Alpha particles	Few centimetres	No penetration	Paper
Beta particles	Few metres	Few millimetres	Aluminium sheet
X-rays/ gamma rays	Kilometres	Passes through	Lead
Neutrons	Kilometres	Passes through	Concrete or thick polythene

'Background radiation' refers to our exposure to naturally occurring radioactivity (e.g. radon gas and cosmic radiation). This produces an average annual individual dose of approximately 2.6 mSv per year, although this varies according to local geology.

Effects of radiation exposure

Effects on the individual are classified as either deterministic or stochastic.

Deterministic effects

Deterministic (threshold) effects occur with increasing severity as the dose of radiation rises above a threshold level. Tissues with actively dividing cells, such as bone marrow and gastrointestinal mucosa, are particularly sensitive to ionising radiation. Lymphocyte depletion is the most sensitive marker of bone marrow injury, and after exposure to a fatal dose, marrow aplasia is a common cause of death. However, gastrointestinal mucosal toxicity may cause earlier death due to profound diarrhoea, vomiting, dehydration and sepsis. The gonads are highly radiosensitive and radiation may result in temporary or permanent sterility. Eye exposure can result in cataracts and the skin is susceptible to radiation burns. Irradiation of the lung and central nervous system may induce acute inflammatory reactions, pulmonary fibrosis and permanent neurological deficit respectively. Bone necrosis and lymphatic fibrosis are characteristic following regional irradiation, particularly for breast cancer. The thyroid gland is not inherently sensitive but its ability to concentrate iodine makes it susceptible to damage after exposure to relatively low doses of radioactive iodine isotopes, such as were released from Chernobyl.

Stochastic effects

Stochastic (chance) effects occur with increasing probability as the dose of radiation increases. Carcinogenesis represents a stochastic effect. With acute exposures, leukaemias may arise after an interval of around 2–5 years and solid tumours after an interval of about 10–20 years. Thereafter the incidence rises with time. An individual's risk of developing cancer depends on the dose received, the time to accumulate the total dose and the interval following exposure.

Management of radiation exposure

The principal problems after large-dose exposures are maintenance of adequate hydration, control of sepsis and the management of marrow aplasia. Associated injuries such as thermal burns need specialist management within 48 hours of active resuscitation. Internal exposure to radioisotopes should be treated with chelating agents (such as Prussian blue used to chelate [137]caesium after ingestion). White cell colony stimulation and bone marrow transplantation may need to be considered for marrow aplasia.

Extremes of temperature

Thermoregulation

Body heat is generated by basal metabolic activity and muscle movement, and lost by conduction (which is more effective in water than in air), convection, evaporation and radiation (most important at lower temperatures when other mechanisms conserve heat) (Box 5.8). Body temperature is controlled in the hypothalamus, which is directly sensitive to changes in core temperature and

5.8 Thermoregulation: responses to hot and cold environments

	Mechanism	Hot environment	Cold environment
Heat production	Basal metabolic rate	$\rightarrow$	↓ in hypothermia
	Muscle activity	↓ by lethargy	↑ by shivering ↓ in severe hypothermia
Heat loss	Conduction*	↑ by vasodilatation	↓ by vasoconstriction ↑↑ in water < 31 °C
	Convection*	↑ by vasodilatation ↓ by lethargy	↓ by vasoconstriction ↑ by wind and movement
	Evaporation*	↑↑ by sweating ↓ by high humidity	↑ by hyperventilation
	Radiation	↑ by vasodilatation	↓ by vasoconstriction (but is the major heat loss in dry cold)

*These losses are dependent on the relative ambient and skin temperatures.

indirectly responds to temperature-sensitive neurons in the skin. The normal 'set-point' of core temperature is tightly regulated within 37 ± 0.5 °C, necessary to preserve the normal function of many enzymes and other metabolic processes. The temperature set-point is increased in response to infection (p. 292).

In a cold environment, protective mechanisms include cutaneous vasoconstriction and shivering; however, any muscle activity which involves movement may promote heat loss by increasing convective loss from the skin, and respiratory heat loss by stimulating ventilation. In a hot environment, sweating is the main mechanism for increasing heat loss. This usually occurs when the ambient temperature rises above 32.5 °C or during exercise.

Hypothermia

Hypothermia exists when the body's normal thermal regulatory mechanisms are unable to maintain heat in a cold environment and core temperature falls below 35 °C (Fig. 5.3).

Whilst infants are susceptible to hypothermia because of their poor thermoregulation and high body surface area to weight ratio, it is the elderly who are at highest risk (Box 5.9). Hypothyroidism is often a contributory factor in old age, while alcohol or other drugs (e.g. phenothiazines) commonly impede the thermoregulatory response in younger people. More rarely, hypothermia is secondary to glucocorticoid insufficiency, stroke, hepatic failure or hypoglycaemia.

Hypothermia also occurs in healthy individuals whose thermoregulatory mechanisms are intact but insufficient to cope with the intensity of the thermal stress. Typical examples include immersion in cold water, when core temperature may fall rapidly (acute hypothermia), exposure to extreme climates such as during hill walking (subacute hypothermia), and slow-onset hypothermia, as develops in an immobilised older individual (subchronic hypothermia). This classification is important, as it determines the method of rewarming.

Clinical features

Diagnosis is dependent on recognition of the environmental circumstances and measurement of core (rectal)

body temperature. Clinical features depend on the degree of hypothermia (see Fig. 5.3).

It is very difficult to diagnose death reliably by clinical means in a cold patient. It has been suggested that, in extreme environmental conditions, irreversible hypothermia is probably present if there is asystole (no carotid pulse for 1 minute), the chest and abdomen are rigid, the core temperature is below 13 °C and serum potassium is > 12 mmol/L. However, in general, resuscitative measures should continue until the core temperature is

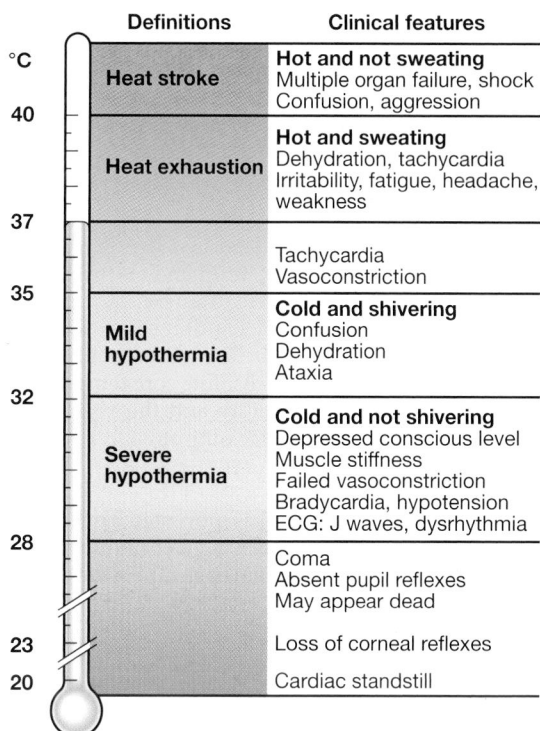

Fig. 5.3 Clinical features of abnormal core temperature. The hypothalamus normally maintains core temperature at 37 °C, but this set-point is altered—for example, in fever (pyrexia, p. 292)—and may be lost in hypothalamic disease (p. 783). In these circumstances the clinical picture at a given core temperature may be different.

5

5.9 Thermoregulation in old age

- **Age-associated changes**: impairments in vasomotor function, skeletal muscle response and sweating mean that older people react more slowly to changes in temperature.
- **Increased comorbidity**: thermoregulatory problems are more likely in the presence of pathology such as atherosclerosis and hypothyroidism, and medication such as sedatives and hypnotics.
- **Hypothermia**: may arise as a primary event, but more commonly complicates other acute illness, e.g. pneumonia, stroke or fracture.
- **Ambient temperature**: financial pressures and older equipment may result in inadequate heating during cold weather.

normal and only then should a diagnosis of brain death be considered (p. 1158).

Investigations

Blood gases, a full blood count, electrolytes, chest X-ray and electrocardiogram (ECG) are all essential investigations. Haemoconcentration and metabolic acidosis are common, and the ECG may show characteristic J waves which occur at the junction of the QRS complex and the ST segment (Fig. 5.4). Cardiac dysrhythmias, including ventricular fibrillation, may occur. Although the arterial oxygen tension may be normal when measured at room temperature, the arterial PO_2 in the blood falls by 7% for each 1°C fall in core temperature. Serum aspartate aminotransferase and creatine kinase may be elevated secondary to muscle damage and the serum amylase is often high due to subclinical pancreatitis. If the cause of hypothermia is not obvious, additional investigations for thyroid and pituitary dysfunction (p. 734), hypoglycaemia (p. 804) and the possibility of drug intoxication (p. 207) should be performed.

Management

Following resuscitation, the objectives of management are to rewarm the patient in a controlled manner while treating associated hypoxia (by oxygenation and ventilation if necessary), fluid and electrolyte disturbance, and cardiovascular abnormalities, particularly dysrhythmias. Careful handling is essential to avoid precipitating the latter. The method of rewarming is dependent not on the absolute core temperature, but on haemodynamic stability and the presence or absence of an effective cardiac output.

Mild hypothermia

Outdoors, continued heat loss is prevented by sheltering the patient from the cold, replacing wet clothing, covering the head and insulating him or her from the ground.

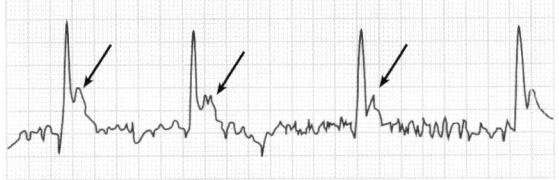

Fig. 5.4 Electrocardiogram showing J waves (arrows) in a hypothermic patient.

Once in hospital, even in the presence of profound hypothermia, if there is an effective cardiac output then forced-air rewarming, heat packs placed in axilla, groin and around the abdomen, inhaled warmed air and correction of fluid and electrolyte disturbances are usually sufficient. Rewarming rates of 1–2°C per hour are effective in leading to a gradual and safe return to physiological normality. Underlying conditions should be treated promptly (e.g. hypothyroidism with triiodothyronine 10 µg i.v. 8-hourly; p. 742).

Severe hypothermia

In the case of severe hypothermia with cardiopulmonary arrest (non-perfusing rhythm), the aim is to restore perfusion, and rapid rewarming at a rate greater than 2°C per hour is required. This is best achieved by cardiopulmonary bypass or extracorporeal membrane oxygenation. If these are unavailable, then veno–veno haemofiltration, and pleural, peritoneal, thoracic or bladder lavage with warmed fluids are alternatives. Monitoring of cardiac rhythm and arterial blood gases, including H^+ (pH) is essential. Significant acidosis may require correction (p. 443).

Cold injury

Freezing cold injury (frostbite)

This represents the direct freezing of body tissues and usually affects the extremities: in particular, the fingers, toes, ears and face. Risk factors include smoking, peripheral vascular disease, dehydration and alcohol consumption. The tissues may become anaesthetised before freezing and, as a result, the injury often goes unrecognised at first. Frostbitten tissue is initially pale and doughy to the touch and insensitive to pain (Fig. 5.5). Once frozen, the tissue is hard.

Rewarming should not occur until it can be achieved rapidly in a water bath. Give oxygen and aspirin 300 mg as soon as possible. Frostbitten extremities should be rewarmed in warm water at 40–42°C, with antiseptic added. Adequate analgesia is necessary, as rewarming is very painful. Vasodilators such as pentoxifylline (a phosphodiesterase inhibitor) have been shown to improve tissue survival. Once thawed, the injured part must not be re-exposed to cold, and should be dressed and rested. Whilst wound débridement may be neces-

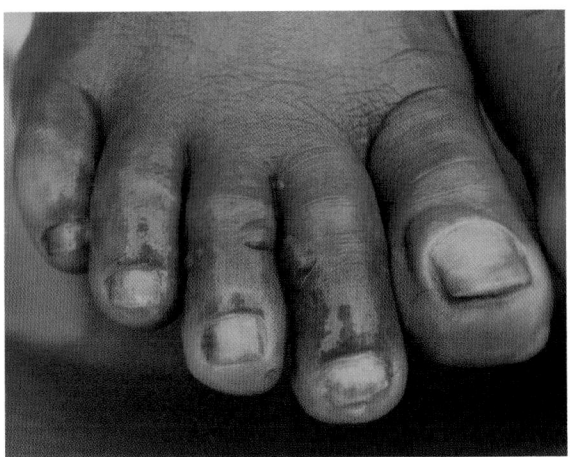

Fig. 5.5 Frostbite in a female Everest sherpa.

sary, amputations should be delayed for 60–90 days, as good recovery may occur over an extended period.

Non-freezing cold injury (trench or immersion foot)

This results from prolonged exposure to cold, damp conditions. The limb (usually the foot) appears cold, ischaemic and numb, but there is no freezing of the tissue. On rewarming, the limb appears mottled and thereafter becomes hyperaemic, swollen and painful. Recovery may take many months, during which there may be chronic pain and sensitivity to cold. The pathology remains uncertain but probably involves endothelial injury. Gradual rewarming is associated with less pain than rapid rewarming. The pain and associated paraesthesia are difficult to control with conventional analgesia and may require amitriptyline (50 mg nocte), best instituted early. The patient is at risk of further damage on subsequent exposure to the cold.

Chilblains

Chilblains are tender, red or purplish skin lesions that occur in the cold and wet. They are often seen in horse riders, cyclists and swimmers, and are more common in women than men. They are short-lived, and although painful, not usually serious.

Heat-related illness

When generation of heat exceeds the body's capacity for heat loss, core temperature rises. Non-exertional heat illness (NEHI) occurs with high environmental temperature in those with attenuated thermoregulatory control mechanisms: the elderly, the young, those with comorbidity or those taking drugs that affect thermoregulation (particularly phenothiazines, diuretics and alcohol). Exertional heat illness (EHI), on the other hand, typically develops in athletes when heat production exceeds the body's ability to dissipate it.

Acclimatisation mechanisms to environmental heat include stimulation of the sweat mechanism with increased sweat volume, reduced sweat sodium content and secondary hyperaldosteronism to maintain body sodium balance. The risk of heat-related illness falls as acclimatisation occurs. Heat illness can be prevented to a large extent by adequate replacement of salt and water, although excessive water intake alone should be avoided because of the risk of dilutional hyponatraemia (p. 435).

A spectrum of illnesses occurs in the heat (see Fig. 5.3). The cause is usually obvious but the differential diagnosis should be considered (Box 5.10).

Heat cramps

These painful muscle contractions occur following vigorous exercise and profuse sweating in hot weather. There is no elevation of core temperature. The mechanism is considered to be extracellular sodium depletion as a result of

persistent sweating, exacerbated by replacement of water but not salt. Symptoms usually respond rapidly to rehydration with oral rehydration salts or intravenous saline.

Heat syncope

This is similar to a vasovagal faint (p. 553) and is related to peripheral vasodilatation in hot weather.

Heat exhaustion

Heat exhaustion occurs with prolonged exertion in hot and humid weather, profuse sweating and inadequate salt and water replacement. There is an elevation in core (rectal) temperature to between 37 °C and 40 °C, leading to the clinical features shown in Figure 5.3. Blood analyses may show evidence of dehydration with mild elevation of the blood urea, sodium and haematocrit. Treatment involves removal of the patient from the heat, and active evaporative cooling using tepid sprays and fanning (strip-spray-fan). Fluid losses are replaced with either oral rehydration mixtures or intravenous isotonic saline. Up to 5 L positive fluid balance may be required in the first 24 hours. Untreated, heat exhaustion may progress to heat stroke.

Heat stroke

Heat stroke occurs when the core body temperature rises above 40 °C and is a life-threatening condition. The symptoms of heat exhaustion progress to include headache, nausea and vomiting. Neurological manifestations include a coarse muscle tremor and confusion, aggression or loss of consciousness. The patient's skin feels very hot, and sweating is often absent due to failure of thermoregulatory mechanisms. Complications include hypovolaemic shock, lactic acidosis, disseminated intravascular coagulation, rhabdomyolysis, hepatic and renal failure, and pulmonary and cerebral oedema.

The patient should be resuscitated with rapid cooling by spraying with water, fanning and ice packs in the axillae and groins. Cold crystalloid intravenous fluids are given but solutions containing potassium should be avoided. Overaggressive fluid replacement must be avoided, as it may precipitate pulmonary oedema or further metabolic disturbance. Appropriate monitoring of fluid balance, including central venous pressure, is important. Investigations for complications include routine haematology and biochemistry, coagulation screen, hepatic transaminases (aspartate aminotransferase and alanine aminotransferase), creatine kinase and chest X-ray. Once emergency treatment is established, heat stroke patients are best managed in intensive care.

With appropriate treatment, recovery from heat stroke can be rapid (within 1–2 hours) but patients who have had core temperatures higher than 40 °C should be monitored carefully for later onset of rhabdomyolysis, renal damage and other complications before discharge from hospital. Clear advice to avoid heat and heavy exercise during recovery is important.

High altitude

The physiological effects of high altitude are significant. On Everest, the barometric pressure of the atmosphere falls from sea level by ~50% at base camp (5400 m) and ~70% at the summit (8848 m). The proportions of oxygen, nitrogen and carbon dioxide in air do not change with the fall in pressure but their partial pressure falls

5.10 Differential diagnosis in patients with elevated core body temperature

- Heat illness (heat exhaustion, heat stroke)
- Sepsis, including meningitis
- Malaria
- Drug overdose
- Malignant hyperpyrexia
- Thyroid storm (p. 741)

in proportion to barometric pressure (Fig. 5.6). Oxygen tension within the pulmonary alveoli is further reduced at altitude because the partial pressure of water vapour is related to body temperature and not barometric pressure, and so is proportionately greater at altitude, accounting for only 6% of barometric pressure at sea level, but 19% at 8848 m.

Physiological effects of high altitude

Reduction in oxygen tension results in a fall in arterial oxygen saturation (see Fig. 5.6). This varies widely between individuals, depending on the shape of the sigmoid oxygen–haemoglobin dissociation curve (see Fig. 8.2, p. 181) and the ventilatory response. Acclimatisation to hypoxaemia at high altitude involves a shift in this dissociation curve (dependent on 2,3-DPG), erythropoiesis, haemoconcentration, and hyperventilation resulting from hypoxic drive (which is then sustained despite hypocapnia by restoration of cerebrospinal fluid pH to normal in prolonged hypoxia). This process takes several days, so travellers need to plan accordingly.

Illnesses at high altitude

Ascent to altitudes up to 2500 m or travel in a pressurised aircraft cabin is harmless to healthy people. Above 2500 m high-altitude illnesses may occur in previously healthy people, and above 3500 m these become common. Sudden ascent to altitudes above 6000 m, as experienced by aviators, balloonists and astronauts, may result in decompression illness with the same clinical features as seen in divers (see below), or even loss of consciousness. However, most altitude illness occurs in travellers and mountaineers.

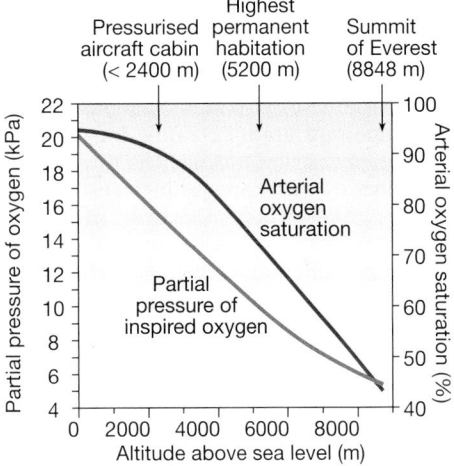

Fig. 5.6 Change in inspired oxygen tension and blood oxygen saturation at altitude. The blue curve shows changes in oxygen availability at altitude and the red curve shows the typical resultant changes in arterial oxygen saturation in a healthy person. Oxygen saturation varies between individuals according to the shape of the oxygen–haemoglobin dissociation curve and the ventilatory response to hypoxaemia. (To convert kPa to mmHg, multiply by 7.5.)

Acute mountain sickness (AMS)

AMS is a syndrome comprised principally of headache, together with fatigue, anorexia, nausea and vomiting, difficulty sleeping or dizziness. Ataxia and peripheral oedema may be present. Its aetiology is not fully understood but it is thought that hypoxaemia increases cerebral blood flow and hence intracranial pressure. Symptoms occur within 6–12 hours of an ascent and vary in severity from trivial to completely incapacitating. The incidence in travellers to 3000 m may be 40–50%, depending on the rate of ascent.

Treatment of mild cases consists of rest and simple analgesia; symptoms usually resolve after 1–3 days at a stable altitude, but may recur with further ascent. Occasionally there is progression to cerebral oedema. Persistent symptoms indicate the need to descend but may respond to acetazolamide, a carbonic anhydrase inhibitor which induces a metabolic acidosis and stimulates ventilation; acetazolamide may also be used as prophylaxis if a rapid ascent is planned.

High-altitude cerebral oedema (HACE)

The cardinal symptoms of HACE are ataxia and altered consciousness. This is rare, life-threatening and usually preceded by AMS. In addition to features of AMS, the patient suffers confusion, disorientation, visual disturbance, lethargy and ultimately loss of consciousness. Papilloedema and retinal haemorrhages are common, and focal neurological signs may be found.

Treatment is directed at improving oxygenation. Descent is essential and dexamethasone (8 mg immediately and 4 mg 6-hourly) should be given. If descent is impossible, oxygen therapy in a portable pressurised bag may be helpful.

High-altitude pulmonary oedema (HAPE)

This life-threatening condition usually occurs in the first 4 days after ascent above 2500 m. Unlike HACE, HAPE may occur de novo without the preceding signs of AMS. Presentation is with symptoms of dry cough, exertional dyspnoea and extreme fatigue. Later, the cough becomes wet and sputum may be blood-stained. Tachycardia and tachypnoea occur at rest and crepitations may often be heard in both lung fields. There may be profound hypoxaemia, pulmonary hypertension and radiological evidence of diffuse alveolar oedema. It is not known whether the alveolar oedema is a result of mechanical stress on the pulmonary capillaries associated with the high pulmonary arterial pressure, or an effect of hypoxia on capillary permeability. Reduced arterial oxygen saturation is not diagnostic but is a marker for disease progression.

Treatment is directed at reversal of hypoxia with immediate descent and oxygen administration. Nifedipine (20 mg 6-hourly) should be given to reduce pulmonary arterial pressure, and oxygen therapy in a portable pressurised bag should be used if descent is delayed.

Chronic mountain sickness (Monge's disease)

This occurs on prolonged exposure to altitude and has been reported in residents of Colorado, South America and Tibet. Patients present with headache, poor concentration and other signs of polycythaemia. They are cyanosed and often have finger clubbing.

High-altitude retinal haemorrhage

This occurs in over 30% of trekkers at 5000 m. The haemorrhages are usually asymptomatic and resolve spontaneously. Visual defects can occur with haemorrhage involving the macula, but there is no specific treatment.

Venous thrombosis

This has been reported at altitudes over 6000 m. Risk factors include dehydration, inactivity and the cold. The use of the oral contraceptive pill at high altitude should be considered carefully, as this is an additional risk factor.

Refractory cough

A cough at high altitude is common and usually benign. It may be due to breathing dry, cold air and increased mouth breathing, with consequent dry oral mucosa. This may be indistinguishable from the early signs of HAPE.

Air travel

Commercial aircraft usually cruise at 10 000–12 000 m, with the cabin pressurised to an equivalent of around 2400 m. At this altitude, the partial pressure of oxygen is 16 kPa (120 mmHg), leading to a PaO_2 in healthy people of 7.0–8.5 kPa (53–64 mmHg). Oxygen saturation is also reduced, but to a lesser degree (see Fig. 5.6). Although well tolerated by healthy people, this degree of hypoxia may be dangerous in patients with respiratory disease.

Advice for patients with respiratory disease

The British Thoracic Society has published guidance on the management of patients with respiratory disease who want to fly. Specialist pre-flight assessment is advised for all patients who have hypoxaemia (oxygen saturation < 95%) at sea level, and includes spirometry and a hypoxic challenge test with 15% oxygen (performed in hospital). Air travel may have to be avoided or undertaken only with inspired oxygen therapy during the flight. Asthmatic patients should be advised to carry their inhalers in their hand baggage. Following pneumothorax, flying should be avoided while air remains in the pleural cavity, but can be considered after proven resolution or definitive (surgical) treatment.

Advice for other patients

Other circumstances in which patients are more susceptible to hypoxia require individual assessment. These include cardiac dysrhythmia, sickle-cell disease and ischaemic heart disease. Most airlines decline to carry pregnant women after the 36th week of gestation. In complicated pregnancies it may be advisable to avoid air travel at an earlier stage. Patients who have had recent abdominal surgery, including laparoscopy, should avoid flying until all intraperitoneal gas is reabsorbed. Divers should not fly for 24 hours after a dive requiring decompression stops.

Ear and sinus pain due to changes in gas volume are common but usually mild, although patients with chronic sinusitis and otitis media may need specialist assessment. A healthy mobile tympanic membrane visualised during a Valsalva manœuvre usually suggests a patent Eustachian tube.

On long-haul flights, patients with diabetes mellitus may need to adjust their insulin or oral hypoglycaemic dosing according to the timing of in-flight and subsequent meals (p. 823). Advice is available from Diabetes UK and other websites. Documentary evidence of the need to carry needles and insulin should be carried.

Deep venous thrombosis

Air travellers have an increased risk of venous thrombosis (p. 1004), due to a combination of factors, including loss of venous emptying because of prolonged immobilisation (lack of muscular activity) and reduced barometric pressure on the tissues, together with haemoconcentration as a result of oedema and perhaps a degree of hypoxia-induced diuresis.

Venous thrombosis can probably be prevented by avoiding dehydration and excess alcohol, and exercising muscles during the flight. Without a clear cost–benefit analysis, prophylaxis with aspirin or heparin cannot be recommended routinely, but may be considered in high-risk cases.

Under water

Drowning and near-drowning

Drowning is defined as death due to asphyxiation following immersion in a fluid, whilst near-drowning is defined as survival for longer than 24 hours after suffocation by immersion. Drowning remains a common cause of accidental death throughout the world and is particularly common in young children (Box 5.11). In about 10% of cases no water enters the lungs and death follows intense laryngospasm ('dry' drowning). Prolonged immersion in cold water, with or without water inhalation, results in a rapid fall in core body temperature and hypothermia (p. 101).

Following inhalation of water, there is a rapid onset of ventilation–perfusion imbalance with hypoxaemia, and the development of diffuse pulmonary oedema. Fresh water is hypotonic and, although rapidly absorbed across alveolar membranes, impairs surfactant function, which leads to alveolar collapse and right-to-left shunting of unoxygenated blood. Absorption of large

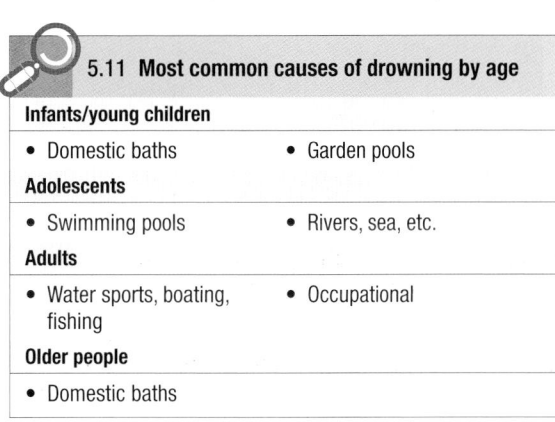

5.11 Most common causes of drowning by age

Infants/young children

• Domestic baths	• Garden pools

Adolescents

• Swimming pools	• Rivers, sea, etc.

Adults

• Water sports, boating, fishing	• Occupational

Older people

• Domestic baths	

amounts of hypotonic fluid can result in haemolysis. Salt water is hypertonic and inhalation provokes alveolar oedema, but the overall clinical effect is similar to that of freshwater drowning.

Clinical features

Those rescued alive (near-drowning) are often unconscious and not breathing. Hypoxaemia and metabolic acidosis are inevitable features. Acute lung injury usually resolves rapidly over 48–72 hours, unless infection occurs (Fig. 5.7). Complications include dehydration, hypotension, haemoptysis, rhabdomyolysis, renal failure and cardiac dysrhythmias. A small number of patients, mainly the more severely ill, progress to develop the acute respiratory distress syndrome (ARDS; p. 187).

Survival is possible after immersion for periods of up to 30 minutes in very cold water, as the rapid development of hypothermia after immersion may be protective, particularly in children. Long-term outcome depends on the severity of the cerebral hypoxic injury and is predicted by the duration of immersion, delay in resuscitation, intensity of acidosis and the presence of cardiac arrest.

Management

Initial management requires cardiopulmonary resuscitation with administration of oxygen and maintenance of the circulation (p. 556). It is important to clear the airway of foreign bodies and protect the cervical spine. Continuous positive airways pressure (CPAP; p. 194) should be considered for spontaneously breathing patients with oxygen saturations below 94%. Observation is required for a minimum of 24 hours. Prophylactic antibiotics are only required if exposure was to obviously contaminated water.

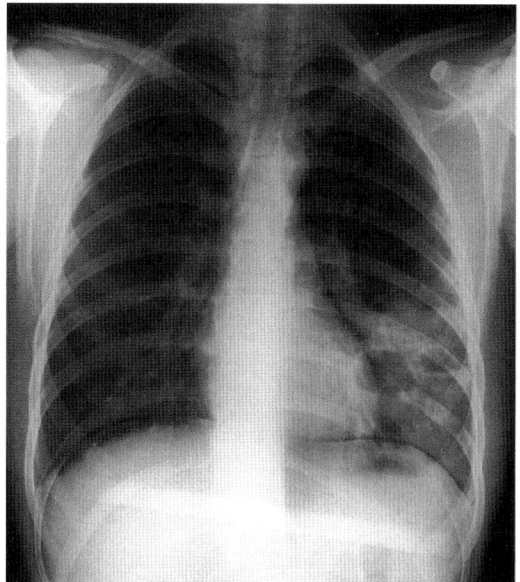

Fig. 5.7 Near-drowning. Chest X-ray of a 39-year-old farmer, 2 weeks after immersion in a polluted freshwater ditch for 5 minutes before rescue. Airspace consolidation and cavities in the left lower lobe reflect secondary staphylococcal pneumonia and abscess formation.

Diving-related illness

The underwater environment is extremely hostile. Other than drowning, most diving illness is related to changes in barometric pressure and its effect on gas behaviour.

Ambient pressure under water increases by 101 kPa (1 atmosphere) for every 10 metres of seawater (msw) depth. As divers descend, the partial pressures of the gases they are breathing increase (Box 5.12), and the blood and tissue concentrations of dissolved gases rise accordingly. Nitrogen is a weak anaesthetic agent, and if the inspiratory pressure of nitrogen is allowed to increase above ~320 kPa (i.e. a depth of ~30 msw), it produces 'narcosis', resulting in impairment of cognitive function and manual dexterity, not unlike alcohol intoxication. For this reason, compressed air can only be used for shallow diving. Oxygen is also toxic at inspired pressures above ~40 kPa (inducing apprehension, muscle twitching, euphoria, sweating, tinnitus, nausea and vertigo), so 100% oxygen cannot be used as an alternative. For dives deeper than ~30 msw, mixtures of oxygen with nitrogen and/or helium are used.

Whilst drowning remains the most common diving-related cause of death, another important group of disorders usually present once the diver returns to the surface: decompression illness (DCI) and barotrauma.

5.12 Physics of breathing compressed air while diving in sea water				
Depth	**Lung volume**	**Barometric pressure**	**PiO_2**	**PiN_2**
Surface	100%	101 kPa (1 atmos)	21 kPa	79 kPa
10 m	50%	202 kPa (2 atmos)	42 kPa	159 kPa
20 m	33%	303 kPa (3 atmos)	63 kPa	239 kPa
30 m	25%	404 kPa (4 atmos)	84 kPa	319 kPa

Clinical features

Decompression illness

This includes decompression sickness (DCS) and arterial gas embolism (AGE). Whilst the vast majority of symptoms of decompression illness present within 6 hours of a dive, they can also be provoked by flying and thus patients may present to medical services at sites far removed from the dive.

Exposure of individuals to increased partial pressures of nitrogen results in additional nitrogen being dissolved in body tissues; the amount dissolved depends on the depth/pressure and on the duration of the dive. On ascent, the tissues become supersaturated with nitrogen, and this places the diver at risk of producing a critical quantity of gas (bubbles) in tissues if the ascent is too fast. The gas so formed may cause symptoms locally, by bubbles passing through the pulmonary vascular bed (Box 5.13) or by embolisation elsewhere. Arterial embolisation may occur if the gas load in the venous system exceeds the lungs' abilities to excrete nitrogen, or when bubbles pass through a patent foramen ovale (present asymptomatically in 25–30% of adults; p. 524). Although DCS and AGE can be indistinguishable, their early treatment is the same.

Barotrauma

During the ascent phase of a dive, the gas in the diver's lungs expands due to the decreasing pressure. The diver

5.13 Assessment of a patient with decompression illness*

Evolution

- Progressive
- Static
- Relapsing
- Spontaneously improving

Manifestations

- Pain: often large joints, e.g. shoulder ('the bends')
- Neurological: any deficit is possible
- Audiovestibular: vertigo, tinnitus, nystagmus; may mimic inner ear barotrauma
- Pulmonary: chest pain, cough, haemoptysis, dyspnoea; may be due to arterial gas embolism
- Cutaneous: itching, erythematous rash
- Lymphatic: tender lymph nodes, oedema
- Constitutional: headache, fatigue, general malaise

Dive profile

- Depth
- Type of gas used
- Duration of dive

*Information required by diving specialists to decide appropriate treatment. See contact details on page 129.

must therefore ascend slowly and breathe regularly; if ascent is rapid or the diver holds his/her breath, the expanding gas may cause lung rupture (pulmonary barotrauma). This can result in pneumomediastinum, pneumothorax or AGE due to gas passing directly into the pulmonary venous system. Other air-filled body cavities may be subject to barotrauma, including the ear and sinuses.

Management

The patient is nursed horizontally and airway, breathing and circulation are assessed. Treatment includes the following:

- *High-flow oxygen* is given by a tight-fitting mask using a rebreathing bag. This assists in the washout of excess inert gas (nitrogen) and may reduce the extent of local tissue hypoxia resulting from focal embolic injury.
- *Fluid replacement* (oral or intravenous) corrects the intravascular fluid loss from endothelial bubble injury and the dehydration associated with immersion. Maintenance of an adequate peripheral circulation is important for the excretion of excess dissolved gas.
- *Recompression* is the definitive therapy. Transfer to a recompression chamber facility may be by surface or air, provided that the altitude remains low (< 300 m) and the patient continues to breathe 100% oxygen. Recompression reduces the volume of gas within tissues and puts nitrogen back into solution.

The majority of patients make a complete recovery with treatment, although a small but significant proportion are left with neurological disability.

PRINCIPLES AND INVESTIGATION OF NUTRITIONAL FACTORS IN DISEASE

Obtaining adequate nutrition is a fundamental requirement for survival of every individual and species. The politics of food provision for humans are complex, and constitute a prominent factor in wars, natural disasters and the global economy. In recent decades, economic success has been rewarded by plentiful nutrition unknown to previous generations, which has led to a pandemic of obesity and its serious consequences for health. Yet in many parts of the world, famine and under-nutrition still represent a huge burden. Quality, as well as quantity, of food influences health. Inappropriate diets have been linked with diseases such as coronary heart disease and cancer. Deficiencies of simple vitamins or minerals lead to avoidable conditions such as anaemia due to iron deficiency or blindness due to severe vitamin A deficiency. A proper understanding of nutrition is therefore essential in dealing with the needs of individual patients and to inform the planning of public policy.

Physiology of nutrition

Nutrients in the diet can be classified into 'macronutrients', which are eaten in relatively large amounts to provide fuel for energy, and 'micronutrients' (e.g. vitamins and minerals), which do not contribute to energy balance but are required in small amounts because they are not synthesised in the body.

Energy balance

The laws of thermodynamics dictate that energy balance is achieved when energy intake = energy expenditure (Fig. 5.8).

Energy expenditure has several components. The basal metabolic rate (BMR) describes the obligatory energy expenditure required to maintain metabolic functions in tissues and hence sustain life. It is most closely predicted by fat-free mass (i.e. total body mass minus fat mass), which is lower in females and older people (Fig. 5.8B). Extra metabolic energy is consumed during growth, pregnancy and lactation, and when febrile. Metabolic energy is also required for thermal regulation, and expenditure is higher in cold or hot environments. The energy required for digestion of food (diet-induced thermogenesis (DIT); Fig. 5.8C) accounts for approximately 10% of total energy expenditure, with protein requiring more energy than other macronutrients. Another component of energy expenditure is governed by the level of muscular activity, which can vary considerably with occupation and lifestyle (Fig. 5.8D). Physical activity levels are usually defined as multiples of BMR.

Energy intake is determined by the 'macronutrient' content of food. Carbohydrates, fat, protein and alcohol provide fuel for oxidation in the mitochondria to generate energy (as adenosine triphosphate (ATP; p. 42). The energy provided by each differs:

- carbohydrates (16 kJ/g)
- fat (37 kJ/g)
- protein (17 kJ/g)
- alcohol (29 kJ/g).

Regulation of energy balance

Energy intake and expenditure are highly regulated (Fig. 5.9). A link with reproductive function ensures that pregnancy is most likely to occur during times of nutritional plenty when both mother and baby have a better chance of survival. Improved nutrition is thought to be

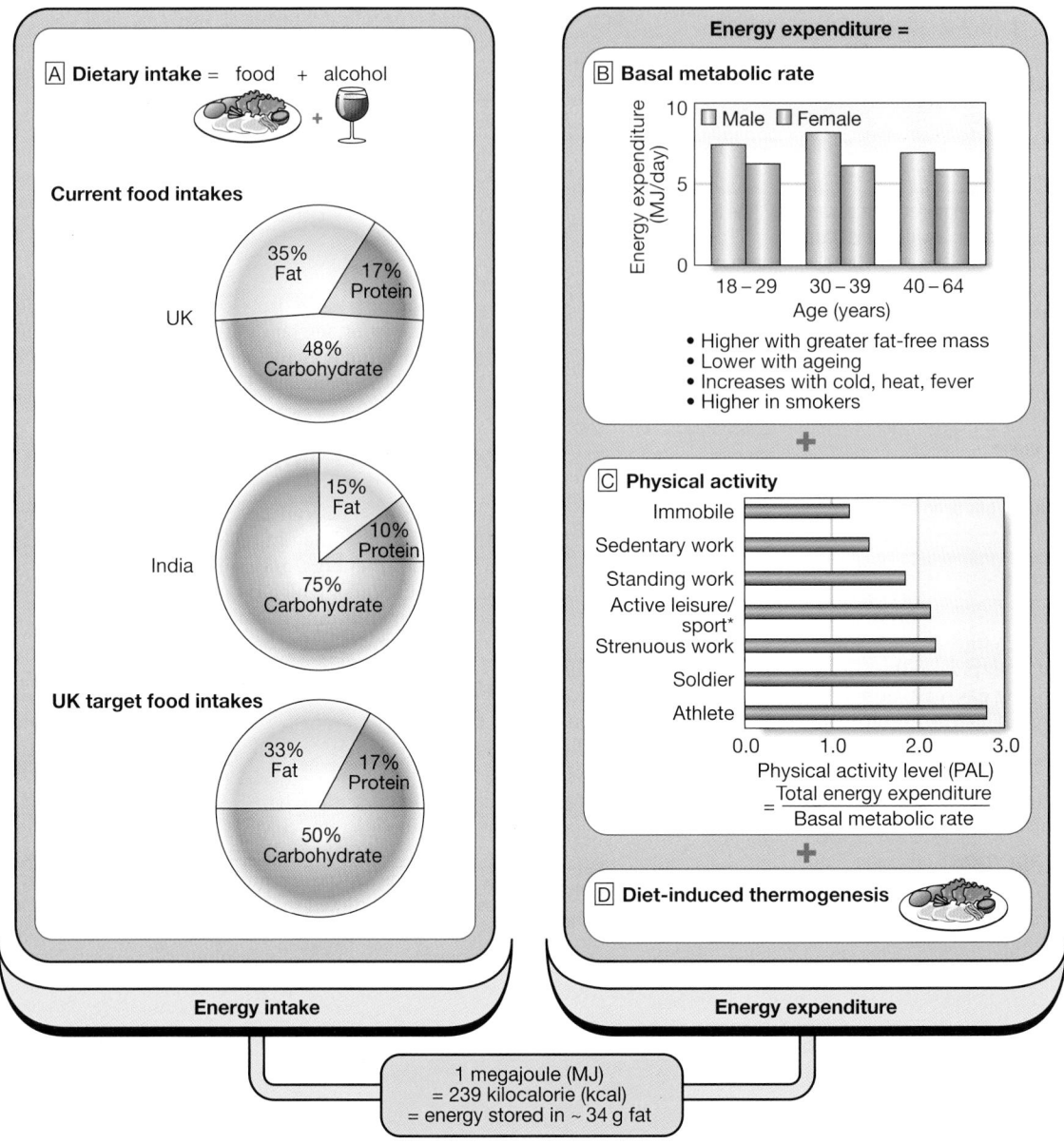

Fig. 5.8 Determinants of energy balance. $\boxed{A}$ Energy intake is shown as national averages, highlighting the differences in sources of energy in different countries (but obscuring substantial regional variations). The targets are recommendations as a percentage of food energy only (Source: Dept of Health 1991). For WHO target, see Box 5.17. In the UK it is assumed that 5% of energy intake will be derived from alcohol. $\boxed{B}$ Data for normal basal metabolic rate (BMR) were obtained from healthy men and women in various countries. BMR declines from middle age and is lower in women, even after adjustment for body size because of differences in fat-free mass. $\boxed{C}$ Energy is required for movement and activity. Physical activity level (PAL) is the multiple of BMR by which total energy expenditure is increased by activity. $\boxed{D}$ Energy is consumed in order to digest food. *Leisure or sport activity increases PAL by ~0.3 for each 30–60 minutes of moderate exercise performed 4–5 times per week.

the reason for the increasingly early onset of puberty in many societies. At the other extreme, anorexia nervosa and excessive exercise can lead to amenorrhoea (p. 249).

Regulation of energy balance is coordinated in the hypothalamus, which receives afferent signals that indicate nutritional status in the short term (e.g. the stomach hormone ghrelin, which falls immediately after eating and rises gradually thereafter, to suppress satiety and signal that it is time for the next meal) and the long term (e.g. the adipose hormone leptin, which increases with growing fat mass and stimulates satiety). The hypothal-

amus responds with changes in many local neurotransmitters that alter activity in a number of pathways which influence energy balance (see Fig. 5.9), including hormones acting on the pituitary gland (see Fig. 20.2, p. 743), and neural control circuits which connect with the cerebral cortex and autonomic nervous system.

Responses to under- and over-nutrition

These complex regulatory pathways allow adaptation to variations in nutrition. In response to starvation, reproductive function is suppressed, BMR is reduced, and there are profound psychological effects, including energy

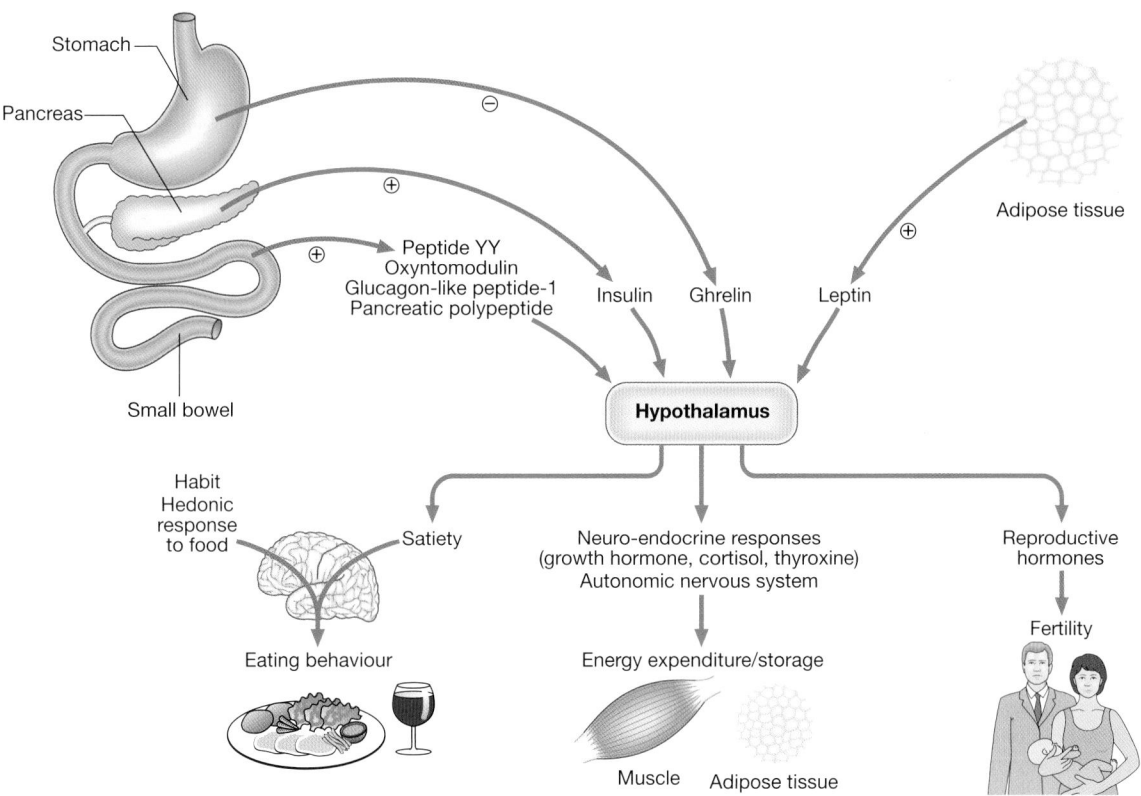

Fig. 5.9 Regulation of energy balance and its link with reproduction. ⊕ indicates factors which are stimulated by eating and induce satiety. ⊖ indicates factors which are suppressed by eating and inhibit satiety.

conservation through lethargy. These adjustments can 'defend' body weight within certain limits. However, in the low-insulin state of starvation (Fig. 21.2, p. 799), fuels are liberated from stores initially in glycogen (in liver and muscle), then in triglyceride (lipolysis in adipose tissue, with excess free fatty acid supply to the liver leading to ketosis) and finally in protein (proteolysis in muscle).

In response to over-nutrition, BMR is increased, and extra energy is consumed in the work of carrying increased fat stores, so that body weight is again 'defended' within certain limits. In the high-insulin state of over-nutrition, excess energy is invested in fatty acids and stored as triglycerides; these are deposited principally in adipose tissue but they may also accumulate in liver (non-alcoholic fatty liver disease; p. 956) and skeletal muscle. In the absence of hypothalamic function (e.g. in those with craniopharyngioma; see Fig. 20.32, p. 792) or in rare patients with mutations in relevant genes (e.g. in leptin or melanocortin-4 receptors), loss of satiety signals, together with loss of adaptive changes in energy expenditure, result in relentless weight gain.

Energy-yielding nutrients (macronutrients)

Carbohydrates

Types of carbohydrate and their dietary sources are listed in Box 5.14. The 'available' carbohydrates (starches and sugars) are broken down to monosaccharides before absorption from the gut (p. 839), and supply over half the energy in a normal, well-balanced diet (see Fig. 5.8A). No individual carbohydrate is an essential nutrient, as car-

bohydrates can be synthesised de novo from glycerol or protein. However, if the available carbohydrate intake is less than 100 g per day, increased lipolysis leads to ketosis (see Fig. 21.5, p. 802).

Dietary guidelines do not restrict the intake of intrinsic sugars in fruit and vegetables or the sugars in milk. However, intake of non-milk extrinsic sugars (sucrose, maltose, fructose), which increase the risk of dental caries and diabetes mellitus, should be limited. Starches in cereal foods, root foods and legumes provide the largest proportion of energy in most diets around the world. All starches are polymers of glucose, linked by the same 1–4 glycosidic linkages. However, some starches are digested promptly by salivary and then pancreatic amylase, producing rapid delivery of glucose to the blood. Other starches are digested more slowly, either because they are protected in the structure of the food, because of their crystal structure, or because the molecule is unbranched (amylose). These differences are the basis for the 'glycaemic index' of foods. This is the area under the curve of the rise in blood glucose concentration in the 2 hours following ingestion of 50 g carbohydrate, expressed as a percentage of the response to 50 g anhydrous glucose. There is emerging evidence linking high glycaemic index foods with obesity and type 2 diabetes (p. 803).

Dietary fibre

Dietary fibre is plant food that is not digested by human enzymes in the gastrointestinal tract. Most dietary fibre is known as the 'non-starch polysaccharides' (NSP) (see Box 5.14). A small percentage of 'resistant' dietary starch may also pass unchanged into the large intestine.

109

i 5.14 Dietary carbohydrates

Class	Components	Examples	Source
Free sugars	Monosaccharides Disaccharides	Glucose, fructose Sucrose, lactose, maltose	Intrinsic: fruits, milks, vegetables Extrinsic (extracted, refined): beet or cane sucrose
Short-chain carbohydrates	Oligosaccharides	Maltodextrins, fructo-oligosaccharides	
Starch polysaccharides	Rapidly digestible Slowly digestible Resistant		Cereals (wheat, rice), root vegetables (potato), legumes (lentils, beans, peas)
Non-starch polysaccharides (NSP, dietary fibre)	Fibrous Viscous	Cellulose Hemicellulose Pectins Gums	Plants

Dietary fibre can be broken down by the resident bacteria in the colon to produce short-chain fatty acids. This is essential fuel for the enterocytes and contributes to bowel health. The extent of flatus formed is dependent on the food source.

Some types of NSP, notably the hemicellulose of wheat, increase the water-holding capacity of colonic contents and the bulk of faeces. They relieve simple constipation, appear to prevent diverticulosis and may reduce the risk of cancer of the colon. Other viscous, indigestible polysaccharides like pectin and guar gum are important in the upper gastrointestinal tract, where they slow gastric emptying, contribute to satiety, and reduce bile salt absorption and hence plasma cholesterol concentration.

Fats

Fat has the highest energy density of the macronutrients (37 kJ/g) and excessive consumption may be an insidious cause of obesity (see Fig. 5.8A). Free fatty acids are absorbed in chylomicrons (p. 449), allowing access of complex molecules into the circulation. Fatty acid structures are shown in Figure 5.10. The principal polyunsaturated fatty acid (PUFA) in plant seed oils is linoleic acid (18:2 ω6). This and alpha-linolenic acid (18:3 ω3) are the 'essential' fatty acids, which humans cannot synthesise de novo. They undergo further desaturation and elongation, to produce e.g. γ-linolenic acid (18:3 ω6) and arachidonic acid (20:4 ω6). These are precursors of prostaglandins and eicosanoids, and form part of the structure of lipid membranes in all cells. Fish oils are rich in ω3 PUFA (e.g. eicosapentaenoic (20:5 ω3) and docosahexaenoic (22:6 ω3), which promote the anti-inflammatory cascade of prostaglandin production and occur in the lipids of the human brain and retina. They inhibit thrombosis by competitively antagonising thromboxane A_2 formation. Substituting saturated fat (i.e. from animal sources: butter, ghee or lard) with PUFA in the diet can lower the concentration of circulating low-density lipoprotein (LDL) cholesterol and may help prevent coronary heart disease. Intake of *trans* fatty acids (TFA) (isomers of the natural *cis* fatty acids) has increased in the UK diet, primarily due to use of oils that have been partially hydrogenated in the food industry. It is recommended that TFAs are limited to < 2% of the dietary fat intake, as they are associated with cardiovascular disease.

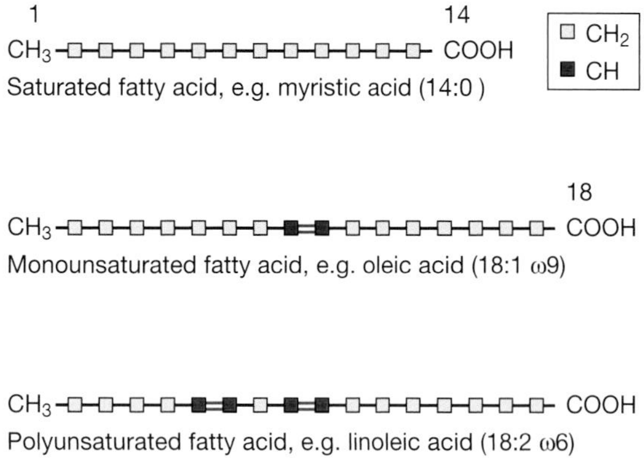

Cholesterol is also absorbed directly from food in chylomicrons and is an important substrate for steroid and sterol synthesis, but not an important source of energy.

Proteins

Proteins are made up of some 20 different amino acids, of which nine are 'essential' (Box 5.15), i.e. they cannot be synthesised in humans but are required for synthesis of important proteins. Another group of five amino acids are termed 'conditionally essential', meaning that they can be synthesised from other amino acids, provided there is an adequate dietary supply. The remaining amino acids can be synthesised in the body by transamination, provided there is a sufficient supply of amino groups.

The nutritive or 'biological' value of different proteins depends on the relative proportions of essential amino acids they contain. Proteins of animal origin, particularly from eggs, milk and meat, are generally of higher biological value than proteins of vegetable origin, which are low in one or more of the essential amino acids. However, when two different vegetable proteins are eaten together (e.g. a cereal and a legume), their

```
 1                              14
CH3 -□-□-□-□-□-□-□-□-□-□-□-□-□- COOH
Saturated fatty acid, e.g. myristic acid (14:0 )
```

□ CH2
■ CH

```
                                18
CH3 -□-□-□-□-□-□-□-■-□-□-□-□-□-□-□-□- COOH
Monounsaturated fatty acid, e.g. oleic acid (18:1 ω9)
```

```
CH3 -□-□-□-□-■-■-□-□-□-■-□-□-□-□-□-□- COOH
Polyunsaturated fatty acid, e.g. linoleic acid (18:2 ω6)
```

Fig. 5.10 Schematic representation of fatty acids. Standard nomenclature specifies the number of carbon atoms and indicates the number and position of the double bond(s) relative to the methyl (–CH₃, ω) end of the molecule after a colon.

5.15 Amino acids

Essential amino acids

- Tryptophan
- Histidine
- Methionine
- Threonine
- Isoleucine
- Valine
- Phenylalanine
- Lysine
- Leucine

Conditionally essential amino acids and their precursors

- Cysteine: methionine, serine
- Tyrosine: phenylalanine
- Arginine: glutamine/glutamate, aspartate
- Proline: glutamate
- Glycine: serine, choline

amino acid contents are complementary and produce an adequate mix, an important principle in vegan diets.

Dietary recommendations for macronutrients

Recommendations for energy intake (Box 5.16) and proportions of macronutrients (Box 5.17) have been calculated to provide a balance of essential nutrients and minimise the risks of excessive refined sugar (dental caries, high glycaemic index/diabetes mellitus), saturated fat or trans fat (obesity, coronary heart disease). Recommended dietary fibre intake is based on avoiding

5.16 Daily adult energy requirements in health

Circumstances	Requirements	
	Females	Males
At rest	6.7 MJ (1600 kcal)	8.4 MJ (2000 kcal)
Light work	8.4 MJ (2000 kcal)	11.3 MJ (2700 kcal)
Heavy work	9.4 MJ (2250 kcal)	14.6 MJ (3500 kcal)

5.17 WHO recommended population macronutrient goals

Nutrient (% of total energy unless indicated)	Target limits for population average intakes	
	Lower	Upper
Total fat	15	30
Saturated fatty acids	0	10
Polyunsaturated fatty acids	6	10
Trans fatty acids	0	2
Dietary cholesterol (mg/day)	0	300
Total carbohydrate	55	75
Free sugars	0	10
Complex carbohydrate	50	70
Dietary fibre (g/day)		
As non-starch polysaccharides	16	24
As total dietary fibre	27	40
Protein	10	15

risks of colonic disease. The usual recommended protein intake for a healthy man doing light work is 65–100 g/day. The minimum requirement is around 40 g of protein with a high proportion of essential amino acids or a high biological value.

Vitamins

Vitamins are organic substances with key roles in certain metabolic pathways, and are categorised into those that are fat-soluble (vitamins A, D, E and K) and those that are water-soluble (vitamins of the B complex group and vitamin C).

Recommended daily intakes of micronutrients (Box 5.18) vary between countries and the nomenclature has become potentially confusing. In the UK, the 'reference nutrient intake' (RNI) has been calculated as the mean plus two standard deviations (SD) of daily intake in the population, which therefore describes normal intake for 97.5% of the population. The lower reference nutrient intake (LRNI) is the mean minus 2 SD, below which would be considered deficient in most of the population. These dietary reference values (DRV) have superseded the terms RDI (recommended daily intakes) and RDA (recommended daily amounts). Other countries use different terminology. Additional amounts of some micronutrients may be required in pregnancy and lactation (Box 5.19).

Vitamin A (retinol)

Preformed retinol is found only in foods of animal origin. Vitamin A can also be derived from carotenes, which are present in green and coloured vegetables and some fruits. Carotenes provide most of the total vitamin A in the UK, and provide the only supply in vegans. Retinol is converted to several other important molecules:

- *11-cis retinaldehyde* is part of the photoreceptor complex in rods of the retina.
- *Retinoic acid* induces differentiation of epithelial cells by binding to specific nuclear receptors, which induce responsive genes. In vitamin A deficiency, mucus-secreting cells are replaced by keratin-producing cells.
- *Retinoids* are necessary for normal growth, fetal development, fertility, haematopoiesis and immune function.

Vitamin D

The natural form of vitamin D, cholecalciferol or vitamin D_3, is formed in the skin by the action of UV light on 7-dehydrocholesterol, a metabolite of cholesterol. Few foods contain vitamin D naturally and skin exposure to sunlight is the main source. Moving away from the equator, the intensity of UV light decreases, so that at a latitude above 50° (including northern Europe), vitamin D is not synthesised from October to March, and even at > 30° there is seasonal variation. The body store accumulated during the summer is consumed during the winter. Vitamin D is converted in the liver to 25-hydroxy vitamin D (25(OH)D), which is further hydroxylated in the kidneys to 1,25-dihydroxy-vitamin D (1,25(OH)$_2$D), the active form of the vitamin (see Fig. 20.17, p. 764). 1,25(OH)$_2$D activates specific intracellular receptors which influence calcium metabolism, bone mineralisation and tissue differentiation. The synthetic form, ergocalciferol or vitamin D_2, is considered to be less effective than the endogenous D_3.

111

i 5.18 Summary of clinically important vitamins

Vitamin	Sources*	Reference nutrient intake (RNI)
Fat-soluble		
A (retinol)	*Rich:* liver	700 µg men
	Important: milk and milk products, eggs, fish oils	600 µg women
D (cholecalciferol)	UV exposure to skin	10 µg if > 65 yrs or no sunlight exposure
	Rich: fish oils	
	Important: egg yolks, margarine, fortified cereals	
E (tocopherol)	*Rich:* sunflower oil	No RNI. Safe intake:
	Important: vegetables, nuts, seed oils	4 mg men
		3 mg women
K (phylloquinone, menaquinone)	*Rich:* green vegetables	No RNI. Safe intake: 1 µg/kg
	Important: soya oil, menaquinones produced by intestinal bacteria	
Water-soluble		
B₁ (thiamin)	*Rich:* pork	0.8 mg per 9.68 MJ (2000 kcal) energy intake
	Important: cereals, grains, beans	
B₂ (riboflavin)	*Rich:* milk	1.3 mg men
	Important: milk and milk products, breakfast cereals, bread	1.1 mg women
B₃ (niacin, nicotinic acid, nicotinamide)	*Rich:* meat, cereals	17 mg men
		13 mg women
B₆ (pyridoxine)	*Rich:* meat, fish, potatoes, bananas	1.4 mg men
	Important: vegetables, intestinal microflora synthesis	1.2 mg women
Folate	*Rich:* liver	200 µg
	Important: green leafy vegetables, fortified breakfast cereals	
B₁₂ (Cobalamin)	*Rich:* animal products	1.5 µg
	Important: bacterial colonisation	
Biotin	*Rich:* egg yolk	No RNI. Safe intake: 10–200 µg
	Important: intestinal flora	
C (ascorbic acid)	*Rich:* citrus fruit	40 mg
	Important: fresh fruit, fresh and frozen vegetables	

*Rich sources contain the nutrient in high concentration but are not generally eaten in large amounts; important sources contain less but contribute most because larger amounts are eaten.

Recommended dietary intakes aim to prevent rickets and osteomalacia (p. 1121). There is increasing evidence that vitamin D is important for immune and muscle function, and may reduce falls in the elderly (p. 170). Margarines are fortified with vitamin D in the UK, and milk is fortified in some parts of Europe and in North America.

Vitamin E

There are eight related fat-soluble substances with vitamin E activity. The most important dietary form is α-tocopherol. Vitamin E has many direct metabolic actions:

- It prevents oxidation of polyunsaturated fatty acids in cell membranes by free radicals.
- It helps maintain cell membrane structure.
- It affects DNA synthesis and cell signalling.
- It is involved in the anti-inflammatory and immune systems.

Vitamin K

Vitamin K is supplied in the diet mainly as vitamin K_1 (phylloquinone) in the UK, or as vitamin K_2 (menaquinone) from fermented products in parts of Asia. Vitamin K_2 is also synthesised by bacteria in the colon. Vitamin K is a co-factor for carboxylation reactions: in particular, the production of γ-carboxyglutamate (gla). Gla residues are found in four of the coagulation factor proteins (II, VII, IX and X; p. 993), conferring their capacity to bind to phospholipid surfaces in the presence of calcium. Other important gla proteins are osteocalcin and matrix gla protein, which are important in bone mineralisation.

Thiamin (vitamin B₁)

Thiamin is widely distributed in foods of both vegetable and animal origin. Thiamin pyrophosphate (TPP) is a co-factor for enzyme reactions involved in the metabolism of macronutrients (carbohydrate, fat and alcohol), including:

- decarboxylation of pyruvate to acetyl-co-enzyme A, which bridges between glycolysis and the tricarboxylic acid (Krebs) cycle
- transketolase activity in the hexose monophosphate shunt pathway
- decarboxylation of α-ketoglutarate to succinate in the Krebs cycle.

Riboflavin (vitamin B₂)

Riboflavin is required for the flavin co-factors involved in oxidation–reduction reactions. It is widely distributed

5.19 Nutrition in pregnancy and lactation

- **Energy requirements**: increased in both the mother and fetus, but can be met through reduced maternal energy expenditure.
- **Micronutrient requirements**: adaptive mechanisms ensure increased uptake of minerals in pregnancy, but extra increments of some are required during lactation (see Box 5.21). Additional increments of some vitamins are recommended during pregnancy and lactation:
  - Vitamin A: for growth and maintenance of the fetus, and to provide some reserve (important in some countries to prevent blindness associated with vitamin A deficiency). Teratogenic in excessive amounts.
  - Vitamin D: to ensure bone and dental development in the infant. Higher incidences of hypocalcaemia, hypoparathyroidisim and defective dental enamel have been seen in infants of women not taking vitamin D supplements at > 52° latitude.
  - Folate: to avoid neural tube defects (Box 5.20).
  - Vitamin B_{12} in lactation only.
  - Thiamin: to meet increased fetal energy demands.
  - Riboflavin: to meet extra demands.
  - Niacin in lactation only.
  - Vitamin C: for the last trimester to maintain maternal stores as fetal demands increase.
  - Iodine: in countries with high consumption of staple foods (e.g. brassicas, maize, bamboo shoots) that contain goitrogens (thiocyanates or perchlorates) which interfere with iodine update, supplements prevent infants being born with cretinism.

5

in animal and vegetable foods. Levels are low in staple cereals but germination increases its content. It is destroyed under alkaline conditions by heat and by exposure to sunlight.

Niacin (vitamin B_3)

Niacin encompasses nicotinic acid and nicotinamide. Nicotinamide is an essential part of the two pyridine nucleotides, nicotinamide adenine dinucleotide (NAD) and nicotinamide adenine dinucleotide phosphate (NADP), which play a key role as hydrogen acceptors and donors for many enzymes. Niacin can be synthesised in the body in limited amounts from the amino acid tryptophan.

Pyridoxine (vitamin B_6)

Pyridoxine, pyridoxal and pyridoxamine are different forms of vitamin B_6 which undergo phosphorylation to produce pyridoxal 5-phosphate (PLP). PLP is the cofactor for a large number of enzymes involved in the metabolism of amino acids. Vitamin B_6 is available in most foods.

Folate (folic acid)

Folates exist in many forms. The main circulating form is 5-methyltetrahydrofolate. The natural forms are prone to oxidation. Folic acid is the stable synthetic form. Folate works as a methyl donor for cellular methylation and protein synthesis. It is directly involved in DNA and RNA synthesis, and requirements increase during embryonic development. The UK Department of Health advises that women who have experienced a pregnancy affected by a neural tube defect should take 5mg of folic acid daily from before conception and throughout the first trimester (Box 5.20). All women planning a pregnancy are advised to include good sources of folate in their diet, and take folate supplements throughout the first trimester. Liver is the richest source of folate but an alternative source (e.g. leafy vegetables) is advised in early pregnancy because of the high vitamin A content of liver (p. 111). In the US, there is mandatory fortification of flour with folic acid and there is voluntary fortification of many foods across Europe. There are now concerns that this may be responsible for the increased incidence of colon cancer through promotion of the growth of polyps.

Hydroxycobalamin (vitamin B_{12})

Vitamin B_{12} is a co-factor in folate co-enzyme recycling and nerve myelination. Vitamin B_{12} and folate are particularly important in DNA synthesis in red blood cells (p. 1020).

Vitamin C (ascorbic acid)

Ascorbic acid is the most active reducing agent in the aqueous phase of living tissues and is involved in intracellular electron transfer. It takes part in the hydroxylation of proline and lysine in protocollagen to hydroxyproline and hydroxylysine in mature collagen. It is very easily destroyed by heat, increased pH and light, and is very soluble in water; hence many traditional cooking methods reduce or eliminate it. Claims that high-dose vitamin C improves immune function (including resistance to the common cold) and cholesterol turnover remain unsubstantiated.

Inorganic nutrients

A number of inorganic elements are essential dietary constituents for humans (Box 5.21).

Calcium and phosphorus

Calcium is the most abundant cation in the body and powerful homeostatic mechanisms control circulating ionised calcium levels (p. 763). World Health Organization (WHO) dietary guidelines for calcium differ between countries, with higher intakes usually recommended in places with higher fracture prevalence. Between 20 and 30% of calcium in the diet is absorbed, depending on vitamin D status and food source. Calcium requirements depend on phosphorus intakes with an optimum molar ratio (Ca:P) of 1:1.

EBM 5.20 Periconceptual folate supplementation and neural tube defects

'Folate supplementation in advance of conception and during the first trimester reduces the incidence of neural tube defects by ~70%.'

- Lumley J, et al. (Cochrane Review). Cochrane Library, issue 3, 2005. Oxford: Update Software.

For further information: www.cochrane.org

5.21 Summary of clinically important minerals

Mineral	Sources[1]	Reference nutrient intake (RNI)
Calcium	*Rich:* milk and milk products, tofu *Important:* milk, boned fish, green vegetables, beans	700 mg[2]
Phosphorus	Most foods contain phosphorus *Rich:* Marmite® and dry-roasted peanuts *Important:* milk, cereal products, bread and meat	550 mg[2]
Magnesium	*Rich:* whole grains, nuts *Important:* unprocessed and wholegrain foods	300 mg men 270 mg women[2]
Iron	*Rich:* liver, red meat (haem iron) *Important:* non-haem iron from vegetables, wholemeal bread	8.7 mg 14.8 mg women < 50 yrs
Zinc	*Rich:* red meat, seafood *Important:* dairy produce, wholemeal bread	9.5 mg men 7 mg women[2]
Iodine	*Rich:* edible seaweeds *Important:* milk and dairy products	140 µg
Selenium	*Rich:* fish, wheat grown in selenium-rich soils *Important:* fish	60 µg women[2] 75 µg men
Copper	*Rich:* shellfish, liver *Important:* bread, cereal products, vegetables	1.2 mg[2]
Fluoride	Drinking water, tea	No RNI. Safe intake: 0.5 mg/kg
Potassium	*Rich:* dried fruit, potatoes, coffee *Important:* fresh fruit, vegetables, milk	3500 mg
Sodium	*Rich:* Table salt, anchovies *Important:* processed foods, bread, bacon	1600 mg

[1]Rich sources contain the nutrient in high concentration but are not generally eaten in large amounts; important sources contain less but contribute most because larger amounts are eaten.
[2]Increased amounts are required in women during lactation.

Excessive phosphorus intakes (e.g. 1–1.5 g/day) with a Ca:P of 1:3 have been shown to cause hypocalcaemia and secondary hyperparathyroidism (p. 765).

Iron

Iron is involved in the synthesis of haemoglobin, and is required for the transport of electrons within cells and in a number of enzyme reactions. Non-haem iron in cereals and vegetables is poorly absorbed, but makes the greater contribution to overall intake, compared to the well-absorbed haem iron from animal products. Fruits and vegetables containing vitamin C enhance iron absorption, while the tannins in tea reduce it. Dietary calcium reduces iron uptake from the same meal, which may precipitate iron deficiency in those with borderline iron stores. There is no physiological mechanism for excretion of iron, so homeostasis depends on the regulation of iron absorption. The normal daily loss of iron is 1 mg, arising from desquamated surface cells and intestinal losses. A regular loss of only 2 mL of blood per day doubles the iron requirement. On average, an additional 20 mg of iron is lost during menstruation, so pre-menopausal women require about twice as much iron as men (and more if menstrual losses are heavy).

Iodine

Iodine is required for synthesis of thyroid hormones (p. 736). It is present in sea fish, seaweed and most plant foods grown near the sea. The amount of iodine in soil and water influences the iodine content of most foods. Iodine is lacking in the highest mountainous areas of the world (e.g. the Alps and the Himalayas) and in the soil of frequently flooded plains (e.g. Bangladesh).

Zinc

Zinc is present in most foods of vegetable and animal origin. It is an essential component of many enzymes, including carbonic anhydrase, alcohol dehydrogenase and alkaline phosphatase.

Selenium

The family of seleno-enzymes includes glutathione peroxidase, which helps prevent free radical damage to cells, and monodeiodinase, which converts thyroxine to triiodothyronine (p. 736). North American soil has a higher selenium content than European and Asian soil, and the decreasing reliance of Europe on imported American food in recent decades has resulted in a decline in dietary selenium intake.

Fluoride

Fluoride helps prevent dental caries, since it increases the resistance of the enamel to acid attack. It is a component of bone mineral and some studies have shown anti-fracture effects at low doses but excessive intakes may compromise bone structure.

Sodium, potassium and magnesium

The roles of these are discussed in Chapter 16. Western diets are high in sodium due to the sodium chloride (salt) that is added to processed food. In the UK it is suggested that daily salt intakes are kept well below 6 g.

Other essential inorganic nutrients

These include chloride (counter-ion to sodium and potassium), cobalt (required for vitamin B12), sulphur (constituent of methionine and cysteine), manganese (required for or activates many enzymes) and chromium (required for insulin action).

Clinical assessment and investigation of nutritional status

The diverse manifestations of inadequate nutrition dictate that its clinical assessment and investigation involve many systems. Energy balance is reflected in body composition, which is most readily assessed by clinical anthropometric measurements. It can also be tested non-invasively by the measurement of body fat by bioimpedance or dual energy X-ray absorptiometry (DEXA) scanning. Abnormal micronutrient status is commonly manifest in clinical signs in the skin and mucous membranes, or in other systems.

A dietary history provides useful information, especially when obtained by a dietitian. A weighed food diary is considered to be the gold standard dietary assessment but is rarely conducted in clinical practice. Body stores of some micronutrients can be assessed by biochemical tests, although many of these provide indicative rather than definitive results (Box 5.22).

Anthropometric measurements

Body mass index (BMI) is useful for categorising under- and over-nutrition. It is the weight in kilograms divided by the height in metres, squared. For example, an adult weighing 70 kg with a height of 1.75 m has a BMI of $70/1.75^2 = 22.9 \,\text{kg/m}^2$. If height cannot be determined (e.g. in older people with kyphosis or in those who cannot stand), a surrogate measure is:

- *the demispan*: measured from the sternal notch to the middle finger; height = $0.73 \times (2 \times \text{demispan}) + 0.43$
- *knee height*:
    females (60–80 years): height (cm) = (knee height (cm) $\times$ 1.91) − (age (years) $\times$ 0.17) + 75.00
    males (60–80 years): height (cm) = (knee height (cm) $\times$ 2.05) + 59.01.

BMI does not discriminate between fat mass and lean body mass and can be increased by muscle mass (e.g. in athletes). Moreover, there are ethnic differences in body fat content; at the same BMI, Asians have more body fat than Europeans. For optimal health, the BMI should be 18.5–24.9 kg/m².

An indication of the degree of abdominal obesity is the waist circumference, measured at the level of the umbilicus. Hip circumference can be measured at the level of the greater trochanters; waist:hip ratios show whether the distribution of fat is android or gynoid (see below). Skinfold measurements can be used to calculate body fat content, whereas relative loss of muscle and subcutaneous fat can be estimated by measuring mid-arm circumference (at the middle of the humerus) and skinfold thickness over the triceps (using special callipers); muscle mass is estimated by subtracting triceps skinfold thickness from mid-arm circumference.

5

5.22 Biochemical assessment of vitamin status

Nutrient	Biochemical assessments of deficiency or excess
Vitamin A	Serum retinol may be low in deficiency Serum retinyl esters: when vitamin A toxicity is suspected
Vitamin D	Plasma/serum 25-hydroxy vitamin D (25(OH)D): reflects liver stores Plasma/serum 1,25(OH)$_2$D: difficult to interpret
Vitamin E	Serum tocopherol:cholesterol ratio
Vitamin K	Coagulation assays (e.g. prothrombin time) Plasma vitamin K
Vitamin B$_1$ (thiamin)	Red blood cell transketolase activity or whole blood vitamin B$_1$
Vitamin B$_2$ (riboflavin)	Red blood cell glutathione reductase activity or whole blood vitamin B$_2$
Vitamin B$_3$ (niacin)	Urinary metabolites: 1-methyl-2-pyridone-5-carboxamide, 1-methylnicotinamide
Vitamin B$_6$	Plasma pyridoxal phosphate or erythrocyte transaminase activation coefficient
Vitamin B$_{12}$	Plasma B$_{12}$: poor measure of overall vitamin B$_{12}$ status but will detect severe deficiency. Alternatives (methylmalonic acid and holotranscobalamin) are not used routinely
Folate	Red blood cell folate Plasma folate: reflects recent intake but also detects unmetabolised folic acid from foods and supplements
Vitamin C	Leucocyte ascorbic acid: assesses vitamin C tissue stores Plasma ascorbic acid: reflects recent (daily) intake

5

PRESENTING PROBLEMS OF ALTERED ENERGY BALANCE

Obesity

Obesity is widely regarded as a pandemic, with potentially disastrous consequences for human health. Nearly one-quarter of adults in the UK were obese (i.e. BMI ≥ 30 kg/m²) in 2006, compared with 7% prevalence in 1980 and 16% in 1995. Moreover, almost two-thirds of the UK adult population are overweight (BMI ≥ 25 kg/m²), although there is considerable regional and age group variation. In developing countries, average national rates of obesity are low, but these figures may disguise high rates of obesity in urban communities; for example, nearly one-quarter of women in urban India are overweight.

There is increasing public awareness of the health implications of obesity. Many patients will seek medical help for their obesity, others will present with one of the complications of obesity, and increasing numbers are being identified during health screening examinations.

Complications of obesity

Obesity has adverse effects on both mortality and morbidity (Box 5.23). Changes in mortality are difficult to analyse due to the confounding effects of lower body weight in cigarette smokers. However, it is clear that the lowest mortality rates are seen in Europeans in the BMI range 18.5–24 kg/m² (and at lower BMI in Asians).

5.23 Complications of obesity

Risk factors	Outcomes
'Metabolic syndrome'	
Type 2 diabetes	Coronary heart disease
Hypertension	Stroke
Hyperlipidaemia	Diabetes complications
Liver fat accumulation	Non-alcoholic steatohepatitis
	Cirrhosis
Restricted ventilation	Exertional dyspnoea
	Sleep apnoea
	Respiratory failure (Pickwickian syndrome)
Mechanical effects of weight	Urinary incontinence
	Osteoarthritis
	Varicose veins
Increased peripheral steroid interconversion in adipose tissue	Hormone-dependent cancers (breast, uterus)
	Polycystic ovary syndrome (infertility, hirsutism; p. 760)
Others	Psychological morbidity (low self-esteem, depression)
	Socioeconomic disadvantage (lower income, less likely to be promoted)
	Gallstones
	Colorectal cancer
	Skin infections (groin and submammary candidiasis; hidradenitis)

It is suggested that obesity at age 40 years can reduce life expectancy by up to 7 years for non-smokers and by 13 years for smokers. Coronary heart disease (Fig. 5.11) is the major cause of death but cancer rates are also increased in the overweight, especially colorectal cancer in males and cancer of the gallbladder, biliary tract, breast, endometrium and cervix in females. Obesity has little effect on life expectancy at > 70 years, but the obese do spend a greater proportion of their active life disabled. Epidemic obesity has been accompanied by an epidemic of type 2 diabetes (p. 803) and osteoarthritis, particularly of the knee. Although an increased body size results in greater bone density through increased mechanical stress, it is not certain whether this translates to a lower incidence of osteoporotic fractures (p. 1116). Obesity may have profound psychological consequences, compounded by stigmatisation of the obese in many societies.

Body fat distribution

For some complications of obesity, the distribution rather than the absolute amount of excess adipose tissue appears to be important. Increased intra-abdominal fat causes 'central' ('abdominal', 'visceral', 'android' or 'apple-shaped') obesity, which contrasts with subcutaneous fat

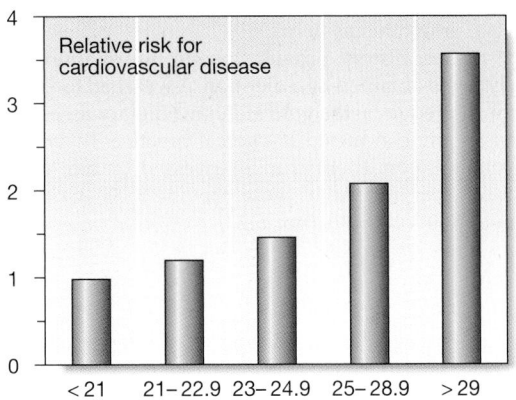

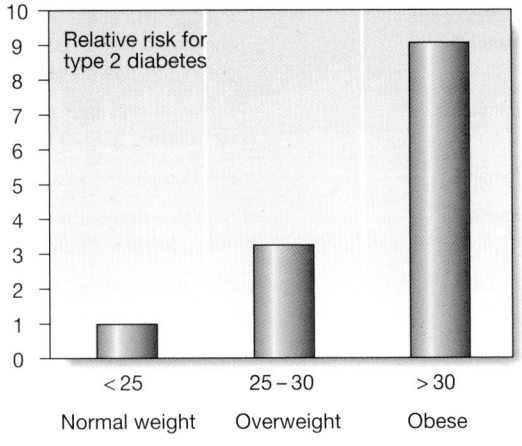

Fig. 5.11 Risks of diabetes and cardiovascular disease in overweight and obese women. Data are from the Nurses' Health Study in the USA, mostly of Caucasian women. In some ethnic groups (e.g. South Asians, Native Americans) and in people with higher waist circumference, the metabolic complications are even more severe at a given level of BMI.

accumulation causing 'generalised' ('gynoid' or 'pear-shaped') obesity; the former is more common in men and is more closely associated with type 2 diabetes, the metabolic syndrome and cardiovascular disease (see Box 5.23). The key difference between these depots of fat may lie in their vascular anatomy, with intra-abdominal fat draining into the portal vein and thence directly to the liver. Thus many factors which are released from adipose tissue (including free fatty acids; 'adipokines', such as tumour necrosis factor-α, adiponectin and resistin; and steroid hormones) may be at higher concentration in the liver and hence induce insulin resistance and promote type 2 diabetes (p. 803).

Aetiology

Accumulation of fat results from a discrepancy between energy consumption and energy expenditure which is too large to be defended by the hypothalamic regulation of BMR. A continuous small daily positive energy balance of only 0.2–0.8 MJ (50–200 kcal; < 10% of intake) would lead to weight gain of 2–20 kg over a period of 4–10 years. Given the cumulative effects of subtle energy excess, body fat content shows 'tracking' with age such that obese children usually become obese adults. Weight tends to increase throughout adult life, as BMR and physical activity decrease (see Fig. 5.8).

The pandemic of obesity reflects changes in both energy intake and energy expenditure (Box 5.24), although both are difficult to measure reliably. The estimated average global daily supply of food energy per person increased from ~9.8 MJ (~2350 kcal) in the 1960s to ~11.7 MJ (~2800 kcal) in the 1990s, but its delivery is unequal. For example, in India it is estimated that 5% of the population receives 40% of the available food energy, leading to obesity in the urban population in parallel with persisting under-nutrition in some rural communities. In affluent societies, a significant proportion of this food supply is discarded. In the US, the average daily energy intake of men reportedly rose from 10.2 MJ (2450 kcal) in 1971 to 11.0 MJ (2618 kcal) in 2000. Portion sizes, particularly of energy-dense foods such as drinks with highly refined sugar content and salty snacks, have increased. However, data in the UK suggest that energy intakes have declined (which may in part be due to deliberate restriction or 'dieting'), but this is apparently insufficient to compensate for the decrease in physical activity levels in recent years. Obesity is correlated positively with the number of hours spent watching television, and inversely with levels of physical activity (e.g. stair climbing). It is suggested that minor activities such as fidgeting and chewing gum may contribute to energy expenditure and protect against obesity.

Susceptibility to obesity

Susceptibility to obesity and its adverse consequences undoubtedly varies between individuals. It is not true that obese subjects have a 'slow metabolism', since their BMR is higher than that of lean subjects. Twin and adoption studies confirm a genetic influence on obesity. The pattern of inheritance suggests a polygenic disorder, with small contributions from a number of different genes, together accounting for 25–70% of variation in weight. Recent results from 'genome-wide' association studies of polymorphisms in large numbers of people (p. 51) have identified a handful of genes that influence obesity, some of which encode proteins known to be involved in the control of appetite or metabolism and some of which have unknown function. However, these genes account for < 5% of variation in body weight.

A few rare single gene disorders have been identified which lead to severe childhood obesity. These include mutations of the melanocortin-4 receptor (MC4R) that accounts for approximately 5% of severe early-onset obesity; defects in the enzymes processing propiomelanocortin (POMC, the precursor for adrenocorticotrophic hormone (ACTH)) in the hypothalamus; and mutations in the leptin gene (see Fig. 5.9). The latter can be cured by injected leptin treatment. Additional genetic conditions in which obesity is a feature include the Prader–Willi (see Box 3.3, p. 51) and Lawrence–Moon–Biedl syndromes.

Reversible causes of obesity and weight gain

In a small minority of patients presenting with obesity, specific causal factors can be identified and treated (Box 5.25). These patients are distinguished from those with idiopathic obesity by their short history, with a recent marked change in the trajectory of their adult weight gain.

5.25 Potentially reversible causes of weight gain

Endocrine factors

- Hypothyroidism
- Cushing's syndrome
- Insulinoma
- Hypothalamic tumours or injury

Drug treatments

- Tricyclic antidepressants
- Sulphonylureas
- Oestrogen-containing contraceptive pill
- Corticosteroids
- Sodium valproate
- β-blockers

Clinical assessment and investigations

In assessing an individual presenting with obesity, the aims are to:
- quantify the problem
- exclude an underlying cause
- identify complications
- reach a management plan.

Severity of obesity can be quantified using the BMI (Box 5.26). A waist circumference of > 102 cm in men or > 88 cm in women indicates that the risk of metabolic and cardiovascular complications of obesity is high.

5.24 Some reasons for the increasing prevalence of obesity—the 'obesogenic' environment

Increasing energy intake

- ↑ Portion sizes
- ↑ Snacking and loss of regular meals
- ↑ Energy-dense food (mainly fat)
- ↑ Affluence

Decreasing energy expenditure

- ↑ Car ownership
- ↓ Walking to school/work
- ↑ Automation; ↓ manual labour
- ↓ Sports in schools
- ↑ Time spent on computer games and watching TV
- ↑ Central heating

i **5.26 Quantifying obesity with body mass index (weight/height²)**

BMI (kg/m²)	Classification*	Risk of obesity comorbidity
18.5–24.9	Normal range	Negligible
25.0–29.9	Overweight	Mildly increased
> 30.0	**Obese**	
30.0–34.9	Class I	Moderate
35.0–39.9	Class II	Severe
> 40.0	Class III	Very severe

*Classification of the World Health Organization (WHO) and International Obesity Task Force. The Western Pacific Region Office of WHO recommends that, amongst Asians, BMI > 23.0 is overweight and > 25.0 is obese.

A dietary history may be helpful in guiding dietary advice, but is notoriously susceptible to under-reporting of food consumption. It is important to consider 'pathological' eating behaviour (such as binge eating, nocturnal eating or bulimia; p. 249), which may be the most important issue to address in some patients. Alcohol is an important source of energy intake and should be considered in detail.

The history of weight gain may help diagnose underlying causes. A patient who has recently gained substantial weight or at a faster rate than previously, and is not taking relevant drugs (see Box 5.25), is more likely to have an underlying disorder such as hypothyroidism (p. 741) or Cushing's syndrome (p. 770). All obese patients should have thyroid function tests performed on one occasion, and an overnight dexamethasone suppression test or 24-hour urine free cortisol if Cushing's syndrome is suspected. Monogenic and 'syndromic' causes of obesity are usually only relevant in children presenting with severe obesity.

Assessment of the diverse complications of obesity (see Box 5.23) requires a thorough history, examination and screening investigations. The impact of obesity on the patient's life and work is a major consideration. Assessment of other cardiovascular risk factors is important. Blood pressure should be measured with a large cuff, if required (p. 605). Associated type 2 diabetes and dyslipidaemia are detected by measuring blood glucose and a serum lipid profile, ideally in a fasting morning sample. Elevated serum transaminases occur in patients with non-alcoholic fatty liver disease (p. 956).

Management

The health risks of obesity are largely reversible. Interventions proven to reduce weight in obese patients also ameliorate cardiovascular risk factors. Lifestyle advice which lowers body weight and increases physical exercise reduces the incidence of type 2 diabetes (p. 818). Given the high prevalence of obesity and the large magnitude of its risks, population strategies to prevent and reverse obesity are high on the priority list for most health organisations. Initiatives include promoting healthy eating in schools, enhancing walking and cycling options for commuters, and liaising with the food industry to reduce energy and fat content and to label foods appropriately. Unfortunately, 'low-fat' foods are often still energy-dense, and current lifestyles with labour-saving devices, sedentary work and passive leisure

activities have much lower energy requirements than the manual labour and household duties of previous generations.

Most patients seeking assistance with obesity are motivated to lose weight but have attempted to do so previously without long-term success. Often weight will have oscillated between periods of successful weight loss and then regain of weight ('recidivism'). They may hold misconceptions that they have an underlying disease, inaccurate perceptions of their energy intake and expenditure, and an unrealistic view of the target weight which they would regard as 'success'. An empathetic explanation of energy balance, which recognises that some individuals are more susceptible to obesity than others and therefore require greater deficits in energy balance in order to lose and sustain body weight, is important. Exclusion of underlying 'hormone imbalance' with simple tests is reassuring and shifts the focus on to consideration of energy balance. Appropriate goals for weight loss should be agreed, recognising that the slope of the relationship between obesity and many of its complications becomes steeper with increasing BMI, so that a given amount of weight loss achieves greater risk reduction at higher levels of BMI. A reasonable goal for most patients is to lose 10% of body weight.

The management plan will vary according to the severity of the obesity (see Box 5.26) and the associated risk factors and complications. It will also be influenced by availability of resources; health-care providers and regulators have generally been careful not to recommend expensive interventions (especially long-term drug therapy and surgery) for everyone who is overweight. Instead, most guidelines focus resources on short-term interventions in those who have high health risks and comorbidities associated with their obesity, and who have demonstrated their capacity to alter their lifestyle to achieve weight loss (Fig. 5.12).

Lifestyle advice

Behavioural modification to avoid some of the effects of the 'obesogenic' environment (see Box 5.24) is the cornerstone of long-term control of weight. Regular eating

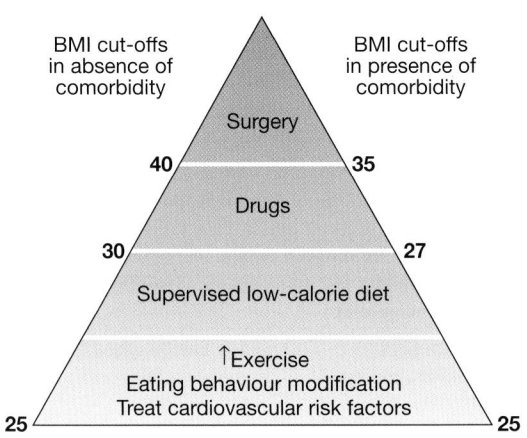

Fig. 5.12 Therapeutic options for obesity. Relevant comorbidities include type 2 diabetes, hypertension, cardiovascular disease, sleep apnoea, and waist circumference > 102 cm in men or 88 cm in women. This is an approximate consensus of the numerous national guidelines which vary slightly in their recommendations and are revised every few years.

5.27 Low-calorie diet therapy for obesity

Diet	% carbohydrate	% fat	% protein	Comment
Normal (typical developed country)	50	30	15	
Moderate fat (e.g. Weight Watchers)	60	25	15	Maintains balance in macronutrients and micronutrients while reducing energy-dense fats
Low carbohydrate (e.g. Atkins)	10	60	30	Induction of ketosis may suppress hunger
High protein (e.g. Zone)	43	30	27	Protein has greater satiety effect than other macronutrients
Low fat (e.g. Ornish)	70	13	17	

patterns and maximising physical activity are advised, with reference to the modest extra activity required to increase PAL ratios (see Fig. 5.8C, p. 108). Where possible, this should be incorporated in the daily routine (e.g. walking rather than driving to work), since this is more likely to be sustained. Alternative exercise (e.g. swimming) may be necessary if musculoskeletal complications prevent walking. Changes in eating behaviour (including food selection, portion size control, avoidance of snacking, regular meals to encourage satiety, and substitution of sugar with artificial sweeteners) should be discussed. Regular support from a dietitian or attendance at a weight loss group may be helpful.

Weight loss diets

In overweight people, adherence to the lifestyle advice above may gradually induce weight loss. In obese patients, more active intervention is usually required to lose weight before conversion to 'weight maintenance' advice above. A significant industry has developed in marketing diets for weight loss. These vary substantially in their balance of macronutrients (Box 5.27), but there is little evidence that they vary in their medium-term (1 year) efficacy. They all involve a reduction of daily total energy intake of ~2.5 MJ (600 kcal) from the patient's normal consumption. The goal is to lose ~0.5 kg/week. Weight loss is highly variable, with patient compliance being the major determinant of success. There is some evidence that weight loss diets are most effective in their early weeks, and that compliance is improved by novelty of the diet; this provides some justification for switching to a different dietary regime when weight loss slows on the first diet. Vitamin supplementation is wise in those diets in which macronutrient balance is markedly disturbed.

In some patients more rapid weight loss is required, e.g. in preparation for surgery. There is no role for starvation diets, which risk profound loss of muscle mass and the development of arrhythmias (and even sudden death) secondary to elevated free fatty acids, ketosis and deranged electrolytes. Very low calorie diets (VLCDs) are recommended for short-term rapid weight loss, producing losses of 1.5–2.5 kg/week compared to 0.5 kg/week on conventional regimes, but require the supervision of an experienced physician and nutritionist. The composition of the diet should ensure a minimum of 50 g of protein each day for men and 40 g for women to minimise muscle degradation. Energy content should be a minimum of 1.65 MJ (400 kcal) for women of height < 1.73 m, and 2.1 MJ (500 kcal) for all men and for women taller than 1.73 m. Side-effects are a problem in the early stages and include orthostatic hypotension, headache, diarrhoea and nausea.

Drugs

A huge investment has been made by the pharmaceutical industry in finding drugs for obesity. The side-effect profile has limited the use of many agents, but a few drugs are currently licensed (Box 5.28). There is no role for diuretics, or for thyroxine therapy without biochemical evidence of hypothyroidism.

Orlistat inhibits pancreatic and gastric lipases and thereby decreases the hydrolysis of ingested triglycerides, reducing dietary fat absorption by ~30%. The drug is not absorbed and adverse side-effects relate to the effect of the resultant fat malabsorption on the gut: namely, loose stools, oily spotting, faecal urgency, flatus and the potential for malabsorption of fat-soluble vitamins. Orlistat is taken with each of the three main meals of the day and the dose can be adjusted (60–120 mg) to minimise side-effects. Its efficacy is shown in Box 5.29 and Figure 5.13; these effects may be explained because patients taking orlistat adhere better to low-fat diets in order to avoid unpleasant gastrointestinal side-effects.

Sibutramine reduces food intake through β_1-adrenoceptor and 5-HT$_{2A/2C}$ (5-hydroxytryptamine,

5.28 Drugs which lower body weight[1]

Status	Drugs	Mechanism of action
Not recommended due to toxicity	Amphetamines	Catecholaminergic in CNS and periphery
	Fenfluramine, dexfenfluramine	Serotonergic in CNS
	Rimonabant[2]	Cannabinoid receptor antagonist
Not recommended as primary treatment; weight loss a useful minor/temporary effect	Fluoxetine	Serotonergic in CNS
	Metformin	Probably inhibits mitochondrial respiratory chain
	Exenatide	Glucagon-like peptide (GLP)-1 analogue
Currently recommended	Orlistat	Pancreatic lipase inhibitor
	Sibutramine	Serotonergic in CNS

[1] Many other approaches are in development, several of which have reached clinical trials.
[2] Rimonabant is not licensed in the USA and its licence in Europe is under threat, due to concerns about its effects on mood.

EBM 5.29 **Efficacy of anti-obesity drugs**

'In a meta-analysis of 30 placebo-controlled RCTs, orlistat reduced body weight by 2.9 kg (95% confidence intervals, 2.5–3.2 kg), sibutramine by 4.2 kg (3.6–4.7 kg), and rimonabant by 4.7 kg (4.1–5.3 kg). Orlistat and rimonabant improved serum lipid profile, blood pressure, and glycaemic control in diabetic patients. However, sibutramine increased blood pressure and rimonabant increased the risk of mood disorders.'

• Rucker D, et al. British Medical Journal 2007 335:1194–1199.

serotonin) receptor agonist activity in the central nervous system. Weight loss with sibutramine is 3–5 kg better than placebo with 6 months' therapy and is associated with an improvement in lipid profile (see Box 5.29). Side-effects include dry mouth, constipation and insomnia. Unfortunately, noradrenergic effects of the drug can increase heart rate and blood pressure; these effects are especially undesirable in obese patients. Sibutramine is thus usually second choice after orlistat and cannot be used in those with hypertension or cardiovascular disease. There is insufficient evidence to recommend co-prescription of orlistat and sibutramine.

Rimonabant is a cannabinoid receptor antagonist which acts in the hypothalamus to reduce appetite and may also have beneficial effects in peripheral tissues. Its efficacy in patients with obesity and type 2 diabetes is similar to orlistat (see Box 5.29), including reducing HbA1c by ~1%. However, rimonabant may exacerbate or induce depression and has been associated with a small increased risk of suicide, which has prevented it being licensed in the US and has limited its use in Europe.

Drug therapy is usually reserved for patients with high risk of complications from obesity (see Fig. 5.12), and its optimum timing and duration are controversial. Although life-long therapy is advocated for many drugs which reduce risk on the basis of relatively short-term research trials (e.g. drugs for hypertension and osteoporosis), patients who continue to take anti-obesity drugs tend to regain weight with time (see Fig. 5.13). This, together with finite health-care resources, has led to the recommendation in some guidelines that anti-obesity drugs are used in the short term to maximise the weight loss achieved with low-calorie diets (so that inevitable regain of weight starts from a lower baseline), but are not used in the long-term maintenance of weight.

Surgery

'Bariatric' surgery to reduce the size of the stomach is by far the most effective long-term treatment for obesity (see Fig. 5.13) and is the only anti-obesity intervention that has been associated with reduced mortality. Several approaches are used (Fig. 5.14) and all can be performed laparoscopically. The mechanism of weight loss may not relate to limiting the stomach or absorptive capacity per se, but rather in disrupting the release of ghrelin from the stomach or of other peptides from the small bowel, thereby enhancing satiety signalling in the hypothalamus. Complications depend upon the approach. Mortality is low in experienced centres, but post-operative respiratory problems, wound infection and dehiscence, staple leaks, stomal stenosis, marginal ulcers and venous thrombosis are common. Additional problems may arise at a later stage, such as pouch and distal oesophageal dilatation, persistent vomiting, 'dumping' (p. 873) and micronutrient deficiencies, particularly of folate, vitamin B_{12} and iron, which are of concern especially to women contemplating pregnancy.

Bariatric surgery should be contemplated in motivated patients who have very high risks of complications of obesity (see Fig. 5.12), in whom extensive dietary and drug therapy has been inadequately effective. Only experienced specialist surgeons should undertake these procedures.

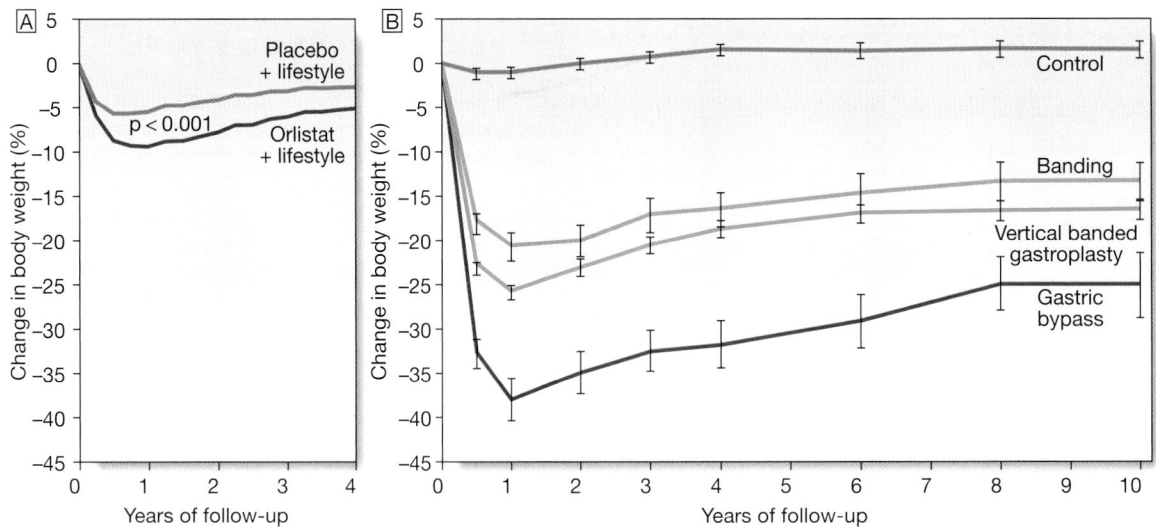

Fig. 5.13 Effects of orlistat and bariatric surgery on weight loss. **A** Data are from Torgerson JS, et al. Diabetes Care 2004; 27:155–161. **B** Data for surgery are from Sjostrom L, et al. New Engl J Med 2004; 351:2683–2693. Each obese subject undergoing surgery was matched with a control subject whose obesity was 'treated' by standard non-operative interventions. Note that the maximum weight loss achieved with orlistat was ~11%; surgery achieves much more substantial and prolonged weight loss.

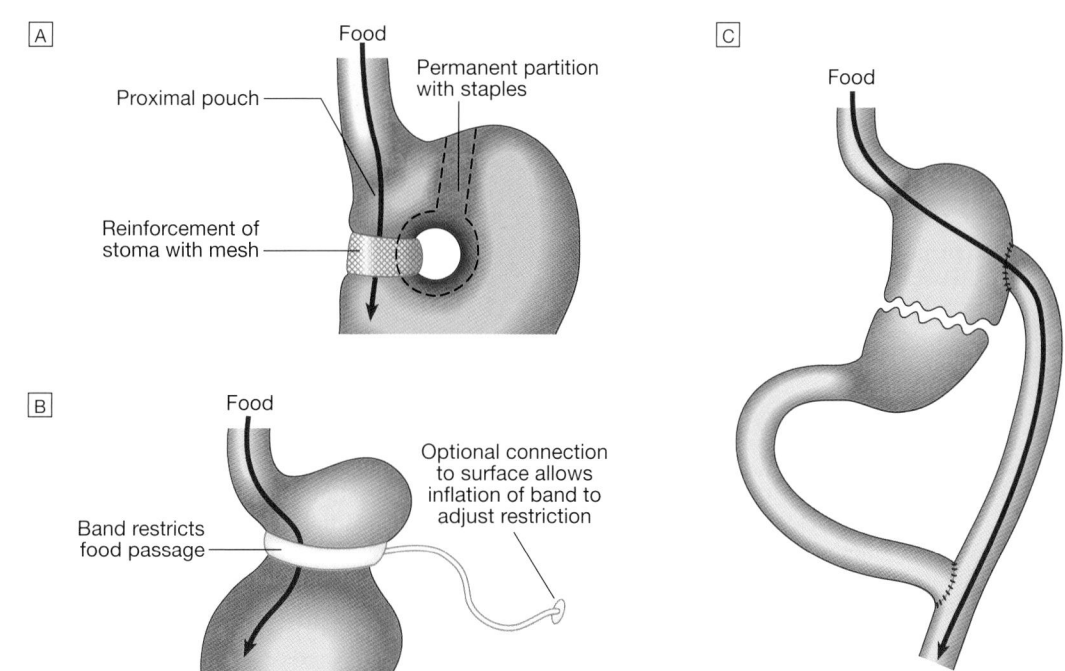

Fig. 5.14 Bariatric surgical procedures. A Vertical banded gastroplasty. B Laparoscopic banding, with the option of a reservoir band and subcutaneous access to restrict the stomach further after compensatory expansion has occurred. C Roux-en-Y gastric bypass.

Cosmetic surgical procedures may be required in obese patients. Apronectomy is usually advocated to remove an overhang of abdominal skin, especially if infected or ulcerated. This operation is of no value for long-term weight reduction if food intake remains unrestricted.

Treatment of additional risk factors

Obesity must not be treated in isolation and other risk factors must be addressed, including smoking, excess alcohol consumption, diabetes mellitus, hyperlipidaemia and hypertension. Treatment of these is discussed in the relevant chapters.

Under-nutrition

Starvation and famine

There remain regions of the world, particularly rural Africa, where under-nutrition due to famine is endemic, the prevalence of BMI < 18.5 kg/m² (Box 5.30) in adults is as high as 20%, and growth retardation due to under-nutrition affects 50% of children.

5.30 Classification of under-nutrition in adults by body mass index (weight/height²)

BMI (kg/m²)	Classification
> 20	Adequate nutrition
18.5–20	Marginal
< 18.5	**Under-nutrition**
17–18.4	Mild
16–17	Moderate
< 16	Severe

WHO reports that under-nutrition is responsible for more than half of all childhood deaths world-wide. Starvation is manifest as marasmus (malnutrition with marked muscle-wasting); or when additional complicating mechanisms, such as oxidative stress, come into play, malnourished children can develop kwashiorkor (malnutrition with oedema). Growth retardation is due to deficiency of key nutrients, e.g. protein, zinc, potassium, phosphorus and sulphur. Treatment of these childhood conditions is not discussed in this adult medicine textbook.

In adults, starvation is the result of chronic under-nutrition, i.e. sustained negative energy (calorie) balance. Causes are shown in Box 5.31. Causes of weight loss are considered further on page 858.

Clinical assessment

In starvation, the severity of malnutrition can be assessed by anthropometric measurements, such as

5.31 Causes of under-nutrition and weight loss in adults

Decreased energy intake

- Famine
- Persistent regurgitation or vomiting
- Anorexia, including anorexia nervosa
- Malabsorption (e.g. small intestinal disease)
- Maldigestion (e.g. pancreatic exocrine insufficiency)

Increased energy expenditure

- Increased BMR (thyrotoxicosis, trauma, fever, cancer cachexia)
- Excessive physical activity (e.g. marathon runners)
- Energy loss (e.g. glycosuria in diabetes)
- Impaired energy storage (e.g. Addison's disease, phaeochromocytoma)

BMI (see Box 5.30). Demispan and mid-arm circumference measurements (p. 115) are most useful in monitoring progress during treatment. The clinical features of severe under-nutrition in adults include:

- weight loss
- thirst, craving for food, weakness and feeling cold
- nocturia, amenorrhoea or impotence
- lax, pale, dry skin with loss of turgor and, occasionally, pigmented patches
- cold and cyanosed extremities, pressure sores
- hair thinning or loss (except in adolescents)
- muscle-wasting, best demonstrated by the loss of the temporalis and periscapular muscles and reduced mid-arm circumference
- loss of subcutaneous fat, reflected in reduced skinfold thickness and mid-arm circumference
- hypothermia, bradycardia, hypotension and small heart
- oedema, which may be present without hypoalbuminaemia ('famine oedema')
- distended abdomen with diarrhoea
- diminished tendon jerks
- apathy, loss of initiative, depression, introversion, aggression if food is nearby
- susceptibility to infections (Box 5.32).

Under-nutrition often leads to vitamin deficiencies, especially of thiamin, folate and vitamin C (see below). Diarrhoea can lead to depletion of sodium, potassium and magnesium. The high mortality rate in famine situations is often due to outbreaks of infection, e.g. typhus or cholera, but the usual signs of infection may not be apparent. In advanced starvation, patients become completely inactive and may assume a flexed, fetal position. In the last stage of starvation, death comes quietly and often quite suddenly. The very old are most vulnerable. All organs are atrophied at necropsy, except the brain, which tends to maintain its weight.

Investigations

In a famine, laboratory investigations may be impractical, but will show that plasma free fatty acids are increased and there is ketosis and a mild metabolic acidosis. Plasma glucose is low but albumin concentration is often maintained because the liver still functions normally. Insulin secretion is diminished, glucagon and cortisol tend to increase, and reverse T_3 replaces normal triiodothyronine (p. 736). The resting metabolic rate falls, partly because of reduced lean body mass and partly because of hypothalamic compensation (see Fig. 5.8, p. 108). The urine has a fixed specific gravity and creatinine excretion becomes low. There may be mild anaemia, leucopenia and thrombocytopenia. The erythrocyte sedimentation rate is normal unless there is infection. Tests of delayed skin hypersensitivity, e.g. to tuberculin, are falsely negative. The electrocardiogram shows sinus bradycardia and low voltage.

Management

Whether in a famine or in wasting secondary to disease, the severity of under-nutrition is graded according to BMI (see Box 5.30). People with mild starvation are in no danger; those with moderate starvation need extra feeding; those who are severely underweight need hospital care.

In severe starvation, there is atrophy of the intestinal epithelium and of the exocrine pancreas, and the bile is dilute. When food becomes available, it should be given by mouth in small, frequent amounts at first, using a suitable formula preparation (Box 5.33). Individual energy requirements can vary by 30%. During rehabilitation, more concentrated formula can be given with additional food that is palatable and similar to the usual staple meal. Salt should be restricted and micronutrient supplements may be essential (e.g. potassium, magnesium, zinc and multivitamins). Between 6.3 and 8.4 MJ/day (1500–2000 kcal/day) will arrest progressive under-nutrition, but additional energy may be required for regain of weight. During refeeding, a weight gain of 5% body weight per month indicates satisfactory progress. Other care is supportive, and includes attention to the skin, adequate hydration, treatment of infections, and careful monitoring of body temperature since thermoregulation may be impaired.

---

i | **5.32 Infections associated with starvation**

- Gastroenteritis and Gram-negative septicaemia
- Respiratory infections, especially bronchopneumonia
- Certain viral diseases, especially measles and herpes simplex
- Tuberculosis
- Streptococcal and staphylococcal skin infections
- Helminthic infestations

5.33 WHO recommended diets for refeeding

Nutrient (per 100 mL)	F-75 diet[1]	F-100 diet[2]
Energy	315 kJ (75 kcal)	420 kJ (100 kcal)
Protein (g)	0.9	2.9
Lactose (g)	1.3	4.2
Potassium (mmol)	3.6	5.9
Sodium (mmol)	0.9	1.9
Magnesium (mmol)	0.43	0.73
Zinc (mg)	2.0	2.3
Copper (mg)	0.25	0.25
Percentage of energy from		
Protein	5	12
Fat	32	53
Osmolality (osmol/L)	333	419
Dose	170 kJ/kg (40 kcal/kg)	630–920 kJ/kg (150–220 kcal/kg)
Rate of feeding by mouth	2.2 (mL/kg/hr)	Gradual increase in volume, 4-hourly

[1] F-75 is prepared from milk powder (25 g), sugar (70 g), cereal flour (35 g), vegetable oil (27 g), and vitamin and mineral supplements, made up to 1 L with water.
[2] F-100 (1 L) contains milk powder (80 g), sugar (50 g), vegetable oil (60 g), and vitamin and mineral supplements (no cereal).

Circumstances and resources are different in every famine, but many problems are non-medical and concern organisation, infrastructure, liaison, politics, procurement, security and ensuring that food is distributed on the basis of need. Lastly, plans must be made for the future for prevention and/or earlier intervention if similar circumstances prevail.

Under-nutrition in hospital

Under-nutrition is a common problem in the hospital setting. In the UK, approximately one-third of patients are affected by moderate or severe undernutrition on admission. The elderly are particularly at risk (Box 5.34). Once in hospital, many patients lose weight due to factors such as poor appetite, poor dental health, concurrent illness and even being kept 'nil by mouth' for investigations. Under-nutrition is poorly recognised in hospital and has serious consequences. Physical effects include impaired immunity and muscle weakness, which in turn affect cardiac and respiratory function, and delayed wound healing after surgery with increased risks of post-operative infection. The undernourished patient is often apathetic and withdrawn, which may be mistaken for a depressive illness and can affect cooperation with treatment and rehabilitation.

This can be averted with proper monitoring and involvement of an appropriate multidisciplinary team. As a minimum standard, all patients should be weighed on admission to hospital and at least weekly until discharge. A scoring system for identifying patients at nutritional risk is shown in Figure 5.15.

Nutritional support of the hospital patient
Normal diet

As a first step, patients should be encouraged to eat a normal and adequate diet. This is often neglected and there is evidence of substantial wastage in hospital food. In patients at risk of under-nutrition (see Fig. 5.15) quantities eaten should be recorded on a food chart. Hospital staff must identify and overcome barriers to adequate food intake, such as unpalatability of food, cultural and religious factors influencing acceptability of food, difficulty with hand dexterity (arthritis, stroke), immobility in bed, or poor oral health. Hospital catering departments have an important role in providing acceptable and adequate meals.

Dietary supplements

If sufficient nutritional intake cannot be achieved from normal diet alone, then dietary supplements should be used. These are drinks with high energy and protein content, and are available in cartons as manufactured, flavoured products or made in the hospital kitchen from milk products and egg. They should be prescribed, and administered by nursing staff, to ensure that they are taken regularly. Dietary supplements do not significantly affect the patient's consumption of normal food.

Enteral tube feeding

Patients who are unable to swallow may require artificial nutritional support: for example, after acute stroke or throat surgery or with long-term neurological problems such as motor neuron disease and multiple sclerosis. The enteral route should always be used if possible, since feeding via the gastrointestinal tract preserves the integrity of the mucosal barrier. This prevents bacteraemia

5.34 Energy balance in old age

- **Body composition**: muscle mass is decreased and percentage body fat increased.
- **Energy expenditure**: with the fall in lean body mass, BMR is decreased and energy requirements are reduced.
- **Weight loss**: after weight gain throughout adult life, weight often falls beyond the age of 70 years. This may reflect decreased appetite, loss of smell and taste, and decreased interest in and financial resources for food preparation, especially after loss of a partner.
- **BMI**: less reliable in old age as height is lost (due to kyphosis, osteoporotic crush fractures, loss of intervertebral disc spaces). Alternative measurements include arm demispan and knee height (p. 115), which can be extrapolated to estimate height.

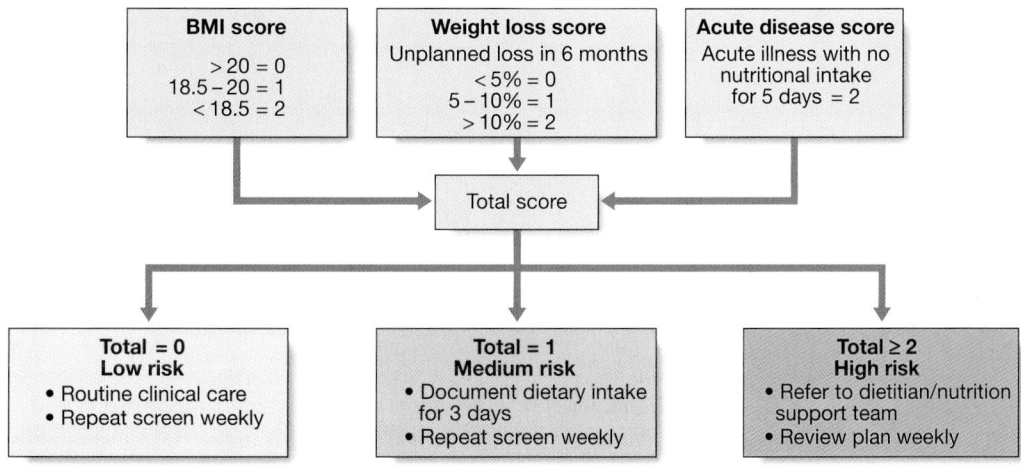

Fig. 5.15 Screening hospitalised patients for risk of malnutrition. Adapted from the British Association of Parenteral and Enteral Nutrition 'Malnutrition Universal Screening Tool' (www.bapen.org.uk).

and, in intensive care patients, reduces the risk of multi-organ failure (p. 199).

If the need for artificial nutritional support is thought to be short-term, then feeding is instituted using a fine-bore nasogastric tube. The position of the tube in the stomach must be confirmed before any fluid is administered, as intrabronchial tube placement is not uncommon and severe respiratory complications can occur if fluid is inadvertently infused into a bronchus. Gastric aspirate has a pH < 4. If there is any doubt about the result of pH testing of the aspirate, then a chest X-ray should be performed to confirm the tube is below the diaphragm. Thereafter, specially prepared liquid feeds are administered either by continuous infusion or using a bolus technique. If the patient fails to absorb the administered feed or vomits it, this may indicate gastric outlet obstruction or gastric stasis, which can be overcome by placing a nasojejunal tube.

If long-term artificial enteral feeding is needed, a percutaneous endoscopic gastrostomy (PEG) should be sited (Fig. 5.16). A PEG tube is more comfortable for the patient, since there is no irritation to the nasal mucosa. The tube is less likely to become displaced or to be pulled out, so the feed can be given more reliably. However, inserting a gastrostomy is an invasive procedure and may be complicated by local infection (30%) and inadvertent puncture of other intra-abdominal organs, causing peritonitis and bleeding. It takes approximately 10 days for a fibrous tract to form around the PEG tube. If the PEG is displaced or removed during that time, there is a high risk of peritonitis. If a problem occurs with food absorption, a jejunal extension can be placed through the PEG tube and liquid feed administered directly into the small bowel.

Parenteral nutrition

Intravenous feeding should only be used when enteral feeding is impossible. Parenteral feeding is expensive and carries higher risks of complications. There is little benefit if parenteral feeding is required for less than 1 week.

There are a number of possible routes for parenteral nutrition:

- *Peripheral venous cannula*. This can only be used for low-osmolality solutions due to the development of thrombophlebitis, and is unsuitable for patients with high nutritional requirements.
- *Peripherally inserted cannula (PIC)*. A 20 cm cannula is placed in a mid-arm vein. Once again, hyperosmolar solutions cannot be used.
- *Peripherally inserted central catheter (PICC)*. A 60 cm cannula is inserted into a vein in the antecubital fossa. The distal end lies in a central vein, allowing hyperosmolar solutions to be used.
- *Central line*. The subclavian route is preferred to the internal jugular vein, due to lower infection rates. Hyperosmolar solutions can be used without difficulty. Lines need to be handled with strict aseptic technique, and a single lumen tube is preferred, to prevent infection.

If access has been gained to a central vein, nutritional support is usually given as an 'all in one' mixture. The main energy source is provided by carbohydrate, usually as glucose. The solution also contains amino acids, lipid emulsion, electrolytes, trace elements and vitamins. These are mixed as a large bag in a sterile environment, with the constituents adjusted according to the results of regular blood monitoring. Relevant tests include:

- daily: urea and electrolytes, glucose
- twice weekly: liver function tests, calcium, phosphate, magnesium
- weekly: full blood count, zinc, triglycerides
- monthly: copper, selenium, manganese.

If the patient develops fever or other features of septicaemia, it should be assumed to be due to a line infection

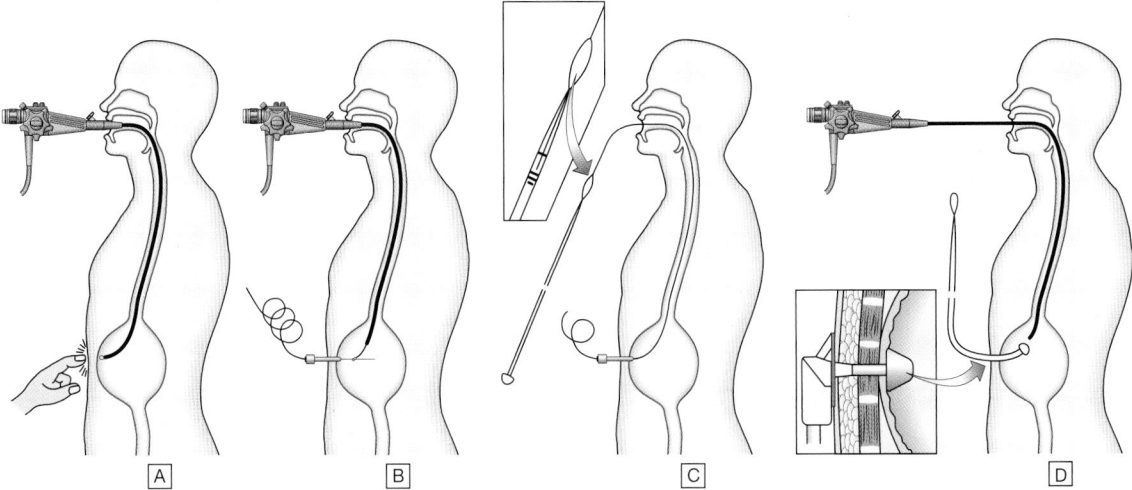

Fig. 5.16 Percutaneous endoscopic gastrostomy (PEG) placement. **A** Finger pressure on the anterior abdominal wall is noted by the endoscopist. **B** Following insertion of a cannula through the anterior abdominal wall into the stomach, a guidewire is threaded through the cannula and grasped by the endoscopic forceps or snare. **C** The endoscope is withdrawn with the guidewire. The gastrostomy tube is then attached to the guidewire. **D** The guidewire and tube are pulled back through the mouth, oesophagus and stomach to exit on the anterior abdominal wall, and the endoscope is repassed to confirm the site of placement of the retention device. The latter closely abuts the gastric mucosa; its position is maintained by an external fixation device (see inset). It is also possible to place PEG tubes using fluoroscopic guidance in patients in whom endoscopy is difficult (radiologically inserted gastrostomy (RIG)).

5.35 Ethical and legal considerations in the management of artificial nutritional support*

- Care of the sick involves the duty of providing adequate fluid and nutrients
- Food and fluid should not be withheld from a patient who expresses a desire to eat and drink, unless there is a medical contraindication (e.g. risk of aspiration)
- A treatment plan should include consideration of nutritional issues and should be agreed by all members of the health-care team
- In the situation of palliative care, tube feeding should only be instituted if it is needed to relieve symptoms
- Tube feeding is usually regarded in law as a medical treatment. Like other treatments, the need for such support should be reviewed on a regular basis and changes made in the light of clinical circumstances
- A competent adult patient must give consent for any invasive procedures, including the passage of a nasogastric tube or the insertion of a central venous cannula
- If a patient is unable to give consent, the health-care team should act in that person's best interests, taking into account any previously expressed wishes of the patient and the views of family
- Under certain specified circumstances (e.g. anorexia nervosa), it will be appropriate to provide artificial nutritional support to the unwilling patient

*Based on British Association for Parenteral and Enteral Nutrition guidelines (www.bapen.org.uk).

5

(p. 189). Blood cultures should be taken, the existing line removed, the tip sent for bacteriological analysis, and a new line inserted.

Refeeding syndrome

When nutritional support is given to an undernourished patient, there is a rapid conversion from a catabolic to an anabolic state. Administration of carbohydrates stimulates release of insulin, leading to cellular uptake of phosphate, potassium and magnesium which may provoke significant falls in serum levels. The resulting electrolyte imbalance can have serious consequences such as cardiac arrhythmias, so careful monitoring is essential. In patients who are thiamin-deficient, Wernicke's encephalopathy can be precipitated by refeeding with carbohydrates (p. 1199); this is prevented by administering thiamin before starting nutritional support.

Legal and ethical aspects of artificial nutritional support

The ability to intervene with artificial nutritional support raises many legal and ethical dilemmas (pp. 9 and 287). Starvation will inevitably lead to death, but inability to eat may be part of the terminal stages of a disease process. Difficult decisions are raised by situations such as strokes which affect swallowing. The instigation of feeding may speed recovery and lead to better functional outcome; on the other hand, feeding might prolong the process of dying in severe stroke. There will be different approaches to these decisions, depending on the local availability of resources as well as legal, cultural and religious influences. Some guidelines are given in Box 5.35.

Cachexia

Cachexia is the weight loss and muscle-wasting associated with chronic illness, which is characteristic of chronic infections such as AIDS, end-stage organ failure and certain cancers (especially of the lung and upper gastrointestinal tract). Although there is decreased energy intake with loss of appetite, the main cause is thought to be increased metabolic rate through the production of key cytokines and other proteolytic factors.

DISEASES OF VITAMINS AND MINERALS

Vitamins

Vitamin deficiency diseases are most prevalent in developing countries but still occur in developed countries. Older people (and alcoholics) are at risk of deficiencies in B vitamins, and vitamins D and C. Nutritional deficiencies in pregnancy can affect either the mother or the developing fetus, and extra increments of vitamins are recommended in the UK (see Boxes 5.19 and 5.20, p. 113). Some nutrient deficiencies are induced by diseases or drugs. Deficiencies of fat-soluble vitamins are seen in conditions of fat malabsorption (e.g. biliary obstruction).

Some vitamins also have pharmacological actions when given at supraphysiological doses, e.g. the use of vitamin A (p. 1268) for acne. Taking vitamin supplements is fashionable in many countries, although there is no evidence of benefit. Toxic effects are most serious with high dosages of vitamins A, B_6 and D.

Investigation of suspected vitamin deficiency or excess may involve biochemical assessment of body stores (see Box 5.22, p. 115). However, measurements in blood should be interpreted carefully in conjunction with the clinical presentation.

Fat-soluble vitamins

Vitamin A

Deficiency

Globally, the most important consequence of vitamin A deficiency is blindness. Each year, approximately 500 000 new cases of blindness occur in young children, mostly in Asia. Adults are not usually at risk because liver stores can supply vitamin A when foods containing vitamin A are unavailable.

Early deficiency causes impaired adaptation to the dark (night blindness). Keratinisation of the cornea (xerophthalmia) causes characteristic Bitot's spots, which progresses to keratomalacia, with corneal ulceration, scarring and irreversible blindness (Fig. 5.17). In countries where vitamin A deficiency is endemic, pregnant

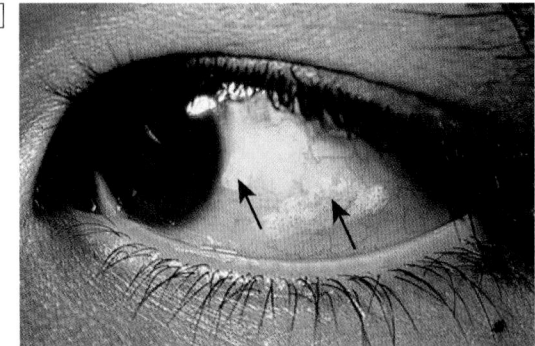

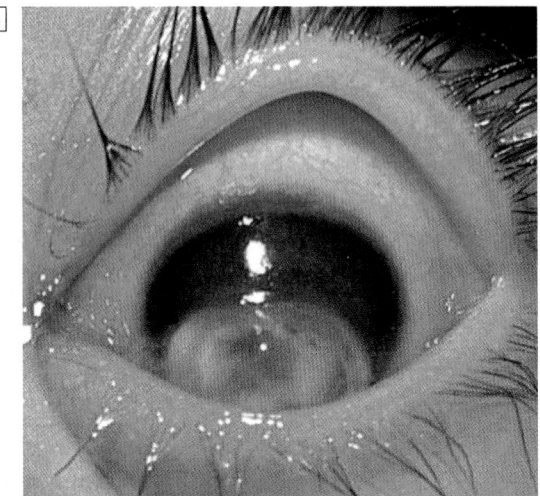

Fig. 5.17 Eye signs of vitamin A deficiency. A Bitot's spots in xerophthalmia, showing the white triangular plaques (arrows). B Keratomalacia in a 14-month-old child. There is liquefactive necrosis affecting the greater part of the cornea, with typical sparing of the superior aspect.

women should be advised to eat dark green leafy vegetables and yellow fruits (to build up stores of retinol in the fetal liver), and infants should be fed the same. WHO is giving high priority to prevention in communities where xerophthalmia occurs, with single prophylactic oral doses of 60 mg retinyl palmitate (providing 200 000 U retinol) given to pre-school children. This also reduces mortality from gastroenteritis and respiratory infections.

Toxicity

Repeated moderate or high doses of retinol can cause liver damage, hyperostosis and teratogenicity. Women in countries where deficiency is not endemic are therefore advised not to take vitamin A supplements in pregnancy. Retinol intake may also be restricted in those at risk of osteoporosis. Acute overdose leads to nausea and headache, increased intracranial pressure and skin desquamation. Excessive intake of carotene can cause pigmentation of the skin (hypercarotenosis); this gradually fades when intake is reduced.

Vitamin D

The effects of vitamin D deficiency (calcium deficiency, rickets and osteomalacia) are described on page 1121. An analogue of vitamin D (calipotriol) is used for treatment of skin conditions such as psoriasis. Excessive doses of cholecalciferol, ergocalciferol or the hydroxylated metabolites cause hypercalcaemia (p. 764).

Vitamin E

Human deficiency is rare and has only been described in premature infants and in malabsorption. It can cause a mild haemolytic anaemia, ataxia and visual scotomas. Vitamin E intakes are considered safe up to 3200 mg/day (1000-fold greater than recommended intakes).

Diets rich in vitamin E are consumed in countries with lower rates of coronary heart disease. However, randomised controlled trials have not demonstrated cardioprotective effects of vitamin E or other antioxidants.

Vitamin K

Vitamin K deficiency leads to delayed coagulation and bleeding. In obstructive jaundice, dietary vitamin K is not absorbed and it is essential to administer the vitamin in parenteral form before surgery. Warfarin and related anticoagulants (p. 993) act by antagonising vitamin K. Vitamin K is given routinely to newborn babies to prevent haemorrhagic disease. Symptoms of excess have been reported only in infants, with synthetic preparations linked to haemolysis and liver damage.

Water-soluble vitamins

Thiamin (vitamin B₁)

In thiamin deficiency, cells cannot metabolise glucose aerobically to generate energy as ATP. Neuronal cells are most vulnerable, since they depend almost exclusively on glucose for energy requirements. Impaired glucose oxidation also causes an accumulation of pyruvic and lactic acids, which produce vasodilatation and increased cardiac output.

Deficiency—beri-beri

In the developed world, thiamin deficiency is mainly encountered in chronic alcoholics. Poor diet, impaired absorption, storage and phosphorylation of thiamin in the liver, and the increased requirements for thiamin to metabolise ethanol all contribute. In the developing world, deficiency usually arises as a consequence of a diet based on polished rice. The body has very limited stores of thiamin, so deficiency is manifest after only 1 month on a thiamin-free diet. There are two forms of the disease in adults:

- *Dry (or neurological) beri-beri* manifests with chronic peripheral neuropathy and with wrist and/or foot drop, and may cause Korsakoff's psychosis and Wernicke's encephalopathy (pp. 246 and 1199).
- *Wet (or cardiac) beri-beri* causes generalised oedema due to biventricular heart failure with pulmonary congestion.

In dry beri-beri, response to thiamin administration is not uniformly good. However, multivitamin therapy seems to produce some improvement, suggesting that other vitamin deficiencies may be involved. Wernicke's encephalopathy and wet beri-beri should be treated without delay with intravenous Pabrinex (pp. 247 and 1199). Korsakoff's psychosis is irreversible and does not respond to thiamin treatment.

Riboflavin (vitamin B₂)

Riboflavin deficiency is rare in developed countries. It mainly affects the tongue and lips and manifests as glossitis, angular stomatitis and cheilosis. The genitals may be affected, as well as the skin areas rich in sebaceous glands, causing nasolabial or facial dyssebacea. Rapid recovery usually follows administration of riboflavin 10 mg daily by mouth.

Niacin (vitamin B₃)

Deficiency—pellagra

Pellagra was formerly endemic among the poor who subsisted chiefly on maize, which contains niacytin, a form of niacin that the body is unable to utilise. Pellagra can develop in only 8 weeks in individuals eating diets that are very deficient in niacin and tryptophan. It remains a problem in parts of Africa, and is occasionally seen in alcoholics and in patients with chronic small intestinal disease in developed countries. Pellagra can occur in Hartnup's disease, a genetic disorder characterised by impaired absorption of several amino acids, including tryptophan. It is also seen occasionally in carcinoid syndrome (p. 782), when tryptophan is consumed in the excessive production of 5-HT.

Pellagra has been called the disease of the three Ds:

- *Dermatitis.* Characteristically, there is erythema resembling severe sunburn, appearing symmetrically over the parts of the body exposed to sunlight, particularly the limbs and especially on the neck, but not the face (Casal's necklace, Fig. 5.18). The skin lesions may progress to vesiculation, cracking, exudation and secondary infection.
- *Diarrhoea.* This is often associated with anorexia, nausea, glossitis and dysphagia, reflecting the presence of a non-infective inflammation that extends throughout the gastrointestinal tract.
- *Dementia.* In severe deficiency, delirium occurs acutely and dementia develops in chronic cases.

Treatment is with nicotinamide, given in a dose of 100 mg 8-hourly by mouth or by the parenteral route. The response is usually rapid. Within 24 hours, the erythema

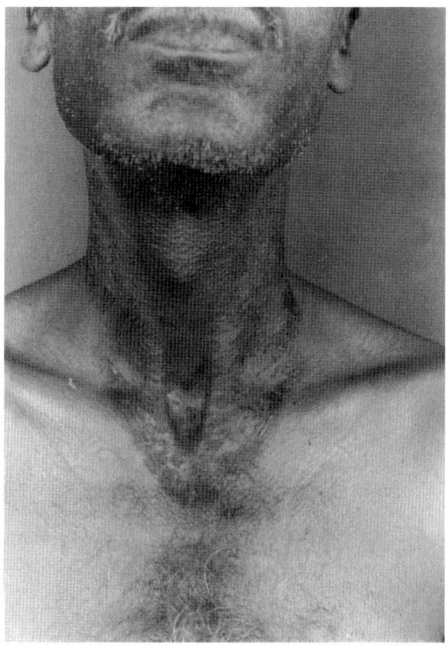

Fig. 5.18 Dermatitis due to pellagra (niacin deficiency). The lesions appear on those parts of the body exposed to sunlight. The classic 'Casal's necklace' can be seen around the neck and upper chest.

5.36 Vitamin deficiency in old age

- **Requirements:** although energy requirements fall with age, those for micronutrients do not. If dietary intake falls, a vitamin-rich diet is required to compensate.
- **Vitamin D:** levels are commonly low due to reduced dietary intake, decreased sun exposure and less efficient skin conversion. This leads to bone loss and fractures. Supplements should be given to those in institutional care and those with recurrent falls.
- **Vitamin B₁₂ deficiency**: a causal relationship with dementia has not been identified, but it does produce neuropsychiatric effects and should be checked in all those with declining cognitive function.

---

diminishes, the diarrhoea ceases and a striking improvement occurs in the patient's mental state.

Toxicity

Excessive intakes of niacin may lead to reversible hepatotoxicity. Nicotinic acid is a lipid-lowering agent, but at doses above 200 mg a day gives rise to vasodilatory symptoms ('flushing' and/or hypotension).

Pyridoxine (vitamin B₆)

Vitamin B₆ deficiency is rare. However, certain drugs, such as isoniazid and penicillamine, act as chemical antagonists to pyridoxine. Pyridoxine administration is effective in isoniazid-induced peripheral neuropathy and some cases of sideroblastic anaemia.

Large doses of vitamin B₆ have an antiemetic effect in radiotherapy-induced nausea. Although vitamin B₆ supplements have become popular in the treatment of nausea in pregnancy, carpal tunnel syndrome and premenstrual syndrome, there is no convincing evidence of benefit. Very high doses of vitamin B₆ taken for several months can cause a sensory polyneuropathy.

Biotin

Biotin deficiency results from consuming very large quantities of raw egg whites (> 30% energy intake) because the avidin they contain binds to and inactivates biotin in the intestine. It may also be seen after long periods of total parenteral nutrition. The clinical features of deficiency include scaly dermatitis, alopecia and paraesthesia.

Vitamin B₁₂ and folate

These vitamins and the haematological disorders (macrocytic or megaloblastic anaemias) due to their deficiency are discussed on pages 1020–1022. Vitamin B₁₂, but not folate, is needed for the integrity of myelin, so that vitamin B₁₂ deficiency is also associated with neurological disease (see Box 24.38, p. 1020). Folate deficiency has been associated with heart disease, dementia and cancer.

Neurological consequences of vitamin B₁₂ deficiency

In older people and chronic alcoholics, vitamin B₁₂ deficiency arises from insufficient intake and/or from malabsorption. Several drugs, including neomycin, can render vitamin B₁₂ inactive. Adequate intake of folate maintains erythropoiesis and there is a concern that

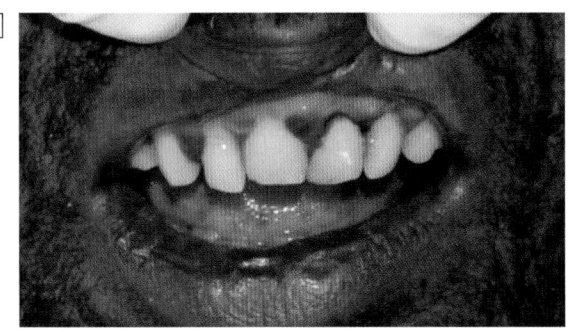
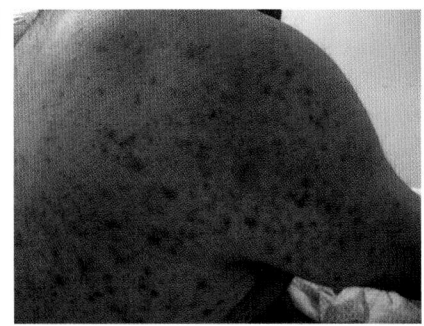

Fig. 5.19 Scurvy. A Gingival swelling and bleeding. B Perifollicular hyperkeratosis.

fortification of foods with folate may mask underlying vitamin B$_{12}$ deficiency. In severe deficiency there is insidious, diffuse and uneven demyelination. It may be clinically manifest as peripheral neuropathy or spinal cord degeneration affecting both posterior and lateral columns ('subacute combined degeneration of the spinal cord'; p. 1225), or there may be cerebral manifestations (resembling dementia) or optic atrophy. Vitamin B$_{12}$ therapy improves symptoms in most cases.

Folic acid in the prevention of neural tube defects

Folate deficiency may cause three major birth defects (spina bifida, anencephaly and encephalocele) resulting from imperfect closure of the neural tube, which takes place 3–4 weeks after conception. Maternal supplementation with folate reduces the risk (see Box 5.20, p. 113).

Vitamin C (ascorbic acid)

Deficiency—scurvy

Vitamin C deficiency causes defective formation of collagen with impaired healing of wounds, capillary haemorrhage and reduced platelet adhesiveness (normal platelets are rich in ascorbate) (Fig. 5.19). Precipitants and clinical features of scurvy are shown in Box 5.37. A dose of 250 mg vitamin C 8-hourly by mouth should saturate the tissues quickly. The deficiencies of the patient's diet also need to be corrected and other vitamin supplements given if necessary.

Daily intakes of more than 1 g/day have been reported to cause diarrhoea and the formation of renal oxalate stones.

5.37 Scurvy—vitamin C deficiency	
Precipitants	
Increased requirement	**Dietary deficiency**
• Trauma, surgery, burns, infections • Smoking • Drugs (corticosteroids, aspirin, indometacin, tetracycline)	• Lack of dietary fruit and vegetables for > 2 months • Infants fed exclusively on boiled milk
Clinical features	
• Swollen gums which bleed easily • Perifollicular and petechial haemorrhages • Ecchymoses	• Haemarthrosis • Gastrointestinal bleeding • Anaemia • Poor wound healing

Inorganic nutrients

Deficiency is seen when there is inadequate dietary intake of minerals or excessive loss from the body. Toxic effects have also been observed from self-medication and disordered absorption or excretion. Examples of clinical toxicity include excess of iron (haemochromatosis or haemosiderosis), fluoride (fluorosis; p. 114), copper (Wilson's disease) and selenium (selenosis, seen in parts of China). For most minerals the available biochemical markers do not accurately reflect dietary intake and dietary assessment is required.

Calcium

Calcium absorption may be impaired in vitamin D deficiency (pp. 764 and 1121) and in malabsorption secondary to small intestinal disease. Calcium deficiency causes impaired bone mineralisation and can lead to osteomalacia in adults. The potential benefits of high calcium intake in osteoporosis are discussed on page 1120. Too much calcium can lead to constipation and toxicity has been observed in 'milk alkali syndrome' (p. 765).

Phosphorus

Dietary deficiency of phosphorus is rare (except in older people with limited diets) since it is present in nearly all foods and phosphates are added to a number of processed foods. Phosphate deficiency in adults occurs:

- in patients with renal tubular phosphate loss (p. 447)
- due to prolonged high dosage of aluminium hydroxide (p. 491)
- sometimes when alcoholics are fed with high-carbohydrate foods
- in patients receiving parenteral nutrition if inadequate phosphate is provided.

Deficiency causes hypophosphataemia (p. 447) and muscle weakness secondary to ATP deficiency.

Iron

The major consequence of iron deficiency is anaemia (p. 1017). This is one of the most important nutritional causes of ill health in all parts of the world. In the UK it is estimated that 10% women are iron-deficient. Dietary iron overload is occasionally observed and results in iron accumulation in the liver and, rarely, cirrhosis. Haemochromatosis results from an inherited increase in iron absorption (p. 959).

Iodine

About a billion people in the world are estimated to have an inadequate iodine intake and are hence at risk of iodine deficiency disorder. Goitre is the most common manifestation, affecting about 200 million people (p. 750).

In those areas where most women have endemic goitre, 1% or more of babies are born with cretinism (characterised by mental and physical retardation). There is a higher than usual prevalence of deafness, slowed reflexes and poor learning in the remaining population. The best way of preventing neonatal cretinism is to ensure adequate levels of iodine during pregnancy. This can be achieved by intramuscular injections with 1–2 mL of iodised poppy seed oil (475–950 mg iodine) to women of child-bearing age every 3–5 years, by administration of iodised oil orally at 6-monthly or yearly intervals to adults and children, or by providing iodised salt for cooking.

Zinc

Acute zinc deficiency has been reported in patients receiving prolonged zinc-free parenteral nutrition and causes diarrhoea, mental apathy, a moist eczematoid dermatitis, especially around the mouth, and loss of hair. Chronic zinc deficiency occurs in dietary deficiency, malabsorption syndromes, alcoholism and its associated hepatic cirrhosis. It causes the clinical features seen in the very rare congenital disorder known as acrodermatitis enteropathica (growth retardation, hair loss and chronic diarrhoea). Zinc deficiency is thought to be responsible for one-third of the world's population not reaching their optimal height. In the Middle East, chronic deficiency has been associated with dwarfism and hypogonadism. In starvation, zinc deficiency causes thymic atrophy, and zinc supplements may accelerate the healing of skin lesions, promote general well-being, improve appetite and reduce the morbidity associated with the undernourished state.

Fluoride

If the local water supply contains more than 1 part per million (ppm) of fluoride, the incidence of dental caries is low. Soft waters usually contain no fluoride, whilst very hard waters may contain over 10 ppm. The benefit of fluoride is greatest when it is taken before the permanent teeth erupt, while their enamel is being laid down. The addition of traces of fluoride (at 1 ppm) to public water supplies is now a widespread practice.

Chronic fluoride poisoning is occasionally seen where the water supply contains > 10 ppm fluoride. It can also occur in workers handling cryolite (aluminium sodium fluoride), used in smelting aluminium. Fluoride poisoning is described on page 221. Pitting of teeth is a result of too much fluoride as a child.

Other minerals

Disease states associated with abnormal intakes or disordered metabolism of sodium, potassium and magnesium are discussed in Chapter 16.

Copper metabolism is abnormal in Wilson's disease (p. 960). Deficiency occasionally occurs but only in young children, causing microcytic hypochromic anaemia, neutropenia, retarded growth, skeletal rarefaction and dermatosis.

Selenium deficiency can cause hypothyroidism, cardiomyopathy in children (Keshan's disease) and myopathy in adults. Excess selenium can cause heart disease.

Chromium facilitates the action of insulin. Deficiency presents as hyperglycaemia and has been reported in adults as a rare complication of prolonged parenteral nutrition.

Further information

Websites

www.foodstandards.gov.uk *Information on food composition and dietary surveys.*

www.hpa.org.uk/radiation *The Health Protection Agency provides information and links on all forms of radiation for patients and professionals.*

www.nice.org.uk *NICE guidelines for nutritional support and obesity.*

www.who.int/nut *WHO recommendations and intervention programmes for macronutrient- and micronutrient-related diseases.*

www.who.int/topics/global_burden_of_disease/en/ *The WHO global burden of disease project.*

Telephone numbers

- In the UK two organisations provide advice on the clinical management of diving illness and the availability of the nearest recompression facility:
    Aberdeen Royal Infirmary +44 (0)1224 681818. *Hyperbaric doctor on call.*
    Royal Navy +44 (0)7831 151523.
- Outside the UK, contact the Divers Alert Network (DAN; www.diversalertnetwork.org).

5

R.P. Hobson
D.H. Dockrell

Principles of infectious disease

6

6

Infection is the establishment of foreign organisms, or 'infectious agents', in or on a human host. This may result in colonisation, if the microorganism exists at an anatomical site without establishing overt tissue injury, or infectious disease, when the interaction between the host and pathogenic organism (or pathogen) induces tissue damage and clinical illness. In clinical practice the term 'infection' is often used interchangeably with 'infectious disease'. Most pathogens are microorganisms, although some are multicellular organisms (parasites).

The interaction between the pathogen and the host is dynamic and complex. Whilst it is rarely in the organism's interest to kill the host (on which it relies for nutrition and protection), the generation of disease manifestations (e.g. diarrhoea, sneezing) may aid its dissemination. Conversely, it is in the host's interests to kill microorganisms likely to cause disease, whilst preserving colonising organisms from which it may derive benefit.

Communicable infectious diseases are caused by organisms transmitted between hosts, whereas endogenous diseases are caused by colonising organisms already established in the host. Opportunistic infections, which may be communicable or endogenous, are those which arise only in individuals with impaired host defence. The chain of infection (Fig. 6.1) describes six essential elements for communicable disease transmission.

Despite dramatic advances in hygiene, immunisation and antimicrobial therapy, infectious diseases are still responsible for a major global health burden. Key challenges remain in tackling the diversity of infection in developing countries and the emergence of new infectious agents and of antimicrobial-resistant microorganisms. This chapter describes the processes underlying infectious diseases and the general approach to their prevention, diagnosis and treatment. Chapters 13–15 describe specific infectious diseases.

INFECTIOUS AGENTS

The concept of an infectious agent was established by Robert Koch in the late 19th century (Box 6.1). Although fulfilment of 'Koch's postulates' became the standard for the definition of an infectious agent, they do not apply to organisms which cannot be grown in culture (e.g. *Mycobacterium leprae*, *Tropheryma whipplei*) or members of the normal human flora (e.g. *Escherichia coli*, *Candida* spp.). The following groups of infectious agents are now recognised.

Prions

Prions are unique amongst infectious agents in that they are devoid of any nucleic acid. They appear to be transmitted by acquisition of a normal mammalian protein (prion protein, PrP^c) which is in an abnormal conformation (PrP^{Sc}, containing an excess of beta-sheet protein); the abnormal protein inhibits the enzyme proteasome 26S, leading to a vicious circle of further accumulation of abnormally configured PrP^{Sc} protein instead of normally configured PrP^c protein. The result is accumulation of protein forming amyloid in the central nervous system (CNS), causing transmissible spongiform encephalopathies in humans, sheep, cows and cats (see Box 13.38, p. 325 and see p. 1214).

Viruses

Viruses are incapable of independent replication, instead subverting the cellular processes of host cells. A virus that infects a bacterium is a bacteriophage (phage). Viruses contain genetic material (genome), which may be single- or double-stranded DNA or RNA. Some viruses copy their RNA into DNA by reverse transcription (retroviruses). The virus genome is enclosed in an antigenically unique protein coat (capsid); together, these form the nucleocapsid. In many viruses the nucleocapsid is packaged within a lipid envelope. Enveloped viruses are less able to survive in the environment and are spread by respiratory, sexual or blood-borne routes, including arthropod-based transmission. Non-enveloped viruses survive better in the environment

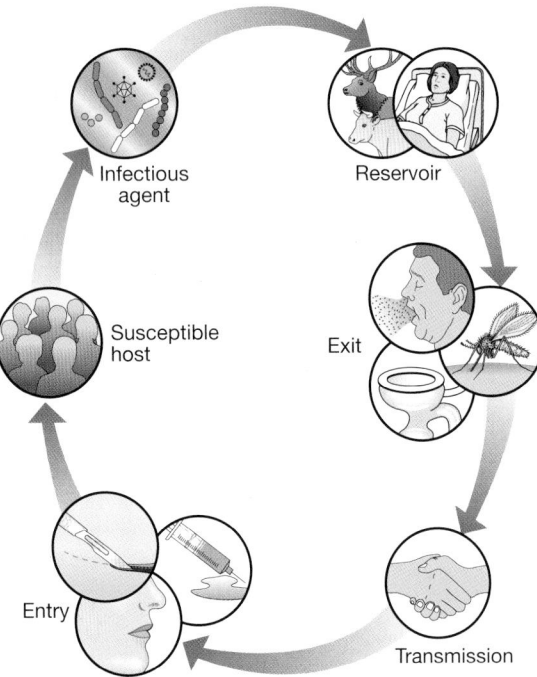

Fig. 6.1 Chain of infection. The infectious agent is the organism that causes the disease. The reservoir is the place where the population of an infectious agent is maintained. The portal of exit is the point from which the infectious agent leaves the reservoir. Transmission is the process by which the infectious agent is transferred from the reservoir to the human host, either directly or via a vector or fomite. The portal of entry is the body site that is first accessed by the infectious agent. Finally, in order for disease to ensue, the person to whom the infectious agent is transmitted must be a susceptible host.

> **i**   6.1 **Definition of an infectious agent: Koch's postulates**
>
> 1. The same organism must be present in every case of the disease
> 2. The organism must be isolated from the diseased host and grown in pure culture
> 3. The isolate must cause the disease, when inoculated into a healthy, susceptible animal
> 4. The organism must be re-isolated from the inoculated, diseased animal

and are predominantly transmitted by faecal–oral or, less often, respiratory routes. The virus life cycle is shown in Figure 6.2.

Prokaryotes: bacteria (including mycobacteria and actinomycetes)

Prokaryotic cells are capable of synthesising their own proteins and nucleic acids, and are able to reproduce autonomously, although they lack a nucleus. The bacterial cell membrane is bounded by a peptidoglycan cell wall, which is thick (20–80nm) in Gram-positive organisms and thin (5–10nm) in Gram-negative ones. The Gram-negative cell wall is surrounded by an outer membrane containing lipopolysaccharide (endotoxin). Many bacteria contain extra-chromosomal DNA in the form of plasmids, which can be transferred between organisms. Bacteria may be embedded in a polysaccharide capsule, and motile bacteria are equipped with flagella. Although many prokaryotes are capable of independent existence, some (e.g. *Chlamydia trachomatis, Coxiella burnetii*) are obligate intracellular organisms. Bacteria that replicate in artificial culture media are classified and identified

using a range of characteristics (Box 6.2), with examples in Figures 6.3 and 6.4.

Eukaryotes: fungi, protozoa and helminths

Eukaryotes contain functional organelles such as nuclei, mitochondria and Golgi apparatus. Eukaryotes involved in human infection include fungi, protozoa (unicellular eukaryotes with a flexible cell membrane, p. 348) and helminths (multicellular complex organisms including nematodes, trematodes and cestodes, p. 364).

Fungi exist as either moulds (filamentous fungi) or yeasts. Dimorphic fungi exist in either form, depending on environmental conditions (see Fig. 13.55, p. 377). The fungal plasma membrane differs from the human cell membrane in that it contains the sterol, ergosterol. Fungi have a cell wall made up of polysaccharides, chitin and mannoproteins. In most fungi the main structural component of the cell wall is β-1, 3-D-glucan, a glucose polymer.

Protozoa and helminths are often referred to as parasites. Many parasites have complex multi-stage

6

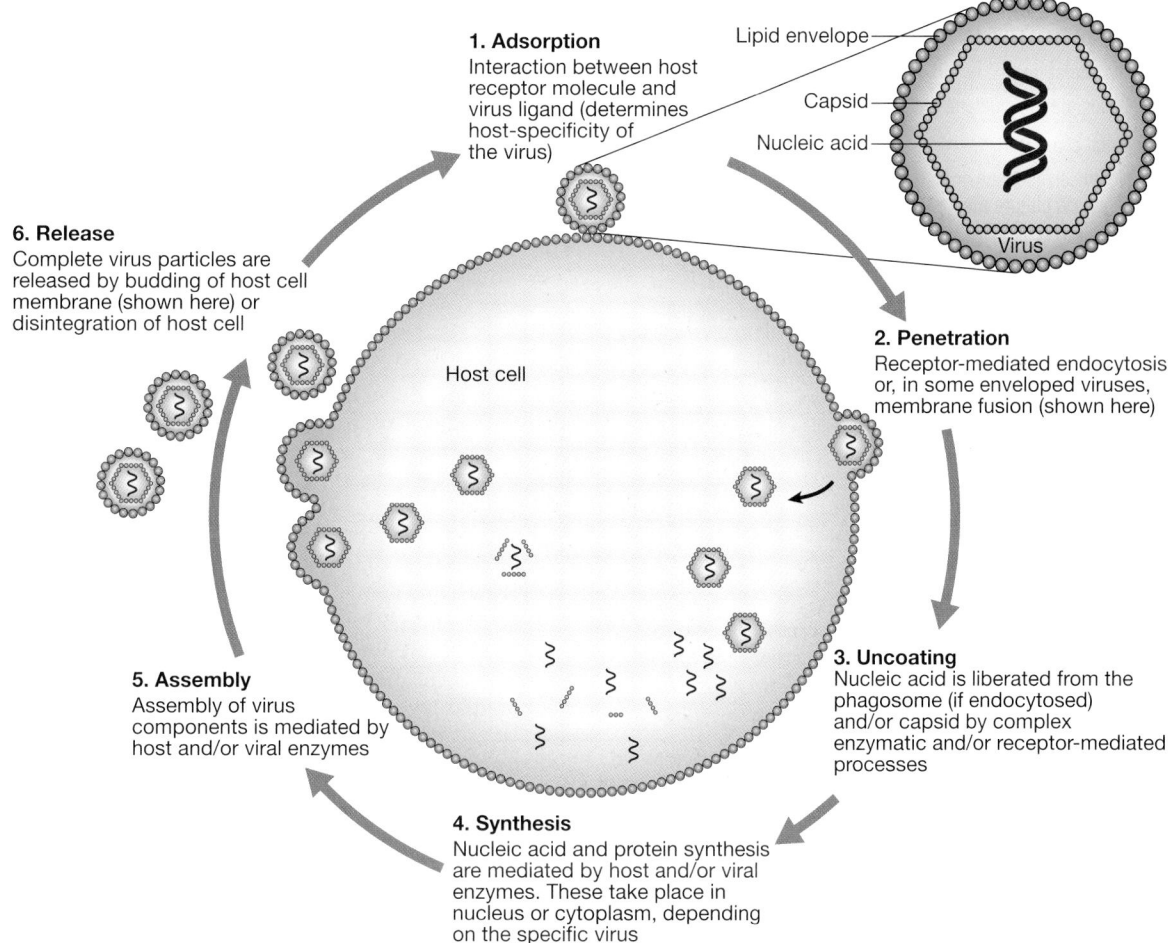

1. Adsorption
Interaction between host receptor molecule and virus ligand (determines host-specificity of the virus)

Lipid envelope
Capsid
Nucleic acid
Virus

6. Release
Complete virus particles are released by budding of host cell membrane (shown here) or disintegration of host cell

Host cell

2. Penetration
Receptor-mediated endocytosis or, in some enveloped viruses, membrane fusion (shown here)

5. Assembly
Assembly of virus components is mediated by host and/or viral enzymes

3. Uncoating
Nucleic acid is liberated from the phagosome (if endocytosed) and/or capsid by complex enzymatic and/or receptor-mediated processes

4. Synthesis
Nucleic acid and protein synthesis are mediated by host and/or viral enzymes. These take place in nucleus or cytoplasm, depending on the specific virus

Fig. 6.2 Virus life cycle. Life cycles vary between viruses. Life cycle components common to most viruses are host cell attachment and penetration, virus uncoating, nucleic acid and protein synthesis, virus assembly and release. Virus release is achieved either by budding, as illustrated, or by lysis of the cell membrane.

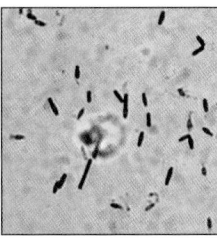
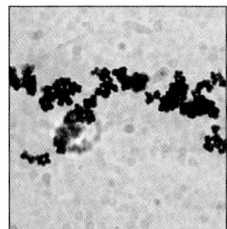
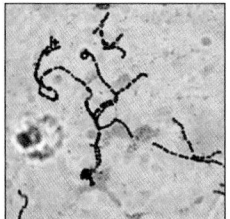
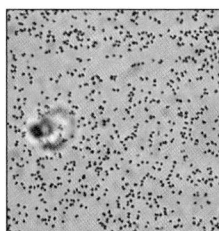
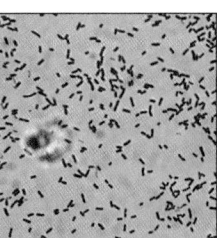

Gram-positive bacilli
- *Clostridium* spp. (shown here)
- *Corynebacterium* spp.
- *Bacillus* spp.

Gram-positive cocci in clusters
- Staphylococci

Gram-positive cocci in chains
- Streptococci

Gram-negative cocci
- *Neisseria* spp. (shown here)
- *Moraxella* spp.

Gram-negative bacilli
- Enterobacteriaceae (shown here)
- *Serratia* spp.
- *Acinetobacter* spp.
- *Bacteroides* spp.

Fig. 6.3 Gram film appearances of bacteria on light microscopy (×100).

6.2 Criteria used in identification of bacteria

Gram stain reaction (Fig. 6.3)
- Gram-positive (thick peptidoglycan layer), Gram-negative (thin peptidoglycan) or unstainable

Microscopic morphology
- Cocci (round cells) or bacilli (elongated cells)
- Presence or absence of capsule

Cell association
- Associated in clusters, chains or pairs

Colonial characteristics
- Colony size, shape or colour
- Effect on culture media (e.g. β-haemolysis of blood agar in haemolytic streptococci; Fig. 6.4)

Atmospheric requirements
- Strictly aerobic (requires O_2), strictly anaerobic (requires absence of O_2), facultatively aerobic (grows with or without O_2) or micro-aerophilic (requires reduced O_2)

Biochemical reactions
- Expression of enzymes (oxidase, catalase, coagulase)
- Ability to ferment or hydrolyse various biochemical substrates

Motility
- Motile or non-motile

Antibiotic susceptibility
- Identifies organisms with invariable susceptibility (e.g. to optochin in *Strep. pneumoniae* or metronidazole in obligate anaerobes)

life cycles, which involve animal and/or plant hosts in addition to humans.

NORMAL FLORA

Every human is host to an estimated 10^{13}–10^{14} colonising microorganisms which constitute the normal flora. Resident flora are able to survive and replicate at a body site, whereas transient flora are present only for short periods. Knowledge of non-sterile body sites

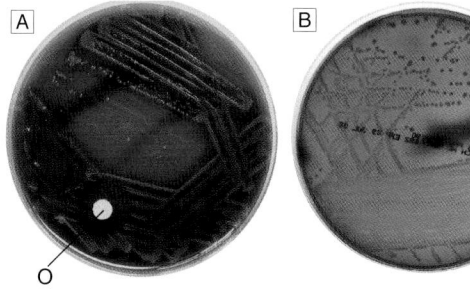

Fig. 6.4 Appearances of α- and β-haemolytic streptococci on blood agar. **A** Alpha-haemolytic streptococci. The colonies cause partial haemolysis, which imparts a green tinge to the agar. The organism shown is *Strep. pneumoniae* from the CSF of a patient with meningitis (note also the susceptibility to optochin (O), which is another feature used to identify this organism). **B** Beta-haemolytic streptococci. The colonies cause complete haemolysis, which renders the agar transparent. The organism shown is *Strep. pyogenes* (group A β-haemolytic streptococci) from a superficial wound swab.

and their specific normal flora is required to interpret microbiological culture results (Fig. 6.5).

The relationship between human host and normal flora is symbiotic (the organisms are in close proximity) and may be:
- mutualistic (both organisms benefit)
- commensal (one organism benefits whilst the other derives neither benefit nor harm)
- parasitic (the parasite benefits at the expense of the host, as in infectious disease).

Maintenance of the normal flora is beneficial to health. For example, lower gastrointestinal tract bacteria synthesise and excrete vitamins (e.g. vitamins K and B_{12}); colonisation with normal flora confers 'colonisation resistance' to infection by pathogenic organisms by altering the local environment (e.g. lowering of pH), producing antibacterial agents (such as bacteriocin peptides, fatty acids and metabolic waste products), and inducing host antibodies which may cross-react with pathogenic organisms.

Conversely it is important to exclude infectious agents from sterile body sites. The mucociliary escalator transports environmental material deposited in the respiratory tract to the nasopharynx. The urethral sphincter prevents flow from the non-sterile urethra to the sterile bladder.

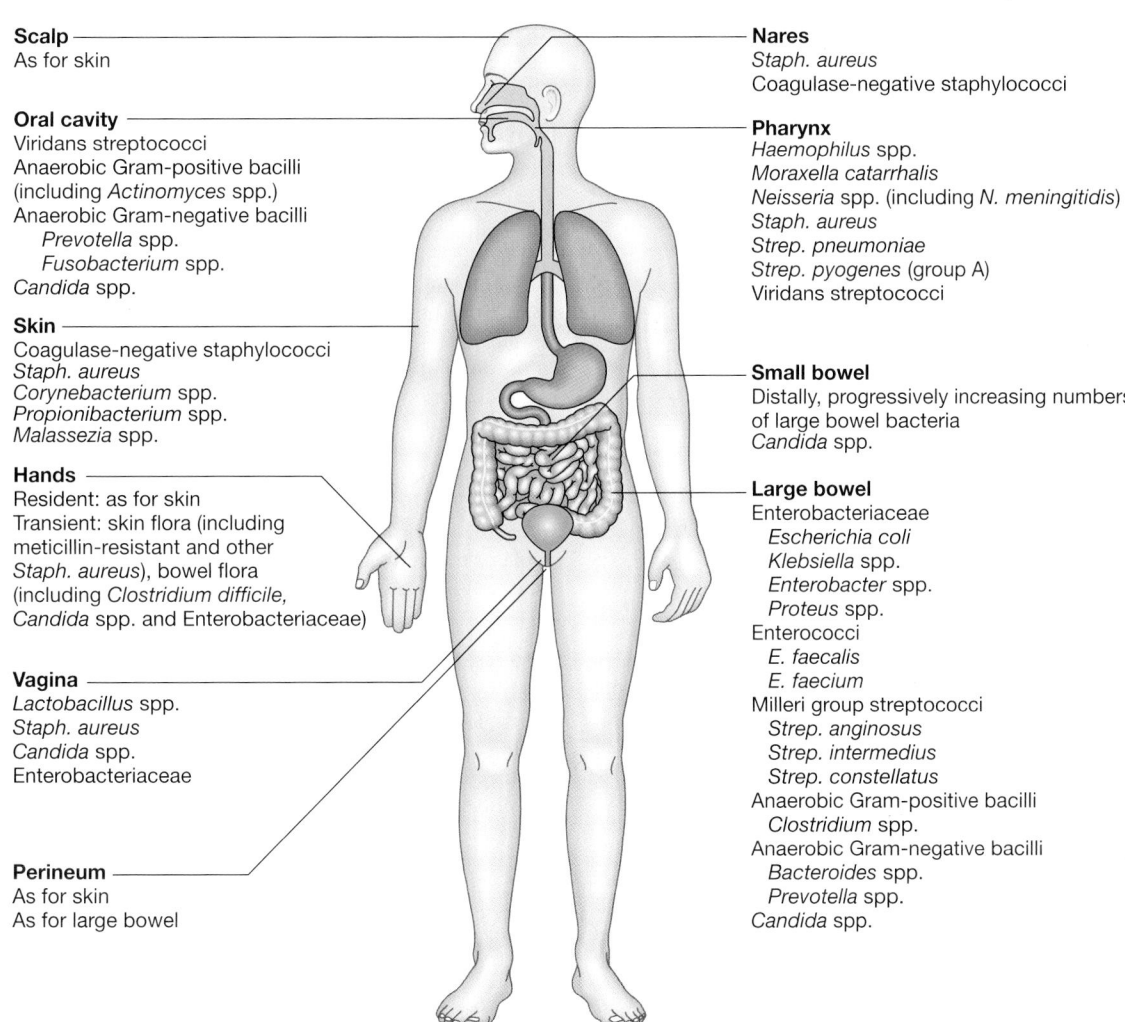

Scalp
As for skin

Oral cavity
Viridans streptococci
Anaerobic Gram-positive bacilli
(including *Actinomyces* spp.)
Anaerobic Gram-negative bacilli
    Prevotella spp.
    Fusobacterium spp.
Candida spp.

Skin
Coagulase-negative staphylococci
Staph. aureus
Corynebacterium spp.
Propionibacterium spp.
Malassezia spp.

Hands
Resident: as for skin
Transient: skin flora (including
meticillin-resistant and other
Staph. aureus), bowel flora
(including *Clostridium difficile*,
Candida spp. and Enterobacteriaceae)

Vagina
Lactobacillus spp.
Staph. aureus
Candida spp.
Enterobacteriaceae

Perineum
As for skin
As for large bowel

Nares
Staph. aureus
Coagulase-negative staphylococci

Pharynx
Haemophilus spp.
Moraxella catarrhalis
Neisseria spp. (including *N. meningitidis*)
Staph. aureus
Strep. pneumoniae
Strep. pyogenes (group A)
Viridans streptococci

Small bowel
Distally, progressively increasing numbers
of large bowel bacteria
Candida spp.

Large bowel
Enterobacteriaceae
    Escherichia coli
    Klebsiella spp.
    Enterobacter spp.
    Proteus spp.
Enterococci
    E. faecalis
    E. faecium
Milleri group streptococci
    Strep. anginosus
    Strep. intermedius
    Strep. constellatus
Anaerobic Gram-positive bacilli
    Clostridium spp.
Anaerobic Gram-negative bacilli
    Bacteroides spp.
    Prevotella spp.
Candida spp.

6

Fig. 6.5 Human non-sterile sites and normal flora in health.

Physical barriers, including the skin, lining of the gastro-intestinal tract and mucous membranes, maintain sterility of the blood stream, peritoneal and pleural cavities, chambers of the eye, subcutaneous tissue etc.

The normal flora contribute to endogenous infectious disease by either excessive growth (overgrowth) at the 'normal' site, or translocation to a sterile site. Overgrowth is exemplified by 'blind loop' syndrome (see p. 881), dental caries and vaginal thrush, in which external factors favour overgrowth of specific components of the normal flora. Translocation results from spread along a surface or penetration of a closed barrier: for example, in urinary tract infection caused by perineal/enteric flora, and in skin and surgical site infections caused by skin flora such as staphylococci. Normal flora also contributes to disease by cross-infection, in which organisms that are colonising one individual cause disease when transferred to another more susceptible individual.

HOST–PATHOGEN INTERACTIONS

Microorganisms capable of causing disease are termed pathogens. The components of pathogenicity are infectivity (the ability to become established in or on a host) and virulence (the ability to cause harm once established). Pathogens produce an array of proteins and other factors, termed virulence factors, which interact with host cells to contribute to disease.

- *Primary pathogens* cause disease in a proportion of individuals to whom they are exposed, regardless of their immunological status.
- *Opportunistic pathogens* cause disease only in individuals whose natural host defences are compromised, for example, by genetic susceptibility, immunosuppressive disease or a medical intervention.

Characteristics of successful pathogens

Successful pathogens have a number of attributes. They compete with host cells and colonising flora by various methods including sequestration of nutrients, use of metabolic pathways not used by competing bacteria, or production of bacteriocins (small antimicrobial peptides/proteins that kill closely related bacteria). Motility enables pathogens to reach their site of infection, often in sterile sites that colonising bacteria do not reach, such as the distal airway. Many microorganisms, including

6.3 Exotoxin-mediated bacterial diseases

Disease	Organism
Antibiotic-associated diarrhoea/ pseudo-membranous colitis	*Clostridium difficile* (p. 304)
Botulism	*Clostridium botulinum* (p. 1214)
Cholera	*Vibrio cholerae* (p. 339)
Diphtheria	*Corynebacterium diphtheriae* (p. 340)
Haemolytic uraemic syndrome	*Escherichia coli* 0157 (and other strains) (p. 498)
Necrotising pneumonia	*Staphylococcus aureus* (p. 686)
Tetanus	*Clostridium tetani* (p. 1213)
Toxic shock syndrome	*Staphylococcus aureus* (p. 326)

viruses, use 'adhesins' to attach to host cells at the site of infection. Other pathogens can invade through tissues.

Pathogens may produce toxins, microbial molecules that cause adverse effects on host cells either at the site of infection or remotely following carriage through the blood stream. Endotoxin is a cell wall component released mainly following bacterial cell damage and has generalised inflammatory effects. Exotoxins are proteins released by living bacteria, which often have specific effects on target organs (Box 6.3.)

Intracellular pathogens, including viruses, bacteria (e.g. *Salmonella* spp., *Listeria monocytogenes* and *Mycobacterium tuberculosis*), parasites (e.g. *Leishmania* spp.) and fungi (e.g. *Histoplasma capsulatum*), have the capacity to survive in intracellular environments, including after phagocytosis by macrophages.

Pathogenic bacteria express different arrays of genes, depending on environmental stress (pH, iron starvation, O_2 starvation etc.) and anatomical location. In quorum sensing, bacteria communicate with one another to adapt their replication or metabolism according to local population density. Bacteria and fungi may respond to the presence of an artificial surface (e.g. prosthetic device, venous catheter) by forming a biofilm, which is a population of organisms encased in a matrix of extracellular molecules. Biofilm-associated organisms are highly resistant to antimicrobial agents.

Genetic diversity enhances the pathogenic capacity of bacteria. Some virulence factor genes are found on plasmids or in phages and are exchanged between different strains or species. The ability to acquire genes from the gene pool of all strains of the species (the 'bacterial supragenome') increases diversity and the potential for pathogenicity. Viruses exploit their rapid reproduction and potential to exchange nucleic acid with host cells to enhance diversity. Once a strain acquires a particularly effective combination of virulence genes, it may become an epidemic strain, accounting for a large subset of infections in a particular region. This phenomenon accounts for influenza pandemics.

The host response

The human host relies on innate and adaptive immune and inflammatory responses to control the normal flora and respond to pathogens. These responses, and the consequences when they are impaired, are reviewed in Chapter 4.

Pathogenesis of infectious disease

The harmful manifestations of infection are determined by a combination of the virulence factors of the organism and the host response to infection, both of which vary at different stages of disease. Despite the obvious benefits of an intact host response, an excessive response is undesirable. Cytokines and antimicrobial factors contribute to tissue injury at the site of infection, and an excessive inflammatory response may lead to hypotension and organ dysfunction (p. 81). The importance of the immune response in determining disease manifestations is exemplified in immune reconstitution inflammatory syndrome (IRIS, or immune reconstitution disease). In this condition—seen, for example, in HIV infection, neutropenia or tuberculosis (which causes suppression of T-cell function)—there is a paradoxical worsening of the clinical condition as the immune dysfunction is corrected.

The febrile response

Thermoregulation (p. 100) is altered in infectious disease. Microbial pyrogens or the endogenous pyrogens released during tissue necrosis stimulate specialised cells such as monocytes/macrophages to release cytokines including IL-1β, tumour necrosis factor (TNF)-α, IL-6 and IFN-γ. Cytokine receptors in the pre-optic region of the anterior hypothalamus activate phospholipase A, releasing arachidonic acid as substrate for the cyclo-oxygenase pathway and producing prostaglandin E2 (PGE_2), which in turn alters the responsiveness of thermosensitive neurons in the thermoregulatory centre. Rigors occur when the body inappropriately attempts to 'reset' core temperature to a higher level by stimulating skeletal muscle activity and shaking.

The role of the febrile response as a defence mechanism requires further study, but there are data to support the hypothesis that raised body temperature interferes with the replication and/or virulence of pathogens.

INVESTIGATION OF INFECTION

Microbiological tests detect either a microorganism (e.g. direct detection and culture) or the host response to the organism (immunological tests) (Box 6.4). They also provide information on responsiveness to antimicrobial therapy. Careful and appropriate sampling increases the chance of useful results (Box 6.5). The results must be interpreted in light of the normal flora in the site from which the sample was obtained and the likely findings in a person without infectious disease. Like all tests, whether a positive test result is diagnostic of disease depends on the specificity and positive predictive value (PPV) of the test (p. 5), and whether a negative test result excludes disease depends on its sensitivity and negative predictive value (NPV). Test sensitivity varies according to the time between infection and testing (there is a 'window of opportunity' during which sensitivity is maximal; see Fig 6.7, p. 140), and the PPV and NPV depend on the prevalence of the condition in the test population.

6.4 Investigation modalities in infectious diseases

Non-microbiological

- e.g. FBC, plasma CRP, cell counts in urine or CSF, CSF protein and glucose

Direct detection

- Microscopy
- Detection of organism components (e.g. antigen, toxin)
- Nucleic acid amplification (e.g. PCR)

Culture

- ± Antimicrobial sensitivity testing

Immunological tests

- Antibody detection
- T-cell stimulation tests

Microbiological results are therefore interpreted in light of other findings consistent with infectious disease, including the clinical scenario and results of other investigations (e.g. neutrophilia, elevated C-reactive protein (CRP)). Given this complexity, effective two-way communication between the clinician and the microbiologist is a vital component of test interpretation.

Direct detection

Direct detection methods provide rapid results, and may be applied to organisms that cannot be grown easily on artificial culture media, such as *Chlamydia* spp. They do not usually provide information on antimicrobial susceptibility or the degree to which organisms are related to each other (which is important in the investigation of possible disease outbreaks) unless relevant specific nucleic acid sequences are detected by polymerase chain reaction (PCR).

Detection of whole organisms

Whole organisms are detected by microscopic examination of biological fluids or tissue using a light or electron microscope.

- *Bright field microscopy* (in which the test sample is interposed between the light source and the objective lens) uses stains to enhance visual contrast between the organism and its background. Examples include Gram-staining of bacteria and Ziehl–Neelsen or auramine staining of acid- and alcohol-fast bacilli (AAFB) in tuberculosis. In histopathological examination of tissue samples multiple stains are used to demonstrate not only the presence of microorganisms, but also features of disease pathology.
- *Dark field microscopy* (in which light is scattered to make organisms appear bright on a dark background) is used, for example, to examine genital chancre fluid in suspected syphilis.
- *Electron microscopy* is used to examine stool and vesicle fluid to detect enteric and herpes viruses, respectively.

6

6.5 How to provide samples for microbiological sampling

Communication

- Discuss samples that may require to be forwarded to another laboratory or processed urgently or by an unusual method with laboratory staff *before* collection
- Communication is the most important requirement for good microbiological sampling. If there is doubt about any aspect of sampling, it is far better to discuss it with laboratory staff beforehand than to risk diagnostic delay by inappropriate sampling or sample handling

Indication

- Screening (e.g. collecting 'routine' urine, i.v. cannulae or sputum) in the absence of clinical evidence of infection is rarely appropriate

Container

- Certain tests (e.g. nucleic acid and antigen detection tests) require proprietary sample collection equipment

Collection

- Follow sample collection instructions precisely (e.g. proper collection of mid-stream, terminal and early morning urine samples, skin decontamination prior to blood culture etc.) to increase diagnostic yield

Labelling

- Label sample containers and request forms according to local policies with demographic identifiers, specimen type and time/date collected
- Include clinical details on request forms
- Identify samples carrying a high risk of infection (e.g. blood liable to contain a blood-borne virus) with a hazard label

Packaging

- Close sample containers tightly and package securely (usually in sealed plastic bags)
- Attach request forms to samples but not in the same compartment (to avoid contamination should leakage occur)

Storage and transport

- Transport samples to the microbiology laboratory as quickly as possible
- If pre-transport storage is required, conditions (e.g. refrigeration, incubation, storage at room temperature) vary with sample type
- Notify the receiving laboratory prior to arrival of samples, to ensure timely processing

6

Detection of components of organisms

Components of microorganisms that are detected for diagnostic purposes include nucleic acids (DNA and RNA), cell wall molecules, toxins and other antigens. Methods to detect non-nucleic acid antigenic components of microorganisms are described under immunological tests (see below), as they share similar methodology. Examples of antigen detection include *Legionella pneumophila* serogroup 1 antigen in urine, HIV p24 antigen in blood and cryptococcal polysaccharide antigen in cerebrospinal fluid (CSF). Non-immunological methods may also be used, e.g. detection of *Clostridium botulinum* toxin in a mouse bioassay. In toxin-mediated disease, detection of toxin may be of greater relevance than identification of organism (e.g. detection of *C. difficile* toxin in stool).

Nucleic acid amplification tests (NAAT)

Specific sequences of microbial DNA and RNA are identified using a nucleic acid primer which is amplified exponentially by enzymes to generate multiple copies of the specific sequence. The most commonly used amplification method is the polymerase chain reaction (PCR; see Fig. 3.10, p. 58). Reverse transcription (RT) PCR is used to detect RNA from organisms such as hepatitis C virus and HIV-1. In modern amplification systems the use of fluorescent-labelled primers and probes allows 'real-time' detection of amplified DNA. Quantification is based on the principle that the time taken to reach the detection threshold is proportional to the initial number of copies of the target nucleic acid sequence.

Determination of nucleic acid sequence is also used to assign microorganisms to specific strains according to their genotype, which may be relevant to treatment and/or prognosis (e.g. in hepatitis C infection, p. 953). Nucleic acid sequences that are relevant to pathogenicity (such as toxin genes) or antimicrobial resistance can also be detected. For example, detection of the *mecA* gene is used to screen for meticillin-resistant *Staphylococcus aureus* (MRSA).

Nucleic acid amplification provides the most sensitive direct detection methods, but their extreme sensitivity can produce false positive results from contamination. PCR techniques are particularly useful when a rapid diagnosis is required. They are used widely in virology, where the possibility of false positive results from colonising or contaminating organisms is remote, and are applied to blood, respiratory samples, stool and urine. In bacteriology, PCR is used mainly to examine samples from normally sterile sites, such as CSF, blood and, increasingly, tissue. The role of PCR in mycology and parasitology is not yet established.

Culture

Organisms in samples of tissue, swabs and body fluids may replicate in culture, allowing their detection and characterisation.

- *In vivo culture* (in a living organism) is not used in routine diagnostic microbiology.
- *Ex vivo culture* (tissue culture) was widely used in the isolation of viruses, but is being gradually supplanted by nucleic acid amplification techniques.
- *In vitro culture* (in artificial culture media) of bacteria and fungi is used for definitive identification, to test for antimicrobial susceptibility and to subtype the organism for epidemiological purposes.

However, culture has its limitations. Results are not immediate, even for organisms which are easy to grow, and negative culture rarely excludes infection completely. Organisms such as *M. tuberculosis* are inherently slow-growing, typically taking 2 weeks to be detectable in the most specialised systems (liquid culture with constant monitoring) and longer when grown on solid media. Certain organisms, such as *M. leprae* and *Tropheryma whipplei*, cannot be cultivated on artificial media, and others (e.g. *Chlamydia* spp. and viruses) grow only in ex vivo systems, which are slow and labour-intensive to use.

Blood culture

Rapid microbiological diagnosis is required for bloodstream infection (BSI). To diagnose BSI, a liquid culture medium is inoculated with freshly drawn blood (Fig. 6.6). Bacterial growth can be detected by serial subculture or the detection of radio-labelled CO_2 produced by bacteria on breakdown of radio-labelled carbon sources provided in the growth media. Modern blood culture systems allow constant monitoring of liquid media for products of microbial respiration (mainly CO_2) using fluorescence. It is likely that constant-monitoring systems will be replaced or enhanced by nucleic acid amplification-based techniques.

Immunological tests

Immunological tests detect the host response to a specific microorganism and can be used to diagnose infection with organisms that are difficult to detect by other methods or are no longer present in the host. The term 'serological' describes tests carried out on serum, and includes both antigen and antibody detection. Immunological tests can also be performed on fluids other than blood (e.g. CSF, urine). Immunological tests require a functional host immune system, and often provide only a retrospective diagnosis.

The diagnostic opportunities afforded by methods that detect organism components and antibodies are illustrated in Figure 6.7.

Antibody detection

Detection of antibodies specific to the antigens of microorganisms is applied mainly to blood (Fig. 6.7). Results are typically expressed as titres: that is, the reciprocal of the highest dilution of the serum at which antibody is detectable (for example, detection at serum dilution of 1:64 gives a titre of 64). 'Seroconversion' is defined as either a change from negative to positive detection or a fourfold rise in titre between acute and convalescent serum samples. An acute sample is usually taken during the first week of disease and the convalescent sample 2–4 weeks later. Earlier diagnosis can be achieved by detection of IgM antibodies, which are produced early in infection (p. 75). Many immunological tests may be adapted to detect antigens instead of antibodies.

6

1 Patient sampling

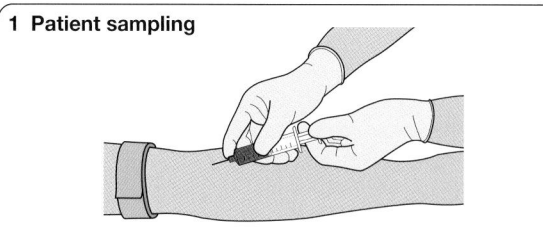

Contamination of blood culture bottles should be minimised by using careful aseptic technique and following local guidelines

2 Sample handling

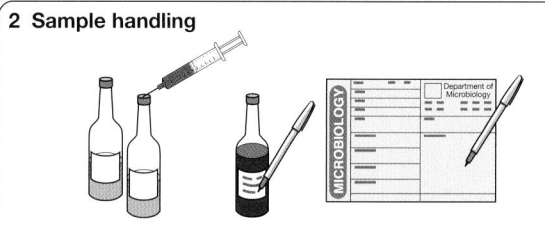

Local instructions should be followed, including safety instructions, labelling requirements, submission of paired vs. single bottles and use of multiple sets of blood cultures

3 Specimen transport

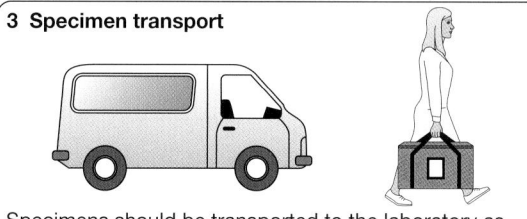

Specimens should be transported to the laboratory as quickly as possible. If there is a delay, the sample must be stored in conditions specified by the manufacturer of the blood culture system in use

4 Incubation

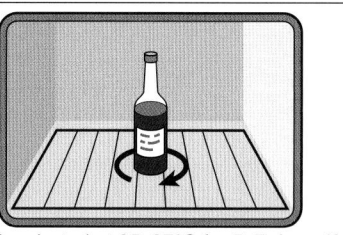

The specimen is incubated at 35–37°C for 5–7 days. If there has been no growth at this time, it is reported as negative and discarded

5 Growth detection

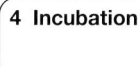

In most systems microbial growth is detected by constant automatic monitoring of CO_2 in the bottle. For significant bacteraemias this usually takes 12–24 hrs. Time to positivity (TTP) may be shorter in overwhelming sepsis and longer with fastidious organisms (e.g. *Brucella* spp.)

6 Preliminary results

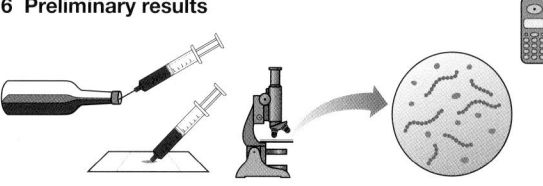

If growth is detected, a Gram film is made from the blood culture medium. The results are communicated immediately to the clinician and used to guide antibiotic therapy

7 Incubation

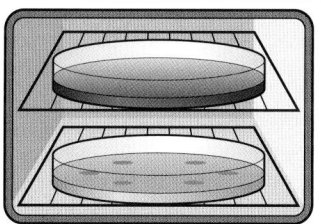

A small amount of the medium is incubated on a range of appropriate culture media. Preliminary susceptibility testing may also be carried out

8 Culture results

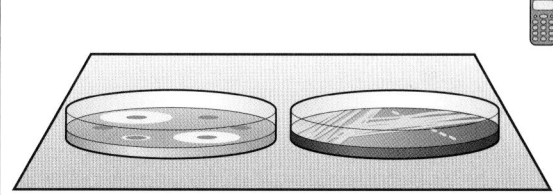

After incubation, presumptive identification and preliminary susceptibility results are communicated to the clinician

9 Definitive results

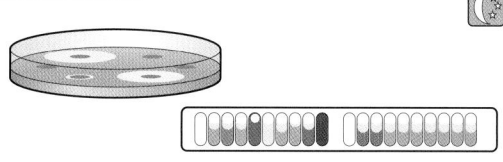

For most organisms definitive identification requires a further overnight incubation to enable confirmatory and/or further biochemical tests. Definitive susceptibility testing may also require further incubation with a range of antimicrobials

10 Reporting

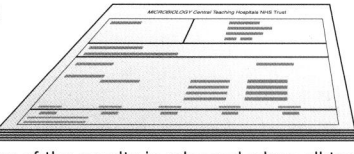

A final summary of the results is released when all testing is complete. For purposes of clinical care, liaison of the interim results (e.g. Gram film, presumptive identification and susceptibility) is usually more important than release of the final result. Effective clinical–laboratory communication is vital

 Overnight incubation required

 Urgent communication required

Fig. 6.6 An overview of the processing of blood cultures.

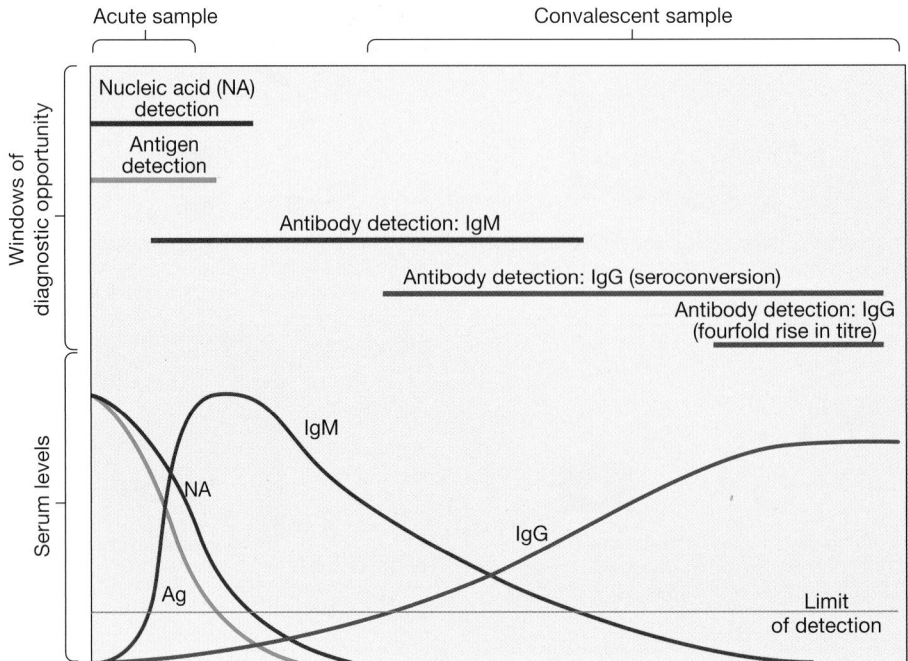

Fig. 6.7 Detection of antigen, nucleic acid and antibody in infectious disease. The acute sample is usually taken during the first week of illness, and the convalescent sample 2–4 weeks later. Detection limits and duration of detectability vary between tests and diseases, although in most diseases IgM is detectable within the first 1–2 weeks.

Enzyme-linked immunosorbent assay (ELISA, EIA)

The principles of ELISA are illustrated in Figure 6.8. These assays rely on linking an antibody with an enzyme which generates a colour change on exposure to a chromogenic substrate. Various configurations allow detection of antigens or specific subclasses of immunoglobulin (e.g. IgG, IgM, IgA). ELISA may also be adapted to detect PCR products, using immobilised oligonucleotide hybridisation probe and various detection systems.

Immunoblot (Western blot)

Microbial proteins are separated according to molecular weight by polyacrylamide gel electrophoresis (PAGE) and transferred (blotted) on to a nitrocellulose membrane, which is incubated with patient serum. Binding of specific antibody is detected with an enzyme-anti-immunoglobulin conjugate similar to that used in ELISA, and specificity is confirmed by its location on the membrane. Immunoblotting is a highly specific test, which may be used to confirm the results of less specific tests, such as ELISA.

Immunofluorescence assays (IFA)

IFAs are highly specific. In indirect immunofluorescence a serum sample is incubated with immobilised antigen (e.g. cells known to be infected with virus on

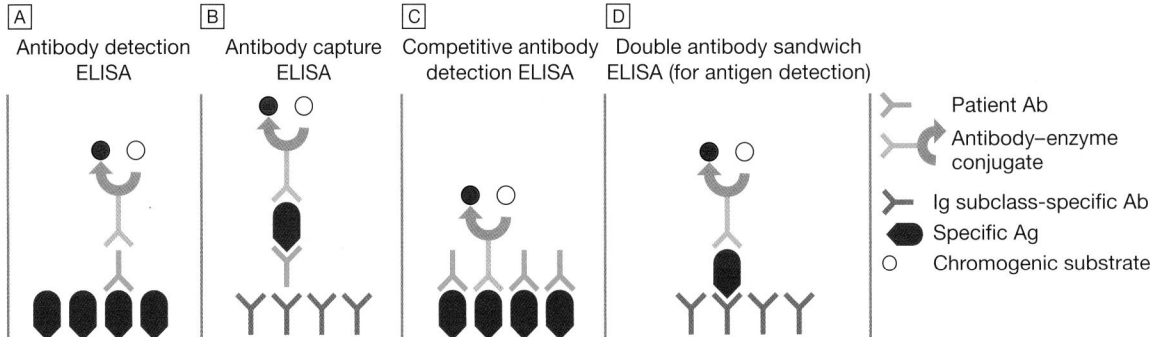

Fig. 6.8 Antibody (Ab) and antigen (Ag) detection by enzyme-linked immunosorbent assay (ELISA). This can be configured in various ways.
A Patient Ab binds to immobilised specific Ag, and is detected by addition of anti-immunoglobulin–enzyme conjugate and chromogenic substrate.
B Patient Ab binds to immobilised Ig subclass-specific Ag, and is detected by addition of specific Ag followed by antibody–enzyme conjugate and chromogenic substrate. **C** Patient Ab and antibody–enzyme conjugate bind to immobilised specific Ag. Magnitude of colour change reaction is inversely proportional to concentration of patient Ab. **D** Patient Ag binds to immobilised Ab, and is detected by addition of antibody–enzyme conjugate and chromogenic substrate. In A the conjugate Ab is specific for human immunoglobulin. In B–D it is specific for Ag from the disease-causing organism.

a glass slide) and antibody binding is detected using a fluorescent-labelled anti-human immunoglobulin (the 'secondary' antibody). This method can also detect organisms in clinical samples (usually tissue or centrifuged cells) using a specific antibody in place of patient serum. In direct immunofluorescence clinical samples are incubated directly with fluorescent-labelled specific antibodies to detect antigen, eliminating the need for secondary antibody.

Complement fixation test (CFT)

In a CFT, patient serum is heat-treated to inactivate complement, and added to specific antigen. Any specific antibody present in the serum will complex with the antigen. Complement is then added to the reaction. If antigen–antibody complexes are present, the complement will be 'fixed' (consumed). Sheep erythrocytes, coated with an anti-erythrocyte antibody, are added. The degree of erythrocyte lysis reflects the remaining complement and is inversely proportional to the level of the specific antigen–antibody complexes.

Agglutination tests

When antigens are present on the surface of particles (e.g. cells, latex particles or microorganisms) and cross-linked with antibodies, visible clumping (or 'agglutination') occurs.

- In *direct agglutination*, patient serum is added to a suspension of organisms that express the test antigen. For example, in the Weil–Felix test, host antibodies to various rickettsial species cause agglutination of *Proteus* bacteria because they cross-react with bacterial cell surface antigens.
- In *indirect (passive) agglutination*, specific antigen is attached to the surface of carrier particles which agglutinate when incubated with patient samples that contain specific antibodies.
- In *reverse passive agglutination* (an antigen detection test), the carrier particle is coated with antibody rather than antigen.

Other tests

Immunodiffusion. This involves antibodies and antigen migrating through gels, with or without the assistance of electrophoresis, and forming insoluble complexes where they meet. The complexes are seen on staining as 'precipitin bands'. Immunodiffusion is used in the diagnosis of chronic and allergic bronchopulmonary aspergillosis.

Immunochromatography. This is used for detection of antigen. The system consists of a porous test strip (e.g. a nitrocellulose membrane), at one end of which there is target-specific antibody, complexed with coloured microparticles. Further specific antibody is immobilised in a transverse narrow line some distance along the strip. Test material (e.g. blood or urine) is added to the antibody-particle complexes, which then migrate along the strip by capillary action. If these are complexed with antigen, they will be immobilised by the specific antibody and visualised as a transverse line across the strip. If the test is negative, the antibody–particle complexes will bind to a line of immobilised anti-immunoglobulin antibody placed further along the strip, which acts as a negative control. Immunochromatographic tests are rapid and relatively cheap to perform, and are appropriate for point-of-care testing, e.g. in HIV 1.

Antibody-independent immunological tests

It is also possible to measure components of the host immune response other than antibody responses. Many investigations in patients with infectious disease reflect the non-specific innate immune response and acute phase response (p. 81), including peripheral blood neutrophil counts and CRP levels. These are used in combination with microbiological tests to assess the likelihood of infectious disease and its severity.

A few tests assess specific cellular immunity. For example, IFN-γ release assays are used to diagnose tuberculosis, since blood lymphocytes from infected individuals produce IFN-γ in response to specific mycobacterial antigens.

Antimicrobial susceptibility testing

If growth of microorganisms in culture is inhibited by the addition of an antimicrobial agent, the organism is considered to be susceptible. This information is often used to select antimicrobial therapy (p. 148). Bacteriostatic agents cause reversible inhibition of growth and bactericidal agents cause cell death. The lowest concentration of antimicrobial agent at which growth is inhibited is the minimum inhibitory concentration (MIC), and the lowest concentration that causes cell death is the minimum bactericidal concentration (MBC) (the terms fungistatic/fungicidal are used for antifungal agents, and virustatic/virucidal for antiviral agents). If the MIC is less than a predetermined threshold, the organism is considered to be susceptible, and if the MIC is greater than or equal to the threshold, the organism is resistant.

Threshold MICs are determined for each antimicrobial agent from a combination of pharmacokinetic and clinical data. In reality, the relationship between antimicrobial susceptibility in culture and clinical response is more complex, as it depends on comorbidities, immune status, pharmacokinetic variability (p. 26) and antibiotic dosing, as well as MIC/MBC. Thus, susceptibility testing does not guarantee therapeutic success, but does indicate its probability.

Susceptibility testing is most often carried out by disc diffusion (Fig. 6.9). Antibiotic-impregnated filter

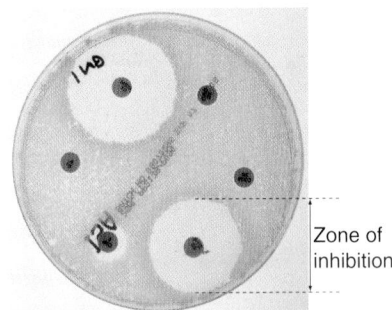

Fig. 6.9 Antimicrobial susceptibility testing by disc diffusion. The test organism is grown as a 'lawn' on an agar plate in the presence of antimicrobial-impregnated discs. The organism is considered susceptible if the diameter of the zone of inhibition exceeds a predetermined threshold.

Zone of inhibition

paper discs are placed on an agar plate containing bacteria. The antibiotic diffuses through the agar, resulting in a concentration gradient centred on the disc. Bacteria are unable to grow where the antibiotic concentration exceeds the MIC, and the size of the resulting zone of inhibition is inversely proportional to the MIC. Susceptibility testing methods using serial dilutions of antimicrobial in liquid media are generally more accurate and reproducible, and are used for generating epidemiological data.

EPIDEMIOLOGY OF INFECTION

The potential of infectious diseases for transmission means that, once a clinician has diagnosed an infectious disease, potential exposure of other patients must be considered. The patient may require treatment in isolation, or an outbreak of disease may need to be investigated in the community (Ch. 5). The approach will be specific to the microorganism involved (Chs 13–15) but the principles are outlined below.

Geographic and temporal patterns of infection

Endemic disease

Endemic disease has a constant presence within a given geographic area or population. The infectious agent may have a reservoir, vector or intermediate host that is geographically restricted, or may itself have restrictive environmental requirements (e.g. temperature range, humidity). The population affected may be geographically isolated, or the disease may be limited to unvaccinated populations. Factors that alter geographical restriction include:

- expansion of an animal reservoir (e.g. Lyme disease from reforestation)
- vector escape (e.g. airport malaria)
- extension of host range (e.g. schistosomiasis from dam construction)
- human migration (e.g. HIV)
- public health service breakdown (e.g. diphtheria in unvaccinated areas)
- climate change.

Emerging and re-emerging disease

An emerging infectious disease is one that has newly appeared in a population, or that has been known for some time but is rapidly increasing in incidence or geographic range. If the disease was previously known and thought to have been controlled or eradicated, it is considered to be re-emerging. Emergence may result from an organism adapting to cause a truly 'new' disease or escaping from a pre-existing restriction. Many emerging diseases are caused by organisms which infect animals and have undergone adaptations that enable them to infect humans. This is exemplified by HIV, which is believed to have originated in higher primates in Africa. The geographical pattern of some recent emerging and re-emerging infections is shown in Figure 6.10.

Reservoirs of infection

The US Centers for Disease Control (CDC) define a reservoir of infection as 'one or more epidemiologically connected populations or environments in which a pathogen can be permanently maintained, and from which infection is transmitted to a defined target population'. Reservoirs of infection may be human, animal or environmental.

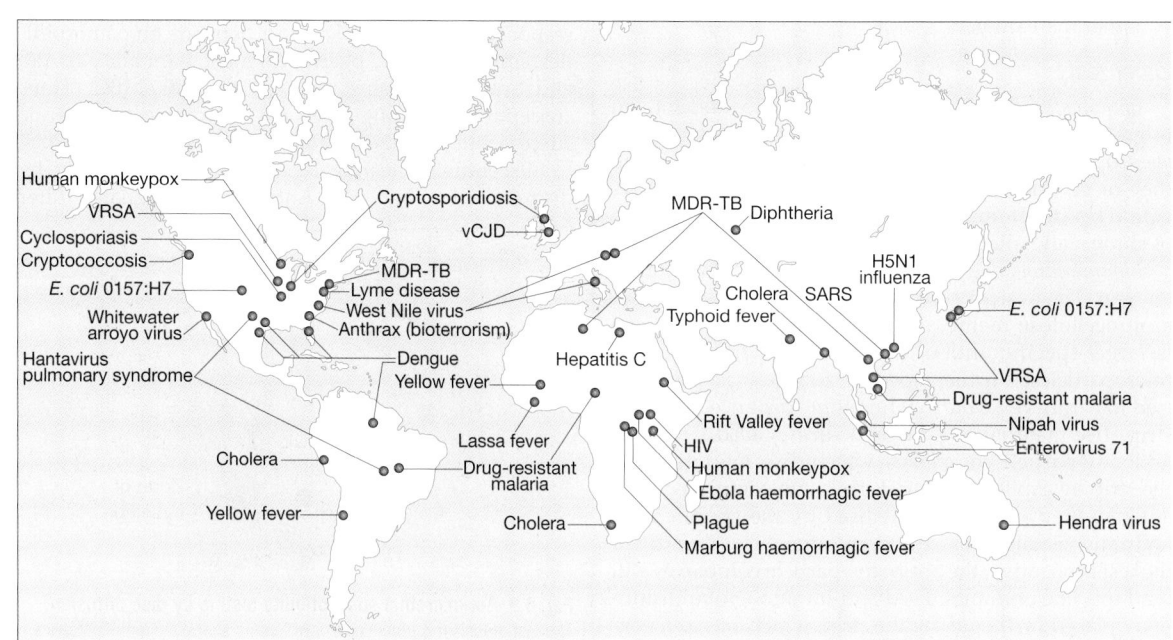

Fig. 6.10 Recent locations of some emerging and re-emerging diseases. (MDR-TB = multidrug-resistant tuberculosis; SARS = severe acute respiratory syndrome; vCJD = variant Creutzfeldt–Jakob disease; VRSA = vancomycin-resistant *Staph. aureus*)

Human reservoirs

Colonised individuals or those with clinical infectious disease may act as reservoirs, e.g. for *Staph. aureus* (including MRSA), which is carried in the nares of 30–40% of humans, and *C. difficile*. For infected humans to act as reservoirs, the infections caused must be long-lasting and/or non-fatal, at least in a proportion of those affected, to enable onward transmission (e.g. tuberculosis, typhoid and sexually transmitted infections). Humans are the only reservoir for some organisms (e.g. smallpox and measles).

Animal reservoirs

The World Health Organisation (WHO) defines a zoonosis as 'a disease or infection that is naturally transmissible from vertebrate animals to humans'. The infection may be asymptomatic in the animal. Zoonotic agents may be transmitted via any of the routes described below. Primary infection with zoonoses may on rare occasions be transmitted onward between humans by sexual contact (e.g. Q fever, brucellosis, Marburg, Ebola), causing secondary disease.

Environmental reservoirs

Many infective pathogens are acquired from an environmental source. However, some of these are maintained in human or animal reservoirs, with the environment acting simply as a conduit for infection.

Transmission of infection

Infectious agents may be transmitted by multiple routes.

- *The respiratory route* refers to acquisition of infection by inhalation.
- *The faecal–oral route* describes acquisition by ingestion of infectious material originating from faecal matter.
- *Sexually transmitted infections* are acquired by direct contact between mucous membranes.
- *Blood-borne infections* are transmitted by direct inoculation of infected blood or body fluids.
- *Direct contact.* Very few organisms are capable of causing infection by direct contact with intact skin.

Most infection by this route requires inoculation or contact with damaged skin.

In many infections there is an intermediary, which bridges the gap between the infected host (or the reservoir) and the uninfected host.

- If the intermediary is animate it is known as a *vector* (e.g. mosquitoes in malaria and dengue, fleas in plague, humans in MRSA).
- Inanimate intermediaries are known as *fomites*, and are particularly associated with health care-associated infection, where fomites include door handles, water taps, ultrasound probes etc.

The likelihood of infection following transmission of an infectious agent depends on both organism factors and host susceptibility. The numbers of organisms required to cause infection or death in 50% of the exposed population

i 6.7 Incubation periods of important infections[1]

Infection	Incubation period
Short incubation periods	
Anthrax, cutaneous[3]	9 hrs–2 weeks
Anthrax, inhalational[3]	2 days[2]
Bacillary dysentery[5]	1–6 days
Cholera[3]	2 hrs–5 days
Dengue haemorrhagic fever[6]	3–14 days
Diphtheria[6]	1–10 days
Gonorrhoea[4]	2–10 days
Influenza[5]	1–3 days
Meningococcaemia[3]	2–10 days
SARS coronavirus[3]	2–7 days[2]
Scarlet fever[5]	2–4 days
Intermediate incubation periods	
Amoebiasis[6]	1–4 weeks
Brucellosis[4]	5–30 days
Chickenpox[5]	11–20 days
Lassa fever[3]	3–21 days
Malaria[3]	10–15 days
Measles[5]	6–19 days
Mumps[5]	15–24 days
Poliomyelitis[6]	3–35 days
Psittacosis[4]	1–4 weeks
Rubella[5]	15–20 days
Typhoid[5]	5–31 days
Whooping cough[5]	5–21 days
Long incubation periods	
Hepatitis A[5]	3–7 weeks
Hepatitis B[4]	6 weeks–6 months
Leishmaniasis, cutaneous[6]	Weeks–months
Leishmaniasis, visceral[6]	Months–years
Leprosy[3]	5–20 years
Rabies[4]	2–8 weeks[2]
Trypanosoma brucei gambiense infection[6]	Months–years
Tuberculosis[5]	1–12 months

[1]Incubation periods are approximate and may differ from local or national guidance.
[2]Longer incubation periods have been reported.

Reference sources:
[3]WHO.
[4]Health Protection Agency, UK.
[5]Richardson M, Elliman D, Maguire H, et al. Pediatr Infect Dis J 2001; 20:380–388.
[6]Centers for Disease Control, USA.

i 6.6 Periods of infectivity in childhood infectious diseases[1]

Disease	Infectious period
Chickenpox	From 4 days before[2] until 5 days after appearance of the rash[3]
Measles	From 1–2 days before onset of rash; duration unknown[3]
Mumps	Unknown[4]
Rubella	Unknown, but most infectious during prodromal illness[3]
Scarlet fever	Unknown[5]
Whooping cough	Unknown[5,6]

[1]From Richardson M, Elliman D, Maguire H, et al. Pediatr Infect Dis J 2001; 20:380–388. These recommendations may differ from local or national guidance.
[2]Transmission before 48 hours prior to the onset of rash is rare.
[3,4,5]Exclude from contact with non-immune and immunocompromised people for 5 days from [3]onset of rash, [4]onset of parotitis or [5]start of antibiotic treatment.
[6]Exclude for 3 weeks if untreated.

6

are referred to as the ID_{50} (infectious dose) and LD_{50} (lethal dose), respectively. The incubation period is the time between exposure and development of disease, and the period of infectivity is the period after exposure during which the patient is infectious to others. Knowledge of incubation periods and periods of infectivity is important in controlling the spread of disease (Boxes 6.6 and 6.7).

Bioterrorism and deliberate release

Infectious agents may be released or transmitted deliberately with the intention of causing disease. The large-scale use of microorganisms for this purpose is known as biological warfare or bioterrorism, depending on the context. Deliberate-release incidents have included a 750-person outbreak of *Salmonella typhimurium* by deliberate contamination of salads in 1984 (Oregon, USA) and 22 cases of anthrax (five fatal) from the mailing of finely powdered (weaponised) anthrax spores

in 2001 (New Jersey, USA). Diseases with high potential for use in bioterrorism include anthrax, plague, tularaemia, smallpox and botulism (through toxin release).

CONTROL AND PREVENTION OF INFECTION

Infection prevention and control (IPC) describes the measures applied to populations with the aim of breaking the chain of infection (see Fig. 6.1, p. 132).

Health care-acquired infection

Admission to a health-care facility in the developed world carries a considerable risk of acquiring infection, estimated by the UK Department of Health as 6–10%. The factors that contribute to health care-acquired (nosocomial) infection in an individual patient are shown in Box 6.8. Many nosocomial bacterial infections are caused by organisms that are resistant to numerous antibiotics

6.8 Risk factors for nosocomial infection

Predisposing factor	Likely infection
Environmental	
Inadequate cleaning of potential fomites (furniture, shared facilities, medical equipment etc.)	Diverse organisms
Building work and dust	*Aspergillus* spp.
Contaminated water supply	*Cryptosporidium* spp., *Legionella pneumophila*, enteric organisms
Contact with health-care staff	*Staph. aureus* including MRSA, Enterobacteriaceae including ESBL, GRE, *C. difficile*, *Candida* spp.
Contact with other patients	Norovirus, respiratory viruses (RSV, influenza, parainfluenza), VZV, *Staph. aureus* including MRSA, *Strep. pyogenes*, *C. difficile*
Personal	
Prolonged admission	Diverse organisms
Immunocompromise due to disease (haematological malignancy, HIV, diabetes mellitus, organ failure etc.) or therapy (e.g. cytotoxic agents, corticosteroids)	Diverse organisms
Antibiotic use, especially broad-spectrum (e.g. cephalosporins)	Multi-resistant organisms (MRSA, ESBL-containing Enterobacteriaceae, multi-resistant *Acinetobacter* spp., *Stenotrophomonas maltophilia*, GRE, *C. difficile*)
Receipt of blood products	Blood-borne infections (p. 1010)
Insertion of prosthesis (joint or cardiac valve) or other device (cannulae, catheters, shunts etc.)	Biofilm-related organisms (coagulase-negative staphylococci, *Staph. aureus* including MRSA, *Candida* spp.)
Surgical procedures	Diverse organisms

(ESBL = extended-spectrum β-lactamase; GRE = glycopeptide-resistant enterococci; RSV = respiratory syncytial virus; VZV = varicella zoster virus)

6.9 Methods used in the prevention and control of infection in hospitals

Institutional
- Handling, storage and disposal of clinical waste
- Containment and safe removal of spilled blood and body fluids
- Cleanliness of environment and medical equipment
- Specialised ventilation (e.g. laminar flow, air filtration, controlled pressure gradients)
- Sterilisation and disinfection of instruments and equipment
- Food hygiene
- Laundry management

Health-care staff
- Education
- Hand hygiene, including hand-washing (see Fig. 6.11)
- Sharps management and disposal
- Use of personal protective equipment (masks, sterile and non-sterile gloves, gowns and aprons)
- Screening health workers for disease (e.g. tuberculosis, hepatitis B virus, MRSA)
- Immunisation and post-exposure prophylaxis

Clinical practice
- Antibiotic stewardship (use only when necessary; avoid drugs known to select multi-resistant organisms or predispose to other infections)
- Aseptic technique (see Box 6.10)
- Perioperative antimicrobial prophylaxis
- Screening patients for colonisation or infection (e.g. MRSA, GRE)

Response to infections
- Surveillance to detect alert organism (see text) outbreaks and antimicrobial resistance
- Antibiotic chemoprophylaxis to infectious disease contacts, if indicated (see Box 6.20, p. 151)
- Isolation (see Box 6.11)
- Reservoir control
- Vector control

(MRSA = meticillin-resistant *Staphyloccus aureus;* GRE = glycopeptide-resistant enterococci)

(multi-resistant bacteria), including meticillin-resistant *Staph. aureus* (MRSA) (p. 326), extended-spectrum β-lactamase (ESBL)-producing Enterobacteriaceae and glycopeptide-resistant enterococci (GRE). Other infections of particular concern in hospitals include *C. difficile* (p. 338) and norovirus (p. 323).

IPC measures are described in Box 6.9. The most important infection control practice is maintenance of good hand hygiene (Fig. 6.11). Hand decontamination or washing is *mandatory* before and after every patient contact. In most cases, decontamination with alcohol gel is adequate. However, hand-washing (with hot water, liquid soap and complete drying) is required after undertaking any procedure that involves more than casual physical contact, or if hands are visibly soiled. In situations where the prevalence of *C. difficile* is high (e.g. a local outbreak), alcohol gel decontamination between patient contacts is inadequate, as it does not kill *C. dif-*

EBM	6.10 Skin antisepsis prior to insertion of central venous catheters

'Skin preparation with chlorhexidine in 70% isopropyl alcohol is more effective than povidone-iodine or aqueous antiseptic solutions in preventing catheter infections.'

• Pratt RJ, et al. J Hosp Infect 2007; 65S: S1–S64.

ficile spores, and hands must be washed with soap and water.

To avoid infection, all invasive procedures must be performed with strict aseptic technique (Box 6.10). Some infections necessitate additional measures to prevent cross-infection (Box 6.11).

Outbreaks of infection

Descriptive terms are defined in Box 6.12. Confirmation of an infectious disease outbreak usually requires evidence from typing (p. 136) that the causal organisms have identical genotypic characteristics. If this is found not to be the case, the term pseudo-outbreak is used. When an outbreak of infection is suspected, a case definition is agreed. The number of cases that meet the case definition is then assessed by case finding, using methods ranging from administration of questionnaires to national reporting systems. Case finding usually includes microbiological testing, at least in the early stages of an outbreak. Temporal changes in cases are noted to plot an outbreak curve, and demographic details are collected to identify possible sources of infection. A case control study, in which recent activities (potential exposures) of affected 'cases' are compared to those of unaffected 'controls', may be undertaken to establish the outbreak source, and measures are taken to manage the outbreak and control its spread. Good communication between relevant personnel during and after the outbreak is important to inform practice in future outbreaks.

Surveillance ensures that disease outbreaks are either pre-empted or identified early. In hospitals, staff are alerted to the isolation of *alert organisms*, which have the propensity to cause outbreaks, and *alert conditions* (infectious diseases), which are likely to be caused by such organisms. Similar systems are used nationally; many countries publish lists of organisms and diseases which, if detected (or suspected), must be reported to public health authorities (Box 6.13).

Principles of food hygiene

'Food poisoning' (p. 302) is largely preventable by food hygiene measures. The main principles are:
• segregation of uncooked food (which may be contaminated with pathogenic microorganisms) from cooked food during storage, handling and preparation
• avoidance of conditions which allow growth of pathogenic bacteria before or after cooking
• adequate bacterial killing during cooking.

Safe storage requires knowledge of the temperatures at which food bacteria are inhibited and destroyed (Fig. 6.12).

Wash hands only when visibly soiled! Otherwise use handrub!

 Duration of the entire procedure: 40–60 sec.

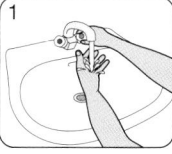

Wet hands with water

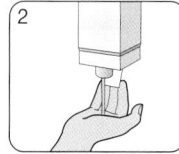

Apply enough soap to cover all hand surfaces

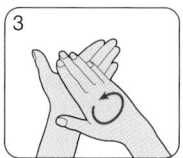

Rub hands palm to palm

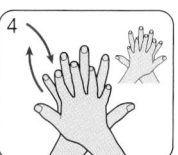

Right palm over left dorsum with interlaced fingers and vice versa

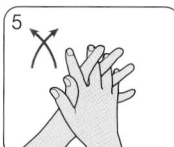

Palm to palm with fingers interlaced

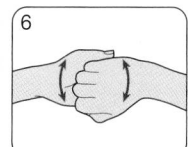

Backs of fingers to opposing palms with fingers interlaced

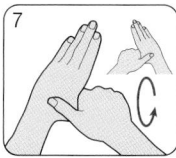

Rotational rubbing of left thumb clasped in right palm and vice versa

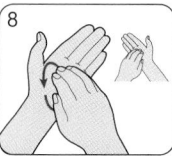

Rotational rubbing, backwards and forwards with clasped fingers of right hand in left palm and vice versa

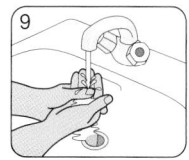

Rinse hands with water

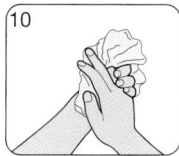

Dry thoroughly with a single-use towel

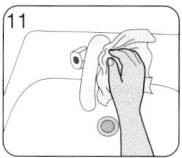

Use towel to turn off tap

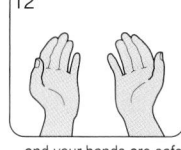

...and your hands are safe

Fig. 6.11 Hand-washing. Good hand hygiene, whether with soap/water or alcohol handrub, includes areas that are often missed, such as fingertips, web spaces, palmar creases and the backs of hands. Adapted from WHO guidance at www.who.int.

6

6.11 Types of isolation precaution[1]

Airborne transmission	Contact transmission	Droplet transmission
Precautions		
Negative pressure room with air exhausted externally or filtered N95 masks or personal respirators for staff; avoid using non-immune staff	Private room preferred (otherwise inter-patient spacing ≥ 1 m) Gloves and gown for staff in contact with patient or contaminated areas	Private room preferred (otherwise inter-patient spacing ≥ 1 m) Surgical masks for staff in close contact with patient
Infections managed with these precautions		
Measles Tuberculosis, pulmonary or laryngeal, confirmed or suspected	Enteroviral infections in young children (diapered or incontinent) Norovirus[2] *C. difficile* infection Multidrug-resistant organisms (e.g. MRSA, ESBL, GRE, VRSA, penicillin-resistant *Strep. pneumoniae*)[3] Parainfluenza in infants and young children Rotavirus RSV in infants, children and immunocompromised Viral conjunctivitis, acute	Diphtheria, pharyngeal *Haemophilus influenzae* type B infection Herpes simplex virus, disseminated or severe Influenza Meningococcal infection Mumps *Mycoplasma pneumoniae* Parvovirus (erythrovirus) B19 (erythema infectiosum, fifth disease) Pertussis Plague, pneumonic/bubonic Rubella *Strep. pyogenes* (group A), pharyngeal

Infections managed with multiple precautions

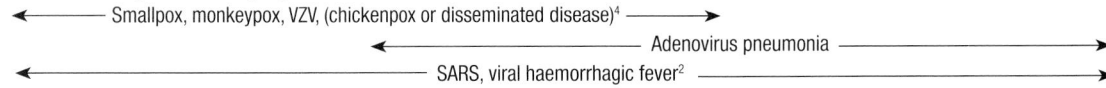

◄—————— Smallpox, monkeypox, VZV, (chickenpox or disseminated disease)[4] ——————►

◄———————————————————— Adenovirus pneumonia ————————————————————►

◄————————————— SARS, viral haemorrhagic fever[2] —————————————►

[1] Recommendations based on 2007 CDC guideline for isolation precautions. May differ from local or national recommendations.
[2] Not a CDC recommendation.
[3] Subject to local risk assessment.
[4] Or in any immunocompromised patient until possibility of disseminated infection excluded.
(VRSA = vancomycin-resistant *Staph. aureus*)

6.12 Terminology in outbreaks of infection

Term	Definition
Classification of related cases of infectious disease*	
Cluster	An aggregation of cases of a disease which are closely grouped in time and place, and may or may not exceed the expected number
Epidemic	The occurrence of more cases of disease than expected in a given area or among a specific group of people over a particular period of time
Outbreak	Synonymous with epidemic. Alternatively, a localised as opposed to generalised epidemic
Pandemic	An epidemic occurring over a very wide area (several countries or continents) and usually affecting a large proportion of the population
Classification of affected patients (cases)	
Index case	The first case identified in an outbreak
Primary cases	Cases acquired from a specific source of infection
Secondary cases	Cases acquired from primary cases
Types of outbreak	
Common source outbreak	Exposure to a common source of infection (e.g. water-cooling tower, medical staff member shedding MRSA). New primary cases will arise until the source is no longer present
Point source outbreak	Exposure to a single source of infection at a specific point in time (e.g. contaminated food at a party). Primary cases will develop disease synchronously
Person-to-person spread	Outbreak with both primary and secondary cases. May complicate point source or common source outbreak

*Adapted from www.cdc.gov.

6.13 Infectious diseases reportable to public health authorities in the UK

- Acute encephalitis[1]
- Anthrax
- Cholera
- Chickenpox[2]
- Continued fever[2]
- Diphtheria
- Dysentery[3]
- Erysipelas[2]
- Food poisoning
- Legionellosis[2]
- Leprosy[1]
- Leptospirosis
- Lyme disease[2]
- Malaria
- Measles
- Membranous croup[2]
- Meningitis[1]
- Meningococcal infection
- Mumps
- Ophthalmia neonatorum[1]
- Paratyphoid fever
- Plague
- Poliomyelitis
- Puerperal fever[2]
- Rabies
- Relapsing fever
- Rubella
- Scarlet fever
- Smallpox
- Tetanus
- Toxoplasmosis[2]
- Tuberculosis
- Typhoid fever
- Typhus fever
- Viral haemorrhagic fever
- Viral hepatitis
- Whooping cough
- Yellow fever[1]

[1]England and Wales only.
[2]Scotland only.
[3]Scotland: bacillary dysentery only.

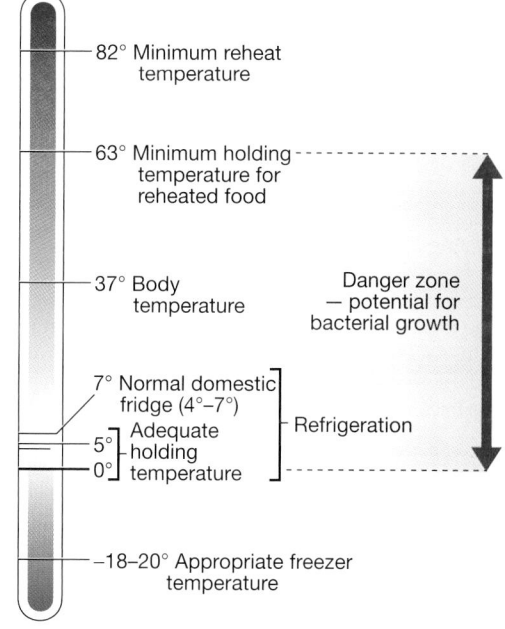

Fig. 6.12 Important temperatures (°C) in food hygiene.

Immunisation

Immunisation may be passive or active. Passive immunisation is achieved by administering antibodies targeted against a specific pathogen. Antibodies are obtained from human blood, so confer some of the risks associated with blood products (p. 1008). The protection afforded by passive immunisation is immediate but of short duration (a few weeks or months); it is used to prevent or attenuate infection before or after exposure (Box 6.14).

Vaccination

Active immunisation is achieved by vaccination with entire organisms or antigenic components such as proteins and polysaccharides. DNA vaccines are also under investigation. Desirable vaccine attributes include:

- minimal vaccine-related adverse effects
- a high level of immunity (i.e. few vaccine failures)
- long-lasting protection
- minimal cost
- ease of delivery.

Types of vaccine

Vaccine types in current use are shown in Box 6.15.

Vaccines may be either live or inactivated. Live vaccines contain organisms with attenuated (reduced)

6.14 Indications for post-exposure prophylaxis with immunoglobulins

Human normal immunoglobulin (pooled immunoglobulin)

- Hepatitis A (unvaccinated contacts*)
- Measles (if exposed child has heart or lung disease)

Human specific immunoglobulin

- Hepatitis B (sexual partners, inoculation injuries, infants born to infected mothers)
- Tetanus (high-risk wounds or when immunisation status is incomplete or unknown)
- Rabies
- Chickenpox (immunosuppressed children and adults, pregnant women)

*Active immunisation is preferred if contact is with a patient who is within 1 week of onset of jaundice.

6.15 Vaccines in current clinical use

Live attenuated vaccines

- Measles, mumps, rubella (MMR)
- Oral poliomyelitis (OPV, not used in UK)
- Tuberculosis (bacille Calmette–Guérin, BCG)
- Typhoid (oral typhoid vaccine)
- Varicella zoster virus

Inactivated (killed) whole-cell vaccines

- Cholera
- Hepatitis A
- Rabies

Toxin/toxoid/polysaccharide vaccines

- Anthrax (adsorbed antigens)
- Diphtheria (adsorbed toxoid)
- Hepatitis B (adsorbed antigen)
- *Haemophilus influenzae* type B (Hib; conjugated polysaccharide)
- Meningococcal, quadrivalent A, C, Y, W135 (polysaccharide)
- Meningococcal, serogroup C (conjugated polysaccharide)
- Pertussis (adsorbed components)
- Pneumococcal conjugate (PCV; conjugated polysaccharide, 7 or more serotypes)
- Pneumococcal polysaccharide (PPV; polysaccharide, 23 serotypes)
- Inactivated poliomyelitis (IPV; adsorbed antigens)
- Tetanus (adsorbed toxoid)
- Typhoid (Vi polysaccharide)

virulence, which result in a fully integrated T lymphocyte and humoral response (p. 75) and are therefore more immunogenic than inactivated vaccines. However, the use of live vaccines in immunocompromised individuals requires careful consideration. Inactivated vaccines consist of whole killed organisms or their antigenic components.

Vaccines consisting only of polysaccharides, such as pneumococcal polyvalent vaccine (PPV), are poor activators of T lymphocytes, and produce a short-lived antibody response without long-lasting memory. Protein antigens are more immunogenic than polysaccharides. Conjugation of a polysaccharide moiety to a protein, as in *Haemophilus influenzae* type B (Hib), *Neisseria meningitidis* serogroup C (MenC) and pneumococcal conjugate (PCV) vaccines, activates T lymphocytes, which results in a sustained response and immunological memory. Toxoids are bacterial toxins that have been modified to reduce toxicity but maintain antigenicity. Response can be improved further by co-administration with mildly pro-inflammatory adjuvants such as aluminium hydroxide.

Use of vaccines

Guidelines for individuals are shown in Box 6.16. Vaccination may be applied to entire populations (as in childhood vaccination schedules) or populations at specific risk through travel, occupation or other risk activities. In ring vaccination, the population immediately surrounding a case or outbreak of infectious disease is vaccinated, to curtail further spread.

Vaccination becomes successful once the number of susceptible hosts in a population falls below the level required to sustain continued transmission of the target organism (herd immunity). Naturally acquired smallpox was declared to have been eradicated world-wide in 1980 through mass vaccination. In 1988 the WHO resolved to eradicate poliomyelitis by vaccination; the number of cases world-wide has since fallen from approximately 350 000 p.a. to 1651 in 2008. Measles virus, however, is very infectious, and over 90% of a population needs to be vaccinated to achieve herd immunity. A recent decline in the uptake of measles vaccination in the UK has been associated with increased prevalence of disease. Recommended vaccination schedules vary between different countries.

6.16 Guidelines for vaccination against infectious disease

- The principal contraindication to inactivated vaccines is an anaphylactic reaction to a previous dose or a component of the vaccine
- Live vaccines should not be given to pregnant women, to the immunosuppressed, or in the presence of an acute infection
- If two live vaccines are required, they should be given either simultaneously in opposite arms or 4 weeks apart
- Live vaccines should not be given for 3 months after an injection of human normal immunoglobulin (HNI)
- HNI should not be given for 2 weeks after a live vaccine
- Hay fever, asthma, eczema, sickle-cell disease, topical corticosteroid therapy, antibiotic therapy, prematurity and chronic heart and lung diseases, including tuberculosis, are not contraindications to vaccination

TREATMENT OF INFECTIOUS DISEASES

The key components of treating infectious disease are:
- Address any identifiable predisposing factor, e.g. diabetes mellitus or known immune deficit (HIV, neutropenia).
- Antimicrobial therapy (see below).
- Adjuvant therapy, without which eradication of infection is unlikely, e.g. removal of an indwelling catheter (urinary or vascular), abscess drainage or débridement of an area of necrotising fasciitis.
- Treatment of the consequences of infection, e.g. the systemic inflammatory response syndrome (SIRS; p. 184), inflammation and pain.

For communicable disease, treatment must also take into account contacts of the infected patient, and may include infection prevention and control activities such as isolation, antimicrobial prophylaxis, vaccination and contact tracing.

Principles of antimicrobial therapy

When infection is diagnosed, it is often important to start antimicrobial therapy promptly. The general principles underlying the use of drugs are discussed in Chapter 2. Factors specific to antimicrobial agents are discussed below. The process of selecting antimicrobial therapy is illustrated in Figure 6.13.

Antimicrobial action and spectrum

Antimicrobial agents bring about killing by inhibiting, damaging or destroying a target that is a required component of the organism. Every antimicrobial agent is able to kill a specific range of microorganisms, and this must be considered in selecting appropriate antimicrobial therapy. The mechanisms of action of the major classes of antibacterial agent are listed in Box 6.17 and appropriate antibiotic choices for a range of common infecting organisms are shown in Box 6.18. In severe infections and/or immunocompromised patients, it is customary to use bactericidal agents in preference to bacteriostatic agents.

Empiric versus targeted therapy

Empiric antimicrobial therapy is selected to treat a clinical syndrome (e.g. meningitis) before a microbiological diagnosis has been made. Targeted therapy is aimed at the causal pathogen(s) of known antimicrobial sensitivity. Ideally, broad-spectrum agents are used in empiric therapy, and narrow-spectrum agents in targeted therapy. Optimum empiric therapy differs according to clinical presentation (e.g. pneumonia versus meningitis), patient groups (e.g. children, immunocompromised hosts) and local antimicrobial resistance patterns. Hospitals should establish local antibiotic policies to guide rational antimicrobial prescribing, maximising efficacy while minimising antimicrobial resistance and cost.

Combination therapy

Antimicrobial combination therapy is usually restricted to three settings:
- to increase efficacy (e.g. enterococcal endocarditis, where a β-lactam/aminoglycoside combination results in better outcomes than a β-lactam alone)

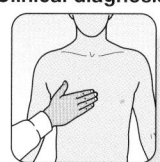

Clinical diagnosis

Information available:

- Organ system involved
- Endogenous or exogenous infection
- Likely pathogens

Antimicrobial spectrum of agent(s) used

1 Empiric therapy
Based on:
- Predicted susceptibility of likely pathogens
- Local antimicrobial policies

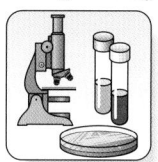

Laboratory investigations: microbiological diagnosis

- Infecting organism(s)
- Likely antimicrobial susceptibility

2 Targeted therapy
Based on:
- Predicted susceptibility of infecting organism(s)
- Local antimicrobial policies

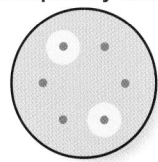

Antimicrobial susceptibility results

- Antimicrobial susceptibility of infecting organism(s)

Level of knowledge of infecting organism(s)

3 Susceptibility-guided therapy
Based on:
- Susceptibility testing results

Fig. 6.13 Stages in the selection and refinement of antimicrobial therapy.

 6.17 Target and mechanism of action of common antibacterial agents

Aminoglycosides, chloramphenicol, macrolides, lincosamides and streptogramins, oxazolidinones (linezolid)

- Inhibition of bacterial protein synthesis by binding to subunit of bacterial ribosomes

Tetracyclines

- Inhibition of protein synthesis by preventing tRNA binding to ribosomes

Beta-lactams

- Inhibition of cell wall peptidoglycan synthesis by competitive inhibition of transpeptidases ('penicillin-binding proteins')

Cyclic lipopeptide (daptomycin)

- Insertion of lipophilic tail into plasma membrane causes depolarisation and cell death

Glycopeptides

- Inhibition of cell wall peptidoglycan synthesis by forming complexes with D-alanine residues on peptidoglycan precursors

Nitroimidazoles

- Reduced drug causes strand breaks in DNA

Quinolones

- Inhibition of DNA replication by binding to DNA topoisomerases (DNA gyrase and topoisomerase IV), preventing supercoiling and uncoiling of DNA

Rifamycins

- Inhibition of DNA synthesis by inhibiting DNA-dependent RNA polymerase

Sulphonamides and trimethoprim

- Inhibition of folate synthesis by pteridine synthase (sulphonamides) and dihydrofolate reductase (trimethoprim) inhibition

---

- when no single agent's spectrum covers all potential pathogens (e.g. in polymicrobial infection or empiric treatment of sepsis)
- to reduce antimicrobial resistance, as the organism would need to develop resistance to multiple agents simultaneously (e.g. antituberculous chemotherapy, highly active anti-retroviral therapy (HAART, p. 403)).

Antimicrobial resistance

Microorganisms have evolved in the presence of antibiotics, which are antimicrobial agents produced naturally by bacteria and fungi. They have therefore developed multiple resistance mechanisms (categorised in Fig. 6.14) to all classes of antimicrobial agent (antibiotics and their derivatives). Resistance may be an innate property of a microorganism (intrinsic resistance) or may be acquired, by either spontaneous mutation or horizontal transfer of genetic material from another organism. For some agents, e.g. penicillins, a degree of resistance occurs in vivo when the bacterial load is high and the molecular target for the antimicrobial is down-regulated (an 'inoculum effect').

The *mecA* gene encodes a low-affinity penicillin-binding protein, which confers resistance to meticillin and other penicillinase-resistant penicillins in *Staph. aureus*. It is common for plasmids to encode resistance to multiple antimicrobials, which may be transferred horizontally. Extended spectrum β-lactamases (ESBL) are encoded on plasmids, which are transferred relatively easily between bacteria including Enterobacteriaceae. Plasmid-mediated carbapenemases have been detected in strains of *Klebsiella pneumoniae*. Glycopeptide resistance in enterococci is also transferred on mobile genetic elements. Strains of MRSA have been described that exhibit intermediate resistance to glycopeptides, through the development of a relatively impermeable cell wall (GISA).

6

6.18 Antimicrobial options for common infecting bacteria

Organism	Antimicrobial options*
Gram-positive organisms	
Enterococcus faecalis	Ampicillin, tigecycline, vancomycin/teicoplanin
Enterococcus faecium	Tigecycline, vancomycin/teicoplanin, linezolid
Glycopeptide-resistant enterococci (GRE)	Linezolid, tigecycline, quinupristin-dalfopristin
MRSA	Clindamycin, vancomycin, rifampicin (never used as monotherapy), linezolid, daptomycin, tetracyclines, tigecycline, co-trimoxazole
Staph. aureus	Flucloxacillin, clindamycin
Strep. pyogenes	Penicillin, clindamycin, erythromycin
Strep. pneumoniae	Penicillin, macrolides, cephalosporins, levofloxacin, vancomycin
Gram-negative organisms	
E. coli, 'coliforms' (enteric Gram-negative bacilli)	Trimethoprim, cefuroxime, ciprofloxacin, co-amoxiclav, amoxicillin (resistance common)
Enterobacter spp., Citrobacter spp.	Ciprofloxacin, meropenem, aminoglycosides
ESBL-producing Enterobacteriaceae	Ciprofloxacin, meropenem, piperacillin-tazobactam, aminoglycosides, tigecycline
Haemophilus influenzae	Amoxicillin, co-amoxiclav, macrolides, cefuroxime, cefotaxime, ciprofloxacin
Legionella pneumophila	Azithromycin, levofloxacin, doxycycline
Neisseria gonorrhoeae	Ceftriaxone/cefixime, spectinomycin
Neisseria meningitidis	Penicillin, cefotaxime, chloramphenicol
Pseudomonas aeruginosa	Ciprofloxacin, piperacillin-tazobactam, aztreonam, meropenem, aminoglycosides, ceftazidime/cefepime
Salmonella typhi	Ciprofloxacin, ceftriaxone, chloramphenicol (resistance common)
Strict anaerobes	
Bacteroides spp.	Metronidazole, clindamycin, co-amoxiclav, piperacillin-tazobactam, meropenem
Clostridium difficile	Metronidazole, vancomycin (oral)
Clostridium spp.	Penicillin, metronidazole, clindamycin
Fusobacterium spp.	Penicillin, metronidazole, clindamycin
Other organisms	
Chlamydia trachomatis	Azithromycin, doxycycline
Treponema pallidum	Penicillin, doxycycline

*Antibiotic selection depends on multiple factors, including local susceptibility patterns. There are many appropriate alternatives to those listed.

Factors implicated in the emergence of antimicrobial resistance include the inappropriate use of antibiotics when not indicated (e.g. in viral infections), inadequate dosage or treatment duration, excessive use of broad-spectrum agents, and use of antimicrobials as growth-promoters in agriculture. However *any* antimicrobial use exerts a selection pressure that favours the development of resistance. Combination antimicrobial therapy may reduce the emergence of resistance. This is recommended in treatment of patients infected with HIV, which is highly prone to spontaneous mutation (p. 406). Despite use of combination therapy for *M. tuberculosis*, multidrug-resistant TB (MDR-TB, resistant to isoniazid and rifampicin) and extremely drug-resistant TB (XDR-TB, resistant to isoniazid and rifampicin, any fluoroquinolone, and at least one injectable antimicrobial antituberculous agent) have been reported worldwide and are increasing in incidence (p. 693).

Duration of therapy

Treatment duration generally reflects severity of infection and the accessibility of the infected site to antimicro-

6.19 Duration of antimicrobial therapy for some common infections*

Infection	Duration of therapy
Viral infections	
Herpes simplex encephalitis	2–3 weeks
Bacterial infections	
Gonorrhoea	Single dose
Infective endocarditis (streptococcal, native valve)	4 weeks ± gentamicin for first 2 weeks
Infective endocarditis (prosthetic valve)	≥6 weeks
Osteomyelitis	4–6 weeks
Pneumonia (community-acquired, severe)	10 days (no organism identified), 14–21 days (Staph. aureus or Legionella spp.)
Septic arthritis	2–4 weeks
Urinary tract infection (male)	2 weeks
Urinary tract infection, upper (female)	7 days
Urinary tract infection, lower (female)	3 days
Mycobacterial infections	
Tuberculosis (meningeal)	12 months
Tuberculosis (pulmonary)	6 months
Fungal infections	
Invasive pulmonary aspergillosis	Until clinical/radiological resolution and reversal of predisposition
Candidaemia (acute disseminated)	2 weeks after last positive blood culture and resolution of signs and symptoms

*All recommendations are indicative. Actual duration takes into account predisposing factors, specific organisms and antimicrobial susceptibility, adjuvant therapies and clinical response.

Active efflux of antimicrobial agent
Tetracycline resistance in Gram-positive and Gram-negative bacteria
Fluconazole resistance in *Candida* spp.

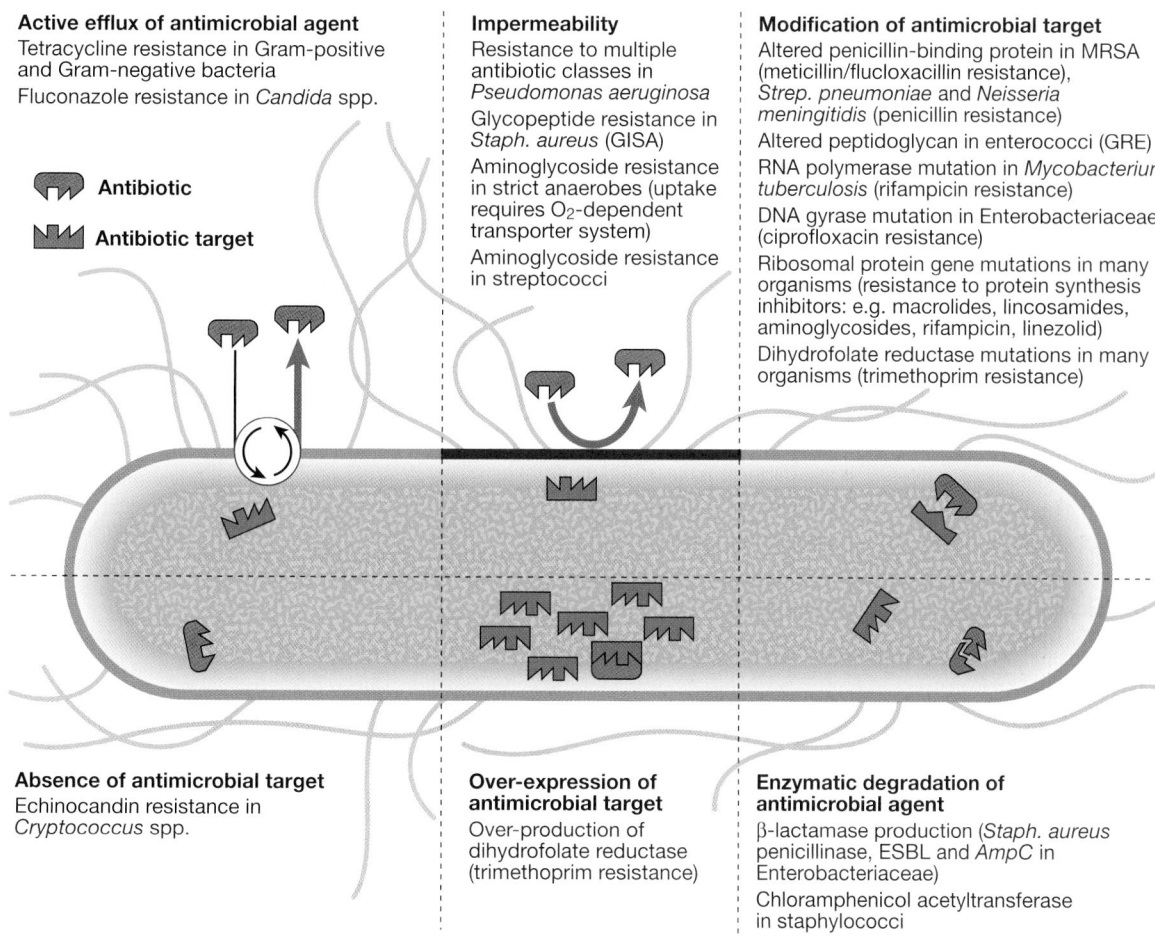

Impermeability
Resistance to multiple antibiotic classes in *Pseudomonas aeruginosa*
Glycopeptide resistance in *Staph. aureus* (GISA)
Aminoglycoside resistance in strict anaerobes (uptake requires O_2-dependent transporter system)
Aminoglycoside resistance in streptococci

Modification of antimicrobial target
Altered penicillin-binding protein in MRSA (meticillin/flucloxacillin resistance), *Strep. pneumoniae* and *Neisseria meningitidis* (penicillin resistance)
Altered peptidoglycan in enterococci (GRE)
RNA polymerase mutation in *Mycobacterium tuberculosis* (rifampicin resistance)
DNA gyrase mutation in Enterobacteriaceae (ciprofloxacin resistance)
Ribosomal protein gene mutations in many organisms (resistance to protein synthesis inhibitors: e.g. macrolides, lincosamides, aminoglycosides, rifampicin, linezolid)
Dihydrofolate reductase mutations in many organisms (trimethoprim resistance)

Antibiotic

Antibiotic target

Absence of antimicrobial target
Echinocandin resistance in *Cryptococcus* spp.

Over-expression of antimicrobial target
Over-production of dihydrofolate reductase (trimethoprim resistance)

Enzymatic degradation of antimicrobial agent
β-lactamase production (*Staph. aureus* penicillinase, ESBL and *AmpC* in Enterobacteriaceae)
Chloramphenicol acetyltransferase in staphylococci

Fig. 6.14 Examples of mechanisms of antimicrobial resistance. (ESBL = extended spectrum β-lactamases; GISA = glycopeptide-intermediate *Staph. aureus*; GRE = glycopeptide-resistant enterococci).

bial agents. For most infections there is limited clinical evidence available to support a specific duration of treatment (Box 6.19). When initial therapy is intravenous, it is often possible to switch to oral therapy after a patient has been apyrexial for approximately 48 hours. In the absence of specific guidance, antimicrobial therapy should be stopped when there is no longer any clinical evidence of infection.

Antimicrobial prophylaxis

Prophylaxis is used when there is a risk of infection from a procedure or exposure (Box 6.20). It may be combined with (or replaced by) passive immunisation (see Box 6.15). Ideally, prophylaxis should be of short duration, have minimal adverse effects and not encourage growth of resistant pathogens.

Pharmacokinetics and pharmacodynamics

Pharmacokinetics of antimicrobial agents determine whether adequate concentrations are obtained at the primary site of infection and likely areas of dissemination. Septic patients often have poor gastrointestinal absorption, so the preferred initial route of therapy is intravenous. Knowledge of anticipated antimicrobial drug concentrations at sites of infection is critical. For example, achieving a 'therapeutic' blood level of gentamicin is of little prac-

tical use in treating meningitis, as CSF penetration of the drug is severely limited. Knowledge of routes of elimination is also critical in antimicrobial therapy; for instance, a urinary tract infection is more appropriately treated with a drug that is excreted unchanged in the urine than one which is fully eliminated by hepatic metabolism.

Pharmacodynamics describes the relationship between antimicrobial concentration and microbial killing. For many agents, antimicrobial effect can be categorised as concentration-dependent or time-dependent. The concentration of antimicrobial achieved after a single dose is illustrated in Figure 6.15. The maximum concentration achieved is C_{max} and the measure of overall exposure is the area under the curve (AUC). The efficacy of antimicrobial agents whose killing is concentration-dependent (e.g. aminoglycosides) increases with the amount by which C_{max} exceeds the minimum inhibitory concentration (C_{max}:MIC ratio). For this reason, it has become customary to administer aminoglycosides (e.g. gentamicin) infrequently at high doses (e.g. 7 mg/kg) rather than frequently at low doses. This has the added advantage of minimising toxicity by reducing the likelihood of drug accumulation. Conversely, the β-lactam antibiotics, macrolides and clindamycin exhibit time-dependent killing, and their efficacy depends on C_{max} exceeding the MIC for a certain time (which

6

6.20 Recommendations for antimicrobial prophylaxis in adults*

Infection risk	Recommended antimicrobial
Bacterial	
Diphtheria (prevention of secondary cases)	Erythromycin
Gas gangrene (after high amputation or major trauma)	Penicillin or metronidazole
Lower gastrointestinal tract surgery	Cefuroxime + metronidazole, gentamicin + metronidazole, or co-amoxiclav (single dose only)
Meningococcal disease (prevention of secondary cases)	Rifampicin or ciprofloxacin
Rheumatic fever (prevention of recurrence)	Phenoxymethylpenicillin or sulfadiazine
Tuberculosis (prevention of secondary cases)	Isoniazid ± rifampicin
Whooping cough (prevention of secondary cases)	Erythromycin
Viral	
HIV, occupational exposure (sharps injury)	Combination tenofovir/ emtricitabine and lopinavir/ ritonavir. Modified if index case's virus known to be resistant
Influenza A (prevention of secondary cases in adults with chronic respiratory, cardiovascular renal disease, immunosuppression or diabetes mellitus)	Oseltamivir
Fungal	
Aspergillosis (in high-risk haematology patients)	Itraconazole or posaconazole
Pneumocystis pneumonia (prevention in HIV and other immunosuppressed states)	Co-trimoxazole, pentamidine or dapsone
Protozoal	
Malaria (prevention of travel-associated disease)	Specific antimalarials depend on travel itinerary (p. 352)

*These are based on current UK practice. Recommendations may vary locally or nationally. There is currently no recommendation in the UK to administer antimicrobial prophylaxis for infective endocarditis during dental procedures.

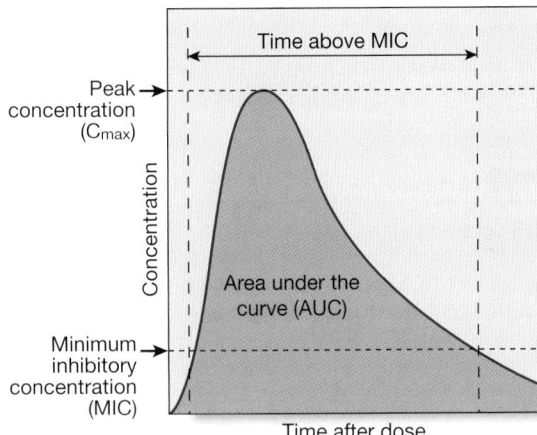

Fig. 6.15 Antimicrobial pharmacodynamics. The curve represents drug concentrations after a single dose of an antimicrobial agent. Factors that determine microbial killing are C_{max}:MIC ratio (concentration-dependent killing), time above MIC (time-dependent killing) and AUC:MIC ratio.

6.21 Antimicrobial agents in pregnancy[1]

Contraindicated

- Chloramphenicol: neonatal 'grey baby' syndrome—collapse, hypotension and cyanosis
- Fluconazole: teratogenic in high doses
- Quinolones, nalidixic acid: arthropathy in animals
- Sulphonamides: neonatal haemolysis and methaemoglobinaemia
- Tetracyclines, glycylcyclines: skeletal abnormalities in animals in 1st trimester; fetal dental discoloration and maternal hepatotoxicity with large parenteral doses in 2nd or 3rd trimesters
- Trimethoprim: teratogenic in 1st trimester

Relatively contraindicated

- Aminoglycosides: potential damage to fetal auditory and vestibular nerves in 2nd and 3rd trimesters
- Metronidazole: avoidance of high dosages is recommended[2]

Not known to be harmful; use only when necessary

- Aciclovir
- Cephalosporins
- Clarithromycin
- Clindamycin
- Erythromycin
- Glycopeptides
- Linezolid
- Meropenem
- Penicillins

[1] Data extracted from Joint Formulary Committee. British National Formulary, 55th edn. London: BMJ and RPS; 2008.
[2] Theoretical risk of teratogenicity, not supported by available clinical evidence.

is different for each class of agent). This is reflected in the dosing interval of benzylpenicillin, which is usually given every 4 hours in severe infection (e.g. meningococcal meningitis), and may be administered by continuous intravenous infusion. For other antimicrobial agents the relationships between MIC, C_{max} and AUC are more complex and often less well understood. With some agents bacterial inhibition persists after antimicrobial exposure (post-antibiotic and post-antibiotic sub-MIC effects).

Therapeutic drug monitoring

Therapeutic drug monitoring is used to confirm non-toxic levels of antimicrobial agents with a low therapeutic index (e.g. aminoglycosides), and to confirm effective levels (if these are known) of agents with marked inter-patient pharmacokinetic variability (e.g. vancomycin, itraconazole). Specific recommendations for monitoring depend on individual drugs and regimens, so specialist advice should be sought. For instance, different pre- and post-dose levels of gentamicin are recommended depending on whether it is being used in traditional divided doses, once daily or for synergy in endocarditis (p. 624).

6.22 Problems with antimicrobial therapy in old age

- **_Clostridium difficile_ infection**: many antibiotics predispose, especially second- and third-generation cephalosporins.
- **Hypersensitivity reactions**: rise in incidence due to increased previous exposure.
- **Renal impairment**: may be significant in old age despite 'normal' creatinine levels (p. 465)
- **Nephrotoxicity** is more likely, e.g. first-generation cephalosporins, aminoglycosides.
- **Accumulation of β-lactam antibiotics**: may result in myoclonus, seizures or coma.
- **Reduced gastric acid production**: gastric pH is higher, which causes increased penicillin absorption.
- **Reduced hepatic metabolism**: results in a higher risk of isoniazid-related hepatotoxicity.
- **Quinolones**: associated with confusion and may increase the risk of seizures.

6.23 Beta-lactam antibiotics

Penicillins

- Natural penicillins: benzylpenicillin, phenoxymethylpenicillin
- Penicillinase-resistant penicillins: meticillin, flucloxacillin, nafcillin, oxacillin
- Aminopenicillins: ampicillin, amoxicillin
- Carboxy- and ureido-penicillins: ticarcillin, piperacillin

Cephalosporins

- See Box 6.24

Monobactams

- Aztreonam

Carbapenems

- Imipenem, meropenem, ertapenem

Beta-lactam antibiotics

These antibiotics have a β-lactam ring structure and exert a bactericidal action by inhibiting enzymes involved in cell wall synthesis (penicillin-binding proteins, PBP). They are classified in Box 6.23.

Pharmacokinetics

- Good drug levels are achieved in lung, kidney, bone, muscle and liver, and in pleural, synovial, pericardial and peritoneal fluids.
- CSF levels are low, except in the presence of inflammation.
- Activity is not inhibited in abscess (e.g. by low pH and PO_2, high protein and polymorphonuclear cells).
- β-lactams are subject to an 'inoculum effect'— activity is reduced in the presence of a high organism burden (PBP expression is down-regulated by high organism density).
- Generally safe in pregnancy (except imipenem/cilastatin).

Adverse reactions

Generalised allergy to penicillin occurs in 0.7–10% of cases and anaphylaxis in 0.004–0.015%. Over 90% of patients with infectious mononucleosis develop a rash if given aminopenicillins; this does not imply lasting allergy. The relationship between allergy to penicillin and allergy to cephalosporins depends on the specific cephalosporin used. Although there is significant cross-reactivity with first-generation cephalosporins, cross-reactivity to second- and third-generation cephalosporins is much less common (and may be negligible with some agents). However, it is usually recommended to avoid cephalosporins in patients who have a type 1 penicillin allergy (e.g. anaphylaxis, urticaria, angio-oedema).

Gastrointestinal upset and diarrhoea are common, and a mild reversible hepatitis is well recognised with many β-lactams. Leucopenia, thrombocytopenia and coagulation deficiencies can occur. Interstitial nephritis and increased renal damage in combination with aminoglycosides are also recognised (p. 504). Seizures and encephalopathy have been reported, particularly with high doses in the presence of renal insufficiency.

Thrombophlebitis occurs in up to 5% of patients receiving parenteral β-lactams. Direct intrathecal injection of a β-lactam is contraindicated.

Drug interactions

Synergism occurs in combination with aminoglycosides. Simultaneous dual β-lactam administration can result in either synergy or antagonism. Ampicillin decreases the biological effect of oral contraceptives and the whole class is significantly affected by concurrent administration of probenecid, producing a 2–4-fold increase in the peak serum concentration.

Penicillins

Natural penicillins are primarily effective against Gram-positive organisms (except staphylococci, most of which produce a penicillinase) and anaerobic organisms. _Strep. pyogenes_ has remained sensitive to natural penicillins world-wide. The prevalence of penicillin resistance in _Strep. pneumoniae_ in Europe in 2006 was 9%. This figure includes both low- and high-level resistance (non-severe infections with low-level resistant strains may be treated with high-dose penicillins).

Penicillinase-resistant penicillins are the mainstay of treatment for infections with _Staph. aureus_, other than meticillin-resistant strains (MRSA). In 2006 24% of invasive _Staph. aureus_ isolates in Europe were meticillin-resistant.

Aminopenicillins have the same spectrum of activity as the natural penicillins, with additional Gram-negative cover against Enterobacteriaceae. Amoxicillin has much better oral absorption than ampicillin. Resistance to these agents is widespread (57% of _E. coli_ in the UK in 2006), mainly due to β-lactamase production, but can be overcome by the addition of β-lactamase inhibitors (clavulanic acid or sulbactam).

Carboxy- and ureidopenicillins are particularly active against Gram-negative organisms, especially _Pseudomonas_ spp. which are resistant to the aminopenicillins. Beta-lactamase inhibitors may be added to extend their spectrum of activity.

Cephalosporins and cephamycins

Cephalosporins are safe and reliable and have a broad spectrum of activity. The more active compounds are only available in intravenous form. They are significantly associated with _C. difficile_ infection (CDI) (p. 338).

6.24 Cephalosporins	
First generation	
• Cefalexin, cefradine (oral)	• Cefazolin (i.v.)
Second generation	
• Cefuroxime (oral/i.v.) • Cefaclor (oral)	• Cefoxitin (i.v.)
Third generation	
• Cefixime (oral) • Cefotaxime (i.v.)	• Ceftriaxone (i.v.) • Ceftazidime (i.v.)
Fourth generation	
• Cefepime (i.v.)	
'Next generation'	
• Ceftobiprole (i.v.)	• Ceftaroline (i.v.)

The group has no activity against *Enterococcus* spp. and little anti-anaerobic activity (with the exception of cephamycins). Cephalosporins are arranged in 'generations' (Box 6.24).

* *First-generation compounds* have excellent activity against Gram-positive organisms and some activity against Gram-negative ones. Many of them are potentially nephrotoxic.
* *Second-generation drugs* retain Gram-positive activity but have extended Gram-negative activity. Cephamycins (e.g. cefoxitin), which are included in this group, have good activity against anaerobic Gram-negative bacilli.
* *Third-generation agents* further improve anti-Gram-negative cover. For some (e.g. ceftazidime), this is extended to include *Pseudomonas* spp. Cefotaxime and ceftriaxone have excellent Gram-negative activity and retain good activity against *Strep. pneumoniae* and β-haemolytic streptococci. Ceftriaxone is administered once daily, and is therefore a suitable agent for outpatient antimicrobial therapy.
* *Fourth-generation agents* have an extremely broad spectrum of activity, including *Pseudomonas* spp., *Staph. aureus* and streptococci.
* *'Next generation' agents* have a fourth-generation spectrum enhanced to include MRSA.

Monobactams

Aztreonam is the only agent available in this class. It has excellent Gram-negative activity but no useful activity against Gram-positive organisms or anaerobes. It is available only as a parenteral preparation. It can be used safely in penicillin-allergic patients.

Carbapenems

These have the broadest antibiotic activity of the β-lactam antibiotics and include activity against anaerobes. They are available in intravenous formulation only.

Macrolide and lincosamide antibiotics

Macrolides (erythromycin, clarithromycin and azithromycin) and lincosamides (lincomycin, clindamycin) have related properties and are bacteriostatic agents.

Both classes bind to the same element of the ribosome so they are potentially competitive and should not be administered together. Macrolides are used in Gram-positive infections in penicillin-allergic patients and in *Mycoplasma* and *Chlamydia* infections. Erythromycin is administered 6-hourly and clarithromycin 12-hourly. The long intracellular half-life of azithromycin allows single-dose/short-course therapy for genitourinary *Chlamydia/Mycoplasma* spp. infections. Clarithromycin and azithromycin are also used to treat legionellosis.

Pharmacokinetics

Macrolides
* Variable bioavailability.
* Short half-life (except azithromycin).
* High protein binding.
* Excellent intracellular accumulation.

Lincosamides (e.g. clindamycin)
* Good bioavailability.
* Food has no effect on absorption.
* Limited CSF penetration.

Adverse effects

* Generally very safe.
* Gastrointestinal upset, especially in young adults (erythromycin 30%).
* Cholestatic jaundice with erythromycin estolate.
* Prolongation of QT interval on ECG, potential for torsades de pointes.
* Clindamycin predisposes to *C. difficile* infection.

Ketolides

The ketolides were developed in response to the emergence of penicillin and macrolide resistance in respiratory pathogens. Cross-resistance with macrolides is uncommon. Telithromycin is administered orally and has useful activity against common bacterial causes of respiratory infection, as well as *Mycoplasma, Chlamydia* and *Legionella* spp.

Aminoglycosides

Aminoglycosides are very effective anti-Gram-negative antibiotics, e.g. in intra-abdominal and urinary tract sepsis. They act synergistically with β-lactam antibiotics and are particularly useful where β-lactam or quinolone resistance occurs in health care-acquired infections. They cause very little local irritation at injection sites and negligible allergic responses. Oto- and nephrotoxicity must be avoided by monitoring of renal function and drug levels and use of short treatment regimens. Aminoglycosides are not subject to an inoculum effect (p. 149) and they all exhibit a post-antibiotic effect (p. 151).

Pharmacokinetics

* Negligible oral absorption, i.v. administration.
* Hydrophilic, so excellent penetration to extracellular fluid in body cavities and serosal fluids.
* Very poor intracellular penetration (except hair cells in cochlea and renal cortical cells).

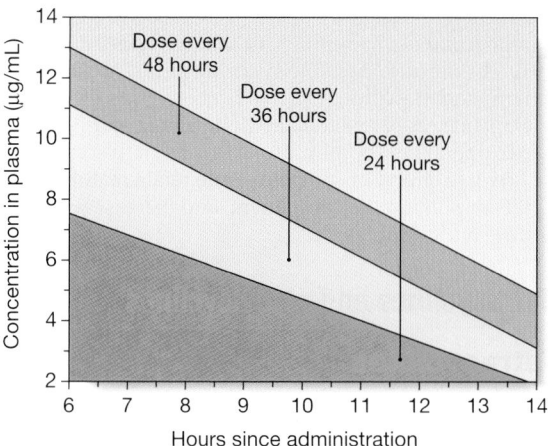

Fig. 6.16 Dosing of aminoglycosides using the Hartford nomogram.
The nomogram is used to determine the dose interval for 7 mg doses of
gentamicin or tobramycin, using measurements of drug levels in plasma
6–14 hours after a single dose.

6.25 Quinolones and fluoroquinolones		
Agent	**Route of administration**	**Typical antimicrobial spectrum**
Quinolones		
Nalidixic acid	Oral	Enteric Gram-negative bacilli (not *Pseudomonas aeruginosa*)
Fluoroquinolones		
Ciprofloxacin	I.v./oral	Enteric Gram-negative bacilli, *P. aeruginosa*, *Haemophilus* spp., 'atypical' respiratory pathogens*
Norfloxacin	Oral	
Ofloxacin	I.v./oral/topical	
Levofloxacin (L-isomer of ofloxacin)	I.v./oral	*Haemophilius* spp., *Strep. pneumoniae*, 'atypical' respiratory pathogens*
Moxifloxacin	Oral	*Strep. pneumoniae*, *Staph. aureus*, 'atypical' respiratory pathogens* and anaerobes

*'Atypical' pathogens include *Mycoplasma pneumoniae* and *Legionella* spp.
Fluoroquinolones have variable activity against *M. tuberculosis* and other
mycobacteria.

- Negligible CSF and corneal penetration.
- Peak plasma levels 30 minutes after infusion.
- Once-daily administration possible in many infections.
- Monitoring of therapeutic levels required.

Gentamicin dosing

- Except in endocarditis, pregnancy, severe burns, end-stage renal disease and paediatric patients, gentamicin may be administered at 7 mg/kg body weight. The appropriate dose interval depends on drug clearance, and is determined by reference to the Hartford nomogram (Fig. 6.16).
- In streptococcal and enterococcal endocarditis, gentamicin is used with a cell wall active agent (usually a β-lactam), to provide synergy. The usual dose is 1 mg/kg/day every 8 or 12 hours. Target pre- and post-dose levels are < 1 mg/L and 3–5 mg/L respectively.
- For other indications, gentamicin is administered 8- or 12-hourly at 3–5 mg/kg/day. Target pre- and post-dose levels are < 2 mg/L and 5–10 mg/L (7–10 mg/L with less sensitive organisms, e.g. *Pseudomonas* spp.) respectively.
- For dosing of other aminoglycosides, consult local guidance.

Adverse reactions

- Renal toxicity (usually reversible) accentuated by other nephrotoxic agents.
- Cochlear toxicity (permanent) more likely in older people and those with a predisposing mitochondrial gene mutation.
- Neuromuscular blockade after rapid i.v. infusion (potentiated by calcium channel blockers, myasthenia gravis and hypomagnesaemia).

Quinolones and fluoroquinolones

These are bactericidal agents that are usually well tolerated and effective. The quinolones have purely anti-Gram-negative activity, whereas the fluoro-
quinolones are broad-spectrum agents (Box 6.25). Ciprofloxacin has anti-pseudomonal activity but resistance emerges rapidly. In Europe in 2006 between 5 and 48% of invasive *E. coli* isolates were resistant to ciprofloxacin.

Pharmacokinetics

- Well absorbed after oral administration but delayed by food, antacids, ferrous sulphate and multivitamins. Excellent anti-Gram-negative activity.
- Wide volume of distribution; tissue concentrations twice those in serum.
- Good intracellular penetration, concentrating in phagocytes.

Adverse reactions

- Gastrointestinal side-effects in 1–5%.
- Rare skin reactions (phototoxicity).
- Achilles tendon rupture is reported, especially in older people.
- CNS effects (confusion, tremor, dizziness and occasional seizures in 5–12%), especially in older people.
- Reduces clearance of xanthines and theophyllines, potentially inducing insomnia and increased seizure potential.
- Reports of prolongation of QT interval on ECG with newer fluoroquinolones.
- Cases of hypo- or hyperglycaemia in association with gatifloxacin, so glucose monitoring is needed in patients with diabetes or those with severe hepatic dysfunction.
- Quinolone use is associated with the acquisition of MRSA and emergence of a highly virulent strain of *C. difficile* (ribotype 027).

6

Glycopeptides

Glycopeptides (vancomycin and teicoplanin) are only effective against Gram-positive organisms, and are used against MRSA and ampicillin-resistant enterococci. Some staphylococci and enterococci demonstrate intermediate sensitivity or resistance. Vancomycin use should be restricted, particularly in the management of *C. difficile* infections, to limit emergence of resistant strains. Teicoplanin is not available in all countries. Neither drug is absorbed after oral administration, but vancomycin is used orally in the treatment of *C. difficile* infection.

Pharmacokinetics

Vancomycin

- Administered by slow i.v. infusion, good tissue distribution and short half-life.
- Enters CSF only in the presence of inflammation.
- Therapeutic monitoring of i.v. vancomycin is recommended, to maintain pre-dose levels of > 10 mg/L (10–20 mg/L in serious staphylococcal infections).

Teicoplanin

- Long half-life allows once-daily dosing.

Adverse effects

- Histamine release due to rapid vancomycin infusion produces a 'red man' reaction (rare with modern preparations).
- Nephrotoxicity is rare, but may occur with concomitant aminoglycoside use.
- Teicoplanin can cause rash, bronchospasm, eosinophilia and anaphylaxis.

Folate antagonists

These bacteriostatic antibiotics interfere with the prokaryotic cell metabolism of para-aminobenzoic acid to folic acid. A combination of a sulphonamide and either trimethoprim or pyrimethamine is most commonly used and interferes with two consecutive steps in the metabolic pathway. Combinations in use include trimethoprim/sulfamethoxazole (co-trimoxazole) and pyrimethamine with either sulfadoxine (used to treat malaria) or sulfadiazine (used in toxoplasmosis). Co-trimoxazole in high dosage (120 mg/kg daily in 2–4 divided doses) is the first-line drug for *Pneumocystis jirovecii* (*carinii*) infection in HIV disease. The clinical use of these agents is limited by adverse effects. Folate supplements should be given if they are used long term or unavoidably in early pregnancy.

Pharmacokinetics

- Well absorbed orally.
- Sulphonamides are hydrophilic, distributing well to the extracellular fluid.
- Trimethoprim is lipophilic with high tissue concentrations.

Adverse reactions

- Trimethoprim is generally well tolerated with few adverse effects.
- Sulphonamides and dapsone may cause haemolysis in glucose-6-phosphate dehydrogenase deficiency (p. 1024).

- Sulphonamides and dapsone cause skin and mucocutaneous reactions including Stevens-Johnson syndrome and 'dapsone syndrome' (rash, fever and lymphadenopathy).
- Dapsone causes methaemoglobinaemia and peripheral neuropathy.
- Adverse effects of co-trimoxazole relate mainly to the sulphonamide component, and increase with dose and duration.

Tetracyclines and glycylcyclines

Tetracyclines

Of this mainly bacteriostatic class, the newer drugs doxycycline and minocycline show better absorption and distribution than older ones. Most streptococci and Gram-negative bacteria are now resistant, in part due to use in animals (which is banned in Europe). Tetracyclines are indicated for *Mycoplasma* spp., *Chlamydia* spp., *Rickettsia* spp., *Coxiella* spp., *Bartonella* spp., *Borrelia* spp., *Helicobacter pylori, Treponema pallidum* and atypical mycobacterial infections. Minocycline is occasionally used in chronic staphylococcal infections.

Pharmacokineticsis

- Best oral absorption is in the fasting state (doxycycline is 100% absorbed unless gastric pH rises).

Adverse reactions

- All tetracyclines except doxycycline are contraindicated in renal failure.
- Dizziness with minocycline.
- Binding to metallic ions in bones and teeth causes discoloration (avoid in children and pregnancy) and enamel hypoplasia.
- Phototoxic skin reactions.

Glycylcyclines (tigecycline)

Chemical modification of tetracycline has produced tigecycline, a broad-spectrum parenteral-only antibiotic with activity against resistant Gram-positive and Gram-negative pathogens such as MRSA and ESBL (but excluding *Pseudomonas* spp.). Tigecycline has prominent gastrointestinal side-effects.

Nitroimidazoles (metronidazole, tinidazole)

Nitroimidazoles are highly active against strictly anaerobic bacteria, especially *B. fragilis, C. difficile* and other *Clostridium* spp. They also have significant anti-protozoal activity against amoebae and *Giardia lamblia*.

Pharmacokinetics

- Almost completely absorbed after oral administration (60% after rectal administration).
- Well distributed, especially to brain and CSF.
- Safe in pregnancy.

Adverse effects

- Metallic taste (dose-dependent).
- Severe vomiting if taken with alcohol—'Antabuse effect'.
- Peripheral neuropathy with prolonged use.

Other antibacterial agents

Chloramphenicol

This is a potent and cheap antibiotic, still widely prescribed throughout the world despite its potential toxicity. Its use, however, is increasingly reserved for severe and life-threatening infections where other antibiotics are either unavailable or impractical. It is bacteriostatic to most organisms but apparently bactericidal to *H. influenzae, Strep. pneumoniae* and *N. meningitidis*. It has a very broad spectrum of activity against aerobic and anaerobic organisms, spirochaetes, *Rickettsia, Chlamydia* and *Mycoplasma* spp. It also has quite useful activity against anaerobes such as *Bacteroides fragilis*. It competes with macrolides and lincosamides for ribosomal binding sites, so should not be used in combination with these agents.

Pharmacokinetics

- Well absorbed after i.v. or oral dose (not i.m.). Good tissue distribution and levels.
- Good CSF levels.
- Crosses placenta and reaches breast milk.

Adverse reactions

- Dose-dependent 'grey baby' syndrome in infants (cyanosis and circulatory collapse due to inability to conjugate drug and excrete active form in urine).
- Reversible dose-dependent bone marrow depression in adults if > 4 g per day administered or cumulative dose > 25 g.
- Severe idiopathic aplastic anaemia in 1:25 000–40 000 exposures (unrelated to dose, duration of therapy or route of administration).

Daptomycin

Daptomycin is a cyclic lipopeptide which has bactericidal activity against Gram-positive organisms (including MRSA and GRE) but no activity against Gram-negatives. It is not absorbed orally, and is used intravenously to treat resistant Gram-positive infections, e.g. soft tissue infections and infective endocarditis, where other options are not available.

Fusidic acid

This antibiotic, active against Gram-positive bacteria, is available in intravenous, oral or topical formulations. It is lipid-soluble and distributes well to tissues. However, its antibacterial activity is unpredictable. Fusidic acid is used in combination, typically with anti-staphylococcal penicillins, or for MRSA with clindamycin or rifampicin. It interacts with coumarin derivatives and oral contraceptives.

Nitrofurantoin

This drug has very rapid renal elimination and is active against aerobic Gram-negative and Gram-positive bacteria, including enterococci. It is used only for treatment of urinary tract infection, being generally safe in pregnancy and childhood. However, it can produce eosinophilic lung infiltrates, fever, pulmonary fibrosis, peripheral neuropathy, hepatitis and haemolytic anaemia.

Linezolid

Linezolid is the only currently licensed member of the oxazolidinone class, which shows excellent oral absorption with good activity against Gram-positive organisms, including MRSA and GRE. It is competitively inhibited by co-administration of chloramphenicol, vancomycin or clindamycin. It appears to be very safe, although mild gastrointestinal side-effects and tongue discoloration are common. Myelodysplasia and peripheral neuropathy can occur with prolonged use. Co-administration with monoamine oxidase inhibitors or serotonin re-uptake inhibitor antidepressants should be avoided, as it may precipitate a serotonin syndrome (neuromuscular effects, autonomic hyperactivity and altered mental status).

Spectinomycin

Chemically similar to the aminoglycosides and given intramuscularly, spectinomycin was developed to treat strains of *N. gonorrhoeae* resistant to β-lactam antibiotics. Unfortunately, resistance to spectinomycin is very common and its only indication is the treatment of gonococcal urethritis in pregnancy or in patients allergic to β-lactam antibiotics.

Streptogramins

Quinupristin/dalfopristin (supplied as a 30:70% combination) is active against MRSA and GRE (*Enterococcus faecium* but not *E. faecalis*), and its use should be reserved for these organisms. It is available in intravenous formulation only and shows good tissue penetration, but does not cross the blood–brain barrier or the placenta. Significant phlebitis occurs at injection sites and a raised serum creatinine and eosinophilia may occur.

Antifungal agents

See Box 6.26.

Azole antifungals

The azoles (imidazoles and triazoles) inhibit synthesis of ergosterol, a key constituent of the fungal cell membrane. Side-effects vary but include gastrointestinal upset, hepatitis and rash. Azoles are amongst the drugs metabolised by cytochrome p450 enzymes, so must be used cautiously if combined with other such drugs with which they may interact (p. 34).

Imidazoles

Miconazole, econazole, clotrimazole and ketoconazole are relatively toxic and therefore mainly administered topically. Clotrimazole is used extensively to treat superficial fungal infections. Ketoconazole may be given orally, but causes severe hepatitis in ~1:15 000 cases and inhibits enzymes involved in steroid biosynthesis in the adrenals and gonads. Triazoles are preferred for systemic administration because of their reduced toxicity.

Triazoles

Fluconazole is effective against yeasts only (*Candida* and *Cryptococcus* spp.). It is well absorbed after oral administration, and has a long half-life (approximately 30 hours) and an excellent safety profile. The drug is highly water-soluble

6

157

6

6.26 Antifungal agents

Agent (usual route(s) of administration)	Clinically relevant antifungal spectrum
Imidazoles	
Miconazole (topical)	
Econazole (topical)	*Candida* spp., dermatophytes
Clotrimazole (topical)	
Ketoconazole (topical, oral)	*Malassezia* spp., dermatophytes, agents of eumycetoma
Triazoles	
Fluconazole (oral, i.v.)	Yeasts (*Candida* and *Cryptococcus* spp.)
Itraconazole (oral, i.v.)	Yeasts, dermatophytes, dimorphic fungi (p. 376), *Aspergillus* spp.
Voriconazole (oral, i.v.)	Yeasts and most filamentous fungi (excluding *Mucorales*)
Posaconazole (oral)	Yeasts and most filamentous fungi (including most *Mucorales*)
Echinocandins	
Anidulafungin (i.v. only)	*Candida* spp., *Aspergillus* spp.
Caspofungin (i.v. only)	(no activity against *Cryptococcus*
Micafungin (i.v. only)	spp. or *Mucorales*)
Polyenes	Yeasts and most dimorphic and
Amphotericin B (i.v.)	filamentous fungi (including
Nystatin (topical)	*Mucorales*)
Others	
5-fluorocytosine (oral, i.v.)	Yeasts
Griseofulvin (oral)	Dermatophytes
Terbinafine (topical, oral)	Dermatophytes

and distributes widely to all body sites and tissues, including CSF.

Itraconazole is lipophilic and distributes extensively, including to toenails and fingernails. CSF penetration is poor. Oral absorption is erratic and formulation-dependent, which necessitates monitoring of blood levels.

Voriconazole is extremely well absorbed (96% oral bioavailability) and is used mainly in the treatment of aspergillosis.

Posaconazole is the broadest-spectrum antifungal azole, and the only one with consistent activity against the *Mucorales*. It is currently available as an oral agent only.

Echinocandins

Anidulafungin, caspofungin and micafungin inhibit β-1,3-glucan synthesis in the fungal cell wall. They do not demonstrate cross-resistance with azoles or polyenes and have very few significant adverse effects. Caspofungin, anidulafungin and micafungin are used to treat candidaemia, and caspofungin is also used in aspergillosis.

Polyenes

Amphotericin B deoxycholate causes cell death by binding to ergosterol and damaging the fungal cytoplasmic membrane. Its use in resource-rich countries is being supplanted by less toxic antifungal agents. It is

lipophilic, insoluble in water and not absorbed orally. Its long half-life enables once-daily administration. CSF penetration is poor.

Adverse reactions include immediate anaphylaxis (a test dose should always be given before infusion), other infusion-related reactions, and nephrotoxicity. Nephrotoxicity may be sufficient to require dialysis, and occurs in most patients who are adequately dosed. It may be ameliorated by concomitant infusion of normal saline. Irreversible nephrotoxicity occurs with large cumulative doses of amphotericin B.

Nystatin has a similar spectrum of antifungal activity to amphotericin B. Its toxicity limits it to topical use, e.g. in oral and vaginal candidiasis.

Lipid formulations of amphotericin B

Lipid formulations of amphotericin B (AmB) have been developed to reduce the toxicity of the parent compound. These consist of AmB encapsulated in liposomes (liposomal AmB, L-AmB) or complexed with phospholipids (AmB lipid complex, ABLC) or cholesteryl sulphate (AmB colloidal dispersion, ABCD). The drug becomes active dissociating from its lipid component after administration. Adverse reactions are similar to, but considerably less frequent than, those with AmB deoxycholate, and efficacy is similar. Lipid formulations of AmB are used as empirical therapy in patients with neutropenic fever (p. 1000), and also in visceral leishmaniasis.

Other antifungal agents

5-fluorocytosine

This drug has particular activity against yeasts. When used as monotherapy, resistance develops rapidly, so it should be administered in combination with another antifungal agent. Oral dosing is effective. Adverse reactions include myelosuppression, gastrointestinal upset and hepatitis.

Griseofulvin

Griseofulvin has been largely superseded by terbinafine and itraconazole for treatment of dermatophyte infections, except in children, for whom these agents remain unlicensed. It demonstrates excellent oral bioavailability and is deposited in keratin precursor cells, which become resistant to fungal invasion. The duration of treatment is 2–4 weeks for tinea corporis/capitis, 4–8 weeks for tinea pedis, and 4–6 months for onychomycosis (fungal nail infections).

Terbinafine

Terbinafine is well absorbed orally, can be given once daily and distributes with high concentration to sebum and skin with a half-life of greater than 1 week. It is used topically for skin infections and orally for onychomycosis (nail infections). The major adverse reaction is hepatic toxicity (approximately 1:50 000 cases). Terbinafine is not recommended for breastfeeding mothers and should not be applied vaginally.

Antiviral agents

Most viral infections in immunocompetent individuals resolve without intervention. Antiviral therapy is available only for a limited number of infections (Boxes 6.27 and 14.23, p. 404).

6.27 Antiviral agents

Drug	Route(s) of administration	Indications	Significant side-effects
Highly active antiretroviral therapy			
(HAART, p. 403)	Oral	HIV infection (including AIDS)	CNS symptoms, anaemia, lipodystrophy
Anti-herpes virus agents			
Aciclovir	Topical Oral I.v.	Herpes zoster Chickenpox (esp. in immunosuppressed) Herpes simplex infections: encephalitis (i.v. only), genital tract, oral, ophthalmic	Significant side-effects rare. Hepatitis, renal impairment and neurotoxicity reported rarely
Valaciclovir	Oral	Herpes zoster, herpes simplex	As for aciclovir
Famciclovir	Oral	Herpes zoster, herpes simplex (genital)	As for aciclovir
Penciclovir	Topical	Labial herpes simplex	Local irritation
Ganciclovir	I.v.	Treatment and prevention of CMV infection in immunosuppressed	Gastrointestinal symptoms, liver dysfunction, neurotoxicity, myelosuppression, renal impairment, fever, rash, phlebitis at infusion sites. Potential teratogenicity
Valganciclovir	Oral	Treatment and prevention of CMV infection in immunosuppressed	As for ganciclovir but neutropenia is predominant
Cidofovir	I.v. Topical	HIV-associated CMV infections and occasionally other viruses (see text)	Renal impairment, neutropenia
Foscarnet	I.v.	CMV and aciclovir-resistant HSV and VZV infections in immunosuppressed	Gastrointestinal symptoms, renal impairment, electrolyte disturbances, genital ulceration, neurotoxicity
Anti-influenza agents			
Zanamivir	Inhalation	Influenza A and B	Allergic reactions (very rare)
Oseltamivir	Oral	Influenza A and B	Gastrointestinal side-effects, rash, hepatitis (very rare)
Amantadine, rimantadine	Oral	Influenza A (but see text)	CNS symptoms, nausea
Other antiviral agents			
Ribavirin	Oral/i.v./inhalation	Hepatitis C infection (with interferons) (oral) Lassa fever (i.v.) RSV infection in infants (inhalation)	Haemolytic anaemia, cough, dyspnoea, bronchospasm and ocular irritation (when given by inhalation)
Interferon-α Pegylated interferon-α	S.c. S.c.	Chronic hepatitis B and (with ribavirin) hepatitis C	Influenza-like syndrome following dose, gastrointestinal symptoms, hepatitis, myelosuppression
Adefovir dipivoxil, entecavir, lamivudine, telbivudine	Oral	Chronic hepatitis B infection	Generally well tolerated with minimal side-effects Creatine kinase elevation (telbivudine only)
Tenofovir	Oral	Hepatitis B in co-infection with HIV (with other antiretroviral agents)	Minimal side-effects Rarely nephrotoxicity

Antiretroviral agents

These agents, used predominantly against HIV, are discussed in Chapter 14.

Anti-herpes virus agents

Aciclovir, valaciclovir, penciclovir and famciclovir

Aciclovir, valaciclovir, penciclovir and famciclovir are acyclic analogues of guanosine, which inhibit viral DNA polymerase after being phosphorylated by virus-derived thymidine kinase (TK). Aciclovir is slowly and incompletely absorbed after oral dosing; much better levels are achieved intravenously or by use of the pro-drug valaciclovir. Famciclovir is the pro-drug of penciclovir. Resistance is mediated by mutations in the viral kinase or polymerase.

Ganciclovir

Chemical modification of the aciclovir molecule allows preferential phosphorylation by protein kinases of CMV and other β-herpesviruses (e.g. HHV6/7) and hence greater inhibition of the DNA polymerase, but at the expense of increased toxicity. Ganciclovir is administered intravenously or as a pro-drug (valganciclovir) orally.

Cidofovir

Cidofovir inhibits viral DNA polymerases with potent activity against CMV, including most ganciclovir-resistant CMV. It also has activity against aciclovir-resistant HSV and VZV, human herpes virus 6 and occasionally adenovirus, pox virus, papillomavirus or polyoma virus, and may be used to treat these infections in immunocompromised hosts.

Foscarnet

This analogue of inorganic pyrophosphate acts as a non-competitive inhibitor of HSV, VZV, HHV6/7 or CMV DNA polymerase. It does not require significant intracellular phosphorylation and so may be effective when HSV or CMV resistance is due to altered phosphorylation of the antiviral substrate. It has variable CSF penetration.

Anti-influenza agents

Zanamivir and oseltamivir

These agents inhibit the neuraminidase enzyme in influenza A and B, which is required for release of virus from infected cells (see Fig. 6.2, p. 133). They are used in treatment and prophylaxis of influenza. Administration within 48 hours of disease onset reduces the duration of symptoms by approximately 1–1½ days. In the UK their use is limited mainly to adults with chronic respiratory or renal disease, significant cardiovascular disease, immunosuppression or diabetes mellitus, during known outbreaks.

Amantadine and rimantadine

These drugs reduce replication of influenza A by inhibition of viral M2 protein ion channel function, which is required for uncoating (see Fig. 6.2, p. 133). Resistance develops rapidly and is widespread, and they should be used only if local prevalence of resistant strains is known to be low. They are no longer recommended for either treatment or prophylaxis in the UK or USA, having been superseded by zanamivir and oseltamivir. However, they may still be indicated to treat oseltamivir-resistant influenza A strains in patients unable to take zanamivir (e.g. ventilated patients).

Other antiviral agents

Ribavirin

Ribavirin is a guanosine analogue that inhibits nucleic acid synthesis in a variety of viruses.

Lamivudine, adefovir dipivoxil, tenofovir, entecavir and telbivudine

These agents have excellent activity against hepatitis B virus DNA polymerase-reverse transcriptase. They are well tolerated after oral administration but resistance develops with monotherapy. Resistance seems to emerge most rapidly for lamivudine (via the tyrosine-methionine-aspartate-aspartate, or YMDD, mutation) and slowly for entecavir (multiple mutations required). Organisms resistant to lamivudine are usually also resistant to telbivudine, but not to adefovir/tenofovir. The role of monotherapy for HBV is currently a matter for debate, and combination therapy, as used in HIV treatment, is likely to be used increasingly. Lamivudine and tenofovir are also used against HIV (p. 403).

Interferon-α

The interferons are naturally occurring cytokines that are produced as an early response to viral infection (p. 72). The addition of a polyethylene glycol (PEG) moiety to the molecule significantly enhances pharmacokinetics and efficacy.

Antiparasitic agents

Drugs used against helminths

Benzimidazoles (albendazole, mebendazole)

These agents act by inhibiting both helminth glucose uptake, causing depletion of glycogen stores, and fumarate reductase. Albendazole is used in hookworm, ascariasis, threadworm, *Strongyloides* infection, trichinellosis, *Taenia solium* (cysticercosis) and hydatid disease. Mebendazole is used for hookworm, ascariasis, threadworm and whipworm. The drugs are administered orally. Absorption is relatively poor, but increased by a fatty meal. Significant adverse reactions are uncommon.

Bithionol

Bithionol is used to treat fluke infections with *Fasciola hepatica*. It is well absorbed orally. Adverse reactions are mild (e.g. nausea, vomiting, diarrhoea, rashes) but relatively common (approximately 30%).

Diethylcarbamazine (DEC)

DEC is an oral agent used to treat filariasis and loiasis. Treatment of filariasis is often followed by fever, headache, nausea, vomiting, arthralgia and prostration. This is caused by the host response to dying microfilariae, rather than the drug, and may be reduced by pre-treatment with corticosteroids.

Ivermectin

Ivermectin binds to helminth nerve and muscle cell ion channels, causing increased membrane permeability. It is an oral agent, used in *Strongyloides* infection, filariasis and onchocerciasis. Significant side-effects are uncommon.

Niclosamide

Niclosamide inhibits oxidative phosphorylation, causing paralysis of helminths. It is an oral agent, used in *Taenia saginata* and intestinal *T. solium* infection. Systemic absorption is minimal, and it has few significant side-effects.

Piperazine

Piperazine inhibits neurotransmitter function, causing helminth muscle paralysis. It is an oral agent, used in ascariasis and threadworm (*Enterobius vermicularis*) infection. Significant adverse effects are uncommon, but include neuropsychological reactions such as vertigo, confusion and convulsions.

Praziquantel

Praziquantel increases membrane permeability to Ca^{++}, causing violent contraction of worm muscle. It is the drug of choice for schistosomiasis, and is also used in *T. saginata*, *T. solium* (cysticercosis), fluke infections (*Clonorchis*, *Paragonimus*) and echinococcosis. It is administered orally and well absorbed. Adverse reactions are usually mild and transient, and include nausea and abdominal pain.

Pyrantel pamoate

This agent causes spastic paralysis of helminth muscle through a suxamethonium-like action. It is used orally in ascariasis and threadworm infection. Systemic absorption is poor, and adverse effects are uncommon.

Thiabendazole

Thiabendazole inhibits fumarate reductase, which is required for energy production in helminths. It is used orally in *Strongyloides* infection and topically to treat cutaneous larva migrans. Significant adverse effects are uncommon.

Antimalarial agents

Artemisinin (quinghaosu) derivatives

Artemisinin originates from a herb (sweet wormwood, *Artemisia annua*), which was used in Chinese medicine to treat fever. Its derivatives, artemether and artesunate, were developed for use in malaria in the 1970s. Their mechanism of action is unknown. They are used in the treatment, but not prophylaxis, of malaria, usually in combination with other antimalarials, and are effective against strains of *Plasmodium* spp. that are resistant to other antimalarials. Artemether is lipid-soluble, and may be administered via intramuscular and oral routes. Artesunate is water-soluble and is administered intravenously or orally. Serious adverse effects are uncommon. Current advice for malaria in pregnancy is that the artemisinin derivatives should be used to treat uncomplicated falciparum malaria in the second and third trimesters, but should not be used in the first trimester until more information becomes available.

Atovaquone

Atovaquone inhibits mitochondrial function. It is an oral agent, used for treatment and prophylaxis of malaria, in combination with proguanil (see below), without which it is ineffective. It is also used in the treatment of *Pneumocystis jirovecii (carinii)* pneumonia where there is intolerance to co-trimoxazole. Significant adverse effects are uncommon.

Folate synthesis inhibitors (proguanil, pyrimethamine-sulfadoxine)

Proguanil inhibits dihydrofolate reductase, and is used for malaria prophylaxis. Pyrimethamine-sulfadoxine is used in the treatment of malaria (p. 352).

Quinoline-containing compounds

Chloroquine and quinine are believed to act by intraparasitic inhibition of haem polymerisation, resulting in toxic build-up of intracellular haem. The mechanisms of action of other agents in this group (quinidine, amodiaquine, mefloquine, primaquine, etc.) may differ. They are used in the treatment and prophylaxis of malaria. Primaquine is used for radical cure of malaria due to *Plasmodium vivax* and *P. ovale* (destruction of liver hypnozoites). Chloroquine is also used in extra-intestinal amoebiasis.

Chloroquine can cause a pruritus sufficient to compromise compliance with therapy. If used in long-term, high-dose regimens, it causes an irreversible retinopathy. Overdosage causes life-threatening cardiotoxicity. The side-effect profile of mefloquine includes neuropsychiatric effects ranging from mood change, nightmares and agitation to hallucinations and psychosis. Quinine may cause hypoglycaemia and cardiotoxicity, especially when administered parenterally. Primaquine causes haemolysis in people with glucose-6-phosphate dehydrogenase deficiency (p. 1024), which should be excluded before therapy. Chloroquine is considered safe in pregnancy, but mefloquine should be avoided in the first trimester.

Lumefantrine

Lumefantrine is used in combination with artemether to treat uncomplicated falciparum malaria, including chloroquine-resistant strains. Its mechanism of action is unknown. Significant adverse effects are uncommon.

Drugs used in trypanosomiasis

Benznidazole

Benznidazole is an oral agent used to treat South American trypanosomiasis (Chagas' disease, p. 354). Significant and common adverse effects include dose-related peripheral neuropathy, purpuric rash and granulocytopenia.

Eflornithine

Eflornithine inhibits biosynthesis of polyamines by ornithine decarboxylase inhibition, and is used in West African trypanosomiasis (*T. brucei gambiense* infection) of the CNS. It is administered as a 6-hourly intravenous infusion, which may be logistically difficult in the geographic areas affected by this disease. Significant adverse effects are common, and include convulsions, gastrointestinal upset and bone marrow depression. Eflornithine is also used (topically) to treat hirsutism (p. 759).

Melarsoprol

This is an arsenical agent, which is used to treat CNS infections in both E. and W. African trypanosomiasis (*T. brucei rhodesiense* and *gambiense*). It is administered intravenously. Melarsoprol treatment is associated with peripheral neuropathy and reactive arsenical encephalopathy (RAE), which carries a significant mortality.

Nifurtimox

Nifurtimox is administered orally to treat South American trypanosomiasis (Chagas' disease). Gastrointestinal and neurological adverse effects are common.

Pentamidine isetionate

Pentamidine is an inhibitor of DNA replication used in West African trypanosomiasis (*T. brucei gambiense*) and, to a lesser extent, in visceral and cutaneous leishmaniasis. It is also used in *Pneumocystis jirovecii (carinii)* pneumonia. It is administered via intravenous or intramuscular routes. It is a relatively toxic drug, commonly causing rash, renal impairment, profound hypotension (especially on rapid infusion), electrolyte disturbances, blood dyscrasias and hypoglycaemia.

Suramin

Suramin is a naphthaline dye derivative, used to treat East African trypanosomiasis (*T. brucei rhodesiense*). It is administered intravenously. Adverse effects are common, and include rash, gastrointestinal disturbance, blood dyscrasias, peripheral neuropathies and renal impairment.

Other antiprotozoal agents

Pentavalent antimonials

Sodium stibogluconate and meglumine antimoniate inhibit protozoal glycolysis by phosphofructokinase inhibition. They are used parenterally (intravenous or intramuscular) to treat leishmaniasis. Adverse effects include arthralgia, myalgias, raised hepatic transaminases, pancreatitis and ECG changes. Severe cardiotoxicity leading to death is not uncommon.

Diloxanide furoate

This oral agent is used to eliminate luminal cysts following treatment of intestinal amoebiasis, or in asymptomatic cyst excreters. The drug is absorbed slowly (enabling luminal persistence) and has no effect in hepatic amoebiasis. It is a relatively non-toxic drug, the most significant adverse effect being flatulence.

Iodoquinol (di-iodohydroxyquinoline)

Iodoquinol is a quinoline derivative (p. 161) with activity against *Entamoeba histolytica* cysts and trophozoites. It is used orally to treat asymptomatic cyst excreters or, in association with another amoebicide (e.g. metronidazole), to treat extra-intestinal amoebiasis. Long-term use of this drug is not recommended, as neurological adverse effects include optic neuritis and peripheral neuropathy.

Nitazoxanide

Nitazoxanide is an inhibitor of pyruvate-ferredoxin oxidoreductase-dependent anaerobic energy metabolism in protozoa. It is a broad-spectrum agent, active against various nematodes, tapeworms and flukes, as well as intestinal protozoa and some anaerobic bacteria and viruses. It is administered orally in giardiasis and cryptosporidiosis. Adverse effects are usually mild, and involve the gastrointestinal tract (e.g. nausea, diarrhoea and abdominal pain).

Paromomycin

Paromomycin is an aminoglycoside (p. 154), which is used to treat visceral leishmaniasis and intestinal amoebiasis. It is not significantly absorbed when administered orally, and is therefore given orally for intestinal amoebiasis and by intramuscular injection for leishmaniasis. It showed early promise in the treatment of HIV-associated cryptosporidiosis, but subsequent trials have demonstrated that this effect is marginal at best.

Further information

www.cdc.gov *Centers for Disease Control, Atlanta, USA.*
Provides information on all aspects of communicable disease, including prophylaxis against malaria.
www.dh.gov.uk *UK Department of Health*
The publications section provides current UK recommendations for immunisation.
www.doctorfungus.org *For information on clinical and laboratory aspects of medical mycology.*
www.hpa.org.uk *Health Protection Agency. Provides information on infectious diseases relating mainly to the UK, including community infection control.*
www.idsociety.org *Infectious Diseases Society of America. Publishes up-to-date, evidence-based guidelines.*
www.who.int *World Health Organisation. Provides up-to-date information on global aspects of infectious disease, including outbreak updates.*

N.R. Colledge

Ageing and disease

7

COMPREHENSIVE GERIATRIC ASSESSMENT

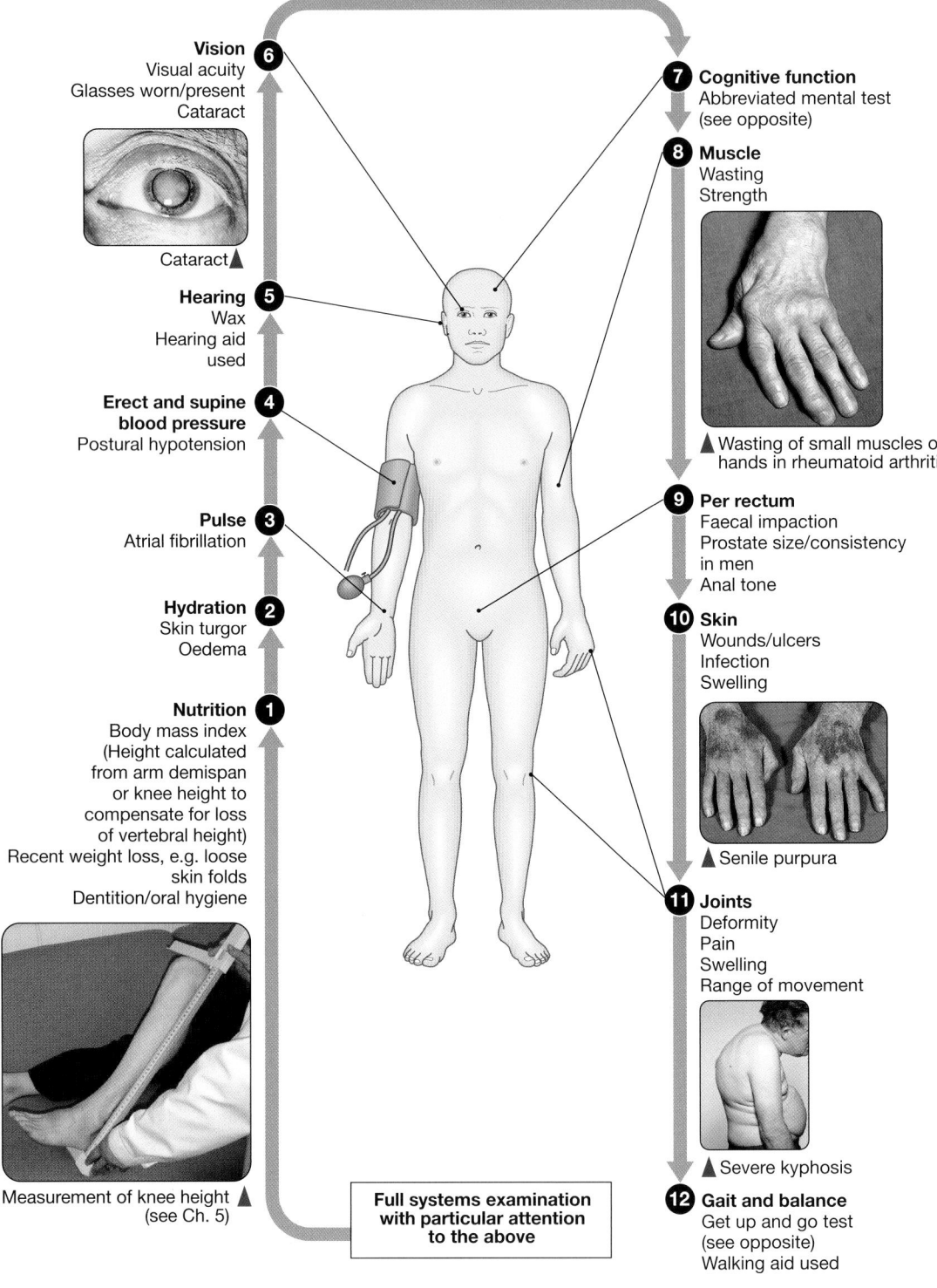

Vision 6
Visual acuity
Glasses worn/present
Cataract

Cataract▲

Hearing 5
Wax
Hearing aid
used

Erect and supine 4
blood pressure
Postural hypotension

Pulse 3
Atrial fibrillation

Hydration 2
Skin turgor
Oedema

Nutrition 1
Body mass index
(Height calculated
from arm demispan
or knee height to
compensate for loss
of vertebral height)
Recent weight loss, e.g. loose
skin folds
Dentition/oral hygiene

Measurement of knee height ▲
(see Ch. 5)

7 **Cognitive function**
Abbreviated mental test
(see opposite)

8 **Muscle**
Wasting
Strength

▲ Wasting of small muscles of
hands in rheumatoid arthritis

9 **Per rectum**
Faecal impaction
Prostate size/consistency
in men
Anal tone

10 **Skin**
Wounds/ulcers
Infection
Swelling

▲ Senile purpura

11 **Joints**
Deformity
Pain
Swelling
Range of movement

▲ Severe kyphosis

12 **Gait and balance**
Get up and go test
(see opposite)
Walking aid used

**Full systems examination
with particular attention
to the above**

History

- **Slow down** the pace.
- **Ensure the patient can hear.**
- Establish the **speed of onset of the illness.**
- If the presentation is vague, carry out a **systematic enquiry**.
- Obtain full details of:
  - **all drugs**, especially any recent prescription changes
  - **past medical history**, even from many years previously
  - **usual function**
    - (a) Can the patient walk normally?
    - (b) Has the patient noticed memory problems?
    - (c) Can the patient perform all household tasks?
- **Obtain a collateral history**: confirm information with a relative or carer and the general practitioner, particularly if the patient is confused or communication is limited by deafness or speech disturbance.

Social assessment

Home circumstances

- Living alone, with another or in a care home.

Activities of daily living (ADL)

- Tasks for which help is needed:
  - domestic ADL: shopping, cooking, housework
  - personal ADL: bathing, dressing, walking.
- Informal help: relatives, friends, neighbours.
- Formal social services: home help, meals on wheels.
- Carer stress.

Examination

- **Thorough** to identify all comorbidities.
- **Tailored to the patient's stamina** and ability to cooperate.
- Includes **functional status**:
  - cognitive function
  - gait and balance
  - nutrition
  - hearing and vision.

7 Abbreviated Mental Test

Each correct answer scores 1 mark.
1. What time is it? (*to the nearest hour*)
2. What year is it?
3. What is the name of this place/hospital?
4. How old are you? (*exact year*)
5. What is your date of birth?

Please memorise the following address: 42 West Street.

6. When did the First World War begin?
7. Who is the present monarch?
8. Please count backwards from 20 down to 1.
9. Can you recognise two people?
   (*e.g. relative or photograph*)
10. Can you tell me the address I asked you to memorise a few minutes ago?

Mini-Mental State Examination is used for more detailed assessment (p. 232).

Multidisciplinary team (MDT) and functional assessment

Team member	Activity assessed and promoted
Physiotherapist	Mobility, balance and upper limb function
Occupational therapist	Activities of daily living (ADL), e.g. dressing, cooking (Assessment of home environment)
Dietitian	Nutrition
Speech and language therapist	Communication and swallowing
Social worker	Care needs
Nurse	Motivation and initiation of activities Feeding Continence Skin care

12 Get up and go test

To assess balance, ask the patient to stand up from a sitting position, walk 10 m, turn and go back to the chair.

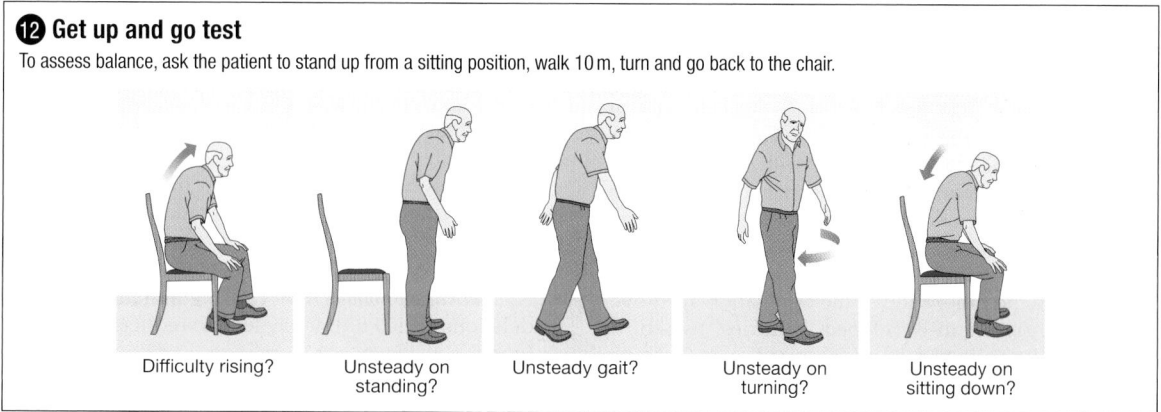

| Difficulty rising? | Unsteady on standing? | Unsteady gait? | Unsteady on turning? | Unsteady on sitting down? |

165

Sweeping demographic change has meant that older people now represent the core practice of medicine in many countries. A good knowledge of the effects of ageing and the clinical problems associated with old age is thus essential in most medical specialties. The older population is extremely diverse; a substantial proportion of 90-year-olds enjoy an active healthy life, while some 70-year-olds are severely disabled by chronic disease. The terms 'chronological' and 'biological' ageing have been coined to describe this phenomenon. Biological rather than chronological age is taken into consideration when making clinical decisions about, for example, the extent of investigation and intervention that is appropriate.

Geriatric medicine is concerned particularly with frail older people, in whom physiological capacity is so reduced that they are incapacitated by even minor illness. They frequently have multiple comorbidities, and acute illness may present in non-specific ways, such as confusion, falls, or loss of mobility and day-to-day functioning. These patients are prone to adverse drug reactions, partly because of polypharmacy and partly because of age-related changes in responses to drugs and their elimination (p. 28). Disability is common, but patients' function can often be improved by the interventions of the multidisciplinary team (p. 165).

Older people have been neglected in research terms and, until recently, were rarely included in randomised controlled clinical trials. There is thus little evidence on which to base practice.

DEMOGRAPHY

The demography of developed countries has changed rapidly in recent decades. In the UK, the total population grew by 8% over the last 35 years, but the number of people aged over 65 years rose by 31%, with the steepest rise in those aged over 85; the population aged under 16 fell by 19%. The proportion of the UK population aged over 65 is projected to increase further from 16% currently to 24% in 2061. This will have a significant impact on the old-age dependency ratio, i.e. the number of people of working age for each person aged over 65. Young people support older members of the population directly (e.g. through living arrangements) and financially (e.g. through taxation and pension contributions), so the consequences of a reduced ratio are far-reaching. However, many older people support the younger population, through care of children and other older people.

Life expectancy in the developed world is now prolonged, even in old age (Box 7.1); women aged 80 years can expect to live for a further 9 years. However, rates of disability and chronic illness rise sharply with ageing and have a major impact on health and social services. In the UK, the reported prevalence of a chronic illness or disability sufficient to restrict daily activities is around 25% in those aged 50–64, but 66% in men and 75% in women aged over 85.

Although the proportion of the population aged over 65 years is greater in developed countries, two-thirds of the world population of people aged over 65 live in developing countries at present, and this is projected to rise to 75% in 2025. The rate of population ageing is much faster in developing countries (Fig. 7.1) so they have less time to adjust to its impact.

7.1 Mean life expectancy in years, UK and India

	Males		Females	
	UK	India	UK	India
At birth	77	62	81	64
At 60 years	20.5	15	24	17
At 70 years	13	10	16	11
At 80 years	7.5	7	9	7

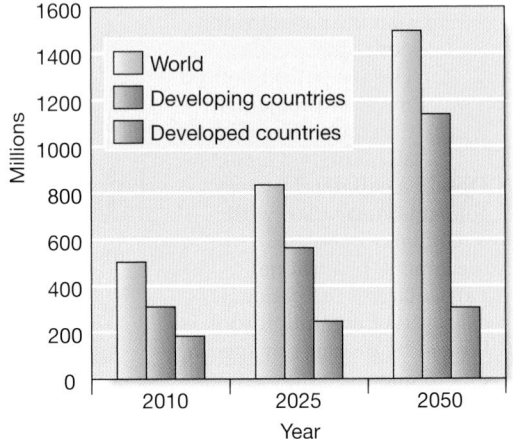

Fig. 7.1 Number of people aged 65 and over projected in the world population.

FUNCTIONAL ANATOMY AND PHYSIOLOGY

Biology of ageing

Ageing can be defined as a progressive accumulation through life of random molecular defects that build up within tissues and cells. Eventually, despite multiple repair and maintenance mechanisms, these result in age-related functional impairment of tissues and organs.

Many genes probably contribute to ageing, with those that determine durability and maintenance of somatic cell lines particularly important. However, genetic factors only account for around 25% of variance in human lifespan; nutritional and environmental factors determine the rest.

A major contribution to random molecular damage is made by reactive oxygen species produced during the metabolism of oxygen to produce cellular energy. They cause oxidative damage at a number of sites:

- *Nuclear chromosomal DNA*, causing mutations and deletions which ultimately lead to reduced gene function.
- *Telomeres*, which are the protective end regions of chromosomes which shorten with each cell division because telomerase (which copies the end of the 3' strand of linear DNA in germ cells) is absent

in somatic cells. When telomeres are sufficiently eroded, cells stop dividing. It has been suggested that telomeres represent a 'biological clock' which prevents uncontrolled cell division and cancer. Telomeres are particularly shortened in patients with premature ageing due to Werner's syndrome, in which DNA is damaged due to lack of a helicase required for DNA repair and messenger RNA formation.

- *Mitochondrial DNA* resulting in reduced cellular energy production and ultimately cell death.
- *Proteins*: for example, those increasing formation of advanced glycosylation end-products from spontaneous reactions between protein and local sugar molecules. These damage the structure and function of the affected protein, which becomes resistant to breakdown. This is the cause of yellowing of ageing nails and cornea.

The rate at which damage occurs is malleable and this is where the interplay with environment, particularly nutrition, takes place. There is evidence in some organisms that this interplay is mediated by insulin signalling pathways.

Physiological changes of ageing

The physiological features of normal ageing have been identified by examining disease-free populations of older people, to separate the effects of pathology from those due to time alone. However, the fraction of older people who age without disease ultimately declines to very low levels so that use of the term 'normal' becomes debatable. There is a marked increase in inter-individual variation in function with ageing; many physiological processes in older people deteriorate substantially when measured across populations, but some individuals show little or no change. Although there is some genetic influence over this, environmental factors such as poverty, nutrition, exercise, cigarette smoking and alcohol misuse play a large part, and a healthy lifestyle should be encouraged even when old age has been reached.

The effects of ageing are usually not enough to interfere with organ function under normal conditions, but reserve capacity is significantly reduced. Some changes of ageing, such as depigmentation of the hair, are of no clinical significance. Figure 7.2 shows many that are clinically important.

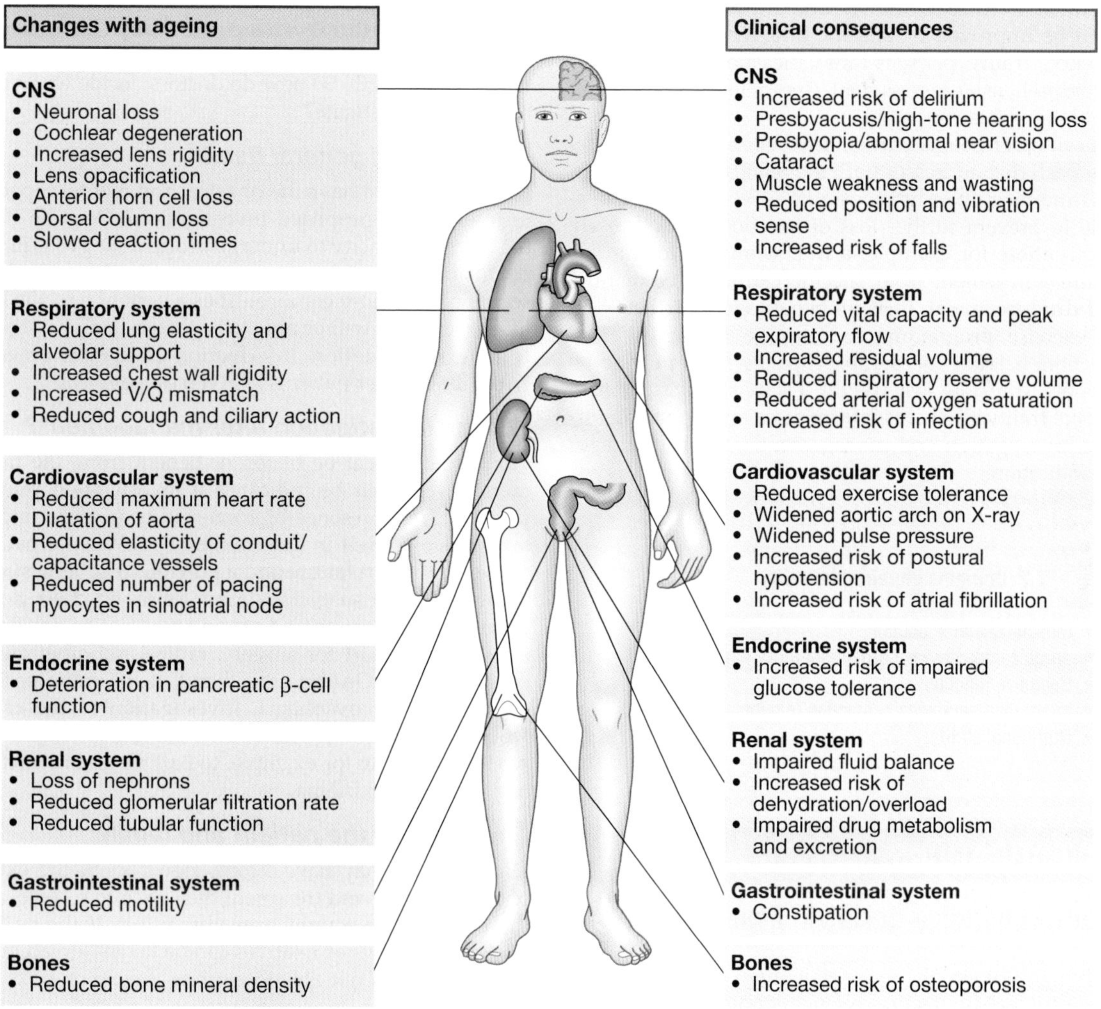

Changes with ageing

CNS
- Neuronal loss
- Cochlear degeneration
- Increased lens rigidity
- Lens opacification
- Anterior horn cell loss
- Dorsal column loss
- Slowed reaction times

Respiratory system
- Reduced lung elasticity and alveolar support
- Increased chest wall rigidity
- Increased V̇/Q̇ mismatch
- Reduced cough and ciliary action

Cardiovascular system
- Reduced maximum heart rate
- Dilatation of aorta
- Reduced elasticity of conduit/ capacitance vessels
- Reduced number of pacing myocytes in sinoatrial node

Endocrine system
- Deterioration in pancreatic β-cell function

Renal system
- Loss of nephrons
- Reduced glomerular filtration rate
- Reduced tubular function

Gastrointestinal system
- Reduced motility

Bones
- Reduced bone mineral density

Clinical consequences

CNS
- Increased risk of delirium
- Presbyacusis/high-tone hearing loss
- Presbyopia/abnormal near vision
- Cataract
- Muscle weakness and wasting
- Reduced position and vibration sense
- Increased risk of falls

Respiratory system
- Reduced vital capacity and peak expiratory flow
- Increased residual volume
- Reduced inspiratory reserve volume
- Reduced arterial oxygen saturation
- Increased risk of infection

Cardiovascular system
- Reduced exercise tolerance
- Widened aortic arch on X-ray
- Widened pulse pressure
- Increased risk of postural hypotension
- Increased risk of atrial fibrillation

Endocrine system
- Increased risk of impaired glucose tolerance

Renal system
- Impaired fluid balance
- Increased risk of dehydration/overload
- Impaired drug metabolism and excretion

Gastrointestinal system
- Constipation

Bones
- Increased risk of osteoporosis

Fig. 7.2 Features and consequences of normal ageing.

7

Frailty

Frailty is defined as the loss of an individual's ability to withstand minor stresses because the reserves in function of several organ systems are so severely reduced that even a trivial illness or adverse drug reaction may result in organ failure and death. The same stresses would cause little upset in a fit person of the same age.

It is important to understand the difference between 'disability' and 'frailty'. Disability indicates established loss of function (e.g. mobility; see Box 7.15, p. 175), while frailty indicates increased vulnerability to loss of function. Disability may arise from a single pathological event (such as a stroke) in an otherwise healthy individual. After recovery, function is largely stable, and the patient may otherwise be in good health. When frailty and disability coexist, function deteriorates markedly even with minor illness, to the extent that the patient can no longer manage independently.

Unfortunately, the term 'frail' is often used rather vaguely, sometimes to justify a lack of adequate investigation and intervention in older people. However, it can be specifically identified by assessing function in a number of domains (Box 7.2). These are all commonly impaired by disease, illness and indeed age, but can often be improved by specific intervention. In clinical practice, 'frailty' per se is rarely measured formally, but a comprehensive assessment (see below) includes an evaluation of each domain.

Frail older people particularly benefit from a clinical approach that addresses both the precipitating acute illness and their underlying loss of reserves. It may be possible to prevent further loss of function through early intervention; for example, a frail woman with cardiac failure will benefit from specific cardiac investigation and drug treatment, but will benefit even further from an exercise programme to improve musculoskeletal function, balance and aerobic capacity, with nutritional support to restore lost weight. Establishing a patient's level of frailty also helps inform decisions regarding further investigation and management, and the need for rehabilitation.

7.2 Domains impaired in frailty

- Musculoskeletal function
- Aerobic capacity, i.e. cardiorespiratory function
- Cognitive function
- Integrative neurological function (e.g. balance and gait)
- Nutritional status

INVESTIGATIONS

Comprehensive geriatric assessment

Although not strictly an investigation, one of the most powerful tools in the management of older people is the Comprehensive Geriatric Assessment, which identifies all the relevant factors contributing to their presentation

EBM 7.3 Comprehensive geriatric assessment

'Inpatient comprehensive geriatric assessment reduces short-term mortality and increases the chance of patients living at home in the long term.'

- Ellis G, Langhorne P. Br Med Bull 2005; 71: 45–59.

(p. 164). In frail patients with multiple pathology, it may be necessary to perform the assessment in stages to allow for their reduced stamina. The outcome should be a management plan that not only addresses the acute presenting problems, but also improves the patient's overall health and function (Box 7.3).

Decisions about investigation

Accurate diagnosis is important at all ages but frail older people may not be able to tolerate lengthy or invasive procedures, and diagnoses may be revealed for which patients could not withstand intensive or aggressive treatment. On the other hand, disability should never be dismissed as due to age alone. For example, it would be a mistake to supply a patient no longer able to climb stairs with a stair lift, when simple tests would have revealed osteoarthritis of a hip and vitamin D deficiency, for which appropriate treatment would have restored his or her strength. So how do doctors decide when and how far to investigate?

The patient's general health

Does this patient have the physical and mental capacity to tolerate the proposed investigation? Does he have the aerobic capacity to undergo bronchoscopy? Will her confusion prevent her from remaining still in the MRI scanner? The more comorbidities a patient has, the less likely he or she will be able to withstand an invasive or complex intervention. Information on the outcomes in critically ill older patients is given on page 202.

Will the investigation alter management?

Would the patient be fit for, or benefit from, the treatment that would be indicated if investigation proved positive? The presence of comorbidity is more important than age itself in determining this. When a patient with severe heart failure and a previous disabling stroke presents with a suspicious mass lesion on chest X-ray, detailed investigation and staging may not be appropriate if he is not fit for surgery, radical radiotherapy or chemotherapy. On the other hand, if the same patient presented with dysphagia, investigation of the cause would be important, as he would be able to tolerate endoscopic treatment: for example, to palliate an obstructing oesophageal carcinoma.

The views of the patient and family

Older people may have strong views about the extent of investigation and treatment they wish to receive, and these should be sought from the outset. If the patient wishes, the views of relatives can be taken into account. If the patient is not able to express a view or lacks the capacity to make decisions, because of cognitive impairment or communication difficulties, then relatives' input becomes particularly helpful. They may be able to give information on views previously expressed by the patient or on what the patient would have wanted under the current circumstances. However, families should never be made to feel responsible for difficult decisions.

Advance directives

Advance directives or 'living wills' are statements made by adults at a time when they have the capacity to decide for themselves about the treatments they would refuse or accept in the future, should they no longer be able to make decisions or communicate them. An advance directive cannot authorise a doctor to do anything that is illegal and doctors are not bound to provide a specific treatment requested, if in their professional opinion it is not clinically appropriate. However, any advance refusal of treatment, made when the patient was able to make decisions based on adequate information about their implications, is legally binding in the UK. It must be respected when it clearly applies to the patient's present circumstances and when there is no reason to believe that the patient has changed his or her mind.

PRESENTING PROBLEMS IN GERIATRIC MEDICINE

Characteristics of presenting problems in old age

Problem-based practice is integral to geriatric medicine. Most problems are multifactorial and there is rarely a unifying diagnosis. All contributing factors have to be taken into account and attention to detail is paramount. Two patients who share the same presenting problem may have completely disparate diagnoses. A wide knowledge of adult medicine is required, as disease in any and often many of the organ systems has to be managed at the same time. There are a number of features that are particular to older patients.

Late presentation

Many people (of all ages) accept ill health as a consequence of ageing and may tolerate symptoms for lengthy periods before seeking medical advice. Comorbidities may also contribute to late presentation; in a patient whose mobility is limited by stroke, angina may only present when coronary artery disease is advanced, as the patient was unable to exercise sufficiently to cause symptoms at an earlier stage.

Atypical presentation

Infection may present with acute confusion and without clinical pointers to the organ system affected. Stroke may present with falls rather than symptoms of focal weakness. Myocardial infarction may present as weakness and fatigue, without the classical symptoms of chest pain or dyspnoea. The reasons for these atypical presentations are not always easy to establish. Perception of pain is altered in old age, which may explain why myocardial infarction presents in other ways. The pyretic response is blunted in old age so that infection may not be obvious at first. Cognitive impairment may limit the patient's ability to give a history of classical symptoms.

Acute illness and changes in function

Atypical presentations in frail elderly patients include 'failure to cope', 'found on floor', 'confusion' and 'off feet', but these are *not* diagnoses. The possibility that an acute illness has been the precipitant must always be considered. It helps to establish whether the patient's current status is a change from his or her usual level of function by asking a relative or carer (by phone if necessary). Investigations aimed at uncovering an acute illness will not be fruitful in a patient whose function has been deteriorating over several months, but if function has suddenly changed, acute illness must be excluded.

Multiple pathology

Presentations in older patients have a more diverse differential diagnosis because multiple pathology is so common. There are frequently a number of causes for any single problem, and adverse effects from medication often contribute. A patient may fall because of osteoarthritis of the knees, postural hypotension due to diuretic therapy for hypertension, and poor vision due to cataracts. All these factors have to be addressed to prevent further falls, and this principle holds true for most of the common presenting problems in old age.

Approach to presenting problems in old age

For the sake of clarity, the common presenting problems are described individually, but in real life, older patients often present with several at the same time, particularly confusion, incontinence and falls. These share some underlying causes and may precipitate each other.

The approach to most presenting problems in old age can be summarised as follows:

- *Obtain a collateral history.* Find out the patient's usual status (e.g. mobility, cognitive state) from a relative or carer. Call these people by phone if they are not present.
- *Check all medication.* Have there been any recent changes?
- *Search for and treat any acute illness.* See Box 7.4.
- *Identify and reverse predisposing risk factors.* These depend on the presenting problem.

7.4 Screening investigations for acute illness

- Full blood count
- Urea and electrolytes, liver function tests, calcium and glucose
- Chest X-ray
- Electrocardiogram
- Urinalysis for leucocytes and nitrites; if positive, urine culture
- C-reactive protein: useful marker for occult infection
- Blood cultures if pyrexial

Falls

Around 30% of those aged over 65 years fall each year, this figure rising to over 40% in those aged over 80. Although only 10–15% of falls result in serious injury, they are the cause of over 90% of hip fractures in this age group, compounded by the rising prevalence of osteoporosis. Falls also lead to loss of confidence and fear, and are frequently the 'final straw' that makes an older person decide to move to institutional care. Management will vary according to the underlying cause.

Acute illness

Falls are one of the classical atypical presentations of acute illness in frail people. The reduced reserves in older people's neurological function mean that they are less able to maintain their balance when challenged by an acute illness. Suspicion should be high when falls have suddenly occurred over a period of a few days. Common underlying illnesses include infection, stroke, metabolic disturbance and heart failure. Thorough examination and investigation are required (see Box 7.4). It is also important to establish whether any drug which precipitates falls, such as a psychotropic or hypotensive agent, has been started recently. Once the underlying acute illness has been treated, falls may no longer be a problem.

Blackouts

A proportion of older people who 'fall' have in fact had a syncopal episode. It is important to ask about loss of consciousness, and if this is a possibility, to perform appropriate investigations (pp. 551 and 1149).

Mechanical and recurrent falls

Amongst patients who have tripped or are uncertain how they fell, those who have fallen more than once in the past year and those who are unsteady during a 'Get up and go' test (p. 165) require further assessment. Patients with recurrent falls are commonly frail, with multiple medical problems and chronic disabilities. Obviously, such patients may present with a fall resulting from an acute illness or syncope, but they will remain at risk of further falls even when the acute illness has resolved. The well-established risk factors for falls (Box 7.5) should be considered. If problems are identified with muscle strength, balance, vision or cognitive function, the causes of these must be identified by specific investigation, and treatment should be commenced if appropriate. Common pathologies identified include cerebrovascular disease (p. 1180), Parkinson's disease (p. 1199) and osteoarthritis of weight-bearing joints (p. 1083). Osteoporosis risk factors should also be sought and DEXA (dual energy X-ray absorptiometry) bone density scanning considered in all

7.5 Risk factors for falls

- Muscle weakness
- History of falls
- Gait or balance abnormality
- Use of a walking aid
- Visual impairment
- Arthritis
- Impaired ADL
- Depression
- Cognitive impairment
- Age over 80 years
- Psychotropic medication

EBM 7.6 Prevention of falls in older people

'Effective interventions to prevent falls in elderly people living in the community include exercise interventions, assessment and multifactorial intervention, withdrawal of psychotropic medication, a prescribing modification programme in primary care, first eye cataract surgery, pacemaker insertion in those with carotid sinus syndrome, and home safety interventions in those with severe visual impairment and in those at high risk of falling.'

- Gillespie LD, et al. Cochrane Database of Systematic Reviews 2009, issue 2. Art. no. CD0071460.

For further information: www.nice.org.uk

7.7 Multifactorial intervention to prevent falls

- Individualised or group exercise training
- Rationalisation of medication, especially psychotropic drugs
- Correction of visual impairment, particularly cataract extraction
- Home environmental hazard assessment and safety education
- Treatment of cardiovascular disorders, including carotid sinus syndrome and postural hypotension

older patients who have recurrent falls, particularly if they have already sustained a fracture (p. 1118).

Prevention of falls and fractures

Falls can be prevented by multiple risk factor intervention (Box 7.6), individualised according to those found in a specific patient (Box 7.7). The most effective intervention is balance and strength training by physiotherapists. An assessment of the patient's home environment for hazards must be delivered by an occupational therapist, who may also provide personal alarms so that patients can summon help should they fall again. Rationalising psychotropic medication may help to reduce sedation, although many older patients are reluctant to stop hypnotics. If postural hypotension is present (defined as a drop in blood pressure of > 20 mmHg systolic or > 10 mmHg diastolic pressure on standing from supine), reducing or stopping hypotensive drugs is helpful. Other measures to address postural hypotension are shown in Box 7.8. Simple interventions, such as new glasses to correct visual acuity, and podiatry, can also have a significant impact on function.

7.8 Management of postural hypotension

- Correction of dehydration
- Head-up tilt of the bed
- Support stockings (older patients may struggle to get these on)
- Non-steroidal anti-inflammatory drugs (NSAIDs; increase circulating volume via salt and water retention; gastric and renal side-effects limit use)
- Fludrocortisone (causes salt and water retention; often poorly tolerated due to fluid overload)
- Midodrine (α-adrenergic agent; not licensed in the UK)

If osteoporosis is diagnosed, specific drug therapy should be commenced (p. 1119). In female patients in institutional care, calcium and vitamin D₃ have been shown to reduce fracture rates, and may also reduce falls by reversing the changes in neuromuscular function associated with vitamin D deficiency. They are not effective in those with osteoporosis living in the community, in whom bisphosphonates are first-line therapy.

In the UK, government policy and National Institute for Health and Clinical Excellence guidelines (www. nice.org.uk) for falls prevention have led to the development of specific Falls and Fracture Prevention Services in many parts of the country.

Delirium (acute confusion)

Delirium is very common, affecting up to 30% of older hospital inpatients either at admission or during their hospital stay. It is associated with high rates of mortality, complication and institutionalisation, and with longer lengths of stay. Characteristic features must be present to make a diagnosis of delirium (Box 7.9), but it may be missed unless routine cognitive testing with an Abbreviated Mental Test (AMT; see p. 165) is performed. Delirium often occurs in patients with dementia, and a history from a relative or carer about the onset and course of confusion is needed to distinguish acute from chronic features. Other risk factors are shown in Box 7.10. More than one of the precipitating causes of delirium (Fig. 7.3) is often present.

7.9 Diagnostic criteria for delirium (DSM IV*)

A patient must show each of features 1–4.

1. Disturbed consciousness with reduced ability to focus, sustain or shift attention
2. A change in cognition (e.g. memory, language, orientation) or the development of a perceptual disturbance (hallucinations) that is not accounted for by a pre-existing or developing dementia
3. Development of the disturbance over a short period (hours or days) and a tendency to fluctuate over the course of the day
4. Evidence from the history, physical examination or laboratory findings that the disturbance is caused by the direct physiological consequences of a general medical condition, or by substance intoxication or withdrawal

*American Psychiatric Association's Diagnostic Statistical Manual Vol. 4 (see also p. 230).

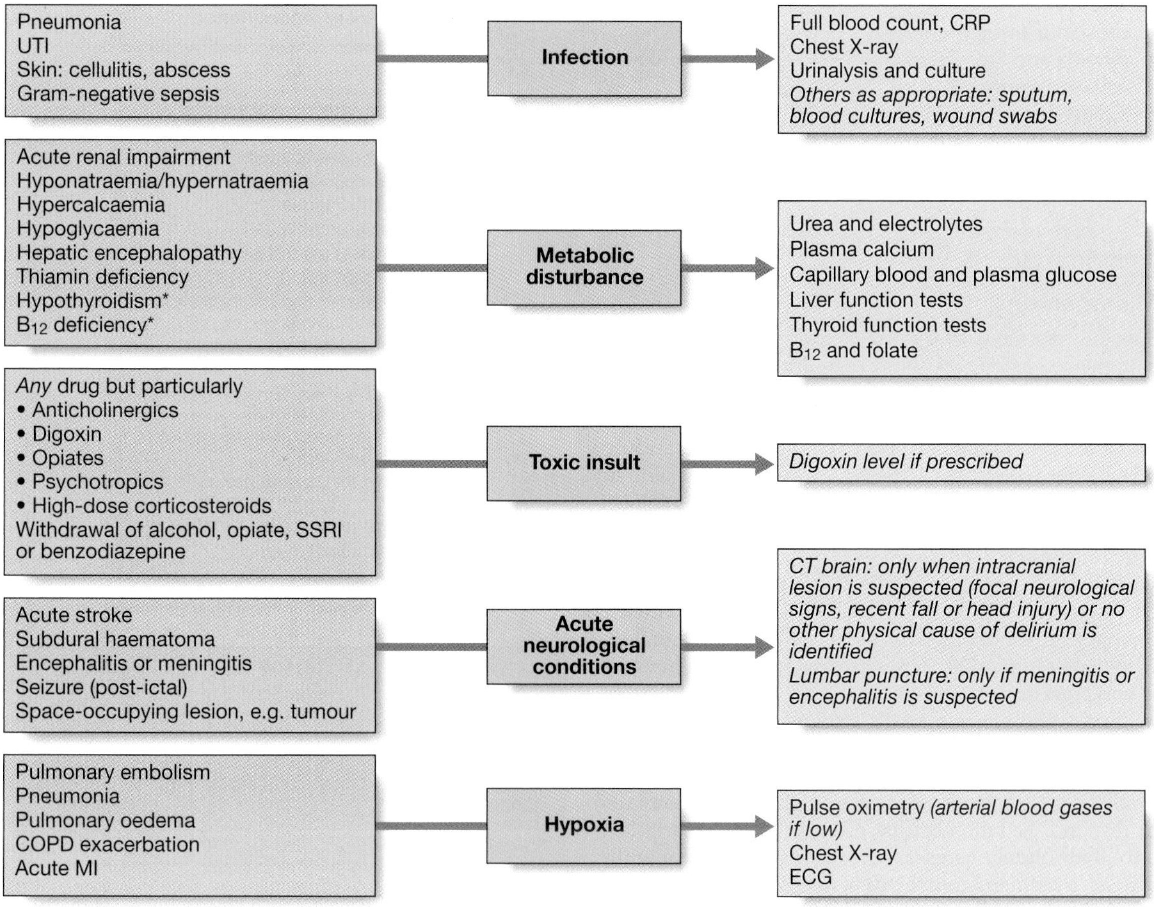

Causes	Category	Investigations
Pneumonia UTI Skin: cellulitis, abscess Gram-negative sepsis	**Infection**	Full blood count, CRP Chest X-ray Urinalysis and culture *Others as appropriate: sputum, blood cultures, wound swabs*
Acute renal impairment Hyponatraemia/hypernatraemia Hypercalcaemia Hypoglycaemia Hepatic encephalopathy Thiamin deficiency Hypothyroidism* B₁₂ deficiency*	**Metabolic disturbance**	Urea and electrolytes Plasma calcium Capillary blood and plasma glucose Liver function tests Thyroid function tests B₁₂ and folate
Any drug but particularly • Anticholinergics • Digoxin • Opiates • Psychotropics • High-dose corticosteroids Withdrawal of alcohol, opiate, SSRI or benzodiazepine	**Toxic insult**	*Digoxin level if prescribed*
Acute stroke Subdural haematoma Encephalitis or meningitis Seizure (post-ictal) Space-occupying lesion, e.g. tumour	**Acute neurological conditions**	*CT brain: only when intracranial lesion is suspected (focal neurological signs, recent fall or head injury) or no other physical cause of delirium is identified* *Lumbar puncture: only if meningitis or encephalitis is suspected*
Pulmonary embolism Pneumonia Pulmonary oedema COPD exacerbation Acute MI	**Hypoxia**	Pulse oximetry *(arterial blood gases if low)* Chest X-ray ECG

Fig. 7.3 Common causes and investigation of delirium. All investigations are performed routinely, except those in italics.* Tend to present over weeks to months rather than hours to days. (COPD = chronic obstructive pulmonary disease; CRP = C-reactive protein; MI = myocardial infarction; SSRI = selective serotonin re-uptake inhibitor; UTI = urinary tract infection)

7.10 Risk factors for delirium

- Old age
- Dementia
- Admission with infection or dehydration
- Surgery, e.g. hip fracture repair
- Alcohol misuse
- Severe physical illness
- Frailty
- Visual impairment
- Polypharmacy
- Renal impairment

Its pathophysiology is unclear; it may be an abnormal reaction of cognitive function to the physiological increase in cortisol release in acute illness, or it may reflect a sensitivity of cholinergic neurotransmission to toxic insults.

Clinical assessment

Confused patients will be unable to give an accurate history and this must be obtained from a relative or carer. Important details are speed of onset, previous mental state and ability to manage day-to-day tasks. Symptoms suggestive of a physical illness, such as an infection or stroke, should be elicited. An accurate drug and alcohol history is required, especially to ascertain whether any drugs have been recently stopped or started.

A full physical examination should be performed, noting in particular:

- conscious level
- pyrexia and any signs of infection in the chest, skin, urine or abdomen
- oxygen saturation
- signs of alcohol withdrawal, such as tremor or sweating
- any neurological signs.

A range of investigations are needed to identify the common causes (see Fig. 7.3).

Management

Specific treatment of the underlying cause(s) must be commenced as quickly as possible. However, the symptoms of delirium also require specific management. To minimise ongoing confusion and disorientation, the environment should be kept well lit and not unduly noisy, with the patient's spectacles and hearing aids in place. Good nursing is needed to preserve orientation, prevent pressure sores and falls, and maintain hydration, nutrition and continence.

The use of sedatives should be kept to a minimum, as they can precipitate delirium; in any case, many confused patients are lethargic and apathetic rather than agitated. However, sedation is appropriate if patients' behaviour is endangering themselves or others, to relieve distress in those who are extremely agitated or hallucinating, and to allow investigation or treatment. Small doses of haloperidol (0.5 mg) or lorazepam (0.5 mg) are tried orally first, and increased doses given if the patient fails to respond. Sedation can be given intramuscularly but only if absolutely necessary. In those with alcohol withdrawal, a reducing course of a benzodiazepine should be prescribed (p. 247).

The resolution of delirium in old age may be slow and incomplete. Delirium may be the first presentation of an underlying dementia, and is also a risk factor for subsequent dementia.

Urinary incontinence

Urinary incontinence is defined as the involuntary loss of urine, and comes to medical attention when sufficiently severe to cause a social or hygiene problem. It occurs in all age groups but becomes more prevalent in old age, affecting about 15% of women and 10% of men aged over 65 years. It may lead to skin damage if severe and can be socially restricting. While age-dependent changes in the lower urinary tract predispose older people to incontinence, it is not an inevitable consequence of ageing and requires investigation and appropriate treatment. Urinary incontinence is frequently precipitated by acute illness in old age and is commonly multifactorial (Fig. 7.4).

Initial management is to identify and address contributory factors. If incontinence fails to resolve, further diagnosis and management should be pursued, as described on pages 476–477.

- *Urge incontinence* is usually due to detrusor overactivity and results in urgency and frequency.

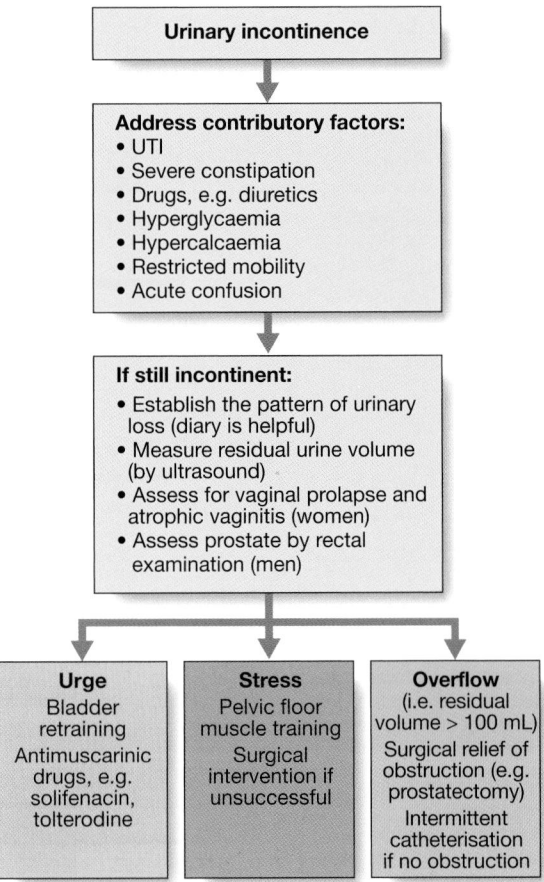

Fig. 7.4 Assessment and management of urinary incontinence in old age. See also Chapter 17 (pp. 476–7) and NICE guideline on the Management of Incontinence in Women: www.nice.org.uk.

- *Stress incontinence* is almost exclusive to women and is due to weakness of the pelvic floor muscles, which allows leakage of urine when intra-abdominal pressure rises, e.g. on coughing. Both may be compounded by atrophic vaginitis, associated with oestrogen deficiency in old age, which can be treated with oestrogen pessaries.
- *Overflow incontinence* is most commonly seen in men with prostatic enlargement, which obstructs bladder outflow and is more common in the elderly.

In patients with severe stroke disease or dementia, treatment may be ineffective, as frontal cortical inhibitory signals to bladder emptying are lost. A timed/prompted toileting programme may help. Other than in overflow incontinence, urinary catheterisation should never be viewed as first-line management but may be required as a final resort if the perineal skin is at risk of breakdown or quality of life is affected by intractable incontinence.

Adverse drug reactions

Adverse drug reactions (ADRs) and the effects of drug interactions are discussed on pages 31–35. They may result in symptoms, abnormal physical signs and altered laboratory test results (Box 7.11). ADRs are the cause of around 5% of all hospital admissions but account for up to 20% of admissions in those aged over 65 years. This is partly because older people receive many more prescribed drugs than younger people. Polypharmacy is defined as the use of four or more drugs but may not always be inappropriate, as many conditions such as hypertension and heart failure dictate the use of several drugs, and older people may have several coexisting medical problems. However, the more drugs that are taken, the greater the risk of an ADR. This risk is compounded by age-related changes in pharmacodynamic and pharmacokinetic factors (pp. 28–29), and by impaired homeostatic mechanisms, such as baroreceptor responses, plasma volume and electrolyte control. Older people are thus especially sensitive to drugs that can cause postural hypotension or volume depletion (see Box 7.11). Non-adherence to drug therapy also rises with the number of drugs prescribed.

The clinical presentations of ADRs are diverse, so for *any* presenting problem in old age the possibility that the patient's medication is a contributory factor should *always* be considered. Failure to recognise this may lead to the use of a further drug to treat the problem, making matters worse, where the better course would be to stop or reduce the dose of the offending drug or to find an alternative.

Several factors contribute to polypharmacy (Box 7.12), and it has been shown that most ADRs are preventable. This is achieved by using as few drugs as possible, at the lowest dose possible in easy-to-take formulations, by ensuring that the patient understands the dosage regime, and by reviewing medication regularly. The patient or carer should be asked to bring all medication for review rather than the doctor relying on previous records. Those drugs that are no longer needed or that are contraindicated can then be discontinued.

7.11 Common adverse drug reactions in old age	
Drug class	**Adverse reaction**
NSAIDs	Gastrointestinal bleeding and peptic ulceration Renal impairment
Diuretics	Renal impairment, electrolyte disturbance Gout Hypotension, PH
Warfarin	Bleeding
ACE inhibitors	Renal impairment, electrolyte disturbance Hypotension, PH
β-blockers	Bradycardia, heart block Hypotension, PH
Opiates	Constipation, vomiting Delirium Urinary retention
Antidepressants	Delirium Hyponatraemia (SSRIs) Hypotension, PH Falls
Benzodiazepines	Delirium Falls
Anticholinergics	Delirium Urinary retention Constipation

(ACE = angiotensin-converting enzyme; NSAID = non-steroidal anti-inflammatory drug; PH = postural hypotension; SSRI = selective serotonin reuptake inhibitor)

7.12 Factors leading to polypharmacy

- Multiple pathology
- Poor patient education
- Lack of routine review of all medications
- Patient expectations of prescribing
- Over-use of drug interventions by doctors
- Attendance at multiple specialist clinics
- Poor communication between specialists

Dizziness

Dizziness is very common, affecting at least 30% of those aged over 65 years in community surveys. It is a good example of the importance of a problem-based rather than an organ-based approach in older people, as it is frequently multifactorial rather than due to a single condition (pp. 551 and 1149). Acute dizziness is relatively straightforward and common causes include:

- hypotension due to arrhythmia, myocardial infarction, gastrointestinal bleed or pulmonary embolism
- onset of posterior fossa stroke
- vestibular neuronitis.

7

Although older people more commonly present with recurrent dizzy spells and often find it difficult to describe the sensation they experience, the most effective way of establishing the cause(s) of the problem is nevertheless to determine which of the following is predominant (even if more than one is present):

- *lightheadedness*, suggestive of reduced cerebral perfusion
- *vertigo*, suggestive of labyrinthine or brain-stem disease
- *unsteadiness/poor balance*, suggestive of joint or neurological disease.

Lightheadedness

Structural cardiac disease (such as left ventricular dysfunction or aortic stenosis) and arrhythmia must be considered, but disorders of autonomic cardiovascular control, such as vasovagal syndrome and postural hypotension, are also very common in old age. Hypotensive medication may exacerbate these. Further investigation and treatment are described on page 1149.

Vertigo

This is most commonly due to benign positional vertigo in old age (p. 1151), but if other brain-stem symptoms or signs are present, magnetic resonance imaging (MRI) of the brain is required to exclude a cerebello-pontine angle lesion.

Unsteadiness

This may be caused by a wide range of joint and neurological conditions. Examination of the gait, joints and neurological system (Box 7.13) guides further specific investigation and treatment. Whatever the cause, gait and balance problems in old age can be improved by physiotherapy. If the patient is falling as a result of dizziness, interventions to prevent falls should be instigated (see Box 7.7, p. 170).

Other problems in old age

There is a vast range of other presenting problems in older people and they present to many medical specialties.

7.13 Abnormal gaits and probable causes

Gait abnormality	Probable cause
Antalgic	Arthropathy
Waddling	Proximal myopathy
Stamping	Sensory neuropathy
Foot drop	Peripheral neuropathy or radiculopathy
Ataxic	Sensory neuropathy or cerebellar disease
Shuffling/festination	Parkinson's disease
Marche à petits pas	Small-vessel cerebrovascular disease
Hemiplegic	Cerebral hemisphere lesion
Apraxic	Bilateral hemisphere lesions

7.14 Other presenting problems in old age

• Hypothermia	p. 101
• Under-nutrition	p. 121
• Infection	pp. 292 and 302
• Fluid balance problems	p. 437
• Heart failure	p. 543
• Hypertension	p. 551
• Dizziness and blackouts	pp. 551 and 1149
• Atrial fibrillation	p. 563
• Diabetes mellitus	p. 804
• Peptic ulceration	p. 874
• Anaemia	p. 997
• Painful joints	p. 1065
• Bone disease and fracture	pp. 1116–1124 and 1068
• Immobility	p. 1154
• Stroke	p. 1180
• Dementia	p. 1197

End-of-life care is an important facet of clinical practice in old age and is discussed in Chapter 12 (pp. 286–287). Relevant sections in other chapters are referenced in Box 7.14.

Within each chapter, 'In Old Age' boxes highlight the areas in which presentation or management differs from that in younger individuals. These are listed on page 176.

REHABILITATION

Rehabilitation aims to improve the ability of people of all ages to perform day-to-day activities, and to restore their physical, mental and social capabilities as far as possible. Acute illness in older people is often associated with loss of their usual ability to walk or care for themselves, and common disabling conditions such as stroke, fractured neck of femur, arthritis and cardio-respiratory disease become increasingly prevalent with advancing age.

Disability is an interaction between factors intrinsic to the individual and the context in which they live, and both medical and social interventions are needed to address this (Box 7.15). Doctors tend to focus on health conditions and impairments, but patients are more concerned with the effect on their activities and ability to participate in everyday life.

The rehabilitation process

Rehabilitation is a problem-solving process focused on improving the patient's physical, psychological and social function. It entails:

- *Assessment*. The nature and extent of the patient's problems are identified using the framework in Box 7.15. Specific assessment scales, such as the Elderly Mobility Scale or Barthel Index of Activities of Daily Living, can be used to quantify components of disability, but do not determine the underlying

7.15 International classification of functioning and disability

Factor	Intervention required
Health condition Underlying disease, e.g. stroke, osteoarthritis	Medical or surgical treatment
Impairment Symptoms or signs of the condition, e.g. hemiparesis, visual loss	Medical or surgical treatment
Activity limitation Resultant loss of function, e.g. walking, dressing	Rehabilitation, assistance, aids
Participation restriction Resultant loss of social function, e.g. cooking, shopping	Adapted accommodation Social services

causes or the interventions required in individual patients.

- *Goal-setting.* Goals should be specific to the patient's problems, realistic, and agreed between the patient and the rehabilitation team.
- *Intervention.* This includes the active treatments needed to achieve the established goals and to maintain the patient's health and quality of life. 'Hard' interventions include hands-on treatment by therapists using a functional, task-orientated approach to improve day-to-day activities. 'Soft' interventions are just as important, and include psychological support and education (Fig. 7.5). The emphasis on the type of intervention will be different, depending on the patient's disabilities, psychological status and progress. The patient and his or her carer(s) must be active participants.

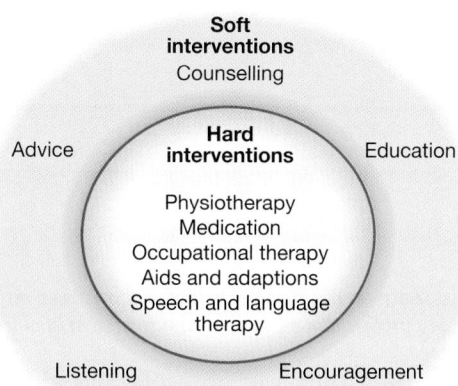

Fig. 7.5 Rehabilitation techniques.

- *Reassessment.* There is ongoing re-evaluation of the patient's function and progress towards the goals by the rehabilitation team, the patient and the carer. Interventions may be modified as a result.

Multidisciplinary team working

The core rehabilitation team includes members from several professional disciplines (Box 7.16). Others may be involved, e.g. audiometry to correct hearing impairment, podiatry for foot problems, and orthotics where a prosthesis or splinting is required. Good communication and mutual respect are essential. Regular team meetings allow sharing of assessments, agreement of rehabilitation goals and interventions, evaluation of progress and planning for the patient's discharge home. Rehabilitation is *not* when the doctor orders 'physio' or 'a home visit', and takes no further role.

Rehabilitation outcomes

There is evidence that rehabilitation improves functional outcomes in older people following acute illness, stroke and hip fracture. It also reduces mortality after stroke and hip fracture. These benefits accrue from complex multi-component interventions, but occupational therapy to improve personal ADLs, and individualised exercise interventions have now been shown to be effective in improving functional outcome in their own right.

7.16 The rehabilitation team

Team member	Role
Physiotherapist	Promotion of balance, mobility and upper limb function
Occupational therapist	Promotion of ADLs, e.g. dressing, cooking Assessment of home environment and care needs
Speech and language therapist	Management of speech and swallowing problems
Dietitian	Management of nutrition
Social worker	Organisation of home support services or institutional care
Nurse	Encouragement towards independent function in all activities Promotion of continence Communication with relatives and other professionals
Doctor	Management of medical problems Coordinator of rehabilitation programme

7

7.17 Index of 'In Old Age' boxes

Further information

Websites

www.bgs.org.uk *British Geriatrics Society: useful publications including a guideline on the diagnosis and management of delirium, and links to other relevant websites.*

www.effectiveolderpeoplecare.org *Collates and summarises the Cochrane evidence for best practice in the health care and rehabilitation of frail older people.*

www.geriatricsyllabus.com *Provides information on the ageing process and on the care and treatment of older people.*

www.profane.eu.org *Prevention of Falls Network Europe: focuses on the prevention of falls and improvement of postural stability in older people.*

Journal articles

Lally F, Crome P. Understanding Frailty. Postgraduate Medical Journal 2007; 83:16–20.

I.S. Grant
G.R. Nimmo

Critical illness

8

CLINICAL EXAMINATION OF THE CRITICALLY ILL PATIENT

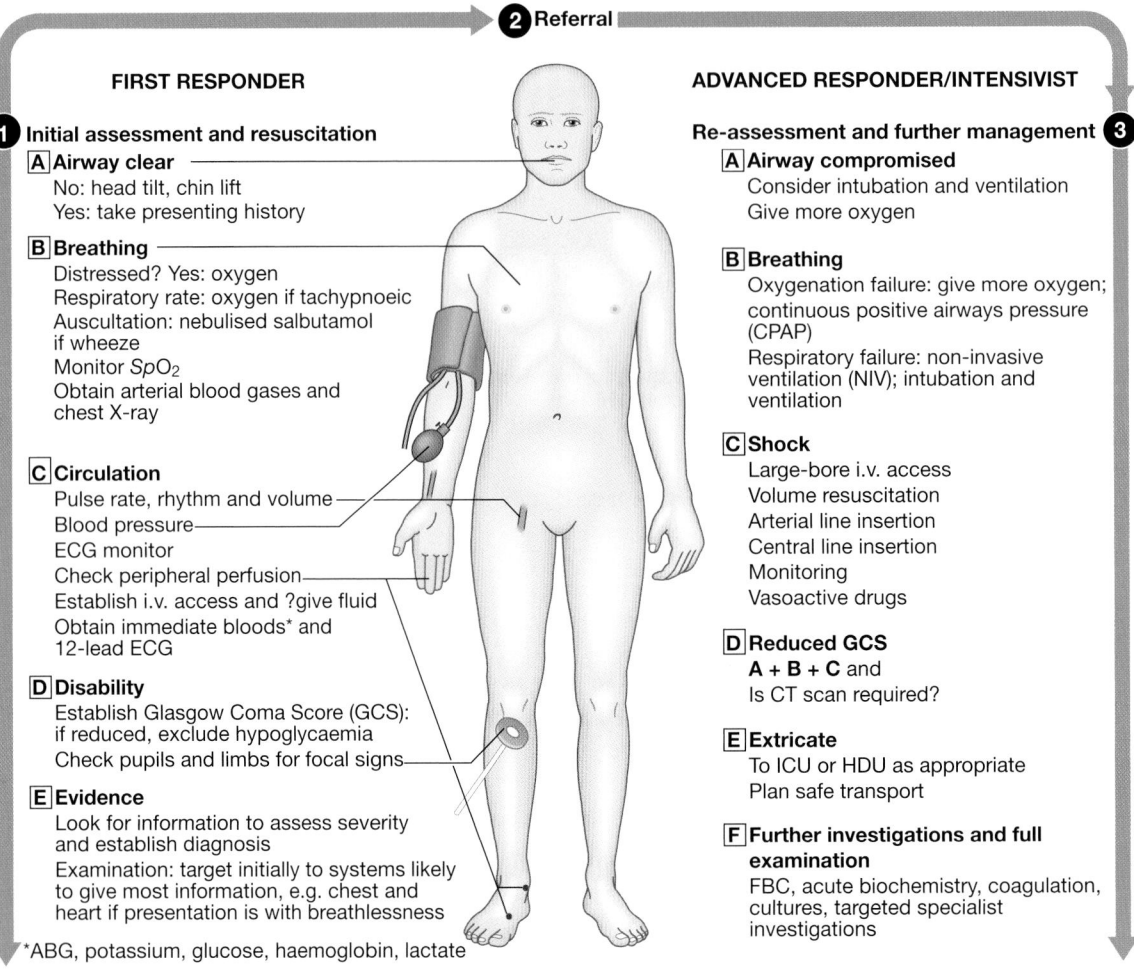

② Referral

FIRST RESPONDER

① **Initial assessment and resuscitation**

A **Airway clear**
No: head tilt, chin lift
Yes: take presenting history

B **Breathing**
Distressed? Yes: oxygen
Respiratory rate: oxygen if tachypnoeic
Auscultation: nebulised salbutamol
if wheeze
Monitor SpO_2
Obtain arterial blood gases and
chest X-ray

C **Circulation**
Pulse rate, rhythm and volume
Blood pressure
ECG monitor
Check peripheral perfusion
Establish i.v. access and ?give fluid
Obtain immediate bloods* and
12-lead ECG

D **Disability**
Establish Glasgow Coma Score (GCS):
if reduced, exclude hypoglycaemia
Check pupils and limbs for focal signs

E **Evidence**
Look for information to assess severity
and establish diagnosis
Examination: target initially to systems likely
to give most information, e.g. chest and
heart if presentation is with breathlessness

*ABG, potassium, glucose, haemoglobin, lactate

ADVANCED RESPONDER/INTENSIVIST

Re-assessment and further management **③**

A **Airway compromised**
Consider intubation and ventilation
Give more oxygen

B **Breathing**
Oxygenation failure: give more oxygen;
continuous positive airways pressure
(CPAP)
Respiratory failure: non-invasive
ventilation (NIV); intubation and
ventilation

C **Shock**
Large-bore i.v. access
Volume resuscitation
Arterial line insertion
Central line insertion
Monitoring
Vasoactive drugs

D **Reduced GCS**
A + B + C and
Is CT scan required?

E **Extricate**
To ICU or HDU as appropriate
Plan safe transport

F **Further investigations and full
examination**
FBC, acute biochemistry, coagulation,
cultures, targeted specialist
investigations

RECOGNISING THE CRITICALLY ILL PATIENT

Respiratory signs
- Respiratory arrest
- Threatened or obstructed airway
- Stridor, intercostal recession, paradoxical breathing (seesaw pattern)
- Respiratory rate < 8 or > 35/min
- Respiratory distress: use of accessory muscles; unable to speak in complete sentences
- SpO_2 < 90% on high-concentration oxygen
- Rising $PaCO_2$ > 7 kPa (52.5 mmHg) or > 2 kPa (> 15 mmHg) above 'normal' with acidosis

Cardiovascular signs
- Cardiac arrest
- Pulse rate < 40 or > 140 bpm
- Systolic blood pressure < 100 mmHg
- Poor peripheral perfusion
- Evidence of inadequate oxygen delivery
  Metabolic acidosis
  Hyperlactataemia
- Poor response to volume resuscitation
- Oliguria < 0.5 mL/kg/hr (check urea, creatinine, K^+)

Neurological signs
- Threatened or obstructed airway
- Absent gag or cough reflex
- Failure to maintain normal PaO_2 and $PaCO_2$
- Failure to obey commands
- GCS < 10
- Sudden fall in level of consciousness (GCS by > 2 points)
- Repeated or prolonged seizures

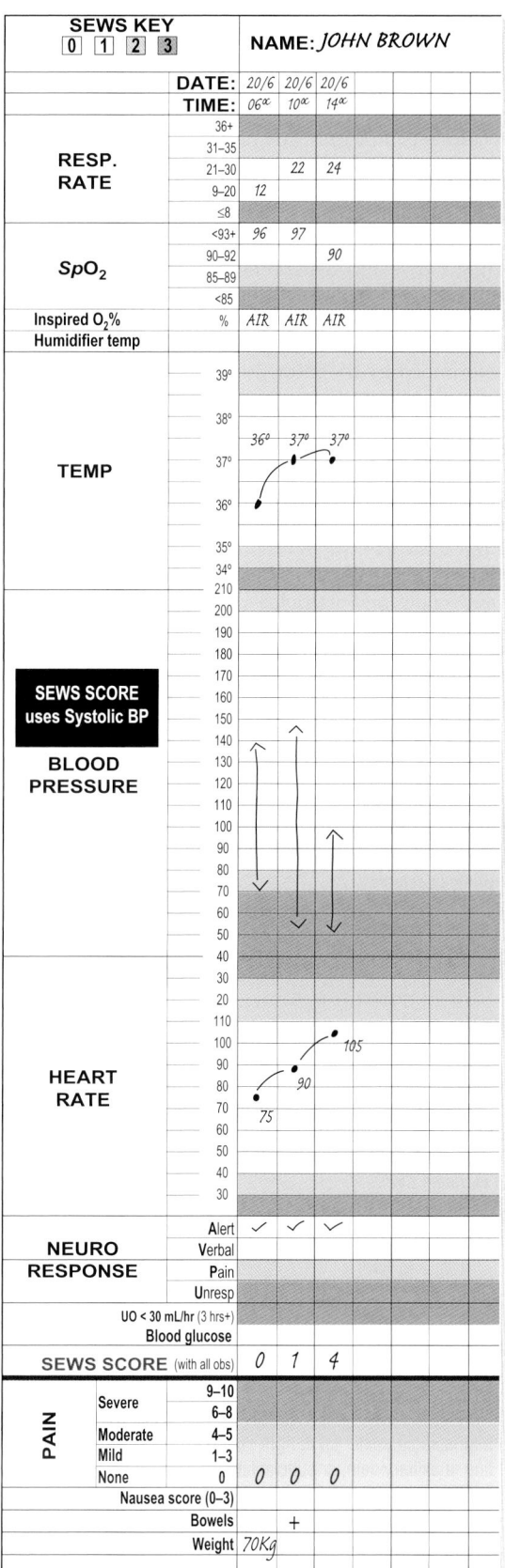

SEWS KEY 0 1 2 3	NAME: *JOHN BROWN*						
DATE:	20/6	20/6	20/6				
TIME:	06ᵒᵒ	10ᵒᵒ	14ᵒᵒ				
RESP. RATE 36+							
31–35							
21–30		22	24				
9–20	12						
≤8							
SpO₂ <93+	96	97					
90–92			90				
85–89							
<85							
Inspired O₂% %	AIR	AIR	AIR				
Humidifier temp							

TEMP (°): $36°$, $37°$, $37°$ plotted

SEWS SCORE uses Systolic BP

BLOOD PRESSURE — plotted arrows

HEART RATE: 75, 90, 105 plotted

NEURO RESPONSE	Alert	✓	✓	✓				
	Verbal							
	Pain							
	Unresp							
UO < 30 mL/hr (3 hrs+)								
Blood glucose								
SEWS SCORE (with all obs)		0	1	4				

PAIN	Severe	9–10						
		6–8						
	Moderate	4–5						
	Mild	1–3						
	None	0	0	0	0			
Nausea score (0–3)								
Bowels			+					
Weight	70Kg							

Standard Early Warning System (SEWS) chart. (UO = urine output)

179

Recognition of critical illness: early warning scores

- Record standard observations:
  Respiratory rate
  SpO₂
  Temperature
  Blood pressure (BP)
  Heart rate
  Neurological response
- Note whether the observation falls in a shaded 'at-risk zone' (see SEWS key)
- Add the points scored and record total SEWS score on chart
- Do not add 'Pain' score to SEWS score

If SEWS score ≥ 4, a doctor should assess the patient within 20 minutes.

If SEWS score ≥ 6, a senior doctor should assess the patient within 10 minutes.

Clinical features of shock

Low-flow shock, e.g. hypovolaemia, cardiogenic shock

- Rapid, shallow respiration
- Cold, clammy skin
- Tachycardia (> 100/min)
- Hypotension (systolic BP < 100 mmHg)
- Drowsiness, confusion, irritability (usually occurs late)
- Oliguria
- Multi-organ failure

Vasodilated shock, e.g. sepsis, anaphylaxis

- Rapid, shallow respiration (very early)
- Warm peripheries*
- Tachycardia (> 100/min)
- Hypotension (systolic BP < 100 mmHg and disproportionately low diastolic BP—early)
- Drowsiness, confusion, irritability (can occur early)
- Oliguria
- Multi-organ failure

*Peripheries may be cool in severe hypovolaemia (low central venous pressure) or if myocardial depression is present (normal or raised central venous pressure).

8

A critically ill patient is one at imminent risk of death. Recognition, assessment and management of critical illness are fundamental to clinical care in any sphere of medicine. Acutely ill patients require rapid but careful assessment, and initiation of treatment often precedes or parallels acquisition of a definitive diagnosis. The principles underpinning intensive care management are the simultaneous assessment of severity of illness and stabilisation of life-threatening physiological abnormalities, with a view to preventing deterioration and effecting improvement as the diagnosis is established and treatment of the underlying definitive disease process(es) is initiated. Slavish attention to *either* resuscitation *or* diagnostic processes in isolation results in suboptimal outcomes and increased mortality; the two processes are inextricably interlinked. At the same time, wherever the clinical environment, appropriate physiological monitoring should be commenced to inform the continuing process of assessment and reassessment, including response to therapy.

PHYSIOLOGY OF CRITICAL ILLNESS

Oxygen transport

The major function of the heart, lungs and circulation is the provision of oxygen (and other nutrients) to the various organs and tissues of the body. During this process, carbon dioxide and other metabolic waste products are removed. The rate of supply and removal should match the specific metabolic requirements of the individual tissues. This requires adequate oxygen uptake in the lungs, global matching of delivery and consumption, and regional control of the circulation. Failure to supply sufficient oxygen to meet the metabolic requirements of the tissues is the cardinal feature of circulatory failure or 'shock', and optimisation of tissue oxygen delivery and consumption is the goal of resuscitation.

Atmospheric oxygen moves down a partial pressure gradient from air, through the respiratory tract, from alveoli to arterial blood and is then transported in the circulation to the capillary beds and cells, diffusing into the mitochondria and being utilised at cytochrome a_3. Clinically important points to note in the management of a critically ill patient are that:

- The movement of oxygen from the left ventricle to the systemic tissue capillaries is referred to as oxygen delivery (DO_2), and is the product of cardiac output (flow) and arterial oxygen content (CaO_2). The latter is calculated from CaO_2 = Hb × arterial oxygen saturation of haemoglobin (SaO_2) × 1.34. By increasing cardiac output, arterial oxygen saturation or haemoglobin concentration, DO_2 will be increased.
- The regional distribution of oxygen delivery is also vital. If skin and muscle receive high blood flows but the splanchnic bed does not, the gut will become hypoxic even if overall DO_2 is high.
- The movement of oxygen from tissue capillary to cell occurs by diffusion and depends on the gradient of oxygen partial pressures, diffusion distance and the ability of the cell to take up and use oxygen. Thus microcirculatory, tissue diffusion and cellular factors, as well as DO_2, influence the oxygen status of the cell.

Cardiovascular component of oxygen delivery: flow

A key determinant of DO_2 is cardiac output, which is determined by the ventricular 'preload', 'afterload', myocardial contractility and heart rate.

Preload

The atrial filling pressures or preload determine the end-diastolic ventricular volume which, according to Starling's Law and depending on the myocardial contractility, defines the force of cardiac contraction and the stroke volume (see Fig. 18.22, p. 544). The predominant factor influencing preload is venous return, which is determined by the intravascular volume, the venous 'tone' and the intrathoracic pressure (Box 8.1).

When volume is lost (e.g. major haemorrhage), venous 'tone' increases and this helps to offset the consequent fall in atrial filling pressure and stroke volume. If the equivalent volume is returned gradually, the right atrial pressure will return to normal as the intravascular volume is restored and the reflex increase in venous tone abates. However, if fluid is infused too rapidly, there will be insufficient time for the venous and arteriolar tone to fall and pulmonary oedema may occur, even though the intravascular volume has only been restored to the pre-morbid level.

If the preload is low, volume loading with intravenous fluids is the priority and this is the most appropriate means of improving cardiac output and tissue

8.1 Factors affecting level and measurement of central venous pressure (CVP)

Physiology-related

- Cardiac function
- Blood volume
- Venoconstriction
- Intrathoracic pressure

Disease-related

- Superior vena cava occlusion
- Chronic obstructive pulmonary disease (COPD)/cor pulmonale
- Pulmonary embolism
- Cardiac tamponade

All increase CVP

Intervention-related

- Positive pressure ventilation and positive end-expiratory pressure (PEEP)
- Fluid resuscitation
- Vasopressors

All increase CVP

- Venodilators *reduce CVP*

Artefactual levels caused by physical aberrations

- Malpositioned line: tip in right ventricle, internal jugular line in axillary vein, or subclavian line in internal jugular vein
- Transducer not in alignment with phlebostatic axis (mid-axillary line)
- Inaccurate calibration of transducer system
- Infusion attached to monitoring line
- Clot/occlusion in line

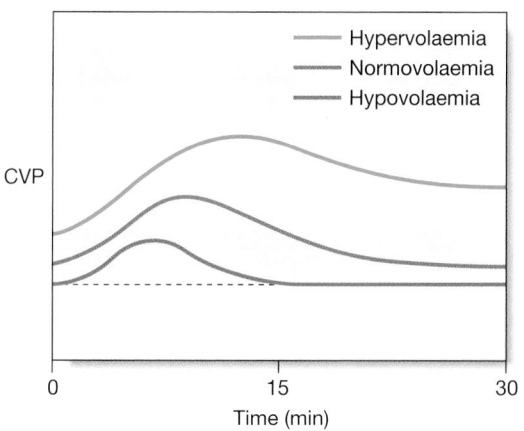

Fig. 8.1 The different responses observed in central venous pressure (CVP) after a fluid challenge of 250 mL, depending on the intravascular volume status of the patient.

perfusion. The choice of fluid for volume loading is controversial. No clear advantage of colloid over crystalloid has ever been demonstrated, but adequate filling is achieved with smaller volumes of colloid. Red cells have traditionally been transfused to achieve and maintain an Hb concentration of 100 g/L, but in the absence of significant heart disease, a target of 70–90 g/L may be preferable (p. 182). Fluid challenges of 200–250 mL should be titrated against clinical signs (heart rate, blood pressure (BP), peripheral circulation) and measurements of central venous pressure (CVP; Fig. 8.1).

When the preload is high due to excessive intravascular volume or impaired myocardial contractility, removing volume from the circulation (diuretics, haemofiltration) or increasing the capacity of the vascular bed using venodilator therapy (glyceryl trinitrate, morphine) often improves stroke volume.

Afterload

The tension in the ventricular myocardium during systole, termed 'afterload', is determined by the resistance to ventricular outflow, which is a function of the peripheral arteriolar resistance.

Understanding the reciprocal relationship between pressure, flow and resistance is crucial for appropriate circulatory management. High resistances produce lower flows at higher pressures for a given amount of ventricular work. Therefore, a systemic vasodilator such as sodium nitroprusside will allow the same cardiac output to be maintained at less ventricular work but with a reduced arterial BP. In hyperdynamic sepsis, the peripheral arteriolar tone and BP are low but the cardiac output is often high; therefore the vasoconstrictor noradrenaline (norepinephrine) is appropriate to restore BP, usually at the price of some reduction in cardiac output.

Myocardial contractility

This determines the work that the ventricle performs under given loading conditions, i.e. the stroke volume that the ventricle will generate against a given afterload for a particular level of preload.

The relationship between stroke work and filling pressure is shown in Figure 18.22 (p. 544). The ventric-

ular stroke work is the external work performed by the ventricle with each beat and is calculated from the stroke volume (SV) multiplied by the difference between afterload and preload pressures.

Consideration of ventricular work is important because it is desirable to maintain satisfactory perfusion and oxygen delivery to all organs at maximum cardiac efficiency, therefore minimising myocardial ischaemia. Myocardial contractility is frequently reduced in critically ill patients due either to pre-existing cardiac disease (usually ischaemic heart disease), drugs (β-blockers, verapamil) or to the disease process itself (particularly sepsis).

Oxygenation component of oxygen delivery: content

The major determinants of the oxygen content of arterial blood (CaO_2) are the arterial oxygen saturation of haemoglobin (SaO_2) and the haemoglobin (Hb) concentration. Over 95% of oxygen carried in the blood is attached to haemoglobin.

The oxyhaemoglobin dissociation curve (Fig. 8.2) describes the relationship between the saturation of haemoglobin (SO_2) and the partial pressure (PO_2) of oxygen in the blood. A shift in the curve will influence the uptake and release of oxygen by the Hb molecule; for example, if the curve moves to the right, the haemoglobin saturation will be lower for any given oxygen tension and therefore less oxygen will be taken up in the lungs but more will be released to the tissues. As capillary PCO_2 rises, the curve moves to the right, increasing unloading of oxygen in the tissues—a phenomenon known as the Bohr effect. In essence, a shift to the right beneficially increases capillary PO_2.

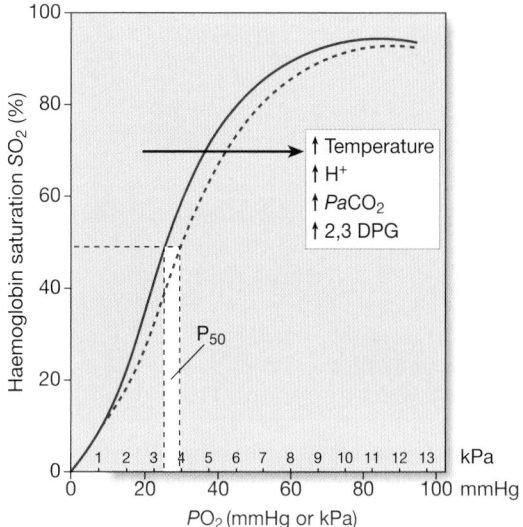

Fig. 8.2 Oxyhaemoglobin dissociation curve: the relationship between oxygen tension (PO_2) and percentage saturation of haemoglobin with oxygen (SO_2). The dotted line illustrates the rightward shift of the curve (i.e. P_{50} increases) caused by increases in temperature, $PaCO_2$, metabolic acidosis and 2,3 diphosphoglycerate (DPG).

Due to the shape of the curve, a small drop in arterial PO_2 (PaO_2) below 8 kPa (60 mmHg) will cause a marked fall in SaO_2. Its position and the effect of various physicochemical factors are defined by the PO_2 at which 50% of the haemoglobin is saturated (P_{50}), which is normally 3.5 kPa (26 mmHg). The shape of the curve also dictates that increases in PaO_2 beyond the level that ensures SaO_2 is > 90% produce relatively small additional increases in CaO_2 (Fig. 8.3). Consider a patient who is both anaemic (Hb 60 g/L) and hypoxaemic (SaO_2 75%) when breathing air (fractional inspired oxygen concentration (FiO_2) 20%). Supplementary oxygen at FiO_2 40% will increase SaO_2 to 93%; CaO_2 will increase by 24% but further increases in FiO_2, while raising PaO_2, cannot produce any further useful increases in SaO_2 or CaO_2. However, increasing Hb to 90 g/L by blood transfusion will result in a further 50% increase in CaO_2.

Traditionally, the optimum haemoglobin concentration for critically ill patients was considered to be approximately 100 g/L, representing a balance between maximising the oxygen content of the blood and avoiding regional microcirculatory problems due to increased viscosity. However, evidence suggests an improved outcome in critically ill patients if the haemoglobin concentration is maintained between 70 and 90 g/L, with the exception of the elderly and patients with coronary artery disease, cardiogenic shock or significant aortic stenosis, in whom 100 g/L remains appropriate.

Oxygen consumption

The sum of the oxygen consumed by the various organs represents the global oxygen consumption (VO_2) and is approximately 250 mL/min for an adult of 70 kg undertaking normal daily activities. VO_2 may be calculated:

- indirectly, from the product of cardiac output and the arterial mixed venous oxygen content difference ($CaO_2 - CvO_2$), as shown in Figure 8.3
- directly, by sampling the inspired and mixed-expired gases from the ventilator and measuring inspired and expired minute volume.

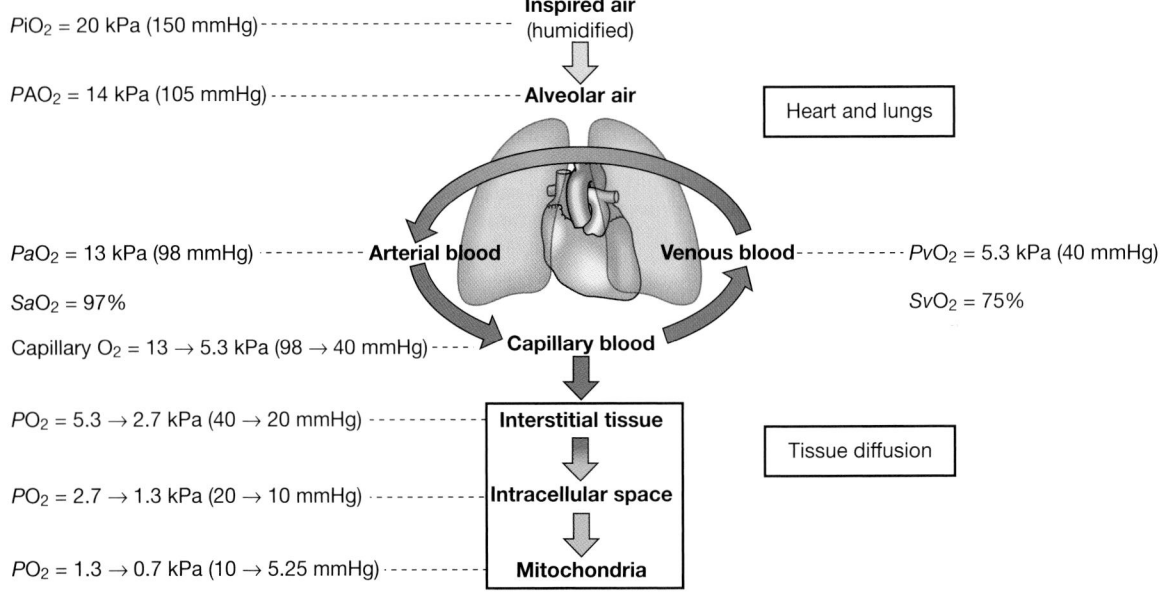

Fig. 8.3 The oxygen cascade in the transport of oxygen from inspired gas to the cell, with equations for calculation of arterial oxygen content, global oxygen delivery, consumption and extraction, and alveolar gas. Values are for a normal 70 kg individual (body surface area: 1.67 m²) breathing air (FiO_2:0.21) at standard atmospheric pressure (P_B: 101 kPa); contents (CaO_2, CvO_2 in mL/L; Hb in g/L; cardiac output in L/min; oxygen delivery (DO_2), VO_2 and VCO_2 in mL/min. To convert kPa to mmHg, multiply by 7.5.

CaO_2 = arterial O_2 content
CO = cardiac output
CvO_2 = mixed venous O_2 content
FiO_2 = fractional inspired oxygen concentration

Hb = haemoglobin
PaO_2 = arterial PO_2
PAO_2 = alveolar PO_2
PiO_2 = inspired PO_2
PO_2 = oxygen partial pressure (kPa)

PvO_2 = venous PO_2
SaO_2 = arterial SO_2
SvO_2 = mixed venous SO_2
VCO_2 = CO_2 production
VO_2 = O_2 consumption

The oxygen saturation in the pulmonary artery, or 'mixed venous oxygen saturation' (SvO_2), is a measure of the oxygen not consumed by the tissues ($DO_2 - VO_2$). The saturation of venous blood from different organs varies considerably; for example, the hepatic venous saturation usually does not exceed 60% but the renal venous saturation may reach 90%, reflecting the great difference in both the metabolic requirements of these organs and the oxygen content of the blood delivered to them. The SvO_2 is a flow-weighted average measured in the mixed effluent blood from all of the perfused tissues, and is influenced by changes in both oxygen delivery (DO_2) and consumption (VO_2). Provided the microcirculation and the mechanisms for cellular oxygen uptake are intact, it can be used to monitor whether global oxygen delivery is adequate to meet overall demand, so is particularly useful in low-flow situations such as cardiogenic shock. Central venous oxygen saturation ($ScvO_2$) has been used in the same way and can be useful, but it only reflects part of the picture and does not represent hepatosplanchnic oxygen consumption, so may be quite different to SvO_2.

The reoxygenation of the blood that returns to the lungs and the resulting arterial saturation (SaO_2) will depend on how closely pulmonary ventilation and perfusion are matched. If part of the pulmonary blood flow perfuses non-ventilated parts of the lung, there will be 'shunting', and the blood entering the left atrium will be desaturated in proportion to the size of this shunt and the level of SvO_2.

Relationship between oxygen consumption and delivery

The tissue oxygen extraction ratio (OER), which is 20–25% in a normal subject at rest, rises as consumption increases or supply diminishes (Fig. 8.4). The maximum OER is approximately 60% for most tissues; at this point no further increase in extraction can occur and any further increase in oxygen consumption or decline in oxygen delivery will cause tissue hypoxia, anaerobic metabolism and increased lactic acid production.

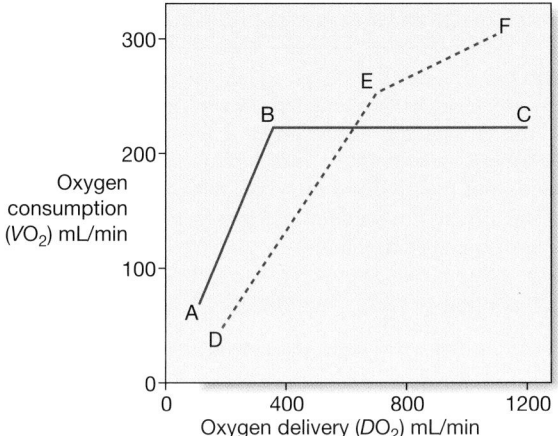

Fig. 8.4 The effects of changing oxygen delivery on consumption. The solid line (ABC) represents the normal relationship and the dotted line (DEF) the altered relationship believed to exist in sepsis.

In sepsis, the slope of maximum OER decreases, reflecting the reduced ability of tissues to extract oxygen (DE cf. AB on Fig. 8.4), but the curve does not plateau and oxygen consumption continues to increase even at 'supranormal' levels of oxygen delivery. Although trials have demonstrated no benefit from pushing oxygen delivery to high levels in those with established organ failure, it may be worthwhile if applied before organ failure supervenes (Box 8.2). In practice, if there is a metabolic acidosis, hyperlactataemia and/or oliguria which could be due to inadequate oxygen delivery, a therapeutic trial of increasing oxygen delivery (with adequate BP secured) may be informative. If oxygen consumption rises, it may indicate an oxygen debt which is being repaid.

EBM 8.2 **Early goal-directed therapy in severe sepsis**

'In patients with severe sepsis or septic shock managed initially in A&E, early goal-directed therapy (EGT) reduced 60-day mortality from 57% to 44%. Both groups were resuscitated with similar targets for CVP, arterial blood pressure and urine output, but in the EGT group additional goals were central venous oxygen saturation > 70% and haematocrit > 30%, resulting in more rapid fluid resuscitation and higher red blood cell transfusion rates in the first 6 hours.'

• Rivers E, et al. N Engl J Med 2001; 345:1368–1377.

Pathophysiology of the inflammatory response

The mediators and clinical manifestations of the inflammatory response are described on pages 81–82. In critically ill patients, these processes have important consequences (Box 8.3).

Fever, tachycardia with warm peripheries, tachypnoea and a raised white cell count traditionally prompt a diagnosis of sepsis with the clinical picture caused by invading microorganisms and their breakdown products. However, other conditions such as pancreatitis, trauma, malignancy, tissue necrosis (e.g. burns), aspiration syndromes, liver failure, blood transfusion and drug reactions can all produce the same clinical picture in the absence of infection.

Local inflammation

The body's initial response to a noxious local insult is to produce a local inflammatory response with sequestration and activation of white blood cells and the release of a variety of mediators to deal with the primary 'insult' and prevent further damage either locally or in distant organs.

Normally, a delicate balance is achieved between pro- and anti-inflammatory mediators. However, if the inflammatory response is excessive, local control is lost and a large array of mediators, including prostaglandins, leukotrienes, free oxygen radicals and particularly pro-inflammatory cytokines (p. 72), are released into the circulation.

The inflammatory and coagulation cascades are intimately related. The process of blood clotting not only involves platelet activation and fibrin deposition but also causes activation of leucocytes and endothelial cells.

8.3 Terminology to describe the inflammatory state

Infection

- Invasion of normally sterile host tissue by microorganisms

Bacteraemia

- Viable bacteria in the blood

Systemic inflammatory response syndrome (SIRS)

- The inflammatory response to both infective and non-infective causes, e.g. pancreatitis, trauma, cardiopulmonary bypass, vasculitis etc.
- Defined by the presence of two or more of:
  Respiratory rate > 20/min
  Heart rate > 90/min
  White blood count > 12×10^9/L or < 4×10^9/L
  Temperature > 38.0°C or < 36.0°C
  $PaCO_2$ < 4.3 kPa (< 32 mmHg) or ventilated
- Hypothermia and septic neutropenia are indicators of more severe infection
- A wide pulse pressure, e.g. 115/42 mmHg, may be an early pointer to systemic sepsis

Sepsis

- Systemic inflammatory response caused by documented infection

Severe sepsis/SIRS

- Sepsis/SIRS with evidence of early organ dysfunction *or* hypotension

Septic/SIRS shock

- Sepsis associated with organ failure *and* hypotension (systolic BP < 90 mmHg or > 40 mmHg fall from baseline) unresponsive to fluid resuscitation

Multiple organ dysfunction syndrome (MODS)

- Development of impaired organ function in critically ill patients with SIRS
- Multiple organ failure (MOF) will ensue if prompt treatment of underlying cause and suitable organ support are not achieved

and proteins, resulting in tissue oedema and inflammation. A vicious circle of endothelial injury, intravascular coagulation, microvascular occlusion, tissue damage and further release of inflammatory mediators ensues.

All organs may become involved. This manifests in the lungs as the acute respiratory distress syndrome (ARDS) and in the kidneys as acute tubular necrosis (ATN), while widespread disruption of the coagulation system results in the clinical picture of DIC.

The endothelium itself produces mediators that control blood vessel tone locally: endothelin 1, a potent vasoconstrictor, and prostacyclin and nitric oxide (NO, p. 82), which are systemic vasodilators. NO (which is also generated outside the endothelium) is implicated in both the myocardial depression and the profound vasodilatation of both arterioles and venules that causes the relative hypovolaemia and systemic hypotension found in septic/systemic inflammatory response syndrome (SIRS) shock.

A major component of the tissue damage in septic/SIRS shock is the inability to take up and use oxygen at mitochondrial level, even if global oxygen delivery is supranormal. This effective bypassing of the tissues results in a reduced arteriovenous oxygen difference, a low oxygen extraction ratio, a raised plasma lactate and a paradoxically high mixed venous oxygen saturation (SvO_2).

Role of splanchnic ischaemia

In shock, splanchnic hypoperfusion plays a major role in initiating and amplifying the inflammatory response, ultimately resulting in multiple organ failure (MOF). The processes involved include:

- increased gut mucosal permeability
- translocation of organisms from the gastrointestinal tract lumen into portal venous and lymphatic circulation
- Kupffer cell activation with production and release of inflammatory mediators.

RECOGNITION AND ASSESSMENT OF THE CRITICALLY ILL PATIENT

Recognition of severity of illness

All clinical staff should be aware of the fundamental physiological criteria which indicate critical illness.

The immediate appearance of the patient yields a wealth of information. Introducing yourself, shaking hands and asking 'How are you?' allows assessment of:

- the airway (for patency and noises, e.g. stridor, snoring, gurgling, none)
- breathing (rate, symmetry, work of breathing including accessory muscle use, paradoxical or seesaw pattern)
- peripheral circulation (temperature of the extremities)
- conscious level (the response of the patient).

Tachypnoea is often the earliest physiological abnormality to appear and the most sensitive to a worsening clinical state, but is the least well documented. A number of approaches have been adopted to improve

Conversely, leucocyte activation induces tissue factor expression and initiates coagulation. Control of the coagulation cascade is achieved through the natural anticoagulants, antithrombin (AT III), activated protein C (APC) and tissue factor pathway inhibitor (TFPI), which not only regulate the initiation and amplification of the coagulation cascade but also inhibit the pro-inflammatory cytokines. Deficiency of AT III and APC (features of disseminated intravascular coagulation (DIC)) facilitates thrombin generation and promotes further endothelial cell dysfunction.

Systemic inflammation

During a severe inflammatory response, systemic release of cytokines and other mediators triggers widespread interaction between the coagulation pathways, platelets, endothelial cells and white blood cells, particularly the polymorphonuclear cells (PMNs). These 'activated' PMNs express adhesion factors (selectins), causing them initially to adhere to and roll along the endothelium, then to adhere firmly and migrate through the damaged and disrupted endothelium into the extravascular, interstitial space together with fluid

the recognition of critical illness, including the use of early warning scores and charts such as the Standard Early Warning System (SEWS, p. 179). This alerts staff to severely ill patients, complements clinical judgement and facilitates the prioritisation of clinical care. A patient with a SEWS score of 4 or greater requires urgent review and appropriate interventions to be commenced. An elevated score correlates with increased mortality.

Assessment and initial resuscitation of the critically ill patient

Airway and breathing

If the patient is talking, the airway is clear and breathing is adequate. A rapid history should be obtained whilst initial assessment is undertaken.

Assess breathing in the same way as the pulse: rate, volume, rhythm, character (work of breathing) and symmetry. Look for accessory muscle use and for the ominous sign of paradoxical chest/abdominal movement, manifest as a seesaw pattern of breathing. Supplemental oxygen should be administered to patients who are breathless, tachypnoeic or bleeding, or who have chest pain or reduced conscious level. The clinical state of the patient will determine how much oxygen to give, but the critically ill should receive at least 60% oxygen initially. High-concentration oxygen is best given using a mask with a reservoir bag which, at 15 L/min, can provide nearly 90% oxygen. Arterial blood gases (ABG) should be checked early to assess oxygenation, ventilation ($PaCO_2$) and metabolic state (pH or H$^+$, HCO$_3$ and base deficit). Oxygen therapy should be adjusted in light of the ABG, remembering that oxygen requirements may subsequently increase or decrease. Early application of pulse oximeter monitoring is ideal, although this may not be reliable if the patient is peripherally shut down. Intubation, while often essential, may be hazardous in the patient with cardiorespiratory failure, and full monitoring and resuscitation facilities must be available.

Circulation

In the collapsed or unconscious patient, the carotid pulse should be palpated first, but in the conscious, peripheral pulses should be sought. The radial, brachial, foot and femoral pulses may disappear as shock progresses, so this gives information on the severity of circulatory compromise.

Venous access for the administration of drugs and/or fluids is pivotal to successful management but is often difficult in sick patients. The gauge of cannula needed is dictated by its purpose. Wide-bore cannulae are required for rapid fluid administration. Ideally, two 16G or larger cannulae should be inserted, one in each arm, in the severely hypovolaemic patient. If the two cannulae are of different sizes, the pulse oximeter should be placed on the same side as the larger, and the BP cuff on the same side as the smaller. This facilitates unimpeded volume resuscitation and uninterrupted oxygen saturation monitoring. Pressure infusors and blood warmers should be utilised for rapid, high-volume fluid resuscitation, particularly of blood products. An 18G cannula is usually adequate for drug administration.

Machine-derived cuff BP is inaccurate at extremes of BP and in tachycardia, especially atrial fibrillation. Manual sphygmomanometer BP readings tend to be more accurate in hypotension. If severe hypotension is not readily corrected with fluid, early consideration should be given to arterial line insertion and vasoactive drug therapy.

Disability

Conscious level should be assessed using the Glasgow Coma Scale (GCS; see Box 26.18, p. 1158). Best eye, verbal and motor responses should be accurately assessed and documented. A score of 8 or less denotes coma with associated airway compromise and loss of airway protection that necessitates intervention. Focal neurological signs may indicate unilateral cerebral pathology. Abnormal pupil size, symmetry or reaction to light may indicate either primary cerebral disease or global cerebral insults induced by drugs (e.g. opioids), hypoxia or hypoglycaemia.

Exposure, evidence and examination

The term exposure indicates the need for targeted clinical examination and evidence, the information provided by any recent investigations, prescription or monitoring charts.

Clinical decision-making and referral to critical care

During the initial assessment and resuscitation period, a number of decisions have to be made regarding ongoing patient care (Box 8.4). A decision about referral to the critical care service is a key part of the assessment of illness severity. It requires local knowledge of the clinical areas providing enhanced care, whether intermediate high-dependency or advanced intensive care, and the mechanism of referral.

- *High-dependency care* allows a greater degree of monitoring, physiological support and nursing/medical input than the standard ward, for patients

8.4 Clinical decision-making and critically ill patients

- How ill is the patient?
- How much help do I need and how quickly?
- Where would the patient be best managed?
- When should we move the patient?
- What do we need to achieve before transporting the patient?
  ABCDE resuscitation, including endotracheal intubation and ventilation where appropriate
  Monitoring, including invasive arterial ± CVP plus volume resuscitation and vasoactive support
  Imaging/diagnostic processes
- Do we need specialist involvement?
  Transfer to another hospital may be necessary for specialised investigations, or to specialist liver, burns, neurosurgical or cardiac surgical units
  Balance the urgency of specialist treatment against the stability of the patient's condition; it may be necessary to admit the patient to the local ICU for stabilisation first
  All critically ill patients require an appropriately trained escort during transfer

8.5 Admission criteria for intensive care units (ICU) and high-dependency units (HDU)

ICU

- Patients requiring/likely to require endotracheal intubation and invasive mechanical ventilatory support
- Patients requiring support of two or more organ systems (e.g. inotropes and haemofiltration)
- Patients with chronic impairment of one or more organ systems (e.g. COPD *or* severe ischaemic heart disease) who *also* require support for acute reversible failure of another organ system

HDU

- Patients who require more detailed observation or monitoring than can be safely provided on a general ward:
  - Direct arterial BP monitoring
  - CVP monitoring
  - Fluid balance
  - Neurological observations, regular GCS recording
- Patients requiring support for a single failing organ system, excluding invasive ventilatory support:
  - CPAP *or* non-invasive (mask) ventilation (NIV)—see Box 8.19, p. 195
  - Moderate inotropic or vasopressor support
  - Renal replacement therapy in an otherwise stable patient
- Patients no longer requiring intensive care but who cannot be safely managed on a general ward

following major surgery, or for the septic patient requiring invasive haemodynamic monitoring and circulatory support alone, or for the patient with respiratory failure manageable with non-invasive ventilation or continuous positive airways pressure (CPAP).

- *Intensive care units* are staffed and equipped to allow management of the sickest patients who require invasive ventilation, multimodal monitoring and multiple organ system support (Box 8.5).

The mechanism of referral to critical care varies between hospitals but clinical staff in all areas and specialties must be aware of the local system and how to access it. Many hospitals have medical emergency or outreach teams to facilitate this.

A clear understanding of what is available in and what is achievable by critical care allows appropriate and early referral, and prevents referral of patients who have no realistic prospect of meaningful survival, due either to the overwhelming nature of their acute condition or to the lack of definitive therapy for the underlying disease process. Patients who do warrant admission should be identified early and admitted without delay, since this improves survival and reduces the length of stay.

PRESENTING PROBLEMS IN CRITICAL ILLNESS

Circulatory failure: 'shock'

The defining feature of 'shock' is a level of oxygen delivery (DO_2) which fails to meet the metabolic requirements of the tissues. 'Shock' is not synonymous with hypotension. While hypotension is a sinister development and

requires urgent attention, it is often a late manifestation of circulatory failure or shock, and also the cardiac output and oxygen delivery may be critically low even though the BP remains normal. The problem should be identified and treated before the BP falls. Objective markers of tissue oxygen delivery, such as base deficit, blood lactate and urine output, may aid earlier identification of shock.

The causes of circulatory failure or 'shock' may be categorised as either low flow (reduced stroke volume) or low peripheral arteriolar resistance (vasodilatation), which are the primary presenting circulatory abnormalities.

Low stroke volume

- *Hypovolaemic*: any condition provoking a major reduction in blood volume, e.g. internal or external haemorrhage, severe burns, salt and water depletion.
- *Cardiogenic*: severe mechanical impairment, e.g. myocardial infarction, acute mitral regurgitation.
- *Obstructive*: obstruction to blood flow around the circulation, e.g. major pulmonary embolism, cardiac tamponade, tension pneumothorax.

Vasodilatation

- *Septic/SIRS*: infection or other causes of a systemic inflammatory response that produce widespread endothelial damage with vasodilatation, arteriovenous shunting, microvascular occlusion, capillary leak and tissue oedema.
- *Anaphylactic*: inappropriate vasodilatation triggered by an allergen (e.g. bee sting), often associated with endothelial disruption and capillary leak.
- *Neurogenic*: caused by major brain or spinal injury which disrupts brain-stem and neurogenic vasomotor control.

Clinical assessment and complications

Clinical features depend upon the primary pathophysiological abnormality (p. 178). Hypovolaemic, cardiogenic and obstructive causes of circulatory failure produce the 'classical' image of shock with cold peripheries, reduced or absent peripheral pulses, weak central pulses and evidence of a low cardiac output. In early haemorrhagic shock, a narrowed pulse pressure, i.e. a raised diastolic (DBP) and reduced systolic (SBP) such as 105/95 mmHg, indicates the combination of hypovolaemia (reduced stroke volume, hence SBP) and activation of the sympathetic nervous system, with noradrenaline (norepinephrine)-induced vasoconstriction raising the DBP.

In contrast, septic shock and anaphylactic shock are usually associated with warm peripheries, bounding pulses and features of a high cardiac output. The BP pattern is again distinctive. In the early stages, peripheral vasodilatation results in a low DBP, but since the left ventricular afterload is reduced, stroke volume and hence systolic BP are maintained, e.g. 115/42 mmHg. These patients are usually warm peripherally. However, in more advanced septic or anaphylactic shock, SBP falls and the peripheries become cool. This is usually due to the hypovolaemia associated with capillary leak and will respond to fluid resuscitation. If it does not, it is possible that myocardial depression is present.

Neurogenic shock often results in vasodilated hypotension with a paradoxically slow heart rate.

All forms of shock require early identification and treatment because, if inadequate regional tissue perfusion and cellular dysoxia persist, multiple organ failure (MOF) will develop. Early institution of invasive haemodynamic monitoring (p. 190) is recommended.

Prognosis

If the precipitating cause and accompanying circulatory failure (hypotension and frequently severe hypovolaemia due to venodilatation and fluid loss through the leaky vascular endothelium) are dealt with promptly before significant organ failure occurs ('early' shock), the prognosis is good. If not, there is progressive deterioration in organ function and MOF ensues ('late' shock).

The mortality of MOF is high and increases with the number of organs that have failed, the duration of organ failure and the patient's age. Failure of four or more organs is associated with a mortality > 80%.

Respiratory failure, including ARDS

The majority of patients admitted to ICU/HDU have respiratory problems either as the primary cause of admission or secondary to pathology elsewhere.

Respiratory failure is classified on the basis of blood gas analysis as:

- *type 1*: hypoxaemia (PaO_2 < 8 kPa (< 60 mmHg) when breathing air) without hypercapnia caused by a failure of gas exchange due to mismatching of pulmonary ventilation and perfusion
- *type 2*: hypoxaemia with hypercapnia ($PaCO_2$ > 6.5 kPa (> 49 mmHg)) due to alveolar hypoventilation which occurs when the respiratory muscles cannot perform sufficient work to clear the carbon dioxide produced by the body.

Although this distinction is conceptually useful, it cannot be applied too rigidly in critically ill patients since they may change from type 1 to 2 as their illness progresses; hypercapnia may develop in pneumonia or pulmonary oedema as the patient tires and can no longer sustain the increased work of breathing.

Pulmonary problems in critically ill patients can also be classified according to the functional residual capacity (FRC, or the lung volume at the end of expiration). Examples of low FRC include lung collapse, pneumonia and pulmonary oedema; examples of high FRC (i.e. over-distended lungs) include asthma, COPD and bronchiolitis. This allows logical management directed at improving lung compliance and reducing the work of breathing.

The more common causes of acute respiratory failure presenting to ICU/HDU for respiratory support are shown in Box 8.6. The presentation, differential diagnosis and initial treatment of the primary respiratory conditions causing acute respiratory failure are covered in Chapter 19.

The assessment of respiratory failure in the critically ill patient should be guided by several important principles:

- The patient's appearance (tachypnoea, difficulty speaking in complete sentences, laboured breathing, exhaustion, agitation or increasing obtundation) is more important than measurement

8.6 Common causes of respiratory failure in critically ill patients	
Type 1 respiratory failure	
• Pneumonia	• Lung collapse*, e.g. retained secretions
• Pulmonary oedema*	
• Pulmonary embolism	• Asthma
• Pulmonary fibrosis	• Pneumothorax
• ARDS*	• Pulmonary contusion (blunt chest trauma)
• Aspiration	
Type 2 respiratory failure	
• Reduced respiratory drive*, e.g. drug overdose, head injury	• COPD
	• Peripheral neuromuscular disease*, e.g. Guillain–Barré, myasthenia gravis
• Upper airway obstruction (oedema, infection, foreign body)	
	• Flail chest injury
	• Exhaustion* (includes all type 1 causes)
• Late severe acute asthma	

*Secondary complications of other diseases.

of blood gases in deciding when it is appropriate to provide mechanical respiratory support or intubation.
- Adequate supplemental oxygen to maintain SpO_2 > 94% should be provided. If the inspired oxygen concentration required exceeds 60%, refer to the critical care team.
- Measurement of SpO_2 and ABGs is essential in monitoring progress.
- Restless patients dependent on supplementary oxygen or with deteriorating conscious level are at risk. If they remove the mask or vomit, the resulting hypoxaemia or aspiration may be catastrophic.
- An attempt should be made to reduce the work of breathing, e.g. by treating bronchoconstriction or using CPAP (see below).

Acute respiratory distress syndrome (ARDS)

This describes the acute, diffuse pulmonary inflammatory response to either direct (via airway or chest trauma) or indirect (blood-borne) insults that originate from extrapulmonary pathology (Box 8.7). It is characterised by:

- neutrophil sequestration in pulmonary capillaries
- increased capillary permeability
- protein-rich pulmonary oedema with hyaline membrane formation
- damage to type 2 pneumocytes leading to surfactant depletion
- alveolar collapse
- reduction in lung compliance.

If this early phase does not resolve with treatment of the underlying cause, a fibroproliferative phase ensues and causes progressive pulmonary fibrosis. It is frequently associated with other organ dysfunction as part of MOF. The term ARDS is often limited to patients requiring ventilatory support on the ICU, but less severe forms, conventionally referred to as acute lung injury (ALI) and with similar pathology, occur on acute medical and surgical wards.

8.7 Conditions predisposing to ARDS

Inhalation (direct)

- Aspiration of gastric contents
- Toxic gases/burn injury
- Pneumonia
- Blunt chest trauma
- Near-drowning

Blood-borne (indirect)

- Sepsis
- Necrotic tissue (particularly bowel)
- Multiple trauma
- Pancreatitis
- Cardiopulmonary bypass
- Severe burns
- Drugs (heroin, barbiturates, thiazides)
- Major transfusion reaction
- Anaphylaxis (wasp or bee stings, snake venom)
- Fat embolism
- Carcinomatosis
- Obstetric crises (amniotic fluid embolus, eclampsia)

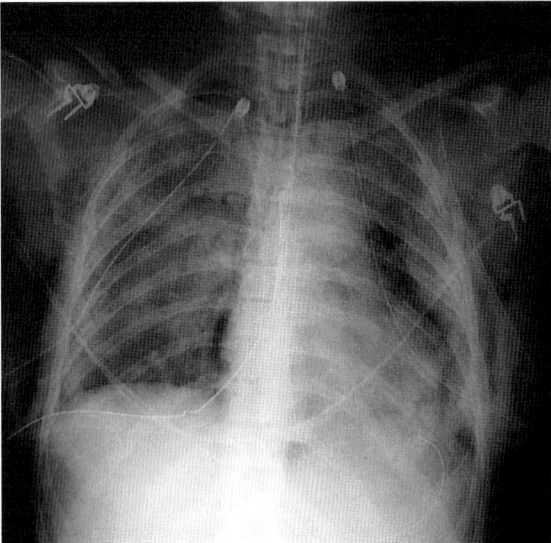

Fig. 8.5 Chest X-ray in acute respiratory distress syndrome (ARDS). This 22-year-old woman was involved in a road traffic accident. Note bilateral lung infiltrates, pneumomediastinum, pneumothoraces with bilateral chest drains, surgical emphysema, and fractures of the ribs, right clavicle and left scapula.

The clinical symptoms and signs are not specific, sharing many features with other pulmonary conditions. The criteria defining ARDS are:

- hypoxaemia, defined as $PaO_2/FiO_2 < 26.7$ kPa (< 200 mmHg) or < 40 kPa (< 300 mmHg) for ALI
- chest X-ray showing diffuse bilateral infiltrates (Fig. 8.5)
- absence of a raised left atrial pressure: pulmonary artery 'wedge' pressure (PAWP) < 15 mmHg
- impaired lung compliance.

The term ARDS has severe limitations as a diagnostic label since, like jaundice or a raised CVP, it represents a response to a variety of primary conditions.

Acute kidney injury

Acute renal failure has been renamed 'acute kidney injury' (AKI), defined as an abrupt and sustained decrease in kidney function (Box 8.8). AKI in the critically ill patient is often due to pre-renal elements such as hypovolaemia, hypotension and ischaemia resulting in reduced renal DO_2. Sepsis is often present. Potentially nephrotoxic drugs liable to contribute to AKI include non-steroidal anti-inflammatory drugs (NSAIDs), angiotensin-converting enzyme (ACE) inhibitors, angiotensin II receptor antagonists, radiological contrast media and some antibiotics. Oliguria is frequently an early sign of systemic problems in critical illness and successful resuscitation is associated with restoration of good urine output, an improving acid–base balance and correction of plasma potassium, urea and creatinine.

Oliguria is also a normal physiological component of the stress response to major surgery, and care should be taken not to overfill the post-operative patient with oliguria who is otherwise cardiovascularly and biochemically well.

In any patient with AKI, renal tract obstruction (including a blocked urinary catheter) must be excluded. Acute glomerulonephritis and vasculitis associated with connective tissue diseases such as microscopic polyarteritis or Goodpasture's disease must always be considered and appropriate investigations such as urine microscopy and immunopathological tests (p. 484) must be carried out early.

8.8 Diagnostic criteria for acute kidney injury*

An abrupt (within 48 hours) decline in kidney function defined as:
- An absolute increase in serum creatinine of ≥ 26.4 μmol/L (0.3 mg/dL)
- A percentage increase in serum creatinine of $\geq 50\%$ (1.5-fold from baseline)
- A reduction in urine output (documented oliguria of < 0.5 mL/kg for > 6 consecutive hours)

*Mehta R, et al. http://ccforum.com/content/11/2/R31.

Neurological failure (coma)

Impaired consciousness or coma is often an early feature of severe systemic illness (Box 8.9). Prompt assessment of conscious level and management of airway, breathing and circulation are essential to prevent further brain injury, to allow diagnosis and to permit definitive treatment to be instituted. Any patient with confusion or reduced conscious level should have blood sugar measured and hypoglycaemia treated.

Impairment of conscious level is graded using the GCS, which is also used to monitor progress. Although necessarily limited, targeted neurological examination is very important in the unconscious patient. Pupil size and reaction to light, presence or absence of neck stiffness, focal neurological signs and evidence of other organ impairment should be noted. After cardiorespiratory stability is achieved, the cause of the coma must be sought from history (family, witness, general practitioner), examination and investigation, particularly computed tomography (CT) of the brain. The possibility of drug overdose should always be considered.

Sepsis

Any or all of the features of SIRS (see Box 8.3, p. 184) may be present, together with an obvious focus of infection, such as purulent sputum with chest X-ray shadowing

8.9 Causes of coma

Systemic causes

Cerebral hypoxia; hypercapnia
- Respiratory failure

Cerebral ischaemia
- Cardiac arrest
- Hypotension

Metabolic disturbance
- Diabetes mellitus
  Hypoglycaemia
  Ketoacidosis
  Hyperosmolar coma
- Hyponatraemia
- Myxoedema coma
- Uraemia
- Hepatic failure
- Hypothermia
- Drugs
- Sepsis

Primary neurological causes

Trauma
- Cerebral contusion
- Extradural haematoma
- Subdural haematoma

Infection
- Cerebral abscess
- Encephalitis
- Meningitis

Cerebrovascular disease
- Intracerebral haemorrhage
- Brain-stem infarction
- Subarachnoid haemorrhage
- Cerebral venous sinus thrombosis

Cerebral tumour

Epilepsy

Hydrocephalus

or erythema around an intravenous line. However, severe sepsis may present with unexplained hypotension (i.e. septic shock), and the speed of onset may mimic a major pulmonary embolus or myocardial infarction.

Box 8.10 gives the common sites of infection in critically ill patients and appropriate investigations to consider. The most important objective is to identify and treat the underlying cause.

The patient may be admitted with infection from home ('community-acquired') or develop infection after admission ('nosocomial'). The likely causative micro-organism and antibiotic sensitivities will depend on this and direct the initial choice of antibiotics. Initial investigations include:
- cultures of blood, sputum, intravascular lines, urine and any wound discharge
- ABGs, plasma lactate, coagulation profile
- urinalysis
- chest X-ray.

Only 10% of ICU patients with a clinical diagnosis of 'septic' shock will have positive blood cultures, due to prior antibiotic treatment and the fact that an inflammatory state is not always due to infection. Specific investigations will be driven by the history and examination (see Box 8.10).

Nosocomial infections are an increasing problem in critical care units (Box 8.11). Cross-infection is a major concern, particularly with meticillin-resistant *Staphylococcus aureus* (MRSA), multidrug-resistant Gram-negative organisms and *Clostridium difficile*. If cross-infection occurs frequently, it should prompt a review of the unit's infection control policies. The most important preventive measure is thorough hand-washing before and after every patient contact (p. 145). The choice of broad-spectrum antibiotics used may influence the development of *C. difficile*-induced pseudomembranous colitis. Limiting antibiotic use helps to prevent the emergence of multidrug-resistant bacteria.

8.10 Sites of infection in critically ill patients

Sites of infection	Investigations and comments
Major	
Intravenous lines (particularly central)	Always suspect; if the patient develops evidence of sepsis and lines have not been changed for > 4 days, they must be replaced
Lungs	High risk of nosocomial pneumonia in intubated patients; after being in ICU for > 3–4 days, particularly if treated with antibiotics, the nasopharynx becomes colonised with Gram-negative bacteria which migrate to the lower respiratory tract. Prophylaxis with both parenteral and enteral antibiotics (selective decontamination of the digestive tract) reduces the incidence of nosocomial pneumonia
Abdomen	Consider intra-abdominal abscess or necrotic gut in patients who have had abdominal surgery. Pancreatitis, acute cholecystitis or perforated peptic ulcer may develop as a complication of critical illness. Ultrasound, CT, aspiration of collections of fluid/pus and laparotomy may be required
Urinary tract	Always culture a catheter specimen of urine in unexplained sepsis, although the lower urinary tract is a relatively unusual source
Other	
Heart valves	Transthoracic or transoesophageal echocardiogram
Meninges	Lumbar puncture but check coagulation and platelet count first
Joints and bones	X-ray, gallium or technetium white cell scan
Nasal sinuses, ears, retropharyngeal space	Clinical examination, plain X-ray, CT
Genitourinary tract (particularly post-partum)	Per vaginam examination, ultrasound
Gastrointestinal tract	Per rectum examination, stool culture, *Clostridium difficile* toxin, sigmoidoscopy

8

8.11 Risk factors for nosocomial infection

- Invasive ventilation
- Trauma
- Invasive catheters: i.v., urinary, nasogastric tubes
- Stress ulcer prophylaxis with H_2-antagonists
- Prolonged length of stay

Disseminated intravascular coagulation (DIC)

Also known as consumptive coagulopathy, this is an acquired disorder of haemostasis (p. 1050); it is common in critically ill patients and often heralds the onset of MOF. It is characterised by an increase in prothrombin time, partial thromboplastin time and fibrin degradation products, and a fall in platelets and fibrinogen. The clinically dominant feature may be widespread bleeding from vascular access points, gastrointestinal tract, bronchial tree and surgical wound sites, or widespread microvascular and even macrovascular thrombosis. Management is supportive with infusions of fresh frozen plasma and platelets, while the underlying cause is treated.

GENERAL PRINCIPLES OF CRITICAL CARE MANAGEMENT

Essential aspects of the management of critically ill patients on admission to the ICU are shown in Box 8.12.

8.12 Management of patients on admission to ICU

- Handover from transferring team to ICU staff
- Full clinical assessment
- Ongoing resuscitation/stabilisation
- Establishment of monitoring
- Review of medical and social history
- Communication (including explanation) with relatives
- Investigations to establish or confirm the definitive diagnosis
- Formulation and implementation of a management plan

Monitoring

Monitoring in ICU represents a mixture of clinical and automated recordings. Electrocardiogram (ECG), SpO_2 (oxygen saturation derived from a pulse oximeter), BP (generally invasive arterial pressure) and usually CVP are established at an early stage, and recordings made at least hourly, on either a 24-hour chart or a computerised system. All invasive haemodynamic monitoring should be referenced to the mid-axillary line as 'zero'. Urine output is a sensitive measure of renal perfusion and early catheterisation is required in most patients. Clinical monitoring is particularly important. Physical signs such as respiratory rate, the appearance of the patient, restlessness, conscious level and indices of peripheral perfusion (pale, cold skin; delayed capillary refill in the nailbed) are just as important as a set of blood gases or monitor readings.

Monitoring the circulation

Electrocardiogram (ECG)

Standard monitors display a single-lead ECG, record heart rate and identify rhythm changes. More sophisticated machines can print out rhythm strips and monitor ST segment shift, which may be useful in patients with ischaemic heart disease.

Blood pressure

In critically ill patients, continuous intra-arterial monitoring is necessary, using a line placed in the radial artery (or the femoral in vasoconstricted patients or where access is difficult). Remember that, when there is systemic vasoconstriction, the mean arterial pressure (MAP) may be normal or even high, although the cardiac output is low. Conversely, if there is peripheral vasodilatation, as in sepsis, the MAP may be low, although the cardiac output is high.

Central venous pressure (CVP)

CVP or right atrial pressure (RAP) is monitored using a catheter inserted via either the internal jugular or the subclavian vein, with the distal end sited in the upper right atrium. The CVP may help in assessing the need for intravascular fluid replacement and the rate at which this should be given (Box 8.13). If the CVP is low in the presence of a low MAP or cardiac output, fluid resuscitation is necessary. However, a raised level does not necessarily mean that the patient is adequately volume-resuscitated. Right heart function, pulmonary artery pressure, intrathoracic pressure and venous 'tone' also influence CVP, and may lead to a raised CVP even when the patient is hypovolaemic (see Box 8.1, p. 180). In addition, positive pressure ventilation raises intrathoracic pressure and causes marked swings in atrial pressures and systemic BP in time with respiration. Pressure measurements should be recorded at end-expiration.

In severe hypovolaemia, the RAP may be sustained by peripheral venoconstriction, and transfusion may initially produce little or no change in the CVP (see Fig. 8.1, p. 181).

8.13 Central venous pressure

Normal	0–5 mmHg
Target (usual) of volume resuscitation	6–10 mmHg
Normal if ventilated	5–10 mmHg
Target of volume resuscitation if ventilated	10–15 mmHg

Pulmonary artery catheterisation and pulmonary artery 'wedge' pressure (PAWP)

In most situations, the CVP is an adequate guide to the filling pressures of both sides of the heart. However, certain conditions, such as pulmonary hypertension or right ventricular dysfunction, may lead to raised CVP levels, even in the presence of hypovolaemia. If this is the case, it may be appropriate to insert a pulmonary artery flotation catheter (Fig. 8.6) so that pulmonary artery pressure and PAWP, which approximates to left atrial pressure, can be measured.

The mean PAWP normally lies between 6 and 12 mmHg (measured from the mid-axillary line), but

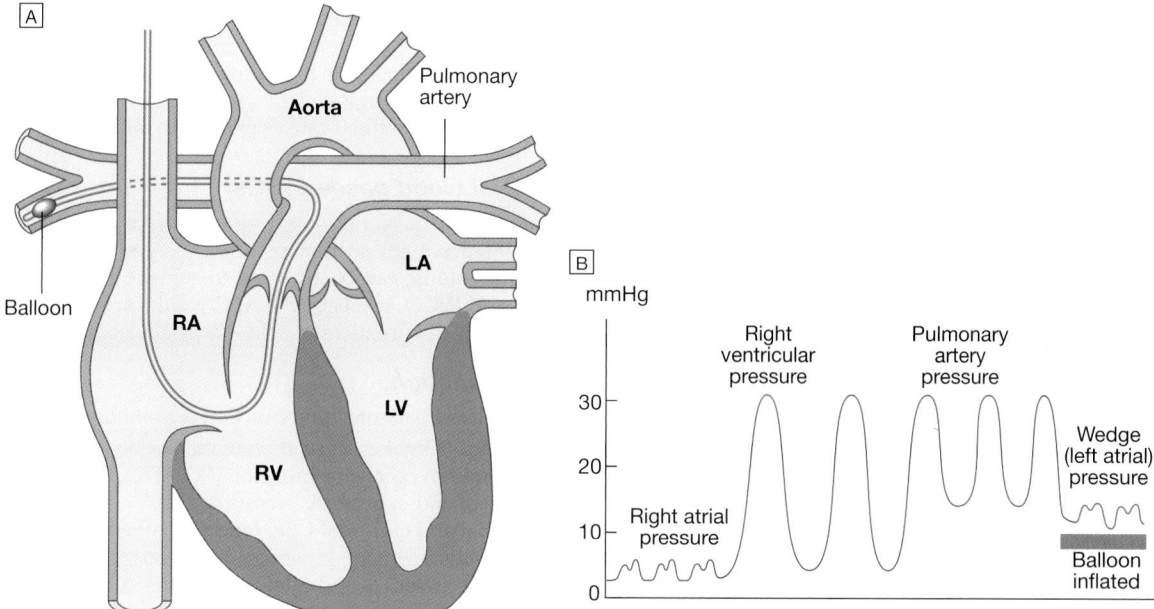

Fig. 8.6 A pulmonary artery catheter. **A** There is a small balloon at the tip of the catheter and pressure can be measured through the central lumen. The catheter is inserted via an internal jugular, subclavian or femoral vein and advanced through the right heart until its tip lies in the pulmonary artery. When the balloon is deflated, the pulmonary artery pressure can be recorded. **B** Advancing the catheter with the balloon inflated will 'wedge' the catheter in the pulmonary artery. In this position blood cannot flow past the balloon, so the tip of the catheter will now record the pressure transmitted from the pulmonary veins and left atrium. This is known as the pulmonary artery wedge pressure and provides an indirect measure of the left atrial pressure. (LA = left atrium; LV = left ventricle; RA = right atrium; RV = right ventricle)

in left heart failure it may be grossly elevated and even exceed 30 mmHg. Provided the pulmonary capillary membranes are intact, the optimum PAWP when managing acute circulatory failure in the critically ill patient is generally 12–15 mmHg because this will ensure good left ventricular filling without risking hydrostatic pulmonary oedema.

Pulmonary artery catheters also allow measurement of cardiac output and sampling of blood from the pulmonary artery ('mixed venous' samples), allowing continuous monitoring of the mixed venous oxygen saturation (SvO_2) by oximetry. Measurement of SvO_2 gives an indication of the adequacy of cardiac output (and hence DO_2) in relation to the body's metabolic requirements and is especially useful in low cardiac output states.

Cardiac output

Measurement of cardiac output is important particularly where large doses of vasopressor are being administered, where there is underlying cardiac disease (acute or chronic), and where volume resuscitation and vasoactive drug therapy are not achieving resolution of lactic acidosis or oliguria. It is most accurately measured by techniques which use an indicator dilution method. Most PA catheters incorporate a heating element, which raises blood temperature at frequent intervals, with the resultant temperature change detected by a thermistor at the tip of the catheter.

Oesophageal Doppler ultrasonography provides a rapid and clinically useful assessment of volume status and cardiac performance to guide early fluid and vasoactive therapy. A 6 mm probe is inserted into the distal oesophagus, allowing continuous monitoring of the aortic flow signal from the descending aorta

(Fig. 8.7). Using the stroke distance (area under velocity/time waveform) and a correction factor that incorporates the patient's age, height and weight, an estimate of left ventricular stroke volume and hence cardiac output can be made. Peak velocity is an indicator of left ventricular performance, while flow time is an indicator of left ventricular filling and peripheral resistance.

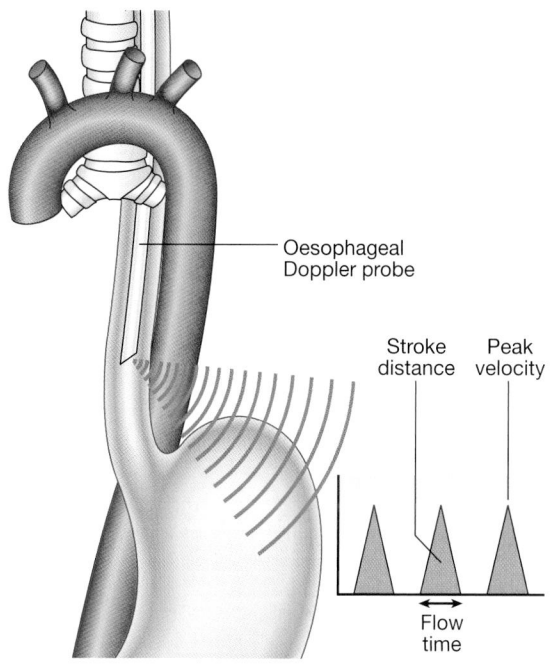

Fig. 8.7 Oesophageal Doppler ultrasonography.

Analysis of arterial pressure waveform is another means of continuously estimating cardiac output, and can be calibrated either by transpulmonary thermodilution (PiCCO) or lithium dilution methods (LidCO). The Vigileo/Flotrac system derives cardiac output from arterial pressure waveform analysis with no external calibration.

Urine output

This is a sensitive measure of renal perfusion, provided that the kidneys are not damaged (e.g. ATN) or affected by drugs (e.g. diuretics, dopamine), and can be monitored accurately if a urinary catheter is in place. Output is measured hourly and the lower limit of normal is 0.5 mL/hr/kg body weight. It is not measured in real time and reflects renal perfusion over the hours preceding measurement.

Peripheral skin temperature

In general, resuscitation is not complete until the patient's feet are warm and well perfused.

Blood lactate, hydrogen ion and base excess/deficit

Acid–base balance is discussed on page 442. Base excess or deficit is calculated as the difference between the patient's bicarbonate and the normal bicarbonate after the PCO_2 has been maintained in the blood gas machine at 5.33 kPa (40 mmHg). This is especially useful in critically ill patients as it describes the underlying metabolic status independently of the current respiratory status. A metabolic acidosis with base deficit > 5 mmol/L requires investigation (p. 443). It often indicates increased lactic acid production in poorly perfused, hypoxic tissues and impaired lactate metabolism due to poor hepatic perfusion. Serial lactate measurements may therefore be helpful in monitoring tissue perfusion and the response to treatment. Other conditions, such as acute renal failure, ketoacidosis and poisoning, may be the cause (p. 443). Large-volume infusions of fluids containing sodium chloride may lead to a hyperchloraemic acidosis.

Monitoring respiratory function

Oxygen saturation (SpO_2)

This is measured by a probe, attached to a finger or earlobe. Spectrophotometric analysis determines the relative proportions of saturated and desaturated haemoglobin.

8.14 Causes of sudden changes in oxygen saturations

Patient factors

- Bronchospasm
- Lung collapse due to thick secretions blocking the proximal bronchial tree
- Pneumothorax
- Circulatory collapse causing a poor signal due to impaired peripheral perfusion

Equipment factors

- Displacement of the endotracheal tube (extubation, endobronchial intubation)
- Blockage of the endotracheal tube
- Disconnection from the ventilator
- Oxygen supply failure
- Error, e.g. detached probe

It is unreliable if peripheral perfusion is poor and may produce erroneous results in the presence of nail polish, excessive movement or high ambient light. In general, arterial oxygenation is satisfactory if SpO_2 is > 90%. Box 8.14 gives the potential causes of sudden falls in SpO_2.

Arterial blood gases (ABGs)

These are usually measured several times a day in a ventilated patient so that inspired oxygen (FiO_2) and minute volume can be adjusted to achieve the desired PaO_2 and $PaCO_2$ respectively. ABG results are also used to monitor disturbances of acid–base balance (Ch. 16).

Lung function

In ventilated patients, lung function is monitored by:

- arterial PO_2 taken in relation to the fractional inspired oxygen concentration (PO_2/FiO_2 ratio) and level of end-expiratory pressure
- arterial and end-tidal CO_2, reflecting alveolar ventilation
- airway pressures and tidal volumes reflecting lung compliance and airways resistance.

Capnography

The CO_2 concentration in inspired gas is zero, but during expiration, after clearing the physiological dead space, it rises progressively to reach a plateau which represents the alveolar or end-tidal CO_2 concentration. This cyclical change in CO_2 concentration, or capnogram, is measured using an infrared sensor inserted between the ventilator tubing and the endotracheal tube. In normal lungs, the end-tidal CO_2 closely mirrors $PaCO_2$, and can be used to assess the adequacy of alveolar ventilation. However, its use is limited, as there may be marked discrepancies in lung disease or impaired pulmonary perfusion (e.g. due to hypovolaemia). In combination with the gas flow and respiratory cycle data from the ventilator, CO_2 production and hence metabolic rate may be calculated. In clinical practice, end-tidal CO_2 is used to confirm correct placement of an endotracheal tube, in the management of head injury, and during the transport of ventilated patients.

Transcutaneous PCO_2

Monitors now exist which measure transcutaneous PCO_2, usually using an earlobe probe which incorporates both pulse oximeter and CO_2 electrode. The transcutaneous PCO_2 closely approximates to $PaCO_2$ and gives continuous monitoring, which is useful in patients with no arterial cannula but who require close monitoring: for example, during ventilatory weaning (see below).

Daily clinical management in the ICU

Regular clinical examination is essential if changes in a patient's condition are to be recognised. Detailed clinical examination is performed at least daily, with additional focused and systematic assessment on ward rounds at least twice daily:

- Review of progress reports from ICU nursing and medical staff, and any specialist opinions.
- Review of 24-hour charts.
- Examination: general (including skin, line sites, wounds etc.) and specific:

cardiovascular, including haemodynamics, fluids and inotropes

respiratory, including ventilator settings and ABGs

gastrointestinal, including nutrition (calorie, protein intake, route), nasogastric aspirate and bowel function

renal, including urine output, overall fluid balance, urea and electrolytes, and renal replacement therapy

neurological, including sedation level, GCS and pupil responses where appropriate.

- Laboratory results: haematology, including coagulation, and biochemistry.
- Microbiology: temperature, white blood count, line sites and other possible sources of infection, results of cultures, antibiotic therapy.
- Drug therapy: review with pharmacist, consider side-effects and interactions, and identify therapy that can be discontinued.
- Imaging: review X-rays and other specialist investigations.
- Monitoring: are all measures still required?
- Management plan: formulate an integrated plan, with specific goals for each organ system.

Sedation and analgesia

Intensive care is an extremely stressful experience for the patient, with pain, discomfort and anxiety related to endotracheal intubation, invasive monitoring and other procedures.

Sedation is required for most patients in order to relieve anxiety, allow tolerance of an endotracheal tube, mechanical ventilation and invasive procedures, and control intracranial pressure in neurological disease. The level of sedation can usually be lightened as the ICU stay progresses. Over-sedation is a common occurrence, and can delay weaning from ventilation and prolong ICU stay. Daily sedation 'pauses' can allow better patient assessment, prevent sedative accumulation and have been shown to reduce ICU stay.

Standard sedation consists of a mixture of either the short-acting anaesthetic agent propofol or the benzodiazepine midazolam, and an opioid analgesic, traditionally morphine. Morphine is metabolised to the active metabolite morphine-6-glucuronide, which accumulates in renal failure; alfentanil is a good alternative in MOF, and for patients in whom frequent neurological assessment is essential.

Analgesia is required to relieve post-operative and other pain.

Muscle relaxants

Muscle relaxants are used less now than previously. They are required to facilitate endotracheal intubation, to facilitate ventilation in patients with critical oxygenation and/or poor lung compliance, and to aid control of critically increased intracranial pressure.

Delirium

Delirium is a feature of severe illness, especially when patients are subjected to major organ dysfunction, metabolic derangement and polypharmacy. Haloperidol in 2.5–5 mg doses (i.v.) and the α_2-adrenergic agonist clonidine are useful in immediate management.

MANAGEMENT OF MAJOR ORGAN FAILURE

Circulatory support

The primary goals (Box 8.15) are to:
- Restore global oxygen delivery (DO_2) by ensuring adequate cardiac output.
- Maintain an MAP that ensures adequate perfusion of vital organs. The target will be patient-specific depending on pre-morbid factors (e.g. hypertension or coronary artery disease) and may range from 60 to 90 mmHg.

The first objective is to ensure that an 'appropriate' ventricular preload is restored. Vasoactive drugs should *not* be used as a substitute for adequate volume resuscitation.

Therapeutic options to optimise cardiac function

If the cardiac output is inadequate and myocardial contractility is poor, the available treatment options are to:

8.15 Initial management of circulatory collapse

Correct hypoxaemia

- Oxygen therapy
- Consider ventilation
  Intractable hypoxaemia
  Hypercapnia: $PaCO_2$ > 6.7 kPa (50 mmHg)
  Respiratory distress
  Impaired conscious level

Assess circulation

- Heart rate
- BP: direct arterial pressure
- CVP
- Peripheral perfusion

Optimise volume status

- Fluid challenge(s)
  CVP < 6 mmHg: 250 mL 0.9% saline or colloid
  CVP > 6 mmHg or poor ventricular function suspected:
  100 mL boluses and consider measuring cardiac output,
  e.g. PA catheter or oesophageal Doppler

Optimise haemoglobin concentration

- 70–90 g/L; 100 g/L if ischaemic heart disease
- Red cells as required
- Septic patients can become profoundly anaemic with crystalloid/colloid resuscitation due to haemodilution and require blood transfusion

Achieve target BP

- Use vasopressor/inotrope once hypovolaemia is corrected

Achieve adequate CO and DO_2

- Inotropic agent if fluid alone inadequate

Other measures

- Establish monitoring, including invasive measures, as resuscitation starts
- Trends in haemodynamics, ABG, H+, base deficit and lactate guide further treatment

- *Reduce afterload.* This can be achieved by using an arteriolar dilator (e.g. nitrates), which may be limited by the consequent fall in systemic pressure. A counterpulsation balloon pump offers the ideal physiological treatment because it reduces LV afterload while increasing cardiac output, diastolic pressure and coronary perfusion; it is particularly valuable in treating myocardial ischaemia.
- *Increase preload.* If there is significant impairment of myocardial contractility, giving intravascular volume to increase filling pressures will only produce a small increase in stroke volume and cardiac output, and risks precipitating pulmonary oedema.
- *Improve myocardial contractility.* An inotrope may be required to ensure adequate cardiac output and peripheral blood flow sufficient to secure adequate oxygen delivery. Box 8.16 lists some characteristics of the commonly used vasoactive agents.
- *Control heart rate and rhythm* (pp. 559–577). The optimum heart rate is usually between 90 and 110 per minute. Correction of low serum potassium and magnesium concentrations should be the first stage in treating tachyarrhythmias in the critically ill. Atrial fibrillation is particularly common and troublesome in septic and critically ill patients; intravenous amiodarone 300 mg over 30–60 minutes, followed by 900 mg over 24 hours, can be successful in controlling ventricular rate and in restoring and maintaining sinus rhythm.

The management of tamponade and pulmonary embolism is described on pages 639 and 719 respectively. Circulatory support in the context of sepsis is described below.

Respiratory support

Respiratory support is indicated to maintain the patency of the airway, correct hypoxaemia and hypercapnia (Boxes 8.17 and 8.18), and reduce the work of breathing. It ranges from oxygen therapy by facemask, through non-invasive techniques such as continuous positive airways pressure (CPAP) and non-invasive positive pressure ventilation (NIV), to invasive ventilation via an endotracheal tube or tracheostomy (Box 8.19).

Oxygen therapy

Oxygen is given to treat hypoxaemia and ensure adequate arterial oxygenation (SpO_2 > 90%). It should initially be given by facemask or nasal cannulae and the inspired oxygen concentration (FiO_2) can then be adjusted according to the results of pulse oximetry and ABG analysis. The risk of progressive hypercapnia in patients with COPD who are dependent on hypoxic drive has been overstated. If administration of oxygen to ensure SpO_2 > 90% results in unacceptable hypercapnia, the patient requires some form of mechanical respiratory support. The theoretical risks of oxygen toxicity are not relevant if the patient is acutely hypoxaemic. It is vital to maintain cerebral oxygenation even at the risk of pulmonary toxicity because hypoxic cerebral damage is irreversible. More detail on oxygen therapy is given on page 660.

Non-invasive respiratory support

If a patient remains hypoxaemic on high-concentration oxygen, other measures are required to improve oxygenation and to reduce the work of breathing. If the patient has respiratory failure associated with decreased lung volume, application of CPAP by mask or hood (see Box 8.19)

8.16 Circulatory effects of commonly used vasoactive drug infusions

Drug	Receptor activity	Cardiac contractility	Heart rate	BP	Cardiac output	Splanchnic blood flow	SVR	PVR
Dopamine								
< 5 µg/kg/min	DA_1, β_1, α	↑	→/↑	→/↑	↑	→/↑	→/↑	→/↑
> 5 µg/kg/min	β_1, α, DA_1, β_2	↑↑	↑	↑	↑↑	→	↑	↑
Adrenaline (epinephrine)	β_1, α, β_2	↑↑	↑	↑↑	↑↑↑	↓	↑	↑
Noradrenaline (norepinephrine)	α, β_1	→/↑	→/↓	↑↑	→/↓	→/↓	↑↑	↑↑
Isoprenaline	β_1, β_2	↑	↑↑	→/↓	↑	→/↑	→/↓	↓
Dobutamine	β_1, β_2, α	↑	↑	→/↓	↑↑	→	↓	↓
Dopexamine	β_2, DA_1, DA_2	↑	↑↑	→/↓	↑	↑	↓	↓
Glyceryl trinitrate	NO	→	↑	↓	↑	↑	↓	↓
Nitroprusside	NO	→	↑	↓	↑	↑	↓	↓
Epoprostenol	Prostacyclin	→	↑	↓	↑	↑	↓	↓
Milrinone	PDEI	→/↑	↑	↓	↑↑	↑	↓	↓

Receptors through which each drug works are listed in order of the extent of receptor stimulation produced. The global circulatory effects listed are guidelines only. The magnitude of the response will depend on the circulatory state of the patient, the dose of the drug administered, and the receptor distribution and density in specific vascular beds. Dopamine acts more like adrenaline at high doses.
(α = α-adrenoceptor; β_1, β_2 = β-adrenoceptors 1 and 2; DA_1, DA_2 = dopaminergic receptors 1 and 2; NO = acts via local nitric oxide release; PDEI = phosphodiesterase inhibitor; PVR = pulmonary vascular resistance; SVR = systemic vascular resistance.)

8.17 Clinical conditions requiring mechanical ventilation*

Post-operative
- e.g. After major abdominal or cardiac surgery

Respiratory failure
- ARDS
- Pneumonia
- COPD
- Acute severe asthma
- Aspiration
- Smoke inhalation, burns

Circulatory failure
- Low cardiac output: cardiogenic shock
- Pulmonary oedema
- Following cardiac arrest

Neurological disease
- Coma of any cause
- Status epilepticus
- Drug overdose
- Respiratory muscle failure (e.g. Guillain–Barré syndrome, poliomyelitis, myasthenia gravis)
- Head injury: to avoid hypoxaemia and hypercapnia, and reduce intracranial pressure
- Bulbar abnormalities causing risk of aspiration (e.g. cerebrovascular accident, myasthenia gravis)

Multiple trauma

* Additional considerations:
  Metabolic rate: ventilatory requirements rise as metabolic rate increases
  Nutritional reserve: low potassium or phosphate reduces respiratory muscle power
  Condition of the abdomen: distension due to surgery or tense ascites causes discomfort and splinting of the diaphragm, compromising spontaneous respiratory effort and promoting bilateral basal lung collapse.

8.18 Indications for tracheal intubation and mechanical ventilation

- Protection of airway
- Respiratory arrest or rate < 8/min
- Tachypnoea > 35/min
- Inability to tolerate oxygen mask/CPAP/NIV, e.g. agitation, confusion
- Removal of secretions
- Hypoxaemia ($PaO_2 < 8$ kPa (< 60 mmHg); $SpO_2 < 90\%$) despite CPAP with $FiO_2 > 0.6$
- Hypercapnia if conscious level impaired or risk of raised intracranial pressure
- Worsening respiratory acidosis
- Vital capacity falling below 1.2 L in patients with neuromuscular disease
- Removing the work of breathing in exhausted patients

8.19 Modes and terms used in mechanical ventilatory support

Intermittent positive pressure ventilation (IPPV)
- Generic term for all types of positive pressure ventilation

Controlled mandatory ventilation (CMV)
- Most basic form of ventilation; may be volume- or pressure-controlled
- Pre-set rate and tidal volume or pressure
- Assist/control mode allows patient triggering of full ventilator breaths
- Appropriate for initial control of patients with little respiratory drive, severe lung injury or circulatory instability

Synchronised intermittent mandatory ventilation (SIMV)
- Pre-set rate of mandatory breaths generally with pre-set tidal volume
- Allows spontaneous breaths between mandatory breaths
- Spontaneous breaths may be pressure-supported (PS)
- Allows patient to settle on ventilator with less sedation

Pressure-controlled ventilation (PCV)
- Pre-set rate; pre-set inspiratory pressure; pre-set inspiratory time
- Tidal volume depends on pre-set pressure, lung compliance and airways resistance
- Used in management of severe acute respiratory failure to avoid high airway pressure, often with prolonged inspiratory to expiratory ratio (pressure-controlled inverse ratio ventilation, PCIRV)

Pressure support ventilation (PSV)/Assisted spontaneous breathing (ASB)
- Breaths are triggered by patient; spontaneous cycling to expiration
- Provides positive pressure to augment patient's breaths; useful for weaning
- Usually combined with CPAP; may be combined with SIMV
- Pressure support is titrated against tidal volume and respiratory rate

Positive end-expiratory pressure (PEEP)
- Positive airway pressure applied during expiratory phase in patients receiving mechanical ventilation
- Improves oxygenation by recruiting atelectatic or oedematous lung

Continuous positive airways pressure (CPAP)
- Positive airway pressure applied throughout the respiratory cycle, via either an endotracheal tube or a tight-fitting facemask or a hood
- Fresh gas flow must exceed patient's peak inspiratory flow (> 30–40 L/min) to maintain positive pressure
- Improves oxygenation by recruitment of atelectatic or oedematous lung
- Mask CPAP discourages coughing and clearance of lung secretions; may increase the risk of aspiration

Bi-level positive airway pressure (BiPAP/BIPAP)
- Two levels of positive airway pressure (higher level in inspiration)
- In fully ventilated patients, BIPAP is essentially the same as PCV with PEEP
- If used non-invasively, BiPAP is essentially PSV with CPAP

Non-invasive positive pressure ventilation (NIPPV/NIV)
- Most modes of ventilation may be applied via a facemask or nasal mask
- Usually PSV/BiPAP (typically 15–20 cmH$_2$O) often with back-up mandatory rate
- Indications include acute exacerbations of COPD

will both improve oxygenation by recruitment of under-ventilated alveoli, and reduce the work of breathing by improving lung compliance. CPAP is most successful in clinical situations where alveoli are readily recruited, such as in pulmonary oedema and post-operative collapse/atelectasis. It is also helpful in correcting hypoxaemia in pneumonia, especially in immunocompromised patients. The risk of nosocomial infection is reduced by avoiding endotracheal intubation. A CPAP mask often becomes uncomfortable and gastric distension may occur; the Castar hood which fits tightly around the neck enclosing the patient's head in a clear plastic hood is much better tolerated (Fig. 8.8). Patients must be cooperative, be able to protect their airway, and have the strength to breathe spontaneously and cough effectively. Failure to improve clinically after 48–72 hours or more of CPAP is a case for consideration of invasive ventilation.

8

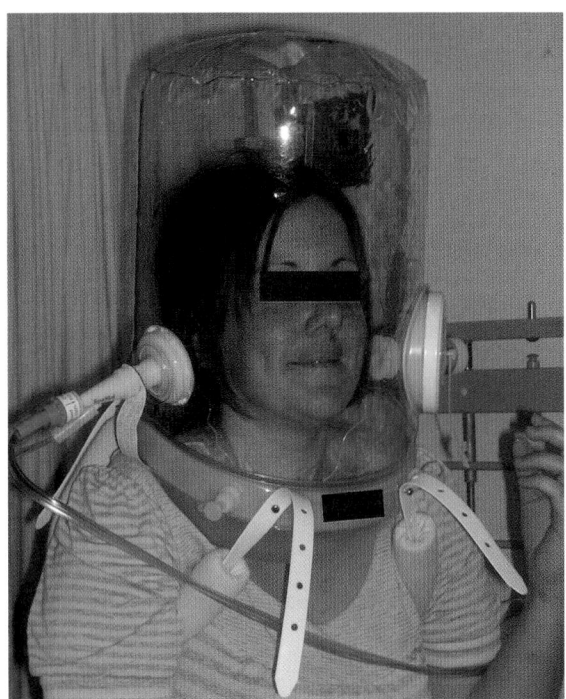

Fig. 8.8 CPAP delivery with a Castar hood.

Non-invasive ventilation (NIV) refers to ventilatory support by nasal or full facemask. NIV can be delivered by a simple bi-level (BiPAP) turbine ventilator which delivers a higher pressure (approximately 15–25 cmH$_2$O) for inspiration and a lower pressure (4–10 cmH$_2$O) to allow expiration. A simple breathing circuit with a leak rather than an expiratory valve is generally used, and ventilation can be spontaneous (PSV) or timed (PCV). In more seriously hypoxaemic patients, NIV can be delivered using a complex ICU ventilator which allows higher oxygen concentrations to be administered. NIV has been shown to improve the outcome of patients with type 2 respiratory failure secondary to acute exacerbation of COPD, and in hypercapnia associated with left ventricular failure and pulmonary oedema. It may also be used during weaning from conventional invasive ventilation, either electively to facilitate earlier extubation, notably in COPD, or after failed extubation with a view to prevention of re-intubation. As with mask CPAP, NIV requires the patient to be conscious and cooperative.

Endotracheal intubation and mechanical ventilation

Over 60% of patients appropriately admitted to ICU require endotracheal intubation and mechanical ventilation, mostly for respiratory failure (see Boxes 8.18 and 8.19). The final decision to perform tracheal intubation and ventilate a patient should be taken on clinical grounds rather than depending on the results of investigations, such as ABG.

In the conscious patient, intubation requires induction of anaesthesia and muscle relaxation, while in more obtunded patients, sedation alone may be adequate. This can be hazardous in the critically ill patient with respiratory and often cardiovascular failure.

Capnography should be used to confirm correct endotracheal tube placement. Continuous monitoring, particularly of heart rate and BP (preferably invasively), is essential and resuscitation facilities and drugs must be immediately available. Hypotension commonly follows sedation or anaesthesia because of direct cardiovascular effects of the drugs and loss of sympathetic drive; positive pressure ventilation may compound this problem by increasing intrathoracic pressure, thereby reducing venous return and hence cardiac output.

There are different types of ventilatory support (Fig. 8.9). Modern ventilators allow flexibility in the level of support from controlled mandatory ventilation to partial ventilatory support modes, and assisted spontaneous breathing which allows the ventilator to respond to patients' demands (see Box 8.19). Use of partial ventilatory support avoids the requirement for and hazards of paralysis and deep sedation, and allows the patient to be conscious and yet comfortable.

General considerations in the management of the ventilated/intubated patient

Beware of the restless patient. Try to establish the cause of the problem before simply administering sedation. Possibilities include pneumothorax, hypoxaemia, hypercapnia due to inadequate ventilation, pain, onset of sepsis, cardiac decompensation (pulmonary oedema, dysrhythmia, infarction) and proximal airway obstruction, e.g. secretions.

Patients who are breathing spontaneously adjust their ventilation to compensate for metabolic derangements; this cannot occur in patients who are ventilated using mandatory modes, so either the underlying metabolic abnormality must be corrected or appropriate changes must be made to the ventilator settings. For example, a patient with severe diabetic ketoacidosis will hyperventilate to compensate for the metabolic acidosis; if mechanical ventilation is instituted,

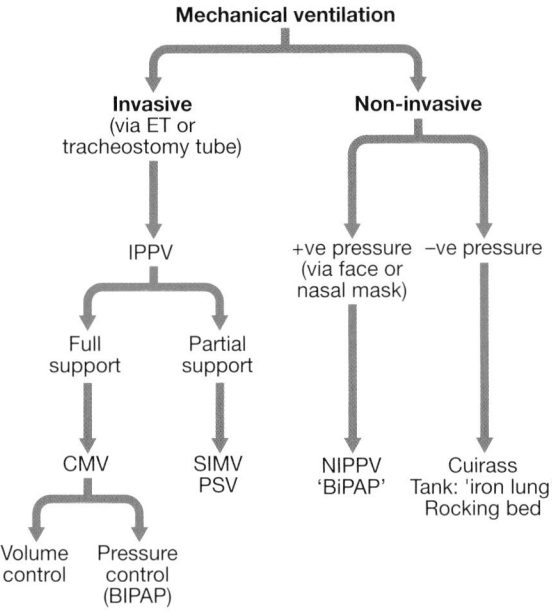

Fig. 8.9 Different types of invasive and non-invasive ventilatory support. (ET = endotracheal; see Box 8.19 for other abbreviations.)

there will be a potentially catastrophic increase in aci-daemia due to reduced minute ventilation, and this should be taken into account when choosing ventila-tor settings.

The ventilator should be set to detect:

- minimum acceptable minute volume to identify inadvertent disconnection
- maximum acceptable airway pressure to prevent barotrauma.

If in PCV mode, a minimum acceptable tidal volume should be an alarm limit.

Humidify and warm inspired gas to prevent inspis-sation of secretions, normally with a heat and moisture exchanger, but occasionally with a hot water humidi-fier. Arrange regular positioning, physiotherapy and suctioning to clear secretions and prevent proximal air-way obstruction and distal alveolar collapse. The patient should be in a 30° head-up position to avoid aspiration. A chest X-ray to check the position of the endotracheal tube following intubation is required (the appropriate position is 4 cm above the carina).

Bronchoscopy should be readily available to:

- investigate upper airways obstruction (plugging of the proximal bronchial tree by inspissated mucus is the most common cause)
- investigate lobar/segmental collapse, and aspirate mucus plug obstructing proximal bronchial tree
- assist in cases of difficult intubation or tracheostomy tube change
- obtain broncho-alveolar lavage specimens for microbiology
- identify the cause of haemoptysis (not always easy)
- exclude tracheobronchial disruption after thoracic trauma.

Ventilation strategy

The selection of ventilator mode and settings for tidal volume, respiratory rate, positive end-expiratory pressure (PEEP) and inspiratory to expiratory ratio is dependent on the cause of the respiratory failure. The objectives are to:

- improve gas exchange
- minimise damage to the lung by avoiding high lung volumes, pressures and FiO_2
- avoid adverse circulatory effects
- make the patient comfortable without heavy sedation or muscle paralysis by reducing the work of breathing and harmonising interaction between patient and ventilator.

In asthma and conditions with increased lung vol-umes (high FRC), a prolonged expiratory phase is nec-essary to prevent progressive lung over-inflation; PEEP and large tidal volumes exacerbate over-distension, produce high alveolar pressures and increase the risk of pneumothorax. High intrathoracic pressures com-promise circulatory function, particularly if there is intravascular volume depletion, so that oxygen deliv-ery may actually fall in spite of improved arterial oxygenation.

In patients with alveolar collapse (low FRC), such as those with ARDS, it is appropriate to use a prolonged inspiratory to expiratory ratio and high levels of PEEP (+10 to +15 cmH$_2$O) to recruit alveoli and improve compliance and gas exchange.

Ventilation and ARDS

Recent studies have shown that, in ARDS, damage to the lungs can be exacerbated by mechanical ventilation, possibly by over-distension of alveoli and repeated open-ing and closure of distal airways. The ventilator strategy for ARDS encompasses limiting tidal volumes and air-way pressures (Boxes 8.20 and 8.21). Other strategies which may be of benefit in severe ARDS include prone ventilation, nitric oxide inhalation and corticosteroids.

Prone positioning improves oxygenation signifi-cantly in two-thirds of patients with ARDS by reducing thoraco-abdominal compliance and the vertical pleu-ral pressure gradient so that ventilation is more evenly distributed and better matched to perfusion. Multicentre trials using manual proning have failed to show a sur-vival benefit, and trials using an automatic rotating bed are under way. Nevertheless it remains a very useful rescue therapy in patients with critical oxygenation.

Nitric oxide is a very short-acting pulmonary vaso-dilator. Delivered to the airway in concentrations of between 1 and 20 parts per million, it improves blood flow to ventilated alveoli, thus improving ventilation–perfusion matching. Oxygenation can be improved markedly in some patients but the evidence indicates that this benefit lasts for only 48 hours and outcome is not improved. Its role, like that of prone ventilation, is as a rescue therapy in patients with critical oxygenation. It may also be useful in patients with severe pulmonary hypertension.

There is conflicting evidence that corticosteroids improve outcome if given in the fibroproliferative stage of ARDS. A trial of corticosteroids may be considered if a patient has consistent gas exchange impairment and ventilator dependence at 7–10 days after diagnosis. The recommended dose of methylprednisolone is 2–3 mg/kg/day, decreasing after 7 days and as gas exchange

---

8.20 Principles of mechanical ventilation in ARDS

- Optimum ventilator settings are:
  Pressure-controlled or limited
  Small tidal volumes (ideally < 6 mL/kg)
  Long inspiratory to expiratory time
  Positive end-expiratory pressure (PEEP)
- Allow $PaCO_2$ to rise (permissive hypercapnia) and tolerate lower oxygen saturations than normal (e.g. 88–90%)
- Avoid:
  Large tidal volumes
  Airway pressure of > 35 cmH$_2$O
  FiO$_2$ of > 0.8 if possible
- Maintain a balance between improving gas exchange, minimising the risk of subsequent pulmonary fibrosis due to lung injury, and avoiding adverse circulatory effects

---

EBM **8.21 Optimal ventilation in ARDS**

'Ventilation using positive end-expiratory pressure but limiting tidal volumes to 5–7 mL/kg and accepting high $PaCO_2$ levels improves outcome in ARDS.'

- Acute Respiratory Distress Syndrome Network. N Engl J Med 2000; 342:1301–1308.

improves. Bronchoscopy and broncho-alveolar lavage should be performed to identify or exclude pulmonary infection before commencing corticosteroid therapy.

Weaning from respiratory support

This is the process of progressively reducing and eventually removing all external ventilatory support and associated apparatus. The majority of patients require mechanical ventilatory support for only a few days and do not need weaning; simple trials of spontaneous breathing via the endotracheal tube will usually indicate whether the patient can be successfully extubated or not.

In contrast, patients who have required long-term ventilatory support for severe lung disease, such as ARDS, may initially be unable to sustain even a modest degree of respiratory work because of residual decreased lung compliance and hence increased work of breathing, compounded by respiratory muscle weakness. These patients require weaning until respiratory muscle strength improves to the point that all support can be discontinued.

Weaning techniques involve the patient breathing spontaneously for increasing periods of the day and a gradual reduction in the level of ventilatory support. This often involves graduation to partial support modes and then non-invasive modes of ventilatory support.

The process of identifying patients able to progress to spontaneous breathing and extubation is carried out according to a 'weaning protocol'. This entails deciding whether a patient can be safely subjected to a spontaneous breathing trial (Box 8.22). If the patient meets these criteria, he/she undergoes the breathing trial for 2–5 minutes. The ratio of the respiratory rate to tidal volume is calculated. If it is < 105 breaths/min/L, the patient continues the trial for a further 30-minute to 2-hour period before extubation.

In the event of failure (increased respiratory rate; decreased tidal volume), gradual weaning of ventilation continues using synchronised intermittent mandatory ventilation (SIMV), pressure support ventilation (PSV) or intermittent periods of spontaneous breathing. Non-invasive ventilation via a facemask can allow earlier extubation in certain groups, such as patients with COPD, with weaning continuing after removal of the endotracheal tube.

Despite the development of objective tests and indices of the patient's ability to sustain spontaneous ventilation, the decision to extubate and the speed of weaning from mechanical ventilation still rely largely on clinical judgement.

8.22 Factors in deciding whether a ventilated patient can be weaned and safely extubated

- Has the original indication for mechanical ventilation resolved?
- Is the patient conscious and able to cough and protect his/her airway?
- Is the circulation stable, with a normal or reasonably low left atrial pressure?
- Is gas exchange satisfactory (PaO_2 > 10 kPa (> 75 mmHg) on FiO_2 < 0.5; $PaCO_2$ < 6 kPa (< 45 mmHg))?
- Is analgesia adequate?
- Are any metabolic problems well controlled?

Tracheostomy

Tracheostomy is usually performed electively when endotracheal intubation is likely to be required for over 14 days. Box 8.23 describes the advantages and disadvantages.

Tracheostomy is usually carried out using a percutaneous technique in the ICU, avoiding the need for transfer to the operating theatre. This has led to its earlier and more frequent use. A recent multicentre RCT found that early tracheostomy (< 3 days) did not lead to earlier weaning or shorter ICU stay.

Mini-tracheostomy

The passage of a smaller (4.5 mm internal diameter) tube through the cricothyroid membrane is a useful technique to clear airway secretions in spontaneously breathing patients with a poor cough effort. It can be particularly useful in the HDU and in post-operative patients.

8.23 Advantages and disadvantages of tracheostomy

Advantages

- Patient comfort
- Improved oral hygiene
- Reduced sedation requirement
- Enables speech with cuff deflated and a speaking valve attached
- Earlier weaning and ICU discharge
- Access for tracheal toilet
- Reduces vocal cord damage

Disadvantages

- Immediate complications: hypoxia, haemorrhage
- Tracheal damage; late stenosis
- Tracheostomy site infection

Renal support

Oliguria (< 0.5 mL/kg/hr for several hours) requires investigation and early intervention to correct hypoxaemia, hypovolaemia, hypotension and renal hypoperfusion. There is little evidence that specific treatments aimed at inducing a diuresis, such as low-dose dopamine, furosemide or mannitol, have renoprotective action or additional beneficial value in restoring renal function beyond aggressive haemodynamic resuscitation to achieve normovolaemia, normotension and an appropriate cardiac output. Sepsis is frequently implicated in the development of AKI, and the focus must be promptly and adequately treated by surgical drainage and antibiotics if renal function is to be restored. Obstruction of the renal tract should always be excluded by abdominal ultrasound and, if present, relieved.

If renal function cannot be restored following resuscitation, renal replacement therapy (p. 492) is indicated (Box 8.24). The preferred renal replacement therapy in ICU patients is pumped venovenous haemofiltration. This is associated with fewer osmotic fluid shifts and hence greater haemodynamic stability than haemodialysis. It is carried out using a double-lumen central venous catheter placed percutaneously. Haemofiltration

8.24 Indications for renal replacement therapy

- Hyperkalaemia: potassium > 6 mmol/L despite medical treatment
- Fluid overload; pulmonary oedema
- Metabolic acidosis: H⁺ > 56 nmol/L (pH < 7.25)
- Uraemia:
    Urea > 30–35 mmol/L (180–210 mg/dL)
    Creatinine > 600 µmol/L (> 6.78 mg/dL)
- Drug removal in overdose
- Sepsis: tentative evidence for mediator removal

should be continuous in the early phase of treatment; higher rates of filtration (preferably > 35 mL/kg/hr) are associated with improved outcome. Intermittent treatment may be used when the patient is recovering from the primary insult and return of normal renal function is expected. Provided the precipitating cause can be successfully treated, renal failure due to ATN usually recovers between 5 days and several weeks later.

Survival rates from MOF including AKI have been around 50% for many years, but evidence suggests that modern haemofiltration techniques are producing better outcomes.

Gastrointestinal and hepatic support

The gastrointestinal tract and liver play an important role in the evolution of MOF, even when the primary diagnosis is not related to the abdomen. Gastrointestinal symptoms, such as nausea, vomiting and large nasogastric aspirates, may be the earliest signs of regional circulatory failure, and when associated with a tender, distended, silent abdomen, indicate the probable site of the primary pathology. Ischaemic bowel is difficult to diagnose in the critically ill patient but in the context of an otherwise unexplained lactic acidosis, hyperkalaemia and coagulopathy, urgent laparotomy must be considered (p. 906).

The gut has a rapid cell turnover rate and fasting alone can produce marked changes in mucosal structure and function. In hypovolaemia and frank shock states, splanchnic vasoconstriction produces gut mucosal ischaemia, damaging the mucosal barrier and allowing toxins to enter the portal circulation and lymphatics. Although equipped to cope with moderate portal toxaemia, the liver may be overwhelmed and then augments the inflammatory response by releasing cytokines into the systemic circulation. For this reason the gut has been described as the 'undrained abscess' or 'motor' of MOF.

Manifestations of MOF within the gastrointestinal tract include loss of gastric acid production, erosive gastritis, stress ulceration, bleeding, ischaemia, pancreatitis and acalculous cholecystitis.

Early institution of enteral nutrition is the most effective strategy for protecting the gut mucosa and providing nutritional support. Evidence suggests that nasogastric feeds supplemented with arginine, omega 3 fatty acids and nucleotides ('immunonutrition') may improve outcome in critical illness. Glutamine supplementation is logical, although not of proven benefit, since it is a 'conditionally essential' amino acid (see Box 5.15, p. 111) and the principal energy substrate used by the gut mucosa in

critical illness. Total parenteral nutrition (TPN) should be started if attempts at implementing enteral feeding fail, but should only be necessary in < 20% of ICU patients.

Tight glycaemic control has been shown to improve outcomes in critically ill surgical patients, but subsequent studies have not replicated this benefit in a mixed critically ill population and have highlighted the dangers of inadvertent hypoglycaemia when using insulin to maintain blood sugars between 4.5 and 6.5 mmol/L (80–120 mg/dL). A rather higher level of glucose, such as 5.5–8 mmol/L (100–144 mg/dL), is thus now the target.

Ranitidine and sucralfate are both used to reduce the risk of gastrointestinal haemorrhage, although ranitidine is the more effective. Both agents are associated with an increased incidence of nosocomial pneumonia. Treatment should be stopped when full enteral nutrition has been established and is probably only necessary in patients with a history of peptic ulcer and those who have evidence of MOF, particularly severe coagulopathy. Proton pump inhibitors are only required if upper GI bleeding due to ulceration occurs.

The hepatic circulation, 80% of which is derived from the portal venous system, is compromised by the same factors which lead to splanchnic vasoconstriction. Hepatic ischaemia leads to impaired filtering of endotoxin from the portal circulation, and as SIRS develops, inflammatory mediators (e.g. cytokines interleukin (IL)-1, IL-6 and tumour necrosis factor (TNF)) are released from activated Kupffer cells (hepatic macrophages) into the systemic circulation, increasing the risk of AKI and the other manifestations of MOF. Increased metabolic activity in the liver as a result of sepsis, and the need for vasoconstricting agents to maintain BP increase hepatic ischaemia. The synthetic inodilator dopexamine, with dopaminergic 1 and 2 and β-adrenergic effects, may enhance splanchnic blood flow but has not been shown to improve outcome.

Three distinctive hepatic dysfunction syndromes occur in the critically ill:

- *Shock liver or ischaemic hepatitis* results from extreme hepatic tissue hypoxia and is characterised by centrilobular hepatocellular necrosis. Transaminase levels are often massively raised (> 1000–5000 U/L) at an early stage, followed by moderate hyperbilirubinaemia (< 100 µmol/L or < 5.8 mg/dL). There is often associated hypoglycaemia, coagulopathy and lactic acidosis. Following successful resuscitation, hepatic function generally returns to normal.
- *Hyperbilirubinaemia ('ICU jaundice')* frequently develops following trauma or sepsis, particularly if there is inadequate control of the inflammatory process. There is a marked rise in bilirubin (predominantly conjugated) but only mild elevation of transaminase and alkaline phosphatase. This results from failure of bilirubin transport within the liver and produces the histological appearance of intrahepatic cholestasis. Extrahepatic cholestasis must be excluded by abdominal ultrasound and potentially hepatotoxic drugs should be stopped. Treatment is non-specific and should include early institution of enteral feeding. Therapy that compromises splanchnic blood flow, particularly high doses of vasoconstrictor agents, should be avoided.
- *Transaminitis* is most commonly due to drug toxicity: for example, antibiotics.

Recognition and management of patients with acute liver failure is described on page 933 .

8

Neurological support

A diverse range of neurological conditions require management in the ICU. These include the various causes of coma, spinal cord injury, peripheral neuromuscular disease and prolonged seizures. Intensive care is required to:

- manage acute brain injury with control of raised intracranial pressure (ICP)
- protect the airway, if necessary by endotracheal intubation
- provide respiratory support to correct hypoxaemia and hypercapnia
- treat circulatory problems, e.g. neurogenic pulmonary oedema in subarachnoid haemorrhage, autonomic disturbances in Guillain–Barré syndrome, spinal shock following high spinal cord injuries
- manage status epilepticus using anaesthetic agents such as thiopental or propofol.

The aim of management in acute brain injury is to optimise cerebral oxygen delivery by maintaining a normal arterial oxygen content and a cerebral perfusion pressure > 60 mmHg. Avoiding secondary insults to the brain, such as hypoxaemia and hypotension, improves outcome in head injury. ICP rises in acute brain injury as a result of haematoma, contusions, oedema or ischaemic swelling. Raised ICP is damaging both directly to the cerebral cortex and by producing downward pressure on the brain stem, and indirectly by reducing cerebral perfusion pressure, thereby threatening cerebral blood flow and oxygen delivery:

Cerebral perfusion pressure (CPP) = mean BP − ICP

ICP is generally measured via pressure transducers inserted directly into the brain tissue. The normal upper limit for ICP is 15 mmHg and management should be directed at keeping ICP < 20 mmHg (Box 8.25). Sustained pressures > 30 mmHg are associated with a poor prognosis.

CPP should be maintained > 60 mmHg by ensuring adequate fluid replacement and, if necessary, by treating hypotension with a vasopressor such as noradrenaline (norepinephrine).

Complex neurological monitoring must be combined with frequent clinical assessment of GCS, pupil response to light and focal neurological signs. The motor response to pain is an important prognostic sign. No response or extension of the upper limbs is associated with severe injury, and unless there is improvement within a few days, prognosis is very poor. A flexor response is encouraging and indicates that a good outcome is still possible.

Neurological complications in intensive care

Neurological complications also occur as a result of systemic critical illness. Sepsis may be associated both with an encephalopathy characterised by delirium and with cerebral oedema and loss of vasoregulation. Hypotension and coagulopathy may provoke cerebral infarction or haemorrhage. Neurological examination is very difficult if patients are sedated or paralysed, and it is important to stop sedation regularly to reassess their underlying level of consciousness. If there is evidence of a focal neurological deficit or a markedly declining level of consciousness, CT of the brain should be performed.

Critical illness polyneuropathy is another potential complication in patients with sepsis and MOF. It is due to peripheral nerve axonal loss and can result in areflexia, gross muscle-wasting and failure to wean from the ventilator, thus prolonging the duration of intensive care. Recovery can take many weeks.

Management of sepsis

Prompt resuscitation with early cultures, administration of appropriate antibiotics and eradication of the source of infection (e.g. surgical drainage) is required. Antibiotics should exhibit a spectrum wide enough to cover probable causative organisms, based on an analysis of the likely site of infection, previous antibiotic therapy and known local resistance patterns. The haemodynamic changes in septic shock are very variable and not specific for the Gram status of the infecting organism. The first feature is often tachypnoea and the early stages are often dominated by hypotension with relative volume depletion due to vasodilatation. Sufficient intravenous fluid should be given to ensure that the intravascular volume is not the limiting factor in determining global oxygen delivery. The type of fluid that should be administered and what constitutes 'adequate' volume resuscitation remain controversial. The response to therapy is crucial and frequently unpredictable, so rigid protocols cannot be used. Depending on haemoglobin concentration, blood or synthetic colloid should be given as 100–200 mL boluses to assess BP response to volume (see Fig. 8.1, p. 181).

Although ventricular function is frequently impaired, the characteristically low SVR usually ensures a high cardiac output (once the patient is adequately volume-resuscitated), albeit with low BP.

The choice of the most appropriate vasoactive drug to use should be based on a full analysis of the circulation

---

8.25 Strategies to control intracranial pressure

- Prevent coughing with sedation, analgesia and occasionally paralysis
- Nurse with 30° head-up tilt and avoid excessive flexion of the head or pressure around the neck that may impair cerebral venous drainage
- Control epileptiform activity with appropriate anticonvulsant therapy; an electroencephalogram (EEG) may be necessary to ensure that this is achieved
- Maintain good glycaemic control with blood glucose between 5.5 and 8 mmol/L (~99–144 mg/dL)
- Aim for a core body temperature of between 36 and 37°C
- Maintain sodium > 140 mmol/L using i.v. 0.9% saline
- Avoid volume depletion or fluid overload
- Provide ventilation aiming to reduce the $PaCO_2$ to 4–4.5 kPa (~30–34 mmHg) for the first 24 hours
- Osmotic diuretic, mannitol 20% 100–200 mL (0.25–0.5 g/kg), coupled with volume replacement
- Hypnotic infusion, thiopental, titrated to 'burst suppression' on EEG
- Surgery: drainage of haematoma or ventricles; lobectomy, decompressive craniectomy

8.26 Factors that increase metabolic rate in critically ill patients

- Fever (10–15% increase in VO_2 for every 1°C rise)
- Sepsis
- Trauma
- Burns
- Surgery
- Sympathetic activation (pain, agitation, shivering)
- Interventions (e.g. nursing procedures, physiotherapy, visitors)
- Drugs (e.g. β-blockers, amphetamines, tricyclics)

N.B. Sedatives, analgesics and muscle relaxants will reduce metabolic rate.

and knowledge of the different inotropic, dilating or constricting properties of these drugs (see Box 8.16, p. 194). In most cases, a vasoconstrictor such as noradrenaline (norepinephrine) is necessary to increase SVR and BP, while an inotrope (dobutamine) may be necessary to maintain cardiac output. In the later stages of severe sepsis, the essential problem is at the microcirculatory level. Oxygen uptake and utilisation are impaired due to failure of the regional distribution of flow and direct cellular toxicity despite adequate global oxygen delivery. Tissue oxygenation may be improved and aerobic metabolism sustained by reducing demand, i.e. metabolic rate (Box 8.26).

Corticosteroids

Assessment of the pituitary–adrenal axis is difficult in the critically ill, but in some series up to 30% of patients have adrenal insufficiency as assessed by baseline cortisol levels and the response to adrenocorticotrophic hormone (ACTH). Corticosteroid replacement therapy is controversial; recent evidence suggests that, although treatment is associated with earlier resolution of shock, it has no effect on survival.

Activated protein C

Administration of activated protein C (levels of which frequently fall in critical illness) may reduce mortality in patients with severe sepsis. Further trials are in progress.

DISCHARGE FROM INTENSIVE CARE

Discharge is appropriate when the original indication for admission has resolved and the patient has sufficient physiological reserve to continue recovery without the facilities available in intensive care. For long-stay ICU patients who have been ventilator-dependent, 'stepdown' to the HDU is appropriate. Discharges from ICU/HDU to standard wards should preferably take place within normal working hours, as there is frequently a lack of sufficient medical and nursing support out of hours and at weekends. The shortage of ICU and HDU beds in most hospitals in the UK creates pressure for early discharge, but it has been shown that readmission rates and hospital mortality increase if discharge occurs prematurely or out of hours.

The critical care team should give the receiving team a detailed handover, a written summary with relevant recent investigations, remain available for advice, and ideally visit the patient on the ward within the 24 hours after discharge.

Withdrawal of care

Withdrawal of support is appropriate when it is clear that the patient has no realistic prospect of recovery or of surviving with a quality of life that he or she would value. In these situations intensive care will only prolong the dying process and is therefore both futile and an inhumane waste of resources. Nevertheless, when intensive support is withdrawn, management should remain active and be directed towards allowing the patient to die with dignity and as free from distress as possible (p. 286).Patients' wishes in this regard are paramount and increasing use is being made of advance directives or 'living wills'. Communication with the patient, if possible, with the family and the referring clinicians, and between members of the critical care team is crucial (p. 175). Failure in this area damages working relations, causes stress and unrealistic expectations, and leads to subsequent unhappiness, anger and litigation.

Brain-stem death

Recent advances in resuscitation and intensive care management of brain-injured patients have inevitably increased the survival of patients who remain ventilated on ICU where progression of brain injury results in brain-stem death. The preconditions for considering brain-stem death and the criteria for establishing the diagnosis are listed on page 1158.

When formal criteria for brain-stem death are met, it is clearly inappropriate to continue supporting life with mechanical ventilation, and the possibility of organ donation should be considered. All intensive care clinicians have a responsibility to approach relatives to seek consent for organ donation, provided there is no contraindication to the use of the organs. This can be very difficult, but is easier if the patient carried an organ donor card or was registered with an organisation such as the UK Organ Donor Register. In the UK, each region has a team of transplant coordinators who provide help with the process of organ donation and care of the potential organ donor.

SCORING SYSTEMS IN INTENSIVE CARE

Admission and discharge criteria vary between units, so it is important to define the characteristics of the patients admitted (case mix) in order to assess the effects of the care provided on the outcome achieved (Box 8.27).

Two systems are widely used to measure severity of illness:
- 'APACHE' II: Acute Physiology Assessment and Chronic Health Evaluation
- 'SAPS' 2: Simplified Acute Physiology Score.

These scores include assessment of certain admission characteristics (e.g. age and pre-existing organ dysfunction) and a variety of routine physiological measurements

8

8

i 8.27 Uses of critical care scoring systems

- Comparison of the performance of different units
- Assessment of new therapies
- Assessment of changes in unit policies and management guidelines
- Measurement of the cost-effectiveness of care

(e.g. temperature, BP, GCS) that reflect the response of the patient to his or her illness. When combined with the admission diagnosis, scoring systems have been shown to correlate well with the risk of hospital death. Such outcome predictions can never be 100% accurate and should be viewed as only one of many factors that the clinician considers when deciding whether or not further intervention is appropriate. Patient age is included in many scoring systems (Box 8.28).

Predicted mortality figures by diagnosis have been calculated from large databases generated from a range of ICUs. These allow a particular unit to evaluate its performance compared to the reference ICUs by calculating standardised mortality ratios (SMRs) for each diagnostic group:

$$SMR = observed\ mortality \div predicted\ mortality$$

8.28 The critically ill older patient

- **ICU demography:** increasing numbers of critically ill older patients are admitted to the ICU; more than 50% of patients in many general ICUs are over 65 years old.
- **Outcome:** affected to some extent by age, as reflected in APACHE II, but age should not be used as the sole criterion for withholding or withdrawing ICU support.
- **Cardiopulmonary resuscitation (CPR):** age does affect outcome. Successful hospital discharge following in-hospital CPR is rare in patients over 70 years old in the presence of significant chronic disease.
- **Functional independence:** tends to be lost during an ICU stay and prolonged rehabilitation may subsequently be necessary.
- **Specific problems:**
  Skin fragility and ulceration
  Poor muscle strength: difficulty in weaning from ventilator and in mobilising
  Delirium: compounded by sedatives and analgesics
  High prevalence of underlying nutritional deficiency.

A value of unity indicates the same performance as the reference ICUs while a value < 1 indicates a better than predicted outcome. If a unit has a high SMR in a certain diagnostic category, this would prompt investigation into how such patients were managed, in order to identify aspects of care that could be improved.

OUTCOME OF INTENSIVE CARE

The most widely used measure to assess outcome from intensive care is mortality. This is quoted at hospital discharge and at 28 days because mortality at the time of discharge from the ICU will be influenced by the unit discharge policy. Mortality is also influenced by case mix, length of stay and organisational issues.

It is important to demonstrate long-term benefit to justify the increasing costs of intensive care provision. Quality of life following discharge should be included but this is difficult to measure and interpret, not least because no objective pre-morbid assessment is possible in emergency admissions. However, several units in the UK now run follow-up clinics and have identified that there is a high incidence of physical and psychological problems affecting patient and family following ICU discharge.

Further information

www.adqi.com *Evidence-based appraisal and consensus recommendations for diagnosis, treatment and research in acute kidney injury.*

www.esicm.org *European Society of Intensive Care Medicine: guidelines, recommendations, consensus conference reports.*

www.ics.ac.uk *Intensive Care Society: clinical guidelines and standards for intensive care.*

www.icudelirium.org *Information on delirium and sedation in intensive care patients.*

www.scottishintensivecare.org.uk/education/index.htm *On-line tutorials, educational materials for learners and teaching support materials for educators.*

www.sicsebm.org.uk *Intensive care evidence-based medicine website. Reviews and critical appraisal of topics.*

www.survivingsepsis.org *Surviving Sepsis website.*

S.H.L. Thomas
J. White

Poisoning

9

COMPREHENSIVE EVALUATION OF THE POISONED PATIENT

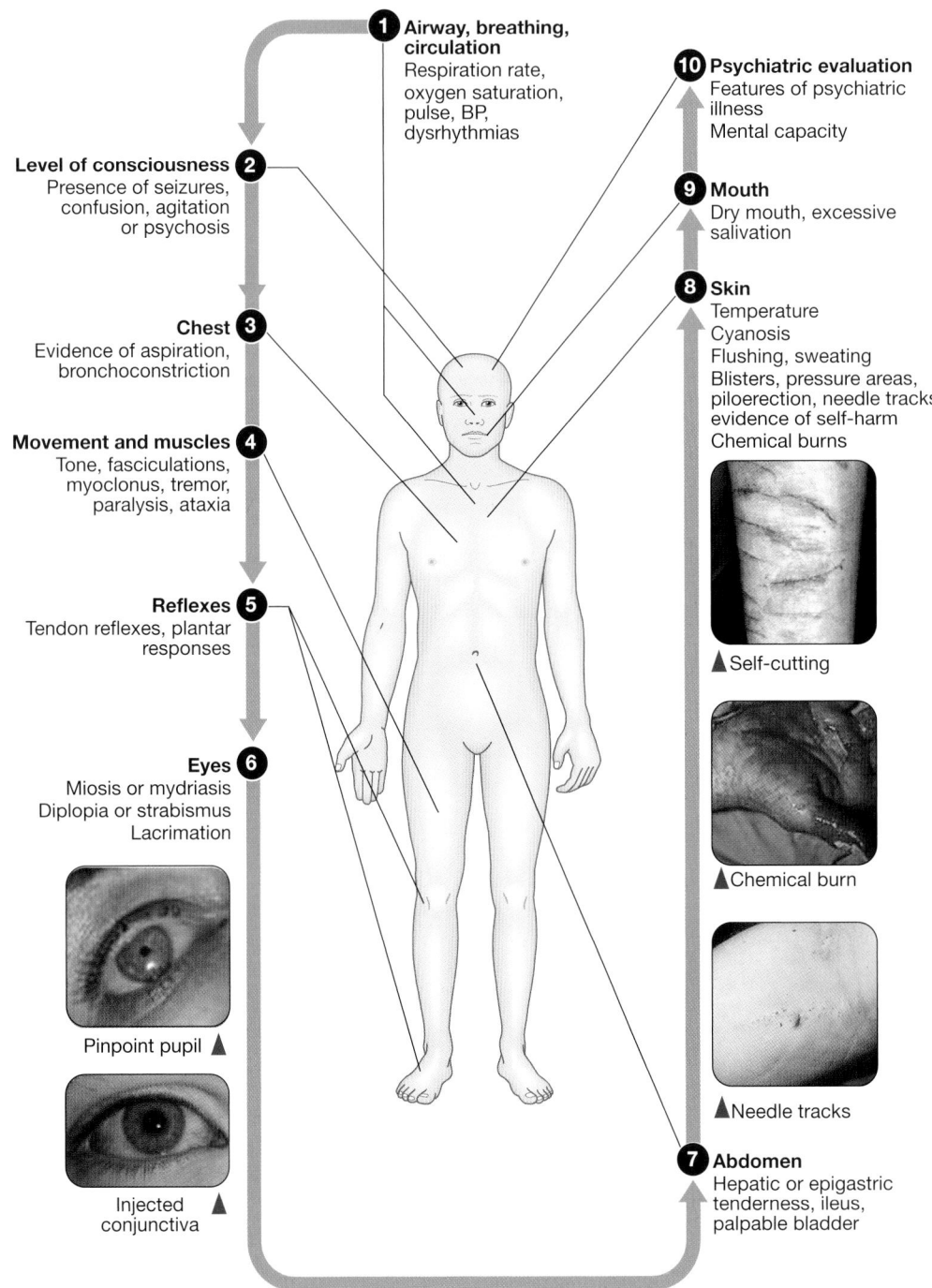

1 Airway, breathing, circulation
Respiration rate, oxygen saturation, pulse, BP, dysrhythmias

Level of consciousness 2
Presence of seizures, confusion, agitation or psychosis

Chest 3
Evidence of aspiration, bronchoconstriction

Movement and muscles 4
Tone, fasciculations, myoclonus, tremor, paralysis, ataxia

Reflexes 5
Tendon reflexes, plantar responses

Eyes 6
Miosis or mydriasis
Diplopia or strabismus
Lacrimation

Pinpoint pupil ▲

Injected ▲
conjunctiva

10 Psychiatric evaluation
Features of psychiatric illness
Mental capacity

9 Mouth
Dry mouth, excessive salivation

8 Skin
Temperature
Cyanosis
Flushing, sweating
Blisters, pressure areas, piloerection, needle tracks, evidence of self-harm
Chemical burns

▲Self-cutting

▲Chemical burn

▲Needle tracks

7 Abdomen
Hepatic or epigastric tenderness, ileus, palpable bladder

Taking a history in poisoning

- What toxin(s) have been taken and how much?
- What time were they taken and by what route?
- Has alcohol or any drug of misuse been taken as well?
- Obtain details of the circumstances of the overdose from family, friends and ambulance personnel
- Ask the general practitioner for background and details of prescribed medication
- Assess suicide risk (full psychiatric evaluation
- when patient has physically recovered)
- Capacity to make decisions about accepting or refusing treatment?
- Past medical history, drug history and allergies, social and family history?
- Record all information carefully

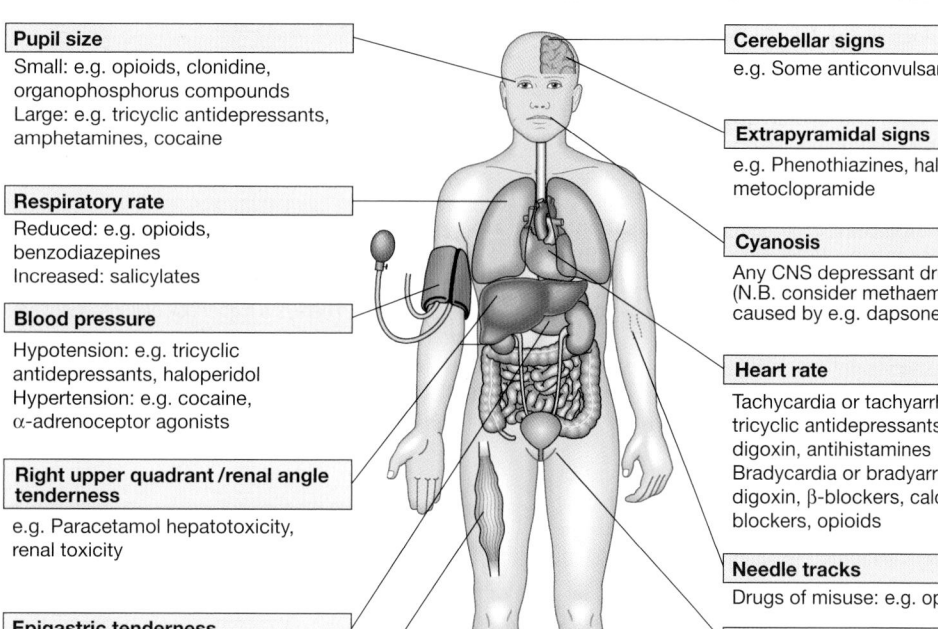

Pupil size
Small: e.g. opioids, clonidine, organophosphorus compounds
Large: e.g. tricyclic antidepressants, amphetamines, cocaine

Respiratory rate
Reduced: e.g. opioids, benzodiazepines
Increased: salicylates

Blood pressure
Hypotension: e.g. tricyclic antidepressants, haloperidol
Hypertension: e.g. cocaine, α-adrenoceptor agonists

Right upper quadrant /renal angle tenderness
e.g. Paracetamol hepatotoxicity, renal toxicity

Epigastric tenderness
e.g. NSAIDs, salicylates

Rhabdomyolysis
e.g. Amphetamines, caffeine

Cerebellar signs
e.g. Some anticonvulsants, alcohol

Extrapyramidal signs
e.g. Phenothiazines, haloperidol, metoclopramide

Cyanosis
Any CNS depressant drug or agent (N.B. consider methaemoglobinaemia caused by e.g. dapsone, amyl nitrite)

Heart rate
Tachycardia or tachyarrhythmias: e.g. tricyclic antidepressants, theophylline, digoxin, antihistamines
Bradycardia or bradyarrhythmias: e.g. digoxin, β-blockers, calcium channel blockers, opioids

Needle tracks
Drugs of misuse: e.g. opioids etc.

Body temperature
Hyperthermia and sweating: e.g. ecstasy, serotonin re-uptake inhibitors, salicylates
Hypothermia: e.g. any CNS depressant drug, e.g. opioids, chlorpromazine

Clinical signs of poisoning by pharmaceutical agents and drugs of misuse.

EVALUATION OF THE ENVENOMED PATIENT

 Assessment of type and extent of envenoming

Neurotoxic paralysis

- 'Sleepy' or drooping eyelids
- Difficulty swallowing, dysarthria and drooling
- Limb weakness
- Respiratory distress

Excitatory neurotoxicity

- Sweating, salivation, piloerection
- Tingling around mouth, tongue or muscle twitching
- Dyspnoea (pulmonary oedema)

Myolysis

- Muscle pain or weakness

Coagulopathy

- Blood oozing from bite site and/or gums
- Bruising
- Melaena, haematemesis

Local effects

- Pain, sweating, blistering, bruising etc.

Taking a history in envenoming

- When was the patient exposed to a bite/sting?
- Was the organism causing it seen and what did it look like (size, colour)?
- What were the circumstances (on land, in water etc.)?
- Was there more than one bite/sting?
- What first aid was used, when and for how long?
- What symptoms has the patient had (local and systemic)?
- Are there symptoms suggesting systemic envenoming (paralysis, myolysis, coagulopathy etc.)?
- Past medical history and medications?
- Past exposure to antivenom/ venom and allergies?

Bites showing puncture marks, blistering, bruising and bleeding.

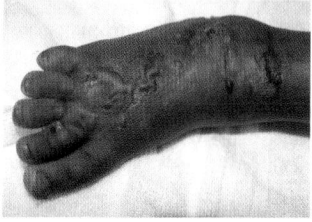
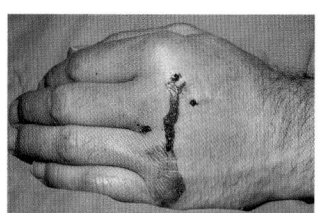
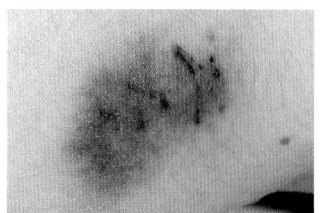

Acute poisoning is common, accounting for about 10% of hospital admissions in the UK. Important substances involved are shown in Box 9.1. In developed countries, the most frequent cause is intentional drug overdose in the context of self-harm and usually involves prescribed or 'over-the-counter' medicines. Accidental poisoning is also common, especially in children and the elderly (Box 9.2). Toxicity also may occur as a result of alcohol or recreational substance use, or following occupational or environmental exposure. Poisoning is a major cause of death in young adults, but most deaths occur before patients reach medical attention, and mortality is much lower than 1% in those admitted to hospital.

In developing countries, the frequency of self-harm is more difficult to estimate because patients may be reticent in admitting to deliberate poisoning. Household and agricultural products such as pesticides and herbicides are more freely available, are common sources of poisoning and are associated with a much higher case fatality. In China and South-east Asia, pesticides account for about 300 000 suicides each year.

9.1 Important substances involved in poisoning

In the UK

- Analgesics, e.g. paracetamol and non-steroidal anti-inflammatory drugs (NSAIDs)
- Antidepressants, e.g. tricyclic antidepressants (TCAs), selective serotonin re-uptake inhibitors (SSRIs) and lithium
- Cardiovascular agents, e.g. β-blockers, calcium channel blockers and cardiac glycosides
- Drugs of misuse, e.g. opiates, benzodiazepines, stimulants (e.g. amphetamines, MDMA, cocaine)
- Carbon monoxide*
- Alcohol

In South and South-east Asia

- Organophosphorus* and carbamate insecticides
- Aluminium and zinc phosphide
- Oleander
- Snake venoms
- Antimalarial drugs, e.g. chloroquine
- Antidiabetic medication

*The most common causes of death by poisoning.

9.2 Poisoning in old age

- **Aetiology:** commonly results from accidental poisoning (e.g. due to confusion or dementia) or drug toxicity as a consequence of impaired renal or hepatic function or drug interaction. Toxic prescription medicines are more likely to be available.
- **Psychiatric illness:** self-harm is less common than in younger adults but more frequently associated with depression and other psychiatric illness, as well as chronic illness and pain. There is a higher risk of subsequent suicide.
- **Severity of poisoning:** increased morbidity and mortality result from reduced renal and hepatic function, reduced functional reserve, increased sensitivity to sedative agents and frequent comorbidity.

GENERAL APPROACH TO THE POISONED PATIENT

A general approach to the poisoned patient is shown on pages 204–205.

Triage and resuscitation

Patients who are seriously poisoned must be identified early so that appropriate management is not delayed. Triage involves:

- immediate measurement of vital signs
- identifying the poison(s) involved and obtaining adequate information about them
- identifying patients at risk of further attempts at self-harm and removing any remaining hazards from them.

Those with possible external contamination with chemical or environmental toxins should undergo appropriate decontamination (Fig. 9.1). Critically ill patients must be resuscitated (p. 178).

The Glasgow Coma Scale (GCS) is commonly employed to assess conscious level, although it has not been specifically validated in poisoned patients. The AVPU (alert/verbal/painful/unresponsive) scale is

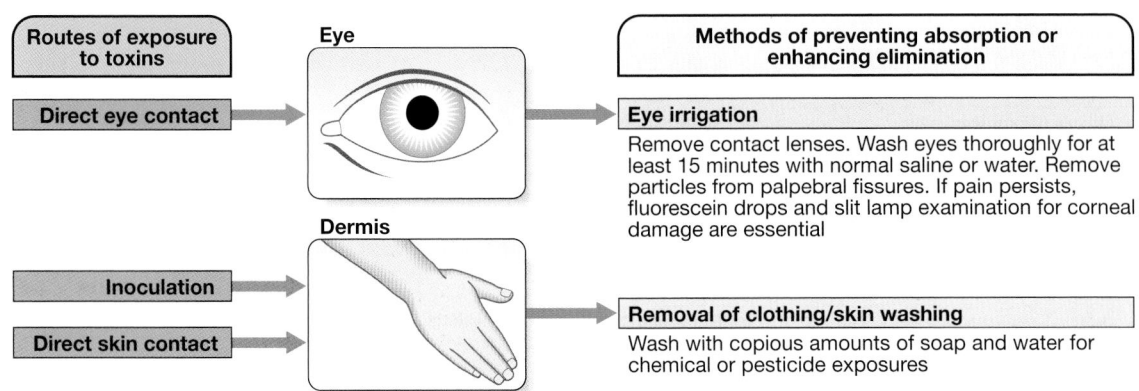

Fig. 9.1 Methods of external decontamination.

9.3 Substances of very low toxicity

- Writing/educational materials
- Decorating products
- Cleaning/bathroom products (except dishwasher tablets which are corrosive)
- Pharmaceuticals: oral contraceptives, most antibiotics (but not tetracyclines and antituberculous drugs), H_2-blockers, proton pump inhibitors, emollients and other skin creams, baby lotion
- Miscellaneous: plasticine, silica gel, household plants, plant food

9.5 Causes of acidosis in the poisoned patient

Cause	Normal lactate*	High lactate
Toxic	Salicylates Methanol Ethylene glycol Paraldehyde	Metformin Iron Cyanide Sodium valproate Carbon monoxide
Other	Renal failure Ketoacidosis Severe diarrhoea	Shock

*Unless circulatory shock is present, when it will be high in any case.

9.6 Anion and osmolar gaps in poisoning

	Anion gap	Osmolar gap
Calculation	$[Na^+ + K^+] - [Cl^- + HCO_3^-]$	Osm (measured) − $[2Na + K + Urea + Glucose]$
Normal range	12–16 mmol/L	< 10 mOsm/kg
Common toxic causes of elevation*	Ethanol Ethylene glycol Methanol Salicylates Iron Cyanide	Ethanol Ethylene glycol Methanol

*Box 16.19 (p. 443) gives non-toxic causes.

also a rapid and simple method. An electrocardiogram (ECG) should be performed and cardiac monitoring instituted in all patients with cardiovascular features or where exposure to potentially cardiotoxic substances is suspected. Patients who may need antidotes should be weighed when this is feasible, so that appropriate doses can be prescribed.

Substances that are unlikely to be toxic in humans should be identified so that inappropriate admission and intervention are avoided (Box 9.3).

Clinical assessment and investigations

History and examination are described on page 204. Occasionally, patients may be unaware or confused about what they have taken, or may exaggerate (or less commonly underestimate) the size of the overdose, but rarely mislead medical staff deliberately. In some parts of the world, such as Asia, patients may not readily admit to deliberate self-poisoning.

Toxic causes of abnormal physical signs are shown on page 205. The patient may have a cluster of clinical features ('toxidrome') suggestive of poisoning with a particular drug type (Box 9.4). Poisoning is a common cause of coma, especially in younger people, but it is important to exclude other potential causes (p. 1158), unless the aetiology is certain.

Urea, electrolytes and creatinine should be measured in most patients. Arterial blood gases should be checked in those with significant respiratory or circulatory compromise, or when poisoning with substances likely to affect acid–base status is suspected (Box 9.5). Calculation of anion and osmolar gaps may help to inform diagnosis and management (Box 9.6).

9.4 Feature clusters in poisoning

Features	Cross-reference
Serotonin syndrome	Box 9.12, p. 211
Anticholinergic	Box 9.12, p. 211
Stimulant	Box 9.13, p. 215
Sedative hypnotic	Box 9.13, p. 215
Opioid	Box 9.13, p. 215
Cholinergic muscarinic	Box 9.15, p. 219
Cholinergic nicotinic	Box 9.15, p. 219

For a limited number of specific substances, management may be facilitated by measurement of the amount of toxin in the blood (Box 9.7). Qualitative urine screens for potential toxins including near-patient testing kits have a limited clinical role. Occasionally, for medico-legal reasons, it is useful to save blood and urine for subsequent measurement of drug concentrations.

Psychiatric assessment

All patients presenting with deliberate drug overdose should undergo psychosocial evaluation by a health professional with appropriate training prior to discharge (p. 236). This should take place once the patient has recovered from any features of poisoning, unless there is an urgent issue such as uncertainty about his or her capacity to decline medical treatment.

General management

Patients presenting with eye or skin contamination should undergo appropriate local decontamination procedures (see Fig. 9.1).

Gastrointestinal decontamination

Patients who have ingested potentially life-threatening quantities of toxins may be considered for gastrointestinal decontamination if poisoning has been

9

9

9.7 Laboratory analysis in poisoning

Acetylcholinesterase

- Plasma cholinesterase is reduced more rapidly but is less specific than red cell cholinesterase (p. 219) in organophosphorus poisoning
- Antidote use should not be delayed pending results

Carboxyhaemoglobin

- > 20% indicates significant carbon monoxide exposure

Digoxin

- Therapeutic range usually 1–2 μg/L
- Concentrations > 4 μg/L usually associated with toxicity, especially with chronic poisoning

Ethanol

- Toxicity at concentrations > 1.8 g/L

Iron

- Take sample at least 4 hrs after overdose or if there are clinical features of toxicity
- Concentrations > 5 mg/L suggest severe toxicity

Lithium

- Take sample at least 6 hrs after overdose or if there are clinical features of toxicity
- Usual therapeutic range 0.4–1.0 mmol/L

Methaemoglobin

- Methaemoglobinaemia associated with toxicity due to nitrites, benzocaine, dapsone, chloroquine, aniline dyes
- Concentrations > 20% may require treatment with methylthioninium chloride (methylene blue)

Paracetamol

- Take sample at least 4 hrs after overdose
- Use nomogram to determine need for antidotal treatment (see Fig. 9.2, p. 211)

Salicylate

- Take sample at least 2 hrs (symptomatic patients) or 4 hrs (asymptomatic patients) after overdose
- Concentrations > 500 mg/L suggest serious toxicity
- Repeat after 2 hrs if severe toxicity is suspected

Theophylline

- Take sample at least 4 hrs after overdose or if there are clinical features of toxicity
- Repeat after 2 hrs if severe toxicity is suspected
- Concentrations > 60 mg/L suggest severe toxicity

EBM 9.8 Use of gastric decontamination methods

Single-dose activated charcoal

'The administration of activated charcoal may be considered if a patient has ingested a potentially toxic amount of a poison (which is known to be adsorbed to charcoal) up to 1 hr previously.'[1]

Multiple-dose activated charcoal

'Multiple-dose activated charcoal should be considered only if a patient has ingested a life-threatening amount of carbamazepine, dapsone, phenobarbital, quinine or theophylline.'[2]

Gastric lavage

'Gastric lavage should not be employed routinely, if ever, in the management of poisoned patients.'[3]

Whole bowel irrigation (WBI)

'WBI should be considered for potentially toxic ingestions of sustained-release or enteric-coated drugs, particularly for those patients presenting more than 2 hrs after drug ingestion. WBI should be considered for patients who have ingested substantial amounts of iron, as the morbidity is high and there is a lack of other options for gastrointestinal decontamination. The use of WBI for the removal of ingested packets of illicit drugs is also a potential indication.'[4]

- American Academy of Clinical Toxicology and European Association of Poison Centres and Clinical Toxicologists Joint Position Statements on Gastric Decontamination Methods:
[1]AACT and EAPCCT. Clin Toxicol 2005; 43:61–87.
[2]AACT and EAPCCT. Clin Toxicol 1999; 37:731–751.
[3]AACT and EAPCCT. Clin Toxicol 2004; 42:933–943.
[4]AACT and EAPCCT. J Toxicol Clin Toxicol 2004; 42843–42854.

bind to activated charcoal (Box 9.9) so it will not affect their absorption. In patients with an impaired swallow or a reduced level of consciousness, the use of activated charcoal, even via a nasogastric tube, carries a risk of aspiration pneumonitis. This risk can be reduced but not completely removed by protecting the airway with a cuffed endotracheal tube.

Multiple doses of oral activated charcoal (50 g every 4 hours) may enhance the elimination of some drugs at any time after poisoning and are recommended for serious poisoning with some substances (see Box 9.8). They achieve their effect by interrupting enterohepatic circulation or by reducing the concentration of free drug in the gut lumen, to the extent that drug diffuses from the blood back into the bowel to be absorbed on to the charcoal: so-called 'gastrointestinal dialysis'. A laxative is generally given with the charcoal to reduce the risk of constipation or intestinal obstruction by charcoal 'briquette' formation in the gut lumen.

9.9 Substances poorly adsorbed by activated charcoal

Medicines

- Iron	- Lithium

Chemicals

- Acids*	- Mercury
- Alkalis*	- Methanol
- Ethanol	- Petroleum distillates*
- Ethylene glycol	

*Gastric lavage contraindicated.

recent (Box 9.8). Induction of emesis using ipecacuanha is now never recommended.

Activated charcoal

Given orally as slurry, activated charcoal absorbs toxins in the bowel as a result of its large surface area. If given sufficiently early, it can prevent absorption of an important proportion of the ingested dose of toxin. However, efficacy decreases with time and current guidelines do not advocate use more than 1 hour after overdose in most circumstances (see Box 9.8). However, use after a longer interval may be reasonable when a delayed-release preparation has been taken or when gastric emptying may be delayed. Some toxins do not

Recent evidence suggests that single or multiple doses of activated charcoal do not improve clinical outcomes after poisoning with pesticides or oleander.

Gastric aspiration and lavage

Gastric aspiration and/or lavage is now very infrequently indicated in acute poisoning, as it is no more effective than activated charcoal, and complications are common, especially aspiration. Use may be justified for life-threatening overdoses of some substances that are not absorbed by activated charcoal (see Box 9.9).

Whole bowel irrigation

This is occasionally indicated to enhance the elimination of ingested packets or slow-release tablets that are not absorbed by activated charcoal (e.g. iron, lithium), but use is controversial. It is performed by administration of large quantities of polyethylene glycol and electrolyte solution (1–2 L/hr for an adult), often via a nasogastric tube, until the rectal effluent is clear. Contraindications include inadequate airway protection, haemodynamic instability, gastrointestinal haemorrhage, obstruction or ileus. Whole bowel irrigation does not cause osmotic changes but may precipitate nausea and vomiting, abdominal pain and electrolyte disturbances.

Urinary alkalinisation

Urinary excretion of weak acids and bases is affected by urinary pH, which changes the extent to which they are ionised. Highly ionised molecules pass poorly through lipid membranes and therefore little tubular reabsorption occurs and urinary excretion is increased. If the urine is alkalinised (pH > 7.5) by the administration of sodium bicarbonate (e.g. 1.5 L of 1.26% sodium bicarbonate over 2 hrs), weak acids (e.g. salicylates, methotrexate and the herbicides 2,4-dichlorophenoxyacetic acid and mecoprop) are highly ionised and so their urinary excretion is enhanced. This technique should be distinguished from forced alkaline diuresis, in which large volumes of fluid with diuretic are given in addition to alkalinisation. This is no longer used because of the risk of fluid overload.

Urinary alkalinisation is currently recommended for patients with clinically significant salicylate poisoning when the criteria for haemodialysis are not met (see below). It is also sometimes used for poisoning with methotrexate. Complications include alkalaemia, hypokalaemia and occasionally alkalotic tetany (p. 444). Hypocalcaemia is rare.

Haemodialysis and haemoperfusion

These can enhance the elimination of poisons that have a small volume of distribution and a long half-life after overdose, and are useful when the episode of poisoning is sufficiently severe to justify invasive elimination methods. The toxin must be small enough to cross the dialysis membrane (haemodialysis) or must bind to activated charcoal (haemoperfusion) (Box 9.10). Haemodialysis may also correct acid–base and metabolic disturbances associated with poisoning (p. 207).

Antidotes

Antidotes are available for some poisons and work by a variety of mechanisms: for example, by specific antagonism (e.g. isoproterenol for β–blockers), chelation (e.g.

9.10 Poisons effectively eliminated by haemodialysis or haemoperfusion	
Haemodialysis	
• Ethylene glycol	• Salicylates
• Isopropanol	• Sodium valproate
• Methanol	• Lithium
Haemoperfusion	
• Theophylline	• Phenobarbital
• Phenytoin	• Amobarbital
• Carbamazepine	

desferrioxamine for iron) or reduction (e.g. methylene blue for dapsone). The use of some antidotes is described in the management of specific poisons below.

Supportive care

For most poisons, antidotes and methods to accelerate elimination are inappropriate, unavailable or incompletely effective. Outcome is dependent on appropriate nursing and supportive care, and on treatment of complications (Box 9.11). Patients should be monitored carefully until the effects of any toxins have dissipated.

POISONING BY SPECIFIC PHARMACEUTICAL AGENTS

Analgesics

Paracetamol

Paracetamol (acetaminophen) is the drug most commonly used in overdose in the UK. Toxicity results from formation of an intermediate reactive metabolite which binds covalently to cellular proteins, causing cell death. This results in hepatic and occasionally renal failure. In therapeutic doses, the toxic intermediate metabolite is detoxified in reactions requiring glutathione, but in overdose, glutathione reserves become exhausted.

Management

Management is summarised in Figure 9.2. Activated charcoal may be used in patients presenting within 1 hour. Antidotes for paracetamol act by replenishing hepatic glutathione. Acetylcysteine given intravenously (or orally in some countries) is highly efficacious if administered within 8 hours of the overdose. However, since efficacy declines thereafter, administration should not be delayed in patients presenting after 8 hours to await a paracetamol blood concentration result. The antidote can be stopped if the paracetamol concentration is shown to be below the appropriate treatment line. The most important adverse effect of acetylcysteine is related to dose-related histamine release, the 'anaphylactoid' reaction, which causes itching and urticaria, and in severe cases, bronchospasm and hypotension. Most cases can be managed by temporary discontinuation of acetylcysteine and administration of an antihistamine. An alternative antidote in paracetamol poisoning is methionine 2.5 g orally 4-hourly to a total of four doses, but it is less effective, especially after delayed

+ 9.11 Complications of poisoning and their management

	Examples of causative agents	Management
Coma	Sedative agents	Appropriate airway protection and ventilatory support Pressure area and bladder care Identification and treatment of aspiration pneumonia
Seizures	NSAIDs Anticonvulsants TCAs Theophylline	Appropriate airway and ventilatory support I.v. benzodiazepine (e.g. diazepam 10–20 mg, lorazepam 2–4 mg) Correction of hypoxia, acid–base and metabolic abnormalities
Acute dystonias	Typical antipsychotics Metoclopramide	Procyclidine, benzatropine or diazepam
Hypotension Due to vasodilatation	Vasodilator antihypertensives Anticholinergic agents TCAs	I.v. fluids Vasopressors (rarely indicated; see pp. 193–194)
Due to myocardial suppression	β-blockers Calcium channel blockers TCAs	Optimisation of volume status Inotropic agents (pp. 193–194)
Ventricular tachycardia Monomorphic, associated with QRS prolongation	Sodium channel blockers	Correction of electrolyte and acid–base abnormalities and hypoxia Sodium bicarbonate
Torsades de pointes, associated with QT_c prolongation	Anti-arrhythmic drugs (quinidine, amiodarone, sotalol) Antimalarials Organophosphate insecticides Antipsychotic agents Antidepressants Antibiotics (erythromycin)	Magnesium sulphate, 2 g i.v. over 1–2 mins, repeated if necessary

presentation. If a patient presents more than 15 hours after ingestion, liver function tests, prothrombin time (or international normalised ratio—INR), renal function tests and a venous bicarbonate should be measured, the antidote started, and a poisons information centre or local liver unit contacted for advice if results are abnormal. An arterial blood gas sample should be taken in patients with severe liver function abnormalities; metabolic acidosis indicates severe poisoning. Liver transplantation should be considered in individuals who develop life-threatening liver failure due to paracetamol poisoning (p. 933).

If multiple ingestions of paracetamol have taken place over several hours or days (i.e. a staggered overdose), acetylcysteine should be given when the paracetamol dose exceeds 150 mg/kg body weight in any one 24-hour period or 75 mg/kg body weight in 'high-risk groups' (see Fig. 9.2).

Salicylates (aspirin)

Clinical features

Salicylate overdose commonly causes nausea, vomiting, sweating, tinnitus and deafness. Direct stimulation of the respiratory centre produces hyperventilation and respiratory alkalosis. Peripheral vasodilatation with bounding pulses and profuse sweating occurs in moderately severe poisoning. Serious salicylate poisoning is associated with metabolic acidosis, hypoprothrombinaemia, hyperglycaemia, hyperpyrexia, renal failure, pulmonary oedema, shock and cerebral oedema. Agitation, confusion, coma and fits may occur, especially in children. Toxicity is enhanced by acidosis, which increases salicylate transfer across the blood–brain barrier.

Management

Activated charcoal should be administered if the patient presents early. Multiple doses of activated charcoal may enhance salicylate elimination but currently are not routinely recommended.

The plasma salicylate concentration should be measured at least 2 (in symptomatic patients) or 4 hours (asymptomatic patients) after overdose and repeated in patients with suspected serious poisoning, since concentrations may continue to rise some hours after overdose. In adults, concentrations above 500 mg/L and 700 mg/L suggest serious and life-threatening poisoning respectively, although clinical status is more important than the salicylate concentration in assessing severity.

Dehydration should be corrected carefully, as there is a risk of pulmonary oedema, and metabolic acidosis should be identified and treated with intravenous sodium bicarbonate (8.4%), once plasma potassium has been corrected. Urinary alkalinisation is indicated for adult patients with salicylate concentrations above 500 mg/L.

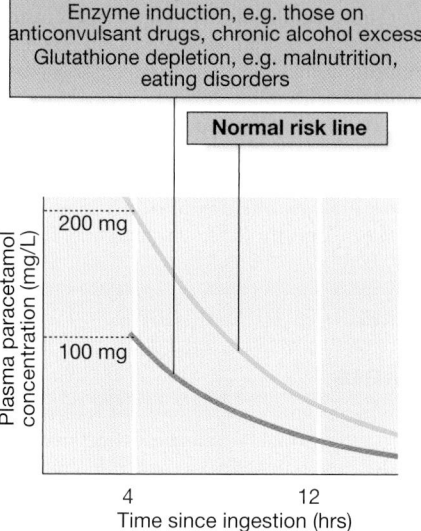

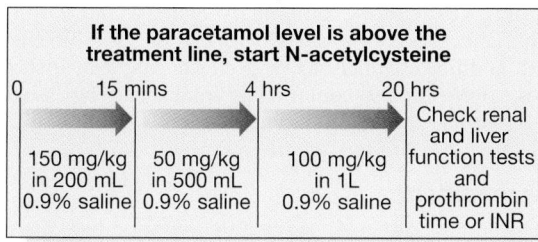

Fig. 9.2 The management of a paracetamol overdose.

Haemodialysis is very effective at removing salicylate and correcting acid–base and fluid balance abnormalities, and should be considered when serum concentrations are above 700 mg/L in adult patients with severe toxic features, or when there is renal failure, pulmonary oedema, coma, convulsions or refractory acidosis.

Non-steroidal anti-inflammatory drugs (NSAIDs)

Clinical features

Overdose of most NSAIDs (e.g. ibuprofen, diclofenac, naproxen, indometacin) usually causes little more than minor abdominal discomfort, vomiting and/or diarrhoea, but convulsions occur occasionally, especially with mefenamic acid. Coma, prolonged seizures,

apnoea, liver dysfunction and renal failure can occur after substantial overdose but are rare. Features of toxicity are unlikely to develop more than 6 hours after overdose.

Management

Electrolytes, liver function tests and a full blood count should be checked in all but the most trivial cases. Activated charcoal may be given if the patient presents sufficiently early. Symptomatic treatment for nausea and gastrointestinal irritation may be necessary.

Antidepressants

Tricyclic antidepressants (TCAs)

TCAs continue to be used frequently in overdose and carry a high morbidity and mortality relating to their sodium channel-blocking, anticholinergic and α-adrenoceptor-blocking effects.

Clinical features

Anticholinergic effects are common (Box 9.12). Life-threatening complications are frequent, including convulsions, coma, arrhythmias (ventricular tachycardia, ventricular fibrillation and, less commonly, heart block) and hypotension, which results from inappropriate vasodilatation or impaired myocardial contractility.

9.12 **Anticholinergic and serotonergic feature clusters**		
	Anticholinergic	**Serotonin syndrome**
Common causes	Benzodiazepines Antipsychotics TCAs Antihistamines Scopolamine Benzatropine Belladonna Jimson weed Mushrooms (some)	SSRIs Monoamine oxidase inhibitors (MAOIs) TCAs Amphetamines Buspirone Bupropion (especially in combination)
Clinical features		
Cardiovascular	Tachycardia, hypertension	Tachycardia, hyper- or hypotension
CNS	Confusion, hallucinations, sedation	Confusion, delirium, hallucinations, sedation, coma
Muscle	Myoclonus	Shivering, tremor, myoclonus, raised creatine kinase
Temperature	Fever	Fever
Eyes	Diplopia, mydriasis	Normal pupil size
Abdomen	Ileus, palpable bladder	Diarrhoea, vomiting
Mouth	Dry	
Skin	Flushing, hot, dry	Flushing, sweating
Complications	Seizures	Seizures Rhabdomyolysis Renal failure Metabolic acidosis Coagulopathies

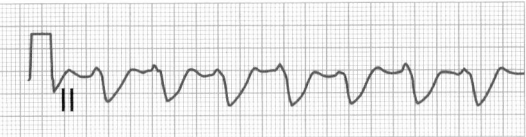

Fig 9.3 ECG in severe tricyclic antidepressant poisoning. This rhythm strip shows a broad QRS complex due to impaired conduction.

Serious complications appear to occur more commonly with dosulepin and amitriptyline.

Management

Activated charcoal should be administered if the patient presents sufficiently early. All patients with possible tricyclic overdose should have a 12-lead ECG and ongoing cardiac monitoring for at least 6 hours. Prolongation of the QRS interval (especially if > 0.16 s) indicates severe sodium channel blockade and is associated with an increased risk of arrhythmia (Fig. 9.3). Arterial blood gases should be measured in patients with suspected severe poisoning.

In patients with arrhythmias, severe ECG effects or acidosis, intravenous sodium bicarbonate (50 mL of 8.4% solution) should be administered and repeated to correct pH. The correction of the acidosis and the sodium loading that result is often associated with rapid improvement in ECG features and arrhythmias. Hypoxia and electrolyte abnormalities should also be corrected. Anti-arrhythmic drugs should only be given on specialist advice. Prolonged convulsions should be treated with intravenous benzodiazepines (see Box 9.11).

Selective serotonin re-uptake inhibitors (SSRIs)

The SSRIs, including fluoxetine, paroxetine, fluvoxamine, sertraline and citalopram, are commonly used to treat depression, in part because they are less toxic than TCAs.

Clinical features and management

Overdose may produce nausea and vomiting, tremor, insomnia and sinus tachycardia. Agitation, drowsiness and convulsions occur infrequently and may be delayed for several hours after ingestion. Occasionally, features of serotonin syndrome may develop (see Box 9.12), especially if SSRIs are taken in combination or with other serotonergic agents. Cardiac arrhythmias, e.g. junctional bradycardias, occur infrequently. Most patients require supportive care only.

Lithium

Severe lithium toxicity is uncommon after intentional overdose and is more often encountered in patients taking therapeutic doses as a result of drug interactions (e.g. with diuretics or NSAIDs), deteriorating renal function or dehydration, or because an excessive dose has been prescribed.

Clinical features

Nausea, diarrhoea, polyuria, dizziness and tremor may progress to muscular weakness, drowsiness, confusion, myoclonus, fasciculations, choreoathetosis and renal failure. Coma, convulsions, ataxia, cardiac dysrhythmias (e.g. heart block), blood pressure disturbances and renal failure may occur in severe poisoning.

Management

Activated charcoal is ineffective. Gastric lavage is of theoretical benefit if used early after overdose, but lithium tablets are likely to remain intact in the stomach and may be too large for aspiration via a lavage tube. Some advocate whole bowel irrigation after substantial overdose but efficacy is unknown.

Lithium concentrations should be measured immediately in symptomatic patients or after at least 6 hours in asymptomatic patients following acute overdose. Adequate hydration should be maintained with intravenous fluids. Convulsions should be treated as in Box 9.11.

In patients with features suggesting severe toxicity associated with high lithium concentrations (e.g. > 4.0 mmol/L after chronic poisoning or > 7.5 mmol/L after acute poisoning), haemodialysis should be considered. Lithium concentrations are lowered substantially during dialysis but rebound increases occur after discontinuation, and multiple sessions may be required.

Cardiovascular medications

β-blockers

These have negative inotropic and chronotropic effects. Some have additional properties that may increase toxicity, such as blockade of sodium channels (e.g. propranolol) or potassium channels (e.g. sotalol).

Clinical features

The major features of toxicity are bradycardia and hypotension. Heart block, pulmonary oedema and cardiogenic shock occur in severe poisoning. Beta-blockers with sodium channel-blocking effects may cause seizures, confusion and coma, while sotalol may be associated with repolarisation abnormalities (including QT_c prolongation) and torsades de pointes (p. 567).

Management

Intravenous fluids may reverse hypotension but care is required to avoid pulmonary oedema. Bradycardia and hypotension may respond to high doses of atropine (up to 3 mg in an adult). The adrenoceptor agonist isoprotereenol (isoprenaline) may also be effective but high doses are often needed. Glucagon (5–10 mg over 10 mins, then 1–5 mg/hr by infusion), which does not act via adrenoceptors, is now more commonly used.

Calcium channel blockers

Calcium channel blockers are highly toxic in overdose via blockade of L-type calcium channels. Dihydropyridines such as nifedipine or amlodipine affect vascular smooth muscle in particular, resulting in vasodilatation. 'Rate-limiting' calcium channel blockers such as diltiazem and verapamil have direct cardiac effects, resulting in bradycardia and reduced myocardial contractility.

Clinical features

Hypotension is associated with vasodilatation and myocardial depression. Bradycardias and heart block may also occur, especially with verapamil and diltiazem.

Non-cardiac effects include gastrointestinal disturbances, confusion, metabolic acidosis, hyperglycaemia
and hyperkalaemia.

Management

Hypotension should be corrected with intravenous fluids, taking care to avoid pulmonary oedema. Persistent
hypotension may respond to intravenous calcium gluconate (10 mg i.v. over 5 mins, repeated as required).
Isoproterenol and glucagon may also be useful.
Successful use of intravenous insulin with glucose (10–
20% dextrose with insulin at 0.5–1.0 U/kg/hr), so-called
'hyperinsulinaemia euglycaemic therapy', has been
reported in patients unresponsive to other strategies.
Cardiac pacing may be needed for severe unresponsive
bradycardias or heart block.

Cardiac glycosides (including oleander)

Poisoning with digoxin is usually accidental, arising
from prescription of an excessive dose, impairment of
renal function or drug interactions. In South Asia, deliberate self-poisoning with yellow oleander (*Thevetia peruviana*), which contains cardiac glycosides, is common.

Clinical features

Characteristic cardiac effects of toxicity are tachyarrhythmias (either atrial or ventricular) and bradycardias, with
or without atrioventricular block. Ventricular bigeminy is common and atrial tachycardia with evidence of
atrioventricular block is highly suggestive of the diagnosis. Severe poisoning is associated with hyperkalaemia. Non-cardiac features include confusion, headache,
nausea, vomiting, diarrhoea and (rarely) altered colour
vision.

Management

Activated charcoal is commonly administered to patients
presenting early after ingestion of an acute overdose,
although evidence of benefit is lacking. Urea, electrolytes and creatinine should be measured, a 12-lead ECG
performed and cardiac monitoring instituted. Hypoxia,
hypokalaemia (sometimes associated with concurrent
diuretic use), hypomagnesaemia and acidosis increase the
risk of arrhythmias and should be corrected. Significant
bradycardias may respond to atropine, although temporary pacing is sometimes needed. Ventricular arrhythmias may respond to intravenous magnesium (see Box
9.11). If available, digoxin-specific antibody fragments
should be administered when there are severe ventricular arrhythmias or unresponsive bradycardias. This antidote has been shown to be effective for both digitalis and
yellow oleander poisoning.

Antimalarials

Chloroquine

Chloroquine is highly toxic; doses of 5 g or more of chloroquine base are likely to be fatal in an adult.

Clinical features

Features of toxicity occur within 1 hour of ingestion
and include nausea, vomiting, agitation, drowsiness,
hypokalaemia, acidosis, headaches and blurred vision.

Coma, convulsions and hypotension may occur in severe
poisoning. ECG changes indicating conduction and
repolarisation delay (prolonged QRS and QT_c intervals)
occur and are associated with ventricular tachycardia
(including torsades de pointes), ventricular fibrillation
and sudden death.

Management

Activated charcoal should be given to all patients presenting within 1 hour of ingestion of chloroquine in
amounts greater than 15 mg/kg. The cardiac rhythm
should be monitored and dysrhythmias managed as
in Box 9.11. The arterial pH should be corrected, but
hypokalaemia is thought to have a protective effect and
should not be corrected in the first 8 hours after poisoning. High-dose diazepam (2 mg/kg body weight i.v.
over 30 mins) has been suggested as having a protective
effect, especially if given in the early stages of severe
chloroquine poisoning, but evidence is limited as yet.
Respiratory support may be required.

Quinine

Quinine salts are widely used for treating malaria and
leg cramps. Deaths have been reported with as little as
1.5 g in an adult and 900 mg in a child.

Clinical features

Features of toxicity include nausea, vomiting, tremor, tinnitus and deafness. Hypotension, haemolysis, renal failure, ataxia, convulsions and coma are features of serious
poisoning. Conduction and repolarisation delay results
in prolonged QRS and QT_c intervals on the ECG, and
ventricular tachycardia (including torsades de pointes),
ventricular fibrillation and sudden death may occur.
Quinine-induced retinal vasoconstriction and retinal
photoreceptor cell toxicity may result in blurred vision
and impaired colour perception. This usually develops a
few hours after overdose and progresses to constriction
of the visual field, scotoma and complete blindness associated with pupillary dilatation and unresponsiveness to
light. Fundoscopy may show retinal artery spasm, disc
pallor and retinal oedema. Although visual loss can be
permanent, some degree of recovery often occurs over
several weeks.

Management

Multiple-dose activated charcoal should be commenced
in patients who have taken quinine in amounts greater
than 15 mg/kg. Gastric lavage may also be considered if
patients have presented within 1 hour. All patients should
have a 12-lead ECG and cardiac monitoring, and their
urea, electrolytes and glucose checked. Dysrhythmias,
hypotension, seizures and coma should be managed as
in Box 9.11.

There are no effective treatments for the visual effects
of quinine. Stellate ganglion block and retrobulbar or
intravenous injections of vasodilators such as nitrates
were previously used but are ineffective, as are haemodialysis and haemoperfusion.

Iron

The toxicity of iron preparations is related to their
elemental iron content.

213

Clinical features

Early clinical features include gastrointestinal disturbance with the passage of grey or black stools. Haematemesis or rectal bleeding may occur. Hyperglycaemia and leucocytosis suggest significant toxicity. Drowsiness, convulsions, coma, metabolic acidosis and cardiovascular collapse may occur in severe poisoning.

Early symptoms may improve or even resolve within 6–12 hours, but hepatocellular necrosis may develop 12–24 hours after overdose and occasionally this progresses to hepatic failure. Gastrointestinal strictures are late complications of iron poisoning.

Management

Gastric lavage may be considered in patients presenting within 1 hour of overdose but efficacy has not been established. Activated charcoal is ineffective since iron is not bound. Serum iron concentration should be measured (see Box 9.7, p. 208). The antidote desferrioxamine chelates iron and should be administered immediately in patients with severe features, without waiting for serum iron concentrations to be available. Symptomatic patients with high serum iron concentrations (e.g. > 5 mg/L) should also receive desferrioxamine. Desferrioxamine may cause hypotension, allergic reactions and occasionally pulmonary oedema. Otherwise treatment is supportive and directed at complications.

Antipsychotic drugs

Antipsychotic drugs (p. 245) are often prescribed for patients at high risk of self-harm or suicide, and are commonly encountered in overdose.

Clinical features

Drowsiness, tachycardia and hypotension are frequently found. Anticholinergic features (see Box 9.12) and acute dystonias (e.g. oculogyric crisis, torticollis and trismus) may occur after overdose with typical antipsychotics such as haloperidol or chlorpromazine. QT interval prolongation and torsades de pointes may occur with some antipsychotics, either typical (e.g. thioridazine, haloperidol) or atypical (e.g. quetiapine, ziprasidone). Convulsions may occur.

Management

Activated charcoal may be of benefit if given sufficiently early. Cardiac monitoring should be undertaken for at least 6 hours. Management is largely supportive, with treatment directed at complications (see Box 9.11, p. 210).

Antidiabetic agents

Antidiabetic agents commonly causing toxicity in overdose include the sulphonylureas (e.g. chlorpropamide, glibenclamide, gliclazide, glipizide and tolbutamide), biguanides (metformin and phenformin) and insulins.

Clinical features

Sulphonylureas and parenteral insulin cause hypoglycaemia when taken in overdose, although insulin is non-toxic if ingested. The duration of hypoglycaemia depends on the half-life or release characteristics of the preparation and may be prolonged over several days with long-acting agents such as chlorpropamide, insulin zinc suspension or insulin glargine.

Features of hypoglycaemia include nausea, agitation, sweating, aggression and behavioural disturbances, confusion, tachycardia, hypothermia, drowsiness, coma or convulsions (p. 812). Permanent neurological damage can occur if the hypoglycaemia is prolonged. Hypoglycaemia can be diagnosed using bedside glucose strips but venous blood should also be sent for laboratory confirmation.

Metformin is uncommonly associated with hypoglycaemia. Its major toxic effect in overdose is lactic acidosis, which can be associated with a high mortality, and is particularly common in older patients and those with renal or hepatic impairment, or when ethanol is co-ingested. Other features of metformin overdose are nausea and vomiting, diarrhoea, abdominal pain, drowsiness, coma, hypotension and cardiovascular collapse.

Management

Activated charcoal should be considered for all patients who present within 1 hour of ingestion of a substantial overdose of an oral hypoglycaemic agent. Venous blood glucose, urea and electrolytes should be measured and tests repeated regularly. Hypoglycaemia should be corrected using oral or intravenous glucose (50 mL of 50% dextrose); an infusion of 10–20% dextrose may be required to prevent recurrence. Intramuscular glucagon can be used as an alternative, especially if intravenous access is unavailable. Failure to regain consciousness within a few minutes of normalisation of the blood glucose can indicate that a central nervous system (CNS) depressant has also been ingested, the hypoglycaemia has been prolonged, or there is another cause for the coma (e.g. cerebral haemorrhage or oedema).

Arterial blood gases should be taken after metformin overdose to assess the extent of acidosis. If present, plasma lactate should be measured and acidosis should be corrected with intravenous sodium bicarbonate (e.g. 250 mL 1.26% solution or 50 mL 8.4% solution, repeated as necessary). In severe cases haemodialysis or haemodiafiltration is used.

DRUGS OF MISUSE

Cannabis

Cannabis is derived from the dried leaves and flowers of *Cannabis sativa*. When smoked, the onset of effect occurs within 10–30 minutes; after ingestion the onset is 1–3 hours. The duration of effect is 4–8 hours. Cannabis produces euphoria, perceptual alterations and conjunctival injection, followed by enhanced appetite, relaxation, and occasionally hypertension, tachycardia, slurred speech and ataxia. High doses may produce anxiety, confusion, hallucinations and psychosis (Box 9.13). Psychological dependence is common, but tolerance and withdrawal symptoms are unusual. Long-term use is thought to increase the lifetime

9.13 Stimulant, sedative and opioid feature clusters

	Stimulant	Sedative hypnotic	Opioid
Common causes	Amphetamines	Benzodiazepines	Heroin
	MDMA ('ecstasy')	Barbiturates	Morphine
	Ephedrine	Ethanol	Methadone
	Pseudoephedrine	Gammahydroxybutyrate (GHB)	Oxycodone
	Cocaine		Dihydrocodeine
	Cannabis		Codeine
	Phencyclidine		Pethidine
			Dipipanone
			Buprenorphine
			Dextropropoxyphene
			Tramadol
Clinical features			
Respiratory	Tachypnoea	Reduced respiratory rate and ventilation[1]	Reduced respiratory rate and ventilation
Cardiovascular	Tachycardia, hypertension	Hypotension[1]	Hypotension, relative bradycardia
CNS	Restlessness, anxiety, anorexia, insomnia	Confusion, hallucinations, slurred speech	Confusion, hallucinations, slurred speech
	Hallucinations	Sedation, coma[1]	Sedation, coma[2]
Muscle	Tremor	Ataxia, reduced muscle tone	Ataxia, reduced muscle tone
Temperature	Fever	Hypothermia	Hypothermia
Eyes	Mydriasis	Diplopia, strabismus, nystagmus Normal pupil size	Miosis
Abdomen	Abdominal pain, diarrhoea	–	Ileus
Mouth	Dry	–	–
Skin	Piloerection	Blisters, pressure sores	Needle tracks[2]
Complications	Seizures	Respiratory failure[1]	Respiratory failure[2]
	Myocardial infarction		
	Dysrhythmias		
	Rhabdomyolysis		
	Renal failure		
	Intracerebral haemorrhage or infarction		

[1]Especially barbiturates.
[2]I.v. use.

risk of developing schizophrenia. Ingestion or smoking of cannabis rarely results in serious poisoning and supportive treatment is all that is required.

Benzodiazepines

Benzodiazepines may be prescribed or used illicitly. They are of low toxicity when taken alone in overdose, but can enhance CNS depression when taken with other sedative agents, including alcohol. They may also cause significant toxicity in the elderly and those with chronic lung or neuromuscular disease.

Clinical features

Clinical features of toxicity include drowsiness, ataxia and confusion (see Box 9.13). Respiratory depression and hypotension may occur with severe poisoning in susceptible groups, especially after intravenous administration of short-acting agents.

Management

Activated charcoal may be useful after ingestion in susceptible patients or after mixed overdose, if given

within 1 hour. Conscious level and oxygen saturation should be monitored for at least 6 hours after substantial overdose.

The specific benzodiazepine antagonist flumazenil increases conscious level in patients with overdose but carries a risk of seizures, and is contraindicated in patients co-ingesting proconvulsant agents such as TCAs and in those with a history of seizures.

Stimulants

Amphetamines, ecstasy and cocaine are sympathomimetic amines and, as a result, some clinical features of poisoning are similar (see Box 9.13).

Cocaine

Cocaine is available as a water-soluble hydrochloride salt suitable for nasal inhalation ('snorting'), or as an insoluble free base ('crack' cocaine) which, unlike the hydrochloride salt, vaporises at high temperature and can be smoked, giving a more rapid and intense effect. Cocaine hydrochloride is usually purchased as a white crystalline powder while crack cocaine is usually sold in 'rocks'.

9

Clinical features

Cocaine's toxic effects appear rapidly after inhalation and especially after smoking. Sympathomimetic stimulant effects are common (see Box 9.13). Serious complications usually occur within 3 hours of use, and include coronary artery spasm which may result in myocardial ischaemia or infarction, even in patients with normal coronary arteries. This may lead to hypotension, cyanosis and ventricular arrhythmias. Cocaine toxicity should be considered in young adults who present with ischaemic chest pain. Hyperpyrexia may be associated with rhabdomyolysis, acute renal failure and disseminated intravascular coagulation.

Management

All patients should be observed with ECG monitoring for a minimum of 4 hours. A 12-lead ECG should be performed, although ECG changes can be misleading. Troponin T estimations are the most sensitive and specific markers of myocardial damage. Benzodiazepines and intravenous nitrates are useful for managing patients with chest pain or hypertension, but β-blockers are best avoided because of the risk of unopposed α-adrenoceptor stimulation. Coronary angiography should be considered in patients with myocardial infarction or acute coronary syndromes. Acidosis should be corrected. Physical cooling measures may be required for hyperthermia (p. 103).

Amphetamines and ecstasy

These include amphetamine sulphate ('speed'), methylamphetamine ('crystal meth') and 3,4-methylenedioxymethamphetamine (MDMA, 'ecstasy'). Tolerance to amphetamines is common, leading regular users to seek progressively higher doses.

Clinical features

Toxic features usually appear within a few minutes of use and last 4–6 hours or substantially longer after a large overdose. Sympathomimetic stimulant effects are common (see Box 9.13). A proportion of ecstasy users develop hyponatraemia as a result of drinking large amounts of water and inappropriate antidiuretic hormone secretion. Muscle rigidity, pain and trismus (jaw-clenching) may occur. Hyperpyrexia, rhabdomyolysis, metabolic acidosis, acute renal failure, disseminated intravascular coagulation, hepatocellular necrosis, acute respiratory distress syndrome (ARDS) and cardiovascular collapse have all been described following MDMA use but these are rare. Strokes, due to either cerebral infarction or haemorrhage, have been reported, especially after intravenous amphetamine use.

Management

Management is supportive and directed at complications (see Box 9.11, p. 210).

Gammahydroxybutyrate (GHB)

GHB is a sedative agent with psychedelic and body-building effects, which is easily manufactured from commonly available industrial chemicals. These include 1,4 butanediol, which is metabolised to GHB in vivo and has similar effects after ingestion. GHB solution is drunk by users, who titrate the dose until the desired effects are achieved.

Clinical features

Toxic features are those of a sedative hypnotic (see Box 9.13). Nausea, diarrhoea, vertigo, tremor, myoclonus, extrapyramidal signs, euphoria, bradycardia, convulsions, metabolic acidosis, hypokalaemia and hyperglycaemia may also occur. As the drug may be produced in batches and shared amongst a number of individuals, several patients may present with coma at the same time. The sedative effects are potentiated by other CNS depressants, e.g. alcohol, benzodiazepines, opioids and neuroleptic drugs. Coma usually resolves spontaneously and abruptly within a few hours, but may occasionally persist for several days.

Management

Activated charcoal is recommended within 1 hour for ingestion of GHB in amounts greater than 20 mg/kg. Urea, electrolytes and glucose should be measured in all but the most trivial of cases. All patients should be observed for a minimum of 2 hours, with monitoring of blood pressure, heart rate, respiratory rate and oxygenation. Patients who remain symptomatic should be observed in hospital until symptoms resolve, but require supportive care only.

LSD

d-Lysergic acid diethylamide (LSD) is a synthetic hallucinogen usually ingested as small squares of impregnated absorbent paper, which are often printed with a distinctive design, or as 'microdots'. The drug causes perceptual effects, such as heightened visual awareness of colours, distortion of images, and hallucinations which may be pleasurable or terrifying ('bad trip') and associated with panic, confusion, agitation or aggression. Dilated pupils, hypertension, pyrexia and metabolic acidosis may occur and psychosis may sometimes last several days.

Patients with psychotic reactions or CNS depression should be observed in hospital, preferably in a quiet, dimly lit room to minimise external stimulation. Where sedation is required, diazepam is the drug of choice. Antipsychotics should be avoided if possible, as they may precipitate cardiovascular collapse or convulsions.

Opioids

Commonly encountered opioids are shown in Box 9.13. Toxicity may result from drug misuse (e.g. heroin) or after overdose of medicinal opiates (e.g. dextropropoxyphene). Intravenous use of heroin or morphine gives a rapid, intensely pleasurable experience, often accompanied by heightened sexual arousal. Physical dependence occurs within a few weeks of regular high-dose injection; as a result, the dose is escalated and the user's life becomes increasingly centred on obtaining and taking the drug. Withdrawal, which can start within 12 hours, presents with intense craving, rhinorrhoea, lacrimation, yawning, perspiration, shivering, piloerection, vomiting, diarrhoea and abdominal cramps. Examination reveals tachycardia, hypertension, mydriasis and facial flushing.

Accidental overdose with prescribed strong opioid preparations is common, especially in the elderly.

Clinical features

These are shown in Box 9.13. Needle tracks may be visible in intravenous drug misusers and drug-related paraphernalia may be found amongst their possessions. Severe poisoning results in respiratory depression, hypotension, non-cardiogenic pulmonary oedema and hypothermia, leading to respiratory arrest or aspiration of gastric contents. Dextropropoxyphene (the opioid component of co-proxamol) may also cause cardiac conduction effects, particularly QRS prolongation, ventricular arrhythmias and heart block. Excess deaths caused by these complications have prompted the withdrawal of co-proxamol (dextropropoxyphene and paracetamol combination) in the UK. Methadone may cause QT_c prolongation and torsades de pointes.

Symptoms of opioid poisoning can be prolonged for up to 48 hours after use of long-acting agents (e.g. methadone, dextropropoxyphene and oxycodone).

Management

The airway should be cleared and, if necessary, respiratory support and oxygen given. Oxygen saturation monitoring and measurement of arterial blood gases should be performed. Prompt use of the specific opioid antagonist naloxone (0.8–2 mg i.v., repeated if necessary) may obviate the need for intubation, although excessive doses may precipitate acute withdrawal in opiate misusers. An infusion may be required in some cases because the half-life of the antidote is short compared to that of most opiates, especially those with prolonged elimination. It is important that patients are monitored for at least 4 hours after the last naloxone dose. Other complications of naloxone therapy include fits and ventricular arrhythmias, although these appear to be rare. Box 9.11 (p. 210) describes the management of coma, fits and hypotension. Non-cardiogenic pulmonary oedema does not usually respond to diuretic therapy, and continuous positive airways pressure (CPAP) or positive end-expiratory pressure (PEEP) ventilatory support (p. 195) may be required.

Bodypackers

Bodypackers ('mules') attempt to smuggle illicit drugs (usually cocaine, heroin or amphetamines) by ingesting multiple small packages wrapped in multiple layers of clingfilm or in condoms. They are at risk of developing severe toxicity if these packages rupture.

Patients suspected of bodypacking should be admitted for observation. A careful history taken in private is important, but for obvious reasons patients may withhold details of the drugs involved. The mouth, rectum and vagina should be examined as possible sites for concealed drugs. Packages may be visible on plain abdominal films (Fig. 9.4), but this is not always the case, and ultrasound and computed tomography (CT) provides more sensitive methods of visualisation.

Antimotility agents are often used by bodypackers to prevent premature passage of packages, so it can take

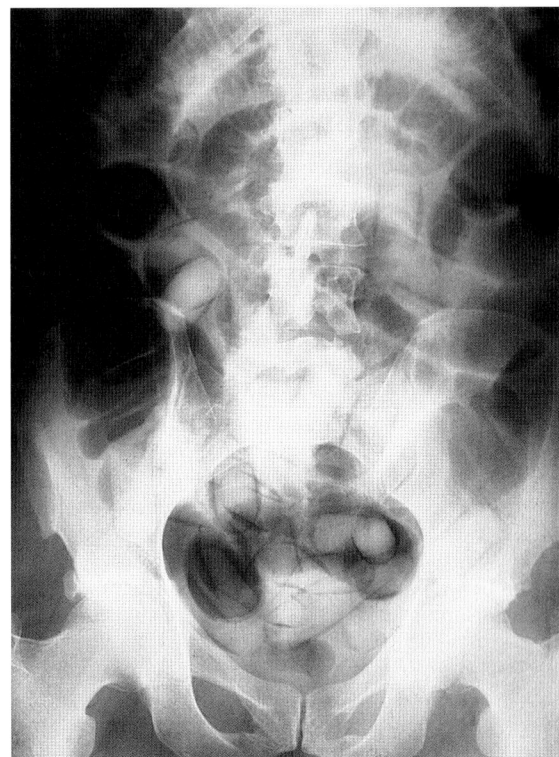

Fig. 9.4 Abdominal X-ray of a bodypacker showing multiple drug-filled condoms.

a number of days for packages to pass spontaneously; during this period the carrier is at risk from package rupture. Whole bowel irrigation is commonly used to accelerate passage and is continued until all packages have passed. Surgery may be required for mechanical bowel obstruction or when evolving clinical features suggest package rupture.

CHEMICALS AND PESTICIDES

Carbon monoxide (CO)

CO is a colourless and odourless gas produced by faulty appliances burning organic fuels. It is also present in vehicle exhaust fumes and sometimes in smoke from house fires. It causes toxicity by binding with haemoglobin and cytochrome oxidase, which reduces tissue oxygen delivery and inhibits cellular respiration. It is a common cause of death by poisoning and most patients who die of CO poisoning do so before reaching hospital.

Clinical features

The early clinical features of acute severe carbon monoxide poisoning are headache, nausea, irritability, weakness and tachypnoea. Because these are non-specific, the correct diagnosis will not be obvious if the exposure is occult, e.g. from a faulty domestic appliance. Subsequently, ataxia, nystagmus, drowsiness and hyper-reflexia may develop, progressing to coma, convulsions, hypotension, respiratory depression, cardiovascular collapse and death. Myocardial ischaemia may occur and result in arrhythmias or myocardial infarction. Cerebral

9

oedema is common and rhabdomyolysis may lead to myoglobinuria and renal failure. In those who recover from acute toxicity, longer-term neuropsychiatric effects are common, such as personality change, memory loss and concentration impairment. Extrapyramidal effects, urinary or faecal incontinence, and gait disturbance may also occur. Poisoning during pregnancy may cause fetal hypoxia and intrauterine death.

Management

Patients should be removed from exposure as soon as possible and the patient resuscitated as necessary. Oxygen should be administered in as high a concentration as possible via a tightly fitting facemask, as this reduces the half-life of carboxyhaemoglobin from 4–6 hours to about 40 minutes. Measurement of carboxyhaemoglobin is useful for confirming exposure (see Box 9.7, p. 208) but results do not correlate well with the severity of poisoning, partly because concentrations fall rapidly after removal of the patient from exposure, especially if supplemental oxygen has been given.

An ECG should be performed in all patients with acute poisoning, especially those with pre-existing heart disease. Arterial blood gas analysis should be checked in those with serious poisoning. Oxygen saturation readings by pulse oximetry are misleading since both carboxyhaemoglobin and oxyhaemoglobin are measured. Excessive intravenous fluid administration should be avoided, particularly in the elderly, because of the risk of pulmonary and cerebral oedema. Convulsions should be controlled with diazepam.

Hyperbaric oxygen therapy is controversial. In theory, at 2.5 atmospheres, it reduces the half-life of carboxyhaemoglobin to 20 minutes and increases the amount of dissolved oxygen by a factor of 10. The logistical difficulties of transporting sick patients to hyperbaric chambers and managing them therein should not be underestimated and recent systematic reviews have shown no improvement in clinical outcomes.

Organophosphorus (OP) insecticides/ nerve agents

OP compounds (Box 9.14) are widely used as pesticides, especially in developing countries. The case fatality rate following deliberate ingestion of OP pesticides in developing countries in Asia is 5–20%.

Nerve agents developed for chemical warfare are derived from OP insecticides but are much more toxic.

ℹ️	**9.14 Organophosphorus compounds**

Nerve agents

- G agents: sarin, tabun, soman
- V agents: VX, VE

Insecticides

Dimethyl compounds	**Diethyl compounds**
• Dichlorvos	• Chlorpyrifos
• Fenthion	• Diazinon
• Malathion	• Parathion-ethyl
• Methamidophos	• Quinalphos

'G' agents are volatile, are absorbed by inhalation or via the skin, and dissipate rapidly after use. 'V' agents are contact poisons unless aerosolised, and contaminate ground for weeks or months.

The toxicology and management of nerve agent and pesticide poisoning are similar.

Mechanism of toxicity

OP compounds phosphonylate the active site of acetylcholinesterase (AChE), inactivating the enzyme and leading to the accumulation of acetylcholine (ACh) in cholinergic synapses (Fig. 9.5). Spontaneous hydrolysis of the OP-enzyme complex allows reactivation of the enzyme. However, loss of a chemical group from the OP-enzyme complex prevents further enzyme reactivation, a process termed 'ageing'. After ageing has taken place, new enzyme needs to be synthesised before function can be restored. The rate of ageing is an important determinant of toxicity and is more rapid with dimethyl compounds (3.7 hours) than diethyl compounds (31 hours), and especially rapid after exposure to nerve agents (soman in particular), which cause ageing within minutes.

Clinical features and management

OP poisoning causes an acute cholinergic phase, which may occasionally be followed by the intermediate syndrome or organophosphate-induced delayed polyneuropathy (OPIDN). The onset, severity and duration of poisoning depend on the route of exposure and agent involved.

Acute cholinergic syndrome

The acute cholinergic syndrome usually starts within a few minutes of exposure. Nicotinic or muscarinic features may be present (Box 9.15). Vomiting and profuse diarrhoea are typical following oral ingestion. Bronchoconstriction, bronchorrhoea and salivation may cause severe respiratory compromise. Miosis is characteristic and the presence of muscle fasciculations strongly suggests the diagnosis, although this feature is often absent, even in serious poisoning. Subsequently, the patient may develop generalised flaccid paralysis which can affect respiratory and ocular muscles and result in respiratory failure. Ataxia, coma and convulsions may occur. In severe poisoning, cardiac repolarisation abnormalities and torsades de pointes may occur. Other early complications of OP poisoning include extrapyramidal features, pancreatitis, hepatic dysfunction and pyrexia.

Management

In the event of external contamination, further exposure should be prevented, contaminated clothing and contact lenses removed, the skin washed with soap and water, and the eyes irrigated. The airway should be cleared of excessive secretions and high-flow oxygen administered. Intravenous access should be obtained. Gastric lavage or activated charcoal may be considered within 1 hour of ingestion. Convulsions should be treated as described in Box 9.11, p. 210. The ECG, oxygen saturation, blood gases, temperature, urea and electrolytes, amylase and glucose should be monitored closely.

Early use of sufficient doses of atropine is potentially life-saving in patients with severe toxicity. Atropine reverses ACh-induced bronchospasm, bronchorrhoea,

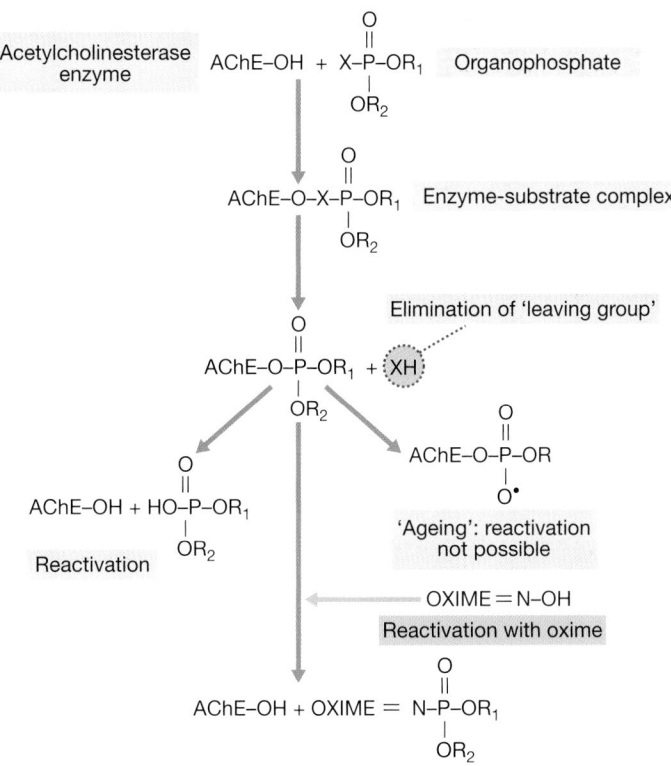

Fig. 9.5 Mechanism of toxicity of organophosphorus compounds and treatment with oxime.

bradycardia and hypotension. When the diagnosis is uncertain, a marked increase in heart rate associated with skin flushing after a 1 mg intravenous dose makes OP poisoning unlikely. In OP poisoning, atropine should be administered in doses of 0.6–2 mg i.v., repeated every 10–25 mins until secretions are controlled, the skin is dry and there is a sinus tachycardia. Large doses may be needed but excessive doses may cause anticholinergic effects (see Box 9.12, p. 211).

In patients requiring atropine, an oxime such as pralidoxime chloride (or obidoxime), if available, should also be administered, as this may reverse or prevent muscle weakness, convulsions or coma, especially if administered rapidly after exposure. The dose for an adult is 2 g i.v. over 4 mins, repeated 4–6-hourly. Oximes work by reactivating AChE that has not undergone 'ageing' and are therefore less effective with dimethyl compounds and nerve agents, especially soman. Oximes may provoke hypotension, especially if administered rapidly.

Ventilatory support should be instituted before the patient develops respiratory failure (p. 194). Benzodiazepines may be used to reduce agitation and fasciculations, treat convulsions and sedate patients during mechanical ventilation.

Exposure is confirmed by measurement of plasma (butyrylcholinesterase) or red blood cell cholinesterase activity. These correlate poorly with the severity of clinical features, although values are usually less than 10% in severe poisoning, 20–50% in moderate poisoning and > 50% in subclinical poisoning.

The acute cholinergic phase usually lasts 48–72 hours, with most patients requiring intensive cardiorespiratory support and monitoring.

The intermediate syndrome

About 20% of patients with OP poisoning develop weakness rapidly spreading from the ocular muscles

9.15 Cholinergic features in poisoning*

	Cholinergic muscarinic	Cholinergic nicotinic
Respiratory	Bronchorrhoea, bronchoconstriction	Reduced ventilation
Cardiovascular	Bradycardia, hypotension	Tachycardia, hypertension
CNS	Confusion	–
Muscle	–	Fasciculation, paralysis
Temperature	Fever	–
Eyes	Diplopia, mydriasis	Lacrimation, miosis
Abdomen	Ileus, palpable bladder	Vomiting, profuse diarrhoea
Mouth	Dry	Salivation
Skin	Flushing, hot, dry	Sweating
Complications	Seizures	Seizures

*Both muscarinic and nicotinic features occur in OP poisoning. Nicotinic features occur in nicotine poisoning and black widow spider bites. Cholinergic features are sometimes seen in poisoning with some mushrooms.

to those of the head and neck, proximal limbs and the muscles of respiration, resulting in ventilatory failure. This 'intermediate syndrome' (IMS) generally develops quite rapidly between 1 and 4 days after exposure, often after resolution of the acute cholinergic syndrome, and may last 2–3 weeks. There is no specific treatment but supportive care, including maintenance of airway and ventilation, is important.

Organophosphate-induced delayed polyneuropathy (OPIDN)

This is a rare complication that usually occurs 2–3 weeks after acute exposure. It is a mixed sensory/motor poly-neuropathy, especially affecting long myelinated neurons, and appears to result from inhibition of enzymes other than AChE. It is a feature of poisoning with some OPs (e.g. trichlorocresylphosphate), while others, including nerve agents, are not thought to have this effect. Early clinical features are muscle cramps followed by numbness and paraesthesiae, proceeding to flaccid paralysis of the lower and subsequently the upper limbs. Paralysis of the lower limbs is associated with foot drop and a high-stepping gait, progressing to paraplegia. Paralysis of the arms leads to wrist drop. Sensory loss may also be present but is variable. Initially, tendon reflexes are reduced or lost, but later mild spasticity may develop.

There is no specific therapy for OPIDN. Regular physiotherapy may limit deformity caused by muscle-wasting. Recovery is often incomplete and may be limited to the hands and feet, although substantial functional recovery after 1–2 years may occur, especially in younger patients.

Carbamate insecticides

Carbamate insecticides (e.g. aldicarb, carbofuran, methomyl) inhibit a number of tissue esterases, including AChE. The mechanism of action, clinical features and management are similar to those of OP compounds. However, clinical features tend to be less severe and of shorter duration, because the carbamate/AChE complex dissociates quickly, with a half-life of 30–40 minutes, and does not undergo ageing. Also, carbamates penetrate the CNS poorly. Pancreatitis has been reported as a sequel, and deaths have occurred.

Atropine may be given intravenously in frequent small doses (0.6–2.0 mg i.v. for an adult) until signs of atropinisation develop. Diazepam may be used to relieve anxiety. The use of oximes is unnecessary.

Methanol and ethylene glycol

Ethylene glycol (1,2-ethanediol) is found in antifreeze, brake fluids and, in lower concentrations, windscreen washes. Methanol is present in some antifreeze products and commercially available industrial solvents, and in low concentrations in some screen washes and methylated spirits. It may also be an adulterant of illicitly produced alcohol. Both are rapidly absorbed after ingestion. Although methanol and ethylene glycol are not of high intrinsic toxicity, they are converted via alcohol dehydrogenase to toxic metabolites that are largely responsible for their clinical effects (Fig. 9.6).

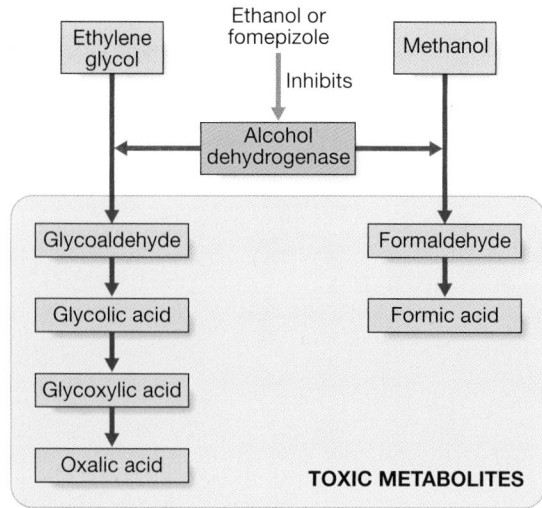

Fig. 9.6 Metabolism of methanol and ethylene glycol.

Clinical features

Early features with either methanol or ethylene glycol include ataxia, drowsiness, dysarthria and nystagmus, often associated with vomiting. As the toxic metabolites are formed, metabolic acidosis, tachypnoea, coma and seizures may develop.

Toxic effects of ethylene glycol toxicity include ophthalmoplegia, cranial nerve palsies, hyporeflexia and myoclonus. Renal pain and acute tubular necrosis occur because of precipitation of calcium oxalate in the kidneys. Hypocalcaemia, hypomagnesaemia and hyperkalaemia are common.

Features of methanol poisoning include headache, confusion and vertigo. Visual impairment and photophobia develop, associated with optic disc and retinal oedema and impaired pupil reflexes. Blindness may be permanent, although some recovery may occur over several months. Pancreatitis and abnormal liver function have also been reported.

Management

Urea, electrolytes, chloride, bicarbonate, glucose, calcium, magnesium, albumin and plasma osmolarity and arterial blood gases should be measured in all patients with suspected methanol or ethylene glycol toxicity. The osmolal and anion gaps should be calculated (see Box 9.6, p. 207). Initially, poisoning is associated with an increased osmolar gap, but as toxic metabolites are produced, an increased anion gap associated with metabolic acidosis will develop. The diagnosis can be confirmed by measurement of ethylene glycol or methanol concentrations, but these assays are not widely available.

An antidote, either ethanol or fomepizole, should be administered to all patients with suspected significant exposure while awaiting the results of laboratory investigations. These block alcohol dehydrogenase and delay the formation of toxic metabolites until the parent drug is eliminated either naturally or by dialysis. The antidote should be continued until ethylene glycol or methanol concentrations are undetectable. Metabolic acidosis should be corrected with sodium bicarbonate (e.g. 250 mL of 1.26% solution, repeated as necessary).

Convulsions should be treated with an intravenous benzodiazepine. In ethylene glycol poisoning, hypocalcaemia should only be corrected if there are severe ECG features or seizures occur, since this may increase calcium oxalate crystal formation.

Haemodialysis or haemodiafiltration should be used in severe poisoning, especially if renal failure is present or there is visual loss in the context of methanol poisoning. It should be continued until acute toxic features are no longer present and ethylene glycol or methanol concentrations are no longer detectable.

Aluminium and zinc phosphide

These rodenticides and fumigants are a common means of self-poisoning in northern India, where the mortality rate has been estimated at 60%. When ingested, both compounds react with gastric water to form phosphine, a potent pulmonary and gastrointestinal toxicant. Clinical features include severe gastrointestinal disturbances, chest tightness, cough and breathlessness progressing to ARDS and respiratory failure, tremor, paraesthesiae, convulsions, coma, tachycardia, metabolic acidosis, electrolyte disturbances, hypoglycaemia, myocarditis, liver and renal failure, and leucopenia. Just a few tablets can be fatal.

Detection of phosphine in the exhaled air or stomach aspirate using either a silver nitrate-impregnated strip or specific phosphine detector tube is diagnostic, but gas chromatography provides the most sensitive indicator. Treatment is supportive and directed at correcting electrolyte abnormalities and treating complications; there is no specific antidote. Early gastric lavage is sometimes used, often with vegetable oil to reduce the release of toxic phosphine, but the benefit is uncertain.

ENVIRONMENTAL POISONING AND ILLNESS

Arsenism

Chronic arsenic exposure from drinking water has been reported in many countries, especially India, Bangladesh, Nepal, Thailand, Taiwan, China, Mexico and South America, where a large proportion of the drinking water (ground water) has a high arsenic content, placing large population groups at risk. The World Health Organization (WHO) guideline value for arsenic content in tube well water is 10 μg/L.

Health effects associated with chronic exposure to arsenic in drinking water are shown in Box 9.16. In exposed individuals, high concentrations of arsenic are present in bone, hair and nails. Specific treatments are of no benefit in chronic arsenic toxicity and recovery from the peripheral neuropathy may never be complete. The emphasis should be on the prevention of exposure to arsenic in drinking water.

Fluorosis

Though water-borne fluorides at levels of 1 part per million (ppm) are associated with significant immunity

9.16 Clinical features of chronic arsenic poisoning

GI tract

- Anorexia, vomiting, weight loss, diarrhoea, increased salivation, metallic taste

Neurological

- Peripheral neuropathy (sensory and motor) with muscle wasting and fasciculation, ataxia

Skin

- Hyperpigmentation, palmar and plantar keratosis, alopecia, multiple epitheliomas, Mee's lines (transverse white lines on finger nails)

Eyes

- Conjunctivitis, corneal necrosis and ulceration

Bone marrow

- Aplastic anaemia

Other

- Low-grade fever, vasospasm and gangrene, jaundice, hepatomegaly, splenomegaly

Increased risk of malignancy

- Lung, liver, bladder, kidney, larynx and lymphoid system

9

to dental caries, the presence of excessive quantities of fluoride (> 10 ppm) in drinking water, e.g. from deep bore wells, leads to characteristic changes in teeth, bone and periarticular tissues. Fluorosis may also result from industrial exposure to fluoride dust and consumption of brick teas. Yellowish-brown staining and pitting of permanent teeth particularly are early and easily recognisable features of chronic toxicity. Damage of the enamel may ensue. Skeletal involvement is not clinically apparent unless advanced, but radiological changes are present at an early stage. Early symptoms include stiffness and back pain. Later, deformities (e.g. kyphosis), calcification of ligaments and joint ankylosis may occur and result in severe disability. Changes in the bones of the thoracic cage may lead to rigidity that causes dyspnoea on exertion. Very high doses of fluoride may cause abdominal pain, nausea, vomiting, seizures and muscle spasm. In calcium-deficient children, the toxic effects of fluoride manifest even at marginally high exposures to fluoride.

In endemic areas, such as Jordan, Turkey, Chile, India, Bangladesh, China and Tibet, fluorosis is a major public health problem. The maximum impact is seen in communities engaged in physically strenuous agricultural or industrial activities. Dental fluorosis is endemic in East Africa and some West African countries.

SUBSTANCES LESS COMMONLY TAKEN IN OVERDOSE

Box 9.17 gives an overview of the clinical features and management for some substances that are less often encountered in overdose.

9.17 Substances taken less commonly in overdose

Drug/substance	Features	Specific management
Anticonvulsants		
Carbamazepine, phenytoin	Cerebellar signs Convulsions Cardiac arrhythmias Coma	Multiple-dose activated charcoal (carbamazepine)
Sodium valproate	Coma Metabolic acidosis	Haemodialysis for severe poisoning
Isoniazid	Peripheral neuropathy Convulsions	Activated charcoal I.v. pyridoxine
Theophylline	Cardiac arrhythmias Convulsions Coma	Multiple-dose activated charcoal
Corrosives and bleach	Injuries to stomach (esp. acids) and oesophagus (esp. alkali) GI perforation and late strictures Aspiration pneumonitis	Gastric lavage and neutralising chemicals are contraindicated Chest X-ray to exclude perforation Consider early endoscopy or Gastrografin studies to assess extent of damage and need for surgery
Lead, e.g. chronic occupational exposure, leaded paint, water contaminated by lead pipes, use of kohl cosmetics	Abdominal pain Microcytic anaemia with basophilic stippling Headache and encephalopathy Motor neuropathy Nephrotoxicity Hypertension Hypocalcaemia	Prevent further exposure Measure blood lead concentration, full blood count and blood film, urea and electrolytes, liver function tests and calcium Abdominal X-ray in children to detect pica Bone X-ray for 'lead lines' Chelation therapy with dimercaprol, DMSA, DMPS or sodium calcium edetate for severe poisoning (esp. in children)
Petroleum distillates, white spirit, kerosene	Vomiting Aspiration pneumonitis	Gastric lavage contraindicated Activated charcoal ineffective Oxygen and nebulised bronchodilators Chest X-ray to assess pulmonary effects
Paraquat	Buccal ulceration Progressive respiratory fibrosis with respiratory failure Renal failure	Urine screen for paraquat Multiple-dose activated charcoal Check blood paraquat concentration and compare with survival curve for prognosis
Organochlorines, e.g. DDT, lindane, dieldrin, endosulfan	Nausea, vomiting Agitation Fasciculation Paraesthesiae (face, extremities) Convulsions Coma Respiratory depression Cardiac arrhythmias Hyperthermia Rhabdomyolysis Pulmonary oedema Disseminated intravascular coagulation	Activated charcoal (with nasogastric aspiration for liquid preparations) within 1 hour of ingestion Cardiac monitoring
Pyrethroid insecticides, e.g. cypermethrin, permethrin, imiprothrin	Skin contact: dermatitis, skin paraesthesiae Eye contact: lacrimation, photophobia and oedema of the eyelids Inhalation: dyspnoea, nausea, headaches Ingestion: epigastric pain, nausea, vomiting, headache, coma, convulsions, pulmonary oedema	Symptomatic and supportive care Washing contaminated skin makes irritation worse
Anticoagulant rodenticides (e.g. brodifacoum, bromodialone) **and warfarin**	Abnormal bleeding (prolonged)	Monitor INR/prothrombin time Vitamin K_1 by slow i.v. injection if coagulopathy Fresh frozen plasma or specific clotting factors for bleeding

(DMPS = 2,3-dimercapto-1-propane sulphonate; DMSA = 2,3-dimercaptosuccinic acid)

ENVENOMING

Envenoming occurs when a venomous animal injects sufficient venom into a prey item or perceived predator. This may be by a bite or a sting, and results in local and/or systemic toxic effects. Venomous animals generally use their venom to acquire and in some cases predigest prey, with defensive use a secondary function. Accidental encounters between venomous animals and humans occur frequently, particularly in the rural tropics, with millions of cases of venomous bites and stings annually. Globally, an increasing number of exotic venomous animals are kept privately, so cases of envenoming may present to hospitals where doctors have insufficient knowledge to manage potentially complex presentations. Doctors everywhere should thus be aware of the basic principles of management of envenoming and how to seek expert support.

Venom

Venom is a complex mixture of diverse components, often with several separate toxins that can cause adverse effects in humans, and each potentially capable of multiple effects (Box 9.18). Venom is produced at considerable metabolic cost, so is used sparingly; thus only some bites/stings by venomous animals result in significant envenoming, the remainder being 'dry bites'. The concept of dry bites is important in understanding approaches to management.

Venomo us animals

There are many animal groups that contain venomous species (Box 9.19). The epidemiology estimates shown reflect the importance of snakes and scorpions as causes of severe or lethal envenoming, and social insect stings (e.g. bees, wasps) as causes of sometimes lethal anaphylaxis. Other venomous animals may commonly envenom humans but cause mostly non-lethal effects. A few rarely envenom humans, but have a high potential for severe or lethal envenoming (e.g. box jellyfish, cone shells, blue-ringed octopus, paralysis ticks, Australian funnel web spiders). Within any given group, particularly snakes, there may be a wide range of clinical presentations. Some are described here but for a more detailed discussion of the types of venomous animal, their venoms and effects on humans see www.toxinology.com.

Clinical effects

With the exception of dry bites where no significant effects occur, venomous bites/stings can result in three broad classes of effect.

Local effects

These vary from trivial to severe (Box 9.20). There may be minimal or no local effects with some snakebites (not even pain), yet lethal systemic envenoming may still be present. For other species, local effects predominate over systemic, and for others, e.g. many snakes, both are important.

General systemic effects

By definition, these are non-specific (see Box 9.20). Shock is an important complication of major local envenoming by some snake species and, if inadequately treated, can prove lethal, especially in children.

Specific systemic effects

These are important in both diagnosis and treatment.
- *Neurotoxic flaccid paralysis* can develop very rapidly, progressing from mild weakness to full respiratory paralysis in less than 30 minutes (blue-ringed octopus bite, cone shell sting), or may develop far more slowly, over hours (some snakes) to days (paralysis tick). For neurotoxic snakes, the cranial nerves are usually involved first, with ptosis a common initial

9.18 Key venom effects*

Venom component	Clinical effects	Type of venomous animal
Neurotoxin Paralytic	Flaccid paralysis	Some snakes Paralysis ticks Cone shells Blue-ringed octopus
Excitatory	Neuroexcitation: autonomic storm, cardiotoxicity, pulmonary oedema	Some scorpions, spiders, jellyfish
Myotoxins	Systemic or local myolysis	Some snakes
Cardiotoxins	Direct or indirect cardiotoxicity	Some snakes, scorpions, spiders, and jellyfish
Haemostasis system toxins	Vary from rapid coagulopathy and bleeding to thrombosis, DVT and pulmonary emboli	Many snakes and a few scorpions Brazilian caterpillars
Nephrotoxins	Renal damage	Some snakes
Necrotoxins	Local tissue injury/necrosis, shock	Some snakes, a few scorpions, spiders, jellyfish and stingrays
Allergic toxins	Induce acute allergic response	Almost all venoms, but particularly those of social insects (i.e. bees, wasps, ants)

*All venom components have lethal potential.

9.19 Venomous animals and human envenoming

Phyla	Principal venomous animal groups	Estimated number of human cases/year	Estimated number of human deaths/year
Chordata	Snakes	> 2.5 million	> 100 000
	Spiny fish	? > 100 000	Close to zero
	Stingrays	? > 100 000	? < 10
Arthropoda	Scorpions	> 1 million	? < 5000
	Spiders	? > 100 000	? < 100
	Paralysis ticks	? > 1000	? < 10
	Insects	? > 1 million	? > 1000*
Mollusca	Cone shells	? < 1000	? < 10
	Blue-ringed octopus	? < 100	? < 10
Coelenterata	Jellyfish	? > 1 million	? < 10

*Social insect stings cause death by anaphylaxis rather than primary venom toxicity, except for massive multiple sting attacks.

9.20 Local and systemic effects of envenoming

Local effects

- Pain
- Sweating
- Swelling
- Erythema
- Bleeding and bruising
- Blistering
- Necrosis
- Major direct tissue trauma (e.g. stingray injuries)

Non-specific systemic effects

- Headache
- Nausea
- Vomiting and diarrhoea
- Abdominal pain
- Tachycardia or bradycardia
- Hypertension or hypotension
- Dizziness
- Collapse
- Convulsions
- Shock
- Cardiac arrest

sign (Fig. 9.7). From this, paralysis may extend to the limbs, with weakness and loss of deep tendon reflexes, then finally respiratory paralysis.

- *Excitatory neurotoxins* cause an 'autonomic storm', with profuse sweating, variable cardiac effects and cardiac failure, sometimes with pulmonary oedema (notably Australian funnel web spider bite). This type of envenoming can be rapidly fatal (many scorpions, funnel web spiders), or may cause distressing symptoms but constitute a lesser risk of death (widow spiders, banana spiders).
- *Myotoxicity* can initially be silent, then present with generalised muscle pain, tenderness, myoglobinuria and huge rises in serum creatine kinase (CK). Secondary renal failure can precipitate potentially lethal hyperkalaemic cardiotoxicity.
- *Cardiotoxicity* is often secondary, and symptoms and signs are non-specific in most cases.
- *Haemostasis system toxins* cause a variety of effects, depending on the type of toxin, and the specific features can be diagnostic. Coagulopathy may present as bruising and bleeding from the bite site, gums and intravenous sites. Surgical interventions are high-risk in such cases. Other venoms cause thrombosis, usually presenting as deep venous thrombosis (DVT), pulmonary embolus or stroke (particularly Caribbean/ Martinique vipers).
- *Renal damage* in envenoming is mostly secondary, although some species can cause primary damage (e.g. Russell's vipers). Presentation is similar, with changes in urine output (polyuria, oliguria or anuria) or rises in creatinine and urea. In cases with intravascular haemolysis, secondary renal damage is likely.

The clinical effects of specific animals in different regions of the world are shown in Boxes 9.21–9.23.

Management

It is important to determine an accurate diagnosis and the degree of risk, so that potentially severe/lethal cases are identified quickly and managed as a priority. With correct care, even severe cases are treatable, but delays in initiating effective treatment can severely compromise outcomes. Expert advice should thus be sought at the earliest opportunity.

First aid

Pre-hospital first aid (Box 9.24) can be critical in major envenoming. It depends on the type of envenoming, but the key principles are:

- supporting vital systems
- delaying or preventing the onset of envenoming
- avoiding harmful 'treatments' (e.g. electric shock, cut and suck, tourniquets, cryotherapy in snakebite).

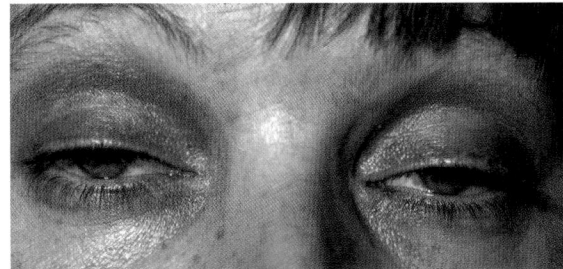

Fig. 9.7 Ptosis following neurotoxin envenomation.

9.21 Important venomous animals in Asia

Scientific name[1]	Common name	Clinical effects	Antivenom/antidote/treatment
Indian subcontinent			
Bungarus spp. (E)	Kraits	Flaccid paralysis[2,3]	Indian PV or specific
Naja spp. (E)	Cobras	Flaccid paralysis[3], local necrosis/blistering, shock	Indian PV or specific
Ophiophagus hannah (E)	King cobra	Flaccid paralysis[3], local blistering, shock	Indian PV or specific
Echis spp. (Vp)	Saw-scaled vipers	Procoagulant coagulopathy, local necrosis/blistering, renal failure	Indian PV or specific
Daboia russelli (Vp)	Russell's viper	Procoagulant coagulopathy, local necrosis/blistering, myolysis, renal failure, shock, flaccid paralysis[2]	Indian PV or specific
Hypnale spp. (Vc)	Hump-nosed vipers	Procoagulant coagulopathy, shock, renal failure	Try Indian PV
Trimeresurus[4] spp. (Vc)	Green pit vipers	Procoagulant coagulopathy, local necrosis, shock	Indian PV or specific
Mesobuthus spp. (Sc)	Indian scorpions	Neuroexcitation, cardiotoxicity	Prazosin
East Asia			
Bungarus spp. (E)	Kraits	Flaccid paralysis[2,3]	Specific AV from country
Naja spp. (E)	Cobras (some spitters)	Flaccid paralysis[3], local necrosis, shock	Specific AV from country
Ophiophagus hannah (E)	King cobra	Flaccid paralysis[3], local necrosis, shock	King cobra AV
Calloselasma rhodostoma (Vc)	Malayan pit viper	Procoagulant coagulopathy, local necrosis/blistering, renal failure, shock	Specific AV from country
Daboia russelli (Vv)	Russell's viper	Procoagulant coagulopathy, local necrosis/blistering, renal failure, shock	Specific AV from country
Gloydius (Vc)	Mamushis, pit vipers	Procoagulant coagulopathy, local necrosis/blistering, shock, renal failure, flaccid paralysis[2]	Specific AV from country
Trimeresurus[4] (Vc)	Green pit vipers, habus	Procoagulant coagulopathy, local necrosis/blistering, shock	Specific AV from country
Tropidolaemus wagleri (Vc)	Wagler's temple viper	Shock, local necrosis, pain and swelling	None available

[1]Family names: A = Atractaspididae; C = Colubridae (mostly non-venomous); E = Elapidae (all venomous); Vv = Viperidae viperinae (Old World vipers); Vc = Viperidae Crotalinae (New World and Asian vipers).
[2]Pre-synaptic.
[3]Post-synaptic.
[4]Genus is subject to major taxonomic change.
(AV = antivenom; PV = polyvalent)

Pre-hospital preventable deaths occur when ineffective cardiorespiratory resuscitation is given to patients with respiratory paralysis or cardiac arrest/failure, which can occur due to either primary envenoming or an anaphylactic reaction (p. 89).

Diagnosis

Envenoming is sometimes but not always obvious. Humans may be bitten/stung by an unseen organism, or fail to be aware of a bite/sting at all. If the latter, the patient may present with a variety of symptoms but no linking history to indicate envenoming, so it should be considered in selected cases of unexplained paralysis, myotoxicity, coagulopathy, nephrotoxicity, cardiotoxicity, pulmonary oedema, necrosis, collapse and convulsions.

History, examination and laboratory findings help to confirm or exclude a diagnosis of envenoming, and its extent. Establish whether a bite/sting is a possibility and, if the organism was seen, obtain a description. Multiple bites/stings are more likely to cause major envenoming. Ask for specific symptoms and search for specific signs that may indicate the type and extent of envenoming (p. 205).

Specific tests for venom are currently only commercially available for Australian snakebite, but are likely to be developed for snakebite in other regions. They are not available for other types of envenoming, where venom concentrations are low. For snakebite, a screen for envenoming includes full blood count, coagulation screen, urea and electrolytes, creatinine, CK and ECG. Lung function tests, peripheral oximetry or arterial blood gases may be indicated in cases with potential or established respiratory failure. In areas without access to routine laboratory tests, the whole blood clotting time (using a glass test tube) is a valuable test for coagulopathy. A derivative of this, the 20-minute whole blood clotting test (are a few millilitres of venous blood clotted at 20 minutes?), is useful.

If patients state that they have been bitten by a particular species, ensure this is accurate. Private keepers of

9.22 Important venomous animals in the Americas and Australia

Scientific name[1]	Common name	Clinical effects	Antivenom/antidote treatment
North America			
Crotalus spp. (Vc)	Rattlesnakes	Procoagulant coagulopathy, local necrosis/blistering (flaccid paralysis[2] rare)	CroFab AV
Sistrurus spp. (Vc)	Massasaugas	Procoagulant coagulopathy, local necrosis/blistering, shock	CroFab AV
Agkistrodon spp. (Vc)	Copperheads and moccasins	Procoagulant coagulopathy, local necrosis/blistering, shock	CroFab AV
Micrurus spp. (E)	Coral snakes	Flaccid paralysis[3]	Coral snake AV
Latrodectus mactans	Widow spider	Neuroexcitation	Widow spider AV
Central and South America			
Crotalus spp. (Vc)	Rattlesnakes	Flaccid paralysis[2], myolysis, procoagulant coagulopathy, shock, renal failure	Specific AV from country
Bothrops spp. (Vc)	Lancehead vipers	Procoagulant coagulopathy, local necrosis/blistering, shock, renal failure	Specific AV from country
Bothriechis spp. (Vc)	Eyelash pit vipers	Shock, pain and swelling	Specific AV from country
Lachesis spp. (Vc)	Bushmasters	Procoagulant coagulopathy, shock, renal failure, local necrosis/blistering	Specific AV from country
Micrurus spp. (E)	Coral snakes	Flaccid paralysis[2,3], myolysis, renal failure	Specific AV from country
Tityus serrulatus	Brazilian scorpion	Neuroexcitation, shock	Instituto Butantan scorpion AV
Loxosceles spp.	Recluse spiders	Local necrosis	Instituto Butantan spider AV
Phoneutria nigriventer	Banana spider	Neuroexcitation, shock	Instituto Butantan spider AV
Potamotrygon, Dasyatis spp.	Freshwater stingrays	Necrosis of bite area, shock	No available AV; good wound care
Australia			
Pseudonaja spp. (E)	Brown snakes	Procoagulant coagulopathy, renal failure, flaccid paralysis[2] (rare)	CSL brown snake AV
Notechis spp. (E)	Tiger snakes	Procoagulant coagulopathy, myolysis, flaccid paralysis[2,3], renal failure	CSL tiger snake AV
Oxyuranus spp. (E)	Taipans	Procoagulant coagulopathy, flaccid paralysis[2,3], myolysis, renal failure	CSL taipan or PV AV
Acanthophis spp. (E)	Death adders	Flaccid paralysis[3]	CSL death adder or PV AV
Pseudechis spp.	Black and mulga snakes	Anticoagulant coagulopathy, myolysis, renal failure	CSL black snake AV
Atrax, Hadronyche spp.	Funnel web spiders	Neuroexcitation, shock	CSL funnel web spider AV
Latrodectus hasseltii	Red back spider	Neuroexcitation	CSL red back spider AV
Chironex fleckeri	Box jellyfish	Neuroexcitation, cardiotoxicity, local necrosis	CSL box jellyfish AV

[1]For family name, see Box 9.21.
[2]Pre-synaptic.
[3]Post-synaptic.

venomous animals may not have accurate knowledge of what they are keeping, and misidentification of a snake, scorpion or spider can have dire consequences if the wrong antivenom is then used.

Treatment

Envenoming is managed on two levels, which must be delivered in tandem:
- treating the effects with specific treatments/antidotes (usually antivenom)
- supportive management of the organ systems affected and of the whole patient.

For a major snakebite such as Russell's viper, the patient might have local effects with oedema, blistering, necrosis, and resultant fluid shifts causing shock, and at the same time have systemic effects such as intractable vomiting, coagulopathy, paralysis and secondary renal failure. Specific treatment with antivenom will be required to reverse the coagulopathy, and may prevent worsening of the paralysis and reduce the vomiting, but will not greatly affect the local tissue damage or the renal failure or shock, which will require intravenous fluid therapy, possibly respiratory support, renal dialysis and local wound care, perhaps including antibiotics.

9.23 Important venomous animals in Africa and Europe

Scientific name[1]	Common name	Clinical effects	Antivenom/antidote/treatment
Africa			
Naja spp. (E)	Cobras		
	Non-spitters	Flaccid paralysis[3] ± local necrosis/blistering	South African PV
	Spitters	Local necrosis/blistering (flaccid paralysis[3] uncommon)	South African PV
Dendroaspis spp. (E)	Mambas	Mamba neurotoxin flaccid paralysis and muscle fasciculation, shock	South African PV
Hemachatus haemachatus (E)	Rinkhals	Flaccid paralysis[3], local necrosis, shock	South African PV
Atheris spp. (Vv)	Bush vipers	Procoagulant coagulopathy, shock, pain and swelling	No available AV (can try South African AV)
Bitis spp. (Vv)	Puff adders etc.	Procoagulant coagulopathy, shock, cardiotoxicity, local necrosis/blistering	South African PV
Causus spp. (Vv)	Night adders	Pain and swelling	No available AV
Echis spp. (Vv)	Carpet vipers	Procoagulant coagulopathy, shock, renal failure, local necrosis/blistering	Specific anti-*Echis* AV
Cerastes spp. (Vv)	Horned desert vipers	Procoagulant coagulopathy, local necrosis, shock	Specific or polyspecific AV covering *Cerastes* from country of origin
Dispholidus typus (C)	Boomslang	Procoagulant coagulopathy, shock	Boomslang AV
Androctonus spp.	North African scorpions	Neuroexcitation	Specific scorpion AV (Algeria, Tunisia)
Lelurus quinquestriatus	Yellow scorpion	Neuro excitation, shock	Specific scorpion AV
Europe			
Vipera spp. (Vv)	Vipers and adders	Shock, local necrosis/blistering, procoagulant coagulopathy (flaccid paralysis[2] rare)	ViperaTab AV or Zagreb AV

[1]For family name, see Box 9.21.
[2]Pre-synaptic.
[3]Post-synaptic.

9.24 First aid for envenoming

Method	Situations where indicated
Immobilisation of bitten limb	All snakebites
Pressure bandage and immobilisation of bitten limb	Non-necrotic snakebites (Australian snakes, sea snakes, some cobras, king cobra, kraits, coral snakes, mambas, a few vipers, Australian funnel web spiders, blue-ringed octopus, cone shell)
Local heat (hot water immersion or shower, to 45°C)	Venomous fish stings, stingray injuries, jellyfish stings (except possibly box jellyfish)
Staunching local bleeding	Traumatic injury with significant bleeding (some stingray injuries)
Cardiorespiratory support	Cardiac or respiratory impairment and particularly if respiratory paralysis is developing (some snakes, paralysis ticks, blue-ringed octopus, cone shells)
No specific first aid	Widow and recluse spider bites

Each venomous animal will cause a particular pattern of envenoming, requiring a tailored response. Listing all of these is beyond the scope of this chapter (see Further information below). Pulse, blood pressure, pulse oximetry and urine output should be monitored in all cases.

Antivenom

This is the most important tool in treating envenoming. It is made by hyperimmunising an animal, usually horses, to produce antibodies against venom. Once refined, these bind to venom toxins and render them impotent or allow their rapid clearance. Antivenom is only available for certain venomous animals and cannot reverse all types of envenoming. With a few exceptions it should be given intravenously, with adrenaline (epinephrine) ready in case of an anaphylactoid reaction. It should only be used when clearly indicated, and indications will vary between venomous animals. It is critical that the correct antivenom is used at the appropriate dose. Doses vary widely between antivenoms; those recommended for North American antivenoms are not applicable to those elsewhere.

Antivenom can sometimes reverse post-synaptic neurotoxic paralysis (α-bungarotoxin-like neurotoxins) but will not usually reverse established pre-synaptic paralysis (β-bungarotoxin-like neurotoxins), so needs to be given before major paralysis has occurred. Coagulopathy is best reversed by antivenom, but even after all venom is neutralised, there may be a delay of hours before normal coagulation is restored. More antivenom should not be given because coagulopathy has failed to normalise fully in the first 1–3 hours (except in very particular circumstances). The role of antivenom in reversing established myolysis and renal failure is uncertain. Antivenom may help reduce local tissue effects/injury in the bitten limb, but this is quite variable and time-dependent. Neuroexcitatory envenoming can respond very well to antivenom (Australian funnel web spider bites, Mexican and South American scorpion stings), but there is controversy about the effectiveness of antivenom for some species (some North African, Middle Eastern and Indian scorpions). The role of antivenom in treating local venom effects, including necrosis, is also controversial; it is most likely to be effective when given early.

All patients receiving antivenom are at risk of both early and late adverse reactions, including anaphylactic/anaphylactoid reactions and serum sickness.

Other treatments

Anticholinesterases are used as an adjunctive treatment for post-synaptic paralysis.

Prazosin (an α-adrenoceptor antagonist) is used in the management of hypertension or pulmonary oedema in scorpion sting cardiotoxicity, particularly for Indian scorpion stings.

Antibiotics are not routinely required for most bites/stings, though a few animals regularly cause significant wound infection/abscess (e.g. some South American pit vipers; stingrays). Tetanus is a risk in some types of bite/sting, such as snakebite, but intramuscular toxoid should not be given until any coagulopathy is reversed.

Mechanical ventilation (p. 196) is vital for established respiratory paralysis that will not reverse with antivenom, and may be required for prolonged periods: up to several months in some cases.

Follow-up

Cases with significant envenoming and those receiving antivenom should be followed up to ensure any complications have resolved and to identify any delayed envenoming.

Further information

Books and journal articles

Thomas SH, Watson ID, on behalf of the National Poisons Information Service and Association of Clinical Biochemists. Laboratory analyses for poisoned patients. Ann Clin Biochem 2002; 39:328–339.

Websites

http://curriculum.toxicology.wikispaces.net/ *Free access to educational material related to poisoning.*

www.toxbase.org *Toxbase, the clinical toxicology database of the UK National Poisons Information Service. Free for UK health professionals but registration is required. Access for overseas users by special arrangement.*

www.toxinology.com *Women's and Children's Hospital Adelaide Toxinology Department.*

www.toxnet.nlm.nih.gov *US National Library of Medicine's Toxnet: a hazardous substances databank, including Toxline for references to literature on drugs and other chemicals.*

Telephone numbers

Australian Poison Centre Network 131126 *From anywhere within Australia.*

UK National Poisons Information Service 0844 892 0111 *UK health professionals or by arrangement only.*

US Poisons Centers 1-800-222-1222 *From anywhere in the USA.*

World Health Organization/International Programme on Chemical Safety (WHO/IPCS) directory of poisons centres available at www.intox.org/databank/index.htm.

M.C. Sharpe
S.M. Lawrie

Medical psychiatry

10

Psychiatric disorders have traditionally been considered as mental rather than as physical illnesses. This is probably because they manifest with disordered functioning in the areas of emotion, perception, thinking and memory, and/or have had no clearly established biological basis. However, as research identifies abnormalities of the brain in an increasing number of psychiatric disorders and an important role for psychological and behavioural factors in many medical ones, a clear distinction between mental and physical illness has become increasingly questionable.

CLASSIFICATION OF PSYCHIATRIC DISORDERS

There are two main classifications of psychiatric disorders in current use:

- the American Psychiatric Association's Diagnostic and Statistical Manual (4th edition), or DSM-IV
- the World Health Organization's International Classification of Disease (10th edition), known as ICD-10.

The two systems are very similar and here we use the ICD-10 classification (Box 10.1).

EPIDEMIOLOGY OF PSYCHIATRIC DISORDERS

Psychiatric disorders are amongst the most common of human illnesses. The relative frequency of each disorder depends on the setting (Box 10.2). In the general population, depression, anxiety disorders and adjustment disorders are most common (10%) and psychosis is rare (1–2%); in general hospitals, organic disorders such as delirium (10%) are prevalent; in specialist psychiatric services psychoses are amongst the most common disorders.

AETIOLOGY OF PSYCHIATRIC DISORDERS

The aetiology of psychiatric disorders is multifactorial, with a combination of biological, psychological and social causes. Each of these factors may predispose, precipitate or perpetuate the illness (Box 10.3).

Biological factors
Genetic

Genetic factors play a role in many psychiatric disorders, including schizophrenia and bipolar affective disorder.

10.1 Classification of psychiatric disorders

Stress-related disorders
- Acute stress disorder
- Adjustment disorder
- Post-traumatic stress disorder

Anxiety disorders
- Generalised anxiety
- Phobic anxiety
- Panic disorder
- Obsessive-compulsive disorder

Affective (mood) disorders
- Depressive disorder
- Mania and bipolar disorder

Schizophrenia and delusional disorders

Substance misuse disorders
- Alcohol
- Drugs

Organic disorders
- Acute, e.g. delirium
- Chronic, e.g. dementia

Disorders of adult personality and behaviour
- Personality disorder
- Factitious disorder

Eating disorders
- Anorexia nervosa
- Bulimia nervosa

Somatoform disorders
- Somatisation disorder
- Dissociative (conversion) disorder
- Pain disorder
- Hypochondriasis
- Body dysmorphic disorder
- Somatoform autonomic dysfunction

Neurasthenia

Puerperal mental disorders

10.2 Prevalence of psychiatric disorders by medical setting

		Medical/surgical		Psychiatric services
	General practice	Outpatients	Inpatients	Psychiatric services
Adjustment disorders	++	++	+++	++
Depression/anxiety	++	++	+++	+++
Alcohol abuse	++	++	+++	+++
Personality disorders	++	++	++	+++
Somatoform disorders	+	+++	++	+
Delirium	–	–	+++	–
Psychosis	–	–	–	+++

(– rare; + uncommon; ++ common; +++ very common)

10.3 Classification of aetiological factors in psychiatric disorders

Predisposing

- Increase susceptibility to psychiatric disorder
- Established in utero or in childhood
- Operate throughout patient's lifetime (e.g. genetic factors, congenital defects, chronic physical illness, disturbed family background)

Precipitating

- Trigger an episode of illness
- Determine its time of onset (e.g. stressful life events, acute physical illness)

Perpetuating

- Delay recovery from illness (e.g. lack of social support, chronic physical illness)

Whilst some disorders such as Huntington's disease are due to mutations in a single gene, the genetic contribution to most psychiatric disorders is polygenic in nature and is mediated by the combined effects of several genetic variants, each with modest effects.

Brain structure and function

Brain structure is normal in most psychiatric disorders, although abnormalities may be observed in some conditions such as generalised atrophy in Alzheimer's disease and enlarged ventricles with a slight decrease in brain size in schizophrenia. The function of the brain is commonly altered, however, with, for example, changes in neurotransmitters such as dopamine, noradrenaline (norepinephrine) and 5-hydroxytryptamine (5-HT, serotonin), and differences in activity of specific areas of the brain, as seen on functional brain scans.

Psychological and behavioural factors

Perceived stress and trauma

Early childhood adversity, such as emotional deprivation or abuse, increases the risk of developing psychiatric illnesses such as depression and eating disorders as an adult. Events in adult life that are perceived as stressful may trigger psychiatric illness, as in post-traumatic stress disorder.

Personality

The relationship between personality and psychiatric illness can be difficult to assess because the development of psychiatric illness can change a patient's personality. Some personality types do predispose to illness; for example, a depressive personality increases the risk of clinical depression. Abnormal personality may also perpetuate psychiatric illness once it is established, leading to a poorer prognosis.

Behaviour

A person's behaviour may predispose to the development of a disorder (e.g. excess alcohol intake leading to dependence, and dieting to anorexia) or perpetuate it, as in persistent avoidance of the feared situation in a phobia.

Social and environmental factors

Social isolation

The lack of a close, confiding relationship predisposes to psychiatric illnesses such as depression. The reduced social support resulting from psychiatric illness may also perpetuate it.

Stressors

Social and environmental stressors can precipitate illness in vulnerable people. Their effect is modified by how they are perceived by the individual, although some may be so severe that they precipitate illness in most people. Losses (such as bereavement) commonly precede the onset of depression, and events perceived as threatening (such as potential loss of employment) commonly precipitate anxiety.

DIAGNOSING PSYCHIATRIC DISORDERS

The key differences between a psychiatric and a medical assessment are:

- a greater emphasis on the history
- a systematic examination of the patient's mental state
- routine interviewing of an informant (usually a relative or friend who knows the patient), especially when the illness affects the patient's ability to give an accurate history.

A full psychiatric history and detailed mental state examination (MSE) may take an hour or more, but a much briefer mental state examination should be part of the assessment of *all* patients.

Psychiatric interview

The aims of the interview are to:

- establish a therapeutic relationship with the patient
- elicit the symptoms, history and background information (Box 10.4)
- examine the mental state
- provide information, reassurance and advice.

Some aspects of the patient's mental state may be observed whilst the history is being taken, but specific enquiry must always be made for important features.

Mental state examination

General appearance and behaviour

Any abnormalities of alertness or motor behaviour, such as restlessness or retardation, are noted. The level of consciousness should be examined, especially in the assessment of possible delirium.

Speech

Speed and fluency should be observed, including slow (retarded) speech and word-finding difficulty. 'Pressure of speech' describes rapid speech that is difficult to interrupt.

Mood

This can be judged by facial expression, posture and movements. Patients should also be asked if they feel sad or depressed, or lack ability to experience pleasure

10

10

10.4 How to structure a psychiatric interview

Presenting problem

Reason for referral
- Why the patient has been referred and by whom

Presenting complaints
- The patient should be asked to describe the symptoms for which help is requested

History of present illness
- The patient should be asked to describe the course of the illness from the time when symptoms were first noticed
- The interviewer asks direct questions to determine the nature, duration and severity of symptoms and any associated factors

Background

Family history
- Description of parents and siblings, and a record of mental illness in relatives

Personal history
- Birth history, major events in childhood, education, occupational history, relationship, marriage, children, current social circumstances

Previous medical and psychiatric history
- Previous health, accidents and operations
- Use of alcohol, tobacco and other drugs
- Direct questions may be needed concerning previous psychiatric history since this may not be volunteered: 'Have you ever been treated for depression or nerves?' or 'Have you ever suffered a nervous breakdown?'

Previous personality
- The characteristic patterns of behaviour and thinking which determine a person's adjustment to the environment, including relationships with other people and reactions to stress
- The most useful information may be obtained from an informant who has known the patient well for many years

(anhedonia). Are they anxious, worried or tense, or is mood elevated with excess energy and a reduced need for sleep, as in mania?

Thoughts

The content of thought can be elicited by asking 'What are your main concerns?' Is thinking negative, guilty or hopeless, suggesting depression? Are there thoughts of self-harm? If so, enquiry should be made about plans. Does the patient think that he or she is especially powerful, important or gifted (grandiose thoughts), suggesting mania, or is he/she excessively worried about many things, suggesting anxiety?

The form of thinking may also be abnormal. For example, in schizophrenia, patients may display loosened associations between ideas, making it difficult to follow their train of thought. There may also be abnormalities of thought possession, when patients experience the intrusion of alien thoughts or the broadcasting of their own (p. 243).

Abnormal beliefs

A delusion is a false belief, out of keeping with a patient's cultural background, which is held with unshakable conviction despite evidence to the contrary (p. 234).

Abnormal perceptions

Illusions are abnormal perceptions of real stimuli. Hallucinations are sensory perceptions which occur in the absence of external stimuli: for example, hearing voices when no one is present (p. 234).

Cognitive function

The Mini-Mental State Examination (MMSE) is a useful screening questionnaire to detect cognitive impairment (Box 10.5). A score of less than 24 out of 30 indicates cognitive impairment. The degree of cognitive impairment

10.5 How to perform a Mini-Mental State Examination (MMSE)

Patient name _____

Date of birth _____ Date of test _____

Max. points	Patient score	
		Orientation
5	( )	What is the (year) (season) (date) (day) (month)?
5	( )	Where are we (country) (county) (town/city) (building) (floor)?
		Registration
3	( )	Name three common objects (e.g. 'apple', 'table', 'penny'). Take 1 second to say each. Then ask the patient to repeat all three after you have said them. Give 1 point for each correct answer. Then repeat them until he/she learns all three. Count trials and record. Trials ( )
		Attention
5	( )	Spell 'world' backwards. The score is the number of letters in the correct order. (D_L_R_O_W_)
		Recall
3	( )	Ask for the three objects repeated above. Give 1 point for each correct answer. (Note: recall cannot be tested if all three objects were not remembered during registration)
		Language
2	( )	Name a 'pencil' and a 'watch'. (2 points)
1	( )	Repeat the following: 'No ifs, ands or buts.' (1 point)
3	( )	Follow a three-stage command: 'Take this paper in your right hand, fold it in half, and put it on the floor.' (3 points)
1	( )	Read and obey the following: (1 point) CLOSE YOUR EYES
1	( )	Write a sentence. (1 point)
1	( )	Copy the following design. Give 1 point if no construction problem

| 30 | ( ) | **Total** |

Examiner _____

in delirium typically fluctuates and may be missed by a single assessment.

- *Concentration.* Serial 7s is a test in which the patient is asked to subtract 7 from 100 and then 7 from the answer, down to 0.
- *Orientation.* This is assessed by asking the patient about place—his or her exact location; time—what day, date, month and year it is now; and person—details of personal identity, such as name, date of birth, marital status and address.
- *Intellectual abilities.* These can be gauged from the history of the patient's educational background and attainments but can also be assessed during the interview from the patient's speech and grasp of the interviewer's questions.
- *Memory.* Registration of memories is tested by asking the patient to repeat simple new information, such as a name and address, immediately. Short-term memory is assessed by asking him/her to repeat it after an interval of 1–2 minutes, during which time the patient's attention should be diverted elsewhere. Long-term memory is checked by assessing the recall of previous events.

Patients' understanding of illness ('insight')

Patients should be asked what they think their symptoms are due to, and whether they warrant treatment. Lack of insight is a failure to accept that one is ill and/or in need of treatment, and is characteristic of acute psychosis.

PRESENTING PROBLEMS IN PSYCHIATRIC ILLNESS

Anxiety symptoms

Anxiety may be transient, persistent, episodic or limited to specific situations. The symptoms of anxiety are both psychological and somatic (Box 10.6). The differential diagnosis of anxiety is shown in Box 10.7. Most commonly it is transient, as an adjustment disorder (p. 240), and subsides with time. Other more persistent forms of anxiety are described in detail on pages 241–242. Anxiety may occasionally be a manifestation of a medical condition such as thyrotoxicosis (see Box 10.7).

10.6 **Symptoms of anxiety disorder**	
Psychological	
• Apprehension	• Fear of impending disaster
• Irritability	• Poor concentration
• Worry	• Depersonalisation
Somatic	
• Palpitations	• Frequent desire to pass urine
• Fatigue	• Chest pain
• Tremor	• Initial insomnia
• Dizziness	• Breathlessness
• Sweating	• Headache
• Diarrhoea	

10.7 **Differential diagnosis of anxiety**
• Normal response to threat
• Adjustment disorder
• Generalised anxiety disorder
• Panic disorder
• Phobic disorder
• Organic (medical) cause
Hyperthyroidism
Paroxysmal arrhythmias
Phaeochromocytoma
Alcohol and benzodiazepine withdrawal
Hypoglycaemia
Temporal lobe epilepsy

Depressed mood

Depressive disorder is common, occurring in a quarter to a half of medical inpatients. The symptoms of depression are both mental and physical (Box 10.8). In the physically ill patient, diagnosis of comorbid depression is based mainly on careful assessment of the core psychological symptoms: namely, persistently lowered mood and anhedonia.

Differential diagnosis

Depressive disorder must be differentiated from an adjustment disorder with depressed mood (p. 240). Adjustment disorders are common, self-limiting reactions to adversity, including physical illness, which are transient and require only general support. On the other hand, depressive disorders (p. 242) are characterised by more severe and persistent mood disturbance and do require specific treatment. In some cases, depression may occur as a result of a direct effect of a medical condition or its treatment on neurotransmitters or neural pathways in the brain, when it is referred to as an 'organic mood disorder' (Box 10.9).

Suicide

Depression is the major risk factor for suicide, especially when it co-occurs with a medical condition or substance misuse. Other risk factors are shown in Box 10.10. When depression is suspected, tactful enquiry should always be made into suicidal thoughts and plans. Asking about suicide does not increase the risk of it occurring, whereas failure to enquire denies the opportunity to prevent it.

10.8 **Symptoms of depressive disorders**	
Psychological	
• Depressed mood	• Loss of interest
• Reduced self-esteem	• Loss of enjoyment (anhedonia)
• Pessimism	
• Guilt	• Suicidal thinking
Somatic	
• Reduced appetite	• Loss of libido
• Weight change	• Bowel disturbance
• Disturbed sleep	• Motor retardation (slowing of activity)
• Fatigue	

10

10.9 Organic affective disorders*

Neurological
- Cerebrovascular disease
- Cerebral tumour
- Multiple sclerosis
- Parkinson's disease
- Huntington's disease
- Alzheimer's disease
- Epilepsy

Endocrine
- Hypothyroidism
- Hyperthyroidism
- Cushing's syndrome
- Addison's disease
- Hyperparathyroidism

Malignant disease

Infections
- Infectious mononucleosis
- Herpes simplex
- Brucellosis
- Typhoid
- Toxoplasmosis

Connective tissue disease
- Systemic lupus erythematosus

Drugs
- Reserpine, methyldopa
- Phenothiazines
- Phenylbutazone
- Corticosteroids, oral contraceptives
- Interferon

*Diseases that may cause organic affective disorders by direct action on the brain.

10.10 Risk factors for suicide

- Psychiatric illness (depressive illness, schizophrenia)
- Older age
- Male sex
- Living alone
- Unemployed
- Recently bereaved, divorced or separated
- Chronic physical ill health
- Drug or alcohol misuse
- Suicide note written
- History of previous attempts (especially if a violent method was used)

Elated mood

Elation, or euphoria, is the converse of depression and is characteristic of mania. It may manifest as infectious joviality, over-activity, lack of sleep and appetite, undue optimism, over-talkativeness, irritability, and recklessness in spending and sexual behaviour. When more severe, psychotic symptoms are often evident, such as delusional degrees of grandiosity. Elevated mood is much less common than depression, and where it arises in medical settings is often secondary to drug or alcohol misuse, an organic disorder or medical treatment. Where none of these applies, the patient may have a bipolar mood disorder (p. 243), a condition which requires specialist treatment.

Delusions and hallucinations

Delusions

Various types of delusion are identified on the basis of their content. They may be:

- persecutory, such as a conviction that others are out to get one
- hypochondriacal, such as an unfounded conviction that one has cancer
- grandiose, such as a belief that one has special powers or status.

The most extreme form of delusion is nihilistic, e.g. 'My head is missing,' 'I have no body,' 'I am dead.' Delusions should be differentiated from overvalued ideas, which are strongly held but not fixed.

Hallucinations

These are perceptions without external stimuli. They can occur in any sensory modality, most commonly visual or auditory. Typical examples are hearing voices when no one else is present, or seeing 'visions'. Hallucinations have the quality of ordinary perceptions and are perceived as originating in the external world, not the patient's own mind (when they are termed pseudo-hallucinations). Those occurring when falling asleep ('hypnagogic') and on waking ('hypnopompic') are not pathological. Hallucinations should be distinguished from illusions, which are misperceptions of real external stimuli (such as mistaking a shrub for a person in poor light).

Differential diagnosis

Agitation, terror or the fear of being thought 'mad' may make patients unable or unwilling to volunteer or describe their abnormal beliefs or experiences. Careful enquiry is therefore required. The nature of hallucinations can be important diagnostically; for example, 'running commentary' voices which discuss the patient in the third person are strongly associated with schizophrenia. In general, auditory hallucinations suggest a 'functional psychosis' such as schizophrenia, while hallucinations in other sensory modalities, especially vision but also taste and smell, suggest an 'organic psychosis' such as delirium or temporal lobe epilepsy.

Hallucinations and delusions often co-occur; if their content is consistent with coexisting emotional symptoms, they are described as 'mood-congruent'. Thus patients with severely depressed mood may believe themselves responsible for all the evils in the world, and hear voices saying 'You're worthless. Go and kill yourself.' In this case, the diagnosis of depressive psychosis is made on the basis of the congruence of different phenomena (mood, delusion and hallucination). Incongruence between hallucinations, delusions and mood suggests schizophrenia.

Where hallucinations and delusions arise within disturbed consciousness and impaired cognition, the diagnosis is usually organic disorder, most commonly delirium and/or dementia (p. 248). This differential diagnosis is made by assessing the nature, extent and time course of any cognitive disturbances, and by investigating for underlying causes.

Disturbed and aggressive behaviour

Disturbed and aggressive behaviour is common in general hospitals, especially in emergency departments. Most behavioural disturbance arises not from medical or psychiatric illness, but from alcohol intoxication and personality. The key principles of management are to establish control of the situation and thereby ensure the safety of the patient and others, and also to assess the cause of the disturbance in order to remedy it. Establishing control requires the presence of an adequate number of trained staff, an appropriate physical environment and sedation, as set out in Figure 10.1. Hospital security staff and sometimes police may be required. In all cases staff behaviour is important; a calm,

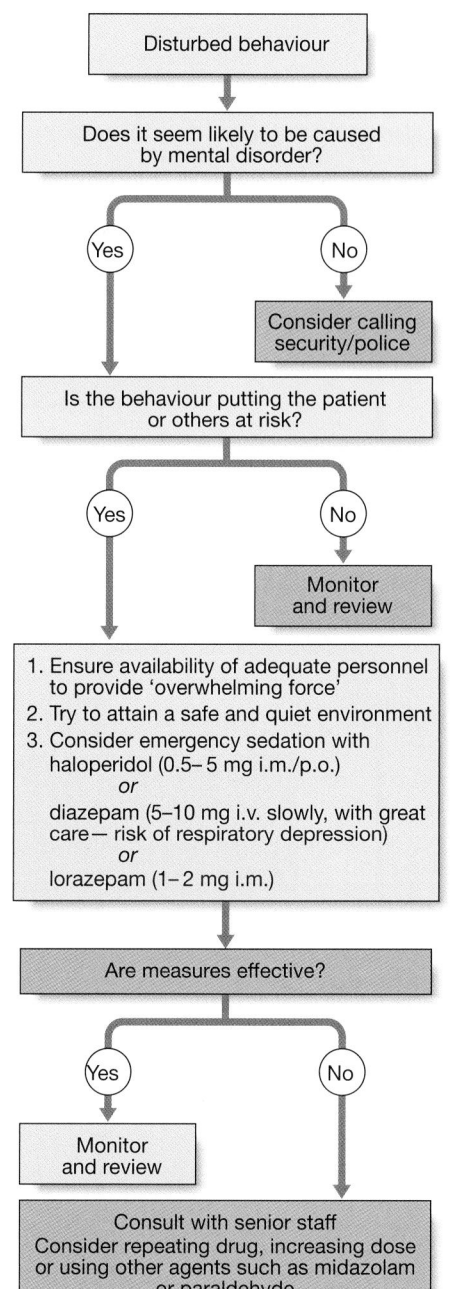

Fig. 10.1 Acute management of disturbed behaviour.

10.11 Psychiatric emergencies

10.11 Psychiatric emergencies

- Intervene as necessary to reduce the risk of harm to the patient and to others
- Adopt a calm, non-threatening approach
- Arrange availability of other staff and parenteral medication
- Consider diagnostic possibilities of drug intoxication, acute psychosis and delirium
- Involve friends and relatives as appropriate

frail elderly woman with emphysema and delirium may be a low dose (0.5 mg) of oral haloperidol, while a strong young man with an acute psychotic episode may need at least 10 mg of intravenous diazepam and a similar dose of haloperidol. A parenterally administered anticholinergic agent, such as procyclidine, should be available to treat extrapyramidal effects arising from haloperidol. When benzodiazepines are used, flumazenil (p. 215) should be on hand to reverse respiratory depression. When benzodiazepines are used in large doses, oxygen and ventilation should be available.

Differential diagnosis

Many factors may contribute to disturbed behaviour, although little may be learned from an attempted interview with an uncooperative patient. Other sources of information about the patient are therefore crucial and include medical and psychiatric records, and discussion with nursing staff, family members and other informants, including the patient's general practitioner. Important information to obtain includes:

- psychiatric, medical (especially neurological) and criminal history
- current psychiatric and medical treatment
- alcohol and drug misuse
- recent stressors
- the time course and accompaniments of the current episode in terms of mood, belief and behaviour.

Simple observation of the patient's behaviour may also yield useful clues. Do they appear to be responding to hallucinations? Are they alert or variably drowsy and confused? Are there physical features suggestive of drug or alcohol misuse or withdrawal? Are there new injuries or old scars, especially on the head? Do they smell of alcohol or solvents? Do they bear the marks of drug injection? Are they grubby and unkempt, suggesting a gradual development of their condition?

If the person is psychiatrically ill, then admission to a psychiatric facility is indicated. If a medical cause is likely, psychiatric transfer is inappropriate and the patient should be managed in a medical setting, with whatever nursing and security support is required. Where it is clear that there is no medical or psychiatric illness, the person should be removed from the hospital, to police custody if necessary.

Measures such as restraint, sedation, the investigation and treatment of medical problems, and psychiatric transfer all raise legal as well as medical issues (p. 252). In most countries, including the UK, the law confers upon doctors the right and indeed the duty to intervene against a patient's wishes in cases of acute behavioural disturbance, if this is necessary to protect the patient or other people.

non-threatening approach by someone who can understand and address the patient's fears is often all that is required to defuse potential aggression (Box 10.11).

The most widely used sedating agents are antipsychotic drugs, such as haloperidol, and benzodiazepines, such as diazepam. The choice of drug, dose, route and rate of administration will depend on the patient's age, sex and physical health, as well as the likely cause of the disturbed behaviour. The benefits of sedation must be balanced against the risks. Haloperidol can cause acute dystonias including oculogyric crises, while the benzodiazepines can precipitate respiratory depression in patients with lung disease, and encephalopathy in those with liver disease. Thus appropriate sedation for a

10

Self-harm

Self-harm (SH) is a common reason for presentation to medical services. The term 'attempted suicide' is potentially misleading, as most such patients are not unequivocally trying to kill themselves. Most cases of SH involve overdose, of either prescribed or non-prescribed drugs (Ch. 9). Less common methods include asphyxiation, drowning, hanging, jumping from a height or in front of a moving vehicle, and the use of firearms. Methods which carry a high chance of being fatal are more likely to be associated with serious psychiatric illness. Self-cutting is common and often repetitive, but rarely leads to contact with medical services.

The incidence of SH has changed over time and varies between countries. In the UK, the lifetime prevalence of suicidal ideation is 15% and that of acts of SH 4%. SH is more common in women than in men, and in young adults than in the elderly. In contrast, completed suicide is more common in men and in the elderly (see Box 10.10). There is a higher incidence among lower socioeconomic groups, particularly those living in crowded, socially deprived urban areas. Self-harming patients often have a deprived family background. There is also an association with alcohol misuse, child abuse, unemployment and recently broken relationships.

Differential diagnosis

The main differential diagnosis is from accidental poisoning and from so-called 'recreational' overdose in drug users. It must be remembered that SH is not a diagnosis but a presentation, and may be associated with any psychiatric diagnosis; the most common are adjustment disorders, substance and alcohol misuse, depressive disorders and personality disorders. In many cases there is no psychiatric diagnosis.

Initial management

A thorough psychiatric and social assessment should be carried out in all cases (Fig. 10.2), although some patients will discharge themselves before this can take place. In most UK hospitals, assessment is usually undertaken by psychiatrists, although other doctors, physicians, nurses and social workers can also be trained to do this. Psychiatric assessment should not delay urgent medical or surgical treatment, and may need to be deferred until the patient is well enough for interview, and the sedating or intoxicating effect of the drugs and any alcohol taken have worn off. The purpose of the psychiatric assessment is to:

- establish the short-term risk of suicide
- identify potentially treatable problems, whether medical, psychiatric or social.

Topics to be covered when assessing a patient are listed in Box 10.12. The history should cover events occurring immediately before and after the act and especially any evidence of planning. The nature and severity of any current psychiatric symptoms must be assessed, along with the personal and social supports available to the patient outside hospital.

Most SH patients have depressive and anxiety symptoms on a background of chronic social and personal difficulties and alcohol misuse, and do not require psychotropic medication or specialised psychiatric treatment. They do need emotional support and practical advice from a GP,

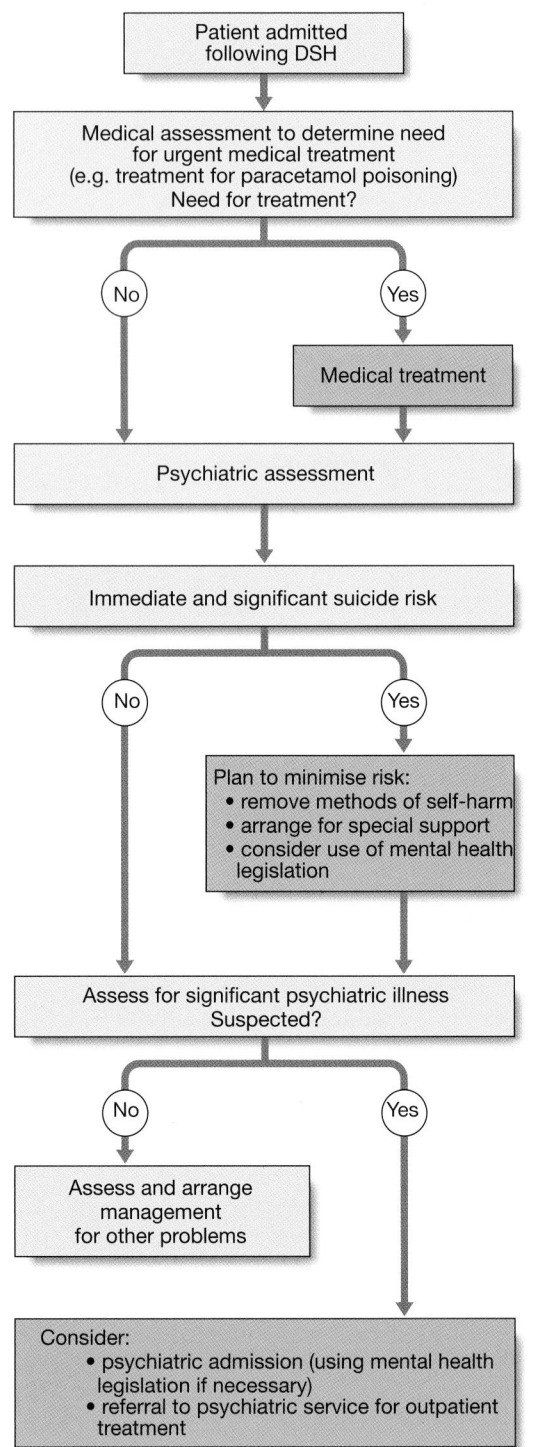

Fig. 10.2 Assessment of patients admitted following self-harm (SH).

social worker or community psychiatric nurse. Admission to a psychiatric ward is necessary only for persons who:

- have major psychiatric illness
- remain intent on suicide
- need temporary respite from intolerable circumstances
- require further assessment of their mental state.

10.12 Assessment of patients after self-harm

Current attempt

- Patient's account
- Degree of intent at the time: preparations, plans, precautions against discovery, note
- Method used, particularly whether violent
- Degree of intent now
- Symptoms of psychiatric illness

Background

- Previous attempts and their outcome
- Family and personal history
- Social support
- Previous response to stress
- Extent of drug and alcohol misuse

Approximately 20% of SH patients make a repeat attempt during the following year and 1–2% kill themselves. Factors associated with suicide after an episode of SH are listed in Box 10.10.

Confusion

This is a vague term used to describe a range of primarily cognitive problems but also includes disturbances in perception, belief and behaviour. 'Confusion' usually presents as a problem when patients cannot comply with medical care; they may repeatedly wander off the ward, pull out essential cannulae and catheters, and hit out at nurses. The apparently confused patient may have deficits in any or all cognitive domains. Cognitive assessments range from simple screening questions to detailed psychometric testing. All doctors should be able to undertake a brief cognitive assessment, as outlined above (p. 232 and Box 10.5).

Differential diagnosis

A history from the patient and informants is essential to establish the time course, variability and functional consequences of any cognitive deficit. Mental state examination is necessary to seek evidence of associated mood disorder, hallucinations, delusions or behavioural abnormalities, and physical examination to identify medical illness. A clinical assessment should distinguish between organic disorders such as delirium, dementia, and focal deficits secondary to brain lesions; psychiatric disorders

10.13 Medical psychiatry in old age

- **Organic psychiatric disorders:** especially common, so cognitive function should always be assessed; if impaired, an associated medical condition or adverse drug effect should be suspected.
- **Disturbed behaviour:** delirium is the most common cause.
- **Depression:** common. Just because a person is old and frail does not mean that depression is 'to be expected' and that it should not be treated.
- **Self-harm:** associated with an increased risk of completed suicide.
- **Medically unexplained symptoms:** common and often associated with depressive disorder.
- **Loneliness, poverty and lack of social support:** must be taken into consideration in management decisions.

such as pseudo-dementia and dissociative disorder; and malingering (p. 252). Further investigation will usually be needed to identify the specific causes of any delirium (Chs 9 and 26).

Alcohol misuse

Misuse of alcohol is a world-wide problem. It presents in a multitude of ways, which are discussed further on page 246 and in Box 10.31 (p. 247). In many cases, the link to alcohol will be all too obvious but in others it may not be. Denial and concealment of alcohol intake is common; consequently, a high index of suspicion is essential. The patient should be asked to describe a typical week's drinking, quantified in terms of units of alcohol (1 unit contains approximately 8 g alcohol and is the equivalent of half a pint of beer, a single measure of spirits or a small glass of wine). Drinking becomes hazardous at levels above 21 units weekly for men and 14 units weekly for women. The history from the patient may need corroboration by the GP, earlier medical records and family members. The mean cell volume (MCV) and γ-glutamyl transferase (GGT) may be raised, but are abnormal in only half of problem drinkers, so normal results do not exclude an alcohol problem. When abnormal, these measures may be helpful in challenging denial and monitoring treatment response. The prevention and management of alcohol-related problems is discussed on pages 246–247.

Substance misuse

The misuse of drugs of all kinds is widespread. As well as the general headings listed for alcohol problems in Box 10.31 (p. 247), there are two additional sets of problems associated with drug misuse:

- problems linked with the route of administration rather than the substance taken
- problems arising from pressure applied to doctors by the patient to prescribe the misused substances (Box 10.14).

Assessment and management are described on pages 247–248.

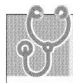

10.14 Substance misuse: additional presenting problems

Complications arising from the route of use

Intravenous
- Local: abscesses, cellulitis, thrombosis
- Systemic: bacterial (endocarditis), viral (hepatitis, human immunodeficiency virus (HIV))

Nasal ingestion
- Erosion of nasal septum, epistaxis

Smoking
- Oral, laryngeal and lung cancer

Inhalation
- Burns, chemical pneumonitis, rashes

Pressure to prescribe misused substance

- Manipulation, deceit and threats
- Factitious description of illness
- Malingering

10

10

Psychological factors affecting medical conditions

Psychological factors influence the presentation, management and outcome of most medical conditions. Specific factors are shown in Box 10.15. The most common psychiatric diagnoses in the medically ill are anxiety and depressive disorders. Often these appear understandable as adjustments to illness and treatment; however, if they are severe and persistent, active management is required. Anxiety may present as an increase in somatic symptoms such as breathlessness, tremor or palpitations, or as the avoidance of treatment. It is most common in those facing difficult or painful treatment, deterioration of their illness or death. Depression may manifest as increased symptoms such as pain or fatigue and disability, as well as with depressed mood and loss of interest and pleasure. It is most common in patients who have suffered actual or anticipated loss, such as receiving a terminal diagnosis or undergoing disfiguring surgery.

Treatment is by psychological and/or pharmacological therapies, as described below. Care is required when prescribing psychotropic drugs to the medically ill in order to avoid exacerbating the medical condition or causing interactions with other prescribed drugs.

10.15 Risk factors for psychological problems associated with medical conditions

- Previous history of depression or anxiety
- Lack of social support
- New diagnosis of a serious medical condition
- Deterioration of or failure of treatment for medical condition
- Unpleasant, disabling or disfiguring treatment
- Change in medical care, e.g. discharge from hospital
- Impending death

Medically unexplained somatic symptoms

Patients commonly present to doctors with somatic symptoms. Whilst these are often clearly associated with a medical condition, in other cases they are not. Symptoms may be disproportionate to, or occur in the absence of, a medical condition and are then often referred to as 'medically unexplained symptoms' (MUS). MUS are very common and occur in a quarter to a half of patients attending general medical outpatient clinics. Almost any symptom can be medically unexplained and common examples include:

- pain (including back, chest, abdominal and headache)
- fatigue
- dizziness
- fits, 'funny turns' and feelings of weakness.

Patients with MUS may receive a medical diagnosis of a so-called functional somatic syndrome, such as irritable bowel syndrome (Box 10.16) and may also merit a psychiatric diagnosis on the basis of the same symptoms. The most frequent psychiatric diagnoses associated with MUS are anxiety or depressive disorders. When these are absent, a diagnosis of somatoform disorder may be applied (Box 10.17).

Differential diagnosis

The main medical differential diagnosis is from symptoms of a medical disease. Diagnostic difficulties are most likely with unusual presentations of common diseases and with rare diseases. A medical and psychiatric assessment should be completed in all cases (Fig. 10.3).

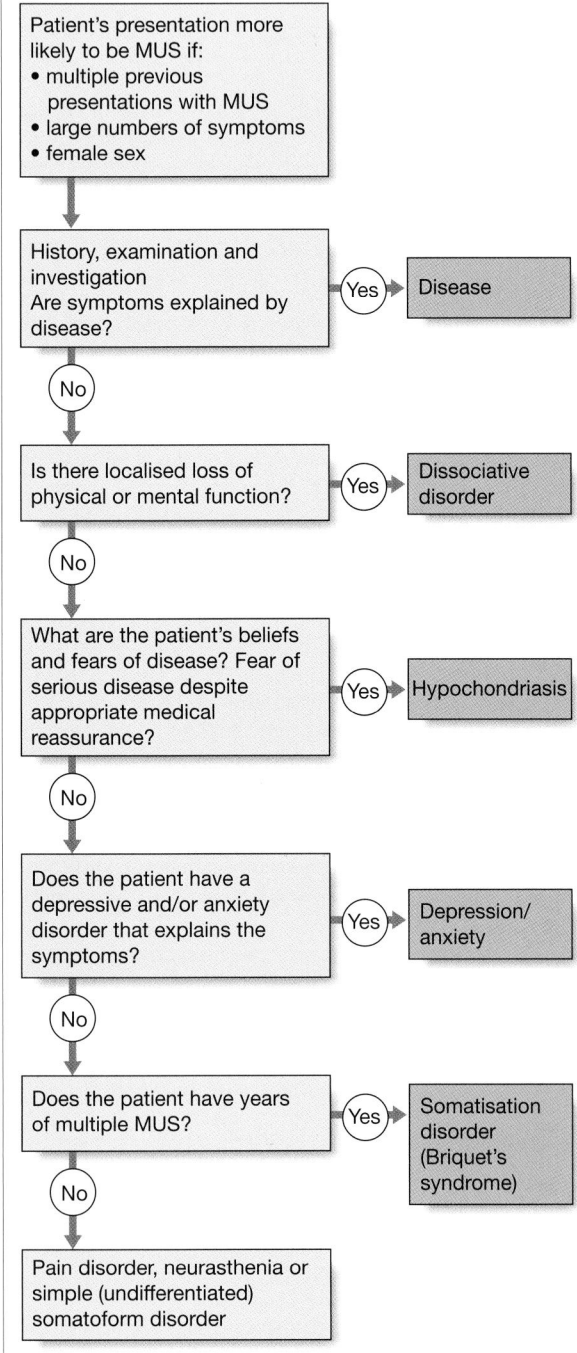

Fig. 10.3 Diagnosis of medically unexplained symptoms (MUS).

10.16 Functional somatic syndromes

- Gastroenterology: irritable bowel syndrome, non-ulcer dyspepsia
- Gynaecology: premenstrual syndrome, chronic pelvic pain
- Rheumatology: fibromyalgia
- Cardiology: atypical or non-cardiac chest pain
- Respiratory medicine: hyperventilation syndrome
- Infectious diseases: chronic (post-viral) fatigue syndrome
- Neurology: tension headache, non-epileptic attacks
- Dentistry: temporomandibular joint dysfunction, atypical facial pain
- Ear, nose and throat: globus syndrome
- Allergy: multiple chemical sensitivity

10.17 Psychiatric diagnoses for medically unexplained somatic symptoms

- Hypochondriasis: predominant concern about disease
- Somatisation: predominant concern about symptoms
- Somatic presentation of depression and anxiety
- Simple somatoform disorders: small number of symptoms
- Somatisation disorder (Briquet's syndrome): chronic multiple symptoms
- Conversion disorder: loss of function
- Body dysmorphic disorder: dislike of body parts

TREATING PSYCHIATRIC DISORDERS

The multifactorial origin of most psychiatric disorders means that there may be multiple potential targets for treatment.

Biological treatments

These aim to relieve psychiatric illness by modifying brain function. Psychotropic drugs are widely used for various purposes; a pragmatic classification is set out in Box 10.18. It should be noted that some drugs have applications to more than one condition; for example, antidepressants are widely used in the treatment of anxiety *and* chronic pain. The specific subgroups of psychotropic drugs are discussed in the sections on the appropriate disorders.

Electroconvulsive therapy (ECT) entails producing a convulsion by the administration of high-voltage, brief direct current impulses to the head while the patient is anaesthetised and paralysed by muscle relaxants. If properly administered it is remarkably safe, has few side-effects, and is of proven efficacy for severe depressive illness. There may be amnesia for events occurring a few hours before ECT (retrograde) and after it (anterograde). Pronounced amnesia can occur but is infrequent and difficult to distinguish from the effects of severe depression. There is a very limited place for psychosurgery in very severe chronic psychiatric illness.

Psychological treatments

These treatments are useful in many psychiatric disorders and non-psychiatric conditions. They are based on talking with patients, either individually or in groups. Sometimes discussion is supplemented by 'homework' or tasks to complete between sessions. Psychological treatments take a number of forms based on the duration and frequency of contact, the specific techniques applied and their underlying theory.

General or supportive psychotherapy

This should form part of all medical treatment. It involves empathic listening, in which the doctor encourages the patient to describe symptoms, express feelings and reflect on associated problems. The doctor should offer an explanation of the symptoms (and, where possible, a diagnosis), practical advice and such reassurance as is appropriate. For patients with incurable or chronic conditions, supportive psychotherapy may be the best treatment that can be offered.

10.18 Classification of psychotropic drugs

Action	Main groups	Clinical use
Antipsychotic	Phenothiazines	Schizophrenia
	Butyrophenones	Bipolar mania
	Second-generation antipsychotics	Acute confusion
Antidepressant	Tricyclics and related drugs	Depression/anxiety
		Obsessive-compulsive disorder
	Monoamine oxidase inhibitors	Depression/anxiety
	Novel noradrenergic or serotonin	Depression/anxiety
	re-uptake inhibitors	Obsessive-compulsive disorder
Mood-stabilising	Lithium	Treatment and prophylaxis of bipolar disorder
	Carbamazepine	Prophylaxis of bipolar disorder
	(Semi)Sodium valproate	Prophylaxis of bipolar disorder
	Lamotrigine	Bipolar depression
Anti-anxiety	Benzodiazepines	Anxiety/insomnia (short term)
		Alcohol withdrawal (short term)
	β-adrenoceptor antagonists	Anxiety (somatic symptoms)

10.19 The negative cognitive triad associated with depression

- Negative view of self, e.g. 'I am no good'
- Negative view of current life experiences, e.g. 'The world is an awful place'
- Negative view of the future, e.g. 'The future is hopeless'

Cognitive therapy

This is based on the observation that some psychiatric disorders are associated with systematic errors in the patient's conscious thinking: for example, a tendency to interpret events in a negative way or see them as unduly threatening. A triad of such cognitive errors has been described in depression (Box 10.19). Cognitive therapy aims to help patients identify recurring negative thoughts and learn how to challenge them. It is widely used for depression, anxiety and bulimia nervosa, and increasingly in the management of somatoform disorders.

Behaviour therapy

This is a practically orientated form of treatment, in which patients are helped to change their behaviour. In conditions such as phobic anxiety, working with the patient through a carefully constructed programme of graded exposure to the feared stimulus is usually remarkably effective.

Cognitive behaviour therapy (CBT)

This combines the methods of behaviour therapy and cognitive therapy. It is the most widely available and most extensively researched psychological treatment.

Problem-solving therapy

This is a simplified brief form of CBT, which helps patients actively tackle problems in a structured way (Box 10.20). It is of benefit in mild to moderate depression, and can be delivered by non-psychiatric doctors and nurses after brief training.

10.20 Stages of problem-solving therapy

- Define and list problems
- Choose one to work on
- List possible solutions
- Evaluate these and choose the best
- Try it out
- Evaluate the result
- Repeat until problems are resolved

Psychodynamic psychotherapy

This treatment, also known as 'interpretive psychotherapy', was pioneered by Freud, Jung and Klein, amongst others. It is based upon the theory that early life experience generates powerful motivating forces, of which the patient is unaware. Psychotherapy aims to help the patient to become aware of these unconscious factors on the assumption that, once identified, their negative effects are reduced. The relationship between therapist and patient is used as a therapeutic tool to identify issues in patients' relationships with others, particularly parents, which may be replicated or transferred to their relationship with the therapist. Explicit discussion of this transference is the basis for the treatment, which traditionally requires frequent sessions over a period of months or even years.

Interpersonal therapy (IPT) is a specific form of brief psychotherapy which focuses on patients' current interpersonal relationships and is an effective treatment for mild to moderate depression.

Social interventions

Factors such as unemployment may not be readily amenable to intervention but others, such as access to benefits and poor housing, are. Patients can be helped to address these problems themselves by being taught a problem-solving approach. Befrienders and day centres can reduce social isolation, benefits advisers can ensure appropriate financial assistance, and medical recommendations can be made to local housing departments to help patients obtain more appropriate accommodation.

PSYCHIATRIC DISORDERS

Stress-related disorders

Acute stress reaction

Following a stressful event such as a serious medical diagnosis or a major accident, some people develop a characteristic pattern of symptoms. These include a sense of bewilderment, anxiety, anger, depression, altered activity and withdrawal. The symptoms are transient and usually resolve completely within a few days.

Adjustment disorder

A more common psychological response to the onset or deterioration of a medical illness is a less severe but more prolonged emotional reaction. The predominant symptom is usually depression and/or anxiety, which is insufficiently persistent or intense to merit a diagnosis of depressive or anxiety disorder. There may also be anger, aggressive behaviour and excessive alcohol use. Symptoms develop within a month of the onset of the stress, and their duration and severity reflect the course of the underlying physical condition, resolution tending to occur with physical recovery.

Grief reactions following bereavement are a particular type of adjustment disorder. They manifest as a brief period of emotional numbing, followed by a period of distress lasting several weeks, during which sorrow, tearfulness, sleep disturbance, loss of interest and a sense of futility are common. Perceptual distortions may occur, including misinterpreting sounds as the dead person's voice. 'Pathological grief' describes a grief reaction that is abnormally intense or persistent.

Management and prognosis

Ongoing contact with and support from a doctor or other who can listen, reassure, explain and advise are helpful and often all that is needed. Most patients do not require psychotropic medication, although benzodiazepines reduce arousal in acute stress reactions and can aid sleep in adjustment disorders. Psychotherapy may be helpful for some patients with abnormal grief reactions. These conditions usually resolve with time but can develop into depressive or anxiety disorders.

Post-traumatic stress disorder (PTSD)

This is a protracted response to a stressful event of an exceptionally threatening or catastrophic nature. Examples include natural disasters, terrorist activity, serious accidents and witnessing violent deaths. PTSD may also occur after distressing medical treatments. There is usually a delay ranging from a few days to several months between the traumatic event and the onset of symptoms. Typical symptoms are recurrent intrusive memories (flashbacks) of the trauma, as well as sleep disturbance, especially nightmares (usually of the traumatic event) from which the patient awakes in a state of anxiety, symptoms of autonomic arousal, emotional blunting and avoidance of situations which evoke memories of the trauma. Anxiety and depression are associated and excessive use of alcohol or drugs frequently complicates the clinical picture.

Management and prognosis

Immediate counselling for those who have survived a major trauma is unnecessary and even potentially harmful if forced on people (Box 10.21). It should only be given to those who request it. The main aims are to provide support, direct advice and the opportunity for emotional catharsis. In established PTSD, structured psychological approaches (particularly cognitive therapy) and antidepressant medication are effective. There is some evidence that a novel therapy called eye movement desensitisation and reprocessing (EMDR) is effective. The condition runs a fluctuating course, with most patients recovering within 2 years. In a small proportion the symptoms become chronic.

EBM **10.21 Early debriefing for post-traumatic stress disorder (PTSD)**

'At present the routine use of individual debriefing in the aftermath of individual trauma cannot be recommended. Early counselling has been found to be unhelpful and possibly even harmful.'

• Rose S, et al. (Cochrane Review). Cochrane Library, issue 2, 2005. Oxford: Update Software.

For further information: www.cochrane.org

Anxiety disorders

These are characterised by the emotion of anxiety, worrisome thoughts, avoidance behaviour and the somatic symptoms of autonomic arousal. Anxiety disorders are divided into three main subtypes: phobic, paroxysmal (panic) and generalised (Box 10.22). The nature and prominence of the somatic symptoms often lead the patient to present initially to medical services. Anxiety may be stress-related and phobic anxiety may follow an unpleasant incident. Patients with anxiety often also have depression.

---

i **10.22 Classification of anxiety disorders**

	Phobic anxiety disorder	Panic disorder	Generalised anxiety disorder
Occurrence	Situational	Paroxysmal	Persistent
Behaviour	Avoidance	Escape	Agitation
Cognitions	Fear of situation	Fear of symptoms	Worry
Symptoms	On exposure	Episodic	Persistent

Phobic anxiety disorder

A phobia is an abnormal or excessive fear of an object or situation, which leads to avoidance of it (such as excessive fear of dying in an air crash leading to avoidance of flying). A generalised phobia of going out alone or being in crowded places is called agoraphobia. Phobic responses can develop to medical interventions such as venepuncture.

Panic disorder

Panic disorder describes repeated attacks of severe anxiety, which are not restricted to any particular situation or circumstances. Somatic symptoms such as chest pain, palpitations and paraesthesiae in lips and fingers are common. The symptoms are in part due to involuntary over-breathing (hyperventilation). Patients often fear they are suffering from a serious illness such as a heart attack or stroke, and may therefore seek emergency medical attention. Panic disorder is often associated with agoraphobia.

Generalised anxiety disorder

This is chronic anxiety associated with uncontrollable worry. Somatic symptoms of muscle tension and bowel disturbance often lead to a medical presentation.

Management of anxiety disorders
Psychological treatment

Explanation and reassurance are essential, especially when patients fear they have a serious medical condition. Specific treatment may be needed. Treatments include relaxation, graded exposure (desensitisation) to feared situations for phobic disorders, and CBT.

Drug treatment

Antidepressants are the drugs of choice. Benzodiazepines are useful in the short term but long-term use can lead to dependence. A β-blocker such as propranolol can help when somatic symptoms are prominent.

Obsessive-compulsive disorder

Obsessive-compulsive disorder (OCD) is characterised by obsessive thoughts, which are recurrent, unwanted and usually anxiety-provoking, and by compulsions, which are repeated acts performed to relieve feelings of tension. An example is repeated hand-washing because of thoughts of contamination. The differential diagnosis is from normal checking behaviour and from delusional beliefs about thought possession. OCD is equally common in men and women.

10

Management and prognosis

OCD usually responds to antidepressant drugs such as clomipramine, and to CBT which helps patients expose themselves to the feared thought or situation without performing the anxiety-relieving compulsions. Relapses are common and the condition often becomes chronic.

Mood disorders

Mood or affective disorders include:

- *unipolar depression*: one or more episodes of low mood and associated symptoms
- *bipolar disorder*: episodes of elevated mood interspersed with episodes of depression
- *dysthymia*: chronic low-grade depressed mood without sufficient other symptoms to count as 'clinically significant' or 'major' depression.

Depression

Major depressive disorder has a prevalence of 5% in the general population and approximately 10% in chronically ill medical out patients. It is a major cause of disability and of suicide. If comorbid with a medical condition, depression magnifies disability, diminishes adherence to medical treatment and rehabilitation, and may even shorten life expectancy. Such comorbid depression may incrementally worsen health more than any combination of chronic diseases without depression.

Aetiology

There is a genetic predisposition to depression, especially when of early onset. The number and identity of the genes are largely unknown but the serotonin transporter gene is a candidate. Adversity and emotional deprivation early in life also predispose to depression. Depressive episodes are often triggered by stressful life events (especially those that involve loss), including medical illnesses. Associated biological factors include hypofunction of monoamine neurotransmitter systems (5-HT and noradrenaline (norepinephrine)) and abnormal hypothalamo-pituitary-adrenal axis (HPA) regulation, which results in elevated cortisol levels that do not suppress with dexamethasone. Exclusion of Cushing's syndrome is described on pages 771–772.

Diagnosis

The symptoms are listed in Box 10.8 (p. 233). Depression may be mild, moderate or severe, and episodic, recurrent or chronic. It can be both a complication of a medical condition and a cause of MUS (see below), so physical examination is essential; and an associated medical condition should always be considered (Box 10.23).

> **10.23 Pointers to an organic cause for psychiatric disorder**
>
> - Late age of onset of psychiatric illness
> - No previous history of psychiatric illness
> - No family history of psychiatric illness
> - No apparent psychological precipitant

Management and prognosis

There is evidence that both drug and psychological treatments work in depression. In practice, the choice is determined by patient preference and local availability. Severe depression complicated by psychosis, dehydration or suicide risk may require ECT.

Drug treatment

Antidepressant drugs are effective in patients whose depression is secondary to medical illness, as well as those in whom it is the primary problem (Box 10.24). These agents are all effective in moderate and severe depression. Commonly used antidepressants are shown in Box 10.25.

- *Tricyclic antidepressants (TCAs)*. These agents inhibit the re-uptake of the amines noradrenaline (norepinephrine) and 5-HT at synaptic clefts. The therapeutic effect is noticeable within 1–2 weeks. Side-effects, such as sedation, anticholinergic effects, postural hypotension, lowering of the seizure threshold and cardiotoxicity can be troublesome during this period. TCAs may be dangerous in overdose and in people who have coexisting heart disease, glaucoma and prostatism.
- *Selective serotonin re-uptake inhibitors (SSRIs)*. These are less cardiotoxic and less sedative, and have fewer

> **EBM 10.24 Antidepressants in the medically ill**
>
> 'There is evidence to support the use of antidepressants in depressed patients who are also physically ill.'
>
> • Evan DL, et al. Biol Psychiatry 2005; 58(3):175–189.

10.25 Antidepressant drugs

Group	Drug	Usual dose*
Tricyclics	Amitriptyline	75–150 mg daily
	Imipramine	75–150 mg daily
	Dosulepin	75–150 mg daily
	Clomipramine	75–150 mg daily
SSRIs	Citalopram	20–40 mg daily
	Escitalopram	10–20 mg daily
	Fluoxetine	20–60 mg daily
	Fluvoxamine	100–300 mg daily
	Sertraline	50–100 mg daily
	Paroxetine	20–50 mg daily
Monoamine oxidase inhibitors (MAOIs)	Phenelzine	45–90 mg daily
	Tranylcypromine	20–40 mg daily
	Moclobemide	300–600 mg daily
Noradrenergic re-uptake inhibitors and SSRIs	Venlafaxine	75–375 mg daily
Selective noradrenaline (norepinephrine) re-uptake inhibitor	Reboxetine	8–12 mg daily
Noradrenergic and specific serotonergic inhibitor	Mirtazapine	15–45 mg daily

*Higher doses may be required: see guidelines.

anticholinergic effects than tricyclics. They are safer in overdose, but can still cause headache, nausea, anorexia and sexual dysfunction.

- *Newer antidepressants.* A variety is available, including venlafaxine, mirtazapine, reboxetine and duloxetine. They have different modes of action and adverse effects but none has been shown to be more effective than the agents listed above.
- *Monoamine oxidase inhibitors (MAOIs).* These drugs increase the availability of neurotransmitters at synaptic clefts by inhibiting metabolism of noradrenaline (norepinephrine) and 5-HT. They are now rarely prescribed in the UK, since they can cause potentially dangerous interactions with drugs such as amphetamines, and foods rich in tyramine such as cheese and red wine. This is due to accumulation of amines in the systemic circulation, causing a potentially fatal hypertensive crisis.
- *Moclobemide.* This is a reversible and selective inhibitor of monoamine oxidase subtype A, which causes minimal potentiation of the pressor response to dietary tyramine.

The different classes of antidepressants have similar efficacy and about three-quarters of patients respond to treatment. Successful treatment requires the patient to take an appropriate dose of an effective drug for an adequate period. In case of non-response it is worth trying a different agent. The patient's progress must be monitored and, after recovery, treatment should be continued for at least 6–12 months to reduce the high risk of relapse; the dose should then be tapered off over several weeks to avoid discontinuation symptoms. In England and Wales, NICE guidelines help with the choice of an antidepressant regimen (www.nice.org.uk).

Psychological treatments

Both CBT and interpersonal psychotherapy are as effective as antidepressants for mild to moderate depression. Antidepressant drugs are, however, preferred for severe depression. Drug and psychological treatments can be used in combination.

Over 50% of people who have had one depressive episode and over 90% of people who have had three or more episodes will have another. The risk of suicide in an individual who has had a depressive disorder is ten times greater than in the general population.

Bipolar disorder

Bipolar disorder is an episodic disturbance with interspersed periods of depressed and elevated mood; the latter is known as hypomania, or mania when severe. The lifetime risk of developing bipolar disorder is approximately 1%. Onset is usually in the teens, and men and women are equally affected. Bipolar disorder has been divided into two types:

- *Bipolar I disorder* has a clinical course characterised by one or more manic episodes or mixed episodes. Often individuals have also had one or more major depressive episodes.
- *Bipolar II disorder* features depressive episodes which are more frequent and more intense than manic episodes, but there is a history of at least one hypomanic episode.

Aetiology

Bipolar disorder is strongly heritable (80%). Relatives of patients have an increased incidence of both bipolar and unipolar affective disorder but life events, such as physical illness and medication, may play a role in triggering episodes.

Diagnosis

Isolated episodes of hypomania or mania do occur but they are usually preceded or followed by an episode of depression. Psychosis may occur in both the depressive and the manic phases, with delusions and hallucinations that are usually in keeping with the mood disturbance. This is described as an affective psychosis. Patients who present with symptoms of both bipolar disorder and schizophrenia may be given a diagnosis of schizoaffective disorder.

Management and prognosis

Depression should be treated, as described above. Manic episodes usually respond well to antipsychotic drugs (see Box 10.28 below). Prophylaxis to prevent recurrent episodes is important. The main drugs used are lithium, carbamazepine and sodium valproate. Lamotrigine and quetiapine are increasingly being used. Caution must be exercised when stopping these, as a relapse may follow.

- *Lithium carbonate* is the drug of choice. It is also used for acute mania, and in combination with a tricyclic as an adjuvant treatment for resistant depression. It has a narrow therapeutic range, so regular blood monitoring is required to maintain a serum level of 0.5–1.0 mmol/L. Toxic effects include nausea, vomiting, tremor and convulsions. With long-term treatment, weight gain, hypothyroidism, nephrogenic diabetes insipidus (p. 792) and renal failure can occur. Thyroid and renal function should be checked before treatment is started and every 6–12 months thereafter. Lithium is teratogenic, as are anti-epileptics, and should never be prescribed during the first trimester of pregnancy.
- *Carbamazepine* and *sodium valproate* are established anticonvulsant drugs that have been used successfully as prophylaxis in bipolar disorder, usually as second-line alternatives to lithium. Both can cause the adverse effects of ataxia, nausea and tremor.

The relapse rate is high, although patients may be perfectly well between episodes. After one episode the annual average risk of relapse is about 10–15%, which doubles after more than three episodes. There is a substantially increased lifetime risk of suicide of 5–10%.

Schizophrenia

Schizophrenia is a psychosis characterised by delusions, hallucinations and lack of insight. Acute schizophrenia may present with disturbed behaviour, marked delusions, hallucinations and disordered thinking, or with insidious social withdrawal and less obvious delusions and hallucinations. The prevalence is similar world-wide at about 1% and the disorder is more common in men. The children of one affected parent have approximately a 10% risk of developing the illness, but this rises to 50%

if an identical twin is affected. The usual age of onset is the mid-twenties.

Aetiology

There is a strong genetic contribution, probably involving many susceptibility genes, each of small effect. The best candidates, such as *disrupted in schizophrenia-1 (DISC1)* and *neuregulin1 (NRG1)*, have supportive linkage, association, animal model and basic neurobiological evidence. Environmental risk factors include obstetric complications and urban birth. Brain imaging techniques have identified subtle structural abnormalities, including an enlargement of the lateral ventricles and an overall decrease in brain size (by about 3% on average), with relatively greater reduction in temporal lobe volume (5–10%). Episodes of acute schizophrenia may be precipitated by social stress and cannabis, which increase dopamine turnover and sensitivity. Consequently, schizophrenia is now viewed as a neurodevelopmental disorder, caused by abnormalities of brain development associated with genetic predisposition and early environmental influences, but precipitated by later triggers.

Diagnosis

Schizophrenia usually presents with an acute episode and may progress to a chronic state. Acute schizophrenia should be suspected in any individual with bizarre behaviour accompanied by delusions and hallucinations that are not due to organic brain disease or substance misuse. The diagnosis is made on clinical grounds, with investigations used principally to rule out organic brain disease. The characteristic clinical features are listed in Box 10.26. Hallucinations are typically auditory, although they can occur in any sensory modality. They commonly involve voices from outside the head that talk to or about the person. Sometimes the voices repeat the person's thoughts. Patients may also describe 'passivity of thought', experienced as disturbances in the normal privacy of thinking; this is expressed in the belief that their thoughts are being 'withdrawn' from them, perhaps 'broadcast' to others, with alien thoughts being 'inserted' into their mind. Other characteristic symptoms are delusions of control: believing that one's emotions, impulses or acts are controlled by others. Another first-rank phenomenon is delusional perception, a delusion which arises suddenly alongside a perception (e.g. 'I saw the moon and I immediately knew he was evil'). Many other less specific symptoms may occur, including thought disorder, as manifest by incomprehensible speech, and abnormalities of movement, such as those in which the patient can become immobile or adopt awkward postures for prolonged periods (catatonia).

The main differential diagnosis of schizophrenia is from:

- *Other functional psychoses*, particularly psychotic depression and mania, in which delusions and hallucinations are congruent with a marked mood disturbance (negative in depression and grandiose in mania). If features of schizophrenia and affective disorder coexist in equal measure, a diagnosis of schizoaffective disorder is made. Schizophrenia must also be differentiated from specific delusional disorders that are not associated with the other typical features of schizophrenia (Box 10.27).
- *Organic psychoses*, including delirium, in which there is impairment of consciousness and loss of orientation (not found in the functional psychoses), with typically visual hallucinations and drug misuse, the latter particularly in young people. Schizophrenia must also be differentiated from other organic psychoses such as temporal lobe epilepsy, in which olfactory and gustatory hallucinations may occur (see Box 10.27).

Some of those who experience acute schizophrenia go on to develop a chronic state. The acute, so-called positive symptoms resolve, or at least do not dominate the clinical picture, leaving so-called negative symptoms which include blunt affect, apathy, social isolation, poverty of speech and poor self-care. Patients with chronic schizophrenia may also manifest positive symptoms, particularly when under stress, and it can be difficult for those who do not know the patient to judge whether or not these are signs of an acute relapse.

10.26 Symptoms of schizophrenia

First-rank symptoms of acute schizophrenia

- A = Auditory hallucinations—second or third person/écho de la pensée
- B = Broadcasting, insertion/withdrawal of thoughts
- C = Controlled feelings, impulses or acts ('passivity' experiences/phenomena)
- D = Delusional perception (a particular experience is bizarrely interpreted)

Symptoms of chronic schizophrenia (negative symptoms)

- Flattened (blunted) affect
- Apathy and loss of drive (avolition)
- Social isolation
- Poverty of speech
- Poor self-care

10.27 Differential diagnosis of schizophrenia

Alternative diagnosis	Distinguishing features
Other functional psychoses	
Delusional disorders	Absence of specific features of schizophrenia
Psychotic depression	Prominent depressive symptoms
Manic episode	Prominent manic symptoms
Schizoaffective disorder	Mood and schizophrenia symptoms both prominent
Puerperal psychosis	Acute onset after childbirth
Organic disorders	
Drug-induced psychosis	Evidence of drug or alcohol misuse
Side-effects of prescribed drugs	Levodopa, methyldopa, corticosteroids, antimalarial drugs
Temporal lobe epilepsy	Other evidence of seizures
Delirium	Visual hallucinations; impaired consciousness
Dementia	Age; established cognitive impairment
Huntington's disease	Family history; choreiform movements; dementia

Management

First-episode schizophrenia usually requires admission to hospital because patients lack insight that they are ill and are unwilling to accept treatment. In some cases, they may be at risk of harming themselves or others. Subsequent acute relapses and chronic schizophrenia are now usually managed in the community.

Drug treatment

Antipsychotic agents are effective against the positive symptoms of schizophrenia in the majority of cases. They take 2–4 weeks to be maximally effective, but have some beneficial effects shortly after administration. Treatment is then ideally continued to prevent relapse. In a patient with a first episode of schizophrenia, this will usually be for 1–2 years, but in patients with multiple episodes, treatment may be required for many years. The benefits of prolonged treatment must be weighed against the adverse effects, which include tardive dyskinesia (abnormal movements, commonly of the face, over which the patient has no voluntary control). For long-term use, antipsychotic agents are often given in slow-release (depot) injected form to improve patient adherence.

A number of antipsychotic agents are available (Box 10.28). These may be divided into conventional (typical, first-generation) drugs such as chlorpromazine and haloperidol, and newer or atypical (also so-called novel or second-generation) drugs such as clozapine. All are believed to work by blocking D_2 dopamine receptors in the brain. Patients who have not responded to conventional drugs may respond to newer agents, which are also less likely to produce unwanted extrapyramidal side-effects but do tend to cause greater weight gain. Clozapine can also cause an agranulocytosis and consequently requires regular monitoring of the white blood cell count, initially on a weekly basis. Details of the side-effects of antipsychotic drugs are listed in Box 10.29.

10.29 Side-effects of antipsychotic drugs

Weight gain due to increased appetite

Effects due to dopamine blockade*
- Parkinsonism
- Akathisia (motor restlessness)
- Acute dystonia
- Tardive dyskinesia
- Gynaecomastia
- Galactorrhoea

Effects due to cholinergic blockade
- Dry mouth
- Blurred vision
- Constipation
- Urinary retention
- Impotence

Hypersensitivity reactions
- Cholestatic jaundice
- Photosensitive dermatitis
- Blood dyscrasias (neutropenia with clozapine)

Ocular complications (long-term use)
- Corneal and lens opacities

*Less severe with clozapine, quetiapine and olanzapine because of strong 5-HT-blocking effect and relatively weak dopamine blockade.

Serious adverse effects of antipsychotic drugs include:

- *Neuroleptic malignant syndrome*, which is rare but serious. It is characterised by fever, tremor and rigidity, autonomic instability and confusion. Characteristic laboratory findings are an elevated creatinine phosphokinase and leucocytosis. Antipsychotic medication must be stopped immediately and supportive therapy provided, often in an intensive care unit. Treatment includes ensuring hydration and reducing hyperthermia. Dantrolene sodium and bromocriptine may be helpful. Mortality is 20% untreated and 5% with treatment.
- *Prolongation of the QT_c interval*, which may be associated with ventricular tachycardia, torsades de pointes and sudden death. Treatment is by stopping the drug, monitoring the ECG and treating serious arrhythmias (p. 559).

Psychological treatment

Psychological treatment, including general support for the patient and his or her family, is now seen as an essential component of the therapeutic plan. CBT may help patients to cope with treatment-resistant symptoms. There is evidence that personal and/or family education reduces the rate of relapse.

Social treatment

After an acute episode of schizophrenia has been controlled by drug therapy, social rehabilitation may be required. Recurrent illness is likely to cause disruption to patients' relationships and their ability to manage their accommodation and occupation; consequently, they may need help to obtain housing and employment. A graded return to employment and sometimes a period of supported accommodation are required.

10.28 Antipsychotic drugs

Group	Drug	Usual dose
Phenothiazines	Chlorpromazine	100–1500 mg daily
	Trifluoperazine	5–30 mg daily
	Fluphenazine	20–100 mg fortnightly
Butyrophenones	Haloperidol	5–30 mg daily
Thioxanthenes	Flupentixol decanoate	20–200 mg fortnightly (depot injection)
Diphenylbutylpiperidines	Pimozide	4–30 mg daily
Substituted benzamides	Sulpiride	200–1800 mg daily
Dibenzodiazepines*	Clozapine	25–900 mg daily
Benzisoxazole*	Risperidone	2–16 mg daily
Thienobenzodiazepines*	Olanzapine	5–20 mg daily
Dibenzothiazepines	Quetiapine	200–800 mg daily

*Second-generation antipsychotics.

Patients with chronic schizophrenia have particular difficulties and may need long-term supervised accommodation. This was previously provided in mental hospitals but now tends to be in sheltered or hostel accommodation in the community. Patients may also benefit from sheltered employment if they are unable to participate effectively in the labour market. Ongoing contact with a health worker allows monitoring for signs of relapse so that treatment can be administered early. This is sometimes called 'assertive outreach', with multidisciplinary teams working to agreed plans (a 'care programme approach'). Partly because of a tendency to inactivity, smoking and a poor diet, patients with chronic schizophrenia are at increased risk of cardiovascular disease, diabetes and tuberculosis, and require medical as well as psychiatric care.

Prognosis

About one-quarter of those who develop an acute schizophrenic episode have a good outcome. One-third develop chronic schizophrenia, and the remainder recover after each episode but suffer relapses. Most will not work or live independently. Prophylactic treatment with antipsychotic drugs reduces the rate of relapse in the first 2 years after an episode of schizophrenia from 70% to 40%. Schizophrenia is associated with suicide, 1 in 10 patients taking their own lives.

Alcohol misuse and dependence

Alcohol consumption associated with social, psychological and physical problems constitutes harmful use. The criteria for alcohol dependence, a more restricted term, are shown in Box 10.30. Approximately one-quarter of male patients in general hospital medical wards in the UK have a current or previous alcohol problem.

Aetiology

Availability of alcohol and social patterns of use appear to be the most important factors. Genetic factors may play some part in predisposition to dependence. The majority of alcoholics do not have an associated psychiatric illness, but a few drink heavily in an attempt to relieve anxiety or depression.

Diagnosis

Alcohol misuse may emerge during the patient's history, although patients may minimise their intake. It may also present via its effects on one or more aspects of the patient's life, listed below. Alcohol dependence commonly presents with withdrawal in those admitted to hospital, as they can no longer maintain their high alcohol intake in this setting.

10.30 Criteria for alcohol dependence

- Narrowing of the drinking repertoire
- Priority of drinking over other activities (salience)
- Tolerance of effects of alcohol
- Repeated withdrawal symptoms
- Relief of withdrawal symptoms by further drinking
- Subjective compulsion to drink
- Reinstatement of drinking behaviour after abstinence

Complications of chronic alcohol misuse

Social problems include absenteeism from work, unemployment, marital tensions, child abuse, financial difficulties and problems with the law, such as violence and traffic offences.

Psychological problems

- *Depression* is common. Alcohol has a direct depressant effect and heavy drinking creates numerous social problems. Attempted suicide and completed suicide are often associated with alcohol misuse.
- *Anxiety* is relieved by alcohol. People who are socially anxious may consequently use alcohol in this way and may develop dependence. Conversely, alcohol withdrawal increases anxiety.
- *Alcoholic hallucinosis* is a rare condition in which alcoholic individuals experience auditory hallucination in clear consciousness.
- *Alcohol withdrawal* is described in Box 10.30. Symptoms usually become maximal about 2 days after the last drink and can include seizures ('rum fits').
- *Delirium tremens* is a form of delirium associated with severe alcohol withdrawal. It has a significant mortality and morbidity (see Box 10.31).

Effects on the brain

The familiar features of drunkenness are ataxia, slurred speech, emotional incontinence and aggression. Very heavy drinkers may experience periods of amnesia for events which occurred during bouts of intoxication, termed 'alcoholic blackouts'. Established alcoholism may lead to alcoholic dementia, a global cognitive impairment resembling Alzheimer's disease, but which does not progress and may even improve if the patient becomes abstinent. Indirect effects on behaviour can result from head injury, hypoglycaemia and encephalopathy (p. 938).

A rare but important effect of chronic alcohol misuse is the Wernicke–Korsakoff syndrome. This organic brain disorder results from damage to the mamillary bodies, dorsomedial nuclei of the thalamus and adjacent areas of periventricular grey matter. It is caused by a deficiency of thiamin (vitamin B_1), which is most commonly caused by long-standing heavy drinking and an inadequate diet. Without prompt treatment (see below), the acute presentation of Wernicke's encephalopathy (nystagmus, ophthalmoplegia, ataxia and confusion) can progress to the irreversible deficits of Korsakoff's syndrome (severe short-term memory deficits and confabulation). In those who die in the acute stage, microscopic examination of the brain shows hyperaemia, petechial haemorrhages and astrocytic proliferation.

Effects on other organs

These are protean and virtually any organ can be involved (see Box 10.31); alcohol has replaced syphilis as the great mimic of disease. These effects are discussed in detail in the relevant chapters.

Management and prognosis

The provision of clear information from a doctor about the harmful effects of alcohol and safe levels of consumption is often all that is needed. In more serious cases, patients may have to be advised to alter leisure activities or change jobs if these are contributing to the problem. Psychological treatment is used for patients who have

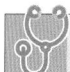

10.31 Consequences of chronic alcohol misuse

Acute intoxication

- Emotional and behavioural disturbance
- Medical problems: hypoglycaemia, aspiration of vomit, respiratory depression
- Complicating other medical problems
- Accidents, and injuries sustained in fights

Withdrawal phenomena

- Psychological symptoms: restlessness, anxiety, panic attacks
- Autonomic symptoms: tachycardia, sweating, pupil dilatation, nausea, vomiting
- Delirium tremens: agitation, hallucinations, illusions, delusions
- Seizures

Harmful use

Medical consequences

- Neurological: peripheral neuropathy, cerebellar degeneration, cerebral haemorrhage, dementia
- Hepatic: fatty change and cirrhosis, liver cancer
- Gastrointestinal: oesophagitis, gastritis, pancreatitis, oesophageal cancer, Mallory–Weiss syndrome, malabsorption, oesophageal varices
- Respiratory: pulmonary TB, pneumonia
- Skin: spider naevi, palmar erythema, Dupuytren's contractures, telangiectasiae
- Cardiac: cardiomyopathy, hypertension
- Musculoskeletal: myopathy, fractures
- Endocrine and metabolic: pseudo-Cushing's syndrome, hypoglycaemia, gout
- Reproductive: hypogonadism, fetal alcohol syndrome, infertility

Psychiatric and cerebral consequences

- Depression
- Alcoholic hallucinosis
- Alcoholic 'blackouts'
- Wernicke's encephalopathy: nystagmus, ophthalmoplegia, ataxia, confusion
- Korsakoff's syndrome: short-term memory deficits, confabulation

---

recurrent relapses and is usually available at specialised centres. Support is also provided by voluntary organisations, such as Alcoholics Anonymous (AA) in the UK.

If alcohol dependence is suspected, withdrawal syndromes can be prevented, or treated once established, with benzodiazepines. Large doses may be required (e.g. diazepam 20 mg 6-hourly), tailed off over a period of 5–7 days as symptoms subside. Prevention of the Wernicke–Korsakoff complex requires the immediate use of high doses of thiamin, which is given parenterally in the form of Pabrinex (p. 1199). There is no treatment for Korsakoff's syndrome once it has arisen. The risk of side-effects, such as respiratory depression with benzodiazepines and anaphylaxis with Pabrinex, is small when weighed against the risks of no treatment.

Disulfiram (200–400 mg daily) can be given as a deterrent to patients who have difficulty resisting the impulse to drink after becoming abstinent. It blocks the metabolism of alcohol, causing acetaldehyde to accumulate.

When alcohol is consumed, an unpleasant reaction follows with headache, flushing and nausea. Disulfiram is always an adjunct to other treatments, especially supportive psychotherapy. Acamprosate (666 mg 8-hourly) has recently been introduced to maintain abstinence by reducing the craving for alcohol. Only rarely are antidepressants required; depressive symptoms, if present, usually resolve with abstinence. Antipsychotics (e.g. chlorpromazine 100 mg 8-hourly) are required for alcoholic hallucinosis.

Many but not all who become dependent on alcohol relapse after treatment. Chronic alcohol misuse greatly increases the risk of death from accidents, disease and suicide.

Substance misuse disorder

Dependence on and misuse of both illegal and prescribed drugs is a major problem world-wide. Drugs of misuse are described in detail in Chapter 9. They can be grouped as follows.

Sedatives

These commonly give rise to physical dependence, the manifestations being tolerance and a withdrawal syndrome. They include benzodiazepines, opiates (including morphine, heroin, methadone and dihydrocodeine) and barbiturates (now rarely prescribed). Overdosage can be dangerous with the opiates and benzodiazepines, primarily as a result of respiratory depression (Ch. 9). Withdrawal from opiates is notoriously unpleasant, and withdrawal from benzodiazepines (Box 10.32) and barbiturates may be dangerous because of seizures.

Intravenous opiate users are prone to bacterial infections, hepatitis B, hepatitis C (pp. 948–954) and HIV infection (Ch. 14) through needle contamination. Accidental overdose is common, mainly because of the varied and uncertain potency of illicit supplies of the drug. The withdrawal syndrome, which can start within 12 hours of the drug's last use, presents with intense craving, rhinorrhoea, lacrimation, yawning, perspiration, shivering, piloerection, vomiting, diarrhoea and abdominal cramps. Examination reveals tachycardia, hypertension, mydriasis and facial flushing.

Stimulants

These include amphetamines and cocaine. They are less dangerous than the sedatives in overdose, although they can cause cardiac and cerebrovascular problems through their pressor effects. With prolonged heavy use, psychiatric disturbance can be prominent. Physical dependence syndromes do not arise, but withdrawal causes a rebound lowering in mood and can give rise to an intense craving for further use, especially in any form of

10.32 Benzodiazepine withdrawal symptoms

- Anxiety
- Heightened sensory perception
- Hallucinations
- Epileptic seizures
- Ataxia
- Paranoid delusions

10

drug with a rapid onset and offset of effect such as crack cocaine. Chronic ingestion can cause a syndrome similar to schizophrenia. A toxic psychosis can occur with high levels of consumption, and tactile hallucinations (formication) may be prominent.

Hallucinogens

The hallucinogens are a disparate group of drugs that cause prominent sensory disturbances. They include cannabis, ecstasy, lysergic acid diethylamide (LSD) and *Psilocybin* (magic mushrooms).

A toxic confusional state can occur after heavy cannabis consumption. Acute psychotic episodes are well recognised, especially in those with a family or personal history of psychotic illness, and there is evidence that prolonged heavy use increases the risk of developing schizophrenia. Paranoid psychoses have been reported in association with ecstasy. A chronic psychotic illness has also been reported after regular LSD use.

Organic solvents

Solvent inhalation (glue sniffing) is popular in some adolescent groups. Solvents produce acute intoxication characterised by euphoria, excitement, dizziness and a floating sensation. Further inhalation leads to loss of consciousness; death can occur from the direct toxic effect of the solvent, or from asphyxiation if the substance is inhaled from a plastic bag.

Aetiology

Many of the aetiological factors for alcohol misuse also apply to drug dependence. The main factors are cultural pressures, particularly within a peer group, and availability of a drug. In the case of some drugs, medical overprescribing has increased their availability, but there has also been a relative decline in the price of illegal drugs. Most drug users take a range of drugs—so-called polydrug misuse.

Diagnosis

As with alcohol, the diagnosis either may be apparent from the history, or may only be made once the patient presents with a complication. Drug screening of samples of urine or blood can be very valuable in confirming the diagnosis, especially if the patient persists in denial.

Management and prognosis

The first step is to determine whether patients wish to stop using the drug. If they do not, they can still benefit from advice about how to minimise harm from their habit: for example, advice to use clean needles for those who inject. For those who are physically dependent on sedative drugs, substitute prescribing (using methadone, for example, in opiate dependence) may help stabilise their lifestyles sufficiently to allow a gradual reduction in dosage until they reach abstinence. Some specialist units offer inpatient detoxification. For details of the medical management of overdose, see Chapter 9.

The drug lofexidine, a centrally acting α-agonist, can be useful in treating the autonomic symptoms of opiate withdrawal, as can clonidine, although this carries a risk of hypotension and is best used by specialists. Long-acting opiate antagonists, such as naltrexone, may also have a place, again in specialist hands, in blocking the euphoriant effects of the opiate, which may aid in breaking patterns of addiction.

In some cases, complete opiate withdrawal is not successful and the patient functions better if maintained on regular doses of oral methadone as an outpatient. This decision should only be taken by a specialist, and long-term supervision requires the patient to attend a specialist drug treatment centre.

Substitute prescribing is neither necessary nor possible for the hallucinogens and stimulants, so the principles of management are the same as those that should accompany prescribing for the sedatives. These include identifying problems associated with the drug misuse which may serve to maintain it, and intervening where possible. Intervention may be directed at physical ill health, psychiatric comorbidity, social problems or family disharmony.

Relapsing patients and those with complications should be referred to specialist drug misuse services. Support can also be provided by self-help groups and voluntary bodies such as Narcotics Anonymous in the UK.

Delirium, dementia and organic disorders

Delirium, dementia and other organic disorders can be thought of as medical conditions rather than psychiatric disorders, but are included in psychiatric classifications and sometimes misdiagnosed because they manifest with disturbed behaviour.

Delirium

Delirium is common in acute medical settings, affecting more than half of patients in high-dependency and intensive care units. Aetiology, assessment and management are described in Chapters 26 and 7.

Dementia

Dementia affects 5% of those over 65 and 20% of those over 85. It is defined as a global impairment of cognitive function, and although memory is most affected in the early stages, deficits in visuo-spatial function, language ability, concentration and attention gradually become apparent. Aetiology and investigation are described in Chapter 26. Management is essentially symptomatic and supportive. The anticholinesterase inhibitors, such as donepezil, may arrest progression for a time in Alzheimer-type dementia, while addressing the underlying vascular risk factors may slow deterioration in vascular dementia, but neither can be reversed. Psychotropic drugs may help where there is associated disturbance of sleep, perception or mood, but should only be used with care, especially since evidence shows increased mortality in patients treated long term with these agents. Sedation is not a substitute for good community support for patients and carers or, in the later stages, attentive residential nursing care. In the UK, incapacity and mental health legislation may be required to manage patients' financial and domestic affairs, as well as to determine safe placement. Most dementias have a progressive course, which may be gradual (as in Alzheimer's disease) or step-wise (as in vascular dementia).

Personality disorders

Personality is the set of characteristics and behavioural traits which best describes an individual's patterns of interaction with the world. The intensity of particular traits varies from person to person, although many, such as shyness or irritability, are displayed to some degree by most people.

A personality disorder is diagnosed when an individual's personality causes persistent and severe problems for the person himself or herself or for others. For example, shyness may be so pronounced that the individual never ventures into any situation where he/she fears scrutiny, so that that person's life becomes narrow and empty. Antisocial traits, such as disregard for the well-being of others and a lack of guilt concerning the adverse effects of one's actions on others, may lead to damage to others and to criminal acts.

Personality disorder is classified into 8–10 types (such as emotionally unstable, antisocial or schizotypal), depending on the particular behavioural traits in question. There are differences between ICD-10 and DSM-IV classifications. A patient who meets diagnostic criteria for one subtype commonly meets criteria for two or three others. As allocation to one particular subtype gives little guidance to management or prognosis, classification is of limited value. Personality disorder commonly accompanies other psychiatric conditions, making treatment of those conditions more difficult and therefore affecting their prognosis.

Aetiology

Some personality disorders appear to have an inherited aspect but most are more clearly related to an unsatisfactory upbringing and childhood abuse.

Management and prognosis

Personality disorder is largely untreatable. There is little evidence of benefit from psychotropics, and limited evidence for the value of psychotherapy. Furthermore, any such treatment has to be intensive and/or long-term if it is to effect any substantial change. By definition, personality disorders tend to persist throughout life, although they may become less extreme with age.

Eating disorders

There are two well-defined eating disorders, anorexia nervosa (AN) and bulimia nervosa (BN), which share some overlapping features. Ninety per cent of cases are female. There is a much higher prevalence of abnormal eating behaviour in the population which does not meet diagnostic criteria for AN or BN. In developed societies, obesity is arguably a much greater problem but is usually considered to be more a disorder of lifestyle or physiology than a psychiatric illness.

Anorexia nervosa

There is marked weight loss, arising from food avoidance, often in combination with bingeing, purging, excessive exercise, or the use of diuretics and laxatives. Body image is profoundly disturbed so that, despite emaciation, patients still feel overweight and are terrified of weight gain. These preoccupations are intense and pervasive, and the false beliefs may be held with a conviction approaching the delusional. Anxiety and depressive symptoms are common accompaniments. Downy hair (lanugo) may develop on the back, forearms and cheeks. Extreme starvation is associated with a wide range of physiological and pathological bodily changes. All organ systems may be affected, although the most serious problems are cardiac and skeletal (Box 10.33).

Aetiology

This is unknown but probably includes genetic and environmental factors, including the social pressure on women to be thin.

Diagnosis

The condition usually emerges in adolescence, with a marked female preponderance. Diagnostic criteria are shown in Box 10.34. Differential diagnosis covers other causes of weight loss, including psychiatric disorders such as depression, and medical conditions such as inflammatory bowel disease, malabsorption, hypopituitarism and cancer. The diagnosis is made on the presence of a pronounced fear of fatness despite being thin, and on the absence of alternative causes of weight loss.

Management and prognosis

The aims of management are to ensure the patient's physical well-being, whilst helping her to increase her weight to the normal range by addressing abnormal beliefs and behaviour. Treatment is usually given on an outpatient basis, inpatient treatment being indicated only if weight loss is intractable and severe (for example, less than 65% of normal), or if there is a risk of death from medical complications or from suicide. There is a limited evidence base for treatment, although individual

 10.33 Physical consequences of eating disorders

Cardiac

- ECG abnormalities: T wave inversion, ST depression and prolonged QT_c interval
- Arrhythmias, including profound sinus bradycardia and ventricular tachycardia

Haematological

- Anaemia, thrombocytopenia and leucopenia

Endocrine

- Pubertal delay or arrest
- Growth retardation and short stature
- Amenorrhoea
- Sick euthyroid state

Metabolic

- Uraemia
- Renal calculi
- Osteoporosis

Gastrointestinal

- Constipation
- Abnormal liver function tests

10

Anorexia nervosa

- Weight loss of at least 15% of total body weight (or body mass index ≤ 17.5)
- Avoidance of high-calorie foods
- Distortion of body image so that patients regard themselves as fat even when grossly underweight
- Amenorrhoea for at least 3 months

Bulimia nervosa

- Recurrent bouts of binge eating
- Lack of self-control over eating during binges
- Self-induced vomiting, purgation or dieting after binges
- Weight maintained within normal limits

psychological treatments, particularly CBT and family therapy, are commonly used. Psychotropic drugs are of little benefit except in those with clear-cut comorbid depressive disorder.

Weight gain is best managed in a collaborative fashion. Compulsory admission and refeeding (including tube feeding) are very occasionally resorted to when patients are at risk of death and other measures have failed. Whilst this may produce a short-term improvement in weight, it probably does not change long-term prognosis. About 20% of patients with anorexia nervosa have a good outcome, a further 20% develop a chronic intractable disorder and the rest have an intermediate outcome. There is a long-term mortality rate of 10–20%, either due to the complications of starvation or from suicide.

Bulimia nervosa

In BN, patients are usually at or near normal weight (unlike in AN), but display a morbid fear of fatness associated with disordered eating behaviour. They recurrently embark on eating binges, often followed by corrective measures such as self-induced vomiting. The prevalence is similar to or slightly greater than that of AN, but only a small proportion of sufferers reach treatment services.

Diagnosis

BN usually begins later in adolescence than AN, and is even more predominantly a female malady. Diagnostic criteria are shown in Box 10.33. Physical signs of repeated self-induced vomiting include pitted teeth (from gastric acid), calluses on knuckles ('Russell's sign') and parotid gland enlargement. There are many associated physical complications, including the dental and oesophageal consequences of repeated vomiting, as well as electrolyte abnormalities, cardiac arrhythmias and renal problems (see Box 10.32).

Management and prognosis

CBT achieves short- and long-term improvements. Guided self-help and interpersonal psychotherapy may also be of value. There is also evidence for benefit from the SSRI, fluoxetine, although high doses (60 mg daily) and long courses (1 year) may be required; this appears to be independent of the antidepressant effect.

Bulimia does not carry the mortality associated with AN, and few sufferers develop anorexia. At 10 years, approximately 10% are still unwell, 20% have a subclinical degree of BN, and the remainder have recovered.

Somatoform disorders

The essential feature of these disorders is somatic symptoms which are not explained by a medical condition (MUS) and not better diagnosed as part of a depressive or anxiety disorder. Several syndromes are described within this category; there is considerable overlap between them in both aetiology and clinical presentation.

Aetiology

The cause of somatoform disorders is incompletely understood but contributory factors include depression or anxiety, the erroneous interpretation of somatic symptoms as evidence of disease, and excessive concern with physical illness. A family history or previous history of a particular condition may have shaped the patient's beliefs about illness. Doctors may exacerbate the problem, either by dismissing the complaints as non-existent or by over-emphasising the possibility of disease.

Somatisation disorder

Somatisation disorder (Briquet's syndrome) is characterised by the occurrence of chronic multiple somatic symptoms for which there is no physical cause. Symptoms start in early adult life and may be referred to any part of the body. It is much more common in women. Common complaints include pain, vomiting, nausea, headache, dizziness, menstrual irregularities and sexual dysfunction. Patients may undergo a multitude of negative investigations and unhelpful operations, particularly hysterectomy and cholecystectomy. There is no proven treatment but minimisation of iatrogenic harm from investigation and attempts at medical treatment is important.

Hypochondriacal disorder

Patients with hypochondriasis have a strong fear or belief that they have a serious, often fatal, disease that persists despite appropriate medical reassurance. They are typically anxious and seek many medical opinions and investigations in futile but repeated attempts to relieve their fears. CBT may be helpful. The condition may become chronic.

In a small proportion of cases, the conviction that disease is present reaches delusional intensity, the best-known example being that of parasitic infestation ('delusional parasitosis'), which leads patients to consult dermatologists. Antipsychotic medication may be effective.

Body dysmorphic disorder

This describes a preoccupation with bodily shape or appearance, with the belief that one is disfigured in some way (previously known as dysmorphophobia). People with this condition may make inappropriate requests for cosmetic surgery. CBT may be helpful. The belief in disfigurement may sometimes be delusional, in which case antipsychotic drugs may help.

Somatoform autonomic dysfunction

This describes somatic symptoms referable to bodily organs which are largely under the control of the autonomic nervous system. The most common examples involve the cardiovascular system (cardiac neurosis), respiratory system (psychogenic hyperventilation) and gut (psychogenic vomiting and irritable bowel syndrome). Antidepressant drugs and CBT may be helpful.

Somatoform pain disorder

This describes severe, persistent pain which cannot be explained by a medical condition. Antidepressant drugs (especially tricyclics and dual action drugs such as duloxetine and mirtazapine) are helpful, as are some of the anticonvulsant drugs, particularly carbamazepine and gabapentin. CBT and multidisciplinary pain management teams are also useful.

Chronic fatigue syndrome

Neurasthenia is characterised by excessive fatigue after minimal physical or mental exertion, poor concentration, dizziness, muscular aches and sleep disturbance. This pattern of symptoms may follow a viral infection such as infectious mononucleosis, influenza or hepatitis. Symptoms overlap considerably with those of depression and anxiety. There is evidence that many patients improve with carefully graded exercise and with CBT.

Dissociative (conversion) disorder

This has replaced the term 'hysteria' in the ICD-10 classification. It is characterised by a loss or distortion of neurological function not fully explained by organic disease. The most common symptoms mimic lesions in the motor or sensory nervous system (Box 10.35). Dissociative disorder can also involve psychological functions, especially memory and general intelligence. The aetiology of dissociation is unknown. It has been considered to be the result of unconscious psychological processes and there is an association with adverse childhood experiences, including physical and sexual abuse. Organic disease may facilitate dissociative mechanisms and provide a model for symptoms; thus, for example, non-epileptic seizures may occur in those with epilepsy. Coexisting depression should be treated with CBT or antidepressant drugs.

10.35 Common presentations of dissociative (conversion) disorder

- Gait disturbance
- Loss of function in limbs
- Aphonia
- Non-epileptic seizures
- Sensory loss
- Blindness

General management of patients with medically unexplained symptoms

Management of the various syndromes of medically unexplained complaints described above is based on general principles (Box 10.36) and specific measures for individual syndromes.

Reassurance

Patients should be asked what they are most worried about. Clearly, it may be unwise to state categorically

10.36 General management principles for medically unexplained symptoms

- Take a full, sympathetic history
- Exclude disease but avoid unnecessary investigation or referral
- Seek specific treatable psychiatric syndromes
- Demonstrate to patients that you believe their complaints
- Establish a collaborative relationship
- Give the patient a positive explanation including but not over-emphasising psychological factors
- Encourage a return to normal functioning

that the patient has no disease but it can be emphasised that the probability of having disease is low. If patients repeatedly ask for reassurance about the same issue, they may have hypochondriasis.

Explanation

Patients need a positive explanation for their symptoms. It is unhelpful to say that symptoms are psychological or 'all in the mind', but useful to describe a plausible physiological mechanism for the symptom that emphasises the link with psychological factors such as stress and which demonstrates that the symptoms are reversible. For example, in irritable bowel syndrome, psychological stress results in increased activation of the autonomic nervous system which leads to constriction of smooth muscle in the gut wall, which in turn causes pain.

Advice

This should focus on how to overcome probable perpetuating factors: for example, by resolving stressful social problems or by practising relaxation. The doctor can offer to review progress, to prescribe (for example) an antidepressant drug and, if appropriate, to refer for physiotherapy or psychological treatments. The attitudes of relatives may need to be addressed if they have adopted an over-protective role, unwittingly reinforcing the patient's disability.

Drug treatment

Antidepressant drugs are often helpful, even if the patient is not depressed (Box 10.37).

Psychological treatment

There is moderate evidence for the effectiveness of CBT (Box 10.38). Other psychological treatments may also have a role.

EBM 10.37 Antidepressants for medically unexplained somatic symptoms

'There is evidence for the efficacy of antidepressant drugs for patients with medically unexplained symptoms.'

- Sumathipala A. Psychosom Med 2007; 69:889–900.

EBM 10.38 CBT for medically unexplained somatic symptoms

'CBT is the best established treatment for a variety of somatoform disorders.'

- Kroenke K. Psychosom Med 2007; 69:881–888.

10

Rehabilitation

Where there is chronic disability, particularly in dissociative disorder, conventional physical rehabilitation may be the best approach.

Shared care with the GP

Ongoing planned care is required for patients with chronic intractable symptoms, especially somatisation disorder. Review by the same specialist, interspersed with visits to the GP, is probably the best way to avoid unnecessary re-referral for investigation, to ensure that treatable aspects of the patient's problems such as depression are actively managed, and also to prevent the GP from becoming demoralised by feelings of helplessness.

Factitious disorders and malingering

It is important to distinguish somatoform disorders from factitious disorder and malingering.

Factitious disorder

This describes the repeated and deliberate production of the signs or symptoms of disease, apparently to obtain medical care. It is uncommon and typically presents in young women who work in paramedical professions. Examples include the dipping of thermometers into hot drinks to fake a fever, or patients with diabetes who deliberately induce hypo- and hyperglycaemic episodes. The factitious disorder is usually medical but may relate to a psychiatric illness, with reports of hallucinations or depressive illness.

Münchausen's syndrome

This refers to a severe chronic form of factitious disorder. Patients are usually older and male, with a solitary, peripatetic lifestyle in which they travel widely, sometimes visiting several hospitals in one day. Although the condition is rare, such patients are memorable because they present so frequently and so dramatically. The history can be convincing enough to persuade doctors to undertake investigations or initiate treatment, including exploratory surgery. It may be possible to trace the patient's history and show that he has presented similarly elsewhere, often changing name several times. Some emergency departments hold lists of such patients.

Management is by gentle but firm confrontation with clear evidence of the fabrication of illness, together with an offer of psychological support. Treatment is usually declined but recognition of the condition may help to avoid further iatrogenic harm.

Malingering

Malingering is a description of a behaviour, not a psychiatric diagnosis. It refers to the conscious simulation of signs of disease and disability. Patients have motives which are clear to them but which they conceal from doctors. Examples include the avoidance of burdensome responsibilities (such as work or court appearances) or the pursuit of financial gain (fraudulent claims for benefits or compensation). Malingering can be hard to detect at clinical assessment, but is suggested by evasion or inconsistency in the history.

Puerperal disorders

There are three common psychiatric complications of childbirth. When managing these conditions, it is important always to consider both the mother and the baby, and their relationship (Box 10.39).

Post-partum blues

These are characterised by irritability, labile mood and tearfulness. Most women are affected to some degree. Symptoms begin soon after childbirth, peak on about the fourth day and then resolve. They may be related to hormonal or psychological changes associated with childbirth. No treatment is required, other than to reassure the mother.

Post-partum depression

This occurs in 10–15% of women and within a month of delivery. Women with a previous history of depression are at risk. Explanation and reassurance are important. The usual psychological and drug treatments for depression should be considered, as well as practical help with childcare. If hospital admission is required, it should ideally be to a mother and baby unit. Further episodes of depression, both after childbirth and in response to other stressors, are likely.

Puerperal psychosis

This has its onset in the first 2 weeks after childbirth. It is a rare but serious complication affecting about 1 in 500 women and usually takes the form of a manic or depressive psychosis, although a schizophrenic psychosis can also occur. Delirium is rare with modern obstetric management but should still be considered in the differential diagnosis. Management depends on the type of psychosis that presents. In addition, it is important to consider the baby, and especially so to establish whether the mother has ideas of harming it. If so, the risk to the baby must be assessed and, if necessary, the baby temporarily removed. Most women recover but are at an increased (25%) risk of puerperal psychosis with the next pregnancy, and a 50% lifetime risk. Admission to a psychiatric mother and baby unit may be required.

 10.39 Psychiatric illness and pregnancy

- Always consider the effects of psychiatric disorder and treatment on mother, fetus and neonate
- Lithium, carbamazepine and valproate are significant teratogens, so minimise their use
- Most cases of post-partum low mood ('blues') are transient
- However, persistent low mood may indicate depressive illness
- Puerperal psychosis usually requires psychiatric admission

PSYCHIATRY AND THE LAW

Medicine takes place in a legal framework, made up of legislation (statute law) drafted by parliament or other governing bodies, and common law (case law) built up from court judgements over time. Psychiatry differs from other branches of medicine in that patients can be subject to legislative requirements to remain in hospital or to undergo treatments they refuse, such as the administration of antipsychotic drugs to a patient with acute schizophrenia who lacks insight, and whose symptoms and/or behaviour pose a risk to himself/herself or to others.

The UK has three different Mental Health Acts, covering England and Wales, Scotland, and Northern Ireland, and all of these have recently been revised. Other countries may have very different provisions. It is important for practitioners to be familiar with the relevant provisions that apply in their jurisdictions, and are likely to arise in the clinical settings in which they work.

Scotland has an Incapacity Act, with detailed provisions covering medical treatments for patients incapable of consenting, whether this incapacity arises from physical or mental illness. Similar legislation is being introduced elsewhere in the UK. In general, the guiding principle in British law is that people should be free to make their own decisions about medical treatment, except where their ability to decide is impaired by mental illness or physical incapacity, and where there are clear risks to the health and safety of themselves or others. Any restrictions or compulsions applied should be the minimum necessary, and they should only be applied for as long as is necessary; there should also be provisions for appeals and oversight.

Further information

Books and journal articles

Abramowitz JS, Taylor S, McKay D. Obsessive–compulsive disorder. Lancet 2009; 374 (9688):491–499.

Belmaker RH. Bipolar disorder. N Engl J Med 2004; 351(5):476–486.

Brown TM, Boyle MF. Delirium. BMJ 2002; 325(7365):644–647.

Harrison P, Geddes J, Sharpe M. Lecture notes on psychiatry. 9th edn. Oxford: Blackwell Science; 2005.

Hatcher S, Arroll B. Assessment and management of medically unexplained symptoms. BMJ 2008; 336(7653):1124–1128.

Henningsen P, Zipfel S, Herzog W. Management of functional somatic syndromes. Lancet 2007; 369(9565):946–955.

Johnstone EC, Owens DGC, Lawrie SM, et al (eds). Companion to psychiatric studies. 8th edn. Edinburgh: Churchill Livingstone; 2009.

Katon WJ. Clinical practice. Panic disorder. N Engl J Med 2006; 354(22):2360–2367.

Levenson JL (ed). American Psychiatric Publishing textbook of psychosomatic medicine. Washington DC: American Psychiatric Publishing; 2005.

Mann JJ. The medical management of depression. N Engl J Med 2005; 353(17): 1819–1834.

Mayou R, Sharpe M, Carson A (eds). ABC of psychological medicine. London: BMJ Books; 2003.

Moussavi S, Chatterji S, Verdes E, et al. Depression, chronic diseases, and decrements in health: results from the World Health Surveys. Lancet 2007; 370(9590):851–858.

Mueser KT, McGurk SR. Schizophrenia. Lancet 2004; 363(9426):2063–2072.

Room R, Babor T, Rehm J. Alcohol and public health. Lancet 2005; 365(9458):519–530.

Tyrer P, Baldwin D. Generalised anxiety disorder. Lancet 2006; 368(9553):2156–2166.

Websites

http://cebmh.warne.ox.ac.uk/cebmh/ *Website of the Centre for Evidence-based Mental Health.*

www.depressionalliance.org *Information on depression.*

www.mja.com.au/public/mentalhealth/articles/singh/sinbox5.html/ *Managing chronic somatisation disorder.*

www.niaaa.nih.gov/ *Information on alcoholism.*

www.nimh.nih.gov/practitioners/ *General information on depression, anxiety etc.*

www.nimh.nih.gov/health/topics/schizophrenia.htm *Information on schizophrenia.*

www.rcpsych.ac.uk/info/index.htm *Royal College of Psychiatrists: mental health information.*

www.who.int/mental_health/ *WHO website on mental health and brain disorders.*

10

G.G. Dark
A.R. Abdul Razak

Oncology

11

CLINICAL EXAMINATION OF THE CANCER PATIENT

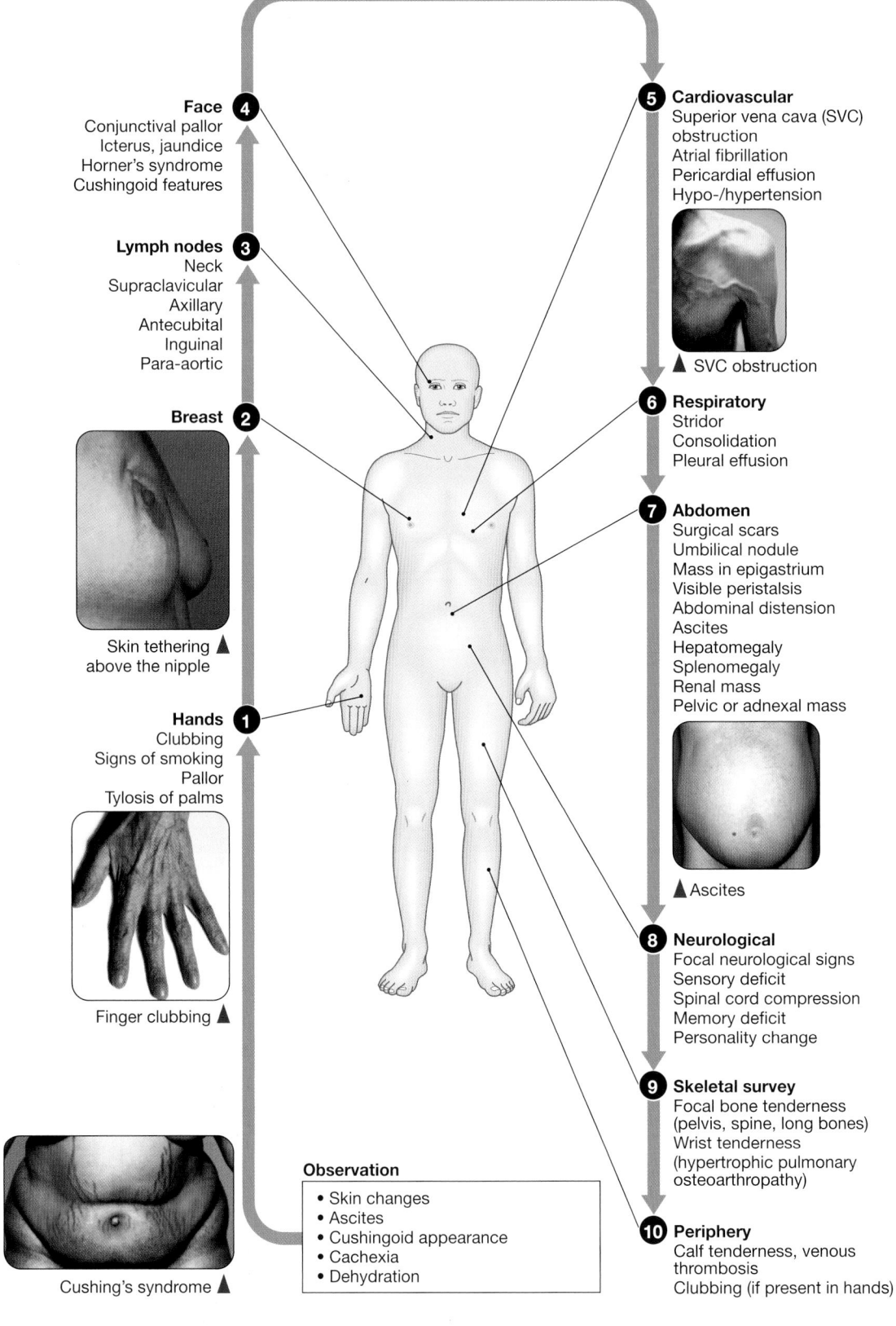

Face 4
Conjunctival pallor
Icterus, jaundice
Horner's syndrome
Cushingoid features

Lymph nodes 3
Neck
Supraclavicular
Axillary
Antecubital
Inguinal
Para-aortic

Breast 2

Skin tethering ▲
above the nipple

Hands 1
Clubbing
Signs of smoking
Pallor
Tylosis of palms

Finger clubbing ▲

Cushing's syndrome ▲

Observation
• Skin changes
• Ascites
• Cushingoid appearance
• Cachexia
• Dehydration

5 **Cardiovascular**
Superior vena cava (SVC)
obstruction
Atrial fibrillation
Pericardial effusion
Hypo-/hypertension

▲ SVC obstruction

6 **Respiratory**
Stridor
Consolidation
Pleural effusion

7 **Abdomen**
Surgical scars
Umbilical nodule
Mass in epigastrium
Visible peristalsis
Abdominal distension
Ascites
Hepatomegaly
Splenomegaly
Renal mass
Pelvic or adnexal mass

▲ Ascites

8 **Neurological**
Focal neurological signs
Sensory deficit
Spinal cord compression
Memory deficit
Personality change

9 **Skeletal survey**
Focal bone tenderness
(pelvis, spine, long bones)
Wrist tenderness
(hypertrophic pulmonary
osteoarthropathy)

10 **Periphery**
Calf tenderness, venous
thrombosis
Clubbing (if present in hands)

Examination of the skin

Important features of skin lesions that should alert suspicion include:
- Asymmetry: irregular shape
- Bleeding
- Border: not a smooth edge
- Colour: uneven, variegated or changing colour
- Diameter: > 6 mm in diameter or growing
- Itching or pain in a pre-existing mole

❼ Abdominal examination
- Are there scars from previous surgery?
- Is the umbilicus everted, suggesting ascites?
- Is there a firm nodule at the umbilicus due to ovarian cancer metastasis, causing a Sister Mary Joseph's nodule?
- Is there smooth hepatomegaly—possibly primary liver cancer or heart failure?
- Is the liver firm or knobbly, suggesting metastasis?
- Is the ascites too tense to demonstrate hepatomegaly?
- Are other masses palpable in the abdomen?
- Are there signs of obstruction or paralytic ileus with absence of bowel sounds?
- Palpate for inguinal nodes (occasionally involved in ovarian cancer)
- Percuss for flank dullness and shifting dullness
- Perform vaginal and rectal examinations to detect adnexal or rectal masses

❸ Examination of the lymph nodes

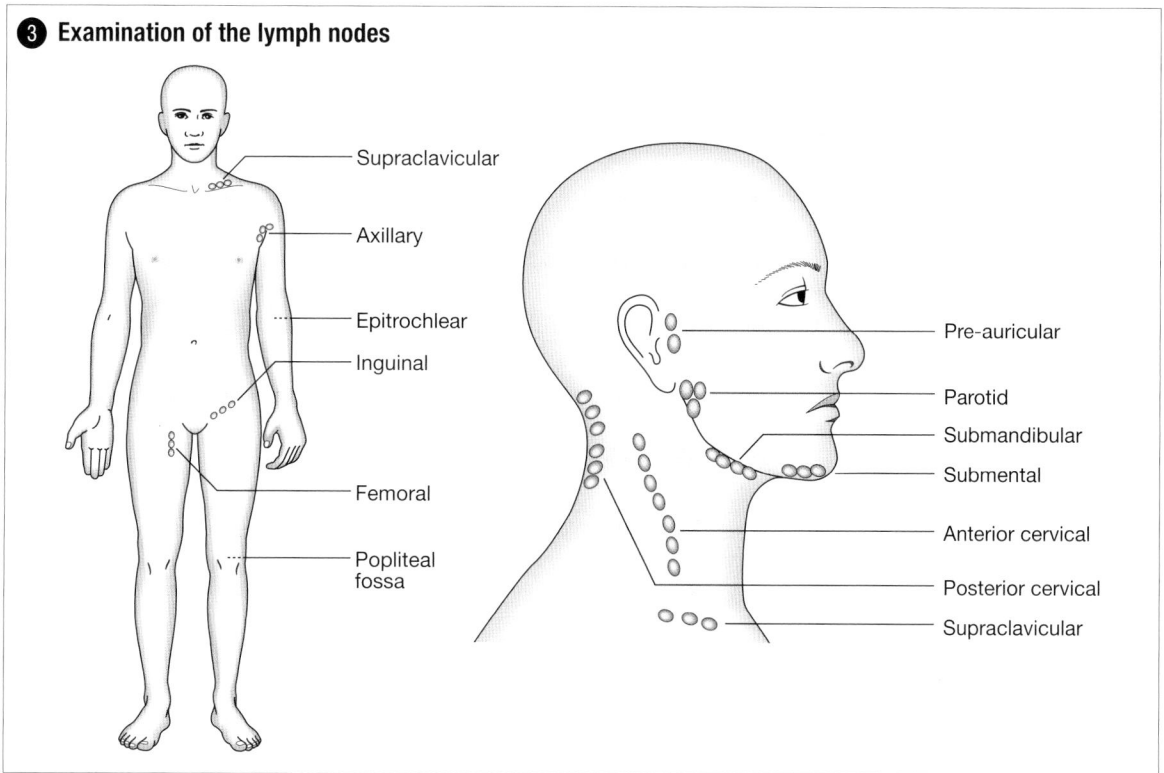

Supraclavicular

Axillary

Epitrochlear

Inguinal

Femoral

Popliteal fossa

Pre-auricular

Parotid

Submandibular

Submental

Anterior cervical

Posterior cervical

Supraclavicular

❻ Malignant pleural effusions

Large right pleural effusion

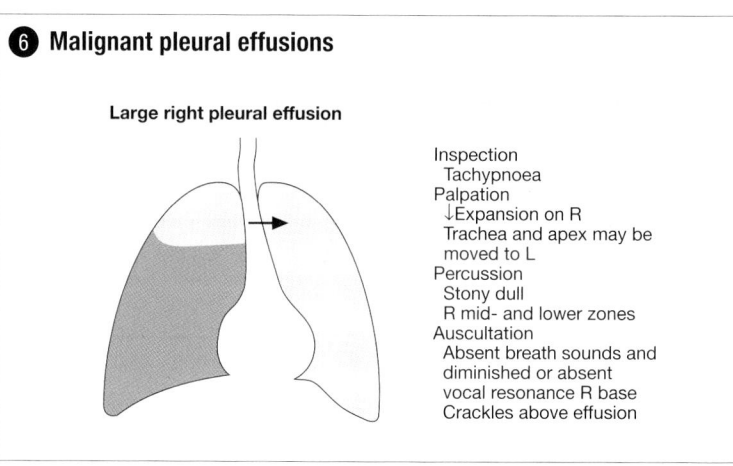

Inspection
  Tachypnoea
Palpation
  ↓Expansion on R
  Trachea and apex may be moved to L
Percussion
  Stony dull
  R mid- and lower zones
Auscultation
  Absent breath sounds and diminished or absent vocal resonance R base
  Crackles above effusion

❺ SVC obstruction
- Venous distension of neck
- Elevated but non-pulsatile JVP
- Venous distension of chest wall
- Facial oedema
- Cyanosis
- Plethora of face
- Oedema of arms

❺ Pericardial effusion
- Tachycardia
- Falling BP
- Rising JVP
- Muffled heart sounds
- Kussmaul's sign

Cancer is a significant global health-care problem, with an estimated world-wide incidence of 10 million new cases per year, 46% of which are in developed countries. Mortality is high, with more than 7 million deaths per year. The global costs and socioeconomic impact are considerable. The most common solid organ malignancies arise in the lung, breast and gastrointestinal tract (Fig. 11.1), but the most common form world-wide is skin cancer. Tobacco is a major factor in the aetiology of 30% of cancers, including those of the lung, nasopharynx, bladder and kidney, and these could be prevented by smoking cessation. Diet and alcohol contribute to a further 30% of cancers, including those of the stomach, colon, oesophagus, breast and liver. Lifestyle modification could reduce these if steps were taken to avoid animal fat and red meat, reduce alcohol, increase fibre, fresh fruit and vegetable intake, and avoid obesity. Infections account for a further 15% of cancers, including those of the cervix, stomach, liver, nasopharynx and bladder, and some of these could be prevented by infection control and vaccination.

FUNCTIONAL ANATOMY AND PATHOPHYSIOLOGY

Cancer cells possess unique characteristics, in that their proliferation is unregulated and in that they have the capacity to invade surrounding tissues and penetrate the walls of blood vessels and lymphatics to spread to other sites. Oncogenesis is a multistage process which often begins with a somatic mutation in a single cell, resulting in a growth advantage (Fig. 11.2).

Subsequently, further mutations occur, selecting a subset of cells for more rapid growth which is mediated by increased growth factor production, constitutive activation of signalling pathways that stimulate cell division, and failure of apoptosis. Angiogenic factors are then produced which provide the growing tumour with a blood supply, and other factors are expressed that break down connective tissues and disturb cell adhesion, resulting in distant spread and the development of metastases. Important factors in the pathophysiology of cancer are discussed in detail below.

The cell cycle

Proliferation of both normal cells and cancer cells is dependent on progression of the cell cycle, which consists of four phases (Fig. 11.3). Briefly, there are two functional (S phase and M phase) and two preparatory phases (G_1 phase and G_2 phase). In the S phase, DNA replication occurs, doubling the number of chromosomes and producing sister chromatids. In the M phase, the nucleus divides and the chromosomes separate into two daughter cells during the process of mitosis. The G_1 phase precedes the S phase, while the G_2 phase precedes the M phase; their function is primarily synthesis of the materials needed for the subsequent phase. Following division, some cells enter a phase called G_0, in which differentiated functions are carried out.

The cell cycle is regulated by two families of molecules known as cyclins and cyclin-dependant kinases (CDKs). Cyclins bind to CDKs, which regulate target proteins required for entry into the next phase of the cell cycle. Multiple checkpoints monitor and regulate the progress of the cell cycle. These checkpoints prevent the cell cycle

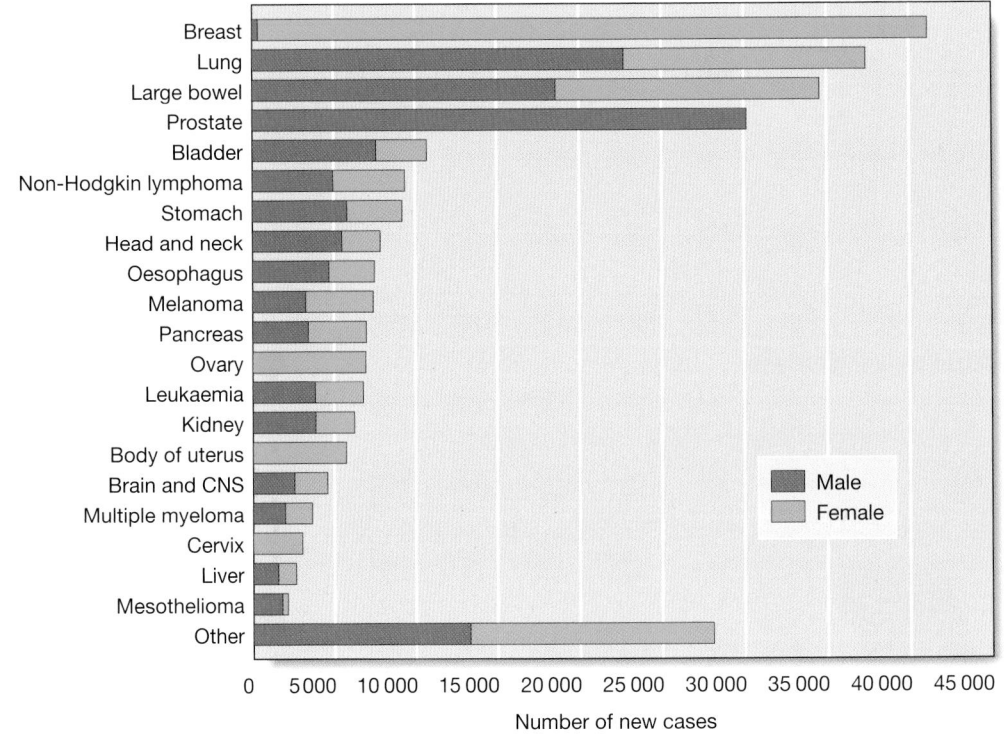

Fig. 11.1 The 20 most commonly diagnosed cancers in the UK.

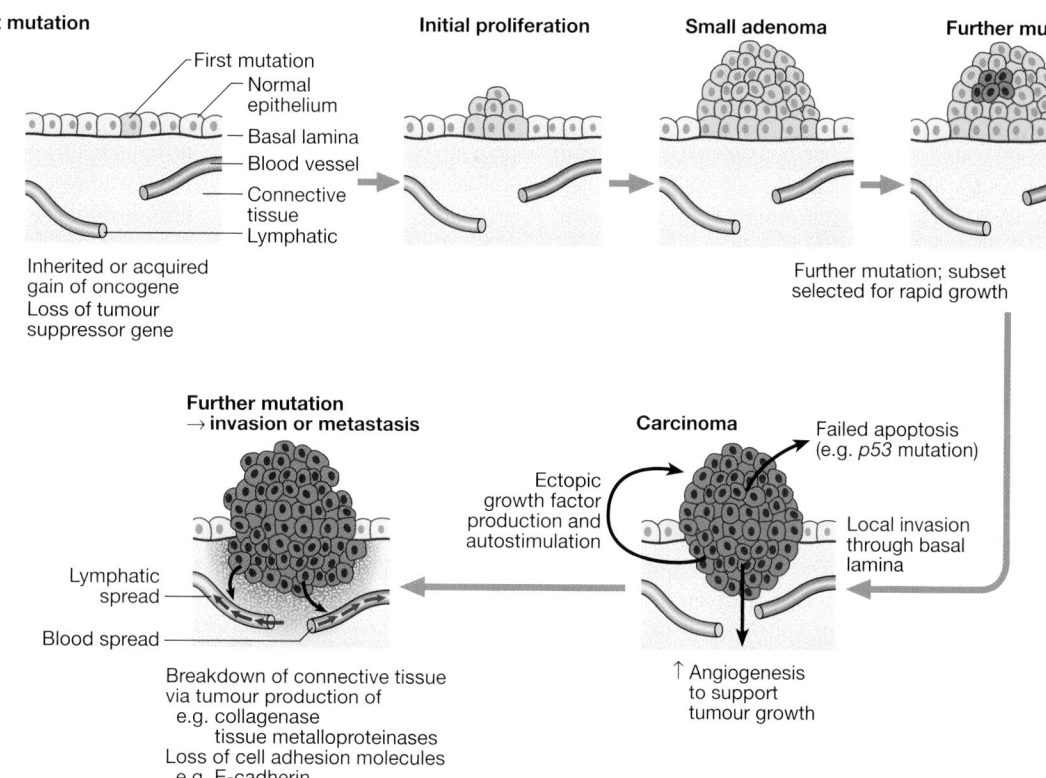

First mutation

First mutation
Normal epithelium
Basal lamina
Blood vessel
Connective tissue
Lymphatic

Inherited or acquired gain of oncogene
Loss of tumour suppressor gene

Initial proliferation

Small adenoma

Further mutation

Further mutation; subset selected for rapid growth

Further mutation → invasion or metastasis

Lymphatic spread
Blood spread

Breakdown of connective tissue via tumour production of
e.g. collagenase
tissue metalloproteinases
Loss of cell adhesion molecules
e.g. E-cadherin

Carcinoma

Ectopic growth factor production and autostimulation

Failed apoptosis (e.g. *p53* mutation)

Local invasion through basal lamina

↑ Angiogenesis to support tumour growth

Fig. 11.2 Oncogenesis. The multistep origin of cancer, showing events implicated in cancer initiation, progression, invasion and metastasis.

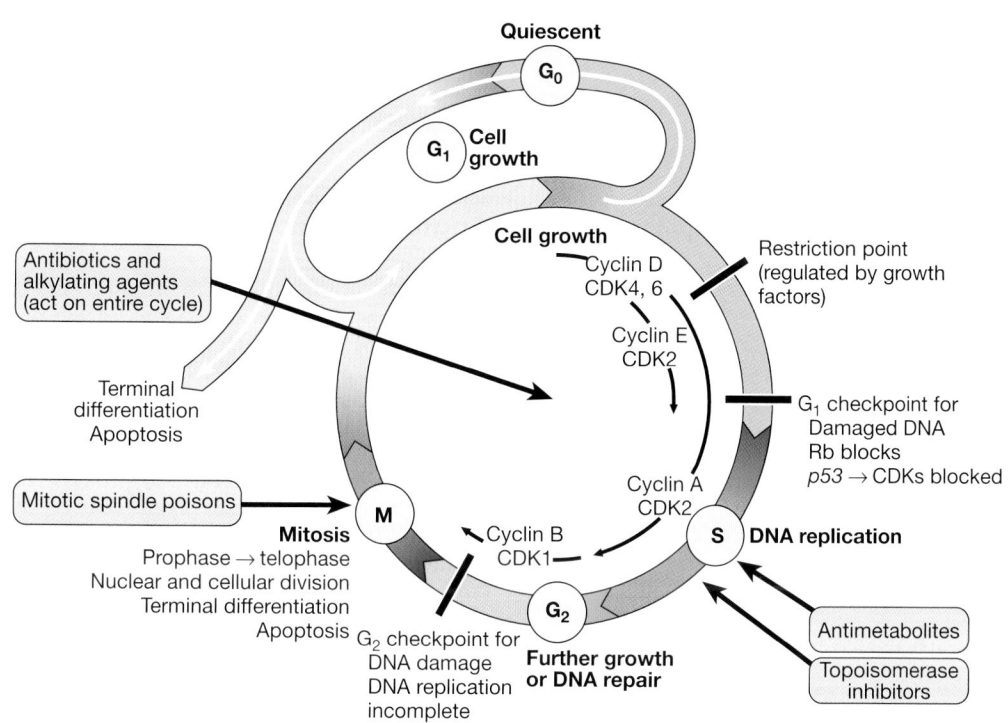

Quiescent

G₀

G₁ Cell growth

Cell growth
Cyclin D
CDK4, 6

Cyclin E
CDK2

Antibiotics and alkylating agents (act on entire cycle)

Restriction point (regulated by growth factors)

G₁ checkpoint for Damaged DNA
Rb blocks
p53 → CDKs blocked

Terminal differentiation Apoptosis

Mitotic spindle poisons

M

Mitosis
Prophase → telophase
Nuclear and cellular division
Terminal differentiation
Apoptosis

Cyclin B
CDK1

G₂

G₂ checkpoint for DNA damage
DNA replication incomplete

Further growth or DNA repair

Cyclin A
CDK2

S DNA replication

Antimetabolites

Topoisomerase inhibitors

Fig. 11.3 The cell cycle and sites of action of chemotherapeutic agents. (Rb = retinoblastoma gene; CDK = cyclin-dependent kinase)

259

from progressing if certain requirements have not been met, allowing verification of the necessary phase processes and repair of defective DNA products. Two main checkpoints exist: namely, the G_1/S checkpoint and the G_2/M checkpoint. The cell cycle is also regulated by genes which prevent its progression, such as *p53*, *p21* and *p16*. These play an important part in tumour prevention, and are known as tumour suppressor genes. They halt the cell cycle by binding to and deactivating cyclin–CDK complexes. Dysregulation of any part of the cell cycle may be associated with increased susceptibility to cancer.

An understanding of the cell cycle has been used to develop chemotherapeutic agents. Actively replicating cells are targeted in cancer therapy, as the DNA during cell division is susceptible to damage or radiation. Examples of chemotherapeutic agents include antimetabolites such as azathioprine and methotrexate, which prevent purines and pyrimidines from becoming incorporated into DNA during the S phase of the cell cycle, thereby arresting cell division. The mitotic spindle poisons vinblastine and vincristine inhibit assembly of tubulin into microtubules, hence disrupting the M phase of the cell cycle. Other anticancer drugs, such as antibiotics and alkylating agents, affect cell division by a variety of mechanisms. The effects of cytotoxic drugs on the cell cycle are depicted in Figure 11.3.

Regulation of cancer cell growth

Abnormal regulation of cell growth in cancer can occur as the result of several mechanisms.

Activation of cell growth

Many cancer cells produce growth factors which drive their own proliferation by a positive feedback loop, a process known as autocrine stimulation. Examples include tumour growth factor-alpha (TGF-α) and platelet-derived growth factor (PDGF) production by hepatocellular cancer and non-small cell lung cancer respectively. Other cancer cells express growth factor receptors at increased levels due to gene amplification, or express abnormal receptors that are permanently activated. This results in abnormal cell growth in response to physiological growth factor stimulation or even in the absence of growth factor stimulation (ligand independent signalling). The epidermal growth factor receptor (EGFR) is often over-expressed in lung and gastrointestinal tumours and the Her2/neu receptor is frequently over-expressed in breast cancer. Both receptors activate the Ras–Raf–MAP kinase pathway which stimulates cell growth. Understanding these effects has been important in the development of novel therapies targeted to these receptors (p. 274). An example of ligand independent signalling occurs in the case of Ras mutations, which are present in about 30% of all cancers and cause constitutive activation of MAP kinase signalling, leading to abnormal cell growth.

Inhibition of tumour suppressor genes

In the normal cell, several proteins inhibit cell growth; these may be inactivated by loss of function mutations or their levels reduced by diverse mechanisms. The retinoblastoma protein (Rb) is an example. This protein sequesters transcription factors essential for cell cycle progression and inhibits cell growth. One mechanism via which Rb function is disrupted in cancer is inactivating mutations in Rb protein, as occur in retinoblastoma. Another is abnormal regulation of the Rb pathway by growth factors. For example, transforming growth factor-β (TGF-β) normally regulates Rb function by producing proteins that block its phosphorylation, causing growth inhibition. Loss of TGF-β responsiveness, downregulation of TGF-β receptors and dysfunctional receptors occur in some types of cancer, leading to disruption of the Rb signalling circuit and rendering cancer cells insensitive to growth inhibition.

Avoidance of apoptosis

Evasion of apoptosis is a common finding in cancer; it can occur through altered activity or loss of function of molecules that take part in the apoptotic process. The molecules involved are numerous and have complex interactions, but the Bcl-2 family plays a critical role. Some members of the Bcl-2 family (Bcl-2, Bcl-X_L) are anti-apoptotic, while others (Bax, Bak) are pro-apoptotic. In some cancer cells, reduced levels of apoptosis are associated with increased levels of Bcl-2/Bcl-X_L or decreased levels of Bax/Bak. Another molecule that plays a key role in apoptosis is PTEN. The PTEN molecule is a phosphatase which dephosphorylates Akt (pAkt), a molecule which stimulates cell growth. PTEN also affects the function of the tumour suppressor gene *p53*, by sequestrating an inhibitory molecule called Mdm-2, allowing *p53* to promote apoptosis of cells with damaged DNA. Inactivating mutations of PTEN have been found in a number of different tumours. They cause activation of pAkt and inhibition of the *p53* pathway, which stimulates cell growth and inhibits apoptosis.

Maintenance of telomeres

When normal cells replicate, there is progressive shortening of the telomeres; eventually, this prevents the cell from dividing further. Cancer cells can replicate an infinite number of times and this is associated with maintenance of telomere length. There are several mechanisms by which this occurs, the best established being up-regulation of the telomerase enzyme, which adds nucleotides to the telomeres and allows cell division to continue.

Angiogenesis

Malignant tumours need to acquire a network of blood vessels for continued growth. This process is known as angiogenesis and is dependent on the production of angiogenic growth factors by the tumour. There are more than 15 angiogenic molecules, the best characterised being vascular endothelial growth factor (VEGF) and PDGF. Both play a central role in producing neovascularisation for the tumour cells and metastasis. The requirement for tumours to promote angiogenesis has been exploited therapeutically in the development of agents that target angiogenic molecules or their receptors. Examples include bevacizumab (an antibody against VEGF) and sunitinib (a small-molecule inhibitor of the PDGF and VEGF receptors). Bevacizumab has been shown to improve survival in metastatic colon, breast and lung cancer, while sunitinib has been shown to be useful in the treatment of renal cell cancer and second-line treatment of gastrointestinal stromal tumour (GIST).

Immune surveillance

The immune system is thought to protect against cancer via a continuous surveillance programme which eliminates cells that have undergone malignant transformation. One of the hallmarks of cancer development is escape from immune surveillance. Tumour cells constantly shed surface antigens into the circulation. Although this would normally evoke a response from the immune system, including the recruitment of cytotoxic T cells, natural killer cells and macrophages, it is thought that tumours escape from immune control for one of three reasons:

- failure of antigen recognition by immune cells
- tumour escape from the activity of cytotoxic lymphocytes
- tumour-induced immune dysfunction.

It has been speculated that the increased risk of some cancers in patients receiving anti-TNF therapy for inflammatory diseases (p. 1092) may be due to impairment of immune surveillance.

Invasion and metastasis

The ability of cancer cells to transgress normal tissue boundaries and to spread to other sites is an important process in cancer progression. Cells are attached to one another and to the extracellular matrix (ECM) by cell adhesion molecules (CAM) such as cadherins and integrins. Cell–cell and cell–matrix interactions are critical for the survival of normal cells. In cancer cells, CAMs are absent or dysfunctional, allowing the cell to detach from the primary site and to replicate, despite not being anchored to another cell or to the ECM (anchorage-independent growth). Cancer cells are also able to penetrate the basement membrane by producing enzymes called matrix metalloproteinases (MMP). The MMP degrade the basement membrane, allowing cancer cells to penetrate blood vessels at the primary site and to develop in new sites.

Anatomical spread of tumours

Tumours can spread both by local invasion and by migration to distant sites. The process of staging determines the extent of the tumour; it entails clinical examination and imaging to establish possible sites or extent of disease involvement. The outcome is recorded using a standard staging system which allows comparisons to be made between different groups of patients. Therapeutic decisions and prognostic predictions can then be made using the evidence base for the disease. One of the most commonly used systems is the T (tumour), N (regional lymph nodes), M (metastatic sites) approach of the International Union against Cancer (UICC, Box 11.1). For some tumours, such as colon cancer, the Dukes system (p. 912) is used rather than the UICC classification.

ENVIRONMENTAL AND GENETIC DETERMINANTS OF CANCER

The majority of cancers do not have a single cause but rather are the result of a complex interaction between genetic factors and exposure to environmental carcinogens. These are often tumour type-specific but some general principles do apply.

11.1 TNM classification

Extent of primary tumour*

TX	Not assessed
T0	Excised tumour
T1 T2 T3	Increases in primary tumour size or depth of invasion

Increased involvement of nodes*

NX	Not assessed
N0	No nodal involvement
N1 N2/3	Increases in involvement

Presence of metastases

MX	Not assessed
M0	Not present
M1	Present

*Exact criteria for size and region of nodal involvement have been defined for each anatomical site.

Environmental factors

Environmental triggers for cancer have mainly been identified through epidemiological studies which examine patterns of distribution of cancers in patients in whom age, sex, presence of other illnesses, social class, geography and so on differ. Sometimes these give strong pointers to the molecular or cellular causes of the disease, such as the association between aflatoxin production within contaminated food supplies and hepatocellular carcinomas. However, for many solid cancers such as breast and colorectal, there is evidence of a multifactorial pathogenesis, even when there is a principal environmental cause (Box 11.2).

Smoking is now established beyond all doubt as a major cause of lung cancer, but there are obviously additional predisposing factors since not all smokers develop cancer. Similarly, most carcinomas of the cervix are related to infection with human papillomavirus (HPV subtype 16 and 18). For carcinomas of the bowel and breast, there is strong evidence of an environmental component. For example, the risk of breast cancer in women of Far Eastern origin remains relatively low when they first migrate to a country with a Western lifestyle, but rises in subsequent generations approach that of the resident population of the host country. The precise environmental factor that causes this change is unclear, but may include diet (higher intake of saturated fat and/or dairy products), reproductive patterns (later onset of first pregnancy) and lifestyle (increased use of artificial light and shift in diurnal rhythm).

Genetic factors

A number of inherited cancer syndromes are recognised which account for 5–10% of all cancers (Box 11.3). The molecular basis of these is discussed in Chapter 3, but in general they occur as the result of inherited mutations in genes which regulate cell growth, cell death and apoptosis. Examples include the *BRCA1*, *BRCA2* and *AT* (ataxia telangiectasia) genes which cause breast cancer and some other cancers, the *FAP* gene which causes bowel cancer,

11.2 Environmental factors that predispose to cancer

Environmental aetiology	Processes	Diseases
Occupational exposure (see also ultraviolet and radiation)	Dye and rubber manufacturing (aromatic amines)	Bladder cancer
	Asbestos mining, construction work, shipbuilding (asbestos)	Lung cancer and mesothelioma
	Vinyl chloride (PVC) manufacturing	Liver angiosarcoma
	Petroleum industry (benzene)	Acute leukaemia
Chemicals	Chemotherapy (e.g. melphalan, cyclophosphamide)	Acute myeloid leukaemia
Cigarette smoking	Exposure to carcinogens from inhaled smoke	Lung and bladder cancer
Viral infection	Epstein–Barr virus	Burkitt's lymphoma and nasopharyngeal cancer
	Human papillomavirus	Cervical cancer
Bacterial infection	*Helicobacter pylori*	Gastric mucosa-associated lymphoid tissue (MALT) lymphomas, gastric cancer
Parasitic infection	Liver fluke *(Opisthorchis sinensis)*	Cholangiocarcinoma
	Schistosoma haematobium	Squamous cell bladder cancer
Dietary factors	Low-roughage/high-fat content diet	Colonic cancer
	High nitrosamine intake	Gastric cancer
	Aflatoxin from contamination of *Aspergillus flavus*	Hepatocellular cancer
Radiation	Ultraviolet (UV) exposure	Basal cell carcinoma
		Melanoma
		Non-melanocytic skin cancer
	Nuclear fallout following explosion (e.g. Hiroshima)	Leukaemia
		Solid tumours
	Diagnostic exposure (e.g. computed tomography (CT))	Cholangiocarcinoma following thorotrast usage
	Occupational exposure (e.g. beryllium and strontium mining)	Lung cancer
	Therapeutic radiotherapy	Medullary thyroid cancer
		Sarcoma
Inflammatory diseases	Ulcerative colitis	Colon cancer
Hormonal	Use of diethylstilboestrol	Vaginal cancer
	Oestrogens	Endometrial cancer
		Breast cancer

and the *Rb* gene which causes retinoblastoma. Although carriers of these gene mutations have a greatly elevated risk of cancer, none has 100% penetrance and additional modulating factors, both genetic and environmental, are likely to be operative. Exploration of a possible genetic contribution is a key part of cancer management, especially with regard to ascertaining the risk for an affected patient's offspring.

INVESTIGATIONS

When a patient is suspected of having cancer, a full history should be taken; specific questions should be included as to potential risk factors such as smoking and occupational exposures. A thorough clinical examination is also essential to identify sites of metastases, and to discover any other conditions that may have a bearing on the management plan. In order to make a diagnosis and to plan the most appropriate management, information is needed on:

• the type of tumour
• the extent of disease, as assessed by staging investigations
• the patient's general condition and any comorbidity.

The overall fitness of a patient is often assessed by the Eastern Cooperative Oncology Group (ECOG) performance scale (Box 11.4). The outcome for patients with a performance status of 3 or 4 is worse in almost all malignancies than for those with a status of 0–2, and this has a strong influence on the approach to treatment in the individual patient.

Histology

Histological analysis of a biopsy or resected specimen is pivotal in clinching the diagnosis and in deciding on the best form of management. The results of histological analysis are most informative when combined with knowledge of the clinical picture, and so biopsy results should ideally be reviewed within the context of a multidisciplinary meeting involving oncologists and pathologists.

Light microscopy

Examination of tumour samples by light microscopy remains the core method of cancer diagnosis and, in cases where the primary site is unclear, may also give clues to the origin of the tumour:

• Signet-ring cells favour a gastric primary.
• Presence of melanin favours melanoma.

11.3 Inherited cancer predisposition syndromes

Syndrome	Malignancies	Inheritance	Gene
Ataxia telangiectasia	Leukaemia, lymphoma, ovarian, gastric, brain, colon	AR	*AT*
Breast/ovarian	Breast, ovarian, colonic, prostatic, pancreatic	AD	*BRCA1, BRCA2*
Bloom syndrome	Leukaemia, tongue, oesophageal, colonic, Wilms' tumour	AR	*BLM*
Cowden syndrome	Breast, thyroid, gastrointestinal tract, pancreatic	AD	*PTEN*
Familial polyposis coli	Colonic, upper gastrointestinal tract	AD	*APC*
Fanconi anaemia	Leukaemia, oesophageal, skin, hepatoma	AR	*FACA, FACC, FACD*
Gorlin syndrome	Basal cell skin, brain	AD	*PTCH*
Hereditary non-polyposis colon cancer (HNPCC)	Colonic, endometrial, ovarian, pancreatic, gastric	AD	*MSH2, MLH1, PMS1, PMS2*
Li–Fraumeni syndrome	Sarcoma, breast, osteosarcoma, leukaemia, glioma, adrenocortical	AD	*p53*
Melanoma	Melanoma	AD	CDK2 (*p16*)
Multiple endocrine neoplasia (MEN)-1	Pancreatic islet cell, pituitary adenoma, parathyroid adenoma and hyperplasia	AD	*MEN1*
MEN-2	Medullary thyroid, phaeochromocytoma, parathyroid hyperplasia	AD	*RET*
Neurofibromatosis 1	Neurofibrosarcoma, phaeochromocytoma, optic glioma	AD	*NF1*
Neurofibromatosis 2	Vestibular schwannoma	AD	*NF2*
Papillary renal cell cancer syndrome	Renal cell cancer	AD	*MET*
Peutz–Jeghers syndrome	Colonic, ileal, breast, ovarian	AD	*STK11*
Prostate cancer	Prostate	AD	*HPC1*
Retinoblastoma	Retinoblastoma, osteosarcoma	AD	*RB1*
von Hippel–Lindau syndrome	Haemangioblastoma of retina and CNS, renal cell, phaeochromocytoma	AD	*VHL*
Wilms' tumour	Nephroblastoma, neuroblastoma, hepatoblastoma, rhabdomyosarcoma	AD	*WT1*
Xeroderma pigmentosa	Skin, leukaemia, melanoma	AR	*XPA, XPC, XPD (ERCC2), XPF*

(AD = autosomal dominant; AR = autosomal recessive)

11.4 Eastern Cooperative Oncology Group (ECOG) performance status scale

0	Fully active, able to carry on all usual activities without restriction and without the aid of analgesics
1	Restricted in strenuous activity but ambulatory and able to carry out light work or pursue a sedentary occupation. This group also contains patients who are fully active, as in grade 0, but only with the aid of analgesics
2	Ambulatory and capable of all self-care but unable to work. Up and about more than 50% of waking hours
3	Capable of only limited self-care, confined to bed or chair more than 50% of waking hours
4	Completely disabled, unable to carry out any self-care and confined totally to bed or chair

- Mucin is common in gut/lung/breast/endometrial cancers, but particularly common in ovarian cancer and rare in renal cell or thyroid cancers.
- Psammoma bodies are a feature of ovarian cancer (mucin +) and thyroid cancer (mucin −).

Immunohistochemistry

Immunohistochemical (IHC) staining for tumour markers can provide useful diagnostic information and can help with treatment decisions. Commonly used examples of IHC in clinical practice include:

- *Oestrogen (ER) and progesterone (PR) receptors.* Positive results indicate that the tumour may be sensitive to hormonal manipulation.
- *Alpha fetoprotein (AFP)* and *human chorionic gonadotrophin (HC) ± placental alkaline phosphatase (PLAP).* These favour germ-cell tumours.

- *Prostate-specific antigen (PSA)* and *prostatic acid phosphatase (PAP)*. These favour prostate cancer.
- *Carcinoembryonic antigen (CEA), cytokeratin* and *epithelial membrane antigen (EMA)*. These favour carcinomas.
- *HER2 receptor*. Breast cancers which have high levels of expression of HER2 indicate that the tumour may respond to trastuzumab (herceptin), an antibody directed against the HER2 receptor.

The pattern of immunoglobulin, T-cell receptor and cluster designation (CD) antigen expression on the surface is also helpful in the diagnosis and classification of lymphomas. This can be achieved by immunohistochemical staining of biopsy samples or flow cytometry.

Electron microscopy

Electron microscopy (EM) can sometimes be of diagnostic value. Examples include the visualisation of melanosomes in amelanotic melanoma and dense core granules in neuroendocrine tumours. EM may also help to distinguish adenocarcinoma from mesothelioma, as the ultrastructural properties of these two diseases are different (mesothelioma appears to have long, narrow, branching microvilli while adenocarcinomas appear to have short, stubby microvilli). EM is also useful for differentiating spindle-cell tumours (sarcomas, melanomas, squamous cell cancers) from small round-cell tumours, again due to their ultrastructural differences.

Cytogenetic analysis

Some tumours demonstrate typical chromosomal changes that help in diagnosis. The utilisation of fluorescent in-situ hybridisation (FISH) techniques can be useful in Ewing's sarcoma and peripheral neuroectodermal tumours where there is a translocation between chromosome 11 and 22—t(11; 22)(q24; q12). In some cases, gene amplification can also be detected via FISH (e.g. determining over-expression of Her2/neu).

Imaging

Imaging plays a critical role in oncology, not only in locating the primary tumour, but also in staging the disease. The imaging modality employed depends primarily on the site of the disease and the likely patterns of spread, but usually more than one modality is required.

Radiography

Plain radiographs remain part of the initial workup, but have a limited role in defining disease extent and have been superseded by more sophisticated techniques.

Ultrasound

Ultrasound is useful in characterising lesions within the liver, kidney, pancreas and reproductive organs. It is also used for guiding the placement of needles during biopsies of tumours in the breast and the liver. Endoscopic ultrasound is useful in staging upper gastrointestinal cancers; it involves using a special endoscope with an ultrasound probe attached.

Computerised tomography

Computerised tomography (CT) is a key investigation in cancer patients and is particularly useful in imaging the thorax and abdomen. With some modern CT scanners it is also possible to visualise the bowel, and in some instances, diagnosis of intestinal cancer is possible.

Magnetic resonance imaging

Magnetic resonance imaging (MRI) has a high resolution and because of this is the preferred technique for brain imaging. It is also used to image structures within the pelvis and is widely employed for staging of rectal, cervical and prostate cancers.

Positron emission tomography

Positron emission tomography (PET) visualises metabolic activity of tumour cells and is widely used, often in combination with CT (PET-CT), to evaluate patients with various cancers, including lung cancer and lymphoma (Fig. 11.4). It can accurately assess the severity and spread of cancer by detecting tumour metabolic activity following injection of small amounts of radioactive tracers such as fluorodeoxyglucose (FDG). In addition to having a role in diagnosis, PET can also be used in some patients to assess treatment response.

Biochemical markers

Many tumours produce substances called tumour markers which can be used in diagnosis and surveillance.

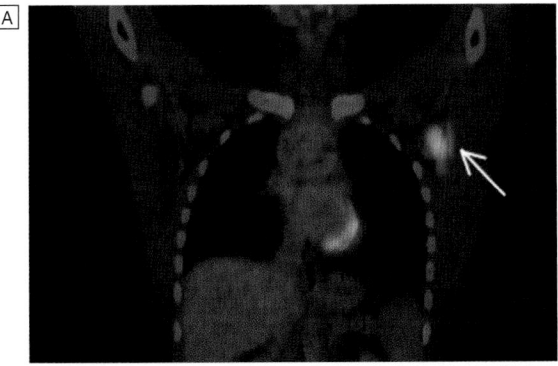
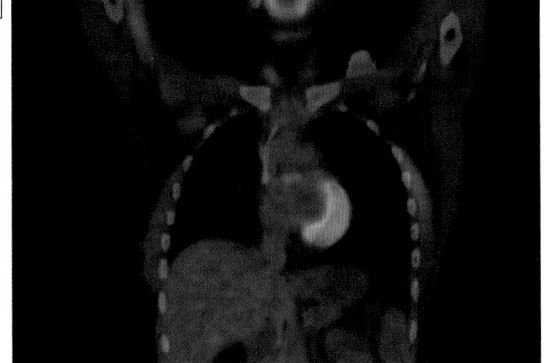

Fig. 11.4 PET-CT images. [A] There is a neoplastic lesion in the left axilla, evidenced by the increased uptake of FDG traces. [B] Imaging after chemotherapy, demonstrating that the abnormal uptake has disappeared and indicating a response to treatment.

11.5 Commonly used serum tumour markers

Name	Natural occurrence	Tumours
Alphafetoprotein (AFP)	Glycoprotein found in yolk sac and fetal liver tissue. Transient elevation in liver diseases. Has a role in screening during pregnancy for the detection of neural tube defects and Down's syndrome	Ovarian non-seminomatous germ cell tumours (80%), hepatocellular cancer (50%)
Calcitonin	32 amino acid peptide from C-cells of thyroid. Used to screen for MEN-2	Medullary cell carcinoma of thyroid
Cancer antigen 125 (CA-125)	Differentiation antigen of coelomic epithelium (Muller's duct). Raised in any cause of ascites, pleural effusion or heart failure. Can be raised in inflammatory conditions	Ovarian epithelial cancer (75%), gastrointestinal cancer (10%), lung cancer (5%) and breast cancer (5%)
Carcinoembryonic antigen (CEA)	Glycoprotein found in intestinal mucosa during embryonic and fetal life. Elevated in smokers, cirrhosis, chronic hepatitis, ulcerative colitis, pneumonia	Colorectal cancer, particularly with liver metastasis, gastric cancer, breast cancer, lung cancer, mucinous cancer of the ovary
Human chorionic gonadotrophin (HCG)	Glycoprotein hormone, 14KD α subunit and 24KD β subunit from placental syncytiotrophoblasts. Used for disease monitoring in hydatidiform mole and as the basis of a pregnancy test	Choriocarcinoma (100%), hydatidiform moles (97%), ovarian non-seminomatous germ cell tumours (50–80%), seminoma (15%)
Placental alkaline phosphatase (PLAP)	Isoenzyme of alkaline phosphatase	Seminoma (40%), ovarian dysgerminoma (50%)
Prostate-specific antigen (PSA)	Glycoprotein member of human kallikrein gene family. PSA is a serine protease that liquefies semen in excretory ducts of prostate. Can be elevated in benign prostatic hypertrophy and prostatitis	Prostate cancer (95%)
Thyroglobulin	Matrix protein for thyroid hormone synthesis in normal thyroid follicles	Papillary and follicular thyroid cancer
β-2-microglobulin	A human leucocyte antigen (HLA) common fragment present on surface of lymphocytes, macrophages and some epithelial cells. Can be elevated in autoimmune disease and renal glomerular disease	Non-Hodgkin's lymphoma, myeloma

Some of these are useful in population screening, diagnosis, prognostication, treatment monitoring, detection of relapse and imaging of metastasis. Unfortunately, most tumour markers are not sufficiently sensitive or specific to be used in isolation and need to be interpreted in the context of the other clinical features. However, some tumour markers can be used for antibody-directed therapy or imaging, where they have a greater role in diagnosis. Tumour markers in routine use are outlined in Box 11.5.

PRESENTING PROBLEMS IN ONCOLOGY

In the early stages of cancer development, the number of malignant cells is small and the patient is usually asymptomatic. With tumour progression, localised signs or symptoms develop due to mass effects and/or invasion of local tissues. With further progression, symptoms may occur at distant sites as a result of metastatic disease or from non-metastatic manifestations due to production of biologically active hormones by the tumour or as the result of an immune response to the tumour. The possible presentations of patients with cancer are summarised in Boxes 11.6 and 11.7, and common presenting features are discussed below. Although the incidence of cancer

11.6 Local features of malignant disease

Symptom	Typical site or possible tumour
Haemorrhage	Stomach, colon, bronchus, endometrium, bladder, kidney
Lump	Breast, lymph node (any site), testicle
Bone pain or fracture	Bone (primary sarcoma, secondary metastasis from breast, prostate, bronchus, thyroid, kidney)
Skin abnormality	Melanoma, basal cell carcinoma (rodent ulcer)
Ulcer	Oesophagus, stomach, anus, skin
Dysphagia	Oesophagus, bronchus, gastric
Increasing constipation, abdominal discomfort or pain	Colon, rectum, ovary
Airway obstruction, stridor, cough, recurrent infection	Bronchus, thyroid
Odynophagia, early satiety, vomiting	Bronchus, stomach, oesophagus, colon, rectum
Abdominal swelling (ascites)	Ovary, stomach, pancreas

11

11.7 Non-metastatic manifestations of malignant disease

Feature	Common cancer site associations
Weight loss and anorexia	Lung, gastrointestinal tract
Fatigue	Any
Hypercalcaemia	Myeloma, breast, kidney
Prothrombotic tendency	Ovary, pancreas, gastrointestinal tract
Syndrome of inappropriate antidiuretic hormone secretion (SIADH) **Ectopic adrenocorticotrophin hormone (ACTH)**	Small cell lung cancer
Lambert–Eaton myasthenia-like syndrome	Small cell lung cancer
Subacute cerebellar degeneration	Small cell lung cancer, ovarian cancer
Acanthosis nigricans	Stomach, oesophagus
Dermatomyositis/polymyositis	Stomach, lung

11.8 Cancer in old age

- **Incidence:** around 50% of cancers occur in the 15% of the population aged over 65 years.
- **Screening:** women aged over 65 in the UK are not invited to breast cancer screening but can request it. Uptake is low despite increasing incidence with age.
- **Presentation:** may be later for some cancers. When symptoms are non-specific, patients (and their doctors) may initially attribute them to age alone.
- **Life expectancy:** an 80-year-old woman can expect to live 8 years, so cancer may still shorten life and an active approach remains appropriate.
- **Prognosis:** histology, stage at presentation and observation for a brief period are better guides to outcome than age alone.
- **Rate of progression:** malignancy may have a more indolent course. This is poorly understood but may be due to reduced effectiveness of angiogenesis with age, inhibiting the development of metastases.
- **Response to treatment:** equivalent to that in younger people. This is well documented for a range of cancers and for surgery, radiotherapy, chemotherapy and hormonal therapy.
- **Treatment selection:** chronological age is of minor importance compared to comorbid illness and patient choice. Although older patients can be treated effectively and safely, aggressive intervention is not appropriate for all individuals. Symptom control may be all that is possible or desired by the patient.

increases with patient age, the approach to investigation and management is similar at all ages (Box 11.8).

Palpable mass

A palpable mass detected by the patient or physician may be the first sign of cancer. Primary tumours of the thyroid, breast, testis and skin are often detected in this way, whereas palpable lymph nodes in the neck, groin or axilla may indicate secondary spread of tumour. Hepatomegaly may be the first sign of primary liver cancer or tumour metastasis, whereas skin cancer may present as an enlarging or changing pigmented lesion.

Weight loss and fever

Unintentional weight loss is a characteristic feature of advanced cancer, but can be due to other causes such as thyrotoxicosis, chronic inflammatory disease and chronic infective disorders. Fever can occur in any cancer secondary to infection, but may be a primary feature in Hodgkin's disease, lymphoma, leukaemia, renal cancer and liver cancer. The presence of unexplained weight loss or fever warrants investigation to exclude the presence of occult malignancy.

Finger clubbing

Finger clubbing is a characteristic feature of lung cancer, and especially non-small cell lung cancer, although benign causes are also recognised. It is often part of the wider process of hypertrophic osteoarthropathy in which there is periosteal new bone formation and arthritis. Recent evidence suggests that this may be due to increased levels of prostaglandin E. The diagnosis is primarily clinical, but X-rays show periosteal reaction and an isotope bone scan shows increased tracer update in the affected digits. The condition responds to antitumour therapy, but if this is not possible, non-steroidal anti-inflammatory drugs (NSAIDs) and corticosteroids should be given.

Ectopic hormone production

In some cases, the first presentation of cancer is with a metabolic abnormality due to ectopic production of hormones by tumour cells, including insulin, ACTH, ADH, FGF23, erythropoietin and parathyroid hormone-related protein (PTHrP). This can result in a wide variety of presentations, as summarised in Box 11.9. Further details on presentation and management of ACTH and ADH-producing tumours are given on page 774, and of FGF23-producing tumours on page 1123. The management of hypercalcaemia associated with malignancy is discussed on page 268.

Neurological paraneoplastic syndromes

These form a group of conditions associated with cancer which are thought to be due to an immunological response to the tumour that results in damage to the nervous system or muscle. The cancers most commonly implicated are those of the lung (small cell and non-small cell), pancreas, breast, prostate, ovary and lymphoma.

11.9 Ectopic hormone production by tumours

Hormone	Consequence	Tumours
ADH	Hyponatraemia	SCLC
ACTH	Cushing's syndrome	SCLC
FGF-23	Hypophosphataemic osteomalacia	Mesenchymal tumours
Insulin	Hypoglycaemia	Insulinoma
Erythropoietin	Polycythaemia	Kidney, hepatoma, cerebellar haemangioblastoma, uterine fibroids
PTHrP	Hypercalcaemia	NSCLC (squamous cell), breast, kidney

(SCLC = small cell lung cancer)

- *Peripheral neuropathy* results from axonal degeneration or demyelination.
- *Encephalomyelitis* can present with diverse symptoms, depending on which region of the brain is involved. Lumbar puncture shows raised protein in the cerebrospinal fluid (CSF) and a pleocytosis, predominantly that of lymphocytes. In some centres, flow cytometry of the CSF is also used to detect carcinomatous cells. MRI shows meningeal enhancement, particularly at the level of the brain stem, and anti-Hu antibodies may be detectable in serum. Encephalomyelitis is due to perivascular inflammation and selective neuronal degeneration. Most cases are caused by small cell lung cancer (75%).
- *Cerebellar degeneration* may be the presenting feature of an underlying malignancy and presents with rapid onset of cerebellar ataxia. Diagnosis is by MRI or CT, which may show cerebellar atrophy. Patients with these neurological paraneoplastic syndromes may be found to have circulating anti-Yo, Tr and Hu antibodies, but these are not completely specific and negative results do not exclude the diagnosis.
- *Retinopathy* is a rare complication of cancer and presents with blurred vision, episodic visual loss and impaired colour vision. If left untreated, it may lead to blindness. The diagnosis should be suspected if the electroretinogram is abnormal and anti-retinal antibodies are detected.
- *Lambert–Eaton syndrome* (LEMS) is due to underlying cancer in about 60% of cases. It presents with proximal muscle weakness which improves on exercise and is caused by the development of antibodies to presynaptic calcium channels (p. 1232). The diagnosis is made by electromyelogram (EMG), which shows a low-amplitude compound muscle action potential that enhances to near normal following exercise.
- *Dermatomyositis* or *polymyositis* may be the first presentation of some cancers. Clinical features and management of these conditions are discussed on page 1111.

Cutaneous manifestations of cancer

Many cancers can present with skin manifestations which are not due to metastases.

- *Pruritus* may be a presenting feature of lymphoma, leukaemia and central nervous system tumours.
- *Acanthosis nigricans* may precede cancers by many years and is particularly associated with gastric cancer.
- *Vitiligo* may be associated with malignant melanoma, and is possibly due to an immune response to melanocytes.
- *Pemphigus* may occur in lymphoma, Kaposi's sarcoma and thymic tumours.
- *Dermatitis herpetiformis* associated with coeliac disease may precede tumour development by many years, and is associated with gastrointestinal lymphoma.

The clinical features and management of these skin conditions is discussed in Chapter 27.

EMERGENCY COMPLICATIONS OF CANCER

Spinal cord compression

Spinal cord compression complicates 5% of cancers and is most common in myeloma, prostate, breast and lung cancers which involve bone. Cord compression often results from posterior extension of a vertebral body mass but intrathecal spinal cord metastases can cause similar signs and symptoms.

Clinical features

The earliest sign is back pain, particularly on coughing and lying flat. Subsequently, sensory changes develop in dermatomes below the level of compression and motor weakness distal to the block occurs. Finally, sphincter disturbance, causing urinary retention and bowel incontinence, is observed. Involvement of the lumbar spine may cause conus medullaris or cauda equina compression (Box 11.10). Physical examination reveals findings consistent with an upper motor neuron lesion, but lower motor neuron findings may predominate early on or in cases of nerve root compression.

Management

Spinal cord compression is a medical emergency which should be treated with analgesia and high-dose steroid therapy (dexamethasone 10 mg i.v. stat and 4 mg 6-hourly orally; Box 11.11). Neurosurgical treatment produces superior outcome and survival compared to radiotherapy alone, and should be considered first for all patients. Radiotherapy is used for the remaining patients and selected tumour types when the cancer is likely to be radiosensitive. The prognosis varies considerably, depending on tumour type, but the degree of neurological dysfunction at presentation is the strongest predictor of outcome irrespective of the underlying diagnosis. Ambulation can be preserved in more than 80% of patients who are ambulatory at presentation, but neurological function is seldom regained in patients with established deficits such as paraplegia.

11

11.10 Comparison of features of neurological deficit

Clinical feature	Spinal cord	Conus medullaris	Cauda equina
Weakness	Symmetrical and profound	Symmetrical and variable	Asymmetrical, may be mild
Reflexes	Increased (or absent) knee and ankle reflexes with extensor plantar reflex	Increased knee reflex, decreased ankle reflex, extensor plantar reflex	Decreased knee and ankle reflexes with flexor plantar reflex
Sensory loss	Symmetrical, sensory level	Symmetrical, saddle distribution	Asymmetrical, radicular pattern
Sphincters	Late loss	Early loss	Spared often
Progression	Rapid	Variable	Variable

11.11 Management of suspected spinal cord compression

- Confirm diagnosis with urgent MRI scan
- Administer high-dose steroids
- Dexamethasone 10 mg i.v. stat
- Dexamethasone 4 mg 6-hourly orally
- Ensure adequate analgesia
- Refer for surgical decompression or urgent radiotherapy

11.12 Common symptoms and physical findings in SVC obstruction (% patients affected)

Symptoms

- Dyspnoea (63%)
- Facial swelling and head fullness (50%)
- Cough (24%)
- Arm swelling (18%)
- Chest pain (15%)
- Dysphagia (9%)

Physical findings

- Venous distension of neck (66%)
- Venous distension of chest wall (54%)
- Facial oedema (46%)
- Cyanosis (20%)
- Plethora of face (19%)
- Oedema of arms (14%)

Superior vena cava obstruction

Superior vena cava obstruction (SVCO) is a common complication of cancer which can occur through extrinsic compression or intravascular blockage. The most common causes of extrinsic compression are lung cancer, lymphoma and metastatic tumours. Patients with cancer can also develop SVCO due to intravascular blockage in association with a central catheter or thrombophilia secondary to the tumour.

Clinical features

The typical presentation is with oedema of the arms and face, distended neck and arm veins and dusky skin coloration over the chest, arms and face. Collaterals may develop over a period of weeks and the flow of blood in the collaterals helps to confirm the diagnosis. Headache secondary to cerebral oedema arising from the backflow pressure may also occur and tends to be aggravated by bending forward, stooping or lying down. The severity of symptoms is related to the rate of obstruction and the development of a venous collateral circulation. Accordingly, symptoms may develop rapidly or gradually. Clinical features are summarised in Box 11.12.

Diagnosis and management

The investigation of choice is CT of the thorax since it can clinch the diagnosis and distinguish between extra- and intravascular causes. A biopsy should be obtained when the tumour type is unknown because tumour type has a major influence on treatment. CT of the brain may be indicated if cerebral oedema is suspected. Patients with suspected cerebral oedema, usually manifesting as a headache, should be started on high-dose steroid therapy (dexamethasone 16–24 mg/24 hours), and mannitol should be considered if the response is inadequate. Tumours that are exquisitely sensitive to chemotherapy, such as germ cell tumours and lymphoma, can be treated with chemotherapy alone, but for most other tumours mediastinal radiotherapy is required. This relieves symptoms within 2 weeks in 50–90% of patients. In most centres, stenting is now increasingly favoured over radiotherapy, as it produces rapid results and can be repeated with reasonable effectiveness. This technique is particularly useful when dealing with tumours that are relatively chemo- or radio-resistant, such as non-small cell lung cancer.

Where possible, these measures should be followed by treatment of the primary tumour, as long-term outcome strongly is dependent on the prognosis of the underlying cancer.

Hypercalcaemia

Hypercalcaemia is the most common metabolic disorder in patients with cancer and has a prevalence of 15–20 cases per 100 000 persons. The incidence is highest in myeloma and breast cancer (approximately 40%), intermediate in non-small cell lung cancer, and uncommon in colon, prostate and small cell lung carcinomas. It is most commonly due to over-production of PTHrP, which binds to the PTH receptor and elevates serum calcium by stimulating osteoclastic bone resorption and increasing renal tubular reabsorption of calcium.

Clinical features

The symptoms of hypercalcaemia are often non-specific and may mimic those of the underlying malignancy. They include drowsiness, confusion, nausea and vomiting, constipation, polyuria, polydipsia and dehydration.

11

11.13 Medical management of severe hypercalcaemia

- I.v. 0.9% saline 2–4 L/day
- I.v. bisphosphonate
- Zoledronic acid 4 mg i.v.

or

- Pamidronate 60–90 mg i.v.

or

- Clodronate 300 mg i.v. daily over 5 days
- I.m./s.c. calcitonin 100 U 8-hourly for first 24–48 hours in life-threatening hypercalcaemia

Diagnosis and management

The diagnosis is made by measuring serum total calcium and adjusting for albumin. It is especially important to correct for albumin in cancer because hypoalbuminaemia is common and total calcium values underestimate the level of ionised calcium. The principles of management are outlined in Box 11.13.

Patients should initially be treated with intravenous 0.9% saline (2–4 L/day) to improve renal function and increase urinary calcium excretion. This alone often results in clinical improvement. Concurrently, intravenous bisphosphonates should be given to inhibit bone resorption. Intravenous pamidronate (60–90 mg i.v.), zoledronic acid (4 mg i.v.) or clodronate (1500 mg i.v. in divided doses) are all effective. Calcitonin (100 U s.c. or i.m. 8-hourly) acts rapidly to increase calcium excretion and to reduce bone resorption and can be combined with fluid and bisphosphonate therapy for the first 24–48 hours in patients with life-threatening hypercalcaemia. Bisphosphonates will usually reduce the serum calcium levels to normal within 5 days, but if not, treatment can be repeated. The duration of action is up to 4 weeks and repeated therapy can be given at 3–4-weekly intervals as an outpatient. Hypercalcaemia is frequently a sign of tumour progression and the patient requires further investigation to establish disease status and review of the anticancer therapy.

Neutropenic sepsis

Neutropenia is a common complication of malignancy. It is usually secondary to chemotherapy but may occur with radiotherapy if large amounts of marrow are irradiated; alternatively, it may be a component of pancytopenia due to malignant infiltration of the marrow. Neutropenic sepsis is defined as a pyrexia of 38°C for over 1 hour in a patient with a neutrophil count $< 1.0 \times 10^9$/L. The risk of sepsis is related to the severity and duration of neutropenia and the presence of other risk factors such as intravenous or bladder catheters.

Clinical features

The typical presentation is with high fever and affected patients are often non-specifically unwell. Examination is usually unhelpful in defining a primary source of the infection. Hypotension is an adverse prognostic feature and may progress to systemic circulatory shutdown and organ failure.

Investigations and management

An infection screen should be performed to include blood cultures (both peripheral and from central lines if present), urine culture, chest X-ray, and swabs for culture (throat, central line, wound). High-dose intravenous antibiotics should then be commenced, pending the results of cultures. Typical first line empirical therapy consists of an antipseudomonal β-lactam (ceftazidime, cefotaxime or meropenem), or a combination of an aminoglycoside and a broad-spectrum penicillin with antipseudomonal activity (gentamicin and piperacillin), but this may need adjusting on the basis of local hospital policy and antibiotic resistance patterns. Metronidazole should be added if anaerobic infection is suspected, and flucloxacillin or vancomycin or teicoplanin where Gram-positive infection is suspected (for example, in patients with central lines). If there is no response after 36–48 hours, treatment with amphotericin-B or voriconazole should be considered to cover fungal infection. Antibiotics should be adjusted according to culture results, though these are often negative. Other supportive therapy, including intravenous fluids, inotropes, ventilation or haemofiltration, may be required.

METASTATIC DISEASE

Metastatic disease is the major cause of death in cancer patients and the principal cause of morbidity. For the majority of patients, the aim of treatment is palliative, but treatment of a solitary metastasis can occasionally be curative.

Brain metastases

Brain metastases occur in 10–30% of adults and 6–10% of children with cancer, and are an increasingly important cause of morbidity. Tumours which typically metastasise to the brain are shown in Box 11.14. Most involve the brain parenchyma but can also affect the cranial nerves, the blood vessels and other intracranial structures. The median survival without treatment is 1 month. Steroids can increase survival to 2–3 months and whole-brain radiotherapy improves survival to 3–6 months. Patients with brain metastases as the only manifestation of an undetected primary tumour have a more favourable prognosis, with an overall median survival of 13.4 months. Tumour type also influences prognosis; breast cancer patients have a better prognosis than those with other types of tumour, and

11.14 Primary tumour sites that metastasise to brain

Primary tumour	Patients (%)
Lung	48
Breast	15
Melanoma	9
Colon	5
Other known primary	13
Unknown primary	11

those with colorectal carcinoma tend to have a poorer prognosis.

Clinical features

The presentation is with headaches (40–50% of patients), focal neurological dysfunction (20–40%), cognitive dysfunction (35%), seizures (10–20%) and papilloedema (< 10% of cases).

Diagnosis and management

The diagnosis can be confirmed by CT or contrast-enhanced MRI. Treatment options include high-dose steroids (dexamethasone 4 mg 6-hourly) for tumour-associated oedema, anticonvulsants for seizures, whole-brain radiotherapy, and chemotherapy. Surgery may be considered for single sites of disease and can be curative; stereotactic radiotherapy may also be considered for patients with solitary site involvement where surgery is not possible.

Lung metastases

These are common in breast cancer, colon cancer, and tumours of the head and neck. The presentation is usually with a lesion on chest X-ray or CT. Solitary lesions require investigation, as single metastases can be difficult to distinguish from a primary lung tumour. Patients with two or more pulmonary nodules can be assumed to have metastases. The approach to treatment depends on the extent of disease in the lung and elsewhere. For solitary lesions, surgery should be considered with a generous wedge resection. Radiotherapy, chemotherapy or endocrine therapy can be used as systemic treatment and is dependent on the underlying primary cancer diagnosis.

Liver metastases

Metastatic cancer in the liver can represent the sole or life-limiting component of disease for many patients with colorectal cancer, ocular melanoma, neuro-endocrine tumours and, less commonly, other tumour types. The most common clinical presentations are with right upper quadrant pain due to stretching of the liver capsule, jaundice, deranged liver function tests or an abnormality detected on imaging. In selected cases, resection of the metastasis can be contemplated. In colorectal cancer, successful resection of a metastasis improves 5-year survival from 3% to 30–40%. Other techniques, such as chemoembolisation or radio-frequency ablation, can also be used, provided the number and size of metastases remain small. If these approaches are not feasible, symptoms may respond to systemic chemotherapy.

Bone metastases

Bone is the third most common organ involved by metastasis, after lung and liver. Bone metastases are a major clinical problem in patients with myeloma and breast or prostate cancers, but other tumours that commonly metastasise to bone include those of the kidney and thyroid. Bone metastases are an increasing management problem in other tumour types which do not classically target bone, due to the prolonged survival of patients generally. Accordingly, effective management of bony metastases has become a focus in the treatment of patients with many incurable cancers.

Clinical features

The main presentations are with pain, pathological fractures and spinal cord compression (p. 267). The pain tends to be worst at night and may be partially relieved by activity, but subsequently becomes more constant in nature and is exacerbated by movement. The majority of pathological fractures occur in patients with metastatic breast cancer (53%); other tumour types associated with fracture include the kidney (11%), lung (8%), thyroid (5%), lymphoma (5%) and prostate (3%).

Diagnosis and management

The most sensitive way of detecting bone metastases is by isotope bone scan, but this may give false negative results in multiple myeloma due to suppression of osteoblast activity so in this situation X-rays are preferred. In patients with a single lesion, it is especially important to perform a biopsy to obtain a tissue diagnosis, since primary bone tumours may look very similar to metastases on X-ray. The main goals of management are as follows:

- pain relief
- preservation and restoration of function
- skeletal stabilisation
- local tumour control (e.g. relief of tumour impingement on normal structure).

Surgical intervention may be warranted where there is evidence of skeletal instability (e.g. anterior or posterior spinal column fracture) or an impending fracture (e.g. large lytic lesion on a weight-bearing bone). Intravenous bisphosphonates (pamidronate, zoledronic acid or ibandronate) are widely used in the treatment of patients with bone metastases and are effective at improving pain and in reducing further skeletal related events, such as fractures and hypercalcaemia (Box 11.15). In certain types of cancer, such as breast and prostate, hormonal therapy may be effective. Radiotherapy, in the form of external beam therapy or systemic radio-nucleotides (strontium treatment) can also be useful for these patients. In some settings (e.g. breast carcinoma) chemotherapy may also be used in the management of bony metastases.

EBM 11.15 **Use of bisphosphonates in bony metastases**

'The use of bisphosphonates in cancer patients with bony metastases results in decreased pain and a decrease in skeletal-related events.'

- Wong R, Wiffen PJ. (Cochrane Review). Cochrane Library, issue 2, 2002.
- Rosen LS, et al. Cancer 2004; 100(12):2613–2621.

For further information: www.ncbi.nlm.nih.gov/pubmed/12136223

Malignant pleural effusion

This is a common complication of cancer and 40% of all pleural effusions are due to malignancy. The most common causes are lung and breast cancers, and the presence of an effusion indicates advanced and incurable disease. The presentation may be with dyspnoea, cough or chest discomfort, which can be dull or pleuritic in nature.

Diagnosis and management

Pleural aspirate is the key investigation and may show the presence of malignant cells. Malignant effusions are

11.16 How to aspirate a malignant pleural effusion

- Ask the patient to sit up and lean forward slightly.
- Identify a suitable site for aspiration. Typically this should be in the midscapular line, below the top of the fluid level and above the diaphragm.
- Confirm that the site is below the fluid level by reviewing the chest X-ray and percussing the chest.
- Infiltrate the skin and the intercostal space immediately above the rib below with 1% lidocaine.
- As you advance the needle, aspirate at each step prior to injecting the local anaesthetic.
- On reaching the pleural cavity, you should be able to aspirate pleural fluid; when you do, note the depth of the needle.
- Insert a thoracentesis needle into the pleural space by advancing it along the same track as was used for the local anaesthetic and connect it to a three-way tap and container to collect the fluid.
- Drain the pleural effusion, to a maximum of 1.5 L. If the effusion is larger than this, repeat the procedure on further occasions as necessary.
- Consider using ultrasound-guided placement of a drainage catheter if the effusion proves difficult to drain.

11.17 Goals of non-surgical treatment

Curative

- Choriocarcinoma
- Teratoma
- Seminoma
- High-grade lymphoma
- Cervical cancer
- Head and neck cancer

Radical, occasionally curative

- Small cell lung cancer
- Stage III ovarian cancer

Adjuvant (following surgery)

- Breast cancer
- Stage I–II ovarian cancer
- Colorectal cancer
- Osteosarcoma

Palliative

- Metastatic breast cancer
- Stage IV ovarian cancer
- Advanced gastrointestinal cancer
- Metastatic sarcoma
- Metastatic prostate cancer
- Advanced lung cancer

commonly blood-stained and are exudates with a raised fluid:serum lactate dehydrogenase (LDH) ratio (> 0.6) and a raised fluid:serum protein ratio (> 0.5).Treatment should focus on palliation of symptoms and be tailored to the patient's physical condition and prognosis. Aspiration alone may be an appropriate treatment in frail patients with a limited life expectancy (Box 11.16). Those who present with malignant pleural effusion as the initial manifestation of breast cancer, small cell lung cancer, germ cell tumours or lymphoma should have the fluid aspirated and should be given systemic chemotherapy to try to treat disease in the pleural space. Treatment options for patients with recurrent pleural effusion include pleurodesis, pleurectomy and pleuroperitoneal shunt. Ideally, pleurodesis should be attempted once recurrence of effusion after initial drainage occurs.

THERAPEUTICS IN ONCOLOGY

Anticancer therapy may be either curative or palliative, and this distinction influences the approach to management of individual patients.

- *Palliation.* The majority of patients who receive chemotherapy for metastatic disease do so for the palliation of symptoms. The aim of palliative chemotherapy is to produce an improvement in quality of life with a minimised impact of toxicity on the patient; there may be a small increase in survival.
- *Adjuvant treatment.* This is administered after surgery and the main aim is to increase the disease-free and overall survival. As impact on survival is the main focus, a greater toxicity is acceptable, sometimes with a significant impact on quality of life. As patients have often had their cancers surgically removed, it is not possible to assess the response to treatment, other than by improvement in survival.

- *Neoadjuvant treatment.* This also has the long-term aim of improved survival but in this case patients receive chemotherapy, radiotherapy or hormonal treatment before surgery. The response of the cancer to the treatment can be assessed and a reduction in the extent of surgery required may be produced. Examples of approach are outlined in Box 11.17.

Surgical treatment

Surgery has a pivotal role in the management of cancer. There are three main situations in which it is necessary.

Biopsy

In the vast majority of cases, a histological or cytological diagnosis of cancer is necessary, and tissue will also provide important information such as tumour type and differentiation, to assist subsequent management. Cytology can be obtained with fine needle aspiration, but a biopsy is usually preferred. This can be a core biopsy, an image-guided biopsy or an excision biopsy.

Excision

The main curative management of most solid cancers is surgical excision. In early localised cases of colorectal, breast and lung cancer, cure rates are high with surgery. There is increasing evidence that outcome is related to surgical expertise, and most multidisciplinary teams include surgeons experienced in the management of a particular cancer. There are some cancers for which surgery is one of two or more options for primary management, and the role of the multidisciplinary team is to recommend appropriate treatment for a specific patient. Examples include prostate and transitional cell carcinoma of the bladder, in which radiotherapy and surgery may be equally effective.

Palliation

Surgical procedures are often the quickest and most effective way of palliating symptoms. Examples include the treatment of faecal incontinence with a defunctioning colostomy; fixation of pathological fractures and decompression of spinal cord compression; and the treatment of fungating skin lesions by 'toilet' surgery. A more specialist role for surgery is in resection of residual masses after chemotherapy and, in very selected cases, resection of metastases.

Systemic chemotherapy

Chemotherapeutic drugs are classified by their mode of action. They have the greatest activity in proliferating cells and this provides the rationale for their use in the treatment of cancer. Chemotherapeutic agents are not specific for cancer cells, however, and the side-effects of treatment are a result of their antiproliferative actions in normal tissues such as the bone marrow, skin and gut.

Combination therapy

In order to overcome drug resistance and to limit the side-effects of different drugs, chemotherapy is most commonly given as a combination of agents. Combinations usually include drugs from different classes, with the aim of targeting several pathways and gaining maximum therapeutic effect. Drugs are conventionally given by intravenous injection every 3–4 weeks, allowing enough time for the patient to recover from short-term toxic effects before the next dose. Between four and eight such cycles of treatment are usually given in total. More recently, other strategies have been developed. For example, 5-fluorouracil (5-FU), which has a very short half-life, has increased efficacy when given by continuous intravenous infusion, using a semi-permanent indwelling intravenous catheter. However, the use of such catheters is not without risk and the potential of oral 5-FU is now being explored, using precursors such as capecitabine. Schedules of administration at weekly or 2-weekly intervals have also found their place in the management of both solid and haematological malignancies. Each tumour type has specific regimens that are used at various stages of the disease.

Mode of administration

Most drugs have to be given intravenously, and many are vesicant or locally irritant if there is an extravasation. Chemotherapy should be administered into a vein in which the infusion is free-flowing to minimise the risk of extravasation. A few patients require central venous catheters due to the nature of their treatment or poor vascular access. Patients who receive chemotherapy through a peripheral line must be carefully observed, and the chemotherapy stopped at the first sign of any extravasation. Chemotherapy is potentially dangerous to the person giving the therapy, because cytotoxics are carcinogenic and teratogenic. In view of this, policies must be in place for the use of gloves and aprons and for the safe disposal of syringes containing cytotoxics. Other oral chemotherapeutic agents have been developed over the past 30 years, although not many have replaced their intravenous counterparts.

Adverse effects

Most cytotoxics have a narrow therapeutic window or index and can have significant adverse effects, as shown in Figure 11.5. Considerable supportive therapy is often required to enable patients to tolerate therapy and achieve benefit. Nausea and vomiting are common,

but with modern antiemetics, regimens such as the combination of dexamethasone and highly selective 5-hydroxytryptamine (5-HT) receptor antagonists such as ondansetron, most patients now receive chemotherapy without any significant problems. Myelosuppression is common to almost all cytotoxics. This not only limits the dose of drug, but also can cause life-threatening complications. The risk of neutropenia can be reduced with the use of specific growth factors that accelerate the repopulation of myeloid precursor cells. The most commonly employed is granulocyte colony-stimulating factor (G–CSF), which is widely used in conjunction with chemotherapy regimens that induce a high rate of neutropenia. More recently, it has also been used to 'accelerate' the administration of chemotherapy, enabling standard doses to be given at shorter intervals where the rate-limiting factor has been the time taken for the peripheral neutrophil count to recover. Accelerated chemotherapy regimens have now been demonstrated to offer therapeutic advantages in small cell lung cancer, lymphoma and possibly breast cancer.

Radiation therapy

Radiation therapy (radiotherapy) involves treating the cancer with ionising radiation; for certain localised cancers it may be curative. Ionising radiation can be delivered by radiation emitted from the decay of radioactive isotopes or by high-energy radiation beams, usually X-rays. Three methods are usually employed:

- *Teletherapy*: application from a distance by a linear accelerator.
- *Brachytherapy*: direct application of a radioactive source on to or into a tumour. This allows the delivery of a very high, localised dose of radiation and is integral to the management of localised cancers of the head and neck and cancer of the cervix and endometrium.
- *Intravenous injection of a radioisotope*: such as ^{131}iodine for cancer of the thyroid and ^{89}strontium for the treatment of bone metastases from prostate cancer.

The majority of treatments are now delivered by linear accelerators which produce electron or X-ray beams of high energy that are used to target tumour tissue. Whatever the method of delivery, the biological effect of ionising radiation is to cause lethal and sublethal damage to DNA. Since normal tissues are also radiosensitive, treatment has to be designed to maximise exposure of the tumour and minimise exposure of normal tissues. This is now possible with modern imaging techniques such as CT and MRI, which allow better visualisation of normal and tumour tissue. In addition, techniques such as conformal radiotherapy, where shaped rather than conventional square or rectangular beams are used, allow much more precise targeting of therapy to the tumour, and reduce the volume of normal tissue irradiated by up to 40% compared to non-conformal techniques.

Biological differences between normal and tumour tissues are also used to obtain therapeutic gain. Fundamental to this is fractionation, which entails delivering the radiation as a number of small doses on a daily basis. This allows normal cells to recover from irradiation damage, but recovery occurs to a lesser degree in malignant cells. Fractionation regimens vary from centre to centre but radical treatments given with curative intent are often

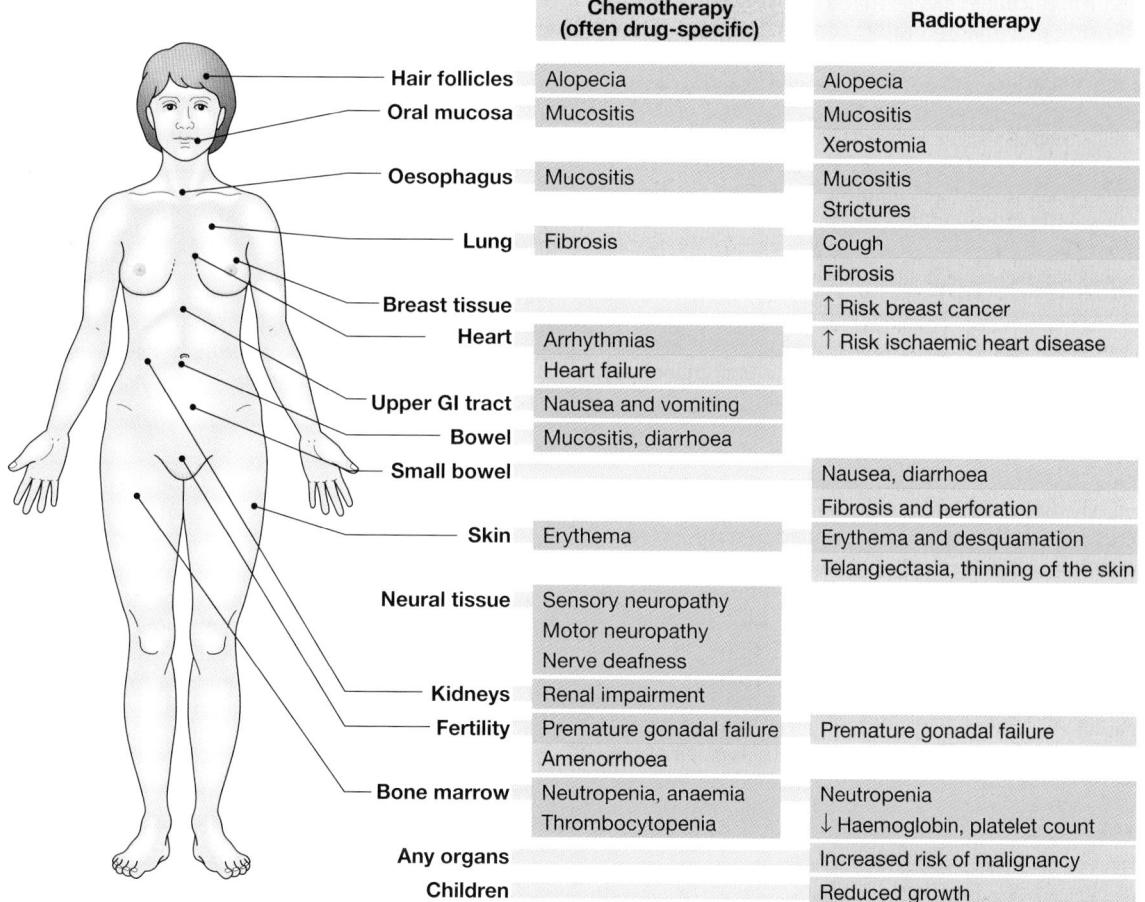

	Chemotherapy (often drug-specific)	Radiotherapy
Hair follicles	Alopecia	Alopecia
Oral mucosa	Mucositis	Mucositis Xerostomia
Oesophagus	Mucositis	Mucositis Strictures
Lung	Fibrosis	Cough Fibrosis
Breast tissue		↑ Risk breast cancer
Heart	Arrhythmias Heart failure	↑ Risk ischaemic heart disease
Upper GI tract	Nausea and vomiting	
Bowel	Mucositis, diarrhoea	
Small bowel		Nausea, diarrhoea Fibrosis and perforation
Skin	Erythema	Erythema and desquamation Telangiectasia, thinning of the skin
Neural tissue	Sensory neuropathy Motor neuropathy Nerve deafness	
Kidneys	Renal impairment	
Fertility	Premature gonadal failure Amenorrhoea	Premature gonadal failure
Bone marrow	Neutropenia, anaemia Thrombocytopenia	Neutropenia ↓ Haemoglobin, platelet count
Any organs		Increased risk of malignancy
Children		Reduced growth

Fig. 11.5 Adverse effects of chemotherapy and radiotherapy. Acute effects are shown in red and late effects in blue.

11

delivered in 20–30 fractions given daily, 5 days a week over 4–6 weeks. Radiotherapy can also be extremely useful for the alleviation of symptoms, and for palliative treatments such as this a smaller number of fractions (1–5) is usually adequate.

Both normal and malignant tissues vary widely in their sensitivity to radiotherapy. Germ cell tumours and lymphomas are extremely radiosensitive and relatively low doses are adequate for cure, but most cancers require doses close to or beyond that which can be tolerated by adjacent normal structures. Normal tissue also varies in its radiosensitivity, the central nervous system, small bowel and lung being amongst the most sensitive. The side-effects of radiotherapy (see Fig. 11.5) depend on the normal tissues treated, their radiosensitivity and the dose delivered.

Adverse effects

An acute inflammatory reaction commonly occurs towards the end of most radical treatments and is localised to the area treated. For example, skin reactions are common with breast or chest wall radiotherapy, and proctitis and cystitis with treatment to the bladder or prostate. These acute reactions settle over a period of a few weeks after treatment, assuming normal tissue tolerance has not been exceeded. Late effects of radiotherapy develop 6 weeks or more after treatment and occur in 5–10% of patients. Examples include brachial nerve

damage and subcutaneous fibrosis after breast cancer treatment, and shrinkage and fibrosis of the bladder after treatment for bladder cancer. There is a risk of inducing cancer after radiotherapy, which varies depending on the site treated and whether the patient has had other treatment such as chemotherapy.

Hormone therapy

Hormone therapy is most commonly used in the treatment of breast cancer and prostate cancer. Breast tumours which are positive for expression of the oestrogen receptor (ER) respond well to anti-oestrogen therapy, and assessment of ER status is now standard in the diagnosis of breast cancer. Several drugs are now available which reduce oestrogen levels or block the effects of oestrogen on the receptor. When targeted appropriately, adjuvant hormone therapy reduces the risk of relapse and death at least as much as chemotherapy, and in advanced cases can induce stable disease and remissions that may last months to years, with acceptable toxicity. Hormonal manipulation may be effective in other cancers. In prostate cancer, hormonal therapy (e.g. luteinising hormone releasing hormone (LHRH) analogues such as goserelin and/or anti-androgens such as bicalutamide) aimed at reducing androgen levels can provide good long-term control of advanced disease, but there is no convincing evidence that it is an effective therapy following potentially curative surgery. Progestogens are active in the treatment of endometrial and breast cancer. In the metastatic setting, progestogen use (e.g. megestrol acetate) is associated with response rates of 20–40% in endometrial cancer. In breast cancer, progestogens are used in patients whose disease has progressed with conventional anti-oestrogen therapy. Their exact mechanism in this setting is not fully understood.

Immunotherapy

A profound stimulus to the patient's immune system can sometimes alter the natural history of a malignancy, and the discovery of interferons stimulated much research. Although solid tumours show little benefit, interferons are active in melanoma and lymphoma, and there is evidence that they are beneficial as adjuvants (after surgery and chemotherapy respectively) to delay recurrence. Whether interferon-induced stimulation of the immune system is capable of eradicating microscopic disease remains unproven. More powerful immune responses can be achieved with potent agents like interleukin-2 (IL-2), but the accompanying systemic toxicity is a problem still to be overcome. The most striking example of successful immunotherapy is with rituximab, an antibody against the common B-cell antigen CD20. It increases complete response rates and improves survival in diffuse large cell non-Hodgkin's lymphoma when combined with chemotherapy, and is also effective in palliating advanced follicular non-Hodgkin's lymphoma (p. 1040).

Biological therapies

Advances in knowledge about the molecular basis of cancer have resulted in the development of a new generation of treatments to block the signalling pathways responsible for the growth of specific tumours. This has created the potential to target cancer cells more selectively, with reduced toxicity to normal tissues. Some examples are discussed below, but in the years to come many more such agents will come into clinical use, with the potential to revolutionise our approach to some cancers.

Gefitinib/erlotinib

These agents inhibit the activity of the epidermal growth factor receptor, which is over-expressed in many solid tumours. However, the drugs' activity does not depend on the amount of receptor over-expression but on factors such as gene copy number and mutation status.

Imatinib

Imatinib was developed to inhibit the *BCR-ABL* gene product tyrosine kinase that is responsible for chronic myeloid leukaemia (p. 1034), which it does extremely effectively. It is also active in gastrointestinal stromal tumour (GIST), a type of sarcoma which has over-expression of another cell surface tyrosine kinase, c-kit. This agent has good tolerability and is particularly useful in GIST, where conventional chemotherapy is less effective.

Trastuzumab

Trastuzumab (herceptin) targets the *Her-2* receptor, which is an oncogene that is over-expressed in around one-third of breast cancers and in a number of other solid tumours. It is effective as a single-agent therapy, but also improves survival in patients with advanced breast cancer when used in conjunction with chemotherapy. Unfortunately, trastuzumab can induce cardiac failure by an unknown biological mechanism, especially in combination with doxorubicin.

SPECIFIC CANCERS

The diagnosis and management of cancers is discussed in more detail elsewhere in the book. Here we discuss the clinical features, pathogenesis and management of common tumours that are not covered elsewhere.

Breast cancer

Globally, the incidence of breast cancer is only second to that of lung cancer and it represents the leading cause of cancer-related deaths among women. Invasive ductal carcinoma with or without ductal carcinoma in situ (DCIS) is the most common histology, accounting for 70%, whilst invasive lobular carcinoma accounts for most of the remaining cases. DCIS constitutes 20% of breast cancers detected by mammography screening. It is multifocal in one-third of women and has a high risk of becoming invasive (10% at 5 years following excision only). Pure DCIS does not cause lymph node metastases, although these are found in 2% of cases where nodes are examined, owing to undetected invasive cancer. Lobular carcinoma in situ (LCIS) is a predisposing risk factor for developing cancer in either breast (7% at 10 years). The survival for breast cancer by stage is outlined in Box 11.18.

Pathogenesis

Both genetic and hormonal factors play a role; about 5–10% of breast cancers are hereditary and occur in patients with mutations of *BRCA1, BRCA2, AT* or *p53* genes. Prolonged oestrogen exposure associated with early menarche, late menopause and HRT use has been associated with an increased risk. Other risk factors include obesity, alcohol intake, nulliparity and late first pregnancy. There is no definite evidence linking use of the contraceptive pill to breast cancer.

Clinical features

The presentation is usually with a painless mass in the breast that persists throughout the menstrual cycle.

i 11.18 **Five-year survival rates for breast cancer by stage**		
Tumour stage	**Stage definition**	**5-year survival (%)**
Stage I	Tumour < 2 cm, no lymph nodes	96
Stage II	Tumour 2–5 cm, and/or mobile axillary lymph nodes	81
Stage III	Chest wall or skin fixation, and/or fixed axillary lymph nodes	52
Stage IV	Metastasis	18

Increasingly, however, patients are diagnosed through mammography screening programmes. Nipple discharge or pain is present in less than 10% of cases. Approximately 40% of patients have axillary lymph nodes at diagnosis and the risk is proportionate to the size of the primary tumour. Distant metastases are uncommon at presentation but the most common sites in those with advanced disease are bone, lung, liver, pleura and the adrenal glands. These patients may present with bone pain, breathlessness, hepatomegaly or jaundice.

Investigations

Following clinical examination, patients should have an imaging procedure in the form of mammography or ultrasound evaluation and a biopsy. Histological assessment should be carried out to assess tumour type and to determine oestrogen and progesterone receptor (ER/PR) status and Her-2 status. If distant spread is suspected, CT of the thorax and abdomen, and a bone scan may be indicated.

Management

Surgery is the mainstay of treatment for most patients, and this can range from a lumpectomy, where only the tumour is removed, to mastectomy, where the whole breast is removed. Lymph node sampling is performed at the time of surgery to obtain prognostic information that may influence the subsequent decision on adjuvant treatment. Radiotherapy is offered to patients who have breast-sparing surgery in which multifocal disease has been demonstrated and those with lymph node involvement. Systemic therapy is offered as adjuvant treatment to patients with adverse prognostic features such as a large primary tumour (≥ 20 mm) and positive axillary lymph nodes (Box 11.19). Patients whose tumours are found to be positive for ER or PR should have anti-oestrogen treatment with either tamoxifen or aromatase inhibitors (e.g. anastrozole, exemestane), or sequential use of the two. It is important to remember that the use of an aromatase inhibitor should be limited to post-menopausal women. In some cases, where Her-2/neu is over-expressed, trastuzumab may be used.

For patients with metastatic disease, the choice of initial systemic therapy would depend on receptor status (ER, PR and Her-2), rapidity of tumour growth and patient symptomatology. ER/PR-positive patients who are relatively asymptomatic or who have slow tumour growth should be given anti-oestrogen treatment, while patients with rapid tumour growth or negative ER/PR status are best treated with chemotherapy with or without trastuzumab (in Her-2/neu over-expressing tumours). Pamidronate or zoledronic acid should be given to patients with bone metastases. Radiotherapy may be indicated for treating specific problems such as brain metastases, painful bone metastasis or spinal cord compression. Surgery has a role in the treatment of certain complications, such as decompression and fixation of the spine in cord compression.

Ovarian cancer

Ovarian cancer is the most common gynaecological tumour in Western countries. Most ovarian cancers are epithelial in origin (90%) and up to 7% of women with ovarian cancer have a positive family history. Patients often present late in ovarian cancer with vague abdominal discomfort, low back pain, bloating, altered bowel habit and weight loss. Occasionally, peritoneal deposits are palpable as an omental 'cake' and nodules in the umbilicus (Sister Mary Joseph nodules).

The 5-year survival for ovarian and other gynaecological cancers is outlined in Box 11.20.

i	11.20 Five-year survival rates for gynaecological cancers	
Tumour type		**5-year survival (%)**
Ovarian cancer		36
Endometrial cancer		73
Cervical cancer		61

Pathogenesis

Genetic and environmental factors play a role. The risk of ovarian cancer is increased in patients with *BRCA1* or *2* mutations, and Lynch type II families (a subtype of hereditary non-polyposis colon cancer (HNPCC)) have ovarian, endometrial, colorectal and gastric tumours due to mutations of mismatch repair enzymes. Advanced age, nulliparity, ovarian stimulation and Caucasian descent all increase the risk of ovarian cancer whilst suppressed ovulation appears to protect, so pregnancy, prolonged breastfeeding and the contraceptive pill have all been shown to reduce the risk of ovarian cancer.

Investigations

Initial workup for patients with suspected ovarian malignancy includes imaging in the form of ultrasound and CT. Serum levels of the tumour marker CA-125 are often measured. Surgery plays a key role in the diagnosis, staging and treatment of ovarian cancer, and in early cases palpation of viscera, intraoperative washing and biopsies are generally performed to define disease extent.

Management

In early disease surgery followed by adjuvant chemotherapy with carboplatin, or carboplatin plus paclitaxel, is the treatment of choice. Surgery should include removal of the tumour along with total hysterectomy, bilateral salpingo-oophorectomy, and omentectomy. Even in advanced tumours, surgery is undertaken to debulk the tumour and is followed by adjuvant chemotherapy, typically using carboplatin and paclitaxel. Monitoring for relapse is achieved through a combination of serum

EBM | **11.19 Use of adjuvant chemotherapy and endocrine therapy in early breast cancer**

'The use of anthracycline-based chemotherapy reduces the annual breast cancer rate from 38% to 20%, while the adjuvant use of tamoxifen for 5 years in early breast cancer for patients with ER-positive disease reduces the annual breast cancer death rate by 31%.'

• Early Breast Cancer Trialists Collaborative Group (EBCTCG). Lancet 2005; 366:2087–2106.

For further information: www.oncoconferences.ch/2007/home/home.htm

11

CA-125 and CT. If the patient relapses, second-line chemotherapy may be tried with either a further platinum/paclitaxel combination or liposomal doxorubicin or topotecan. These regimens are associated with a response rate of 10–40%. The best responses are observed in patients with a treatment-free interval of more than 12 months.

Endometrial cancer

Endometrial cancer accounts for 4% of all female malignancies, producing a 1 in 73 lifetime risk. The majority of patients are post-menopausal, with a peak incidence at 50–60 years of age. Mortality from endometrial cancer is currently falling. The most common presentation is with post-menopausal bleeding, which often results in detection of the disease before distant spread has occurred.

Pathogenesis

Oestrogen plays an important role in the pathogenesis of endometrial cancer, and factors that increase the duration of oestrogen exposure, such as nulliparity, early menarche, late menopause and unopposed hormone replacement therapy (HRT), increase the risk. Endometrial cancer is 10 times more common in obese women, and this is thought to be due to elevated levels of oestrogens.

Investigations

The diagnosis is confirmed by endometrial biopsy.

Management

Surgery is the treatment of choice and is also used for staging. A hysterectomy and bilateral salpingo-oophorectomy are performed with peritoneal cytology, and in some cases, lymph node dissection. Where the tumour extends beyond the inner 50% of the myometrium, adjuvant pelvic radiotherapy is recommended. Chemotherapy and hormonal therapies have not demonstrated a sufficient survival advantage to be recommended for routine use.

Cervical cancer

This is the second most common gynaecological tumour world-wide. The incidence is decreasing in developed countries but continues to rise in developing nations. Cervical cancer is the leading cause of death from gynaecological cancer. The most common presentation is with an abnormal smear test, but with locally advanced disease the presentation is with vaginal bleeding, discomfort, discharge or symptoms attributable to involvement of adjacent structures, such as bladder, or rectal or pelvic wall. Occasionally, patients present with distant metastases to bone and lung.

Pathogenesis

There is a strong association between cervical cancer and sexual activity that includes sex at a young age and multiple sexual partners. Infection with HPV has an important causal role, and this has underpinned the introduction of programmes to immunise teenagers against HPV in an effort to prevent the later development of cervical cancer (p. 423).

Investigations

Diagnosis is made by smear or cone biopsy. Dilatation and curettage is also used diagnostically, with cystoscopy and rectosigmoidoscopy if there are symptoms referable to the bladder, colon or rectum. In contrast to other gynaecological malignancies, cervical cancer is a clinically staged disease. MRI is often used to characterise the primary tumour. A routine chest X-ray should be obtained to help rule out pulmonary metastasis. CT of the abdomen and pelvis is performed to look for metastasis in the liver and lymph nodes and to exclude hydronephrosis and hydroureter.

Management

This depends on the stage of disease. Pre-malignant disease can be treated with laser ablation or diathermy, whereas in microinvasive disease cone biopsy or a simple hysterectomy is employed. Invasive but localised disease requires radical surgery, while chemotherapy and radiotherapy may be given as primary treatment, especially in patients with adverse prognostic features such as bulky or locally advanced disease, or lymph node or parametrium invasion. In metastatic disease, cisplatin-based chemotherapy may be beneficial in improving symptoms but does not improve survival significantly.

Head and neck tumours

Head and neck cancers are typically squamous tumours which arise in the nasopharynx, hypopharynx and larynx. They are most common in elderly males, but now occur with increasing frequency in a younger cohort, as well as in women. Presentation depends on the location of the primary tumour and the extent of disease. For example, early laryngeal cancers may present with hoarseness, while more extensive local disease may present with pain due to invasion of local structures or with a lump in the neck. Patients who present late often have pulmonary symptoms, as this is the most common site of distant metastases (Box 11.21).

Pathogenesis

The tumours are strongly associated with a history of smoking and excess alcohol intake, but other recognised risk factors include Epstein–Barr virus and HPV infection.

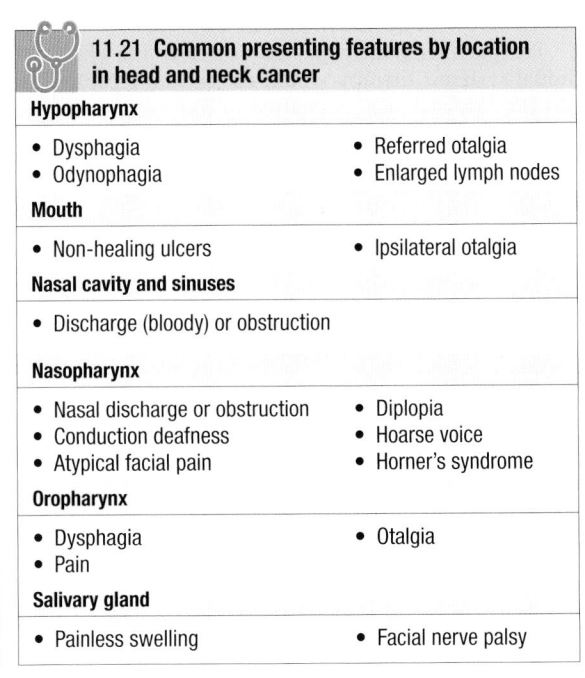

11.21 Common presenting features by location in head and neck cancer	
Hypopharynx	
• Dysphagia	• Referred otalgia
• Odynophagia	• Enlarged lymph nodes
Mouth	
• Non-healing ulcers	• Ipsilateral otalgia
Nasal cavity and sinuses	
• Discharge (bloody) or obstruction	
Nasopharynx	
• Nasal discharge or obstruction	• Diplopia
• Conduction deafness	• Hoarse voice
• Atypical facial pain	• Horner's syndrome
Oropharynx	
• Dysphagia	• Otalgia
• Pain	
Salivary gland	
• Painless swelling	• Facial nerve palsy

Investigations

Careful inspection of the primary site is required as part of the staging process, and most patients will require endoscopic evaluation and examination under anaesthesia. Tissue biopsies should be taken from the most accessible site. CT of the primary site and the thorax is the investigation of choice for visualising the tumour, while MRI may be useful in certain cases.

Management

In localised disease where there is no involvement of the lymph nodes, long-term remission can be achieved in 60–70% of patients with surgery or radiotherapy. The choice of surgery versus radiotherapy often depends on patient preference, as surgical treatment can be mutilating with an adverse cosmetic outcome. Patients with lymph node involvement or metastasis are treated with a combination of surgery and radiotherapy (often with chemotherapy as a radiosensitising agent), and this produces long-term remission in approximately 30% of patients. Recurrent or metastatic tumour may be palliated with further surgery or radiotherapy to aid local control, and systemic chemotherapy has a response rate of around 30%. Second malignancies are common (3% per year) following successful treatment for primary disease, and all patients should be encouraged to give up smoking and drinking alcohol to lower their risk.

Carcinoma of unknown origin

Some patients are found to have evidence of metastatic disease at their initial presentation prior to diagnosis of a primary site. In many cases, a subsequent biopsy reveals adenocarcinoma but the primary site is not always clear.

Investigations

In this situation, there is a temptation to investigate the patient endlessly in order to determine the original primary site. However, there is a compromise between exhaustive investigation and obtaining sufficient information to plan appropriate management. For all patients, histological examination of an accessible site of metastasis is required. The architecture of the tissue can assist the pathologist in determining the likely primary site, and therefore it is better to perform a biopsy rather than fine needle aspiration. The greater volume of tissue also permits the use of immunohistochemistry. Extensive imaging to search for the primary is rarely indicated; a careful history to identify symptoms and risk factors (including familial) will often permit a judicious choice of imaging.

Management

Management of the patient will depend on that person's circumstances, as well as on the site(s) involved and the likely primary sites. The overriding principle is to ensure that a curable diagnosis has not been overlooked. For example, lung metastases from a testicular teratoma do not preclude cure; nor do one or two liver metastases from a colorectal cancer. Early discussion with an oncologist within a multidisciplinary team is essential and avoids unnecessary investigation; for example, a single hCG-based pregnancy test in a young man with lung metastases might confirm the presence of a teratoma and allow rapid administration of potentially curative chemotherapy. Treatment should not necessarily wait for a definitive diagnosis; appropriate analgesia, radiotherapy and surgical palliation can all be helpful. Some patients remain free of cancer for some years after resection of a single metastasis of an adenocarcinoma of unknown primary, justifying this approach in selected patients.

In those with no obvious primary, systemic chemotherapy may achieve some reduction in tumour burden and alleviation of symptoms, but long-term survival is rare.

Further information

Books and journal articles

Cannistra SA. Cancer of the ovary. N Engl J Med 2004; 351:2519–2529.

DeVita V, Hellman S, Rosenberg S. Cancer: principles and practice of oncology. 8th edn. Philadelphia: Lippincott Williams & Wilkins; 2008.

Dixon JM (ed.). ABC of breast diseases. 2nd edn. London: BMJ Books; 2001.

Forastiere A, Koch W, Trotti A, Sidransky D. Head and neck cancer. N Engl J Med 2001; 345:1890–1900.

Hanahan D, Weinberg RA. The hallmarks of cancer. Cell 2000; 100:57–70.

Websites

http://info.cancerresearchuk.org/cancerstats/ *A wide range of cancer statistics that can be sorted by type or geographical location.*

www.cancer.gov/cancerinformation/ *National Cancer Institute (NCI) with Cancernet.*

www.cancer.org *American Cancer Society; clinical practice guidelines.*

www.cebm.net *Centre for Evidence-Based Medicine.*

www.guideline.gov *National Guideline Clearinghouse.*

www.mondofacto.com/dictionary/ *An online medical dictionary of terminology.*

www.nice.org.uk *A location of the health technology assessments related to cancer services in the UK.*

www.who.int/research/en/

www.york.ac.uk/inst/crd/ *NHS Centre for Reviews and Dissemination.*

11

D. Oxenham

Pain management and palliative care

12

Palliative care is the active total care of patients with far advanced, rapidly progressive and ultimately fatal disease. Its focus is quality of life rather than cure, and it encompasses a distinct body of knowledge and skills that all good physicians must possess to allow them to care effectively for patients at the end of life. In palliative care, there is a fundamental change of emphasis in decision-making, with investigations and treatments kept appropriate to the stage of the patient's disease and the prognosis. The principles of palliative care may be applied not only to cancer but to any chronic disease state. In this chapter, the management of cancer and non-malignant pain control are described, along with other issues in palliative care.

PAIN

The International Association for the Study of Pain (IASP) has defined pain as 'an unpleasant sensory and emotional experience associated with actual or potential tissue damage or described in terms of such damage'. It follows that severity of pain does not correlate with the degree of tissue damage, and that each patient's experience and expression of pain are different. Effective pain treatment facilitates recovery from injury or surgery, aids rapid recovery of function, and may minimise chronic pain and disability. Unfortunately, obstacles to the delivery of good pain relief may include poor assessment and concerns about the use of opioid analgesia.

Pain classification and mechanisms

Pain can be classified into two types:
- *nociceptive*: due to direct stimulation of peripheral nerve endings (e.g. wounds, fractures, burns, angina)
- *neuropathic*: due to dysfunction of the pain perception system within the peripheral or central nervous system as a result of injury, disease or surgical damage (e.g. continuing pain experienced from a limb which has been amputated—'phantom limb pain'). This should be identified early (Box 12.1) because it is more difficult to treat once established.

The pain perception system is described on page 1140. There is considerable plasticity (changeability) in all the peripheral and central components of the pain pathway. It is not therefore a simple hard-wired circuit of nerves connecting tissue pain receptors to the brain, but a dynamic system in which a continuing pain stimulus can cause central changes that lead to an increase in pain

perception. Early and appropriate treatment of pain reduces the potential for these changes to develop.

Assessment and measurement of pain

Accurate assessment of the patient is the first step in providing good analgesia.

History and measurement of pain

A full pain history should be taken, to establish its causes and the underlying diagnoses. Patients may have more than one pain; for example, bone and neuropathic pain may arise from skeletal metastases (Box 12.2).

A diagram of the body on which the patient can mark the pain site can be helpful. When patients are asked to score pain, they consistently rate it higher than their physicians and nurses, so if they are able, they should always be asked to rate it. Methods include:
- *Verbal rating scale*. Different verbal descriptions are used to rate pain—'no pain', 'mild pain', 'moderate pain' and 'severe pain'.
- *11-point scale*. A question is used, such as 'Over the past 24 hours, how would you rate your pain, if 0 is no pain and 10 is the worst pain you could imagine?'
- *Behavioural rating scale*. It can be particularly difficult to decide whether a patient with cognitive impairment is suffering pain. A variety of measures are available which assess how a patient is behaving to estimate whether he or she has pain, e.g. agitation, withdrawn posture. Changes in behavioural rating pain scores can indicate whether drug measures have been successful.

Regular recording of formal pain assessment and patient-rated pain scores improves pain management and reduces the time taken to achieve pain control.

Psychological aspects of chronic pain

Perception of pain is influenced by many factors other than the painful stimulus, and pain cannot therefore be easily classified as wholly physical or psychogenic in any individual (Fig. 12.1). Patients who suffer chronic pain will be affected emotionally and, conversely, emotional distress can exacerbate physical pain (p. 238). Full assessment for symptoms of anxiety and depression is fundamental to effective pain management.

Examination

This should include careful assessment of the painful area, looking for signs of neuropathic pain (see Box 12.1) or bony tenderness suggestive of bone metastases. In patients with cancer, it should not be assumed that all pains are due to the cancer or its metastases.

Appropriate investigations

Investigations should be directed towards diagnosis of an underlying cause, remembering that reversible causes are possible even in patients with terminal cancer. Imaging may be indicated, such as plain X-ray for fracture or magnetic resonance imaging (MRI) for spinal cord compression.

12.1 Features of neuropathic pain

- Burning, stabbing or pulsing pain
- Spontaneous pain, without ongoing tissue damage
- Pain in an area of sensory loss
- The presence of a major neurological deficit (e.g. spinal cord trauma)
- Pain in response to non-painful stimuli: 'allodynia'
- Increased pain in response to painful stimuli: 'hyperalgesia'
- Unpleasant abnormal sensations: 'dysaesthesias'
- Poor relief from opioids alone

12.2 Types of pain

Type of pain	Features	Management options
Bone pain	Tender area over bone Possible pain on movement	Non-steroidal anti-inflammatory drugs (NSAIDs) Bisphosphonates Radiotherapy
Increased intracranial pressure	Headache, worse in the morning, associated with vomiting and occasionally confusion	Corticosteroids Radiotherapy Codeine
Abdominal colic	Intermittent severe spasmodic, associated with nausea or vomiting	Antispasmodics, e.g. hyoscine butylbromide
Liver capsule pain	Right upper quadrant abdominal pain, often associated with tender enlarged liver	Corticosteroids (Poor relief with opioids)
Neuropathic pain	See Box 12.1	Anticonvulsants, e.g. gabapentin, valproate Antidepressants, e.g. amitriptyline Ketamine
Ischaemic pain	Diffuse severe aching pain associated with evidence of poor perfusion	Poorly responsive to opioids NSAIDs Ketamine
Incident pain	Episodic pain usually related to movement or bowel spasm	Intermittent short-acting opioids Nerve block

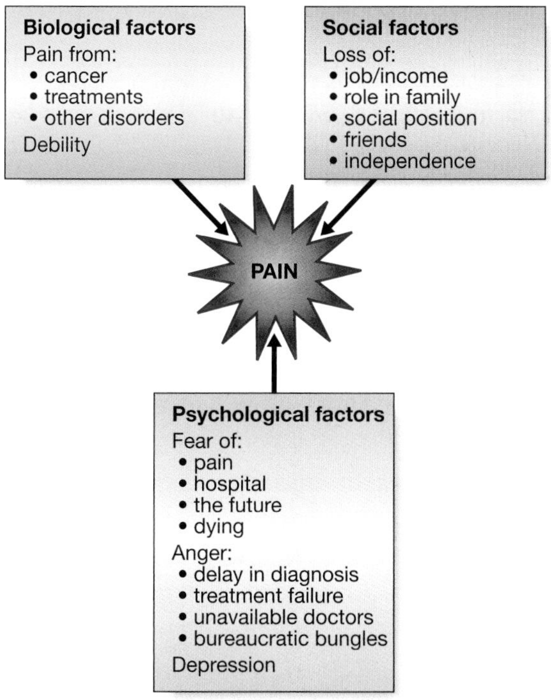

Fig. 12.1 Components of pain.

Management of pain

Many of the principles of pain management apply to any painful condition. Some interventions, such as strong opioids, have (or are perceived to have) a greater potential for harm in patients with a good prognosis. Acute pain post-surgery or following trauma should be controlled with medication without causing unnecessary side-effects or risk to the patient (Fig. 12.2). Chronic, non-malignant pain is more difficult and it may be impossible to relieve pain completely. There is a greater emphasis on non-pharmacological treatments and on enabling the patient to cope with pain. Strong opioids may help chronic pain but need to be used with caution after full assessment.

Two-thirds of patients with cancer experience moderate or severe pain, and a quarter will have three or more different pains. Many of these are of mixed aetiology and 50% of pain from cancer has a neuropathic element. Careful evaluation to identify the likely pain mechanism facilitates appropriate treatment (see Box 12.2). It is vital that the patient's concerns about opioids are explored and reassurance given that, when they are used for pain, psychological dependence and tolerance are not a concern (Box 12.3).

12.3 Opioid myths

Myth	Fact
Pain is inevitable in cancer and many other diseases	**Pain can usually be controlled**
Opioids should be avoided because of dangerous side-effects	**Opioids can cause side-effects and sometimes the therapeutic window is narrow. However, side-effects are treatable and reversible**
The use of opioids commonly leads to addiction	**Addiction is very rare in patients who have pain and no previous history of addiction**
Taking opioids leads to more rapid decline and earlier death	**Opioids do not cause organ damage or serious harm. NSAIDs and paracetamol are more likely to cause irreversible damage**

281

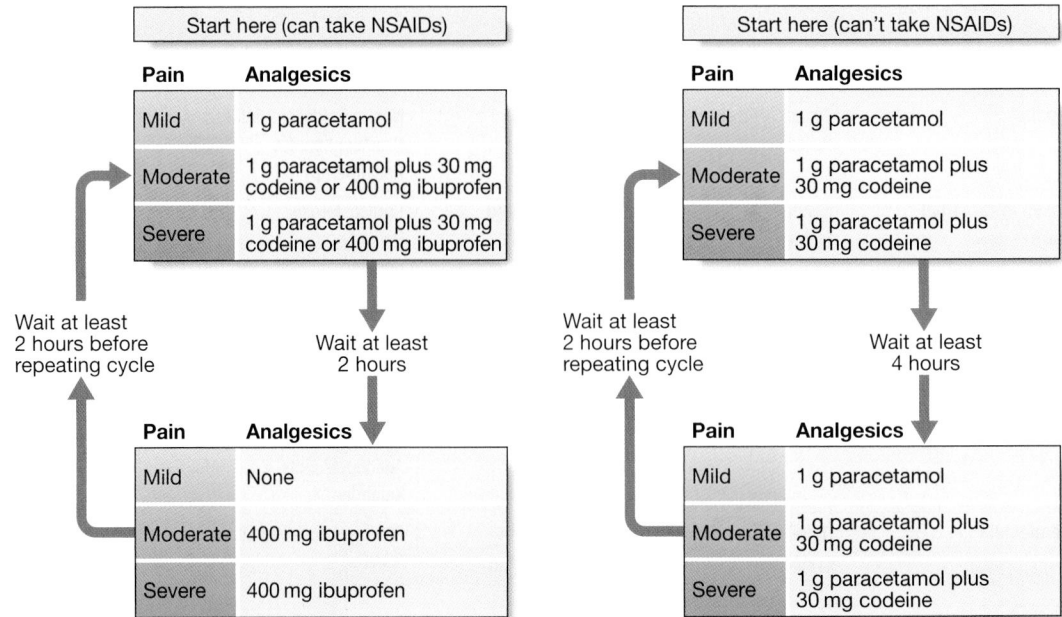

Fig. 12.2 Acute pain management. NSAIDs cannot be taken by those with renal impairment or peptic ulceration. This includes many older people.

Nearly all types of pain respond to morphine to some degree. Some are completely opioid-responsive but others, e.g. neuropathic and ischaemic pains, are relatively unresponsive. Opioid-unresponsive or poorly responsive pain will only be relieved by opioids at a dose which causes significant side-effects. In this situation, effective pain relief can only be achieved with the use of adjuvant analgesics (see below).

Pharmacological treatments
The WHO analgesic ladder
The basic principle of the WHO ladder (Fig. 12.3) is that analgesia which is appropriate for the degree of pain should be prescribed and the dose increased until pain is controlled. If pain is severe or remains poorly controlled, strong opioids should be prescribed.

A patient with mild pain is started on a non-opioid analgesic drug, e.g. paracetamol 1 g 6-hourly (step 1). If the maximum recommended dose is not sufficient or the patient has moderate pain, a weak opioid, e.g. codeine 60 mg 6-hourly, is added (step 2). If adequate pain relief is still not achieved with the maximum recommended dosages or if the patient has severe pain, a strong opioid is substituted for the weak opioid (step 3). It is important not to move 'sideways' (change from one drug to another of equal potency) on a particular step of the ladder. All patients with severe pain should receive a full trial of strong opioids with appropriate adjuvant analgesia, as described below.

Non-opioids
• *Paracetamol.* This is often effective for mild to moderate pain. For severe pain, it is inadequate alone, but remains a useful and well-tolerated adjunct.

• *NSAIDs.* These are effective in the treatment of mild to moderate pain, and are also useful adjuncts in the treatment of severe pain. Adverse effects may be serious, especially in the elderly (p. 173).

Weak opioids
Codeine and dihydrocodeine are weak opioids. They have lower analgesic efficacy than strong opioids and a ceiling dose. They are effective for mild to moderate pain.

Strong opioids
Immediate-release (IR) oral morphine takes about 20 minutes to have an effect and usually provides pain relief for 4 hours. Most patients with continuous pain

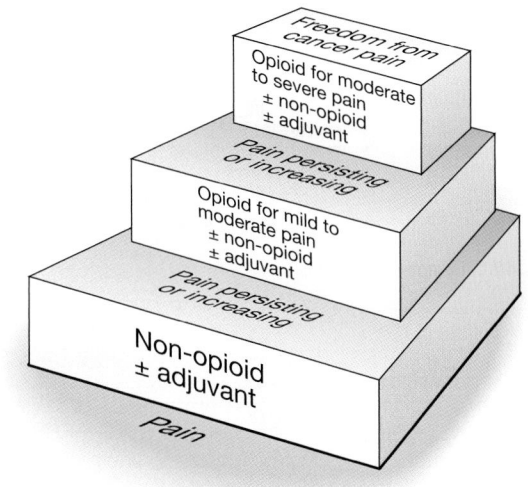

Fig. 12.3 The WHO analgesic ladder.

should be prescribed IR oral morphine every 4 hours (i.e. six times daily) initially, which will provide continuous pain relief over the whole 24-hour period. Controlled-release (CR) morphine lasts for 12 or 24 hours but takes much longer to take effect. It should only be used once the correct dose has been found through dose titration with IR morphine until adequate pain relief is achieved.

In addition to the regular dose, an extra dose of IR morphine should be prescribed 'as required' for when the patient has pain that is not controlled by the regular prescription ('breakthrough' pain). This should be the same as the regular 4-hourly dose. The frequency of breakthrough doses should be dictated by their efficacy and any side-effects, rather than by a fixed time interval. A patient may require breakthrough analgesia hourly if pain is severe, but this should lead to early review of the regular prescription. The patient and/or carer should note the timing of any breakthrough doses and the reason for them. These should be reviewed daily and the regular 4-hourly dose increased for the next 24 hours on the basis of:

- frequency of and reasons for breakthrough analgesia
- degree and acceptability of side-effects.

The regular 24-hour dose should then be increased by adding on the total of the breakthrough doses over the previous 24 hours, unless there are significant problems with unacceptable side-effects. When the correct dose has been established, a CR preparation can be prescribed, usually twice daily.

World-wide, the most effective and appropriate route of administration is oral, though transdermal preparations of strong opioids (usually fentanyl) are extremely useful in certain situations (e.g. patients with dysphagia or reluctance to take regular tablets). Diamorphine is a highly soluble strong opioid used for subcutaneous infusions, particularly in the last few days of life, but is only available in certain countries.

Common side-effects of opioids are shown in Box 12.4. Nausea and vomiting occur initially but usually settle after a few days. Confusion and drowsiness are dose-related and reversible. In acute dosing, respiratory depression can occur but this is rare in those on regular opioids.

Opioid toxicity

All patients will develop dose-related side-effects such as nausea, drowsiness, confusion or myoclonus at some point; the dose at which this occurs varies from 10 to 5000 mg of morphine, depending on the patient and the type of pain. This is termed opioid toxicity, and is managed by reducing the dose and returning to IR morphine so that dose adjustments can be made rapidly. Parenteral rehydration may be necessary. Pain should be reassessed to ensure that appropriate adjuvants are being used, and switching to an alternative strong opioid may be helpful. These include oxycodone, transdermal fentanyl, alfentanyl, hydromorphone and occasionally methadone, any of which may produce a better balance of benefit against side-effects. Fentanyl and alfentanyl have no renally excreted active metabolites and may be particularly useful in patients with renal failure. Pethidine is used in acute pain management but not for chronic or cancer pain because of its short half-life and ceiling dose.

Adjuvant analgesics

An adjuvant analgesic is a drug with a primary indication other than pain but which is analgesic in some painful conditions and may enhance the effect of primary analgesia. At each step of the WHO analgesic ladder, an adjuvant analgesic should be considered, the choice depending on the type of pain (Boxes 12.5 and 12.6).

> **EBM 12.5 Treatment of neuropathic pain**
>
> 'Tricyclic antidepressants, a variety of anticonvulsants, and gabapentin are effective treatments for neuropathic pain.'
>
> • Guideline 106. Scottish Intercollegiate Guidelines Network; 2008.
>
> For further information: www.sign.ac.uk

Non-pharmacological and complementary treatments

Radiotherapy

Radiotherapy has a place in the management of bone metastases (see Box 12.2).

Physiotherapy

This helps to alleviate pain and restore function, through active mobilisation and specific physiotherapy techniques such as spinal manipulation, massage, application of heat or cold, and exercise. Immediate cold application (e.g. ice packs) reduces subsequent swelling and inflammation after sports injury.

Psychological techniques

These include simple relaxation, hypnosis, cognitive behavioural therapies and biofeedback (pp. 239–240), which train the patient to use coping strategies and behavioural techniques. This is more relevant in chronic non-malignant pain than in cancer pain.

12.4 Opioid side-effects

Side-effect	Management
Constipation	Regular laxative, e.g. co-danthramer or co-danthrusate (starting dose 2 capsules daily and titrate as needed)
Dry mouth	Frequent sips of iced water, soft white paraffin to lips, chlorhexidine mouthwashes 12-hourly, sugar-free gum, water or saliva sprays
Nausea/vomiting	Haloperidol 1.5–3 mg nocte or metoclopramide/domperidone 10 mg 8-hourly. If constant, a parenteral antiemetic is necessary to break the nausea cycle
Sedation	Explanation very important. Usually settles in 2–3 days. Avoid other sedating medication where possible. Ensure appropriate use of adjuvant analgesics which can have an opioid-sparing effect

12.6 Adjuvant analgesics

Drug	Dosage	Indications	Side-effects*
NSAIDs (e.g. diclofenac)	50 mg oral 8-hourly (SR 75 mg 12-hourly) 100 mg per rectum once a day	Bone metastases, soft tissue infiltration, liver pain, inflammatory pain	Gastric irritation and bleeding, fluid retention, headache; caution in renal impairment
Corticosteroids (e.g. dexamethasone)	8–16 mg per day (titrate down to lowest dose which controls pain)	Raised intracranial pressure, nerve compression, soft tissue infiltration, liver pain	Gastric irritation if used together with NSAID, fluid retention, confusion, Cushingoid appearance, candidiasis, hyperglycaemia
Gabapentin	100–300 mg nocte (starting dose; titrate to 600 mg 8-hourly)	Neuropathic pain of any aetiology	Mild sedation, tremor, confusion
Carbamazepine (evidence for all anticonvulsants)	100–200 mg nocte (starting dose)	Neuropathic pain of any aetiology	Vertigo, sedation, constipation, rash
Amitriptyline (evidence for all tricyclics)	25 mg nocte (starting dose) 10 mg (elderly)	Neuropathic pain of any aetiology	Sedation, dizziness, confusion, dry mouth, constipation, urinary retention; avoid in cardiac disease
Ketamine	10–60 mg 6-hourly	Severe neuropathic pain (only under specialist supervision)	Confusion, anxiety, agitation, hypertension

*In old age, all drugs can cause confusion.

Stimulation therapies

Acupuncture (Fig. 12.4) has been used successfully in Eastern medicine for centuries. It causes release of endogenous analgesics (endorphins) within the spinal cord. Transcutaneous electrical nerve stimulation (TENS) may have a similar mechanism of action to acupuncture and can be used in both acute and chronic pain.

Herbal medicine and homeopathy

These are widely used for pain, but often with little evidence for efficacy (p. 15). Safety regulations for these treatments are limited compared with conventional drugs, and the doctor should be wary of unrecognised side-effects which may result.

PALLIATIVE CARE

There is a growing recognition that the principles of, and some specific interventions developed in the palliative care of patients with cancer are equally applicable to other conditions. The challenge is recognising when patients have entered this phase of their illness, as there are fewer clear markers and the course of the illness is much more variable. Different chronic disease states progress at different rates, allowing some general trajectories of illness or dying to be defined (Fig. 12.5). Traditionally, palliative care has been associated with cancer because the latter is typified by a progressive decline in function which is more predictable than

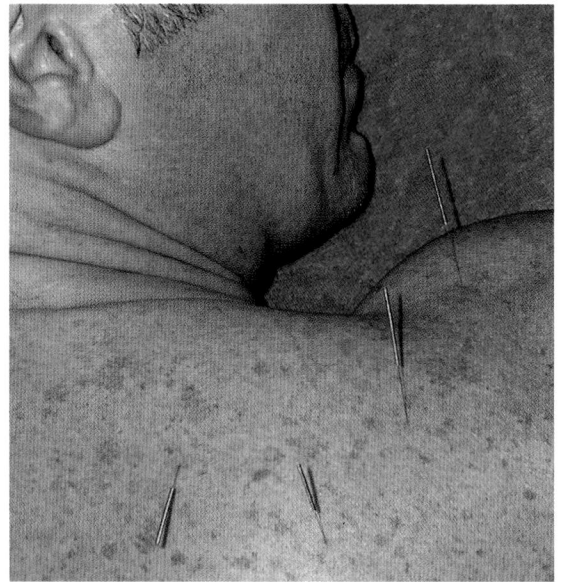

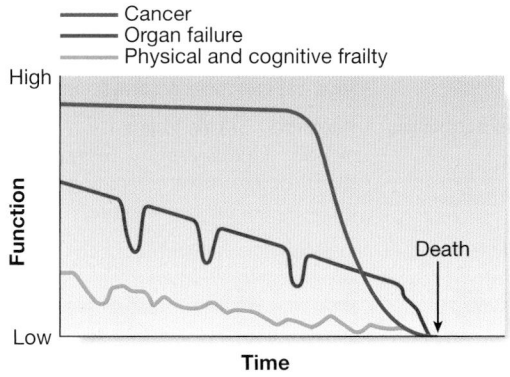

Fig. 12.4 Acupuncture.

Fig. 12.5 Archetypal trajectories of dying.

in many other disease states, but provision of palliative care should be on the basis of need rather than diagnosis. It is relatively easy to provide palliative care to patients with illnesses other than cancer which fit this progressively deteriorating trajectory of dying: for example, motor neuron disease, or AIDS where highly active antiretroviral therapy (HAART) is not available.

Many chronic diseases other than cancer carry as high a burden of symptoms, as well as psychological and family distress. The 'palliative phase' of these illnesses (e.g. chronic obstructive pulmonary disease (COPD) or heart failure) may be more difficult to identify because of periods of relative stability interspersed with acute episodes of severe illness. However, it is still possible to recognise those patients who are close to the end of their lives and to adjust their treatment accordingly. The challenge is that symptom management needs to be delivered at the same time as treatment for acute exacerbations. This leads to difficult decisions as to the balance between symptom relief and aggressive management of the underlying disease.

The third major trajectory is categorised by years of very poor function and frailty before a relatively short terminal period, and is exemplified by dementia. As medical advances extend survival, this mode of dying is being experienced by increasing numbers. The main challenge lies in providing nursing care and ensuring that plans are agreed for the time when medical intervention is no longer beneficial.

Clearly, many of the principles of palliative care are applicable to all these disease states. Breathlessness from any cause can be alleviated, even when there is no reversible 'cause', appropriate drugs can be prescribed for nausea, and any predicted death can be managed effectively and compassionately.

Presenting problems in palliative care

Breathlessness

The sensation of breathlessness is the result of a complex interaction between different factors at the levels of production (the pathophysiological cause), perception (the severity of breathlessness perceived by the patient) and expression (the symptoms expressed by an individual patient). Perception and expression of breathlessness can be significantly improved, even if there is no reversible 'cause' (Box 12.7). Assessment and treatment should therefore be targeted at modifying this, particularly when there is no reversible pathophysiology.

Clearly reversible causes of breathlessness (p. 654) should be identified and managed, but investigation and treatment should be appropriate to the prognosis and stage of disease. A therapeutic trial of corticosteroids (dexamethasone 8 mg for 5 days) and/or nebulised salbutamol may be helpful.

EBM 12.7 **Palliative treatment of breathlessness**

'Interventions based on psychosocial support, breathing control and coping strategies can help patients to cope with the symptom of breathlessness and reduce physical and emotional distress.'

• Bredin M, et al. BMJ 1999; 318:901.

Perception of breathlessness may be affected by specific anxieties and beliefs about breathlessness, which should be explored. For patients with advanced disease, a common fear is that they will die during an attack of breathlessness. Although this is understandable, reassurance can be given that it is unlikely. Another frequently expressed fear is that breathlessness will continue to worsen until it is continuous and unbearable, leading to a distressing and undignified death. Reassurance should again be given that this is uncommon and can be effectively managed with opioids and benzodiazepines.

Some patients have specific panic–breathlessness cycles in which breathlessness leads to panic, which leads to worsening breathlessness and worsening panic. These should be identified and explained to the patient. A rapidly acting benzodiazepine such as sublingual lorazepam or non-drug measures such as relaxation techniques may help. Discussion with a physiotherapist about energy conservation and pacing of activity may also be useful.

Perception of breathlessness may also be improved by night-time or regular morphine, or by regular benzodiazepines. Oxygen may be no more effective than a fan or piped air for non-hypoxic breathlessness, and again the patient's perception of the need for oxygen can be gently explored and modified.

Cough

Intractable cough is a difficult symptom to manage. There are many causes (p. 652) in cancer and other intractable illnesses, e.g. motor neuron disease, cardiac failure and COPD. The underlying condition should be specifically treated. Antitussives, such as codeine linctus, are sometimes effective, particularly for cough at night.

Nausea and vomiting

Different causes of nausea and vomiting (p. 852) are associated with different clinical presentations. Large-volume vomiting with little nausea is common in intestinal obstruction, whereas constant nausea with little or no vomiting is often due to metabolic abnormalities or drugs. Vomiting related to raised intracranial pressure is worse in the morning.

Different receptors are activated, depending on the cause or causes of the nausea (Fig. 12.6). For example, dopamine receptors in the chemotactic trigger zone in the fourth ventricle are stimulated by metabolic and drug causes of nausea, whereas gastric irritation stimulates histamine receptors in the vomiting centre via the vagus nerve.

Reversible causes (e.g. hypercalcaemia, constipation) should be treated appropriately. Potential drug culprits should be considered and stopped if possible. As different classes of antiemetic drug act at different receptors, antiemetic therapy should be based on a careful assessment of the probable causes and a rational decision to use a particular class of drug (Box 12.8). The subcutaneous route is often required initially to overcome gastric stasis and poor absorption of oral medicines.

Gastrointestinal obstruction

Gastrointestinal obstruction is a frequent complication of intra-abdominal cancer. Patients may have multiple levels of obstruction and symptoms may vary greatly in nature and severity. Surgical mortality is high in patients

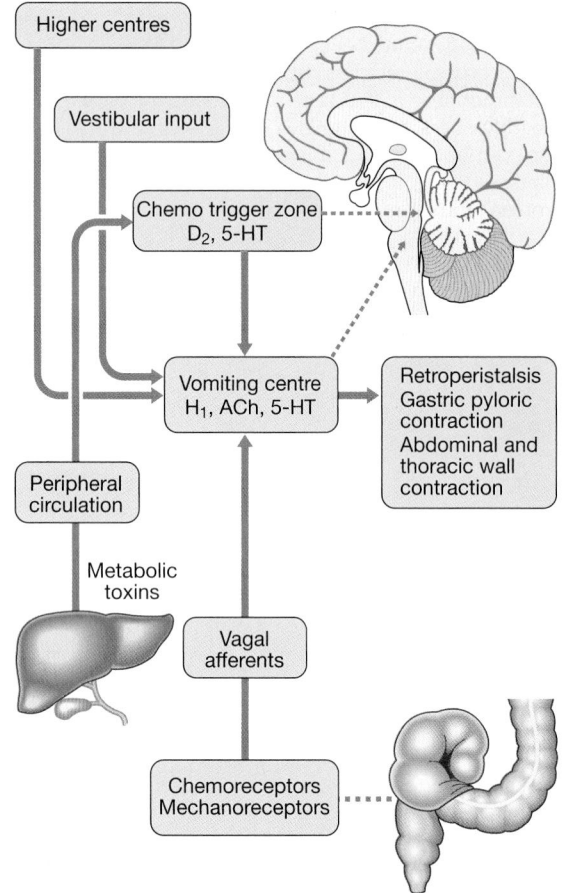

Fig. 12.6 Mechanisms of nausea. (ACh = acetylcholine; D_2 = dopamine; 5-HT = 5-hydroxytryptamine, serotonin; H_1 = histamine)

12.8 Receptor site activity of antiemetic drugs

Area	Receptors	Drugs
Chemo trigger zone	Dopamine₂ 5-HT	Haloperidol Metoclopramide
Vomiting centre	Histamine₁ Acetylcholine	Cyclizine Levomepromazine Hyoscine
Gut (gastric stasis)		Metoclopramide
Gut distension (vagal stimulation)	Histamine₁	Cyclizine
Gut (chemoreceptors)	5-HT	Levomepromazine

with advanced disease and obstruction may be effectively managed without surgery.

The key to effective management is to address the presenting symptoms—colic, abdominal pain, nausea, vomiting, intestinal secretions—individually or in combination, using drugs which do not cause or worsen other symptoms. Colic responds well to anticholinergic agents such as hyoscine butylbromide, and somatostatin analogues such as octreotide will reduce intestinal secretions and therefore large-volume vomits. Nausea will improve with metoclopramide, although this is contraindicated in the presence of colic because of its prokinetic effect. Cyclizine will improve nausea but may reduce gut motility. There is some evidence that corticosteroids (dexamethasone 8 mg) shorten the length of obstructive episodes.

Weight loss and general weakness

Patients with cancer lose weight due to an alteration of metabolism by the tumour known as the cancer cachexia syndrome. NSAIDs and megestrol may be helpful in early-stage disease but are unlikely to be effective in advanced cancer. Corticosteroids can temporarily boost appetite and general well-being, but may cause false weight gain by promoting fluid retention. Their benefits in this situation need to be carefully weighed against the risk of side-effects.

Anxiety and depression

Even in patients with far advanced disease, anxiety and depression may still respond to treatment with a combination of drugs and psychotherapeutic approaches (p. 242). It should not be assumed that depression is 'understandable' because of an unpleasant physical symptom and therefore has no solution other than removing the symptom. It may improve with specific treatment, even if the underlying physical problem remains.

Delirium and terminal agitation

Many patients become confused or agitated in the last days of life. It is important to identify and treat potentially reversible causes (pp. 171 and 248), unless the patient is too close to death for this to be feasible. Effective management of any distressing confusion is extremely important. Patients should be prescribed a neuroleptic agent (haloperidol) for confusion and adequate doses of benzodiazepines (diazepam or midazolam) to relieve distress. If there is profound distress, large doses of benzodiazepines can be used. Opioids are not useful.

THE DYING PHASE

Talking about dying

Talking about dying is difficult for health professionals, as they may feel a sense of failure or a fear of causing distress and loss of hope. Some patients have a great fear of death and never wish to discuss the possibility; others welcome the chance to talk about death and the dying process, express their wishes and gain reassurance that these will be respected. In general, people wish for a dignified and peaceful death. Most people prefer to die at home and early discussion allows this to be planned. Families also are grateful for the chance to prepare themselves for the death of a relative, by timely and gentle discussion with their doctor or other health professionals.

Diagnosing dying

There comes a time when death is predictable and inevitable, and when further active intervention will be futile and will cause distress rather than benefit. At least two-thirds of patients dying in hospital have a death that is predictable, and measures should be taken to plan good care for the patient and family.

When patients with cancer become bed-bound, semi-comatose, unable to take tablets and only able to take sips of water, they are likely to be dying and many will have died within 2 days. Patients with other conditions also reach a stage where death is predictable and imminent. Doctors are sometimes poor at recognising this, and should be alert to the views of other members of the multidisciplinary team. A clear decision that the patient is dying should be agreed and recorded.

Management

Once a decision has been reached, there is a significant shift in management. Symptom control, relief of distress and care for the family are the most important elements of care (Box 12.9). Medication and investigation are only justifiable if they contribute to these ends. When patients can no longer drink because they are dying, intravenous fluids are not necessary and may cause worsening of bronchial secretions. Medicines should always be prescribed for the relief of pain (e.g. morphine or diamorphine), nausea (e.g. levomepromazine), confusion (e.g. haloperidol), distress (e.g. diazepam or midazolam) and respiratory secretions (e.g. hyoscine hydrobromide). If these cause side-effects, such as drowsiness, it is reasonable to continue them none the less, if the principal aim of relieving distress is achieved.

Ethical issues at the end of life

In Europe, between 25 and 50% of all deaths are associated with some form of decision which may affect the length of a patient's life. The most common form of decision involves withdrawing or withholding further treatment: for example, not treating a chest infection in a patient who is clearly dying from advanced cancer. Occasionally, medicines are given which shorten a patient's life utilising the principle of double effect (see below). It is important to have a framework for considering such decisions (such as the four ethical principles: autonomy, beneficence, non-maleficence and justice, p. 10), which balances degrees of importance when there is conflict: for example, when a patient wishes to

12.9 Checklist for the dying phase

- Stop non-essential medication (i.e. that does not contribute to symptom control)
- Stop inappropriate investigations and interventions (e.g. parenteral fluids)
- Complete Do Not Attempt Resuscitation (DNAR) form
- Stop routine observations
- Ensure availability of parenteral medication for symptom relief
- Assess patient and family's awareness of condition
- Assess religious and spiritual needs
- Ensure family understands plan of care and provide ongoing support
- Ensure continued assessment and management of symptoms
- Arrange appropriate care after death

receive treatment which a doctor judges to be harmful or which is illegal. A decision has to be taken as to which principle is most important. Is it better to respect a patient's wishes even if it causes harm, or to prevent harm by not respecting them?

A futile treatment is one which has no chance of achieving worthwhile benefit, i.e. it cannot achieve a result that the patient would consider, now or in the future, to be worthwhile. Doctors are not required to institute a futile treatment, such as resuscitation in the event of cardiac arrest in a patient with terminal cancer.

Incapacity and advance directives

Patients' wishes are very important in Western countries, although this is not true in all cultures. If a patient is unable to express his or her view because of communication or cognitive impairment, that person lacks 'capacity'. In order to decide what the patient would have wished, as much information as possible should be gained about any previously expressed wishes, along with the views of relatives and other health professionals. An advance directive is a previously recorded, written document of a patient's wishes (p. 169). It should carry the same weight in decision-making as a patient's contemporaneously expressed wishes, but may not be sufficiently specific to be used in a particular clinical situation.

Rehydration

Deciding whether to give intravenous fluids can be difficult when a patient is very unwell and the prognosis is uncertain. If a patient is clearly dying and has a prognosis of a few days, rehydration may cause harm by increasing bronchial secretions, and will not benefit the patient by prolonging life or relieving symptoms. A patient with a major stroke, who is unable to swallow but expected to survive the event, will develop renal impairment and thirst if not given fluids and should be hydrated, unless this is considered futile.

Double effect

At the end of life, the principle of double effect allows symptom control to be given to patients, even though it may shorten their life, provided the 'good' effect (control of symptoms) outweighs the 'bad' effect (shortening of life), and there is no other means to achieve the same result. The intention must be to control symptoms rather than shorten life and no more medication should be given than achieves symptom control.

Euthanasia

In the UK and Europe between 3 and 6% of dying patients ask a doctor to end their life. Many of these requests are transient; some are associated with poor control of physical symptoms or a depressive illness. All expressions of a wish to die are an opportunity to help the patient discuss and address unresolved issues and problems.

Reversible causes, such as pain or depression, should be treated. Sometimes patients may choose to discontinue life-prolonging treatments, such as angiotensin-converting enzyme (ACE) inhibitors or anticoagulation, following discussion and the provision of adequate alternative symptom control. However, there remain a small number of patients who have a sustained, competent wish to end their lives, despite good control of physical symptoms. Public ethical and legal debate over this issue is likely to continue.

12

Further information

www.anaesthetist.com/ *Information on pain physiology and acute management of pain.*

www.helpthehospices.org.uk/elearning/clip/index.htm *Useful online tutorials on all aspects of palliative symptom control.*

www.mcpcil.org.uk/liverpool_care_pathway *Further information on end-of-life care pathways.*

www.palliativedrugs.co.uk *Information for health professionals about the use of drugs in palliative care. It highlights drugs given for unlicensed indications or by unlicensed routes, and the administration of multiple drugs by continuous subcutaneous infusion.*

D.H. Dockrell
S. Sundar
B.J. Angus
R.P. Hobson

Infectious disease

13

CLINICAL EXAMINATION OF PATIENTS WITH INFECTIOUS DISEASE

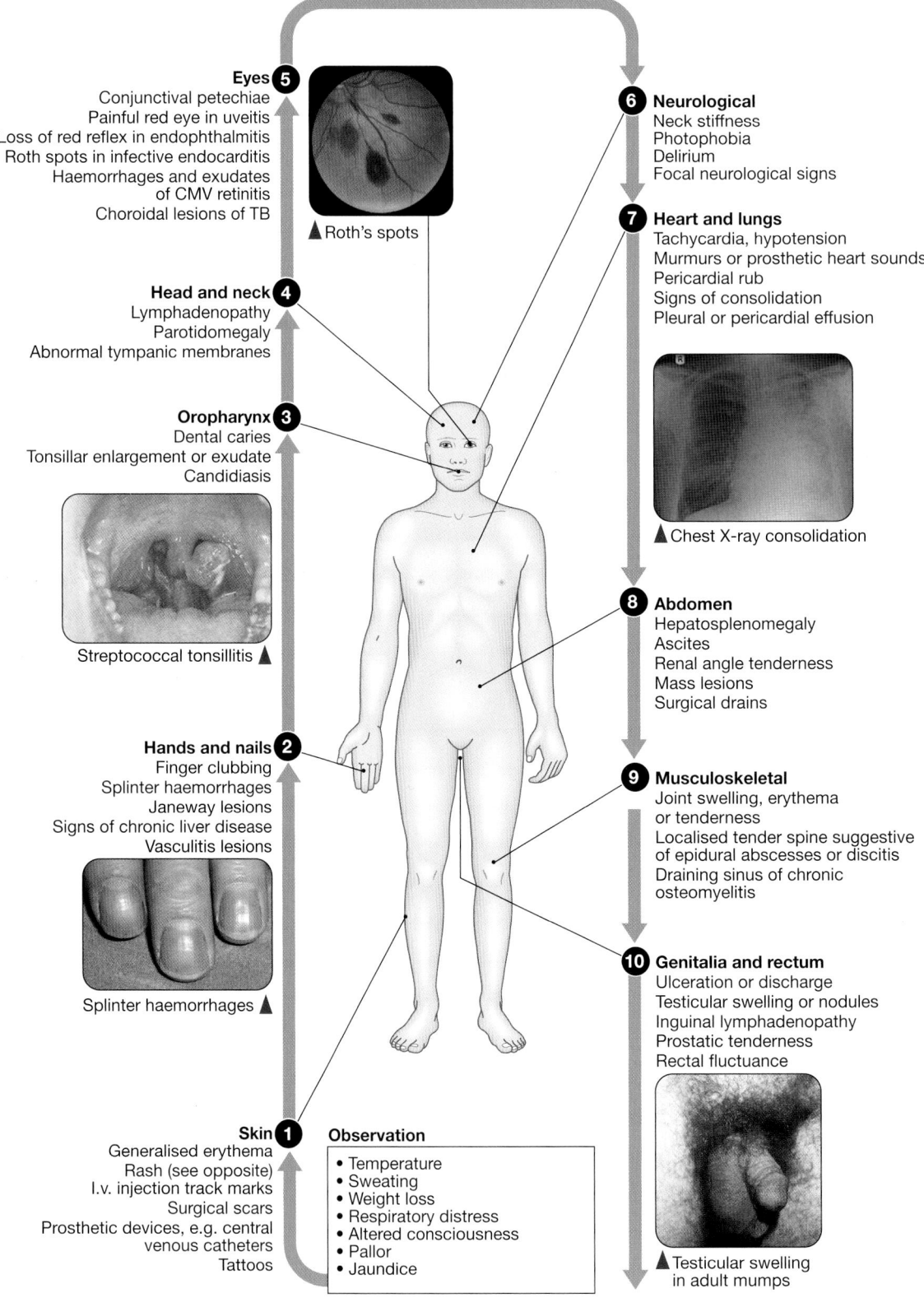

Eyes 5
Conjunctival petechiae
Painful red eye in uveitis
Loss of red reflex in endophthalmitis
Roth spots in infective endocarditis
Haemorrhages and exudates
of CMV retinitis
Choroidal lesions of TB

▲ Roth's spots

4 Head and neck
Lymphadenopathy
Parotidomegaly
Abnormal tympanic membranes

Oropharynx 3
Dental caries
Tonsillar enlargement or exudate
Candidiasis

Streptococcal tonsillitis ▲

Hands and nails 2
Finger clubbing
Splinter haemorrhages
Janeway lesions
Signs of chronic liver disease
Vasculitis lesions

Splinter haemorrhages ▲

Skin 1
Generalised erythema
Rash (see opposite)
I.v. injection track marks
Surgical scars
Prosthetic devices, e.g. central
venous catheters
Tattoos

Observation
• Temperature
• Sweating
• Weight loss
• Respiratory distress
• Altered consciousness
• Pallor
• Jaundice

6 Neurological
Neck stiffness
Photophobia
Delirium
Focal neurological signs

7 Heart and lungs
Tachycardia, hypotension
Murmurs or prosthetic heart sounds
Pericardial rub
Signs of consolidation
Pleural or pericardial effusion

▲ Chest X-ray consolidation

8 Abdomen
Hepatosplenomegaly
Ascites
Renal angle tenderness
Mass lesions
Surgical drains

9 Musculoskeletal
Joint swelling, erythema
or tenderness
Localised tender spine suggestive
of epidural abscesses or discitis
Draining sinus of chronic
osteomyelitis

10 Genitalia and rectum
Ulceration or discharge
Testicular swelling or nodules
Inguinal lymphadenopathy
Prostatic tenderness
Rectal fluctuance

▲ Testicular swelling
in adult mumps

Fever

- *Documentation of fever.* 'Feeling hot' or sweaty is not synonymous with fever. Body temperature must be documented: > 38.0°C is a fever. Axillary and aural measurement is less accurate than oral or rectal. Outpatients may be trained to keep a temperature chart.
- *Rigors.* Shivering (followed by excessive sweating) implies a rapid rise in body temperature but rarely gives a clue to aetiology.
- *Night sweats.* These are characteristic of several infections (e.g. tuberculosis (TB), infective endocarditis), but sweating from any cause is worse at night.
- *Excessive sweating.* Alcohol, anxiety, thyrotoxicosis, diabetes mellitus, acromegaly, lymphoma and excessive environmental heat all cause sweating without temperature elevation.
- *Recurrent fever.* There are various causes of recurrent fever, e.g. *Borrelia recurrentis*, bacterial abscess.
- *Accompanying features*
  Headache. Severe headache and photophobia, although characteristic of meningitis, may accompany other infections.
  Delirium. Mental confusion during fever is more common in young children or the elderly.
  Muscle pain. Myalgia may occur with viral infections, such as influenza, and with septicaemia including meningococcal sepsis.
  Shock. Shock may accompany severe infections and sepsis (Ch. 8).

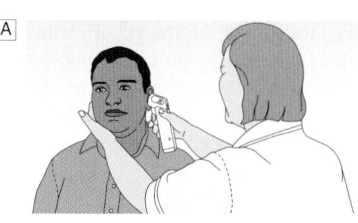
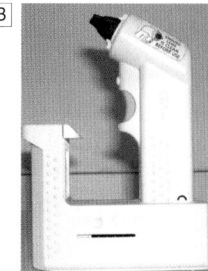

Documentation of temperature.
A Body temperature should be accurately recorded.
B Hand-held tympanic thermometer.

History-taking in suspected infectious disease (ID)*

Presenting complaint

- Diverse manifestations of ID make accurate assessment of features and duration critical; e.g. fever and cough lasting for 2 days imply an acute respiratory tract infection and for 2 months suggest TB

Review of systems

- Must be comprehensive

Past medical history

- Define the 'host' and likelihood of infection(s)
- Include surgical and dental procedures involving prosthetic materials
- Document previous infections

Medication history

- Include non-prescription drugs, use of antimicrobials and immunosuppressive drugs

Allergy history

- Especially to antimicrobials, noting the allergic manifestation (e.g. rash versus anaphylaxis)

Family and contact history

- Note infections and their time course
- Sensitively explore exposure to key infections, e.g. TB and human immunodeficiency virus (HIV)-1

Travel history

- Include countries visited and where previously resident (relevant to exposure and likely vaccination)

Occupation

- e.g. Anthrax in leather tannery workers

Recreational pursuits

- e.g. Leptospirosis in windsurfers

Animal exposures

- Include pets, e.g. dog exposure and hydatid disease

Dietary history

- Consider undercooked meats, shellfish, unpasteurised dairy products or well water

- Establish who else was exposed, e.g. to potential food-borne diarrhoea

History of intravenous drug injection or receipt of blood products

- Risks for blood-borne viruses, such as HIV-1 and hepatitis B and C viruses (HBV and HCV)

Sexual history

- Explore in a confidential, polite and non-threatening way (Ch. 15), remembering that the most common mechanism of HIV-1 transmission is heterosexual contact (Ch. 14)

Vaccination history and use of prophylactic medicines

- Consider occupation- or age-related vaccines
- In a traveller or infection-predisposed patient, establish compliance with prophylactic treatments

*Always consider whether a non-infectious aetiology explains the clinical syndrome.

---

① Skin lesions in infectious diseases

- Diffuse erythema, e.g. panel A
- Migrating erythema, e.g. enlarging rash of erythema migrans in Lyme disease (see Fig. 13.19, p. 330)
- Purpuric or petechial rashes, e.g. panel B
- Macular or papular rashes, e.g. primary infection with HIV (see Box 14.3, p. 389)
- Vesicular or blistering rash, e.g. panel C
- Erythema multiforme (see Fig. 27.48 and Box 27.38, p. 1284)
- Nodules or plaques, e.g. Kaposi's sarcoma (p. 384)
- Erythema nodosum (panel D and Box 27.39, p. 1285)

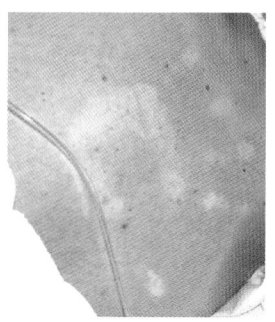
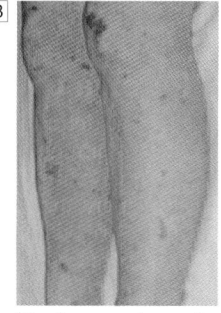
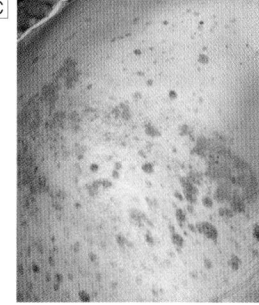
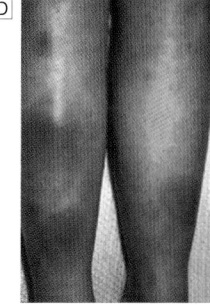

Streptococcal toxic shock syndrome

Meningoccal sepsis

Shingles

Erythema nodosum

13

The principles of infection and its investigation and therapy are described in Chapter 6. This chapter and the following chapters on human immunodeficiency virus/acquired immunodeficiency syndrome (HIV/AIDS) and sexually transmitted infection (STI) describe the approach to patients with potential infectious disease, the individual infections and the syndromes they produce.

PRESENTING PROBLEMS IN INFECTIOUS DISEASES

Infectious diseases present with myriad clinical manifestations. Many of these are described in other chapters of this book. The most common scenarios presenting to specialists in infectious disease are described below.

Fever

'Fever' implies an elevated core body temperature > 38.0 °C, i.e. above the normal daily variation (p. 136). Fever is a response to cytokines and acute phase proteins (pp. 72 and 81) and is a common manifestation of infection, although it also occurs in other conditions.

Clinical assessment

The differential diagnosis is very broad and there is a long list of potential investigations, so any clues from the clinical features which help to focus the investigations are extremely valuable. The systematic approach described on pages 290–291 should be followed. Box 13.1 describes the assessment of elderly patients.

Investigations

If the cause is not obvious, e.g. in a patient with purulent sputum or symptoms of urinary tract infection, then initial screening investigations should include:

- a full blood count (FBC) with differential, including eosinophil count

13.1 Fever in old age

- **Temperature measurement**: fever may be missed because oral temperatures are unreliable in older people. Rectal measurement may be needed but core temperature is increasingly measured using eardrum reflectance.
- **Associated acute confusion**: common with fever, especially in those with underlying cerebrovascular disease or other causes of dementia.
- **Prominent causes of PUO**: include tuberculosis and intra-abdominal abscesses, complicated urinary tract infection and infective endocarditis. Non-infective causes include polymyalgia rheumatica/temporal arteritis and tumours. A smaller fraction of cases remain undiagnosed.
- **Pitfalls in the elderly**: certain conditions such as cerebrovascular accident/thromboembolic disease can cause fever but every effort must be made to exclude concomitant infection.
- **Common infectious diseases in the very frail** (e.g. nursing home residents): include pneumonia, urinary infection, soft tissue infection and gastroenteritis.

- urea and electrolytes, liver function tests (LFTs), blood glucose and muscle enzymes
- inflammatory markers, erythrocyte sedimentation rate (ESR) and C-reactive protein (CRP)
- autoantibodies, including antinuclear antibodies (ANA)
- chest X-ray and electrocardiogram (ECG)
- urinalysis and urine culture
- blood culture (a minimum of 20 mL blood in three sets of blood culture bottles)
- throat swab for culture
- other specimens, as indicated by history and examination, e.g. wound swab; sputum culture; stool culture, microscopy for ova and parasites and *Clostridium difficile* toxin assay; if relevant, malaria films on 3 consecutive days or a malaria rapid diagnostic test (antigen detection by lateral flow immunochromatography, see Ch. 6).

Subsequent investigations in patients with HIV-related (p. 389), immune-deficient (p. 298), nosocomial or travel-related (p. 305) pyrexia, and in patients with associated symptoms or signs of involvement of the respiratory, gastrointestinal or neurological systems are described elsewhere.

Management

Fever and its associated systemic symptoms can be treated with paracetamol, and by tepid sponging to cool the skin. Replacement of salt and water is important in patients with drenching sweats. Further management is focused on the underlying cause.

Fever with localising symptoms or signs

In most patients, the potential site of infection is apparent after clinical evaluation (pp. 290–291), and the likelihood of infection may be reinforced by typical abnormalities on the initial screening investigations (e.g. neutrophilia and raised ESR and CRP in bacterial infections). Not all apparently localising symptoms are reliable, however; headache, breathlessness and diarrhoea can occur in sepsis without localised infection in the central nervous system (CNS), respiratory tract or gastrointestinal tract. Careful evaluation of the constellation of clinical features is vital (e.g. severe headache associated with photophobia, rash and neck stiffness suggests meningitis, whereas moderate headache with cough and rhinorrhoea is consistent with a viral upper respiratory tract infection).

Common infections that present with fever are shown in Figure 13.1. Many are described elsewhere in the book. Further investigation and management is specific to the cause, but may include empirical antimicrobial therapy (p. 148) pending confirmation of the microbiological diagnosis.

Pyrexia of unknown origin (PUO)

PUO is defined as a temperature persistently above 38.0 °C for more than 3 weeks, without diagnosis despite initial investigation during 3 days of inpatient care or after more than two outpatient visits. Subsets of PUO are described by medical setting: HIV-related, immune-deficient or nosocomial. Up to one-third of cases of PUO remain undiagnosed.

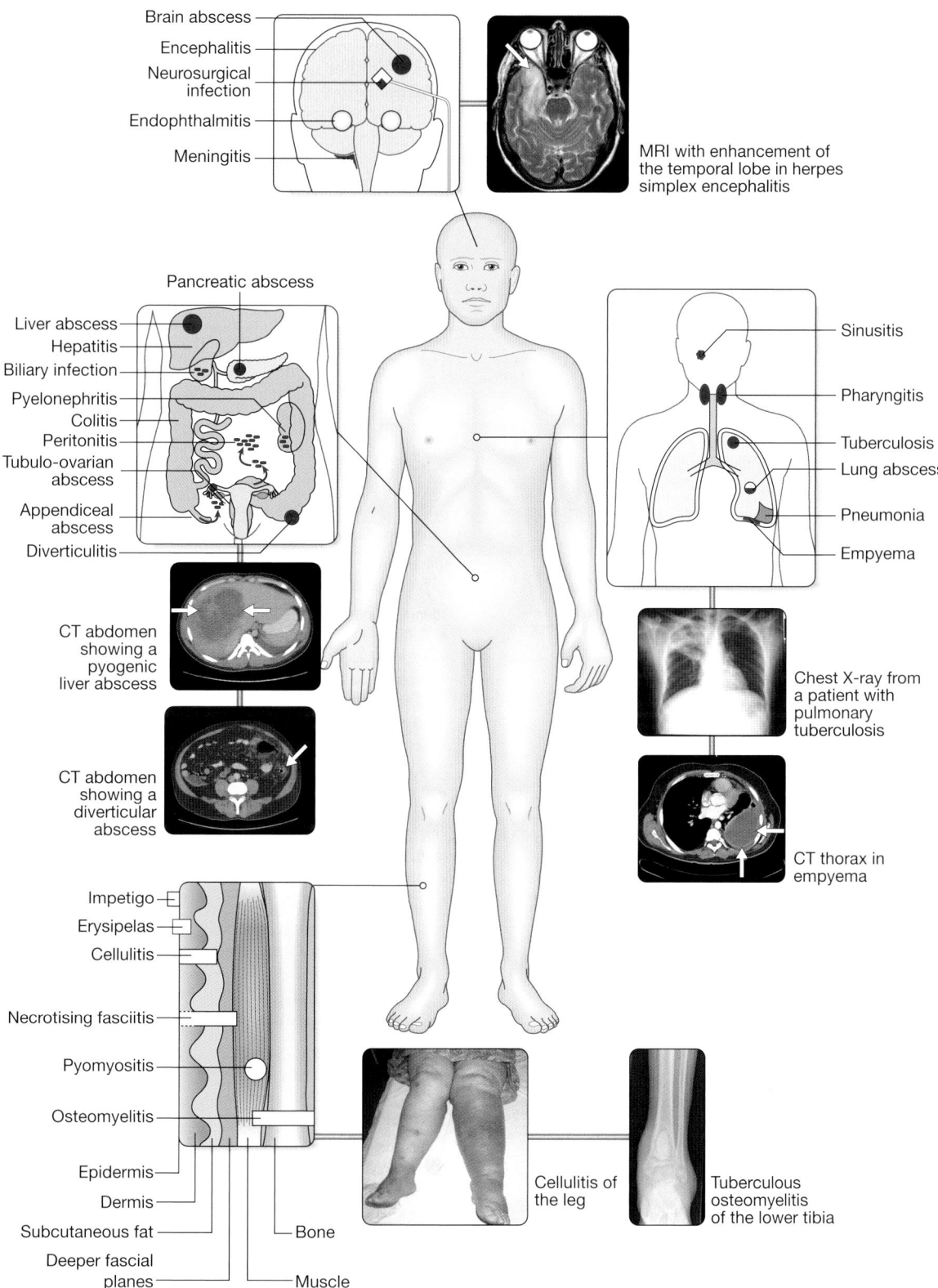

Fig. 13.1 Common infectious syndromes presenting with fever and localised features. Major causes are grouped by approximate anatomical location and include central nervous system infection; respiratory tract infections; abdominal, pelvic or urinary tract infections; and skin and soft tissue infections (SSTI) or osteomyelitis. For each site of infection particular syndromes and their common causes are described elsewhere in the book. The causative organisms vary, depending on host factors, which include whether the patient has lived or resided in a tropical country or particular geographical location, has acquired the infection in a health-care environment or is immunocompromised.

Clinical assessment

Major causes of PUO are outlined in Box 13.2. Rare causes, such as periodic fever syndromes (p. 83), should be considered in those with a positive family history. Children and younger adults are more likely to have infectious causes, in particular viral infections. Older adults are more likely to have certain infections and non-infectious causes (see Box 13.1). Detailed examination should be repeated at regular intervals to detect emerging features, such as rashes, signs of infective endocarditis (p. 624) or features of vasculitis. In men the prostate deserves careful consideration as a potential source of infection.

Clinicians should be alert to the possibility of factitious fever, in which high temperature recordings are engineered by the patient (Box 13.3).

Investigations

If initial investigation of fever (see above) is negative, a series of further microbiological and non-microbiological investigations should be considered (Boxes 13.4 and 13.5). These will usually include:

- induced sputum or other specimens for mycobacterial stains and culture
- serological tests
- imaging of the abdomen by ultrasonography or computed tomography (CT)
- echocardiography.

Lesions identified on imaging should usually be biopsied to obtain material for culture, including for the diagnosis of tuberculosis, and histopathology, including special stains for pathogens associated with

---

13.2 Aetiology of pyrexia of unknown origin

Infections (~30%)

Specific locations
- Abscesses: hepatobiliary*, diverticular*, urinary tract* (including prostate), pulmonary, CNS
- Infections of oral cavity (including dental), head and neck (including sinuses)
- Bone and joint infections
- Infective endocarditis*

Specific organisms
- Tuberculosis (particularly extrapulmonary)*
- HIV-1 infection
- Other viral infections (cytomegalovirus (CMV), Epstein–Barr virus (EBV))
- Fungal infections (e.g. *Aspergillus* spp., *Candida* spp. or dimorphic fungi)
- Infections with fastidious organisms (e.g. *Bartonella* spp., *Tropheryma whipplei*)

Specific patient groups
- Imported infections
  Malaria, dengue, rickettsial infections, *Brucella* spp., amoebic liver abscess, enteric fevers, *Leishmania* spp. (southern Europe, India, Africa and Latin America), *Burkholderia pseudomallei* (South-east Asia)
  HIV and respiratory tract infections
- Nosocomial infections
  Infections related to prosthetic materials and surgical procedures
- HIV-positive individuals
  Acute retroviral syndrome
  AIDS-defining infections (disseminated *Mycobacterium avium* complex (DMAC), *Pneumocystis jirovecii* (*carinii*) pneumonia (PCP), CMV and others)

Malignancy (~20%)

Haematological malignancy
- Lymphoma*, leukaemia and myeloma

Solid tumours
- Renal, liver, colon, stomach, pancreas, kidney

Connective tissue disorders (~15%)

Older adults
- Temporal arteritis/polymyalgia rheumatica*

Younger adults
- Still's disease (juvenile rheumatoid arthritis)*
- Systemic lupus erythematosus (SLE)
- Vasculitic disorders (including polyarteritis nodosa, rheumatoid disease with vasculitis and Wegener's granulomatosis)
- Polymyositis
- Behçet's disease

Geographically restricted
- Rheumatic fever

Miscellaneous (~20%)

Cardiovascular
- Atrial myxoma, aortitis, aortic dissection

Respiratory
- Sarcoidosis, pulmonary embolism and other thromboembolic disease, extrinsic allergic alveolitis

Gastrointestinal
- Inflammatory bowel disease, granulomatous hepatitis, alcoholic liver disease, pancreatitis

Endocrine/metabolic
- Thyrotoxicosis, thyroiditis, hypothalamic lesions, phaeochromocytoma, adrenal insufficiency, hypertriglyceridaemia

Haematological
- Haemolytic anaemia, paroxysmal nocturnal haemoglobinuria, thrombotic thrombocytopenic purpura, myeloproliferative disorders, Castleman's disease, graft-versus-host disease (after allogeneic bone marrow transplantation)

Inherited
- Familial Mediterranean fever and periodic fever syndromes

Drug reactions*,
- e.g. Antibiotic fever, drug hypersensitivity reactions etc.

Factitious fever*

Idiopathic (~15%)

---

*Most common causes within each group.

13.3 Clues to the diagnosis of factitious fever

- A patient who looks well
- Bizarre temperature chart with absence of diurnal variation and/or temperature-related changes in pulse rate
- Temperature > 41°C
- Absence of sweating during defervescence
- Normal ESR and CRP despite high fever
- Evidence of self-injection or self-harm
- Normal temperature during supervised (observed) measurement and of freshly voided urine

the clinical scenario. The chance of a successful diagnosis is greatest if procedures for obtaining and transporting the correct samples in the appropriate media are carefully planned in advance; this requires discussion between the clinical team, the radiologist or surgeon performing the procedure, and the local microbiologist and histopathologist. Liver biopsy may be justified, e.g. to identify idiopathic granulomatous hepatitis, if there are biochemical or radiological abnormalities. Bone marrow biopsies have a diagnostic yield of up to 15%. A biopsy is most useful in revealing haematological malignancy, myelodysplasia or tuberculosis, and may also identify brucellosis, typhoid fever or visceral leishmaniasis. Bone marrow should always be sent for culture as well as microscopy. Laparoscopy is occasionally undertaken with biopsy of abnormal tissues. Splenic aspiration in specialist centres is the diagnostic test of choice for suspected leishmaniasis. Temporal artery biopsy should be considered in patients over the age of 50 years, even in the absence of physical signs or a raised ESR. 'Blind' biopsy of other structures in the absence of localising signs, or laboratory or radiology results is unhelpful.

 13.5 Additional investigations in PUO

Serological tests for connective tissue disorders
- Autoantibody screen
- Complement levels
- Immunoglobulins
- Cryoglobulins

Echocardiography

Ultrasound of abdomen

CT/MRI of thorax, abdomen and/or brain

Imaging of the skeletal system
- Plain X-rays
- CT/MRI spine
- Isotope bone scan

Labelled white cell scan

Positron emission tomography (PET)/single photon emission computed tomography (SPECT)

Biopsy
- Bronchoscopy and lavage ± transbronchial biopsy
- Lymph node aspirate or biopsy
- Biopsy of radiological lesion
- Biopsy of liver
- Bone marrow aspirate and biopsy
- Lumbar puncture
- Laparoscopy and biopsy
- Temporal artery biopsy

Prognosis

The overall mortality of PUO is 30–40%, mainly attributable to malignancy in older patients. If no cause is found, the long-term mortality is low and fever often settles spontaneously.

13

 13.4 Microbiological investigation of PUO

Microscopy

- Blood for atypical lymphocytes (EBV, CMV, HIV-1, hepatitis viruses or *Toxoplasma gondii*), trypanosomiasis, malaria, *Borrelia* spp.
- Respiratory samples for mycobacteria, fungi
- Stool for ova, cysts and parasites
- Biopsy for light microscopy (bacteria, mycobacteria, fungi, *Leishmania* and other parasites) and/or electron microscopy (viruses, protozoa (e.g. microsporidia) and other fastidious organisms (e.g. *T. whipplei*))
- Urine for white or red blood cells, schistosome ova, mycobacteria (early morning urine × 3)

Culture

- Aspirates and biopsies (e.g. joint, deep abscess, debrided tissues)
- Blood, including prolonged culture and special media conditions
- Cerebrospinal fluid (CSF)
- Gastric aspirate for mycobacteria
- Stool

- Swabs
- Urine ± prostatic massage in older men

Antigen detection

- Blood
- CSF for cryptococcal antigen
- Nasopharyngeal aspirate/throat swab for respiratory viruses
- Urine, e.g. for *Legionella* antigen

Nucleic acid detection

- Blood for *Bartonella* spp. and viruses
- CSF for viruses and key bacteria (meningococcus, pneumococcus)
- Nasopharyngeal aspirate/throat swab for respiratory viruses
- Tissue specimens, e.g. for *Tropheryma whipplei*
- Urine, e.g. for *Chlamydia trachomatis, Neisseria gonorrhoeae*
- Stool, e.g. for norovirus, rotavirus

Immunological tests

- Serology (antibody detection) for viruses, dimorphic fungi and some bacteria and protozoa
- Interferon-γ release assay for diagnosis of tuberculosis

Note This list does not apply to every patient with a PUO. Appropriate tests should be selected in a stepwise manner, according to specific predisposing factors, epidemiological exposures and local availability, and should be discussed with a microbiologist.

13

Fever in the injection drug-user

Intravenous injection of drugs of abuse is endemic in many parts of the world (p. 237). Infective organisms are introduced by non-sterile (often shared) injection equipment (Fig. 13.2), while host defences against infection are overcome by direct access to the normally sterile blood stream and by immune deficiencies in poorly nourished addicts. The risks increase with prolonged drug use and injection into large veins of the groin and neck because of progressive thrombosis of superficial peripheral veins. A varied and unusual constellation of infectious diseases is encountered in this group of patients. Although the differential diagnosis of fever is wide, the most common causes are soft tissue or respiratory infections.

Clinical assessment

The history should include consideration of the following risk factors:

- *Site of injection.* Femoral vein injection is associated with vascular complications such as deep venous thrombosis (50% of which are septic) and accidental arterial injection with false aneurysm formation or a compartment syndrome due to swelling within the fascial sheath. Local

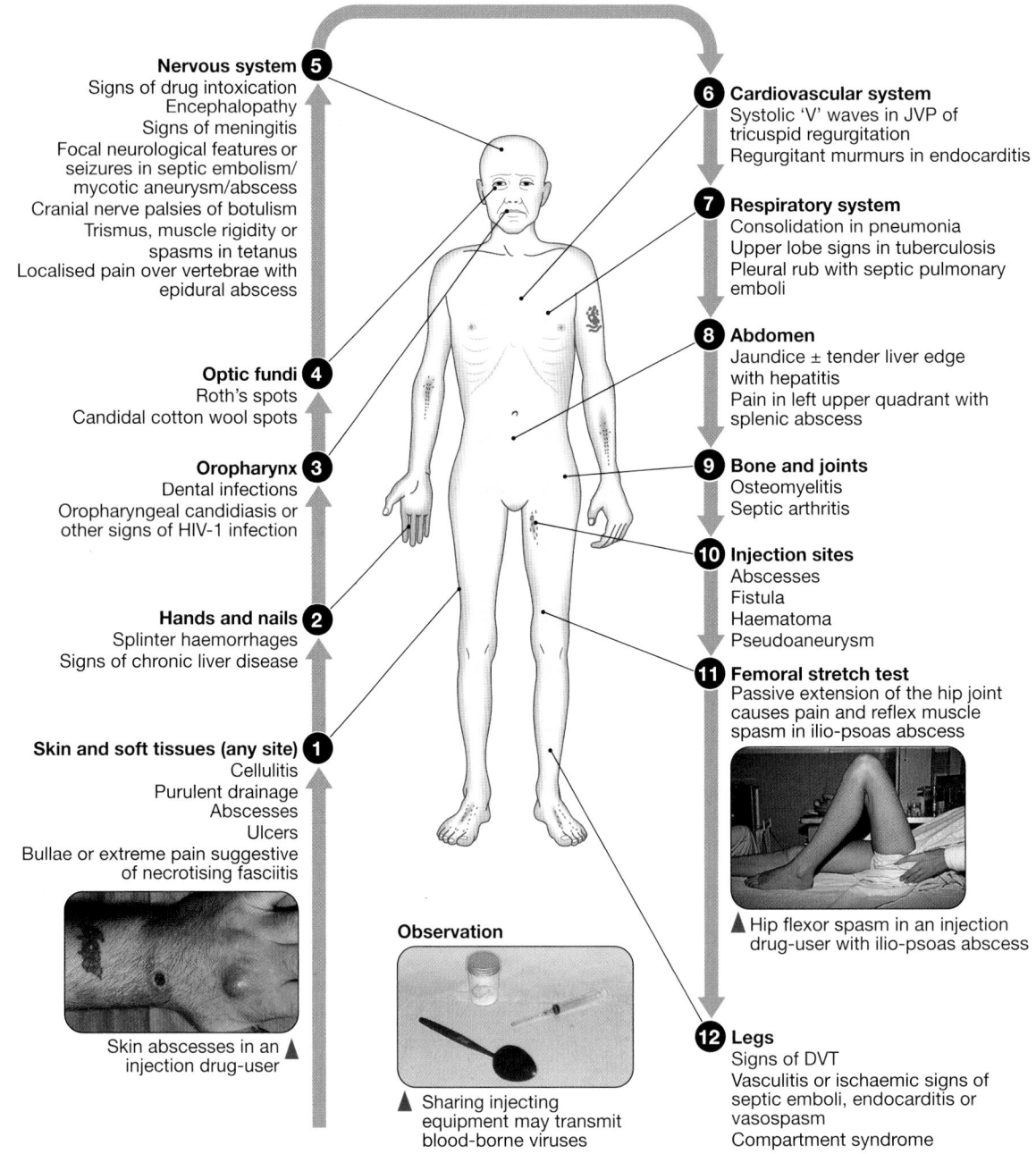

Nervous system ⑤
Signs of drug intoxication
Encephalopathy
Signs of meningitis
Focal neurological features or
seizures in septic embolism/
mycotic aneurysm/abscess
Cranial nerve palsies of botulism
Trismus, muscle rigidity or
spasms in tetanus
Localised pain over vertebrae with
epidural abscess

Optic fundi ④
Roth's spots
Candidal cotton wool spots

Oropharynx ③
Dental infections
Oropharyngeal candidiasis or
other signs of HIV-1 infection

Hands and nails ②
Splinter haemorrhages
Signs of chronic liver disease

Skin and soft tissues (any site) ①
Cellulitis
Purulent drainage
Abscesses
Ulcers
Bullae or extreme pain suggestive
of necrotising fasciitis

▲ Skin abscesses in an
injection drug-user

Observation
▲ Sharing injecting
equipment may transmit
blood-borne viruses

⑥ **Cardiovascular system**
Systolic 'V' waves in JVP of
tricuspid regurgitation
Regurgitant murmurs in endocarditis

⑦ **Respiratory system**
Consolidation in pneumonia
Upper lobe signs in tuberculosis
Pleural rub with septic pulmonary
emboli

⑧ **Abdomen**
Jaundice ± tender liver edge
with hepatitis
Pain in left upper quadrant with
splenic abscess

⑨ **Bone and joints**
Osteomyelitis
Septic arthritis

⑩ **Injection sites**
Abscesses
Fistula
Haematoma
Pseudoaneurysm

⑪ **Femoral stretch test**
Passive extension of the hip joint
causes pain and reflex muscle
spasm in ilio-psoas abscess

▲ Hip flexor spasm in an injection
drug-user with ilio-psoas abscess

⑫ **Legs**
Signs of DVT
Vasculitis or ischaemic signs of
septic emboli, endocarditis or
vasospasm
Compartment syndrome

Fig. 13.2 Fever in the injection drug-user: key features of clinical examination. Full examination (p. 290) is required but features most common amongst injection drug-users are shown here.

complications include ilio-psoas abscess, and septic arthritis of the hip joint or sacro-iliac joint. Injection of the jugular vein can be associated with cerebrovascular complications. Subcutaneous and intramuscular injection has been associated with infection by clostridial species, the spores of which contaminate heroin. *Clostridium novyi* causes a local lesion with significant toxin production leading to shock and multi-organ failure. Tetanus, wound botulism and gas gangrene also occur.

- *Technical details of injection.* Sharing of needles and other injecting paraphernalia (including spoons and filters) greatly increases the risk of blood-borne virus infection. Some users lubricate their needles by licking them prior to injection, thus introducing mouth organisms such as anaerobic streptococci, *Fusobacterium* spp. and *Prevotella* spp. Contamination of commercially available lemon juice, used to dissolve heroin before injection, has been associated with blood-stream infection with *Candida* spp.
- *Substances injected.* Injection of cocaine is associated with a variety of vascular events. Certain formulations of heroin have been associated with particular infections, e.g. wound botulism with black tar heroin. Drugs are often mixed with other substances, e.g. talc.
- *Blood-borne virus status.* Results of previous hepatitis B virus (HBV), HCV and HIV tests or vaccinations for HAV/HBV should be recorded.
- *Surreptitious use of antimicrobials.* Addicts may use antimicrobials to self-treat infections, masking initial blood culture results.

Key findings on clinical examination are shown in Figure 13.2. It can be difficult to distinguish effects of infection from the effects of drugs themselves or the agitated state of drug withdrawal (excitement, tachycardia, sweating, marked myalgia, confusion). Stupor and delirium may result from drug administration but may also signal meningitis or encephalitis. Non-infected venous thromboembolism is also common in this group.

Investigations

The initial investigations are as for any fever (see above), including a chest X-ray and blood cultures. Since blood sampling may be difficult, contamination is often a problem. Echocardiography to detect infective endocarditis should be performed in all injection drug-users: with bacteraemia due to *Staph. aureus* or other organisms associated with endocarditis (Fig. 13.3A); with thrombo-embolic phenomena; or with a new or previously undocumented murmur. Endovascular infection should also be suspected if lung abscesses or pneumatocoeles are detected radiologically. Additional imaging should be focused on sites of symptoms and signs (Fig. 13.3B). Any pathological fluid collections should be sampled either under radiological guidance or by surgical means. In patients with suspected compartment syndrome (leg swelling and pain with neurological and ischaemic features), serum creatine kinase and urine myoglobin are useful.

Urinary toxicology may suggest a non-infectious cause of the presenting complaint. While being investigated, all injection drug-users should be offered testing for HBV, HCV and HIV-1.

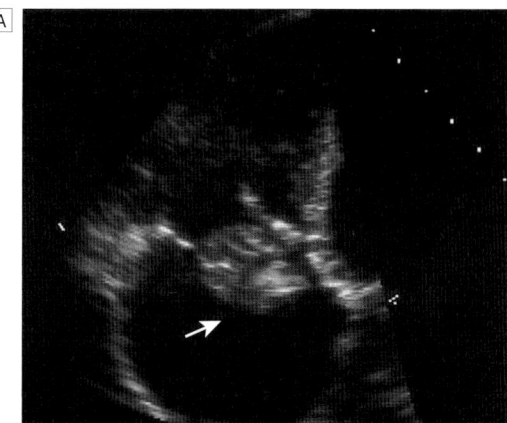

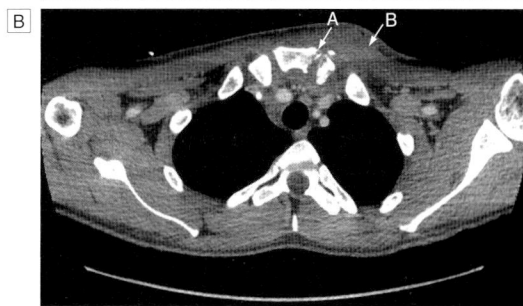

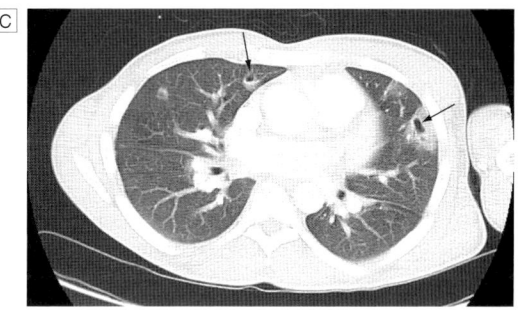

Fig. 13.3 Causes of fever in the injection drug-user. [A] Endocarditis in an injection drug-user. Large vegetation on the tricuspid valve (arrow). [B] Septic arthritis of the left sternoclavicular joint (arrow A) (note the erosion of the bony surfaces at the sternoclavicular joint) with overlying soft tissue collection (arrow B) . [C] CT of the thorax from an injection drug-user with haemoptysis, showing multiple embolic lesions with cavitation (arrows). The patient had *Staph. aureus* endocarditis of the tricuspid valve.

Microbiological results are crucial in guiding therapy. Injection drug-users may have more than one infection. Skin and soft tissue infections are most often due to *Staph. aureus* or streptococci, and sometimes to *Clostridium* spp. or anaerobes. Pulmonary infections are most often due to community-acquired pneumonia, pulmonary tuberculosis or septic pulmonary emboli (Fig. 13.3C). Endocarditis with septic emboli commonly involves *Staph. aureus* and viridans streptococci, but *Pseudomonas aeruginosa* and *Candida* spp. are also encountered.

Management

Empirical therapy of fever in the injection drug user includes an antistaphylococcal penicillin (e.g. flucloxacillin) or, if meticillin-resistant *Staph. aureus* (MRSA) is prevalent in the community, a glycopeptide. Once a particular pathogen is identified, specific therapy is commenced, with modification when antimicrobial susceptibility is available. In injection drug-users, right-sided endocarditis due to *Staph. aureus* is customarily treated with high-dose intravenous flucloxacillin. In left-sided *Staph. aureus* endocarditis, aminoglycoside therapy may be added. Right-sided endocarditis caused by MRSA is usually treated with 4 weeks of vancomycin plus gentamicin for the first week. Specialist advice should be sought.

For localised infections of the skin and soft tissues, oral therapy with agents active against staphylococci, streptococci and anaerobes is appropriate (e.g. co-amoxiclav or clindamycin).

Fever in the immunocompromised host

Immunocompromised hosts include those with congenital immunodeficiency (p. 76), HIV infection (Ch. 14) and iatrogenic immunosuppression induced by chemotherapy (p. 94), transplantation (p. 1013) or immunosuppressant medicines, including high-dose corticosteroids. Metabolic abnormalities such as under-nutrition or hyperglycaemia may also contribute. Multiple elements of the immune system are potentially compromised. A patient may have impaired neutrophil function from chemotherapy, impaired T cell and/or B cell responses due to underlying malignancy, T cell and phagocytosis defects due to corticosteroids, mucositis from chemotherapy and an impaired skin barrier due to insertion of a central venous catheter.

Fever may result from infectious or from non-infectious causes, including drugs, vasculitis, neoplasm, organising pneumonitis, lymphoproliferative disease, graft-versus-host disease (in recipients of haematopoietic bone marrow transplants; p. 1013) and Sweet's syndrome (reddish nodules or plaques with fever and leucocytosis, in association with haematological malignancy).

Clinical assessment

The following should be addressed in the history:

- Identification of the immunosuppressant factors, and nature of the immune defect.
- Any past infections and their treatment. Infections may recur and antimicrobial resistance may have been acquired in response to prior therapy.
- Evidence of microbial colonisation, especially with antimicrobial-resistant organisms, in past surveillance cultures.
- Exposure to infections, including opportunistic infections that would not cause disease in an immunocompetent host.
- Prophylactic medicines and vaccinations administered.

Examination should include inspection of the normal physical barriers provided by skin and mucosal surfaces, in particular central venous catheters, the mouth, sinuses, ears and perianal area (though avoid digital rectal examination). Disseminated infections can manifest as cutaneous lesions; the areas around finger and toenails should be closely inspected.

Investigations

Initial screening tests are as described above (p. 292). Immunocompromised hosts often have decreased signs of inflammation. This manifests as attenuation of physical signs, such as neck stiffness with meningitis, or of radiological and laboratory abnormalities, such as leucocytosis. In patients with respiratory symptoms, a high-resolution chest CT scan should be considered in addition to chest X-ray. Abdominal imaging may also be warranted, particularly if there is right lower quadrant pain. Blood cultures through the central venous catheter, urine cultures, and stool cultures if diarrhoea is present may also be helpful.

Additional investigations are shown in Box 13.4. (p. 295) Nasopharyngeal aspirates are sometimes diagnostic, as immunocompromised hosts may shed respiratory viruses for prolonged periods. Skin lesions should be biopsied if nodules are present and investigation should include fungal stains. Useful molecular techniques include polymerase chain reaction (PCR) for CMV and *Aspergillus* spp. DNA, and antigen assays (e.g. cryptococcal antigen (CrAg) for *Cryptococcus neoformans*, and galactomannan for *Aspergillus* spp. in blood or *Legionella pneumophila* type 1 in urine). Antibody detection is rarely useful in immunocompromised patients. Patients with respiratory signs or symptoms should be considered for a bronchoscopy to obtain bronchoalveolar lavage fluid for investigation of pathogens, including *Pneumocystis jirovecii* (*carinii*) as well as bacteria, fungi and viruses.

Neutropenic fever

Neutropenic fever is strictly defined as a neutrophil count of less than $0.5 \times 10^9/L$ (p. 999) and a single axillary temperature $> 38.5\,°C$ or three recordings $> 38.0\,°C$ over a 12-hour period, although the infection risk increases progressively as the neutrophil count drops below $1.0 \times 10^9/L$. Patients with neutropenia are particularly prone to bacterial or fungal infection. Gram-positive organisms are the most common pathogens, particularly in association with in-dwelling catheters. Empirical broad-spectrum antimicrobial therapy is commenced as soon as neutropenic fever occurs and cultures have been obtained.

The most common regimens for neutropenic sepsis are broad-spectrum penicillins such as piperacillin-tazobactam i.v. Although aminoglycosides are commonly used in combination, this practice is not supported by trial data (Box 13.6). If fever has not resolved after 3–5 days, empirical antifungal therapy (e.g. an amphotericin B preparation or caspofungin) is added (p. 157). An alternative antifungal strategy, which is gaining favour, is to use azole prophylaxis in high-risk patients, and to employ sensitive markers of early fungal infection to guide treatment initiation (a 'pre-emptive approach').

EBM 13.6 **Treatment of neutropenic fever**

'Broad spectrum β-lactam monotherapy is equivalent to β-lactam-aminoglycoside combination therapy for neutropenic fever in many settings.'

- Paul M, et al. BMJ 2003; 326:1111.
- Del Favero A, et al. Clin Infect Dis 2001; 33:1295–1301.

Post-transplantation fever

Fever in transplant recipients may be due to infection, or to episodes of graft rejection in solid organ transplant recipients or graft-versus-host disease in bone marrow transplant recipients.

13.7 Infections in transplant recipients

Time post-transplantation	Infections
Solid organ recipients	
0–1 month	Bacterial or fungal infections related to the underlying condition or surgical complications
1–6 months	CMV, other opportunistic infections (e.g. PCP)
> 6 months	Bacterial pneumonia, other bacterial community-acquired infections, shingles, cryptococcal infection, post-transplant lymphoproliferative disorder (PTLD)
Bone marrow recipients	
Pre-engraftment (typically 0–4 weeks)	Bacterial and fungal infections (including moulds) or respiratory viruses
Post-engraftment	CMV, PCP, moulds, other opportunistic infections
Late (> 100 days)	Community-acquired bacterial infections, shingles, CMV, PTLD

13.8 Common causes of blood-stream infection

Community-acquired

- *Staph. aureus* including MRSA
- *Strep. pneumoniae*
- Other streptococci
- *Escherichia coli*

Nosocomial

- *Staph. aureus* including MRSA
- Coagulase-negative staphylococci
- Enterococci including VRE
- Gram-negative bacteria
- *Candida* spp.

(MRSA = meticillin-resistant *Staph. aureus;* VRE = vancomycin-resistant enterococci)

Infections in solid transplant recipients are grouped according to the time of onset (Box 13.7). Those in the first month are related to the underlying condition or surgical complications. Those occurring 1–6 months after transplantation are characteristic of impaired T cell function. Risk factors for CMV infection have been identified and patients commonly receive either prophylaxis or intensive monitoring involving regular testing for CMV DNA by PCR and early initiation of anti-CMV therapy using intravenous ganciclovir or oral valganciclovir if tests become positive.

For bone marrow transplant recipients (p. 1013), infections in the first four weeks are more common in patients receiving a myeloablative conditioning regimen (see Box 13.7). Later infections are more common if an allogeneic procedure is performed.

Post-transplant lymphoproliferative disorder (PTLD) is an Epstein–Barr virus (EBV)-associated lymphoma that can complicate transplantation, particularly when primary EBV infection occurs after transplantation.

Positive blood culture

Blood-stream infection (BSI) or bacteraemia is a frequent presentation of infection. This can be community-acquired or may arise in hospital ('nosocomial'), although with increasing outpatient treatment 'community-acquired' BSI is more precisely 'community-onset' BSI since it may arise after hospital-based interventions. The most common causes are shown in Box 13.8. In immunocompromised hosts a wider range of microorganisms may be isolated, e.g. fungi in neutropenic hosts.

Primary bacteraemia refers to cases in which the site of infection is unknown; this applies in approximately 10% of community-acquired cases and approximately 30% of nosocomial cases, and is more common in *Staph. aureus* bacteraemias. In community-acquired *Staph. aureus* bacteraemia, 20–30% of cases are associated with infectious endocarditis and up to 10% are due to osteomyelitis. Peripheral and central venous catheter-related infections are an important source of nosocomial BSI.

BSI has an associated mortality of 15–40%, depending on the setting, host and microbial factors.

Clinical assessment

The history should determine the setting in which BSI has occurred. Host factors predisposing to infection include skin disease, diabetes mellitus, injection drug use, the presence of a central venous, urinary or haemodialysis catheter, and surgical procedures, especially involving implantation of prosthetic materials (in particular, endovascular prostheses).

Physical examination should focus on signs of endocarditis (p. 624), evidence of bone or joint infection (tenderness or restriction of movement), and abdominal or flank tenderness. Central venous catheters should be examined for erythema or purulence at the exit site. Particularly in cases with *Candida* spp. infection or suspected infectious endocarditis, fundoscopy after pupil dilatation should be performed.

Investigations

Positive blood cultures may be caused by contaminants. When isolated from only one bottle or from all bottles from one venesection, coagulase-negative staphylococci often represent contamination. Repeated isolation of this organism, however, should raise suspicion of infective endocarditis or, in a patient with any form of prosthetic material, prosthesis infection. Viridans streptococci occasionally contaminate blood cultures but, in view of their association with infective endocarditis, significant infection must always be excluded clinically. *Bacillus* spp. ('aerobic spore bearers') and *Clostridium* spp. often represent incidental transient bacteraemia or contamination, but certain species (e.g. *C. septicum*) may be genuine pathogens.

Further investigations are influenced by the causative organism and setting. Initial screening tests are similar to those for fever (p. 292) and should include chest X-ray, urine culture and, in many cases, ultrasound or other imaging of the abdomen. Imaging should also include any areas of bone or joint pain and any prosthetic material, e.g. a prosthetic joint or an aortic graft.

Echocardiography should be considered for patients with BSI who are at risk of endocarditis from underlying valvular heart disease, those with clinical features of endocarditis (including a heart murmur), those whose cultures reveal an organism that is a common cause of endocarditis (e.g. *Staph. aureus*, viridans streptococci or enterococci), and those in whom multiple blood cultures are positive for the same organism. The sensitivities of

13

transthoracic echocardiography (TTE) and transoesophageal echocardiography (TOE) for the detection of vegetations are 50–90% and > 95%, respectively. Therefore, if TTE is negative, TOE should be used (see Box 18.117, p. 626).

Certain rare causes of BSI have specific associations that warrant further investigation. Endocarditis caused by *Strep. bovis* and infection caused by *C. septicum* are both associated with colonic carcinoma and their isolation is considered to be an indication for colonoscopy.

Management

BSI requires antimicrobial therapy and attention to the source of infection, including surgical drainage if appropriate. Two weeks of therapy may be sufficient for *Staph. aureus* BSI from central and peripheral venous catheter infections when the source is identified and removed, for uncomplicated skin and soft tissue infections and for selected cases of uncomplicated right-sided infective endocarditis. Other *Staph. aureus* BSI is usually treated for 4–6 weeks.

Central venous catheter infections

Infections of central venous catheters typically involve the catheter lumen and are associated with fever, positive blood cultures and, in some cases, signs of purulence or exudate at the site of insertion. Infection is more common in temporary catheters inserted into the groin or jugular vein than those in the subclavian vein. Tunnelled catheters, e.g. Hickman catheters, may also develop tunnel site infections.

Staphylococci account for 70–90% of catheter infections, with coagulase-negative staphylococci more common than *Staph. aureus*. Other causes include enterococci and Gram-negative bacilli. Unusual Gram-negative organisms, such as *Citrobacter freundii* and *Pseudomonas fluorescens*, cause pseudo-outbreaks and raise the possibility of non-sterile infusion equipment or infusate. *Candida* spp. are a common cause of line infections, particularly in association with total parenteral nutrition. Non-tuberculous mycobacteria may cause tunnel infections.

Investigations and management

In bacteraemic patients with fever and no other obvious source of infection, a catheter infection is likely. Local evidence of erythema, purulence or thrombophlebitis supports the diagnosis. However, microbiological confirmation is essential (p. 139). Catheter-related infection is suggested by higher colony counts or shorter time to positivity in blood cultures obtained through the catheter than in peripheral blood cultures. If the line is removed, a semi-quantitative culture of the tip should confirm the presence of 15 or more colony-forming units, but this is retrospective and does not detect luminal infection.

For coagulase-negative staphylococcal line infections, the options are to remove the line or, in the case of tunnelled catheters, to treat empirically with a glycopeptide antibiotic, e.g. vancomycin, with or without the use of antibiotic-containing lock therapy to the catheter for approximately 14 days. For *Staph. aureus* infection, the chance of curing an infection with the catheter in situ is low, and the risks from infection are high. Therefore, unless the risks of catheter removal outweigh the benefits, treatment should involve catheter removal followed by 14 days of appropriate antimicrobial therapy; the same applies to infections with *Candida* spp. or *Bacillus* spp.

Infection prevention is a key component of the management of vascular catheters. Measures include strict attention to hand hygiene, optimal siting, full aseptic technique on insertion and subsequent interventions, skin antisepsis with chlorhexidine and isopropyl alcohol, daily assessment of catheter sites (e.g. with visual infusion phlebitis (VIP) score (p. 326)), and daily consideration of the continuing requirement for catheterisation. The use of catheters impregnated with antimicrobials such as chlorhexidine or silver is advocated in some settings.

Sepsis

Sepsis is defined and discussed on pages 188–190. It describes patients with signs of the systemic inflammatory response syndrome (SIRS: two of temperature > 38 °C or < 36 °C, pulse rate > 90 beats per minute, respiratory rate > 20 per minute or PCO_2 < 4.3 kPa (32.5 mmHg), and white blood cell count > 12 or < 4 × 10^9/L—see Box 8.3, p. 184) and evidence of infection. Septic shock describes sepsis plus hypotension (systolic blood pressure < 90 mmHg systolic or a fall of > 40 mmHg from baseline that is not responsive to fluid challenge or due to another cause). It may be complicated by multi-organ failure and requires intensive care unit admission.

Sepsis largely results from host responses to microbial lipopolysaccharide, peptidoglycans, lipoproteins or superantigens, and there are many infectious causes (Box 13.9). The results of blood cultures and known host factors allow an initial assessment of likely sources of infection which should be the target of initial investigations. Patients who are immunocompromised may have a sepsis syndrome in association with a broader range of pathogens which may be harder to culture, including mycobacteria and fungi. In any individual who has recently visited the tropics, malaria must also be considered.

Severe skin and soft tissue infections (SSTI)

SSTIs are an important cause of sepsis. Cases can be classified as in Box 13.10, according to the clinical features and microbiological findings. In some cases severe systemic features may be out of keeping with mild local features.

Necrotising fasciitis

In this condition, cutaneous involvement with erythema and oedema progresses to bullae or areas of necrosis. However, in contrast to cellulitis, the cutaneous features are often minimal while the pain is severe. The infection spreads quickly along the fascial plane. It is a medical emergency, which requires immediate débridement in addition to antimicrobial therapy (Fig. 13.4). Although the infection may be diagnosed by imaging studies, its rapid spread means that surgical inspection of the involved muscle groups is urgently required to facilitate prompt diagnosis and treatment. Type 1 necrotising fasciitis is a mixed infection with Gram-negative bacteria and anaerobes, often seen post-operatively in diabetic or immunocompromised hosts. Subcutaneous gas may be present. Type 2 necrotising fasciitis is caused by group A or other

13.9 Causes of sepsis

Infection	Setting
Bacterial	
Staph. aureus, coagulase-negative staphylococci	Bacteraemia may be associated with endocarditis, intravascular cannula infection, or skin or bone foci
Strep. pneumoniae	Invasive pneumococcal disease, usually with pneumonia or meningitis
Other streptococci	Invasive streptococcal disease, especially necrotising fasciitis. *Viridans* streptococci in neutropenic host with severe mucositis
Staphylococcal or streptococcal toxic shock syndrome	Toxin-mediated, blood cultures negative; clues include erythrodermic rash and epidemiological setting
Enterococci	Most often with abdominal focus
Neisseria meningitidis	Sepsis in children or young adults with petechial rash and/or meningitis
E. coli, other Gram-negative bacteria	Urinary or biliary tract infection, or other abdominal infections
Pseudomonas aeruginosa, multidrug-resistant Gram-negative bacteraemia	Nosocomial infection
Yersinia pestis	In plague
Burkholderia pseudomallei	Endemic in areas of Thailand; more likely to involve patients with diabetes mellitus or immunocompromised
Capnocytophaga canimorsus	Associated with dog bites and asplenic individuals
C. difficile	Severe colitis, particularly in the elderly
Polymicrobial infection with Gram-negatives and anaerobes	Bowel perforation
Mycobacterium tuberculosis, *M. avium complex* (MAC)	HIV-positive or immunocompromised with miliary TB or disseminated MAC
Fungal	
Candida spp.	Line infection or post-operative complication, nosocomial or immunocompromised host
Histoplasma capsulatum, other dimorphic fungi	Immunocompromised host
Parasitic	
Falciparum malaria	Malaria with high-level parasitaemia and multi-organ failure or as a complication of bacterial superinfection
Babesia microti	Asplenic individual
Strongyloides stercoralis hyperinfection syndrome	Gram-negative infection complicating *Strongyloides* infection in immunocompromised host

 13.10 Severe necrotising soft tissue infections

- Necrotising fasciitis (primarily confined to subcutaneous fascia and fat)
- Clostridial anaerobic cellulitis (confined to skin and subcutaneous tissue)
- Non-clostridial anaerobic cellulitis
- Progressive bacterial synergistic gangrene (*Staph. aureus* + micro-aerophilic streptococcus) ('Meleney's gangrene', primarily confined to skin)
- Pyomyositis (discrete abscesses within individual muscle groups)
- Clostridial myonecrosis (gas gangrene)
- Anaerobic streptococcal myonecrosis (non-clostridial infection mimicking gas gangrene)
- Group A streptococcal necrotising myositis

13

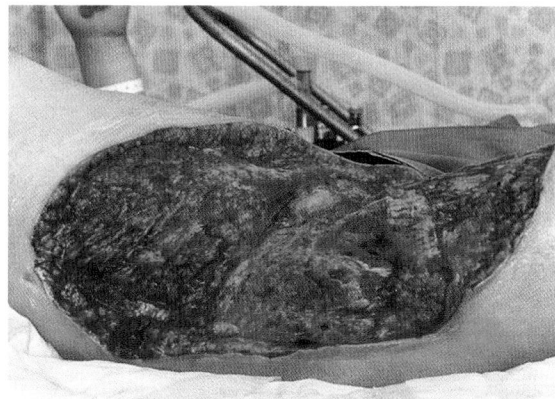

Fig. 13.4 Excision following necrotising fasciitis in an injection drug-user.

streptococci. Approximately 60% of cases are associated with streptococcal toxic shock syndrome (p. 328).

Empiric treatment is with broad-spectrum agents (e.g. piperacillin-tazobactam plus clindamycin plus ciprofloxacin; meropenem monotherapy; or third-generation cephalosporin plus metronidazole) and surgical débridement. Hyperbaric oxygen therapy may be considered for polymicrobial infection. Group A streptococcal infection is treated with benzylpenicillin plus clindamycin, and often immunoglobulin.

Gas gangrene

Although *Clostridium* spp. may colonise or contaminate wounds, no action is required unless there is evidence of spreading infection. In anaerobic cellulitis, usually due to *C. perfringens* or other strains infecting devitalised tissue following a wound, gas forms locally and extends along tissue planes, but bacteraemia and invasion of healthy tissue are not found. Prompt surgical débridement of devitalised tissue and therapy with penicillin or clindamycin usually result in an excellent outcome.

Gas gangrene (clostridial myonecrosis) is defined as acute invasion of healthy living muscle undamaged by previous trauma, and is most commonly caused by *C. perfringens*. In at least 70% of cases it follows deep penetrating injury sufficient to create an anaerobic (ischaemic) environment and allow clostridial introduction and proliferation. Severe pain at the site of the injury progresses rapidly over 18–24 hours. Skin colour changes from pallor to bronze/purple discoloration and the skin is tense, swollen, oedematous and exquisitely tender. Gas in tissues may be obvious with crepitus on clinical examination, or visible on X-ray, CT or ultrasound. Signs of systemic toxicity develop rapidly, with high leucocytosis, multi-organ dysfunction, raised creatine kinase and evidence of disseminated intravascular coagulation and haemolysis. Antibiotic therapy with high-dose intravenous penicillin and clindamycin is recommended, coupled with aggressive surgical débridement of the affected tissues. Alternative agents include cephalosporins and metronidazole. Hyperbaric oxygen has a putative but controversial role.

Other SSTIs

'Synergistic gangrene' is a combined infection with anaerobes and other bacteria (*Staph. aureus* or Gram-negatives). When this affects the genital/perineal area it is known as 'Fournier's gangrene'. Severe gangrenous cellulitis in immunocompromised hosts may involve Gram-negative bacteria or fungi. *Entamoeba histolytica* can cause soft tissue necrosis following abdominal surgery in areas of the world where infection is common. Contact with shellfish in tropical areas and regions such as the Gulf of Mexico can lead to infection with *Vibrio vulnificus*, which causes soft tissue necrosis and bullae. Patients with chronic liver disease are particularly susceptible.

Acute diarrhoea and vomiting

Acute diarrhoea (p. 856), sometimes with vomiting, is the predominant symptom in infective gastroenteritis (Box 13.11). Acute diarrhoea may also be a symptom of other infectious and non-infectious diseases (Box 13.12). Stress, whether psychological or physical, can also produce loose stools.

13.11 Causes of infectious gastroenteritis

Toxin in food: < 6 hours incubation

• *Bacillus cereus* (p. 336)	• *Clostridium* spp.
• *Staph. aureus* (p. 336)	enterotoxin (p. 336)

Bacterial: 12–72 hours incubation

• *Vibrio cholerae* (p. 339)	• *Salmonella** (p. 337)
• Enterotoxigenic *E. coli* (ETEC, p. 337)	• *Shigella** (p. 339)
	• *Campylobacter** (p. 336)
• Shiga toxin-producing *E. coli* (EHEC, p. 337)*	• *Clostridium difficile** (p. 338)
• Enteroinvasive *E. coli* (EIEC, p. 337)*	

Viral: short incubation

• Rotavirus (p. 323)	• Norovirus (p. 323)

Protozoal: long incubation

• Giardiasis (p. 363)	• Amoebic dysentery
• *Cryptosporidium* (pp. 363 and 393)	(p. 362)*
	• Isosporiasis (p. 394)
• Microsporidiosis (p. 393)	

*Associated with bloody diarrhoea.

13.12 Differential diagnosis of acute diarrhoea and vomiting

Infectious causes

• Gastroenteritis	• Pelvic inflammatory disease
• *C. difficile* infection (p. 338)	(p. 415)
• Acute diverticulitis (p. 913)	• Meningococcaemia (p. 1206)
• Sepsis (p. 300)	• Pneumonia (especially 'atypical disease', p. 670)
	• Malaria (p. 348)

Non-infectious causes

Gastrointestinal

• Inflammatory bowel disease (p. 895)	• Overflow from constipation (p. 913)
• Bowel malignancy (p. 907)	

Metabolic

• Diabetic ketoacidosis (p. 809)	• Uraemia (p. 487)
	• Neuroendocrine tumours
• Thyrotoxicosis (p. 738)	releasing (e.g.) VIP or 5-HT

Drugs and toxins

• NSAIDs	• Heavy metals (p. 304)
• Cytotoxic agents	• Ciguatera fish poisoning
• Antibiotics	(p. 304)
• Proton pump inhibitors	• Scombrotoxic fish poisoning
• Dinoflagellates (p. 304)	(p. 304)
• Plant toxins (p. 304)	

The World Health Organization (WHO) estimates that there are more than 1000 million cases of acute diarrhoea annually in developing countries, with 3–4 million deaths, most often in infants and young children. In developed countries diarrhoea remains an important problem and the elderly are most vulnerable (Box 13.13). The majority of episodes are due to infections spread by the faecal–oral route and transmitted either on fomites, on contaminated hands, or in food or water. Measures such as the provision of clean drinking water, appropriate disposal of human and animal sewage, and simple principles of food hygiene all limit gastroenteritis.

The clinical features of food-borne gastroenteritis depend on the pathogenic mechanisms involved. Some organisms (*Bacillus cereus*, *Staph. aureus* and *Vibrio cholerae*) elute exotoxins, which exert their major effects on the stomach and small bowel, and produce vomiting and/or so-called 'secretory' diarrhoea, which is watery diarrhoea without blood or faecal leucocytes. In general, the time from ingestion to the onset of symptoms is short and, other than dehydration, little systemic upset occurs. Other organisms, such as *Shigella* spp., *Campylobacter*

13.13 Infectious diarrhoea in old age

- **Incidence**: not increased, but the impact is greater.
- **Mortality**: most deaths due to gastroenteritis in the developed world are in adults aged over 70 years. Most are presumed to be caused by dehydration leading to organ failure.
- *C. difficile* infection (CDI): old age is associated with CDI, especially in hospital and nursing home settings, usually following antibiotic exposure.

spp. and enterohaemorrhagic *E. coli* (EHEC), may directly invade the mucosa of the small bowel or produce cytotoxins that cause mucosal ulceration, typically affecting the terminal small bowel and colon. The incubation period is longer and more systemic upset occurs, with prolonged bloody diarrhoea. *Salmonella* spp. are capable of invading enterocytes, and of causing both a secretory response and invasive disease with systemic features. This is seen with *Salmonella typhi* and *S. paratyphi* (enteric fever), and, in the immunocompromised host, with non-typhoidal *Salmonella* spp.

Clinical assessment

The history should include questioning about foods ingested (Box 13.14), the duration and frequency of diarrhoea, the presence of blood or steatorrhoea, abdominal pain and tenesmus, and whether family or community members have been affected. Fever and bloody diarrhoea suggest an invasive, colitic, dysenteric process. Incubation periods of less than 18 hours suggest toxin-mediated food poisoning; a period longer than 5 days suggests diarrhoea caused by protozoa or helminths.

Examination includes assessment of the degree of dehydration by skin turgor, with pulse and blood pressure measurement. The urine output and ongoing stool losses should be monitored.

Investigations

These include stool inspection for blood and microscopy for leucocytes, and also an examination for ova, cysts and parasites if the history indicates former tropical residence or travel. Stool culture should be performed, if possible. FBC and serum electrolytes indicate the degree of inflammation and dehydration. In a malarious area, a blood film for malaria parasites should be obtained. Blood and urine cultures and a chest X-ray may identify alternative sites of infection, particularly if the clinical examination is suggestive of a syndrome other than gastroenteritis.

Management

All patients with acute, potentially infective diarrhoea should be appropriately isolated to minimise person-to-person spread of infection. If the history suggests a food-borne source, public health measures must be implemented to identify the source and whether other linked cases exist (p. 144).

Fluid replacement

Replacement of fluid losses in diarrhoeal illness is crucial and may be life-saving.

Although normal daily fluid intake in an adult is only 1–2 L, there is considerable additional fluid movement in and out of the gut in secretions (see Fig. 22.7, p. 842). Infective and toxic processes in the gut disturb or reverse resorption in the small intestine and colon, potentially resulting in substantial fluid loss. Cholera is the archetype of this process, in which 10–20 L of fluid may be lost in 24 hours.

The fluid lost in diarrhoea is isotonic, so both water and electrolytes need to be replaced. Absorption of electrolytes from the gut is an active process requiring energy. Infected mucosa is capable of very rapid fluid and electrolyte transport if carbohydrate is available as an energy source. Oral rehydration solutions (ORS) therefore contain sugars, as well as water and electrolytes (Box 13.15). ORS can be just as effective as intravenous replacement fluid, even in the management of cholera. In mild to moderate gastroenteritis, adults should be encouraged to drink fluids and, if possible, continue normal dietary food intake. If this is impossible, e.g. due to vomiting, intravenous fluid administration will be required. In very sick patients, or those with cardiac or renal disease, monitoring of urine output and central venous pressure may be necessary.

The volume of fluid replacement required should be estimated based on the following considerations.

- *Replacement of established deficit.* After 48 hours of moderate diarrhoea (6–10 stools per 24 hours) the average adult will be 1–2 L depleted from diarrhoea alone. Associated vomiting will compound this. Adults with this symptomatology should therefore be given rapid replacement of 1–1.5 L, either orally (ORS) or by intravenous infusion (normal saline), within the first 2–4 hours of presentation.

13

13.14 Foods associated with infectious illness, including gastroenteritis

Raw seafood

- Norovirus
- *Vibrio* spp.
- Hepatitis A

Raw eggs

- *Salmonella* spp.

Undercooked meat or poultry

- *Salmonella* spp.
- *Campylobacter* spp.
- EHEC
- *C. perfringens*

Unpasteurised milk or juice

- *Salmonella* spp.
- *Campylobacter* spp.
- EHEC
- *Y. enterocolitica*

Unpasteurised soft cheeses

- *Salmonella* spp.
- *Campylobacter* spp.
- ETEC
- *Y. enterocolitica*
- *L. monocytogenes*

Home-made canned goods

- *C. botulinum*

Raw hot dogs, pâté

- *L. monocytogenes*

13.15 Composition of oral rehydration solution and other replacement fluids*

Fluid	Na	K	Cl	Energy
WHO	90	20	80	54
Dioralyte	60	20	60	71
Pepsi®	6.5	0.8	–	400
7UP®	7.5	0.2	–	320
Apple juice	0.4	26	–	480
Orange juice	0.2	49	–	400
Breast milk	22	36	28	670

*mmol/L for electrolyte and Kcal/L for energy components.

Longer symptomatology or more persistent/severe diarrhoea rapidly produces fluid losses comparable to diabetic ketoacidosis and is a metabolic emergency requiring active intervention.

- *Replacement of ongoing losses*. The average adult's diarrhoeal stool accounts for a loss of 200 mL of isotonic fluid. Stool losses should be carefully charted and an estimate of ongoing replacement fluid calculated. Commercially available rehydration sachets are conveniently produced to provide 200 mL of ORS; one sachet per diarrhoea stool is an appropriate estimate of supplementary replacement requirements.
- *Replacement of normal daily requirement*. The average adult has a daily requirement of 1–1.5 L of fluid in addition to the calculations above. This will be increased substantially in fever or a hot environment.

Antimicrobial agents

In non-specific gastroenteritis, antibiotics have been shown to shorten symptoms by only 1 day in an illness usually lasting 1–3 days. This benefit, when related to the potential for the development of antimicrobial resistance or side-effects, does not justify treatment, except if there is systemic involvement and a host with immunocompromise or significant comorbidity.

Evidence suggests that, in EHEC infections, the use of antibiotics may make the complication of haemolytic uraemic syndrome (HUS; p. 498) more likely due to increased toxin release. Antibiotics should therefore not be used routinely in bloody diarrhoea.

Conversely, antibiotics are indicated in *Sh. dysenteriae* infection and in invasive salmonellosis, in particular typhoid fever. Antibiotics may also be advantageous in cholera epidemics, reducing infectivity and controlling the spread of infection.

Antidiarrhoeal, antimotility and antisecretory agents

In general, these agents are not recommended in acute infective diarrhoea and their use may even be contraindicated. Loperamide, diphenoxylate and opiates are potentially dangerous in dysentery in childhood, causing intussusception. Antisecretory agents such as bismuth and chlorpromazine may be effective but can cause significant sedation. They do not reduce stool fluid losses, although the stools may appear more bulky. Adsorbents such as kaolin or charcoal have little effect.

Non-infectious causes of food poisoning

Whilst acute food poisoning and gastroenteritis are most frequently caused by bacteria or their toxins, a number of non-infectious causes must be considered in the differential diagnosis.

Plant toxins

Legumes and beans produce oxidants which are toxic to people with glucose-6-phosphate dehydrogenase (G6PD) deficiency (p. 1024). Consumption produces headache, nausea and fever, progressing to potentially severe haemolysis, haemoglobinuria and jaundice (favism). Red kidney beans, if incompletely cooked, cause acute abdominal pain and diarrhoea from their lectin content. Adequate cooking abolishes this.

Alkaloids develop in potato tubers exposed to light, causing green discoloration. Ingestion induces acute vomiting and anticholinesterase-like activity.

Fungi and mushrooms of the *Psilocybe* spp. produce hallucinogens. Many fungal species induce a combination of gastroenteritis and cholinergic symptoms of blurred vision, salivation, sweating and diarrhoea. *Amanita phalloides* ('death cap') causes acute abdominal cramps and diarrhoea, followed by inexorable hepatorenal failure, often fatal.

Chemical toxins

Paralytic shellfish toxin

Saxitoxin from dinoflagellates, responsible for 'red tides', is concentrated in bivalve molluscs, e.g. mussels, clams, oysters, cockles and scallops. Consumption produces gastrointestinal symptoms within 30 minutes, followed by perioral paraesthesia and even respiratory paralysis. The UK water authorities ban the harvesting of molluscs at times of the year associated with excessive dinoflagellate numbers.

Ciguatera fish poisoning

Warm-water coral reef fish acquire ciguatoxin from dinoflagellates in their food chain. Consumption produces gastrointestinal symptoms 1–6 hours later, with associated paraesthesiae of the lips and extremities, distorted temperature sensation, myalgia and progressive flaccid paralysis. Autonomic dysfunction with hypotension may occur. In the South Pacific and Caribbean there are 50 000 cases per year, with a case fatality of 0.1%. The gastrointestinal symptoms resolve rapidly but the neuropathic features may persist for months.

Scombrotoxic fish poisoning

Under poor storage conditions, histidine in scombroid fish—tuna, mackerel, bonito, skipjack and the canned dark meat of sardines—may be converted by bacteria to histamine and other chemicals. Consumption produces symptoms within minutes, with flushing, burning, sweating, urticaria, pruritus, headache, colic, nausea and vomiting, diarrhoea, bronchospasm and hypotension. Management is with salbutamol and antihistamines. Occasionally, intravenous fluid replacement is required.

Heavy metals

Thallium and cadmium can cause acute vomiting and diarrhoea resembling staphylococcal enterotoxin poisoning.

Antibiotic-associated diarrhoea (AAD)

AAD is a common complication of antibiotic therapy, especially with broad-spectrum agents. It is most common in the elderly but can occur at all ages. Although the specific mechanism is unknown in most AAD, *C. difficile* is implicated in 20–25% of cases and is the most common cause amongst patients with evidence of colitis. Infection is diagnosed by detection of *C. difficile* toxins and is usually treated with metronidazole or vancomycin (p. 338). *C. perfringens* is a rarer cause which usually remains undiagnosed, and *Klebsiella oxytoca* is an occasional cause of antibiotic-associated haemorrhagic colitis.

Infections acquired in the tropics

Recent decades have seen unprecedented increases in long-distance business and holiday travel, as well as extensive migration. Although certain diseases retain their relatively fixed geographical distribution, being dependent on specific vectors or weather conditions, many travel with their human hosts and some may then be transmitted to other people. This means that the pattern of infectious diseases seen in each country changes constantly and travel history is crucial.

In general, the diversity of infectious diseases is greater in tropical than in temperate countries, and people in temperate countries have less immunity to many infections, so that the most common travel-associated infections are those which are acquired by residents of temperate countries during visits to the tropics.

Most travel-associated infections can be prevented. Pre-travel advice is tailored to the destination and the traveller (Box 13.16). It includes avoidance of insect bites (using at least 20% diethyltoluamide (DEET), sun protection (sunscreen with a sun protection factor (SPF) of at least 15), food and water hygiene ('Boil it, cook it, peel it or forget it!'), how to respond to travellers' diarrhoea (seek medical advice if bloody or lasts more than 48 hours) and, if relevant, safe sex (condom use).

Fever in travellers returning from the tropics

Presentation with unexplained fever is common in returning travellers. Frequent final diagnoses in such patients are malaria, typhoid fever, viral hepatitis and dengue fever. Travellers returning from West Africa may have viral haemorrhagic fevers (VHF), such as Lassa fever, Crimean–Congo haemorrhagic fever, Marburg and Ebola (Box 13.37, p. 320). Those from South-east Asia may have avian influenza (H5N1), which may pose an infection control risk and require special isolation precautions to be taken.

Clinical assessment

The approach to unexplained fever is described above. Vital questions to ask anyone returning from the tropics are listed in Box 13.17. Note that medicines purchased while travelling may not be reliable, e.g. for malaria prophylaxis. Consult reliable up-to-date sources about resistance to antimalarial drugs in the country in question. Vaccinations against yellow fever and hepatitis A and B are sufficiently effective to virtually rule out these infections. Oral and injectable typhoid vaccinations are 70–90% effective.

Specific exposures worth documenting are shown in Box 13.18. The incubation period of important pathogens, together with the clinical scenario, also guides the differential diagnosis (Box 13.19). *Falciparum* malaria tends to present between 7 and 28 days after return from an endemic area. VHF, dengue and rickettsial infection can usually be excluded if more than 21 days have passed between return from the affected area and the onset of illness.

Clinical examination is summarised on pages 290–291. Particular attention should be paid to the skin, throat, eyes, nail beds, lymph nodes, abdomen and heart. Patients may be unaware of tick bites or eschars (p. 345). Body temperature should be measured at least twice daily.

13

13.16 How to assess health needs in travellers before departure*

- Destination
- Personal details, including previous travel experience
- Dates of trip
- Itinerary and purpose of trip
- Personal medical history, including pregnancy, medication and allergies (e.g. to eggs, vaccines, antibiotics)
- Past vaccinations
   Childhood schedule followed? Diphtheria, tetanus, pertussis, polio, *N. meningitidis* type C, *Haemophilus influenzae* B (HiB)
   Travel-related? Typhoid, yellow fever, hepatitis A, hepatitis B, meningococcal ACW135Y, rabies, Japanese B encephalitis, tick-borne encephalitis
- Malaria prophylaxis: questions influencing the choice of antimalarial drugs are destination, past experience with antimalarials, history of epilepsy or psychiatric illness

*Further information is available at www.fitfortravel.nhs.uk/

13.17 How to obtain a history from travellers to the tropics with fever

Questions	Factors to ascertain
Countries visited and dates of travel	Relate travel to known outbreaks of infection or antimicrobial resistance
Determine the environment visited	Travel to rural environments, forests, rivers or lakes
Clarify where the person slept	Sleeping in huts, use of bed nets, sleeping on the ground
Establish what he/she was doing	Exposure to people with medical illness, animals, soil, lakes or rivers
History of insect bites	Type of insect responsible, circumstances (location, time of day etc.), preventive measures
Dietary history	Ingestion of uncooked foods, salads and vegetables, meats (especially if undercooked), shellfish, molluscs, unpasteurised dairy products, unbottled water and sites at which food prepared
Sexual history	History of sexual intercourse with commercial sex workers, local population
Malaria prophylaxis	Type of prophylaxis
Vaccination history	Receipt of pre-travel vaccines and appropriateness to area visited
History of any treatments received while abroad	Receipt of medicines, local remedies, blood transfusions or surgical procedures

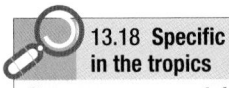

13.18 Specific exposures and causes of fever in the tropics

Exposure	Infection or disease
Mosquito bite	Malaria, dengue fever, Chikungunya, filariasis, tularaemia
Tsetse fly bite	African trypanosomiasis
Tick bite	Rickettsial infections, including typhus, Lyme disease, tularaemia, Crimean–Congo haemorrhagic fever, Kyasanur forest disease, babesiosis, tick-borne encephalitis
Louse bite	Typhus
Flea bite	Plague
Sandfly bite	Leishmaniasis, arbovirus infection
Reduviid bug	Chagas' disease
Animal contact	Q fever, brucellosis, anthrax, plague, tularaemia, viral haemorrhagic fevers, rabies
Fresh-water swimming	Schistosomiasis, leptospirosis, *Naegleria fowleri*
Exposure to soil	Inhalation: dimorphic fungi Inhalation or inoculation: *Burkholderia pseudomallei* Inoculation (most often when barefoot): hookworms, *Strongyloides stercoralis*
Raw or undercooked fruit and vegetables	Enteric bacterial infections, hepatitis A or E virus, *Fasciola hepatica*, *Toxocara* spp., *Echinococcus granulosus* (hydatid disease), *Entamoeba histolytica*
Undercooked pork	*Taenia solium* (cysticercosis)
Crustaceans or molluscs	Paragonimiasis, gnathostomiasis, *Angiostrongylus cantonensis* infection, hepatitis A virus, cholera
Unpasteurised dairy products	Brucellosis, salmonellosis, abdominal tuberculosis, listeriosis
Untreated water	Enteric bacterial infections, giardiasis, *Cryptosporidium* spp. (chronic in immunocompromised), hepatitis A or E virus

Investigations and management

Initial investigations should start with thick and thin blood films for malaria parasites, FBC, urinalysis and chest X-ray if indicated. Box 13.20 gives the diagnoses and further investigations that should be considered in acute fever in the absence of strong clues from the clinical assessment.

Management is directed at the underlying cause. In patients with suspected VHF (p. 319), strict infection control measures with isolation and barrier nursing should be implemented to prevent any contact with the patient's body fluids. The risk of VHF should be determined using epidemiological risk factors and clinical signs (Fig. 13.5), and further management undertaken as described on page 321.

Diarrhoea acquired in the tropics

Gastrointestinal illness is the most commonly reported imported infection, with *Salmonella* spp., *Campylobacter* spp. and *Cryptosporidium* spp. infections common world-

13.19 Incubation times and illnesses in travellers*

< 2 weeks

Non-specific fever
- Malaria
- Chikungunya
- Dengue
- Scrub typhus
- Spotted group rickettsiae
- Acute HIV
- Acute hepatitis C virus
- *Campylobacter*
- Salmonellosis
- Shigellosis
- East African trypanosomiasis
- Leptospirosis
- Relapsing fever
- Influenza
- Yellow fever

Fever and coagulopathy (usually thrombocytopenia)
- Malaria
- Viral haemorrhagic fever (VHF)
- Meningococcaemia
- Enteroviruses
- Leptospirosis and other bacterial pathogens associated with coagulopathy

Fever and central nervous system involvement
- Malaria
- Typhoid fever
- Rickettsial typhus (epidemic caused by *Rickettsia prowazekii*)
- Meningococcal meningitis
- Arboviral encephalitis
- East African trypanosomiasis
- Encephalitis or meningitis
- Angiostrongyliasis
- Rabies

Fever and pulmonary involvement
- Influenza
- Pneumonia due to atypical pathogens
- *Legionella* pneumonia
- Acute histoplasmosis
- Acute coccidioidomycosis
- Q fever
- Severe acute respiratory syndrome (SARS)

Fever and rash
- Viral exanthems (rubella, measles, varicella, mumps, human herpes virus 6 (HHV-6), enteroviruses)
- Chikungunya
- Dengue
- Spotted or typhus group rickettsiosis
- Typhoid fever
- Parvovirus B19

2–6 weeks
- Malaria
- Tuberculosis
- Hepatitis A, B, C and E viruses
- Visceral leishmaniasis
- Acute schistosomiasis
- Amoebic liver abscess
- Leptospirosis
- African trypanosomiasis
- Viral haemorrhagic fever (VHF)
- Q fever
- Acute American trypanosomiasis
- Viral causes of mononucleosis syndromes

> 6 weeks
- Non-*falciparum* malaria
- Tuberculosis
- Hepatitis B and E viruses
- Visceral leishmaniasis
- Filariasis
- Onchocerciasis
- Schistosomiasis
- Amoebic liver abscess
- Chronic mycoses
- African trypanosomiasis
- Rabies
- Typhoid fever

*Adapted from Traveller's Health Yellow Book, CDC Health Information for International Travel 2008.

wide, including in Europe (Box 13.21). For typhoid, paratyphoid, *Shigella* spp. and *Entamoeba histolytica* (amoebiasis), the Indian subcontinent and sub-Saharan and southern Africa are the most commonly reported regions of travel.

13.20 Further investigations in the absence of localising signs in acute fever acquired in the tropics

Features on FBC	Further investigations
Neutrophil leucocytosis	
Bacterial sepsis	Blood culture
Leptospirosis	Culture of blood and urine, serology
Borreliosis (tick- or louse-borne relapsing fever)	Blood film
Amoebic liver abscess	Ultrasound
Normal white cell count and differential	
Typhoid fever	Blood, stool and culture
Typhus	Serology
Arboviral infection	Serology (PCR and viral culture)
Lymphocytosis	
Viral fevers	Serology
Infectious mononucleosis	Monospot test
Rickettsial fevers	Serology

13.21 Most common causes of travellers' diarrhoea

- Enterotoxigenic *E. coli* (ETEC)
- *Shigella* spp.
- *Campylobacter jejuni*
- *Salmonella* spp.
- *Plesiomonas shigelloides*
- Non-cholera *Vibrio* spp.
- *Aeromonas* spp.

EBM 13.22 Antibiotics in travellers' diarrhoea

'Antibiotics reduce the duration of acute non-bloody diarrhoea in patients over 5 years old, but with a risk of side-effects.'

For further information: www.cochrane.org

13.23 Causes of chronic diarrhoea in the tropics

- *Giardia lamblia*
- Strongyloidiasis
- Hypolactasia (primary and secondary)
- Enteropathic *E. coli*
- Tropical sprue
- Chronic calcific pancreatitis
- HIV enteropathy
- Intestinal flukes
- Chronic intestinal schistosomiasis

13

The approach to patients with acute diarrhoea is described on pages 302–304. The benefits of treating travellers' diarrhoea with antimicrobials are marginal (Box 13.22). The differential diagnosis of diarrhoea persisting for more than 14 days is wide (Box 22.21, p. 856). Parasitic and bacterial causes, tropical malabsorption, inflammatory bowel disease and neoplasia should all be considered. Box 13.23 lists causes encountered particularly in the tropics. The work-up should include tests for parasitic causes of chronic diarrhoea, e.g. examination of stool and duodenal aspirates for ova and parasites, and serological investigation.

Tropical sprue is a malabsorption syndrome (p. 881) with no defined aetiology. It was typically associated with a long period of residence in the tropics or with overland travel but is now rarely seen. *Giardia lamblia* infection may progress to a malabsorption syndrome that mimics tropical sprue. If no cause is found, empirical treatment for *Giardia lamblia* infection with metronidazole is often helpful.

HIV has now emerged as a major cause of chronic diarrhoea. This may be due to HIV enteropathy or infection with agents such as *Cryptosporidium* spp., *Isospora belli* or microsporidia (pp. 393–395). However, many other causes of chronic AIDS-associated diarrhoea seen in the developed world are less common in tropical settings, e.g. CMV or disseminated *Mycobacterium avium* complex infections.

Eosinophilia acquired in the tropics

Eosinophilia occurs in a variety of haematological, allergic and inflammatory conditions discussed on pages 1000–1001. It may also occur in HIV and human T cell lymphotropic virus (HTLV)-1 infection. However, eosinophils are important in the immune response to parasitic infections, in particular those parasites with a tissue migration phase. In the context of travel or residence in the tropics, a patient with an eosinophil count of > 0.4 × 10^9/L should be investigated for both non-parasitic (see Box 24.10, p. 1000) and parasitic causes (Box 13.24).

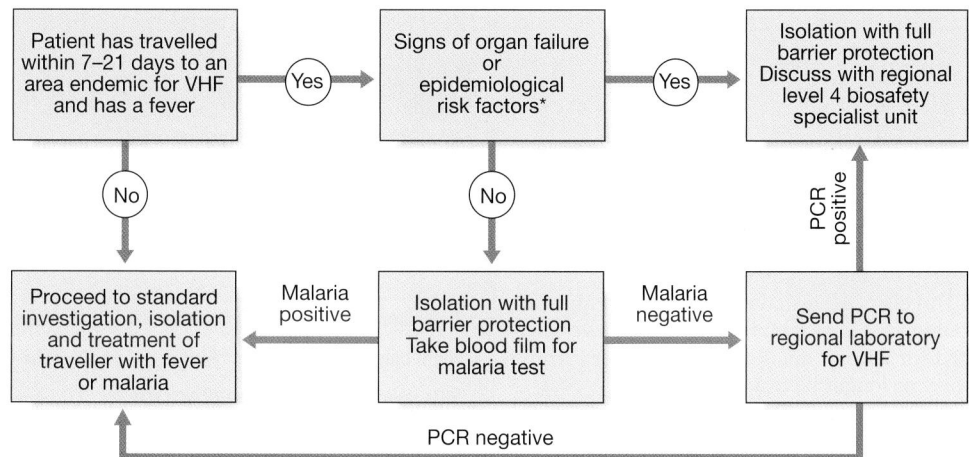

Fig. 13.5 Approach to the patient with suspected viral haemorrhagic fever (VHF). See pages 319–321. *Epidemiological risk factors: staying with a febrile individual, caring for a sick individual or contact with body fluids from a suspected human or animal case of VHF. (PCR = polymerase chain reaction).

13.24 Parasite infections that cause eosinophilia

Infestation	Pathogen	Clinical syndrome with eosinophilia
Strongyloidiasis	*Strongyloides stercoralis*	Larva currens
Soil-transmitted helminthiases		
Hookworm	*Necator americanus*	Anaemia
	Ancylostoma duodenale	Anaemia
Ascariasis	*Ascaris lumbricoides*	Löffler's syndrome
Toxocariasis	*Toxocara canis*	Visceral larva migrans
Schistosomiasis	*Schistosoma haematobium*	Katayama fever
	S. mansoni, S. japonicum	Chronic infection
Filariases		
Loiasis	*Loa loa*	Skin nodules
Wuchereria bancrofti	*W. bancrofti*	Lymphangitis, lymphadenopathy orchitis, intermittent bouts of cellulitis, lymphoedema and elephantiasis
Brugia malayi	*B. malayi*	Brugian elephantiasis similar but typically less severe than that caused by *W. bancrofti*
Mansonella perstans	*M. perstans*	Asymptomatic infection, occasionally subconjunctival nodules
Onchocerciasis	*Onchocerca volvulus*	Visual disturbance, dermatitis
Other nematode infections	*Trichinella spiralis*	Myositis
Cestode infections	*Taenia saginata, T. solium*	Usually asymptomatic; eosinophilia associated with migratory phase
	Echinococcus granulosus	Lesions in liver or other organ; eosinophilia associated with leakage from cyst
Liver flukes	*Fasciola hepatica*	Hepatic symptoms; eosinophilia associated with migratory phase
	Clonorchis sinensis	As for fascioliasis
	Opisthorchis felineus	As for fascioliasis
Lung fluke	*Paragonimus westermani*	Lung lesions

The response to parasite infections is often different when travellers to and residents of endemic areas are compared. Travellers often have recent and light infections associated with eosinophilia. Residents have often been infected for a long time, have evidence of chronic pathology and no longer have an eosinophilia.

Clinical assessment

Comparison of where the patient has travelled and the known endemic areas for diseases such as schistosomiasis, onchocerciasis and the filariases will indicate possible causes. Establish how long patients have spent in endemic areas and take a thorough history, including all the elements in Box 13.17.

Physical signs or symptoms that suggest a parasitic cause for eosinophilia include transient rashes (schistosomiasis or strongyloidiasis), fever (Katayama syndrome—p. 371), pruritus (onchocerciasis) or migrating subcutaneous swellings (loiasis, gnathostomiasis) (see Box 13.24). Paragonimiasis can give rise to haemoptysis and the migratory phase of intestinal nematodes or lymphatic filariasis to cough, wheezing and transient pulmonary infiltrates. Schistosomiasis induces transient respiratory symptoms with infiltrates in the acute stages and, when eggs reach the pulmonary vasculature in chronic infection, can result in shortness of breath with features of right heart failure due to pulmonary hypertension. Fever and hepatosplenomegaly are seen in schistosomiasis, *Fasciola hepatica* and toxocariasis (visceral larva migrans). Intestinal worms such as *Ascaris lumbricoides* and *Strongyloides stercoralis* can cause abdominal symptoms, including intestinal obstruction and diarrhoea. In the case of heavy infestation with ascaris this may be due to fat malabsorption and there may be associated nutritional deficits. *Schistosoma haematobium* can cause haematuria or haematospermia. *Toxocara* spp. can give rise to choroidal lesions with visual field defects. *Angiostrongylus cantonensis* and gnathostomiasis induce eosinophilic meningitis, and the hyperinfection syndrome caused by *Strongyloides stercoralis* in immunocompromised hosts induces meningitis due to Gram-negative bacteria. Myositis is a feature of trichinellosis and cysticercosis, while periorbital oedema is a feature of trichinellosis.

Investigations

To establish the diagnosis of a parasitic infestation, direct visualisation of adult worms, larvae or ova is required. Serum antibody detection may not distinguish between active and past infection and is often unhelpful in those born in endemic areas. Radiological investigations may provide circumstantial evidence of parasite infestation. Box 13.25 describes initial investigations for eosinophilia.

Management

A specific diagnosis guides therapy. In the absence of a specific diagnosis, many clinicians will give an empirical

13.25 Initial investigation of eosinophilia

Investigation	Pathogens sought
Stool microscopy	Ova, cysts and parasites
Terminal urine	Ova of *Schistosoma haematobium*
Duodenal aspirate	Filariform larvae of *Strongyloides*, liver fluke ova
Day bloods	Microfilariae *Brugia malayi*, *Loa loa*
Night bloods	Microfilariae *Wuchereria bancrofti*
Skin snips	*Onchocerca volvulus*
Slit lamp examination	*Onchocerca volvulus*
Serology	Schistosomiasis, filariasis, strongyloidiasis, hydatid, trichinosis etc.

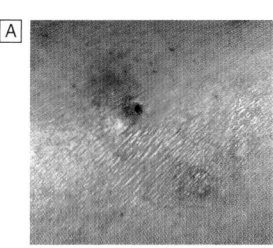 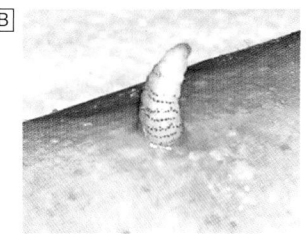 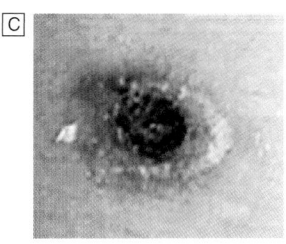 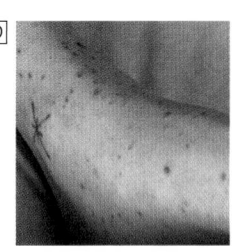

Fig. 13.6 Examples of skin lesions in patients with fever in the tropics. A Subcutaneous nodule due to botfly infection. B Emerging larva after treatment with petroleum jelly. C Eschar of scrub typhus. D Rat bite fever.

13.26 Rash in tropical travellers/residents

Maculopapular rash

- Dengue
- HIV-1
- Typhoid
- *Spirillum minus*
- Rickettsial infections
- Measles

Petechial or purpuric rash

- VHF
- Yellow fever
- Meningococcal sepsis
- Leptospirosis
- Rickettsial spotted fevers
- Malaria

Vesicular rash

- Monkeypox
- Insect bites
- Rickettsial pox

Urticarial rash

- Katayama fever (schistosomiasis)
- *Toxocara* spp.
- *Strongyloides stercoralis*
- Fascioliasis

Ulcers

- Leishmaniasis
- *Mycobacterium ulcerans* (Buruli ulcer)
- Dracunculosis
- Tropical ulcer (*Fusobacterium ulcerans and Treponema vincentii*)
- Anthrax
- Rickettsial eschar
- Ecthyma (staphylococci streptococci)

Papules

- Scabies
- Insect bites
- Prickly heat
- Ringworm
- Onchocerciasis

Nodules or plaques

- Leprosy
- Chromoblastomycosis
- Dimorphic fungi
- Trypanosomiasis
- Onchocerciasis
- Myiasis (larvae of Tumbu or bot fly)
- Tungiasis (*Tunga penetrans*)

Migratory linear rash

- Cutaneous larva migrans (dog hookworms)
- *Strongyloides stercoralis*

Migratory papules/nodules

- Loa loa
- Gnathosomiasis
- Schistosomiasis

Thickened skin

- Elephantiasis (filariasis)
- Mycetoma (fungi/*Nocardia* spp.)

course of praziquantel if the individual has been potentially exposed to schistosomiasis, or with albendazole/ivermectin if strongyloidiasis or intestinal nematodes are likely causes.

Skin conditions acquired in the tropics

Community-based studies in the tropics consistently show that skin infections (bacterial and fungal), scabies and eczema are the most common skin problems (Box 13.26). Scabies and eczema are discussed on pages 1273 and 1256. Cutaneous leishmaniasis and onchocerciasis have defined geographical distributions (pp. 356 and 368). In travellers, secondarily infected insect bites, pyoderma, cutaneous larva migrans and non-specific dermatitis are common.

When investigating skin lesions, enquire about habitation, activities undertaken and regions visited (see Box 13.17). Examples of skin lesions in tropical disease are shown in Figure 13.6.

Skin biopsies are helpful in diagnosing fungal or parasitic infections and persistent reactions to insect bites. Culture of biopsy material may be needed to diagnose bacterial, fungal, parasitic and mycobacterial infections.

Infections in pregnancy

Box 13.27 shows some of the common infections encountered in pregnancy, with their consequences and management.

VIRAL INFECTIONS

Systemic viral infections with exanthem

Exanthem is the term classically used to describe a widespread rash associated with fever in childhood. Maternal antibody gives protection for the first 6–12 months of life and infection occurs thereafter. Comprehensive immunisation programmes have eradicated many of these conditions but lapses in vaccination result in continued infections, which now often present in older children and adults.

Measles

Before immunisation campaigns, measles occurred in almost 100% of children world-wide. The WHO has set the objective of eradicating measles globally by 2010, using the live attenuated vaccine. However, vaccination of only 70–80% of the population, as is currently the case in the UK, for example, is insufficient to prevent outbreaks in older children and adults, who are more

13.27 Infections during pregnancy

Infection	Consequence	Prevention and management
Rubella	Congenital malformation	Vaccination of non-immune mothers
Cytomegalovirus	Neonatal infection, congenital malformation	Limited prevention strategies
Varicella zoster virus	Neonatal infection, congenital malformation, severe infection in mother	VZ immune globulin (see Box 13.33, p. 314), or aciclovir if exposure > 4 days previously
Herpes simplex virus	Congenital or neonatal infection	Aciclovir and consideration of caesarean section for mothers who shed HSV from the genital tract at the time of delivery. Aciclovir for infected neonates
Hepatitis B virus	Chronic infection of neonate	Hepatitis B immune globulin and active vaccination of newborn
HIV	Chronic infection of neonate	Antiretrovirals to mother and infant and consideration of caesarean section if HIV viral load detectable. Avoidance of breastfeeding
Parvovirus B19	Congenital infection	Avoid contact with individuals with acute infection if pregnant
Measles	More severe infection in mother and neonate	Immunisation of mother
Syphilis	Congenital malformation	Serological testing in pregnancy with prompt treatment of infected mothers
Neisseria gonorrhoeae* and *Chlamydia trachomatis	Neonatal conjunctivitis (*ophthalmia neonatorum*)	Treatment of infection in mother and neonate
Listeriosis	Neonatal meningitis or bacteraemia, bacteraemia or PUO in mother	Avoidance of unpasteurised cheeses and other dietary sources
Brucellosis	Possibly increased incidence of fetal loss	Avoidance of unpasteurised dairy products
Group B streptococcal infection	Neonatal meningitis and sepsis. Sepsis in mother after delivery	Risk- or screening-based antimicrobial prophylaxis in labour (recommendations vary between countries)
Toxoplasmosis	Congenital malformation	Diagnosis and prompt treatment of cases, avoidance of undercooked meat while pregnant
Malaria	Fetal loss, intrauterine growth retardation, severe malaria in mother	Avoidance of insect bites. Intermittent preventative treatment during pregnancy to decrease incidence in high-risk countries

susceptible to complications. Natural illness produces lifelong immunity.

Clinical features

Infection is by respiratory droplets with an incubation period of 6–19 days. A prodromal illness, 1–3 days before the rash, occurs with upper respiratory symptoms, conjunctivitis and the presence of Koplik's spots on the internal buccal mucosa (Fig. 13.7A). These small white spots surrounded by erythema are pathognomonic of measles. As natural antibody develops, the maculopapular rash appears, spreading from the face to the extremities (Fig. 13.7B). Generalised lymphadenopathy and diarrhoea are common, with otitis media and bacterial pneumonia recognised complications. Clinical encephalitis occurs in approximately 0.1% of children. A rare late complication is

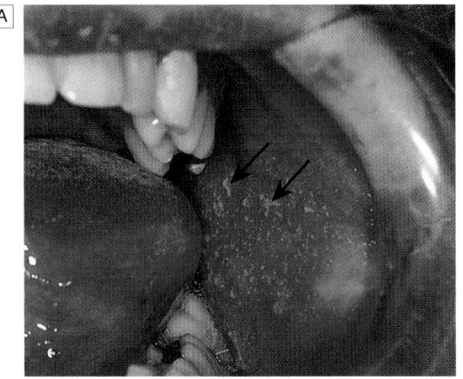
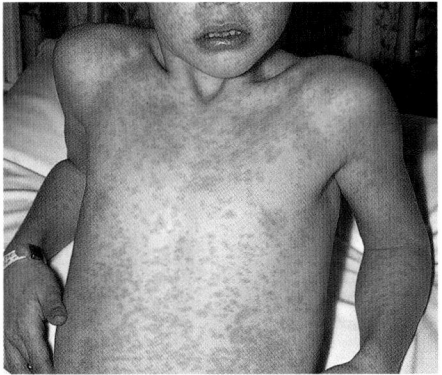

Fig. 13.7 Measles. [A] Koplik's spots (arrows) seen on buccal mucosa in the early stages of clinical measles. [B] Typical measles rash.

subacute sclerosing panencephalitis (SSPE), which occurs up to 7 years after infection. Diagnosis is clinical (although this is unreliable in areas where measles is no longer common) and by detection of antibody (serum IgM, seroconversion or salivary IgM).

Disease is more severe and prolonged in adults and complications include pneumonitis, hepatitis and encephalitis. Measles is a serious disease in the malnourished, vitamin-deficient or immunocompromised, in whom the typical rash may be missing and persistent infection with a giant cell pneumonitis or encephalitis may occur. In tuberculosis infection, measles suppresses cell-mediated immunity and may exacerbate disease; for this reason, measles vaccination should be deferred until after commencing antituberculous treatment. Measles does not cause congenital malformation but may be more severe in pregnant women.

Mortality clusters at the extremes of age, averaging 1:1000 in developed countries and up to 1:4 in developing countries. Death usually results from bacterial superinfection such as pneumonia, diarrhoeal disease or noma/cancrum oris.

Management and prevention

Normal immunoglobulin attenuates the disease in the immunocompromised (regardless of vaccination status) and in non-immune pregnant women, but must be given within 6 days of exposure. Vaccination can be used in outbreaks and vitamin A may improve the outcome in uncomplicated disease. Antibiotic therapy is reserved for bacterial complications.

All children aged 12–15 months (when maternal antibody will no longer be present) should receive measles vaccination (as combined measles, mumps and rubella (MMR), a live attenuated vaccine), and a further MMR dose at the age of 4 years.

Rubella (German measles)

Rubella is an endemic exanthem in countries without universal vaccination. In non-immunised communities 80–85% of young adults have evidence of past infection.

Clinical features

Rubella is spread by respiratory droplet, with infectivity from up to 10 days before to 2 weeks after the onset of the rash. The incubation period is 15–20 days. In childhood, most cases are subclinical, although clinical features may include fever, maculopapular rash spreading from the face, and lymphadenopathy. Complications are rare but include thrombocytopenia and hepatitis. Encephalitis and haemorrhage are occasionally reported. In adults, arthritis involving hands or knees is relatively common, especially in women.

If transplacental infection takes place in the first trimester or later, persistence of the virus is likely and severe congenital disease may result (Box 13.28). Even if normal at birth, the infant has an increased incidence of other diseases developing later, such as diabetes mellitus.

Diagnosis

Laboratory confirmation of rubella is required if there has been contact with a pregnant woman. This is achieved either by detection of rubella IgM in serum or by IgG seroconversion. In the exposed pregnant woman, absence of rubella-specific IgG confirms the potential for congenital infection.

Prevention

MMR should be administered as for measles. Rubella is one of a number of infections that can occur during pregnancy with potentially serious consequences to mother or child (see Box 13.27). All women of child-bearing age should also be tested for rubella and vaccinated if seronegative.

Parvovirus B19 (erythrovirus B19)

This virus causes a variety of clinical syndromes (Box 13.29). Approximately 50% of children and 60–90% of older adults are seropositive world-wide. Most infections are spread by the respiratory route, although spread via contaminated blood is also possible. The virus has particular tropism for red cell precursors.

13.28 Rubella infection: risk of congenital malformation

Stage of gestation	Likelihood of malformations
1–2 months	65–85% chance of illness, multiple defects/spontaneous abortion
3 months	30–35% chance of illness, usually a single congenital defect (most frequently deafness, cataract, glaucoma, mental retardation, congenital heart disease, especially pulmonary stenosis, patent ductus arteriosus)
4 months	10% risk of congenital defects, most commonly deafness
> 20 weeks	Occasional deafness

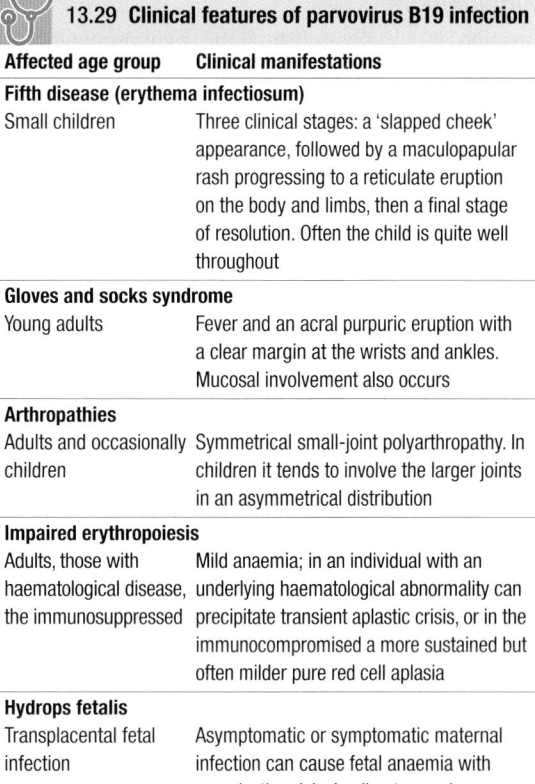

13.29 Clinical features of parvovirus B19 infection

Affected age group	Clinical manifestations
Fifth disease (erythema infectiosum)	
Small children	Three clinical stages: a 'slapped cheek' appearance, followed by a maculopapular rash progressing to a reticulate eruption on the body and limbs, then a final stage of resolution. Often the child is quite well throughout
Gloves and socks syndrome	
Young adults	Fever and an acral purpuric eruption with a clear margin at the wrists and ankles. Mucosal involvement also occurs
Arthropathies	
Adults and occasionally children	Symmetrical small-joint polyarthropathy. In children it tends to involve the larger joints in an asymmetrical distribution
Impaired erythropoiesis	
Adults, those with haematological disease, the immunosuppressed	Mild anaemia; in an individual with an underlying haematological abnormality can precipitate transient aplastic crisis, or in the immunocompromised a more sustained but often milder pure red cell aplasia
Hydrops fetalis	
Transplacental fetal infection	Asymptomatic or symptomatic maternal infection can cause fetal anaemia with an aplastic crisis, leading to non-immune hydrops fetalis and spontaneous abortion

13

Clinical features

Many infections are subclinical. Clinical manifestations result after an incubation period of 14–21 days (see Box 13.29). The classic exanthem (erythema infectiosum) is preceded by a prodromal fever and coryzal symptoms. A 'slapped cheek' rash is characteristic but the rash is very variable (Fig. 13.8). In adults, polyarthropathy is common. Infected individuals have a transient block in erythropoiesis for a few days, which is of no clinical consequence, except in individuals with increased red cell turnover due to haemoglobinopathy or haemolytic anaemia. These individuals develop an acute anaemia which may be severe (transient aplastic crisis; p. 1028). Erythropoiesis usually recovers spontaneously after 10–14 days. Immunocompromised individuals, including those with congenital immunodeficiency or AIDS, can develop a more sustained block in erythropoiesis in response to the chronic viraemia that results from their inability to clear the infection. Infection during the first two trimesters of pregnancy can result in intrauterine infection and impact on fetal bone marrow; it causes 10–15% of non-immune (non-Rhesus-related) hydrops fetalis, a rare complication of pregnancy.

Diagnosis

IgM responses to parvovirus B19 suggest recent infection but may persist for months and false positives occur. Seroconversion to IgG positivity confirms infection but in isolation a positive IgG is of little diagnostic utility. Detection of parvovirus B19 DNA in blood is particularly useful in the immunocompromised host. Giant pronormoblasts or haemophagocytosis may be demonstrable in the bone marrow.

Management

Infection is usually self-limiting. Symptomatic relief for arthritic symptoms may be required. Severe anaemia requires transfusion. Immunocompromised hosts should have immunosuppression decreased, if possible, and if viraemia persists should receive immunoglobulin to aid clearance.

Pregnant women should avoid contact with cases of parvovirus B19 infection; if they are exposed, serology should be performed to establish whether they are non-immune. Passive prophylaxis with normal immunoglobulin has been suggested for non-immune pregnant women exposed to infection but there are limited data to support this recommendation. The pregnancy should be closely monitored by ultrasound scanning, so that hydrops fetalis can be treated by fetal transfusion.

Human herpesvirus 6 and 7 (HHV-6 and HHV-7)

Herpesviruses are classified in Box 13.30.

HHV-6 is a lymphotropic virus that causes a childhood viral exanthem (exanthem subitum), rare cases of an infectious mononucleosis-like syndrome and infection in the immunocompromised host. Infection is almost universal, with approximately 95% of children acquiring this virus by 2 years of age. Transmission is via saliva.

HHV-7 is very closely related to HHV-6, and is believed to be responsible for a proportion of cases of exanthem subitum. Like HHV-6, HHV-7 causes an almost universal infection in childhood, with subsequent latent infection and occasional infection in the immunocompromised host.

13.30 **Herpesvirus infections**	
Virus	**Infection**
Herpesvirus hominis **(herpes simplex, HSV)**	
HSV-1 (p. 321)	Herpes labialis ('cold sores')
	Stomatitis, pharyngitis
	Corneal ulceration
	Finger infections ('whitlows')
	Eczema herpeticum
HSV-2 (p. 321)	Genital ulceration and neonatal infection (acquired during vaginal delivery)
	Encephalitis, acute meningitis or transverse myelitis
Varicella zoster virus (VZV) (p. 313)	Chickenpox (varicella)
	Shingles (herpes zoster)
Cytomegalovirus (CMV) (p. 317)	Congenital infection
	Infectious mononucleosis (heterophile antibody-negative)
	Hepatitis
	Disease in immunocompromised patients: retinitis, encephalitis, pneumonitis, hepatitis, enteritis
	Fever with abnormalities in haematological parameters
Epstein–Barr virus (EBV) (p. 316)	Infectious mononucleosis
	Burkitt's lymphoma
	Nasopharyngeal carcinoma
	Oral hairy leucoplakia (AIDS patients)
	Other lymphomas
Human herpesvirus 6 and 7 (HHV-6, HHV-7)	Exanthem subitum
	Disease in immunocompromised patients
Human herpesvirus 8 (HHV-8) (p. 322)	Kaposi's sarcoma, primary effusion lymphoma, multicentric Castleman's disease

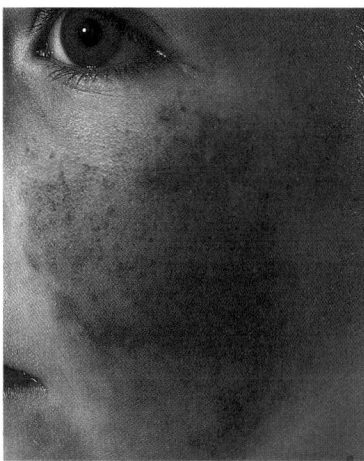

Fig. 13.8 Slapped cheek syndrome. The typical facial rash of parvovirus B19 infection.

Clinical features

Exanthem subitum is also known as roseola infantum or sixth disease (Box 13.30). A high fever is followed by a maculopapular rash as the fever resolves. Fever and/or febrile convulsions may also occur without a rash. Rarely, older children or adults may develop an infectious mononucleosis-like illness, hepatitis or rash. In the immunocompromised infection is rare but can cause fever, rash, hepatitis, cytopenia or encephalitis.

Diagnosis and management

Exanthem subitum is usually a clinical diagnosis. Laboratory diagnosis can be made by antibody and/or DNA detection, although these tests are not widely available. The disease is self-limiting. Treatment with ganciclovir has been used in immunocompromised hosts infected with HHV-6.

Chickenpox (varicella)

Varicella zoster virus (VZV) is a dermotropic and neurotropic virus that produces primary infection, usually in childhood, which may reactivate in later life. VZV is spread by aerosol and direct contact. It is highly infectious to non-immune individuals. Disease in children is usually well tolerated. Manifestations are more severe in adults, pregnant women and the immunocompromised.

Clinical features

The incubation period is 11–20 days, after which a vesicular eruption begins (Fig. 13.9), often on mucosal surfaces first, followed by rapid dissemination in a centripetal distribution (most dense on trunk and sparse on limbs). New lesions occur every 2–4 days and each crop is associated with fever. The rash progresses from small pink macules to vesicles and pustules within 24 hours. Infectivity lasts from up to 4 days (but usually 48 hours) before the lesions appear until the last vesicles crust over. Due to intense itching, secondary bacterial infection from scratching is the most common complication of primary chickenpox. Self-limiting cerebellar ataxia and encephalitis are rare complications.

Adults, pregnant women and the immunocompromised are at increased risk of visceral involvement, which presents as pneumonitis, hepatitis or encephalitis. Pneumonitis can be fatal and is more likely to occur in smokers. Maternal infection in early pregnancy carries a 3% risk of neonatal damage with developmental abnormalities of eyes, CNS and limbs. Chickenpox within 5 days of delivery leads to severe neonatal varicella with visceral involvement and haemorrhage.

Diagnosis

Diagnosis is primarily clinical, by recognition of the rash. If necessary, this can be confirmed by detection of antigen (direct immunofluorescence), DNA (PCR) or by viral culture of aspirated vesicular fluid. Serology is used to identify seronegative individuals at risk of infection.

Management and prevention

Antivirals, although effective if commenced within 48 hours of rash appearance, are not licensed in the UK for uncomplicated primary VZV infection, since published evidence suggests the benefits are marginal (Box 13.31). They are, however, widely used around the world for uncomplicated chickenpox in adults. Treatment is required in individuals with complications and those who are immunocompromised, including pregnant women (Box 13.32). More severe disease, particularly in immunocompromised hosts, requires initial parenteral therapy. Immunocompromised patients may have prolonged viral shedding and may require prolonged treatment until all lesions crust over.

Human VZ immunoglobulin (VZIG) is used to attenuate infection in people who have had significant contact with VZV, are susceptible to infection (i.e. have no history of chickenpox or shingles and are negative for serum VZV IgG) and are at risk of severe disease (e.g. immunocompromised, steroid-treated or pregnant) (Box 13.33). Ideally, VZIG should be given within 7 days of exposure, but it may attenuate disease even if given up to 10 days afterwards. Susceptible contacts who

EBM 13.31 **Aciclovir for chickenpox/shingles**

'Aciclovir shortens symptoms in chickenpox by an average of 1 day. In shingles aciclovir reduces pain by 10 days and the risk of post-herpetic neuralgia by 8%. Aciclovir is therefore cost-effective in shingles but not chickenpox.'

• Nathwani D, et al. Infect Dis Clin Prac 1995; 4:138–145.
• Trying SK. Arch Fam Med; 2000; 9:863–869.

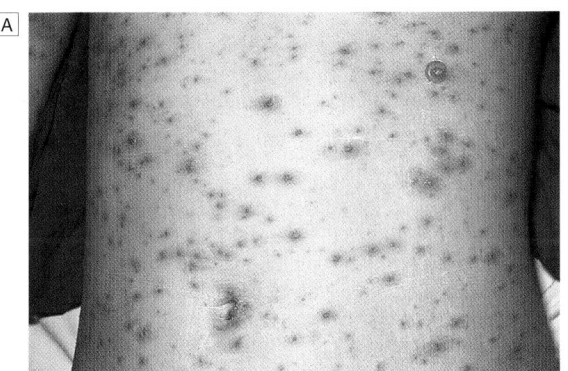 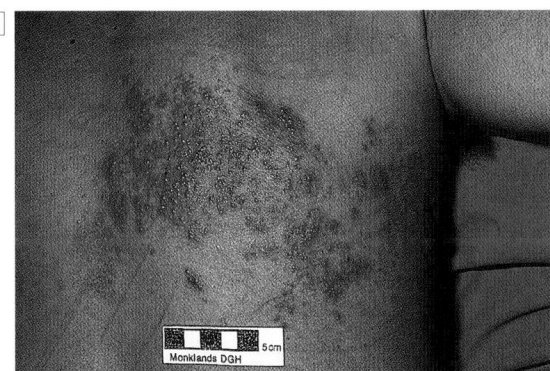

Fig. 13.9 Varicella zoster virus infection. A Chickenpox. B Shingles in a thoracic dermatome.

13.32 Therapy for herpes simplex and varicella zoster virus infection

Disease state	Treatment options
Primary genital HSV	Famciclovir 250 mg 8-hourly for 7–10 days Valaciclovir 1 g 12-hourly for 7–10 days Oral aciclovir 200 mg 5 times daily or 400 mg 8-hourly for 7–10 days
Severe and preventing oral intake	Aciclovir 5 mg/kg 8-hourly i.v. until patient can tolerate oral therapy
Recurrent genital HSV-1 or 2	Oral aciclovir 200 mg 5 times daily or 400 mg 8-hourly for 5 days Famciclovir 125 mg 12-hourly for 5 days Valaciclovir 500 mg 12-hourly for 5 days
Primary or recurrent oral HSV	Usually no treatment If required, usually shorter duration and lower dose than for genital lesions, e.g. valaciclovir 500 mg 12-hourly for 3–5 days
Mucocutaneous HSV infection in immuno-compromised host	Aciclovir 5 mg/kg 8-hourly i.v. for 7–10 days Oral aciclovir 400 mg 6-hourly for 7–10 days Famciclovir 500 mg 8-hourly for 7–10 days Valaciclovir 1 g 12-hourly for 7–10 days
Chickenpox in adult or child	Oral aciclovir 800 mg 5 times a day for 5 days Famciclovir 500 mg 8-hourly for 5 days Valaciclovir 1 g 8-hourly for 5 days
Immunocompromised host/pregnant woman	Aciclovir 5 mg/kg 8-hourly i.v. until patient is improving, then complete therapy with oral therapy until all lesions crusting over
Shingles	Treatment and doses as for chickenpox but duration typically 7–10 days
Visceral involvement (non-CNS) in HSV	Aciclovir i.v. 5 mg/kg 8-hourly for 14 days
Visceral involvement (non-CNS) in VZV	Aciclovir i.v. 5 mg/kg 8-hourly for 7 days
Severe complications (encephalitis, disseminated infection)	Aciclovir i.v. 10 mg/kg 8-hourly (up to 20 mg/kg in neonates) for 14–21 days
HSV disease suppression	Aciclovir 400 mg 12-hourly Famciclovir 250 mg 12-hourly Valaciclovir 500 mg daily

develop severe chickenpox after receiving VZIG should be treated with aciclovir.

A live, attenuated VZV vaccine is available and in routine use in the USA and other countries. Children receive one dose after 1 year of age and seronegative adults two doses. The vaccine may also be used in patients prior to planned iatrogenic immunosuppression, e.g. before a transplant procedure.

Shingles (herpes zoster)

After initial infection VZV persists in latent form in the dorsal root ganglion of sensory nerves and can reactivate in later life as a localised rash or with other clinical manifestations. Commonly seen in the elderly, shingles

13.33 Indications for varicella zoster immunoglobulin (VZIG) in adults

An adult should satisfy all three of the following conditions.

1. Significant contact

With exposed zoster, disseminated zoster, localised zoster (if index case is immunocompromised) or chickenpox, defined as:
- Prolonged household contact, sharing a room for ≥ 15 minutes or face-to-face contact (includes direct contact with zoster lesions) at any time from 48 hrs before development of rash to crusting of lesions (chickenpox) or from development of rash to crusting (zoster)
- Hospital contact with chickenpox in another patient, health-care worker or visitor
- Intimate contact (e.g. touching) with person with shingles lesions
- Newborn whose mother develops chickenpox no more than 5 days before delivery or 2 days after delivery

2. Susceptible contact

- Individual with no history of chickenpox, ideally confirmed by negative test for VZV IgG

3. Predisposition to severe chickenpox

- Immunocompromised due to disease (e.g. acute leukaemia, HIV, other primary or secondary immunodeficiency)
- Medically immunosuppressed (e.g. following solid organ transplant or other indication, current or recent (≤ 6 months) cytotoxic chemotherapy or radiotherapy, current or recent (≤ 3 months) high-dose corticosteroids, bone marrow transplant
- Pregnant (any stage)
- Infants: newborn whose mother has had chickenpox as above, premature infants < 28 weeks

may also present in younger patients with immune deficiency.

Clinical features

Burning discomfort occurs in the affected dermatome, where discrete vesicles appear 3–4 days later. This is associated with a brief viraemia and can produce distant satellite 'chickenpox' lesions. Severe disease, a prolonged duration of rash, multiple dermatomal involvement or recurrence suggests underlying immune deficiency, including HIV. Chickenpox may be contracted from a case of shingles but not vice versa.

Although thoracic dermatomes are most commonly involved (Fig. 13.9B), the ophthalmic division of the trigeminal nerve is also frequently affected; vesicles may appear on the cornea and lead to ulceration. This condition can lead to blindness and urgent ophthalmology review is required. Geniculate ganglion involvement causes the Ramsay Hunt syndrome of facial palsy, ipsilateral loss of taste and buccal ulceration, plus a rash in the external auditory canal. This may be mistaken for Bell's palsy (p. 1228). Bowel and bladder dysfunction occur with sacral nerve root involvement. The virus occasionally causes myelitis or encephalitis. Granulomatous cerebral angiitis is a cerebrovascular complication that leads to a stroke-like syndrome in association with shingles, especially in an ophthalmic distribution.

Post-herpetic neuralgia causes troublesome persistence of pain for 1–6 months or longer, following healing of the rash. It is more common with advanced age.

Management and prevention

Early therapy with aciclovir or related agents has been shown to reduce both early- and late-onset pain, especially in patients over 65 years (see Box 13.31, p. 313). Post-herpetic neuralgia requires aggressive analgesia, along with agents such as amitriptyline 25–100 mg daily or gabapentin (commencing at 300 mg daily and building slowly to 300 mg 12-hourly or more). Capsaicin cream (0.075%) may be helpful. Studies are investigating the role of corticosteroids to reduce post-herpetic neuralgia.

Enteroviral exanthems

Coxsackie or echovirus infections can lead to a maculopapular eruption or roseola-like rash that occurs after fever falls. Enteroviral infections are discussed further under viral infections of the skin (see below).

Systemic viral infections without exanthem

Other systemic viral infections present with features other than a rash suggestive of exanthem. Rashes may occur in these conditions but differ from those seen in exanthems or are not the primary presenting feature.

Mumps

Mumps is a systemic viral infection characterised by swelling of the parotid glands. Infection is endemic world-wide and peaks at 5–9 years of age. Vaccination has reduced the incidence in children but incomplete coverage has increased susceptibility amongst older non-immune adults. Infection is spread by respiratory droplets.

Clinical features

The median incubation period is 19 days, with a range of 15–24 days. Classical tender parotid enlargement, which is bilateral in 75%, follows a prodrome of pyrexia and headache (Fig. 13.10). In non-vaccinated communities, mumps is the most common cause of sporadic viral meningitis, and meningitis complicates up to 10% of cases. The cerebrospinal fluid (CSF) reveals a lymphocytic pleocytosis, or less commonly neutrophils. Rare

complications include encephalitis, transient hearing loss, labyrinthitis, electrocardiographic abnormalities, pancreatitis and arthritis.

Approximately 25% of post-pubertal males with mumps develop epididymo-orchitis but, although testicular atrophy occurs, sterility is unlikely. Oophoritis is much less common. Abortion may occur if infection takes place in the first trimester of pregnancy. Complications may occur in the absence of parotitis.

Diagnosis

The diagnosis is usually clinical. In atypical presentations without parotitis, serology for mumps-specific IgM or IgG seroconversion (four-fold rise in IgG convalescent titre) confirms the diagnosis. Virus can also be cultured from urine in the first week of infection or detected by PCR in urine, saliva or CSF.

Management and prevention

Treatment is with analgesia. There is no evidence that corticosteroids are of value for orchitis. Mumps vaccine is one of the components of the combined MMR vaccine.

Influenza

Influenza is an acute systemic viral infection that primarily affects the respiratory tract (p. 671); it carries a significant mortality. It is caused by influenza A virus or, in milder form, influenza B virus. Infection is seasonal, and variation in the haemagglutinin (H) and neuraminidase (N) glycoproteins on the surface of the virus leads to disease of variable intensity each year. Minor changes in haemagglutinin are known as 'genetic drift', whereas a switch in the haemagglutinin or neuraminidase antigen is termed 'genetic shift'. Nomenclature of influenza strains is based on these glycoproteins, e.g. H1N1, H3N2 etc. Genetic shift results in the circulation of a new influenza strain within a community to which few people are immune, potentially initiating an influenza epidemic or pandemic in which there is a high attack rate and there may be increased disease severity.

Clinical features

After an incubation period of 1–3 days, uncomplicated disease leads to fever, malaise and cough. Viral pneumonia may occur, although pulmonary complications are most often due to superinfection with *Strep. pneumoniae*, *Staph. aureus* or other bacteria. Rare extrapulmonary manifestations include myositis, myocarditis, pericarditis and neurological complications (Reye's syndrome in children, encephalitis or transverse myelitis).

Diagnosis

Acute infection is diagnosed by viral culture, or by antigen or RNA detection (reverse transcription (RT)-PCR) in a nasopharyngeal sample. The disease may also be diagnosed retrospectively on the basis of seroconversion.

Management and prevention

Administration of the neuraminidase inhibitors, oral oseltamivir (75 mg 12-hourly) or inhaled zanamivir (10 mg 12-hourly) for 5 days can reduce the severity of symptoms if started within 48 hours of symptom onset (or possibly later in immunocompromised individuals). These agents have superseded amantadine and

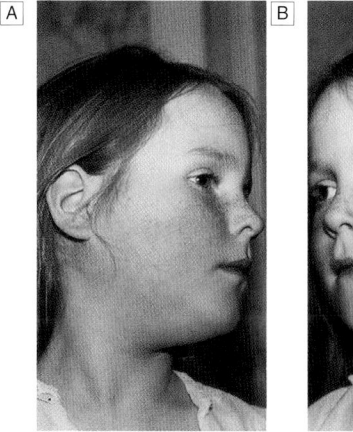
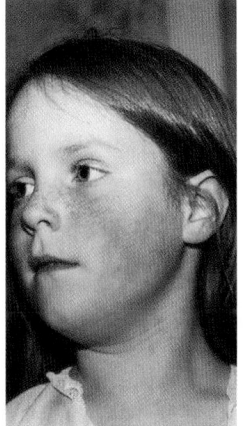

Fig. 13.10 Typical unilateral mumps. [A] Note the loss of angle of the jaw on the affected (right) side. [B] Comparison showing normal (left) side.

13

rimantadine. Antiviral drugs can also be used as prophylaxis in high-risk individuals during the 'flu' season. Resistance can emerge to all of these agents.

The major mechanism of prevention is seasonal vaccination of the elderly and of individuals with chronic medical illnesses which place them at increased risk of the complications of influenza, such as chronic cardiopulmonary diseases or immune compromise. Healthcare workers should also receive annual vaccination. The vaccine composition changes each year to reflect the predominant strains circulating but is of limited efficacy when a new pandemic strain emerges.

Avian influenza

Avian influenza is caused by influenza A viruses with alternative haemagglutinin antigens, including the H5N1 strain. These viruses have an increased ability to bind to lower respiratory tract epithelium, causing more severe disease with increased incidence of viral pneumonia and respiratory failure. The majority of cases have occurred in individuals with a history of exposure to poultry, predominantly in South-east Asia. However, in recent 'flu' seasons, cases have spread further west and infection has been identified in Europe in migrating birds and imported poultry. Existing strains have been associated with infrequent person-to-person transmission but there is a concern that adaptation of an avian strain to allow effective person-to-person transmission is likely to lead to a global pandemic of life-threatening influenza.

Vaccination against seasonal 'flu' does not adequately protect against avian influenza. Cases are diagnosed by recognising the relevant epidemiological factors and should be confirmed with specific tests. Avian strains are susceptible to the neuraminidase inhibitors, although strains resistant to oseltamivir have been reported.

Swine influenza

Occasional cases of influenza are transmitted from pigs to humans. An outbreak of swine 'flu' began in 2009, initially in Mexico and then spreading around the world. The causative strain was shown to be an H1N1 strain which showed significant genetic variation from human strains of H1N1. Clinical features of infections with this strain are typical of influenza A infection, although some cases have more pronounced enteric features. Mortality can occur, in particular in individuals with medical comorbidities. Management of such an outbreak involves good infection control with an emphasis on hand hygiene and preventing dissemination of infection by coughing and sneezing. Neuraminidase inhibitors (oseltamivir and zanamivir), but not amantadine or rimantadine, were active against the initial strains of swine flu isolated in 2009 and have been used for treatment and prophylaxis of key contacts.

Infectious mononucleosis (IM) and Epstein–Barr virus (EBV)

IM is an acute viral illness characterised by pharyngitis, cervical lymphadenopathy, fever and lymphocytosis. A variety of medical complications may ensue. It is most often caused by EBV infection, but a variety of other viral infections (CMV, HHV-6, HIV-1) and toxoplasmosis can produce a similar clinical syndrome.

EBV is a gamma herpesvirus. In developing countries, subclinical infection in childhood is virtually universal. In developed countries, primary infection may be delayed until adolescence or early adult life. Under these circumstances about 50% of infections result in typical IM. The virus is usually acquired from asymptomatic excreters via saliva, either by droplet infection or environmental contamination in childhood, or by kissing among adolescents and adults. EBV is not highly contagious and isolation of cases is unnecessary.

Clinical features

IM has a prolonged and undetermined incubation period, followed in some cases by a prodrome of fever, headache and malaise. This is followed by severe pharyngitis, which may include tonsillar exudates, and non-tender anterior and posterior cervical lymphadenopathy. Palatal petechiae, periorbital oedema, splenomegaly, inguinal or axillary lymphadenopathy, and macular, petechial or erythema multiforme rashes may occur. In most cases fever resolves over 2 weeks, and fatigue and other abnormalities settle over a further few weeks. Complications are listed in Box 13.34. Death is rare but can occur due to respiratory obstruction, haemorrhage from splenic rupture or thrombocytopenia, or encephalitis.

The diagnosis of IM outside the usual age in adolescence and young adulthood is difficult. In children under 10 years the illness is mild and short-lived, but in adults over 30 years of age it can be severe and prolonged. In both groups pharyngeal symptoms are often absent. IM may present with jaundice, as a PUO or with a complication.

13.34 Complications of infectious mononucleosis	
Common	
• Severe pharyngeal oedema	• Prolonged post-viral fatigue (10%)
• Antibiotic-induced rash (80–90% with ampicillin)	• Hepatitis (80%)
	• Jaundice (< 10%)
Uncommon	
Neurological	
• Cranial nerve palsies	• Transverse myelitis
• Polyneuritis	• Meningoencephalitis
Haematological	
• Haemolytic anaemia	• Thrombocytopenia
Renal	
• Abnormalities on urinalysis	• Interstitial nephritis
Cardiac	
• Myocarditis	• Pericarditis
• ECG abnormalities	
Rare	
• Ruptured spleen	• X-linked lymphoproliferative syndrome
• Respiratory obstruction	
• Agranulocytosis	
EBV-associated malignancy	
• Nasopharyngeal carcinoma	• Hodgkin's disease (certain subtypes only)
• Burkitt's lymphoma	• Lymphoproliferative disease in immunocompromised
• Primary CNS lymphoma	

Long-term complications of EBV infection

Lymphoma complicates EBV infection in immuno-compromised hosts, and some forms of Hodgkin's disease are EBV-associated (p. 1037). The endemic form of Burkitt's lymphoma complicates EBV infection in areas of sub-Saharan Africa where *falciparum* malaria is endemic. Nasopharyngeal carcinoma is a geographically restricted tumour seen in China and Alaska that is associated with EBV infection. X-linked lymphoproliferative (Duncan's) syndrome is a familial lymphoproliferative disorder that follows primary EBV infection in boys without any other history of immunodeficiency. The course is frequently fatal due to liver failure, haemophagocytosis, lymphoma or progressive agammaglobulinaemia, complicated by infection. The disorder is due to mutation of the *SAP* gene, involved in cell signalling in lymphocytes, and results in failure to contain EBV infection.

Investigations

Atypical lymphocytes are common in EBV infection but also occur in other causes of IM, acute retroviral syndrome with HIV infection, viral hepatitis, mumps and rubella (Fig. 13.11A). A 'heterophile' antibody is present during the acute illness and convalescence, which is detected by the Paul–Bunnell or 'Monospot' test. Sometimes antibody production is delayed, so an initially negative test should be repeated. However, many children and 10% of adolescents with IM do not produce heterophile antibody at any stage.

Specific EBV serology (immunofluorescence) can be used to confirm the diagnosis if necessary. Acute infection is characterised by IgM antibodies against the viral capsid, antibodies to EBV early antigen and the initial absence of antibodies to EBV nuclear antigen (anti-EBNA). Seroconversion of anti-EBNA at approximately 1 month after the initial illness may confirm the diagnosis in retrospect. CNS infections may be diagnosed by detection of viral DNA in cerebrospinal fluid.

Management

Treatment is largely symptomatic. If a throat culture yields a β-haemolytic streptococcus, a course of penicillin should be prescribed. Administration of ampicillin or amoxicillin in this condition commonly causes an itchy macular rash, and should be avoided (Fig. 13.11B). When pharyngeal oedema is severe, a short course of corticosteroids, e.g. prednisolone 30 mg daily for 5 days, may help. Antivirals are not sufficiently active against EBV.

Return to work or school is governed by the patient's physical fitness rather than laboratory tests. However, contact sports should be avoided until splenomegaly has completely resolved because of the danger of splenic rupture. Unfortunately, about 10% of patients with IM suffer a chronic relapsing syndrome.

Cytomegalovirus (CMV)

CMV, like EBV, circulates readily among children. A second period of virus acquisition occurs among teenagers and young adults, peaking between the ages of 25 and 35 years, rather later than with EBV infection. CMV infection is persistent, and is characterised by subclinical cycles of active virus replication and by persistent low-level virus shedding. Most post-childhood infections are therefore acquired from asymptomatic excreters who shed virus in saliva, urine, semen and genital secretions. Sexual transmission and oral spread are common among adults, but infection may also be acquired by women caring for children with asymptomatic infections.

Clinical features

Most post-childhood CMV infections are subclinical, although some young adults develop an IM-like syndrome and some have a prolonged influenza-like illness lasting 2 weeks or more. Physical signs resemble those of IM, but in CMV mononucleosis hepatomegaly is relatively more common, while lymphadenopathy, splenomegaly, pharyngitis and tonsillitis are found less often. Jaundice is uncommon and usually mild. Unusual complications include meningoencephalitis, Guillain–Barré syndrome, autoimmune haemolytic anaemia, thrombocytopenia, myocarditis and skin eruptions such as ampicillin-induced rash. Immunocompromised patients can develop hepatitis, oesophagitis, colitis, pneumonitis, retinitis, encephalitis and polyradiculitis.

Women who develop a primary CMV infection during pregnancy have about a 40% chance of passing CMV to the fetus, causing congenital infection and disease at any stage of gestation. Features include petechial rashes, hepatosplenomegaly and jaundice; 10% of infected infants will have long-term CNS sequelae such as microcephaly, cerebral calcifications, chorioretinitis and deafness. Infections in the newborn usually are asymptomatic or have features of an IM-like illness, although some studies suggest subtle sequelae affecting hearing or mental development may occur.

13

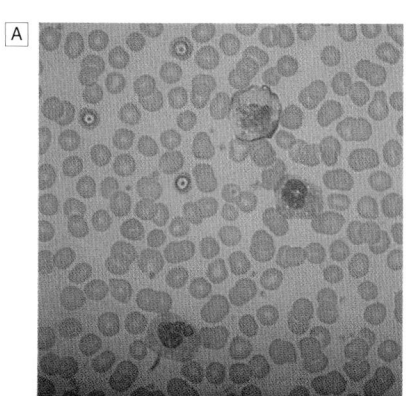

Fig. 13.11 Features of infectious mononucleosis. A Atypical lymphocytes in peripheral blood. B Skin reaction to ampicillin.

Investigations

Atypical lymphocytosis is not as prominent as in IM and heterophile antibody tests are negative. LFTs are often abnormal, with an alkaline phosphatase level raised out of proportion to transaminases. Serological diagnosis depends on the detection of CMV-specific IgM antibody plus a four-fold rise or seroconversion of IgG. In the immunocompromised, antibody detection is unreliable and detection of CMV in an involved organ by PCR, culture or histopathology establishes the diagnosis. A positive culture of CMV in the blood may be useful in transplant populations but not in HIV-positive individuals, since in HIV infection CMV reactivates at regular intervals but these episodes do not correlate well with episodes of clinical disease. Detection of CMV in urine is not helpful in diagnosing infection, except in neonates, since viruses are intermittently shed in the urine throughout life following infection.

Management

Only symptomatic treatment is required in the immunocompetent patient. Immunocompromised individuals are treated with ganciclovir 5 mg/kg i.v. 12-hourly or with oral valganciclovir 900 mg 12-hourly for at least 14 days. Foscarnet or cidofovir is also used in CMV treatment of immunocompromised patients who are resistant or intolerant of ganciclovir-based therapy.

Dengue

The dengue flavivirus is a common cause of fever and acute systemic illness in the tropics. It is endemic in South-east Asia and India, and is also seen in Africa, the Caribbean and the Americas (Fig. 13.12). The principal vector is the mosquito *Aedes aegypti*, which breeds in standing water; collections of water in containers, water-based air coolers and tyre dumps are a good environment for the vector in large cities. *Aedes albopictus* is a vector in some South-east Asian countries. There are four serotypes of dengue virus, all producing a similar clinical syndrome; homotypic immunity after infection with one of the serotypes is life-long, but heterotypic immunity against the other serotypes lasts only a few months after infection.

Clinical features

The incubation period from being bitten by an infected mosquito is usually 2–7 days. Clinical features are listed in Box 13.35. Asymptomatic infections are common but the disease is more severe in infants and the elderly. A morbilliform rash, which characteristically blanches under pressure, may occur, often as the fever is settling.

A more severe illness, called dengue haemorrhagic fever or dengue shock syndrome, occurs mainly in children in South-east Asia (see Box 13.35). In mild forms, there is thrombocytopenia and haemoconcentration. In the most severe form, after 3–4 days of fever, hypotension and circulatory failure develop with pleural effusions, ascites, hypoalbuminaemia and features of acute respiratory distress syndrome (ARDS, p. 187). Minor

13.35 Clinical features of dengue fever

Prodrome

- 2 days of malaise and headache

Acute onset

- Fever, backache, arthralgias, headache, generalised pains ('break-bone fever'), pain on eye movement, lacrimation, anorexia, nausea, vomiting, relative bradycardia, prostration, depression, lymphadenopathy, scleral injection

Fever

- Continuous or 'saddle-back', with break on 4th or 5th day and then recrudescence; usually lasts 7–8 days

Rash

- Initial flushing faint macular rash in first 1–2 days. Maculopapular, scarlet morbilliform rash from days 3–5 on trunk, spreading centrifugally and sparing palms and soles, onset often with fever defervescence. May desquamate on resolution or give rise to petechiae on extensor surfaces

Convalescence

- Slow

Complications

- Minor bleeding from mucosal sites, hepatitis, cerebral haemorrhage or oedema, rhabdomyolysis

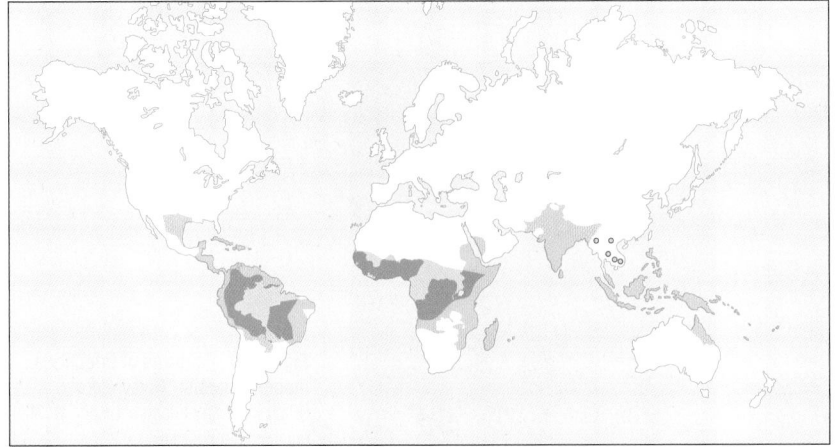

Dengue
Yellow fever
Dengue + yellow fever
Outbreaks of dengue haemorrhagic fever

Fig. 13.12 Endemic zones of yellow fever and dengue.

(petechiae, ecchymoses, epistaxis) or major (gastrointestinal or cerebrovascular) haemorrhagic signs may occur. The pathogenesis is unclear but pre-existing active or passive immunity to a dengue virus serotype different to the one causing the current infection is a predisposing factor; these heterotypic antibodies cause enhanced virus entry and replication in monocytes in vitro. Cytokine release is thought to be the cause of capillary leak causing effusions, and disseminated intravascular coagulation (DIC, p. 190) may contribute to haemorrhage. Adults rarely have classical dengue shock syndrome but they may have a stormy and fatal course characterised by elevated liver enzymes, haemostatic abnormalities and gastrointestinal bleeding.

Diagnosis

Diagnosis of dengue is easier in an endemic area when a patient has the characteristic symptoms and signs. However, mild cases may have a similar presentation to other viral infections. Leucopenia is usual and thrombocytopenia common. The diagnosis is confirmed by either a fourfold rise in IgG antibody titres, isolation of dengue virus from blood or detection of dengue virus RNA by PCR (p. 138). Serological tests may detect cross-reacting antibodies against other flaviviruses, including yellow fever vaccine.

Management and prevention

Treatment is symptomatic. Aspirin should be avoided due to bleeding risk. Volume replacement and blood transfusions may be indicated in patients with shock. With intensive care support, mortality rates are 1% or less. Corticosteroids have not been shown to help. No existing antivirals are effective.

Breeding places of *Aedes* mosquitoes should be abolished and the adults destroyed by insecticides. There is no licensed vaccine available.

Yellow fever

Yellow fever is a haemorrhagic fever of the tropics, caused by a flavivirus. It is a zoonosis of monkeys in West and Central African, and South and Central American tropical rainforests, where it may cause devastating epidemics (see Fig. 13.12). Transmission is by tree-top mosquitoes *Aedes africanus* (Africa) and *Haemagogus* spp. (America). The infection is introduced to humans either by infected mosquitoes when trees are felled, or by monkeys raiding human settlements. In towns, yellow fever may be transmitted between humans by *Aedes aegypti*, which breeds efficiently in small collections of water. The distribution of this mosquito is far wider than that of yellow fever and more widespread infection is a continued threat.

Yellow fever causes between 200 000 and 300 000 deaths each year, mainly in sub-Saharan Africa, where it remains a major public health problem. Overall mortality is around 15%, although this varies widely. Humans are infectious during the viraemic phase, which starts 3–6 days after the bite of the infected mosquito and lasts for 4–5 days.

Clinical features

After an incubation period of 3–6 days, yellow fever is often a mild febrile illness lasting less than 1 week with headache, myalgia, conjunctival erythema and bradycardia. This is followed by fever resolution (defervescence), but in some cases fever recurs after a few hours to days. In more severe disease, fever recrudescence is associated

13.36 Diagnosis of yellow fever

- Clinical features in endemic area
- Virus isolation from blood in first 24 days
- IgM or fourfold rise in IgG antibody titre
- Post-mortem liver biopsy
- Differentiation from malaria, typhoid, viral hepatitis, leptospirosis, haemorrhagic fevers, aflatoxin poisoning

with lower back pain, abdominal pain and somnolence, prominent nausea and vomiting, bradycardia and jaundice. Liver damage and DIC lead to bleeding with petechiae, mucosal haemorrhages and gastrointestinal bleeding. Shock, hepatic failure, renal failure, seizures and coma may ensue.

Diagnosis

Diagnostic procedures are listed in Box 13.36. Leucopenia is characteristic. Liver biopsy should be avoided in life due to the risk of fatal bleeding. Post-mortem features, such as acute mid-zonal necrosis and Councilman bodies with minimal inflammation in the liver, are suggestive but not specific. Immunohistochemistry for viral antigens improves specificity.

Management and prevention

Treatment is supportive, with meticulous attention to fluid and electrolyte balance, urine output and blood pressure. Blood transfusions, plasma expanders and peritoneal dialysis may be necessary. Patients should be isolated, as their blood and body products may contain virus particles.

A single vaccination with a live attenuated vaccine gives full protection for at least 10 years. Potential side-effects include hypersensitivity, encephalitis and systemic features of yellow fever caused by the attenuated virus. Vaccination is not recommended in people who are significantly immunosuppressed. The risk of vaccine side-effects must be balanced against the risk of infection for less immunocompromised hosts, pregnant women and older patients. An internationally recognised certificate of vaccination is sometimes necessary when crossing borders.

Viral haemorrhagic fevers (VHF)

VHF are zoonoses caused by several different viruses (Box 13.37). They are geographically restricted and occur in rural settings or in health-care facilities.

Serological surveys have shown that Lassa fever is widespread in West Africa and may lead to up to 500 000 infections annually. Mortality overall may be low, as 80% of cases are asymptomatic, but in hospitalised cases mortality averages 15%. Ebola outbreaks have occurred at a rate of approximately 1 outbreak per year, involving up to a few hundred cases. The largest outbreaks have been in the Democratic Republic of Congo, Uganda and Sudan. Marburg has been documented less frequently, with outbreaks in the Democratic Republic of Congo and Uganda, but the largest outbreak to date involved 163 cases in Angola in 2005. Mortality rates of Ebola and Marburg are high.

VHF have extended into Europe, with an outbreak of Congo–Crimean haemorrhagic fever in Turkey in 2006, and cases of haemorrhagic fever with renal syndrome in

13

13

Disease	Reservoir	Transmission	Incubation period	Geography	Mortality rate	Clinical features of severe disease[1]
Lassa fever	Multimammate rats (*Mastomys natalensis*)	Urine from rat Body fluids from patients	6–21 days	West Africa	15%	Haemorrhage, shock, encephalopathy, ARDS (responds to ribavirin) Deafness in survivors
Ebola fever	Undefined (?bats)	Body fluids from patients Handling infected primates	2–21 days	Central Africa Outbreaks as far north as Sudan	25–90%	Haemorrhage, hepatic and renal failure
Marburg fever	Undefined	Body fluids from patients Handling infected primates	3–9 days	Central Africa Outbreak in Angola	25–90%	Haemorrhage, diarrhoea, encephalopathy, orchitis
Yellow fever	Monkeys	Mosquitoes	3–6 days	Tropical Africa, South and Central America	~15%	Hepatic failure, renal failure, haemorrhage
Dengue	Humans	*Aedes aegypti*	2–7 days	Tropical and subtropical coasts; Asia, Africa, Americas	< 10%[2]	Haemorrhage, shock
Crimean–Congo haemorrhagic fever	Small vertebrates Domestic and wild animals	*Ixodes* tick Body fluids	1–3 days up to 9 days 3–6 days up to 13 days	Africa, Asia, Eastern Europe	30%	Encephalopathy, haemorrhage, hepatic or renal failure, ARDS
Rift Valley fever	Domestic livestock	Contact with animals, mosquito or other insect bites	2–6 days	Africa, Arabian peninsular	1%	Haemorrhage, blindness, meningoencephalitis (complications only in a minority)
Kyasanur fever	Monkeys	Ticks	3–8 days	Karnataka State, India	5–10%	Haemorrhage, pulmonary oedema, neurological features Iridokeratitis in survivors
Bolivian and Argentinian haemorrhagic fever (Junin and Machupo viruses)	Rodents (*Calomys* spp.)	Urine, aerosols Body fluids from case (rare)	5–19 days (3–6 days for parenteral)	South America	15–30%	Haemorrhage, shock, cerebellar signs (may respond to ribavirin)
Haemorrhagic fever with renal syndrome (Hantaan fever)	Rodents	Aerosols from faeces	5–42 days (typically 14 days)	Northern Asia, northern Europe, Balkans	5%	Acute renal impairment, cerebrovascular accidents, pulmonary oedema, shock (hepatic failure and haemorrhagic features only in some variants)

[1] All potentially have circulatory failure.
[2] Mortality of uncomplicated and haemorrhagic dengue fever, respectively.

the Balkans and Russia. These conditions remain very rare in the UK, with about 1 case of Lassa fever arriving in the country every 2 years.

Kyasanur forest disease is a tick-borne VHF currently confined to a small focus in Karnataka, India; there are about 500 cases annually. Monkeys are the principal hosts, but with forest felling there are fears that this disease will increase.

All of these viral illnesses, except Ebola and Marburg, have mild self-limiting forms. Details on recent disease outbreaks can be found at the WHO website (www.who.int).

Clinical features

All VHF have similar non-specific presentations with fever, malaise, body pains, sore throat and headache. On examination conjunctivitis, throat injection, an erythematous or petechial rash, haemorrhage, lymphadenopathy and bradycardia may be noted. The viruses cause endothelial dysfunction with the development of capillary leak. Bleeding is due to endothelial damage and platelet dysfunction. Hypovolaemic shock and ARDS may develop (p. 187).

Haemorrhage is a late feature of VHF and most patients present with earlier features. In Lassa fever, joint and abdominal pain are prominent. A macular blanching rash may be present but bleeding is unusual, occurring in only 20% of hospitalised patients. Encephalopathy may develop and deafness affects 30% of survivors.

The clue to the viral aetiology comes from the travel and exposure history. Travel to an outbreak area, activity in a rural environment and contact with sick individuals or animals within 21 days all increase the risk of VHF. Enquiry should be made about insect bites, hospital visits and attendance at ritual funerals (Ebola virus infection). For Lassa fever retrosternal pain, pharyngitis and proteinuria have a positive predictive value of 80% in West Africa.

Investigations and management

Non-specific findings include leucopenia, thrombocytopenia and proteinuria. In Lassa fever an aspartate aminotransferase (AST) > 150 U/L is associated with a 50% mortality. It is important to exclude other causes of fever, especially malaria, typhoid and respiratory tract infections. Most patients suspected of having a VHF in the UK turn out to have malaria.

In patients with suspected VHF, strict infection control is important (see Fig. 13.5, p. 307). The diagnosis of VHF must be considered in all individuals who present with fever within 21 days of leaving an endemic area or who present with haemorrhage or organ failure. A febrile patient from an endemic area within the incubation period, who has specific epidemiological risk factors (see Fig. 13.5, p. 307) or who has signs of organ failure or haemorrhage, should be treated as being at high risk of VHF. These patients must be transferred to a centre with the appropriate biosafety facilities to care for them. Individuals with a history of travel within 21 days and fever, but without the relevant epidemiological features or signs of VHF, are classified as medium-risk and should have an initial blood sample tested to exclude malaria. If this is negative, relevant specimens (blood, throat swab, urine and pleural fluid (if available)) are collected and sent to an appropriate reference laboratory for nucleic acid detection (PCR), virus isolation, and serology. If patients are felt to be at high risk of VHF or if infection is confirmed, they should be transferred to a specialised high-security infectious disease unit. All further laboratory tests should be performed at biosafety level 4. Transport requires an ambulance with biosafety level 3 facilities.

In addition to general supportive measures, ribavirin is given intravenously (100 mg/kg, then 25 mg/kg daily for 3 days and 12.5 mg/kg daily for 4 days) when Lassa fever or South American haemorrhagic fevers are suspected.

Prevention

Ribavirin has been used as prophylaxis in close contacts in Lassa fever but there are no formal trials of its efficacy.

Viral infections of the skin

Herpes simplex virus 1 and 2 (HSV)

These cause widespread recurrent mucocutaneous infection; HSV-1 typically involves the mucocutaneous surfaces of the head and neck (Fig. 13.13), whilst HSV-2 predominantly involves the genital mucosa (pp. 416 and 421), although there is overlap (see Box 13.30, p. 312). The seroprevalence of HSV-1 is 30–100%, varying by socioeconomic status, while that of HSV-2 is 20–60%. Infection is acquired by inoculation of viruses shed by an infected individual on to a mucosal surface in a susceptible person. The virus infects sensory and autonomic neurons and establishes latent infection in the nerve ganglia. Primary infection is followed by episodes of reactivation throughout life.

Clinical features

Primary HSV-1 or 2 infection is more likely to be symptomatic later in life, causing gingivostomatitis, pharyngitis or painful genital tract lesions. The primary attack may be associated with fever and regional lymphadenopathy.

Recurrence

Recurrent attacks occur throughout life, most often in association with concomitant medical illness, menstruation, mechanical trauma, immunosuppression, psychological stress or, for oral lesions, ultraviolet light exposure. HSV reactivation in the oral mucosa produces the classical 'cold sore' or 'herpes labialis'. Prodromal hyperaesthesia is followed by rapid vesiculation, pustulation and crusting. Recurrent HSV genital disease is a common cause of recurrent painful genital ulceration (p. 421). An inoculation lesion on the finger gives rise to

13

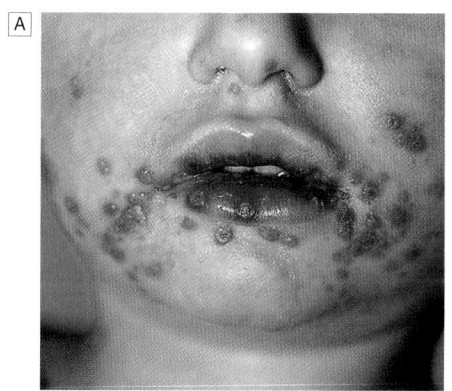 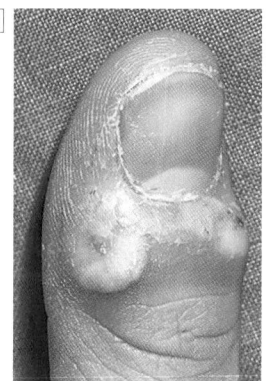 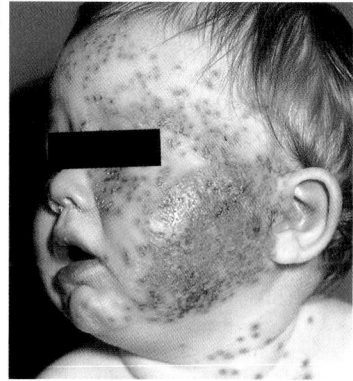

Fig. 13.13 Cutaneous manifestations of herpes simplex virus-1 (HSV-1). [A] Acute HSV-1. There were also vesicles in the mouth—herpetic stomatitis. [B] Herpetic whitlow. [C] Eczema herpeticum. HSV-1 infection spreads rapidly in eczematous skin.

a paronychia termed a 'whitlow' in contacts of patients with herpetic lesions (Fig. 13.13B). It was formerly seen in health-care workers and dentists, but is prevented by protective gloves.

Complications

Complications include disseminated cutaneous lesions in individuals with underlying dermatological diseases such as eczema (eczema herpeticum) (Fig. 13.13C). Herpes keratitis presents with pain and blurring of vision; characteristic dendritic ulcers are visible on slit-lamp examination and may produce corneal scarring and permanent visual impairment.

Primary HSV-2 can cause meningitis or transverse myelitis. HSV is the leading cause of sporadic viral encephalitis (p. 1209); this serious complication may occur following either primary or secondary disease, usually with HSV-1. A haemorrhagic necrotising temporal lobe cerebritis produces temporal lobe epilepsy and altered consciousness/coma. Without treatment, mortality is 80%. HSV is also implicated in the pathogenesis of Bell's palsy with a lower motor neuron VII nerve palsy.

Neonatal HSV disease is usually associated with primary infection of the mother at term (see Box 13.27, p. 310). In excess of two-thirds of cases develop disseminated disease with cutaneous lesions, hepatitis, pneumonitis and frequently encephalitis.

Immunocompromised hosts can develop visceral disease with oesophagitis, hepatitis, pneumonitis, encephalitis or retinitis.

Diagnosis

Differentiation from other vesicular eruptions is achieved by demonstration of virus in vesicular fluid by direct immunofluorescence or culture, or of virus DNA by PCR. HSV encephalitis is diagnosed by detection of virus DNA in CSF. Serology is of limited value, only confirming whether an individual has had previous infection.

Management

The acyclic antivirals are the treatment of choice for HSV infection (see Box 13.32, p. 314). Therapy must commence in the first 48 hours of clinical disease (primary or recurrent); thereafter it is unlikely to influence clinical outcome. Oral lesions in an immunocompetent individual may be treated with topical aciclovir. All severe manifestations should be treated, regardless of the time of presentation. Any reasonable suspicion of HSV encephalopathy is an indication for immediate empiric antiviral therapy. Aciclovir resistance is encountered occasionally in immunocompromised hosts, in which case foscarnet is the treatment of choice.

Human herpesvirus 8 (HHV-8)

This virus (see Box 13.30, p. 421) causes Kaposi's sarcoma in both AIDS-related and endemic non-AIDS-related forms (p. 402). HHV-8 is spread via saliva and men who have sex with men have increased incidence of infection. Seroprevalence varies widely, being highest in sub-Saharan Africa. HHV-8 also causes two rare haematological malignancies: primary effusion lymphoma and multicentric Castleman's disease. Current antivirals are not effective.

Enterovirus infections

Hand, foot and mouth disease

This systemic infection is usually caused by Coxsackie viruses or occasionally echoviruses. It affects children and occasionally adults, resulting in local or household outbreaks, particularly in the summer months. A relatively mild illness with fever and lymphadenopathy develops after an incubation period of approximately 10 days; 2–3 days later a painful papular or vesicular rash appears on palmoplantar surfaces of hands and feet, with associated oral lesions on the buccal mucosa and tongue that ulcerate rapidly. A papular erythematous rash may appear on buttocks and thighs. Antiviral treatment is not available and management consists of symptom relief with analgesics.

Herpangina

This infection, caused by Coxsackie viruses, primarily affects children and teenagers in the summer months. It is characterised by a small number of vesicles at the soft/hard palate junction, often associated with high fever, an extremely sore throat and headache. The lesions are short-lived, rupturing after 2–3 days and rarely persisting for more than 1 week. Treatment is with analgesics if required. Culture of the virus from vesicles or DNA detection by PCR differentiates herpangina from HSV.

Poxviruses

These DNA viruses are rare but potentially important pathogens.

Smallpox (variola)

This severe disease, which has high mortality, was eradicated world-wide by a global vaccination programme. Interest in the disease has re-emerged due to its potential as a bioweapon. The virus is spread by the respiratory route or contact with lesions, and is highly infectious.

The incubation period is 7–17 days. A prodrome with fever, headache and prostration leads in 1–2 days to the rash, which develops through macules and papules to vesicles and pustules, worst on the face and distal extremities. Lesions in one area are all at the same stage of development with no cropping (unlike chickenpox). Vaccination can lead to a modified course of disease with milder rash and lower mortality.

If a case of smallpox is suspected, national public health authorities must be contacted. Electron micrography (like Fig. 13.14) and DNA detection tests (PCR) are used to confirm smallpox or, using specific primers, an alternative poxvirus.

Monkeypox

Despite the name, the animal reservoirs for this virus are probably small squirrels and rodents. It causes a rare zoonotic infection in communities in the rainforest belt of central Africa, producing a vesicular rash indistinguishable from smallpox, but differentiated by the presence of lymphadenopathy. Little person-to-person transmission occurs. Recent outbreaks outside Africa have been linked to importation of African animals as exotic pets. Diagnosis is by EM and/or DNA detection (PCR).

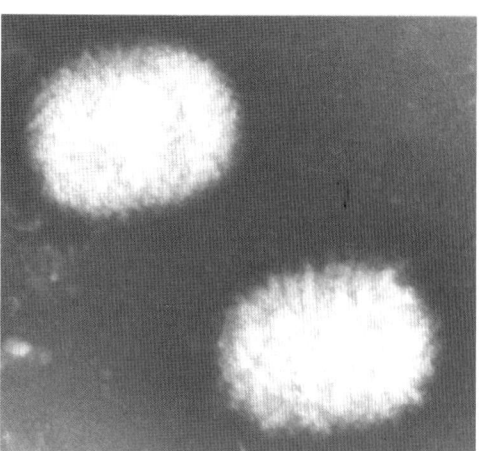

Fig. 13.14 Electron micrograph of molluscum contagiosum, a poxvirus.

Cowpox

Humans in contact with infected cows develop large vesicles, usually on the hands or arms and associated with fever and regional lymphadenitis. The reservoir is thought to be wild rodents, and the virus also produces symptomatic disease in cats and a range of other animals.

Vaccinia virus

This laboratory strain is the basis of the existing vaccine to prevent smallpox. Widespread vaccination is no longer recommended due to the likelihood of local spread from the vaccination site (potentially life-threatening in those with eczema (eczema vaccinatum) or immune deficiency) and of encephalitis. However, vaccination may still be recommended for key medical staff.

Orf

See page 1273.

Molluscum contagiosum

See page 1273 and Figure 13.14.

Gastrointestinal viral infections

Norovirus (Norwalk agent)

Noroviruses have been associated with outbreaks of gastroenteritis in closed communities such as long-stay hospital wards, cruise ships and military camps. Food handlers may also transmit this virus, which is relatively resistant to decontamination procedures. Incubation periods are 24–48 hours. High attack rates and prominent vomiting are characteristic. Diagnosis is by electron microscopy, antigen or DNA detection (PCR) in stool samples.

Astrovirus

Astroviruses cause diarrhoea in small children and occasionally in immunocompromised adults.

Rotavirus

Rotaviruses are the major cause of diarrhoeal illness in young children world-wide and cause 10–20% of deaths due to gastroenteritis in developing countries. There are winter epidemics in developed countries, particularly in nurseries. Adults are less often infected but those in close contact with cases may develop disease. The virus infects enterocytes, causing decreased surface absorption. The incubation period is 48 hours and patients present with watery diarrhoea, vomiting, fever and abdominal pain. Dehydration is prominent. Diagnosis is aided by commercially available enzyme immunoassay kits, which require fresh or refrigerated stool samples. Immunity develops to natural infection. A licensed vaccine is effective but is associated with increased rates of intussusception and so its use is not recommended. Other vaccines are in development.

Hepatitis viruses (A–E)

See Chapter 23.

Other viruses

Adenoviruses are frequently identified from stool culture and implicated as a cause of diarrhoea in children. They have also been linked to cases of intussusception.

Respiratory viral infections

These infections are described on pages 680–681.

Adenoviruses, rhinoviruses and enteroviruses (Coxsackie viruses and echoviruses) (Box 19.40, p. 680) often produce non-specific symptoms. Parainfluenza and respiratory syncytial viruses cause upper respiratory tract disease, croup and bronchiolitis in small children and pneumonia in the immunocompromised. Respiratory syncytial virus also causes pneumonia in nursing home residents and may be associated with nosocomial pneumonia. Metapneumovirus and bocavirus have emerged as new causes of upper respiratory tract infection and occasionally lower respiratory tract infection. They may also cause pneumonia in immunosuppressed individuals, such as recipients of allogeneic bone marrow transplants. The severe acute respiratory syndrome (SARS) caused by the SARS coronavirus emerged as a major respiratory pathogen during an outbreak in 2002–3, with 8000 cases and 10% mortality (p. 682).

Viral infections with neurological involvement

See also page 1209.

Japanese B encephalitis

This flavivirus is an important cause of endemic encephalitis in Japan, China, Russia, South-east Asia, India and Pakistan; outbreaks also occur elsewhere. There are 10 000–20 000 cases reported to the WHO annually. Pigs and aquatic birds are the virus reservoirs and transmission is by mosquitoes. Exposure to rice paddies is a recognised risk factor.

Clinical features

The incubation period is 4–21 days. Most infections are probably subclinical in childhood and only around 1% of infections lead to encephalitis. There is an initial

13

systemic illness with fever, malaise and anorexia, followed by photophobia, vomiting, headache and changes in brain-stem function. Neurological features other than encephalitis include meningitis, seizures, cranial nerve palsies, flaccid or spastic paralysis, and extrapyramidal features. Mortality with neurological disease is 25%. Most children die from respiratory failure with infection of brain-stem nuclei. Approximately 50% of survivors are left with neurological sequelae.

Investigations, management and prevention

Other infectious causes of encephalitis should be excluded (p. 1209). There is neutrophilia and often hyponatraemia. CSF analysis reveals lymphocytosis and elevated protein. Serological testing may be helpful and there is a CSF antigen test.

Treatment is supportive, anticipating and treating complications. Vaccination for travellers to endemic areas during the monsoon period is effective prophylaxis. Some endemic countries include this vaccination in their childhood schedules.

West Nile virus

This flavivirus has emerged as an important cause of neurological disease in an area that extends from Australia, India and Russia through Africa and Southern Europe and across to North America. The disease has an avian reservoir and a mosquito vector. The elderly are at increased risk of neurological disease.

Clinical features

Most infections are asymptomatic. After 2–6 days' incubation, a mild febrile illness and arthralgia constitute the most common clinical presentation. A prolonged incubation may be seen in immunocompromised individuals. Children may develop a maculopapular rash. Neurological disease is seen in 1% and is characterised by encephalitis, meningitis or asymmetric flaccid paralysis with 10% mortality.

Diagnosis and management

Diagnosis is by serology or detection of viral RNA in blood or CSF. Serological tests may show cross-reactivity with other flaviviruses, including vaccine strains. Treatment is supportive.

Enterovirus 71

Enterovirus 71 has caused outbreaks around the globe of enteroviral disease with hand, foot and mouth disease (p. 322) and aseptic meningitis. Some cases have been complicated by encephalitis with flaccid paralysis or by brain-stem involvement and death. The virus can be isolated from vesicle fluid, stool or CSF, and viral RNA can be detected in CSF by RT-PCR.

Nipah virus encephalitis

In 1999 a newly discovered paramyxovirus in the Hendra group, the Nipah virus, caused an epidemic of encephalitis amongst Malaysian pig farmers. Infection is through direct contact with pig secretions. Mortality is around 30%. Antibodies to the Hendra virus are present in 76% of cases.

Human T cell lymphotropic virus type I (HTLV-1)

HTLV-I is a retrovirus which causes chronic infection with development of adult T-cell leukaemia/lymphoma or HTLV-1-associated myelopathy (HAM) in a subset of those infected (p. 1039). It is found mainly in Japan, the Caribbean, Central and South America, and the Seychelles. HAM or tropical spastic paraparesis occurs in < 5% of those with chronic infection, and presents with gait disturbance, spasticity of the lower extremities, urinary incontinence, impotence and sensory disturbance. Myositis and uveitis may also occur with HTLV-1 infection. Serology confirms the diagnosis. Treatment is supportive.

Viral infections with rheumatological involvement

Rheumatological syndromes characterise a variety of viral infections ranging from exanthems, such as rubella and parvovirus B19 (p. 311), to blood-borne viruses, such as HBV and HIV-1.

Chikungunya virus

Chikungunya is an alphavirus that causes fever, rash and arthropathy. It is found principally in Africa and Asia, including India. Humans and non-human primates are the main reservoir and the main vector is the *Aedes aegypti* mosquito. Cases occur in epidemics on a background of sporadic cases. In 2007 an outbreak extended as far north as Italy.

The incubation period is 2–12 days. A period of fever may be followed by an afebrile phase and then recrudescence of fever. Children may develop a maculopapular rash. Adults are susceptible to arthritis, which causes early morning pain and swelling, most often in the small joints. Arthritis can persist for months and may become chronic in HLA-B27-positive individuals. Related alphaviruses causing similar syndromes include Sindbis virus (Scandinavia and Africa), O'nyong-nyong virus (Central Africa), Ross River virus (Australia) and Mayaro virus (Caribbean and South America).

Diagnosis is by serology but cross-reactivity between alphaviruses occurs. Treatment is symptomatic.

PRION DISEASES

Prions (p. 132) cause spongiform encephalopathies in humans, sheep, cows and cats (Box 13.38 and see p. 1214). The prion protein is not inactivated by cooking or conventional sterilisation, and transmission is thought to occur by consumption of infected CNS tissue or by inoculation (e.g. via depth EEG electrodes, corneal grafts, cadaveric dura mater grafts and pooled cadaveric growth hormone preparations). The same diseases can occur in an inherited form, due to mutations in the PrP gene.

The apparent transmission of bovine spongiform encephalopathy (BSE) to humans following an outbreak of BSE in the UK beginning in the late 1980s has caused great concern, leading to precautionary measures in the UK, such as leucodepletion of all blood used for transfusion, and the mandatory use

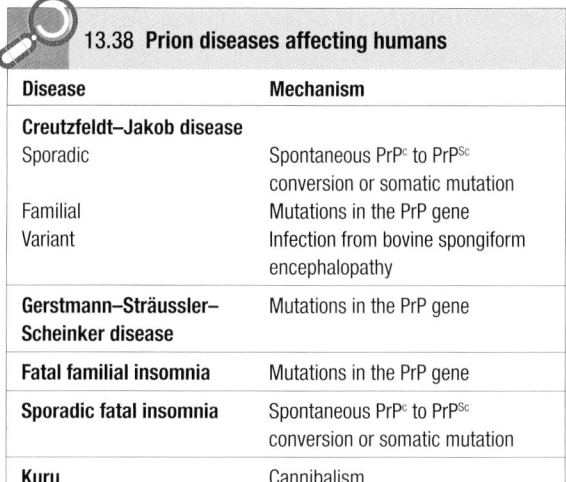

13.38 Prion diseases affecting humans

Disease	Mechanism
Creutzfeldt–Jakob disease	
Sporadic	Spontaneous PrP^c to PrP^{Sc} conversion or somatic mutation
Familial	Mutations in the PrP gene
Variant	Infection from bovine spongiform encephalopathy
Gerstmann–Sträussler–Scheinker disease	Mutations in the PrP gene
Fatal familial insomnia	Mutations in the PrP gene
Sporadic fatal insomnia	Spontaneous PrP^c to PrP^{Sc} conversion or somatic mutation
Kuru	Cannibalism

of disposable surgical instruments wherever possible for tonsillectomy, appendicectomy and ophthalmological procedures.

BACTERIAL INFECTIONS

Bacterial infections of the skin, soft tissues and bones

Most infections of the skin, soft tissues and bone are caused by either staphylococci (mainly *Staph. aureus*) or streptococci (mainly *Strep. pyogenes*). Clinical manifestations are also described in Chapters 25 and 27.

Staphylococcal infections

Staphylococci are usually found colonising the anterior nares and skin. Traditionally, staphylococci were divided into two groups according to their ability to produce coagulase, an enzyme that converts fibrinogen to fibrin in rabbit plasma, causing it to clot. *Staph. aureus* is coagulase-positive, and most other species coagulase-negative. The coagulase test is now less commonly undertaken, with identification of *Staph. aureus* often achieved by other methods.

Staph. aureus is the main cause of staphylococcal infections. *Staph. intermedius* is another coagulase-positive staphylococcus, which causes infection following dog bites. Among coagulase-negative organisms, *Staph. epidermidis* is the predominant commensal organism of the skin, and can cause severe infections in those with central venous catheters or implanted prosthetic materials. *Staph. saprophyticus* is part of the normal vaginal flora and causes urinary tract infections in sexually active young women. Others implicated in human infections include *Staph. lugdunensis*, *Staph. schleiferi*, *Staph. haemolyticus* and *Staph. caprae*. Coagulase-negative staphylococci are not usually identified to species level.

Staphylococci are particularly dangerous if they gain access to the blood stream, having the potential to cause disease in many sites (Fig. 13.15). In any patient with staphylococcal bacteraemia, especially injection drug-users, the possibility of endocarditis must be considered (p. 624). Growth of *Staph. aureus* in blood cultures should not be dismissed as a 'contaminant' unless

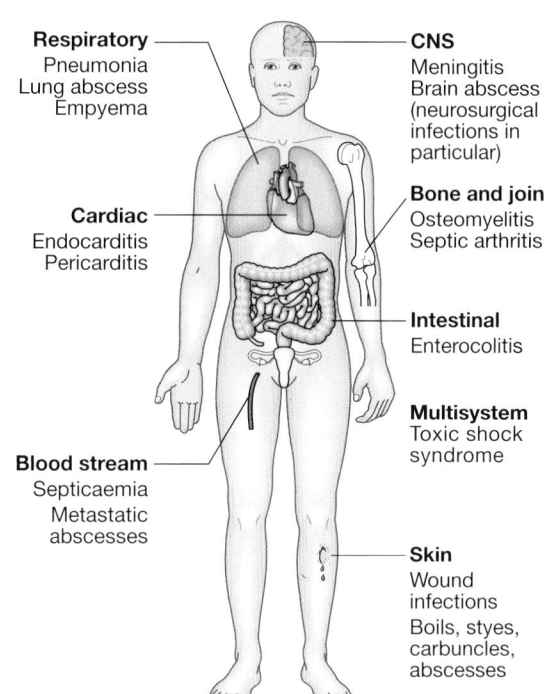

Respiratory
Pneumonia
Lung abscess
Empyema

Cardiac
Endocarditis
Pericarditis

Blood stream
Septicaemia
Metastatic abscesses

CNS
Meningitis
Brain abscess
(neurosurgical infections in particular)

Bone and joint
Osteomyelitis
Septic arthritis

Intestinal
Enterocolitis

Multisystem
Toxic shock syndrome

Skin
Wound infections
Boils, styes, carbuncles, abscesses

Fig. 13.15 Infections caused by *Staphylococcus aureus*.

all possible underlying sources have been excluded and repeated blood culture is negative. Any evidence of spreading cellulitis indicates the urgent need for an antistaphylococcal antibiotic such as flucloxacillin. This is particularly true for mid-facial cellulitis, which can result in cavernous sinus thrombophlebitis.

In addition, *Staph. aureus* can cause severe systemic disease due to the effects of toxin produced at superficial sites in the absence of tissue invasion by bacteria.

Skin infections

Staphylococcal infections cause ecthyma, folliculitis, furuncles, carbuncles, bullous impetigo and the scalded skin syndrome (pp. 1269–1270). They may also be involved in necrotising infections of the skin and subcutaneous tissues (p. 300).

Wound infections

Many wound infections are caused by staphylococci and may significantly prolong hospital stays in otherwise uncomplicated surgery (Fig. 13.16A). Prevention involves paying careful attention to hand hygiene, skin preparation and aspetic technique, and the use of topical and systemic antibiotic prophylaxis.

Treatment is by drainage of any abscesses plus adequate dosage of antistaphylococcal antibiotics. These should be instituted early, particularly if prosthetic implants of any kind have been inserted.

Cannula-related infection

Staphylococcal infection associated with cannula sepsis (Fig. 13.16B and see p. 300) and thrombophlebitis is an important and, unfortunately, extremely common reason for morbidity following hospital admission. The Visual Infusion Phlebitis (VIP) score is a useful way of monitoring cannulae (Box 13.39). Staphylococci have a predilection for plastic, rapidly forming a biofilm

13

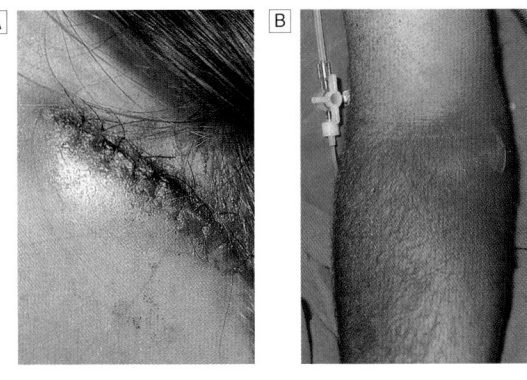

Fig. 13.16 Manifestations of skin infection with *Staph. aureus*.
A Wound infection. B Cannula-related infection.

which remains as a source of bacteraemia as long as the plastic is in situ. Local poultice application may relieve symptoms but cannula removal and antibiotic treatment with flucloxacillin (or a glycopeptide if MRSA is suspected) are necessary if there is any suggestion of spreading infection.

	13.39 How to assess an i.v. cannula using the Visual Infusion Phlebitis score (VIP)		
Clinical features	**Score**	**Assessment and management**	
I.v. site appears healthy	0	No signs of phlebitis Observe cannula	
One of the following is evident: 　Slight pain near i.v. site 　Slight redness near i.v. site	1	Possible first signs of phlebitis Observe cannula	
Two of the following are evident: 　Pain near i.v. site 　Erythema 　Swelling	2	Early stage of phlebitis Resite cannula	
ALL of the following are evident and extensive: 　Pain along path of cannula 　Erythema 　Induration	3	Medium stage of phlebitis Resite cannula Consider treatment	
ALL of the following are evident and extensive: 　Pain along path of cannula 　Erythema 　Induration 　Palpable venous cord	4	Advanced stage of phlebitis or start of thrombophlebitis Resite cannula Consider treatment	
ALL of the following are evident: 　Pain along path of cannula 　Erythema 　Induration 　Palpable venous cord 　Pyrexia	5	Advanced stage of thrombophlebitis Initiate treatment Resite cannula	

*Adapted from Jackson A, Nursing Times 1997; 94:68–71.

Meticillin-resistant Staph. aureus (MRSA)

Resistance to meticillin, due to a penicillin-binding protein mutation, has been recognised in *Staph. aureus* for more than 30 years. The recent recognition of resistance to vancomycin/teicoplanin (glycopeptides) in either glycopeptide intermediate *Staph. aureus* (GISA) or, rarely, vancomycin-resistant (VRSA) strains threatens the ability to manage serious infections produced by such organisms. MRSA is now a major world-wide health care-acquired pathogen, accounting for up to 40% of staphylococcal bacteraemia in developed countries. Community-acquired MRSA (c-MRSA) currently accounts for 50% of all MRSA infections in the USA. These organisms have also acquired other virulence factors such as Panton–Valentine leukocidin (PVL), which can cause rapidly fatal infection in young people. Clinicians must be aware of the potential danger of these infections and be prepared to take whatever appropriate infection control measures are locally advised (p. 143–144).

Treatment options for MRSA are shown in Box 6.18 (p. 150). Treatment should always be based on the results of antimicrobial susceptibility testing since resistance to all these agents occurs. Milder MRSA infections may be treated with clindamycin, tetracyclines or co-trimoxazole. Glycopeptides, linezolid and daptomycin are reserved for treatment of more severe infections. PVL-producing *Staph. aureus* infections should be treated with protein-inhibiting antibiotics (clindamycin, linezolid).

Staphylococcal toxic shock syndrome (TSS)

This serious and life-threatening disease is associated with infection by *Staph. aureus*, which produces a specific toxin (toxic shock syndrome toxin 1, TSST1). It was commonly seen in young women associated with the use of highly absorbent intravaginal tampons but can occur with any *Staph. aureus* infection involving a relevant toxin-producing strain. The toxin acts as a 'superantigen', triggering significant T-helper cell activation and massive cytokine release.

TSS has an abrupt onset with high fever, generalised systemic upset (myalgia, headache, sore throat and vomiting), a generalised erythematous blanching rash resembling scarlet fever, and hypotension. It rapidly

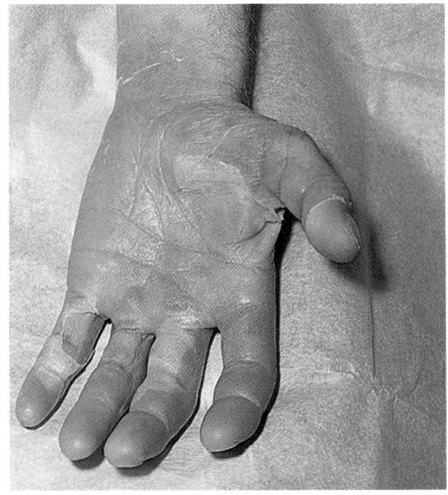

Fig. 13.17 Full-thickness desquamation after staphylococcal toxic shock syndrome.

progresses over a matter of hours to multisystem involvement with cardiac, renal and hepatic compromise, leading to death in 10–20%. Recovery is accompanied at 7–10 days by desquamation (Fig. 13.17).

The diagnosis is clinical and may be confirmed in menstrual cases by vaginal examination, the finding of a retained tampon and microbiological examination by Gram stain demonstrating typical staphylococci. Subsequent culture and demonstration of toxin production are confirmatory.

Management

Treatment is with immediate and aggressive fluid resuscitation and an intravenous antistaphylococcal antibiotic (flucloxacillin or vancomycin), usually with the addition of a protein synthesis inhibitor (e.g. clindamycin) to inhibit toxin production. Intravenous immunoglobulin is occasionally added in the most severe cases on the basis of efficacy in streptococcal toxic shock. Women who recover should be advised not to use tampons for at least 1 year and should also be warned that, due to an inadequate antibody response to TSST1, the condition can recur.

Streptococcal infections

Streptococci are nasopharyngeal and gut commensals, which appear as Gram-positive cocci in chains (Fig. 6.3, p. 134). They are classified by the haemolysis they produce on blood agar (Fig. 6.4, p. 134) and by their serotypes (Box 13.40). Some streptococci (e.g. *milleri* group) defy simple classification.

Skin presentations of streptococcal infections

Group A streptococci (GAS) are the major cause of cellulitis, erysipelas and impetigo (p. 1269–1271). Groups C and G streptococci cause cellulitis in particular in elderly, diabetic or immunocompromised patients. Group B streptococcal (GBS) infection is an increasing problem at the extremes of age.

Streptococcal scarlet fever

Group A (or occasionally groups C and G) streptococci causing pharyngitis, tonsillitis or other infection may lead to scarlet fever, if the infecting strain produces a

13.40 Streptococcal and related infections

β-haemolytic group A (*Strep. pyogenes*)

- Skin and soft tissue infection (including erysipelas, impetigo, necrotising fasciitis)
- Streptococcal toxic shock syndrome
- Puerperal sepsis
- Scarlet fever
- Glomerulonephritis
- Rheumatic fever
- Bone and joint infection
- Tonsillitis

β-haemolytic group B (*Strep. agalactiae*)

- Neonatal infections, including meningitis
- Septicaemia
- Female pelvic infections
- Cellulitis

β-haemolytic group C (various zoonotic streptococci)

- Septicaemia
- Cellulitis

α, β- or non-haemolytic group D enterococci (*E. faecalis/faecium*)

- Endocarditis
- Intra-abdominal infections
- Urinary tract infection

α, β- or non-haemolytic group D streptococci (*Strep. bovis*)

- Septicaemia
- Liver abscess
- Brain abscess

β-haemolytic group G streptococci

- Septicaemia
- Cellulitis
- Liver abscess

α-haemolytic viridans group (*Strep. mitis, sanguis, mutans, salivarius*)

- Septicaemia in immunosuppressed
- Endocarditis

α-haemolytic optochin-sensitive (*Strep. pneumoniae*)

- Pneumonia
- Meningitis
- Endocarditis
- Otitis media
- Septicaemia
- Spontaneous bacterial peritonitis

Anaerobic streptococci (*Peptostreptococcus* spp.)

- Peritonitis
- Dental infections
- Liver abscess
- Pelvic inflammatory disease

N.B. All streptococci can cause septicaemia.

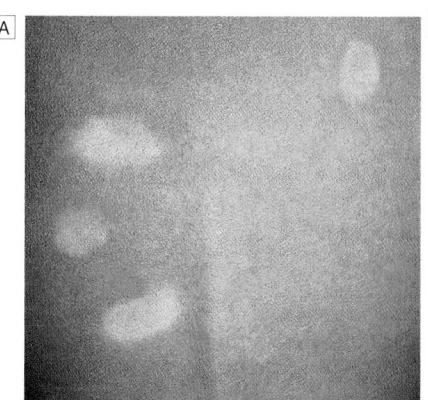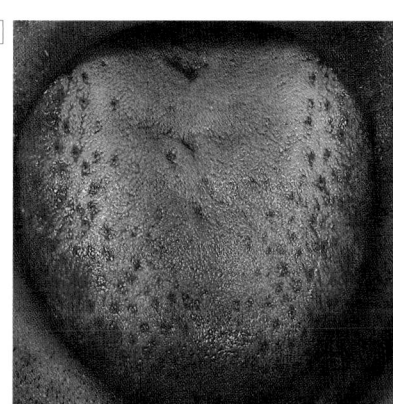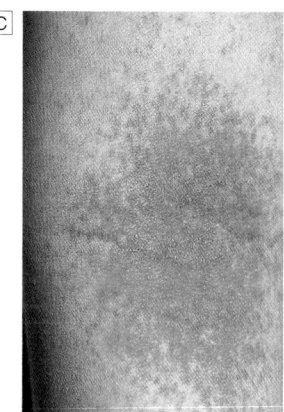

Fig. 13.18 Clinical features of scarlet fever. [A] Characteristic rash with blanching on pressure. [B] 'Strawberry tongue'. [C] Pastia's sign: a petechial rash in the cubital fossa.

streptococcal pyrogenic exotoxin. Common in school-age children, scarlet fever can occur in young adults who have contact with young children. A diffuse erythematous rash occurs, which blanches on pressure (Fig. 13.18A), classically with circumoral pallor. The tongue, initially coated, becomes red and swollen ('strawberry tongue'— Fig. 13.18B). The disease lasts about 7 days, the rash disappearing in 7–10 days followed by a fine desquamation. Residual petechial lesions in the antecubital fossa may be seen ('Pastia's sign'—Fig. 13.18C).

Treatment involves active therapy for the underlying infection (benzylpenicillin or orally available penicillin) plus symptomatic measures.

Streptococcal toxic shock syndrome

This is associated with severe group A (or occasionally group C or G) streptococcal skin infections producing one of a variety of toxins such as pyogenic exotoxin A. Like staphylococcal toxic shock syndrome toxin (see above), these act as superantigens, stimulating T-helper cells and a dramatic cytokine response. Initially, an influenza-like illness occurs with, in 50% of cases, signs of localised infection, most often involving the skin and soft tissues. A faint erythematous rash, mainly on the chest, rapidly progresses to circulatory shock. Without aggressive management, multi-organ failure will develop.

Fluid resuscitation must be undertaken, with parenteral antistreptococcal antibiotic therapy, usually with benzylpenicillin and a protein inhibitor such as clindamycin to inhibit toxin production. Intravenous immunoglobulin is usually administered in addition. If necrotising fasciitis is present, it should be treated as described on page 300 with urgent débridement.

Treponematoses

Syphilis

This disease is described on page 417.

Endemic treponematoses

Yaws

Yaws is a granulomatous disease, mainly involving the skin and bones, which is caused by *Treponema pertenue*, morphologically and serologically indistinguishable from the causative organisms of syphilis and pinta. It is important to establish the geographical origin and sexual history of patients to exclude a false-positive syphilis serology due to the endemic treponemal infections. WHO campaigns between 1950 and 1960 treated over 60 million people and eradicated yaws from many areas, but the disease has persisted patchily throughout the tropics; there was resurgence in the 1980s and 1990s in West and Central Africa and the South Pacific.

Organisms are transmitted by bodily contact from a patient with infectious yaws through minor abrasions of the skin of another patient, usually a child. After an incubation period of 3–4 weeks, a proliferative granuloma containing numerous treponemes develops at the site of inoculation. This primary lesion is followed by secondary eruptions. In addition, there may be hypertrophic periosteal lesions of many bones, with underlying cortical rarefaction. Lesions of late yaws are characterised by destructive changes which closely resemble the osteitis and gummas of tertiary syphilis and which heal with much scarring and deformity. Investigations and management are outlined in Box 13.41.

13.41 Diagnosis and treatment of yaws, pinta and bejel
Diagnosis of early stages
• Detection of spirochaetes in exudate of lesions by dark ground microscopy
Diagnosis of latent and early stages
• Positive serological tests, as for syphilis (Box 15.7, p. 419)
Treatment of all stages
• Single intramuscular injection of 1.2 g long-acting (e.g. benzathine) benzylpenicillin

The disease disappears with improved housing and cleanliness. In few fields of medicine have chemotherapy and improved hygiene achieved such dramatic success as in the control of yaws.

Pinta and bejel

These two treponemal infections occur in poor rural populations with low standards of domestic hygiene, but are found in separate parts of the world. They have features in common, notably that they are transmitted by contact, usually within the family and not sexually, and in the case of bejel, through common eating and drinking utensils. Their diagnosis and management are as for yaws (see Box 13.41).

• *Pinta.* Pinta is probably the oldest of the human treponemal infections. It is found only in South and Central America, where its incidence is declining. The infection is confined to the skin. The early lesions are scaly papules or dyschromic patches on the skin. The late lesions are often depigmented and disfiguring.

• *Bejel.* Bejel is the Middle Eastern name for non-venereal syphilis, which has a patchy distribution across sub-Saharan Africa, the Middle East, Central Asia and Australia. It has been eradicated from Eastern Europe. Transmission is most commonly from the mouth of the mother or child and the primary mucosal lesion is seldom seen. The early and late lesions resemble those of secondary and tertiary syphilis (pp. 417–418) but cardiovascular and neurological disease are rare.

Tropical ulcer

Tropical ulcer is due to a synergistic bacterial infection caused by a fusobacterium (*F. ulcerans*, an anaerobe) and *Treponema vincentii*. It is common in hot humid regions. The ulcer is most common on the lower legs and develops as a papule that rapidly breaks down to a sharply defined, painful ulcer. The base of the ulcer has a foul slough. Penicillin and metronidazole are useful in the early stages but rest, elevation and dressings are the mainstays of treatment.

Buruli ulcer

This ulcer is caused by *Mycobacterium ulcerans* and occurs widely in tropical rainforests. In 1999 a survey in Ghana found 6500 cases; there are an estimated 10 000 cases in West Africa as a whole.

The initial lesion is a small subcutaneous nodule on the arm or leg. This breaks down to form a shallow, necrotic ulcer with deeply undermined edges which extends rapidly. Healing may occur after 6 months, but granuloma formation and the accompanying fibrosis cause contractures and deformity. Clumps of acid-fast bacilli can be detected in the ulcer floor.

A combination of rifampicin and streptomycin can cure the infection. Infected tissue should be removed surgically. Health campaigns in Ghana have successfully focused on early removal of the small, pre-ulcerative nodules.

Systemic bacterial infections

Brucellosis

Brucellosis is an enzootic infection (i.e. endemic in animals). Although six species of *Brucella* Gram-negative bacilli are known, only four are important to humans: *B. melitensis* (goats, sheep and camels in Europe, especially the Mediterranean basin, the Middle East, Africa, India, Central Asia and South America), *B. abortus* (cattle, mainly in Africa, Asia and South America), *B. suis* (pigs in South Asia) and *B. canis* (dogs). *B. melitensis* causes the most severe disease; *B. suis* is often associated with abscess formation.

Infected animals may excrete *Brucella* spp. in their milk for prolonged periods and human infection is acquired by ingesting contaminated dairy products, uncooked meat or offal. Animal urine, faeces, vaginal discharge and uterine products may act as sources of infection through abraded skin or via splashes and aerosols to the respiratory tract and conjunctiva.

Clinical features

Brucella spp. are intracellular organisms that survive for long periods within the reticulo-endothelial system. This explains many of the clinical features, including the chronicity of disease and tendency to relapse even after antimicrobial therapy.

Acute illness is characterised by a high swinging temperature, rigors, lethargy, headache, joint and muscle pains, and scrotal pain. Occasionally, there is delirium, abdominal pain and constipation. Physical signs are non-specific, e.g. enlarged lymph nodes. Enlargement of the spleen may lead to hypersplenism and thrombocytopenia.

Localised infection (Box 13.42), which occurs in about 30% of patients, is more likely if diagnosis and treatment are delayed.

Diagnosis

Definitive diagnosis of brucellosis depends on the isolation of the organism. Blood cultures are positive in 75–80% of infections caused by *B. melitensis* and 50% of those caused by *B. abortus*. Bone marrow culture should not be used routinely but may increase the diagnostic yield, particularly if antibiotics have been given before specimens are taken. CSF culture in neurobrucellosis is positive in about 30% of cases. The laboratory should be alerted to a suspected diagnosis of brucellosis, as the organism has a propensity for infecting laboratory workers and must be cultured at an enhanced containment level.

Serum tests are also used to detect brucellosis antibodies. In endemic areas a single high titre of > 1/320 or a fourfold rise in titre is needed to support a diagnosis

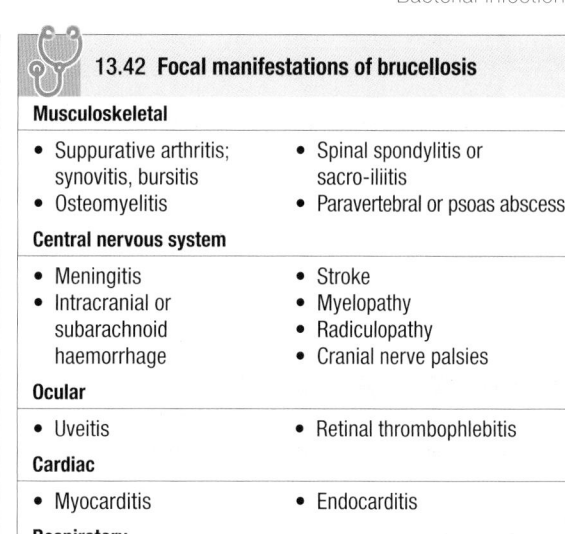

13.42 Focal manifestations of brucellosis

Musculoskeletal
- Suppurative arthritis; synovitis, bursitis
- Osteomyelitis
- Spinal spondylitis or sacro-iliitis
- Paravertebral or psoas abscess

Central nervous system
- Meningitis
- Intracranial or subarachnoid haemorrhage
- Stroke
- Myelopathy
- Radiculopathy
- Cranial nerve palsies

Ocular
- Uveitis
- Retinal thrombophlebitis

Cardiac
- Myocarditis
- Endocarditis

Respiratory
- Pneumonitis or abscesses
- Hilar adenopathy

Abdominal
- Splenic abscesses or calcification
- Hepatitis

Genitourinary
- Epididymo-orchitis

Haematological
- Pancytopenia

of acute infection. The test usually takes several weeks to become positive but should eventually detect 95% of acute infections.

Management

Aminoglycosides show synergistic activity with tetracyclines against brucellae; standard therapy in acute infection consists of doxycycline 100 mg 12-hourly for 6 weeks, with streptomycin 1 g i.m. daily for the first 2 weeks. The relapse rate with this treatment is about 5%. An alternative oral regimen consists of doxycycline 100 mg 12-hourly plus rifampicin 900 mg (15 mg/kg) daily for 6 weeks, but failure and relapse rates are higher, particularly with spondylitis. Rifampicin may antagonise doxycycline activity by reducing serum levels through enzyme induction. Rifampicin and co-trimoxazole are potential agents to use in pregnancy. Endocarditis is often treated with three active drugs, usually doxycycline, rifampicin and streptomycin, but surgery is often required.

Chronic illness or neurobrucellosis should be treated for a minimum of 3 months and many authorities would extend this to 6 months, depending upon the response.

Borrelia infections

Borrelia are flagellated spirochaetal bacteria which infect humans after bites from ticks or lice. They cause a variety of human infections world-wide (Box 13.43).

Lyme disease

Lyme disease (named after the town of Old Lyme in Connecticut, USA) is caused by *B. burgdorferi*, which

13.43 Clinical diseases caused by *Borrelia* spp.

Species	Vector	Geographic distribution
Lyme disease		
B. burgdorferi sensu stricto	Tick: *Ixodes scapularis*	Northern and eastern USA
	I. pacificus	Western USA
B. afzelii	*I. ricinus*	Europe
	I. persulcatus	Asia
B. garinii	*I. ricinus*	Europe
	I. persulcatus	Asia
Louse-borne relapsing fever		
B. recurrentis	Human louse: *Pediculus humanus corporis*	World-wide
Tick-borne relapsing fever		
B. hermsii	Tick: *Ornithodoros hermsii*	Western North America
B. turicatae	*O. turicatae*	Southwestern North America and northern Mexico
B. venezuelensis	*O. rudis*	Central America and northern South America
B. hispanica	*O. erraticus*	Iberian peninsula and northwestern Africa
B. crocidurae	*O. erraticus*	North Africa and Mediterranean region
B. duttonii	*O. moubata*	Central, eastern and southern Africa
B. persica	*O. tholozani*	Western China, India, central Asia, Middle East
B. latyschewii	*O. tartakovskyi*	Tajikistan, Uzbekistan

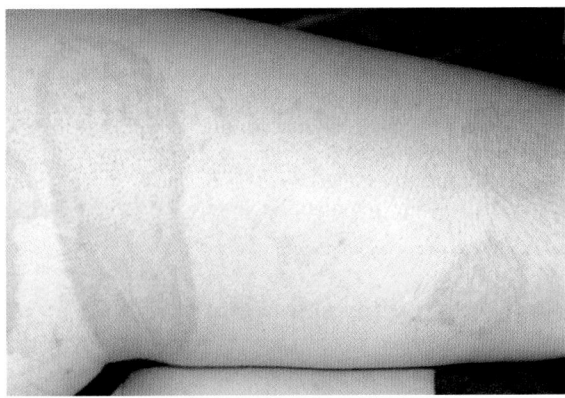

Fig. 13.19 Rash of erythema migrans in Lyme disease with metastatic secondary lesions.

occurs in the USA, Europe, Russia, China, Japan and Australia. In Europe two additional genospecies are also encountered, *B. afzelii* and *B. garinii*. The reservoir of infection is ixodid (hard) ticks that feed on a variety of large mammals, particularly deer. Birds may spread ticks over a wide area. The organism is transmitted to humans via the bite of infected ticks; larval, nymphal and adult forms are all capable of spreading infection.

Ehrlichiosis is a common co-infection with Lyme disease (*Anaplasma phagocytophila*, human granulocytic anaplasmosis (HGA); *Ehrlichia chaffeensis*, human monocytic ehrlichiosis (HME)).

Clinical features

There are three stages of disease. Progression may be arrested at any stage.

- *Early localised disease*: The characteristic feature is a skin reaction around the site of the tick bite, known as erythema migrans (Fig. 13.19). Initially, a red 'bull's eye' macule or papule appears 2–30 days after the bite. It then enlarges peripherally with central clearing, and may persist for months. Atypical forms are fairly common. The lesion is not pathognomonic of Lyme disease since similar lesions can occur after tick bites in areas where Lyme disease does not occur. Other acute manifestations such as fever, headache and regional lymphadenopathy may develop with or without the rash.

- *Early disseminated disease*: Dissemination occurs via the blood stream and lymphatics. There may be a systemic reaction with malaise, arthralgia, and occasionally metastatic areas of erythema migrans (see Fig. 13.19). Neurological involvement may follow weeks or months after infection. Common features include lymphocytic meningitis, cranial nerve palsies (especially unilateral or bilateral facial nerve palsy) and peripheral neuropathy. Radiculopathy, often painful, may present a year or more after initial infection. Carditis, sometimes accompanied by atrioventricular conduction defects, is not uncommon in the USA but appears to be rare in Europe.

- *Late disease*: Late manifestations include arthritis, polyneuritis and encephalopathy. Prolonged arthritis, particularly affecting large joints, and brain parenchymal involvement causing neuropsychiatric abnormalities may occur, but are rare in the UK. Acrodermatitis chronica atrophicans is an uncommon late complication seen more frequently in Europe than North America. Doughy, patchy discoloration occurs on the peripheries, eventually leading to shiny atrophic skin. The lesions are easily mistaken for those of peripheral vascular disease. In patients from an endemic area or with risk factors, who have facial nerve palsy, Lyme disease should be considered.

Diagnosis

The diagnosis of early Lyme borreliosis is often clinical. Culture from biopsy material is not generally available, has a low yield, and may take longer than 6 weeks. Antibody detection is frequently negative early in the course of the disease, but sensitivity increases to 90–100% in disseminated or late disease. Immunofluorescence or ELISA can give false positive reactions in a number of conditions, including other spirochaetal infections, infectious mononucleosis, rheumatoid arthritis and systemic lupus erythematosus (SLE). Immunoblot (Western blot) techniques are more specific and, although technically demanding, should be used to confirm the diagnosis. Microorganism DNA detection by PCR has been applied to blood, urine, CSF, and biopsies of skin and synovium.

Management

Recent evidence suggests that asymptomatic patients with positive antibody tests should not be treated. However, erythema migrans always requires therapy because organisms may persist and cause progressive disease, even if the skin lesions resolve. Standard therapy consists of a 14-day course of doxycycline (200 mg daily) or amoxicillin (500 mg 8-hourly). Some 15% of patients with early disease will develop a mild Jarisch–Herxheimer reaction (JHR) during the first 24 hours of therapy (p. 419). In pregnant women and small children, or in those allergic to amoxicillin and doxycycline, 14-day treatment with cefuroxime axetil (500 mg 12-hourly) or erythromycin (250 mg 6-hourly) may be used.

Disseminated disease and arthritis require therapy for a minimum of 28 days. Arthritis may respond poorly, and prolonged or repeated courses may be necessary. Neuroborreliosis is treated with parenteral β-lactam antibiotics for 3–4 weeks; the cephalosporins may be superior to penicillin in this situation.

Prevention

Protective clothing and insect repellents should be used in tick-infested areas. Since the risk of borrelial transmission is lower in the first few hours of a blood feed, prompt removal of ticks is advisable. Unfortunately, larval and nymphal ticks are tiny and may not be noticed. Where risk of transmission is high, a single 200 mg dose of doxycycline, given within 72 hours of exposure, has been shown to prevent erythema migrans. A recombinant vaccine, OspA, in adjuvant was developed but withdrawn due to side-effects.

Louse-borne relapsing fever

The human body louse, *Pediculus humanus*, causes itching. Borreliae (*B. recurrentis*) are liberated from the infected lice when they are crushed during scratching, which also inoculates the borreliae into the skin. The disease occurs world-wide, with epidemic relapsing fever most often seen in Central and East Africa, and in South America.

The borreliae multiply in the blood, where they are abundant in the febrile phases, and invade most tissues, especially the liver, spleen and meninges. Hepatitis and thrombocytopenia are common.

Clinical features

Onset is sudden with fever. The temperature rises to 39.5–40.5°C, accompanied by a tachycardia, headache, generalised aching, injected conjunctivae (Fig. 13.20)

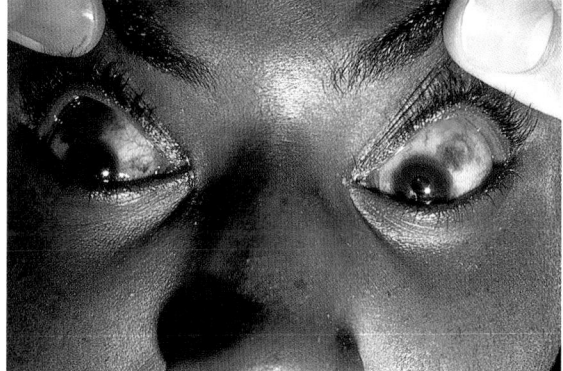

Fig. 13.20 Louse-borne relapsing fever. Injected conjunctivae.

and, frequently, a petechial rash, epistaxis and herpes labialis. As the disease progresses, the liver and spleen frequently become tender and palpable, and jaundice is common. There may be severe serosal and intestinal haemorrhage, mental confusion and meningism. The fever ends in crisis between the 4th and 10th days, often associated with profuse sweating, hypotension, and circulatory and cardiac failure. There may be no further fever but, in a proportion of patients, after an afebrile period of about 7 days, there are one or more relapses, which are usually milder and less prolonged. In the absence of specific treatment, the mortality rate is up to 40%, especially among the elderly and malnourished.

Investigations and management

The organisms are demonstrated in the blood during fever either by dark ground microscopy of a wet film or by staining thick and thin films.

The problems of treatment are to eradicate the organism, to minimise the severe Jarisch–Herxheimer reaction which inevitably follows successful chemotherapy, and to prevent relapses. The safest treatment is procaine penicillin 300 mg i.m., followed the next day by 0.5 g tetracycline. Tetracycline alone is effective and prevents relapse, but may give rise to a worse reaction. Doxycycline 200 mg once by mouth in place of tetracycline has the advantage of also being curative for typhus, which often accompanies epidemics of relapsing fever. JHR is best managed in a high-dependency unit with expert nursing and medical care.

The patient, clothing and all contacts must be freed from lice as in epidemic typhus.

Tick-borne relapsing fever

Soft ticks (*Ornithodoros* spp.) transmit *B. duttoni* (and several other borrelia species) through saliva while feeding on their host. Those sleeping in mud houses are at risk, as the tick hides in crevices during the day and feeds on humans during the night. Rodents are the reservoir in all parts of the world except East Africa, where humans are the reservoir. Clinical manifestations are similar to the louse-borne disease but spirochaetes are detected in fewer patients on dark field microscopy. A 7-day course (due to a higher relapse rate than louse-borne relapsing fever) of treatment with either tetracycline (500 mg 6-hourly) or erythromycin (500 mg 6-hourly) is needed.

Leptospirosis
Microbiology and epidemiology

Leptospirosis is one of the most common zoonotic diseases, favoured by a tropical climate and flooding during the monsoon but occurring world-wide. Leptospires are tightly coiled, thread-like organisms about 5–7 μm in length which are actively motile; each end is bent into a hook. *Leptospira interrogans* is pathogenic for humans. The genus can be separated into more than 200 serovars (subtypes) belonging to 23 serogroups.

Leptospirosis appears to be ubiquitous in wildlife and in many domestic animals. The organisms persist indefinitely in the convoluted tubules of the kidney and are shed into the urine in massive numbers, but infection is asymptomatic in the host. The most frequent hosts are rodents, especially the common rat (*Rattus norvegicus*). Particular leptospiral serogroups are associated with characteristic animal hosts; *L. ictero-haemorrhagiae* is the classical parasite of rats, *L. canicola* of dogs, *L. hebdomadis* of cattle, and *L. pomona* of pigs. There is nevertheless considerable overlap in host–serogroup associations.

Leptospires can enter their human hosts through intact skin or mucous membranes, but entry is facilitated by cuts and abrasions. Prolonged immersion in contaminated water will also favour invasion, as the spirochaete can survive in water for months. Leptospirosis is common in the tropics and also in freshwater sports enthusiasts.

Clinical features

After a relatively brief bacteraemia, invading organisms are distributed throughout the body, mainly in kidneys, liver, meninges and brain. The incubation period averages 1–2 weeks. Four main clinical syndromes can be discerned.

Bacteraemic leptospirosis

Bacteraemia with any serogroup can produce a non-specific illness with high fever, weakness, muscle pain and tenderness (especially of the calf and back), intense headache and photophobia, and sometimes diarrhoea and vomiting. Conjunctival congestion is the only notable physical sign. The illness comes to an end after about 1 week, or else merges into one of the other forms of infection.

Aseptic meningitis

Classically associated with *L. canicola* infection, this illness is very difficult to distinguish from viral meningitis. The conjunctivae may be congested but there are no other differentiating signs. Laboratory clues include a neutrophil leucocytosis, abnormal LFTs, and the occasional presence of albumin and casts in the urine.

Icteric leptospirosis (Weil's disease)

Less than 10% of symptomatic infections result in severe icteric illness. Weil's disease is a dramatic life-threatening event, characterised by fever, haemorrhages, jaundice and renal impairment. Conjunctival hyperaemia is a frequent feature. The patient may have a transient macular erythematous rash, but the characteristic skin changes are purpura and large areas of bruising. In severe cases there may be epistaxis, haematemesis and melaena, or bleeding into the pleural, pericardial or subarachnoid spaces. Thrombocytopenia, probably related to activation of endothelial cells with platelet adhesion and aggregation, is present in 50% of cases. Jaundice is deep and the liver is enlarged, but there is usually little evidence of hepatic failure or encephalopathy. Renal failure, primarily caused by impaired renal perfusion and acute tubular necrosis, manifests as oliguria or anuria, with the presence of albumin, blood and casts in the urine.

Weil's disease may also be associated with myocarditis, encephalitis and aseptic meningitis. Uveitis and iritis may appear months after apparent clinical recovery.

Pulmonary syndrome

This syndrome has long been recognised in the Far East, and has been described during an outbreak of leptospirosis in Nicaragua. It is characterised by haemoptysis, patchy lung infiltrates on chest X-ray, and respiratory failure. Total bilateral lung consolidation and ARDS (p. 187) with multi-organ dysfunction may develop, with a high mortality (> 50%).

Diagnosis

A polymorphonuclear leucocytosis is accompanied in severe infection by thrombocytopenia and elevated blood levels of creatine kinase. In jaundiced patients there is mild hepatitis and the prothrombin time may be a little prolonged. The CSF in leptospiral meningitis shows a variable cellular response, a moderately elevated protein level and normal glucose content.

In the tropics, dengue, malaria, typhoid fever, scrub typhus and hantavirus infection are important differential diagnoses.

Definitive diagnosis of leptospirosis depends upon isolation of the organism, serological tests or the detection of specific DNA.

- Blood cultures are most likely to be positive if taken before the 10th day of illness. Special media are required and cultures may have to be incubated for several weeks.
- Leptospires appear in the urine during the 2nd week of illness, and in untreated patients may be recovered on culture for several months.
- Serological tests are diagnostic if seroconversion or a fourfold increase in titre is demonstrated. The microscopic agglutination test (MAT) is the test of choice and can become positive by the end of the first week. IgM ELISA and immunofluorescent techniques are, however, easier to perform, while rapid immunochromatographic tests are specific but of only moderate sensitivity in the 1st week of illness.
- Detection of leptospiral DNA by PCR is possible in blood in early symptomatic disease, and in urine from the 8th day of illness and for many months thereafter.

Management and prevention

The general care of the patient is critically important. Blood transfusion for haemorrhage and careful attention to renal failure, the usual cause of death, are especially important. Renal failure is potentially reversible with adequate support such as dialysis. The optimal antimicrobial regimen has not been established. Most infections are self-limiting. Therapy with either oral doxycycline (100 mg 12-hourly for 1 week) or intravenous penicillin (900 mg 6-hourly for 1 week) is effective but may not prevent the development of renal failure. Parenteral ceftriaxone (1 g daily) is as effective as penicillin. A Jarisch–Herxheimer reaction may occur during treatment but is usually mild. Uveitis is treated with a combination of systemic antibiotics and local corticosteroids.

Trials in military personnel have shown that infection with *L. interrogans* can be prevented by taking prophylactic doxycycline 200 mg weekly.

Plague

Plague is caused by *Yersinia pestis*, a small Gram-negative bacillus that is spread between rodents by their fleas. If domestic rats become infected, infected fleas may bite humans. Hunters and trappers can contract plague from handling rodents. In the late stages of human plague, *Y. pestis* may be expectorated and spread between humans by droplets, causing 'pneumonic plague'.

Epidemics of plague, such as the 'Black Death', have occurred since ancient times. It is often said that the first sign of plague is the appearance of dead rats. Plague foci are widely distributed throughout the world, including the USA; human cases are reported from about ten countries per year (Fig. 13.21).

Y. pestis is a potential bioweapon because of its capacity for mass production and aerosol transmission, and the high fatality rate associated with pneumonic plague.

Clinical features

Organisms inoculated through the skin are taken rapidly to the draining lymph nodes, where they elicit a severe inflammatory response that may be haemorrhagic. If the infection is not contained, septicaemia ensues and necrotic, purulent or haemorrhagic lesions develop in many organs. Oliguria and shock follow, and disseminated intravascular coagulation may result in widespread haemorrhage. Inhalation of Y. pestis causes alveolitis. The incubation period is 3–6 days, but shorter in pneumonic plague.

Bubonic plague

In this, the most common form of the disease, onset is usually sudden, with a rigor, high fever, dry skin and severe headache. Soon, aching and swelling at the site of the affected lymph nodes begin. The groin is the most common site of this 'bubo', made up of the swollen lymph nodes and surrounding tissue. Some infections are relatively mild but in the majority of patients toxaemia quickly increases, with a rapid pulse, hypotension and mental confusion. The spleen is usually palpable.

Septicaemic plague

Those not exhibiting a bubo usually deteriorate rapidly and have a high mortality. The elderly are more prone to this form of illness. The patient is toxic and may have gastrointestinal symptoms such as nausea, vomiting, abdominal pain and diarrhoea. DIC may occur, manifested by bleeding from various orifices or puncture sites, along with ecchymoses. Hypotension, shock, renal failure and ARDS may lead to further deterioration. Meningitis, pneumonia and expectoration of blood-stained sputum containing Y. pestis may complicate septicaemic, or occasionally bubonic, plague.

Pneumonic plague

Following primary infection in the lung, the onset of disease is very sudden, with cough and dyspnoea. The patient soon expectorates copious blood-stained, frothy, highly infective sputum, becomes cyanosed and dies. Chest radiology reveals bilateral infiltrates which may be nodular and progress to an ARDS-like picture.

Investigations

The organism may be cultured from blood, sputum and bubo aspirates. For rapid diagnosis Gram, Giemsa and Wayson's stains (the latter containing methylene blue) are applied to smears from these sites. Y. pestis is seen as bipolar staining coccobacilli, sometimes referred to as having a 'safety pin' appearance. Smears are also subjected to antigen detection by immunofluorescence, using Y. pestis F1 antigen-specific antibodies. The diagnosis may be confirmed by seroconversion or a single high titre (> 128) of anti-F1 antibodies in serum. DNA detection by PCR is under evaluation.

Plague is a notifiable disease under international health regulations (Box 6.13, p. 147).

Management

If the diagnosis is suspected on clinical and epidemiological grounds, treatment must be started as soon as, or even before, samples have been collected for laboratory diagnosis. Streptomycin (1 g 12-hourly) or gentamicin (1 mg/kg 8-hourly) is the drug of choice. Tetracycline (500 mg 6-hourly) and chloramphenicol (12.5 mg/kg 6-hourly) are alternatives. Fluoroquinolones (ciprofloxacin and levofloxacin) may be as effective, but there is less clinical experience. Treatment may also be needed for acute circulatory failure, DIC and hypoxia.

Prevention and infection control

Rats and fleas should be controlled. In endemic areas, people should avoid handling and skinning wild animals. The patient should be isolated for the first 48 hours or until clinical improvement begins. Attendants must wear gowns, masks and gloves. Exposed symptomatic or asymptomatic people who have been in close contact with a patient with pneumonic plague should receive post-exposure antibiotic prophylaxis (doxycycline 100 mg or ciprofloxacin 500 mg 12-hourly) for 7 days.

A formalin-killed vaccine is available for those at occupational risk but offers little protection against

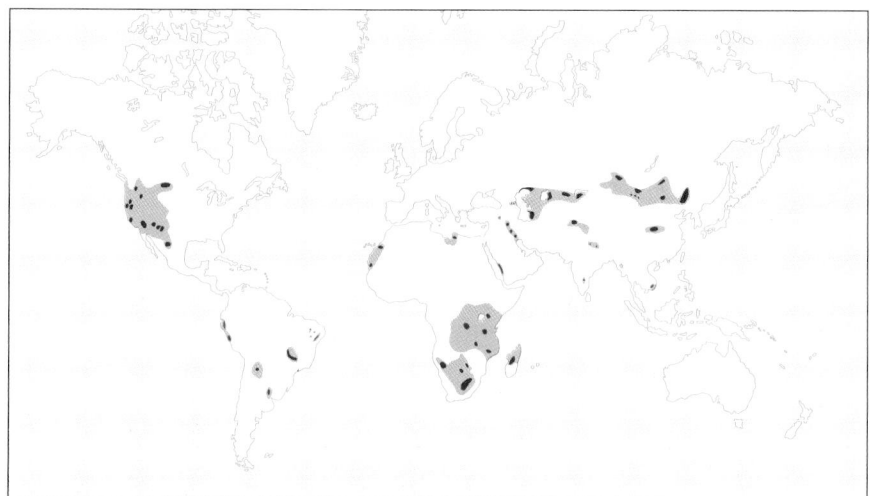

Frequent transmission

Infrequent or suspected transmission

Fig. 13.21 Foci of the transmission of plague.

pneumonic plague. A recombinant subunit vaccine (protein antigens F1 + V) is in development.

Listeriosis

Listeria monocytogenes is an environmental Gram-positive bacillus which can contaminate food. Outbreaks have been associated with raw vegetables, soft cheeses, undercooked chicken, fish, meat and pâtés. The bacterium demonstrates 'cold enrichment', outgrowing other contaminating bacteria during refrigeration. Although food-borne outbreaks of gastroenteritis have been reported in immunocompetent individuals, *Listeria* causes more significant invasive infection especially in pregnancy, the elderly and the immunocompromised.

In pregnancy, in addition to systemic symptoms of fever and myalgia, listeriosis causes chorioamnionitis, fetal deaths, abortions and neonatal infection. In other susceptible individuals, it causes systemic illness due to bacteraemia without focal symptoms. Meningitis, similar to other bacterial meningitis but with normal CSF glucose, is the next most common presentation; CSF usually shows increased neutrophils but occasionally only the mononuclear cells are increased (p. 1205).

Investigations and management

Diagnosis is made by blood and CSF culture. The organism grows readily in culture media.

The most effective regimen consists of a combination of an intravenous aminopenicillin (amoxicillin or ampicillin) plus an aminoglycoside. A sulfamethoxazole/trimethoprim combination can be used in those with penicillin allergy. Cephalosporins are of no use in this infection, as the organism is inherently resistant, an important consideration when empirically treating meningitis.

Proper treatment of foods before eating is the key to preventing listeriosis. Pregnant women are advised to avoid high-risk products, including soft cheeses.

Typhoid and paratyphoid (enteric) fevers

Typhoid and paratyphoid fevers, which are transmitted by the faecal–oral route, are important causes of fever in India, sub-Saharan Africa and Latin America. Elsewhere they are relatively rare. Enteric fevers are caused by infection with *Salmonella typhi* and *S. paratyphi* A and B. After a few days of bacteraemia, the bacilli localise, mainly in the lymphoid tissue of the small intestine, resulting in typical lesions in the Peyer's patches and follicles. These swell at first, then ulcerate and usually heal. After clinical recovery, about 5% of patients become chronic carriers; the bacilli may live in the gallbladder for months or years and pass intermittently in the stool and less commonly in the urine.

Clinical features

Typhoid fever

Clinical features are outlined in Box 13.44. The incubation period is about 10–14 days and the onset may be insidious. The temperature rises in a stepladder fashion for 4 or 5 days with malaise, increasing headache, drowsiness and aching in the limbs. Constipation may be present, although in children diarrhoea and vomiting may be prominent early in the illness. The pulse is often

13.44 Clinical features of typhoid fever	
1st week	
• Fever	• Relative bradycardia
• Headache	• Constipation
• Myalgia	• Diarrhoea and vomiting in children
End of 1st week	
• Rose spots on trunk	• Abdominal distension
• Splenomegaly	• Diarrhoea
• Cough	
End of 2nd week	
• Delirium, complications, then coma and death (if untreated)	

slower than would be expected from the height of the temperature, i.e. a relative bradycardia.

At the end of the first week, a rash may appear on the upper abdomen and on the back as sparse, slightly raised, rose-red spots, which fade on pressure. It is usually visible only on white skin. Cough and epistaxis occur. Around the 7th–10th day the spleen becomes palpable. Constipation is then succeeded by diarrhoea and abdominal distension with tenderness. Bronchitis and delirium may develop. If untreated, by the end of the 2nd week the patient may be profoundly ill.

Paratyphoid fever

The course tends to be shorter and milder than that of typhoid fever and the onset is often more abrupt with acute enteritis. The rash may be more abundant and the intestinal complications less frequent.

Complications

These are given in Box 13.45. Haemorrhage from, or a perforation of, the ulcerated Peyer's patches may occur at the end of the 2nd week or during the 3rd week of the illness. A drop in temperature to normal or subnormal levels may be falsely reassuring in patients with intestinal haemorrhage. Additional complications may involve almost any viscus or system because of the septicaemia present during the 1st week. Bone and joint infection is common in children with sickle-cell disease.

Investigations

In the first week the diagnosis may be difficult because in this invasive stage with bacteraemia the symptoms are

13.45 Complications of typhoid fever	
Bowel	
• Perforation	• Haemorrhage
Septicaemic foci	
• Bone and joint infection	• Cholecystitis
• Meningitis	
Toxic phenomena	
• Myocarditis	• Nephritis
Chronic carriage	
• Persistent gallbladder carriage	

those of a generalised infection without localising features. A white blood count may be helpful, as there is typically a leucopenia. Blood culture is the most important diagnostic method. The faeces will contain the organism more frequently during the 2nd and 3rd weeks.

Management

Antibiotic therapy must be guided by in vitro sensitivity testing. Chloramphenicol (500 mg 6-hourly), ampicillin (750 mg 6-hourly) and co-trimoxazole (2 tablets or i.v. equivalent 12-hourly) are losing their effect due to resistance in many areas of the world, especially India and South-east Asia. The fluoroquinolones are the drugs of choice (e.g. ciprofloxacin 500 mg 12-hourly) if the organism is susceptible, but resistance is common, especially in the Indian subcontinent; 40% of cases in the UK are now resistant. Extended-spectrum cephalosporins (ceftriaxone and cefotaxime) are useful alternatives but have a slightly increased treatment failure rate. Azithromycin (500 mg once daily) is an alternative where fluoroquinolone resistance is present but has not been validated in severe disease. Treatment should be continued for 14 days. Pyrexia may persist for up to 5 days after the start of specific therapy. Even with effective chemotherapy there is still a danger of complications, recrudescence of the disease and the development of a carrier state.

Chronic carriers are treated for 4 weeks with ciprofloxacin; cholecystectomy may be necessary.

Prevention

Improved sanitation and living conditions reduce the incidence of typhoid. Travellers to countries where enteric infections are endemic should be inoculated with one of the three available typhoid vaccines (two inactivated injectable and one oral live attenuated).

Tularaemia

Tularaemia is primarily a zoonotic disease of the northern hemisphere. It is caused by a highly infectious Gram-negative bacillus, *Francisella tularensis*. *F. tularensis* is passed transovarially (ensuring transmission from parent to progeny) in ticks, which allows persistence in nature without the absolute requirement for an infected animal reservoir. It is a potential weapon for bioterrorism. Wild rabbits, rodents, and domestic dogs or cats are some of the many potential reservoirs, and ticks, mosquitoes or other biting flies are the vectors.

Infection is introduced either through an arthropod or animal bite or via contact with infected animals, soil or water through skin abrasions. This results in the most common 'ulceroglandular' variety of the disease (70–80%), characterised by skin ulceration with regional lymphadenopathy. There is also a purely 'glandular' form. Alternatively, inhalation of the infected aerosols may result in pulmonary tularaemia, presenting as pneumonia. Rarely, the portal of entry of infection may be the conjunctiva, leading to a nodular, ulcerated conjunctivitis with regional lymphadenopathy (an 'oculoglandular' form).

Investigations and management

Demonstration of a single high titre ($\geq$ 1:160) or a fourfold rise in 2–3 weeks in the tularaemia tube agglutination test confirms the diagnosis. Bacterial yield from the lesions is extremely poor. DNA detection methods to enable rapid diagnosis are in development.

Treatment consists of a 7–10-day course of parenteral aminoglycosides, streptomycin (7.5–10 mg/kg 12-hourly) or gentamicin (1.7 mg/kg 8-hourly). *F. tularensis* is not susceptible to most other antibiotics.

Melioidosis

Melioidosis is caused by *Burkholderia pseudomallei*, a saprophyte found in soil and water (rice paddy fields). Infection is by inoculation or inhalation leading to bacteraemia, which is followed by the formation of abscesses in the lungs, liver and spleen. Patients with diabetes, renal stones, thalassaemia or severe burns are particularly susceptible. The disease is most common in South India, East Asia and northern Australia, and carries a significant mortality. Disease may present many years or decades after the initial exposure.

Clinical features

There is high fever, prostration and sometimes diarrhoea, with signs of pneumonia and enlargement of the liver and spleen. The chest X-ray resembles that of acute caseous tuberculosis. In more chronic forms multiple abscesses occur in subcutaneous tissue and bone, and profound wasting is a major problem.

Investigations and management

Culture of blood, sputum or pus may yield *B. pseudomallei*. Indirect haemagglutination testing can be helpful in travellers; however, most people in endemic areas are seropositive.

In the acute illness prompt treatment, without waiting for confirmation by culture, may be life-saving. Ceftazidime 100 mg/kg (2 g 8-hourly), imipenem 50 mg/kg (1 g 6-hourly) or meropenem (0.5–1 g 8-hourly) is given for 2–3 weeks. This is followed by maintenance therapy of doxycycline 200 mg daily, plus co-trimoxazole (sulfamethoxazole 1600 mg plus trimethoprim 320 mg 12-hourly) for a minimum of 12 weeks. Abscesses should be drained surgically.

Actinomycete infections

Nocardiosis

Nocardiosis is an uncommon Gram-positive bacterial infection caused by aerobic actinomycetes of the genus *Nocardia*. They can cause localised or systemic suppurative disease in immunocompromised humans and animals, especially lung and brain abscesses. On microscopy, nocardia appear as long filamentous branching Gram-positive rods which are also weakly acid-fast. They are easily grown in culture but require prolonged incubation.

Co-trimoxazole is the treatment of choice but third-generation cephalosporins and carbapenems have also been used successfully. For severe infections an aminoglycoside such as amikacin is usually added. Surgical drainage of large abscesses may be necessary. Oral treatment is usually continued for a year if there is CNS involvement.

Actinomyces israelii

Actinomyces israelii can cause deep infection in the head and neck, and also suppurating disease in the pelvis associated with intrauterine contraceptive devices (IUCDs). Treatment is usually with penicillin or doxycycline.

13

Gastrointestinal bacterial infections

The differential diagnosis and approach to patients presenting with acute gastroenteritis is described on pages 302–303.

Staphylococcal food poisoning

Staph. aureus transmission takes place via the hands of food handlers to foodstuffs such as dairy products, including cheese, and cooked meats. Inappropriate storage of these foods allows growth of the organism and production of one or more heat-stable enterotoxins which cause the symptoms.

Nausea and profuse vomiting develop within 1–6 hours. Diarrhoea may not be marked. The toxins which cause the syndrome act as 'super-antigens', inducing a significant neutrophil leucocytosis which may be clinically misleading. Super-antigens are secreted proteins (exotoxins) that exhibit highly potent lymphocyte-transforming (mitogenic) activity directed towards T lymphocytes. Most cases settle rapidly but severe dehydration can occasionally be life-threatening.

Antiemetics and appropriate fluid replacement are the mainstays of treatment. Suspect food should be cultured for staphylococci and demonstration of toxin production. The public health authorities should be notified if food vending is involved.

Bacillus cereus food poisoning

Ingestion of the pre-formed heat-stable exotoxins of *B. cereus* causes rapid onset of vomiting and some diarrhoea within hours of food consumption, which resolves within 24 hours. Fried rice and freshly made vanilla sauces are frequent sources; the organism grows and produces enterotoxin during storage (Fig. 13.22). If viable bacteria are ingested and toxin formation takes place within the gut lumen, then the incubation period is longer (12–24 hours) and watery diarrhoea and cramps are the predominant symptoms. The disease is self-limiting but can be quite severe.

Rapid and judicious fluid replacement and appropriate notification of the public health authorities are all that is required.

Clostridium perfringens food poisoning

Spores of *C. perfringens* are widespread in the guts of large animals and in soil. If contaminated meat products are incompletely cooked and stored in anaerobic conditions, *C. perfringens* spores germinate and viable organisms multiply to give large numbers. Subsequent reheating of the food causes heat-shock sporulation of the organisms, during which they release an enterotoxin. Symptoms (diarrhoea and cramps) occur some 6–12 hours following ingestion. The illness is usually self-limiting.

Clostridial enterotoxins are potent and most people who ingest them will be symptomatic. 'Point source' outbreaks, in which a number of cases all become symptomatic following ingestion, classically occur after school or canteen lunches where meat stews are served.

Clostridial necrotising enteritis (CNE) or pigbel is an often fatal type of food poisoning caused by a β-toxin of *C. perfringens*, type C. It occurs in association with protein malnutrition or food containing trypsinases

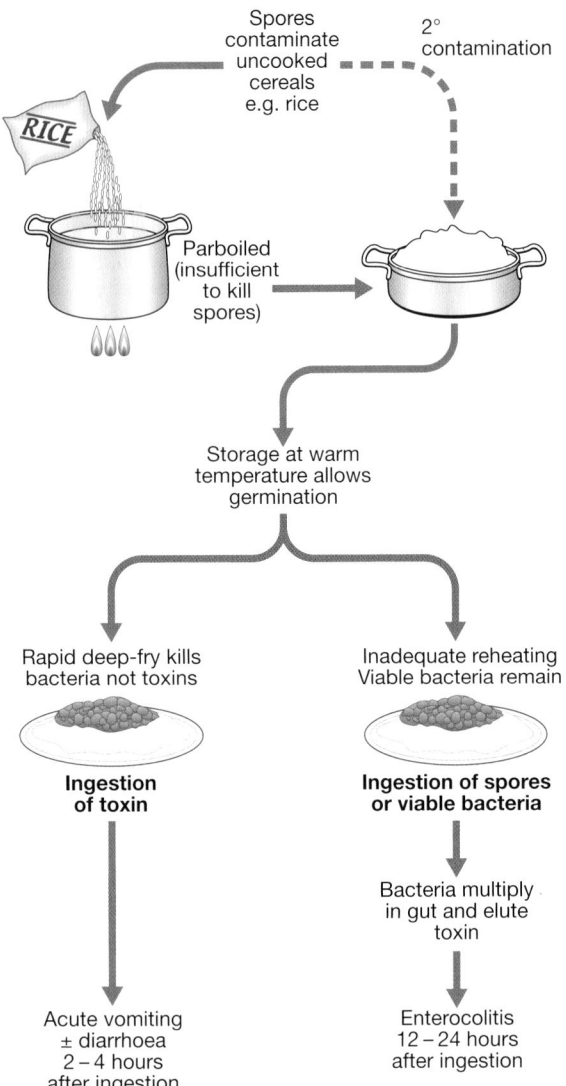

Fig. 13.22 *Bacillus cereus* food poisoning.

such as sweet potatoes. The toxin is normally inactivated by proteolytic enzymes and by normal cooking, but when these protections are impeded, the disease emerges.

Campylobacter jejuni infection

This infection is essentially a zoonosis, although contaminated water may be implicated, as the organism can survive for many weeks in fresh water. The most common sources of the infection are chicken, beef and contaminated milk products. There has been an association with pet puppies. *Campylobacter* infection is now the most common cause of bacterial gastroenteritis in the UK, accounting for some 100 000 cases per annum, most of which are sporadic.

The incubation period is 2–5 days. Colicky abdominal pain, which may be quite severe and mimic surgical pathology, occurs with nausea, vomiting and significant diarrhoea, frequently containing blood. The majority of *Campylobacter* infections affect fit young adults and are self-limiting after 5–7 days. About 10–20% will have prolonged symptomatology, occasionally meriting treatment with antibiotics such as ciprofloxacin.

Approximately 1% of cases will develop bacteraemia and possible distant foci of infection. *Campylobacter* species have been linked to Guillain–Barré syndrome and post-infectious reactive arthritis (pp. 1229 and 1094).

Salmonella spp. infection

Salmonella serotypes other than *S. typhi* and *S. paratyphi* (see p. 334), of which there are more than 2000, are subdivided into five distinct subgroups which produce gastroenteritis. They are widely distributed throughout the animal kingdom. Two serotypes are most important world-wide: *S. enteritidis* phage type 4 and *S. typhimurium* dt.104. The latter may be resistant to commonly used antibiotics such as ciprofloxacin. Some strains have a clear relationship to particular animal species, e.g. *S. arizonae* and pet reptiles. Transmission is by contaminated water or food, particularly poultry, egg products and related fast foods, direct person-to-person spread or the handling of exotic pets such as salamanders, lizards or turtles. The incidence of *Salmonella* enteritis is falling in the UK due to an aggressive culling policy in broiler chicken stocks, coupled with vaccination.

The incubation period of *Salmonella* gastroenteritis is 12–72 hours and the predominant feature is diarrhoea. Vomiting may be present at the outset and blood is quite frequently noted in the stool. Approximately 5% of cases are bacteraemic. Reactive (post-infective) arthritis occurs in approximately 2%.

Antibiotics are not indicated for uncomplicated *Salmonella* gastroenteritis (Box 13.46). However, evidence of bacteraemia is a clear indication for antibiotic therapy, as salmonellae are notorious for persistent infection and often colonise endothelial surfaces such as an atherosclerotic aorta or a major blood vessel. Mortality, as with other forms of gastroenteritis, is higher in the elderly (see Box 13.13, p. 302).

EBM 13.46 **Antibiotics in *Salmonella* gastroenteritis**

'In otherwise healthy adults or children with non-severe *Salmonella* diarrhoea, antibiotics have no clinical benefit over placebo, increase side-effects and prolong *Salmonella* detection.'

- Sirinavin S, Garner P (Cochrane Review). Cochrane Library, issue 1, 2001. Oxford:Update Software.

For further information: www.cochrane.org

Escherichia coli infection

Many serotypes of *E. coli* are present in the human gut at any given time. Production of disease depends on either colonisation with a new or previously unrecognised strain, or the acquisition by current colonising bacteria of a particular pathogenicity factor for mucosal attachment or toxin production. Travel to unfamiliar areas of the world allows contact with different strains of endemic *E. coli* and the development of travellers' diarrhoea. Enteropathogenic strains may be found in the gut of healthy individuals and, if these people move to a new environment, close contacts may develop symptoms.

At least five different clinico-pathological patterns of diarrhoea are associated with specific strains of *E. coli* with characteristic virulence factors.

Enterotoxigenic E. coli (ETEC)

These cause the majority of cases of travellers' diarrhoea in developing countries, although there are other causes (see Box 13.21, p. 307). The organisms produce either a heat-labile or a heat-stable enterotoxin, causing marked secretory diarrhoea and vomiting after 1–2 days' incubation. The illness is usually mild and self-limiting after 3–4 days. Antibiotics, such as ciprofloxacin, have been used to limit the duration of symptoms (see Box 13.22, p. 307) but are of questionable value.

Entero-invasive E. coli (EIEC)

This illness is very similar to *Shigella* dysentery (see p. 339) and is caused by invasion and destruction of colonic mucosal cells. No enterotoxin is produced. Acute watery diarrhoea, abdominal cramps and some scanty blood-staining of the stool are common. The symptoms are rarely severe and are usually self-limiting.

Enteropathogenic E. coli (EPEC)

These organisms are very important in infant diarrhoea. They are able to attach to the gut mucosa, inducing a specific 'attachment and effacement' lesion, and causing destruction of microvilli and disruption of normal absorptive capacity. The symptoms vary from mild non-bloody diarrhoea to quite severe illness, but without bacteraemia.

Entero-aggregative E. coli (EAEC)

These strains adhere to the mucosa but also produce a locally active enterotoxin and demonstrate a particular 'stacked brick' aggregation to tissue culture cells when viewed by microscopy. They have been associated with prolonged diarrhoea in children in South America, South-east Asia and India.

Enterohaemorrhagic E. coli (EHEC)

A number of distinct 'O' serotypes of *E. coli* possess both the genes necessary for adherence (see 'EPEC' above) and plasmids encoding for two distinct enterotoxins (verotoxins) which are identical to the toxins produced by *Shigella* ('shiga-toxins 1 and 2'). *E. coli* O157:H7 is perhaps the best known of these verotoxin-producing *E. coli* (VTEC), but others, including types O126 and O11, are also implicated. Although the incidence is considerably lower than *Campylobacter* and *Salmonella* infection, it is increasing in the developing world.

The reservoir of infection is in the gut of herbivores. The organism has an extremely low infecting dose (10–100 organisms). Runoff water from pasture lands where cattle have grazed which is used to irrigate vegetable crops, as well as contaminated milk, meat products (especially hamburgers which have been incompletely cooked), lettuce, radish shoots and apple juice, have all been implicated as sources (Fig. 13.23).

The incubation period is between 1 and 7 days. Initial watery diarrhoea becomes frankly and uniformly blood-stained in 70% of cases and is associated with severe and often constant abdominal pain. There is little systemic upset, vomiting or fever.

Enterotoxins have both a local effect on the bowel and a distant effect on particular body tissues such as glomerular apparatus, heart and brain. The potentially life-threatening haemolytic uraemic syndrome (HUS, p. 498) occurs in 10–15% of sufferers from this infection, arising

13

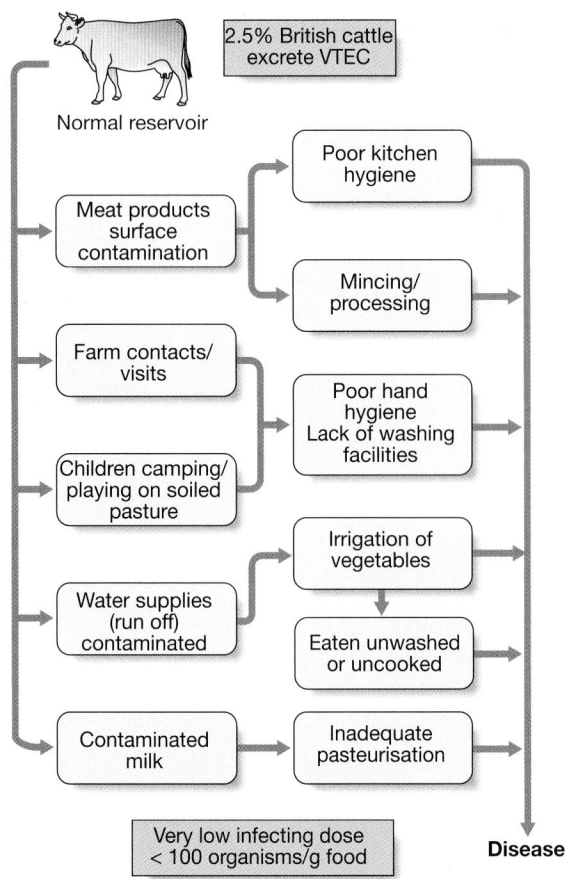

Fig. 13.23 Verocytotoxigenic *E. coli* (VTEC) infections.

5-7 days after the onset of symptoms. It is most likely at the extremes of age, is heralded by a high peripheral leucocyte count and may be induced, particularly in children, by antibiotic therapy.

HUS is treated by dialysis if necessary and may be averted by plasma exchange. Antibiotics should be avoided since they can stimulate toxin release.

Clostridium difficile infection

C. difficile is the most commonly diagnosed cause of antibiotic-associated diarrhoea (p. 304), and is an occasional constituent of the normal intestinal flora. *C. difficile* is capable of producing two toxins (A and B). *C. difficile* infection (CDI) usually follows antimicrobial therapy. It has been assumed that disease results from abolition of colonisation resistance following broad-spectrum antibiotic therapy. However, antibiotic exposure itself can also stimulate toxin production. The combination of toxin production and the ability to produce environmentally stable spores accounts for the clinical features and transmissibility of CDI. A hypervirulent strain of *C. difficile*, ribotype 027, has emerged, which produces more toxin than other *C. difficile* strains and thus more severe disease.

Clinical features

Disease manifestations range from diarrhoea to life-threatening pseudomembranous colitis. Around 80% of cases occur in people over 65 years of age, many of whom are frail with comorbid diseases. Symptoms usually begin in the first week of antibiotic therapy but can occur at any time up to 6 weeks after treatment has finished. The onset is often insidious, with lower abdominal pain and diarrhoea which may become profuse and watery. The presentation may resemble acute ulcerative colitis with bloody diarrhoea, fever and even toxic dilatation and perforation. Ileus is also seen in pseudomembranous colitis.

Investigations

C. difficile can be isolated from stool culture in 30% of patients with antibiotic-associated diarrhoea and over 90% of those with pseudomembranous colitis, but also from 5% of healthy adults and up to 20% of elderly patients in residential care. The diagnosis of CDI therefore rests on detection of toxins A or B in the stool using ELISA or tissue culture cytotoxicity assays.

The rectal appearances at sigmoidoscopy may be characteristic, with erythema, white plaques or an adherent pseudomembrane (Fig. 13.24). Appearances may also resemble those of ulcerative colitis. In some cases, the rectum is spared and abnormalities are observed in the proximal colon. Patients who are ill may require abdominal and erect chest X-rays to exclude perforation or toxic dilatation, respectively. CT may be useful when the diagnosis is in doubt.

Management

The precipitating antibiotic should be stopped and the patient should be isolated. Supportive therapy with intravenous fluids and resting of the bowel is often needed. CDI is treated with antibiotics. Traditionally, metronidazole (500 mg orally 8-hourly for 10 days) was used as first-line therapy, with a switch to vancomycin (125 mg orally 6-hourly for 7–10 days) if there was a relapse (15–30% of patients), failure of initial response or evidence of more fulminant infection. However, some authorities now recommend vancomycin as initial therapy, in view of reports of metronidazole resistance and better efficacy of vancomycin against hypervirulent *C. difficile* strains. Fusidic acid, nitazoxanide and rifaximin have been used successfully in some studies, while intravenous immunoglobulin is sometimes given in the most severe cases.

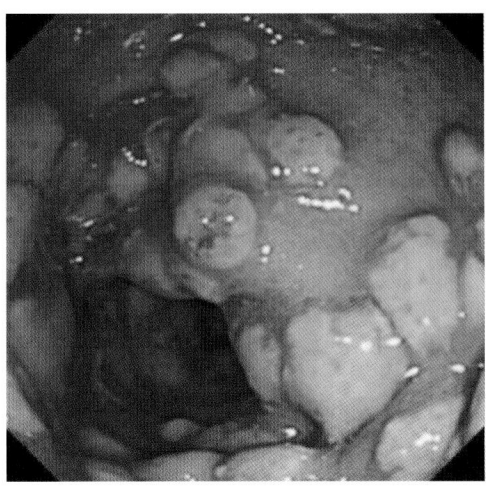

Fig. 13.24 *Clostridium difficile* infection. Colonoscopic view showing numerous adherent 'pseudomembranes' on the mucosa.

Yersinia enterocolitica infection

This organism, commonly found in pork, causes mild to moderate gastroenteritis and can produce significant mesenteric adenitis after an incubation period of 3–7 days. It predominantly causes disease in children but adults may also be affected. The illness resolves slowly, with 10–30% of cases complicated by persistent arthritis or Reiter's syndrome (p. 1094).

Cholera

Cholera, caused by *Vibrio cholerae* serotype 01, is the archetypal toxin-mediated bacterial cause of acute watery diarrhoea. The enterotoxin activates adenylate cyclase in the intestinal epithelium, inducing net secretion of chloride and water. Following its origin in the Ganges valley, devastating epidemics have occurred, often in association with large religious festivals, and pandemics have spread world-wide. The seventh pandemic, due to the El Tor biotype, began in 1961 and spread via the Middle East to become endemic in Africa. In 1990 it reached Peru and spread throughout South and Central America. Since 2005 numbers of cases of cholera have been increasing. There are recurrent outbreaks and epidemics in Africa, often related to flooding. El Tor is more resistant to commonly used antimicrobials than classical *Vibrio*, and causes prolonged carriage in 5% of infections. A new classical toxigenic strain, serotype 0139, established itself in Bangladesh in 1992 and started a new pandemic.

Infection spreads via the stools or vomit of symptomatic patients or of the much larger number of subclinical cases. Organisms survive for up to 2 weeks in fresh water and 8 weeks in salt water. Transmission is normally through infected drinking water, shellfish and food contaminated by flies, or on the hands of carriers.

Clinical features

Severe diarrhoea without pain or colic begins suddenly and is followed by vomiting. Following the evacuation of normal gut faecal contents, typical 'rice-water' material is passed, consisting of clear fluid with flecks of mucus. Classical cholera produces enormous loss of fluid and electrolytes, leading to intense dehydration with muscular cramps. Shock and oliguria develop but mental clarity remains. Death from acute circulatory failure may occur rapidly unless fluid and electrolytes are replaced. Improvement is rapid with proper treatment.

The majority of infections, however, cause mild illness with slight diarrhoea. Occasionally, a very intense illness, 'cholera sicca', occurs, with loss of fluid into dilated bowel, killing the patient before typical gastrointestinal symptoms appear. The disease is more dangerous in children.

Diagnosis and management

Clinical diagnosis is easy during an epidemic. Otherwise the diagnosis should be confirmed bacteriologically. Stool dark-field microscopy shows the typical 'shooting star' motility of *V. cholerae*. Rectal swab or stool cultures allow identification. Cholera is notifiable under international health regulations.

Maintenance of circulation by replacement of water and electrolytes is paramount (p. 303). Ringer-Lactate is the best fluid for intravenous replacement. Vomiting usually stops once the patient is rehydrated, and fluid should then be given orally up to 500 mL hourly. Early intervention with oral rehydration solutions that include resistant starch shortens the duration of diarrhoea and improves prognosis. Total fluid requirements may exceed 50 L over a period of 2–5 days. Accurate records are greatly facilitated by the use of a 'cholera cot', which has a reinforced hole under the patient's buttocks beneath which a graded bucket is placed.

Three days' treatment with tetracycline 250 mg 6-hourly, a single dose of doxycycline 300 mg or ciprofloxacin 1 g in adults reduces the duration of excretion of *V. cholerae* and the total volume of fluid needed for replacement.

Prevention

Strict personal hygiene is vital and drinking water should come from a clean piped supply or be boiled. Flies must be denied access to food. Parenteral vaccination with a killed suspension of *V. cholerae* provides some protection. Oral vaccines containing killed *V. cholerae* and the B subunit of cholera toxin are available but are of limited efficacy.

In epidemics, public education and control of water sources and population movement are vital. Mass single-dose vaccination and treatment with tetracycline are valuable. Disinfection of discharges and soiled clothing, and scrupulous hand-washing by medical attendants reduce the danger of spread.

Vibrio parahaemolyticus infection

This marine organism produces a disease similar to enterotoxigenic *E. coli* (see above). It is acquired from raw seafood and is very common where ingestion of such food is widespread (e.g. Japan). After an incubation period of approximately 20 hours, explosive diarrhoea, abdominal cramps and vomiting occur. Systemic symptoms of headache and fever are frequent but the illness is self-limiting after 4–7 days. Rarely, a severe septicaemic illness arises; in this case *V. parahaemolyticus* can be isolated using specific halophilic culture.

Bacillary dysentery (shigellosis)

Shigellae are Gram-negative rods, closely related to *E. coli*, that invade the colonic mucosa. There are four main groups: *Sh. dysenteriae*, *flexneri*, *boydii* and *sonnei*. In the tropics bacillary dysentery is usually caused by *Sh. flexneri*, whilst in the UK most cases are caused by *Sh. sonnei*. Shigellae are often resistant to multiple antibiotics, especially in tropical countries. The organism only infects humans and its spread is facilitated by its low infecting dose of around 10 organisms.

Spread may occur via contaminated food or flies, but transmission by unwashed hands after defecation is by far the most important factor. Outbreaks occur in mental hospitals, residential schools and other closed institutions, and dysentery is a constant accompaniment of wars and natural catastrophes, which bring crowding and poor sanitation in their wake. *Shigella* infection may spread rapidly amongst men who have sex with men.

Clinical features

Disease severity varies from mild *Sh. sonnei* infections that may escape detection to more severe *Sh. flexneri* infections, while those due to *Sh. dysenteriae* may be fulminating and cause death within 48 hours.

In a moderately severe illness, the patient complains of diarrhoea, colicky abdominal pain and tenesmus. Stools are small, and after a few evacuations contain blood and purulent exudate with little faecal material. Fever, dehydration and weakness occur, with tenderness over the colon. Arthritis or iritis may occasionally complicate bacillary dysentery (Reiter's syndrome, p. 1094), associated with HLA-B27.

Management and prevention

Oral rehydration therapy or, if diarrhoea is severe, intravenous replacement of water and electrolyte loss is necessary. Antibiotic therapy with ciprofloxacin (500 mg 12-hourly for 3 days) is effective in known shigellosis and appropriate in epidemics. The use of antidiarrhoeal medication should be avoided.

The prevention of faecal contamination of food and milk and the isolation of cases may be difficult, except in limited outbreaks. Hand-washing is very important.

Respiratory bacterial infections

Most of these infections are described in Chapter 19.

Diphtheria

Infection with *Corynebacterium diphtheriae* occurs most commonly in the upper respiratory tract and is usually spread by droplet infection from cases or carriers. Infection may also complicate skin lesions, especially in those who misuse alcohol. The organisms remain localised at the site of infection but serious consequences result from the absorption of a soluble exotoxin which damages the heart muscle and the nervous system.

Diphtheria has been eradicated from many parts of the world by mass vaccination using a modified exotoxin but remains important in areas where vaccination has been incomplete, e.g. in Russia and South-east Asia. The disease is notifiable in all countries of Europe and North America and international guidelines have been issued by the WHO for the management of infection.

Clinical features

The average incubation period is 2–4 days. The disease begins insidiously with a sore throat (Box 13.47). Despite modest fever there is usually marked tachycardia. The diagnostic feature is the 'wash-leather' elevated greyish-green membrane on the tonsils. It has a well-defined edge, is firm and adherent, and is surrounded by a zone of inflammation. There may be swelling of the neck ('bull-neck') and tender enlargement of the lymph nodes.

13.47 Clinical features of diphtheria
Acute infection
• Membranous tonsillitis
• *or* Nasal infection
• *or* Laryngeal infection
• *or* Skin/wound/conjunctival infection (rare)
Complications
• Laryngeal obstruction or paralysis
• Myocarditis
• Peripheral neuropathy

In the mildest infections, especially in the presence of a high degree of immunity, a membrane may never appear and the throat is merely slightly inflamed.

With anterior nasal infection there is nasal discharge, frequently blood-stained. In laryngeal diphtheria a husky voice and high-pitched cough signal potential respiratory obstruction requiring urgent tracheostomy. If infection spreads to the uvula, fauces and nasopharynx, the patient is gravely ill.

Death from acute circulatory failure may occur within the first 10 days. Late complications occur as a result of toxin action on the heart or nervous system. About 25% of survivors of the early toxaemia may later develop myocarditis with arrhythmias or cardiac failure. These are usually reversible with no permanent damage other than heart block in survivors.

Neurological involvement occurs in 75% of cases. After tonsillar or pharyngeal diphtheria it usually starts after 10 days with palatal palsy. Paralysis of accommodation often follows, manifest by difficulty in reading small print. Generalised polyneuritis with weakness and paraesthesia may follow in the next 10–14 days. Recovery from such neuritis is always ultimately complete.

Management

A clinical diagnosis of diphtheria must be notified to the public health authorities and the patient sent urgently to a specialist infectious diseases unit. Treatment should begin once appropriate swabs have been taken before waiting for microbiological confirmation.

Diphtheria antitoxin is produced from hyperimmune horse serum. It neutralises circulating toxin, but has no effect on toxin already fixed to tissues, so it must be injected intramuscularly without awaiting the result of a throat swab. However, reactions to this foreign protein include a potentially lethal immediate anaphylactic reaction (p. 89) and a 'serum sickness' with fever, urticaria and joint pains, which occurs 7–12 days after injection. A careful history of previous horse serum injections or allergic reactions should be taken and a small test injection of serum should be given half an hour before the full dose in every patient. Adrenaline (epinephrine) solution must be available to deal with any immediate type of reaction (0.5–1.0 mL of 1/1000 solution i.m.). An antihistamine is also given. In a severely ill patient the risk of anaphylactic shock is outweighed by the mortal danger of diphtheritic toxaemia, and up to 100 000 U of antitoxin are injected intravenously if the test dose has not given rise to symptoms. For disease of moderate severity, 16 000–40 000 U i.m. will suffice, and for mild cases 4000–8000 U.

Penicillin (1200 mg 6-hourly i.v.) or amoxicillin (500 mg 8-hourly) should be administered for 2 weeks to eliminate *C. diphtheriae*. Patients allergic to penicillin can be given erythromycin. Due to poor immunogenicity of primary infection all sufferers should be immunised with diphtheria toxoid following recovery.

Patients must be managed in strict isolation attended by staff with a clearly documented immunisation history until three swabs 24 hours apart are culture-negative.

Prevention

Active immunisation should be given to all children. If diphtheria occurs in a closed community, contacts should be given erythromycin, which is more effective than penicillin in eradicating the organism in carriers.

All contacts should also be immunised or given a booster dose of toxoid. Booster doses are required every 10 years to maintain immunity.

Pneumococcal infection

Strep. pneumoniae (the pneumococcus) is the leading cause of community-acquired pneumonia globally (p. 670) and one of the leading causes of infection-related mortality. Otitis media, meningitis and sinusitis are also frequently due to *Strep. pneumoniae*. Occasional patients present with bacteraemia without obvious focus. Asplenic individuals are at risk of fulminant pneumococcal disease with purpuric rash.

Increasing rates of penicillin resistance have been reported for *Strep. pneumoniae*, and strains with high-level resistance require treatment with glycopeptides rather than with penicillins or cephalosporins. Newer quinolones are also used but rates of resistance are rising.

Vaccination of infants with the protein conjugate pneumococcal vaccine decreases *Strep. pneumoniae* infection in infants and in their relatives. The polysaccharide pneumococcal vaccine is used in individuals predisposed to *Strep. pneumoniae* infection and the elderly, but only modestly reduces pneumococcal bacteraemia and does not prevent pneumonia. All asplenic individuals should receive vaccination against *Strep. pneumoniae*.

Anthrax

Anthrax is an endemic zoonosis in many countries; it causes human disease following inoculation of the spores of *Bacillus anthracis*. *B. anthracis* was the first recognised bacterial pathogen described by Koch and became the model pathogen for 'Koch's postulates' (see Box 6.1, p. 132). It is a Gram-positive organism with a central spore. The spores can survive for years in soil. Infection is commonly acquired from contact with animals, particularly herbivores. The ease of production of *B. anthracis* spores makes this infection a candidate for biological warfare or bioterrorism. *B. anthracis* produces a number of toxins which mediate the clinical features of disease.

Clinical features

These depend on the route of entry of the anthrax spores.

Cutaneous anthrax

This skin lesion is associated with occupational exposure to anthrax spores during processing of hides and bone products, or with bioterrorism. It accounts for the vast majority of clinical cases. Animal infection is a serious problem in Africa, India, Pakistan and the Middle East.

Spores are inoculated into exposed skin. A single lesion develops as an irritable papule on an oedematous haemorrhagic base. This progresses to a depressed black eschar. Despite extensive oedema, pain is infrequent.

Gastrointestinal anthrax

This is associated with the ingestion of meat products that have been contaminated or incompletely cooked. The caecum is the seat of the infection, which produces nausea, vomiting, anorexia and fever, followed in 2–3 days by severe abdominal pain and bloody diarrhoea. Toxaemia and death can develop rapidly thereafter.

Inhalational anthrax

This form of the disease is extremely rare, unless associated with bioterrorism. Without rapid and aggressive therapy at the onset of symptoms, the mortality is 50–90%. Fever, dyspnoea, cough, headache and symptoms of septicaemia develop 3–14 days following exposure. Typically, the chest X-ray shows only widening of the mediastinum and pleural effusions which are haemorrhagic. Meningitis may occur.

Management

B. anthracis can be cultured from skin swabs from lesions. Skin lesions are readily curable with early antibiotic therapy. Treatment is with ciprofloxacin (500 mg 12-hourly) until penicillin susceptibility is confirmed; the regimen can then be changed to benzylpenicillin with doses up to 2.4 g i.v. given 4-hourly or phenoxy-methylpenicillin 500–1000 mg 6-hourly administered for 10 days. The addition of an aminoglycoside may improve the outlook in severe disease. In view of concerns about concomitant inhalational exposure, particularly in the era of bioterrorism, a further 2-month course of ciprofloxacin 500 mg 12-hourly or doxycycline 100 mg 12-hourly orally is added. Prophylaxis with ciprofloxacin (500 mg 12-hourly) is recommended for anyone at high risk of exposure to anthrax spores.

Bacterial infections with neurological involvement

Infections affecting the CNS, including bacterial meningitis, botulism and tetanus, are described on pages 1205–1214.

Mycobacterial infections

Tuberculosis is predominantly, although by no means exclusively, a respiratory disease and is described on page 688.

Leprosy

Leprosy (Hansen's disease) is a chronic granulomatous disease affecting skin and nerves, caused by *Mycobacterium leprae*, a slow-growing mycobacterium which cannot be cultured in vitro. The clinical manifestations are determined by the degree of the patient's cell-mediated immunity (CMI, p. 76) towards *M. leprae* (Fig. 13.25). High levels of CMI with elimination of leprosy bacilli produce tuberculoid leprosy, whereas absent CMI results in lepromatous leprosy. The complications of leprosy are due to nerve damage, immunological reactions and bacillary infiltration. Leprosy patients are frequently stigmatised and using the word 'leper' is inappropriate.

Epidemiology and transmission

Some 4 million people have leprosy and around 750 000 new cases are detected annually. About 70% of the world's leprosy patients live in India, with the disease endemic in Brazil, Indonesia, Mozambique, Madagascar, Tanzania and Nepal.

Untreated lepromatous patients discharge bacilli from the nose. Infection occurs through the nose, followed by haematogenous spread to skin and nerve. The

13

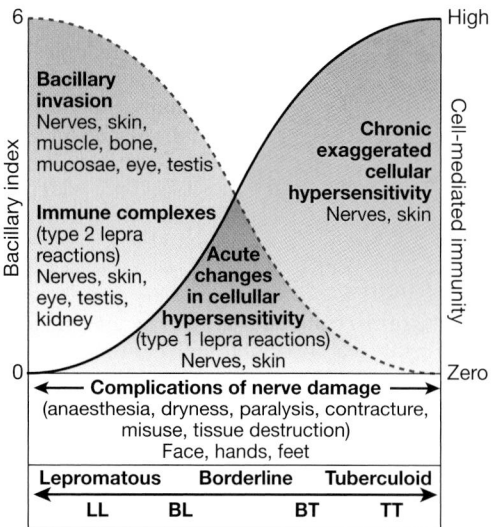

Fig. 13.25 Leprosy: mechanisms of damage and tissue affected.
Mechanisms under the broken line are characteristic of disease near the lepromatous end of the spectrum, and those under the solid line are characteristic of the tuberculoid end. They overlap in the centre where, in addition, instability predisposes to type 1 lepra reactions. At the peak in the centre neither bacillary growth nor cell-mediated immunity has the upper hand. (BL = borderline lepromatous; BT = borderline tuberculoid)

incubation period is 2–5 years for tuberculoid cases and 8–12 years for lepromatous cases. Leprosy incidence peaks at 10–14 years, and is more common in males and in those with close household exposure to leprosy cases.

Pathogenesis

M. leprae has a predilection for infecting Schwann cells and skin macrophages. In tuberculoid leprosy, effective CMI controls bacillary multiplication ('paucibacillary') but organised epithelioid granulomas are formed. In lepromatous leprosy, there is abundant bacillary multiplication ('multibacillary'), e.g. in Schwann cells and perineurium. Between these two extremes is a continuum, varying from patients with moderate CMI (borderline tuberculoid) to patients with little cellular response (borderline lepromatous).

In addition, immunological reactions to the infection occur as the immune response develops and the antigenic stimulus from the bacilli varies, particularly in borderline patients. Delayed hypersensitivity reactions produce type 1 (reversal) reactions, while immune complexes contribute to type 2 (erythema nodosum leprosum) reactions.

HIV/leprosy co-infected patients have typical lepromatous and tuberculoid leprosy skin lesions and typical leprosy histology and granuloma formation. Surprisingly, even with low circulating CD4 counts, tuberculoid leprosy may be observed and there is not an obvious shift to lepromatous leprosy.

Clinical features

Box 13.48 gives the cardinal features of leprosy. Types of leprosy are compared in Box 13.49.

- *Skin.* The most common skin lesions are macules or plaques. Tuberculoid patients have few, hypopigmented lesions. In lepromatous leprosy,

13.48 Cardinal features of leprosy

- Skin lesions, typically anaesthetic at tuberculoid end of spectrum
- Thickened peripheral nerves
- Acid-fast bacilli on skin smears or biopsy

13.49 Clinical characteristics of the polar forms of leprosy

Clinical and tissue-specific features	Lepromatous	Tuberculoid
Skin and nerves		
Number and distribution	Widely disseminated	One or a few sites, asymmetrical
Skin lesions		
Definition		
Clarity of margin	Poor	Good
Elevation of margin	Never	Common
Colour		
Dark skin	Slight hypopigmentation	Marked hypopigmentation
Light skin	Slight erythema	Coppery or red
Surface	Smooth, shiny	Dry, scaly
Central healing	None	Common
Sweat and hair growth	Impaired late	Impaired early
Loss of sensation	Late	Early and marked
Nerve enlargement and damage	Late	Early and marked
Bacilli (bacterial index)	Many (5 or 6+)	Absent (0)
Natural history	Progressive	Self-healing
Other tissues	Upper respiratory mucosa, eye, testes, bones, muscle	None
Reactions	Immune complexes (type 2)	Cell-mediated (type 1)

papers, nodules or diffuse infiltration of the skin occur. The earliest lesions are ill defined; gradually, the skin becomes infiltrated and thickened. Facial skin thickening leads to the characteristic leonine facies (Fig. 13.26B).

- *Anaesthesia.* In skin lesions the small dermal sensory and autonomic nerve fibres are damaged, causing local sensory loss and loss of sweating within that area. Anaesthesia may also occur in the distribution of a damaged large peripheral nerve. A 'glove and stocking' sensory neuropathy is also common in lepromatous leprosy.
- *Nerve damage.* Peripheral nerve trunks are affected at 'sites of predilection'. These are the ulnar (elbow), median (wrist), radial (humerus), radial cutaneous (wrist), common peroneal (knee), posterior tibial and sural nerves (ankle), facial nerve (zygomatic arch) and great auricular nerve (posterior triangle

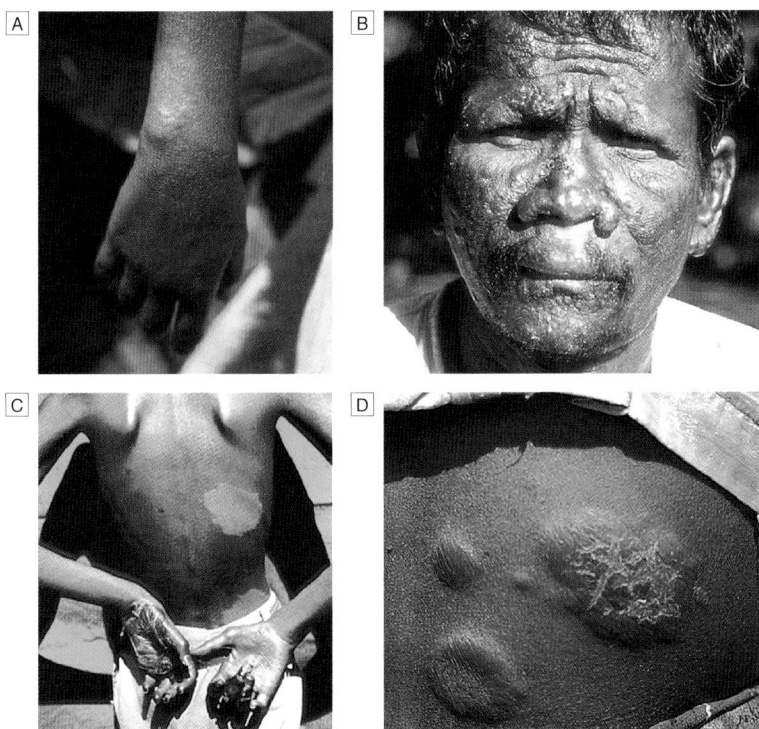

Fig. 13.26 Clinical features of leprosy. **A** Tuberculoid leprosy. Single lesion with a well-defined active edge and anaesthesia within the lesion. **B** Lepromatous leprosy. Widespread nodules and infiltration, with loss of the eyebrows. This man also has early collapse of the nose. **C** Borderline tuberculoid leprosy with severe nerve damage. This boy has several well-defined, hypopigmented, macular, anaesthetic lesions. He has severe nerve damage affecting both ulnar and median nerves bilaterally and has sustained severe burns to his hands. **D** Reversal (type 1) reactions. Erythematous, oedematous lesions.

of the neck). Damage to peripheral nerve trunks produces characteristic signs with regional sensory loss and muscle dysfunction (Fig. 13.26C). All these nerves should be examined for enlargement and tenderness and tested for motor and sensory function. The CNS is not affected.

- *Eye involvement.* Blindness is a devastating complication for a patient with anaesthetic hands and feet. Eyelid closure is impaired when the facial nerve is affected. Damage to the trigeminal nerve causes anaesthesia of the cornea and conjunctiva. The cornea is then susceptible to trauma and ulceration.
- *Other features.* Many organs can be affected. Nasal collapse occurs secondary to bacillary destruction of the bony nasal spine. Diffuse infiltration of the testes causes testicular atrophy and the acute orchitis that occurs with type 2 reactions. This results in azoospermia and hypogonadism.

Leprosy reactions

Leprosy reactions (Box 13.50) are events superimposed on the cardinal features shown in Box 13.48.

- *Type 1 (reversal) reactions*: These occur in 30% of borderline patients (BT, BB or BL) and are delayed hypersensitivity reactions. Skin lesions become erythematous (Fig. 13.26D). Peripheral nerves become tender and painful, with sudden loss of nerve function. These reactions may occur spontaneously, after starting treatment and also after completion of multidrug therapy.
- *Type 2 (erythema nodosum leprosum—ENL) reactions*: These are partly due to immune complex deposition

and occur in BL and LL patients who produce antibodies and have a high antigen load. They manifest with malaise, fever and crops of small pink nodules on the face and limbs. Iritis and episcleritis

	13.50 Reactions in leprosy	
	Lepra reaction type 1 (reversal)	**Lepra reaction type 2 (erythema nodosum leprosum, ENL)**
Mechanism	Cell-mediated hypersensitivity	Immune complexes
Clinical features	Painful tender nerves, loss of function Swollen skin lesions New skin lesions	Tender papules and nodules; may ulcerate Painful tender nerves, loss of function Iritis, orchitis, myositis, lymphadenitis Fever, oedema
Management	Prednisolone 40 mg, reducing over 3–6 months[1]	Moderate: prednisolone 40 mg daily Severe: thalidomide[2] or prednisolone 40–80 mg daily, reducing over 1–6 months; local if eye involved[3]

[1]Indicated for any new impairment of nerve or eye function.
[2]Contraindicated in fertile women.
[3]1% hydrocortisone drops or ointment and 1% atropine drops.

are common. Other signs are acute neuritis, lymphadenitis, orchitis, bone pain, dactylitis, arthritis and proteinuria. ENL may continue intermittently for several years.

Borderline cases

In borderline tuberculoid (BT) cases, skin lesions are more numerous than in tuberculoid (TT) cases, and there is more severe nerve damage and a risk of type 1 reactions. In borderline leprosy (BB) cases, skin lesions are numerous and vary in size, shape and distribution; annular lesions are characteristic and nerve damage is variable. In borderline lepromatous (BL) cases, there are widespread small macules in the skin and widespread nerve involvement; both type 1 and type 2 reactions occur.

Pure neural leprosy (i.e. without skin lesions) occurs principally in India and accounts for 10% of patients. There is asymmetrical involvement of peripheral nerve trunks and no visible skin lesions. On nerve biopsy all types of leprosy have been found.

Investigations

The diagnosis is clinical, made by finding a cardinal sign of leprosy and supported by finding acid-fast bacilli in slit-skin smears or typical histology in a skin biopsy. Slit-skin smears are obtained by scraping dermal material on to a glass slide. The smears are then stained for acid-fast bacilli, the number counted per high-power field and a score derived on a logarithmic scale (0–6): the bacterial index (BI). Smears are useful for confirming the diagnosis and monitoring response to treatment. Neither serology nor PCR testing for *M. leprae* DNA is sensitive or specific enough for diagnosis.

Management

The principles of treatment are outlined in Box 13.51. All leprosy patients should be given multidrug treatment (MDT) with an approved first-line regimen (Box 13.52).

Rifampicin is a potent bactericidal for *M. leprae* but should always be given in combination with other antileprotics since a single-step mutation can confer resistance. Dapsone is bacteriostatic. It commonly causes mild haemolysis but rarely anaemia. Clofazimine is a red, fat-soluble crystalline dye, weakly bactericidal for *M. leprae*. Skin discoloration (red to purple-black) and ichthyosis are troublesome side-effects, particularly on pale skins. New drugs that are bactericidal for *M. leprae* have been identified, notably the fluoroquinolones pefloxacin and ofloxacin, minocycline and clarithromycin. These agents are now established second-line drugs. Minocycline causes a grey pigmentation of skin lesions.

13.51 Principles of leprosy treatment

- Stop the infection with chemotherapy
- Treat reactions
- Educate the patient about leprosy
- Prevent disability
- Support the patient socially and psychologically

13.52 Modified WHO-recommended multidrug therapy (MDT) regimens in leprosy

Type of leprosy[1]	Monthly supervised treatment	Daily self-administered treatment	Duration of treatment[2]
Paucibacillary	Rifampicin 600 mg	Dapsone 100 mg	6 mths
Multibacillary	Rifampicin 600 mg Clofazimine 300 mg	Clofazimine 50 mg Dapsone 100 mg	12 mths
Paucibacillary single-lesion	Ofloxacin 400 mg Rifampicin 600 mg Minocycline 100 mg		Single dose

[1]Classification uses the bacillary index (BI) in slit-skin smears or, if BI is not available, the number of skin lesions:
- paucibacillary single-lesion leprosy (one skin lesion)
- paucibacillary (2–5 skin lesions)
- multibacillary (> 5 skin lesions).

[2]Studies from India have shown that multibacillary patients with an initial BI > 4 need longer treatment, for at least 24 months.

Although single-dose treatment is less effective than the conventional 6-month treatment for paucibacillary leprosy, it is an operationally attractive field regimen and has been recommended for use by the WHO.

Lepra reactions are treated as shown in Box 13.50. Chloroquine can also be used.

Patient education

Educating leprosy patients about their disease is vital. Patients should be reassured that after 3 days of chemotherapy they are not infectious and can lead a normal social life. It should be emphasised that gross deformities are not inevitable.

Patients with anaesthetic hands or feet need to take special care to avoid and treat burns and other minor injuries. Good footwear is important. Physiotherapy may be required to maintain range of movement of affected muscles and neighbouring joints.

Prognosis

Untreated, tuberculoid leprosy has a good prognosis; it may self-heal and peripheral nerve damage is limited. Lepromatous leprosy (LL) is a progressive condition with high morbidity if untreated.

After treatment, the majority of patients, especially those who have no nerve damage at the time of diagnosis, do well, with resolution of skin lesions. Borderline patients are at risk of developing type 1 reactions which may result in devastating nerve damage.

Prevention and control

The previous strategy of centralised leprosy control campaigns has now been superseded by integrated programmes, with primary health-care workers in many countries now responsible for case detection and provision of MDT. It is not yet clear how successful this will be, especially in the time-consuming area of disability prevention.

BCG vaccination has been shown to give good but variable protection against leprosy; adding killed *M. leprae* to BCG does not enhance protection.

Rickettsial and related intracellular bacterial infections

Rickettsial fevers

The rickettsial fevers are the most common tick-borne infections. Patients present acutely with headache, rash and sometimes neurological disturbance. It is important to ask about exposures that would put patients at risk of bites or contact with ticks, lice or fleas. There are two main groups of rickettsial fevers: spotted fevers and typhus (Box 13.53).

Pathogenesis

The rickettsiae are intracellular Gram-negative organisms which parasitise the intestinal canal of arthropods. Infection is usually conveyed to humans through the skin from the excreta of arthropods, but the saliva of some biting vectors is infected. The organisms multiply in capillary endothelial cells, producing lesions in the skin, CNS, heart, lungs, liver, kidneys and skeletal muscles. Endothelial proliferation, associated with a perivascular reaction, may cause thrombosis and purpura. In epidemic typhus the brain is the target organ; in scrub typhus the cardiovascular system and lungs in particular are attacked. An eschar, a black necrotic crusted sore, is often found in tick- and mite-borne typhus (see Fig. 13.6C, p. 309). This is due to vasculitis following immunological recognition of the inoculated organism. Regional lymph nodes often enlarge.

Spotted fever group

Rocky Mountain spotted fever

Rickettsia rickettsii is transmitted by tick bites. It is widely distributed and increasing in western and south-eastern states of the USA and also in Central and South America. The incubation period is about 7 days. The rash appears on about the 3rd or 4th day of illness, looking at first

13

---

i | **13.53 Features of rickettsial infections**

Disease	Organism	Reservoir	Vector	Geographical area	Rash	Gangrene	Target organs	Mortality
Spotted fever group								
Rocky Mountain spotted fever	*R. rickettsii*	Rodents, dogs, ticks	*Ixodes* tick	North, Central and South America	Morbilliform Haemorrhagic	Often	Bronchi, myocardium, brain, skin	2–12%[2]
Boutonneuse fever	*R. conorii*	Rodents, dogs, ticks	*Ixodes* tick	Mediterranean, Africa, South-west Asia, India	Maculopapular	–	Skin, meninges	2.5%[3]
Siberian tick typhus	*R. siberica*	Rodents, birds, domestic animals, ticks	Various ticks	Siberia, Mongolia, northern China	Maculopapular	–	Skin, meninges	Rare[3]
Australian tick typhus	*R. australis*	Rodents, ticks	Ticks	Australia	Maculopapular	–	Skin, meninges	Rare[3]
Oriental spotted fever	*R. japonica*	Rodents, dogs, ticks	Ticks	Japan	Maculopapular	–	Skin, meninges	Rare[3]
African tick bite fever[1]	*R. africae*	Cattle, game, ticks	*Ixodes* tick	South Africa	Can be spotless	–	Skin, meninges	Rare[3]
Typhus group								
Scrub typhus	*Orientia tsutsugamushi*	Rodents	*Trombicula* mite	SE Asia	Maculopapular	Unusual	Bronchi, myocardium, brain, skin	Rare[3]
Epidemic typhus	*R. prowazekii*	Humans	Louse	World-wide	Morbilliform Haemorrhagic	Often	Brain, skin, bronchi, myocardium	Up to 40%
Endemic typhus	*R. typhi*	Rats	Flea	World-wide	Slight	–	–	Rare[3]

[1]Eschar at bite site and local lymphadenopathy
[2]Highest in adult males.
[3]Except in infants, older people and the debilitated.

like measles, but in a few hours a typical maculopapular eruption develops. The rash spreads in 24–48 hours from wrists, forearms and ankles to the back, limbs and chest, and then to the abdomen, where it is least pronounced. Larger cutaneous and subcutaneous haemorrhages may appear in severe cases. The liver and spleen become palpable. At the extremes of life the mortality is 2–12%.

Other spotted fevers

R. conorii (boutonneuse fever) and *R. africae* (African tick fever) cause Mediterranean and African tick typhus, which also occurs on the Indian subcontinent. The incubation period is approximately 7 days. Infected ticks may be picked up by walking on grasslands or dogs may bring ticks into the house. Careful examination might reveal a diagnostic eschar, and the maculopapular rash on the trunk, limbs, palms and soles. There may be delirium and meningeal signs in severe infections but recovery is usual. *R. africae* can be associated with multiple eschars. Some cases, particularly those with *R. africae*, present without rash ('spotless spotted fever'). Other spotted fevers are shown in Box 13.53.

Typhus group

Scrub typhus fever

Scrub typhus is caused by *Orientia tsutsugamushi* (formerly *Rickettsia tsutsugamushi*), transmitted by mites. It occurs in the Far East, Myanmar, Pakistan, Bangladesh, India, Indonesia, the South Pacific islands and Queensland, particularly where patches of forest cleared for plantations have attracted rats and mites.

In many patients one eschar or more develops, surrounded by an area of cellulitis (see Fig. 13.6C, p. 309) and enlargement of regional lymph nodes. The incubation period is about 9 days.

Mild or subclinical cases are common. The onset of symptoms is usually sudden, with headache (often retro-orbital), fever, malaise, weakness and cough. In severe illness the general symptoms increase, with apathy and prostration. An erythematous maculopapular rash often appears on about the 5th–7th day and spreads to the trunk, face and limbs, including the palms and soles, with generalised painless lymphadenopathy. The rash fades by the 14th day. The temperature rises rapidly and continues as a remittent fever (i.e. the difference between maximum and minimum temperature exceeds 1°C) remaining above normal with sweating until it falls on the 12th–18th day. In severe infection the patient is prostrate with cough, pneumonia, confusion and deafness. Cardiac failure, renal failure and haemorrhage may develop. Convalescence is often slow and tachycardia may persist for some weeks.

Epidemic (louse-borne) typhus

Epidemic typhus is caused by *R. prowazekii* and is transmitted by infected faeces of the human body louse, usually through scratching the skin. Patients suffering from epidemic typhus infect the lice, which leave when the patient is febrile. In conditions of overcrowding the disease spreads rapidly. It is prevalent in parts of Africa, especially Ethiopia and Rwanda, and in the South American Andes and Afghanistan. Large epidemics have occurred in Europe, usually as a sequel to war. The incubation period is usually 12–14 days.

There may be a few days of malaise but the onset is more often sudden with rigors, fever, frontal headaches, pains in the back and limbs, constipation and bronchitis. The face is flushed and cyanotic, the eyes are congested and the patient becomes confused. The rash appears on the 4th–6th day. In its early stages it disappears on pressure but soon becomes petechial with subcutaneous mottling. It appears first on the anterior folds of the axillae, sides of the abdomen or backs of hands, then on the trunk and forearms. The neck and face are seldom affected. During the 2nd week symptoms increase in severity. Sores develop on the lips. The tongue becomes dry, brown, shrunken and tremulous. The spleen is palpable, the pulse feeble and the patient stuporous and delirious. The temperature falls rapidly at the end of the 2nd week and the patient recovers gradually. In fatal cases the patient usually dies in the 2nd week from toxaemia, cardiac or renal failure, or pneumonia.

Endemic (flea-borne) typhus

Flea-borne or 'endemic' typhus caused by *R. typhi* is endemic world-wide. Humans are infected when the faeces or contents of a crushed flea, which has fed on an infected rat, are introduced into the skin. The incubation period is 8–14 days. The symptoms resemble those of a mild louse-borne typhus. The rash may be scanty and transient.

Investigation of rickettsial infection

Routine blood investigations are not diagnostic but malaria must be excluded by blood film examination in most cases, and there is usually hepatitis and thrombocytopenia. Diagnosis is made on clinical grounds and response to treatment. Species-specific antibodies may be detected in specialised laboratories. Differential diagnoses include malaria, typhoid, meningococcal sepsis and leptospirosis.

Management of rickettsial fevers

The different rickettsial fevers vary greatly in severity but all respond to tetracycline 500 mg 6-hourly, doxycycline 200 mg daily or chloramphenicol 500 mg 6-hourly for 7 days. Louse-borne typhus and scrub typhus can be treated with a single dose of 200 mg doxycycline, repeated for 2–3 days to prevent relapse. Chloramphenicol and doxycycline-resistant strains of *O. tsutsugamushi* have been reported from Thailand and patients here may need treatment with rifampicin.

Nursing care is important, especially in epidemic typhus. Sedation may be required for delirium and blood transfusion for haemorrhage. Relapsing fever and typhoid are common intercurrent infections in epidemic typhus, and pneumonia in scrub typhus. They must be sought and treated. Convalescence is usually protracted, especially in older people.

To prevent rickettsial infection, lice, fleas, ticks and mites need to be controlled with insecticides.

Q fever

Q fever occurs world-wide and is caused by the rickettsia-like organism *Coxiella burnetii*, an obligate intracellular organism that can survive in the extracellular environment. Cattle, sheep and goats are important reservoirs and the organism is transmitted by inhalation of aerosolised particles. An important characteristic of

C. burnetii is its antigenic variation, called phase variation, due to a change of lipopolysaccharide (LPS). When isolated from animals or humans, *C. burnetii* express phase I antigen and are very infectious (a single bacterium is sufficient to infect a human). In culture there is an antigenic shift to the phase II form, which is not infectious. This antigenic shift can be measured and is valuable for the differentiation of acute and chronic Q fever.

Clinical features

The incubation period is 3–4 weeks. The initial symptoms are non-specific with fever, headache and chills; in 20% of cases a maculopapular rash occurs. Other presentations include pneumonia and hepatitis. Chronic Q fever may present with osteomyelitis, encephalitis and endocarditis.

Investigations and management

Diagnosis is usually serological and the stage of the infection can be distinguished by isotype tests and phase-specific antigens. Phase I and II IgM titres peak at 4–6 weeks. In chronic infections IgG titres to phase I and II antigens may be raised.

Prompt treatment of acute Q fever with doxycycline reduces fever duration. Treatment of Q fever endocarditis is problematic, requiring prolonged therapy with doxycycline and rifampicin or ciprofloxacin; even then, organisms are not always eradicated. Valve surgery is often required (p. 628).

Bartonellosis

This group of diseases are caused by intracellular Gram-negative bacilli closely related to the rickettsiae and have been found to be important causes of 'culture-negative' endocarditis. They are found in many domestic pets, such as cats, although for several the host is ill defined (Box 13.54). The principal human pathogens are *Bartonella quintana*, *B. henselae* and *B. bacilliformis*. *Bartonella* infections are associated with the following clinical conditions:

- *Trench fever*. This is a relapsing fever with severe leg pain and is due to *B. quintana*. The disease is not fatal but is very debilitating.
- *Bacteraemia and endocarditis in the homeless.* The endocarditis due to *B. quintana* or *henselae* is associated with severe damage to the heart valves.

- *Cat scratch disease*. *B. henselae* causes this common benign lymphadenopathy in children and young adults. A vesicle or papule develops on the head, neck or arms after a cat scratch. The lesion resolves spontaneously but there may be regional lymphadenopathy that persists for up to 4 months before also resolving spontaneously.
- *Bacillary angiomatosis*. This is an HIV-associated disease due to *B. quintana* or *henselae* (p. 391).
- *Oroya fever and verruga peruana (Carrion's disease)*. This is endemic in areas of Peru. It is a biphasic disease caused by *B. bacilliformis* and is transmitted by sandflies of the genus *Phlebotomus*. Fever, haemolytic anaemia and microvascular thrombosis with end-organ ischaemia are features. It is frequently fatal if untreated.

Investigations and management

Bartonellae can be grown from the blood but this requires prolonged incubation using enriched media. Serum antibody detection is possible.

Bartonella species are susceptible to β-lactams, rifampicin, erythromycin and tetracyclines. Antibiotic use is guided by clinical need. Cat scratch disease usually resolves spontaneously but *Bartonella* endocarditis requires valve replacement and combination antibiotic therapy.

Chlamydial infections

These are listed in Box 13.55 and are also described in Chapters 15 and 19.

Trachoma

Trachoma is a chronic keratoconjunctivitis caused by *Chlamydia trachomatis*, and is the most common cause of avoidable blindness. The classic trachoma environment is dry and dirty, causing children to have eye and nose discharges. Transmission occurs through flies, on fingers and within families. In endemic areas the disease is most common in children.

Pathology and clinical features

The onset is usually insidious and infection may be asymptomatic. The infection lasts for years, may be latent over long periods and may recrudesce. The conjunctiva of the upper lid is first affected with vascularisation and cellular infiltration. Early symptoms include conjunctival irritation and blepharospasm. The early follicles of

13

13.54 Clinical diseases caused by bartonellosis

Reservoir	Vector	Organism	Disease
Cats	Flea	*B. henselae*	**Cat scratch disease, bacillary angiomatosis, endocarditis**
Undefined	Lice	*B. quintana*	**Trench fever, bacillary angiomatosis, endocarditis**
Undefined	Sandfly	*B. bacilliformis*	**Carrion's disease: Oroya fever and verruga peruana**
Undefined	Flea	*B. rochalimae*	**Fever, rash, anaemia, splenomegaly**

13.55 Chlamydial infections

Organism	Disease caused
Chlamydia trachomatis	Trachoma Lymphogranuloma venereum (Box 15.11, p. 422) Cervicitis, urethritis, proctitis (pp. 421–422)
Chlamydia psittaci	Psittacosis (Box 19.43, p. 682)
Chlamydophila (Chlamydia) pneumoniae	Atypical pneumonia (Box 19.43, p. 682) Acute/chronic sinusitis

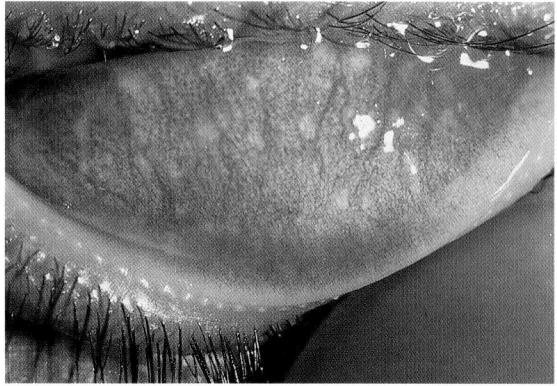

Fig. 13.27 Trachoma. Trachoma is characterised by hyperaemia and numerous pale follicles.

trachoma are characteristic (Fig. 13.27), but clinical differentiation from conjunctivitis due to other viruses may be difficult. Scarring causes inversion of the lids (entropion) so that the lashes rub against the cornea (trichiasis). The cornea becomes vascularised and opaque. The problem may not be detected until vision begins to fail.

Investigations and management

Intracellular inclusions may be demonstrated in conjunctival scrapings by staining with iodine or immunofluorescence. Chlamydia may be isolated in chick embryo or cell culture.

A single dose of azithromycin (20 mg/kg) has been shown to be superior to 6 weeks of 12-hourly tetracycline eye ointment for individuals in mass treatment programmes. Deformity and scarring of the lids, and corneal opacities, ulceration and scarring require surgical treatment after control of local infection.

Prevention

Personal and family cleanliness should be improved. Proper care of the eyes of newborn and young children is essential. Family contacts should be examined. The WHO is promoting the SAFE strategy for trachoma control (**s**urgery, **a**ntibiotics, **f**acial cleanliness and **e**nvironmental improvement).

PROTOZOAL INFECTIONS

Protozoa are responsible for many important infectious diseases. They can be categorised according to whether they cause systemic or local infection. Trichomoniasis is described on page 415.

Systemic protozoal infections

Malaria

Malaria in humans is caused by *Plasmodium falciparum*, *P. vivax*, *P. ovale*, *P. malariae* and the predominantly simian parasite, *P. knowlesi*. It is transmitted by the bite of female anopheline mosquitoes and occurs throughout the tropics and subtropics at altitudes below 1500 metres (Fig. 13.28). Recent estimates have put the number of episodes of clinical malaria at 515 million cases per year, with two-thirds of these occurring in sub-Saharan Africa, especially amongst children and pregnant women. Following previous WHO-sponsored campaigns focusing on prevention and effective treatment, the incidence of malaria was greatly reduced between 1950 and 1960, but since 1970 there has been resurgence. Furthermore, *P. falciparum* has now become resistant to chloroquine and sulfadoxine-pyrimethamine, initially in South-east Asia and now throughout Africa. The WHO's Millennium Development Goal 6 aims to halt the spread of the disease by 2015, and its 'Roll Back Malaria' campaign is designed to halve mortality by 2010 by utilising the 'best evidence' vector and disease control methods, such as artemisinin combination therapy (ACT).

Travellers are susceptible to malaria (p. 305). Due to increased travel, over 2000 cases are imported annually into the UK. Most are due to *P. falciparum*, usually from Africa, and of these 1% die because of late diagnosis. Immigrants returning home after visiting family and friends overseas but who have long-term residence in the UK are particularly at risk. They have lost their partial immunity and do not realise that they should be taking malaria prophylaxis. A few people living near airports in Europe have acquired malaria from accidentally imported mosquitoes.

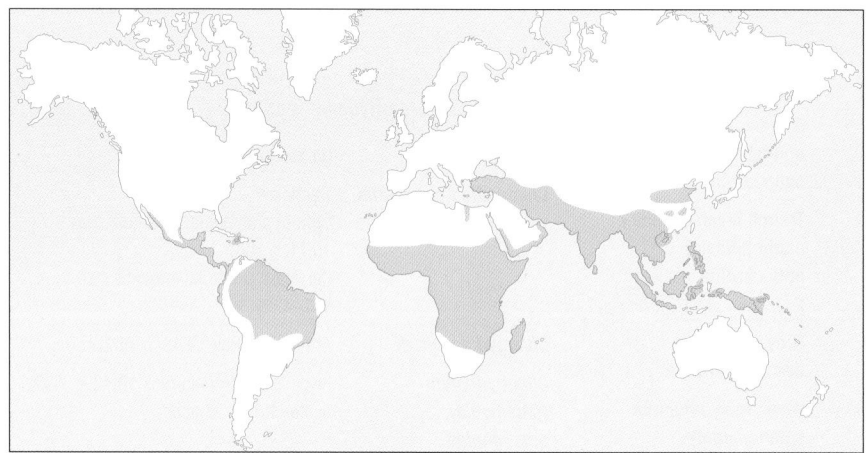

Fig. 13.28 Distribution of malaria. (For up-to-date information see the Malaria Atlas Project (MAP): www.map.ox.ac.uk).

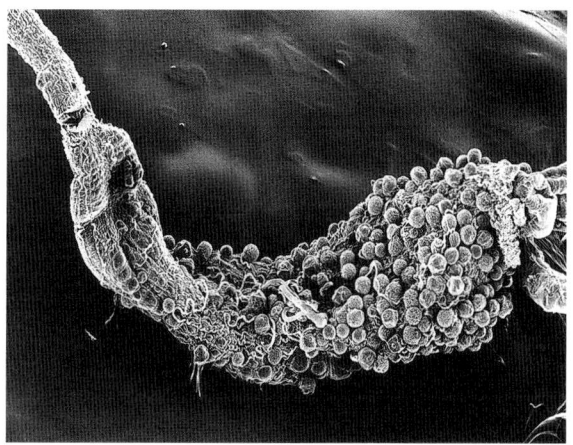

Fig. 13.29 Scanning electron micrograph of *P. falciparum* oöcysts lining an anopheline mosquito's stomach.

Pathogenesis

Life cycle of the malarial parasite

The female anopheline mosquito becomes infected when it feeds on human blood containing gametocytes, the sexual forms of the malarial parasite (Figs 13.29 and 13.30). Development in the mosquito takes from 7 to 20 days, and results in sporozoites accumulating in the salivary glands which are inoculated into the human blood stream. Sporozoites disappear from human blood within half an hour and enter the liver. After some days merozoites leave the liver and invade red blood cells, where further asexual cycles of multi-

plication take place, producing schizonts. Rupture of the schizont releases more merozoites into the blood and causes fever, the periodicity of which depends on the species of parasite.

P. vivax and *P. ovale* may persist in liver cells as dormant forms, hypnozoites, capable of developing into merozoites months or years later. Thus the first attack of clinical malaria may occur long after the patient has left the endemic area, and the disease may relapse after treatment if drugs that kill only the erythrocytic stage of the parasite are given.

P. falciparum and *P. malariae* have no persistent exo-erythrocytic phase but recrudescence of fever may result from multiplication of parasites in red cells which have not been eliminated by treatment and immune processes (Box 13.56).

Pathology

Red cells infected with malaria are prone to haemolysis. This is most severe with *P. falciparum*, which invades red cells of all ages but especially young cells; *P. vivax* and *P. ovale* invade reticulocytes, and *P. malariae* normoblasts, so that infections remain lighter. Anaemia may be profound and is worsened by dyserythropoiesis, splenomegaly and depletion of folate stores.

In *P. falciparum* malaria, red cells containing trophozoites adhere to vascular endothelium in post-capillary venules in brain, kidney, liver, lungs and gut. The vessels become congested, resulting in widespread organ damage which is exacerbated by rupture of schizonts, liberating toxic and antigenic substances (see Fig 13.30).

P. falciparum has influenced human evolution, with the appearance of protective mutations such as sickle-cell

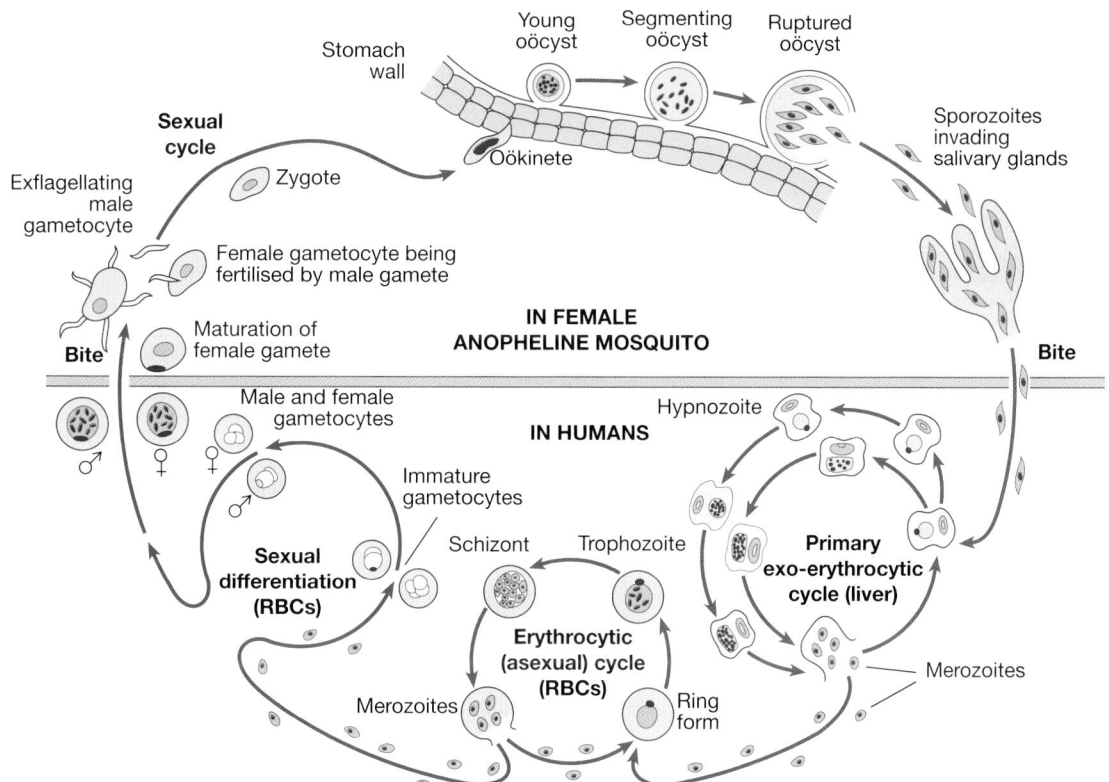

Fig. 13.30 **Malarial parasites: life cycle.** Hypnozoites(*) are present only in *P. vivax* and *P. ovale* infections.

13.56 Relationships between life cycle of parasite and clinical features of malaria

Cycle/feature	P. vivax, P. ovale	P. malariae	P. falciparum
Pre-patent period (minimum incubation)	8–25 days	15–30 days	8–25 days
Exo-erythrocytic cycle	Persistent as hypnozoites	Pre-erythrocytic only	Pre-erythrocytic only
Asexual cycle	48 hrs synchronous	72 hrs synchronous	< 48 hrs asynchronous
Fever periodicity	Alternate days	Every third day	None
Delayed onset	Common	Rare	Rare
Relapses	Common up to 2 yrs	Recrudescence many years later	Recrudescence up to 1 yr

(HbS; p. 1028), thalassaemia (p. 1029), G6PD deficiency (p. 1024) and HLA-B53. *P. falciparum* does not grow well in red cells that contain haemoglobin F, C or especially S. Haemoglobin S heterozygotes (AS) are protected against the lethal complications of malaria. *P. vivax* cannot enter red cells that lack the Duffy blood group; therefore many West Africans and African-Americans are protected.

Clinical features

The clinical features of malaria are non-specific and the diagnosis must be suspected in anyone returning from an endemic area who has features of infection.

P. falciparum infection

This is the most dangerous of the malarias and patients are either 'killed or cured'. The onset is often insidious, with malaise, headache and vomiting. Cough and mild diarrhoea are also common. The fever has no particular pattern. Jaundice is common due to haemolysis and hepatic dysfunction. The liver and spleen enlarge and may become tender. Anaemia develops rapidly, as does thrombocytopenia.

A patient with *falciparum* malaria, apparently not seriously ill, may rapidly develop dangerous complications (Fig. 13.31 and Box 13.57). Cerebral malaria is manifested

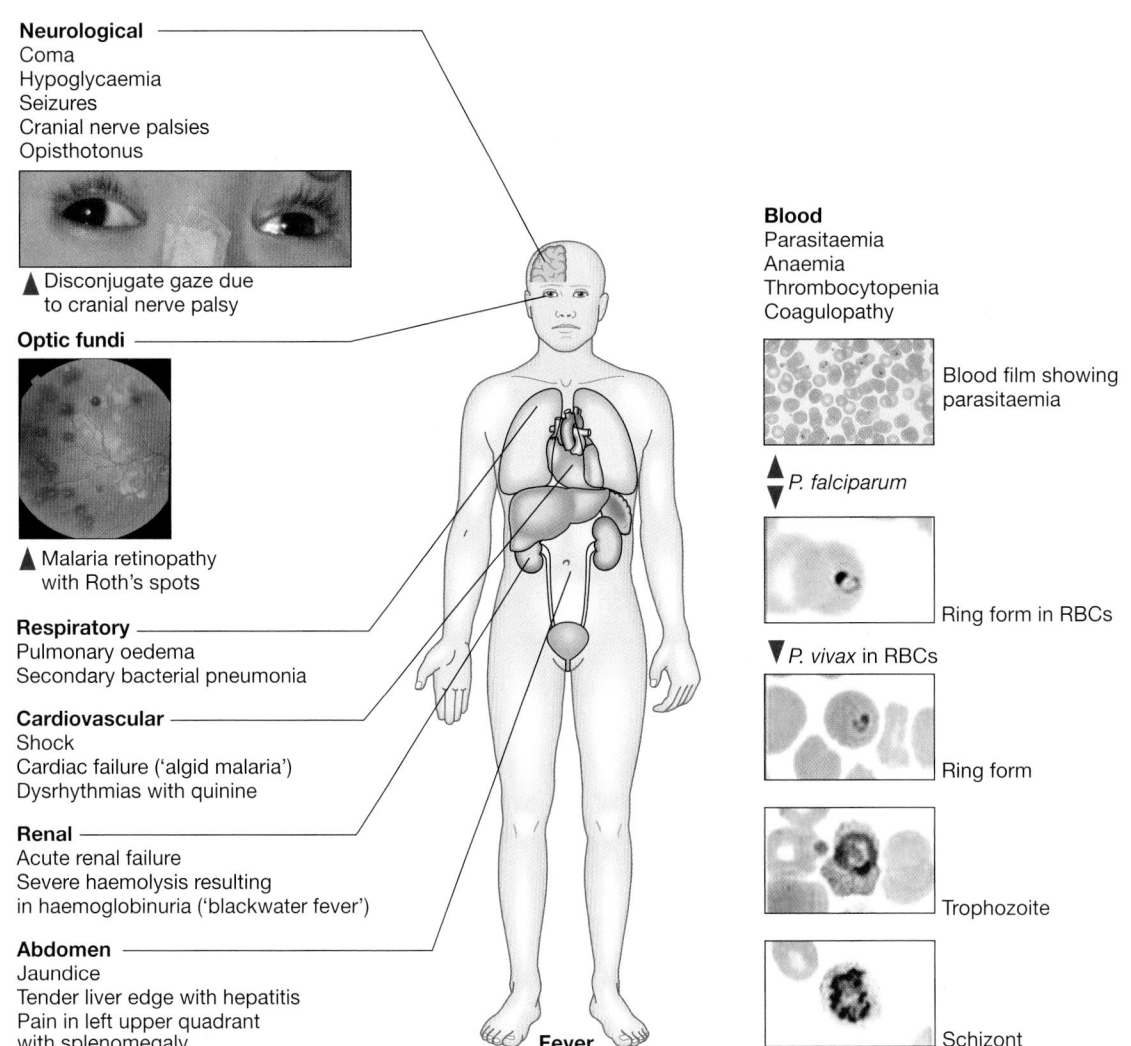

Neurological
Coma
Hypoglycaemia
Seizures
Cranial nerve palsies
Opisthotonus

▲ Disconjugate gaze due to cranial nerve palsy

Optic fundi

▲ Malaria retinopathy with Roth's spots

Respiratory
Pulmonary oedema
Secondary bacterial pneumonia

Cardiovascular
Shock
Cardiac failure ('algid malaria')
Dysrhythmias with quinine

Renal
Acute renal failure
Severe haemolysis resulting in haemoglobinuria ('blackwater fever')

Abdomen
Jaundice
Tender liver edge with hepatitis
Pain in left upper quadrant with splenomegaly

Fever

Blood
Parasitaemia
Anaemia
Thrombocytopenia
Coagulopathy

Blood film showing parasitaemia

▲ ▼ *P. falciparum*

Ring form in RBCs

▼ *P. vivax* in RBCs

Ring form

Trophozoite

Schizont

Fig. 13.31 Features of *P. falciparum* infection.

13.57 Severe manifestations/complications of *falciparum* malaria and their immediate management

Coma (cerebral malaria)

- Maintain airway
- Nurse on side
- Exclude other treatable causes of coma (e.g. hypoglycaemia, bacterial meningitis)
- Avoid harmful ancillary treatments such as corticosteroids, heparin and adrenaline (epinephrine)
- Intubate if necessary

Hyperpyrexia

- Tepid sponging, fanning, cooling blanket
- Antipyretic drug (paracetamol)

Convulsions

- Maintain airway
- Treat promptly with diazepam or paraldehyde injection

Hypoglycaemia

- Measure blood glucose
- Give 50% dextrose injection followed by 10% dextrose infusion (glucagon may be ineffective)

Severe anaemia (packed cell volume < 15%)

- Transfuse fresh whole blood or packed cells if pathogen screening of donor blood is available

Acute pulmonary oedema

- Nurse at 45°, give oxygen, venesect 250 mL of blood, give diuretic, stop intravenous fluids
- Intubate and add PEEP/CPAP (p. 195) in life-threatening hypoxaemia
- Haemofilter

Acute renal failure

- Exclude pre-renal causes
- Fluid resuscitation if appropriate
- Peritoneal dialysis (haemofiltration or haemodialysis if available)

Spontaneous bleeding and coagulopathy

- Transfuse screened fresh whole blood (cryoprecipitate/fresh frozen plasma and platelets if available)
- Vitamin K injection

Metabolic acidosis

- Exclude or treat hypoglycaemia, hypovolaemia and Gram-negative septicaemia
- Fluid resuscitation
- Give oxygen

Shock ('algid malaria')

- Suspect Gram-negative septicaemia
- Take blood cultures
- Give parenteral antimicrobials
- Correct haemodynamic disturbances

Aspiration pneumonia

- Give parenteral antimicrobial drugs
- Change position
- Physiotherapy
- Give oxygen

Hyperparasitaemia

- Consider exchange or partial exchange transfusion, manual or haemophoresis (e.g. > 10% of circulating erythrocytes parasitised in non-immune patient with severe disease)

Specific therapy

- Intravenous artesunate
- Mefloquine should be avoided due to increased risk of post-malaria neurological syndrome

13

by confusion, seizures or coma, usually without localising signs. Children die rapidly without any special symptoms other than fever. Immunity is impaired in pregnancy and the parasite can preferentially bind to a placental protein known as chondroitin sulphate A. Abortion and intrauterine growth retardation from parasitisation of the maternal side of the placenta are frequent. Previous splenectomy increases the risk of severe malaria.

P. vivax and P. ovale infection

In many cases the illness starts with several days of continued fever before the development of classical bouts of fever on alternate days. Fever starts with a rigor. The patient feels cold and the temperature rises to about 40 °C. After half an hour to an hour the hot or flush phase begins. It lasts several hours and gives way to profuse perspiration and a gradual fall in temperature. The cycle is repeated 48 hours later. Gradually the spleen and liver enlarge and may become tender. Anaemia develops slowly. Relapses are frequent in the first 2 years after leaving the malarious area and infection may be acquired from blood transfusion.

P. malariae infection

This is usually associated with mild symptoms and bouts of fever every third day. Parasitaemia may persist for many years with the occasional recrudescence of fever, or without producing any symptoms. Chronic *P. malariae* infection causes glomerulonephritis and long-term nephrotic syndrome in children.

Investigations

Giemsa-stained thick and thin blood films should be examined whenever malaria is suspected. In the thick film erythrocytes are lysed, releasing all blood stages of the parasite. This, as well as the fact that more blood is used in thick films, facilitates the diagnosis of low-level parasitaemia. A thin film is essential to confirm the diagnosis, to identify the species of parasite and, in *P. falciparum* infections, to quantify the parasite load (by counting the percentage of infected erythrocytes). *P. falciparum* parasites may be very scanty, especially in patients who have been partially treated. With *P. falciparum*, only ring forms are normally seen in the early stages (see Fig. 13.31); with the other species all stages of the erythrocytic cycle may be found. Gametocytes appear after about 2 weeks, persist after treatment and are harmless, except that they are the source by which more mosquitoes become infected.

Immunochromatographic tests for malaria antigens, such as OptiMal® (which detects the *Plasmodium* lactate dehydrogenase of several species) and ParasightF® (which detects the *P. falciparum* histidine-rich protein 2), are extremely sensitive and specific for *falciparum* malaria but less so for other species. They should be used in parallel with blood film examination but are especially useful where the microscopist is less experienced in examining blood films (e.g. in the UK).

DNA detection (PCR) is used mainly in research and is useful for determining whether a patient has a recrudescence of the same malaria parasite or a reinfection with a new parasite.

Management

Mild P. falciparum malaria

Since *P. falciparum* is now resistant to chloroquine and sulfadoxine-pyrimethamine (Fansidar) almost worldwide, an artemisinin-based treatment is recommended. Co-artemether (CoArtem® or Riamet®) contains artemether and lumefantrine and is given as 4 tablets at 0, 8, 24, 36, 48 and 60 hours. Alternatives are quinine by mouth (600 mg of quinine salt every 8 hours for 5–7 days), together with or followed by either doxycycline (200 mg once daily for 7 days) or clindamycin (450 mg every 8 hours for 7 days) or atovaquone-proguanil (Malarone®, 4 tablets once daily for 3 days). Doxycycline and artemether should be avoided in pregnancy.

WHO policy in Africa is moving towards always using artemisinin-based combination therapy (ACT), e.g. co-artemether or artesunate-amodiaquine. A combination of chloroproguanil and dapsone (Lapdap) is in clinical trials in uncomplicated malaria in sub-Saharan African children and has also been combined with artesunate. In India and other areas, artesunate (200 mg orally daily for 3 days) and mefloquine (1 g orally on day 2 and 500 mg orally on day 3) may be used.

Complicated P. falciparum malaria

Severe malaria should be considered in any non-immune patient with a parasite count greater than 2% and is a medical emergency (see Box 13.57). Management includes early and appropriate antimalarial chemotherapy, active treatment of complications, correction of fluid, electrolyte and acid–base balance, and avoidance of harmful ancillary treatments.

The treatment of choice is intravenous artesunate given as 2.4 mg/kg i.v. at 0, 12 and 24 hours and then once daily for 7 days. However, as soon as the patient has recovered sufficiently to swallow tablets, oral artesunate 2 mg/kg once daily is given instead of i.v. therapy, to complete a total cumulative dose of 17–18 mg/kg. Rectal administration of artesunate is also being developed to allow administration in remote rural areas.

Quinine salt can also be used and is started with a loading dose infusion of 20 mg/kg over 4 hours up to a maximum of 1.4 g. This is followed by maintenance doses of 10 mg/kg quinine salt given as 4-hour infusions 2–3 times daily up to a maximum of 700 mg per dose, until the patient can take drugs orally. The loading dose should *not* be given if the patient has received quinine, quinidine or mefloquine during the previous 24 hours. Patients should be monitored by ECG, with special attention to QRS duration and QT interval. Mefloquine should not be used for severe malaria since no parenteral form is available.

Exchange transfusion has not been tested in randomised controlled trials but may be beneficial for non-immune patients with persisting high parasitaemias (> 10% circulating erythrocytes).

Management of non-falciparum malaria

P. vivax, *P. ovale* and *P. malariae* infections should be treated with oral chloroquine: 600 mg chloroquine base followed by 300 mg base in 6 hours, then 150 mg base 12-hourly for 2 more days. Some chloroquine resistance has been reported from Indonesia.

Late relapses can be prevented by prescribing antimalarial drugs in suppressive doses. However, 'radical cure' is now achieved in most patients with *P. vivax* or *P. ovale* malaria using a course of primaquine (15 mg daily for 14 days), which destroys the hypnozoite phase in the liver. Haemolysis may develop in those who are G6PD-deficient. Cyanosis due to the formation of methaemoglobin in the red cells is more common but not dangerous.

Prevention

Clinical attacks of malaria may be preventable with chemoprophylaxis using chloroquine, atovaquone plus proguanil (Malarone), doxycycline or mefloquine. Box 13.58 gives the recommended doses for protection of the non-immune. The risk of malaria in the area to be visited and the degree of chloroquine resistance guide the recommendations for prophylaxis. Updated recommendations are summarised at www.fitfortravel.nhs.uk. Fansidar should not be used for chemoprophylaxis, as deaths have occurred from agranulocytosis or Stevens–Johnson

13.58 Chemoprophylaxis of malaria[1]		
Antimalarial tablets	**Adult prophylactic dose**	**Regimen**
Chloroquine resistance high		
Mefloquine[2]	250 mg weekly	Started 2–3 wks before travel and continued until 4 wks after
or Doxycycline[3,4]	100 mg daily	Started 1 wk before and continued until 4 wks after travel
or Malarone[4]	1 tablet daily	From 1–2 days before travel until 1 wk after return
Chloroquine resistance absent		
Chloroquine[5]	300 mg base weekly	Started 1 wk before and continued until 4 wks after travel
and proguanil	100–200 mg daily	

[1]Choice of regimen is determined by area to be visited, length of stay, level of malaria transmission, level of drug resistance, presence of underlying disease in the traveller and concomitant medication taken.
[2]Contraindicated in the first trimester of pregnancy, lactation, cardiac conduction disorders, epilepsy, psychiatric disorders; may cause neuropsychiatric disorders.
[3]Causes photosensitisation and sunburn if high-protection sunblock is not used.
[4]Avoid in pregnancy.
[5]British preparations of chloroquine usually contain 150 mg base, French preparations 100 mg base and American preparations 300 mg base.

EBM 13.59 Prevention of malaria

Insecticide-treated bed nets (ITNs)

'Five RCTs provided strong evidence that widespread use of ITNs reduces overall mortality by about one-fifth in Africa. For every 1000 children aged 1–5 years protected, ~5.5 lives can be saved every year. In Africa, full ITN coverage could prevent 370 000 child deaths per year.'

Electronic mosquito repellents (EMRs)

'EMRs are not effective.'

Intermittent preventive treatment in pregnancy

'Antimalarial drugs reduce antenatal parasitaemia and fever in pregnant women living in areas with endemic malaria. For women in their first or second pregnancy, this reduces the instances of severe antenatal anaemia, antenatal parasitaemia and perinatal deaths, and increases birth weight.'

Intermittent preventive treatment in children

'Antimalarial drugs reduce clinical malaria, severe anaemia and hospital admissions. Effects on mortality and on health, if prophylaxis is stopped, are unknown.'

For further information: www.cochrane.org

syndrome (p. 1285). Mefloquine is useful in areas of multiple drug resistance, such as East and Central Africa and Papua New Guinea. Experience shows it to be safe for at least 2 years, but there are several contraindications to its use (see Box 13.58).

Expert advice is required for individuals unable to tolerate the first-line agents listed, or in whom they are contraindicated. Mefloquine should be started 2–3 weeks before travel to give time for assessment of side-effects. Chloroquine should not be taken continuously as a prophylactic for more than 5 years without regular ophthalmic examination, as it may cause irreversible retinopathy. Pregnant and lactating women may take proguanil or chloroquine safely.

Prevention also involves advice about the use of high-percentage diethyltoluamide (DEET), covering up extremities when out after dark and sleeping under permethrin-impregnated mosquito nets (Box 13.59).

Malaria control in endemic areas

There are major initiatives under way to reduce malaria in endemic areas and it is estimated that these would be cost-effective, even at a cost of $3 billion per year. Successful programmes have involved a combination of vector control, including indoor residual spraying, use of long-lasting insecticide-treated bed nets (ITNs) and intermittent preventative therapy (IPT) (repeated dose of prophylactic drugs in high-risk groups such as children and pregnant women) (see Box 13.59).

Development of a fully protective malaria vaccine is still some way off, which is not surprising considering that natural immunity is incomplete and not long-lived. There is, however, some evidence that vaccination can reduce the incidence of severe malaria in populations. Trial vaccines are being evaluated in Africa.

Babesiosis

This is caused by a tick-borne intra-erythrocytic protozoon parasite. There are more than 100 species of *Babesia*, all of which have an animal reservoir, typically either rodents or cattle, and are transmitted to humans via the tick vector *Ixodes scapularis*. Most cases of babesiosis in

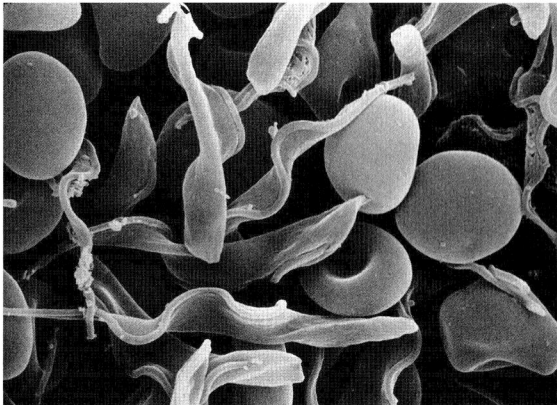

Fig. 13.32 Trypanosomiasis. Scanning electron micrograph showing trypanosomes swimming among erythrocytes.

the USA are due to *B. microti* and most in Europe due to *B. divergens*. Patients present with fever and malaise 1–4 weeks after a tick bite. Illness may be complicated by haemolytic anaemia. Severe illness is seen in splenectomised patients. The diagnosis is made by blood-film examination. Treatment is with quinine and clindamycin.

African trypanosomiasis (sleeping sickness)

African sleeping sickness is caused by trypanosomes (Fig. 13.32) conveyed to humans by the bites of infected tsetse flies, and is unique to sub-Saharan Africa. *Trypanosoma brucei gambiense* trypanosomiasis has a wide distribution in West and Central Africa. *T. brucei rhodesiense* trypanosomiasis is found in parts of East and Central Africa, where it is currently on the increase (Fig. 13.33). In West Africa transmission is mainly at the riverside, where the fly rests in the shade of trees; no animal reservoir has been identified for *T. gambiense*. *T. rhodesiense* has a large reservoir in numerous wild animals and transmission takes place in the shade of woods bordering grasslands. Rural populations earning their livelihood from agriculture, fishing and animal husbandry are susceptible. Local people and tourists visiting forests infested with tsetse flies and animal reservoirs may become infected.

Clinical features

A bite by a tsetse fly is painful and commonly becomes inflamed, but if trypanosomes are introduced, the site may again become painful and swollen about 10 days

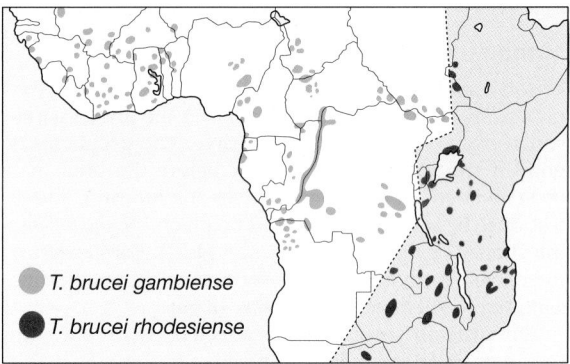

● *T. brucei gambiense*
● *T. brucei rhodesiense*

Fig. 13.33 Geographical distribution of African trypanosomiasis.

13

13

later ('trypanosomal chancre') and the regional lymph nodes enlarge ('Winterbottom's sign'). Within 2–3 weeks of infection the trypanosomes invade the blood stream. The disease is characterised by an early haematolymphatic stage and a late encephalitic stage in which the parasite crosses the blood–brain barrier and chronic encephalopathy develops.

Rhodesiense infections

In these infections the disease is more acute and severe than in *gambiense* infections, so that within days or a few weeks the patient is usually severely ill and may have developed pleural effusions and signs of myocarditis or hepatitis. There may be a petechial rash. The patient may die before there are signs of involvement of the CNS. If the illness is less acute, drowsiness, tremors and coma develop.

Gambiense infections

The distinction between early and late stages may not be apparent in *gambiense* infections. The disease usually runs a slow course over months or years, with irregular bouts of fever and enlargement of lymph nodes. These are characteristically firm, discrete, rubbery and painless, and are particularly prominent in the posterior triangle of the neck. The spleen and liver may become palpable. After some months without treatment, the CNS is invaded. This is shown clinically by headache and changed behaviour, blunting of higher mental functions, insomnia by night and sleepiness by day, mental confusion and eventually tremors, pareses, wasting, coma and death.

Investigations

Trypanosomiasis should be considered in any febrile patient from an endemic area. In *rhodesiense* infections thick and thin blood films, stained as for the detection of malaria, will reveal trypanosomes. The trypanosomes may be seen in the blood or from puncture of the primary lesion in the earliest stages of *gambiense* infections, but it is usually easier to demonstrate them by aspiration of a lymph node. Concentration methods include buffy coat microscopy and miniature anion exchange chromatography.

Due to the cyclical nature of parasitaemia, the diagnosis is often made by demonstration of antibodies using a simple, rapid card agglutination trypanosomiasis test (CATT). If the CNS is affected, the cell count (> 20 × 10⁹ leucocytes per litre) and protein content of the CSF are increased and the glucose is diminished. Very high levels of serum IgM or the presence of IgM in the CSF are suggestive of trypanosomiasis. Recognition of CNS involvement is critical, as failure to treat it might be fatal.

Management

Unfortunately, therapeutic options for African trypanosomiasis are limited and most of the antitrypanosomal drugs are toxic and expensive. The prognosis is good if treatment is begun early before the brain has been invaded. At this stage intravenous suramin, after a test dose of 100–200 mg, should be given for *rhodesiense* infections (1 g on days 1, 3, 7, 14 and 21). For *gambiense* infections, intramuscular or intravenous pentamidine 4 mg/kg for 10 days is given (Box 13.60).

Once the nervous system is affected, treatment with melarsoprol (an arsenical) is effective for both East and West African diseases. It is used in a dose of 2–3.6 mg/

13.60 Drugs used to treat human African trypanosomiasis
***Gambiense* trypanosomiasis**
Stage 1 • First-line: pentamidine • Second-line: eflornithine or melarsoprol
Stage 2 • First-line: eflornithine • Second-line: melarsoprol
***Rhodesiense* trypanosomiasis**
Stage 1 • First-line: suramin • Second-line: melarsoprol
Stage 2 • First-line: melarsoprol • Second-line: nifurtimox combined with melarsoprol

kg/day i.v. for the first course and 3.6 mg/kg/day thereafter. Three 3-day treatment courses are given, separated by 7 days and by 10–21 days. Melarsoprol should be given with prednisolone 1 mg/kg up to 40 mg started 1–2 days before, continued during and tapered after treatment to reduce side-effects. Treatment-related mortality with melarsoprol is 4–12% due to reactive encephalopathy. For CNS infections due to *gambiense*, eflornithine (DFMO), an irreversible inhibitor of ornithine decarboxylase (100 and 150 mg/kg i.v. 6-hourly for 14 days for adults and children, respectively), is considered to be a safer and cost-effective option. Combinations of either melarsoprol or eflornithine with oral nifurtimox (used for the treatment of Chagas' disease; see below) in lesser dosage and duration have been shown to decrease relapses, deaths and drug toxicity.

Prevention

In endemic *gambiense* areas, various measures may be taken against tsetse flies, and field teams help to detect and treat early human infection. In *rhodesiense* areas control is difficult.

American trypanosomiasis (Chagas' disease)

Chagas' disease occurs widely in South and Central America. The cause is *Trypanosoma cruzi*, transmitted to humans from the faeces of a reduviid (triatomine) bug in which the trypanosomes have a cycle of development before becoming infective to humans. These bugs live in wild forests in crevices, burrows and palm trees. The *Triatoma infestans* bug has become domesticated in the Southern Cone countries (Argentina, Brazil, Chile, Paraguay and Uruguay). It lives in the mud and wattle walls and thatched roofs of simple rural houses, and emerges at night to feed and defecate on the sleeping occupants. Infected faeces are rubbed in through the conjunctiva, mucosa of mouth or nose, or abrasions of the skin. Over one hundred species of mammal, domestic, peridomestic and wild, may serve as reservoirs of infection. In some areas, blood transfusion accounts for about 5% of cases. Congenital transmission occasionally occurs.

Pathology

The trypanosomes migrate via the blood stream, develop into amastigote forms in the tissues and multiply intracellularly by binary fission. In the acute phase (primarily cell-mediated), inflammation of parasitised as well as non-parasitised cardiac muscles and capillaries occurs, resulting in acute myocarditis. In the chronic phase focal myocardial atrophy, signs of chronic passive congestion and thromboembolic phenomena, cardiomegaly and apical cardiac aneurysm are salient findings. In the digestive form of disease, focal myositis and discontinuous lesions of the intramural myenteric plexus, predominantly in the oesophagus and colon, are seen.

Clinical features

Acute phase

Clinical manifestations of the acute phase are seen in only 1–2% of individuals who are infected before the age of 15 years. Young children (1–5 years) are most commonly affected. The entrance of *T. cruzi* through an abrasion produces a dusky-red firm swelling and enlargement of regional lymph nodes. A conjunctival lesion, although less common, is characteristic; the unilateral firm reddish swelling of the lids may close the eye and constitutes 'Romaña's sign'. In a few patients an acute generalised infection soon appears, with a transient morbilliform or urticarial rash, fever, lymphadenopathy and enlargement of the spleen and liver. In a small minority of patients acute myocarditis and heart failure or neurological features, including personality changes and signs of meningoencephalitis, may be seen. The acute infection may be fatal to infants.

Chronic phase

About 50–70% of infected patients become seropositive and develop an indeterminate form when no parasitaemia is detectable. They have a normal lifespan with no symptoms, but are a natural reservoir for the disease and maintain the life cycle of parasites. After a latent period of several years, 10–30% of chronic cases develop low-grade myocarditis, and damage to conducting fibres causes a cardiomyopathy characterised by cardiac dilatation, arrhythmias, partial or complete heart block and sudden death. In nearly 10% of patients, damage to Auerbach's plexus results in dilatation of various parts of the alimentary canal, especially the colon and oesophagus, so-called 'mega' disease. Dilatation of the bile ducts and bronchi is also a recognised sequela. Autoimmune processes may be responsible for much of the damage. There are geographical variations of the basic pattern of disease. Reactivation of Chagas' disease can occur in patients with HIV if the CD4 count falls lower than 200 cells/mm³ (p. 390).

Investigations

T. cruzi is easily detectable in a blood film in the acute illness. In chronic disease it may be recovered in up to 50% of cases by xenodiagnosis, in which infection-free, laboratory-bred reduviid bugs are allowed to feed on the patient; subsequently, the hind gut or faeces of the bug are examined for parasites. Parasite DNA detection by PCR in the patient's blood is a highly sensitive method for documentation of infection and, in addition, can be employed in faeces of bugs used in xenodiagnosis tests to improve sensitivity. Antibody detection is also highly sensitive (99%).

Management and prevention

Parasiticidal agents are used to treat the acute phase, congenital disease and early chronic phase (within 10 years of infection). Nifurtimox is given orally. The dose, which has to be carefully supervised to minimise toxicity while preserving parasiticidal activity, is 10 mg/kg divided into three equal doses, daily by mouth for 60–90 days. The paediatric dose is 15 mg/kg daily. Cure rates of 80% in acute disease are obtained. Benznidazole is an alternative, given at a dose of 5–10 mg/kg daily by mouth, in two divided doses for 60 days; children receive 10 mg/kg daily. Both nifurtimox and benznidazole are toxic, with adverse reaction rates of 30–55%. Specific drug treatment of the chronic form is now increasingly favoured, but in the cardiac or digestive 'mega' diseases it does not reverse established tissue damage. Surgery may be needed.

Preventative measures include improving housing and destruction of reduviid bugs by spraying of houses with insecticides. Blood donors should be screened.

Toxoplasmosis

Toxoplasma gondii is an intracellular parasite. The sexual phase of the parasite's life cycle (Fig. 13.34) occurs in the small intestinal epithelium of the domestic cat. Oöcysts are shed in cat faeces and are spread to intermediate hosts (pigs, sheep and also humans) through widespread contamination of soil. Oöcysts may survive in moist conditions for weeks or months. Once they are ingested, the parasite transforms into rapidly dividing tachyzoites through cycles of asexual multiplication.

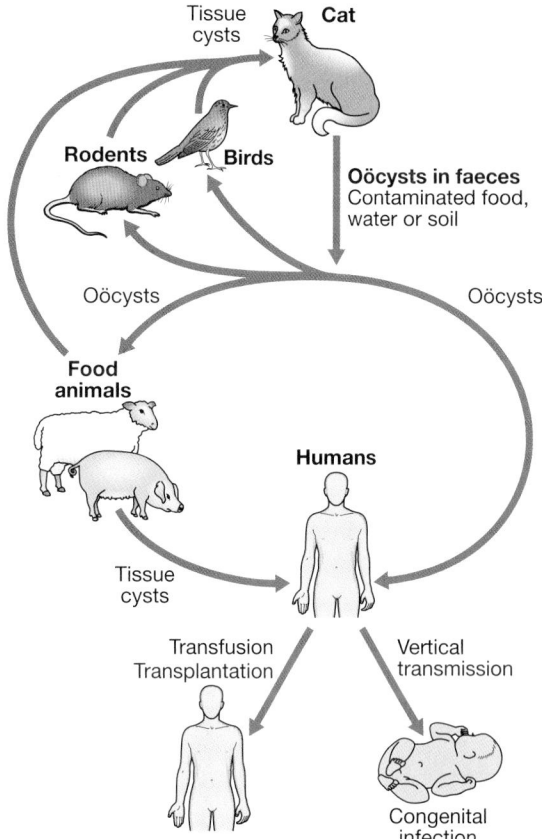

Fig. 13.34 Life cycle of *Toxoplasma gondii*.

13

This leads to the formation of microscopic tissue cysts containing bradyzoites, which persist for the lifetime of the host. Cats become infected or reinfected by ingesting tissue cysts in prey such as rodents and birds.

Human acquisition of infection occurs via oöcyst-contaminated soil, salads and vegetables, or by the ingestion or tasting of raw or undercooked meats containing tissue cysts. Sheep, pigs and rabbits are the most common meat sources. Outbreaks of toxoplasmosis have been linked to the consumption of unfiltered water. In developed countries, toxoplasmosis is the most common protozoal infection; around 22% of adults in the UK are seropositive. Most primary infections are subclinical; however, toxoplasmosis is thought to account for about 15% of heterophile antibody-negative glandular fever (p. 316). In India or Brazil, approximately 40–60% of pregnant females are seropositive for *Toxoplasma*. In HIV infection (p. 397), toxoplasmosis is an important opportunistic infection with considerable morbidity and mortality. Generalised toxoplasmosis has been described after accidental laboratory infection with highly virulent strains.

Clinical features

In most immunocompetent individuals, including children and pregnant women, the infection goes unnoticed. In approximately 10% of patients it causes a self-limiting illness, most common in adults aged 25–35 years. The most common presenting feature is painless lymphadenopathy, either local or generalised. In particular, the cervical nodes are involved, but mediastinal, mesenteric or retroperitoneal groups may be affected. The spleen is seldom palpable. Most patients have no systemic symptoms, but some complain of malaise, fever, fatigue, muscle pain, sore throat and headache. Complete resolution usually occurs within a few months, although symptoms and lymphadenopathy tend to fluctuate unpredictably and some patients do not recover completely for a year or more. Very infrequently, patients may develop encephalitis, myocarditis, polymyositis, pneumonitis or hepatitis. Retinochoroiditis (Fig. 13.35) is nearly always the result of congenital infection but has also been reported in acquired disease.

Congenital toxoplasmosis

Acute toxoplasmosis, mostly subclinical, affects 0.3–1% of pregnant women, with an approximately 60%

transmission rate to the fetus which increases with increasing gestation. Seropositive females infected 6 months before conception have no risk of fetal transmission. Congenital disease affects approximately 40% of infected fetuses, and is more likely and more severe with infection early in gestation (see Box 13.27, p. 310). Many fetal infections are subclinical at birth but long-term sequelae include retinochoroiditis, microcephaly and hydrocephalus.

Investigations

In contrast to immunocompromised patients, in whom the diagnosis often requires direct detection of parasites, serology is often used in immunocompetent individuals. The Sabin–Feldman dye test (indirect fluorescent antibody test), which detects IgG antibody. Recent infection is indicated by a fourfold or greater increase in titre when paired sera are tested in parallel. Peak titres of 1/1000 or more are reached within 1–2 months of the onset of infection, and the dye test then becomes an unreliable indicator of recent infection. The detection of significant levels of *Toxoplasma*-specific IgM antibody may be useful in confirming acute infection. False positives or persistence of IgM antibodies for years after infection make interpretation difficult; however, negative IgM antibodies virtually rule out acute infection.

During pregnancy it is critical to differentiate between recent and past infection; the presence of high-avidity IgG antibodies excludes infection acquired in the preceding 3–4 months.

If necessary, the presence of *Toxoplasma* organisms in a lymph node biopsy can be sought by staining sections histochemically with *T. gondii* antiserum, or by the use of PCR to detect *Toxoplasma*-specific DNA.

Management

In immunocompetent subjects uncomplicated toxoplasmosis is self-limiting and responds poorly to antimicrobial therapy. Treatment with pyrimethamine, sulfadiazine and folinic acid is therefore usually reserved for rare cases of severe or progressive disease, and for infection in immunocompromised patients.

In a pregnant woman with an established recent infection, spiramycin (3 g daily in divided doses) should be given until term. Once fetal infection is established, treatment with sulfadiazine and pyrimethamine plus calcium folinate is recommended (spiramycin does not cross the placental barrier). The cost/benefit of routine *Toxoplasma* screening and treatment in pregnancy is being debated in many countries. There is insufficient evidence to determine the effects on mother or baby of current antiparasitic treatment for women who seroconvert in pregnancy.

Leishmaniasis

Leishmaniasis is caused by unicellular flagellate intracellular protozoa belonging to the genus *Leishmania* (order Kinetoplastidae). There are 21 leishmanial species which cause several diverse clinical syndromes, which can be placed into three broad groups:

- visceral leishmaniasis (VL, kala-azar)
- cutaneous leishmaniasis (CL)
- mucosal leishmaniasis (ML).

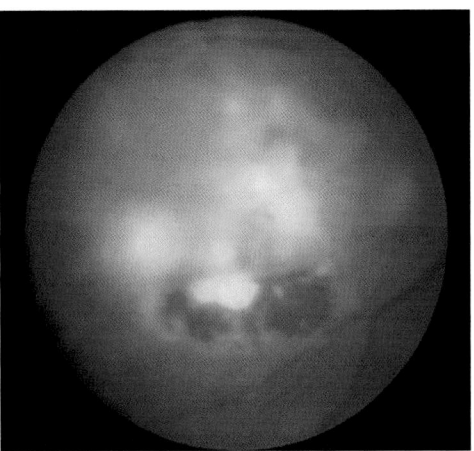

Fig. 13.35 Retinochoroiditis due to toxoplasmosis.

Epidemiology and transmission

Although most clinical syndromes are caused by zoonotic transmission of parasites from animals (chiefly canine and rodent reservoirs) to humans through phlebotomine sandfly vectors (Fig. 13.36A), humans are the only known reservoir (anthroponotic) in major VL foci in India and for transmission of leishmaniasis between injection drug-users (Fig. 13.36B and C). Leishmaniasis occurs in 88 countries around the world, with an estimated annual incidence of 2 million new cases (500 000 for VL, and 1.5 million for CL).

The life cycle of *Leishmania* is shown in Figure 13.37. Flagellar promastigotes (10–20 μm) are introduced by the feeding female sandfly. The promastigotes are taken up by macrophages, in which they lose their flagellae and transform into amastigotes (2–4 μm; Leishman–Donovan body). These multiply, ultimately causing lysis of the macrophages and infection of other cells. Sandflies pick up amastigotes when feeding on infected patients or animal reservoirs. In the sandfly, the parasite transforms into a flagellar promastigote, which multiplies by binary fission in the gut of the vector and migrates to the proboscis to infect a new host.

Sandflies live in hot and humid climates in the cracks and crevices of mud or straw houses and lay eggs in

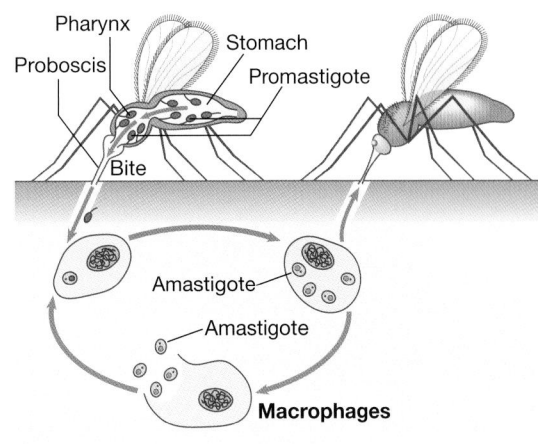

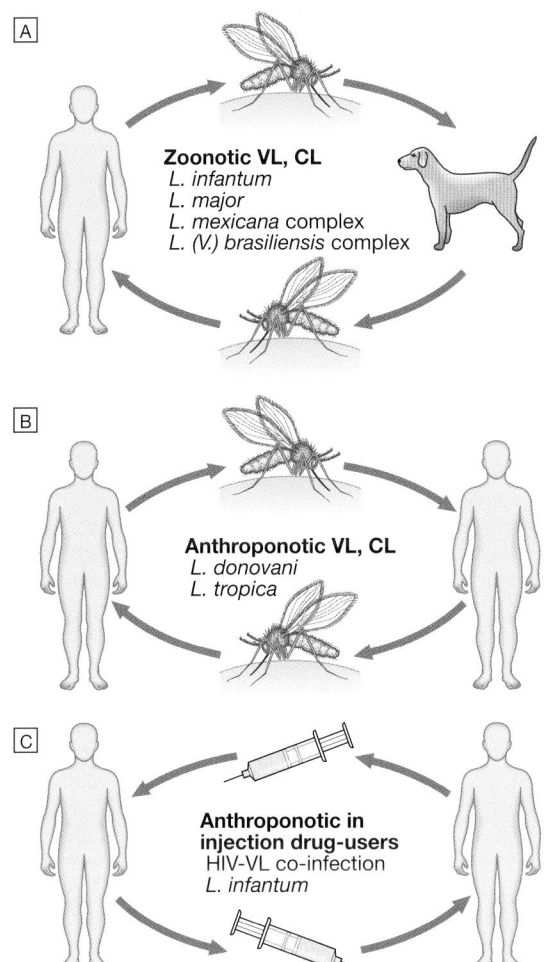

Fig. 13.36 Transmission of leishmaniasis. [A] Zoonotic transmission. [B] Anthroponotic transmission. [C] Anthroponotic transmission in the injection drug-user.

Fig. 13.37 Life cycle of *Leishmania*.

organic matter. People living in such conditions are more prone to acquire the disease. Female sandflies bite during the night and preferentially feed on animals; humans are incidental hosts.

Visceral leishmaniasis (VL, kala-azar)

VL is caused by the protozoon *Leishmania donovani* complex (comprising *L. donovani*, *L. infantum* and *L. chagasi*). India, Sudan, Bangladesh and Brazil account for 90% of cases of VL, while other affected regions include the Mediterranean, East Africa, China, Arabia, Israel and other South American countries (Fig. 13.38). In addition to sandfly transmission, VL has also been reported to follow blood transfusion and disease can present unexpectedly in immunosuppressed patients—for example, after renal transplantation and in HIV infection.

The great majority of people infected remain asymptomatic. In visceral diseases the spleen, liver, bone marrow and lymph nodes are primarily involved.

Clinical features

On the Indian subcontinent adults and children are equally affected; on other continents VL is predominantly a disease of small children and infants, except in adults with HIV co-infection. The incubation period ranges from weeks to months (occasionally several years).

The first sign of infection is high fever, usually accompanied by rigor and chills. Fever intensity decreases over time and patients may become afebrile for intervening periods ranging from weeks to months. This is followed by a relapse of fever, often of lesser intensity. Splenomegaly develops quickly in the first few weeks and becomes massive as the disease progresses. Moderate hepatomegaly occurs later. Lymphadenopathy is seen in the majority of

13

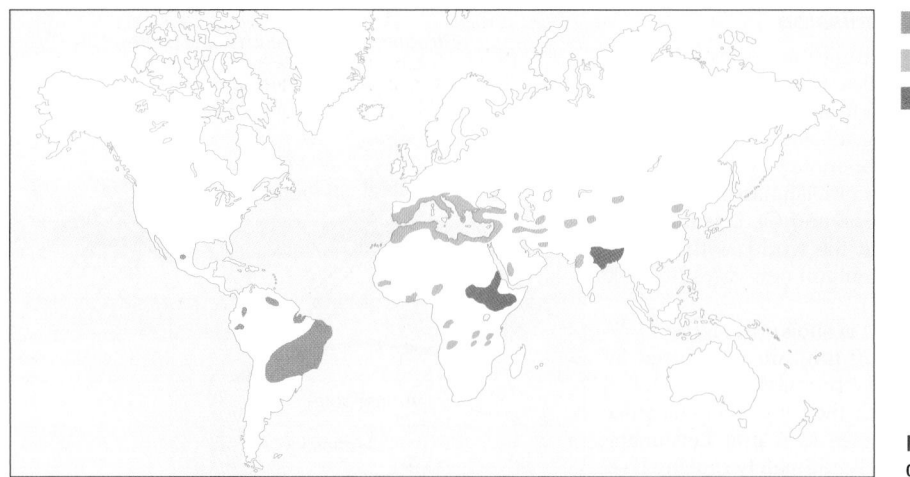

L. *chagasi*

L. *infantum*

L. *donovani*

Fig. 13.38 World distribution of visceral leishmaniasis.

cases in Africa, the Mediterranean and South America, but is rare on the Indian subcontinent. Blackish discoloration of the skin, from which the disease derived its name, kala-azar (the Hindi word for 'black fever'), is a feature of advanced illness and is now rarely seen. Pancytopenia is a common feature. Moderate to severe anaemia develops rapidly, and can result in congestive cardiac failure and associated clinical features. Thrombocytopenia, often compounded by hepatic dysfunction, may result in bleeding from the retina, gastrointestinal tract and nose. In advanced illness, hypoalbuminaemia may manifest as pedal oedema, ascites and anasarca (gross generalised oedema and swelling).

As the disease advances, there is profound immunosuppression and secondary infections are very common. These include tuberculosis, pneumonia, severe amoebic or bacillary dysentery, gastroenteritis, herpes zoster and chickenpox. Skin infections, boils, cellulitis and scabies are common. Without adequate treatment most patients with clinical VL die.

Investigations

Pancytopenia is the most dominant feature, with granulocytopenia and monocytosis. Polyclonal hypergammaglobulinaemia, chiefly IgG followed by IgM, and hypoalbuminaemia are seen later.

Demonstration of amastigotes (Leishman–Donovan bodies) in splenic smears is the most efficient means of diagnosis, with 98% sensitivity (Fig. 13.39); however, it carries a risk of serious haemorrhage in inexperienced hands. Safer methods, such as bone marrow or lymph node smears, are not as sensitive. Parasites may be demonstrated in buffy coat smears, especially in immunosuppressed patients. Sensitivity can be improved by culturing the aspirate material or by PCR for DNA detection and species identification, but these tests can only be performed in specialised laboratories.

Serodiagnosis, by ELISA or immunofluorescence antibody test, is employed in developed countries. In endemic regions, a highly sensitive and specific direct agglutination test using stained promastigotes and an equally efficient rapid immunochromatographic k39 strip test have become popular. These tests remain positive for several months after cure has been achieved, so do not predict response to treatment or relapse. A significant proportion of the healthy population in an endemic region will be positive for these tests due to past exposure. Formal gel (aldehyde) or other similar tests based on the detection of raised globulin have limited value and should not be employed for the diagnosis of VL.

Differential diagnosis

This includes malaria, typhoid, tuberculosis, schistosomiasis and many other infectious and neoplastic conditions, some of which may coexist with VL. Fever, splenomegaly, pancytopenia and non-response to antimalarial therapy may provide clues before specific laboratory diagnosis is made.

Management
Pentavalent antimonials

Antimony (Sb) compounds were the first drugs to be used for the treatment of leishmaniasis and remain the mainstay of treatment in most parts of the world. The exception is the Indian subcontinent, especially Bihar state, where almost two-thirds of cases are refractory to Sb treatment. Traditionally, pentavalent antimony is available as sodium stibogluconate (100 mg/mL) in English-speaking countries and meglumine antimoniate (85 mg/mL) in French-speaking ones. The daily dose is 20 mg/kg body weight, given either intravenously or intramuscularly for 28–30 days. Side-effects are common and include arthralgias, myalgias, raised hepatic

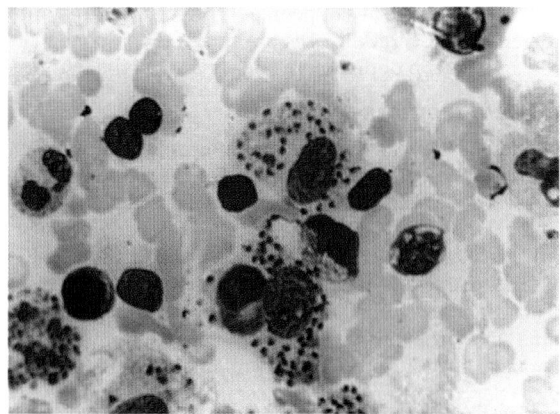

Fig. 13.39 Splenic smear showing numerous intracellular, and a few extracellular, amastigotes.

transaminases, pancreatitis (especially in patients co-infected with HIV) and ECG changes (T wave inversion and reduced amplitude). Severe cardiotoxicity, manifest by concave ST segment elevation, prolongation of QT_c > 0.5 msec, and ventricular dysrythmias, is not uncommon. The incidence of cardiotoxicity and death can be very high with improperly manufactured Sb.

Amphotericin B

The antifungal drug, amphotericin B deoxycholate, given once daily or on alternate days at a dose of 0.75–1.00 mg/kg for 15–20 doses, is used as a first-line drug in many regions with a significant level of Sb unresponsiveness. It has a cure rate of nearly 100%. Infusion-related side-effects, e.g. high fever with rigor, thrombophlebitis, diarrhoea and vomiting, are extremely common. Serious adverse events, such as renal or hepatic toxicity, hypokalaemia and thrombocytopenia are not uncommon.

Lipid formulations of amphotericin B (p. 158) are less toxic and have been tested widely for the treatment of VL. AmBisome is approved by the US Food and Drug Administration and is first-line therapy in Europe for VL. Drug doses vary according to geographical location. On the Indian subcontinent a total dose of 10–15 mg/kg is considered adequate, whereas in Africa 14–18 mg, and in South America and Europe 21–24 mg, is needed for immunocompetent patients. High daily doses (5–7.5 mg/kg) of the lipid formulations are well tolerated, thus reducing hospital stay, but the high price of lipid formulations has limited their use in endemic regions. AmBisome has been made available at a preferential low price for developing countries, and greater use of this drug for treatment of VL is expected.

Other drugs

The oral drug miltefosine, an alkyl phospholipid, has been approved in several countries for the treatment of VL. A daily dose of 50 mg (patient's body weight < 25 kg) to 100 mg (≥ 25 kg), or 2.5 mg/kg body weight for children, for 28 days cures over 90% of patients. Side-effects include mild to moderate vomiting and diarrhoea, and rarely skin allergy or renal or liver toxicity. Since it is a teratogenic drug, it cannot be used in pregnancy; female patients are advised not to become pregnant for the duration of treatment and 3 months thereafter, because of its half-life of nearly 1 week.

Paromomycin is an aminoglycoside that has undergone trials in India and Africa, and is highly effective if given intramuscularly at 11 mg/kg body weight of paromomycin base, daily for 3 weeks. No significant auditory or renal toxicity is seen. The drug has been approved in India for the treatment of VL.

Pentamidine isetionate was used to treat Sb-refractory patients with VL. However, declining efficacy and serious side-effects, such as type 1 diabetes mellitus, hypoglycaemia and hypotension, have led to it being abandoned.

Response to treatment

A good response results in abatement of fever, a feeling of well-being, gradual decrease in spleen size, weight gain and recovery of blood counts. Patients should be followed regularly for a period of 6–12 months, as a small minority may experience a relapse of the disease during this period, irrespective of the treatment regimen.

HIV-visceral leishmaniasis co-infection

HIV-induced immunosuppression (Ch. 14) increases the risk of contracting VL 100–1000 times. Most cases of HIV-VL co-infection have been reported from Spain, France, Italy and Portugal. Highly active antiretroviral therapy (HAART) has led to a remarkable decline in the incidence of VL co-infection in Europe. However, numbers are increasing in Africa (mainly Ethiopia) and Brazil and on the Indian subcontinent.

The clinical triad of fever, splenomegaly and hepatomegaly is found in fewer than half of patients with a CD4 count < 50 cells/mm³. Atypical clinical presentations of VL pose a diagnostic challenge. VL may present with gastrointestinal involvement (stomach, duodenum or colon), ascites, pleural or pericardial effusion, or involvement of lungs, tonsil, oral mucosa or skin. Diagnostic principles remain the same as those in non-HIV patients. Parasites are numerous and easily demonstrable, even in buffy coat preparations. Sometimes amastigotes are found in unusual sites, such as bronchoalveolar lavage fluid, pleural fluid or biopsies of the gastrointestinal tract. Immunofluorescence, Western blot, ELISA and other serological tests used singly have low sensitivity. DNA detection by PCR of the blood or its buffy coat are ≥ 95% sensitive, and accurately track recovery and relapse.

Treatment of VL with HIV co-infection is essentially the same as in immunocompetent patients but there are some differences in outcome. Conventional amphotericin B (0.7 mg/kg/day for 28 days) may be more effective in achieving initial cure than Sb (20 mg/kg/day for 28 days). Using high-dose AmBisome (4 mg/kg on days 1–5, 10, 17, 24, 31 and 38), a high cure rate is possible. However, these co-infected patients have a tendency to relapse within 1 year. For prevention of relapse, maintenance chemotherapy with monthly liposomal amphotericin B is useful.

Post-kala-azar dermal leishmaniasis (PKDL)

After treatment and apparent recovery from the visceral disease in India and Sudan, some patients develop dermatological manifestations due to local parasitic infection.

Clinical features

In India dermatological changes occur in a small minority of patients 6 months to ≥ 3 years after the initial infection. They are seen as macules, papules, nodules (most frequently) and plaques which have a predilection for the face, especially the area around the chin. The face often appears erythematous (Fig. 13.40A). Hypopigmented macules can occur over all parts of the body and are highly variable in extent and location. There are no systemic symptoms and no spontaneous healing.

In Sudan approximately 50% of patients with VL develop PKDL, experiencing skin manifestations concurrently with VL or within 6 months afterwards. In addition to the dermatological features described above, a measles-like micropapular rash (Fig. 13.40B) may be seen all over the body. In Sudan, children are more frequently affected than in India. Spontaneous healing occurs in about three-quarters of cases within 1 year.

Investigations and management

The diagnosis is clinical, supported by demonstration of scanty parasites in lesions by slit-skin smear and culture.

13

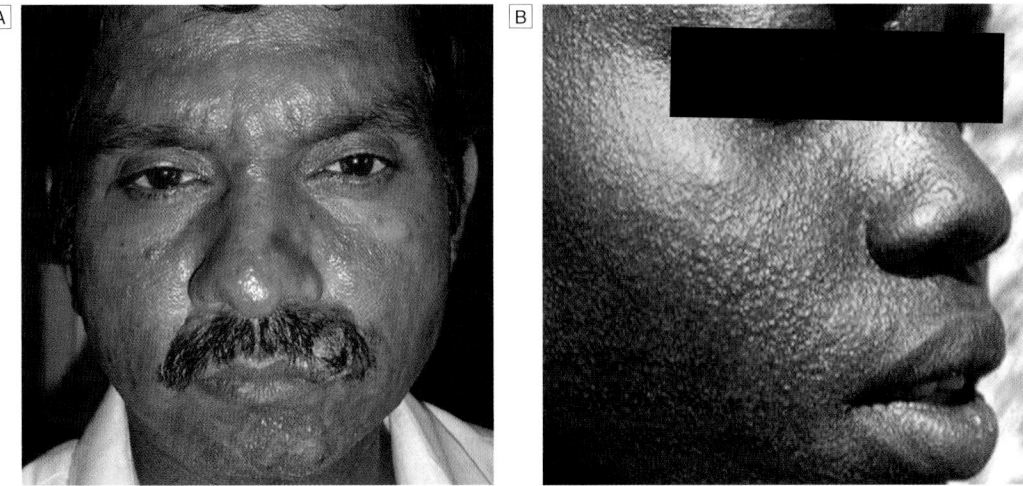

Fig. 13.40 **Post-kala-azar dermal leishmaniasis.** [A] In India, with macules, papules, nodules and plaques. [B] In Sudan, with micronodular rash.

Immunofluorescence and immunohistochemistry may demonstrate the parasite in skin tissues. In the majority of patients serological tests (direct agglutination test or k39 strip tests) are positive.

Treatment of PKDL is difficult. In India, Sb for 120 days or several courses of amphotericin B infusions are required. In Sudan, Sb for 2 months is considered adequate. In the absence of a physical handicap, most patients are reluctant to complete the treatment. PKDL patients are a human reservoir, and focal outbreaks have been linked to patients with PKDL in areas previously free of VL.

Prevention and control

Sandflies are extremely sensitive to insecticides, and vector control through insecticide spray is very important. Mosquito nets or curtains treated with insecticides will keep out the tiny sandflies. In endemic areas with zoonotic transmission, infected or stray dogs should be destroyed.

In areas with anthroponotic transmission, early diagnosis and treatment of human infections, to reduce the reservoir and control epidemics of VL, is extremely important. Serology is useful in diagnosis of suspected cases in the field. No vaccine is currently available.

Cutaneous and mucosal leishmaniasis

Cutaneous leishmaniasis (CL)

CL (oriental sore) occurs in both the Old World and the New World (the Americas). Transmission is described on page 357.

In the Old World, CL is mild. It is found around the Mediterranean basin, throughout the Middle East and Central Asia as far as Pakistan, and in sub-Saharan West Africa and Sudan (Fig. 13.41). The causative organisms for Old World zoonotic CL are *L. major, L. tropica* and *L. aethiopica* (Box 13.61). Anthroponotic CL is caused by *L. tropica*, and is confined to urban or suburban areas of the Old World. Afghanistan is currently the biggest focus, but infection is endemic in Pakistan, the western deserts of India, Iran, Iraq, Syria and other areas of the Middle East. In recent years there has been an increase in the incidence of zoonotic CL in both the Old and the New World due to urbanisation and deforestation which led to peridomestic transmission (in and around human dwellings).

New World CL is a more significant disease, which may disfigure the nose, ears and mouth, and is caused

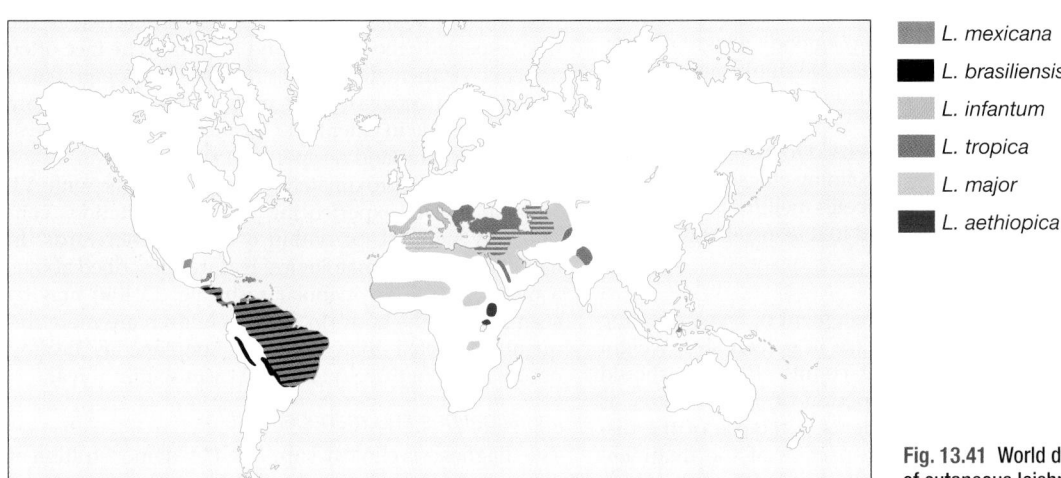

L. mexicana
L. brasiliensis
L. infantum
L. tropica
L. major
L. aethiopica

Fig. 13.41 World distribution of cutaneous leishmaniasis.

13.61 Types of Old World *Leishmania*

Leishmania spp.	Host	Clinical features
L. tropica	Dogs	Slow evolution, less severe
L. major	Gerbils, desert rodents	Rapid necrosis, wet sores
L. aethiopica	Hyraxes	Solitary facial lesions with satellites

by the *L. mexicana* complex (comprising *L. mexicana*, *L. amazonensis* and *L. venezuelensis*) and by the *Viannia* subgenus *L. (V.) brasiliensis* complex (comprising *L. (V.) guyanensis*, *L. (V.) panamensis*, *L. (V.) brasiliensis* and *L. (V.) peruviana*).

CL is commonly imported and should be considered in the differential diagnosis of an ulcerating skin lesion, especially in travellers who have visited endemic areas of the Old World or forests in Central and South America.

Pathogenesis

Inoculated parasites are taken up by dermal macrophages, in which they multiply and form a focus for lymphocytes, epithelioid cells and plasma cells. Self-healing may occur with necrosis of infected macrophages, or the lesion may become chronic with ulceration of the overlying epidermis, depending upon the aetiological pathogen.

Clinical features

The incubation period is typically 2–3 months (range 2 weeks to 5 years). In all types of CL, the common feature is development of a papule followed by ulceration of the skin with raised borders, usually at the site of the bite of the vector. Lesions, single or multiple, start as small red papules that increase gradually in size, reaching 2–10 cm in diameter. A crust forms, overlying an ulcer with a granular base (Fig. 13.42). These ulcers develop a few weeks or months after the bite. There can be satellite lesions, especially in *L. major* and occasionally in *L. tropica* infections. Regional lymphadenopathy, pain, pruritus and secondary bacterial infections may occur.

Clinically, lesions of *L. mexicana* and *L. peruviana* closely resemble those seen in the Old World, but lesions on the pinna of the ear are common, and are chronic and destructive. *L. mexicana* is responsible for chiclero ulcers, the self-healing sores of Mexico.

If immunity is good, there is usually spontaneous healing in *L. tropica*, *L. major* and *L. mexicana* lesions. In some patients with anergy to *Leishmania*, the skin lesions of *L. aethiopica*, *L. mexicana* and *L. amazonensis* infections progress to the development of diffuse CL; this is characterised by spread of the infection from the initial ulcer, usually on the face, to involve the whole body in the form of non-ulcerative nodules. Occasionally, in *L. tropica* infections, sores that have apparently healed relapse persistently (recidivans or lupoid leishmaniasis).

Mucosal leishmaniasis (ML)

The *Viannia* subgenus extends widely from the Amazon basin as far as Paraguay and Costa Rica, and is responsible for deep sores and ML. In *L. (V.) brasiliensis* complex infections, cutaneous lesions may be followed by mucosal spread of the disease simultaneously or even years later. Young men with chronic lesions are particularly at risk, and between 2% and 40% of infected persons develop 'espundia', metastatic lesions in the mucosa of the nose or mouth. This is characterised by thickening and erythema of the nasal mucosa, typically starting at the junction of the nose and upper lip. Later, ulceration develops. The lips, soft palate, fauces and larynx may also be invaded and destroyed, leading to considerable suffering and deformity. There is no spontaneous healing, and death may result from severe respiratory tract infections due to massive destruction of the pharynx.

Investigations in CL and ML

CL is often diagnosed on the basis of clinical characteristics of the lesions. However, parasitological confirmation is important because clinical manifestations may be mimicked by other infections. Amastigotes can be demonstrated on a slit-skin smear with Giemsa staining; alternatively, they can be cultured from the sores early during the infection. Parasites seem to be particularly difficult to isolate from sores caused by *L. brasiliensis*, responsible for the vast majority of cases in Brazil. Touch preparations from biopsies and histopathology usually have a low sensitivity. Culture of fine needle aspiration material has been reported to be the most sensitive method.

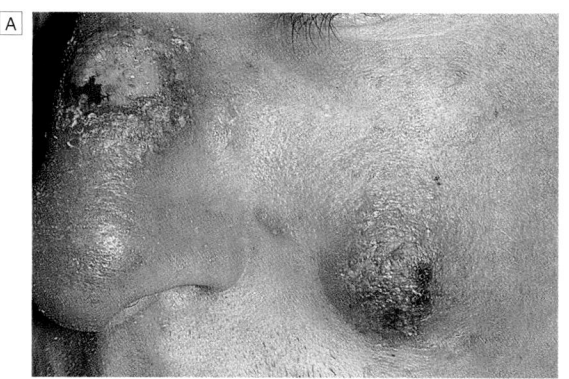

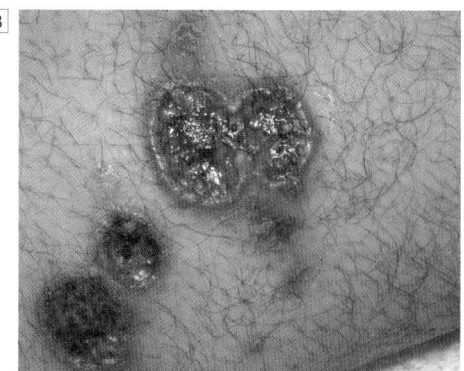

Fig. 13.42 Cutaneous leishmaniasis. **A** Papule. **B** Ulcer.

ML is more difficult to diagnose parasitologically. The leishmanin skin test measures delayed-type hypersensitivity to killed *Leishmania* organisms. A positive test is defined as induration > 5 mm 48 hours after intradermal injection. The test is positive, except in diffuse CL and during active VL. PCR is used increasingly for diagnosis and speciation, which is useful in selecting therapy.

Management of CL and ML

Small lesions may self-heal or are treated by freezing with liquid nitrogen or curettage. There is no ideal antimicrobial therapy. Treatment should be individualised on the basis of the causative organism, severity of the lesions, availability of drugs, tolerance of the patient for toxicity, and local resistance patterns.

In CL, topical application of paromomycin 15% plus methylbenzethonium chloride 12% is beneficial. Intralesional antimony (Sb: 0.2–0.8 mL/lesion) up to 2 g seems to be rapidly effective in suitable cases, well tolerated and economic, and is safe in patients with cardiac, liver or renal diseases.

In ML, and in CL when the lesions are multiple or in a disfiguring site, it is better to treat with parenteral Sb in a dose of 20 mg/kg/day (usually given for 20 days for CL and 28 days for ML), or with conventional or liposomal amphotericin B (see treatment of VL above). Sb is also indicated to prevent the development of mucosal disease, if there is any chance that a lesion acquired in South America is due to an *L. brasiliensis* strain. Refractory CL or ML should be treated with an amphotericin B preparation.

Other regimens may be effective. Two to four doses (2–4 mg/kg) of alternate-day administration of pentamidine are effective in New World CL. In ML, 8 injections of pentamidine (4 mg/kg on alternate days) cure the majority of patients. Ketoconazole 600 mg daily for 4 weeks has shown some potential against *L. mexicana* infection. In Saudi Arabia, fluconazole 200 mg daily for 6 weeks reduced healing times and cured 79% of patients with CL due to *L. major*. In India itraconazole 200 mg daily for 6 weeks produced good results in CL.

Prevention of CL and ML

Personal protection against sandfly bites is important. No effective vaccine is yet available.

Gastrointestinal protozoal infections

Amoebiasis

Amoebiasis is caused by *Entamoeba histolytica*, which is spread between humans by its cysts. It is one of the leading parasitic causes of morbidity and mortality in the tropics and is occasionally acquired in other countries, such as the UK. Two non-pathogenic *Entamoeba* species (*E. dispar* and *E. moshkovskii*) are morphologically identical to *E. histolytica*, and are distinguishable only by molecular techniques, isoenzyme studies or monoclonal antibody typing. However, only *E. histolytica* causes amoebic dysentery or liver abscess. The life cycle of the amoeba is shown in Figure 13.43A.

Pathology

Cysts of *E. histolytica* are ingested in water or uncooked foods contaminated by human faeces. Infection may also be acquired through anal/oral sexual practices. In the colon, vegetative trophozoite forms emerge from the cysts. The parasite may invade the mucous membrane of the large bowel, producing lesions that are maximal in the caecum but found as far down as the anal canal. These are flask-shaped ulcers, varying greatly in size and surrounded by healthy mucosa. A localised granuloma

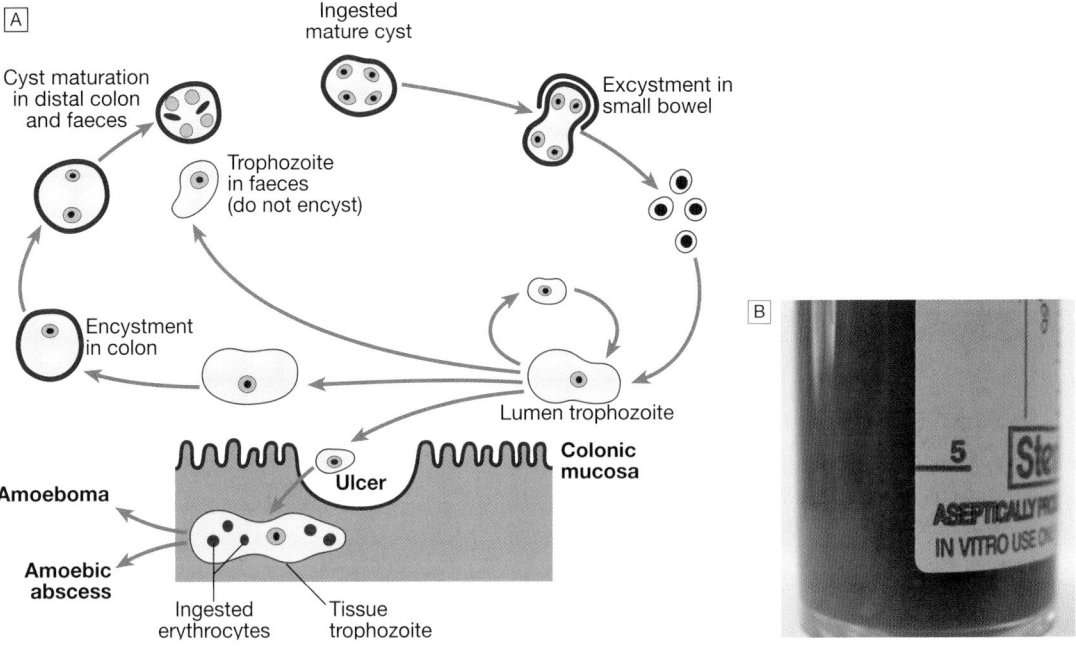

Fig. 13.43 Amoebiasis. **A** The life cycle of *Entamoeba histolytica*. **B** The chocolate-brown appearance of aspirated material from an amoebic liver abscess.

(amoeboma), presenting as a palpable mass in the rectum or a filling defect in the colon on radiography, is a rare complication which should be differentiated from colonic carcinoma. Amoebic ulcers may cause severe haemorrhage but rarely perforate the bowel wall.

Amoebic trophozoites can emerge from the vegetative cyst from the bowel and be carried to the liver in a portal venule. They can multiply rapidly and destroy the liver parenchyma, causing an abscess (see also p. 972). The liquid contents at first have a characteristic pinkish colour which may later change to chocolate brown (like anchovy sauce).

Cutaneous amoebiasis, though rare, causes progressive genital, perianal or peri-abdominal surgical wound ulceration.

Clinical features

Intestinal amoebiasis—amoebic dysentery

Most amoebic infections are asymptomatic. The incubation period of amoebiasis ranges from 2 weeks to many years, followed by a chronic course with abdominal pains and two or more unformed stools a day. Offensive diarrhoea alternating with constipation, and blood or mucus in the stool, are common. There may be abdominal pain, especially right lower quadrant (which may simulate acute appendicitis). A dysenteric presentation with passage of blood, simulating bacillary dysentery or ulcerative colitis, occurs particularly in older people, in the puerperium and with superadded pyogenic infection of the ulcers.

Amoebic liver abscess

The abscess is usually found in the right hepatic lobe. There may not be associated diarrhoea. Early symptoms may be local discomfort only and malaise; later, a swinging temperature and sweating may develop, usually without marked systemic symptoms or associated cardiovascular signs. An enlarged, tender liver, cough and pain in the right shoulder are characteristic, but symptoms may remain vague and signs minimal. A large abscess may penetrate the diaphragm and rupture into the lung, from where its contents may be coughed up. Rupture into the pleural cavity, the peritoneal cavity or pericardial sac is less common but more serious.

Investigations

The stool and any exudate should be examined at once under the microscope for motile trophozoites containing red blood cells. Movements cease rapidly as the stool preparation cools. Several stools may need to be examined in chronic amoebiasis before cysts are found. Sigmoidoscopy may reveal typical flask-shaped ulcers, which should be scraped and examined immediately for *E. histolytica*. In endemic areas one-third of the population are symptomless passers of amoebic cysts.

An amoebic abscess of the liver is suspected on clinical grounds; there is often a neutrophil leucocytosis and a raised right hemidiaphragm on chest X-ray. Confirmation is by ultrasonic scanning. Aspirated pus from an amoebic abscess has the characteristic anchovy sauce or chocolate brown appearance but only rarely contains free amoebae (Fig. 13.43B).

Serum antibodies are detectable by immunofluorescence in over 95% of patients with hepatic amoebiasis and intestinal amoeboma, but in only about 60% of dysenteric amoebiasis. DNA detection by PCR has been shown to be useful in diagnosis of *E. histolytica* infections but is not generally available.

Management

Intestinal and early hepatic amoebiasis responds quickly to oral metronidazole (800 mg 8-hourly for 5–10 days) or other long-acting nitroimidazoles like tinidazole or ornidazole (both in doses of 2 g daily for 3 days). Nitaxozanide (500 mg 12-hourly for 3 days) is an alternative drug. Either diloxanide furoate or paromomycin, in doses of 500 mg orally 8-hourly for 10 days after treatment, should be given to eliminate luminal cysts.

If a liver abscess is large or threatens to burst, or if the response to chemotherapy is not prompt, aspiration is required and is repeated if necessary. Rupture of an abscess into the pleural cavity, pericardial sac or peritoneal cavity necessitates immediate aspiration or surgical drainage. Small serous effusions resolve without drainage.

Prevention

Personal precautions against contracting amoebiasis consist of not eating fresh uncooked vegetables or drinking unclean water.

Giardiasis

Infection with *Giardia lamblia* is found world-wide and is common in the tropics. It particularly affects children, tourists and immunosuppressed individuals, and is the parasite most commonly imported into the UK. In cystic form it remains viable in water for up to 3 months and infection usually occurs by ingesting contaminated water. Its flagellar trophozoite form attaches to the duodenal and jejunal mucosa, causing inflammation.

Clinical features and investigations

After an incubation period of 1–3 weeks, there is diarrhoea, abdominal pain, weakness, anorexia, nausea and vomiting. On examination there may be abdominal distension and tenderness.

Stools obtained at 2–3-day intervals should be examined for cysts. Duodenal or jejunal aspiration by endoscopy gives a higher diagnostic yield. The 'string test' may be used, in which one end of a piece of string is passed into the duodenum by swallowing, retrieved after an overnight fast, and expressed fluid examined for the presence of *G. lamblia* trophozoites. A number of stool antigen detection tests are available. Jejunal biopsy specimens may show *G. lamblia* on the epithelial surface.

Management

Treatment is with a single dose of tinidazole 2 g, or metronidazole 400 mg 8-hourly for 10 days.

Cryptosporidiosis

Cryptosporidium spp. are coccidian protozoal parasites of humans and domestic animals. Infection is acquired by the faecal–oral route through contaminated water supplies. The incubation period is approximately 7–10 days, and is followed by watery diarrhoea and abdominal cramps. The illness is usually self-limiting, but in immunocompromised patients, especially those with HIV, the

13

illness can be devastating, with persistent severe diarrhoea and substantial weight loss (p. 393).

Cyclosporiasis

Cyclospora cayetanensis is a globally distributed coccidian protozoal parasite of humans. Infection is acquired by ingestion of contaminated water. The incubation period is approximately 2–11 days, and is followed by acute onset of diarrhoea with abdominal cramps, which may remit and relapse. Although usually self-limiting, the illness may last as long as 6 weeks with significant associated weight loss and malabsorption, and is more severe in immunocompromised individuals. Diagnosis is by detection of oöcysts on faecal microscopy. Treatment may be necessary in a few cases, and the agent of choice is co-trimoxazole 960 mg 12-hourly for 7 days.

INFECTIONS CAUSED BY HELMINTHS

Helminths (from the Greek *Helmins*, meaning worm) include three groups of parasitic worm (Box 13.62), large multicellular organisms with complex tissues and organs.

Intestinal human nematodes

Diseases are caused by adult nematodes living in the human gut. There are two types:

- the hookworms, which have a soil stage in which they develop into larvae that then penetrate the host
- a group of nematodes which survive in the soil merely as eggs that have to be ingested for their life cycle to continue.

The geographical distribution of hookworms is limited by the larval requirement for warmth and humidity. Soil-transmitted nematode infections can be prevented

13.62 Classes of helminth that parasitise humans

Nematodes or roundworms

- Intestinal human nematodes: *Ancylostoma duodenale, Necator americanus, Strongyloides stercoralis, Ascaris lumbricoides, Enterobius vermicularis, Trichuris trichiura*
- Tissue-dwelling human nematodes: *Wuchereria bancrofti, Brugia malayi, Loa loa, Onchocerca volvulus, Dracunculus medinensis, Mansonella perstans, Dirofilaria immitis*
- Zoonotic nematodes: *Trichinella spiralis*

Trematodes or flukes

- Blood flukes: *Schistosoma haematobium, S. mansoni, S. japonicum, S. mekongi, S. intercalatum*
- Lung flukes: *Paragonimus* spp.
- Hepatobiliary flukes: *Clonorchis sinensis, Fasciola hepatica, Opisthorchis felineus*
- Intestinal flukes: *Fasciolopsis buski*

Cestodes or tapeworms

- Intestinal tapeworms: *Taenia saginata, T. solium, Diphyllobothrium latum, Hymenolepis nana*
- Tissue-dwelling cysts or worms: *Taenia solium, Echinococcus granulosus*

by avoidance of faecal soil contamination (adequate sewerage disposal) or skin contact (wearing shoes), and by strict personal hygiene.

Ancylostomiasis (hookworm)

Ancylostomiasis is caused by parasitisation with *Ancylostoma duodenale* or *Necator americanus*. The complex life cycle is shown in Figure 13.44. The adult hookworm is 1 cm long and lives in the duodenum and upper jejunum. Eggs are passed in the faeces. In warm, moist, shady soil the larvae develop into rhabditiform and then the infective filariform stages; they then penetrate human skin and are carried to the lungs. After entering the alveoli they ascend the bronchi, are swallowed and mature in the small intestine, reaching maturity 4–7 weeks after infection. The worms attach themselves to the mucosa of the small intestine by their buccal capsule (Fig. 13.45) and withdraw blood. The mean daily

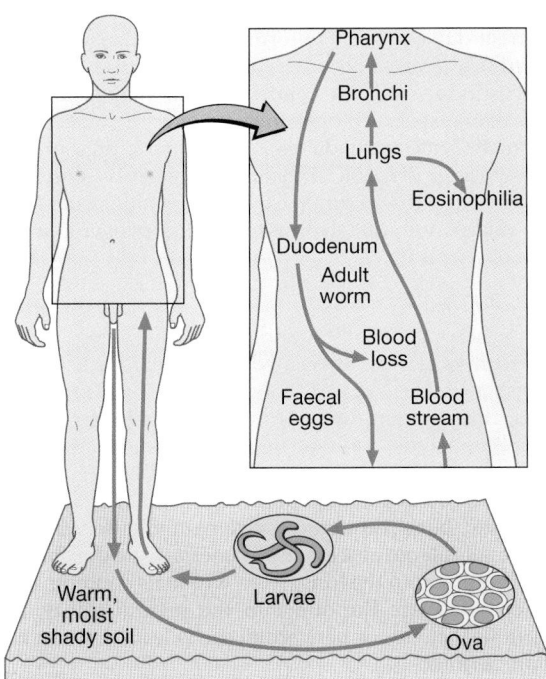

Fig. 13.44 Ancylostomiasis. Life cycle of *Ancylostoma*.

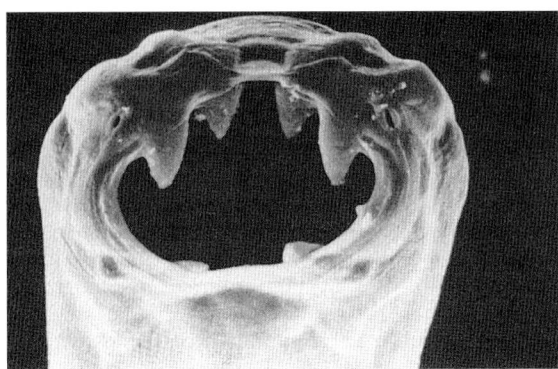

Fig. 13.45 *Ancylostoma duodenale.* Electron micrograph showing the ventral teeth.

loss of blood from one *A. duodenale* is 0.15 mL and from *N. americanus* 0.03 mL.

Hookworm infection is one of the main causes of anaemia in the tropics and subtropics. *A. duodenale* is endemic in the Far East and Mediterranean coastal regions, and is also present in Africa, while *N. americanus* is endemic in West, East and Central Africa, and Central and South America, as well as in the Far East.

Clinical features

An allergic dermatitis, usually on the feet (ground itch), may be experienced at the time of infection. The passage of the larvae through the lungs in a heavy infection causes a paroxysmal cough with blood-stained sputum, associated with patchy pulmonary consolidation and eosinophilia. When the worms have reached the small intestine, vomiting and epigastric pain resembling peptic ulcer disease may occur. Sometimes frequent loose stools are passed. The degree of iron and protein deficiency which develops depends not only on the load of worms but also on the nutrition of the patient and especially on the iron stores. Anaemia with high-output cardiac failure may result. The mental and physical development of children may be retarded in severe infection.

Investigations

There is eosinophilia. The characteristic ovum can be recognised in the stool. If hookworms are present in numbers sufficient to cause anaemia, faecal occult blood testing will be positive and many ova will be present.

Management

A single dose of albendazole (400 mg) is the treatment of choice. Alternatively, mebendazole 100 mg 12-hourly for 3 days may be used. Anaemia and heart failure associated with hookworm infection respond well to oral iron, even when severe; blood transfusion is rarely required.

Strongyloidiasis

Strongyloides stercoralis is a very small nematode (2 mm × 0.4 mm) which parasitises the mucosa of the upper part of the small intestine, often in large numbers, causing persistent eosinophilia. The eggs hatch in the bowel but only larvae are passed in the faeces. In moist soil they moult and become the infective filariform larvae. After penetrating human skin, they undergo a development cycle similar to that of hookworms, except that the female worms burrow into the intestinal mucosa and submucosa. Some larvae in the intestine may develop into filariform larvae, which may then penetrate the mucosa or the perianal skin and lead to autoinfection and persistent infection. Patients with *Strongyloides* infection persisting for more than 35 years have been described. Strongyloidiasis occurs in the tropics and subtropics, and is especially prevalent in the Far East.

Clinical features

These are shown in Box 13.63. The classic triad of symptoms consists of abdominal pain, diarrhoea and urticaria. Cutaneous manifestations, either urticaria or larva currens (a highly characteristic pruritic, elevated, erythematous lesion advancing along the course of larval migration), are characteristic and occur in 66% of patients.

13.63 Clinical features of strongyloidiasis
Penetration of skin by infective larvae
• Itchy rash
Presence of worms in gut
• Abdominal pain, diarrhoea, steatorrhoea, weight loss
Allergic phenomena
• Urticarial plaques and papules, wheezing, arthralgia
Autoinfection
• Transient itchy linear urticarial weals across abdomen and buttocks (larva currens)
Systemic (super)infection
• Diarrhoea, pneumonia, meningoencephalitis, death

Systemic strongyloidiasis (the *Strongyloides* hyperinfection syndrome), with dissemination of larvae throughout the body, occurs in association with immune suppression (intercurrent disease, HIV and HTLV-1 infection, corticosteroid treatment). Patients present with severe, generalised abdominal pain, abdominal distension and shock. Massive larval invasion of the lungs causes cough, wheeze and dyspnoea; cerebral involvement has manifestations ranging from subtle neurological signs to coma. Gram-negative sepsis frequently complicates the picture.

Investigations

There is eosinophilia. Serology (ELISA) is helpful, but definitive diagnosis depends upon finding the larvae. The faeces should be examined microscopically for motile larvae; excretion is intermittent so repeated examinations may be necessary. Larvae can also be found in jejunal aspirate or detected using the string test (p. 363). Larvae may also be cultured from faeces.

Management

Ivermectin 200 µg/kg as a single dose, or two doses of 200 µg/kg on successive days, is effective. Alternatively, albendazole is given orally in a dose of 15 mg/kg body weight 12-hourly for 3 days. A second course may be required. For the *Strongyloides* hyperinfection syndrome, ivermectin is given at 200 µg/kg on days 1, 2, 15 and 16.

Ascaris lumbricoides (roundworm)

This pale yellow nematode is 20–35 cm long. Humans are infected by eating food contaminated with mature ova. *Ascaris* larvae hatch in the duodenum, migrate through the lungs, ascend the bronchial tree, are swallowed and mature in the small intestine. This tissue migration can provoke both local and general hypersensitivity reactions, with pneumonitis, eosinophilic granulomas, bronchial asthma and urticaria.

Clinical features

Intestinal ascariasis causes symptoms ranging from occasional vague abdominal pain through to malnutrition. The large size of the adult worm and its tendency to aggregate and migrate can result in obstructive complications. Tropical and subtropical areas are endemic for ascariasis, and in these areas it causes up to 35% of all intestinal obstructions, most commonly in the terminal ileum. Obstruction can be complicated further by intussusception, volvulus, haemorrhagic infarction and perforation. Other complications include blockage of the bile or pancreatic duct and obstruction of the appendix by adult worms.

Investigations

The diagnosis is made microscopically by finding ova in the faeces. Adult worms are frequently expelled rectally or orally. Occasionally, the worms are demonstrated radiographically by a barium examination. There is eosinophilia.

Management

A single dose of albendazole (400 mg), pyrantel pamoate (11 mg/kg; maximum 1 g), piperazine (4 g) or mebendazole (100 mg 12-hourly for 3 days) is effective for intestinal ascariasis. Patients should be warned that they might expel numerous whole, large worms. Obstruction due to ascariasis should be treated with nasogastric suction, piperazine and intravenous fluids.

Prevention

Community chemotherapy programmes have been used to reduce *Ascaris* infection. The whole community can be treated every 3 months for several years. Alternatively, schoolchildren can be targeted; treating them lowers the prevalence of ascariasis in the community.

Enterobius vermicularis (threadworm)

This helminth is common throughout the world. It affects mainly children. After the ova are swallowed, development takes place in the small intestine, but the adult worms are found chiefly in the colon.

Clinical features

The gravid female worm lays ova around the anus, causing intense itching, especially at night. The ova are often carried to the mouth on the fingers and so reinfection or human-to-human infection takes place (Fig. 13.46). In females the genitalia may be involved. The adult worms may be seen moving on the buttocks or in the stool.

Investigations

Ova are detected by applying the adhesive surface of cellophane tape to the perianal skin in the morning. This is then examined on a glass slide under the microscope. A perianal swab, moistened with saline, is an alternative sampling method.

Management

A single dose of mebendazole (100 mg), albendazole (400 mg), pyrantel pamoate (11 mg/kg) or piperazine (4 g) is given and may be repeated after 2 weeks to control auto-reinfection. If infection recurs in a family, each member should be treated as above. During this period all nightclothes and bed linen are laundered. Fingernails must be kept short and hands washed carefully before meals. Subsequent therapy is reserved for those family members who develop recurrent infection.

Trichuris trichiura (whipworm)

Infections with whipworm are common all over the world under unhygienic conditions. Infection is contracted by

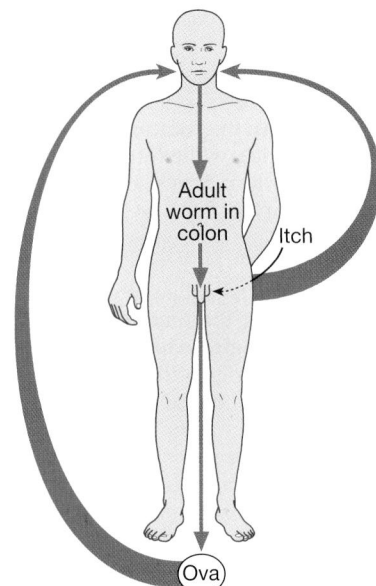

Fig. 13.46 Threadworm. Life cycle of *Enterobius vermicularis*.

the ingestion of earth or food contaminated with ova which have become infective after lying for 3 weeks or more in moist soil. The adult worm is 3–5 cm long and has a coiled anterior end resembling a whip. Whipworms inhabit the caecum, lower ileum, appendix, colon and anal canal. There are usually no symptoms, but intense infections in children may cause persistent diarrhoea or rectal prolapse, and growth retardation. The diagnosis is readily made by identifying ova in faeces. Treatment is with mebendazole in doses of 100 mg 12-hourly for 3–5 days or a single dose of albendazole 400 mg.

Tissue-dwelling human nematodes

Filarial worms are tissue-dwelling nematodes. The larval stages are inoculated by biting mosquitoes or flies, each specific to a particular filarial species. The larvae develop into adult worms (2–50 cm long) which, after mating, produce millions of microfilariae (170–320 μm long) that migrate in blood or skin. The life cycle is completed when the vector takes up microfilariae while feeding on humans. In the insect, ingested microfilariae develop into infective larvae for inoculation in humans, normally the only host.

Disease is due to the host's immune response to the worms (both adult and microfilariae), particularly dying worms, and its pattern and severity vary with the site and stage of each species (Box 13.64). The worms are long-lived; microfilariae survive 2–3 years and adult worms 10–15 years. The infections are chronic and worst in individuals constantly exposed to reinfection.

Lymphatic filariasis

Infection with the filarial worms *Wuchereria bancrofti* and *Brugia malayi* is associated with clinical outcomes ranging from subclinical infection to hydrocele and elephantiasis.

W. bancrofti is transmitted by night-biting culicine or anopheline mosquitoes in most areas (Fig. 13.47). The adult worms, 4–10 cm in length, live in the lymphatics,

13.64 Pathogenicity of filarial infections depending on site and stage of worms

Worm species	Adult worm	Microfilariae
Wuchereria bancrofti and *Brugia malayi*	Lymphatic vessels+++	Blood⁻ Pulmonary capillaries++
Loa loa	Subcutaneous+	Blood+
Onchocerca volvulus	Subcutaneous+	Skin+++ Eye+++
Mansonella perstans	Retroperitoneal⁻	Blood⁻
Mansonella streptocerca	Skin+	Skin++

(+++ severe; ++ moderate; + mild; − rarely pathogenic)

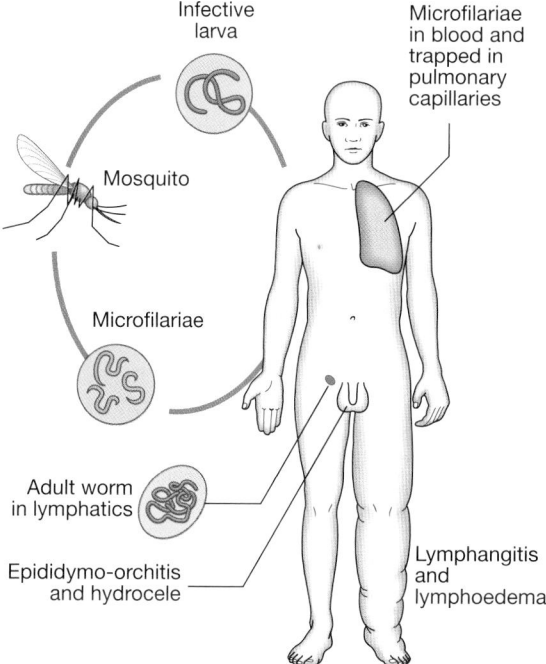

Fig. 13.47 *Wuchereria bancrofti* and *Brugia malayi*. Life cycle of organisms and pathogenesis of lymphatic filariasis.

Labels: Infective larva; Microfilariae in blood and trapped in pulmonary capillaries; Mosquito; Microfilariae; Adult worm in lymphatics; Epididymo-orchitis and hydrocele; Lymphangitis and lymphoedema

and the females produce microfilariae which circulate in large numbers in the peripheral blood, usually at night. The infection is widespread in tropical Africa, the North African coast, coastal areas of Asia, Indonesia and northern Australia, the South Pacific islands, the West Indies and also in North and South America.

B. malayi is similar to *W. bancrofti* and is found in Indonesia, Borneo, Malaysia, Vietnam, South China, South India and Sri Lanka.

Pathology

Several factors contribute to the pathogenesis of lymphatic filariasis. Toxins released by the adult worm cause lymphangiectasia; this dilatation of the lymphatic vessels leads to lymphatic dysfunction and the chronic clinical manifestations of lymphatic filariasis, lymphoedema and hydrocele. Death of the adult worm results

in acute filarial lymphangitis. The filariae are symbiotically infected with rickettsia-like bacteria (*Wolbachia* spp.) and release of lipopolysaccharide from these bacteria contributes to inflammation. Lymphatic obstruction persists after death of the adult worm. Secondary bacterial infections cause tissue destruction. The host response to microfilariae is central to the pathogenesis of tropical pulmonary eosinophilia.

Clinical features

Acute filarial lymphangitis presents with fever, pain, tenderness and erythema along the course of inflamed lymphatic vessels. Inflammation of the spermatic cord, epididymis and testis is common. The whole episode lasts a few days but may recur several times a year. Temporary oedema becomes more persistent and regional lymph nodes enlarge. Progressive enlargement, coarsening, corrugation, fissuring and bacterial infection of the skin and subcutaneous tissue develop gradually, causing irreversible 'elephantiasis'. The scrotum may reach an enormous size. Chyluria and chylous effusions are milky and opalescent; on standing, fat globules rise to the top.

The acute lymphatic manifestations of filariasis must be differentiated from thrombophlebitis and infection. The oedema and lymphatic obstructive changes must be distinguished from congestive cardiac failure, malignancy, trauma and idiopathic abnormalities of the lymphatic system. Silicates absorbed from volcanic soil can also cause non-filarial elephantiasis.

Tropical pulmonary eosinophilia is a complication seen mainly in India and is likely to be due to microfilariae trapped in the pulmonary capillaries and destroyed by allergic inflammation. Patients present with paroxysmal cough, wheeze and fever. If untreated, this progresses to debilitating chronic interstitial lung disease.

Investigations

In the earliest stages of lymphangitis the diagnosis is made on clinical grounds, supported by eosinophilia and sometimes by positive filarial serology. Filarial infections cause the highest eosinophil counts of all helminthic infections.

Microfilariae can be found in the peripheral blood at night, and either are seen moving in a wet blood film or are detected by microfiltration of a sample of lysed blood. They are usually present in hydrocele fluid, which may occasionally yield an adult filaria. By the time elephantiasis develops, microfilariae become difficult to find. Calcified filariae may sometimes be demonstrable by radiography. Movement of adult worms can be seen on scrotal ultrasound. PCR-based tests for detection of *W. bancrofti* and *B. malayi* DNA from blood have been developed.

Indirect fluorescence and ELISA detect antibodies in over 95% of active cases and 70% of established elephantiasis. The test becomes negative 1–2 years after cure. Serological tests cannot distinguish the different filarial infections. Highly sensitive and specific immunochromatographic card tests for detection of filarial infection are now commercially available; finger prick blood taken at any time of the day can be used for these.

In tropical pulmonary eosinophilia, serology is strongly positive and IgE levels are massively elevated, but circulating microfilariae are not found. The chest X-ray shows miliary changes or mottled opacities. Pulmonary function tests show a restrictive picture.

Management

Treatment of the individual is aimed at reversing and halting disease progression. Diethylcarbamazine (DEC) kills microfilariae and adult worms. The dose is 6 mg/kg daily orally in three divided doses for 12 days. Most adverse effects seen with DEC treatment are due to the host response to dying microfilariae, and the reaction intensity is directly proportional to the microfilarial load. The main symptoms are fever, headache, nausea, vomiting, arthralgia and prostration. These usually occur within 24–36 hours of the first dose of DEC. Antihistamines or corticosteroids may be required to control these allergic phenomena. Both the 12-day course and a single dose of DEC reduce microfilaria levels by about 90% 6–12 months after treatment. No carefully controlled trials have evaluated the effects of DEC treatment alone on the chronic manifestations of lymphatic filariasis.

A single dose of either ivermectin (200 μg/kg) or albendazole (400 mg) in combination with DEC (300 mg) also eliminates microfilariae for 1 year. With the discovery of an endosymbiotic bacterium, *Wolbachia*, in most of the filarial worms, there is a possible role for doxycycline in eliminating the bacteria; the drug leads to interruption of embryogenesis and hence the production of microfilariae.

For tropical pulmonary eosinophilia, DEC (6 mg/kg daily orally in three divided doses for 14 days) is the treatment of choice.

Chronic lymphatic pathology

Experience in India and Brazil shows that active management of chronic lymphatic pathology can alleviate symptoms. Patients should be taught meticulous skin care of their lymphoedematous limbs to prevent secondary bacterial and fungal infections. Tight bandaging, massage and bed rest with elevation of the affected limb may help to control the lymphoedema. Prompt diagnosis and antibiotic therapy of bacterial cellulitis are important in preventing further lymphatic damage and worsening of existing elephantiasis. Plastic surgery may be indicated in established elephantiasis. Great relief can be obtained by removal of excess tissue but recurrences are probable unless new lymphatic drainage is established. Hydroceles and chyluria can be repaired surgically.

Prevention

Treatment of the whole population in endemic areas with annual single-dose DEC (6 mg/kg), either alone or in combination with albendazole or ivermectin, can reduce filarial transmission. This mass treatment should be combined with mosquito control programmes.

Loiasis

Loiasis is caused by infection with the filaria *Loa loa*. The adults, 3–7 cm × 4 mm, chiefly parasitise the subcutaneous tissue of humans, releasing larval microfilariae into the peripheral blood in the daytime. The vector is *Chrysops*, a forest-dwelling, day-biting fly.

The host response to *Loa loa* is usually absent or mild, so that the infection may be harmless. From time to time a short-lived, inflammatory, oedematous swelling (a Calabar swelling) is produced around an adult worm. Heavy infections, especially when treated, may cause encephalitis.

Clinical features

The infection is often symptomless. The incubation period is commonly over a year but may be just 3 months. The first sign is usually a Calabar swelling, an irritating, tense, localised swelling that may be painful, especially if it is near a joint. The swelling is generally on a limb; it measures a few centimetres in diameter but sometimes is more diffuse and extensive. It usually disappears after a few days but may persist for 2 or 3 weeks. A succession of such swellings may appear at irregular intervals, often in adjacent sites. Sometimes there is urticaria and pruritus elsewhere. Occasionally, a worm may be seen wriggling under the skin, especially that of an eyelid, and may cross the eye under the conjunctiva, taking many minutes to do so.

Investigations

Diagnosis is by demonstrating microfilariae in blood taken during the day, but they may not always be found in patients with Calabar swellings. Antifilarial antibodies are positive in 95% of patients and there is massive eosinophilia. Occasionally, a calcified worm may be seen on X-ray.

Management

DEC (see above) is curative, in a dose of 9–12 mg/kg daily which is continued for 21 days. Treatment may precipitate a severe reaction in patients with a heavy microfilaraemia characterised by fever, joint and muscle pain, and encephalitis; microfilaraemic patients should be given corticosteroid cover.

Prevention

Protection is afforded by building houses away from trees and by having dwellings wire-screened. Protective clothing and insect repellents are also useful. DEC in a dose of 5 mg/kg daily for 3 days each month is partially protective.

Onchocerciasis (river blindness)

Onchocerciasis is the result of infection by the filarial *Onchocerca volvulus*. The infection is conveyed by flies of the genus *Simulium*, which breed in rapidly flowing, well-aerated water. Adult flies inflict painful bites during the day, both inside and outside houses. While feeding, they pick up the microfilariae, which mature into the infective larva and are transmitted to a new host in subsequent bites. Humans are the only known hosts (Fig. 13.48).

Onchocerciasis is endemic in sub-Saharan Africa, Yemen, and a few foci in Central and South America. It is estimated that 17.7 million people are infected, of whom 500 000 are visually impaired and 270 000 blind. Due to onchocerciasis huge tracts of fertile land lie virtually untilled, and individuals and communities are impoverished.

Pathology

After inoculation of larvae by a bite from an infected fly, the worms mature in 2–4 months and live for up to

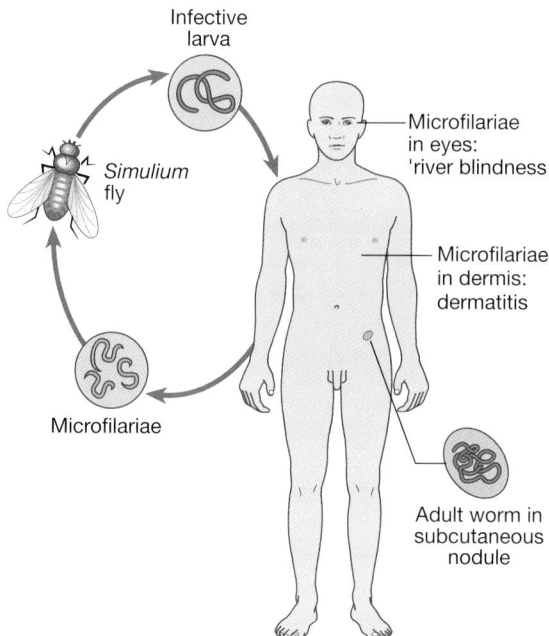

Fig. 13.48 *Onchocerca volvulus.* Life cycle of organism and pathogenesis of onchocerciasis.

17 years in subcutaneous and connective tissues. At sites of trauma, over bony prominences and around joints, fibrosis may form nodules around adult worms which otherwise cause no direct damage. Innumerable microfilariae, discharged by the female *O. volvulus*, move actively in these nodules and in the adjacent tissues, are widely distributed in the skin, and may invade the eye. Live microfilariae elicit little tissue reaction, but dead ones may cause severe allergic inflammation leading to hyaline necrosis and loss of collagen and elastin. Death of microfilariae in the eye causes inflammation and may lead to blindness.

Clinical features

The infection may remain symptomless for months or years. The first symptom is usually itching, localised to one quadrant of the body and later becoming generalised and involving the eyes. Transient oedema of part or all of a limb is an early sign, followed by papular urticaria spreading gradually from the site of infection. This is difficult to see on dark skins, in which the most common signs are papules excoriated by scratching, spotty hyperpigmentation from resolving inflammation, and more chronic changes of a rough, thickened or inelastic, wrinkled skin. Both infected and uninfected superficial lymph nodes enlarge and may hang down in folds of loose skin at the groins. Hydrocele, femoral hernias and scrotal elephantiasis can occur. Firm subcutaneous nodules > 1 cm in diameter (onchocercomas) occur in chronic infection.

Eye disease is most common in highly endemic areas and is associated with chronic heavy infections and nodules on the head. Early manifestations include itching, lacrimation and conjunctival injection. These lead to conjunctivitis, sclerosing keratitis with pannus formation, uveitis which may lead to glaucoma and cataract, and, less commonly, choroiditis and optic neuritis.

Classically, 'snowflake' deposits are seen in the edges of the cornea.

Investigations

The finding of nodules or characteristic lesions of the skin or eyes in a patient from an endemic area, associated with eosinophilia, is suggestive. Skin snips or shavings, taken with a corneoscleral punch or scalpel blade from calf, buttock and shoulder, are placed in saline under a cover slip on a microscope slide and examined after 4 hours. Microfilariae are seen wriggling free in all but the lightest infections. Slit-lamp examination may reveal microfilariae moving in the anterior chamber of the eye or trapped in the cornea. A nodule may be removed and incised, showing the coiled, thread-like adult worm.

Filarial antibodies may be detected in up to 95% of patients. Several promising rapid strip tests based on antibody or antigen detection are under clinical evaluation. In patients with strong suspicion of onchocerciasis but negative tests, a provocative Mazzotti test, in which administration of 0.5–1.0 mg/kg of DEC exacerbates pruritus or dermatitis, strongly suggests onchocerciasis.

Management

Ivermectin, in a single dose of 100–200 µg/kg, repeated several times at 3-monthly intervals to prevent relapses, is recommended. It kills microfilariae, and is non-toxic and does not trigger severe reactions. In the rare event of a severe reaction causing oedema or postural hypotension, prednisolone 20–30 mg may be given daily for 2 or 3 days. Eradication of *Wolbachia* with doxycycline (100 mg daily for 6 weeks) prevents reproduction of the worm.

Prevention

Mass treatment with ivermectin is practised. It reduces morbidity in the community and prevents eye disease from getting worse. *Simulium* can be destroyed in its larval stage by the application of insecticide to streams. Long trousers, skirts and sleeves discourage the fly from biting.

Dracunculiasis (Guinea worm)

Infestation with the Guinea worm *Dracunculus medinensis* manifests itself when the female worm, over a metre long, emerges from the skin. Humans are infected by ingesting a small crustacean, *Cyclops*, which inhabits wells and ponds, and contains the infective larval stage of the worm. The worm was widely distributed across Africa and the Middle East but after a successful eradication programme is now seen only in sub-Saharan Africa.

Management and prevention

Traditionally, the protruding worm is extracted by winding it out gently over several days on a matchstick. The worm must never be broken. Antibiotics for secondary infection and prophylaxis of tetanus are also required.

A global elimination campaign is based on the provision of clean drinking water and eradication of water fleas from drinking water. The latter is being achieved by simple filtration of water through a plastic mesh filter and chemical treatment of water supplies.

13

Other filariases

Mansonella perstans

This filarial worm is transmitted by the midges *Culicoides austeni* and *C. grahami*. It is common throughout equatorial Africa as far south as Zambia, and also in Trinidad and parts of northern and eastern South America.

M. perstans has never been proven to cause disease but it may be responsible for a persistent eosinophilia and occasional allergic manifestations. *M. perstans* is resistant to ivermectin and DEC, and the infection may persist for many years.

Dirofilaria immitis

This dog heart worm infects humans, causing skin and lung lesions. It is not uncommon in the USA, Japan and Australia.

Zoonotic nematodes

Trichinosis (trichinellosis)

Trichinella spiralis is a nematode that parasitises rats and pigs, and is only transmitted to humans if they eat partially cooked infected pork, usually as sausage or ham. Bear meat is another source. Symptoms result from invasion of intestinal submucosa by ingested larvae, which develop into adult worms, and the secondary invasion of striated muscle by fresh larvae produced by these adult worms. Outbreaks have occurred in the UK, as well as in other countries where pork is eaten.

Clinical features

The clinical features of trichinosis are determined by the larval numbers. A light infection with a few worms may be asymptomatic; a heavy infection causes nausea and diarrhoea 24–48 hours after the infected meal. A few days later, the symptoms associated with larval invasion predominate: there is fever and oedema of the face, eyelids and conjunctivae; invasion of the diaphragm may cause pain, cough and dyspnoea; and involvement of the muscles of the limbs, chest and mouth causes stiffness, pain and tenderness in affected muscles. Larval migration may cause acute myocarditis and encephalitis. An eosinophilia is usually found after the 2nd week. An intense infection may prove fatal but those who survive recover completely.

Investigations

Commonly, a group of people who have eaten infected pork from a common source develop symptoms at about the same time. Biopsy from the deltoid or gastrocnemius after the 3rd week of symptoms in suspected cases may reveal encysted larvae. Serological tests are also helpful.

Management

Treatment is with albendazole 20 mg/kg daily for 7 days. Given early in the infection, this may kill newly formed adult worms in the submucosa and thus reduce the number of larvae reaching the muscles. Corticosteroids are necessary to control the serious effects of acute inflammation.

Cutaneous larva migrans (CLM)

CLM is the most common linear lesion seen in travellers (Fig. 13.49). Intensely pruritic, linear, serpiginous lesions

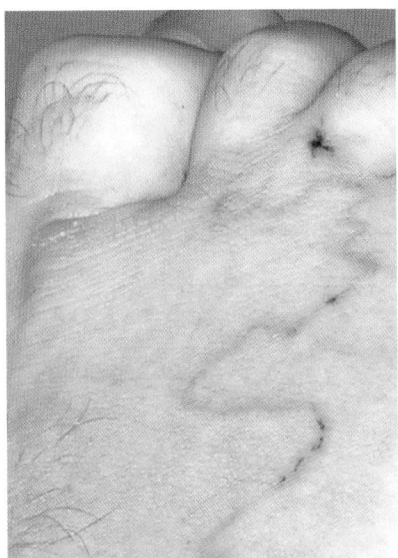

Fig. 13.49 Cutaneous larva migrans.

result from the larval migration of the dog hookworm (*Ancylostoma caninum*). The track moves across the skin at a rate of 2–3 cm/day. This contrasts with the rash of *Strongyloides* (p. 365), which is fast-moving and transient. Although the larvae of dog hookworms frequently infect humans, they do not usually develop into the adult form. The most common site for CLM is the foot but elbows, breasts and buttocks may be affected. Most patients with CLM have recently visited a beach where the affected part was exposed. The diagnosis is clinical. Treatment may be local with 12-hourly application of 15% thiabendazole cream, or systemic with a single dose of albendazole (400 mg) or ivermectin (150–200 µg/kg).

Trematodes (flukes)

These leaf-shaped worms are parasitic to humans and animals. Their complex life cycles may involve one or more intermediate hosts, often freshwater molluscs.

Schistosomiasis

Schistosomiasis is one of the most important causes of morbidity in the tropics. There are five species of the genus *Schistosoma* which commonly cause disease in humans: *S. haematobium*, *S. mansoni*, *S. japonicum*, *S. mekongi* and *S. intercalatum*. *S. haematobium* was discovered by Theodor Bilharz in Cairo in 1861 and the disease is sometimes called bilharzia or bilharziasis. Schistosome eggs have been found in Egyptian mummies dated 1250 BC.

The life cycle is shown in Figure 13.50A. The ovum is passed in the urine or faeces of infected individuals and gains access to fresh water, where the ciliated miracidium inside it is liberated; it enters its intermediate host, a species of freshwater snail, in which it multiplies. Large numbers of fork-tailed cercariae are then liberated into the water, where they may survive for 2–3 days. Cercariae can penetrate the skin or the mucous membrane of the mouth of humans. They transform into schistosomulae and moult as they pass through the lungs; thence they are carried by the blood stream to the liver, and so to the portal vein, where they mature. The

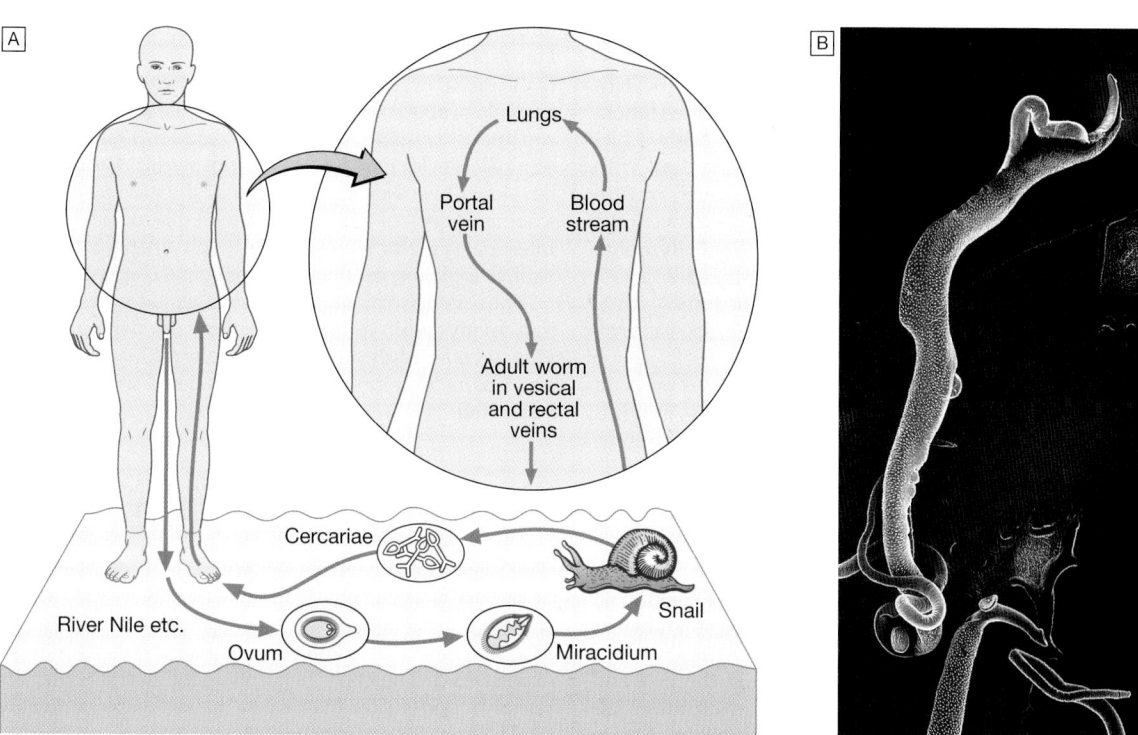

Fig. 13.50 *Schistosoma.* [A] Life cycle. [B] Scanning electron micrograph of adult schistosome worms showing the larger male worm embracing the thinner female.

male worm is up to 20 mm in length and the more slender cylindrical female, usually enfolded longitudinally by the male, is rather longer (Fig. 13.50B). Within 4–6 weeks of infection they migrate to the venules draining the pelvic viscera, where the females deposit ova.

Pathology

This depends on the species and the stage of infection (Box 13.65). Most disease is due to the passage of eggs through mucosa and to the granulomatous reaction to eggs deposited in tissues. The eggs of *S. haematobium* pass mainly through the wall of the bladder, but may also involve rectum, seminal vesicles, vagina, cervix and uterine tubes. *S. mansoni* and *S. japonicum* eggs pass mainly through the wall of the lower bowel or are carried to the liver. The most serious, although rare, site of ectopic deposition of eggs is in the CNS. Granulomas are composed of macrophages, eosinophils, and epithelioid and giant cells around an ovum. Later there is fibrosis and eggs calcify, often in sufficient numbers to become radiologically visible. Eggs of *S. haematobium* may leave the vesical plexus and be carried directly to the lung. Those of *S. mansoni* and *S. japonicum* may also reach the lungs after the development of portal hypertension and consequent portasystemic collateral circulation. In both circumstances egg deposition in the pulmonary vasculature, and the resultant host response, can lead to the development of pulmonary hypertension.

Clinical features

Recent travellers, especially those overlanding through Africa, may present with allergic manifestations and eosinophilia; residents of schistosomiasis-endemic areas

13.65 Pathogenesis of schistosomiasis

Time	*S. haematobium*	*S. mansoni* and *S. japonicum*
Cercarial penetration		
Days	Papular dermatitis at site of penetration	As for *S. haematobium*
Larval migration and maturation		
Weeks	Pneumonitis, myositis, hepatitis, fever, 'serum sickness', eosinophilia, seroconversion	As for *S. haematobium*
Early egg deposition		
Months	Cystitis, haematuria	Colitis, granulomatous hepatitis, acute portal hypertension
	Ectopic granulomatous lesions: skin, CNS etc. Immune complex glomerulonephritis	As for *S. haematobium*
Late egg deposition		
Years	Fibrosis and calcification of ureters, bladder: bacterial infection, calculi, hydronephrosis, carcinoma	Colonic polyposis and strictures, periportal fibrosis, portal hypertension
	Pulmonary granulomas and pulmonary hypertension	As for *S. haematobium*

are more likely to present with chronic urinary tract pathology or portal hypertension.

During the early stages of infection there may be itching lasting 1–2 days at the site of cercarial penetration. After a symptom-free period of 3–5 weeks, acute schistosomiasis (Katayama syndrome) may present with allergic manifestations such as urticaria, fever, muscle aches, abdominal pain, headaches, cough and sweating. On examination hepatomegaly, splenomegaly, lymphadenopathy and pneumonia may be present. These allergic phenomena may be severe in infections with *S. mansoni* and *S. japonicum*, but are rare with *S. haematobium*. The features subside after 1–2 weeks.

Chronic schistosomiasis is due to egg deposition and occurs months to years after infection. The symptoms and signs depend upon the intensity of infection and the species of infecting schistosome (see Box 13.65).

Schistosoma haematobium

Humans are the only natural hosts of *S. haematobium*, which is highly endemic in Egypt and East Africa, and occurs throughout Africa and the Middle East (Fig. 13.51). Infection can be acquired after a brief exposure, such as swimming in freshwater lakes in Africa.

Painless terminal haematuria is usually the first and most common symptom. Frequency of micturition follows, due to bladder neck obstruction. Later the disease may be complicated by frequent urinary tract infections, bladder or ureteric stone formation, hydronephrosis, and ultimately renal failure with a contracted calcified bladder. Pain is often felt in the iliac fossa or in the loin, and radiates to the groin. In several endemic areas there is a strong epidemiological association of *S. haematobium* infection with squamous cell carcinoma of the bladder. Disease of the seminal vesicles may lead to haemospermia. Females may develop schistosomal papillomas of the vulva, and schistosomal lesions of the cervix may be mistaken for cancer. Intestinal symptoms may follow involvement of the bowel wall. Ectopic worms cause skin or spinal cord lesions.

The severity of *S. haematobium* infection varies greatly, and many with a light infection are asymptomatic. However, as adult worms can live for 20 years or more and lesions may progress, these patients should always be treated.

Schistosoma mansoni

S. mansoni is endemic throughout Africa, the Middle East, Venezuela, Brazil and the Caribbean (see Fig. 13.51).

Characteristic symptoms begin 2 months or more after infection. They may be slight, no more than malaise, or consist of abdominal pain and frequent stools which contain blood-stained mucus. With severe advanced disease, increased discomfort from rectal polyps may be experienced. The early hepatomegaly is reversible, but portal hypertension may cause massive splenomegaly, fatal haematemesis from oesophageal varices, or progressive ascites (p. 945). Liver function is initially preserved because the pathology is fibrotic rather than cirrhotic.

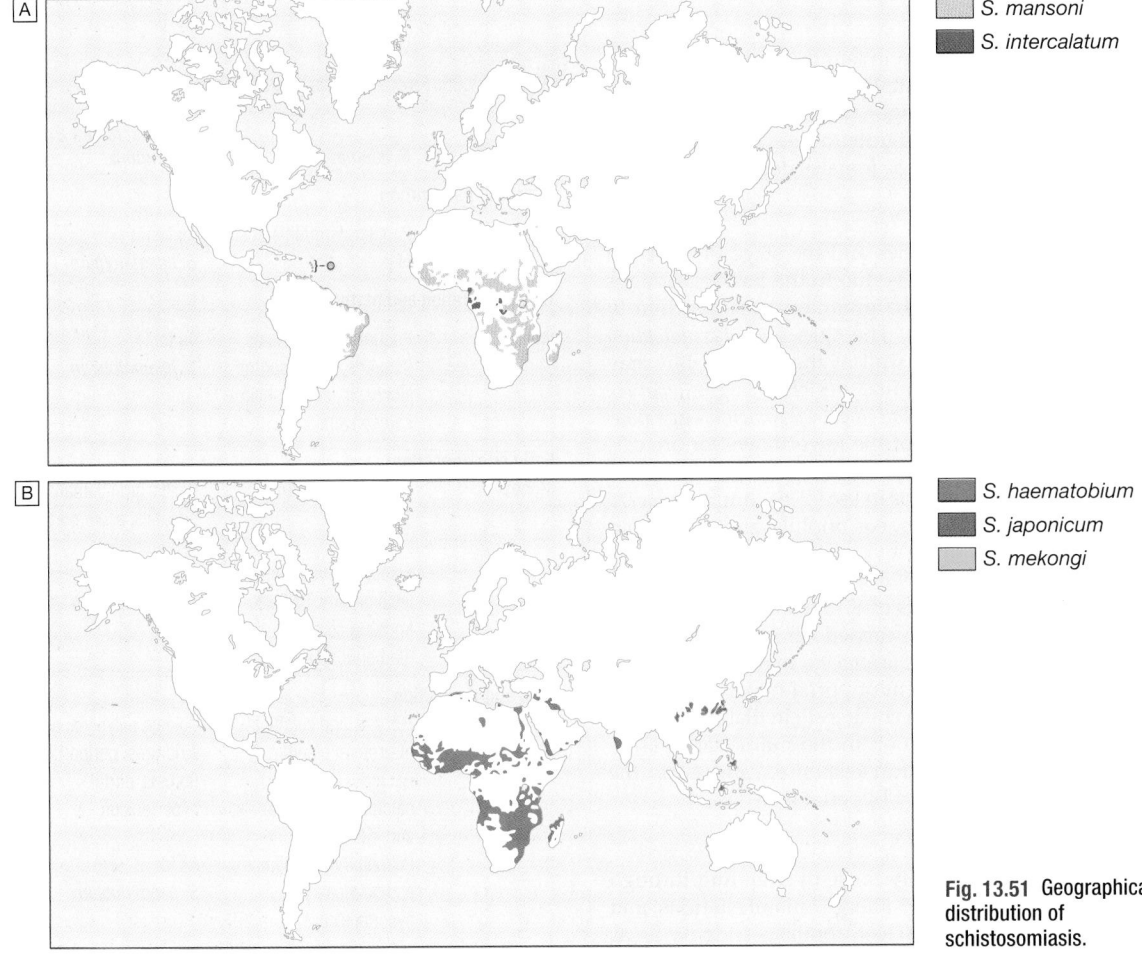

A
- S. mansoni
- S. intercalatum

B
- S. haematobium
- S. japonicum
- S. mekongi

Fig. 13.51 Geographical distribution of schistosomiasis.

S. mansoni and other schistosoma infections predispose to the carriage of *Salmonella*, in part because *Salmonella* may attach to the schistosomes and in part because shared antigens on schistosomes may induce immunological tolerance to *Salmonella*.

Schistosoma japonicum, S. mekongi and S. intercalatum

In addition to humans, the adult worm of *S. japonicum* infects the dog, rat, field mouse, water buffalo, ox, cat, pig, horse and sheep. Although other *Schistosoma* spp. can infect species other than humans, the non-human reservoir seems to be particularly important in transmission for *S. japonicum* but not for *S. haematobium* or *S. mansoni*. *S. japonicum* is prevalent in the Yellow River and Yangtze–Jiang basins in China, where the infection is a major public health problem. It also has a focal distribution in the Philippines, Indonesia and Thailand (see Fig. 13.51). The related *S. mekongi* occurs in Laos, Thailand and Myanmar, and *S. intercalatum* in West and Central Africa.

The pathology of *S. japonicum* is similar to that of *S. mansoni*, but as this worm produces more eggs, the lesions tend to be more extensive and widespread. The clinical features resemble those of severe infection with *S. mansoni*, with added neurological features. The small and large bowel may be affected, and hepatic fibrosis with splenic enlargement is usual. Deposition of eggs or worms in the CNS, especially in the brain or spinal cord, causes symptoms in about 5% of infections, notably epilepsy, blindness, hemiplegia or paraplegia.

Investigations

There is marked eosinophilia. Serological tests (ELISA) are useful as screening tests but remain positive after chemotherapeutic cure.

In *S. haematobium* infection, dipstick urine testing shows blood and albumin. The eggs can be found by microscopic examination of the centrifuged deposit of terminal stream urine Fig. 13.52. Ultrasound is useful for assessing the urinary tract; bladder wall thickening, hydronephrosis and bladder calcification can be detected. Cystoscopy reveals 'sandy' patches, bleeding mucosa and later distortion.

In a heavy infection with *S. mansoni* or *S. japonicum* the characteristic egg with its lateral spine can usu-

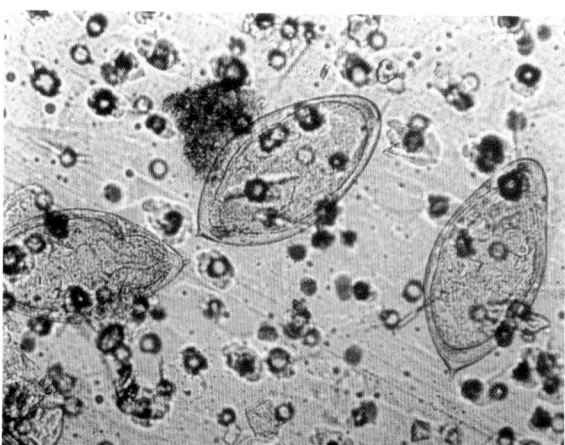

Fig. 13.52 Ova of *Schistosoma haematobium* in urine. Note the terminal spike.

ally be found in the stool. When the infection is light or of long duration, a rectal biopsy can be examined. Sigmoidoscopy may show inflammation or bleeding. Biopsies should be examined for ova.

Management

The object of specific treatment is to kill the adult schistosomes and so stop egg-laying. Praziquantel is the drug of choice for all forms of schistosomiasis. The drug produces parasitological cure in 80% of treated individuals and over 90% reduction in egg counts in the remainder. Side-effects are uncommon but include nausea and abdominal pain. Praziquantel therapy in early infection reverses pathologies such as hepatomegaly and bladder wall thickening and granulomas.

Surgery may be required to deal with residual lesions such as ureteric stricture, small fibrotic urinary bladders, or granulomatous masses in the brain or spinal cord. Removal of rectal papillomas by diathermy or by other means may provide symptomatic relief.

Prevention

So far no satisfactory single means of controlling schistosomiasis has been established. The life cycle is terminated if the ova in urine or faeces are not allowed to contaminate fresh water containing the snail host. The provision of latrines and of a safe water supply, however, remains a major problem in rural areas throughout the tropics. Furthermore, *S. japonicum* has so many hosts besides humans that latrines would be of little avail. Annual mass treatment of the population helps against *S. haematobium* and *S. mansoni*, but this method has so far had little success with *S. japonicum*. Attack on the intermediate host, the snail, presents many difficulties and has not on its own proved successful on any scale. For personal protection, contact with infected water must be avoided.

Liver flukes

Liver flukes infect at least 20 million people and remain an important public health problem in many endemic areas. They are associated with abdominal pain, hepatomegaly and relapsing cholangitis. *Clonorchis sinensis* is a major aetiological agent of bile duct cancer. The three major liver flukes have similar life cycles and pathologies, as outlined in Box 13.66.

Other flukes of medical importance include lung and intestinal flukes (see Box 13.62, p. 364).

Cestodes (tapeworms)

Cestodes are ribbon-shaped worms which inhabit the intestinal tract. They have no alimentary system and absorb nutrients through the tegumental surface. The anterior end, or scolex, has suckers for attaching to the host. From the scolex arises a series of progressively developing segments, the proglottides, which, when shed, may continue to show active movements. Cross-fertilisation takes place between segments. Ova, present in large numbers in mature proglottides, remain viable for weeks and during this period they may be consumed by the intermediate host. Larvae liberated from the ingested ova pass into the tissues, forming larval cysticerci.

Tapeworms cause two distinct patterns of disease, either intestinal infection or systemic cysticercosis (Fig. 13.53).

ℹ **13.66 Diseases caused by flukes in the bile duct**

	Clonorchiasis	Opisthorchiasis	Fascioliasis
Parasite	*Clonorchis sinensis*	*Opisthorchis felineus*	*Fasciola hepatica*
Other mammalian hosts	Dogs, cats, pigs	Dogs, cats, foxes, pigs	Sheep, cattle
Mode of spread	Ova in faeces, water	As for *C. sinensis*	Ova in faeces on to wet pasture
1st intermediate host	Snails	Snails	Snails
2nd intermediate host	Freshwater fish	Freshwater fish	Encysts on vegetation
Geographical distribution	Far East, especially S. China	Far East, especially NE Thailand	Cosmopolitan, including UK
Pathology	*E. coli* cholangitis, abscesses, biliary carcinoma	As for *C. sinensis*	Toxaemia, cholangitis, eosinophilia
Symptoms	Often symptom-free, recurrent jaundice	As for *C. sinensis*	Unexplained fever, tender liver, may be ectopic, e.g. subcutaneous fluke
Diagnosis	Ova in stool or duodenal aspirate	As for *C. sinensis*	As for *C. sinensis*, also serology
Prevention	Cook fish	Cook fish	Avoid contaminated watercress
Treatment	Praziquantel 25 mg/kg 8-hourly for 2 days	As for *C. sinensis* but for 1 day only	Triclabendazole 10 mg/kg single dose; repeat treatment may be required*

*In the UK, available from the Hospital for Tropical Diseases, London.

Taenia saginata (beef tapeworm) and *Diphyllobothrium latum* (fish tapeworm) cause only intestinal infection, following human ingestion of intermediate hosts that contain cysticerci (the larval stage of the tapeworm). *Taenia solium* causes intestinal infection if a cysticerci-containing intermediate host is ingested, and cysticercosis (systemic infection from larval migration) if ova are ingested. *Echinococcus granulosus* (dog tapeworm) does not cause human intestinal infection, but causes hydatid disease (which is analogous to cysticercosis) following ingestion of ova and subsequent larval migration.

Intestinal tapeworm

Humans acquire tapeworm by eating undercooked beef infected with the larval stage of *T. saginata*, undercooked pork containing the larval stage of *T. solium*, or undercooked freshwater fish containing larvae of *D. latum*. Usually only one adult tapeworm is present in the gut but up to ten have been reported. The ova of *T. saginata* and *T. solium* are indistinguishable microscopically. However, examination of scolex and proglottides can differentiate between them. *T. solium* has a rostellum and two rows of hooklets on the scolex, and discharges multiple proglottides (3–5) attached together with lower degrees of uterine branching (approximately 10); *T. saginata* has only four suckers in its scolex, and discharges single proglottids with greater uterine branching (up to 30).

Taenia saginata

Infection with *T. saginata* occurs in all parts of the world. The adult worm may be several metres long and produces little or no intestinal upset in human beings, but knowledge of its presence, by noting segments in the faeces or on underclothing, may distress the patient. Ova may be found in the stool. Praziquantel is the drug of choice; niclosamide or nitazoxanide are alternatives. Prevention depends on efficient meat inspection and the thorough cooking of beef.

Taenia solium

T. solium, the pork tapeworm, is common in central Europe, South Africa, South America and parts of Asia. It is not as large as *T. saginata*. The adult worm is found

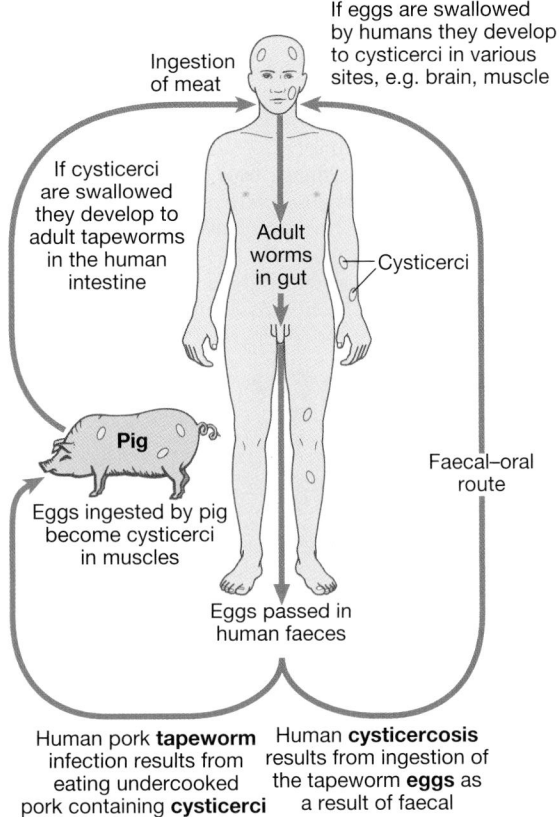

If eggs are swallowed by humans they develop to cysticerci in various sites, e.g. brain, muscle

Ingestion of meat

If cysticerci are swallowed they develop to adult tapeworms in the human intestine

Adult worms in gut — Cysticerci

Pig

Eggs ingested by pig become cysticerci in muscles

Eggs passed in human faeces

Faecal–oral route

Human pork **tapeworm** infection results from eating undercooked pork containing **cysticerci**

Human **cysticercosis** results from ingestion of the tapeworm **eggs** as a result of faecal contamination of food

Fig. 13.53 Cysticercosis. Life cycle of *Taenia solium*.

only in humans following the eating of undercooked pork containing cysticerci. Niclosamide, followed by a mild laxative (after 1–2 hours) to prevent retrograde intestinal autoinfection, is effective for intestinal infection. Cooking pork well prevents intestinal infection. Great care must be taken by nurses and other adults while attending a patient harbouring an adult worm to avoid ingestion of ova or segments.

Cysticercosis

Human cysticercosis is acquired by ingesting *T. solium* tapeworm ova, from either contaminated fingers or food (see Fig. 13.53). The larvae are liberated from eggs in the stomach, penetrate the intestinal mucosa and are carried to many parts of the body where they develop and form cysticerci, 0.5–1 cm cysts that contain the head of a young worm. They do not grow further or migrate. Common locations are the subcutaneous tissue, skeletal muscles and brain.

Clinical features

When superficially placed, cysts can be palpated under the skin or mucosa as pea-like ovoid bodies. Here they cause few or no symptoms, and will eventually die and become calcified.

Heavy brain infections, especially in children, may cause features of encephalitis. More commonly, however, cerebral signs do not occur until the larvae die, 5–20 years later. Epilepsy, personality changes, staggering gait or signs of hydrocephalus are the most common features.

Investigations

Calcified cysts in muscles can be recognised radiologically. In the brain, however, less calcification takes place and larvae are only occasionally visible by plain X-ray; usually CT or MRI will show them. Epileptic fits starting in adult life suggest the possibility of cysticercosis if the patient has lived in or travelled to an endemic area. The subcutaneous tissue should be palpated and any nodule excised for histology. Radiological examination of the skeletal muscles may be helpful. Antibody detection is available for serodiagnosis.

Management and prevention

Albendazole, 15 mg/kg daily for a minimum of 8 days, has now become the drug of choice for parenchymal neurocysticercosis. Praziquantel is another option, 50 mg/kg in three divided doses daily for 10 days. Prednisolone, 10 mg 8-hourly, is also given for 14 days, starting 1 day before the albendazole or praziquantel. In addition, anti-epileptic drugs should be given until the reaction in the brain has subsided. Operative intervention is indicated for hydrocephalus. Studies from India and Peru suggest that most small solitary cerebral cysts will resolve without treatment.

Echinococcus granulosus (Taenia echinococcus) and hydatid disease

Dogs are the definitive hosts of the tiny tapeworm *E. granulosus*. The larval stage, a hydatid cyst, normally occurs in sheep, cattle, camels and other animals that are infected from contaminated pastures or water. By handling a dog or drinking contaminated water, humans may ingest eggs (Fig. 13.54). The embryo is liberated from the ovum in the small intestine and gains access to the blood stream and thus to the liver. The resultant cyst grows very slowly, sometimes intermittently. It is composed of an enveloping fibrous

13

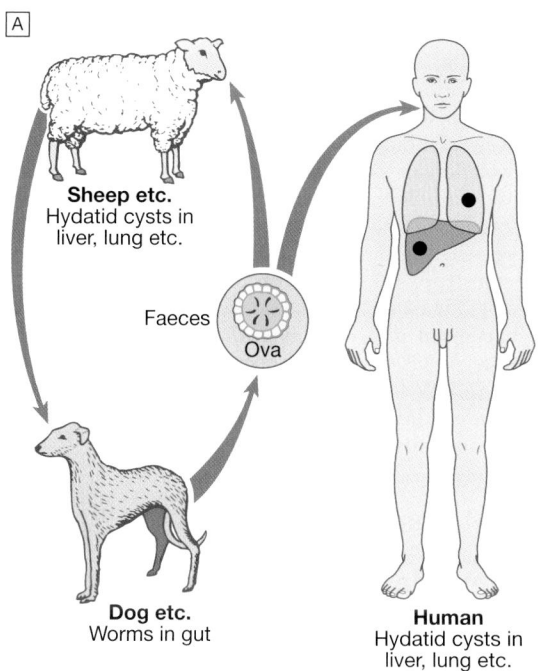

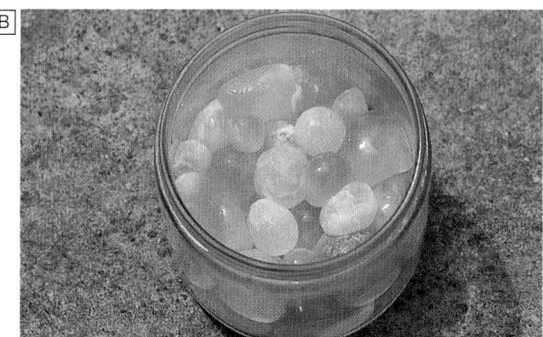

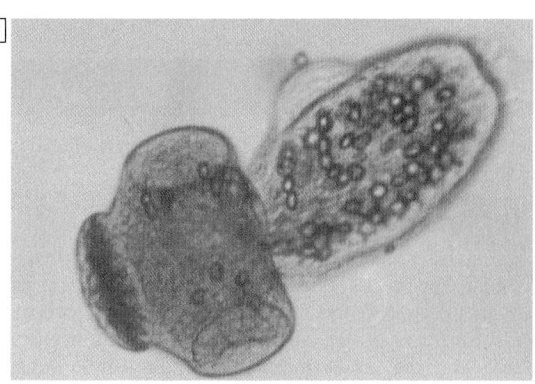

Fig. 13.54 Hydatid disease. A Life cycle of *Echinococcus granulosus*. B Daughter cysts removed at surgery. C Within the daughter cysts are the protoscolices.

pericyst, laminated hyaline membrane (ectocyst) and inner germinal layers (endocyst) which gives rise to daughter cysts, or germinating cystic brood capsule in which larvae (protoscolices) develop. Over time some cysts may calcify and become non-viable. The disease is common in the Middle East, North and East Africa, Australia and Argentina. Foci of infection persist in rural Wales and Scotland. *E. multilocularis*, which has a cycle between foxes and voles, causes a similar but more severe infection, 'alveolar hydatid disease', which invades the liver like cancer.

Clinical features

A hydatid cyst is typically acquired in childhood and may, after growing for some years, cause pressure symptoms. These vary, depending on the organ or tissue involved. In nearly 75% of patients with hydatid disease the right lobe of the liver is invaded and contains a single cyst (p. 972). In others a cyst may be found in lung, bone, brain or elsewhere.

Investigations

The diagnosis depends on the clinical, radiological and ultrasound findings in a patient who has lived in close contact with dogs in an endemic area. Complement fixation and ELISA are positive in 70–90% of patients.

Management and prevention

Hydatid cysts should be excised wherever possible. Great care is taken to avoid spillage and cavities are sterilised with 0.5% silver nitrate or 2.7% sodium chloride. Albendazole (400 mg 12-hourly for 3 months) should also be used. The drug is now often combined with PAIR (**p**ercutaneous puncture, **a**spiration, **i**njection of scolicidal agent and **r**e-aspiration) to good effect. Praziquantel 20 mg/kg 12-hourly for 14 days also kills protoscolices perioperatively.

Prevention is difficult in situations where there is a close association with dogs and sheep. Personal hygiene, satisfactory disposal of carcasses, meat inspection and deworming of dogs can greatly reduce the prevalence of disease.

Other tapeworms

There are many other cestodes whose adult or larval stages may infect humans. Sparganosis is a condition in which an immature worm develops in humans, usually subcutaneously, as a result of eating or applying to the skin the secondary or tertiary intermediate host.

ECTOPARASITES

Ectoparasites only interact with the outermost surfaces of the host; see also pages 1273–1274

Jiggers (tungiasis)

This is widespread in tropical America and Africa, and is caused by the sand flea *Tunga penetrans*. The pregnant flea burrows into the skin around toes and produces large numbers of eggs. The burrows are intensely irritating and the whole inflammatory nodule should be removed with a sterile needle. Secondary infection of tunga lesions is common.

Myiasis

Myiasis is due to skin infestation with larvae of the South American botfly, *Dermatobia hominis*, or the African Tumbu fly, *Cordylobia anthropophaga*. The larvae develop in a subcutaneous space with a central sinus. This orifice is the air source for the larvae, and periodically the larval respiratory spiracles protrude through the sinus. Patients with myiasis feel movement within the larval burrow and can experience intermittent sharp, lancinating pains. Myiasis is diagnosed clinically and should be suspected with any furuncular lesion accompanied by pain and a crawling sensation in the skin. The larva may be suffocated by blocking the respiratory orifice with petroleum jelly and gently removing it with tweezers. Secondary infection of myiasis is remarkably infrequent and rapid healing follows removal of intact larvae.

FUNGAL INFECTIONS

Fungal infections, or mycoses, are classified as superficial, subcutaneous or systemic (deep), depending on the degree of invasion of the host. They are also classified by the kind of fungus which causes the infection, which may be a filamentous fungus (mould) or a yeast, or may vary between these two forms depending on the environmental conditions (dimorphic fungi; Fig. 13.55).

Superficial mycoses

Superficial cutaneous fungal infections caused by dermatophyte fungi are described in Chapter 27.

Candidiasis (thrush)

Superficial candidiasis is caused by *Candida* spp. yeasts (mainly *C. albicans*). Common disease manifestations include oropharyngeal (pp. 863 and 392) and vaginal candidiasis ('thrush'), intertrigo and chronic paronychia. Oral and vaginal thrush often follow treatment with broad-spectrum antibiotics. Intertrigo is characterised by inflammation in skin folds with surrounding 'satellite lesions'. Chronic paronychia is associated with occupations involving frequent wetting of the hands. Treatment of superficial candidiasis is mainly with topical antifungal azoles (pp. 157–158), with oral azoles reserved for refractory or recurrent disease (mainly thrush). Severe oropharyngeal and oesophageal candidiasis is a consequence of CD4+ T lymphocyte depletion/dysfunction, as in HIV infection (p. 392), and recurrent vaginal or penile candidiasis may be an early manifestation of diabetes mellitus.

Subcutaneous mycoses

Chromoblastomycosis

Chromoblastomycosis is a predominantly tropical or subtropical fungal disease caused by environmental dematiaceous (dark-pigmented) fungi, most commonly *Fonsecaea pedrosoi*. Other causes include *F. compacta*, *Cladophialophora carrionii* and *Phialophora verrucosa*. The disease is a cutaneous/subcutaneous mycosis acquired by traumatic inoculation. Consequently, the most

Filamentous fungi (moulds)	Dimorphic fungi	Yeasts

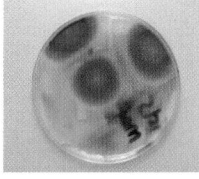 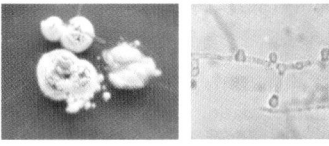 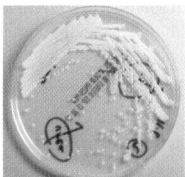

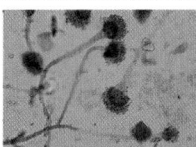 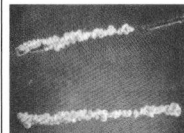 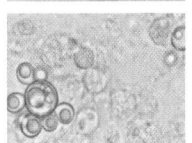 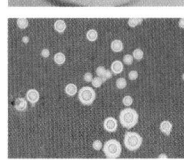

Characterised by the production of elongated, cylindrical, often septate cells (hyphae) and conidia (spores)	Exist in filamentous (top) or yeast (bottom) form, depending on environmental conditions	Characterised by the production of oval or round cells, which reproduce by binary fission (budding)
Examples: • *Aspergillus* spp. (*A. fumigatus* shown here) • *Fusarium* spp. • Dermatophyte fungi (*Tricophyton* spp., *Microsporum* spp. etc.) • Mucorales	Examples: • *Histoplasma capsulatum, Coccidioides immitis, Paracoccidioides brasiliensis* (shown here), *Blastomyces dermatidis* • *Sporothrix schenkii* • *Penicillium marneffei* • *Malassezia* spp.	Examples: • *Candida* spp.* • *Cryptococcus* spp. (*C. neoformans* shown here)

13

Fig. 13.55 Classification of medically important fungi. Fungal classification is based on simple morphological characteristics. *Pneumocystis jirovecii* (*carinii*) is morphologically distinct from other fungi and does not fit into this classification. *Candida albicans* is capable of hypha production and therefore is technically 'dimorphic'. However, in this classification scheme, 'dimorphic' is reserved for fungi for which transformation from hypha to yeast is associated with infection.

commonly affected areas are the foot, ankle and lower leg. Lesions may start several months after the initial injury, and medical attention is often sought several years later. The initial lesion is a papule. Further papules develop, and coalesce to form irregular plaques. Nodular lesions may produce a characteristic 'cauliflower' appearance.

Diagnosis is by histopathological examination of infected material, which shows dematiaceous, rounded, thick-walled 'sclerotic bodies' with septa at right angles to each other. The aetiological agent is confirmed by culture. Many therapeutic approaches have been explored, including antifungal agents, cryosurgery and surgical excision, alone or in combination, but the optimal therapy is unknown. Of the antifungal agents, itraconazole and terbinafine are considered to be the most effective. However, posaconazole has also been used with a good outcome.

Mycetoma

Mycetoma is a chronic suppurative infection of the deep soft tissues and bones, most commonly of the limbs but also of the abdominal or chest wall or head. It is caused by either aerobic or anaerobic branching Gram-positive bacilli, *Actinomycetales* (actinomycetoma—60%), or by true fungi, Eumycetes (eumycetoma—40%). Many fungi cause eumycetomas, the most common being *Madurella mycetomatis, M. grisea, Leptosphaera senegalensis* and *Scedosporium apiospermum*. Actinomycetomas are caused by *Actinomadura, Nocardia* and *Streptomyces* spp. Both groups produce characteristically coloured grains, the colour depending on the organism (black grains—eumycetoma, red and yellow grains—actinomycetoma,

white grains—either). The disease occurs mostly in the tropics and subtropics.

Clinical features

The disease is acquired by inoculation (e.g. from a thorn) and most commonly affects the foot (Madura foot). The mycetoma begins as a painless swelling at the site of implantation, which grows and spreads steadily within the soft tissues, causing further swelling and eventually penetrating bones. Nodules develop under the epidermis and these rupture, revealing sinuses through which grains (*Actinomycete*/fungal colonies) may be discharged. Some sinuses may heal with scarring while fresh sinuses appear elsewhere. Deeper tissue invasion and involvement of bone are rapid and greater in actinomycetoma than eumycetoma. There is little pain and usually no fever or lymphadenopathy, but there is progressive disability.

Investigations

Diagnosis is confirmed by demonstration of fungal grains in pus, and/or histopathological examination of tissue. Culture is necessary for species identification and (for actinomycetoma) susceptibility testing. Serological tests are not available.

Management

Eumycetoma is generally treated with surgery plus antifungal therapy, and actinomycetoma with antibacterial therapy alone. Antifungal therapy for eumycetoma depends on the specific fungus isolated. Itraconazole and ketoconazole (both 200–400mg/day) are used commonly, and success has also been reported with voriconazole and posaconazole. Therapy is continued for 6–12 months. In extreme cases amputation may be required.

In general actinomycetoma is treated with co-trimoxazole for several months. Disease caused by *Nocardia* spp. is treated with dapsone plus co-trimoxazole. In extensive disease amikacin or netilmicin may be added. Other agents, including minocycline, co-amoxiclav, streptomycin, imipenem and rifampicin, have been used successfully.

Phaeohyphomycosis

Phaeohyphomycosis is a heterogenous group of fungal diseases caused by a large number (> 70) of dematiaceous fungi. In phaeohyphomycosis the tissue form of the fungus is predominantly mycelial (filamentous), as opposed to eumycetoma (grain) or chromoblastomycosis (sclerotic body). Disease may be superficial, subcutaneous or deep. The most serious manifestation is cerebral phaeohyphomycosis, which presents with a ring-enhancing, space-occupying cerebral lesion. Optimal therapy for this condition has not been established, but treatment usually consists of neurosurgical intervention and antifungal (usually triazole) therapy. Causative agents are *Cladophialophora bantiana*, *Fonsecaea* spp. and *Rhinocladiella* (formerly *Ramichloridium*) *mackenziei*, which occurs in the Middle East and is usually fatal.

Sporotrichosis

Sporotrichosis is caused by *Sporothrix schenckii*, a dimorphic fungal saprophyte of plants in tropical and subtropical regions. Disease is caused by accidental dermal inoculation of the fungus, usually from a thorn (occasionally from a cat scratch). In fixed cutaneous sporotrichosis a subcutaneous nodule develops at the site of infection and subsequently ulcerates, with a purulent discharge. The disease may then spread along the cutaneous lymphatic channels, resulting in multiple cutaneous nodules along their route, which ulcerate and discharge (lymphocutaneous sporotrichosis). Rarer forms of disease are seen, for example, in patients with cutaneous disease presenting with arthritis. Later, draining sinuses may form. Pulmonary sporotrichosis occurs as a result of inhalation of the conidia and manifests itself as chronic cavitary fibronodular disease with haemoptysis and constitutional symptoms. Disseminated disease may occur, especially in patients with HIV.

Investigations

Typical yeast forms detected on histology of the biopsy confirm the diagnosis but are rarely seen; the fungus can be grown from the specimen in culture. A latex agglutination test is available to detect *S. schenkii* antibodies in serum.

Management

Cutaneous and lymphocutaneous disease is treated with oral itraconazole (200–400 mg daily, best absorbed as the oral solution formulation) for 3–6 months. Alternative agents include a saturated solution of potassium iodide (SSKI, given orally), initiated with 5 drops and increased to 40–50 drops 8-hourly, or terbinafine (500 mg 12-hourly). Localised hyperthermia may be used in pregnancy (to avoid azole use). Osteoarticular disease requires a longer course of therapy (≥ 12 months). Severe

or life-threatening disease is treated with amphotericin B (lipid formulation preferred).

Systemic mycoses

Aspergillosis

Aspergillosis is an opportunistic systemic mycosis, which affects predominantly the respiratory tract. It is described on page 696.

Candidiasis

Systemic candidiasis is an opportunistic mycosis caused by *Candida* spp. The most common cause is *C. albicans*. Other agents include *C. dubliniensis*, *C. glabrata*, *C. krusei*, *C. parapsilosis* and *C. tropicalis*. Species distribution varies geographically. *Candida* species identification often enables prediction of susceptibility to fluconazole; *C. krusei* is universally resistant, many *C. glabrata* isolates are either 'susceptible-dose dependent' (S-DD) or resistant, and other species are mostly susceptible. Candidiasis is usually an endogenous disease that originates from oropharyngeal, genitourinary or skin colonisation, although nosocomial spread has been reported.

Syndromes of systemic candidiasis

Acute disseminated candidiasis

This usually presents as candidaemia (isolation of *Candida* spp. from the blood). The main predisposing factor is the presence of a central venous catheter. Other major factors include recent abdominal surgery, total parenteral nutrition (TPN), recent antibiotic therapy and localised *Candida* colonisation. Up to 40% of cases will have ophthalmic involvement, with characteristic retinal 'cotton wool' exudates. As this is a sight-threatening condition, candidaemic patients should be assessed by detailed ophthalmoscopy. Skin lesions (non-tender pink/red nodules) may be seen. Although predominantly a disease of intensive care and surgical patients, acute disseminated candidiasis and/or *Candida* endophthalmitis is seen occasionally in injection drug-users, thought to be due to candidal contamination of citric acid or lemon juice used to dissolve heroin.

Chronic disseminated candidiasis (CDC, hepatosplenic candidiasis)

In this condition a neutropenic patient has a persistent fever despite antibacterial therapy. The fever persists despite neutrophil recovery, and is associated with the development of abdominal pain, raised alkaline phosphatase and multiple lesions in abdominal organs (e.g. liver, spleen and/or kidneys) on radiological imaging. CDC may represent an immune reconstitution inflammatory syndrome (IRIS, p. 136), and usually lasts for several months despite appropriate therapy.

Other manifestations

Renal tract candidiasis, osteomyelitis, septic arthritis, peritonitis, meningitis and endocarditis are all well recognised, and are usually sequelae of acute disseminated disease. Diagnosis and treatment of these conditions require specialist mycological advice.

Management

Blood cultures positive for *Candida* spp. must never be ignored. Acute disseminated candidiasis is treated with antifungal therapy, removal of any in-dwelling central venous catheter (whether known to be the source of infection or not) and removal of any known source. Initial therapy is usually with fluconazole, unless the patient has recently received this agent, is known to be colonised with a resistant *Candida* strain, or is considered to be unstable (i.e. exhibiting signs of sepsis); in this case, an echinocandin (p. 158) is preferred. Therapy is adjusted according to clinical response, species involved and susceptibility testing, and continues for at least 14 days. Other appropriate therapies include voriconazole and amphotericin B formulations.

CDC is treated with fluconazole or other agents, depending on species and clinical response, and is prolonged (several months). There is some evidence that duration may be reduced by adjuvant therapy with systemic corticosteroids.

Cryptococcosis

Cryptococcosis is an opportunistic systemic mycosis caused by two environmental yeast species, *Cr. neoformans* and *Cr. gattii*. *Cr. neoformans* is distributed worldwide and causes opportunistic disease associated with many immunosuppressed states, predominantly HIV infection (p. 400). *Cr. gattii* is a primary pathogen, mainly of the tropics and subtropics.

Although the disease is acquired by inhalation of yeasts, isolated pulmonary disease is rare. The fungus may disseminate to any organ, most commonly the CNS (cryptococcal meningitis/cryptococcoma; Fig. 13.56) and skin. Cryptococcal meningitis is characterised by an indolent presentation with headache and visual loss. CSF is predominantly lymphocytic, although there may be few or no white blood cells, and frequently an elevated

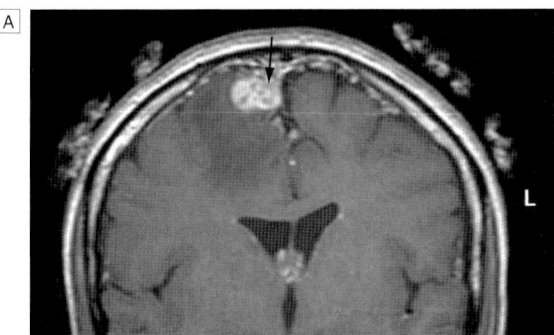

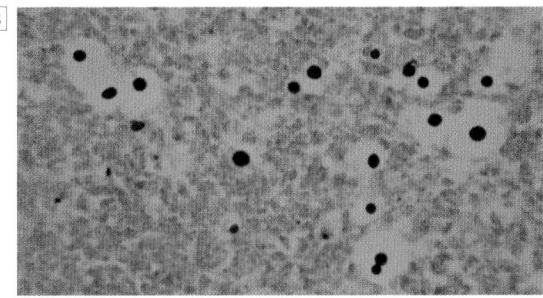

Fig. 13.56 Cryptococcal disease. A 23-year-old HIV-positive male developed headache and left-sided weakness. **A** MRI scan of the brain showed a space-occupying lesion (arrow) with surrounding oedema. **B** Histopathological examination of the lesion stained with Grocott's silver stain showed encapsulated yeasts. *Cryptococcus neoformans* was cultured from the lesion.

opening pressure. Diagnosis is by direct detection or culture. Microscopy of infected specimens shows encapsulated yeasts (India ink test); cryptococcal antigen (capsular polysaccharide) may be detected in blood and/or CSF; or the organism may be cultured from blood, CSF or lesions (e.g. skin nodules, bone). Serological testing (i.e. antibody detection) is not appropriate.

Antifungal treatment of cryptococcal meningitis consists of induction therapy with intravenous amphotericin B (lipid formulation if available) and oral 5-flucytosine (5-FC), followed by consolidation therapy with an azole (usually fluconazole). Therapy with fluconazole is continued for as long as the patient has significant immunosuppression. If CSF pressure is elevated, regular lumbar drainage may be used to prevent features of raised intracranial pressure. Monitoring of recovery by changes in antigen titre is unreliable, and is not recommended.

Fusariosis

Fusarium spp. cause disseminated disease in patients with profound or prolonged neutropenia. The disease presents with antibiotic-resistant fever and evidence of dissemination (e.g. skin nodules, endophthalmitis, septic arthritis, pulmonary disease; Fig. 13.57). In contrast to *Aspergillus* spp., *Fusarium* spp. is often recovered from blood cultures. Treatment is challenging, because of resistance to several antifungal agents. Voriconazole, posaconazole and lipid-formulated amphotericin B are the most commonly used antifungal agents.

Mucormycosis

Mucormycosis is a severe but uncommon opportunistic systemic mycosis caused by any of the Mucorales, mainly *Myocladus (formerly Absidia)* spp., *Rhizomucor* spp., *Mucor* spp. and *Rhizopus* spp. Disease patterns include rhinocerebral/craniofacial, pulmonary, cutaneous and systemic disease. All are characterised by the rapid development of severe tissue necrosis, which is almost always fatal if left untreated. The major predisposing factors are uncontrolled diabetes mellitus, iron chelation therapy with desferrioxamine, severe burns and, most commonly, profound immunosuppression from neutropenia or bone marrow transplant in association with the use of broad-spectrum azole prophylaxis with agents like voriconazole.

Diagnosis is by culture, but histopathological confirmation is required as the fungi may be environmental contaminants. Treatment requires a combination of antifungal therapy and surgical débridement, with correction of predisposing factor(s) if possible. High-dose lipid-formulated amphotericin B is used most commonly, although posaconazole is active in vitro and has been used successfully.

Penicillium marneffei infection

P. marneffei is a thermally dimorphic pathogen (filamentous in environmental conditions and yeast at body temperature), which causes disease in South-east Asia, mainly in association with HIV infection (although immunocompetent patients may also be infected). Acquisition is most likely to be by inhalation of environmental spores, with primary lung infection followed by haematogenous dissemination. A generalised papular rash, which progresses to widespread necrosis and

13

379

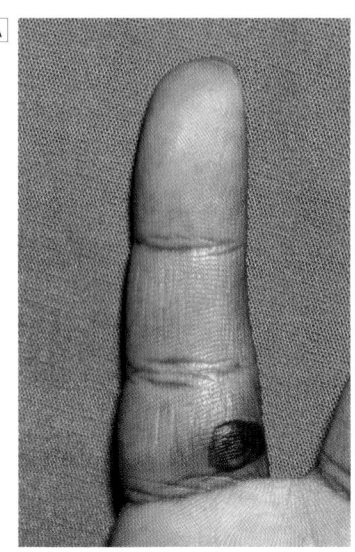
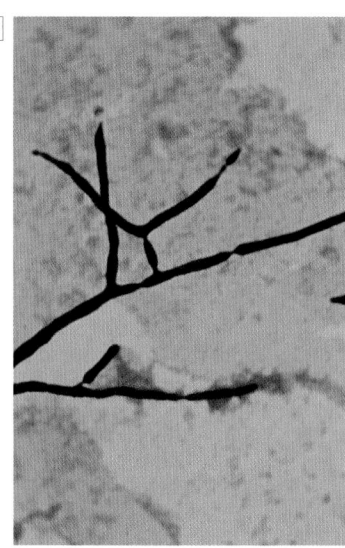

Fig. 13.57 *Fusarium* infection. A patient presented with fever and skin nodules after a prolonged severe neutropenia secondary to acute myeloid leukaemia. **A** Skin nodule on her hand. **B** *Fusarium* sp. was cultured from skin scrapings and blood cultures (Gram's stain of blood culture medium).

ulceration, is a characteristic feature. Skin lesions may resemble those of molluscum contagiosum. Diagnosis is by histopathology and/or culture of respiratory secretions, blood or any infected clinical material (e.g. skin lesions, bone marrow, biopsies). Recommended treatment is with an amphotericin B formulation (in severe infection), followed by itraconazole.

Histoplasmosis

Histoplasmosis is a primary systemic mycosis caused by *Histoplasma capsulatum*, a dimorphic fungus. *H. capsulatum* is considered to consist of two variants, var. *capsulatum* and var. *duboisii*. *H. capsulatum* var. *capsulatum* is endemic to the Mississippi and Ohio river valleys and found throughout east-central USA. Less commonly, it is found in Latin America from Mexico to Argentina, Europe, Africa, India, Malaysia, Indonesia and Australia. *H. capsulatum* var. *duboisii* is found mainly in tropical parts of West Africa and Madagascar. The taxonomic status of *H. capsulatum* is subject to ongoing re-evaluation.

Habitat

The primary reservoir of *H. capsulatum* is soil enriched by bird and bat droppings, in which the fungus remains viable for many years. Infection is by inhalation of dust from such soil. Natural infections are found in bats, which represent a secondary reservoir of infection (via bat faeces). Histoplasmosis is a specific hazard for explorers of caves and people who clear out bird (including chicken) roosts.

Pathology

The organism is inhaled in the form of conidia (spores) or hyphal fragments and transforms to the yeast phase during infection. Conidia or yeasts are phagocytosed by alveolar macrophages and neutrophils, and this may be followed by haematogenous dissemination to any organ. Subsequent development of a T-lymphocyte response brings the infection under control, resulting in a latent state in most exposed individuals.

Clinical features

Disease severity depends on the quantity of spores inhaled and the immune status of the host. In most cases infection is asymptomatic. Pulmonary symptoms are the most common disease presentation, with fever, non-productive cough and an influenza-like illness. Erythema nodosum, myalgia and joint pain are common, and chest radiography may reveal a pneumonitis with hilar or mediastinal lymphadenopathy.

Patients with pre-existing lung disease, such as chronic obstructive pulmonary disease (COPD) or emphysema, may develop chronic pulmonary histoplasmosis. The predominant features of this condition, which may easily be mistaken for tuberculosis, are fever, cough, dyspnoea, weight loss and night sweats. Radiological findings include fibrosis, nodules, cavitation and hilar/mediastinal lymphadenopathy.

Disease caused by *H. capsulatum* var. *duboisii* presents more commonly with papulonodular and ulcerating lesions of the skin and underlying subcutaneous tissue and bone (sometimes referred to as 'African histoplasmosis'). Multiple lesions of the ribs are common and the bones of the limbs may be involved. Lung involvement is relatively rare. Radiological examination may show rounded foci of bone destruction, sometimes associated with abscess formation. Other disease patterns include a visceral form with liver and splenic invasion, and disseminated disease.

Acute disseminated histoplasmosis is seen in association with immunocompromise, including HIV infection. Features include fever, pancytopenia, hepatosplenomegaly, lymphadenopathy and often a papular skin eruption. Chronic disseminated disease presents with fever, anorexia and weight loss. Cutaneous and mucosal lesions, lymphadenopathy, hepatosplenomegaly and meningitis may also develop.

Investigations

In areas where the disease occurs, histoplasmosis should be suspected in every undiagnosed infection in which there are pulmonary signs, enlarged lymph nodes, hepatosplenomegaly or characteristic cutaneous/bony lesions. Radiological examination in long-standing cases may show calcified lesions in the lungs, spleen or other organs. In the more acute phases of the disease, single or multiple soft pulmonary shadows with enlarged tracheobronchial nodes are seen on chest X-ray.

Laboratory diagnosis is by direct detection (histopathology or antigen detection), culture and serology, with antigen and antibody detection being most effective (antigen detection, however, is not widely available). Antibody is detected by complement fixation testing or immunodiffusion; the pattern of antibody production is complex, and the results require specialist interpretation. *Histoplasma* antigen may be detectable in blood or urine. Culture is definitive but slow (up to 12 weeks). Histopathology may show characteristic intracellular yeasts. Diagnosis of subcutaneous or bony infection is mainly by histopathological examination and/or culture.

Management

Mild pulmonary disease does not require treatment. However, if prolonged, it may be treated with itraconazole. More severe pulmonary disease is treated with an amphotericin B formulation for 2 weeks, followed by itraconazole for 12 weeks, with methylprednisolone added for the first 2 weeks of therapy if there is hypoxia or ARDS. Chronic pulmonary histoplasmosis is treated with itraconazole (ideally the oral solution, which has better bio-availability than the capsule formulation) for 12–24 months, and disseminated histoplasmosis with an amphotericin B formulation followed by itraconazole. Lipid formulations of amphotericin B are preferred, but their use is subject to availability. Treatment should be guided by current evidence-based guidelines (e.g. Infectious Diseases Society of America practice guidelines; www.idsociety.org). In subcutaneous and bone infection patterns of remission and relapse are more common than cure. A solitary bony lesion may require only local surgical treatment.

Coccidioidomycosis

This is a primary systemic mycosis caused by the dimorphic fungi *Coccidioides immitis* and *C. posadasii*, found in the south-western USA, and Central and South America. The disease is acquired by inhalation of conidia (arthrospores). In 60% of cases it is asymptomatic, but in the remainder it affects the lungs, lymph nodes and skin. Rarely (approx. 0.5%), it may spread haematogenously to bones, adrenals, meninges and other organs.

Pulmonary coccidioidomycosis has two forms: primary and progressive. If symptomatic, primary coccidioidomycosis presents with cough, fever, chest pain, dyspnoea and (commonly) arthritis and a rash (erythema multiforme). Progressive disease presents with systemic upset (e.g. fever, weight loss, anorexia) and features of lobar pneumonia, and may resemble tuberculosis.

Coccidioides meningitis (which may be associated with CSF eosinophils) is the most severe disease manifestation, which is fatal if untreated, and requires life-long suppressive therapy with antifungal azoles.

Investigations and management

Diagnosis is by direct detection (histopathological examination of infected tissue), culture of infected tissue or fluids, or antibody detection. IgM may be detected after 1–3 weeks of disease by precipitin tests. IgG appears later and is detected with the complement fixation test. Change in IgG titre may be used to monitor clinical progress.

Treatment depends on specific disease manifestations, and ranges from regular clinical re-assessment without antifungal therapy (in mild pulmonary, asymptomatic cavitary or single nodular disease) to high-dose treatment with an antifungal azole, which may be continued indefinitely (e.g. in meningitis). Amphotericin B is used in diffuse pneumonia, disseminated disease and, intrathecally, in meningitis. Posaconazole has been used successfully in refractory disease.

Paracoccidioidomycosis

This is a primary systemic mycosis caused by inhalation of the dimorphic fungus *Paracoccidioides brasiliensis* which is restricted to South America. The disease affects the lungs, mucous membranes (painful destructive ulceration in 50% of cases), skin, lymph nodes and adrenal glands (hypoadrenalism). Diagnosis is by microscopy and culture of lesions, and antibody detection. Oral itraconazole solution 200 mg/day has demonstrated 98% efficacy, and is currently the treatment of choice (mean duration 6 months). Ketoconazole, fluconazole and voriconazole have also been used, as have long (2–3-year) courses of sulphonamides. Amphotericin B may be used in severe or refractory disease, followed by an azole or sulphonamide.

Blastomycosis

Blastomyces dermatitidis is a dimorphic fungus endemic to restricted parts of North America, mainly around the Mississippi and Ohio rivers. Very occasionally, it is reported from Africa. The disease usually presents as a chronic pneumonia similar to pulmonary tuberculosis. Bones, skin and the genitourinary tract may also be affected. Diagnosis is by culture of the organism or identification of the characteristic yeast form in a clinical specimen. Antibody detection is rarely helpful. Treatment is with amphotericin B (severe disease) or itraconazole.

Further information

www.britishinfectionsociety.org *British Infection Society. Source of general information on communicable diseases.*

www.cdc.gov *Centers for Disease Control, USA.Source of general information about infectious diseases.*

www.fitfortravel.scot.nhs.uk *Scottish site with valuable information for travellers.*

www.hpa.org.uk *Health Protection Agency. Information on infectious diseases in the UK.*

www.idsociety.org *Infectious Diseases Society of America. Source of general information relating to infectious diseases and of authoritative practice guidelines.*

www.who.int *World Health Organization. Invaluable links on travel medicine with updates on outbreaks of infections, changing resistance patterns and vaccination requirements.*

13

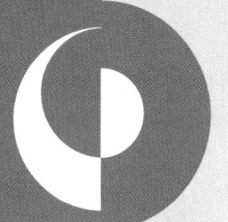

E.G.L. Wilkins

HIV infection and AIDS

14

CLINICAL EXAMINATION IN HIV INFECTION

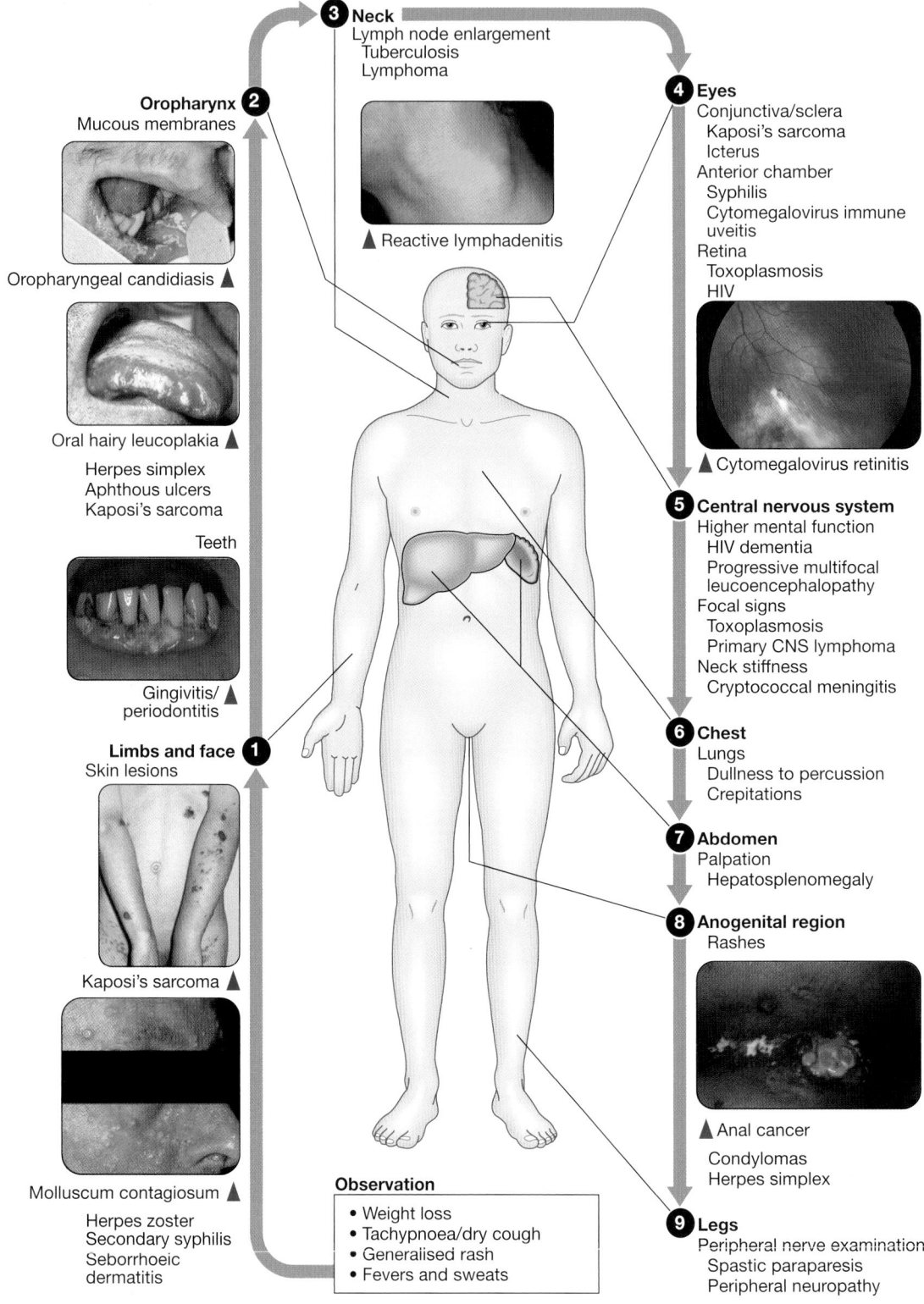

3 Neck
Lymph node enlargement
Tuberculosis
Lymphoma

▲ Reactive lymphadenitis

2 Oropharynx
Mucous membranes

Oropharyngeal candidiasis ▲

Oral hairy leucoplakia ▲

Herpes simplex
Aphthous ulcers
Kaposi's sarcoma

Teeth

Gingivitis/ ▲
periodontitis

1 Limbs and face
Skin lesions

Kaposi's sarcoma ▲

Molluscum contagiosum ▲

Herpes zoster
Secondary syphilis
Seborrhoeic
dermatitis

4 Eyes
Conjunctiva/sclera
Kaposi's sarcoma
Icterus
Anterior chamber
Syphilis
Cytomegalovirus immune
uveitis
Retina
Toxoplasmosis
HIV

▲ Cytomegalovirus retinitis

5 Central nervous system
Higher mental function
HIV dementia
Progressive multifocal
leucoencephalopathy
Focal signs
Toxoplasmosis
Primary CNS lymphoma
Neck stiffness
Cryptococcal meningitis

6 Chest
Lungs
Dullness to percussion
Crepitations

7 Abdomen
Palpation
Hepatosplenomegaly

8 Anogenital region
Rashes

▲ Anal cancer

Condylomas
Herpes simplex

9 Legs
Peripheral nerve examination
Spastic paraparesis
Peripheral neuropathy

Observation
• Weight loss
• Tachypnoea/dry cough
• Generalised rash
• Fevers and sweats

1 HIV indicator presentations

- Herpes zoster, severe seborrhoeic dermatitis or psoriasis
- Tuberculosis, recurrent bacterial pneumonia (especially pneumococcal)
- Hepatitis B or hepatitis C
- Recurrent oral or vaginal candidiasis
- Anal cancer, lymphoma (Hodgkin or non-Hodgkin), Castleman's disease
- Aseptic meningitis, dementia
- Other HIV symptomatic disease (see Box 14.4, p. 390)
- Other AIDS-defining disease (see Box 14.5, p. 390)

Unexplained presentation

- Lymphadenopathy
- Pyrexia of unknown origin (PUO)
- Weight loss

Abnormal investigations

- Thrombocytopenia, lymphopenia or neutropenia

2 Pre-test counselling

- Discuss purpose of test
- Carry out risk assessment
- Explore knowledge and explain natural history of HIV
- Discuss transmission and risk reduction
- Assess likely coping strategy
- Explain test procedure
- Obtain informed consent

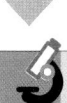

3 Laboratory confirmation

Serology using commercial ELISA screening test[1]

- Test result negative:
  Second test 3 months after last exposure
- Test result positive:
  Result confirmed using two different immunoassays and/or Western blot
  Second sample checked

Nucleic acid amplification test[2] if:

- Seroconversion suspected
- Confirming vertical transmission

[1] Commonly for HIV-1 antibody, HIV-2 antibody and p24 antigen.
[2] E.g. PCR or branched-chain DNA assay.
(ELISA = enzyme-linked immunosorbent assay;
PCR = polymerase chain reaction)

6 Clinical examination

- See opposite.

5 Key history points

HIV (assessing time of HIV acquisition/ likelihood of resistance)

- Previous negative HIV test
- History consistent with seroconversion
- Known HIV-infected ex-/current partner
- Episodes of 'unsafe' sex in high-risk situations (e.g. saunas)
- Previous antenatal screening
- Presence of 'HIV indicator disease'

General

- Birthplace, residence, occupation
- Tuberculosis: past history or contact
- Travel history/animal contacts
- Immunisation history (BCG, hepatitis A and B)
- Recreational drug use
- Past STIs
- Partner and children
- Others' knowledge of status (to contact if needed)
- GP awareness and permission to inform

4 Post-test counselling

Test result negative

- Discuss transmission and need for behaviour modification
    e.g. Safer sex
    Needle exchange
- Advise second test 3 months after last exposure
- Support if uninfected partner

Test result positive

- Explain significance and implications of result
- Organise urgent medical follow-up
- Assess coping strategy
    e.g. Fear of disclosure
    Discrimination/social rejection
- Provide verbal and written information
- Discuss confidentiality issues
- Organise emotional and practical support (provide names/phone numbers)

7 Baseline investigations

All

- CD4 count
- Viral load
- Hepatitis B (HBV) status
- Hepatitis C (HCV) antibody
- HIV resistance test
- Hepatitis A (HAV) IgG antibody
- *Toxoplasma* and cytomegalovirus (CMV) IgG antibody
- *Treponema* serology
- HLA-B*5701 screen for hypersensitivity to abacavir (p. 406)
- Lipid profile and urinalysis
- Cervical smear in women
- STI screen

Consider depending on ethnicity, exposure risk, CD4 count and baseline laboratory results

- Chest X-ray
- HCV-RNA
- Cryptococcal antigen
- CMV-PCR
- Dilated fundoscopy

8 Other issues

Immunisations

- Hepatitis A and hepatitis B if non-immune
- Pneumovax (at initial diagnosis and then 3–5-yearly)
- Influenza (yearly)
- Consider tetanus booster (if injection drug-user)

Counselling

- Safe sex/behaviour modification
- Cryptosporidial risk: need to boil water
- *Toxoplasma* risk: safe handling of cats/litter, avoidance of undercooked meat
- Live vaccines and travel
- Avoiding over-the-counter medicines if on highly active antiretroviral therapy (HAART)
- Planning pregnancy

Repeat tests

- Treponemal antibody 3–4 times/yr
- HBV markers every 1–2 yrs
- HCV antibody every 1–2 yrs
- HBV surface antibody in those immunised, to assess need for booster
- Cervical smear yearly
- *Toxoplasma* and CMV serology: if negative initially, check annually

14

EPIDEMIOLOGY AND BIOLOGY OF HIV

The acquired immunodeficiency syndrome (AIDS) was first recognised in 1981, although the earliest documented case has been traced to a blood sample from 1959. It is caused by the human immunodeficiency virus (HIV-1), which has evolved a number of mechanisms to elude immune control and has thereby prevented effective control of the epidemic. HIV-2 causes a similar illness to HIV-1 but is less aggressive and restricted mainly to western Africa. The origin of HIV is a non-human primate simian virus which probably passed from chimpanzees to humans via bush hunters. AIDS remains the second leading cause of disease burden world-wide and the leading cause of death in Africa, although downward trends in prevalence are occurring in several countries, partly as a result of effective prevention measures and partly due to scaling up of antiretroviral access. Highly active retroviral therapy (HAART) with three or more drugs has improved life expectancy to near normal in the majority of patients receiving it, with an 80% reduction of mortality since its introduction.

Global epidemic and regional patterns

In 2007, the World Health Organization (WHO) estimated that there were 33.2 million people living with HIV/AIDS, 2.5 million new infections and 2.1 million deaths (Fig. 14.1). The cumulative death toll since the epidemic began is over 20 million, the vast majority of cases occurring in sub-Saharan Africa where over 11.4 million children are now orphaned. In eight Southern African countries (Botswana, South Africa, Swaziland, Mozambique, Lesotho, Namibia, Zaire and Zimbabwe) the prevalence exceeds 15%, and for many others, such as Cameroon, Central African Republic and Cote d'Ivoire, it is over 5%. Between 2001 and 2007, the steepest increases have been seen in Asia (> 90%) and Eastern Europe/Central Asia (150%), predominantly India, China, Russia and Ukraine. In South-east Asia, the epidemic is well developed but prevalence is falling in Thailand, Cambodia and Myanmar, although still increasing in Vietnam and Indonesia. In India, the national prevalence is 0.36% (varying from 0.07% in Uttar Pradesh to 1.13% in Manipur) and

it is estimated that 2.5 million persons were infected in 2006. Given that Asia is home to 60% of the world's population, these changes have huge implications.

Many different cultural, social and behavioural aspects determine the regional characteristics of HIV disease. Historically, the epidemic in North America and northern Europe has been in men who have sex with men (MSM), whereas in southern and Eastern Europe, Vietnam, Malaysia, Indonesia, North-east India and China the incidence has been greatest in injection drug-users. In Africa, the Caribbean and much of South-east Asia the dominant route of transmission remains heterosexual and from mother to child. However, the epidemic in many nations is changing. Heterosexual transmission has become a significant and often dominant route with racial and ethnic minorities representing an increasing fraction, largely as a consequence of the influx of migrants from high-prevalence countries. In the European Union (EU) in 2006, more than half of patients were infected heterosexually, with a doubling of new cases in the UK over the last 5 years. Additionally, there has been a 50% increase in reported new diagnoses in MSM, although some of this may be accounted for by an increased uptake in testing. It is of concern that around 30% of patients are unaware of their diagnosis and one-quarter of these present with late disease. This underlies the importance of having a low threshold to test individuals, especially when they present with any condition that has been associated with HIV.

The economic and demographic impact of HIV infection in developing countries is profound, as it affects those at their most economically productive and fertile age, and is also eroding the health and economic advances made in the last few decades. Although roll-out of drugs and access to care has improved dramatically recently, less than one-quarter of patients in many resource-poor countries are able to access antiretrovirals.

Modes of transmission

HIV is present in blood, semen and other body fluids such as breast milk and saliva. Exposure to infected fluid leads to a risk of contracting infection, which is dependent on

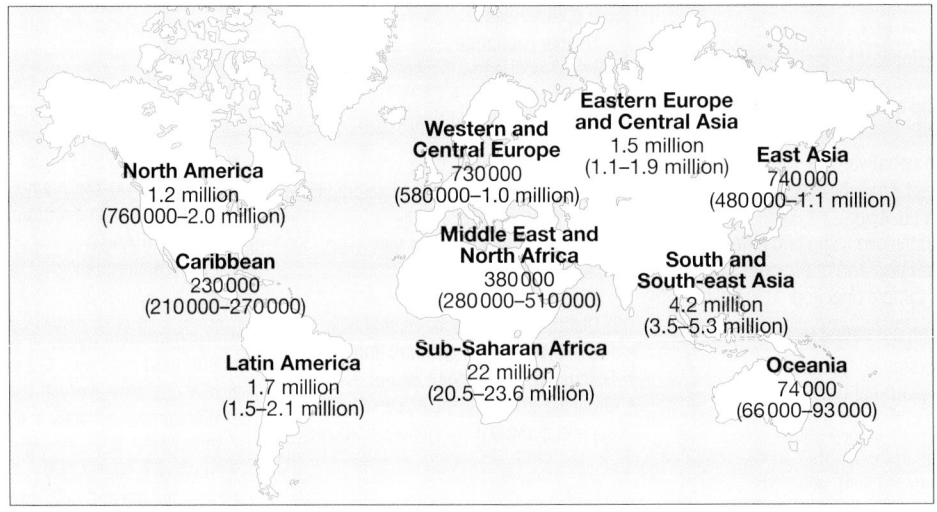

North America
1.2 million
(760 000–2.0 million)

Caribbean
230 000
(210 000–270 000)

Latin America
1.7 million
(1.5–2.1 million)

Western and
Central Europe
730 000
(580 000–1.0 million)

Eastern Europe
and Central Asia
1.5 million
(1.1–1.9 million)

East Asia
740 000
(480 000–1.1 million)

Middle East and
North Africa
380 000
(280 000–510 000)

South and
South-east Asia
4.2 million
(3.5–5.3 million)

Sub-Saharan Africa
22 million
(20.5–23.6 million)

Oceania
74 000
(66 000–93 000)

Fig. 14.1 World-wide distribution of HIV infection.

the integrity of the exposed site, the type and volume of body fluid, and the viral load. HIV can enter either as free virus or within cells. The modes of spread are sexual (man to man, heterosexual and oral), parenteral (blood or blood product recipients, injection drug-users and those experiencing occupational injury) and vertical. The transmission risk after exposure is over 90% for blood or blood products, 15–40% for the vertical route, 0.5–1.0% for injection drug use, 0.2–0.5% for genital mucous membrane spread and under 0.1% for non-genital mucous membrane spread. Box 14.1 outlines the important factors increasing the risk of acquisition and Box 14.2 how this information is used to target HIV testing.

World-wide, the major route of transmission (> 75%) is heterosexual. About 5–10% of new HIV infections are in children and more than 90% of these are infected during pregnancy, birth or breastfeeding. The rate of mother-to-child transmission is higher in developing countries (25–44%) than in industrialised nations (13–25%). Postnatal transmission via breast milk accounts for some of this increased risk. Of those infected vertically, 80% are infected close to the time of delivery and 20% in utero. Around 70% of patients with haemophilia A and 30% of those with haemophilia B had been infected through contaminated blood products by the time HIV antibody screening was adopted in the USA and Europe in 1985. In developed nations, because of routine antibody screening, the likelihood of acquiring HIV from blood products is now less than 1:500 000 and arises from donors in the seroconverting phase of infection. However, the WHO estimates that because of the lack of adequate screening

14.2 HIV testing

Services where testing is recommended to all

- Genitourinary medicine or sexual health
- Antenatal
- Termination of pregnancy
- Drug dependency
- Hepatitis B, hepatitis C, tuberculosis and lymphoma

Individuals to whom testing is routinely offered and recommended

- People known to be from a country of high HIV prevalence (> 1%), or their sexual partners
- Men who have sex with men (MSM)
- Commercial sex workers
- Patients with a sexually transmitted infection (STI)
- Sexual partners of HIV-positive individuals
- Health-care workers or transfusion recipients from a country of high HIV prevalence (> 1%)
- Those with possible primary HIV infection (e.g. mononucleosis-like syndrome)
- Those with history of injection drug use

Settings where testing should be considered

- Areas where diagnosed HIV prevalence exceeds 2 in 1000 population

facilities in resource-poor countries, 5–10% of blood transfusions globally are with HIV-infected blood. There have been approximately 100 definite and 200 possible cases of HIV acquired occupationally in health-care workers. Such infections are substantially more frequent in developing nations, where it is estimated that 40% of syringes/needles used in injections are reused without sterilisation.

Virology and immunology

HIV is a single-stranded RNA retrovirus from the Lentivirus family. After mucosal exposure, HIV is transported to the lymph nodes via dendritic, CD4 T lymphocytes or Langerhans cells, where infection becomes established. Dendritic cells express various receptors (e.g. DC–SIGN) that facilitate capture and transport of HIV-1. Free or cell-associated virus is then disseminated widely through the blood with seeding of 'sanctuary' sites (e.g. central nervous system (CNS)) and latent CD4 cell reservoirs.

Each mature virion is spherical and has a lipid membrane lined by a matrix protein that is studded with glycoprotein (gp) 120 and gp41 spikes surrounding a cone-shaped protein core. This core houses two copies of the single-stranded RNA genome and viral enzymes. The virus infects the CD4 cell in a complicated sequence of events beginning with engagement of the viral gp120 and the CD4 cell receptor (stage 1, Fig. 14.2), which results in a conformational change in gp120. This permits interaction with one of two chemokine co-receptors (CXCR4 or CCR5: stage 2), which is followed by membrane fusion and cellular entry involving gp41 (stage 3). Monocyte-macrophages, follicular dendritic cells and microglial cells in the central nervous system also express the CD4 cell receptor and are permissive to infection.

After penetrating the cell and uncoating, a DNA copy is transcribed from the RNA genome by the reverse transcriptase (RT) enzyme (stage 4) that is carried by the

14.1 Factors increasing the risk of acquisition of HIV

Common to all transmission categories

- High viral load
- Lower CD4 cell count
- AIDS
- Seroconversion

Vertical transmission

- Older gestational age
- Prolonged rupture of membranes
- Chorioamnionitis
- Fetal trauma (e.g. scalp electrodes)
- Lower birth weight
- Vaginal vs. elective caesarean delivery
- No peripartum prophylaxis
- First-born twin

Breastfeeding

- Longer-duration feeding
- Lower parity
- Younger age
- Mastitis

Sexual transmission

- STIs, especially genital ulcers
- Cervical ectopy
- Receptive vs. insertive anal sex
- Rectal or vaginal trauma
- Menstruation
- Male–male vs. heterosexual sex
- Non-circumcised
- Increased number of partners

Injection drug use transmission

- Sharing equipment
- Frequency of use
- Linked commercial sex
- Lower income
- Intravenous use
- Cocaine use
- Incarceration

Occupational transmission

- Deep injury
- Visible blood on device
- Previous arterial or venous device siting

14

Stage	Steps in replication	Drug targets
1	Attachment to CD4 receptor	
2	Binding to co-receptor CCR5 or CXCR4	CCR5/CXCR4 receptor inhibitors
3	Fusion	Fusion inhibitors
4	Reverse transcription	Nucleoside and non-nucleoside reverse transcription inhibitors
5	Integration	Integrase inhibitors
6	Transcription	
7	Translation	
8	Cleavage of polypeptides and assembly	Protease inhibitors
9	Viral release	

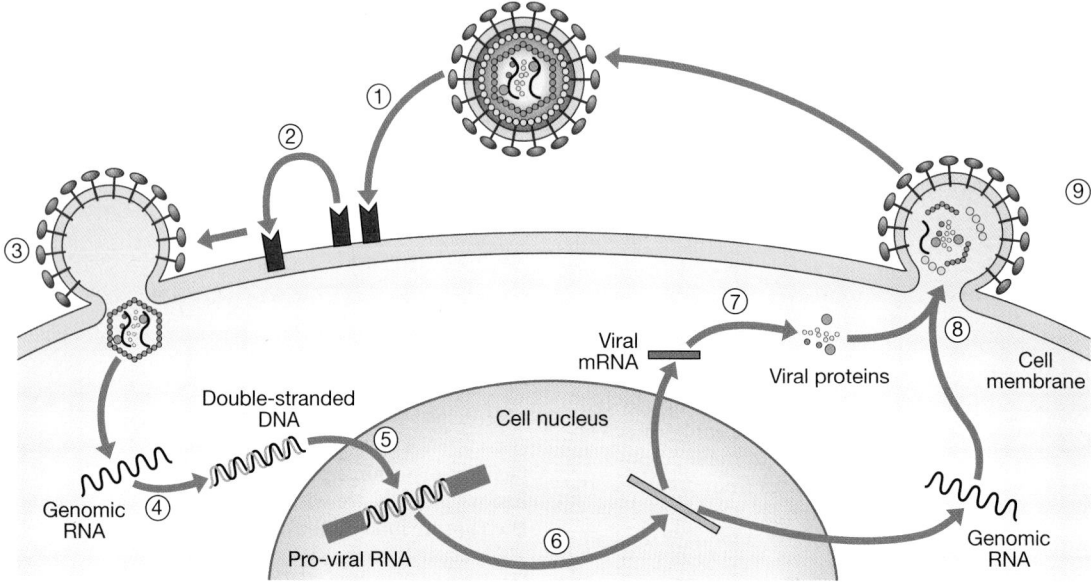

Fig. 14.2 Life cycle of HIV.

infecting virion. Reverse transcription is an error-prone process and multiple mutations arise with ongoing replication (hence the rapid generation of viral resistance to drugs). This DNA is transported into the nucleus and integrated randomly within the host cell genome via integrase enzyme (stage 5). Integrated virus is known as proviral DNA. On host-cell activation, this DNA copy is used as a template to transcribe new RNA copies (stage 6), which are processed and exported from the nucleus, viral mRNA then being translated into viral peptide chains (stage 7). The precursor polyproteins are then cleaved by the viral protease enzyme to form new viral structural proteins and viral enzymes such as the reverse transcriptase and protease. These then migrate to the cell surface and are assembled using the host cellular apparatus to produce infectious viral particles. These bud from the cell surface, incorporating the host cell membrane as their own lipid bilayer coat, and cell lysis occurs (stage 9). Once maturation is complete, the new infectious virus (virion) is then available to infect uninfected cells and repeat the process. All of these processes are enabled by three viral genes (*Gag*, *Pol* and *Env*), as well as the products of six regulatory genes (*Vif, Vpr, Vpu, Nef, Tat* and *Rev*). It has been calculated that each day more than 10^{10} virions are produced and 10^9 CD4 cells destroyed. This represents a daily turnover of 30% of the total viral burden and 6–7% of the total body CD4 cells.

A small percentage of T cells (< 0.01%) either produce small quantities of virus or enter a post-integration latent phase and represent the main reservoir of HIV. Together with virion-associated immune complexes bound to follicular dendritic cells, they can refuel infection if host defences fail or HAART is discontinued. There is ongoing low-level replication within these cells, even when plasma levels of HIV are below the level of detection as a result of antiretroviral treatment. They are important as sanctuary sites from antiviral therapy, as continuing sources of virus (including the generation of drug-resistant strains) and as eventual targets for eradication strategies. The half-life of the virus is 1–2 hours in plasma, 1.5 days in productively infected CD4 cells and over 12 months in latently infected CD4 cells.

With time, there is gradual attrition of the CD4 cell population and, as CD4 cells are pivotal in orchestrating the immune response, any depletion renders the body susceptible to opportunistic infections and oncogenic virus-related tumours. The predominant opportunist infections seen in HIV disease are intracellular parasites (e.g. *Mycobacterium tuberculosis*) or pathogens susceptible to cell-mediated rather than antibody-mediated immune responses. The exact mechanism underlying the CD4 decline is not fully understood, but it is not restricted to virus-infected cells and is linked to the height of plasma viral load. Both are monitored closely in patients and used as measures of disease progression. Virus-specific CD8 cytotoxic T lymphocytes develop rapidly after infection and are crucial in recognising, binding and lysing infected CD4 cells, thus controlling HIV replication after infection and the subsequent rate of disease progression.

On the basis of DNA sequencing, HIV-1 can be subdivided into group M ('major', world-wide distribution), group O ('outlier', divergent from group M) and group N ('non-major and non-outlier', highly divergent) types. Groups O and N are restricted to West Africa and may screen weakly positive or negative on routine antibody testing. Group M can be subdivided further into subtypes; 9 are currently recognised (A–K), with numerous subsubtypes (e.g. A1–A4) and circulating recombinant forms (e.g. CRF01_AE). Globally, subtype C (Africa and India) accounts for half of strains. Subtype A (Africa, Asia and Eastern Europe) and subtype B (Western Europe, the Americas and Australia) are responsible for approximately 10% each, and in many countries, more than one subtype or recombinant exists, or is emerging in restricted groups (e.g. West Africa, South-east Asia, southern Europe, and Russia). Increased HIV diversity has implications for diagnostic tests, treatments and vaccine development. It may also influence transmission (more frequent with subtype C), disease progression (faster with subtypes A and D), co-receptor usage (CXCR4 used early with subtype D) and emergent resistance patterns (subtype C). In Europe, the prevalence of non-B subtypes is increasing because of migrants (predominantly from Africa) and now accounts for a significant proportion of newly diagnosed infection. HIV-2 is an important but separate retrovirus which has at least five subtypes. The virus differs from HIV-1 in that patients have lower viral loads, slower CD4 decline, lower rates of vertical transmission and 12-fold lower progression to AIDS.

14.3 Clinical features of primary infection

- Fever with rash
- Pharyngitis with cervical lymphadenopathy
- Myalgia/arthralgia
- Headache
- Mucosal ulceration

(e.g. oropharyngeal candidiasis, *Pneumocystis jirovecii* pneumonia (PCP)) may rarely occur. Symptomatic recovery parallels the return of the CD4 count (although this rarely recovers to its previous value) and fall in the viral load. In many patients, the illness is mild and only identified on retrospective enquiry at later presentation.

Diagnosis is made by detecting HIV-RNA in the serum or by immunoblot assay (which shows antibodies developing to early proteins). The appearance of specific anti-HIV antibodies in serum (seroconversion) takes place later at 3–12 weeks (median 8 weeks). Factors likely to indicate faster disease progression are the presence and duration of symptoms, evidence of candidiasis, and neurological involvement. The level of the viral load post-seroconversion correlates with subsequent progression of disease. The differential diagnosis of primary HIV includes acute Epstein–Barr virus (EBV), cytomegalovirus (CMV), streptococcal pharyngitis, toxoplasmosis and secondary syphilis.

Asymptomatic infection

Asymptomatic infection (category A disease in the Centers for Disease Control (CDC) classification) follows and lasts for a variable period, during which the infected individual remains well with no evidence of disease except for the possible presence of persistent generalised lymphadenopathy (PGL, defined as enlarged glands at ≥ 2 extra-inguinal sites). At this stage the bulk of virus replication takes place within lymphoid tissue (e.g. follicular dendritic cells). There is sustained viraemia with a decline in CD4 count dependent on the height of the viral load but usually between 50 and 150 cells/year (see Fig. 14.3).

Mildly symptomatic disease

Mildly symptomatic disease (CDC classification category B disease) then develops in the majority, indicating

NATURAL HISTORY AND CLASSIFICATION OF HIV

Primary infection

Primary infection is symptomatic in 70–80% of cases and usually occurs 2–6 weeks after exposure. The major clinical manifestations are listed in Box 14.3. Rarely, presentation may be with neurological features (pp. 397–401). This coincides with high plasma HIV-RNA levels and a fall in the CD4 count to 300–400 cells/mm³, but occasionally to below 200 (Fig. 14.3) when opportunistic infections

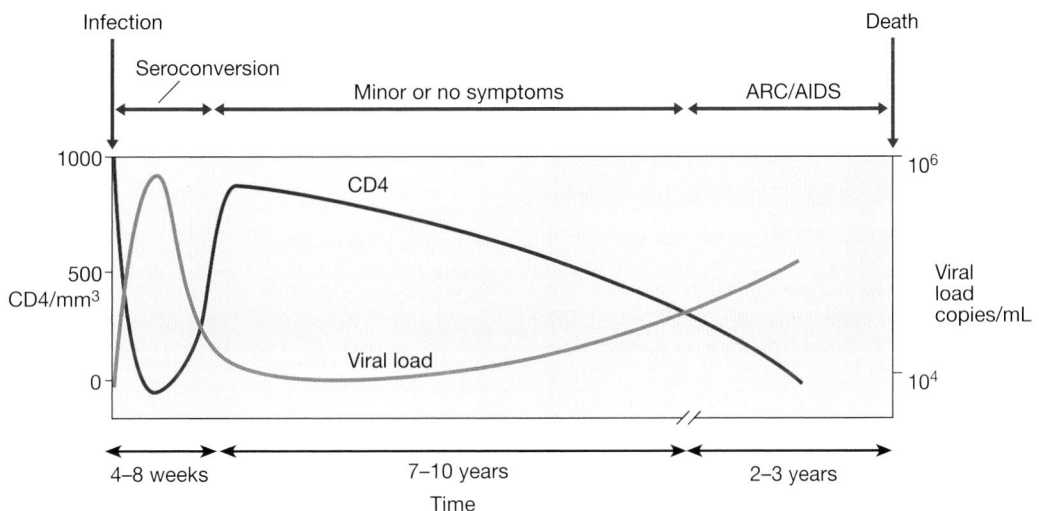

Fig. 14.3 Virological and immunological progression of HIV infection. (ARC = AIDS-related complex)

14.4 HIV symptomatic/indicator diseases

- Oral hairy leucoplakia
- Recurrent oropharyngeal candidiasis
- Recurrent vaginal candidiasis
- Severe pelvic inflammatory disease
- Bacillary angiomatosis
- Cervical dysplasia
- Idiopathic thrombocytopenic purpura
- Weight loss
- Chronic diarrhoea
- Herpes zoster
- Peripheral neuropathy
- Low-grade fever/night sweats

14.5 AIDS-defining diseases

- Oesophageal candidiasis
- Cryptococcal meningitis
- Chronic cryptosporidial diarrhoea
- Cerebral toxoplasmosis
- CMV retinitis or colitis
- Chronic mucocutaneous herpes simplex
- Disseminated *Mycobacterium avium intracellulare* (MAI)
- Pulmonary or extrapulmonary tuberculosis
- *Pneumocystis jirovecii* (*carinii*) pneumonia
- Progressive multifocal leucoencephalopathy
- Recurrent non-typhi *Salmonella* septicaemia
- Extrapulmonary coccidioidomycosis
- Invasive cervical cancer
- Extrapulmonary histoplasmosis
- Kaposi's sarcoma
- Non-Hodgkin lymphoma
- Primary cerebral lymphoma
- HIV-associated wasting
- HIV-associated dementia

14.6 Correlations between CD4 count and HIV-associated diseases

> 500 cells/mm³

- Acute primary infection
- Recurrent vaginal candidiasis
- Persistent generalised lymphadenopathy

< 500 cells/mm³

- Pulmonary tuberculosis
- Pneumococcal pneumonia
- Herpes zoster
- Oropharyngeal candidiasis
- Oral hairy leucoplakia
- Extra-intestinal salmonellosis
- Kaposi's sarcoma
- HIV-associated idiopathic thrombocytopenic purpura
- Cervical intra-epithelial neoplasia II–III
- Lymphoid interstitial pneumonitis

< 200 cells/mm³

- *Pneumocystis jirovecii* pneumonia
- Mucocutaneous herpes simplex
- Cryptosporidium
- Microsporidium
- Oesophageal candidiasis
- Miliary/extrapulmonary tuberculosis
- HIV-associated wasting
- Peripheral neuropathy

< 100 cells/mm³

- Cerebral toxoplasmosis
- Cryptococcal meningitis
- Non-Hodgkin lymphoma
- HIV-associated dementia
- Progressive multifocal leucoencephalopathy

< 50 cells/mm³

- CMV retinitis/gastrointestinal disease
- Primary CNS lymphoma
- Disseminated MAI

Mucocutaneous disease

Mucocutaneous manifestations are common in HIV and range from the trivial to markers of significant systemic infection (Boxes 14.7 and 14.8). Most patients are affected at some point and for many it is a major problem. Dermatological problems may present atypically, coexist

14.7 Differential diagnosis of HIV-related skin disease

Early HIV

Infection

- Herpes simplex
- Varicella zoster
- Human papillomavirus (HPV)
- Impetigo
- Dermatophytosis
- Scabies
- Syphilis
- HIV seroconversion

Other

- Xeroderma
- Pruritus
- Seborrhoeic dermatitis
- Drug reaction (e.g. co-trimoxazole, nevirapine)
- Itchy folliculitis
- Psoriasis
- Acne
- Papular pruritic eruption

Late HIV

Common

- Kaposi's sarcoma
- Molluscum contagiosum
- Chronic mucocutaneous herpes simplex

Rare

- Bacillary angiomatosis
- CMV
- Non-Hodgkin lymphoma
- *Cryptococcus*
- Histoplasmosis
- Mycobacteria

some impairment of cellular immunity but which is not AIDS-defining (Box 14.4). The median interval from infection to the development of symptoms is around 7–10 years, although subgroups of patients exhibit 'fast' or 'slow' rates of progression.

Acquired immunodeficiency syndrome (AIDS)

AIDS (CDC classification category C disease) is defined by the development of specified opportunistic infections, tumours and presentations (Box 14.5). Box 14.6 outlines the correlation between CD4 count and HIV-related diseases.

PRESENTING PROBLEMS IN HIV INFECTION

Before discussion of these, it is important to understand the principles of HAART, described in detail on pages 404–407. Initial HAART is introduced when the CD4 count falls below 350 cells/mm³ or an AIDS-defining illness develops. Over 85% of cases achieve complete virological suppression by 3 months, a steady increase in CD4 count and a return to good health. Occasionally, patients with low CD4 counts can experience immune reconstitution disease (IRD). This indicates either subclinical infection which has become manifest with HAART, or an enhanced reaction to dying or dead microorganisms which results in clinical illness.

14.8 Differential diagnosis of HIV-related oral disease

Early HIV

- Oral hairy leucoplakia
- Herpes simplex
- Oropharyngeal candidiasis
- Aphthous ulcers
- Gingivitis/periodontitis
- Syphilis
- HPV
- Herpes zoster

Late HIV

- Kaposi's sarcoma
- Drug reaction
- Lymphoma
- CMV

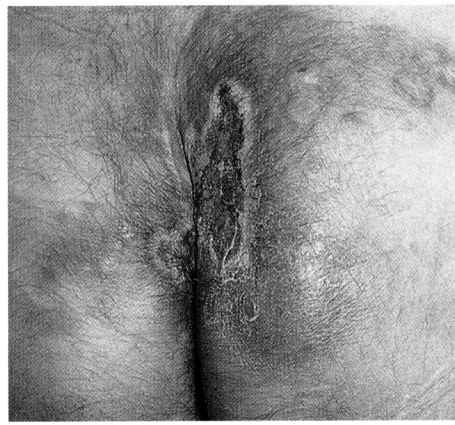

Fig. 14.4 Severe mucocutaneous herpes simplex. Perianal or perioral infection is not uncommon in later-stage HIV infection.

with other pathologies and be harder to manage than in an HIV-negative patient. Type and severity of rash are often dependent upon the level of CD4 count. The presence of either oropharyngeal candidiasis or oral hairy leucoplakia in a young person is suggestive of HIV infection. Anyone with an unusual rash, especially one persistent and unresponsive to topical antifungal/corticosteroid combinations, or in the presence of severe immune compromise (CD4 < 50 cells/mm³), merits a skin biopsy for histology and culture.

Specific skin conditions

Fungal infections

Early HIV-associated skin diseases include xerosis with pruritus, seborrhoeic dermatitis, and an itchy folliculitic rash which may be fungal (*Malassezia furfur*), staphylococcal or eosinophilic in aetiology. Dermatophyte infection affecting skin (feet, body and face) and nails is also common, and may be extensive and difficult to treat. Seborrhoeic dermatitis is very common in HIV and is present in up to 80% of patients with AIDS; severity increases as the CD4 count falls. It presents as dry scaly red patches on the face (typically on the cheeks, in the nasolabial folds, around the eyebrows, behind the ears and on the scalp). The cause is multifactorial but *M. furfur* is important. It responds well to a combined topical antifungal/steroid.

Viral infections

The major viral infections affecting the skin are herpes simplex, varicella zoster (VZV), human papillomavirus (HPV) and molluscum contagiosum.

Herpes simplex (type 1 or 2). This may affect the lips, mouth and skin or anogenital area and is seen in 20% of cases. In later-stage HIV, the lesions are usually chronic, extensive, harder to treat and recurrent. Persistent and severe anogenital ulceration is usually herpetic and a marker for underlying HIV (Fig. 14.4).

VZV. This usually presents with a dermatomal vesicular rash on an erythematous base, and may be the first clue to a diagnosis of HIV infection. It can occur at any stage but is more frequent with failing immunity. In patients with a CD4 count < 100 cells/mm³, the rash may be more severe, multidermatomal, persistent or recurrent, or may become disseminated. Involvement of the trigeminal nerve, scarring on recovery and associated motor defects are probably also more common. Diagnosis of herpetic infection can be confirmed by culture, smear preparations showing characteristic inclusion bodies, electron microscopy or biopsy. Treatment should be given for all cases of active disease, irrespective of the time since onset of rash. In patients with severe mucocutaneous herpes simplex or herpes zoster which is disseminated, multiderma-

tomal, ophthalmic or very dense, or when the CD4 count is < 200 cells/mm³, parenteral aciclovir must be used.

HPV infection. This is frequent amongst HIV patients and is usually anogenital; disease may be extensive and very difficult to manage. Warts on the hands and feet (especially periungual) are also common and may attain considerable size, requiring surgery. Occasionally, myriads of flat-topped papules occur over the body and face. Both oncogenic (16, 18, 31, 33) and non-oncogenic (6, 11) genotypes are found. There is often improvement on HAART.

Molluscum contagiosum. This is an epidermal poxvirus infection. It is found in approximately 10% of AIDS patients. The lesions are usually 2–5mm diameter papules with a central umbilicus and most frequently affect the face, neck, scalp and genital region (p. 384). Lesions may become widespread and attain a large size (giant mollusca). Treatment is with curettage or cryotherapy, and with improvement in CD4 counts, lesions usually disappear.

Bacterial and parasitic infections

Bacterial infections include *Staphylococcus aureus* (folliculitis, cellulitis and abscesses), bacillary angiomatosis and syphilis (primary and secondary, p. 417). Bacillary angiomatosis is a bacterial infection due to the cat-scratch bacillus, *Bartonella henselae*. Skin lesions range from solitary superficial reddish-purple lesions resembling Kaposi's sarcoma or pyogenic granuloma, to multiple subcutaneous nodules or even hyperpigmented plaques. Lesions are painful and may bleed or ulcerate. The infection may become disseminated with fevers, lymphadenopathy and hepatosplenomegaly. Diagnosis is made by biopsy of a lesion and Warthin–Starry silver staining which reveals aggregates of bacilli. Treatment with doxycycline or azithromycin is effective.

In HIV, scabies (due to the mite *Sarcoptes scabiei*, p. 1273) may cause intensely pruritic, encrusted papules affecting most areas. Classically, the interdigital web spaces, wrists, periumbilical area, buttock and sides of the feet are involved. Commonly in HIV the infestation may be heavy, the rash hyperkeratotic (Norwegian scabies) and the patient highly infectious. Uniquely, the face and neck are often affected.

Rarely, cutaneous disease may be a manifestation of mycobacterial infection (tuberculosis or an atypical mycobacterium) or disseminated fungal infection.

Papular pruritic eruption is an itchy symmetrical rash affecting the extremities and resulting in

14

hyper-/hypopigmentation. It is seen mainly in those from sub-Saharan Africa where it is the most common skin manifestation of HIV, and is highly indicative of HIV when present. Topical steroids, emollients and antihistamines are useful but response is variable.

Specific oral conditions

Candidiasis

Candida infection in HIV is almost exclusively mucosal, affecting nearly all patients with CD4 counts < 200 cells/mm³. In early disease, it is nearly always caused by *C. albicans* (p. 376). Pseudomembranous candidiasis describes white patches on the buccal mucosa that can be scraped off to reveal a red raw surface (p. 384). The tongue, palate and pharynx may also be involved. Less common is erythematous candidiasis; patients present with a sore mouth, reddened mucosa and a smooth shiny tongue. Hypertrophic candidiasis (leucoplakia-like lesions which do not scrape off but respond to antifungal treatment) and angular cheilitis may also be present.

Diagnosis is clinical but it is important to perform a mouth swill for culture, speciation and sensitivities in patients unresponsive to fluconazole or other azole drugs. The cause is usually *C. albicans*. Prophylaxis is not recommended and therapeutic courses of azoles should be given with each attack.

Oesophageal infection may coexist, although no oropharyngeal candidiasis is visible in up to 30%. Up to 80% of patients with pain on swallowing have *Candida* oesophagitis (see Fig. 14.6 below for differential diagnosis), with pseudomembranous plaques visible on barium swallow and endoscopy (Fig. 14.5). The pain is usually associated with dysphagia and, when untreated, leads to weight loss. Treatment is with an oral azole drug,

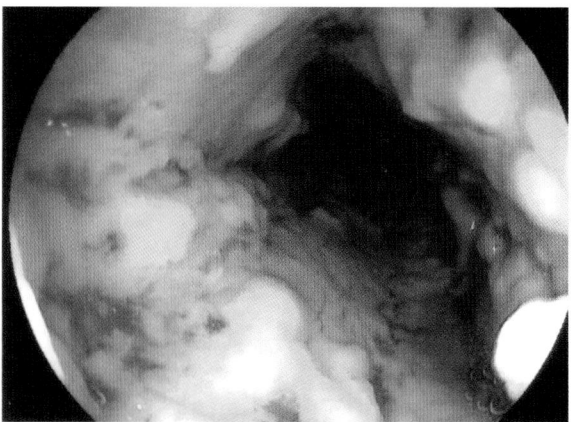

Fig. 14.5 Oesophageal candidiasis. Endoscopy may show pseudomembranous plaques or extensive confluent infection.

usually fluconazole. Where azole-resistant candida is present, caspofungin or amphotericin can be used.

Oral hairy leucoplakia

Oral hairy leucoplakia appears as corrugated white plaques running vertically on the side of the tongue, and is virtually pathognomonic of HIV disease in the context of HIV risk factors (p. 385). It is usually asymptomatic and does not require treatment. The aetiology is closely associated with EBV. High-dose aciclovir or valaciclovir is sometimes effective in eradicating the infection but relapse often follows cessation of treatment.

Kaposi's sarcoma

This is discussed on page 402.

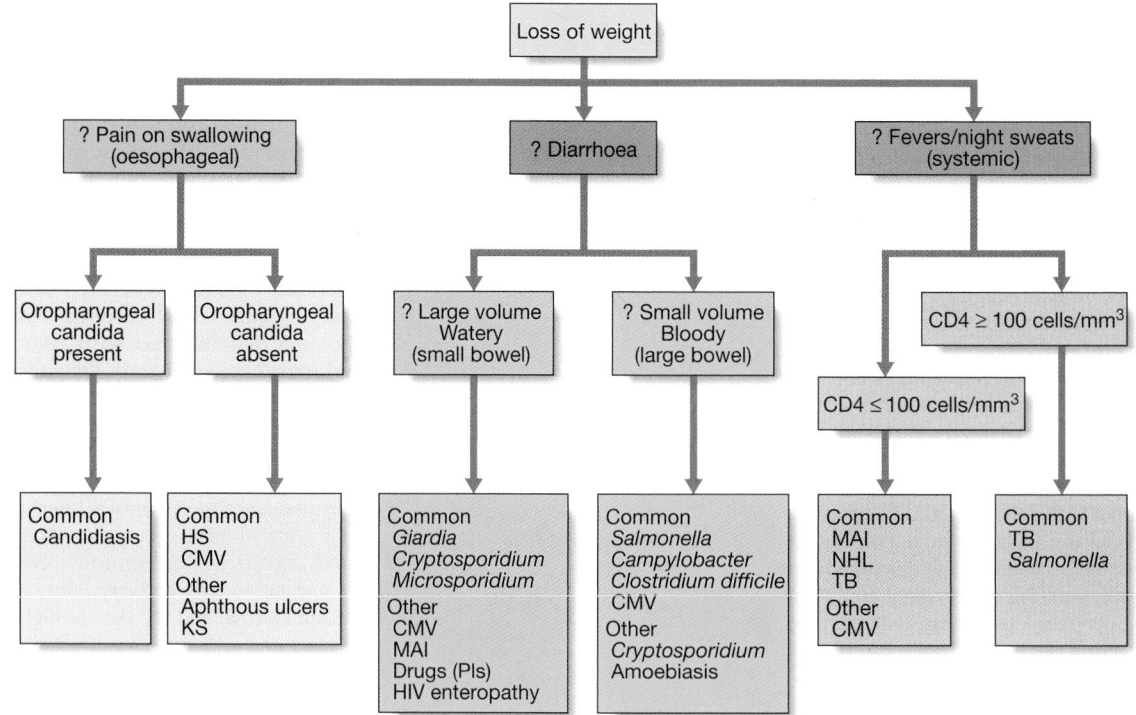

Fig. 14.6 Presentation and differential diagnosis of HIV-related gastrointestinal disorders. (CMV = cytomegalovirus; HS = herpes simplex; KS = Kaposi's sarcoma; MAI = *Mycobacterium avium intracellulare*; NHL = non-Hodgkin lymphoma; PI = protease inhibitor; TB = tuberculosis)

Gastrointestinal disease

Pain on swallowing, weight loss and chronic diarrhoea are common presenting features of later-stage HIV. A range of opportunistic organisms and HIV-related tumours may be responsible (Fig. 14.6).

Specific conditions

Cytomegalovirus (CMV) (Box 14.9)

Gastrointestinal CMV is now infrequent and is only seen if the CD4 count is < 100 cells/mm³ (usually < 50). It may cause disease throughout the entire gastrointestinal tract, including the liver and biliary tree, but most commonly affects the oesophagus, where it accounts for 10–20% of disease, and the colon.

Cryptosporidium and Microsporidium

Cryptosporidium (Box 14.10 and Fig. 14.6) is a highly contagious zoonotic protozoal enteric pathogen that infects a wide range of animals.

Microsporidia are water-borne zoonoses, of which four main species infect humans: *Encephalitozoon bieneusi*, *E. hellem*, *E cuniculi* and *E. intestinalis*. They are intracellular spore-forming protozoa which cause a mild inflammatory infiltrate and are carried by a wide range of animals, birds and fish.

Both *Cryptosporidium* and *Microsporidium* complete their life cycle in a single host. Together they account for 10–20% of cases of diarrhoea in HIV patients. This may vary from a mild illness to severe diarrhoea, and may be complicated by malabsorption and biliary disease. Encephalitis, sinusitis, and ocular and disseminated infection may rarely occur with *E. intestinalis*.

14

14.9 CMV oesophagitis and colitis

Epidemiology	Reactivation of latent herpes virus infection Develops in < 5% of patients
At-risk CD4 count	< 100 cells/mm³
Pathology	Intracellular and intracytoplasmic 'owl's-eye' inclusion bodies pathognomonic

Clinical features

Presentation	2–4-wk history *Oesophageal*: gradual onset of localised pain on swallowing, retrosternal pain, dysphagia, fever and weight loss *Colitis*: watery diarrhoea often accompanied by blood, colicky abdominal pain, weight loss and fever
Suspect if	*Oesophageal*: empirical fluconazole fails *Colitis*: pathogen-negative bloody diarrhoea or thickened dilated bowel on X-ray
Differential diagnosis	*Oesophageal*: *Candida*, herpes simplex, aphthous ulcers, lymphoma, KS *Colitis*: standard enteric pathogens
Complications	*Oesophageal*: strictures *Colitis*: toxic megacolon, haemorrhage and perforation

Key investigations and diagnosis

Endoscopy	*Oesophageal*: large shallow erosions/ulcers distally with inflammation at ulcer edge *Colitis*: generalised hyperaemia to segmental or confluent shallow or deep ulcers. 20% have disease proximal to splenic flexure so colonoscopy preferable
Blood	CMV viraemia in high titre
Tissue biopsy	Evidence of inclusion bodies and CMV on immunofluorescence/PCR. May be seen in the absence of clinical disease

Management

Treatment	*Induction*: First-line: i.v. ganciclovir or oral valganciclovir for 3 wks *Maintenance*: valganciclovir Commence/optimise HAART (p. 404) Consider stopping CMV therapy when CD4 > 100 cells/mm³, CMV and HIV viral loads undetectable, and on HAART
Prophylaxis	Not recommended; consider if recurrent relapses with persistently low CD4 count
Prognosis	Good if uncomplicated and immune restoration

14.10 Cryptosporidiosis

Epidemiology	Most common species are *C. hominis*, *C. parvum* and *C. meleagridis*. Transmitted through ingestion of *Cryptosporidium* oöcysts from animals or contaminated water. Resistant to standard chlorination
At-risk CD4 count	< 100 cells/mm³
Pathology	Intracellular extracytoplasmic protozoan on brush border

Clinical features

Presentation	History is acute or subacute Large-volume watery stools, vomiting, abdominal pain and weight loss
Suspect if	Watery stools negative for standard pathogens
Differential diagnosis	Giardiasis, microsporidiosis
Complications	Cholera-like illness and malabsorption. Rarely, acalculous cholecystitis, sclerosing cholangitis, pancreatitis and pneumonitis

Key investigations and diagnosis

Faeces	Oöcysts by acid-fast stain or antigen testing on microscopy in 90%. Electron microscopy increases yield
Other	Duodenal biopsy if stools negative (see Fig. 14.7) ERCP or MRCP if sclerosing cholangitis possible

Management

Treatment	Commence/optimise HAART Some effect with nitazoxanide or azithromycin and paromomycin Anti-motility agents Stop therapy on completion of treatment course and CD4 restoration > 200 cells/mm³
Prevention/prophylaxis	Boil water if CD4 < 200 cells/mm³
Prognosis	Good with immune restoration

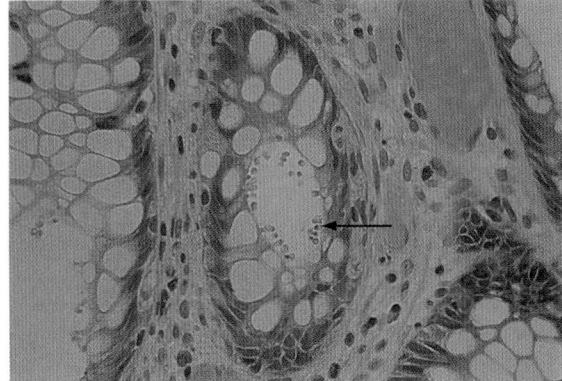

Fig. 14.7 Cryptosporidial infection. Duodenal biopsy may be necessary to confirm cryptosporidiosis or microsporidiosis.

Diagnosis is usually made by stool microscopy, although duodenal biopsy (Fig. 14.7) is occasionally necessary. Electron microscopy is essential for speciation of microsporidia. Although treatment for cryptosporidiosis (see Box 14.10) and microsporidiosis (albendazole ± itraconazole for *E. intestinalis* and nitazoxanide or fumagillin for *E. bieneusi*) may be effective, reconstitution of the immune system with HAART is the most important component of treatment and offers the best chance of cure.

Other infections

Isospora (Africa and Latin America) and *Cyclospora* (Asia) cause watery diarrhoea, weight loss and malabsorption akin to *Cryptosporidium*, accounting overall for 2–4% of cases in the UK. Diagnosis is by stool microscopy and treatment for both is co-trimoxazole. *Giardia, Entamoeba histolytica*, adenovirus and bacterial overgrowth also occur more frequently in HIV patients. Of the standard enteric pathogens, *Salmonella* is important because of the increased probability of bacteraemia and recurrent disease.

Mycobacterium avium intracellulare (MAI)

Until the introduction of HAART and primary prophylaxis, disseminated MAI (Box 14.11) occurred in up to 35% of all patients. Like other opportunistic infections, the incidence has now fallen but it remains a problem in late-stage AIDS, especially those cases that are newly diagnosed. Patients present with fever and weight loss. Combination antibacterial therapy is essential to prevent resistance, but reconstitution of the immune system with HAART is necessary for cure.

Liver disease

Hepatitis B and hepatitis C

The importance of hepatitis B and C co-infection is increasingly recognised. For both HBV and HCV, co-infection is associated with higher HBV or HCV viral loads, accelerated natural progression to cirrhosis (5–8 years after infection), an increased rate of hepatoma and higher mortality. Hepatitis B and C are further described on pages 948–954.

Hepatitis B

The majority of those with HIV have evidence of HBV exposure. HBV carriage rate depends on the mode of

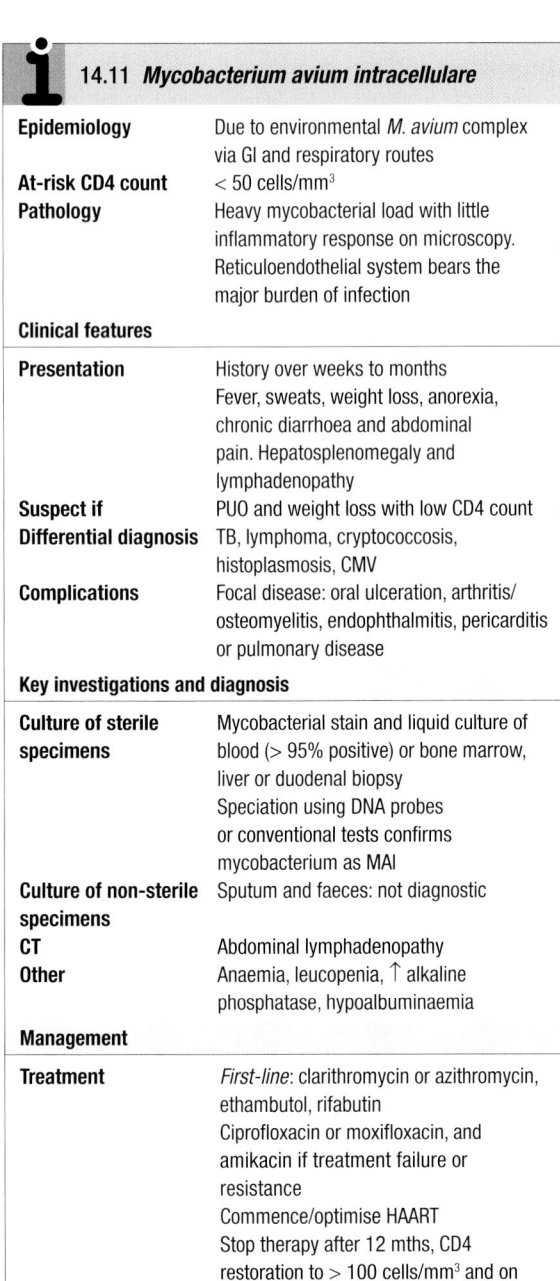

14.11 *Mycobacterium avium intracellulare*	
Epidemiology	Due to environmental *M. avium* complex via GI and respiratory routes
At-risk CD4 count	< 50 cells/mm³
Pathology	Heavy mycobacterial load with little inflammatory response on microscopy. Reticuloendothelial system bears the major burden of infection
Clinical features	
Presentation	History over weeks to months Fever, sweats, weight loss, anorexia, chronic diarrhoea and abdominal pain. Hepatosplenomegaly and lymphadenopathy
Suspect if	PUO and weight loss with low CD4 count
Differential diagnosis	TB, lymphoma, cryptococcosis, histoplasmosis, CMV
Complications	Focal disease: oral ulceration, arthritis/ osteomyelitis, endophthalmitis, pericarditis or pulmonary disease
Key investigations and diagnosis	
Culture of sterile specimens	Mycobacterial stain and liquid culture of blood (> 95% positive) or bone marrow, liver or duodenal biopsy Speciation using DNA probes or conventional tests confirms mycobacterium as MAI
Culture of non-sterile specimens	Sputum and faeces: not diagnostic
CT	Abdominal lymphadenopathy
Other	Anaemia, leucopenia, ↑ alkaline phosphatase, hypoalbuminaemia
Management	
Treatment	*First-line*: clarithromycin or azithromycin, ethambutol, rifabutin Ciprofloxacin or moxifloxacin, and amikacin if treatment failure or resistance Commence/optimise HAART Stop therapy after 12 mths, CD4 restoration to > 100 cells/mm³ and on suppressive HAART
Immune restoration syndrome	Common on starting HAART. Usually focal disease, particularly lymphadenitis
Prophylaxis	*Primary*: CD4 < 50 cells/mm³ *First-line*: azithromycin weekly
Prognosis	5% mortality

acquisition, place of birth and ethnic group (reflecting vertical transmission), immunisation history (although response rates are lower in HIV patients) and likelihood of immune clearance after infection. Although HBV co-infected patients have more aggressive disease, the immunosuppression seen in more advanced HIV affords some protection because hepatic damage is immune-mediated. Treatment with antivirals should be considered for all patients who have active viral replication (HBVeAg-positive or HBV-DNA > 2000 U/mL) and/or evidence of inflammation, fibrosis or scarring on liver biopsy. When the CD4 is ≥500 cells/mm³ and in the absence of cirrhosis, pegylated interferon or adefovir can be considered. Otherwise, antivirals should ordinarily be used. A combination of either tamivudine (3TC) or emtricitabine (FTC) with tenofovir and an additional anti-HIV drug provides effective anti-HIV and anti-HBV treatment. A flare of hepatitis may be associated with improved immune function consequent to HAART or interruption of therapy and rebound HIV viraemia. All patients should be immunised against HAV.

Hepatitis C

Most patients with HCV have acquired their infection from injection drug use but increasingly acute infection is being seen in MSM. The major determinant of co-infection rate is the mode of acquisition: > 80% for haemophiliacs, 70–80% for injection drug-users, 10–15% for MSM and 3–5% for heterosexuals. Only 15–20% of patients ever clear their initial infection, but this rate is higher in females, those with higher CD4 counts, and those with raised transaminases. Response to 12 months' combination therapy with pegylated α-interferon and weight-based ribavirin is dependent on the HCV genotype (approximately 65% with genotypes 2 or 3 as opposed to approximately 27% with other genotypes), HCV viral load, CD4 count and the presence of cirrhosis; those acutely infected also have an improved response rate. HIV treatment is usually initiated first to optimise the CD4 count to ≥ 350 cells/mm³. Because of interactions with ribavirin, some nucleotide reverse transcriptase inhibitors (ZDV, didanosine (ddI) and possibly abacavir, p. 404) should be avoided if HAART is being co-administered. Therapy may be associated with a flare of hepatitis because of improved immune responsiveness. All patients should be screened for HBV and HAV, and immunised if not protected.

Respiratory disease

Many patients with HIV will develop pulmonary disease at some time. Several factors influence the likely cause, including CD4 count, ethnicity, age, risk group, prophylactic history and geographical location. The history is vital in discriminating acute bacterial pneumonia (rapid onset, pleuritic chest pain, rigors) from *Pneumocystis jirovecii* pneumonia (subacute onset, breathlessness, dry cough), a common differential in later-stage disease. The chest X-ray is also important in distinguishing presenting syndromes (Box 14.12).

14.12 Differential diagnosis of HIV-related pulmonary disease: chest X-ray findings

Appearance	Major causes
Diffuse infiltrate	PCP pneumonia, tuberculosis, Kaposi's sarcoma, non-Hodgkin lymphoma, atypical bacterial pneumonia, lymphoid interstitial pneumonitis
Nodules/focal consolidation	Tuberculosis, Kaposi's sarcoma, non-Hodgkin lymphoma, *Cryptococcus*, *Histoplasma*
Hilar lymphadenopathy	Tuberculosis, Kaposi's sarcoma, non-Hodgkin lymphoma; *Cryptococcus*, *Histoplasma*
Pleural effusion	Kaposi's sarcoma, tuberculosis, pyogenic bacterial pneumonia, primary effusion lymphoma

Specific conditions
Pneumocystis jirovecii

Pneumocystis jirovecii (previously *carinii*) pneumonia (PCP, Box 14.13) was the first major indicator disease for HIV at the beginning of the epidemic, and still

14.13 *Pneumocystis* pneumonia

Epidemiology	Caused by *P. jirovecii*. Likely to represent reinfection from other humans by respiratory transmission
At-risk CD4 count	< 200 cells/mm³, with risk increasing as count falls
Pathology	Extracellular fungus with cyst, merozoite and trophozoite morphology. Cannot be cultured but cyst and trophozoite can be visualised by (e.g.) Giemsa, silver or immunofluorescence stains. Causes interstitial plasma cell pneumonia with 'foamy' exudates in the alveoli

Clinical features

Presentation	History over days to weeks. Progressive and disproportionate exertional dyspnoea, fever, dry cough and difficulty in taking deep breath. Few signs on auscultation
Suspect if	Subacute history of fever, cough and breathlessness, or failure to respond to antibiotics
Differential diagnosis	TB, Kaposi's sarcoma, unusual fungi (*Histoplasma*, *Penicillium*, *Cryptococcus*, *Coccidioides*), atypical pneumonia, *Nocardia* and lymphoma
Complications	Respiratory failure, pneumothorax, bacterial superinfection, extrapulmonary disease (rare)

Key investigations and diagnosis

Chest X-ray	Normal early. *Moderate disease*: perihilar interstitial haze. *Severe disease*: white-out with relative sparing of apices and costophrenic angles
Sputum	Positive cytology or PCR on induced sputum (50–90%), or bronchoalveolar lavage (90–95%)
Other	Raised lactate dehydrogenase (LDH); O₂ saturations < 90% on exercise. *Pa*O₂ reduced (mild > 11 kPa; moderate 8.1–11 kPa; severe < 8 kPa)

Management

Treatment	*First-line*: co-trimoxazole for 3 wks. *Second-line*: clindamycin and primaquine. Steroids for moderate to severe disease. CPAP and ventilation/ICU may be necessary. Commence/optimise HAART. Stop therapy when CD4 > 200 cells/mm³ for 3 mths on HAART
Immune restoration syndrome	Rare but described
Prophylaxis	Primary prophylaxis when CD4 < 200/mm³. *First-line*: co-trimoxazole. *Second-line*: dapsone or atovaquone
Prognosis	10% mortality, 5% morbidity

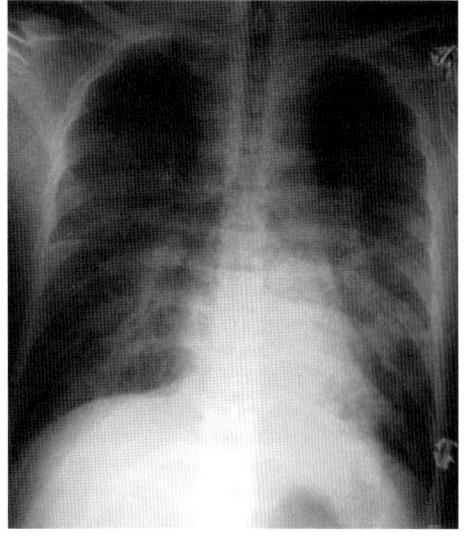

Fig. 14.8 *Pneumocystis* pneumonia: typical chest X-ray appearance. Note the sparing at the apex and base of both lungs.

accounts for 25% of AIDS-defining illness. The incidence of PCP has fallen dramatically with HAART and primary prophylaxis. Presentation is with fever, breathlessness, and dry cough, and other markers of

HIV (e.g. oropharyngeal candidiasis or mucocutaneous herpes simplex) may be present. The chest X-ray is usually typical (Fig. 14.8), but 20% are atypical with unilateral infiltration, upper lobe disease (often when on inhaled pentamidine prophylaxis), focal consolidation, cavitation or nodular shadows. Clinical and radiological deterioration within the first 48 hours of treatment is not uncommon.

Mycobacterium tuberculosis

Tuberculosis (TB) is the most common global infection (p. 688), affecting up to one-third of the estimated 40 million HIV patients (Boxes 14.14 and 14.15). Estimated annual new case and death rates (8 million and 2 million respectively) are expected to continue

 14.14 Tuberculosis in HIV

Patients with HIV are at greater risk of:
- Infection after exposure
- Progressive primary disease after infection
- Reactivation of latent infection
- Reinfection with new strain
- Disseminated and extrapulmonary (e.g. meningeal and pericardial) disease
- Adverse drug reactions

14.15 Pulmonary tuberculosis

Epidemiology	Due to *M. tuberculosis*, *M. bovis* or *M. africanum* *Mycobacterium* enhances HIV replication and acceleration of the disease; HIV causes immunosuppression and increases risk of reactivation and susceptibility to infection	**Sputum**	Organisms seen on Ziehl–Neelsen and auramine stains, and grown by radiometric culture Nucleic acid amplification allows rapid speciation and identification of rifampicin resistance; also used in smear-negative samples to increase diagnostic yield
At-risk CD4 count	Any, with risk increasing as count falls		
Pathology	Granulomas and caseating necrosis	**Other**	Positive mycobacterial cultures from blood identified in 50% of those with CD4 < 200 cells/mm³
Clinical features			
		Management	
Presentation	History over weeks to months Fever, night sweats and weight loss *CD4 count > 200 cells/mm³*: reactivated upper-lobe cavitatory disease is more likely with cough and haemoptysis *CD4 count ≤ 200 cells/mm³*: miliary, atypical pulmonary and extrapulmonary TB become more common	**Treatment**	*First-line*: rifampicin, isoniazid, ethambutol and pyrazinamide for 2 mths, then rifampicin and isoniazid for 4 mths. Drug reactions more common Consider steroids for moderate to severe disease Commence/optimise HAART. Efavirenz (with two NRTIs) first line because metabolism of protease inhibitors (PIs) is induced by rifampicin (p. 404) Stop therapy when complete
Suspect if	PUO, pneumonia failing to respond to antibiotics, exudative pleural effusion, unexplained weight loss, or TB is endemic in patient's country of origin		
Differential diagnosis	PCP, Kaposi's sarcoma, unusual fungi (*Histoplasma*, *Penicillium*, *Cryptococcus*, *Coccidioides*), atypical pneumonia, *Nocardia* and lymphoma	**Immune restoration syndrome**	Occurs in 10–15%. Most common in those with a nadir CD4 < 50 cells/mm³ and a brisk CD4 response to HAART. Commonly presents as focal disease Treatment: NSAIDS or steroids
Complications	Massive haemoptysis, empyema, acute respiratory distress syndrome (ARDS), cor pulmonale, aspergilloma	**Prophylaxis**	Isoniazid (with or without rifampicin) reduces the risk of TB by 60% in patients with positive tuberculin skin tests (less in those with negative tests) Protection limited to 2–4 yrs probably because of reinfection
Key investigations and diagnosis			
Chest X-ray	Cavities, miliary shadowing, pleural effusion, mediastinal lymphadenopathy, collapse and consolidation (see Fig. 14.8) 5% with smear-positive disease have a normal chest X-ray	**Prognosis**	Mortality 5%

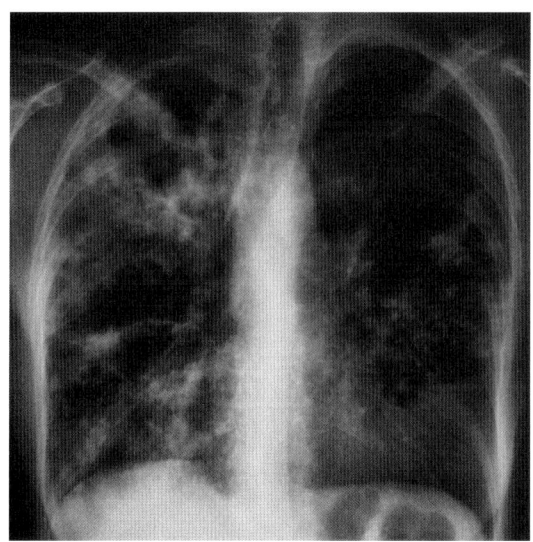

Fig. 14.9 Chest X-ray of pulmonary tuberculosis in HIV infection. Appearances are often atypical but in this case there are multiple cavities and focal consolidation.

to rise inexorably. In some countries up to 30% of patients presenting with TB are co-infected with HIV. Presentation is invariably with fever, weight loss and site-specific symptoms (pulmonary, meningeal, pericardial, etc.). Diagnosis may be difficult, as smear-positive rates are reduced in pulmonary TB, and chest X-ray appearances may be atypical with less cavitation (Fig. 14.9). Standard quadruple therapy (see Box 14.15) is curative in the majority, with mortality often being attributable to other disseminated bacterial infections (e.g. *Salmonella* and pneumococcus). If compliance is likely to be a problem, daily or thrice-weekly directly observed therapy (DOT) should be considered. Multidrug-resistant TB (MDRTB) presents a seri-

ous clinical and public health problem in many areas of the world (e.g. Eastern Europe, South Africa). In addition, extensively drug-resistant TB (XDRTB) has now been reported from South Africa, where it has become a significant problem, and also in small numbers from over 100 countries. MDRTB and XDRTB are described in detail on pages 693–694. Treatment often entails hospital admission and 6–7 drug combinations.

Bacterial infections

Bacterial pneumonia is a common cause of morbidity and mortality in HIV. The incidence, severity, likelihood of bacteraemia and recurrent pneumonia, and mortality rate are all increased compared to non-HIV-infected patients. Susceptibility to particular respiratory pathogens is influenced by risk group, level of immune depletion, age and presence of neutropenia. There is a 150-fold greater risk of pneumococcal pneumonia in advanced HIV, when it is the cause of 40% of all pneumonias in which a pathogen is identified, and 70% of those with bacteraemia. *Pseudomonas* (5%) and *Nocardia* infections are more likely in later-stage disease. *Legionella* is also found more frequently. Chest X-ray appearances may be atypical. Infection usually responds to standard antibiotic therapy.

Nervous system and eye disease

Disease of the central and peripheral nervous system is common in HIV. It may be a direct consequence of HIV infection or an indirect result of CD4 cell depletion. Presentations are outlined in Box 14.16 and Figure 14.10.

Toxoplasma gondii

Toxoplasma infection results in a mild or subclinical illness in immunocompetent individuals, with the formation of latent tissue cysts that persist for life (Box 14.17).

14

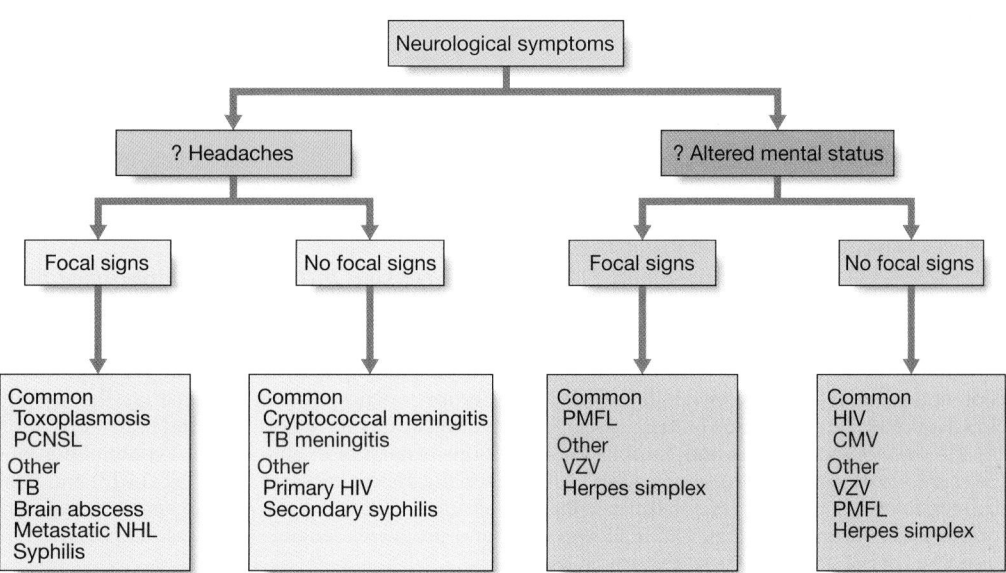

Fig. 14.10 Presentation and differential diagnosis of HIV-related neurological disorders. (CMV = cytomegalovirus; NHL = non-Hodgkin lymphoma; PCNSL = primary CNS lymphoma; PML = progressive multifocal leucoencephalopathy; TB = tuberculosis; VZV = varicella zoster virus)

14.16 Differential diagnosis of HIV-related disorders of the nervous system

Presentation	Main causes
Space-occupying lesion(s)	Toxoplasmosis, primary CNS lymphoma, progressive multifocal leucoencephalopathy (PML), TB
Cognitive impairment	AIDS dementia, PML, CMV, syphilis
Encephalitis	HIV, varicella zoster virus, herpes simplex, syphilis
Meningitis	HIV seroconversion, *Cryptococcus*, TB, syphilis
Spastic paraparesis	HIV-vacuolar myelopathy, transverse myelitis from varicella zoster, herpes simplex, human T-cell lymphotropic virus 1, syphilis
Polyradiculitis	CMV, non-Hodgkin lymphoma
Peripheral neuropathy	HIV, drugs (e.g. d4T, ddl, p. 404)
Retinitis	CMV, toxoplasmosis, retinal necrosis, HIV, syphilis

14.17 Cerebral toxoplasmosis

Epidemiology	Reactivation of latent primary CNS infection. Acquired from ingestion of food contaminated by cat's faeces or undercooked meat Prevalence age- and region-dependent
At-risk CD4 count	< 100 cells/mm³
Pathology	Spherical tachyzoites within inflammatory granulomas and surrounding oedema

Clinical features

Presentation	History < 2 wks Headache, fever, drowsiness, fits (33%) and focal neurological signs. Retinitis may coexist
Suspect if	Short history of headache, fever, fits and focal signs
Differential diagnosis	Primary CNS lymphoma, PML, TB, *Cryptococcus*
Complications	Raised intracranial pressure (ICP)

Key investigations and diagnosis

MRI	Multiple ring-enhancing lesions in cortical grey–white matter interface, basal ganglia or brain stem. Associated oedema and mass effect
Other	85% are *Toxoplasma* IgG antibody-positive Brain biopsy PCR positive on CSF (but lumbar puncture often contraindicated) Response to empirical anti-*Toxoplasma* therapy

Management

Treatment	*First-line*: sulphadiazine or clindamycin with pyrimethamine and folinic acid for 6 wks, with dexamethasone if mass effect Commence/optimise HAART *Maintenance*: same drugs at lower dose Stop therapy when CD4 > 200 cells/mm³ for 3 mths on suppressive HAART
Immune restoration syndrome	Well recognised but uncommon
Prophylaxis	*Primary*: co-trimoxazole *Secondary*: sulphadiazine or clindamycin with pyrimethamine and folinic acid
Prognosis	5% acute mortality, 15% neurological morbidity

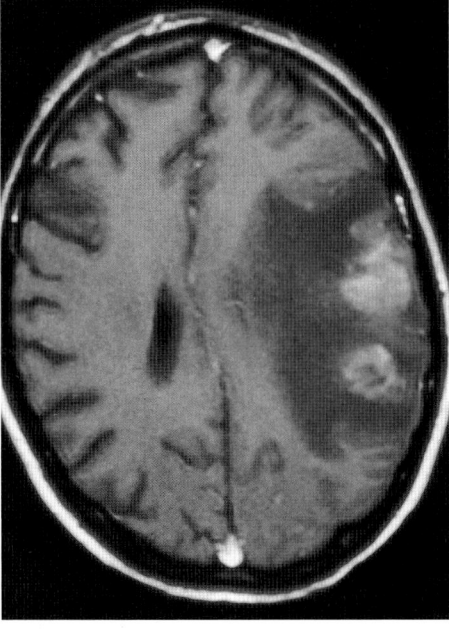

Fig. 14.11 Cerebral toxoplasmosis. Multiple cortical ring-enhancing lesions with surrounding oedema are characteristic.

The infection rate, as judged by seroconversion, is 0.5–1% per year. In advanced HIV, reactivation of these cysts may occur with the development of cerebral toxoplasmosis. Despite the characteristic findings on imaging (Fig. 14.11), it is often impossible to distinguish *Toxoplasma* encephalitis from primary CNS lymphoma (Fig. 14.12). However, the response to a trial of anti-*Toxoplasma* therapy is usually diagnostic, with clinical improvement within 1 week in 50% and 2 weeks in 90%; shrinkage of lesions on MRI is usual by 2–4 weeks.

Progressive multifocal leucoencephalopathy (PML)

PML (Box 14.18) is a demyelinating disease caused by the JC papovavirus; it occurs at very low CD4 counts. Seroprevalence studies demonstrate that up to 90% of young adults have been exposed to JC virus, most infections occurring in childhood. A combination of characteristic appearances on MRI (Fig. 14.13) and positive JC virus in CSF is diagnostic. No specific treatment exists and prognosis remains poor despite HAART.

Primary CNS lymphoma (PCNSL)

PCNSLs are high-grade, diffuse, B-cell lymphomas which usually complicate late-stage HIV (CD4 < 50 cells/mm³).

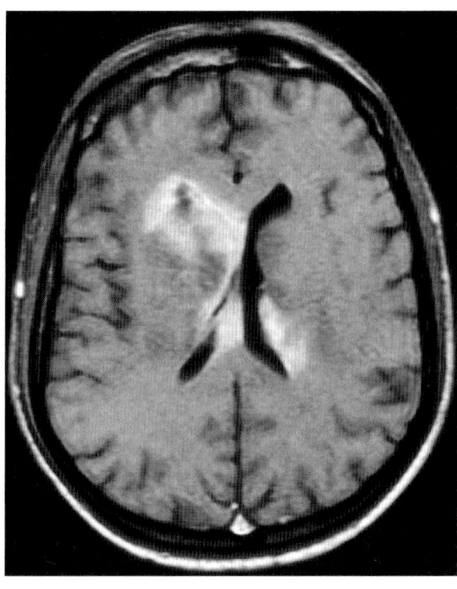

Fig. 14.12 Primary CNS lymphoma. A single enhancing periventricular lesion with moderate oedema is typical.

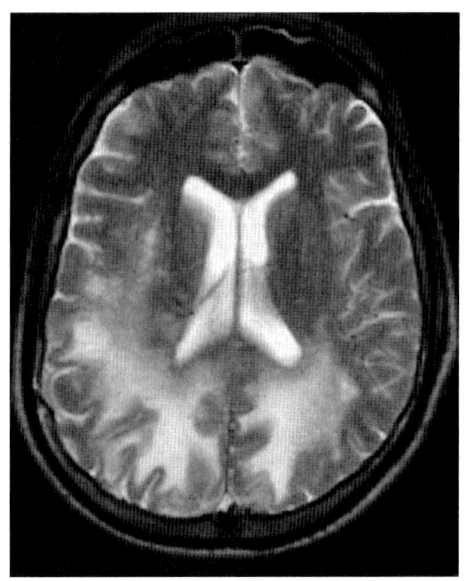

Fig. 14.13 Progressive multifocal leucoencephalopathy. Non-enhancing white matter lesions without surrounding oedema are seen.

14.18 Progressive multifocal leucoencephalopathy (PML)

Epidemiology	Reactivation of latent virus with transport to brain, where it infects oligodendrocytes via serotonin receptor
At-risk CD4 count	< 50 cells/mm^3
Pathology	Multifocal demyelination and enlarged oligodendrocytes with nuclear inclusions at edges
Clinical features	
Presentation	History over weeks to months Hemiparesis, visual/speech defects (25%), altered mental/mood status, ataxia. Seizures rare and fever absent
Suspect if	Gradual-onset focal neurology without fever
Differential diagnosis	HIV encephalopathy, CMV, herpes simplex, VZV, toxoplasmosis, primary CNS lymphoma
Key investigations and diagnosis	
MRI	Bilateral, asymmetric, well-demarcated, non-enhancing lesions, predominantly affecting the white matter. No oedema or shift
CSF	JC papovavirus PCR-positive
Management	
Treatment	Commence/optimise HAART
Immune restoration syndrome	Well characterised and may be presenting diagnosis
Prophylaxis	Nil
Prognosis	50% mortality at 3–12 mths. 35% neurological disability

They occur in approximately 5% of AIDS patients and account for 20% of all focal CNS lesions. The history is 2–8 weeks of headache, focal features and sometimes confusion; seizures occur in 15% but fever is absent. Characteristically, imaging demonstrates a large, single, homogeneously enhancing periventricular lesion with mild to moderate surrounding oedema and mass effect. Multiple lesions may occur on MRI (see Fig. 14.12) but a solitary lesion is four times more likely to be PCNSL than *Toxoplasma*. The presence of EBV-DNA in the CSF has a high sensitivity and specificity for PCNSL. Biopsy is definitive, but carries a small risk of morbidity and may be non-diagnostic in up to one-third. Failure to improve clinically or on scanning with a trial of anti-*Toxoplasma* therapy after 2–4 weeks is consistent with PCNSL and is an indication for brain biopsy. Treatment can be tried with HAART and high-dose methotrexate, but the prognosis is poor.

Other focal brain disease

M. tuberculosis, *Cryptococcus neoformans* and *Treponema pallidum* predominantly affect the meninges but can produce mass lesions with focal neurology. A less frequent cause of focal disease is CMV, which presents with a subacute history of progressive disorientation, withdrawal, apathy, cranial nerve palsies and nystagmus. Bilateral enhancing periventricular changes on MRI are characteristic and retinitis is present in over half. Diagnosis is made by identifying CMV-DNA in the CSF.

HIV-associated encephalopathy

HIV is a neurotropic virus and infects the CNS early during infection. Aseptic meningitis or encephalitis may occur at seroconversion, and minor cognitive defects such as mental slowness and poor memory may develop as the disease progresses. The incidence has fallen dramatically as a result of HAART. Dementia occurs in late disease and is characterised by global deterioration of cognitive function, severe psychomotor retardation, paraparesis, ataxia, and urinary and faecal incontinence. Changes in affect are common, and depression or psychosis may be the predominant feature. Higher plasma and CSF HIV viral load, lower CD4 count and age are predictors. Investigations show diffuse cerebral atrophy with widened sulci and enlarged ventricles on imaging, and a raised protein in the CSF. Combination therapy using agents providing optimal CNS penetration may slow or even reverse the progression of HIV-associated dementia. Appropriate psychotropic medication may also be necessary.

Cryptococcosis

Cryptococcus neoformans (Box 14.19) is the most important cause of meningitis associated with late-stage HIV and occurs in up to 5% of patients, who usually present with a 2–3-week history of headache, fever, vomiting and mild confusion. Neck stiffness is present in less than 25% of patients, and around 10% are asymptomatic. Diagnosis is made by CSF antigen detection and culture. Between 10% and 20% of patients require treatment for raised intracranial pressure with repeated lumbar punctures, a lumbar drain or shunting.

Spinal cord, nerve root and peripheral nerve disease

A variety of neuropathies occur in HIV infection. At seroconversion, Guillain–Barré syndrome, transverse myelitis, facial palsy, brachial neuritis, polyradiculitis and peripheral neuropathy have all rarely been described.

Vacuolar myelopathy is a slowly progressive myelitis resulting in paraparesis with no sensory level. Ataxia and incontinence occur in advanced cases. The CSF may show a raised protein but is frequently normal; MRI of the spine is normal, and the diagnosis is by exclusion of other causes.

A predominantly distal HIV-related sensory neuropathy of the lower limbs affects up to 30% of patients. It is associated with a lower CD4 (usually < 200 cells/mm³), higher viral load, older age and wasting, and results from axonal degeneration. Hyperaesthesia, pain in the soles of the feet and paraesthesia, with diminished pin-prick, light touch and vibration sensation, and loss of ankle reflexes (75%) are typical. The nucleoside reverse transcriptase inhibitor (NRTI) drugs, especially d4T and didanosine (ddI), can produce an identical picture but this remits if the offending agent is withdrawn early. Treatment is often difficult, although amitriptyline, lamotrigine and topical capsaicin cream may help symptoms. HAART has minimal effect on halting or reversing the process.

Polyradiculitis occurs in late-stage HIV (CD4 count < 50 cells/mm³) and is nearly always a result of CMV. It causes rapidly progressive flaccid paraparesis, saddle anaesthesia, absent reflexes and sphincter dysfunction. Pain in the legs and back is an early symptom. Nerve root involvement on nerve conduction studies, a neutrophil CSF pleocytosis and the presence of CMV-DNA demonstrated by PCR confirm the diagnosis. Despite treatment, functional recovery may not occur. CMV is discussed in more detail on page 317.

Lastly, proximal myopathy can result from HIV, when it may occur at any stage, or rarely from zidovudine (ZDV) (< 1% of patients).

---

i | **14.19 Cryptococcal meningitis**

Epidemiology	Caused by *C. neoformans var. grubii* (serotype A) and *C. neoformans var. neoformans* (serotype D). Found in soil and spread by birds. Infection through inhalation with rapid spread to meninges
At-risk CD4 count	< 200 cells/mm³
Pathology	Budding encapsulated yeasts in clusters with limited inflammatory response
Clinical features	
Presentation	History < 4 wks Headache, fever, drowsiness, confusion, photophobia and blurred vision, and seizures. Meningism may be absent and papilloedema uncommon. 10% are asymptomatic Non-meningeal (lung or skin) and disseminated disease are rare
Consider if	Recent-onset headache with fever
Differential diagnosis	TB meningitis
Complications	Blindness and deafness due to raised ICP, arachnoiditis and direct cryptococcal nerve infiltration
Key investigations and diagnosis	
MRI	Meningeal enhancement and evidence of raised ICP, with occasional masses in the basal ganglia
CSF	Lymphocytic, raised protein, low glucose typical but may be normal High pressure on manometry India ink stain positive for organisms (60%), cryptococcal antigen (> 95%) and fungal culture (> 95%)
Blood	Cryptococcal antigen positive > 99%, culture > 95%
Other	Urine/sputum/skin fungal culture may rarely be positive Chest X-ray may be abnormal
Management	
Treatment	*Induction*: *First-line*: liposomal amphotericin B and 5-flucytosine for 2 wks *Maintenance*: *First-line*: fluconazole for 8 wks Commence/optimise HAART Raised ICP must be managed actively to maintain CSF pressure < 20 cm H₂O Stop therapy when CD4 > 200 cells/mm³, for 3 mths on suppressive HAART and negative cultures
Immune restoration syndrome	Well described
Prophylaxis	*Primary*: not recommended *Secondary*: fluconazole
Prognosis	5–10% acute mortality. 10% morbidity

Psychiatric disease

Significant psychiatric morbidity is not uncommon. Anxiety and mood disturbance may be caused by pre-test issues such as worries about being infected and disclosure, receiving a positive result (e.g. confidentiality, discrimination and stigmatisation), concerns about life expectancy, or facing up to death. Mild cognitive dysfunction is a common occurrence in later-stage disease and usually improves with HAART (see above). Disorders of mental state may also result from drugs directly (e.g. depression with efavirenz, p. 405) or indirectly (e.g. those affecting sexual dysfunction). Psychiatric morbidity is a major risk factor for poor compliance with drug treatment, which is a critical component of HAART management.

Retinitis

Since the advent of HAART, there has been a 90% fall in the incidence of CMV infections. Patients usually present with field defects and well-demarcated areas of retinal disease (Box 14.20 and p. 384). Macular dis-

ease is rare but constitutes the most sight-threatening feature. Diagnosis is usually clinical. Treatment needs to be prompt, as the leading edge will progressively advance; no recovery of vision occurs in affected areas. Some patients may develop immune recovery uveitis in response to HAART, with intra-ocular inflammation, macular oedema and cataract formation that requires prompt treatment with oral and intra-ocular corticosteroids to prevent visual loss.

Miscellaneous conditions

Haematological conditions

Disorders of all three major cell lines may occur in HIV and are most frequent in later-stage disease (anaemia 70%, leucopenia 50% and thrombocytopenia 40%), when pancytopenia may also be seen. Numerous causes for anaemia exist, including marrow infiltration with opportunistic infections (MAI or TB) or neoplasms (non-Hodgkin lymphoma); bone marrow suppression from drugs (ZDV) or as a direct effect of HIV; and chronic blood loss (Kaposi's sarcoma) or malabsorption (chronic protozoal infections) in gastrointestinal tract disease. Haemolytic anaemia is uncommon but is seen with lymphoma. Leucopenia is usually seen in the context of marrow infiltration, as above, or drug toxicity (e.g. ZDV, co-trimoxazole, ganciclovir). Lymphopenia ($< 1.0 \times 10^9/L$) is a good marker of HIV. Thrombocytopenia may appear early (5–10%) and be the first indicator of HIV, or in later-stage disease. Its behaviour is very similar to idiopathic thrombocytopenic purpura, with detectable platelet antibodies and short-lived response to intravenous immunoglobulin. However, the treatment of choice is HAART.

Renal, cardiac and endocrine conditions

With the advent of HAART, opportunistic infections have declined substantially, and non-HIV-related illnesses of the cardiovascular, liver and renal systems have emerged as more important causes of morbidity and mortality.

Acute renal failure may be associated with acute infection or medication-related nephrotoxicity; this usually resolves with appropriate management. HIV-associated nephropathy (HIVAN) is the most important cause of chronic renal failure and is seen most frequently in patients of African descent and those with low CD4 counts. Other important HIV-associated renal diseases include HIV immune complex kidney diseases and thrombotic microangiopathy. Several drugs used in HIV management are also associated with renal disease, including indinavir (causes renal stones), tenofovir, pentamidine, cidofovir and co-trimoxazole. HIVAN usually presents with nephrotic syndrome, chronic renal failure or a combination of both. With the overall improvement in life expectancy, conditions such as diabetes mellitus, hypertension and vascular disease add to the burden of chronic kidney disease. HAART has some effect in slowing progression of renal disease. Doses of NRTIs must be adjusted according to creatinine clearance. Those who progress to end-stage renal disease while receiving HAART may be eligible for renal transplant.

14

---

i | **14.20 CMV retinitis**

Epidemiology	Reactivation of primary herpes virus infection
	< 1% end-organ CMV disease
At-risk CD4 count	< 50 cells/mm³
Pathology	Necrosis and haemorrhage
Clinical features	
Presentation	Subacute history with flashing lights, floaters, field defects and reduced visual acuity
	Occasionally asymptomatic and picked up on screening
	Well-demarcated haemorrhagic exudates usually peripheral and along vessels. 10% bilateral
Consider if	Field defect with peripheral retinitis
Differential diagnosis	Retinal necrosis (acute and progressive outer, PORN), toxoplasmosis, syphilis
Complications	Macular involvement and detached retina. CNS involvement rare
Key investigations and diagnosis	
Other	Clinical diagnosis. CMV PCR vitreous (rarely done)
Blood	Quantitative CMV PCR
Management	
Treatment	*First-line*: valganciclovir (oral) or ganciclovir (i.v.) for 3 wks
	If central disease, consider additional ganciclovir implant or intravitreal injections
	Ganciclovir resistance may rarely occur
	Maintenance: valganciclovir
	Commence/optimise HAART
	Stop therapy when on suppressive HAART, CD4 > 100 cells/mm³ and CMV viral load undetectable
Immune restoration syndrome	Immune recovery uveitis well recognised
	More common when > 25% retina affected
Prophylaxis	Not recommended
Prognosis	Blindness 5%, permanent deficit in affected areas

With increasing life expectancy, cardiac disease has become important. Although HIV-related dilated cardiomyopathy can be detected in 25–40% of AIDS patients, symptomatic heart disease is rare (3–6%) and zidovudine-induced cardiomyopathy rarely seen. Nevertheless, patients on certain antiretrovirals (e.g. protease inhibitors, abacavir and ddI) and those with CD4 counts < 350 cells/mm³ not taking HAART have increased rates of coronary artery disease. Moreover, there is a small but additional effect of drug-induced hyperlipidaemia with protease inhibitors and stavudine.

Patients with fatigue and low CD4 counts should be screened for hypoadrenalism, which is seen in up to one-quarter of patients, and hypogonadism (p. 757). Hypopituitarism has also been described (p. 785).

HIV-related cancers

Malignancies in HIV can be divided into AIDS-defining and non-AIDS-defining cancers. AIDS-defining cancers are characterised by a strong inverse association with CD4 count, which is also seen but to a lesser extent in many of the non-AIDS malignancies. Kaposi's sarcoma and non-Hodgkin lymphoma are the most important AIDS-defining malignancies, with anal cancer and Hodgkin disease becoming increasingly important non-AIDS-defining malignancies.

Specific conditions

Kaposi's sarcoma (KS)

Together with PCP, KS has become a hallmark of AIDS (Box 14.21 and Fig. 14.14); it is due to the herpes virus HHV-8. Prior to HIV, KS was a rare tumour restricted to elderly Mediterranean or Jewish males, immunosuppressed transplant recipients, and children and young adults in sub-Saharan Africa. Typical presentation is with raised non-pruritic papules, often found incidentally on examination in a newly diagnosed patient. As the disease progresses, the skin lesions become more numerous and larger. Visceral disease occurs in only 10% at presentation. With the widespread use of HAART, which is also the mainstay of treatment, there has been a 70% fall in incidence.

Primary-effusion lymphoma (< 2% of cases of non-Hodgkin lymphoma) and multicentric Castleman's disease, which is a rare lymphoproliferative disorder affecting mainly HIV patients who present with anaemia, fevers and multifocal lymphadenopathy, are other HHV-8-associated conditions seen rarely with HIV.

HIV-associated lymphoma

In the majority of patients, non-Hodgkin lymphoma (NHL, Box 14.22) represents a late manifestation of HIV, with risk increasing as CD4 count falls. The risk is > 50-fold greater than in HIV-negative individuals, with a lifetime risk of developing NHL of 5–10%. Over the last 10 years, the incidence of NHL has fallen by > 40% but has increased as a proportion of AIDS-defining illnesses. By comparison, the incidence of Hodgkin disease (HD) has a definite but less marked association with HIV (10–20-fold greater than in HIV-negative individuals) and CD4 count fall. For both, extranodal and advanced presentation is more likely, with the majority having B symptoms (p. 1038). Histologically, HD is more likely

14.21 Kaposi's sarcoma (KS)

Epidemiology	Due to HHV-8 and predominantly sexually transmitted (MSM) Non-sexual and non-parenteral horizontal routes of transmission (possibly salivary) more important in sub-Saharan Africa In HHV-8 co-infected, 10-yr cumulative risk for KS is 30–50% with 3–5 yrs median time to development
At-risk CD4 count	Any, but visceral and more aggressive disease more likely at lower CD4 counts
Pathology	Characteristic spindle cells

Clinical features

Presentation	History: months to years *Cutaneous*: purple non-pruritic papules anywhere on skin but especially nose, legs and genitals; crease-line distribution over trunk. Satellite lesions, bruising, local lymphadenopathy and oedema typical *Oral and GI tract*: purple raised lesions; favoured sites palate, gums and fauces; oesophagus, stomach and large bowel. Hepatosplenomegaly *Pulmonary*: (15%) breathlessness, cough, haemoptysis, chest pain and fever
Suspect if	Raised purple spots on skin, in mouth or on endoscopy/bronchoscopy
Differential diagnosis	Bacillary angiomatosis, pyogenic granuloma for cutaneous lesions
Complications	Ulceration and chronic lymphoedema from skin lesions Anaemia and bleeding from GI tract

Key investigations and diagnosis

Skin	Biopsy for single or atypical lesions
Chest X-ray	Typically, disease affects middle and lower zones with patchy coarse reticulonodular shadowing and mediastinal lymphadenopathy Pleural effusion in ~25%
Other	CT, bronchoscopy and endoscopy if indicated by symptoms

Management

Treatment	*Cutaneous/oral: First-line*: commence/optimise HAART (75% response). Radiotherapy valuable for localised disease, where lymphoedema is prominent or there is mass effect *Visceral, widespread or HAART-unresponsive mucocutaneous*: First-line: cyclical liposomal doxorubicin (response rate 60%). Paclitaxel for refractory or relapsed disease Stop therapy after completion of treatment course
Immune restoration syndrome	Uncommon but described
Prognosis	Poor if low CD4, age >50 yrs, and visceral disease Majority with skin disease only enter prolonged remission

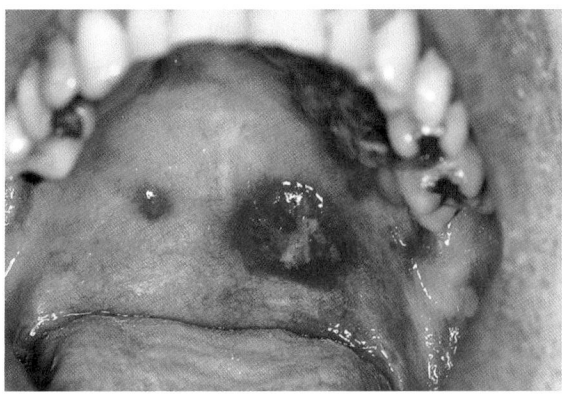

Fig. 14.14 Oral Kaposi's sarcoma. A full examination is important to detect disease that may affect the palate, gums, fauces or tongue.

14.22 Non-Hodgkin lymphoma

Epidemiology	Increased risk if not on HAART, increasing age and low CD4 count. Most are EBV-related
	Initial AIDS-defining illness in 2–3% of patients
At-risk CD4 count	< 50 cells/mm³
Pathology	> 95% are of B-cell lineage with several histological types: diffuse large B-cell, Burkitt's, primary CNS and primary effusion (HHV-8)

Clinical features

Presentation	Typically with fevers, sweats and weight loss over several months; extranodal disease (GI tract, liver, oral cavity, skin, lungs) and bone marrow involvement
	20% with leptomeningeal CNS NHL are asymptomatic
	Primary effusion lymphoma accounts for < 1%
Suspect if	Persistent lymphadenopathy, PUO, weight loss with low CD4
Differential diagnosis	Mycobacterial infection (tuberculosis or MAI), cryptococcaemia
Complications	Progression of lymphoma, drug-induced neutropenia

Key investigations and diagnosis

Biopsy	Tissue diagnosis essential
Staging	Ann Arbor/Cotswold modification (p. 1038)
	Patients are usually stage B4 at presentation (p. 1038)

Management

Treatment	Cycles of multi-agent chemotherapy, e.g. CHOP ± rituximab
	HAART initiation/optimisation and prophylaxis for opportunist infections
	Stop therapy on completion of treatment course
Prognosis	Median survival 50%
	Poor prognostic factors: CD4 < 100 cells/mm³, more advanced stage, high LDH, age > 35 yrs, number of extranodal sites, injection drug-user and cell type

to show mixed cellularity or lymphocyte-depleted sub-types, as opposed to nodular sclerosis; a high percentage stain EBV-positive.

After diagnosis of NHL or Hodgkin lymphoma, a staging evaluation is required (p. 1038). For both, HAART therapy is associated with improved overall response, disease-free survival and complete remission rates, so its introduction should not be delayed. Multi-agent chemotherapy is the mainstay of treatment but intrathecal chemoprophylaxis, support of bone marrow reserves and prevention of infection are also key elements. Additional rituximab may improve response, depending on tumour cell markers. More intensive regimens are required for Burkitt's lymphoma. For HD, first-line treatment is as standard. Use of HAART with chemotherapy is safe, although drugs that have overlapping side-effects with cytotoxics should be avoided (e.g. ZDV and marrow suppression). Following chemotherapy, it may take up to 1 year for the CD4 count to return to pre-treatment levels.

Other non-AIDS-defining cancers

HIV-infected patients have a greater risk of developing anogenital (vulval/vaginal, anal, penile) and in situ cervical cancer (cervical intra-epithelial neoplasia (CIN) III), all of which are closely associated with HPV co-infection. This is more frequently observed in HIV (60% of females; 90% of males), including the most oncogenic genotypes (HPV-16, 18, 31, 33, 35). Patients are more likely to have multiple genotypes which persist with time, and to progress more rapidly from dysplasia to in situ cancer. Both a higher viral load and a lower CD4 count are associated with higher co-infection rates. Invasive cervical cancer is an AIDS-defining diagnosis, although it is unrelated to CD4 count and the risk is much lower than that for KS and NHL; by contrast, CIN is more common and more likely to recur. Disease tends to present late and is more aggressive. Annual cervical smears should be taken from all HIV-infected women.

The incidence of anal cancer is increasing (37-fold for men and 6.8-fold for women), particularly for MSM. Most are squamous cell carcinomas and tend to be advanced at presentation; treatment is with chemo- and radiotherapy. Survival rate is around 50% at 2 years.

MANAGEMENT OF HIV

Management of HIV involves both treatment of the virus and prevention of opportunistic infections. The aims of HIV treatment are to:

- reduce the viral load to an undetectable level for as long as possible
- improve the CD4 count to > 200 cells/mL so that severe HIV-related disease is unlikely
- improve the quantity and quality of life without unacceptable drug-related side-effects or lifestyle alteration
- reduce transmission.

The drugs that are most commonly used are shown in Box 14.23. The principle of combining drugs serves to provide additive antiviral activity with a reduction in the emergence of viral resistance. This is known as highly active antiretroviral therapy (HAART) and is the cornerstone of management.

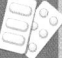

14.23 Antiretroviral drugs and recommended combinations for therapy in treatment-naïve and experienced patients

NAÏVE			EXPERIENCED		
(Regimen should consist of one drug from each column)			(Regimen should include two fully active new agents from different classes)		
PIs and *NNRTIs*	NRTI-1	NRTI-2	PIs and *NNRTIs*	Entry inhibitors	Integrase inhibitors
Preferred					
Efavirenz[1]	Tenofovir[1]	Lamivudine(3TC)[1]	Darunavir/r	Maraviroc	Raltegravir
	Abacavir[1]	Emtricitabine (FTC)[1]	Tipranavir/r[2]	Enfuvirtide (T-20)	
			Etravirine		
Alternative					
Lopinavir/r[1]	Didanosine (ddI)				
Fosamprenavir/r[1,]	Zidovudine (ZDV)[1]				
Darunavir/r					
Atazanavir/r					
Saquinavir/r					
Nevirapine					

Notes With the exception of zidovudine, all drugs listed for naïve patients can be given once daily although lopinavir, fosamprenavir, saquinavir and nevirapine are usually given twice daily.
[1]Fixed-dose combinations available: efavirenz/tenofovir/emtricitabine; tenofovir/emtricitabine; abacavir/lamivudine; zidovudine/lamivudine; zidovudine/lamivudine/abacavir; lopinavir/ritonavir.
[2]Tipranavir cannot be given with etravirine or darunavir.
(NRTI = nucleoside reverse transcriptase inhibitor; NNRTI = non-nucleoside reverse transcriptase inhibitor (shown in italics); PI = protease inhibitor; r = ritonavir in low dose)

Drugs

Nucleoside reverse transcriptase inhibitors (NRTIs)

The drugs in this class are zidovudine (ZDV), didanosine (ddI), lamivudine (3TC), stavudine (d4T), abacavir and emtricitabine (FTC), which have been developed sequentially. The NRTIs act through intracellular phosphorylation to the triphosphate form and incorporation into the DNA, where they inhibit further lengthening of the complementary strand to the viral RNA template (see step 4, Fig. 14.2, p. 388). Each drug specifically competes with a natural nucleoside (e.g. ZDV with thymidine). CNS penetration is good with all NRTIs, and ZDV has been demonstrated to be of benefit in AIDS dementia. Tenofovir is a nucleotide drug which only requires two phosphorylation steps to the triphosphate form. Its activity and characteristics are similar to the NRTIs. The inclusion of two NRTIs, or one NRTI and tenofovir, remains the cornerstone of HAART.

Resistance occurs to all NRTIs unless they are part of a maximally suppressive HAART regimen; resistance to 3TC and FTC is rapid and high-level. Occasionally, certain single mutations in the viral reverse transcriptase may result in broad resistance to several or all of the NRTIs and tenofovir. These can be selected out by combining drugs that have overlapping resistance profiles and a low genetic barrier to resistance.

Early side-effects are uncommon with current recommended NRTIs. Abacavir can result in a hypersensitivity reaction in 3% of patients with rash, fever and an influenza-like illness, but this only occurs in those with the genetic allele HLAB57*01; this can be screened for prior to use of abacavir and the drug avoided if it is present. Abacavir also appears to be associated with a small risk of coronary heart disease, and tenofovir with bone demineralisation and rarely renal tubular toxicity. They should be avoided if possible in those with existing cardiovascular risk factors or renal impairment respectively.

ZDV is occasionally used (mainly during pregnancy), which can result in nausea and macrocytic anaemia. In resource-poor countries, ZDV and d4T are important first-line drugs. However, lipoatrophy (fat loss from the face, limbs and buttocks, Fig. 14.15) is a frequent long-term complication, and peripheral neuropathy and lactic acidosis (ddI and d4T) may occur due to inhibition of mitochondrial DNA synthesis.

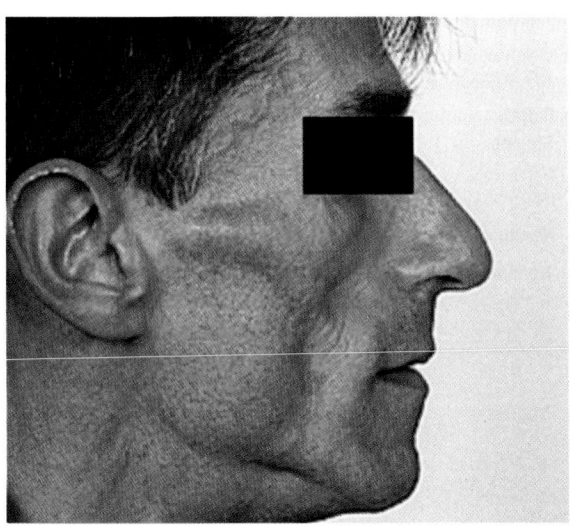

Fig. 14.15 Fat loss seen with certain NRTIs.

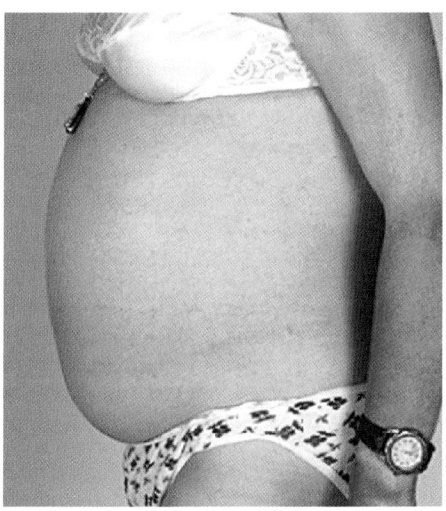

Fig. 14.16 Fat gain seen with PI-based HAART.

Protease inhibitors (PIs)

The first PI developed was saquinavir followed by indinavir, ritonavir, lopinavir and tipranavir; more recently, atazanavir, fosamprenavir and darunavir have become available. Currently used PIs should always be boosted by low-dose ritonavir, which is a potent inhibitor of liver metabolism. This increases drug exposure, thereby prolonging the PI's half-life, allowing reduction in pill burden and dosing frequency and so optimising adherence. It also limits the development of resistance. PIs prevent post-translational cleavage of polypeptides into functional virus proteins (see step 8, Fig. 14.2, p. 388). When they are given with two NRTIs, the combination controls viral replication in plasma and tissues, and allows reconstitution of the immune system.

Early and late side-effects are common. PI use has been linked with fat accumulation which is characterised by central adiposity and localised collections (buffalo hump, peripheral lipomatosis, and breast enlargement in women, Fig. 14.16). In addition, their use may be associated with hyperlipidaemia (mainly total cholesterol and triglyceride), and abnormal glucose tolerance; this is less marked for atazanavir and darunavir. An increased risk of myocardial infarction has been linked to certain PIs that is not explained by dyslipidaemia. Individual PI side-effects include diarrhoea (lopinavir), renal stones (indinavir), hyperbilirubinaemia (atazanavir) and rash (fosamprenavir and darunavir).

PIs are metabolised by the P450 cytochrome system (mainly the CYP3A4 isoenzyme), giving rise to the potential for multiple drug interactions. Commonly used drugs that interact with PIs (in particular ritonavir) are rifampicin, midazolam and simvastatin. Monitoring plasma levels and dose adjustments may be necessary to optimise the antiviral effect and reduce toxicity.

Non-nucleoside reverse transcriptase inhibitors (NNRTIs)

There are two main NNRTIs used in drug-naïve patients (nevirapine and efavirenz) and one in drug-experienced (etravirine). Activity is through inhibiting reverse transcriptase by binding near to the active enzyme site (see stage 4, Fig. 14.2, p, 388). NNRTIs do not require intracellular activation and are not active against HIV-1 subtype O or HIV-2. All have good bioavailability and, for efavirenz and nevirapine, low daily tablet number and apparent freedom from long-term side-effects.

Hypersensitivity rash and hepatitis are the major class-specific side-effects. The rash is usually mild and self-limiting but Stevens–Johnson syndrome may occur (0.3% with nevirapine, 0.1% with efavirenz). Similarly, hepatitis occurs more frequently with nevirapine, when it is gender- and CD4 count-dependent (11% in women with CD4 counts of > 250 cells/mm³), and may be fulminant. Hence its use is restricted to CD4 count thresholds of 250 cells/mm³ for women and 400 cells/mm³ for men. CNS side-effects, including dizziness, vivid dreams, insomnia, somnolence and poor concentration, are described in half the patients treated with efavirenz. These usually resolve by 2–4 weeks and are only sufficiently severe to require discontinuation in 2–5%.

The major disadvantage of efavirenz and nevirapine is the rapid development of resistance in patients with virological failure, although they usually remain susceptible to etravirine. This is commonly used in combination with boosted darunavir and/or an integrase or entry inhibitor in patients with triple-class treatment failure. Nevirapine and efavirenz reduce methadone levels by approximately 50% and may precipitate opiate withdrawal.

Entry inhibitors

Currently, two classes of entry inhibitor exist: those that interfere with fusion by binding to gp41 (see stage 3, Fig. 14.2, p. 388: e.g. enfuvirtide) and those that bind to the CCR5 co-receptor blocking attachment of the virus (see stage 2, Fig. 14.2: e.g. maraviroc). Both are given twice daily and used in patients with advanced disease and few other options. However, enfuvirtide has to be injected subcutaneously, and maraviroc can only be used in patients whose virus is CCR5-tropic (only 50% of patients with advanced disease). Together with boosted darunavir, etravirine and raltegravir (see below), these drugs have transformed the management of patients with triple-class failure or resistant virus. In these highly treatment-experienced patients, it is imperative to use two and preferably three active agents in the new regimen. Because 95% of patients with early disease harbour CCR5-tropic virus, maraviroc has also been evaluated as a drug option for treatment-naïve patients.

Integrase inhibitors

This class of drug inhibits the third and final step of proviral DNA integration: that of strand transfer (see step 5, Fig. 14.2, p. 388). Raltegravir is the first in this class and has shown high potency in heavily experienced patients irrespective of existing resistance, subtype and tropism. It is primarily metabolised by glucuronidation and therefore is not affected by co-administration with other antiviral drugs and has no major side-effects.

Treatment

The naïve patient

The decision to start therapy is a major one; it is influenced by several factors but predominantly by the CD4 count. The risk of HIV-related disease with

14

14

14.24 Indications to start HAART

CD4 count (cells/mm³)	Decision
Seroconversion	Consider treatment[1]
≥ 350	Monitor 3–6-monthly[2]
201–350	Treat as soon as patient ready
< 200	Treat as soon as possible
AIDS-defining diagnosis	Treat as soon as possible[3]

[1] If neurological presentation, CD4 count < 200 cells/mm³ for > 3 mths or AIDS diagnosis.
[2] Consider treatment if hepatitis B or C co-infected or > 55 yrs of age.
[3] Except for TB, if CD4 > 350 cells/mm³.

opportunistic infection and malignancy increases, treatment is less effective and side-effects are more common when the CD4 count is < 200 cells/mm³. When to start therapy and what to start with are outlined in Boxes 14.23, 14.24 and 14.25. Prior to commencing treatment, all patients should have hepatitis B and C status checked, along with HIV viral resistance (5–10% incidence of primary resistance in the UK and Europe) and *HLA-B*5701* tests (if abacavir is being considered as an option). With careful and appropriate choice of HAART, over 80% of patients have an undetectable viral load (VL) (i.e. < 50 copies/mL) at 4–6 months (Box 14.26). The factors that reduce the probability of achieving prolonged viral suppression include low CD4 count (< 50 cells/mm³) and high VL (> 100 000 copies/mL), poor adherence, pre-existing or emergent resistance, and drug interaction or toxicity. The presence of active opportunistic infection or other HIV-related disease should not delay the introduction of HAART, which usually should be commenced as soon as the patient's condition has stabilised.

14.25 Factors to consider when choosing HAART

- Fit of the drug regimen around the patient's lifestyle
- Wishes of the patient
- Comorbidities and drug toxicity
- Potential for drug interactions with HIV and non-HIV medications
- CNS penetration
- Possibility of acquisition of resistant virus

EBM 14.26 Combination therapy for patients naïve to drugs

'Combination antiretroviral therapy (ART) containing either efavirenz or boosted lopinavir together with two NRTIs results in effective and durable virological suppression with limited side-effects. Efavirenz provides improved virological control but failure is more likely to be associated with resistance. Equivalent results are demonstrated with several first-line PIs; all protect against the development of resistance.'

- Riddler SA, et al. N Engl J Med 2008; 358:2095.
- Ortiz R, et al. AIDS 2008; 22:1389.

The drug-experienced patient

A change in antiretroviral therapy may be necessary because of drug side-effects (early or late), difficulties in adherence or virological failure (defined as detectable VL despite treatment). In a patient with a previously undetectable VL, treatment failure is indicated by viral rebound. With increasing time on a failing regimen, the VL rises towards baseline levels, resistance mounts, the CD4 count falls and clinical progression occurs. In essence, most early failures are related to adherence difficulties (sometimes resulting from toxicity) and most late failures are a result of virological resistance. A resistance test should always be obtained before switching drugs, with a new active regimen being introduced as soon as possible and guided by this result. Account should also be taken of prior drug exposure. In certain situations, therapeutic drug monitoring may be helpful in confirming that virological failure is not related to inadequate PI or NNRTI levels. The new combination should include a minimum of two fully active new agents (see Box 14.23). Occasionally, HAART must be stopped because of life-threatening drug toxicity or overriding medical problems where predicted drug interactions will occur. In this situation, the prolonged half-life of the NNRTIs should be covered by substitution of a PI or continuation of the other components of HAART for 2 weeks. Treatment interruption is associated with an increased risk of progression and non-HIV-related complications (Box 14.27).

EBM 14.27 Continuous vs. intermittent treatment strategies for managing HIV

'CD4 count-guided interruption of HAART is inferior to continuous HAART. It demonstrates significantly higher rates of death, opportunistic disease, and renal, hepatic and cardiovascular events when compared to those maintained on continuous treatment.'

- El-Sadr W, et al. N Engl J Med 2006; 355:2283.

Special situations

Children

The general principles of management are the same as those for adults, although the CD4 percentage is a more accurate marker of immunological health until 5 years of age. All infants should receive PCP prophylaxis and commence HAART, irrespective of CD4 count or VL. CD4 counts (cells/mm³) and CD4 percentage thresholds to initiate HAART are:

- < 1000 cells and/or < 25% at 1–2 years
- < 500 cells and/or < 20% at 3–4 years
- < 350 cells and/or < 15% if above 5 years and in any child with advanced clinical disease.

It should also be considered in those with a VL > 100 000 copies/mL. After 1 year of age, PCP prophylaxis should be given to children until they are 5 with a CD4 percentage of < 15%, and then at the same CD4 levels as for adults.

Not all antiretroviral drugs are available in a suitable formulation for children, e.g. suspension, powder, crushable tablet or a capsule that can be opened. First-line preferred choices include boosted lopinavir, nevirapine (< 3 years) and efavirenz (> 3 years) with two NRTIs. Coordinated, comprehensive, family-centred systems of care are necessary to support the child and parents and to optimise compliance with medications.

Maternal HIV

All pregnant women should routinely be recommended for HIV testing at an early stage in pregnancy, with rapid tests considered for those presenting in or just after labour. Pre-HAART, the rate of mother-to-child transmission was 26% with rates being influenced by several factors (see Box 14.1, p. 387). The likelihood of transmission at delivery is decreased to the order of 8% with single-dose nevirapine to mother and child, 6–8% for ZDV alone, < 1% for ZDV and caesarean section, and < 1% for HAART and planned vaginal delivery when the viral load is < 50 copies/mL.

Treatment in pregnancy is outlined in Box 14.28. Single-dose nevirapine is used in resource-poor nations, but in the absence of other drugs is associated with a 30–50% chance of NNRTI resistance in mother and infected child.

Mothers should formula-feed their babies exclusively. Screening for HIV in the baby by proviral DNA should be performed at birth (not on cord blood), 6 weeks and 3 months. If negative, vertical transmission has not occurred. In discordant couples (i.e. only one partner is HIV-positive) who desire a family, self-insemination of the partner's semen is recommended to protect the uninfected male and sperm-washing is recommended to protect the uninfected female partner.

Post-exposure prophylaxis

Post-exposure prophylaxis with combination therapy (boosted lopinavir, tenofovir and FTC) is recommended when the risk is deemed to be significant after a careful risk assessment, in both occupational and non-occupational settings. The first dose should be given as soon as possible, preferably within 6–8 hours. However, protection is not absolute and seroconversion may occur. Non-occupational settings include condom breakage in HIV-serodiscordant partners, victims of rape, and sharps-related home exposures in families of injection drug-users or HIV patients. Many individuals experience side-effects and only half complete the recommended 4 weeks of therapy.

Prevention of opportunistic infection

Patients should be immunised with hepatitis A and hepatitis B vaccines if there is no evidence of naturally acquired infection. HBV surface antibody levels need to be monitored and boosters given when < 100 U/mL. Pneumococcal vaccine (every 3–5 years) and influenza vaccine (annually) should be given to all patients. Response to all immunisations is lower when the CD4 count is < 200 cells/mm³, although some protection is afforded. Live attenuated vaccines (BCG, oral polio) should be avoided or restricted to those with high CD4 counts (yellow fever). Nevertheless, MMR (measles/mumps/rubella) vaccine is safe and can be given.

Prophylaxis against infection is another vital aspect of management. Primary prophylaxis is to prevent the initial disease occurring, and secondary to prevent recurrence of infection. Primary prophylaxis is introduced at specified CD4 counts at which there is a risk of infection. Secondary prophylaxis is started after successful treatment of the opportunistic infection, usually with the same drug(s) that was used to treat it, but at lower doses. Drugs can usually be stopped when the CD4 threshold at which primary prophylaxis is introduced is reached. Specific details of these thresholds for each infection is given in the relevant section above.

Prevention of HIV

HIV vaccine development is slow. An effective, safe and cheap vaccine would radically alter the future global epidemic of HIV. Despite advances in the understanding of HIV pathogenesis and immunology, prototype HIV-1 vaccine candidates aimed at eliciting humoral and cellular immune responses have so far failed. Challenges include the extensive subtype and sequence diversity of HIV, the early establishment of reservoirs, the lack of a safe attenuated virus, the lack of a small animal model, and the inability of vaccines to generate protection across different viral strains. Alternative measures for the prevention of HIV transmission are shown in Boxes 14.29 and 14.30. The United Nations' aim is universal access to comprehensive prevention programmes, treatment, care and support by 2010. To achieve this, access to HIV testing needs to be widened, and strategies are required to protect the HIV non-infected person (e.g. promoting consistent condom use, improved STI management, male circumcision), for effective mother-to-child prevention programmes, and for scaling up of antiretroviral drug access.

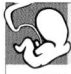 **14.28 Treatment of HIV in pregnancy**

- **Ritonavir-boosted PI (e.g. lopinavir) with zidovudine and lamivudine from 20 weeks**: all mothers, with PI plasma level monitoring. Nevirapine can be used cautiously (risk of hypersensitivity hepatitis) but only when CD4 counts < 250 cells/mm³.
- **Zidovudine monotherapy**: those with viral loads < 10 000 copies/mL and wild-type virus who are willing to have Caesarean section.
- **ZDV i.v. infusion at onset of labour**: those on ZDV alone or those on HAART but with detectable virus, undergoing normal vaginal delivery.

EBM 14.29 Male circumcision for prevention of HIV transmission

'Circumcision is effective in reducing HIV infection rates in men without increasing high-risk behaviour. In a setting of low circumcision and high HIV prevalence, this is likely to provide an effective method for reducing HIV transmission.'

- Gray RH, et al. Lancet 2007; 369:657–666.

14

14.30 Prevention measures for HIV transmission

Sexual

- Comprehensive sex education programmes in schools
- Public awareness campaigns for HIV
- Easily accessible/discreet testing centres
- Safe sex practices (avoiding penetrative intercourse, delaying sexual debut, condom use, fewer sexual partners)
- Targeting safe sex methods to high-risk groups
- Control of STIs
- Effective treatment of HIV-infected individuals
- Post-sexual exposure prophylaxis

Parenteral

- Blood product transmission: donor questionnaire, routine screening of donated blood, blood substitute use
- Injection drug use: education, needle/syringe exchange, avoidance of 'shooting galleries', sharing and support for methadone maintenance programmes

Perinatal

- Routine 'opt-out' antenatal HIV antibody testing
- Preconception family planning if HIV-seropositive
- Measures to reduce vertical transmission (p. 407)

Occupational

- Education/training: universal precautions, needlestick avoidance
- Post-exposure prophylaxis

Further information

Websites

www.bhiva.org *Guidelines on all aspects of HIV and conference reports.*

www.hivandhepatitis.com *Conference reports, important journal articles, and HIV and hepatitis co-infection news.*

www.i-base.org.uk *Conference reports and latest information.*

www.medscape.com *Conference reports and expert topic reviews.*

G.R. Scott

Sexually transmitted infections

15

CLINICAL EXAMINATION IN MEN

Skin of penis 5
(Retract prepuce if present)
Genital warts
Ulcers
Be aware of normal anatomical
features such as coronal papillae,
or prominent sebaceous or
parafrenal glands

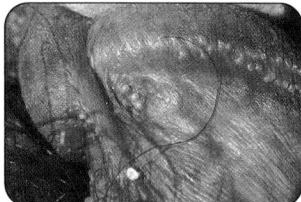

Coronal papillae ▲

Scrotal contents 4
Abnormal masses or tenderness
(epididymo-orchitis)

Pubic area 3
Pthirus pubis (crab louse)

Skin around groin 2
and scrotum
Warts
Tinea cruris

Inguinal glands 1
Significant enlargement

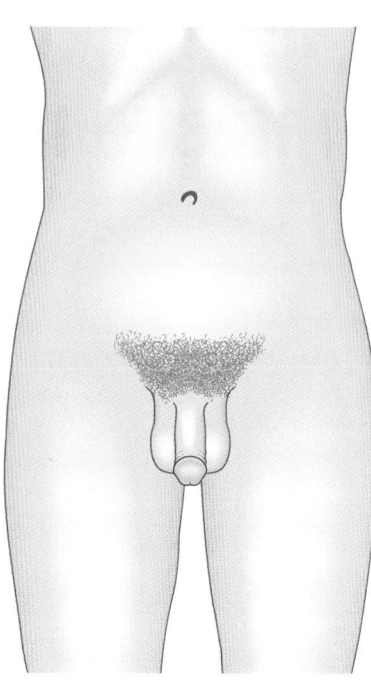

Observation
- Mouth
- Eyes
- Joints
- Skin:
  Rash of secondary syphilis
  Scabies
  Manifestations of HIV
  infection (Ch. 14)

6 **Urethral meatus**
▼ Discharge

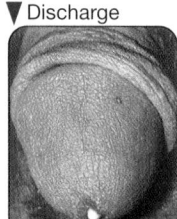

7 **Perianal area**
(Men who have sex with men,
and heterosexual men)
▼ Warts

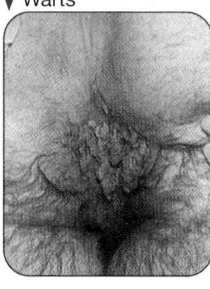

8 **Rectum**
(men who have sex with men
practising receptive anal intercourse)

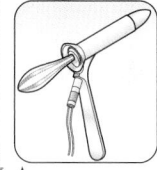

▲ Proctoscope

**Investigations for STIs in
heterosexual males**

- Urethral swab for gonococci—either
  plated directly on a selective medium
  such as modified New York City
  (MNYC), or sent in appropriate transport
  medium for either culture or nucleic
  acid amplification test (NAAT) according
  to local laboratory protocol
- Urethral swab or first void urine (FVU)
  for chlamydia
- Serological test for syphilis (STS), e.g.
  enzyme immunoassay (EIA) for antitreponemal IgG antibody
- HIV test (see note)

**Investigations for STIs in
men who have sex with men**

- Pharyngeal, urethral and rectal
  swabs for gonococci
- Urethral swab or FVU, and rectal
  swab for chlamydia
- STS (repeat testing may be
  necessary in the event that there
  are negative tests results in the
  first few weeks following
  exposure)
- Serological tests for hepatitis
  A/B (with a view to vaccination if
  seronegative)
- HIV test (see note)

HIV testing

It should be standard practice to offer
HIV testing as part of STI screening
because the benefits of early diagnosis outweigh other considerations.
Extensive pre-test counselling is not
required in most instances, but it is
important to establish efficient pathways for referral of patients at high
risk in whom the clinician wishes
specialist support, and for those
diagnosed HIV-positive.

CLINICAL EXAMINATION IN WOMEN

Labia majora and minora **4**
Ulcers
Vulvitis
Warts ▼

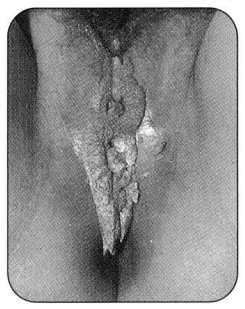

Perineum and perianal skin **5**
Warts
Ulcers

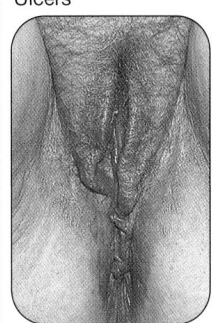

▲ Inflammation

Pubic area **3**
Pthirus pubis (crab louse) ▼

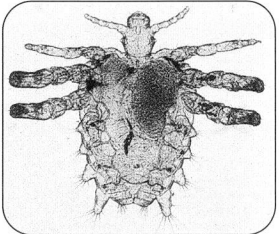

Vagina and cervix **6**
Abnormal discharge
Warts
Ulcers
Inflammation
In women with lower abdominal
pain, bimanual examination for
adnexal tenderness
(pelvic inflammatory disease)

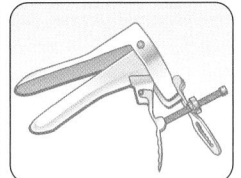

▲ Speculum

Inguinal glands **2**
Significant enlargement

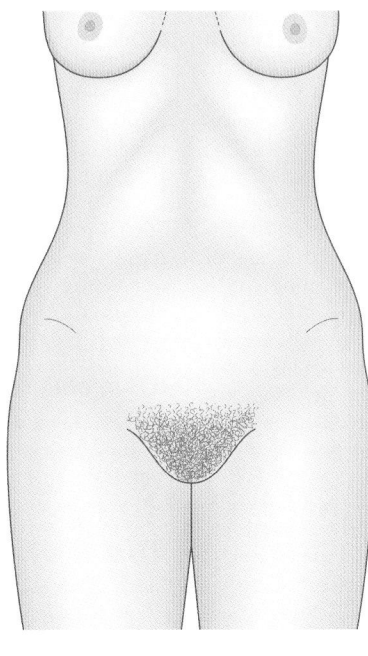

Abdomen **1**
Abnormal masses or tenderness

Observation
- Mouth
- Eyes
- Joints
- Skin:
  Rash of secondary syphilis
  Scabies
  Manifestations of HIV
  infection (Ch. 14)

Investigations for STIs in women

- Urethral and cervical swabs for gonococci
- Cervical swab for chlamydia
- Wet mount for microscopy or high vaginal swab (HVS) for culture of *Trichomonas*
- STS
- HIV test (see note)

Management goals in suspected STI

- Relief of any symptoms
- Screening for treatable STI that may not be causing symptoms
- Tracing and treatment of sexual contacts who may also be infected
- Advice to reduce risk of infection in the future

Those at particular risk from STIs*

- Sex workers, male and female
- Clients of sex workers
- Men who have sex with men
- Injecting drug users (sex for money or drugs) and their partners
- Frequent travellers

*Adapted from WHO/UNAIDS, 1997.

15

Sexually transmitted infections (STIs) are a group of contagious conditions whose principal mode of transmission is by intimate sexual activity involving the moist mucous membranes of the penis, vulva, vagina, cervix, anus, rectum, mouth and pharynx, along with their adjacent skin surfaces. A wide range of infections may be sexually transmitted, including syphilis, gonorrhoea, human immunodeficiency virus (HIV), genital herpes, genital warts, chlamydia and trichomoniasis. Bacterial vaginosis and genital candidiasis are not regarded as STIs, although they are common causes of vaginal discharge in sexually active women. Chancroid, lymphogranuloma venereum and granuloma inguinale are usually seen in tropical countries. Hepatitis viruses A, B, C and D (pp. 947–954) may be acquired sexually, as well as by other routes.

The World Health Organization estimates that 340 million curable STIs occur each year, including 170 million cases of *Trichomonas vaginalis*, 92 million cases of *Chlamydia trachomatis*, 62 million cases of gonorrhoea and 12 million cases of syphilis. In the UK in 2007, the most common treatable STIs diagnosed were chlamydia (more than 120 000 cases) and gonorrhoea (18 000 cases). Genital warts are the second most common complaint seen in genitourinary medicine (GUM) departments.

As coincident infection with more than one STI is frequently seen, GUM clinics routinely offer a full set of investigations at the patient's first visit (pp. 410–411), regardless of the reason for attendance. In other settings, less comprehensive investigation may be appropriate.

The extent of the examination largely reflects the likelihood of HIV infection or syphilis. Most heterosexuals in the UK are at such low risk of these infections that routine extragenital examination is unnecessary. This is not the case in parts of the world where HIV is endemic, or for men who have sex with men (MSM) in the UK. In other words, the extent of the examination is determined by the sexual history.

APPROACH TO PATIENTS WITH A SUSPECTED STI

Patients concerned about the possible acquisition of an STI are often anxious. Staff must be friendly, sympathetic and reassuring; they should have the ability to put patients at ease, whilst emphasising that clinic attendance is confidential. The history focuses on genital symptoms, with reference to genital ulceration, rash, irritation, pain, swelling and urinary symptoms, especially dysuria. In men, the clinician should ask about urethral discharge, and in women, vaginal discharge, pelvic pain or dyspareunia. Enquiry about general health should include menstrual and obstetric history, cervical cytology, recent medication, especially with antimicrobial or antiviral agents, previous STI and allergy. Immunisation status for hepatitis A and B should be noted, as should information about recreational drug use.

A detailed sexual history is imperative, as this informs the clinician of the degree of risk for certain infections as well as specific sites that should be sampled; for example, rectal samples should be taken from men who have had unprotected anal sex with other men. Sexual partners, whether male or female, and casual or regular, should be recorded. Sexual practices—insertive or receptive vaginal, anal, orogenital or oroanal—should be noted. Choice of contraception should be recorded for women, together with condom use for both sexes.

STI in children

The presence of an STI in a child may be indicative of sexual abuse, although vertical transmission may explain some presentations in the first 2 years. In an older child, STI may be the result of voluntary sexual activity.

STI during pregnancy

Many STIs can be transmitted from mother to child in pregnancy, either transplacentally or during delivery. Possible outcomes are highlighted in Box 15.1.

PRESENTING PROBLEMS IN MEN

Urethral discharge

In the UK the most important causes of urethral discharge are gonorrhoea and chlamydia. In a significant minority of cases, tests for both of these infections are negative, a scenario often referred to as non-specific urethritis (NSU). Some of these cases may be caused by *Trichomonas vaginalis*, herpes simplex virus (HSV), mycoplasmas or ureaplasmas. A small minority seem not to have an infectious aetiology.

15.1 Possible outcomes of STI in pregnancy

Organism	Mode of transmission	Outcome for fetus/neonate	Outcome for mother
Treponema pallidum	Transplacental	Ranges from no effect to severe stigmata or miscarriage/stillbirth	None directly relating to the pregnancy
Neisseria gonorrhoeae	Intrapartum	Severe conjunctivitis	Possibility of ascending infection postpartum
Chlamydia trachomatis	Intrapartum	Conjunctivitis, pneumonia	Possibility of ascending infection postpartum
Herpes simplex	Usually intrapartum, but transplacental infection may occur rarely	Ranges from no effect to severe disseminated infection	Rarely, primary infection during 2nd/3rd trimesters becomes disseminated, with high maternal mortality
Human papillomaviruses	Intrapartum	Anogenital warts or laryngeal papillomas are very rare	Warts may become more florid during pregnancy, but usually regress postpartum

Gonococcal urethritis usually causes symptoms within 7 days of exposure. The discharge is typically profuse and purulent. Chlamydial urethritis has an incubation period of 1–4 weeks, and tends to result in milder symptoms than gonorrhoea; there is overlap, however, and microbiological confirmation should always be sought.

Investigations

A presumptive diagnosis of urethritis can be made from a Gram-stained smear of the urethral exudate (Fig. 15.1), which will demonstrate significant numbers of polymorphonuclear leucocytes (≥ 5 per high-power field). A working diagnosis of gonococcal urethritis is made if Gram-negative intracellular diplococci (GNDC) are seen; if no GNDC are seen, a label of non-specific urethritis is applied.

If microscopy is not available, swabs and/or urine samples should be taken and empirical antimicrobials prescribed.

A urethral swab should always be sent for culture of *Neisseria gonorrhoeae*; in addition, a first void urine (FVU) sample or a specific urethral swab should be sent for detection of chlamydial DNA by a nucleic acid amplification test (NAAT) such as polymerase chain reaction (PCR). NAATs are likely to replace the need for routine culture for gonorrhoea. Tests for other potential causes of urethritis are not performed routinely.

A swab should also be taken from the pharynx because gonococcal infection at this site is not reliably eradicated by single-dose therapy. In MSM swabs for gonorrhoea and chlamydia should be taken from the rectum.

Management

This depends upon local epidemiology and the availability of diagnostic resources. Treatment is often presumptive, with prescription of multiple antimicrobials to cover the possibility of gonorrhoea and/or chlamydia. This is likely to include a single-dose treatment for gonorrhoea, which is desirable because it eliminates the risk of non-adherence. The recommended agents for treating gonorrhoea vary according to local antimicrobial resistance patterns (p. 420). Appropriate treatment for chlamydia (p. 421) should also be prescribed because concurrent infection is present in up to 50% of men with

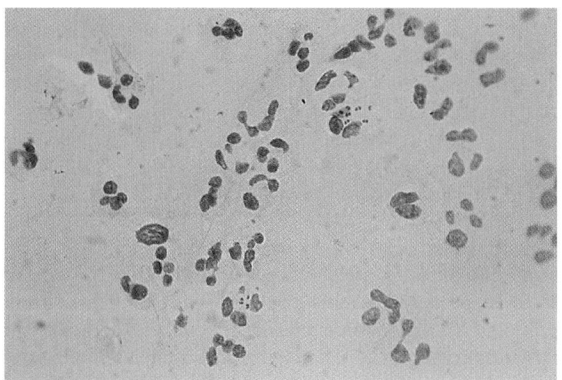

Fig. 15.1 A Gram-stained urethral smear from a man with gonococcal urethritis. Gram-negative diplococci are seen within polymorphonuclear leucocytes.

gonorrhoea. Non-gonococcal, non-chlamydial urethritis is treated as for chlamydia.

Patients should be advised to avoid sexual contact until it is confirmed that any infection has resolved, and whenever possible, recent sexual contacts should be traced. The task of contact tracing—also called partner notification—is best performed by trained nurses based in GUM clinics; it is standard practice in the UK to treat current sexual partners of men with gonococcal or non-specific urethritis without waiting for microbiological confirmation.

If symptoms clear, a routine test of cure is not necessary, but patients should be re-interviewed to confirm that there was no immediate vomiting or diarrhoea after treatment, that there has been no risk of re-infection, and that traceable partners have sought medical advice.

Genital itch and/or rash

Patients may present with many combinations of penile/genital symptoms that may be acute or chronic, and infectious or non-infectious. Box 15.2 provides a guide to diagnosis.

Balanitis refers to inflammation of the glans penis, often extending to the under-surface of the prepuce when it is called balanoposthitis. Tight prepuce and poor hygiene may be aggravating factors. Candidiasis is sometimes associated with immune deficiency, diabetes mellitus, and the use of broad-spectrum antimicrobials, corticosteroids or antimitotic drugs. Local saline bathing is usually helpful, especially when no cause is found.

Genital ulceration

The most common cause of ulceration is genital herpes. Classically, multiple painful ulcers affect the glans, coronal sulcus or shaft of penis (Fig. 15.2), but solitary lesions occur rarely. Perianal ulcers may be seen in MSM. The diagnosis is made by gently scraping material from lesions and sending this in an appropriate transport medium for culture or detection of HSV DNA by PCR.

In the UK, the possibility of any other ulcerating STI is remote unless the patient is an MSM and/or has had a sexual partner from a region where tropical STIs are more common. The classic lesion of primary syphilis (chancre) is single, painless and indurated; however, multiple lesions are seen rarely and anal chancres are often painful. Diagnosis is made in GUM clinics by dark-ground microscopy, but in other settings by serological tests for syphilis (p. 418). Other rare infective causes seen in the UK include varicella zoster virus (p. 313) and trauma with secondary infection. Tropical STI such as chancroid, lymphogranuloma venereum (LGV) and granuloma inguinale are described in Box 15.11 (p. 422). Inflammatory causes include Stevens–Johnson syndrome (p. 1285), Behçet's syndrome (p. 1114) and fixed drug reactions. In older patients, malignant and pre-malignant conditions such as squamous cell carcinoma and erythroplasia of Queyrat (intra-epidermal carcinoma) should be considered.

15.2 Differential diagnosis of genital itch and/or rash in men

Likely diagnosis	Acute or chronic	Itch	Pain	Discharge (non-urethral)	Specific characteristics	Diagnostic test	Treatment
Subclinical urethritis	Either	±	−	±	Often intermittent	Gram stain and urethral swabs	As for urethral discharge
Candida	Acute	✓	−	White	Postcoital	Microscopy	Antifungal cream, e.g. clotrimazole
Anaerobic (erosive) balanitis	Acute	±	−	Yellow	Offensive	Microscopy	Saline bathing ± metronidazole
Pthirus pubis ('crab lice')	Either	✓	−	−	Lice and nits seen attached to pubic hairs	Can be by microscopy, but usually visual	According to local policy–often permethrin
Lichen planus (p. 1265)	Either	±	−	−	Violaceous papules ± Wickham's striae	Clinical	None or mild topical corticosteroid, e.g. hydrocortisone
Lichen sclerosus	Chronic	±	−	−	Ivory white plaques, scarring	Clinical or biopsy	Strong topical corticosteroid, e.g. clobetasol
Plasma cell balanitis of Zoon	Chronic	−	−	±	Shiny, inflamed circumscribed areas	Clinical or biopsy	Strong topical corticosteroid, e.g. clobetasol
Dermatoses, e.g. eczema or psoriasis	Either	✓	−	−	Similar to lesions elsewhere on skin	Clinical	Mild topical corticosteroid, e.g. hydrocortisone
Genital herpes	Acute	±	✓	−	Atypical ulcers are not uncommon	Swab for HSV PCR	Oral antiviral, e.g. aciclovir
Circinate balanitis	Either	−	−	−	Painless erosions with raised edges; usually as part of Reiter's syndrome (p. 1094)	Clinical	Mild topical steroid, e.g. hydrocortisone

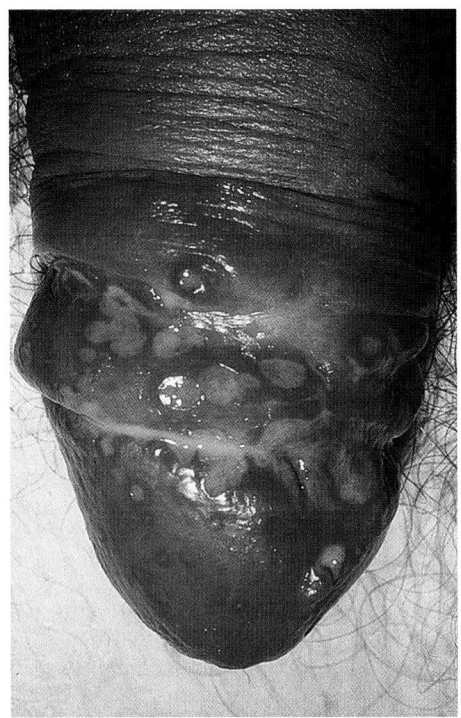

Fig. 15.2 Penile herpes simplex (HSV-2) infection.

Genital lumps

The most common cause of genital 'lumps' is warts (p. 423). These are classically found in areas of friction during sex such as the parafrenal skin and prepuce of the penis. Warts may also be seen in the urethral meatus, and less commonly on the shaft or around the base of the penis. Perianal warts are surprisingly common in men who do not have anal sex.

The differential diagnosis includes molluscum contagiosum and skin tags. Adolescent boys may confuse normal anatomical features such as coronal papillae (p. 410), parafrenal glands or sebaceous glands (Fordyce spots) with warts.

Proctitis in men who have sex with men

STIs that may cause proctitis in MSM include gonorrhoea, chlamydia, herpes and syphilis. The substrains of *Chlamydia trachomatis* that cause LGV (L1–3) have been associated with outbreaks of severe proctitis in the Netherlands and the UK. Symptoms include mucopurulent anal discharge, rectal bleeding, pain and tenesmus.

Examination may show mucopus and erythema with contact bleeding (Fig. 15.3). In addition to the diagnostic tests on page 410, a PCR test for HSV and a request

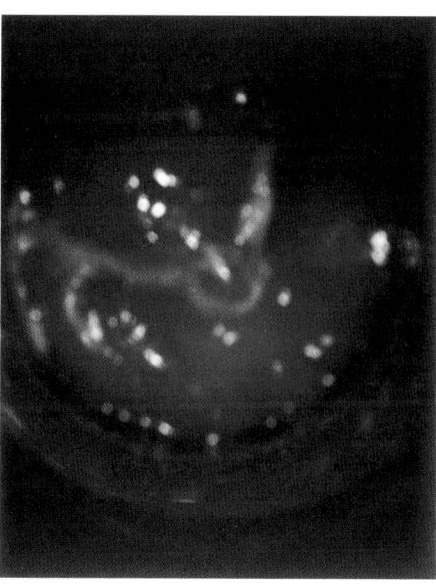

Fig. 15.3 Proctitis showing mucopus in the lumen of the rectum.

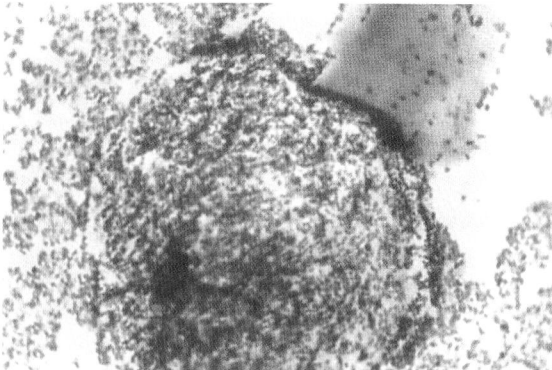

Fig. 15.4 Gram stain of a Clue cell from a patient with bacterial vaginosis. The margin of this vaginal epithelial cell is obscured by a coating of anaerobic organisms.

for identification of LGV substrain should be arranged if chlamydial infection is detected. Treatment is directed at the individual infections (see below).

MSM may also present with gastrointestinal symptoms from infection with organisms such as *Entamoeba histolytica* (p. 358), *Shigella* spp. (p. 339), *Campylobacter* spp. (p. 336) and *Cryptosporidium* spp. (p. 363).

PRESENTING PROBLEMS IN WOMEN

Vaginal discharge

The natural vaginal discharge may vary considerably, especially under differing hormonal influences such as puberty, pregnancy or prescribed contraception. A sudden or recent change in discharge, especially if associated with alteration of colour and/or smell, or vulval itch/irritation is more likely to indicate an infective cause than a gradual or long-standing change.

Local epidemiology is particularly important when assessing possible causes. In the UK, most cases of vaginal discharge are not sexually transmitted, being due to either candidal infection or bacterial vaginosis (BV). World-wide, the most common treatable STI causing vaginal discharge is trichomoniasis; other possibilities include gonorrhoea and chlamydia. HSV may cause increased discharge, although vulval pain and dysuria are usually the predominant symptoms. Non-infective causes include retained tampons, malignancy and/or fistulae.

Speculum examination often allows a relatively accurate diagnosis to be made. In BV, the discharge is characteristically homogeneous and off-white in colour. Vaginal pH is greater than 4.5, and Gram stain microscopy reveals scanty or absent lactobacilli with significant numbers of Gram-variable organisms, some of which may be coating vaginal squames (so-called Clue cells, Fig. 15.4). In candidiasis, there may be vulval and vaginal erythema, and the discharge is typically curdy

in nature. Vaginal pH is usually less than 4.5, and Gram stain microscopy reveals fungal spores and pseudohyphae. Trichomoniasis tends to cause a profuse yellow or green discharge and is usually associated with significant vulvovaginal inflammation. Diagnosis is made by observing motile flagellate protozoa on a wet-mount microscopy slide of vaginal material.

If examination reveals the discharge to be cervical in origin, the possibility of chlamydial or gonococcal infection is increased and appropriate cervical swabs should be taken (p. 411). In addition, Gram stain of cervical and urethral material may reveal GNDC, allowing presumptive treatment for gonorrhoea to be given. If gonococcal cervicitis is suspected, swabs should also be taken from the pharynx and rectum; infections at these sites are not reliably eradicated by single-dose therapy and a test of cure will therefore be required.

GUM clinics in the UK routinely offer sexually active women presenting with vaginal discharge an STI screen (p. 411). In other settings such as primary care or gynaecology, testing for chlamydia and gonorrhoea should be strongly considered in young women (< 25 years old), those who have changed partner recently, and those not using a barrier method of contraception, even if a non-STI cause of discharge is suspected clinically.

Treatment of infections causing vaginal discharge is shown in Box 15.3.

Lower abdominal pain

Pelvic inflammatory disease (PID, infection or inflammation of the Fallopian tubes and surrounding structures) is part of the extensive differential diagnosis of lower abdominal pain in women, especially those who are sexually active. The possibility of PID is increased if, in addition to acute/subacute pain, there is dyspareunia, abnormal vaginal discharge and/or bleeding. There may also be systemic features such as fever and malaise. On examination, lower abdominal pain is usually bilateral, and vaginal examination reveals adnexal tenderness with or without cervical excitation. Unfortunately, a definitive diagnosis can only be made by laparoscopy. A pregnancy test should be performed (in addition to the diagnostic tests listed on page 411) because the differential diagnosis includes ectopic pregnancy.

15

415

15.3 Infections that cause vaginal discharge

Cause	Clinical features	Treatment (in pregnancy seek specialist advice)
Candidiasis	Vulval and vaginal inflammation Curdy white discharge adherent to walls of vagina Low vaginal pH	Clotrimazole[1] 500 mg pessary once at night and clotrimazole cream 12-hourly *or* Econazole[1] pessary 150 mg for 3 nights and econazole cream 12-hourly (topical creams for 7 days) *or* Fluconazole[2] 150 mg orally stat
Trichomoniasis	Vulval and vaginal inflammation Frothy yellow/green discharge	Metronidazole[3] 400 mg 12-hourly orally for 5–7 days *or* Metronidazole[3] 2 g orally as a single dose
Bacterial vaginosis	No inflammation White homogeneous discharge High vaginal pH	Metronidazole[3] 2 g stat or 400 mg 12-hourly orally for 5–7 days Metronidazole[3] vaginal gel 0.75% daily for 5 days Clindamycin[1,4] vaginal cream 2% daily for 7 days
Streptococcal/staphylococcal infection	Purulent vaginal discharge	Choice of antibiotic depends on sensitivity tests

[1] Clotrimazole, econazole and clindamycin damage latex condoms and diaphragms.
[2] Avoid in pregnancy and breastfeeding.
[3] Avoid alcoholic drinks until 48 hours after finishing treatment. Avoid high-dose regimens in pregnancy or breastfeeding.
[4] Pseudomembranous colitis has been reported with the use of clindamycin cream.

Broad-spectrum antibiotics, including those active against gonorrhoea and chlamydia such as ofloxacin and metronidazole, should be prescribed if PID is suspected, along with appropriate analgesia. Delaying treatment increases the likelihood of adverse sequelae such as abscess formation, and tubal scarring that may lead to ectopic pregnancy or infertility. Hospital admission may be indicated in women with severe symptoms.

Genital ulceration

The most common cause of ulceration is genital herpes. Classically, multiple painful ulcers affect the introitus, labia and perineum, but solitary lesions occur rarely. Inguinal lymphadenopathy and systemic features such as fever and malaise are more common than in men. Diagnosis is made by gently scraping material from lesions and sending this in an appropriate transport medium for culture or detection of HSV DNA by PCR. In the UK, the possibility of any other ulcerating STI is unlikely unless the patient has had a sexual partner from a region where tropical STIs are more common (see Box 15.11, p. 422).

Inflammatory causes include lichen sclerosus, Stevens–Johnson syndrome (p. 1285), Behçet's syndrome (p. 1114) and fixed drug reactions. In older patients,

malignant and pre-malignant conditions such as squamous cell carcinoma should be considered.

Genital lumps

The most common cause of genital 'lumps' is warts. These are classically found in areas of friction during sex, such as the fourchette and perineum. Perianal warts are surprisingly common in women who do not have anal sex.

The differential diagnosis includes molluscum contagiosum, skin tags and normal papillae or sebaceous glands.

Chronic vulval pain and/or itch

Women may present with a range of chronic symptoms that may be intermittent or continuous (Box 15.4).

Recurrent candidiasis may lead to hypersensitivity to candidal antigens, with itch and erythema becoming more prominent than increased discharge. Effective treatment may require regular oral antifungals, e.g. fluconazole 150 g once every 2–4 weeks plus a combined antifungal/corticosteroid cream such as Daktacort or Canesten HC.

PREVENTION OF STI

Case-finding

Early diagnosis and treatment facilitated by active case-finding will help to reduce the spread of infection by limiting the period of infectivity; tracing and treating sexual partners will also reduce the risk of re-infection. Unfortunately, the majority of individuals with an STI are asymptomatic and therefore unlikely to seek medical attention. Improving access to diagnosis in primary care or non-medical settings, especially through opportunistic testing, may help. However, the impact of medical intervention through improved access alone is likely to be small.

Changing behaviour

The prevalence of STIs is driven largely by sexual behaviour. Primary prevention encompasses efforts to delay the onset of sexual activity and limit the number of sexual partners thereafter. Encouraging the use of barrier methods of contraception will also help to reduce the risk of transmitting or acquiring STIs. This is especially important in the setting of 'sexual concurrency', where sexual relationships overlap.

Unfortunately, there is contradictory evidence as to which (if any) interventions can reduce sexual activity. Knowledge alone does not translate into behaviour change, and broader issues such as poor parental role modelling, low self-esteem, peer group pressure in the context of the increased sexualisation of our societies, gender power imbalance and homophobia all need to be addressed. Throughout the world there is a critical need to enable women to protect themselves from indisciplined and coercive male sexual activity. Economic collapse and the turmoil of war regularly lead to situations where women are raped or must turn to prostitution to feed themselves and their children, and an inability to negotiate safe sex increases their risk of acquiring STI, including HIV.

15.4 Chronic vulval pain and/or itch

Likely diagnosis	Itch	Pain	Specific characteristics	Diagnostic test	Treatment
Candida	✓	±	Usually cyclical	Microscopy	Oral antifungal, e.g. fluconazole 150 mg
Lichen planus	±	–	Violaceous papules ± Wickham's striae	Clinical	No treatment, or mild topical corticosteroid, e.g. hydrocortisone
Lichen sclerosus	±	–	Ivory white plaques, scarring ± labial resorption	Clinical or biopsy	Strong topical corticosteroid, e.g. clobetasol
Vestibulitis	–	✓	Dyspareunia common, pain on touching erythematous area	Clinical	Refer to specialist vulva clinic
Vulvodynia	–	✓	Pain usually neuropathic in nature	Clinical	Refer to specialist vulva clinic
Dermatoses, e.g. eczema or psoriasis	✓	–	Similar to lesions elsewhere on skin	Clinical	Mild topical corticosteroid, e.g. hydrocortisone
Genital herpes	±	✓	Atypical ulcers are not uncommon	Swab for HSV PCR	Oral antiviral, e.g. aciclovir

SEXUALLY TRANSMITTED BACTERIAL INFECTIONS

Syphilis

Syphilis is caused by infection, through abrasions in the skin or mucous membranes, with the spirochaete *Treponema pallidum*. In adults the infection is usually sexually acquired; however, transmission by kissing, blood transfusion and percutaneous injury has been reported. Transplacental infection of the fetus can occur.

The natural history of untreated syphilis is variable. Infection may remain latent throughout, or clinical features may develop at any time. The classification of syphilis is shown in Box 15.5. All infected patients should be treated. Penicillin remains the drug of choice for all stages of infection.

Acquired syphilis

Early syphilis

Primary syphilis

The incubation period is usually between 14 and 28 days with a range of 9–90 days. The primary lesion or chancre (Fig. 15.5) develops at the site of infection, usually in the genital area. A dull red macule develops, becomes papular and then erodes to form an indurated ulcer (chancre). The draining inguinal lymph nodes may become moderately enlarged, mobile, discrete and rubbery. The chancre and the lymph nodes are both painless and non-tender, unless there is concurrent or secondary infection. Without treatment, the chancre will resolve within 2–6 weeks to leave a thin atrophic scar.

Chancres may develop on the vaginal wall and on the cervix. Extragenital chancres are found in about 10% of patients, affecting sites such as the finger, lip, tongue, tonsil, nipple, anus or rectum. Anal chancres often resemble fissures and may be painful.

Secondary syphilis

This occurs 6–8 weeks after the development of the chancre when treponemes disseminate to produce a multisystem disease. Constitutional features such as mild fever, malaise and headache are common. Over 75% of patients present with a rash on the trunk and limbs that may later involve the palms and soles; this is initially macular but evolves to maculopapular or papular forms, which are generalised, symmetrical and

15.5 Classification of syphilis

Stage	Acquired	Congenital
Early	Primary Secondary Latent	Clinical and latent
Late	Latent Benign tertiary Cardiovascular Neurosyphilis	Clinical and latent

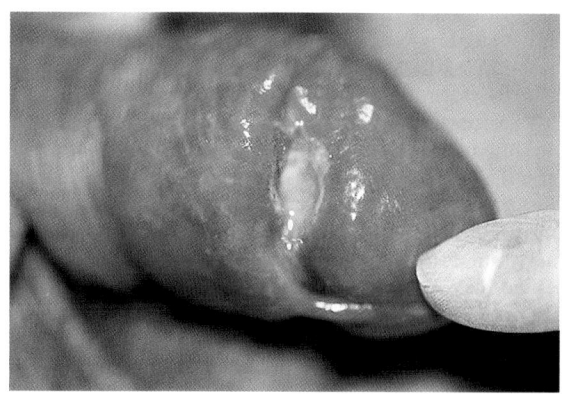

Fig. 15.5 Primary syphilis. A painless ulcer (chancre) is shown in the coronal sulcus of the penis. This is usually associated with inguinal lymphadenopathy.

non-irritable. Scales may form on the papules later. Without treatment, the rash may last for up to 12 weeks. Condylomata lata (papules coalescing to plaques) may develop in warm, moist sites such as the vulva or peri-anal area. Generalised non-tender lymphadenopathy is present in over 50% of patients. Mucosal lesions, known as mucous patches, may affect the genitalia, mouth, pharynx or larynx and are essentially modified papules, which become eroded. Rarely, confluence produces characteristic 'snail track ulcers' in the mouth.

Other features such as meningitis, cranial nerve palsies, anterior or posterior uveitis, hepatitis, gastritis, glomerulonephritis or periostitis are sometimes seen.

The differential diagnosis of secondary syphilis can be extensive, but in the context of a suspected STI, primary HIV infection is the most important alternative condition to consider (Ch. 14).

The clinical manifestations of secondary syphilis will resolve without treatment but relapse may occur, usually within the first year of infection. Thereafter, the disease enters the phase of latency.

Latent syphilis

This phase is characterised by the presence of positive syphilis serology or the diagnostic cerebrospinal fluid (CSF) abnormalities of neurosyphilis in an untreated patient with no evidence of clinical disease. It is divided into early latency (within 2 years of infection), when syphilis may be transmitted sexually, and late latency, when the patient is no longer sexually infectious. Transmission of syphilis from a pregnant woman to her fetus, and rarely by blood transfusion, is possible for several years following infection.

Late syphilis

Late latent syphilis

This may persist for many years or for life. Without treatment over 60% of patients might be expected to suffer little or no ill health. Coincidental prescription of antibiotics for other illnesses such as respiratory tract or skin infections may treat latent syphilis serendipitously.

Benign tertiary syphilis

This may develop between 3 and 10 years after infection but is now rarely seen in the UK. Skin, mucous membranes, bone, muscle or viscera can be involved. The characteristic feature is a chronic granulomatous lesion called a gumma, which may be single or multiple. Healing with scar formation may impair the function of the structure affected. Skin lesions may take the form of nodules or ulcers whilst subcutaneous lesions may ulcerate with a gummy discharge. Healing occurs slowly with the formation of characteristic tissue paper scars. Mucosal lesions may occur in the mouth, pharynx, larynx or nasal septum, appearing as punched-out ulcers. Of particular importance is gummatous involvement of the tongue, healing of which may lead to leucoplakia with the attendant risk of malignant change. Gummas of the tibia, skull, clavicle and sternum have been described, as has involvement of the brain, spinal cord, liver, testis and, rarely, other organs. Resolution of active disease should follow treatment, though some tissue damage may be permanent. Paroxysmal cold haemoglobinuria (p. 1026) may be seen.

Cardiovascular syphilis

This may present many years after initial infection. Aortitis which may involve the aortic valve and/or the coronary ostia is the key feature. Clinical features include aortic incompetence, angina and aortic aneurysm (p. 602). The condition typically affects the ascending aorta and sometimes the aortic arch; aneurysm of the descending aorta is rare. Treatment with penicillin will not correct anatomical damage and surgical intervention may be required.

Neurosyphilis

This may also take years to develop. Asymptomatic infection is associated with CSF abnormalities in the absence of clinical signs. Meningovascular disease, tabes dorsalis and general paralysis of the insane constitute the symptomatic forms (p. 1212). Neurosyphilis and cardiovascular syphilis may coexist and are sometimes referred to as quaternary syphilis.

Congenital syphilis

Congenital syphilis is rare where antenatal serological screening is practised. Antisyphilitic treatment in pregnancy treats the fetus, if infected, as well as the mother.

Treponemal infection may give rise to a variety of outcomes after 4 months of gestation when the fetus becomes immunocompetent:

- miscarriage or stillbirth, premature or at term
- birth of a syphilitic baby (a very sick baby with hepatosplenomegaly, bullous rash and perhaps pneumonia)
- birth of a baby who develops signs of early congenital syphilis during the first few weeks of life (Box 15.6)
- birth of a baby with latent infection who either remains well or develops congenital syphilis/ stigmata later in life (see Box 15.6).

Investigations in adult cases

T. pallidum may be identified in serum collected from chancres, or from moist or eroded lesions in secondary syphilis using a dark-field microscope, a direct fluorescent antibody test or PCR.

The serological tests for syphilis are listed in Box 15.7. Many centres use treponemal enzyme immunoassays (EIAs) for IgG and IgM antibodies to screen for syphilis. EIA for antitreponemal IgM becomes positive at approximately 2 weeks, whilst non-treponemal tests become positive about 4 weeks after primary syphilis. All positive results in asymptomatic patients must be confirmed by repeat tests.

Biological false positive reactions occur occasionally; these are most commonly seen with Venereal Diseases Research Laboratory (VDRL) or rapid plasma reagin (RPR) tests (when treponemal tests will be negative). Acute false positive reactions may be associated with infections such as infectious mononucleosis, chickenpox and malaria, and may also occur in pregnancy. Chronic false positive reactions may be associated with autoimmune diseases. False negative results for non-treponemal tests may be found in secondary syphilis because extremely high antibody levels can prevent the formation of the antibody–antigen lattice necessary for the visualisation of the flocculation reaction (the prozone phenomenon).

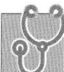

15.6 Clinical features of congenital syphilis

Early congenital syphilis (neonatal period)

- Maculopapular rash
- Condylomata lata
- Mucous patches
- Fissures around mouth, nose and anus
- Rhinitis with nasal discharge (snuffles)
- Hepatosplenomegaly
- Osteochondritis/periostitis
- Generalised lymphadenopathy
- Choroiditis
- Meningitis
- Anaemia/thrombocytopenia

Late congenital syphilis

- Benign tertiary syphilis
- Periostitis
- Paroxysmal cold haemoglobinuria
- Neurosyphilis
- 8th nerve deafness
- Interstitial keratitis
- Clutton's joints (painless effusion into knee joints)

Stigmata

- Hutchinson's incisors (anterior–posterior thickening with notch on narrowed cutting edge)
- Mulberry molars (imperfectly formed cusps/deficient dental enamel)
- High arched palate
- Maxillary hypoplasia
- Saddle nose (following snuffles)
- Rhagades (radiating scars around mouth, nose and anus following rash)
- Salt and pepper scars on retina (from choroiditis)
- Corneal scars (from interstitial keratitis)
- Sabre tibia (from periostitis)
- Bossing of frontal and parietal bones (healed periosteal nodes)

In benign tertiary and cardiovascular syphilis, examination of CSF should be considered because asymptomatic neurological disease may coexist. The CSF should also be examined in patients with clinical signs of neurosyphilis (p. 1212) and in both early and late congenital syphilis. Chest X-ray, ECG and echocardiogram are useful in the investigation of cardiovascular syphilis. Biopsy may be required to diagnose gumma.

Endemic treponematoses such as yaws, endemic (non-venereal) syphilis (bejel) and pinta (pp. 327–328)

15.7 Serological tests for syphilis

Non-treponemal (non-specific) tests

- Venereal Diseases Research Laboratory (VDRL) test
- Rapid plasma reagin (RPR) test

Treponemal (specific) antibody tests

- Treponemal antigen-based enzyme immunoassay (EIA) for IgG and IgM
- *T. pallidum* haemagglutination assay (TPHA)
- *T. pallidum* particle agglutination assay (TPPA)
- Fluorescent treponemal antibody-absorbed (FTA-ABS) test

are caused by treponemes morphologically indistinguishable from *T. pallidum* that cannot be differentiated by serological tests. A VDRL or RPR test may help to elucidate the correct diagnosis because adults with late yaws usually have low titres.

Investigations in suspected congenital syphilis

Passively transferred maternal antibodies from an adequately treated mother may give rise to positive serological tests in her baby. In this situation, non-treponemal tests should become negative within 3–6 months of birth. A positive EIA test for antitreponemal IgM suggests early congenital syphilis. A diagnosis of congenital syphilis mandates investigation of the mother, her partner and any siblings.

Management

Penicillin is the drug of choice. Specific regimens depend on the stage of infection. Longer courses are required in late syphilis. Doxycycline is indicated for patients allergic to penicillin, except in pregnancy (see below). Azithromycin is a further alternative. All patients must be followed up to ensure cure, and partner notification is of particular importance. Resolution of clinical signs in early syphilis with declining titres for non-treponemal tests, usually to undetectable levels within 6 months for primary syphilis and 12–18 months for secondary syphilis, are indicators of successful treatment. Specific treponemal antibody tests may remain positive for life. In patients who have had syphilis for many years there may be little serological response following treatment.

Pregnancy

Penicillin is the treatment of choice in pregnancy. Erythromycin stearate can be given if there is penicillin hypersensitivity, but crosses the placenta poorly; the newborn baby must therefore be treated with a course of penicillin and consideration given to retreating the mother. Some specialists recommend penicillin desensitisation for pregnant mothers so that penicillin can be given during temporary tolerance. The author has successfully prescribed ceftriaxone 250mg i.m. for 10 days in this situation. Babies should be treated in hospital with the help of a pediatrician.

Treatment reactions

- *Anaphylaxis.* Penicillin is a common cause; on-site facilities should be available for management (p. 89).
- *Jarisch–Herxheimer reaction.* This is an acute febrile reaction that follows treatment and is characterised by headache, malaise and myalgia; it resolves within 24 hours. It is common in early syphilis and rare in late syphilis. Fetal distress or premature labour can occur in pregnancy. The reaction may also cause worsening of neurological (cerebral artery occlusion) or ophthalmic (uveitis, optic neuritis) disease, myocardial ischaemia (inflammation of the coronary ostia) and laryngeal stenosis (swelling of a gumma). Prednisolone 10–20mg orally 8-hourly for 3 days is recommended to prevent the reaction in patients with these forms of the disease; antisyphilitic treatment can be started 24 hours after introducing corticosteroids. In high-risk situations it is wise to initiate therapy in hospital.

- *Procaine reaction*. Fear of impending death occurs immediately after the accidental intravenous injection of procaine penicillin and may be associated with hallucinations or fits. Symptoms are short-lived, but verbal assurance and sometimes physical restraint are needed. The reaction can be prevented by aspiration before intramuscular injection to ensure the needle is not in a blood vessel.

Gonorrhoea

Gonorrhoea is caused by infection with *Neisseria gonorrhoeae* and may involve columnar epithelium in the lower genital tract, rectum, pharynx and eyes. Transmission is usually the result of vaginal, anal or oral sex. Gonococcal conjunctivitis may be the result of accidental infection from contaminated fingers. Untreated mothers may infect their babies during delivery, resulting in ophthalmia neonatorum (Fig. 15.6). Infection of children beyond the neonatal period is usually indicative of sexual abuse.

Clinical features

The incubation period is usually 2–10 days. In men the anterior urethra is commonly infected, causing urethral discharge and dysuria, but symptoms are absent in about 10% of cases. Examination will usually show a mucopurulent or purulent urethral discharge. Rectal infection in MSM is usually asymptomatic but may present with anal discomfort, discharge or rectal bleeding. Proctoscopy may reveal either no abnormality, or clinical evidence of proctitis (see Fig. 15.3, p. 415) such as inflamed rectal mucosa and mucopus.

In women, the urethra, paraurethral glands/ducts, Bartholin's glands/ducts or endocervical canal may be infected. The rectum may also be involved either due to contamination from a urogenital site or as a result of anal sex. Occasionally, the rectum is the only site infected. About 80% of women who have gonorrhoea are asymptomatic. There may be vaginal discharge or dysuria but these symptoms are often due to additional infections such as chlamydia (see below), trichomoniasis or candidiasis, making full investigation essential (p. 411). Lower abdominal pain, dyspareunia and intermenstrual bleeding may be indicative of PID. Clinical examination may show no abnormality or pus may be expressed from urethra, paraurethral ducts or Bartholin's ducts. The cervix may be inflamed, with mucopurulent discharge and contact bleeding.

Pharyngeal gonorrhoea is the result of receptive orogenital sex and is usually symptomless. Gonococcal conjunctivitis is an uncommon complication, presenting with purulent discharge from the eye(s), severe inflammation of the conjunctivae and oedema of the eyelids, pain and photophobia. Gonococcal ophthalmia neonatorum presents similarly with purulent conjunctivitis and oedema of the eyelids. Conjunctivitis must be treated urgently to prevent corneal damage.

Disseminated gonococcal infection (DGI) is seen rarely, and typically affects women with asymptomatic genital infection. Symptoms include arthritis of one or more joints, pustular skin lesions and fever. Gonococcal endocarditis has been described.

Investigations

GNDC may be seen on microscopy of smears from infected sites (see Fig. 15.1, p. 413). Pharyngeal smears are difficult to analyse due to the presence of other diplococci, so the diagnosis must be confirmed by culture or NAAT.

Management of adults

Uncomplicated gonorrhoea responds to a single adequate dose of a suitable antimicrobial (many UK centres currently use oral cefixime 400 mg, Box 15.8); cure rates

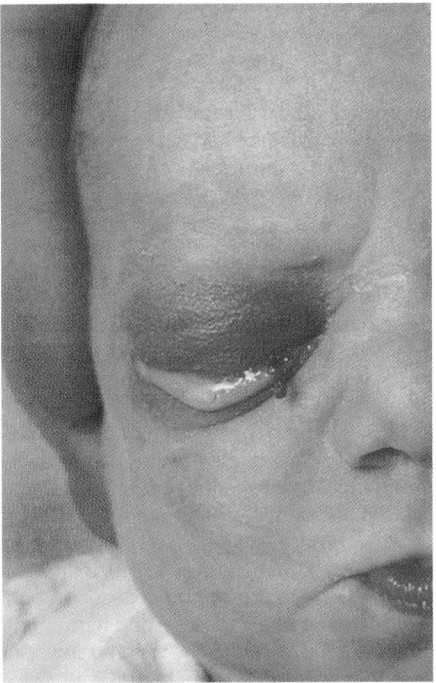

Fig. 15.6 Gonococcal ophthalmia neonatorum.

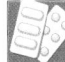 **15.8 Treatment of uncomplicated anogenital gonorrhoea**

Uncomplicated infection

- Cefixime 400 mg stat *or*
- Ciprofloxacin 500 mg orally stat[1,2] *or*
- Ofloxacin 400 mg orally stat[1,2] *or*
- Amoxicillin 3 g *plus* probenecid 1 g orally stat[3]

Quinolone resistance

- Ceftriaxone 250 mg i.m. stat *or*
- Spectinomycin 2 g i.m. stat[4]

Pregnancy and breastfeeding

- Cefixime 400 mg stat *or*
- Ceftriaxone 250 mg i.m. stat *or*
- Amoxicillin 3 g *plus* probenecid 1 g orally stat[3] *or*
- Spectinomycin 2 g i.m. stat[4]

Pharyngeal gonorrhoea

- Cefixime 400 mg stat *or*
- Ceftriaxone 250 mg i.m. stat *or*
- Ciprofloxacin 500 mg[1,2] orally stat *or*
- Ofloxacin 400 mg[1,2] orally stat

[1]Contraindicated in pregnancy and breastfeeding.
[2]If prevalence of quinolone resistance for *N. gonorrhoeae* < 5%.
[3]If prevalence of penicillin resistance for *N. gonorrhoeae* < 5%.
[4]May only be available in specialist clinics.

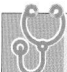

15.9 Complications of delayed therapy in gonorrhoea

- Acute prostatitis
- Epididymo-orchitis
- Bartholin's gland abscess
- PID (may lead to infertility or ectopic pregnancy)
- Disseminated gonococcal infection

should exceed 95%. Longer courses of antibiotics are required for complicated infection. Partner(s) of patients with gonorrhoea should be seen as soon as possible.

Delay in treatment may lead to complications (Box 15.9).

Chlamydial infection

Chlamydial infection in men

Chlamydia is transmitted and presents in a similar way to gonorrhoea; however, urethral symptoms are usually milder and may be absent in over 50% of cases. Conjunctivitis is also milder than in gonorrhoea; pharyngitis does not occur. The incubation period varies from 1 week to a few months. Without treatment, symptoms may resolve but the patient remains infectious for several months. Complications such as epididymo-orchitis and Reiter's syndrome, or sexually acquired reactive arthropathy (SARA, p. 1094) are rare. Sexually transmitted pathogens such as chlamydia or gonococci are usually responsible for epididymo-orchitis in men aged less than 35 years, whereas bacteria such as Gram-negative enteric organisms are more commonly implicated in older men.

Treatments for chlamydia are listed in Box 15.10. Non-specific urethritis is treated identically. The partner(s) of men with chlamydia should be treated even if laboratory tests for chlamydia are negative. Investigation is not mandatory, but serves a useful epidemiological purpose; moreover, positive results encourage further attempts at contact-tracing.

Chlamydial infection in women

The cervix and urethra are commonly involved. Infection is asymptomatic in about 80% of patients but may cause vaginal discharge, dysuria, intermenstrual and/or post-coital bleeding. Lower abdominal pain and dyspareunia are features of PID. Examination may reveal mucopuru-lent cervicitis, contact bleeding from cervix, evidence of PID or no obvious clinical signs. Treatment options are

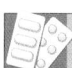

15.10 Treatment of chlamydial infection

Standard regimens

- Azithromycin 1 g orally as a single dose[1] *or*
- Doxycycline 100 mg 12-hourly orally for 7 days[2]

Alternative regimens

- Erythromycin 500 mg 6-hourly orally for 7 days *or* 500 mg 12-hourly for 2 weeks *or*
- Ofloxacin 200 mg 12-hourly orally for 7 days[2]

[1]Safety in pregnancy and breastfeeding has not been fully assessed.
[2]Contraindicated in pregnancy and breastfeeding.

listed in Box 15.10. The patient's male partner(s) should be investigated and treated.

Some infections may clear spontaneously but others persist. PID, with the risk of tubal damage and subsequent infertility or ectopic pregnancy, is an important long-term complication. Other complications include perihepatitis, chronic pelvic pain, conjunctivitis and Reiter's syndrome or SARA. Perinatal transmission may lead to ophthalmia neonatorum and/or pneumonia in the neonate.

Other sexually transmitted bacterial infections

Chancroid, granuloma inguinale and LGV as causes of genital ulcers in the tropics are described in Box 15.11. LGV is also a cause of proctitis in MSM (p. 414).

SEXUALLY TRANSMITTED VIRAL INFECTIONS

15

Genital herpes simplex

Infection with herpes simplex virus type 1 (HSV-1) or type 2 (HSV-2) produces a wide spectrum of clinical problems (p. 321). Transmission is usually sexual (vaginal, anal, orogenital or oroanal), but perinatal infection of the neonate may also occur. Primary infection at the site of HSV entry, which may be symptomatic or asymptomatic, establishes latency in local sensory ganglia. Recurrences, either symptomatic or asymptomatic viral shedding, are a consequence of HSV reactivation. The first symptomatic episode is usually the most severe. Although HSV-1 is classically associated with orolabial herpes and HSV-2 with anogenital herpes, HSV-1 now accounts for more than 50% of anogenital infections in the UK.

Clinical features

The first symptomatic episode presents with irritable vesicles that soon rupture to form small, tender ulcers on the external genitalia (see Figs 15.7 and 15.2, p. 414). Lesions at other sites (e.g. urethra, vagina, cervix, peri-anal area, anus or rectum) may cause dysuria, urethral or vaginal discharge, or anal, perianal or rectal pain. Constitutional symptoms such as fever, headache and malaise are common. Inguinal lymph nodes become enlarged and tender, and there may be nerve root pain in the 2nd and 3rd sacral dermatomes.

Extragenital lesions may develop at other sites such as the buttock, finger or eye due to auto-inoculation. Oropharyngeal infection may result from orogenital sex. Complications such as urinary retention due to autonomic neuropathy, and aseptic meningitis are occasionally seen.

First episodes usually heal within 2–4 weeks without treatment; recurrences are usually milder and of shorter duration than the initial attack. They occur more often in HSV-2 infection and their frequency tends to decrease with time. Prodromal symptoms such as irritation or burning at the subsequent site of recurrence, or neuralgic pains affecting buttocks, legs or hips are commonly seen. The first symptomatic episode may be a recurrence of a previously undiagnosed primary infection. Recurrent episodes of asymptomatic viral shedding are important in the transmission of HSV.

15.11 Salient features of lymphogranuloma venereum, chancroid and granuloma inguinale (Donovanosis)

Infection and distribution	Organism	Incubation period	Genital lesion	Lymph nodes	Diagnosis	Management
Lymphogranuloma venereum (LGV)						
East/West Africa, India, South-east Asia, South America, Caribbean	*Chlamydia trachomatis* types L1,2,3	3–30 days	Small, transient, painless ulcer, vesicle, papule; often unnoticed	Tender, usually unilateral, matted, adherent, multilocular, suppurative bubo; inguinal/femoral nodes involved; there may be late sequelae[1]	Serological tests for L1–3 serotypes; swab from ulcer or bubo pus for *Chlamydia*	Doxycycline[2] 12-hourly orally for 21 days *or* Erythromycin 500 mg 6-hourly orally
Chancroid						
Africa, Asia, Central and South America	*Haemophilus ducreyi* (short Gram-negative bacillus)	3–10 days	Single or multiple painful ulcers with ragged undermined edges	As above but unilocular, suppurative bubo; inguinal nodes involved in ~50%	Microscopy and culture of scrapings from ulcer or pus from bubo	Azithromycin[3] 1 g orally once *or* Ceftriaxone 250 mg i.m. once *or* Ciprofloxacin[2] 500 mg 12-hourly orally for 3 days *or* Erythromycin 500 mg 6-hourly orally for 7 days
Granuloma inguinale						
Australia, Caribbean, India, South Africa, South America, Papua New Guinea	*Klebsiella granulomatis* (Donovan bodies)	3–40 days	Ulcers or hypertrophic granulomatous lesions; usually painless[4]	Initial swelling of inguinal nodes, then spread of infection to form abscess or ulceration through adjacent skin	Microscopy of cellular material for intracellular bipolar-staining Donovan bodies	Azithromycin[3] 1 g weekly orally *or* 500 mg daily orally *or* Doxycycline[2] 100 mg 12-hourly orally *or* Ceftriaxone 1 g i.m. daily *or* Erythromycin 500 mg 6-hourly orally Treatment for at least 3 weeks and until lesions have healed

[1]The genito-ano-rectal syndrome is a late manifestation of LGV.
[2]Doxycycline and ciprofloxacin are contraindicated in pregnancy and breastfeeding.
[3]The safety of azithromycin in pregnancy and breastfeeding has not been fully assessed.
[4]Mother-to-baby transmission of granuloma inguinale may rarely occur.
N.B. Partners of patients with LGV, chancroid and granuloma inguinale should be investigated and treated, even if asymptomatic.

Diagnosis

Swabs are taken from vesicular fluid or ulcers for detection of DNA by PCR or tissue culture and typing. Electron microscopy of such material will only give a presumptive diagnosis, as herpes group viruses appear similar. Type-specific antibody tests are available but are not sufficiently accurate for general use.

Management

First episode

The following 5-day oral regimens are all recommended and should be started within 5 days of the beginning of the episode, or whilst lesions are still forming:

- aciclovir 200 mg five times daily
- famciclovir 250 mg 8-hourly
- valaciclovir 500 mg 12-hourly.

Analgesia may be required and saline bathing can be soothing. Treatment may be continued for longer than 5 days if new lesions develop. Occasionally intravenous therapy may be indicated if oral therapy is poorly tolerated or aseptic meningitis occurs.

Catheterisation via the suprapubic route is advisable for urinary retention due to autonomic neuropathy because the transurethral route may introduce HSV into the bladder.

Recurrent genital herpes

Symptomatic recurrences are usually mild and may require no specific treatment other than saline bathing. For more severe episodes patient-initiated treatment at onset, with one of the following 5-day oral regimens, should reduce the duration of the recurrence:

- aciclovir 200 mg five times daily
- famciclovir 125–150 mg 12-hourly
- valaciclovir 500 mg 12-hourly.

In a few patients, treatment started at the onset of prodromal symptoms may abort recurrence.

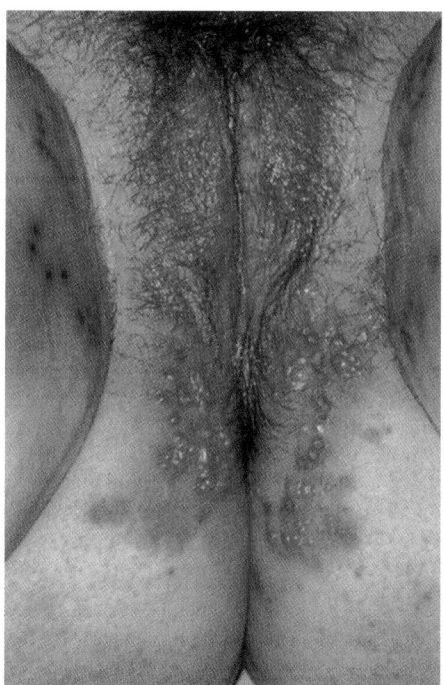

Fig. 15.7 Herpetic ulceration of the vulva.

Suppressive therapy may be required for patients with frequent recurrences, especially if these occur at intervals of less than 4 weeks. Treatment should be given for a minimum of 1 year before stopping to assess recurrence rate. About 20% of patients will experience reduced attack rates thereafter, but for those whose recurrences remain unchanged, resumption of suppressive therapy is justified. Aciclovir 400 mg 12-hourly is most commonly prescribed.

Management in pregnancy

If her partner is known to be infected with HSV, a pregnant woman with no previous anogenital herpes should be advised to protect herself during sexual intercourse because the risk of disseminated infection is increased in pregnancy. Consistent condom use during pregnancy may reduce transmission of HSV. Genital herpes acquired during the first or second trimester of pregnancy is treated with aciclovir as clinically indicated. Although aciclovir is not licensed for use in pregnancy in the UK, there is considerable clinical evidence to support its safety. Third-trimester acquisition has been associated with life-threatening haematogenous dissemination and should be treated with aciclovir.

Vaginal delivery should be routine in women who are symptomless in late pregnancy. Caesarean section (CS) is sometimes considered if there is a recurrence at the beginning of labour, although the risk of neonatal herpes through vaginal transmission is very low. CS is often recommended if primary infection occurs after 34 weeks because the risk of viral shedding is very high in labour.

Human papillomavirus (HPV) and anogenital warts

HPV DNA typing has demonstrated over 90 genotypes (p. 1271), of which HPV-6, HPV-11, HPV-16 and HPV-18 most commonly infect the genital tract through sex-

ual transmission. It is important to differentiate between the benign genotypes (HPV-6 and 11) that cause anogenital warts, and genotypes such as 16 and 18 that are associated with dysplastic conditions and cancers of the genital tract but are not a cause of benign warts. All genotypes usually result in subclinical infection of the genital tract rather than clinically obvious lesions affecting penis, vulva, vagina, cervix, perineum or anus.

Clinical features

Anogenital warts caused by HPV may be single or multiple, exophytic, papular or flat. Perianal warts (p. 410), whilst being more commonly found in MSM, are also found in heterosexual men and in women. Rarely, a giant condyloma (Buschke–Lewenstein tumour) develops with local tissue destruction. Atypical warts should be biopsied. In pregnancy warts may dramatically increase in size and number, making treatment difficult. Rarely, they are large enough to obstruct labour and in this case delivery by CS will be required. Perinatal transmission of HPV rarely leads to anogenital warts, or possibly laryngeal papillomas, in the neonate.

Management

The use of condoms can help prevent the transmission of HPV to non-infected partners, but HPV may affect parts of the genital area not protected by condoms. Vaccination against HPV infection has been introduced and is in routine use in several countries. There are two types of vaccine:

- *A bivalent vaccine* offers protection against HPV types 16 and 18, which account for approximately 75% of cervical cancers in the UK.
- *A quadrivalent vaccine* offers additional protection against HPV types 6 and 11, which account for over 90% of genital warts.

Both types of vaccine have been shown to be highly effective in the prevention of cervical intraepithelial neoplasia in young women, and the quadrivalent vaccine has also been shown to be highly effective in protecting against HPV-associated genital warts (Box 15.12). It is currently recommended that HPV vaccination should be administered prior to the onset of sexual activity, typically at age 11–13, in a course of three injections. In the UK, only girls are being offered vaccination, although it should be noted that this approach will not protect HPV transmission for MSM. As neither vaccine protects against all oncogenic types of HPV, cervical screening programmes will still be necessary.

A variety of treatments are available for established disease, including the following:

- *Podophyllotoxin, 0.5% solution or 0.15% cream* (contraindicated in pregnancy) applied 12-hourly for 3 days, followed by 4 days' rest, for up to 4 weeks is suitable for home treatment of external warts.

EBM **15.12 HPV vaccination and precancerous cervical intraepithelial neoplasia**

'Prophylactic HPV vaccination in women aged 15–25 years is highly effective at preventing precancerous cervical intraepithelial neoplasia in young women who have not previously been infected with HPV.'

- Garland SM, et al. New Engl J Med 2007; 356:1928–1943.
- Paavonen J, et al. Lancet 2007; 369:2161–2170.

- *Imiquimod* cream (contraindicated in pregnancy) applied 3 times weekly (and washed off after 6–10 hours) for up to 16 weeks is also suitable for home treatment of external warts.
- *Cryotherapy* using liquid nitrogen to freeze warty tissue is suitable for external and internal warts but often requires repeated clinic visits.
- *Hyfrecation*—electrofulguration that causes superficial charring—is suitable for external and internal warts. Hyfrecation results in smoke plume which contains HPV DNA and the potential to cause respiratory infection in the operator/patient. Masks should be worn during the procedure and adequate extraction of fumes should be provided.
- *Surgical removal.* Refractory warts, especially pedunculated perianal lesions, may be excised under local or general anaesthesia.

Molluscum contagiosum

Infection by molluscum contagiosum virus, both sexual and non-sexual, produces flesh-coloured umbilicated hemispherical papules usually up to 5 mm in diameter after an incubation period of 3–12 weeks (Fig. 15.8). Larger lesions may be seen in HIV infection (p. 391). Lesions are often multiple and, once established in an individual, may spread by auto-inoculation. They are found on the genitalia, lower abdomen and upper thighs when sexually acquired. Facial lesions are highly suggestive of underlying HIV infection. Diagnosis is made on clinical grounds and by expression of the central core, in which the typical pox-like viral particles can be seen on electron microscopy (differentiating molluscum contagiosum from genital warts). Typically, lesions persist for an average of 2 years before spontaneous reso-

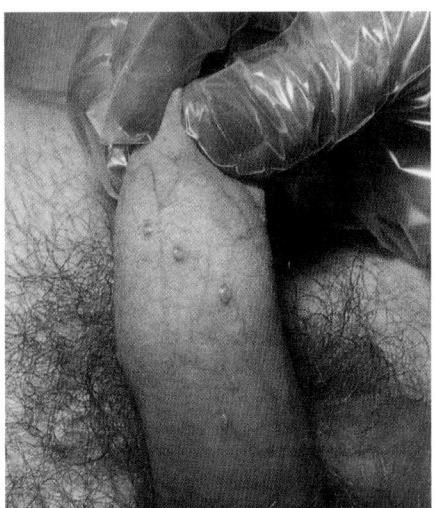

Fig. 15.8 Molluscum contagiosum of the shaft of the penis.

lution occurs. Treatment regimens are therefore cosmetic; they include cryotherapy, hyfrecation, topical applications of 0.15% podophyllotoxin cream (contraindicated in pregnancy) or expression of the central core.

Viral hepatitis

The hepatitis viruses A–D (pp. 947–954) may be sexually transmitted:

- *Hepatitis A (HAV).* Insertive oroanal sex, insertive digital sex, insertive anal sex and multiple sexual partners have been linked with HAV transmission in MSM. HAV transmission in heterosexual men and women is also possible through oroanal sex.
- *Hepatitis B (HBV).* Insertive oroanal sex, anal sex and multiple sexual partners are linked with HBV infection in MSM. Heterosexual transmission of HBV is well documented and commercial sex workers are at particular risk. Hepatitis D (HDV) may also be sexually transmitted.
- *Hepatitis C.* Sexual transmission of HCV is well documented in MSM, but less so in heterosexuals. Sexual transmission is less efficient than for HBV.

The sexual partner(s) of patients with HAV and HBV should be seen as soon as possible and offered immunisation where appropriate. Patients with HAV should abstain from all forms of unprotected sex until non-infectious. Those with HBV should likewise abstain from unprotected sex until they are non-infectious or until their partners have been vaccinated successfully. No active or passive immunisation is available for protection against HCV but the consistent use of condoms is likely to protect susceptible partners. Active immunisation against HAV and HBV should be offered to susceptible people at risk of infection. Many STI clinics offer HAV immunisation to MSM along with routine HBV immunisation; a combined HAV and HBV vaccine is available.

Further information

Books and journal articles

Adler M, Cowan F, French P, et al. ABC of sexually transmitted infections. London: BMJ Books; 2004.

Clutterbuck D. Specialist training in sexually transmitted infections and HIV. London: Mosby; 2004.

Low N, Aral S, Cassell J (eds). Global aspects of STI and HIV. Sex Transm Inf 2007; 83:501–589.

McMillan A, Young H, Ogilvie MM, Scott GR. Clinical practice in sexually transmissible infections. London: Saunders; 2002.

Websites

www.bashh.org/guidelines *Updates on treatment of all STIs.*

M.J. Field
L. Burnett
D.R. Sullivan
P. Stewart

Clinical biochemistry and metabolism

16

16

There is a world-wide trend towards increased use of laboratory-based diagnostic investigations, and biochemical investigations in particular. In health-care systems of developed countries, it has been estimated that 60–70% of all critical decisions taken in regard to patients, and over 90% of data stored in electronic medical records systems, involve a laboratory service or result.

This chapter covers a diverse group of disorders affecting adults not considered elsewhere in this book, whose primary manifestation is in abnormalities of biochemistry laboratory results, or whose underlying pathophysiology involves disturbance in specific biochemical pathways.

BIOCHEMICAL INVESTIGATIONS

There are three broad reasons why a clinician may request a biochemical laboratory investigation:

* to screen an asymptomatic subject for the presence of disease
* to assist in diagnosis of a patient's presenting complaint
* to monitor changes in test results, as a marker of disease progression or response to treatment.

Contemporary medical practice has become increasingly reliant on laboratory investigation, and in particular, on biochemical investigation. This has been associated with extraordinary improvements in the ana-lytical capacity and speed of laboratory instrumentation and the following operational trends:

* Large central biochemistry laboratories feature extensive use of automation and information technology. Specimens are transported from clinical areas to the laboratory using high-speed transport systems (such as pneumatic tubes), and identified with machine-readable labels (such as bar codes). Laboratory instruments have been miniaturised and integrated with robot transport systems to enable multiple rapid analyses of a single sample. Statistical process control techniques are used to assure the quality of analytical results, and increasingly to monitor other aspects of the laboratory, such as the time taken to complete the analysis ('turn-around time').
* Point-of-care testing (POCT) brings selected laboratory analytical systems into clinical areas, to the patient's bedside, or even connected to an individual patient. These systems allow the clinician to receive results almost instantaneously, although with less precision and often at greater cost than using a central laboratory.
* The diversity of analyses has widened considerably with the introduction of many techniques borrowed from the chemical or other industries (Box 16.1).

Good medical practice involves appropriate ordering of laboratory investigations and correct interpretation of test results. The key principles, including the concepts of sensitivity and specificity, are described in Chapter 1

16.1 Range of analytical modalities used in the clinical biochemistry laboratory

Analytical modality	Analyte	Typical applications
Ion-selective electrodes	Blood gases, electrolytes (e.g. Na, K, Cl)	Point-of-care testing (POCT) High-throughput analysers
Colorimetric chemical reaction or coupled enzymatic reaction	Simple mass or concentration measurement (e.g. creatinine, phosphate) Simple enzyme activity	High-throughput analysers
Ligand assay (usually immunoassay)	Specific proteins Hormones Drugs	Increasingly available for POCT or high-throughput analysers
Chromatography: gas chromatography (GC), high-pressure liquid chromatography (HPLC), thin-layer chromatography (TLC)	Organic compounds	Therapeutic drug monitoring (TDM)
Mass spectroscopy (MS)		Drug screening (e.g. drugs of misuse) Vitamins Biochemical metabolites
Spectrophotometry, turbidimetry, nephelometry, fluorimetry	Haemoglobin derivatives Specific proteins Immunoglobulins	Xanthochromia Lipoproteins Paraproteins
Electrophoresis	Proteins Some enzymes	Paraproteins Isoenzyme analysis
Atomic absorption (AA) Inductively coupled plasma/mass spectroscopy (ICP-MS)	Trace elements and metals	Quantitation of heavy metals
Molecular diagnostics	Nucleic acid quantification and/or sequence	Inherited and somatic cell mutations (Ch. 3) Genetic polymorphisms (Ch. 3) Variations in rates of drug metabolism (Ch. 2) Microbial diagnosis (Ch. 6)

(pp. 5–6). Reference ranges for laboratory results are discussed in Chapter 28. Many laboratory investigations can be subject to variability arising from incorrect patient preparation (e.g. fasting or fed state), timing of sample collection (e.g. in relation to diurnal variation of hormone levels, or dosage regimens for therapeutic agents), or analytical factors (e.g. serum vs. plasma sample, use of the correct anticoagulant, or POCT vs. central analyser). It is therefore important for clinical and laboratory staff to communicate effectively and for clinicians to follow local recommendations concerning collection and transport of samples in the appropriate container and with appropriate labelling.

INTEGRATED WATER AND ELECTROLYTE BALANCE

One of the most common uses of the clinical biochemistry laboratory is to monitor electrolyte and acid–base status. The diverse clinical consequences of these biochemical disorders are illustrated in Box 16.2. Some whole-body electrolyte disturbances (notably of sodium) result in major clinical problems with minimal disturbance in measured biochemical parameters. However, these will also be considered for convenience in this section.

Before considering individual electrolytes and acid–base balance in turn, it is important to review the relationships between them.

16.2 Manifestations of disordered water, electrolyte and acid–base status

Primary disturbance	Altered physiology	Clinical effect
Sodium	ECF volume	Circulatory changes
Water	ECF osmolality	Cerebral changes
Potassium	Action potential in excitable tissues	Neuromuscular weakness, cardiac effects
Hydrogen ion	Acid–base balance (pH)	Altered tissue function, respiratory compensation
Magnesium	Cell membrane stability	Neuromuscular, vascular and cardiac effects
Phosphate	Cellular energetics	Widespread tissue effects

(ECF = extracellular fluid)

Water and electrolyte distribution

The following basic concepts are relevant to understanding the origin, consequences and therapy of many of the fluid and electrolyte disturbances discussed in this chapter.

In a typical adult male, total body water (TBW) is approximately 60% of body weight (somewhat more for infants and less for women). Of a TBW of 40 L, more than half is located inside cells (the intracellular fluid or ICF) while the remainder, some 15 L, is in the extracellular fluid (ECF) compartment (Fig. 16.1). Of the ECF, the plasma is itself a small fraction (some 3 L) while the

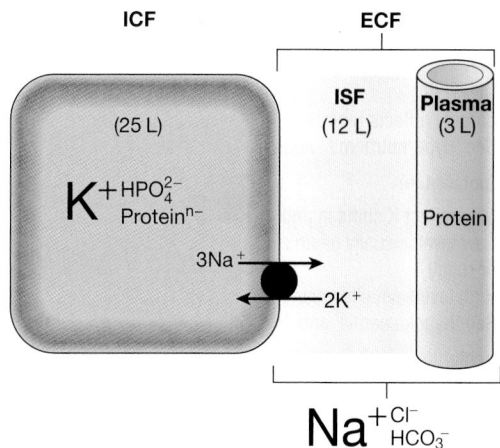

Fig. 16.1 Normal distribution of body water and electrolytes. Schematic representation of volume (L = litres) and composition (dominant ionic species only shown) of the intracellular fluid (ICF) and extracellular fluid (ECF) in a 70 kg male. The main difference in composition between the plasma and interstitial fluid (ISF) is the presence of appreciable concentrations of protein in the plasma but not the ISF.

remainder is interstitial fluid, within the tissues but outside the cells.

Figure 16.1 illustrates some of the major differences in composition between the main body fluid compartments. The dominant cation in the ICF is potassium, while the dominant cation in the ECF is sodium. Phosphates and negatively charged proteins constitute the major intracellular anions, while chloride and, to a lesser extent, bicarbonate dominate the ECF anions. An important difference between the plasma and interstitial compartments of the ECF is that only plasma contains significant concentrations of protein.

The major force maintaining the difference in cation concentration between the ICF and ECF is the activity of the sodium–potassium pump (Na,K-activated ATPase) integral to all cell membranes. Maintenance of the cation gradients across cell membranes is essential for many cell processes, including the excitability of conducting tissues such as nerve and muscle. The difference in protein content between the plasma and the interstitial fluid compartment is maintained by the impermeability of the capillary wall to protein. This protein concentration gradient (the colloid osmotic, or oncotic, pressure of the plasma) contributes to the balance of forces across the capillary wall that favour fluid retention within the circulating plasma.

Investigation of water and electrolytes

The most common biochemical test in plasma is called the urea and electrolytes ('U&Es') test in some parts of the world and the electrolytes/urea/creatinine ('EUC') test in others. A guide to its interpretation is shown in Box 16.3. Because the blood consists of both intracellular (red cell) and extracellular (plasma) components, it is important to avoid haemolysis during or after collection of the sample, which causes contamination of the plasma compartment by intracellular elements, particularly potassium. Blood should not be

16.3 How to interpret 'U&Es' (urea and electrolytes) or 'EUC' (electrolytes, urea, creatinine) results

Na⁺ (sodium)

- Largely reflects reciprocal changes in body water content
- See 'Hypernatraemia' and 'Hyponatraemia', pp. 435–437

K⁺ (potassium)

- May reflect K shifts in and out of cells
- Low levels usually mean excessive losses (gastrointestinal or renal)
- High levels usually mean renal dysfunction
- See 'Hypokalaemia' and 'Hyperkalaemia', pp. 438–440

Cl⁻ (chloride)

- Generally changes in parallel with plasma Na
- Low in metabolic alkalosis
- High in some forms of metabolic acidosis

HCO₃⁻ (bicarbonate)

- Abnormal in acid–base disorders
- See Box 16.18, p. 443

Urea

- Increased with a fall in glomerular filtration rate (GFR), reduced renal perfusion or urine flow rate, and in high protein intake or catabolic states
- See Fig. 17.3, p. 465

Creatinine

- Increased with a fall in GFR, in individuals with high muscle mass, and with some drugs
- See Fig. 17.3, p. 465

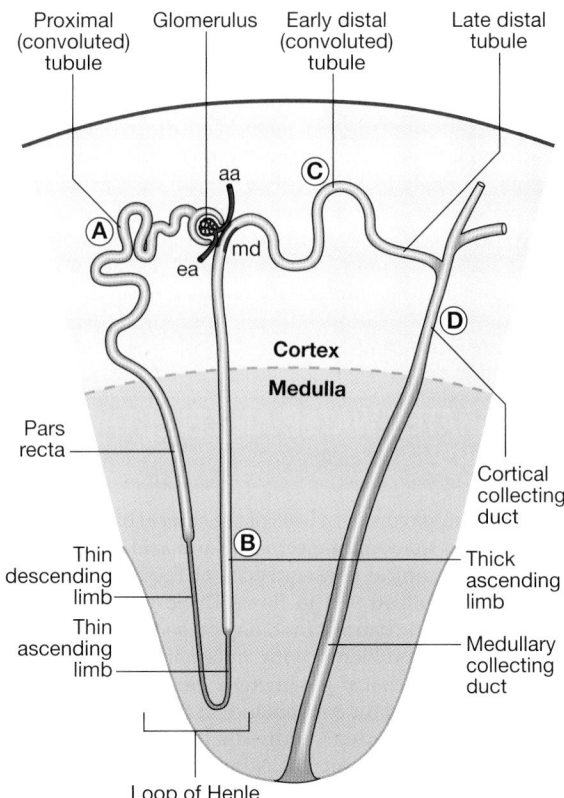

Fig. 16.2 The nephron. Letters A–D refer to tubular segments shown in more detail in Figure 16.3. (aa = afferent arteriole; ea = efferent arteriole; md = macula densa)

drawn from an arm into which an intravenous infusion is being given, to avoid contamination by the infused fluid. Repeated measurements of plasma electrolytes are frequently necessary when a marked abnormality has been detected and corrective therapy instituted.

Since the kidney maintains the constancy of body fluids by adjusting urine volume and composition, it is frequently helpful to obtain a sample of urine ('spot' specimen or 24-hour collection) at the time of blood analysis. An example of the use of urine biochemistry is given for the differential diagnosis of hyponatraemia in Box 16.14 (p. 436).

DISORDERS OF SODIUM BALANCE

Functional anatomy and physiology of renal sodium handling

Since the great majority of the body's sodium content is located in the ECF, where it is by far the most abundant cation, total body sodium is a principal determinant of ECF volume. Regulation of sodium excretion by the kidney is crucially important in maintaining normal ECF volume, and hence plasma volume, in the face of wide variations in sodium intake, typically in the range 50–250 mmol/day.

The functional unit for renal excretion is the nephron (Fig. 16.2). The glomerulus is the site of ultrafiltration of the blood, resulting in the generation of a cell- and protein-free fluid, resembling plasma in electrolyte composition, that is delivered into the initial part of the tubular system (more detail on the structure

and function of the glomerulus is given in Ch. 17). The glomerular filtration rate (GFR) is approximately 125 mL/min (equivalent to 180 L/day) in a typical adult. Over 99% of this filtered fluid is reabsorbed into the blood in the peritubular capillaries during its passage through successive segments of the nephron, largely as a result of tubular reabsorption of sodium. The processes mediating this sodium reabsorption, and the factors which regulate it, are key to understanding clinical disturbances and pharmacological interventions.

Nephron segments

At least four different functional segments of the nephron can be defined in terms of their mechanism for sodium reabsorption (Fig. 16.3).

Proximal tubule

This is responsible for the reabsorption of some 65% of the filtered sodium load. The cellular mechanism is complex but some of the key features are shown in Figure 16.3A. The basolateral membrane contains a high density of Na,K-ATPase pump units which remove sodium from the cell into the blood. The filtered sodium in the luminal fluid enters the cell via several transporters in the apical membrane. Cotransporters couple sodium to the entry of glucose, amino acid, phosphate and other organic molecules. A quantitatively more significant mechanism is the entry of sodium by countertransport with H⁺ ions, using the sodium–hydrogen exchanger (NHE-3).

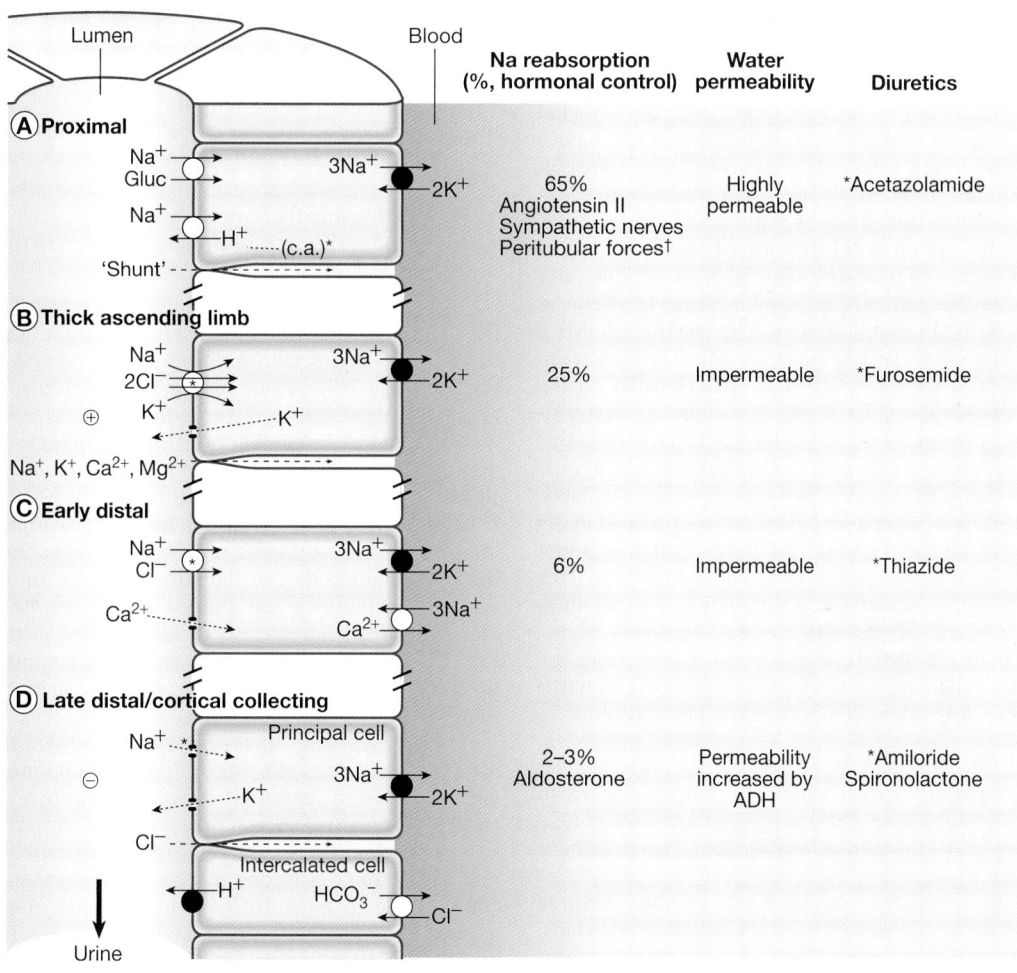

Fig. 16.3 Principal transport mechanisms in segments of the nephron. See text for further details. Black circles indicate primary active transport pumps; open circles are carrier molecules without direct linkage to adenosine triphosphate (ATP) hydrolysis. *Site of diuretic action in each segment. †Peritubular forces refers to the hydrostatic and oncotic pressures in the peritubular capillaries. (ADH = antidiuretic hormone; c.a. = carbonic anhydrase)

Intracellular H^+ ions are generated from carbonic acid, the product of the enzyme carbonic anhydrase, which hydrates carbon dioxide. In addition, a large component of the transepithelial flux of sodium, water and other dissolved solutes occurs through the gaps *between* the cells (the 'shunt' pathway). Overall, fluid and electrolyte reabsorption is almost isotonic in this segment, as water reabsorption is matched very closely to sodium fluxes. A component of this water flow also passes *through* the cells, via aquaporin-1 (AQP-1) water channels, which are not sensitive to hormonal regulation.

The loop of Henle

The thick ascending limb of the loop of Henle (Fig. 16.3B) reabsorbs a further 25% of the filtered sodium but is impermeable to water, resulting in dilution of the luminal fluid. Again, the primary driving force for sodium reabsorption is the Na,K-ATPase on the basolateral cell membrane, but in this segment sodium enters the cell from the lumen via a specific carrier molecule, the Na,K,2Cl cotransporter ('triple cotransporter', or NKCC2), which allows electroneutral entry of these ions. Some of the potassium accumulated inside the cell recirculates across the apical membrane back into the

lumen through a specific potassium channel (ROMK), providing a continuing supply of potassium to match the high concentrations of sodium and chloride available in the lumen. A small positive transepithelial potential difference exists in the lumen of this segment relative to the interstitium and this serves to drive cations such as sodium, potassium, calcium and magnesium between the cells, forming a reabsorptive shunt pathway.

Early distal tubule

Some 6% of filtered sodium is reabsorbed in the early distal (also called distal convoluted) tubule (Fig. 16.3C), again driven by the activity of the basolateral Na, K-ATPase. In this segment, entry of sodium into the cell from the luminal fluid is via a sodium–chloride cotransport carrier (NCCT). This segment is also impermeable to water, resulting in further dilution of the luminal fluid. There is no significant transepithelial flux of potassium in this segment, but calcium is reabsorbed through the mechanism shown in Figure 16.3C; a basolateral sodium–calcium exchanger leads to low intracellular concentrations of calcium, promoting calcium entry from the luminal fluid through a calcium channel.

Late distal tubule and collecting ducts

The late distal tubule and cortical collecting duct are anatomically and functionally continuous (Fig. 16.3D). Here sodium entry from the luminal fluid is via the epithelial sodium channel (ENaC) through which sodium passes alone, generating a substantial lumen-negative transepithelial potential difference. This sodium reabsorptive flux is balanced by excretion of potassium and hydrogen ions and by reabsorption of chloride ions. Potassium is accumulated in the cell by the basolateral Na,K-ATPase, and passes into the luminal fluid down its electrochemical gradient, through an apical potassium channel (ROMK). Chloride ions pass largely between cells. Hydrogen ion secretion is mediated by an H^+-ATPase located on the luminal membrane of the intercalated cells, which constitute approximately one-third of the epithelial cells in this nephron segment. This part of the nephron has a variable permeability to water, depending on the availability of antidiuretic hormone (ADH, or vasopressin) in the circulation. All ion transport processes in this segment are stimulated by the steroid hormone aldosterone. This can increase the sodium reabsorption in this segment to a maximum of 2–3% of the filtered sodium load.

Less than 1% of sodium reabsorption occurs in the medullary collecting duct, where it is inhibited by natriuretic peptides such as ANP (atrial) and BNP (brain).

Regulation of sodium transport

A large number of interrelated mechanisms serve to maintain whole body sodium balance and hence ECF volume by matching urinary sodium excretion to sodium intake (Fig. 16.4).

Important sensing mechanisms include volume receptors in the cardiac atria and the intrathoracic veins, as well as pressure receptors located in the central arterial tree (aortic arch and carotid sinus) and the afferent arterioles within the kidney. A further afferent signal

is generated within the kidney itself; the enzyme renin is released from specialised smooth muscle cells in the walls of the afferent and efferent arterioles, at the point where they make contact with the early distal tubule (at the macula densa) to form the juxtaglomerular apparatus. Renin release is stimulated by:

- reduced perfusion pressure in the afferent arteriole
- increased sympathetic nerve activity
- decreased sodium chloride concentration in the distal tubular fluid.

Renin released into the circulation activates the effector mechanisms for sodium retention which are components of the renin–angiotensin–aldosterone (RAA) system (see Fig. 20.19, p. 769). Renin acts on the peptide substrate angiotensinogen (manufactured in the liver), producing angiotensin I in the circulation. This in turn is cleaved by angiotensin-converting enzyme (ACE) into angiotensin II, largely in the pulmonary capillary bed. Angiotensin II has multiple actions: stimulation of proximal tubular sodium reabsorption, release of aldosterone from the zona glomerulosa of the adrenal cortex, and direct vasoconstriction of small arterioles. Aldosterone acts to amplify sodium retention by its action in the cortical collecting duct. The net effect is to restore ECF volume and blood pressure towards normal, thereby correcting the initiating hypovolaemic stimulus.

The sympathetic nervous system also increases sodium retention, both through haemodynamic mechanisms (afferent arteriolar vasoconstriction and GFR reduction) and by direct stimulation of proximal tubular sodium reabsorption. Other humoral mediators, such as the natriuretic peptides, inhibit sodium reabsorption, contributing to natriuresis during periods of sodium and volume excess. Hypovolaemia also has haemodynamic effects which reduce GFR and alter the peritubular physical forces around the proximal tubule, thereby decreasing sodium excretion. Conversely, increased renal perfusion in hypervolaemia and hypertension results in a compensatory increase in sodium excretion.

Presenting problems in disorders of sodium balance

When the balance of sodium intake and excretion is disturbed, any tendency for plasma sodium concentration to change is usually corrected by the osmotic mechanisms controlling water balance (p. 434). As a result, disorders in sodium balance present chiefly as altered ECF volume rather than altered sodium concentration. Clinical manifestations of altered volume are illustrated in Box 16.4.

Sodium depletion (usually associated with hypovolaemia)
Aetiology and clinical assessment

Sodium depletion can occur occasionally under extreme environmental conditions as a result of inadequate intake of salt, but it is much more commonly due to pathological losses of sodium-containing fluids (Box 16.5). Loss of whole blood, as in acute haemorrhage, is also an obvious cause of hypovolaemia, and elicits the same mechanisms for the conservation of sodium and water.

Diagnosis of hypovolaemia is based on characteristic symptoms and signs (see Box 16.4) in the context of a

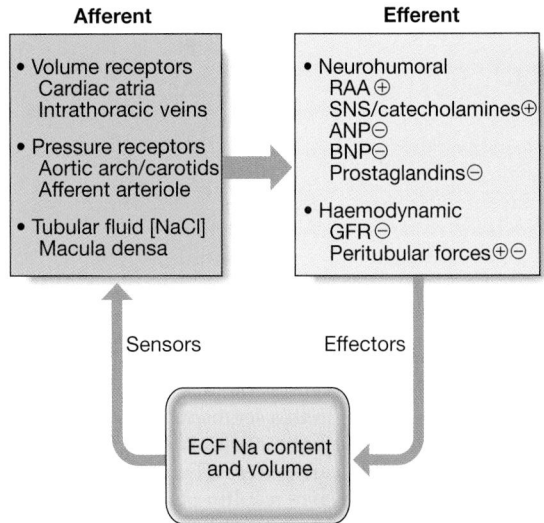

Fig. 16.4 Mechanisms involved in the regulation of sodium transport. (ANP = atrial natriuretic peptide; BNP = brain natriuretic peptide; ECF = extracellular fluid; GFR = glomerular filtration rate; RAA = renin–angiotensin–aldosterone system; SNS = sympathetic nervous system. ⊕ indicates an effect to reduce Na excretion, while ⊖ indicates an effect to increase Na excretion)

16.4 Clinical features of hypovolaemia and hypervolaemia

	Hypovolaemia	Hypervolaemia
Symptoms	Thirst	Ankle swelling
	Dizziness on standing	Abdominal swelling
	Weakness	Breathlessness
Signs	Low JVP	Peripheral oedema
	Postural hypotension	Raised JVP
	Tachycardia	Pulmonary crepitations
	Dry mouth	Pleural effusion
	Reduced skin turgor	Ascites
	Reduced urine output	Weight gain
	Weight loss	Hypertension (sometimes)
	Confusion, stupor	

(JVP = jugular venous pressure)

16.5 Causes of sodium and water depletion

Mechanism	Examples
Inadequate intake	Environmental deprivation, inadequate therapeutic replacement
Gastrointestinal sodium loss	Vomiting, diarrhoea, nasogastric suction, external fistula
Skin sodium loss	Excessive sweating, burns
Renal sodium loss	Diuretic therapy, mineralocorticoid deficiency, tubulointerstitial disease (sometimes)
Internal sequestration*	Bowel obstruction, peritonitis, pancreatitis, crush injury

*A cause of circulatory volume depletion, although total body sodium and water may be normal or increased.

relevant precipitating illness. Supportive evidence may be obtained the clinical biochemistry laboratory. Although plasma sodium concentration may not be reduced if salt and water are lost in equal proportions, a number of other parameters are altered during appropriate renal, hormonal and haemodynamic responses to hypovolaemia. In early hypovolaemic states, GFR is maintained while urinary flow rate is reduced as a consequence of activation of sodium- and water-retaining mechanisms in the nephron. Thus, plasma creatinine, which reflects GFR, may be relatively normal, but the plasma urea concentration is typically elevated, since urea excretion is affected by both GFR and urine flow rate. Plasma uric acid may also rise, reflecting activation of compensatory proximal tubular reabsorption. With avid retention of sodium and water, the urine osmolality increases while the urine sodium concentration falls. Under these circumstances, sodium excretion may fall to less than 0.1% of the filtered sodium load.

Management

Management of sodium and water depletion has two main components:

- treat the cause where possible, to stop ongoing salt and water losses
- replace the salt and water deficits, and provide ongoing maintenance requirements, usually by intravenous fluid replacement when depletion is severe.

Intravenous fluid therapy

Box 16.6 shows the daily maintenance requirements for water and electrolytes in a typical adult, and Box 16.7 summarises the composition of some widely available intravenous fluids. The choice of fluid and the rate of administration depend on the clinical circumstances, as assessed at the bedside and from laboratory data, and described in Box 16.8.

16.6 Basic daily water and electrolyte requirements

	Requirement per kg	Typical 70 kg adult
Water	35–45 mL/kg	2.5–3.0 L/day
Sodium	1.5–2 mmol/kg	100–140 mmol/day
Potassium	1.0–1.5 mmol/kg	70–100 mmol/day

16.7 Composition of some isotonic intravenous fluids (mmol/L except D-glucose)

Fluid	D-glucose	Calories	Na⁺	Cl⁻	Other
5% dextrose	50 g	200	0	0	0
Normal (0.9%) saline	0	0	154	154	0
Hartmann's solution	0	0	131	111	K⁺ 5, Ca²⁺ 2, Lactate⁻ 29

16.8 How to assess fluid and electrolyte balance in hospitalised patients

Step 1: assess clinical volume status

- Examine patient for signs of hypovolaemia or hypervolaemia (see Box 16.4)
- Check daily weight change

Step 2: review fluid balance chart

- Check total volumes IN and OUT on previous day (IN–OUT is positive ~400 mL in normal balance, reflecting insensible fluid losses of ~800 mL and metabolic water generation of ~400 mL)
- Check cumulative change in daily fluid balance over previous 3–5 days
- Correlate chart figures with weight change and clinical volume status to estimate net fluid balance

Step 3: assess ongoing pathological process

- Check losses from GI tract and surgical drains
- Estimate increased insensible losses (e.g. in fever) and internal sequestration ('third space')

Step 4: check plasma U&Es (see Box 16.3)

- Check plasma Na as marker of relative water balance
- Check plasma K as a guide to extracellular K balance
- Check HCO₃ as a clue to acid–base disorder
- Check urea and creatinine to monitor renal function

Step 5: prescribe appropriate i.v. fluid replacement therapy

- Replace basic water and electrolytes each day (see Box 16.6)
- Allow for anticipated oral intake and pathological fluid loss
- Adjust amounts of water (if i.v., usually given as isotonic 5% dextrose), sodium and potassium according to plasma electrolyte results

16

In the absence of normal oral intake (as in a fasting or post-operative patient in hospital), maintenance quantities of fluid, sodium and potassium should be provided. If any deficits or continuing pathological losses are identified, additional fluid and electrolytes will be required. In prolonged periods of fasting (greater than a few days), attention also needs to be given to providing sufficient caloric and nutritional intake to prevent excessive catabolism of body energy stores (p. 121).

The choice of intravenous fluid therapy in the treatment of significant hypovolaemia relates to the concepts in Figure 16.1 (p. 427). If fluid containing neither sodium nor protein is given, it will distribute in the body fluid compartments in proportion to the normal distribution of total body water. Thus, giving 1 L of 5% dextrose will contribute relatively little (approximately 3/40 of the infused volume) towards expansion of the plasma volume. This makes 5% dextrose ineffective at restoring the circulation and perfusion of vital organs. Intravenous infusion of an isotonic (normal) saline solution, on the other hand, results in more effective expansion of the extracellular fluid, although again a minority of the infused volume (some 3/15) will contribute to plasma volume.

Carrying this reasoning further, it might be expected that a solution containing plasma proteins would be largely retained within the plasma, thus maximally expanding the circulating fluid volume and improving tissue perfusion. Recent clinical studies have not verified any overall advantage of infusions containing albumin (Box 16.9). Resuscitation fluids containing synthetic colloids (based on carbohydrate polymers or gelatin) may be more effective in the short-term resuscitation

EBM 16.9 **Albumin infusions in hypovolaemia**

'For patients with hypovolaemia there is no evidence that albumin reduces mortality when compared with cheaper alternatives such as saline.'

• The Albumin Reviewers (Cochrane Review). Cochrane Library, issue 4, 2000. Oxford: Update Software.

For further information: www.cochrane.org

of volume-depleted patients than solutions containing sodium chloride alone (p. 180).

Sodium excess (usually associated with hypervolaemia)

Aetiology and clinical assessment

In the presence of normal function of the heart and kidneys, an excessive intake of salt and water is compensated for by increased excretion and so is unlikely to lead to clinically obvious features of hypervolaemia. However, diseases affecting the heart, kidneys or liver frequently set in train a sequence of events leading to hypervolaemia (Fig. 16.5). This volume expansion does not always involve an increase in circulating blood volume, since in conditions where fluid leaks out of the capillaries due to hypoproteinaemia (e.g. nephrotic syndrome and chronic liver disease), retention of sodium and water may expand the ECF predominantly in the interstitial rather than intravascular compartment. Important causes of sodium excess are given in Box 16.10.

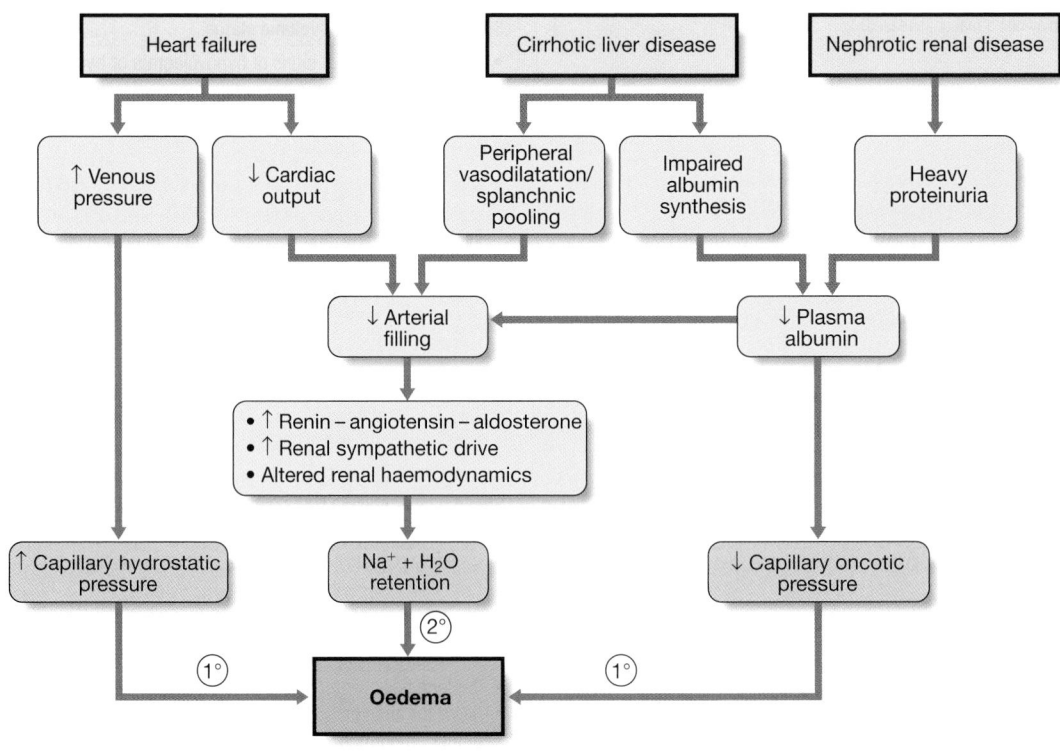

Fig. 16.5 Secondary mechanisms causing sodium excess and oedema in cardiac failure, cirrhosis and nephrotic syndrome. Primary renal retention of Na and water may also contribute to oedema formation when GFR is significantly reduced (see Box 16.10 and p. 481).

16.10 Causes of sodium and water excess

Mechanism	Examples
Impaired renal function (Ch. 17)	Primary renal disease
Primary hyperaldosteronism* (p. 777)	e.g. Conn's syndrome

Secondary hyperaldosteronism (see Fig. 16.5)	Congestive cardiac failure
	Cirrhotic liver disease
	Nephrotic syndrome
	Other hypoalbuminaemic states
	    Protein-losing enteropathy
	    Malnutrition
	Idiopathic/cyclical oedema
	Renal artery stenosis*

*Conditions in this table *other than* primary hyperaldosteronism and renal artery stenosis are typically associated with generalised oedema.

Peripheral oedema is the most common physical sign associated with ECF volume expansion (p. 481). In the three most common systemic disorders associated with sodium and fluid overload (cardiac failure, cirrhosis and nephrotic syndrome), sodium retention is largely a secondary response to circulatory insufficiency caused by the primary disorder, as illustrated in Figure 16.5. The pathophysiology is different in renal failure, when the primary cause of volume expansion is the profound reduction in GFR impairing sodium and water excretion, and secondary tubular mechanisms are of less importance. Further detail on each of these conditions is given in other chapters of this book.

Management

The management of ECF volume overload involves a number of components:

- specific treatment (where available) directed at the cause, e.g. ACE inhibitors in heart failure, corticosteroids in minimal change nephropathy
- restriction of dietary sodium to match more closely the diminished excretory capacity, e.g. 50–80 mmol/day
- treatment with diuretic drugs.

Diuretic therapy

Diuretics are important in the treatment of conditions of ECF expansion due to salt and water retention and in hypertension (p. 609). They act by inhibiting sodium reabsorption at various locations along the nephron (see Fig. 16.3, p. 429). Their potency and adverse effects relate to their mechanism and site of action.

Mechanisms of action

In the proximal tubule, carbonic anhydrase inhibitors (e.g. acetazolamide) inhibit the intracellular production of H^+ ions, thereby reducing the fraction of sodium reabsorption which is exchanged for H^+ by the apical membrane sodium–hydrogen exchanger. These drugs have limited usefulness, however, since only a small fraction of proximal sodium reabsorption uses this mechanism, and much of the unreabsorbed sodium can be reabsorbed by downstream segments of the nephron.

In the thick ascending limb of the loop of Henle, loop diuretics (e.g. furosemide) inhibit sodium reabsorption by blocking the action of the apical membrane Na,K,2Cl cotransporter. Because this segment reabsorbs a significant fraction of the filtered sodium, these drugs are potent diuretics, in common use in diseases causing significant oedema.

In the early distal (distal convoluted) tubule, thiazide drugs inhibit sodium reabsorption by blocking the sodium–chloride cotransporter in the apical membrane. Since this segment reabsorbs a much smaller fraction of the filtered sodium, thiazide drugs are less potent than loop diuretics, but are widely used in the treatment of hypertension and less severe oedema.

All diuretic drugs acting in the proximal, loop and early distal segments cause excretion not only of sodium (and with it water), but also of potassium. This occurs largely as a result of delivery of increased amounts of sodium to the late distal/cortical collecting ducts, where sodium reabsorption is associated with excretion of potassium, and is amplified if circulating aldosterone levels are high. By contrast, drugs acting to inhibit sodium reabsorption in the late distal/cortical collecting duct segment are associated with reduced potassium secretion, and are described as 'potassium-sparing'. One target of drug action in this segment is the apical sodium channel in the principal cells (see Fig. 16.3), which is blocked by drugs such as amiloride and triamterene. Another is the mineralocorticoid receptor, to which binding of aldosterone is blocked by spironolactone and eplerenone.

An important feature of the most commonly used diuretic drugs (furosemide, thiazides and amiloride) is that they act on their target transport molecules from the luminal side of the tubular epithelium. Since they are highly protein-bound in the plasma, very little reaches the urinary fluid by glomerular filtration, but there are active transport mechanisms for secreting organic acids and bases, including these drugs, across the proximal tubular wall, resulting in adequate drug concentrations being delivered to later tubular segments. This secretory process may be impaired by certain other drugs, and also by accumulated organic anions as occurs in chronic renal failure and chronic liver failure, leading to resistance to diuretics.

Osmotic diuretics are a further class of drug which act independently of any specific transport mechanism. These substances are freely filtered but are not reabsorbed by any part of the tubular system. They thus entrain fluid osmotically within the tubular lumen and limit the extent of sodium reabsorption in multiple segments. Mannitol is the most commonly used such drug, given by intravenous infusion to achieve short-term diuresis in conditions associated with cell swelling, such as cerebral oedema.

Clinical use of diuretics

In the selection of a diuretic drug for hypertension or oedema disorders, the following principles should be observed:

- Use the minimum effective dose.
- Use for as short a period of time as necessary.
- Monitor regularly for adverse effects.

The choice of diuretic drug class will be determined by the required potency of action, the presence

16

16.11 Adverse effects of loop-acting and thiazide diuretics

Renal side-effects

- Hypovolaemia
- Hyponatraemia
- Hypokalaemia
- Metabolic alkalosis
- Hyperuricaemia
- Hypomagnesaemia
- Hypercalciuria (loop)
- Hypocalciuria (thiazide)

Metabolic side-effects

- Glucose intolerance/hyperglycaemia
- Hyperlipidaemia

Miscellaneous side-effects

- Hypersensitivity reactions
- Erectile dysfunction
- Acute pancreatitis/cholecystitis (thiazides)

of coexistent conditions, and the anticipated side-effect profile.

The adverse effects encountered with the most commonly used classes of diuretic (loop drugs and thiazide drugs) are summarised in Box 16.11. Volume depletion and electrolyte disorders occur, as predicted from their mechanism of action. The metabolic side-effects listed are rarely of clinical significance and may reflect effects on K^+ channels which influence insulin secretion (p. 798). Since most drugs from these classes are sulphonamides, there is a relatively high incidence of hypersensitivity reactions, and occasional idiosyncratic side-effects in a variety of organ systems.

The side-effect profile of the potassium-sparing diuretics differs in a number of important respects from other diuretics. The disturbances in potassium, magnesium and acid–base balance are in the opposite direction, so that normal or increased levels of potassium and magnesium are found in the blood, and there is a tendency to metabolic acidosis, especially when renal function is impaired.

Diuretic resistance is encountered under a variety of circumstances, including impaired renal function, activation of sodium-retaining mechanisms, impaired oral bioavailability (e.g. due to gastrointestinal disease) and decreased renal blood flow. In these circumstances short-term intravenous therapy with a loop-acting agent such as furosemide may be useful. Combinations of diuretics administered orally may also increase potency. Either a loop or a thiazide drug can be combined with a potassium-sparing drug, and all three classes can be used together for short periods, with carefully supervised clinical and laboratory monitoring.

DISORDERS OF WATER BALANCE

Daily water intake can vary over a wide range, from 500 mL to several litres a day. While a certain amount of water is lost ('insensible losses', approximately 800 mL/day) through the stool, sweat and the respiratory tract, and some water is generated by oxidative metabolism ('metabolic water', approximately 400 mL/day), the kidneys are chiefly responsible for adjusting water excretion to maintain constancy of body water content and body fluid osmolality (normal range 280–295 mmol/kg).

Functional anatomy and physiology of renal water handling

While regulation of total ECF volume is largely achieved through the kidneys' control of sodium excretion, there must also be mechanisms to allow for the excretion of a 'pure' water load when free water intake is high, and for the avid retention of water by the kidneys when access to water is restricted.

These functions are largely achieved by the properties of the loop of Henle and the collecting ducts. The counter-current configuration of flow in adjacent limbs of the loop (see Fig. 16.2, p. 428), involving osmotic water movement from the descending limbs and solute reabsorption from neighbouring ascending limbs, sets up a gradient of tissue osmolality from isotonic (like plasma) in the renal cortex through to hypertonic (around 1200 mmol/kg) in the inner part of the medulla. At the same time, the fluid emerging from the thick ascending limb is hypotonic compared to plasma, because it has been diluted by the reabsorption of sodium, but not water, from the thick ascending limb and early distal tubule. As this dilute fluid passes from the cortex through the collecting duct system to the renal pelvis, it traverses the medullary interstitial gradient of osmolality set up by the operation of the loop of Henle, and water is avidly reabsorbed.

Further changes in the urine osmolality on passage through the collecting ducts depend on the level in the plasma of the peptide ADH, which is released by the posterior pituitary gland under conditions of increased plasma osmolality or other stimuli such as hypovolaemia (Ch. 20).

- When ADH levels are minimal, such as during adequate water intake and low–normal plasma osmolality, the collecting ducts remain impermeable to water and the luminal fluid osmolality remains low, resulting in the excretion of a dilute urine (minimum osmolality approximately 50 mmol/kg in a healthy young person).
- When ADH levels are elevated (during water restriction and high plasma osmolality, or severe volume depletion), the water permeability of the collecting ducts is greatly increased through the action of ADH on its V2 receptor, which enhances collecting duct water permeability via the insertion of aquaporin AQP-2 channels into the luminal cell membrane. This results in osmotic reabsorption of water along the entire length of the collecting duct, with maximum urine osmolality approaching that in the medullary tip (up to 1200 mmol/kg).

Parallel to these changes in ADH release are changes in water-seeking behaviour triggered by the sensation of thirst, which also becomes activated as plasma osmolality rises from normal to above normal levels.

In summary, for adequate dilution of the urine there must be:

- adequate solute delivery to the loop of Henle and early distal tubule
- normal function of the loop of Henle and early distal tubule
- no ADH in the circulation.

If any of these processes is faulty, water retention and hyponatraemia may result.

Conversely, to achieve concentration of the urine there must be:

- adequate solute delivery to the loop of Henle
- normal function of the loop of Henle
- ADH release into the circulation
- ADH action on the collecting ducts.

Failure of any of these steps may result in inappropriate water loss and hypernatraemia.

Presenting problems in disorders of water balance

Disturbances in body water balance, in the absence of changes in sodium balance, alter plasma sodium concentration and hence plasma osmolality. When extracellular osmolality changes abruptly, water flows rapidly across cell membranes with resultant cell swelling (during hypo-osmolality) or shrinkage (during hyper-osmolality). Cerebral cell function is very sensitive to such volume changes, particularly during cell swelling, when an increase in intracerebral pressure occurs due to the constraints imposed by the bony skull, thereby reducing cerebral perfusion.

Hyponatraemia

Aetiology and clinical assessment

Hyponatraemia (plasma Na < 135 mmol/L) is a common electrolyte abnormality, often detected asymptomatically, but it may also be associated with profound disturbances of cerebral function, manifesting as anorexia, nausea, vomiting, confusion, lethargy, seizures and coma. The degree of cerebral symptomatology depends more on the rate of development of the electrolyte abnormality than on its severity. When plasma osmolality falls rapidly, water flows into cerebral cells which become swollen and ischaemic. However, when hyponatraemia develops gradually, cerebral neurons have time to respond by reducing intracellular osmolality, through excreting potassium and reducing synthesis of intracellular organic osmolytes (Fig. 16.6). The osmotic gradient favouring water movement into the cells is thus reduced and cerebral symptomatology avoided.

The causes of hyponatraemia are best categorised according to any associated change in ECF volume status, i.e. the total body sodium (Box 16.12). In all cases, there is retention of water relative to sodium, and it is the clinical examination rather than the electrolyte test results which gives clues to the underlying cause.

Artefactual causes of apparent hyponatraemia should be remembered. This can occur in the presence of severe hyperlipidaemia or hyperproteinaemia, when the aqueous fraction of the plasma specimen is reduced because of the volume occupied by the macromolecules (although this artefact is dependent on the assay technology). Transient hyponatraemia may also occur due to osmotic shifts of water out of cells during hyperosmolar states caused by acute hyperglycaemia or by mannitol infusion.

Hyponatraemia with hypovolaemia

Patients with hyponatraemia in association with a sodium deficit ('depletional hyponatraemia') have clinical features of hypovolaemia (see Box 16.4, p. 431)

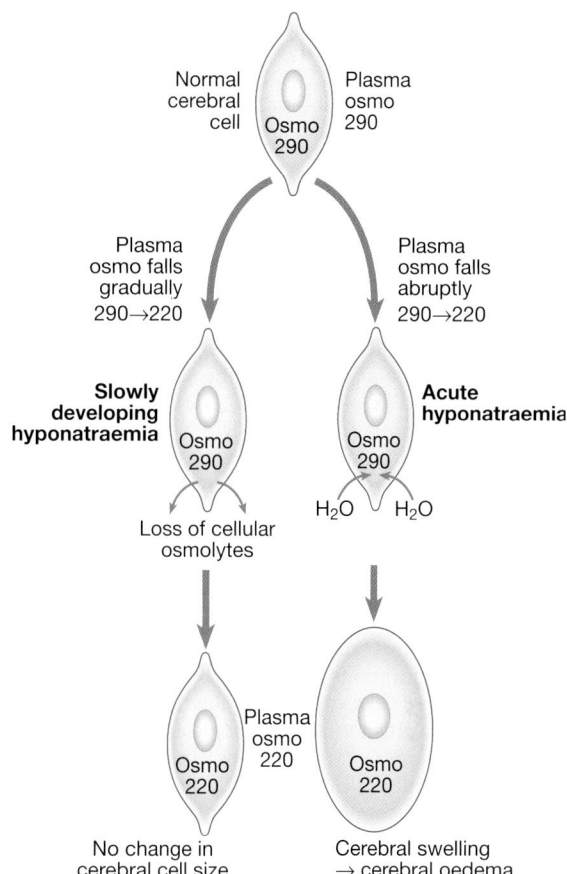

Fig. 16.6 Hyponatraemia and the brain. Numbers represent osmolality in mmol/kg. (Osmo = osmolality)

16.12 Causes of hyponatraemia

Volume status	Examples
Hypovolaemic (sodium deficit with a relatively smaller water deficit)	Renal Na losses Diuretic therapy (especially thiazides) Adrenocortical failure Gastrointestinal Na losses Vomiting Diarrhoea Skin Na losses Burns
Euvolaemic (water retention alone)	Primary polydipsia Excessive electrolyte-free water infusion SIADH* Hypothyroidism
Hypervolaemic (sodium retention with relatively greater water retention)	Congestive cardiac failure Cirrhosis Nephrotic syndrome Chronic renal failure (during free water intake)

*SIADH = syndrome of inappropriate antidiuretic hormone secretion (Box 16.13).

and supportive laboratory findings, including low urinary sodium concentration (< 30 mmol/L) and elevated plasma renin activity. The cause of sodium loss is usually apparent; common examples are shown in Box 16.12.

Hyponatraemia with euvolaemia

Patients in this group ('dilutional hyponatraemia') have no major disturbance of body sodium content and are clinically euvolaemic. Excess body water may be the result of abnormally high intake, either orally (primary polydipsia) or as a result of medically infused fluids (as intravenous dextrose solutions, or by absorption of sodium-free bladder irrigation fluid after prostatectomy).

Water retention also occurs in the syndrome of inappropriate secretion of ADH (SIADH). In this condition an endogenous source of ADH (either cerebral or tumour-derived) promotes renal water retention in the absence of an appropriate physiological stimulus (Box 16.13). The clinical diagnosis requires the patient to be euvolaemic, with no evidence of organ system disease potentially associated with hyponatraemia (heart, liver, kidney). Other non-osmotic stimuli to release of ADH (pain, stress, nausea) should also be excluded. Supportive laboratory findings are shown in Box 16.13. The plasma has low concentrations of sodium, chloride, urea and uric acid, with a correspondingly low osmolality. Urine osmolality, which should physiologically be maximally dilute (approximately 50 mmol/kg) in the face of low plasma osmolality, is higher than at least 100 mmol/kg and indeed is typically higher than the plasma osmolality. The urine sodium concentration is typically high (> 30 mmol/L), consistent with euvolaemia and lack of compensatory factors promoting sodium retention.

Hyponatraemia with hypervolaemia

In the third pattern of hyponatraemia, excess water retention is associated with sodium retention and volume expansion, as in heart failure and other oedematous disorders.

16.13 Syndrome of inappropriate antidiuretic hormone secretion (SIADH): causes and diagnosis

Causes

- Tumours, e.g. lung or colon cancer
- CNS disorders: stroke, trauma, infection, psychosis
- Pulmonary disorders: pneumonia, tuberculosis, obstructive lung disease
- Drugs
  Anticonvulsants, e.g. carbamazepine
  Psychotropics, e.g. haloperidol
  Antidepressants, e.g. amitriptyline, fluoxetine
  Cytotoxics, e.g. cyclophosphamide, vincristine
  Hypoglycaemics, e.g. chlorpropamide
  Opiates, e.g. morphine
- Idiopathic

Diagnosis

- Low plasma sodium concentration (typically < 130 mmol/L)
- Low plasma osmolality (< 270 mmol/kg)
- Urine osmolality not minimally low (typically > 150 mmol/kg)
- Urine sodium concentration not minimally low (> 30 mmol/L)
- Low–normal plasma urea, creatinine, uric acid
- Exclusion of other causes of hyponatraemia (see Box 16.12)
- Appropriate clinical context (above)

Investigations

Plasma and urine electrolytes and osmolality (Box 16.14) are usually the only tests required to classify the hyponatraemia. Doubt about clinical signs of ECF volume may be resolved with measurement of plasma renin activity.

Note that measuring plasma ADH is not generally helpful in distinguishing between these categories of hyponatraemia. This is because ADH is activated both in hypovolaemic states and in most chronic hypervolaemic states, as the impaired circulation in those disorders activates ADH release through non-osmotic mechanisms. Indeed, these disorders may have higher circulating ADH levels than patients with SIADH. The only disorders listed in Box 16.12 in which ADH is not normal or elevated are primary polydipsia and iatrogenic water intoxication, in which the hypo-osmolar plasma suppresses ADH release.

16.14 Urine Na and osmolality in the differential diagnosis of hyponatraemia*

Urine Na (mmol/L)	Urine osmolality (mmol/kg)	Possible diagnoses
Low (< 30)	Low (< 100)	Primary polydipsia Malnutrition Beer excess
Low	High (> 150)	Salt depletion Hypovolaemia
High (> 40)	Low	Diuretic action (acute phase)
High	High	SIADH Cerebral salt-wasting Adrenal insufficiency

*Note that intermediate urine results are of indeterminate significance, and diagnosis depends on a comprehensive clinical assessment.

Management

The treatment for hyponatraemia is critically dependent on the rate of development, severity and underlying cause. In general, if hyponatraemia has developed rapidly (over hours to days), morbidity due to cerebral oedema is more likely, and it is generally safe to correct the plasma sodium relatively rapidly. This can include infusion of hypertonic (3%) sodium chloride solutions, especially when the patient is obtunded or convulsing.

On the other hand, rapid correction of hyponatraemia which has developed slowly (over weeks to months) can itself be hazardous to the brain. This is because cerebral cells adapt to slowly developing hypo-osmolality by reducing the intracellular osmolality, thus maintaining normal cell volume (see Fig. 16.6). Under these conditions, an abrupt increase in extracellular osmolality can lead to water shifting out of the cerebral neurons, abruptly reducing their volume and risking detachment from their myelin sheaths. The resulting 'myelinolysis' can produce permanent structural and functional damage to mid-brain structures, and is generally fatal. The rate of correction of the plasma Na concentration in chronic asymptomatic hyponatraemia should not exceed 10 mmol/L/day, and an even slower rate is generally safer.

The underlying cause should be treated. For hypovolaemic patients, this involves controlling the source of sodium loss, and administering intravenous saline if clinically warranted. Patients with dilutional hyponatraemia will generally respond to fluid restriction in the range 600–1000 mL/day, accompanied where possible by withdrawal of the precipitating stimulus (e.g. a drug causing SIADH). If an inadequate rise in plasma Na results, treatment with demeclocycline (600–900 mg/day) may enhance water excretion, by interfering with collecting duct responsiveness to ADH. An effective alternative for subjects with persistent hyponatraemia due to prolonged SIADH is oral urea therapy (30–45 g/day), which provides a solute load to promote water excretion. Where available, oral vasopressin receptor antagonists (vaptans) may be used to block the ADH-mediated component of water retention in a range of hyponatraemic conditions. Hypervolaemic patients with hyponatraemia need optimal treatment of the underlying condition, accompanied by cautious use of diuretics in conjunction with strict fluid restriction. Potassium-sparing diuretics may be particularly useful in this context where there is significant secondary hyperaldosteronism.

Hypernatraemia

Aetiology and clinical assessment

Just as hyponatraemia represents a failure of the mechanisms for diluting the urine during free access to water, so hypernatraemia (plasma Na > 148 mmol/L) reflects inadequate concentration of the urine in the face of restricted water intake. This can be due to failure to generate an adequate medullary concentration gradient (low GFR states, loop diuretic therapy), but more commonly it is due to failure of the ADH system, either because no ADH is released from the pituitary (central or 'cranial' diabetes insipidus, p. 792) or because the collecting duct cells are unable to respond to circulating ADH (nephrogenic diabetes insipidus, either inherited or acquired).

Patients with hypernatraemia generally have reduced cerebral function, either as a primary problem or as a consequence of the hypernatraemia itself, which results in dehydration of cerebral neurons and brain shrinkage. In the presence of an intact thirst mechanism and preserved capacity to obtain and ingest water, hypernatraemia may not progress very far. If adequate water is not obtained, dizziness, confusion, weakness and ultimately coma and death can result.

Like hyponatraemia, the causes of hypernatraemia are best grouped according to the associated disturbance, if any, in total body sodium content (Box 16.15). It is important to note the risk of iatrogenic induction of hypernatraemia, and to reiterate that, whatever the underlying cause, sustained or severe hypernatraemia must reflect an impaired thirst mechanism or responsiveness to thirst, which would otherwise lead to sufficient water being ingested to prevent this disorder progressing.

Management

Treatment of hypernatraemia depends on both the rate of development and the underlying cause. If there is reason to think that the condition has developed rapidly,

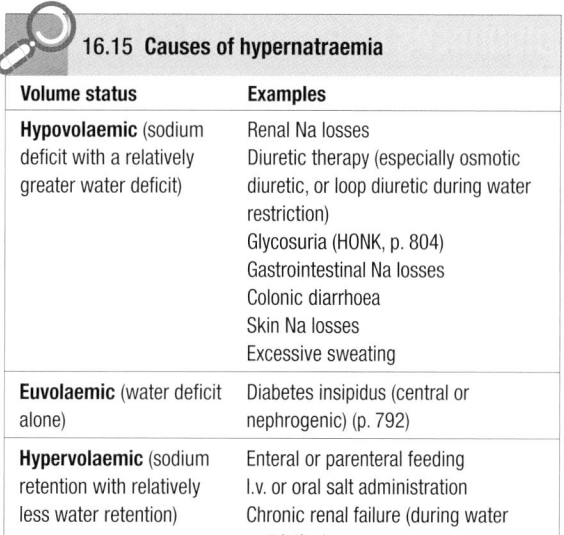

16.15 Causes of hypernatraemia

Volume status	Examples
Hypovolaemic (sodium deficit with a relatively greater water deficit)	Renal Na losses Diuretic therapy (especially osmotic diuretic, or loop diuretic during water restriction) Glycosuria (HONK, p. 804) Gastrointestinal Na losses Colonic diarrhoea Skin Na losses Excessive sweating
Euvolaemic (water deficit alone)	Diabetes insipidus (central or nephrogenic) (p. 792)
Hypervolaemic (sodium retention with relatively less water retention)	Enteral or parenteral feeding I.v. or oral salt administration Chronic renal failure (during water restriction)

cerebral shrinkage may be acute, and relatively rapid correction with appropriate volumes of intravenous fluid (isotonic 5% dextrose or hypotonic 0.45% saline) may be attempted. However, in older, institutionalised patients it is more likely that the disorder has developed slowly, and extreme caution should be used to lower the plasma sodium slowly, to avoid the risk of cerebral oedema in the osmotically adapted cerebral neurons. Where possible, the underlying cause should also be addressed (see Box 16.15).

Elderly patients are predisposed, in different circumstances, to both hyponatraemia and hypernatraemia, and a high index of suspicion of these electrolyte disturbances is appropriate in aged patients with recent alterations in behaviour (Box 16.16).

16.16 Hyponatraemia and hypernatraemia in old age

- **Decline in GFR**: older patients are predisposed to both hyponatraemia and hypernatraemia, mainly because, as GFR declines with age, the capacity of the kidney to dilute or concentrate the urine is impaired.
- **Hyponatraemia**: occurs when free water intake continues in the presence of a low dietary salt intake and/or diuretic drugs (particularly thiazides).
- **ADH release**: water retention is aggravated by any condition which stimulates ADH release, especially heart failure. Moreover, the ADH response to non-osmotic stimuli may be brisker in older subjects. Appropriate water restriction may be a key part of the management.
- **Hypernatraemia**: occurs when water intake is inadequate, due to physical restrictions preventing access to drinks and/or blunted thirst. Both are frequently present in patients with advanced dementia or following a severe stroke.
- **Dietary salt**: hypernatraemia is aggravated if dietary supplements or medications with a high sodium content (especially effervescent preparations) are administered. Appropriate prescription of fluids is a key part of the management.

16

DISORDERS OF POTASSIUM BALANCE

Potassium is the major intracellular cation (see Fig. 16.1, p. 427), and the steep concentration gradient for potassium across the cell membrane of excitable cells plays an important part in generating the resting membrane potential and allowing the propagation of the action potential which is crucial to normal functioning of nerve, muscle and cardiac tissues. Control of body potassium balance is described below.

Factors influencing the distribution of potassium between the ICF and ECF compartments can alter plasma potassium concentration, without any overall change in total body potassium content. Potassium is driven into the cells from the plasma by extracellular alkalosis and by a number of hormones, including insulin, catecholamines (through the β_2 receptor) and aldosterone. These influences alone can produce hypokalaemia, while the contrary changes (extracellular acidosis, lack of insulin, insufficiency or blockade of catecholamines or aldosterone) can contribute to hyperkalaemia due to redistribution of potassium outside the cells.

Functional anatomy and physiology of renal potassium handling

In the steady state, the kidneys excrete some 90% of the daily intake of potassium, typically 80–100 mmol/day. Potassium is freely filtered at the glomerulus; around 65% is reabsorbed in the proximal tubule and a further 25% in the thick ascending limb of the loop of Henle. However, in the early distal tubule little potassium is transported, while in the late distal/cortical collecting duct tubule a significant secretory flux of potassium into the urine ensures that this cation is removed from the blood in proportion to the ingested load.

The mechanism for potassium secretion in the distal parts of the nephron is shown in Figure 16.3D (p. 429). Movement of potassium from blood to lumen is dependent on active uptake across the basal cell membrane by the Na,K-ATPase, followed by diffusion of potassium through a luminal membrane potassium channel (ROMK) into the tubular fluid. The electrochemical gradient for potassium movement into the lumen is contributed to both by the high intracellular potassium concentration and by the negative luminal potential difference relative to the blood.

A number of factors influence the rate of potassium secretion. Luminal influences include the rate of sodium delivery and fluid flow through the late distal/cortical collecting ducts, and this is a major factor in the increased potassium loss during therapy with diuretics acting earlier in the nephron. Agents interfering with the generation of the negative luminal potential impair potassium secretion, and this is the basis of reduced potassium secretion during therapy with potassium-sparing diuretics such as amiloride. Factors acting from the blood side of this tubule segment include plasma potassium and pH, such that hyperkalaemia and alkalosis stimulate potassium secretion directly. However, the most important factor in the acute and chronic adjustment of potassium secretion to match metabolic potassium load is the corticosteroid hormone aldosterone.

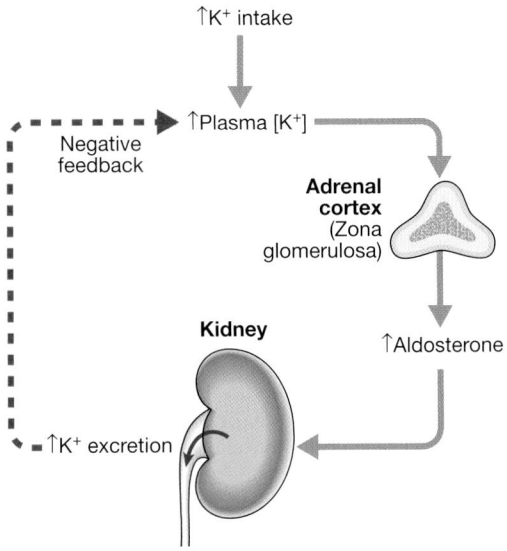

Fig. 16.7 Feedback control of plasma potassium concentration.

As shown in Figure 16.7, a negative feedback relationship exists between the plasma potassium concentration and aldosterone. In addition to its regulation by the renin–angiotensin system (see Fig. 20.19, p. 769), aldosterone is released from the adrenal cortex in direct response to an elevated plasma potassium, and aldosterone acts on the kidney to stimulate potassium secretion, as well as hydrogen secretion and sodium reabsorption, in the late distal/cortical collecting duct segment. The resulting increased potassium excretion serves to dampen the accumulation of potassium in the plasma, keeping plasma concentrations tightly controlled within a narrow normal range (3.3–4.7 mmol/L). Since the plasma aldosterone concentration is the net effect of two different stimuli, factors reducing angiotensin II levels may indirectly impair potassium balance by blunting the rise in aldosterone which would otherwise be provoked by hyperkalaemia. This is the basis for the risk of hyperkalaemia during therapy with ACE inhibitors and related drugs.

Presenting problems in disorders of potassium balance

Hypokalaemia
Aetiology and clinical assessment
Patients with mild hypokalaemia (plasma K 3.0–3.5 mmol/L) are generally asymptomatic, but with more severe falls in the plasma potassium there is often muscular weakness and associated tiredness. Cardiac effects include ventricular ectopic beats or more serious arrhythmias, and potentiation of the adverse effects of digoxin. Typical ECG changes occur, affecting the T wave in particular (Fig. 16.8). Functional bowel obstruction may occur due to paralytic ileus. Long-standing hypokalaemia damages renal tubular structures (hypokalaemic nephropathy) and interferes with the tubular response to

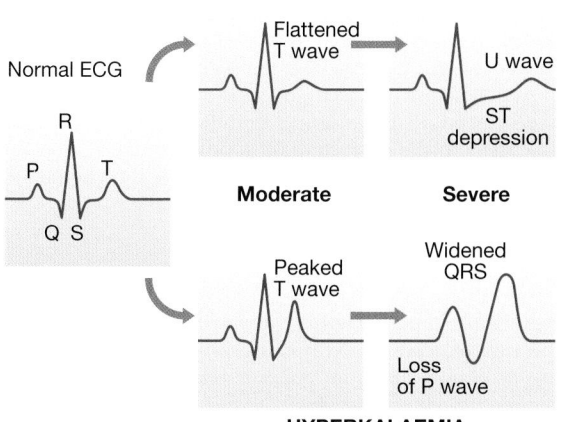

HYPOKALAEMIA

Normal ECG

Flattened T wave → U wave, ST depression

Moderate   **Severe**

Peaked T wave → Widened QRS, Loss of P wave

HYPERKALAEMIA

Fig. 16.8 The ECG in hypokalaemia and hyperkalaemia.

ADH (acquired nephrogenic diabetes insipidus), resulting in polyuria and polydipsia.

The main causes of hypokalaemia and an approach to the differential diagnosis are shown in Figure 16.9. Redistribution of potassium into cells should be considered, since correction of the factors involved (see above) may be sufficient to correct the plasma concentration. An inadequate intake of potassium can contribute to hypokalaemia but is unlikely to be the only cause, except in extreme cases. Generally, hypokalaemia implies abnormal potassium loss from the body, through either the kidney or the gastrointestinal tract. When there is no obvious clinical clue to which pathway is involved, measurement of urinary potassium may be helpful; if the kidney is the route of potassium loss, the urine potassium is relatively high (> 30 mmol/day), whereas potassium loss through the gastrointestinal tract is usually associated with renal potassium retention, resulting in a lower urinary potassium (generally < 20 mmol/day, although paradoxically, if gastrointestinal fluid loss is also associated with hypovolaemia, activation of the renin–angiotensin–aldosterone system may cause loss of potassium through the kidney as well).

The renal causes can be divided into those with or without hypertension. Hypertensive disorders with hypokalaemia may be due to excess mineralocorticoid activity such as aldosterone oversecretion in Conn's syndrome (p. 778). Apparent mineralocorticoid excess can be produced by excess liquorice intake or treatment with carbenoxolone, which inhibit the renal 11βHSD2 enzyme which normally inactivates cortisol and prevents inappropriate activation of mineralocorticoid receptors. Liddle's syndrome produces a similar phenotype, due to a genetic defect causing overactivity of epithelial sodium channels in the distal nephron.

If blood pressure is normal or low, renal potassium loss can be classified according to the associated acid–base change. If hypokalaemia is associated with alkalosis and diuretic use has been excluded, an inherited tubular transport defect may be suspected. In Bartter's syndrome there is a defect in sodium reabsorption in the thick ascending limb of Henle, usually due to a mutation causing malfunction of the NKCC2 transporter. The clinical and biochemical features are similar to chronic treatment with furosemide. In Gitelman's syndrome there is a mutation causing malfunction of

16

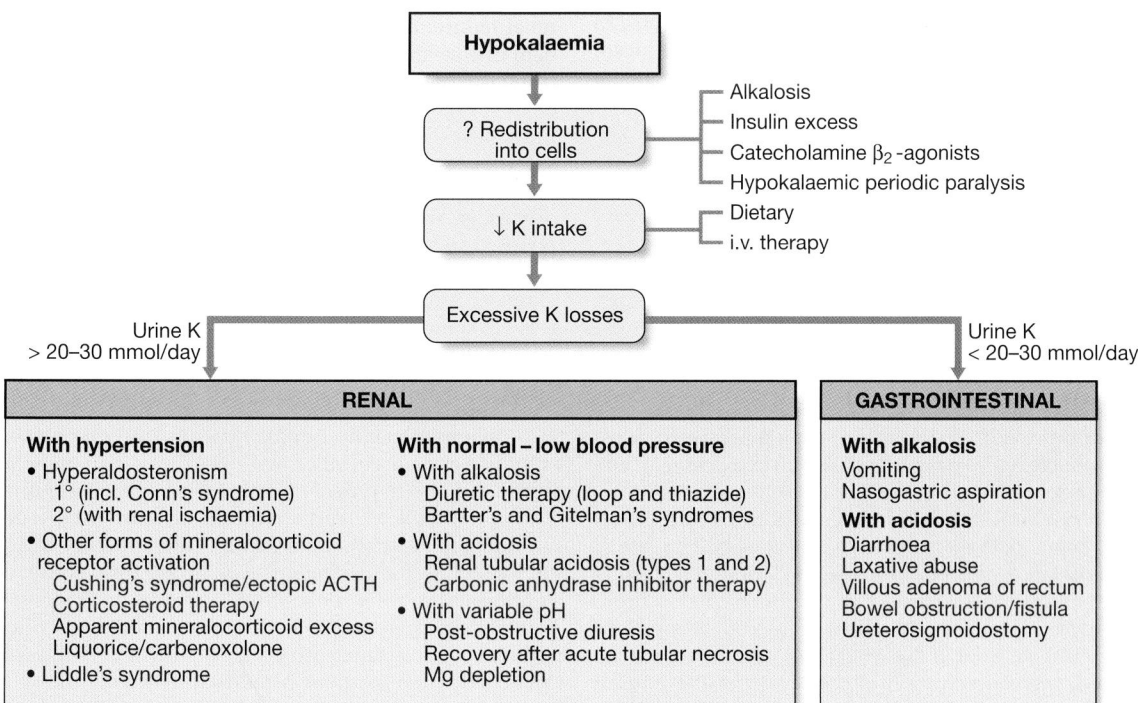

Fig. 16.9 Diagnostic decision tree for hypokalaemia. (ACTH = adrenocorticotrophic hormone)

the NCCT carrier in the early distal tubule. The clinical and biochemical features are similar to chronic thiazide treatment. Note that while both Bartter's and Gitelman's syndromes are characterised by hypokalaemia and hypomagnesaemia, urinary calcium excretion is increased in Bartter's syndrome but decreased in Gitelman's syndrome, analogous to the effects of the loop and thiazide diuretics, respectively, on calcium transport (see Box 16.11, p. 434).

If hypokalaemia is associated with a normal blood pressure but with metabolic acidosis, renal tubular acidosis (proximal or 'classical' distal) should be suspected (p. 444).

When hypokalaemia is due to potassium wasting through the gastrointestinal tract, the cause is usually obvious clinically. In some cases, when there is occult induction of vomiting or surreptitious use of aperients, a useful generalisation is that upper gastrointestinal losses (above the pylorus) are characteristically associated with metabolic alkalosis, whereas losses below the pylorus are associated with metabolic acidosis. In both cases, the urinary potassium excretion would be expected to be low (but see the qualification mentioned above regarding high aldosterone states).

Investigations

Measurement of plasma electrolytes, bicarbonate, urine potassium and sometimes of plasma calcium and magnesium is usually sufficient to establish the diagnosis. Plasma renin activity is low in patients with primary hyperaldosteronism (p. 777) and other forms of mineralocorticoid excess; in other causes of hypokalaemia renin is elevated.

Occasionally the cause of hypokalaemia is obscure, especially when the history is incomplete or unreliable, and the urine potassium is indeterminate. Many such cases are associated with metabolic alkalosis, and in this setting the measurement of urine chloride concentration can be helpful. A low urine chloride (< 30 mmol/L) is characteristic of vomiting (spontaneous or self-induced, in which chloride is lost in HCl in the vomit), while a urine chloride > 40 mmol/L suggests diuretic therapy (acute phase) or a tubular disorder such as Bartter's or Gitelman's syndrome. Differentiation between these latter possibilities can be assisted by performing a screen of urine for diuretic drugs.

Management

Treatment of hypokalaemia involves first determining the cause and then correcting this where possible. If the problem is mainly one of redistribution of potassium into cells, reversal of this influence (e.g. correction of alkalosis) may be sufficient to restore plasma potassium without providing potassium supplements. In most cases, however, a form of potassium replacement will be required. This can generally be achieved with slow-release KCl tablets, but in more acute circumstances intravenous potassium chloride is necessary. The rate of administration depends on the severity of hypokalaemia and the presence of cardiac or neuromuscular complications, but should generally not exceed 10 mmol of potassium per hour. If higher rates of administration are needed, the concentration of potassium in the infused fluid may be increased to 40 mmol/L if a peripheral vein is used, but higher concentrations must be infused into a large 'central' vein with continuous cardiac monitoring.

In the less common situation of hypokalaemia being associated with systemic acidosis, alkaline salts of potassium, such as potassium bicarbonate, can be given by mouth. If magnesium depletion is also present, replacement of magnesium may be necessary to allow correction of hypokalaemia to occur. In appropriate circumstances, use of a potassium-sparing diuretic such as amiloride can assist in the correction of hypokalaemia, hypomagnesaemia and metabolic alkalosis, especially when these are due to use of a loop or thiazide diuretic.

Hyperkalaemia

Aetiology and clinical assessment

Significant hyperkalaemia can be dangerous, because of the risk of cardiac arrest caused by the marked slowing of action potential conduction in the presence of potassium levels above 7 mmol/L. Patients typically present with progressive muscular weakness, but sometimes there are no symptoms until cardiac arrest occurs. Typical ECG changes are shown in Figure 16.8. Peaking of the T wave is an early ECG sign, but widening of the QRS complex presages a dangerous cardiac arrhythmia.

An approach to defining the cause of hyperkalaemia is shown in Figure 16.10. It is important to exclude artefacts due to in vitro haemolysis of blood specimens, but if there is doubt about this and there are consistent changes present in the ECG, treatment for hyperkalaemia should be initiated. Redistribution of potassium from the ICF to the ECF may occur in the presence of systemic acidosis, or when the relevant hormones (insulin, catecholamines and aldosterone) are reduced or blocked (p. 438). While a high potassium intake may contribute to hyperkalaemia, it is unlikely to be the only explanation if renal excretion mechanisms are intact.

Impaired excretion of potassium into the urine may be associated with a reduced GFR, as in acute or chronic renal failure. Acute renal failure is associated with particularly severe hyperkalaemia when there is a concomitant potassium load, such as in rhabdomyolysis or in sepsis, particularly when acidosis is also present. In chronic renal failure, adaptation to a moderately elevated plasma potassium commonly develops, but a further rise can occur during intercurrent events which destabilise the new steady state, e.g. a dietary load of potassium, hypovolaemia or drugs (see below).

Hyperkalaemia can also develop when tubular potassium secretory processes are impaired, even if the GFR is well maintained. In some cases, this is due to inadequate circulating aldosterone, as in Addison's disease, ACE inhibitor therapy, or other situations where the renin–angiotensin–aldosterone system is inactivated (e.g. hyporeninaemic hypoaldosteronism, which typically occurs in association with neuropathy in diabetes and is thought to reflect impaired β-adrenergic stimulation of renin release; or therapy with angiotensin receptor antagonists, non-steroidal anti-inflammatory drugs (NSAIDs) or β-blocking drugs). In another group of conditions, tubular potassium secretion is impaired, even in the presence of high aldosterone levels. Such aldosterone resistance can occur in a variety of diseases involving inflammation in the tubulointerstitium (e.g. systemic lupus erythematosus (SLE), renal transplant), during therapy with potassium-sparing diuretics, and in a number of inherited disorders of tubular transport.

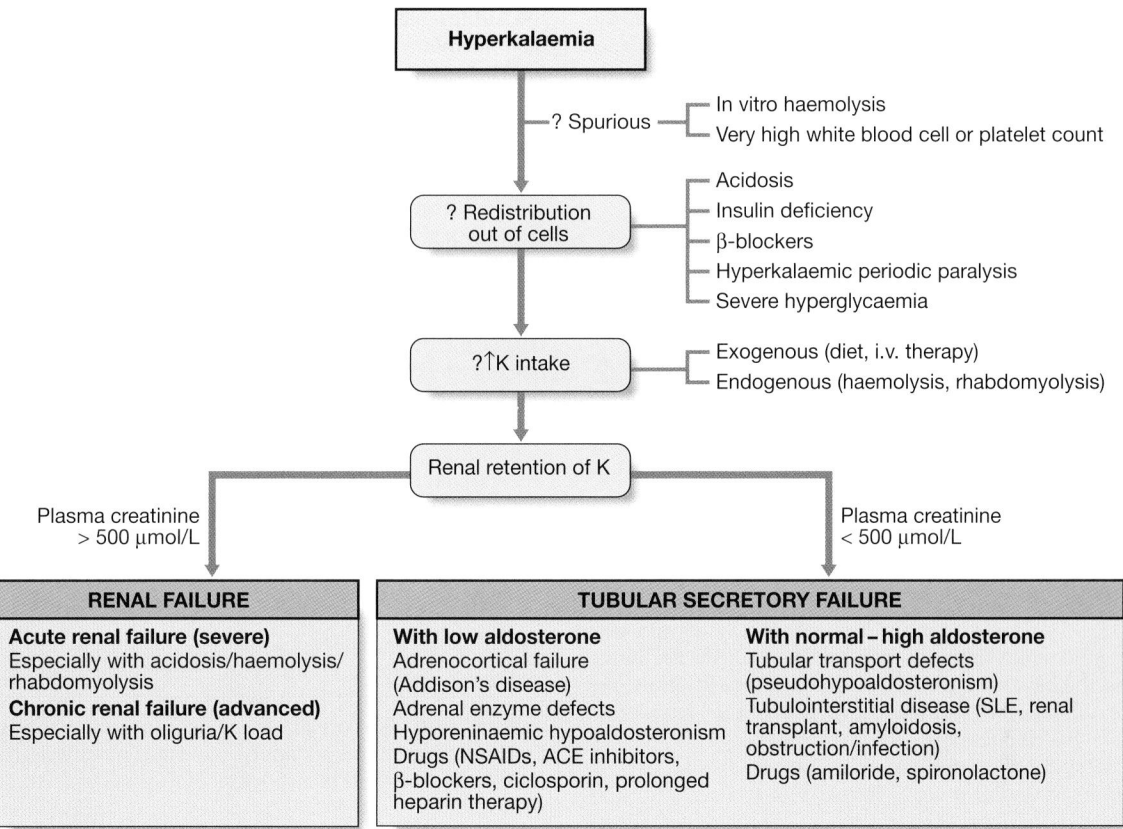

Fig. 16.10 **Diagnostic decision tree for hyperkalaemia.** Creatinine of 500 μmol/L = 5.67 mg/dL.

In all conditions of aldosterone deficiency or aldosterone resistance, hyperkalaemia may be associated with acid retention, giving rise to the pattern of hyperkalaemic distal ('type 4') renal tubular acidosis (p. 444).

Investigations

Results for plasma electrolytes, creatinine and bicarbonate, together with consideration of the clinical scenario, will usually provide the explanation for hyperkalaemia. In aldosterone deficiency, plasma sodium concentration is characteristically low, although this can occur in many causes of hyperkalaemia. Addison's disease should be excluded unless there is an obvious alternative diagnosis, as described on page 775.

Management

Treatment of hyperkalaemia depends on the severity and the rate of development. In the absence of neuromuscular symptoms or ECG changes, reduction of potassium intake and correction of underlying abnormalities may be sufficient. However, in acute and/or severe hyperkalaemia (plasma K > 6.5–7.0 mmol/L) more urgent measures must be taken (Box 16.17).

If ECG changes are present, the first step should be infusion of calcium gluconate to stabilise conductive tissue membranes (calcium has the opposite effect to potassium on conduction of an action potential). Measures to shift potassium from the ECF to the ICF should also be taken, as they generally act rapidly and may avert arrhythmia. Ultimately, a means of removing potassium from the body is generally necessary. When renal function

16.17 Treatment of severe hyperkalaemia

Mechanism	Therapy
Stabilise cell membrane potential[1]	I.v. calcium gluconate (10 mL of 10% solution)
Shift K into cells	Inhaled β_2 agonist, e.g. salbutamol I.v. glucose (50 mL of 50% solution) and insulin (5 U Actrapid) Intravenous sodium bicarbonate[2]
Remove K from body	I.v. furosemide and normal saline[3] Ion-exchange resin (e.g. Resonium) orally or rectally Dialysis

[1]If ECG changes suggestive of hyperkalaemia (K typically > 7 mmol/L).
[2]If acidosis present.
[3]If adequate residual renal function.

is reasonably preserved, loop diuretics (accompanied by intravenous saline if hypovolaemia is present) may be effective; in established renal failure, ion-exchange resins acting through the gastrointestinal tract and urgent dialysis may be required.

DISORDERS OF ACID–BASE BALANCE

The pH of the arterial plasma is normally 7.40, corresponding to a H^+ concentration of 40 nmol/L. An increase in H^+ concentration corresponds to a decrease in pH. To

441

preserve function of many pH-sensitive enzymes, this parameter is under tight homeostatic regulation, such that the H$^+$ concentration does not vary outside the range 36–44 nmol/L (pH 7.44–7.36) under normal circumstances. Abnormal acid–base balance occurs in a wide range of diseases.

Functional anatomy and physiology of acid–base homeostasis

A variety of physiological mechanisms maintain the pH of the ECF. The first is the action of blood and tissue buffers, of which the most important involves reaction of H$^+$ ions with bicarbonate to form carbonic acid, which, under the influence of the enzyme carbonic anhydrase (c.a.), dissociates to form CO_2 and water:

$$CO_2 + H_2O \overset{c.a.}{\rightleftharpoons} H_2CO_3 \rightleftharpoons H^+ + HCO_3^-$$

This buffer system is important because bicarbonate is present in relatively high concentration in the ECF (21–28 mmol/L), and two of its key components are under physiological control: the CO_2 by the lungs, and the bicarbonate by the kidneys. These relationships are illustrated in Figure 16.11 (a form of the Henderson–Hasselbalch equation).

Respiratory compensation for acid–base disturbances can occur quickly. In response to acid accumulation, pH changes in the brain stem stimulate ventilatory drive, serving to reduce the PCO_2 and hence drive up the pH (p. 651). Conversely, systemic alkalosis leads to inhibition of ventilation (although this is limited because hypoxia provides an alternative stimulus to ventilation).

The kidney provides a third line of defence against disturbances of arterial pH. When acid accumulates due to chronic respiratory or metabolic (non-renal) causes,

the kidney has the long-term capacity to enhance urinary excretion of acid, effectively increasing the plasma bicarbonate.

Renal control of acid–base balance

There are several components to the kidneys' contribution to maintaining acid–base balance. First, the proximal tubule reabsorbs some 85% of the filtered bicarbonate ions, through the mechanism for H$^+$ secretion illustrated in Figure 16.3A (p. 429). This is dependent on the enzyme carbonic anhydrase both in the cytoplasm of the proximal tubular cells and on the luminal surface of the brush border membranes. The system has a high capacity but does not lead to significant acidification of the luminal fluid.

Distal nephron segments have an important role in determining net acid excretion by the kidney. In the intercalated cells of the cortical collecting duct and the outer medullary collecting duct cells, acid is secreted into the lumen by an H$^+$-ATPase. This excreted acid is generated in the tubular cell from the hydration of CO_2 to form carbonic acid, which dissociates into an H$^+$ ion secreted luminally, and a bicarbonate ion which passes across the basolateral membrane into the blood. The secreted H$^+$ ions contribute to the reabsorption of any residual bicarbonate present in the luminal fluid, but also contribute net acid for removal from the body, bound to a variety of urinary buffers. The first is filtered non-bicarbonate buffer, such as phosphate (HPO_4^{2-}) which is titrated in the distal lumen to dihydrogen phosphate ($H_2PO_4^-$), excreted in the urine with sodium. The second significant buffer is ammonia, which is generated within tubular cells by the action of the enzyme glutaminase on glutamine. NH_3 reacts with secreted acid to form ammonium (NH_4^+), which becomes trapped in the luminal fluid and is excreted with chloride ions.

The net removal of acid by the kidney, using these latter two mechanisms, amounts to some 1 mmol/kg/day of hydrogen ions, which equals the non-volatile acid load arising from the metabolism of dietary protein. Thus a slightly alkaline plasma pH of 7.4 (H$^+$ 40 nmol/L) is maintained by the kidney's capacity to generate an acidic urine (pH typically 5–6) in which the net daily excess of metabolic acid can be excreted.

Presenting problems in disorders of acid–base balance

Patients with disturbances of acid–base balance may present clinically either with the effects of tissue malfunction due to disturbed pH (such as altered cardiac and central nervous system function), or with secondary changes in respiration as a response to the underlying metabolic change (e.g. Kussmaul respiration during metabolic acidosis). The clinical picture is often dominated by the cause of the acid–base change, such as uncontrolled diabetes mellitus or primary lung disease. Frequently the acid–base disturbance only becomes evident when the venous plasma bicarbonate concentration is noted to be abnormal, or when a full arterial blood gas analysis shows abnormalities in the pH, PCO_2 or bicarbonate. The 'base excess' or 'base deficit' may also be provided with these data; this is the difference

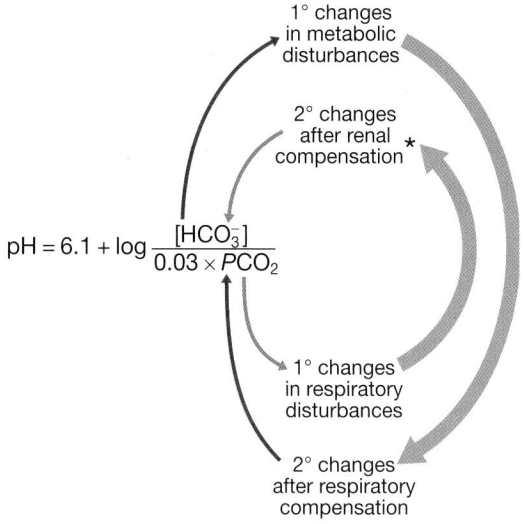

Fig. 16.11 Relationship between pH, PCO_2 (in mmHg) and plasma bicarbonate concentration (in mmol/L). *Note that changes in HCO$_3^-$ concentration are also part of the renal correction for sustained metabolic acid–base disturbances as long as the kidney itself is not the cause of the primary disturbance.

16.18 Principal patterns of acid–base disturbance

Disturbance	Blood H+	Primary change	Compensatory response	Predicted compensation
Metabolic acidosis	> 40[1]	$HCO_3 < 24$ mmol/L	$PCO_2 < 5.33$ kPa[2]	PCO_2 fall in kPa = 0.16 × HCO_3 fall in mmol/L
Metabolic alkalosis	< 40[1]	$HCO_3 > 24$ mmol/L	$PCO_2 > 5.33$ kPa[2,3]	PCO_2 rise in kPa = 0.08 × HCO_3 rise in mmol/L
Respiratory acidosis	> 40[1]	$PCO_2 > 5.33$ kPa[2]	$HCO_3 > 24$ mmol/L	Acute: HCO_3 rise in mmol/L = 0.75 × PCO_2 rise in kPa Chronic: HCO_3 rise in mmol/L = 2.62 × PCO_2 rise in kPa
Respiratory alkalosis	< 40[1]	$PCO_2 < 5.33$ kPa[2]	$HCO_3 < 24$ mmol/L	Acute: HCO_3 fall in mmol/L = 1.50 × PCO_2 fall in kPa Chronic: HCO_3 fall in mmol/L = 3.75 × PCO_2 fall in kPa

[1]H+ of 40 nmol/L = pH of 7.40.
[2]PCO_2 of 5.33 kPa = 40 mmHg.
[3]PCO_2 does not rise above 7.33 kPa (55 mmHg) because hypoxia then intervenes to drive respiration.

between the patient's bicarbonate level and the normal bicarbonate, measured in vitro with the PCO_2 adjusted to 5.33 kPa (40 mmHg), and is particularly useful in patients with combined respiratory and metabolic disorders (p. 192).

The common patterns of abnormality in the blood gas parameters in acid–base disturbances are shown in Box 16.18. (Note that the terms acidosis and alkalosis strictly refer to the underlying direction of the acid–base change, while acidaemia and alkalaemia more correctly refer to the net change present in the blood.) Interpretation of arterial blood gases is also described on page 651.

In metabolic disturbances, respiratory compensation is almost immediate, so that the predicted compensatory change in PCO_2 is achieved soon after the onset of the metabolic disturbance. In respiratory disorders, on the other hand, a small initial change in bicarbonate occurs as a result of chemical buffering of CO_2, largely within red blood cells, but over days and weeks the kidney achieves further compensatory changes in bicarbonate concentration as a result of long-term adjustments in acid secretory capacity. When clinically obtained acid–base parameters do not accord with the predicted compensation shown, a mixed acid–base disturbance should be suspected (p. 445).

Metabolic acidosis

Aetiology and assessment

Metabolic acidosis occurs when an acid other than carbonic acid (due to CO_2 retention) accumulates in the body, resulting in a fall in the plasma bicarbonate. The pH fall which would otherwise occur is blunted by hyperventilation, resulting in a reduced PCO_2. If the kidneys are intact (i.e. not the cause of the initial disturbance), renal excretion of acid can be gradually increased over days to weeks, raising the plasma bicarbonate and hence the pH towards normal in the new steady state.

Two patterns of metabolic acidosis can be defined (Box 16.19), depending on the nature of the accumulating acid:

- In pattern A, when a mineral acid (HCl) accumulates, or when there is a primary loss of bicarbonate buffer from the ECF, there is no addition to the plasma of a new acidic anion. In this case, the 'anion gap' (calculated as the difference between the

16.19 Causes of metabolic acidosis

Disorder	Mechanism
A. Normal anion gap	
Inorganic acid addition	Therapeutic infusion of or poisoning with NH_4Cl, HCl
Gastrointestinal base loss	Loss of HCO_3 in diarrhoea, small bowel fistula, urinary diversion procedure
Renal tubular acidosis (RTA)	Urinary loss of HCO_3 in proximal RTA; impaired tubular acid secretion in distal RTA
B. Increased anion gap	
Endogenous acid load	
Diabetic ketoacidosis	Accumulation of ketones[1] with hyperglycaemia
Starvation ketosis	Accumulation of ketones without hyperglycaemia
Lactic acidosis	Tissue hypoxia (e.g. shock) or liver disease
Renal failure	Accumulation of organic acids
Exogenous acid load	
Aspirin poisoning	Accumulation of salicylate[2]
Methanol poisoning	Accumulation of formate
Ethylene glycol poisoning	Accumulation of glycolate, oxalate

[1]Ketones include the acid anions acetoacetate and β-hydroxybutyrate (p. 805).
[2]Salicylate poisoning is also associated with respiratory alkalosis due to direct ventilatory stimulation.

main measured cations ($Na^+ + K^+$) and the anions ($Cl^- + HCO_3^-$)) is normal, since the plasma chloride increases to replace the depleted bicarbonate levels. This 'gap', normally around 15 mmol/L, is made up of anions such as phosphate, sulphate and multiple negative charges on plasma protein molecules. Normal anion gap metabolic acidosis (pattern A) is usually due either to diarrhoea, where the clinical diagnosis is generally obvious, or to renal tubular acidosis (see below).

- In pattern B, an accumulating acid is accompanied by its corresponding anion, which adds to the unmeasured anion gap, while the chloride concentration remains normal. The cause is usually apparent from associated clinical features such as uncontrolled diabetes mellitus, renal failure or shock, or may be suggested by associated symptoms, such as visual complaints in methanol poisoning (p. 220). It is noteworthy that a number of causes of increased anion gap acidosis are associated with alcoholism, including starvation ketosis, lactic acidosis and intoxication by methanol or ethylene glycol.

Lactic acidosis

Lactic acidosis may be confirmed by the measurement of plasma lactate, which will be increased over the normal maximal level of 2 mmol/L by as much as tenfold. Two types of lactic acidosis have been defined:

- Type 1, due to tissue hypoxia and peripheral generation of lactate, as in patients with circulatory failure and shock.
- Type 2, due to impaired metabolism of lactate as in liver disease. A number of drugs and toxins also impair lactate metabolism, including metformin.

Renal tubular acidosis (RTA)

This condition should be suspected when there is a hyperchloraemic (normal anion gap) acidosis with no evidence of gastrointestinal disturbance, and the urine pH is inappropriately high (i.e. > 5.5 in the presence of systemic acidosis). The defect can affect one of three tubular processes: reabsorption of bicarbonate in the proximal tubule (proximal RTA), acid secretion in the late distal/cortical collecting duct intercalated cells (classical distal RTA), or sodium reabsorption in the principal cells of this nephron segment, with secondary effects to reduce secretion of both potassium and acid (hyperkalaemic distal RTA).

Typical causes of each type of RTA are shown in Box 16.20. Inherited causes are due to defects in the molecular mechanisms mediating acid or bicarbonate transport in the respective tubular segments (see Fig. 16.3, p. 429). However, many causes are acquired, and the metabolic acidosis may serve as an early clue to their diagnosis.

Sometimes distal RTA is 'incomplete' and the plasma bicarbonate concentration is normal under resting conditions. However, in incomplete distal RTA the urine pH fails to fall below 5.3 after an acid challenge test, involving the ingestion of ammonium chloride sufficient to lower the plasma bicarbonate.

A number of features allow differentiation of types of RTA. The proximal form is frequently associated with urinary wasting of amino acids, phosphate and glucose (Fanconi's syndrome), as well as bicarbonate and potassium. In severe acidosis, patients with proximal RTA can lower the urine pH once the plasma bicarbonate has fallen below 16 mmol/L and leakage of bicarbonate has subsided, since distal H^+ secretion mechanisms are intact. In classical distal RTA, by contrast, acid accumulation is relentless and progressive, resulting in mobilisation of calcium from bone and consequent osteomalacia with hypercalciuria, stone formation and nephrocalcinosis. Potassium is also lost in classical distal RTA, while it is retained in hyperkalaemic distal RTA.

Management

The first step in management of metabolic acidosis is to identify and correct the cause when possible (see Box 16.19). This may involve control of diarrhoea, treatment of diabetes mellitus, correction of shock, cessation of drug administration, or dialysis to remove toxins. Since metabolic acidosis is frequently associated with sodium and water depletion, resuscitation with appropriate intravenous fluids is often needed. Use of intravenous bicarbonate in this setting is controversial. Because rapid correction of acidosis has some inherent risks (e.g. induction of hypokalaemia or reduced plasma ionised calcium), use of bicarbonate infusions is best reserved for situations where the underlying disorder cannot be readily corrected and the acidosis is critical (H^+ > 100 nmol/L, pH < 7.00) and associated with evidence of tissue dysfunction.

In RTA, the acidosis can sometimes be controlled by treating the underlying cause (see Box 16.20). Usually, however, supplements of sodium and potassium bicarbonate are necessary to achieve the target of a plasma bicarbonate level above 18 mmol/L with normokalaemia in types 1 and 2 RTA, while diuretics of the loop or thiazide classes or fludrocortisone (as appropriate to the underlying diagnosis) may be effective in increasing acid secretion in type 4 RTA.

Metabolic alkalosis
Aetiology and clinical assessment

Metabolic alkalosis is characterised by an increase in the plasma bicarbonate concentration and the plasma pH (see Box 16.18). There is a compensatory rise in PCO_2 due to hypoventilation, but this is limited by the need to avoid hypoxia. The causes are best classified by the accompanying disturbance of ECF volume.

Hypovolaemic metabolic alkalosis is the most common pattern, typified by disorders such as sustained vomiting in which acid-rich fluid is lost directly from the body. This pattern also occurs during treatment with most diuretic drugs (other than carbonic anhydrase inhibitors and potassium-sparing drugs), since the diuretic action involves increased acid loss into the urine. In the case of sustained vomiting, the loss of acid is the immediate trigger for generating metabolic alkalosis, but several factors act to sustain or amplify

16.20 Causes of renal tubular acidosis (RTA)

Proximal RTA ('type 2')
- Congenital, e.g. Fanconi's syndrome, cystinosis, Wilson's disease
- Paraproteinaemia, e.g. myeloma
- Amyloidosis
- Hyperparathyroidism
- Heavy metal toxicity, e.g. Pb, Cd, Hg
- Drugs, e.g. carbonic anhydrase inhibitors, ifosfamide

Classical distal RTA ('type 1')
- Congenital
- Hyperglobulinaemia
- Autoimmune connective tissue diseases, e.g. SLE
- Toxins and drugs, e.g. toluene, lithium, amphotericin

Hyperkalaemic distal RTA ('type 4')
- Hypoaldosteronism (primary or secondary)
- Obstructive nephropathy
- Drugs, e.g. amiloride, spironolactone
- Renal transplant rejection

metabolic alkalosis in the context of volume depletion (Fig. 16.12). Loss of sodium and fluid leads to hypo-volaemia and secondary hyperaldosteronism, triggering both proximal sodium bicarbonate reabsorption and further distal acid secretion. Hypokalaemia, due to potassium loss in the vomitus as well as through the kidney under the influence of aldosterone, itself stimulates distal acid excretion. Additionally, the compensatory rise in PCO_2 enhances tubular acid secretion. The net result is an inappropriately acid urine and a failure of the kidney to effect long-term correction of the systemic pH disturbance, at least until adequate replenishment of the circulating volume and hence reversal of secondary hyperaldosteronism.

Normovolaemic (or hypervolaemic) metabolic alkalosis occurs when both bicarbonate retention and volume expansion occur simultaneously. Classical causes include corticosteroid excess states such as primary hyperaldosteronism (Conn's syndrome, p. 778), Cushing's syndrome (p. 770) and corticosteroid therapy (p. 774). Occasionally, overuse of antacid salts for treatment of dyspepsia produces a similar pattern.

Clinically, apart from manifestations of the underlying cause, there may be few symptoms or signs related to alkalosis itself. When the rise in systemic pH is abrupt, plasma ionised calcium falls and signs of increased neuromuscular irritability such as tetany may develop (p. 765).

Management

In metabolic alkalosis with hypovolaemia, treatment involves provision of adequate intravenous fluid, specifically isotonic sodium chloride and sufficient potassium to correct the hypokalaemia, which interrupts the volume-conserving mechanisms and allows the kidney to excrete the excess alkali in the urine.

In metabolic alkalosis with normal or increased volume, treatment should focus on the underlying endocrine cause (Ch. 20).

Respiratory acidosis

Respiratory acidosis occurs when there is accumulation of CO_2 due to reduced effective alveolar ventilation (type II respiratory failure, p. 660). This results in a rise in the PCO_2, with a compensatory increase in plasma bicarbonate concentration, particularly when the disorder is of long duration and the kidney has fully developed its capacity for increased acid excretion.

This acid–base disturbance can arise from lesions anywhere along the neuromuscular pathways from the brain to the respiratory muscles that result in impaired ventilation. It can also arise during intrinsic lung disease if there is significant mismatching of ventilation and perfusion.

Clinical features of respiratory acidosis are dominated by the cause of hypoventilation (e.g. obtundation, paralysis, chest wall injury, chronic obstructive lung disease), but the CO_2 accumulation itself leads to drowsiness which itself further depresses respiratory drive.

Management involves correction of causative factors where possible, but ultimately external ventilatory support may be necessary.

Respiratory alkalosis

Respiratory alkalosis develops when there is a period of sustained hyperventilation resulting in a reduction of PCO_2 and increase in plasma pH. If the condition is sustained, renal compensation occurs such that tubular acid secretion is reduced and the plasma bicarbonate falls.

This acid–base disturbance is frequently of short duration, as in anxiety states or over-vigorous assisted ventilation. It can be prolonged in the context of pregnancy, pulmonary embolism, chronic liver disease, and ingestion of certain drugs which stimulate the brainstem respiratory centre (e.g. salicylates).

Clinical features are those associated with the cause, but there is frequently also agitation associated with perioral and digital tingling, due to a reduction in ionised calcium concentration caused by increased binding of calcium to albumin in the alkalotic ECF. In severe cases, Trousseau's sign and Chvostek's sign may be positive, and tetany or seizures may develop (p. 766).

Management involves correction of identifiable causes, reduction of anxiety, and sometimes a period of rebreathing into a closed bag to allow CO_2 levels to rise.

Mixed acid–base disorders

In patients with complex illnesses, it is not uncommon for more than one independent disturbance of acid–base metabolism to be present at the same time. In these situations, the arterial pH will represent the net effect of all primary and compensatory changes. Indeed, the pH may be normal, but the presence of underlying acid–base disturbances can be gauged from concomitant abnormalities in the PCO_2 and bicarbonate concentration.

In assessing these disorders, all clinical influences on the patient's acid–base status should be identified, and reference should be made to the table of predicted

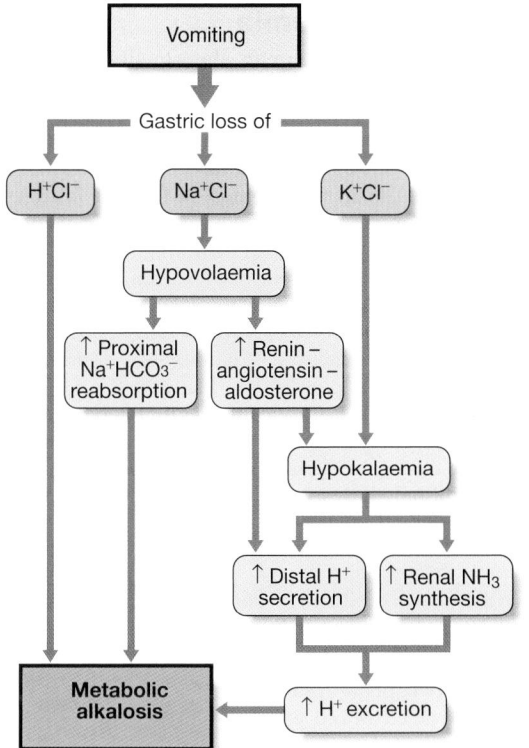

Fig. 16.12 Generation and maintenance of metabolic alkalosis during prolonged vomiting. Loss of H⁺Cl⁻ generates metabolic alkalosis which is maintained by renal changes.

compensation given in Box 16.18 (p. 443). If the compensatory change is discrepant from the rules of thumb provided, the presence of more than one disturbance of acid–base metabolism may be suspected.

DISORDERS OF DIVALENT ION METABOLISM

The present section excludes discussion of calcium disorders, which are considered in Chapters 20 (pp. 764–765) and 25 (p. 1121).

Functional anatomy and physiology of magnesium metabolism

Like potassium, magnesium is mainly an intracellular cation. It is important to the function of many enzymes, including the Na,K-ATPase, and can regulate both potassium and calcium channels. Its overall effect is to stabilise excitable cell membranes.

Renal handling of magnesium involves filtration of free plasma magnesium (about 70% of the total) with extensive reabsorption (50–70%) in the loop of Henle, although significant reabsorption also occurs in the proximal and distal tubules. Reabsorption is enhanced by parathyroid hormone (PTH).

Presenting problems in disorders of magnesium metabolism

Hypomagnesaemia

Aetiology and clinical assessment

A plasma magnesium concentration below the normal range (0.75–1.0 mmol/L; 1.5–2.0 meq/L) is usually a reflection of magnesium depletion (Box 16.21). Reduced

16.21	Causes of hypomagnesaemia
Mechanism	**Examples**
Inadequate intake	Starvation, malnutrition (esp. alcoholism), parenteral alimentation
Excessive losses	
Gastrointestinal	Prolonged vomiting/nasogastric aspiration, chronic diarrhoea/laxative abuse, malabsorption, small bowel bypass surgery, fistulas
Urinary	Diuretic therapy (loop, thiazide), alcohol, tubulotoxic drugs (gentamicin, cisplatin), volume expansion (e.g. primary hyperaldosteronism), diabetic ketoacidosis, post-obstructive diuresis, recovery from acute tubular necrosis, inherited tubular transport defect (Bartter's syndrome, Gitelman's syndrome, primary renal magnesium wasting)
Miscellaneous	Acute pancreatitis, foscarnet therapy, hungry bone syndrome, diabetes mellitus

intake alone is rarely sufficient to cause magnesium depletion, and generally there is excessive loss from either the gastrointestinal tract (notably in chronic diarrhoea) or the kidney (during prolonged use of loop diuretics). Excessive alcohol ingestion can cause magnesium depletion through both gut and renal losses. Some inherited tubular transport disorders result in urinary magnesium wasting, notably Gitelman's syndrome (p. 439).

Hypomagnesaemia is frequently associated with hypocalcaemia, probably because magnesium is required for the normal secretion of PTH in response to a fall in serum calcium, and because hypomagnesaemia induces resistance to PTH in bone. Clinical features of hypomagnesaemia and hypocalcaemia are similar; there may be tetany, cardiac arrhythmias (notably torsades de pointes, p. 567), central nervous excitation and seizures, as well as vasoconstriction and hypertension. Magnesium depletion is also associated (through uncertain mechanisms) with hyponatraemia and hypokalaemia, which may mediate some of the clinical manifestations.

Management

Treatment involves identification and correction of the cause where possible. Oral magnesium salts have limited effectiveness due to poor absorption and may cause diarrhoea. When symptoms are present, treatment should be with intravenous magnesium chloride at a rate not exceeding 0.5 mmol/kg in the first 24 hours. When intravenous access is not available, magnesium sulphate can be given intramuscularly. If hypomagnesaemia is due to diuretic treatment, adjunctive use of a potassium-sparing agent will also reduce magnesium loss into the urine.

Hypermagnesaemia

This is a much less common abnormality than hypomagnesaemia. The cause nearly always involves acute or chronic renal failure, but adrenocortical insufficiency also predisposes to magnesium retention. An increased intake, either through medications containing magnesium (antacids, laxatives, enemas) or through iatrogenic parenteral therapy, greatly increases the risk of hypermagnesaemia in patients with renal impairment.

Clinical features include bradycardia, hypotension, reduced consciousness and respiratory depression.

Management involves ceasing all magnesium intake, improving renal function if possible, and promoting urinary magnesium excretion using a loop diuretic with intravenous hydration, if residual renal function allows. Calcium gluconate may be given intravenously to reverse overt cardiac effects. Ultimately, if renal function is minimal, dialysis may be necessary to remove the magnesium load.

Functional anatomy and physiology of phosphate metabolism

Inorganic phosphate (mainly present as HPO_4^{2-}) is intimately involved in cell energy metabolism, intracellular signalling and bone and mineral balance (Ch. 25). The normal plasma concentration is 0.8–1.4 mmol/L (2.48–4.34 mg/dL). It is freely filtered at the glomerulus and approximately 65% is reabsorbed by the proximal tubule, via an apical sodium-phosphate cotransport carrier.

A further 10–20% is reabsorbed in the distal tubules, leaving a fractional excretion of some 10% to pass into the urine, usually as $H_2PO_4^-$. Proximal reabsorption is decreased by PTH, volume expansion and glucose infusion.

Presenting problems in disorders of phosphate metabolism

Hypophosphataemia

The causes of a reduced plasma phosphate concentration are shown in Box 16.22. Phosphate may redistribute into cells during periods of increased energy utilisation (as in refeeding after a period of starvation) and during systemic alkalosis. However, severe hypophosphataemia usually represents an overall body deficit due either to inadequate intake or absorption through the gut, or to excessive renal losses, notably in primary hyperparathyroidism (p. 766) or in diuresis involving inhibition of proximal tubular reabsorption (e.g. acute volume expansion, osmotic diuresis and proximally acting diuretics). An inherited defect of proximal sodium-phosphate cotransport causes familial hypophosphataemic rickets.

Clinical manifestations of phosphate depletion reflect the widespread involvement of phosphate in tissue metabolism. Defects appear in the blood (impaired function and survival of all cell lines), skeletal muscle (weakness, respiratory failure), cardiac muscle (congestive cardiac failure), smooth muscle (ileus), central nervous system (decreased consciousness, seizures and coma) and bone (osteomalacia in severe prolonged hypophosphataemia, p. 1121).

Management involves administering oral phosphate supplements and high-protein/high-dairy dietary supplements which are rich in naturally occurring phosphate. Intravenous treatment with sodium or potassium phosphate salts can be used in critical situations, but there is a risk of precipitating hypocalcaemia and metastatic calcification.

16.22 Causes of hypophosphataemia	
Mechanism	**Examples**
Redistribution into cells	Refeeding after starvation, respiratory alkalosis, treatment for diabetic ketoacidosis
Inadequate intake or absorption	Malnutrition, malabsorption, chronic diarrhoea, phosphate binders (antacids), vitamin D deficiency or resistance
Increased renal excretion	Hyperparathyroidism, ECF volume expansion with diuresis, osmotic diuresis, proximal tubular transport defect (Fanconi's syndrome, familial hypophosphataemic rickets, cancer-induced hypophosphataemia)

Hyperphosphataemia

Phosphate accumulation is usually the result of acute or chronic renal failure (pp. 482–492, and p. 765). Phosphate excretion is also reduced in hypoparathyroidism and pseudohypoparathyroidism (p. 768). Redistribution of phosphate from cells into the plasma can be a contributing factor to hyperphosphataemia in the 'tumour lysis' syndrome and in catabolic states. Phosphate accumulation is aggravated in any of these conditions if the patient takes phosphate-containing preparations or inappropriate vitamin D therapy.

The clinical features relate to hypocalcaemia and metastatic calcification, particularly in chronic renal failure with tertiary hyperparathyroidism (when a high calcium–phosphate product occurs).

Management involves volume expansion with intravenous normal saline which promotes phosphate excretion if renal function is normal. In the presence of renal failure, dietary phosphate restriction and the use of oral phosphate binders (such as calcium carbonate) are important (p. 490).

DISORDERS OF AMINO ACID METABOLISM

Congenital disorders of amino acid metabolism usually present in the neonatal period and may involve life-long treatment regimens. However, some disorders, particularly those involved in amino acid transport, may not present until later in life.

Phenylketonuria

Phenylketonuria (PKU) is inherited as an autosomal recessive disorder which causes deficiency of enzymatic activity of phenylalanine hydroxylase. As a result, phenylalanine accumulates to high levels in the neonate's blood, causing mental retardation.

Diagnosis of PKU is almost always made by routine neonatal screening. Treatment involves life-long adherence to a low-phenylalanine diet. Early and adequate dietary treatment prevents major mental retardation, although there may still be a slight reduction in IQ.

Homocystinuria

Homocystinuria is caused by cystathionine β-synthase deficiency and inherited as an autosomal recessive trait. This results in increased urinary excretion of homocystine and methionine. Many cases of homocystinuria are diagnosed through newborn screening programmes.

There is a wide spectrum of clinical manifestations, involving the eyes (ectopia lentis—displacement of the lens), central nervous system (mental retardation, delayed developmental milestones, seizures, psychiatric disturbances), skeleton (resembling Marfan's syndrome, and also with generalised osteoporosis), vascular system (thrombotic lesions of arteries and veins) and skin (hypopigmentation).

Treatment is dietary, involving a methionine-restricted, cystine-supplemented diet, as well as large doses of pyridoxine.

DISORDERS OF CARBOHYDRATE METABOLISM

The most common disorder of carbohydrate metabolism is diabetes mellitus, which is discussed in Chapter 21. There are also some rare inherited defects.

Galactosaemia

Galactosaemia is caused by a mutation in the gene encoding galactose-1-phosphate uridylyltransferase (*GALT*) and is usually inherited as an autosomal recessive disorder. The neonate is unable to metabolise galactose, one of the hexose sugars contained in lactose.

Vomiting or diarrhoea usually begins within a few days of ingestion of milk, and the neonate may become jaundiced. Failure to thrive is the most common clinical presentation. The classic form of the disease results in hepatomegaly, cataracts and mental retardation, and fulminant infection with *Escherichia coli* is a frequent complication. Treatment involves life-long avoidance of galactose- and lactose-containing foods.

The widespread inclusion of galactosaemia in newborn screening programmes has resulted in the identification of a number of milder variants (e.g. 'Duarte' variant).

Glycogen storage diseases

Glycogen provides a rapidly mobilisable storage form of glucose, enabling glucose to be released as needed during exercise or between meals. Glycogen storage diseases (GSD, or glycogenoses) result from an inherited defect in one of the many enzymes responsible for the formation or breakdown of glycogen.

There are about eleven major types of GSD which are classified by a number, by the name of the defective enzyme or eponymously after the physician who first described the condition (Box 16.23). Most forms of GSD are inherited as autosomal recessive disorders.

A diagnosis of GSD is made on the basis of the patient's symptoms, a physical examination and the results of biochemical tests. Occasionally, a muscle or liver biopsy is required to confirm the enzyme defect. Different types of GSD present at different ages, and some may require life-long modifications of diet and lifestyle.

16.23 Glycogen storage diseases (GSD)

GSD	Eponym	Enzyme deficiency	Clinical features and complications
I	Von Gierke	Glucose-6-phosphatase	Childhood presentation, hypoglycaemia, hepatomegaly
II	Pompe	α-glucosidase (acid maltase)	Classical presentation in infancy, muscle weakness (may be severe)
III	Cori	Debrancher enzyme	Childhood presentation, hepatomegaly, mild hypoglycaemia
IV	Andersen	Brancher enzyme	Presentation in infancy, severe muscle weakness (may affect heart), cirrhosis
V	McArdle	Muscle glycogen phosphorylase	Exercise-induced fatigue and myalgia
VI	Hers	Liver phosphorylase	Mild hepatomegaly
VII	Tarui	Muscle phosphofructokinase	Exercise-induced fatigue and myalgia
VIII		Liver phosphorylase kinase	Very mild disease; hepatomegaly, growth retardation, elevated hepatic enzymes, hyperlipidaemia, fasting hyperketosis
IX		Liver glycogen phosphorylase kinase	Mild hepatomegaly. Inheritance can be autosomal or X-linked recessive
0		Hepatic glycogen synthase	Fasting hypoglycaemia, post-prandial hyperglycaemia

16.24 Lysosomal storage diseases

Lysosomal storage disease	Clinical features	Enzyme deficiency	Human enzyme replacement therapy
Fabry disease	Variable age of onset Neurological (pain in extremities) Dermatological (hypohidrosis, angiokeratomas) Cerebrovascular (renal, cardiac, CNS)	α-galactosidase A	In clinical practice
Gaucher disease (various types)	Splenic and liver enlargement, with variable severity of disease Some types also have neurological involvement	Glucocerebrosidase	In clinical practice for some types
Mucopolysaccharidosis (MPS) (various types, including Hurler's, Hunter's, Sanfilippo's, Morquio's syndromes)	Vary with syndrome. Can cause mental retardation, skeletal and joint abnormalities, abnormal facies, obstructive respiratory diseases and recurrent respiratory infections	Each MPS type has a different enzyme deficiency	In clinical practice for some types; clinical trials underway for other types
Niemann–Pick disease	Most common presentation is as a progressive neurological disorder, accompanied by organomegaly Some variants do not have neurological symptoms	Acid sphingomyelinase	Clinical trials planned for some types
GM2-gangliosidosis (various types, including Tay–Sachs, Sandhoff's diseases)	Severe progressive neurological disorder. Sandhoff's disease also characterised by organomegaly	Hexosaminidase A, B	

DISORDERS OF COMPLEX LIPID METABOLISM

Complex lipids are key components of the cell membrane (p. 44). They are normally catabolised in organelles called lysosomes. The lysosomal storage diseases are a heterogeneous group of disorders in which there is a missing enzyme in the lysosomes (Box 16.24), resulting in an inability to break down complex glycolipids or other intracellular macromolecules. These disorders have diverse clinical manifestations, typically including mental retardation. Some are becoming treatable using human enzyme replacement therapy, while others (such as Tay–Sachs disease) can be prevented through community participation in genetic carrier screening programmes.

DISORDERS OF BLOOD LIPIDS AND LIPOPROTEINS

The term 'lipid' refers to substances with poor water solubility. Biologically important lipids include sterols (including cholesterol), which are composed of hydrocarbon rings, and glycerides (including triglyceride (TG) and phospholipid), which are chiefly composed of hydrocarbon chains (including fatty acids). Despite their poor water solubility, these materials must be assimilated from the diet and transported in the body; this is achieved by incorporating lipids within lipoproteins. Plasma cholesterol and TG are clinically important mainly because they are major treatable risk factors for cardiovascular disease, whilst severe hypertriglyceridaemia also predisposes to acute pancreatitis.

Functional anatomy, physiology and investigation of lipid metabolism

Lipids can be transported and metabolised in vivo by virtue of the detergent-like properties of apolipoproteins. The laws of physical chemistry dictate that in the aqueous in vivo environment of the blood and tissue fluids, apolipoproteins combine with lipids to form spherical or disc-shaped lipoproteins, which consist of a hydrophobic core and a less hydrophobic coat (Fig. 16.13). The structure of some apolipoproteins also enables them to act as enzyme co-factors or cell receptor ligands. Variations in lipid and apolipoprotein composition result in distinct classes of lipoprotein that perform specific metabolic functions.

Dietary lipid

The intestinal absorption of dietary lipid is described on page 838 (see also Fig. 16.14). Enterocytes lining the gut extract monoglyceride and free fatty acids from micelles and re-esterify them into TG. TG is combined with a truncated form of apolipoprotein B (Apo B48) as it is synthesised. Intestinal cholesterol derived from dietary and biliary sources is also absorbed via a specific intestinal membrane transporter (NPC1L1). These processes produce chylomicrons containing TG and cholesterol

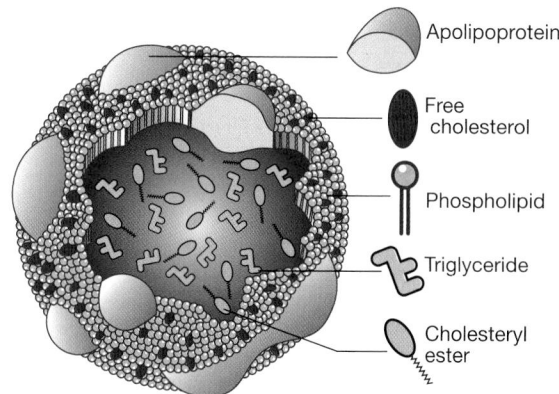

Fig. 16.13 Structure of lipoproteins.

ester that are secreted basolaterally into lymphatic lacteals then carried to the circulation via the thoracic duct. Newly secreted chylomicrons are remodelled by the transfer of additional apolipoproteins. Chylomicron TG is hydrolysed by lipoprotein lipase located on the endothelium of tissue capillary beds. This releases fatty acids that may be used locally for energy or stored in tissues such as muscle or adipose tissue. The residual 'remnant' chylomicron particle is avidly cleared by low-density lipoprotein (LDL)-receptors in the liver which recognise Apo E on the remnant lipoproteins. Complete absorption of dietary lipids takes about 6–10 hours, so chylomicrons are undetectable in the plasma after a 12-hour fast.

The main dietary determinants of plasma cholesterol concentrations are the intakes of saturated and transunsaturated fatty acids, which reduce LDL receptor activity (see below). Dietary cholesterol has surprisingly little effect on fasting cholesterol levels. Plant sterols and drugs that inhibit cholesterol absorption are effective because they also reduce the re-utilisation of biliary cholesterol. Dietary determinants of plasma TG concentrations are complex. Excessive intakes of carbohydrate, fat or alcohol may each contribute to increased plasma TG by different mechanisms.

Endogenous lipid

In the fasting state, the liver is the major source of plasma lipids (see Fig. 16.14). The liver may acquire lipids by uptake, synthesis or conversion from other macronutrients. These lipids are transported to other tissues by secretion of TG-rich very low-density lipoproteins (VLDL), which differ from chylomicrons in that they contain full-length Apo B100. Following secretion into the circulation, VLDL undergo a metabolic process similar to that of chylomicrons. Hydrolysis of VLDL TG releases fatty acids to tissues and converts VLDL into 'remnant' particles, referred to as intermediate-density lipoproteins (IDL). Most IDL are rapidly cleared by LDL receptors in the liver, but some are processed by hepatic lipase, which converts the particle to an LDL by removing most materials other than Apo B100, and free and esterified cholesterol.

LDL is a source of cholesterol for cells and tissues (see Fig. 16.14). LDL cholesterol is internalised by receptor-mediated endocytosis via the LDL receptor. Delivery

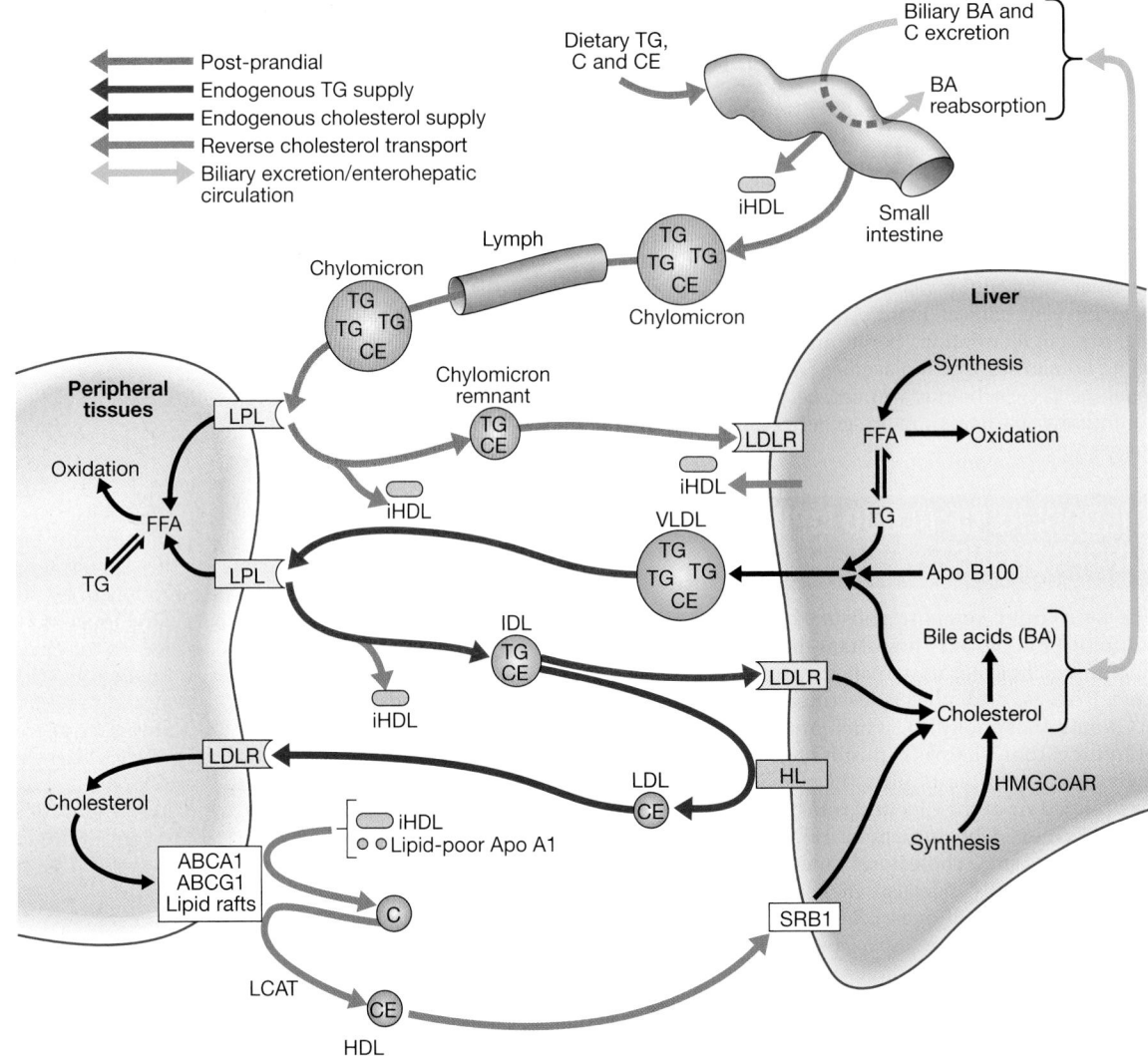

Fig. 16.14 Absorption, transport and storage of lipids. Pathways of lipid transport are shown; in addition cholesterol ester transfer protein exchanges triglyceride and cholesterol ester between VLDL/chylomicrons and HDL/LDL, and free fatty acids released from peripheral lipolysis can be taken up in the liver. (ABCA1, ABCG1 = ATP-binding cassette A1, G1; Apo = apolipoprotein; BA = bile acids; C = cholesterol; CE = cholesterol ester; FFA = free fatty acids; HDL = mature high-density lipoprotein; iHDL = immature high-density lipoprotein; HL = hepatic lipase; HMGCoAR = hydroxy-methyl-glutaryl-coenzyme A reductase; IDL = intermediate-density lipoprotein; LCAT = lecithin cholesterol acyl transferase; LDL = low-density lipoprotein; LDLR = low-density lipoprotein receptor (Apo B100 receptor); LPL = lipoprotein lipase; SRB1 = scavenger receptor B1; TG = triglyceride; VLDL = very low-density lipoprotein)

of cholesterol via this pathway down-regulates further expression of the LDL receptor gene and reduces the synthesis and activity of the rate-limiting enzyme for cholesterol synthesis, HMGCoA reductase. These negative feedback pathways, together with the modulation of cholesterol esterification, control the intracellular free cholesterol level within a narrow range.

Reverse cholesterol transport

Peripheral tissues are further guarded against excessive cholesterol accumulation by high-density lipoproteins (HDL; see Fig. 16.14). Lipid-poor Apo A1 (derived from the liver, intestine and the outer layer of chylomicrons and VLDL) accepts cellular cholesterol and phospholipid from a specific membrane transporter known as the ATP-binding cassette A1 transporter (ABC A1). This produces small HDLs that are able to accept more free cholesterol from cholesterol-rich regions of the cell

membrane via another membrane transporter (ABC G1). The cholesterol that has been accepted by these small HDLs is esterified by lecithin cholesterol acyl transferase (LCAT), thus maintaining an uptake gradient and remodelling the particle into a mature spherical HDL. These HDL release their cholesterol to the liver and other cholesterol-requiring tissues via the scavenger receptor B1 (SRB1).

The cholesterol ester transfer protein (CETP) in plasma allows transfer of cholesterol from HDL or LDL to VLDL or chylomicrons in exchange for TG. When TG is elevated, the action of CETP may reduce HDL cholesterol and remodel LDL into 'small, dense' LDL particles that appear to be more atherogenic in the blood vessel wall. Animal species that lack CETP are resistant to atherosclerosis, suggesting that this process may have a detrimental effect on progression of cardiovascular disease.

Lipids and cardiovascular disease

Plasma lipoprotein levels are major modifiable risk factors for cardiovascular disease. Increased levels of atherogenic lipoproteins (especially LDL, but also IDL, lipoprotein (a) and possibly chylomicron remnants) contribute to the development of atherosclerosis (p. 577). Increased plasma concentration and reduced diameter favour subendothelial accumulation of these lipoproteins. Following chemical modifications such as oxidation, these Apo B-containing lipoproteins are no longer cleared by normal mechanisms. They trigger a self-perpetuating inflammatory response during which they are taken up by macrophages to form foam cells, a hallmark of atherosclerotic lesions. These processes also have an adverse effect on endothelial function.

Conversely, HDL removes cholesterol from the tissues to the liver, where it is metabolised and excreted in bile. HDL may also counteract some components of the inflammatory response, such as the expression of vascular adhesion molecules by the endothelium. Consequently, low HDL cholesterol levels, which are often associated with triglyceride elevation, also predispose to atherosclerosis.

Lipid measurement

Abnormalities of lipid metabolism most commonly come to light following routine blood testing. Measurement of plasma cholesterol alone is not sufficient for comprehensive assessment. Levels of total cholesterol (TC), triglyceride (TG) and HDL cholesterol (HDL-C) need to be obtained after a 12-hour fast to permit accurate calculation of LDL cholesterol (LDL-C) according to the Friedewald formula (LDL-C = TC − HDL-C − (TG/2.2) mmol/L). (Before the formula is applied, lipid levels in mg/dL can be converted to mmol/L by dividing by 38 for cholesterol and 88 for triglycerides.) The formula becomes unreliable when TG levels exceed 4 mmol/L (350 mg/dL). However, non-fasting samples are often used to guide therapeutic decisions since they are unaffected in terms of TC and measured LDL-C, albeit that they differ from fasting samples in terms of TG, HDL-C and, to some extent, calculated LDL-C. Consideration must be given to confounding factors, such as recent illness, after which cholesterol levels temporarily decrease in proportion to severity. Results that will affect major decisions, such as initiation of drug therapy, should be confirmed with a repeat measurement.

Elevated TG is common in obesity, diabetes and insulin resistance (Chs 5 and 21), and is frequently associated with low HDL and increased 'small, dense' LDL. Under these circumstances, LDL-C may underestimate risk. This is one situation in which measurement of Apo B may provide additional useful information.

Presenting problems in disorders of lipids

Lipid measurements are usually performed for the following reasons:

- screening for primary or secondary prevention of cardiovascular disease

- investigation of patients with clinical features of lipid disorders (Fig. 16.15)
- testing relatives of patients with one of the single gene defects causing dyslipidaemia.

Aetiology and clinical assessment

The first step is to consider the effect of other diseases and drugs (Box 16.25). Overt or subclinical hypothyroidism (p. 741) may cause hypercholesterolaemia, so measurement of thyroid-stimulating hormone is warranted in most cases, even in the absence of typical symptoms and signs.

16.25 Causes of secondary hyperlipidaemia

Secondary hypercholesterolaemia

Moderately common
- Hypothyroidism
- Pregnancy
- Cholestatic liver disease
- Drugs (diuretics, ciclosporin, corticosteroids, androgens)

Less common
- Nephrotic syndrome
- Anorexia nervosa
- Porphyria
- Hyperparathyroidism

Secondary hypertriglyceridaemia

Common
- Diabetes mellitus (type 2)
- Chronic renal disease
- Abdominal obesity
- Excess alcohol
- Hepatocellular disease
- Drugs (β-blockers, retinoids, corticosteroids)

Once secondary causes are excluded, primary lipid abnormalities may be diagnosed. The Fredrickson classification (types I–V) adds little to clinical decision-making. Alternatively, primary lipid abnormalities can be classified according to the predominant lipid problem: hypercholesterolaemia, hypertriglyceridaemia or mixed hyperlipidaemia (Box 16.26). Although single gene disorders are encountered in all three categories, the most common cause is an interaction between numerous genetic and environmental factors (i.e. 'polygenic'). Clinical consequences of dyslipidaemia vary somewhat between these categories (see Fig. 16.15).

Predominant hypercholesterolaemia

Polygenic hypercholesterolaemia is the most common cause of a mild to moderate increase in LDL-C (see Box 16.26). Physical signs such as corneal arcus and xanthelasma may be found in this as well as other forms of lipid disturbance (see Fig. 16.15). The risk of cardiovascular disease is proportional to the degree of LDL-C elevation, but is modified by other major risk factors, particularly low HDL-C.

Familial hypercholesterolaemia (FH) causes moderate to severe hypercholesterolaemia with a prevalence of at least 0.2% in most populations. It is usually due to an autosomal dominantly inherited mutation of the LDL receptor gene, but a similar syndrome can arise with defects in Apo B100 or a sterol-sensitive protease known as PCSK-9. Most patients with these abnormalities exhibit LDL levels that are approximately twice as high as in unaffected subjects of the same age and gender.

16

16.26 Classification of hyperlipidaemia

Disease	Elevated lipid results	Elevated lipoprotein	CHD risk	Pancreatitis risk
Predominant hypercholesterolaemia				
Polygenic (majority)	TC ± TG	LDL ± VLDL	+	–
Familial hypercholesterolaemia (LDL receptor defect, defective Apo B100, increased function of PCSK-9)	TC ± TG	LDL ± VLDL	+++	–
Hyperalphalipoproteinaemia	TC ± TG	HDL	–	–
Predominant hypertriglyceridaemia				
Polygenic (majority)	TG	VLDL ± LDL	Variable	+
Lipoprotein lipase deficiency	TG > TC	Chylo	?	+++
Familial hypertriglyceridaemia	TG ± TC	VLDL ± Chylo	?	++
Mixed hyperlipidaemia				
Polygenic (majority)	TC + TG	VLDL + LDL	Variable	+
Familial combined hyperlipidaemia*	TC and/or TG	LDL and VLDL	++	+
Dysbetalipoproteinaemia*	TC and/or TG	IDL	+++	+

*Familial combined hyperlipidaemia and dysbetalipoproteinaemia may also present as predominant hypercholesterolaemia or predominant hypertriglyceridaemia. (Chylo = chylomicrons; CHD = coronary heart disease; TC = total cholesterol; TG = triglycerides)

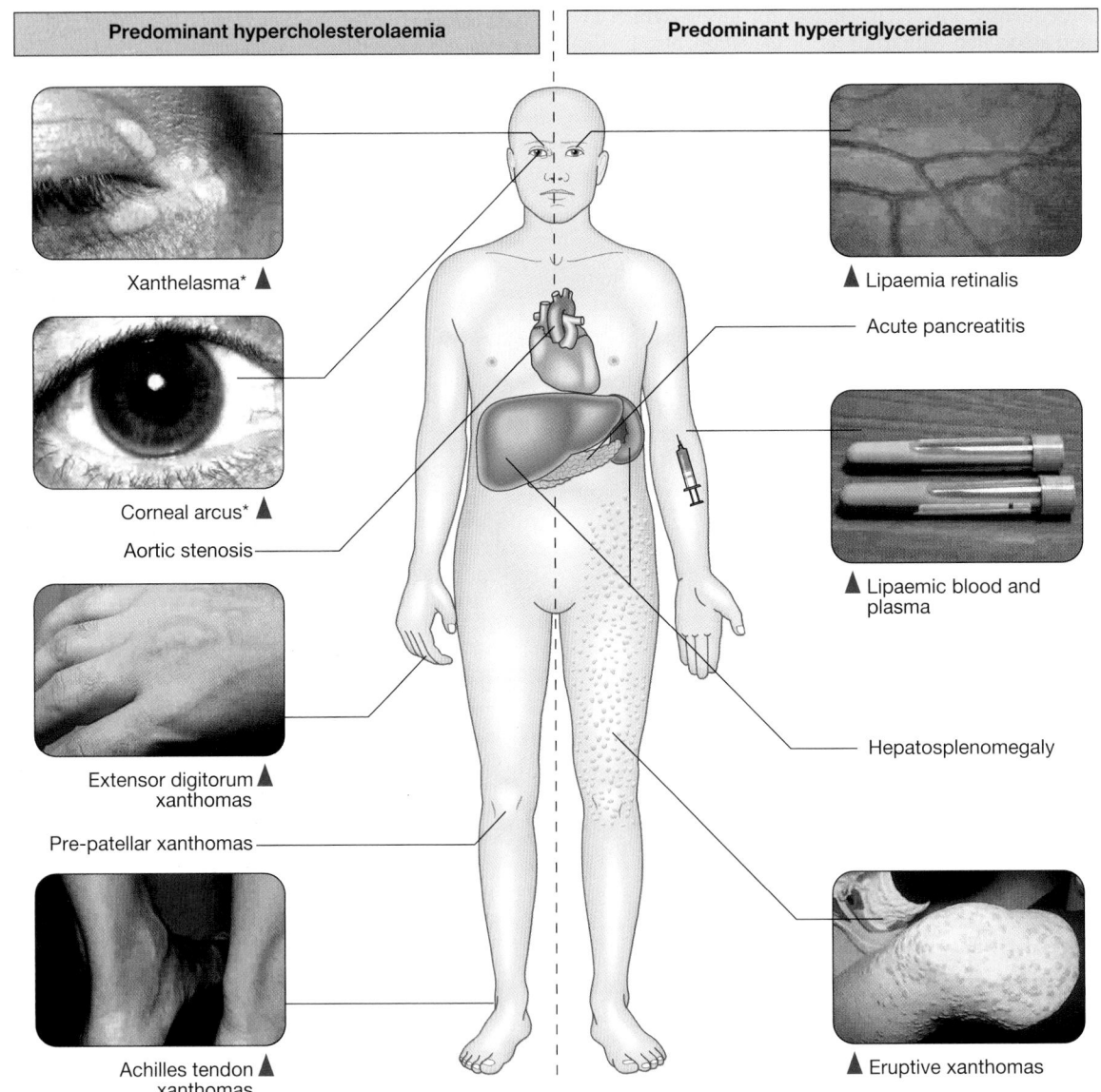

Predominant hypercholesterolaemia

Predominant hypertriglyceridaemia

Xanthelasma* ▲

Corneal arcus* ▲

Aortic stenosis

Extensor digitorum ▲ xanthomas

Pre-patellar xanthomas

Achilles tendon ▲ xanthomas

▲ Lipaemia retinalis

Acute pancreatitis

▲ Lipaemic blood and plasma

Hepatosplenomegaly

▲ Eruptive xanthomas

Fig. 16.15 Clinical manifestations of hyperlipidaemia. *Note that xanthelasma and corneal arcus may be non-specific, especially in later life.

Family history reveals that approximately 50% of each generation suffers hypercholesterolaemia, often with very premature cardiovascular disease. FH may be accompanied by xanthomas of the Achilles or extensor digitorum tendons (see Fig. 16.15), which are strongly suggestive of (but not pathognomonic for) FH. The onset of corneal arcus before age 40 is also suggestive of this condition.

In populations in which there is a 'founder gene' effect or consanguineous marriage, homozygous FH occasionally occurs, resulting in more extensive xanthomas and precocious cardiovascular disease in childhood. A recessive form of this condition has also been described recently.

Hyperalphalipoproteinaemia refers to increased levels of HDL-C. In the absence of an increase in LDL-C, this condition does not cause cardiovascular disease, so it should not be regarded as pathological.

Familial combined hyperlipidaemia, and dysbetalipoproteinaemia, may present with the pattern of predominant hypercholesterolaemia (see 'mixed hyperlipidaemia' below).

Predominant hypertriglyceridaemia

Polygenic hypertriglyceridaemia is the most common primary cause of TG elevation (see Box 16.26). It also commonly occurs secondary to excess alcohol, medications, type 2 diabetes, impaired glucose tolerance, central obesity or other manifestations of the insulin resistance syndrome (p. 802). It is often accompanied by post-prandial hyperlipidaemia and reduced HDL-C, both of which may contribute to cardiovascular risk. Excessive dietary fat intake or other exacerbating factors may precipitate a massive increase in TG levels, which, if they exceed 10 mmol/L (880 mg/dL), may pose a risk of acute pancreatitis.

Lipoprotein lipase deficiency is an infrequent autosomal recessive disorder due to hereditary deficiency of this enzyme or of its co-factor Apo C2. It causes massive hypertriglyceridaemia that is not amenable to drug treatment. It may commence in childhood and is associated with episodes of acute abdominal pain and pancreatitis. In common with other causes of severe hypertriglyceridaemia, it may result in hepatosplenomegaly, lipaemia retinalis and eruptive xanthomas (see Fig. 16.15).

Familial hypertriglyceridaemia refers to dominant inheritance of pure hypertriglyceridaemia. Some cases may be due to a secondary response to impaired bile acid resorption which may not be associated with increased risk of cardiovascular disease, or deficiency of Apo A5. Familial hypertriglyceridaemia also predisposes to levels of hypertriglyceridaemia that are sufficient to pose a risk of pancreatitis.

Familial combined hyperlipidaemia, and dysbetalipoproteinaemia, may present with the pattern of predominant hypertriglyceridaemia (see 'mixed hyperlipidaemia', below).

Mixed hyperlipidaemia

It is difficult to define quantitatively the distinction between predominant hyperlipidaemias and mixed hyperlipidaemia. The term 'mixed' usually implies the presence of hypertriglyceridaemia as well as an increase in LDL or IDL. Treatment of massive hypertriglyceridaemia may improve TG faster than cholesterol, thus temporarily mimicking mixed hyperlipidaemia.

Primary mixed hyperlipidaemia is usually polygenic and, like predominant hypertriglyceridaemia, often occurs in association with type 2 diabetes, impaired glucose tolerance, central obesity or other manifestations of the insulin resistance syndrome (p. 802). Both components of mixed hyperlipidaemia may contribute to the risk of cardiovascular disease.

Familial combined hyperlipidaemia is a dominantly inherited disorder caused by overproduction of atherogenic Apo B-containing lipoproteins. It results in elevation of cholesterol, TG or both in different family members at different times. It is associated with an increased risk of cardiovascular disease but it does not produce any pathognomonic physical signs. In practice, this relatively common condition is substantially modified by factors such as age and weight. It may not be a monogenic condition, but rather one end of a heterogeneous spectrum that overlaps with the insulin resistance syndrome.

Dysbetalipoproteinaemia (also referred to as type 3 hyperlipidaemia, broad-beta dyslipoproteinaemia or remnant hyperlipidaemia) involves accumulation of roughly equimolar levels of cholesterol and TG. It is caused by homozygous inheritance of the Apo E2 allele, which is the isoform least avidly recognised by the LDL receptor. In conjunction with other exacerbating factors, such as obesity and diabetes, it leads to accumulation of atherogenic IDL and chylomicron remnants. Premature cardiovascular disease is common and it may also result in the formation of palmar xanthomas, tuberous xanthomas or tendon xanthomas.

Rare dyslipidaemias

Several rare disturbances of lipid metabolism have been described (Box 16.27). They provide important insights into lipid metabolism and its impact on risk of cardiovascular disease.

Fish eye disease and Apo A1 Milano demonstrate that very low HDL levels do not necessarily cause cardiovascular disease, but Apo A1 deficiency, Tangier disease and LCAT deficiency demonstrate that low HDL-C can be atherogenic under some circumstances. Sitosterolaemia and cerebrotendinous xanthomatosis demonstrate that sterols other than cholesterol can cause xanthomas and cardiovascular disease, while abetalipoproteinaemia and hypobetalipoproteinaemia suggest that low levels of Apo B-containing lipoproteins reduce the risk of cardiovascular

16

🛈 16.27 **Miscellaneous and rare forms of hyperlipidaemia**		
Condition	**Lipoprotein pattern**	**CVD risk**
Tangier disease	Very low HDL, low TC	+
Apo A1 deficiency	Very low HDL	++
Apo A1 Milano	Very low HDL	−
Fish eye disease	Very low HDL, high TG	−
LCAT deficiency	Very low HDL, high TG	?
Sitosterolaemia	High plant sterols including sitosterol	+
Cerebrotendinous xanthomatosis	Bile acid defect (cholestanol accumulation)	+

(CVD = cardiovascular disease; HDL = high-density lipoprotein; LCAT = lecithin cholesterol acyl transferase; TC = total cholesterol; TG = triglycerides)

disease at the expense of fat-soluble vitamin deficiency, leading to retinal lesions and peripheral neuropathy.

Management of dyslipidaemia

Lipid-lowering therapies have a key role in the secondary and primary prevention of cardiovascular diseases (p. 578). Assessment of absolute risk, treatment of all modifiable risk factors and optimisation of lifestyle, especially diet and exercise, are central to management in all cases.

Patients with the greatest absolute risk of cardiovascular disease will derive the greatest benefit from treatment. Public health organisations recommend thresholds for the introduction of lipid-lowering therapy based on the identification of patients in very high-risk categories, or those calculated to be at high absolute risk according to algorithms or tables such as the Joint British Societies Coronary Risk Prediction Chart (see Fig. 18.61, p. 580). These tables, which are based on large epidemiological studies, should be recalibrated for the local population, if possible. In general, patients who already have cardiovascular disease, diabetes mellitus, chronic renal impairment or an absolute risk of cardiovascular disease of greater than 20% in the ensuing 10 years are arbitrarily regarded as having sufficient risk to justify drug treatment.

Public health organisations also recommend target levels for patients receiving drug treatment. High-risk patients should aim for HDL-C > 1 mmol/L (38 mg/dL) and fasting TG < 2 mmol/L (approximately 180 mg/dL), whilst target levels for LDL-C have been reduced from 2.5 to 2.0 mmol/L (76 mg/dL) or less. In general, total cholesterol should be < 5 mmol/L (190 mg/dL) during treatment, and < 4 mmol/L (approximately 150 mg/dL) in high-risk patients and in secondary prevention of cardiovascular disease.

Non-pharmacological management

Patients with lipid abnormalities should receive medical advice and, if necessary, dietary counselling to:

- reduce intake of saturated and trans-unsaturated fat to less than 7–10% of total energy
- reduce intake of cholesterol to < 250 mg/day
- replace sources of saturated fat and cholesterol with alternative foods such as lean meat, low-fat dairy products, polyunsaturated spreads and low glycaemic index carbohydrates
- reduce energy-dense foods such as fats and soft drinks, whilst increasing activity and exercise to maintain or lose weight
- increase consumption of cardioprotective and nutrient-dense foods such as vegetables, unrefined carbohydrates, fish, pulses, nuts, legumes, fruit etc.
- adjust alcohol consumption, reducing intake if excessive or if associated with hypertension, hypertriglyceridaemia or central obesity
- achieve additional benefits with supplementary intake of foods containing lipid-lowering nutrients such as n-3 fatty acids, dietary fibre and plant sterols

Response to diet is usually apparent within 3–4 weeks but dietary adjustment may need to be introduced gradually. Although hyperlipidaemia in general, and hypertriglyceridaemia in particular, can be very responsive to these measures, LDL-C reductions are often only modest in routine practice. Explanation, encouragement and persistence are often required to induce patient compliance. Even minor weight loss can substantially reduce cardiovascular risk, especially in centrally obese patients (p. 117).

All other modifiable cardiovascular risk factors should be assessed and treated. If possible, intercurrent drug treatments that adversely affect the lipid profile should be replaced.

Pharmacological management

The main diagnostic categories provide a useful framework for management and the selection of first-line pharmacological treatment (Fig. 16.16).

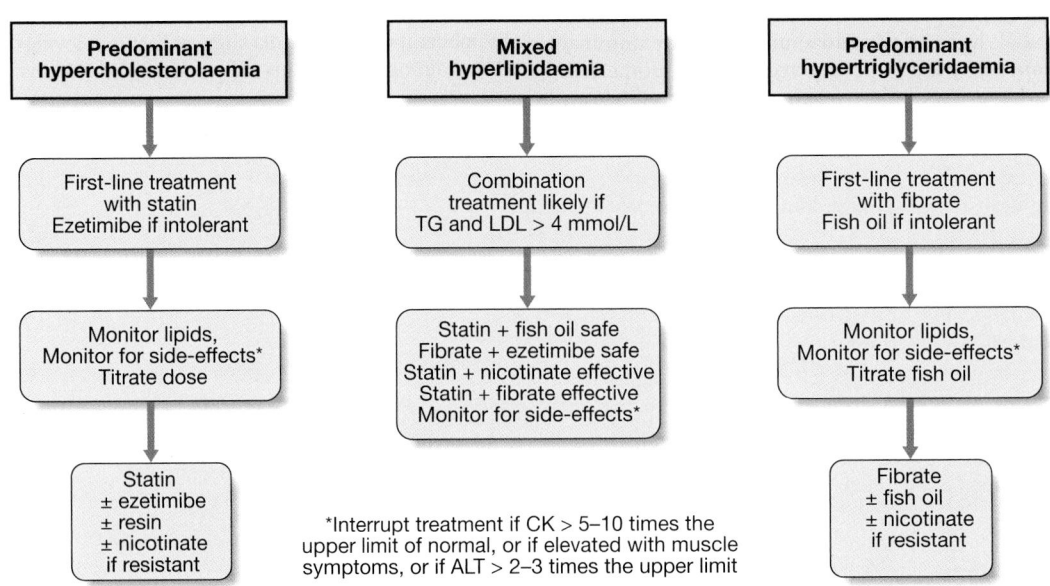

Fig. 16.16 Flow chart for the drug treatment of hyperlipidaemia. To convert TG in mmol/L to mg/dL, multiply by 88. To convert LDL-C in mmol/L to mg/dL, multiply by 38. (ALT = alanine aminotransferase; CK = creatine kinase)

Predominant hypercholesterolaemia

Predominant hypercholesterolaemia is treated with one or more of the cholesterol-lowering drugs.

HMGCoA reductase inhibitors (statins). Statins inhibit cholesterol synthesis, thereby up-regulating activity of the LDL receptor. This increases clearance of LDL and its precursor, IDL, resulting in a secondary reduction in LDL synthesis. Statins reduce LDL-C by up to 60%, reduce TG by up to 40% and increase HDL-C by up to 10%. They also reduce the concentration of intermediate metabolites such as isoprenes, which may lead to other effects such as suppression of the inflammatory response. There is clear evidence of protection against total and coronary mortality, stroke and cardiovascular events in high-risk patients (Box 16.28).

Statins are generally well tolerated and serious side-effects are rare (well below 2%). Liver function test abnormalities and muscle problems such as myalgia, asymptomatic increase in creatine kinase (CK), myositis and, infrequently, rhabdomyolysis are the most common. Side-effects are more likely in patients who are elderly, debilitated or receiving other drugs that interfere with statin degradation, which usually involves cytochrome P450 3A4 or glucuronidation.

EBM   16.28 Benefits of treating patients with hypercholesterolaemia with statins

'Meta-analysis of major RCTs involving over 90 000 subjects receiving statins for an average of 5 years showed reduced mortality from coronary artery disease, 19% (95% confidence interval 15–24%), stroke, 17% (12–22%) and all causes, 12% (9–16%) per 1 mmol/L reduction in LDL-C.'

• Baigent C, et al. Lancet 2005; 366:1267–1278.

Cholesterol absorption inhibitors, such as ezetimibe. These inhibit the intestinal mucosal transporter NPC1L1 that absorbs dietary and biliary cholesterol. Depletion of hepatic cholesterol up-regulates hepatic LDL receptor activity. This mechanism of action is synergistic with the effect of statins. Monotherapy with the standard 10 mg/day dose reduces LDL-C by 15–20%. Slightly greater (17–25%) incremental LDL-C reduction occurs when ezetimibe is added to statins. Ezetimibe is well tolerated, but its effect on cardiovascular disease endpoints is yet to be determined. Plant sterol-supplemented foods, which also reduce cholesterol absorption, lower LDL-C by 7–15%.

Bile acid sequestering resins, such as colestyramine, colestipol and colesevalam. These prevent the reabsorption of bile acids, thereby increasing de novo bile acid synthesis from hepatic cholesterol. As with ezetimibe, the resultant depletion of hepatic cholesterol up-regulates LDL receptor activity and reduces LDL-C in a manner that is synergistic with the action of statins. High doses (24 g/day colestyramine) can achieve substantial reductions in LDL-C and modest increases in HDL-C, but TG may rise. Resins are safe, but they may interfere with bioavailability of other drugs. Colesevalam may cause fewer gastrointestinal effects than older preparations. Development of specific inhibitors of the intestinal bile acid transporter may further improve tolerability of this class of agent.

Nicotinic acid (vitamin B3). In pharmacological doses, this reduces peripheral fatty acid release with the result that cholesterol and TG decline whilst HDL-C increases. Randomised clinical trials suggest a beneficial effect on atherosclerosis and cardiovascular events. Side-effects include flushing, gastric irritation, liver function disturbances, and exacerbation of gout and hyperglycaemia. Slow-release formulations and low-dose aspirin may reduce flushing. Combination therapy with the prostaglandin D2 receptor inhibitor laropiprant to further reduce flushing is being evaluated.

Routine treatment of predominant hypercholesterolaemia generally requires continuation of diet plus the use of a statin in sufficient doses to achieve target LDL-C levels. Patients who do not reach LDL targets on the highest tolerated statin dose, or who are intolerant of statins, may receive ezetimibe, plant sterols, nicotinic acid or resins. Nicotinic acid is very effective in combination with a statin, but caution is required because the risk of side-effects is increased.

Predominant hypertriglyceridaemia

Predominant hypertriglyceridaemia is treated with one of the triglyceride-lowering drugs (see Fig. 16.16).

Fibrates. These stimulate peroxisome proliferator activated receptor (PPAR) alpha, which controls the expression of gene products that mediate the metabolism of triglyceride and HDL. As a result, synthesis of fatty acids, triglyceride and VLDL is reduced, whilst that of lipoprotein lipase, which catabolises TG, is enhanced. In addition, production of Apo A1 and ATP binding cassette A1 is up-regulated, leading to increased reverse cholesterol transport via HDL. Consequently, fibrates reduce TG by up to 50% and increase HDL-C by up to 20%, but LDL-C changes are variable.

Fewer large-scale trials have been conducted with fibrates than with statins and the results are less conclusive, but reduced rates of cardiovascular disease have been reported with fibrate therapy in patients with low HDL-C levels and in subgroups of patients with the clinical picture of insulin resistance (e.g. TG > 2.3 mmol/L (200 mg/dL)). Fibrates are usually well tolerated, but share a similar side-effect profile to statins, including myalgia, myopathy and abnormal liver function tests. In addition, they may increase the risk of cholelithiasis and prolong the action of anticoagulants.

Highly polyunsaturated long-chain n-3 fatty acids. Eicosapentaenoic acid (EPA) and docosahexaenoic acid (DHA) comprise approximately 30% of the fatty acids in fish oil. EPA and DHA are potent inhibitors of VLDL TG formation. Intakes of greater than 2 g n-3 fatty acid (equivalent to 6 g of most forms of fish oil) per day lower TG in a dose-dependent fashion. Up to 50% reduction in TG may be achieved with 15 g fish oil per day. Changes in LDL-C and HDL-C are variable. Fish oil fatty acids have also been shown to inhibit platelet aggregation and improve cardiac arrhythmia in animal models. Dietary and pharmacological trials indicate that n-3 fatty acids reduce mortality from coronary heart disease. Fish oils appear to be safe and well tolerated.

Patients with predominant hypertriglyceridaemia who do not respond to lifestyle intervention can be treated with fibrates, fish oil or nicotinic acid, depending on individual response and tolerance. If target levels are not achieved, the fibrates or nicotinic acid and fish oil can be combined. Massive hypertriglyceridaemia may require more aggressive limitation of dietary

16

16

16.29 Management of hyperlipidaemia in the elderly

- **Prevalence of atherosclerotic cardiovascular disease:** greatest in old age.
- **Associated cardiovascular risk:** lipid levels become less predictive, as do other risk factors apart from age itself.
- **Benefit of statin therapy:** maintained up to the age of 80 years but evidence is lacking beyond this.
- **Life expectancy and statin therapy:** lives saved by intervention are associated with shorter life expectancy than in younger patients, and so the impact of statins on quality-adjusted life years is smaller in old age.

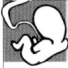

16.30 Dyslipidaemia in pregnancy

- **Lipid metabolism:** lipid and lipoprotein levels increase during pregnancy. This includes an increase in LDL-C which resolves post-partum. Remnant dyslipidaemia and hypertriglyceridaemia may be exacerbated during pregnancy.
- **Treatment:** dyslipidaemia is rarely thought to warrant urgent treatment so pharmacological therapy is usually contraindicated when conception or pregnancy is anticipated. Teratogenicity has been reported with systemically absorbed agents, and non-absorbed agents may interfere with nutrient bioavailability.
- **Monitoring:** cardiovascular disease is very unlikely amongst women of child-bearing age, but is possible in women with severe risk factor profiles or familial hypercholesterolaemia, when pre-conception cardiovascular review can be considered to ensure that the patient will be able to withstand the demands of pregnancy and labour.

fat intake (< 10–20% energy as fat). Any degree of insulin deficiency should be corrected because insulin is required for optimal activity of lipoprotein lipase. The initial target for patients with massive hypertriglyceridaemia is TG < 10 mmol/L (880 mg/dL), to reduce the risk of acute pancreatitis.

Mixed hyperlipidaemia

Mixed hyperlipidaemia can be difficult to treat. Statins alone are less effective first-line therapy once fasting TG exceeds around 4 mmol/L (350 mg/dL). Fibrates alone are first-line therapy for dysbetalipoproteinaemia, but they may not control the cholesterol component in other forms of mixed hyperlipidaemia. Combination therapy is often required. Effective combinations include: statin plus fish oil when TG is not too high; fibrate plus ezetimibe; statin plus nicotinic acid; or statin plus fibrate. Fibrates are effective in combination with statins but the risk of myopathy is increased. There is some evidence that fenofibrate is safer than gemfibrozil in this regard.

Monitoring of therapy

The effect of drug therapy can be assessed after 6 weeks (12 weeks for fibrates), and it is prudent to review side-effects, lipid response (see target levels above), CK and liver function tests at this stage. Follow-up should encourage continued compliance (especially diet and

exercise), and include monitoring for side-effects and cardiovascular symptoms or signs, and measurement of weight, blood pressure and lipids, as well as review of absolute cardiovascular disease risk status. Further assessment of CK and liver function tests is required only if relevant symptoms occur, or if statins are used in combination with fibrates, nicotinic acid or other drugs that may interfere with their clearance. If myalgia or weakness is associated with CK elevation > 5–10 times the upper limit of normal, or if sustained alanine aminotransferase (ALT) elevation > 2–3 times the upper limit of normal (and not accounted for by fatty liver, p. 956) is detected, treatment should be interrupted and alternative therapy sought.

DISORDERS OF HAEM METABOLISM— THE PORPHYRIAS

The porphyrias are rare disorders of the haem biosynthetic pathway (Fig. 16.17). Most of the described forms are due to partial enzyme deficiencies with a dominant mode of inheritance and mutations in the relevant genes. They are commonly classified as either hepatic or erythropoietic, depending on whether the major site of excess porphyrin production is in the liver or the red cell.

The porphyrias show a low penetrance in the order of 25%. Environmental factors are important in modifying disease expression in some forms. In the most common of these conditions, porphyria cutanea tarda (PCT), these include alcohol, excess iron, exogenous oestrogens and exposure to various chemicals. Many cases are now associated with hepatitis C infection.

Clinical features

The clinical features of porphyria fall into two broad categories, causes of which are shown in Figure 16.17.

Photosensitive skin manifestations, attributable to excess production and accumulation of porphyrins in the skin, cause pain, erythema, bullae, erosions, hirsutism and hyperpigmentation, and occur predominantly on areas of the skin that are exposed to sunlight (see Fig. 27.6, p. 1250). The skin also becomes especially sensitive to damage from minimal trauma.

The other pattern of presentation is with an acute relapsing and remitting neurological syndrome. This presents invariably with acute abdominal pain together with features of autonomic dysfunction such as tachycardia, hypertension and constipation. Other frequent associations include neuropsychiatric manifestations, hyponatraemia due to inappropriate ADH release (p. 436), and acute neuropathy (p. 1225), which is usually motor and sometimes causes respiratory failure.

There is no proven explanation for the episodic pattern of these attacks. However, they are often precipitated by alcohol, fasting, or drugs such as anticonvulsants, sulphonamides, oestrogen and progesterone, especially the oral contraceptive pill. In a significant number of cases, no precipitant can be identified.

Diagnosis

The diagnosis of porphyria and categorisation into various forms have traditionally relied on the pattern of the porphyrins and porphyrin precursors found in blood, urine and faeces (Box 16.31). This is straightfor-

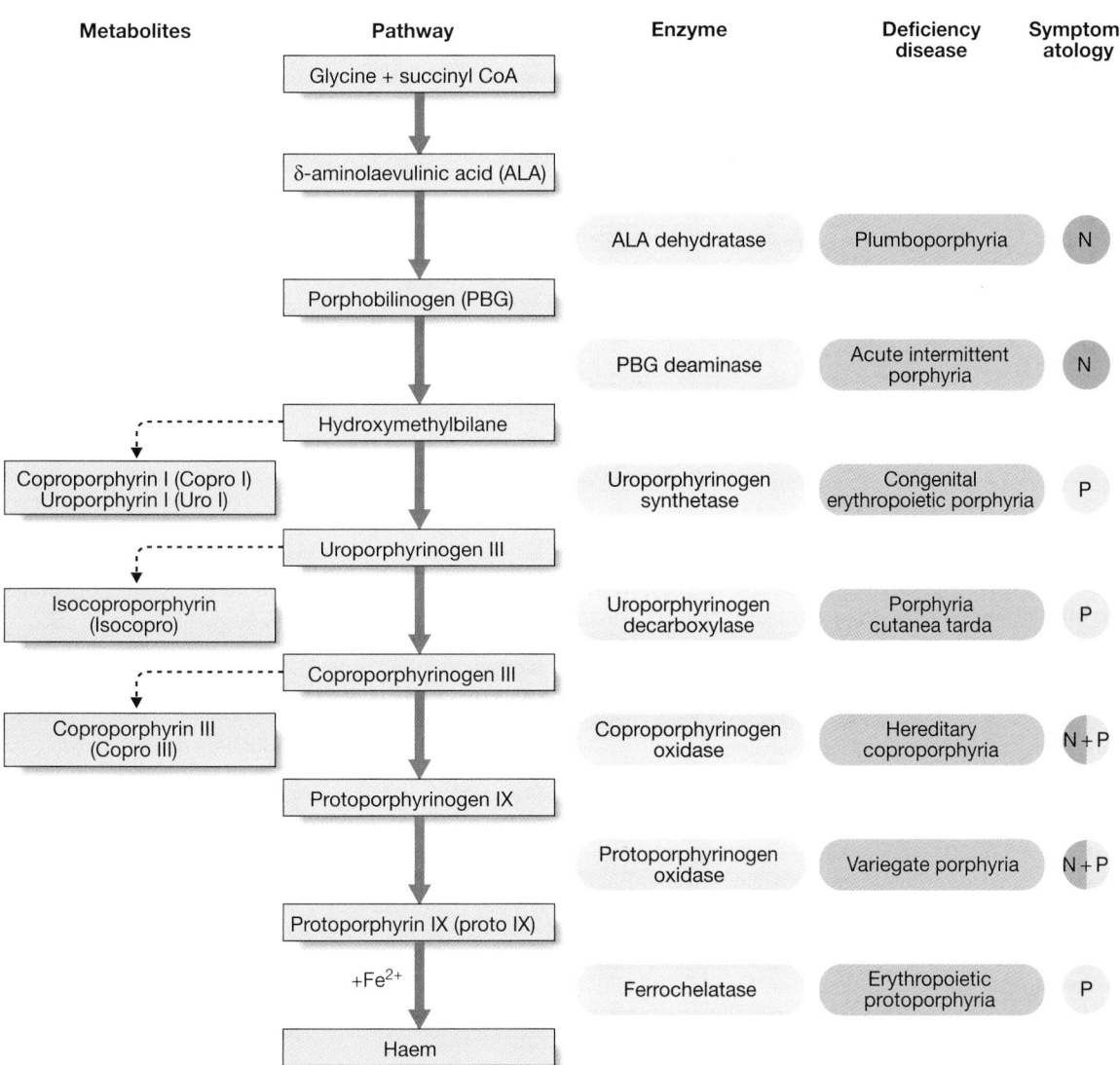

Fig. 16.17 Haem biosynthetic pathway and enzyme defects responsible for the porphyrias. (N = neurovisceral; P = photosensitive)

ward when the metabolites are significantly elevated, but this is not always the case.

More recently, measurement of the enzymes that are deficient in the various porphyrias has provided further important diagnostic information (e.g. PBG deaminase activity in red blood cells to diagnose acute intermittent porphyria). However, there is often considerable overlap between enzyme activities in normal and abnormal populations. Furthermore, some of the enzymes occur in the cell mitochondria, for which it is more difficult to obtain suitable specimens for analysis.

All the genes of the haem biosynthetic pathway have now been characterised. This has made it possible to identify affected individuals in families with known mutations, a significant advance considering that penetrance of porphyria is low and the majority of attacks do not occur without an identified precipitant. At this time, well over 150 mutations have been found to cause acute intermittent porphyria alone.

In the clinical situation if there are active cutaneous manifestations of porphyria, or when a subject pres-

ents in an acute attack, metabolite excretory patterns are always grossly abnormal and diagnostic of the particular porphyria. A normal metabolite profile in this circumstance effectively excludes porphyria. Furthermore, metabolites usually remain abnormal for long periods after an acute attack, and in some individuals never return to normal. The diagnosis may not be so straightforward in patients in remission, and investigation can be very difficult in patients with a positive family history but no clinical or metabolite manifestations. Porphyria rarely manifests before puberty, nor can it be readily diagnosed from metabolite patterns after menopause. In those circumstances, demonstration of a disease-specific mutation can now clarify the situation.

Management

For patients predisposed to neurovisceral attacks, general management includes avoidance of any agents known to precipitate acute porphyria. Specific management includes intravenous glucose, as provision of 5000 kilojoules per day can terminate acute attacks

16.31 Diagnostic biochemical findings in the porphyrias

Condition	Elevated porphyrins and precursors		
	Blood	Urine	Faeces
ALA dehydratase deficiency (plumboporphyria)	Proto IX*	ALA, Copro III*	
Acute intermittent porphyria (AIP)		ALA, PBG	
Congenital erythropoietic porphyria (CEP)	Uro I	Uro I	Copro I
Porphyria cutanea tarda (PCT)		Uro I	Isocopro
Hereditary coproporphyria (HCP)		ALA, PBG, Copro III	Copro III
Variegate porphyria (VP)		ALA, PBG, Copro III	Proto IX
Erythropoietic protoporphyria (EPP)	Proto IX		Proto IX

*The paradoxical rise in coproporphyrin III (Copro III) and protoporphyrin (Proto) in this very rare condition is poorly understood.
Refer to Figure 16.17 for metabolic pathways.

through a reduction in ALA synthetase activity. More recently, administration of haem (in various forms such as haematin or haem arginate) has been shown to reduce metabolite excretory rates, relieve pain and accelerate recovery. Cyclical acute attacks in women sometimes respond to suppression of the menstrual cycle using gonadotrophin-releasing hormone analogues.

There are few specific or effective measures to treat the photosensitive manifestations. The primary goal is to avoid sun exposure and skin trauma. Barrier sun creams containing zinc or titanium oxide are the most effective products. New colourless zinc creams have improved patient acceptance. Beta-carotene is used in some patients with erythropoietic porphyria with some efficacy. In porphyria cutanea tarda, a course of venesections to remove iron can result in long-lasting clinical and biochemical remission, especially if exposure to identified precipitants such as alcohol or oestrogens is reduced. Alternatively, a prolonged course of chloroquine therapy may be effective.

Further information

www.emedicine.com *The Nephrology link on this site contains a useful compendium of articles.*

www.kidneyatlas.org *See especially Vol. 1, Section 1: Disorders of water, electrolytes, and acid–base.*

www.lipidsonline.org *Summarises management strategies for dyslipidaemia.*

www.ncbi.nlm.nih.gov *The link to OMIM (Online Mendelian Inheritance in Man) provides updated information on the genetic basis of metabolic disorders.*

www.porphyria-europe.com and www.drugs-porphyria.org *An excellent resource on drug safety in porphyria.*

J. Goddard
A.N. Turner
L.H. Stewart

Kidney and urinary tract disease

17

CLINICAL EXAMINATION OF THE KIDNEY AND URINARY TRACT

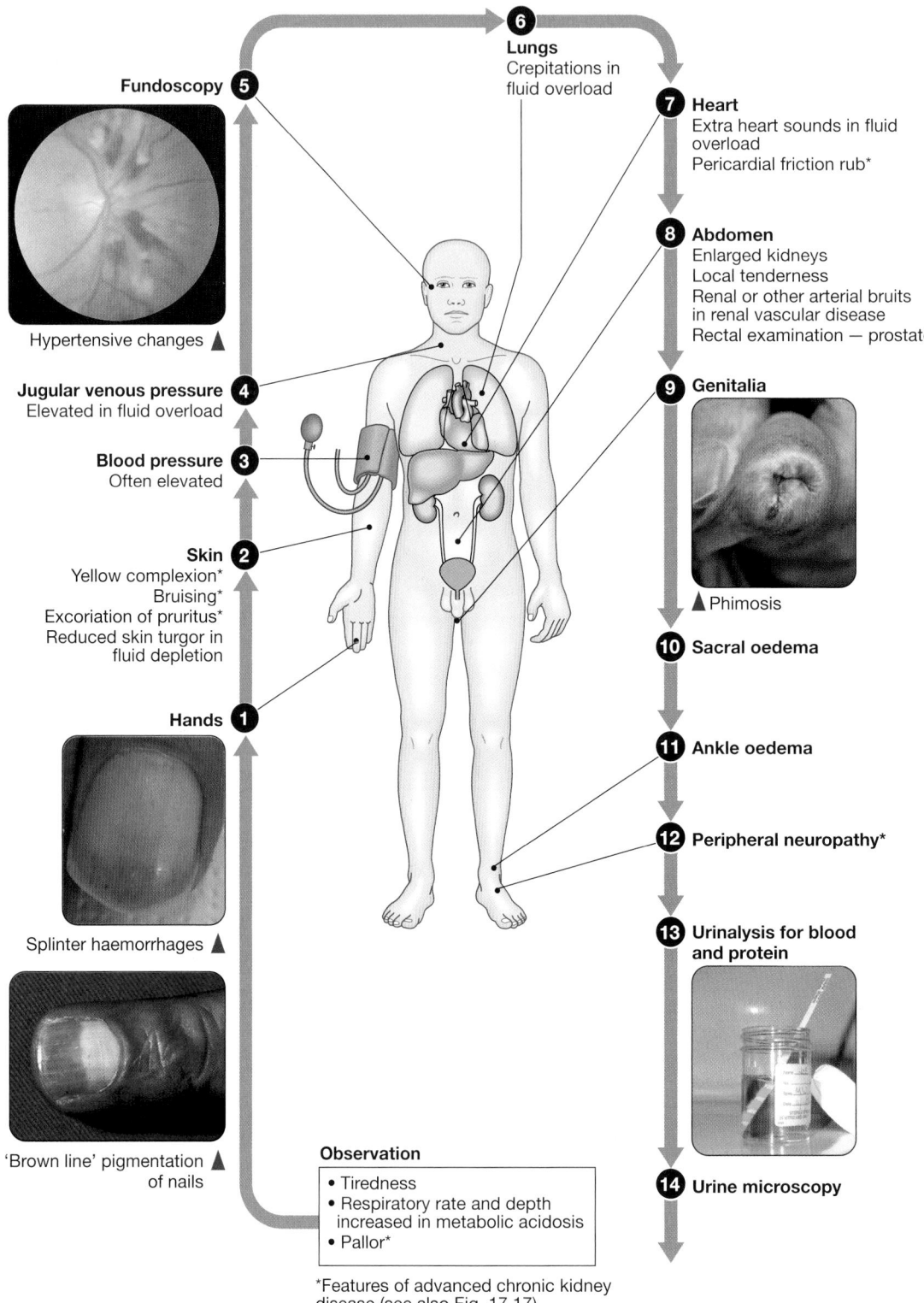

6 Lungs
Crepitations in fluid overload

Fundoscopy 5

Hypertensive changes ▲

7 Heart
Extra heart sounds in fluid overload
Pericardial friction rub*

8 Abdomen
Enlarged kidneys
Local tenderness
Renal or other arterial bruits in renal vascular disease
Rectal examination — prostate

Jugular venous pressure 4
Elevated in fluid overload

Blood pressure 3
Often elevated

9 Genitalia

▲ Phimosis

Skin 2
Yellow complexion*
Bruising*
Excoriation of pruritus*
Reduced skin turgor in fluid depletion

10 Sacral oedema

11 Ankle oedema

Hands 1

Splinter haemorrhages ▲

12 Peripheral neuropathy*

13 Urinalysis for blood and protein

'Brown line' pigmentation ▲
of nails

Observation
- Tiredness
- Respiratory rate and depth increased in metabolic acidosis
- Pallor*

14 Urine microscopy

*Features of advanced chronic kidney disease (see also Fig. 17.17)

Diseases of the kidneys and urinary tract are often clinically 'silent' and may be detected by biochemical testing, e.g. measurement of plasma creatinine or testing of urine. Severe renal disease may present with non-specific symptoms, e.g. tiredness or breathlessness due to renal failure and associated anaemia, or oedema due to fluid retention. In end-stage kidney disease, a wide range of physical signs may be present, as seen opposite.

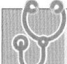
Cardinal features of kidney and urinary tract disease

Lower urinary tract symptoms

- *Dysuria, frequency, urgency:* lower urinary tract infection
- *Impaired urinary flow, hesitancy, dribbling of urine, incomplete emptying of bladder:* bladder outflow obstruction
- *Urinary retention, incontinence/ enuresis:* sphincter or bladder wall dysfunction

Upper urinary tract symptoms

- *Loin pain/tenderness:* renal infection, renal infarction or rarely obstruction and glomerulonephritis
- *Severe loin pain (renal or ureteric colic) ± radiation to iliac fossa, groin and genitalia:* acute obstruction of the renal pelvis and ureter by calculus or blood clot

Abnormal urine volume

- *Anuria or oliguria:* acute renal failure or obstruction to urine flow
- *Polyuria or nocturia:* failure to concentrate urine (e.g. diabetes insipidus, chronic kidney disease)

Abnormal urinary constituents

- *Proteinuria:* suggests glomerular disease; massive proteinuria causes oedema
- *Haematuria:* disease anywhere in the urinary tract

Hypertension

- Acute or chronic parenchymal disease or renovascular disease

Uraemia

- A group of symptoms and signs of advanced kidney disease

Diseases of the testes and epididymis

- Local swelling, pain and tenderness sometimes causing abdominal pain, inflammation and torsion

8 Abdomen

Technique for palpating the kidneys

- Lie the patient flat with abdominal muscles relaxed
- Place one hand posteriorly just below the lower ribs and the other anteriorly over the upper quadrant
- Push the hands towards each other as the patient breathes out; feel for the lower pole of the kidney moving down between the hands as the patient breathes in
- To confirm a palpable kidney, push the kidney backwards and forwards between the hands ('ballotting')
- Assess the size, surface and consistency of a palpable kidney; e.g. polycystic kidneys are often massively enlarged with an irregular, nodular surface

Possible findings

- Normal findings: the right kidney and lower pole of the left kidney may be palpable in normal slim adults
- Enlarged kidneys: polycystic kidney disease, hydronephrosis/pyonephrosis, solitary cyst, compensatory hypertrophy in a single kidney, renal tumours and renal amyloid
- Tender kidneys: may reflect infection or inflammation
- Transplanted kidney: palpable in the iliac fossa, with an overlying scar
- Distended bladder: smooth midline mass arising from the pelvis, dull to percussion
- Arterial bruits: on either side of the epigastrium, may indicate renal artery stenosis
- Testicular mass
- Prostate enlargement on rectal examination: benign enlargement is characteristically smooth and regular; an enlarged, hard, irregular prostate suggests prostatic cancer

14 Urine microscopy

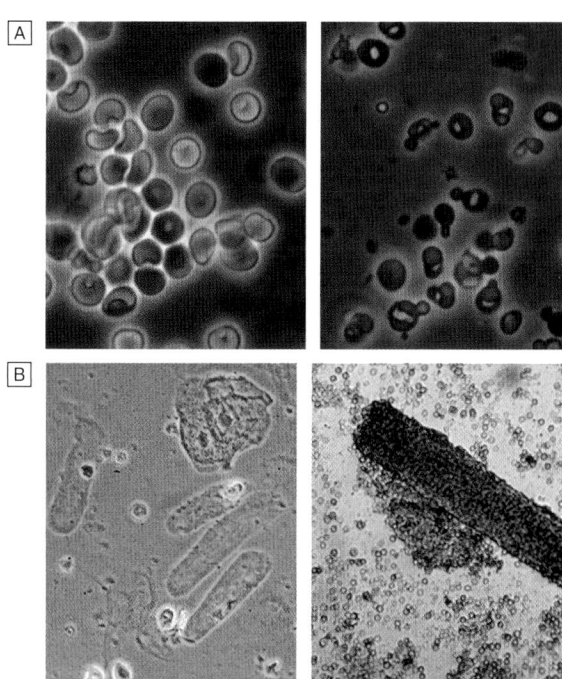

Urine microscopy. **A** Phase contrast images of red blood cells (× 400) showing on the right glomerular bleeding with many dysmorphic forms including acanthocytes (teardrop forms), and on the left bleeding from lower in the urinary tract. **B** On the left, phase contrast images show hyaline casts, a normal feature of urine (× 160). On the right, numerous red cells and a large red cell cast in acute glomerular inflammation (× 100, not phase contrast).

17

Renal medicine ranges from the management of common conditions (e.g. urinary tract infection) to the use of complex technology to replace renal function (e.g. dialysis and transplantation). There are close links with the surgical specialties of urology and transplantation. This chapter describes the common disorders of the kidneys and urinary tract which are encountered in everyday practice, as well as giving an overview of the highly specialised field of renal replacement therapy. Selective disorders of renal tubular function, which cause alterations in electrolyte and acid-base balance, are described in Chapter 16.

FUNCTIONAL ANATOMY AND PHYSIOLOGY

Functions of the kidneys

The kidneys are largely responsible for regulating the volume and composition of body fluids. This is achieved by making large volumes of an ultrafiltrate of plasma (120 mL/min, 170 L/day) at the glomerulus, and selectively reabsorbing components of this ultrafiltrate at points along the nephron. The rates of filtration and reabsorption are controlled by many hormonal and haemodynamic signals.

The kidney is primarily responsible for excretion of many metabolic breakdown products (including ammonia, urea and creatinine from protein, and uric acid from nucleic acids), drugs and toxins. These metabolites either are not reabsorbed from the filtrate, or are actively secreted into it.

In addition, the kidney has a number of hormonal functions. Three of these are particularly important:

- Erythropoietin is produced by interstitial peritubular cells in response to hypoxia. Replacement of erythropoietin reverses the anaemia of chronic kidney disease (p. 490).
- In vitamin D metabolism, the kidneys hydroxylate 25-hydroxycholecalciferol to the active form, 1,25-dihydroxycholecalciferol. Failure of this process contributes to the hypocalcaemia and bone disease of chronic kidney disease (p. 490).
- Renin is secreted from the juxtaglomerular apparatus in response to reduced afferent arteriolar pressure, stimulation of sympathetic nerves, and changes in sodium content of fluid in the distal convoluted tubule at the macula densa. Renin generates angiotensin II (see Fig. 20.19, p. 769), which causes aldosterone release from the adrenal cortex, constricts the efferent arteriole of the glomerulus and thereby increases glomerular filtration pressure (Fig. 17.1D). Angiotensin II also induces systemic vasoconstriction. By these mechanisms, the kidneys 'defend' circulating blood volume, blood pressure and glomerular filtration during circulatory shock. However, the same mechanisms lead to systemic hypertension in renal ischaemia.

Anatomy of the kidneys

Adult kidneys are 11–14 cm (three lumbar vertebral bodies) in length, and are located retroperitoneally on either side of the aorta and inferior vena cava. The right kidney is usually a few centimetres lower because the liver lies above it. Both kidneys rise and descend several centimetres with respiration.

Each kidney contains approximately 1 million functional units, or 'nephrons'. These consist of the glomerulus (where filtration of plasma occurs), proximal convoluted tubule, loop of Henle and distal convoluted tubule (where selective reabsorption of fluid and solutes from the filtrate occurs), and the collecting duct (see Fig. 16.2, p. 428). Of the daily filtrate of over 150 L, typically 99% is reabsorbed in the tubules. The collecting ducts of multiple nephrons drain into the renal pelvis and ureter (Fig. 17.1B). There is a rich blood supply (20–25% of cardiac output). Intralobular branches of the renal artery give rise to the glomerular afferent arterioles which supply the capillaries within the glomerulus. The efferent arteriole, leading from the glomerulus, supplies the distal nephron and medulla in a 'portal' circulation.

Glomeruli

Filtration occurs across the glomerular basement membrane (GBM), produced by fusion of the basement membranes of epithelial and endothelial cells (Fig. 17.1D). The glomerular capillary endothelial cells contain pores (fenestrae) which allow access of circulating molecules to the underlying GBM. On the outer side of the GBM, glomerular epithelial cells (podocytes) put out multiple long foot processes which interdigitate with those of adjacent epithelial cells (Fig. 17.1E). As well as maintaining the filtration barrier, podocytes are involved in the regulation of filtration and of GBM turnover. The third cell type, mesangial cells, lie in the central region of the glomerulus. They have similarities to vascular smooth muscle cells (e.g. contractility), but also some macrophage-like properties.

The filtration barrier at the glomerulus is normally almost absolute to proteins the size of albumin (67 kDa) or larger, while proteins of 20 kDa or smaller are able to filter freely. Between these sizes the ability of individual molecules to cross the GBM varies, e.g. according to charge. Little lipid is filtered.

Filtration pressure at the GBM is controlled by afferent and efferent arteriolar tone. Autoregulation maintains a constant glomerular filtration rate (GFR) by altering arteriolar tone over a wide range of systemic blood pressure and renal perfusion pressure. In response to a reduction in perfusion pressure, angiotensin II mediates constriction of the efferent arteriole, which restores filtration pressure as above.

Tubules and interstitium

Tubular cells are polarised, with a brush border (proximal tubular cells) and specialised functions at both basal and apical surfaces. As described on pages 428–429, different parts of the tubule serve distinct functions and carry a specific complement of transporter, channel and receptor molecules. Interstitial cells between tubules are less well understood. Fibroblast-like cells in the cortex produce erythropoietin in response to hypoxia.

Collecting system and lower urinary tract

The key functions of this part of the urinary system (Fig. 17.2) are to allow free passage of urine to the bladder, and to store urine in the bladder for controlled voiding (i.e. to maintain urinary continence).

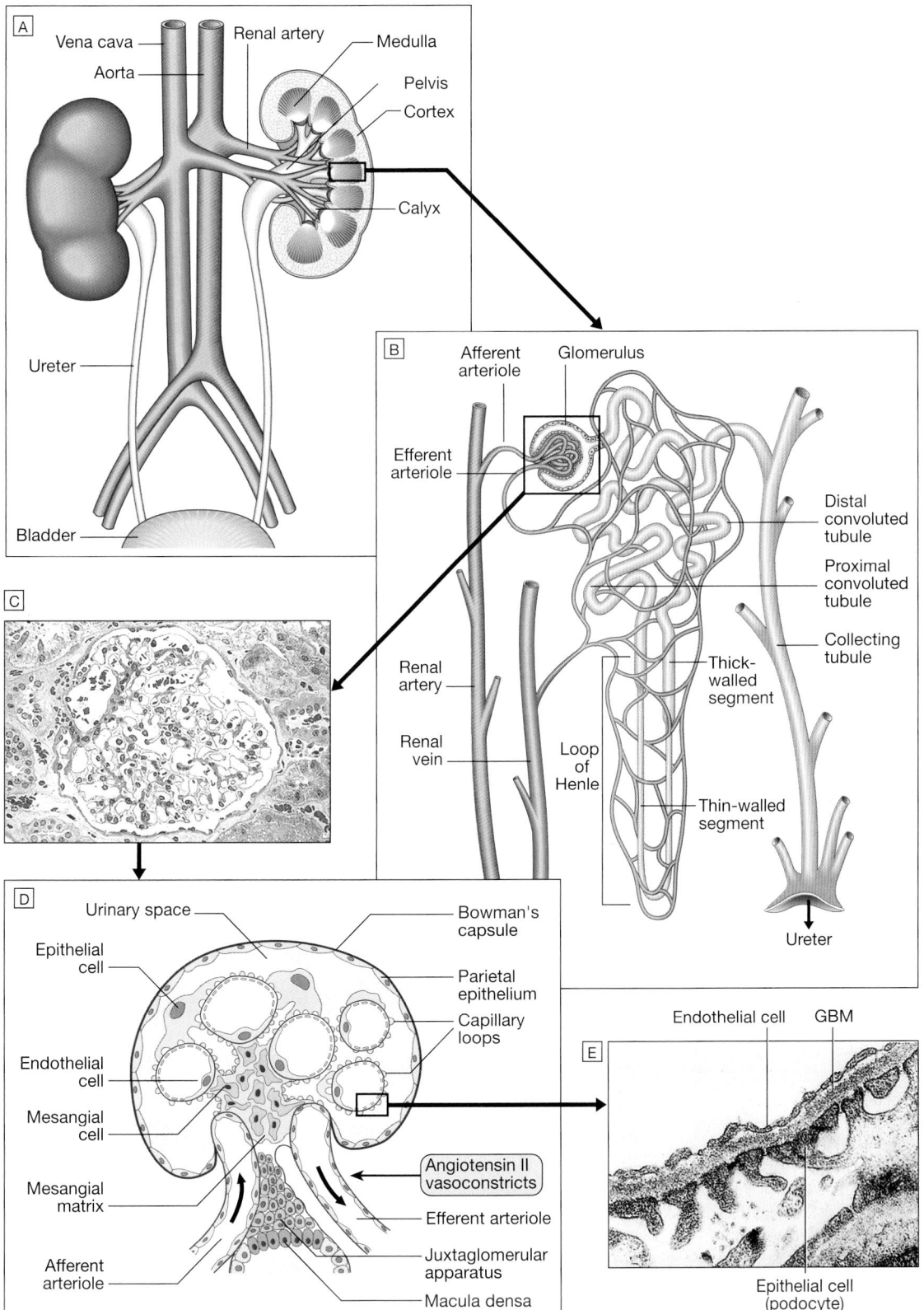

Fig. 17.1 Functional anatomy of the kidney. **A** Anatomical relationships of the kidney. **B** A single nephron. For the functions of different segments, see Figures 16.2 and 16.3 (pp. 428–429). **C** Histology of a normal glomerulus. **D** Schematic cross-section of a glomerulus showing five capillary loops, to illustrate structure and show cell types. **E** Electron micrograph of the filtration barrier. (GBM = glomerular basement membrane)

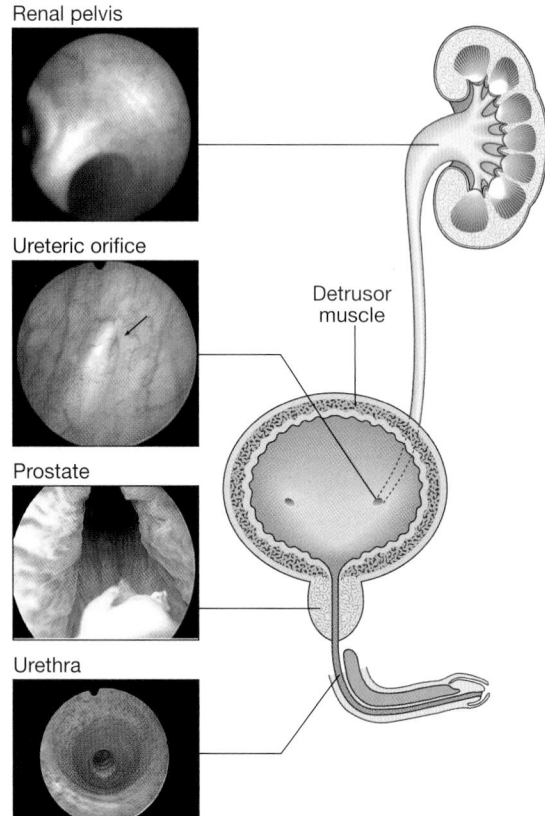

Renal pelvis

Ureteric orifice

Prostate

Urethra

Detrusor muscle

Fig. 17.2 Endoscopic views of the male urinary tract.

Mechanisms of micturition and urinary continence

Continence is dependent on anatomical structures (see Fig. 17.2) and on neurological and muscle (sphincter and detrusor) function. Parasympathetic nerves arising from S2–4 stimulate detrusor contraction, resulting in micturition. Sympathetic nerves arising from T10–L2 relay in the pelvic ganglia and produce detrusor relaxation and contraction of the bladder neck (both via α-adrenoceptors). The distal sphincter mechanism is innervated by somatic motor fibres from sacral segments S2–4 which reach the sphincter either by the pelvic plexus or via the pudendal nerves. Afferent sensory impulses pass to the cerebral cortex, from where reflex-increased sphincter tone and associated suppression of detrusor contraction inhibit micturition until it is appropriate.

These factors operate in a coordinated fashion in the micturition cycle, which has a 'storage' (or 'filling') phase and a 'voiding' (or 'micturition') phase (see Fig. 17.11, p. 476). During the filling phase, the high compliance of the detrusor muscle allows the bladder to fill steadily without a rise in intravesical pressure. As bladder volume increases, stretch receptors in its wall cause reflex bladder relaxation and increased sphincter tone. At approximately 75% bladder capacity there is a desire to void. Voluntary control is now exerted over the desire to void, which disappears temporarily. Compliance of the detrusor allows further increase in capacity until the next desire to void. Just how often this desire needs to be inhibited depends on many factors, not the least of which is finding a suitable place in which to void.

The act of micturition is initiated first by voluntary and then by reflex relaxation of the pelvic floor and distal sphincter mechanism, followed by reflex detrusor contraction. These actions are coordinated by the pontine micturition centre. Intravesical pressure remains greater than urethral pressure until the bladder is empty.

Erectile function

Blood inflow into the corpus cavernosum of the penis is under tonic sympathetic control via nerves from the thoracolumbar plexus which maintain smooth muscle contraction. In response to afferent input from the glans penis and from higher centres, pelvic splanchnic parasympathetic nerves actively relax the cavernosal smooth muscle via neurotransmitters such as nitric oxide, acetylcholine, vasoactive intestinal polypeptide (VIP) and prostacyclin, with consequent dilatation of the lacunar space. At the same time, draining venules are compressed, and possibly actively constricted, trapping blood in the lacunar space with consequent elevation of pressure and tumescence of the penis.

Prostate function

Exocrine glands within the prostate produce fluid which comprises about 20% of the volume of ejaculated seminal fluid and is rich in lipids and phospholipids. Seminal vesicle secretions account for about 60% and contain fructose and prostaglandins. The remainder of the ejaculate is formed in the testes.

Smooth muscle fibres within the prostate, under sympathetic control, contract at orgasm to move seminal fluid via ejaculatory ducts into the bulbar urethra (emission). Contraction of the bulbocavernosus muscle (via a spinal muscle reflex) then ejaculates the semen out of the urethra. These smooth muscle fibres can also effect some control over urine flow through the bulbar urethra.

INVESTIGATION OF RENAL AND URINARY TRACT DISEASE

Tests of function

Glomerular filtration rate (GFR)

GFR is the rate at which fluid passes into nephrons after filtration and measures renal excretory function. GFR is proportionate to body size so the reference range is usually expressed after correction for body surface area as 120 ± 25 mL/min/1.73 m^2. Direct measurement of GFR (Box 17.1) by injecting and measuring the clearance of compounds that are completely filtered and not reabsorbed by the nephron (inulin, radiolabelled ethylenediaminetetraacetic acid (EDTA)) is inconvenient and is usually reserved for special circumstances (e.g. for potential live kidney donors).

Serum levels of endogenous compounds excreted by the kidney give useful information. Blood urea is not the best test, as it increases with high protein intake (including absorption of blood from the gut after a gastrointestinal haemorrhage) and in catabolic states, and is reduced in liver failure (low production from protein) and anorexia or malnutrition (low protein intake). Furthermore, tubular reabsorption of urea is increased when concentrated urine is produced, elevating blood levels. However, variations in blood urea can be useful when combined with other estimates of renal function.

Serum creatinine reflects GFR more reliably than urea, as it is produced from muscle at a constant rate and almost completely filtered at the glomerulus. If muscle mass remains constant, changes in creatinine concentration reflect changes in GFR (Fig. 17.3). However, the reference range for creatinine values is wide because of variations in muscle mass; in patients with low muscle mass (e.g. the elderly) serum creatinine may not be above the reference range until GFR is reduced by > 50%.

A more accurate measurement of GFR can be obtained by creatinine clearance measurements, in which serum level is related to 24-hour urinary creatinine excretion, but 24-hour urine collections are difficult and often inaccurate. Alternatively, equations that estimate creatinine clearance or GFR from serum creatinine are available (see Box. 17.1). The MDRD equation has now become the accepted standard for 'estimated GFR' (eGFR). Although eGFR has important limitations (Box 17.2), its routine reporting by laboratories has enhanced recognition of moderate kidney damage, encouraged early deployment of protective therapies, and facilitated widespread adoption of the staging of chronic kidney disease (CKD), as shown in Box 17.3. This CKD staging recognises lesser degrees of renal damage than would previously have been labelled chronic renal failure (CRF). However, the advanced stages

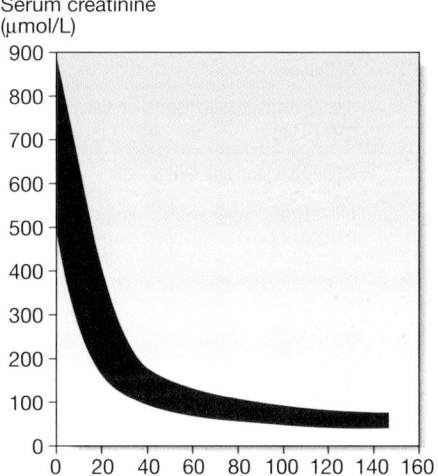

Fig. 17.3 Serum creatinine and the glomerular filtration rate (GFR). The inverse reciprocal relationship between GFR and serum creatinine is shown for a group of patients with renal disease. The red band indicates the range of values obtained. Note that some individuals have a GFR as low as 30–40 mL/min without serum creatinine rising out of the reference range.

of CKD are still often referred to as CRF despite the wide acceptance of CKD stages and terminology.

Urinalysis

Examination of an aliquot of urine provides important information on kidney function. Dipsticks may be used to screen for blood and protein semi-quantitatively (p. 479). Urine microscopy (p. 461) can detect red cells of glomerular origin and red cell casts, indicative of intrinsic renal disease. Flow cytometry can also be used to screen for white blood cells and bacteria. Crystals

---

17.1 How to estimate glomerular filtration rate (GFR)

Measuring GFR

- Direct measurement using labelled EDTA or inulin
- Creatinine clearance (CrCl)
    Minor tubular secretion of creatinine causes CrCl to exaggerate GFR when renal function is poor, and can be affected by drugs (e.g. trimethoprim, cimetidine)
    Needs 24-hr urine collection (inconvenient and often unreliable)

$$CrCl(mL/min) = \frac{\text{urine creatinine concentration } (\mu mol/L) \times \text{volume } (mL)}{\text{plasma creatinine concentration } (\mu mol/L) \times \text{time } (min)}$$

Estimating GFR with equations

- Cockcroft and Gault (C&G) equation
    Reasonably accurate at normal to moderately impaired renal function
    Estimates CrCl, not GFR
    Requires patient weight

$$CrCl \text{ (C\&G)} = \frac{(140 - \text{age in yrs}) \times \text{lean body weight (kg)} \times (1.22 \text{ males or } 1.04 \text{ females})}{\text{serum creatinine } (\mu mol/L)}$$

- The Modification of Diet in Renal Disease (MDRD) study equation (see www.renal.org/eGFR)
    Performs better than C&G at reduced GFR
    Requires knowledge of age and sex only
    Can be reported automatically by laboratories
    For limitations, see Box 17.2

    $eGFR = 186* \times (\text{creatinine in } \mu mol/L/88.4)^{-1.154} \times (\text{age in yrs})^{-0.203} \times (0.742 \text{ if female}) \times (1.21 \text{ if black})$

- No equations perform well in unusual circumstances, such as extremes of body (and muscle) mass, or in acutely unwell patients (see Box 17.2)

*A correction factor, either a value recommended by the laboratory/assay manufacturer or a default value of 186; see www.renal.org/ckd.
To convert creatinine in mg/dL to μmol/L, multiply by 88.4.

17.2 Limitations of eGFR

- It is only an estimate, least reliable at extremes of body composition (e.g. malnourished, amputees etc.) and in hospital inpatients (as it was derived from outpatients)
- Confidence intervals are wide (e.g. 90% of patients will have eGFR within 30% of their measured GFR, and 98% within 50%)
- Values are consistent in individuals, so changes mean more than absolute values
- Creatinine level must be stable over days; eGFR is not valid in assessing acute renal failure
- It tends to underestimate normal or near-normal function, so slightly low values should not be over-interpreted. Many laboratories report only up to > 60 mL/min/1.73 m² for this reason
- In the elderly, who constitute the majority of those with low eGFR, there is controversy about categorising people as having chronic kidney disease (CKD; Box 17.3) on the basis of eGFR alone, particularly at stage 3A, since there is little evidence of adverse outcomes when eGFR is > 50 unless there is also proteinuria
- eGFR is not valid in under-18s or during pregnancy
- The equation was originally validated in US patients and eGFR for any given creatinine was 21% higher in blacks. Performance in other racial groups is under investigation

17

ⓘ **17.3 Stages of chronic kidney disease (CKD)**

Stage[1]	Definition[2]	Description	Prevalence[3]	Clinical presentation[4]
1	Kidney damage with normal or high GFR (> 90)	Mild CKD	6.5%	Asymptomatic
2	Kidney damage and GFR 60–89			
3A[5] 3B[5]	GFR 45–59 GFR 30–44	Moderate CKD	4.5%	Usually asymptomatic Anaemia in some patients at 3B Most are non-progressive or progress very slowly
4	GFR 15–29	Severe CKD	0.4%	First symptoms often at GFR < 20 Electrolyte problems likely as GFR falls
5	GFR < 15 or on dialysis	Kidney failure		Significant symptoms and complications usually present Dialysis initiation varies but usually at GFR < 10

[1] Stages of CKD 1–5 were originally defined by the US National Kidney Foundation Kidney Disease Quality Outcomes Initiative 2002.
[2] Kidney damage means pathological abnormalities or markers of damage, including abnormalities in urine tests or imaging studies. Two GFR values 3 mths apart are required to assign a stage. All GFR values are mL/min/1.73 m².
[3] From the NHANES III study of > 15 000 US adults (Am J Kid Dis 2003; 41:1–12).
[4] For further information, see page 487.
[5] 3A/3B split recommended for UK in 2007/8, plus a suffix indicating presence of proteinuria (Albumin:creatinine ratio (ACR) > 30 or protein:creatinine ratio (PCR) > 50 mg/mmol), e.g. 3Ap, in view of the prognostic importance of proteinuria.

(e.g. of calcium oxalate, cysteine or urate) may be seen in renal calculus disease, although calcium oxalate and urate crystals are also sometimes found in normal urine that has been left to stand. Urine pH can provide diagnostic information in the assessment of renal tubular acidosis (p. 444), and a persistently low specific gravity may be found in diabetes insipidus (p. 792).

Timed (usually 24-hour) urine collections are now used less often to measure GFR or protein excretion (p. 480), but are still required to measure excretion rates of sodium and of solutes that can form renal calculi such as calcium, oxalate and urate (p. 510).

Other dynamic tests of tubular function, including concentrating ability (p. 792), ability to excrete a water load (p. 436) and ability to excrete acid (p. 426), are valuable in some circumstances.

Simple measurement of tubular excretory function can be made by comparison of blood and urine ratios of electrolytes to creatinine. Fractional excretion of sodium (= urinary Na/plasma Na × plasma creatinine/urine creatinine) is reduced in volume depletion when the tubules are avidly conserving sodium, and increased in the tubular damage associated with acute tubular necrosis.

Imaging techniques

Plain X-rays may show the renal outlines (if perinephric fat and bowel gas shadows permit), opaque calculi and calcification within the renal tract.

Ultrasound

This quick, non-invasive technique is the first and often the only method required for renal imaging. It can show renal size and position, detect dilatation of the collecting system (suggesting obstruction, Fig. 17.4), distinguish tumours and cysts, and show other abdominal, pelvic and retroperitoneal pathology. In addition, it can image the prostate and bladder, and estimate completeness

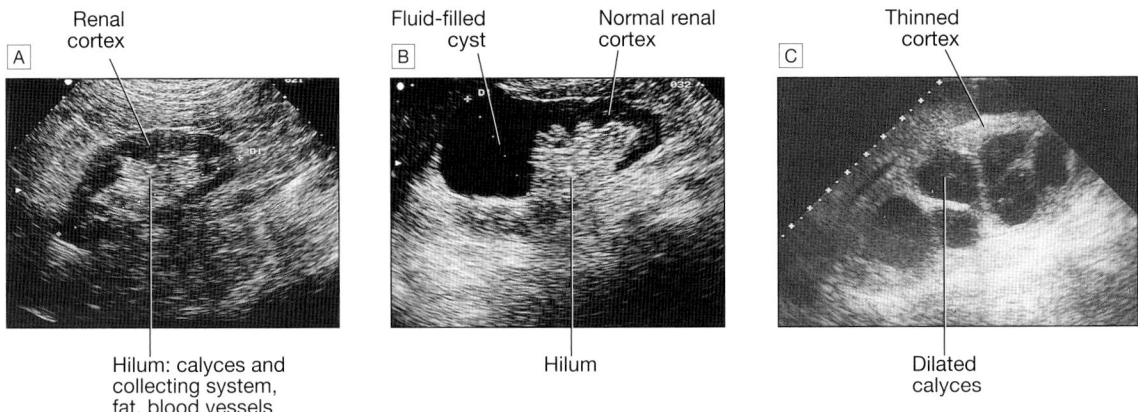

Fig. 17.4 Renal ultrasound. **A** Normal kidney. The normal cortex is less echo-dense (blacker) than the adjacent liver. **B** A simple cyst occupies the upper pole of an otherwise normal kidney. **C** The renal pelvis and calyces are dilated by a chronic obstruction to urinary outflow. The thinness and increased density of the remaining renal cortex indicate chronic changes.

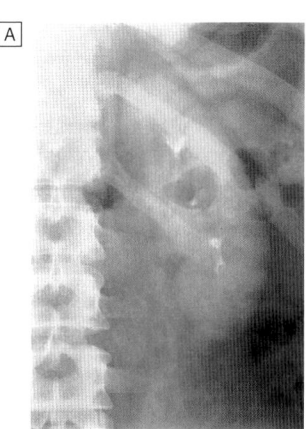 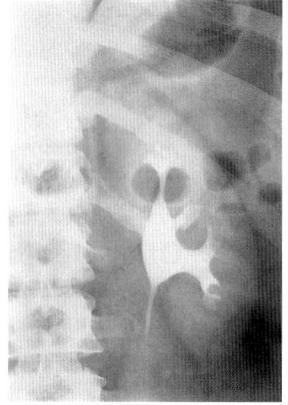 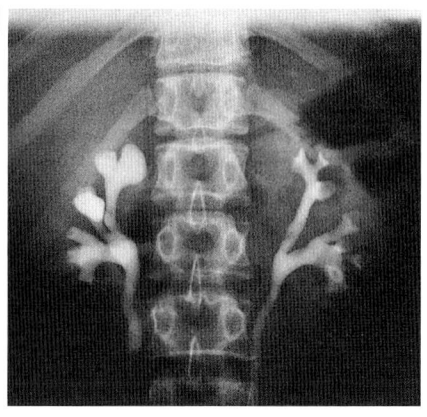

Fig. 17.5 Intravenous urography (IVU). A Normal nephrogram phase at 1 minute. B Normal collecting system at 5 minutes. C Bilateral reflux nephropathy (and chronic pyelonephritis) showing clubbing of the calyces which is particularly marked in the upper right pole.

of emptying in suspected bladder outflow obstruction. In CKD ultrasonographic density of the renal cortex is increased and corticomedullary differentiation is lost.

Doppler techniques can show blood flow in extra-renal and larger intrarenal vessels. The resistivity index is the ratio of peak systolic and diastolic velocities, and is influenced by the resistance to flow through small intrarenal arteries. It may be elevated in various diseases, including acute glomerulonephritis and rejection of a renal transplant. High peak velocities can also occur in severe renal artery stenosis.

However, renal ultrasound is operator-dependent, its stored images convey only a fraction of the information gained during the investigation, and it is often less clear in obese patients.

Intravenous urography (IVU)

While intravenous urography has been largely replaced by ultrasound and/or CT urography for routine renal imaging, the technique provides excellent definition of the collecting system and ureters, and remains superior to ultrasound for examining renal papillae, stones and urothelial malignancy (Fig. 17.5). X-rays are taken at intervals following administration of an intravenous bolus of an iodine-containing compound that is excreted by the kidney. An early image (1 minute after injection) demonstrates the nephrogram phase of renal perfusion in patients with an adequate renal arterial supply. This is followed by contrast filling the collecting system, ureters and bladder. The disadvantages of this technique are the need for an injection, time requirement, dependence on adequate renal function, and exposure to irradiation and contrast medium (Box 17.4).

Pyelography

Pyelography involves direct injection of contrast medium into the collecting system from above or below. It offers the best views of the collecting system and upper tract, and is commonly used to identify the cause of urinary tract obstruction (p. 475). Antegrade pyelography requires the insertion of a fine needle into the pelvicalyceal system under ultrasound or radiographic control. This approach is much more difficult and hazardous in a non-obstructed kidney. In the presence of

17.4 Renal complications of radiological investigations

Contrast nephrotoxicity

- An acute deterioration in renal function, sometimes life-threatening, commencing < 48 hrs after administration of i.v. radiographic contrast media

Risk factors

- Pre-existing renal impairment
- Use of high-osmolality, ionic contrast media and repetitive dosing in short time periods
- Diabetes mellitus
- Myeloma

Prevention

- Hydration, e.g. free oral fluids plus i.v. isotonic saline 500 mL then 250 mL/hr during procedure
- Avoid nephrotoxic drugs; withhold non-steroidal anti-inflammatory drugs (NSAIDs). Omit metformin for 48 hrs after procedure in case renal impairment occurs
- N-acetyl cysteine may provide weak additional protection (Box 17.5)
- If the risks are high, consider alternative methods of imaging

Cholesterol atheroembolism

- Typically follows days to weeks after intra-arterial investigations or interventions (p. 499)

Nephrogenic sclerosing fibrosis after MRI contrast agents

- Chronic progressive sclerosis of skin, deeper tissues and other organs, associated with gadolinium-based contrast agents
- Only reported in patients with renal impairment, typically on dialysis or with GFR < 15 mL/min/1.73m^2, but caution is advised in patients with GFR < 30 mL/min/1.73m^2

EBM **17.5 N-acetylcysteine and radiocontrast-induced nephropathy**

'Despite multiple randomised controlled trials and meta-analyses, the issue of whether N-acetylcysteine can prevent radiocontrast-induced nephropathy is still not resolved.'

- Bagshaw SM. Arch Int Med 2006; 166(2):161–166.

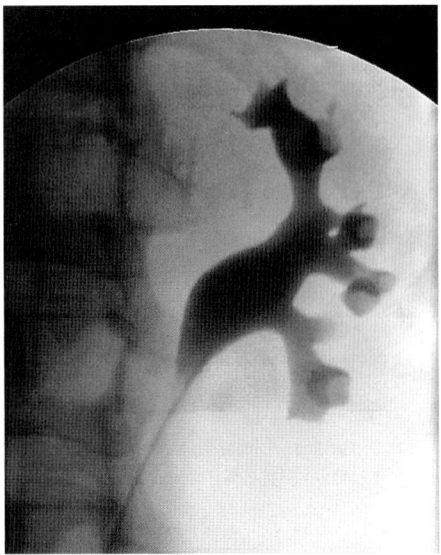

Fig. 17.6 Retrograde pyelography. The best views of the normal collecting system are shown by pyelography. A catheter has been passed into the left renal pelvis at cystoscopy. The anemone-like calyces are sharp-edged and normal. (Compare with the obstructed system shown in Fig. 17.9.)

obstruction, percutaneous nephrostomy drainage can be established, and often stents can be passed through any obstruction. Retrograde pyelography can be performed by inserting catheters into the ureteric orifices at cystoscopy (Fig. 17.6).

Renal arteriography and venography

The main indication for renal arteriography is to investigate suspected renal artery stenosis (p. 496) or haemorrhage. Therapeutic balloon dilatation and stenting of the renal artery may be undertaken, and bleeding vessels or arteriovenous fistulae occluded.

Computed tomography (CT)

CT is particularly useful for characterising mass lesions within the kidney (see Fig. 17.38A, p. 514), or combinations of cysts with masses. It gives clear definition of retroperitoneal anatomy regardless of obesity. Even without contrast medium it is better than IVU for demonstrating renal stones. In CT urography, after a first scan without contrast, scans are repeated during nephrogram and excretory phases. This gives more information but entails a substantially larger radiation dose than IVU.

CT arteriograms are reconstructed using a rapid-sequence technique in which images are obtained immediately following a large bolus injection of intravenous contrast medium. This produces high-quality images of the main renal vessels and is of value in trauma, renal haemorrhage and the investigation of possible renal artery stenosis. The speed of image acquisition also enables functional assessment and enhancement of vascular structures, e.g. angiomyolipomas. However, relatively large doses of contrast medium (see Box 17.4) are required.

Magnetic resonance imaging (MRI)

MRI offers excellent resolution and distinction between different tissues (see Fig. 17.32, p. 507). Magnetic resonance angiography (MRA) uses gadolinium-based contrast media, which may carry risks for patients with very low GFR (see Box 17.4). MRA can produce good images of main renal vessels but may miss branch artery stenoses.

Other tests
Radionuclide studies

These are functional studies requiring the injection of gamma ray-emitting radiopharmaceuticals which are taken up and excreted by the kidney, a process which can be monitored by an external gamma camera.

Diethylenetriamine-pentaacetic acid labelled with technetium (^{99m}Tc-DTPA) is excreted by glomerular filtration. DTPA injection and analysis of uptake and excretion provides information regarding the arterial perfusion of each kidney. Delayed peak activity and reduced excretion is seen in renal artery stenosis but the test is insufficiently reliable to use as a screening technique. In patients with significant obstruction of the outflow tract, DTPA persists in the renal pelvis (see Fig. 17.9, p. 473), and a loop diuretic fails to accelerate its disappearance. This can be useful in determining the functional significance of a 'baggy' or equivocally obstructed collecting system without undertaking pyelography.

Dimercaptosuccinic acid labelled with technetium (^{99m}Tc-DMSA) is filtered by glomeruli and partially bound to proximal tubular cells. Following intravenous injection, images of the renal cortex show the shape, size and relative function of each kidney (Fig. 17.7). This is a sensitive method for showing cortical scarring that is of particular value in children with vesico-ureteric reflux and pyelonephritis.

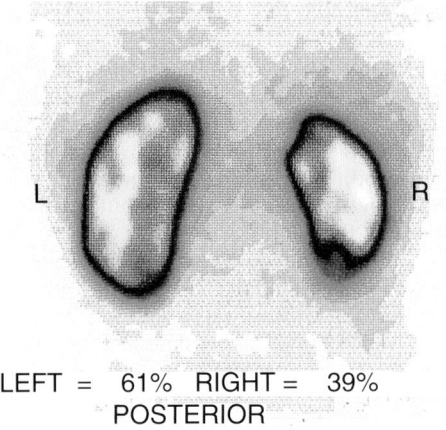

LEFT = 61% RIGHT = 39%
POSTERIOR

Fig. 17.7 DMSA isotope renogram. A posterior view is shown of a normal left kidney and a small right kidney (with evidence of cortical scarring at upper and lower poles) that contributes only 39% of total renal function.

Renal biopsy

Renal biopsy is used to establish the nature and extent of renal disease in order to judge the prognosis and need for treatment (Box 17.6). The procedure is performed transcutaneously with ultrasound or contrast radiography

17.6 Renal biopsy

Indications

- Acute renal failure that is not adequately explained
- CKD with normal-sized kidneys
- Nephrotic syndrome or glomerular proteinuria in adults
- Nephrotic syndrome in children that has atypical features or is not responding to treatment
- Isolated haematuria or proteinuria with renal characteristics or associated abnormalities

Contraindications

- Disordered coagulation or thrombocytopenia. Aspirin and other antiplatelet agents increase bleeding risk
- Uncontrolled hypertension
- Kidneys < 60% predicted size
- Solitary kidney (except transplants) (relative contraindication)

Complications

- Pain, usually mild
- Bleeding into urine, usually minor but may produce clot colic and obstruction
- Bleeding around the kidney, occasionally massive and requiring angiography with intervention, or surgery
- Arteriovenous fistula, rarely significant clinically

guidance to ensure accurate needle placement into a renal pole. Light microscopy, electron microscopy and immunohistological assessment of the specimen may all be required.

PRESENTING PROBLEMS IN RENAL AND URINARY TRACT DISEASE

The broad categories of renal and urinary tract disease, and their typical manifestations, are shown in Figure 17.8. It is convenient to divide these into pre-renal, renal and post-renal disorders.

Urinary tract infection (UTI)

In health, bacterial colonisation is confined to the lower end of the urethra and the remainder of the urinary tract is sterile (see Ch. 6). UTI is the most common bacterial infection managed in general medical practice and accounts for 1–3% of consultations. Up to 50% of women have a UTI at some time. The prevalence of UTI in women is about 3% at the age of 20, increasing by about 1% in each subsequent decade. In males UTI is uncommon, except in the first year of life and in men over 60, in

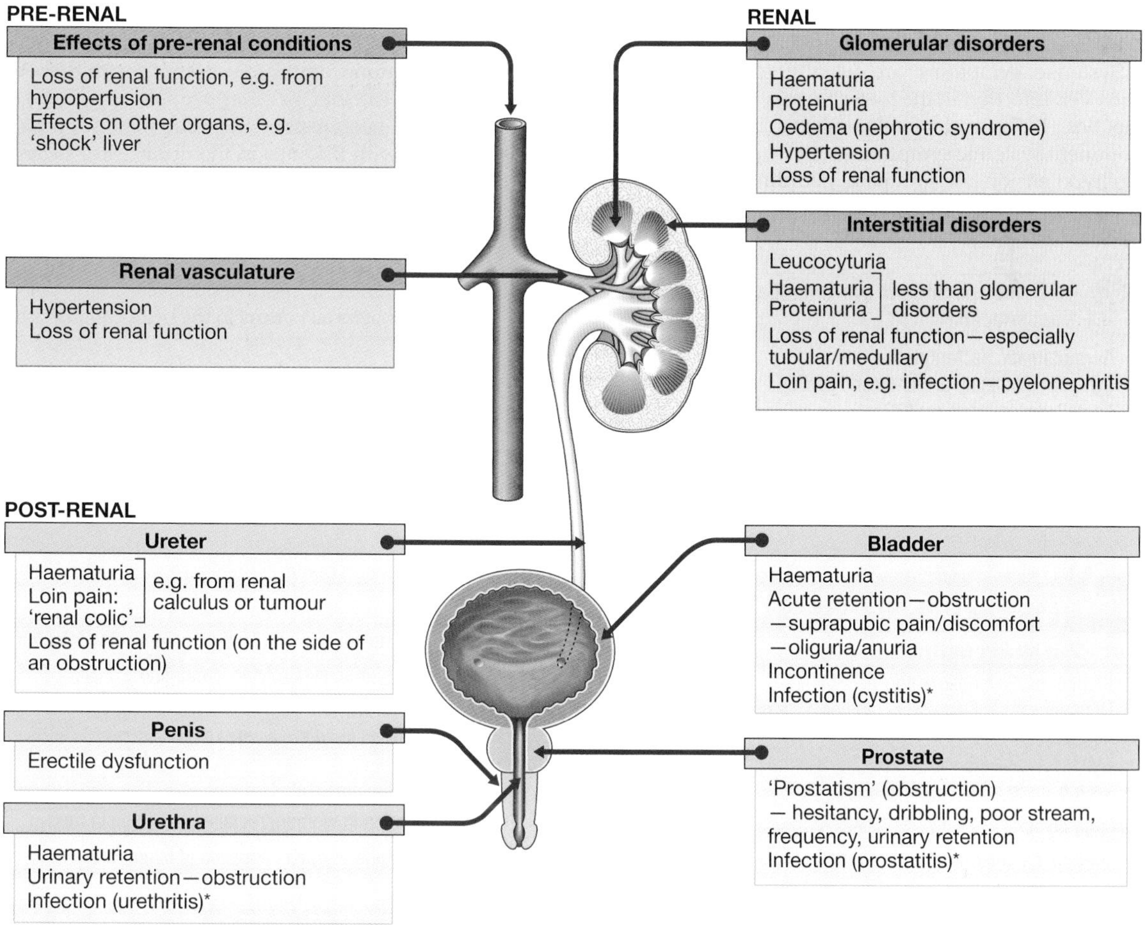

17

PRE-RENAL

Effects of pre-renal conditions

Loss of renal function, e.g. from hypoperfusion
Effects on other organs, e.g. 'shock' liver

Renal vasculature

Hypertension
Loss of renal function

RENAL

Glomerular disorders

Haematuria
Proteinuria
Oedema (nephrotic syndrome)
Hypertension
Loss of renal function

Interstitial disorders

Leucocyturia
Haematuria ⎤ less than glomerular
Proteinuria ⎦ disorders
Loss of renal function—especially tubular/medullary
Loin pain, e.g. infection—pyelonephritis

POST-RENAL

Ureter

Haematuria ⎤ e.g. from renal
Loin pain: ⎦ calculus or tumour
'renal colic'
Loss of renal function (on the side of an obstruction)

Penis

Erectile dysfunction

Urethra

Haematuria
Urinary retention—obstruction
Infection (urethritis)*

Bladder

Haematuria
Acute retention—obstruction
— suprapubic pain/discomfort
— oliguria/anuria
Incontinence
Infection (cystitis)*

Prostate

'Prostatism' (obstruction)
— hesitancy, dribbling, poor stream, frequency, urinary retention
Infection (prostatitis)*

Fig. 17.8 Classification and manifestations of renal and urinary tract disease. Consequences of loss of renal function and effects on other organs are described on pages 482–492. (*Lower urinary tract infection: haematuria, dysuria, frequency, urgency, cloudy and smelly urine.)

whom urinary tract obstruction due to prostatic hypertrophy may occur. The most common presentation is with acute urethritis and cystitis, although this is part of a spectrum of severity (Box 17.7).

Aetiology and risk factors

Urine is an excellent culture medium for bacteria; in addition, the urothelium of susceptible persons may have more receptors to which virulent strains of *Escherichia coli* become adherent. In women, the ascent of organisms into the bladder is easier than in men; the urethra is shorter and absence of bactericidal prostatic secretions may be relevant. Sexual intercourse may cause minor urethral trauma and transfer bacteria from the perineum into the bladder. Instrumentation of the bladder may also introduce organisms. Multiplication of organisms then depends on a number of factors, including the size of the inoculum and virulence of the bacteria. Conditions which predispose to UTI are shown in Box 17.8.

Clinical assessment

Typical features of cystitis and urethritis include:
- abrupt onset of frequency of micturition and urgency
- scalding pain in the urethra during micturition (dysuria)
- suprapubic pain during and after voiding
- intense desire to pass more urine after micturition, due to spasm of the inflamed bladder wall (strangury)
- urine that may appear cloudy and have an unpleasant odour
- microscopic or visible haematuria.

Systemic symptoms are usually slight or absent. However, infection in the lower urinary tract can spread (see Box 17.7); acute pyelonephritis is suggested by prominent systemic symptoms with fever, rigors, vomiting, hypotension and loin pain, guarding or tenderness, and may be an indication for hospitalisation. Only about

30% of patients with acute pyelonephritis have associated symptoms of cystitis or urethritis. Prostatitis is suggested by systemic symptoms and prostatic tenderness on rectal examination.

The differential diagnosis of lower urinary tract symptoms includes urethritis due to sexually transmitted disease, notably chlamydia (p. 412) or Reiter's syndrome. Some patients, usually female, have symptoms suggestive of urethritis and cystitis but no bacteria are cultured from the urine (the 'urethral syndrome'). Possible explanations include infection with organisms not readily cultured by ordinary methods (e.g. *Chlamydia*, certain anaerobes), intermittent or low-count bacteriuria, reaction to toiletries or disinfectants, symptoms related to sexual intercourse, or post-menopausal atrophic vaginitis.

The differential diagnosis of acute pyelonephritis includes acute appendicitis, diverticulitis, cholecystitis, salpingitis, ruptured ovarian cyst or ectopic pregnancy. In perinephric abscess, there is marked pain and tenderness, and often bulging of the loin on the affected side. Patients are extremely ill, with fever, leucocytosis and positive blood cultures, but urinary symptoms are absent and urine contains neither pus cells nor organisms.

Investigations

An approach to investigation is shown in Box 17.9.

In an otherwise healthy woman with a single lower urinary tract infection, urine culture prior to treatment is not mandatory. It is necessary, however, in patients with recurrent infection or after failure of initial treatment, during pregnancy, or in patients susceptible to serious infection (e.g. the immunocompromised, those with diabetes or an indwelling catheter, or older people—Box 17.10).

Definitive diagnosis rests on the combination of typical clinical features with findings in the urine. Most urinary pathogens can reduce nitrate to nitrite, and neutrophils and nitrites can usually be detected in symptomatic infections by urine dipstick tests for leucocyte esterase and nitrite, respectively. The absence of both nitrites and leucocyte esterase in the urine makes UTI unlikely. Interpretation of bacterial counts in the urine, and of what

---

17.7 The spectrum of presentations of urinary tract infection

- Asymptomatic bacteriuria
- Symptomatic acute urethritis and cystitis
- Acute pyelonephritis (p. 472)
- Acute prostatitis (p. 514)
- Septicaemia (usually Gram-negative bacteria)

17.8 Risk factors for urinary tract infection

Incomplete bladder emptying

- Bladder outflow obstruction
- Neurological problems (e.g. multiple sclerosis, diabetic neuropathy)
- Gynaecological abnormalities (e.g. uterine prolapse)
- Vesico-ureteric reflux (p. 509)

Foreign bodies

- Urethral catheter or ureteric stent

Loss of host defences

- Atrophic urethritis and vaginitis in post-menopausal women
- Diabetes mellitus

17.9 Investigation of patients with urinary tract infection

All patients

- Dipstick* estimation of nitrite, leucocyte esterase and glucose
- Microscopy/cytometry of urine for white blood cells, organisms
- Urine culture

Infants, children, and anyone with fever or complicated infection

- Full blood count; urea, electrolytes, creatinine
- Blood cultures

Pyelonephritis; males; children; women with recurrent infections

- Renal tract ultrasound or CT
- Pelvic examination in women, rectal examination in men

Continuing haematuria or other suspicion of bladder lesion

- Cystoscopy

*May substitute for microscopy and culture in simple uncomplicated infection.

17.10 Urinary infection in old age

- **Prevalence of asymptomatic bacteriuria**: rises with age. Amongst the most frail in institutional care it rises to 40% in women and 30% in men.
- **Contributory factors**: include an increased prevalence of underlying structural abnormalities, post-menopausal oestrogen deficiency and increased residual urine in women, and prostatic hypertrophy with reduced bactericidal activity of prostatic secretions in men.
- **Decision to treat**: there is little evidence of benefit from treating asymptomatic bacteriuria in old age. It does not improve chronic incontinence or decrease mortality or morbidity from symptomatic urinary infection. It risks adverse effects from the antibiotic and promoting the emergence of resistant organisms.
- **Source of infection**: the urinary tract is the most frequent source of bacteraemia in older patients admitted to hospital.
- **Incontinence**: new or increased incontinence is a common presentation of UTI in older women.
- **Treatment**: post-menopausal women with acute lower urinary tract symptoms may require longer than 3 days' therapy.

is a 'significant' culture result, is based on probabilities. Urine taken by suprapubic aspiration should be sterile, so the presence of any organisms is significant. If the patient has symptoms and there are neutrophils in the urine, a small number of organisms is significant. In asymptomatic patients, $> 10^5$ organisms/mL is usually regarded as significant (asymptomatic bacteriuria, see below).

Typical organisms causing UTI in the community include *E. coli* derived from the gastrointestinal tract (about 75% of infections), *Proteus* spp., *Pseudomonas* spp., streptococci and *Staphylococcus epidermidis*. In hospital, *E. coli* still predominates, but *Klebsiella* or streptococci are more common. Certain strains of *E. coli* have a particular propensity to invade the urinary tract.

Investigations to detect underlying predisposing factors for UTI are used selectively, most commonly in patients with recurrent infections (see Box 17.9).

Management

Antibiotics are recommended in all cases of proven UTI (Box 17.11). If urine culture has been performed, treatment may be started while awaiting the result. For infection of the lower urinary tract treatment for 3 days

17

17.11 Antibiotic regimens for urinary tract infection (UTI) in adults

Scenario	Drug	Regimen	Duration
Cystitis and uncomplicated UTI			
First choice	Trimethoprim	200 mg 12-hourly	
Second choices*	Amoxicillin	250 mg 8-hourly	
	Nitrofurantoin	50 mg 6-hourly	3 days in women, 10 days in men
	Cefalexin	250 mg 6-hourly	
	Ciprofloxacin	100 mg 12-hourly	
	Co-amoxiclav	250/125 mg 8-hourly	
In pregnancy	Cephalexin	250 mg 6-hourly	7 days
	Amoxicillin	250 mg 8-hourly	
	(Avoid trimethoprim and quinolones)		
Prophylactic therapy			
First choice	Trimethoprim	100 mg at night	
Second choices	Nitrofurantoin	50 mg at night	Continuous
	Co-amoxiclav	250/125 mg at night	
Pyelonephritis and complicated UTI (i.e. with associated systemic toxicity)			
First choices	Co-amoxiclav	500/125 mg 8-hourly	10 days
	Ciprofloxacin	500 mg 12-hourly	
Second choices*	In seriously ill patients start i.v. treatment, e.g.		
	Cefuroxime	750 mg 8-hourly	7–14 days
	Gentamicin	Dose adjusted to renal function and plasma gentamicin levels	
Epididymo-orchitis			
First choice	Ciprofloxacin	500 mg 12-hourly	14 days
Second choice	Consider screening and treatment for chlamydia (p. 421) in young men		
Acute prostatitis			
First choice	Trimethoprim	200 mg 12-hourly	28 days
Second choice*	Ciprofloxacin	500 mg 12-hourly	

*Guided by sensitivities of organism on culture.

is the norm and is less likely to induce significant alterations in bowel flora than more prolonged therapy. Trimethoprim is the usual choice for initial treatment; however, between 10% and 40% of organisms causing UTI are resistant to trimethoprim, the lower rates being seen in community-based practice. Nitrofurantoin, quinolone antibiotics such as ciprofloxacin and norfloxacin, and cefalexin are also generally effective. Co-amoxiclav or amoxicillin should only be used when the organism is known to be sensitive. Penicillins and cephalosporins are safe to use in pregnancy but trimethoprim, sulphonamides, quinolones and tetracyclines should be avoided.

In more severe infection, antibiotics are continued for 7–14 days and may require intravenous therapy with a cephalosporin, quinolone or gentamicin (see Box 17.11), later switching to an oral agent.

A fluid intake of at least 2 L/day is usually recommended, although this is not based on evidence and may make matters worse for patients with severe dysuria. Urinary alkalinising agents such as potassium citrate may help symptomatically but are not of proven efficacy.

Persistent or recurrent UTI

If the causative organism persists on repeat culture despite treatment, or if there is reinfection with any organism after an interval, then an underlying cause is more likely to be present (see Box 17.8) and more detailed investigation is justified (see Box 17.9). In women, recurrent infections are common and further investigation is only justified if infections are frequent (three or more per year) or unusually severe. Recurrent UTI, particularly in the presence of an underlying cause, may result in permanent renal damage, whereas uncomplicated infections rarely (if ever) do so (see chronic pyelonephritis, p. 509).

If an underlying cause cannot be removed, suppressive antibiotic therapy (see Box 17.11) can be used to prevent recurrence and reduce the risk of septicaemia and renal damage. Urine is cultured at regular intervals; a regime of two or three antibiotics in sequence, rotating every 6 months, is often used in an attempt to reduce the emergence of resistant organisms. Other simple measures may help to prevent recurrence (Box 17.12).

17.12 Prophylactic measures to be adopted by women with recurrent urinary infections

- Fluid intake of at least 2 L/day
- Regular complete emptying of bladder
- Good personal hygiene
- Emptying of the bladder before and after sexual intercourse
- Cranberry juice may be effective

Asymptomatic bacteriuria

This is defined as > 10^5 organisms/mL in the urine of apparently healthy asymptomatic patients. Approximately 1% of children under the age of 1, 1% of schoolgirls, 0.03% of schoolboys and men, 3% of non-pregnant adult women and 5% of pregnant women have asymptomatic bacteriuria. It is increasingly common in those aged over 65. There is no evidence that this condition causes renal scarring in adults who are

not pregnant and have a normal urinary tract, and in general, treatment is not indicated. However, up to 30% will develop symptomatic infection within 1 year. Treatment is required in infants, pregnant women and those with urinary tract abnormalities.

Catheter-related bacteriuria

In patients with a urethral catheter, bacteriuria increases the risk of Gram-negative bacteraemia fivefold. However, bacteriuria is common, and almost universal during long-term catheterisation. Treatment is usually avoided in asymptomatic patients, as this may promote antibiotic resistance. Careful sterile insertion technique is important, and the catheter should be removed as soon as it is not required.

Acute pyelonephritis

The kidneys are infected in a minority of patients with UTI. Acute renal infection (pyelonephritis) presents as a classic triad of loin pain, fever and tenderness over the kidneys. The renal pelvis is inflamed and small abscesses are often evident in the renal parenchyma (see Fig. 17.31C, p. 505).

Renal infection is almost always caused by organisms ascending from the bladder, and the bacterial profile is the same as for lower urinary tract infection (p. 471). Rarely, bacteraemia may give rise to renal or perinephric abscesses, most commonly due to staphylococci. Predisposing factors such as cysts or renal scarring facilitate infection.

Rarely, acute pyelonephritis is associated with papillary necrosis. Fragments of renal papillary tissue are passed per urethra and can be identified histologically. They may cause ureteric obstruction and, if this occurs bilaterally or in a single kidney, may cause acute renal failure. Predisposing factors include diabetes mellitus, chronic urinary obstruction, analgesic nephropathy and sickle-cell disease. A necrotising form of pyelonephritis with gas formation, 'emphysematous pyelonephritis', is occasionally seen in patients with diabetes mellitus. Xanthogranulomatous pyelonephritis is a chronic infection that can resemble a tumour. It is usually associated with obstruction, is characterised by accumulation of foamy macrophages and generally requires nephrectomy. Infection of cysts in polycystic kidney disease (p. 506) requires prolonged antibiotic treatment.

Appropriate investigations are shown in Box 17.9 and management is described above and in Box 17.11. Intravenous rehydration may be required in severe cases. If complicated infection is suspected or response to treatment is not prompt, urine should be recultured and renal tract ultrasound performed to exclude urinary tract obstruction or a perinephric collection. If obstruction is present, drainage by a percutaneous nephrostomy should be considered.

Loin pain

Dull ache in the loin is rarely due to renal disease but the differential diagnosis includes renal stone, renal tumour, acute pyelonephritis or urinary tract obstruction. Causes of obstruction are shown in Figure 17.9. Upper urinary tract obstruction is most commonly caused by a congenital abnormality of the pelvi-ureteric junction (PUJ,

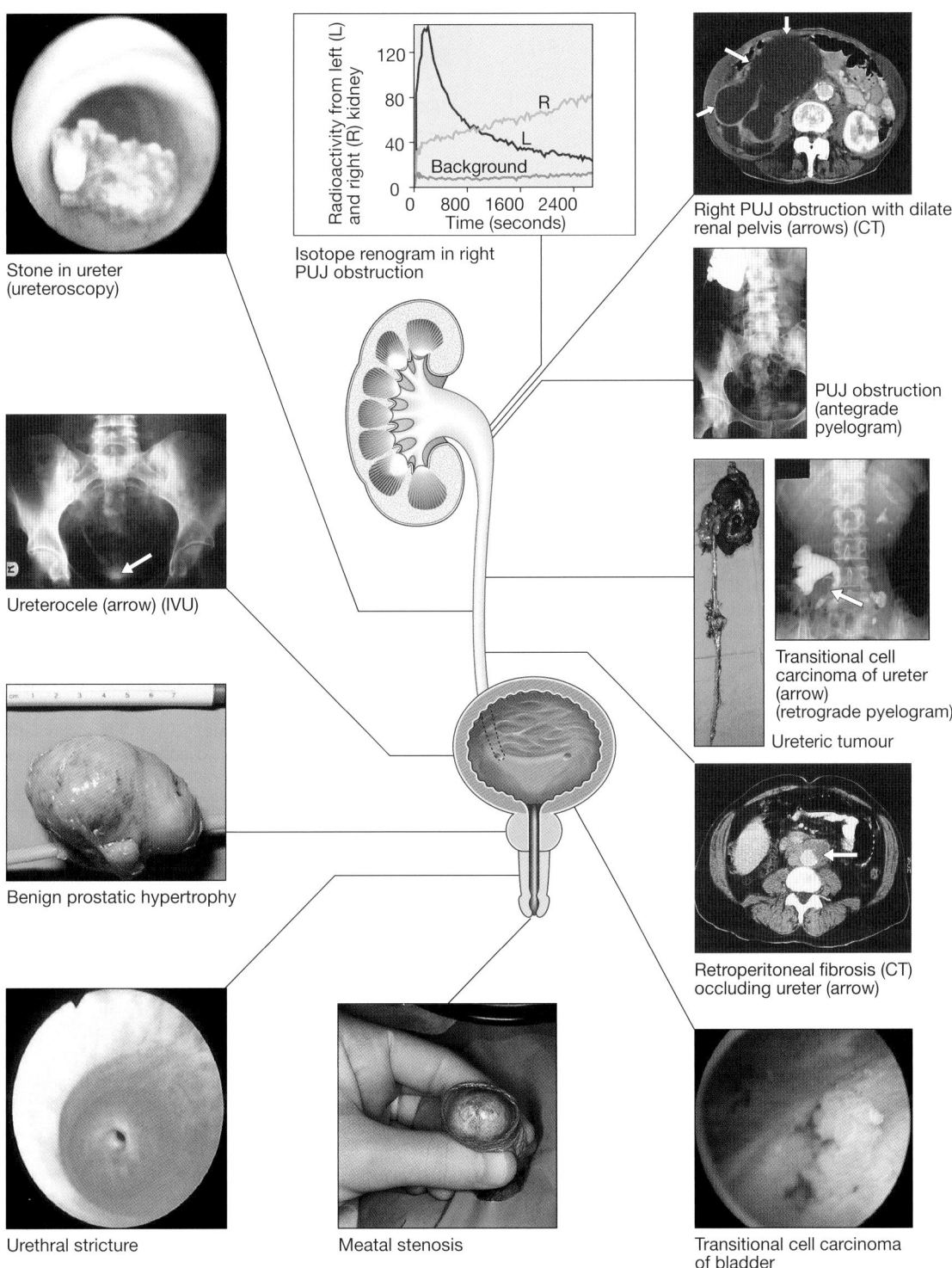

Stone in ureter
(ureteroscopy)

Isotope renogram in right
PUJ obstruction

Right PUJ obstruction with dilated
renal pelvis (arrows) (CT)

PUJ obstruction
(antegrade
pyelogram)

Ureterocele (arrow) (IVU)

Transitional cell
carcinoma of ureter
(arrow)
(retrograde pyelogram)

Ureteric tumour

Benign prostatic hypertrophy

Retroperitoneal fibrosis (CT)
occluding ureter (arrow)

Urethral stricture

Meatal stenosis

Transitional cell carcinoma
of bladder

Fig. 17.9 Urinary tract obstruction. Some common causes and their locations. (PUJ = pelvi-ureteric junction)

p. 509), when typically loin pain is precipitated by a large fluid intake. Lower urinary tract obstruction usually presents with oliguria/anuria (p. 474).

Renal colic

Acute loin pain radiating anteriorly and often to the groin ('renal colic'), together with haematuria, is typical of ureteric obstruction most commonly due to calculi (or 'stones', p. 510), although a sloughed renal papilla, tumour or blood clot may be responsible.

Clinical assessment

Renal colic occurs when a stone becomes impacted in the ureter. The patient is suddenly aware of pain in the loin, which radiates round the flank to the groin and often into the testis or labium, in the sensory distribution of the first

17

lumbar nerve. The pain steadily increases in intensity to reach a peak in a few minutes. The patient is restless and generally tries unsuccessfully to obtain relief by changing position or pacing the room. There is pallor, sweating and often vomiting, and the patient may groan in agony. Frequency, dysuria and haematuria may occur. The intense pain usually subsides within 2 hours, but may continue unabated for hours or days. It is usually constant during attacks, although slight fluctuations in severity may occur. Contrary to general belief, attacks rarely consist of intermittent severe pains coming and going every few minutes. Subsequent to an attack of renal colic there may be intermittent dull pain in the loin or back.

Investigations

The diagnosis of renal colic is usually made easily from the history and by finding red cells in the urine. Investigations are required to confirm the presence of a stone, and to identify the site of the stone and degree of obstruction. About 90% of stones contain calcium and are seen on a plain abdominal X-ray. When the stone is in the ureter an IVU shows delayed excretion of contrast from the kidney and a dilated ureter down to the stone (Fig. 17.10). IVU remains the most commonly used investigation world-wide, but spiral CT gives the most accurate assessment and will identify non-opaque stones (e.g. uric acid). Ultrasound may show dilatation of the ureter if the stone is obstructing urine flow. The stone may also cast an acoustic shadow.

Patients with a first renal stone should have a minimum set of investigations (Box 17.13); the yield of more detailed investigation is low, and hence usually reserved for those with recurrent or multiple stones, or those

	17.13 Investigations for renal stones		
Sample	**Test**	**First stone**	**Recurrent stone**
Stone	Chemical composition—most valuable test when possible	✓	✓
Blood	Calcium	✓	✓
	Phosphate	✓	✓
	Uric acid	✓	✓
	Urea and electrolytes	✓	✓
	Parathyroid hormone—only if calcium or calcium excretion high		(✓)
Urine	Dipstick test for protein, blood, glucose	✓	✓
	Amino acids		✓
24-hour urine	Urea		✓
	Creatinine clearance		✓
	Sodium		✓
	Calcium		✓
	Oxalate		✓
	Uric acid		✓

with complicated or unexpected presentations (e.g. in the very young). Chemical analysis of stones is helpful. Since most stones pass spontaneously through the urinary tract, urine should be sieved for a few days after an episode of colic in order to collect the calculus for analysis.

Management

The immediate treatment of renal pain or renal colic is bed rest and application of warmth to the site of pain. Renal colic is often unbearably painful and demands powerful analgesia, e.g. morphine (10–20 mg), pethidine (100 mg) intramuscularly or diclofenac as a suppository (100 mg). Patients are advised to drink 2 L per day. Around 90% of stones < 4 mm in diameter will pass spontaneously, but only 10% of stones of > 6 mm will pass and these may require endoscopic surgical intervention. All stones are potentially infected and surgery should be covered with appropriate antibiotics. Immediate action is required if there is anuria or if severe infection occurs in the stagnant urine proximal to the stone (pyonephrosis).

Attempts to develop drugs that dissolve stones have so far been unsuccessful. However, most stones can now be fragmented by extracorporeal shock wave lithotripsy (ESWL; see Fig. 17.37, p. 511), in which shock waves generated outside the body are focused on the stone, breaking it into small pieces which can pass easily down the ureter. This requires free drainage of the distal urinary tract.

Further measures to prevent recurrent stone formation are discussed on page 511.

Abnormal micturition

Oliguria/anuria

On an average diet, between 300 and 500 mL/day of urine is required to excrete the solute load at maximum

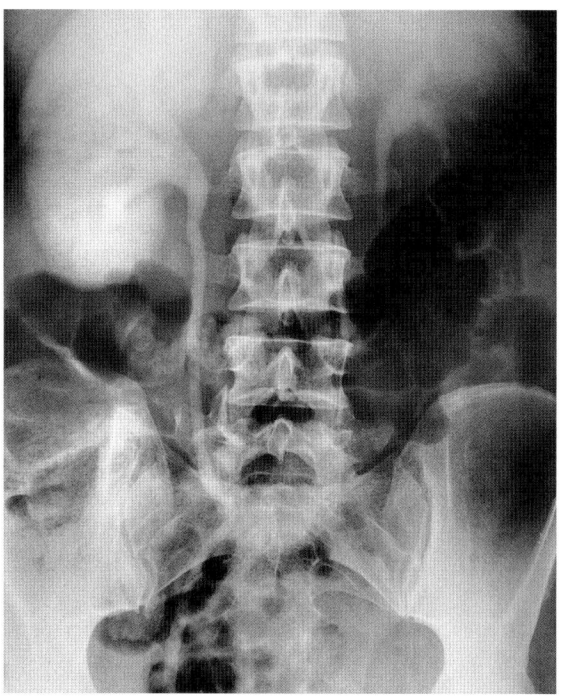

Fig. 17.10 Unilateral obstruction. Intravenous urogram of a patient with a stone (not visible) at the lower end of the right ureter. This film, taken 2 hours post-contrast injection, demonstrates persistence of contrast medium in the right kidney, pelvicalyceal system and ureter, whereas only a small amount remains visible in the normal left pelvicalyceal system.

concentration. Volumes below this are termed oliguria. Anuria is the (almost) total absence of urine (< 50 mL/day). A low measured urine volume is an important finding, as it suggests reduced production of urine or obstruction to urine flow.

Reduced urine production

The volume of urine produced is determined by the difference between glomerular filtration and tubular reabsorption. When GFR is very low, urine volumes may still be normal if tubular reabsorption is correspondingly low; hence urine volume is a poor indicator of CKD. Oliguria/anuria may be caused by a reduction in urine production, as typically seen in pre-renal acute renal failure, when GFR is reduced but intact tubular homeostatic mechanisms increase reabsorption to conserve salt and water. A high solute load or associated tubular dysfunction may, however, produce normal or high urine volumes in such cases until the pre-renal insult becomes severe and GFR is minimal, e.g. in diabetic ketoacidosis with marked glycosuria. Urine volumes are variable in acute renal failure due to intrinsic renal disease, but a rapid decline in urine volume occurs in renal infarction, if bilateral or in a single functioning kidney, and often in rapidly progressive glomerulonephritis.

Urinary tract obstruction

The most common causes of lower urinary tract obstruction causing reduced volume of micturition are urinary calculi (p. 510), prostatic enlargement (benign or malignant, p. 512), or pelvic and retroperitoneal tumours in an older age group. About 50% of cases of acute urinary retention are seen after general anaesthesia, particularly in those with pre-existing prostatic enlargement. In young men, bladder neck dyssynergia may also cause obstruction. Urethral strictures (more likely if there is a history of instrumentation), trauma or urethral infection, urethral valves, phimosis and meatal stenosis are other common causes (see Fig. 17.9, p. 473). Poor flow and post-micturition residual bladder volume are also seen in atonic bladders (e.g. in neurological disorders such as multiple sclerosis and spina bifida), when there is reduced/absent detrusor muscle activity and a failure of the distal sphincter to relax.

Obstruction may be acute or chronic, and partial or complete. Acute obstruction is often associated with pain due to distension of the urinary tract that may be exacerbated by a fluid load. The site of the pain can indicate the site of the obstruction. Obstruction at the bladder neck (acute urinary retention) is associated with lower midline abdominal discomfort due to bladder dilatation. Ureteric obstruction, e.g. from a renal calculus, typically presents as loin pain radiating to the groin. Higher obstructions, e.g. at the level of the renal pelvis, may present as flank pain. Chronic obstruction rarely produces pain but may produce a dull ache.

To produce oliguria/anuria, the obstruction must be complete and distal to the bladder neck, bilateral, or unilateral on the side of a single functioning kidney. If an obstruction is not relieved, the pressure transmitted back to the nephrons will result in cessation of glomerular filtration. All patients with acutely reduced urinary volumes should be palpated/percussed for a full bladder and catheterised. If oliguria persists without another clear explanation, radiological assessment, typically by ultrasound, should be undertaken promptly. Rarely, in acute renal failure due to obstruction, urinary tracts may not be particularly dilated because of lack of urine production. Relief of an acute obstruction is usually accompanied by a rapid return of renal function, although tubular function may be impaired, resulting in polyuria and failure to conserve electrolytes.

Partial obstruction can be associated with normal or even high urine volumes due to chronic tubular injury, with a loss of tubular concentrating ability. This chronic tubular injury can also produce a type 1 renal tubular acidosis (p. 444). Over time, even partial obstruction will cause tubular atrophy and irreversible renal failure.

Polyuria

An inappropriately high urine volume (> 3 L/day) may result from increased urinary solute excretion (osmotic diuresis) or pure water diuresis (Box 17.14). In primary (or psychogenic) polydipsia, the increased urine output is an appropriate response to increased water intake; plasma sodium concentration is typically low–normal in such patients. In diabetes insipidus (p. 492), there is impaired urinary concentrating ability causing increased free water clearance (i.e. water free of solute); plasma sodium will usually be normal in such patients, since increased thirst will usually prevent high plasma sodium concentrations. However, restricted access to water may precipitate hypernatraemia. Free water clearance is calculated by measuring osmotic clearance:

$$\text{Osmotic clearance} = \text{urine flow rate} \times \frac{\text{urine osmolality}}{\text{plasma osmolality}}$$

Free water clearance = urine flow rate − osmotic clearance

Investigation of polyuria includes measurement of plasma electrolytes, glucose and calcium. A 24-hour urine collection may be helpful to confirm the severity of polyuria. Investigation of suspected diabetes insipidus is described on page 493.

17.14 Causes of polyuria

- Excess fluid intake
- Osmotic, e.g. hyperglycaemia, hypercalcaemia
- Cranial diabetes insipidus (reduced antidiuretic hormone (ADH) secretion)
    Idiopathic (50%), mass lesion, trauma, infection
- Nephrogenic diabetes insipidus (tubular dysfunction)
    Genetic tubular defects
    Drugs/toxins, e.g. lithium, diuretics
    Interstitial renal disease
    Hypokalaemia, hypercalcaemia

Nocturia

Waking up at night to void urine may be a consequence of polyuria but may also result from fluid intake or diuretic use in the late evening. Nocturia also occurs in CKD, and in prostatic enlargement when it is associated with poor stream, hesitancy, incomplete bladder emptying, terminal dribbling and urinary frequency due to partial urethral obstruction (p. 512 and Fig. 17.11). Nocturia may also occur in sleep disturbance without functional abnormalities of the urinary tract.

Frequency

Frequency describes micturition more often than a patient's expectations. It may be a consequence of polyuria, most commonly due to diuretic therapy, when volumes passed are normal or high. It is also a symptom of UTIs (urethritis, cystitis, prostatitis) or urethral syndrome when urine volumes are typically low and associated with dysuria, urgency and a feeling of incomplete emptying.

Urinary incontinence

Urinary incontinence is defined as any involuntary leakage of urine. Urinary tract pathology causing incontinence is described below. It may also occur with a normal urinary tract, e.g. in association with poor cognition or poor mobility, or transiently during an acute illness or hospitalisation, especially in older people (Box 17.15). Diuretics (medication, alcohol or caffeine) may worsen incontinence.

Clinical assessment and investigations

The pattern of micturition is important in classifying incontinence and patients should be encouraged to keep a voiding diary, including the estimated volume voided, frequency of voiding, precipitating factors and associated features, e.g. urgency.

Examination includes an assessment of cognitive function and mobility, and of perineal sensation and anal sphincter tone since the innervation is from the same

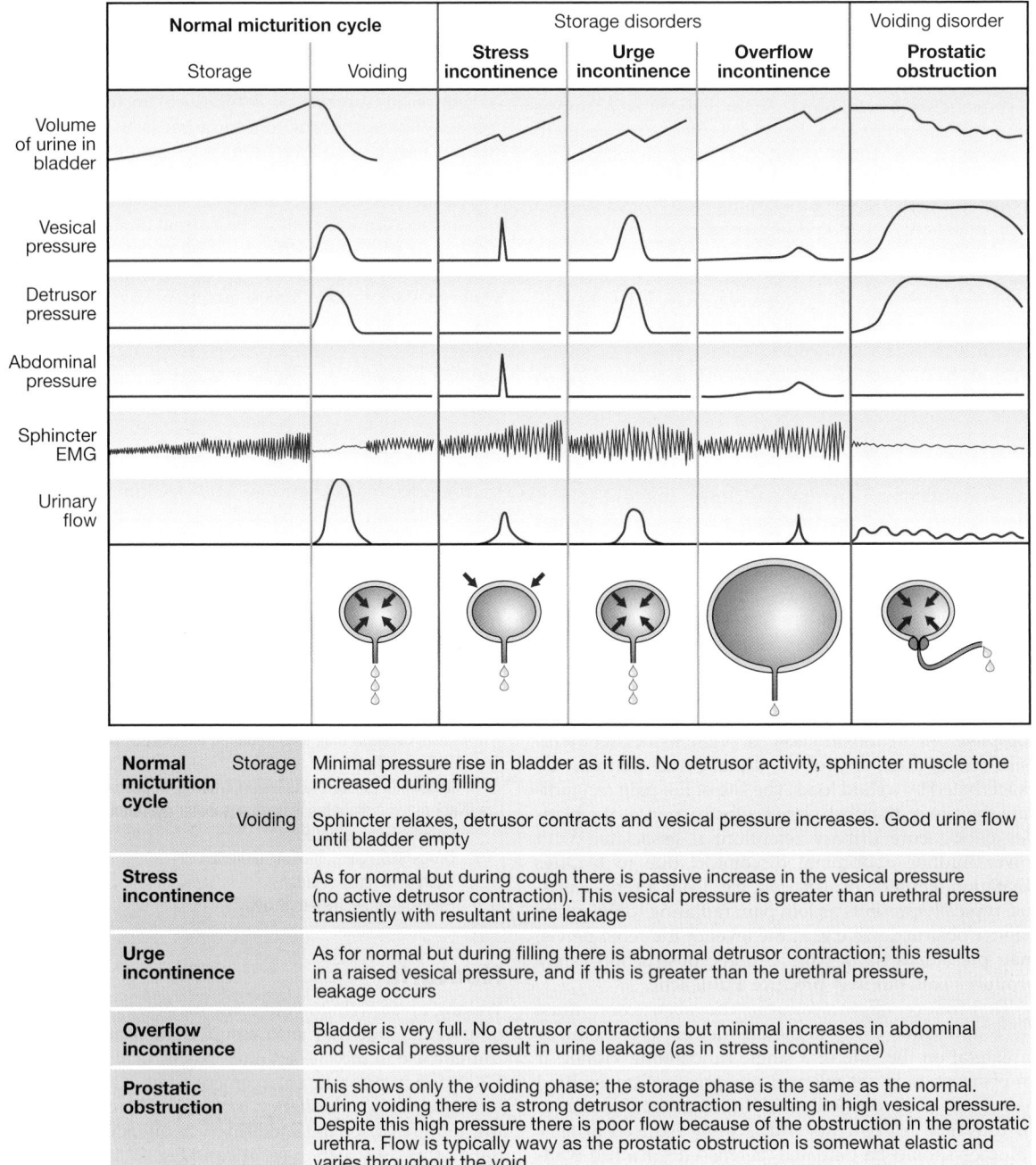

| | Normal micturition cycle | | Storage disorders | | | Voiding disorder |
	Storage	Voiding	Stress incontinence	Urge incontinence	Overflow incontinence	Prostatic obstruction
Volume of urine in bladder						
Vesical pressure						
Detrusor pressure						
Abdominal pressure						
Sphincter EMG						
Urinary flow						

Normal micturition cycle	Storage	Minimal pressure rise in bladder as it fills. No detrusor activity, sphincter muscle tone increased during filling
	Voiding	Sphincter relaxes, detrusor contracts and vesical pressure increases. Good urine flow until bladder empty
Stress incontinence		As for normal but during cough there is passive increase in the vesical pressure (no active detrusor contraction). This vesical pressure is greater than urethral pressure transiently with resultant urine leakage
Urge incontinence		As for normal but during filling there is abnormal detrusor contraction; this results in a raised vesical pressure, and if this is greater than the urethral pressure, leakage occurs
Overflow incontinence		Bladder is very full. No detrusor contractions but minimal increases in abdominal and vesical pressure result in urine leakage (as in stress incontinence)
Prostatic obstruction		This shows only the voiding phase; the storage phase is the same as the normal. During voiding there is a strong detrusor contraction resulting in high vesical pressure. Despite this high pressure there is poor flow because of the obstruction in the prostatic urethra. Flow is typically wavy as the prostatic obstruction is somewhat elastic and varies throughout the void

Fig. 17.11 Urodynamic abnormalities in patients with urinary incontinence. (EMG = electromyogram)

17.15 Incontinence in old age

- **Prevalence**: Urinary incontinence affects 15% of women and 10% of men aged over 65 years.
- **Cause**: incontinence may be transient due to an acute confusional state, urinary infection, medication (such as diuretics), faecal impaction or restricted mobility, and these should be treated before embarking on further specific investigation.
- **Detrusor over-activity**: established incontinence in old age is most commonly due to detrusor over-activity which may be caused by damage to central inhibitory centres or local detrusor muscle abnormalities.
- **Catheterisation**: poor manual dexterity or cognitive impairment may necessitate the help of a carer to assist with intermittent catheterisation.

sacral nerve roots that supply the bladder and urethral sphincter. A general neurological assessment is required to detect disorders such as multiple sclerosis that may affect the nervous supply of the bladder, and the lumbar spine should be inspected for features of spina bifida occulta. Rectal examination is needed to assess the prostate in men and to exclude faecal impaction as a cause of incontinence. Genital examination should identify phimosis and paraphimosis in men, and vaginal mucosal atrophy, cystoceles or rectoceles in women.

Urinalysis and culture should be performed in all patients. An assessment of post-micturition volume should be made, either by post-micturition ultrasound or catheterisation. Urine flow rates and full urodynamic assessment may also be helpful in selected cases (see Fig. 17.11).

Incontinence syndromes

Stress incontinence

In stress incontinence leakage occurs because passive bladder pressure exceeds the urethral pressure, due to either poor pelvic floor support or a weak urethral sphincter. Most often there is an element of both. This is very common in women and most often seen following childbirth. It is rare in men and then usually follows surgery to the prostate. Urine leaks when abdominal pressure rises, e.g. when coughing or sneezing. In women, perineal inspection may reveal leakage of urine when the patient coughs, and sometimes also a prolapse. Females in particular respond well to physiotherapy but if incontinence is persistent and troublesome, surgical treatment is indicated.

Urge incontinence

In urge incontinence leakage usually occurs because of detrusor over-activity producing an increased bladder pressure which overcomes the urethral sphincter (motor urgency). Urgency with or without incontinence may also be driven by a hypersensitive bladder (sensory urgency) resulting from UTI or bladder stone. The incidence of urge incontinence increases with age, occurring in 17% of the population aged over 65 years and around 50% of those requiring nursing home care. It is also seen in men with lower urinary tract obstruction and most often remits after the obstruction is relieved.

The diagnosis is often made simply on the basis of symptoms and the exclusion of urinary retention by bladder ultrasound; confirmation requires urodynamic testing (see Fig. 17.11). The mainstay of treatment is bladder retraining, teaching patients to hold more urine voluntarily in their bladder, assisted by anticholinergic medication. Surgery is restricted to patients who have severe day-time incontinence despite such treatment.

Continual incontinence

This suggests the presence of a fistula, usually between the bladder and vagina (vesicovaginal) or the ureter and vagina (ureterovaginal). This is most common following gynaecological surgery but is also seen in patients with gynaecological malignancy or following radiotherapy. In parts of the world where obstetric services are scarce, prolonged obstructed labour can be a common cause of vesicovaginal fistulas. Continual incontinence may also be seen in infants with congenital ectopic ureters. Occasionally, stress incontinence is so severe that the patient leaks continuously. Diagnosis is confirmed by inspection of the perineum and by IVU. Treatment is surgical.

Overflow incontinence

This occurs when the bladder becomes chronically over-distended. It is most commonly seen in men with benign prostatic hyperplasia or bladder neck obstruction (p. 512), but may occur in either sex as a result of failure of the detrusor muscle (atonic bladder). The latter may be idiopathic but more commonly is the result of damage to the pelvic nerves, either from surgery (commonly, hysterectomy or rectal excision), trauma or infection, or from compression of the cauda equina from disc prolapse, trauma or tumour. Incomplete bladder emptying can be identified by ultrasound, which reveals a significant post-micturition volume (> 100 mL). Obstructed bladders should be treated surgically. Unobstructed bladders need to be drained, preferably by intermittent self-catheterisation. Urodynamic testing may help clarify the aetiology.

Post-micturition dribble

This is very common in men, even in the relatively young. It is due to a small amount of urine becoming trapped in the U-bend of the bulbar urethra, which leaks out when the patient moves. It is more pronounced if associated with a urethral diverticulum or urethral stricture. It may occur in females with a urethral diverticulum and may mimic stress incontinence.

Neurological causes

Neurological disease resulting in abnormal bladder function is almost always associated with obvious neurological signs; these are described on page 1167.

Erectile dysfunction

Causes of erectile failure are shown in Box 17.16. Vascular, neuropathic and psychological causes are most common. With the exception of diabetes mellitus, endocrine causes are relatively uncommon and are characterised by loss of libido as well as erectile dysfunction. Erectile dysfunction and reduced libido occur in over 50% of men with advanced CKD or on dialysis. Judging from experience gained in diabetes clinics, erectile dysfunction is a markedly under-diagnosed problem. It is important to be able to discuss matters frankly with the patient, and to establish whether there are associated features of hypogonadism (p. 757) and whether

17

17.16 Causes of erectile dysfunction

With reduced libido

- Hypogonadism
- Depression

With intact libido

- Psychological problems, including anxiety
- Vascular insufficiency (atheroma)
- Neuropathic causes (e.g. diabetes mellitus, alcohol excess, multiple sclerosis)
- Drugs (e.g. β-blockers, thiazide diuretics)

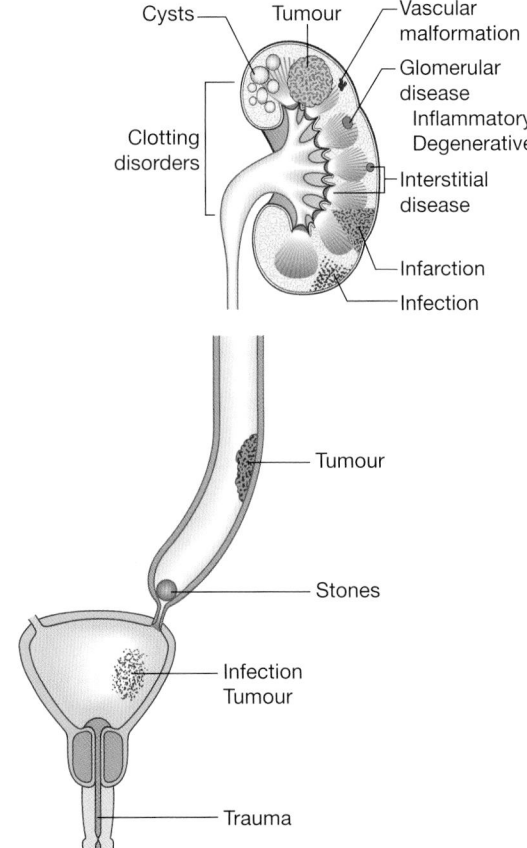

Fig. 17.12 Causes of haematuria.

erections occur at any other time (e.g. if the patient has erections on wakening in the morning, vascular and neuropathic causes are much less likely).

Investigations

Blood should be taken for glucose, prolactin, testosterone, luteinising hormone (LH) and follicle-stimulating hormone (FSH). A number of further tests are available but are rarely employed because they do not usually influence management. These include nocturnal tumescence monitoring (using a plethysmograph placed around the shaft of the penis overnight) to establish whether blood supply and nerve function are sufficient to allow erections to occur during sleep; intracavernosal injection of papaverine or prostaglandin E1 to test the adequacy of blood supply; internal pudendal artery angiography; and tests of autonomic and peripheral sensory nerve conduction.

Management

Psychotherapy which includes the sexual partner is most useful for psychological problems. Neuropathy and vascular disease are unlikely to improve but several treatments are available. First-line therapy is usually with oral phosphodiesterase inhibitors (e.g. sildenafil) which potentiate the vasodilator action of nitric oxide on cyclic guanosine monophosphate (cGMP). Coadministration of phosphodiesterase inhibitors with nitric oxide donors ('nitrate' drugs) is contraindicated because of the risk of severe hypotension. Caution should also be exercised in patients with chronic disease including ischaemic heart disease. Other treatments for impotence include self-administered intracavernosal injection or urethral gel administration of prostaglandin E1; vacuum devices which achieve an erection which is maintained by a tourniquet around the base of the penis; and prosthetic implants, either of a fixed rod or inflatable reservoir. Hypogonadism should be managed as described on page 757.

Haematuria

Haematuria may be visible and reported by the patient (macroscopic haematuria), or invisible and detected on dipstick testing of urine (microscopic haematuria). It indicates bleeding from anywhere in the renal tract (Fig. 17.12).

Microscopy shows that normal individuals have occasional red blood cells (rbc) in the urine (up to 12 500 rbc/mL). The detection limit for dipstick testing is 15–20 000 rbc/mL, which is sufficiently sensitive to detect all significant bleeding. However, dipstick tests

are also positive in the presence of free haemoglobin or myoglobin. Urine microscopy (p. 461) can be valuable in confirming haematuria and in establishing the cause of bleeding (Box 17.17). Other causes of red or dark urine may sometimes be confused with haematuria but produce negative dipstick tests and microscopy (Box 17.18). True positive tests may occur during menstruation, infection or strenuous exercise, but persistent haematuria requires further investigation to exclude malignancy.

Glomerular bleeding is characteristic of inflammatory, destructive or degenerative processes that disrupt the glomerular basement membrane (GBM) to cause microscopic or macroscopic haematuria. In glomerulonephritis, one or more other features of the 'nephritic syndrome' (Box 17.19) may be present, but the full syndrome is rare (p. 500).

Macroscopic (visible) haematuria is more likely to be caused by tumours (p. 514 and Box 17.20). Severe infections or renal infarction can also cause macroscopic haematuria, usually accompanied by pain.

Investigations and management

Investigation of haematuria (Fig. 17.13), whether microscopic or macroscopic, should be directed first at the exclusion of an anatomical bleeding lesion, particularly in older patients or others at risk of carcinoma of the bladder or other malignancy (see Box 17.20). If haematuria

17.17 Interpretation of dipstick-positive haematuria

Dipstick test positive	Urine microscopy	Suggested cause
Haematuria	White blood cells	Infection
	Abnormal epithelial cells	Tumour
	Red cell casts Dysmorphic erythrocytes (phase contrast microscopy)	Glomerular bleeding*
Haemoglobinuria	No red cells	Intravascular haemolysis
Myoglobinuria (brown urine)	No red cells	Rhabdomyolysis

*Glomerular bleeding implies that the GBM is fractured. It can occur physiologically following very strenuous exertion but usually indicates intrinsic renal disease and is an important feature of the nephritic syndrome (see Box 17.19).

17.18 Dipstick-negative dark urine

Cause	Urine colour
Food dyes e.g. Acanthocyanins (beetroot)	Red
Drugs	
e.g. Phenolphthalein	Pink when alkaline
Senna/other anthaquinones	Orange
Rifampicin	Orange
Levodopa	Darkens on standing
Porphyria	Darkens on standing
Alkaptonuria	
Bilirubinuria e.g. Obstructive jaundice	Dark Dipstick-positive for bilirubin, negative for haemoglobin

17.19 Nephritic and nephrotic syndromes

Nephritic syndrome[1]

- Haematuria (red or brown urine)
- Oedema and generalised fluid retention
- Hypertension
- Oliguria

Nephrotic syndrome[2]

- Overt proteinuria: usually > 3.5 g/24 hrs (urine may be frothy)
- Hypoalbuminaemia (< 30 g/L)
- Oedema and generalised fluid retention
- Intravascular volume depletion with hypotension, or expansion with hypertension, may occur

[1]The complete form is classically seen in post-infectious glomerulonephritis, may occur in acute IgA nephropathy, and occasionally occurs in other types of glomerulonephritis. The presence of one or more features is common to many types of glomerular disease.
[2]Classically seen in non-inflammatory and subacute inflammatory/proliferative glomerular disorders (see Fig. 17.27, p. 500).

EBM 17.20 Haematuria and urothelial malignancy

'Macroscopic haematuria has a positive predictive value of 83% for bladder cancer and 22% for all urothelial tumours, rising to 41% in patients over the age of 40.'

- Buntinx F, et al. Fam Pract 1997; 14(1):63–68.

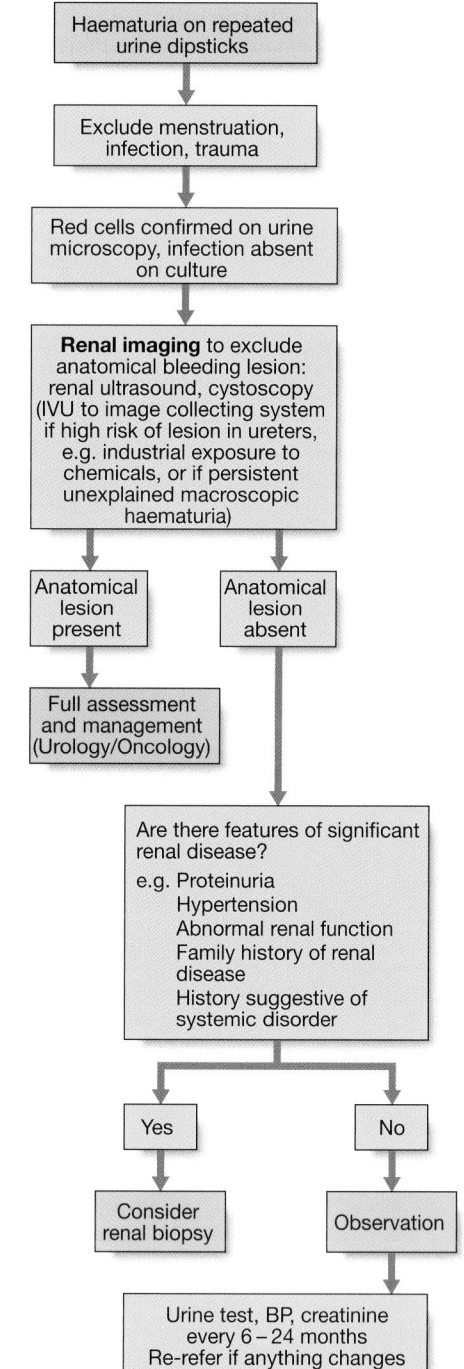

Fig. 17.13 Investigation of haematuria.

occurs with proteinuria or clinical features of kidney disease (see Box 17.19), inflammatory renal disease (p. 500) should be considered and a renal biopsy may be indicated. Where there are no features of significant kidney disease and malignancy has been excluded, patients with isolated microscopic haematuria may be managed by observation alone and biopsy is rarely warranted. Although this scenario occasionally precedes significant renal disease (e.g. Alport's syndrome, IgA nephropathy), it is commonly caused by the usually benign condition of thin basement membrane disease (p. 504), insignificant vascular malformations, renal cysts or renal stones. In 'loin pain-haematuria' syndrome, benign glomerular bleeding is associated with loin pain.

Management of haematuria depends upon the cause.

Proteinuria

Moderate amounts of low molecular weight protein pass through the healthy GBM. These proteins are normally reabsorbed by receptors on tubular cells. Less than 150 mg/day of protein normally appears in urine, and a proportion of that is Tamm–Horsfall protein secreted by the tubules.

Relatively minor leakage of albumin into the urine may occur transiently after vigorous exercise, during fever or UTI, and in heart failure. Tests should be repeated once the stimulus is no longer present. Occasionally, proteinuria occurs only during the day, and the first morning sample is negative. In the absence of other signs of renal disease, such 'orthostatic proteinuria' is usually regarded as benign.

As shown in Box 17.21, larger amounts of protein in the urine indicate renal damage; any renal disease or injury may cause proteinuria. Proteinuria is usually asymptomatic, although large amounts may make urine froth easily. The amount of protein in urine should be quantified to guide further investigations (Fig. 17.14). Quantification in a 24-hour urine collection has been the traditional standard, but collections are arduous and often inaccurate. Use of the protein/creatinine ratio (PCR) in single samples makes allowance for the variable degree of urinary dilution and can allow extrapolation to 24 hour values (see Box 17.21). Changes in PCR give valuable information about the progression of renal disease. Albumin/creatinine ratio (ACR) requires a more expensive immunoassay. At significant levels of glomerular dysfunction, albumin accounts for 70% of serum protein, so ACR values are a little lower than comparable PCR values. Greater consistency in results can be achieved by using first morning urine samples but this is not essential for routine clinical use.

It is sometimes helpful to identify the type of protein in the urine. Low molecular weight proteins may appear in the urine in larger quantities than 150 mg/day, indicating failure of reabsorption by damaged tubular cells, i.e. 'tubular proteinuria'. This can be demonstrated by analysis of the size of excreted proteins or by specific assays for such proteins (e.g. β_2-microglobulin, molecular weight 12 kDa). The amounts of such protein rarely exceed 1.5–2 g/24 hours (maximum PCR 150–200 mg/mmol), and proteinuria greater than this almost always indicates significant glomerular disease.

In many types of renal disease, the severity of proteinuria is a marker for an increased risk of progressive loss of renal function. Treatments that are effective

17.21 Quantifying proteinuria in random urine samples

ACR[1]	PCR[2]	Typical dipstick results[3]	Significance
< 3.5 (female) < 2.5 (male)		–	Normal
~3.5–15		–	Microalbuminuria
~15–50	~15–50	+ to ++	Dipsticks positive; equivalent to 24-hr protein excretion < 0.5 g
50–200	> 250	++ to +++	Glomerular disease more likely
> 200	> 300	+++ to ++++	Nephrotic range: always glomerular disease, equivalent to 24-hr protein excretion > 3 g

[1]Urinary albumin (mg/L)/urine creatinine (mmol/L).
[2]Urine protein (mg/L)/urine creatinine (mmol/L).
[3]Dipstick results are affected by urine concentration and are occasionally weakly positive on normal samples.

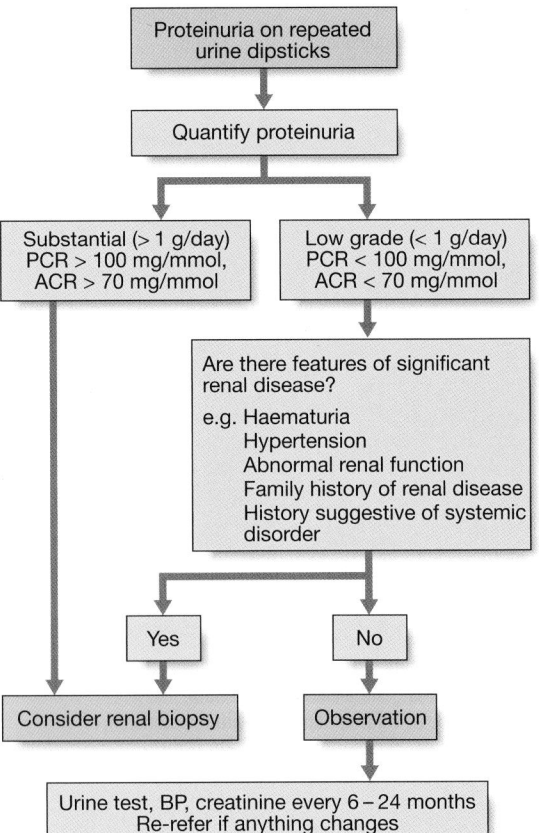

Fig. 17.14 Investigation of proteinuria. (ACR = albumin:creatinine ratio; PCR = protein:creatinine ratio.)

at lowering the risk of progression of kidney disease (e.g. angiotensin-converting enzyme (ACE) inhibitors in diabetic nephropathy) also reduce proteinuria.

Microalbuminuria

Microalbuminuria describes the urinary excretion of small amounts of albumin. The presence of albumin in the urine is a clear sign of glomerular abnormality and can identify the very early stages of progressive glomerular disease, e.g. in diabetic nephropathy (p. 829). Because significant renal damage will have occurred before dipstick tests become positive, patients with diabetes mellitus should be screened regularly for microalbuminuria. Persistent microalbuminuria has also been associated with an increased risk of atherosclerosis and cardiovascular mortality; neither the mechanism of proteinuria nor an explanation of these associations has yet been established.

Bence Jones proteinuria

Patients with a clone of B lymphocytes secreting free immunoglobulin light chains (molecular weight 25 kDa) filter these freely into the urine, and this can be identified as 'Bence Jones protein' in fresh urine samples. This may occur in amyloidosis (p. 84) and in B cell disorders, but is particularly important as a marker for myeloma (p. 1041). Bence Jones protein is poorly identified by dipstick tests and relatively low quantities of protein may be associated with significant pathology, so specific immunodetection methods are required when Bence Jones proteinuria is suspected. Highly sensitive serum assays for free light chains are becoming available for monitoring treatment.

Nephrotic syndrome

Nephrotic syndrome refers to the secondary phenomena that occur when substantial amounts of protein are lost in the urine (see Box 17.19, p. 479). The consequences are shown in Box 17.22.

Dependent oedema accumulates predominantly in the lower limbs in adults, extending to the genitalia and lower abdomen as it becomes more severe. In the morning, the upper limbs and face may be more affected. In children, ascites occurs early and oedema is often seen only in the face. Blood volume may be normal, reduced or increased. Avid renal sodium retention is an early and universal feature; the mechanisms are shown in Figure 16.5 (p. 432).

The diseases that cause nephrotic syndrome all affect the glomerulus (see Fig. 17.27, p. 500), affecting podocytes either directly, or indirectly by causing scarring or deposition of exogenous material (e.g. matrix proteins or amyloid deposits). In children, because minimal change glomerulonephritis is the most common diagnosis, initial management usually includes administration of high-dose corticosteroids. In older patients, and in children where this therapy is unsuccessful, a renal biopsy is required unless there is strong evidence for a specific aetiology (e.g. a long history of diabetes with other microvascular complications and a demonstrated progression from microalbuminuria, and with hypertension but no haematuria). Supportive management in patients with nephrotic syndrome is described in Box 17.22.

Oedema

Accumulation of interstitial fluid causes 'pitting' oedema, that leaves an indentation after pressure on the affected area. This results from disruption of the Starling forces dictating fluid transit across capillary basement membranes (Box 17.23). It is usually influenced by the effect of gravity on venous hydrostatic pressure and so accumulates in the ankles during the day and improves overnight ('dependent' oedema). Non-pitting oedema may reflect protein deposition—for example, in myxoedema associated with hypothyroidism (p. 741)—and also occurs in chronic

17

17.22 Consequences of the nephrotic syndrome and their management

Feature	Mechanism	Consequence	Management
Hypoalbuminaemia	Urinary protein losses exceed synthetic capacity of liver	Reduced oncotic pressure Oedema	Diuretics and a low-sodium diet*
Avid sodium retention	Secondary hyper-aldosteronism Additional poorly characterised intra-renal mechanisms	Oedema	
Hypercholesterolaemia	Non-specific increase in lipoprotein synthesis by liver in response to low oncotic pressure	High rate of atherosclerosis	Lipid-lowering drugs (e.g. HMG CoA reductase inhibitors, p. 455)
Hypercoagulability	Relative loss of inhibitors of coagulation (e.g. antithrombin III, protein C and S) and increase in liver synthesis of procoagulant factors	Venous thromboembolism	Consider prophylaxis in all patients with chronic or severe nephrotic syndrome
Infection	Hypogammaglobulinaemia (urinary losses)	Pneumococcal infection	Consider vaccination

*Severe nephrotic syndrome may need very large doses of combinations of diuretics acting on different parts of the nephron (e.g. loop diuretic plus thiazide plus amiloride). In occasional patients with hypovolaemia, intravenous salt-poor albumin infusions may help to establish a diuresis, although efficacy is controversial. Over-diuresis risks secondary impairment of renal function through hypovolaemia.

17.23 Causes of oedema

Increased total extracellular fluid

- Congestive heart failure
- Renal failure
- Other hypervolaemic states: iatrogenic, Conn's syndrome etc.

High local venous pressure

- Deep venous thrombosis or venous insufficiency
- Pregnancy
- Pelvic tumour

Low plasma oncotic pressure/serum albumin

- Increased loss: nephrotic syndrome
- Decreased synthesis: liver failure
- Malnutrition/malabsorption

Increased capillary permeability

- Leakage of proteins into the interstitium, reducing the osmotic pressure gradient which draws fluid into the lymphatics and blood
- Local: infection/inflammation
- Systemic: severe sepsis
- Drug-related, e.g. calcium channel blockers

Lymphatic obstruction

- Infection: filariasis, lymphogranuloma venereum (pp. 366 and 422)
- Malignancy
- Radiation injury
- Congenital abnormality

lymphoedema. In developed countries the most common causes of oedema are local venous problems and heart failure (p. 543), but it is important to identify other causes.

Lower limb oedema is common in morbid obesity. Although venous obstruction often contributes, the oedema may be multifactorial: for example, being exacerbated by right heart failure caused by sleep apnoea.

Clinical assessment

A substantial volume (litres) of extracellular fluid may accumulate without any clinical signs. In adults dependent regions or immobile limbs are usually the first site of oedema formation, where it is easy to mistake the early signs of generalised oedema for a local problem. Ankle swelling is characteristic, but oedema develops over the sacrum in bed-bound patients. It rises higher up the lower limbs with increasing severity, to affect the genitalia and abdomen. Ascites is common and often an earlier feature in children or young adults, and in liver disease. Pleural effusions are common and can be a feature of any cause of generalised oedema. Facial oedema on waking is common in adults with low oncotic pressure oedema and in young patients. Features of intravascular volume depletion (tachycardia, postural hypotension) may occur when oedema is due to decreased oncotic pressure or increased capillary permeability. If oedema is localised—for example, to one ankle but not the other—then features of venous thrombosis, inflammation and lymphatic disease should be sought.

Investigations

The cause of oedema is usually apparent from the history and examination of the cardiovascular system and abdomen, combined with testing the urine for protein and measuring the serum albumin level. Where ascites or pleural effusions in isolation are causing diagnostic difficulty, aspiration of fluid with measurement of protein and glucose, and microscopy for cells, will usually clarify the diagnosis (p. 659).

Management

Specific causes (e.g. venous thrombosis) should be treated. Diuretics are commonly used for oedema but are also commonly abused. When there is sodium retention and generalised oedema, restriction of sodium (and sometimes fluid) intake, along with diuretic treatment, is rational. Mild fluid retention will respond to a thiazide or to a low dose of a loop diuretic such as furosemide or bumetanide. However, in oedema caused by venous or lymphatic obstruction or by increased capillary permeability, diuretics are likely to be hazardous, as they will cause hypovolaemia with secondary hyperaldosteronism and rebound exaggeration of oedema. Local treatments, such as the use of compression either continuously (e.g. compression stockings) or intermittently (with a mechanical device), can be useful in these circumstances.

In nephrotic syndrome, renal failure and severe cardiac failure, very large doses of diuretics, sometimes in combination, may be required to achieve a negative sodium and fluid balance.

Hypertension

Hypertension is a very common feature of renal disease, and a particularly early manifestation of renovascular and some glomerular diseases. Renal mechanisms seem to be important in essential hypertension (p. 605), and most genetic disorders of blood pressure have been attributed to altered salt and water handling by the kidney. In renal interstitial disorders, increased sodium loss (through reduced reabsorption from glomerular filtrate) may lead to hypotension. However, as GFR declines, hypertension becomes an increasingly common feature. When renal function is replaced by dialysis, control of hypertension often becomes easier as salt and volume balance are controlled. Control of hypertension is very important in patients with renal impairment because of its close relationship with further decline of renal function (p. 490) and because of the exaggerated cardiovascular risk associated with CKD.

Acute renal failure

Acute renal failure (ARF; also referred to as acute kidney injury, or AKI) describes a sudden and usually reversible loss of renal function, which develops over days or weeks and is usually accompanied by a reduction in urine volume. When faced with an abnormally high creatinine it is important to establish if this is acute, acute on chronic, or chronic kidney disease. Previous measurements of renal function should be sought for comparison. A renal ultrasound demonstrating two small kidneys indicates chronicity.

There are many possible causes of ARF (Fig. 17.15) and it is frequently multifactorial. The clinical picture is

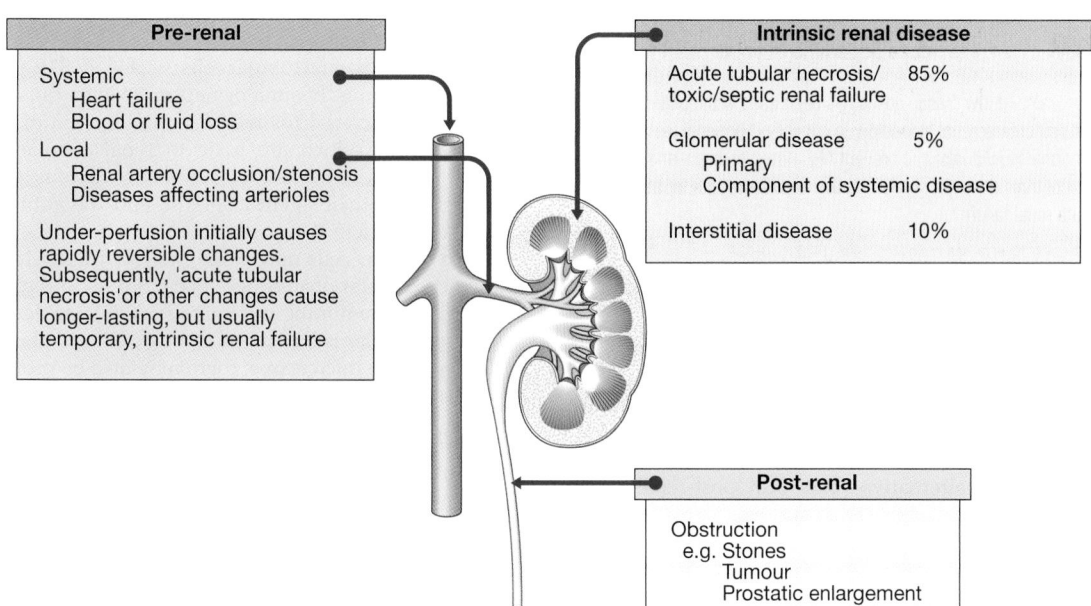

Pre-renal

Systemic
    Heart failure
    Blood or fluid loss
Local
    Renal artery occlusion/stenosis
    Diseases affecting arterioles

Under-perfusion initially causes
rapidly reversible changes.
Subsequently, 'acute tubular
necrosis'or other changes cause
longer-lasting, but usually
temporary, intrinsic renal failure

Intrinsic renal disease

Acute tubular necrosis/   85%
toxic/septic renal failure

Glomerular disease   5%
   Primary
   Component of systemic disease

Interstitial disease   10%

Post-renal

Obstruction
  e.g. Stones
     Tumour
     Prostatic enlargement

Fig. 17.15 Causes of acute renal failure.

often dominated by the underlying condition (e.g. septic shock, trauma). If the cause cannot be rapidly corrected and renal function restored, temporary renal replacement therapy may be required (p. 492).

Reversible pre-renal acute renal failure

Haemodynamic disturbances can produce acute renal dysfunction that may be reversed rapidly by prompt recognition and treatment.

Pathogenesis

The kidney can regulate its own blood flow and GFR over a wide range of perfusion pressures. When the perfusion pressure falls—as in hypovolaemia, shock, heart failure or narrowing of the renal arteries—the resistance vessels in the kidney dilate to facilitate flow. Vasodilator prostaglandins are important, and this mechanism is markedly impaired by NSAIDs (p. 518). If autoregulation of blood flow fails, the GFR can still be maintained by selective constriction of the post-glomerular (efferent) arteriole. This is mediated through the release of renin and generation of angiotensin II, which preferentially constricts this vessel. ACE inhibitors interfere with this response (p. 518).

More severe or prolonged underperfusion of the kidneys may lead to failure of these compensatory mechanisms and hence an acute decline in GFR. This leads to the formation of a low volume of urine which is concentrated (osmolality > 600 mOsm/kg) but low in sodium (< 20 mmol/l). These urinary changes may be absent in patients with pre-existing renal impairment or those who have received diuretics.

Clinical assessment

There may be marked hypotension and signs of poor peripheral perfusion, such as delayed capillary return. However, pre-renal ARF may occur without systemic hypotension, particularly in patients taking NSAIDs or ACE inhibitors (see above). Postural hypotension (a fall in blood pressure > 20/10 mmHg from lying to standing) is a valuable sign of early hypovolaemia.

The cause of the reduced renal perfusion may be obvious, but concealed blood loss can occur into the gastrointestinal tract, following trauma (particularly where there are fractures of the pelvis or femur) and into the pregnant uterus. Large volumes of intravascular fluid are lost into tissues after crush injuries or burns, or in severe inflammatory skin diseases or sepsis. Metabolic acidosis and hyperkalaemia are often present.

In sepsis most patients, once volume-resuscitated, have a vasodilated systemic circulation; this leads to a relative underfilling of the arterial tree and the kidney responds as it would to absolute hypovolaemia. When it is severe or prolonged, sepsis is an important cause of established ARF with acute tubular necrosis. The combination of sepsis with nephrotoxins such as NSAIDs is a common cause of ARF.

Management

- Establish and correct the underlying cause of the ARF.
- If hypovolaemia is present, restore blood volume as rapidly as possible (with blood, plasma or isotonic saline (0.9%), depending on what has been lost).
- Optimise systemic haemodynamics. Monitoring of the central venous pressure or pulmonary wedge pressure may aid in determining the rate of administration of fluid. Critically ill patients may require inotropic drugs to restore an effective blood pressure. Trials do not support a specific role for low-dose dopamine (Box 17.24).
- Correct metabolic acidosis:
    Restoration of blood volume will correct acidosis by restoring kidney function.
    Sodium bicarbonate (e.g. 50 mL of 8.4%) may be used if acidosis is severe to lessen hyperkalaemia.

Prognosis

If treatment is given sufficiently early, renal function will usually improve rapidly; in such circumstances residual renal impairment is unlikely. In some cases, however, treatment is ineffective and renal failure becomes established.

17

EBM 17.24 Low-dose dopamine in acute renal failure

'Dopamine at low, 'renal' doses has been used in the belief that it may increase renal blood flow in critically ill patients (as it does in normal individuals) and prevent ARF. However, meta-analysis of clinical trials does not support its use in patients with, or at risk of, acute renal failure.'

• Friedrich JO, et al. Ann Intern Med. 2005; 142(7):510–524.

Established acute renal failure

Established ARF may develop following severe or prolonged underperfusion of the kidney (pre-renal ARF), when the histological pattern of acute tubular necrosis is usually seen. In patients without an obvious cause of pre-renal ARF, alternative 'renal' and 'post-renal' causes must be considered (Box 17.25 and Fig. 17.15).

17.25 Differential diagnosis of acute renal failure in a haemodynamically stable, non-septic patient

Urinary tract obstruction (see Fig. 17.9, p. 473)

• Suggested by a history of loin pain, haematuria, renal colic or difficulty in micturition but often clinically silent
• Can usually be excluded by renal ultrasound: essential in any patient with unexplained ARF
• Prompt relief of the obstruction restores renal function

Drugs and toxins

• Poisoning, e.g. paraphenylenediamine hair dye, *Cortinarius* mushrooms, snake bite, paraquat, paracetamol
• Therapeutic agents: direct toxicity (aminoglycosides, amphotericin); or haemodynamic effects (NSAIDs, ACE inhibitors), often with other factors
• Auto-toxins: rhabdomyolysis releasing myoglobin; myeloma cast nephropathy

Vascular event

• Due to major vascular occlusion or small-vessel diseases (pp. 496–499), notably malignant hypertension and haemolytic uraemic syndrome/thrombotic thrombocytopenic purpura
• May be precipitated by ACE inhibitors in critical renal artery stenosis (p. 497)
• Urine usually shows minimal abnormalities but there may be haematuria in renal infarction

Rapidly progressive glomerulonephritis (RPGN) (p. 504)

• Typically, significant (dipsticks 3+) haematuria and minor proteinuria (often with red cell casts or 'glomerular' red cells)
• Sometimes associated with systemic features (e.g. systemic vasculitis, systemic lupus erythematosus (SLE), Goodpasture's (anti-GBM) disease)
• Useful blood tests include: antineutrophil cytoplasmic antibodies (ANCA), antinuclear antibodies (ANA), anti-GBM antibodies, complement, immunoglobulins
• Renal biopsy shows aggressive glomerular inflammation, usually with crescent formation

Acute interstitial nephritis (p. 504)

• Usually caused by an adverse drug reaction
• Characterised by small amounts of blood and protein in urine, often with leucocyturia
• Kidneys are normal size
• Requires cessation of drug and often prednisolone treatment

Acute tubular necrosis (ATN)

Acute necrosis of renal tubular cells (see Fig. 17.31B, p. 505) may result from ischaemia or nephrotoxicity, caused by chemical or bacterial toxins, or a combination of these factors. Drugs which are toxic to renal tubular cells include the aminoglycoside antibiotics, such as gentamicin, the cytotoxic agent cisplatin, and the antifungal drug amphotericin B.

Dead tubular cells may shed into the tubular lumen, leading to tubular obstruction. Focal breaks in the tubular basement membrane and interstitial oedema develop. Although tubular cell damage is the dominant phenomenon under the microscope, there may also be profound alterations in the renal microcirculation.

Recovery from ATN

Fortunately, tubular cells can regenerate and re-form the basement membrane. If the patient is supported during the regeneration phase, kidney function usually returns. During recovery, depending on the severity of the renal damage and the rate of recovery, there is often a diuretic phase in which urine output increases rapidly and remains excessive for several days before returning to normal. This is due in part to temporary loss of the medullary concentration gradient, which normally allows concentration of the urine in the collecting duct, and which depends on continued delivery of filtrate to the ascending limb of the loop of Henle and active tubular transport.

Features of established ARF

These reflect the causal condition, such as trauma, septicaemia or systemic disease, together with features of renal failure.

Urea and creatinine

The rate of rise in plasma urea and creatinine is determined by the rate of protein catabolism (tissue breakdown). In ARF associated with catabolic states, such as severe infections, major surgery or trauma, the daily rise in plasma urea often exceeds 5 mmol/L (30 mg/dL). At first the patient may feel well but, unless dialysis is instituted, the clinical features described below eventually appear.

Alterations in urine volume

Patients are usually oliguric (urine volume < 500 mL daily). Anuria (complete absence of urine) is rare and usually indicates acute urinary tract obstruction or vascular occlusion. In about 20% of cases, the urine volume is normal or increased, but with a low GFR and a reduction of tubular reabsorption (non-oliguric ARF). Excretion is inadequate despite good urine output, and the plasma urea and creatinine increase.

Disturbances of fluid, electrolyte and acid–base balance

Hyperkalaemia is common, particularly with massive tissue breakdown, haemolysis or metabolic acidosis (p. 443). Dilutional hyponatraemia occurs if the patient has continued to drink freely despite oliguria or has received inappropriate amounts of intravenous dextrose. Metabolic acidosis develops unless prevented by loss of hydrogen ions through vomiting or aspiration of gastric contents. Hypocalcaemia, due to reduced renal production of 1,25-dihydroxycholecalciferol, is common.

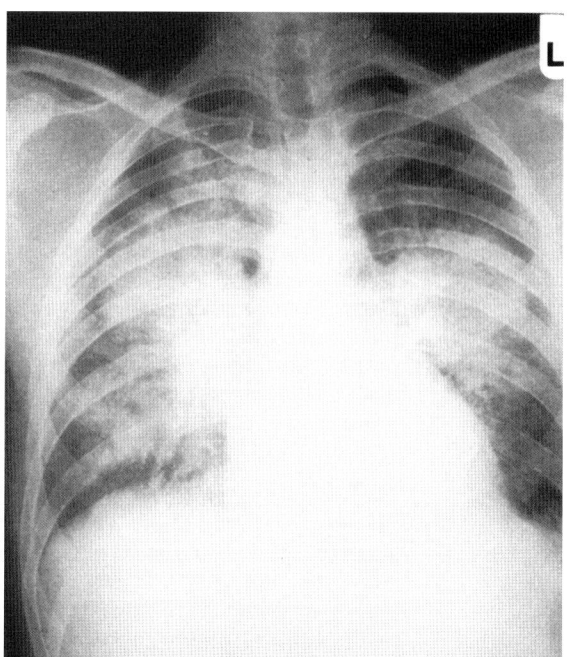

Fig. 17.16 Pulmonary oedema in acute renal failure. The appearances are indistinguishable from left ventricular failure but the heart size is usually normal. Blood pressure is often high.

Other features

- 'Uraemic' features include initial anorexia, nausea and vomiting followed by drowsiness, apathy, confusion, muscle-twitching, hiccups, fits and coma.
- Respiratory rate may be increased due to acidosis, pulmonary oedema or respiratory infection. Pulmonary oedema (Fig. 17.16) may result from the administration of excessive amounts of fluids relative to urine output and because of increased pulmonary capillary permeability.
- Anaemia is common, due to excessive blood loss, haemolysis or decreased erythropoiesis. Bleeding is more likely because of disordered platelet function and disturbances of the coagulation cascade. Spontaneous gastrointestinal haemorrhage may occur, often late in the illness, although this is less common with effective dialysis and the use of agents that reduce gastric acid production.
- Severe infections may complicate ARF because humoral and cellular immune mechanisms are depressed.

Management

In the absence of dialysis, the most common causes of death are hyperkalaemia and pulmonary oedema, followed by infection and uraemia itself. Initial management is targeted at these priorities.

Hyperkalaemia

Hyperkalaemia (a plasma K^+ concentration > 6 mmol/L) must be treated immediately, as described in Box 16.17 (p. 441), to prevent life-threatening cardiac arrhythmias.

Immediate fluid management

Circulating blood volume should be optimised to ensure adequate renal perfusion, with monitoring of central venous pressure as required. Patients with pulmonary oedema or anuria usually require dialysis to remove sodium and water. Temporary respiratory support (continuous positive airways pressure (CPAP), intermittent positive pressure ventilation (IPPV)) may be life-saving. Severe acidosis can be ameliorated with sodium bicarbonate if volume status allows.

Addressing the underlying cause of the ARF

This may be obvious or revealed by simple initial investigations (e.g. ultrasound showing urinary tract obstruction). If not, a range of investigations, including renal biopsy, may be necessary (Boxes 17.27 and 17.28). In many cases, more than one factor contributes to the renal dysfunction.

There is no specific treatment for ATN, other than restoring renal perfusion. Intrinsic renal disease may require specific therapy; for example, immunosuppressive drugs are of value in some causes of rapidly progressive glomerulonephritis (p. 504), and plasma infusion and plasma exchange may be indicated in microangiopathic diseases (p. 498).

'Post-renal' obstruction should be relieved urgently. If pelvic or ureteric dilatation is found and not explained by bladder outlet obstruction, percutaneous nephrostomy is undertaken to decompress the urinary system (p. 467). Injection of dye through the nephrostomy tube (antegrade pyelography) reveals the site of the obstruction. Once obstruction has been relieved and blood chemistry is returning to normal, the underlying cause is treated whenever possible.

Fluid and electrolyte balance

After initial resuscitation, daily fluid intake should equal urine output plus an additional 500 mL to cover insensible losses; such losses are higher in febrile patients and in tropical climates. If abnormal losses occur, as in diarrhoea, additional fluid and electrolyte replacement is required. Measurement of fluid intake and urine output is subject to error so the patient should be weighed daily. Large changes in body weight, the development of oedema or signs of fluid depletion indicate that fluid intake should be reassessed.

17.26 Acute renal failure in old age

- **Physiological change**: nephrons decline in number with age and average GFR falls progressively.
- **Creatinine**: as muscle mass falls with age, less creatinine is produced each day. Serum creatinine can be misleading as a guide to renal function.
- **Renal tubular function**: declines with age, leading to loss of urinary concentrating ability.
- **Drugs**: increased drug prescription in older people (e.g. diuretics, ACE inhibitors and NSAIDs) may contribute to risk of ARF.
- **Causes**: infection, renal vascular disease, prostatic obstruction, hypovolaemia and severe cardiac dysfunction are common.
- **Mortality**: rises with age, primarily because of comorbid conditions.

17.27 Suggested investigations in all patients with established acute renal failure

Initial test	Interpretation and further tests	Initial test	Interpretation and further tests
Urea and creatinine	Compare to previous results. Chronically abnormal in CKD (see Box 17.30)	**Urine microscopy**	Casts or dysmorphic red cells suggest glomerulonephritis Leucocytes suggest infection/interstitial nephritis Crystals can be characteristic of drugs or uric acid
Electrolytes	If potassium > 6 mmol/L, treat urgently (p. 441)		
Calcium and phosphate	Low calcium with high phosphate may indicate CKD (see Box 17.30) Abnormal in rhabdomyolysis: measure creatine kinase	**Renal ultrasound**	Hydronephrosis ± enlarged bladder in post-renal obstruction: request prostate-specific antigen (PSA) and imaging of prostate and urinary tract Small kidneys suggest CKD (see Box 17.30) Asymmetric kidneys in renovascular or developmental disease: consider renal artery imaging
Albumin	Low albumin in nephrotic syndrome (see urinalysis below) Low albumin in sepsis: take blood cultures		
Full blood count Clotting screen	Anaemia may indicate CKD (see Box 17.30) or haemolysis in thrombotic microangiopathy: request blood film and lactate dehydrogenase (LDH) Low platelets and abnormal coagulation in disseminated intravascular coagulation, including in sepsis: take blood cultures	**Cultures**	Blood, urine, wounds etc. as appropriate Treat all infections
		Chest X-ray	Pulmonary oedema in fluid overload Globular heart in pericardial (uraemic) effusion: perform echocardiogram 'Bat wing' appearance with normal heart size (± low Hb) may suggest pulmonary haemorrhage: measure CO transfer factor Fibrotic change in systemic inflammatory disease with lung and kidney involvement: request pulmonary function and high-resolution CT
C-reactive protein (CRP)	Erythrocyte sedimentation rate (ESR) is misleading in renal failure High CRP may indicate sepsis or inflammatory disease		
Urinalysis	Less reliable in an oliguric catheterised patient. Seek earlier results if possible Marked haematuria suggests severe glomerulonephritis or bladder/obstructive lesion Heavy proteinuria in glomerular disease: measure PCR or ACR	**Serology**	HIV and hepatitis serology is urgent if dialysis is needed
		ECG	If patient is > 40 yrs or has electrolyte abnormalities or risk of cardiac disease

17.28 Suggested investigations in established acute renal failure in particular circumstances

Possibility	Consider
Vascular occlusion (Of aorta, or renal artery to single kidney); pointers include newly missing pulses, complete anuria	Kidney size may be normal if occlusion acute Urgent arteriography Doppler ultrasound
Malignant hypertension/scleroderma If very high blood pressure; often some rbc fragments on blood film and haemolysis	Clinical features; examine fundi, previous BP values Autoantibodies to extractable nuclear antigens
Systemic inflammatory disease Pointers include suggestive history, multi-organ involvement, rash and evidence of glomerular disease	Infection as a differential diagnosis, especially endocarditis or tuberculosis Opportunity for urgent treatment; discuss with nephrologist Complement (see Box 17.41), antineutrophil cytoplasmic antibodies (ANCA), antinuclear factor (ANF), anti-GBM, cryoglobulins and tissue biopsy
Glomerular disease Pointers include substantial haematuria or proteinuria	All tests for systemic inflammatory disease above *Plus* urgent renal biopsy, unless cause is already known
Interstitial nephritis Consider if urinary abnormalities minor but leucocytes present, exposure to possible causes, usually non-oliguric in early stages	Detailed history and timing of drug exposures Eosinophilia and urinary eosinophils Renal biopsy Uric acid if tumour lysis possible
Myeloma kidney Features of interstitial disease but cast formation often acute, so patients often oliguric	Other evidence of myeloma: blood count, serum calcium, skeletal lesions, bone marrow. However, renal disease can occur without overt myeloma Urinary light chains (serum paraproteins are very common and usually incidental unless at very high level) Renal biopsy
Other infections E.g. leptospirosis, hantavirus, syphilis, post-streptococcal glomerulonephritis	Serology, e.g. anti-streptolysin O titre

Since sodium and potassium are retained, intake of these should be restricted.

Protein and energy intake

In patients in whom dialysis is likely to be avoided, accumulation of urea is slowed by dietary protein restriction (to about 40 g/day) and by suppression of protein catabolism by giving as much energy as possible in the form of fat and carbohydrate. Patients treated by dialysis may have more dietary protein (e.g. 1 g/kg protein daily, 10–12 g nitrogen).

It is important to give adequate energy and nitrogen to hypercatabolic patients (e.g. sepsis, burns). Enteral or parenteral nutrition (pp. 123–124) may be required. However, tube or parenteral feeding may require large fluid volumes.

Infection control

Patients with ARF are at substantial risk of intercurrent infection. Regular clinical examination and microbiological investigation (Ch. 6), as clinically indicated, are required to diagnose and treat this complication promptly.

Drugs

Vasoactive drugs such as NSAIDs and ACE inhibitors may prolong ARF and they should usually be avoided. Many drugs are excreted by the kidneys and dose adjustment may be required.

Renal replacement therapy (p. 492)

This may be required as supportive management in ARF.

Recovery from ARF

This is usually heralded by a gradual return of urine output and subsequently a steady improvement in plasma biochemistry. Some patients, primarily those with ATN or after relief of chronic urinary obstruction, develop a 'diuretic phase'. Fluid should be given to replace the urine output as appropriate. Supplements of sodium chloride, sodium bicarbonate, potassium chloride, and sometimes phosphate, may be needed to compensate for increased urinary losses. After a few days urine volume falls to normal as the concentrating mechanism and tubular reabsorption are restored.

Prognosis

In uncomplicated ARF, such as that due to simple haemorrhage or drugs, mortality is low even when renal replacement therapy is required. In ARF associated with serious infection and multiple organ failure, mortality is 50–70%. Outcome is usually determined by the severity of the underlying disorder and other complications, rather than by renal failure itself.

Chronic kidney disease (chronic renal failure)

Chronic kidney disease (CKD) refers to an irreversible deterioration in renal function which classically develops over a period of years (see Box 17.3, p. 466). Initially, it is manifest only as a biochemical abnormality. Eventually, loss of the excretory, metabolic and endocrine functions of the kidney leads to the clinical symptoms and signs of renal failure, which are referred to as uraemia. When death is likely without renal replacement therapy, it is called end-stage renal disease/failure (ESRD or ESRF). The social and economic consequences of CKD are considerable. In the UK, over 44 000 patients (725 per million) were kept alive by renal replacement therapy at the end of 2006 and over 110 new patients per million of the adult population are accepted for long-term dialysis treatment each year. Of these, 50% were aged over 65. The incidence of CKD is much higher in some countries due to differences in regional and racial incidences of disease, as well as differences in medical practice. For example, in the USA, incident rates are over 350 per million population, with nearly half of these patients having a primary diagnosis of diabetes mellitus.

Aetiology

Common causes of ESRD are shown in Box 17.29. The underlying diagnosis is not always established, especially amongst the large number of elderly patients with moderate GFR reductions (stage 3 CKD; see Box 17.3, p. 466). Many patients diagnosed at a late stage have bilateral small kidneys; renal biopsy is rarely undertaken in this group since it is more risky, less likely to provide a histological diagnosis because of the severity of damage, and unlikely to indicate treatment that would improve renal function.

17.29 Common causes of end-stage renal failure

Disease	Proportion	Comments
Congenital and inherited	5%	E.g. polycystic kidney disease, Alport's syndrome
Renal artery stenosis	5%	
Hypertension	5–20%	
Glomerular diseases	10–20%	IgA nephropathy is most common
Interstitial diseases	20–30%	
Systemic inflammatory diseases	5–10%	e.g. SLE, vasculitis
Diabetes mellitus	20–40%	Large racial and geographical differences
Unknown	5–20%	

Clinical assessment

Chronic kidney disease may present as a raised blood urea and creatinine found during routine examination, often accompanied by hypertension, proteinuria or anaemia. The great majority of patients with slowly progressive disease are asymptomatic until GFR falls below 30 mL/min/1.73 m^2 (stage 4 or 5). Nocturia, due to the loss of concentrating ability and increased osmotic load per nephron, can be an early symptom. Thereafter, symptoms and signs may develop in almost every body system (Fig. 17.17), and typically include tiredness or breathlessness. In ESRD (stage 5) there may be pruritus, anorexia, nausea and vomiting. Later, hiccups, unusually deep respiration related to metabolic acidosis (Kussmaul's respiration), muscular twitching, fits, drowsiness and coma ensue.

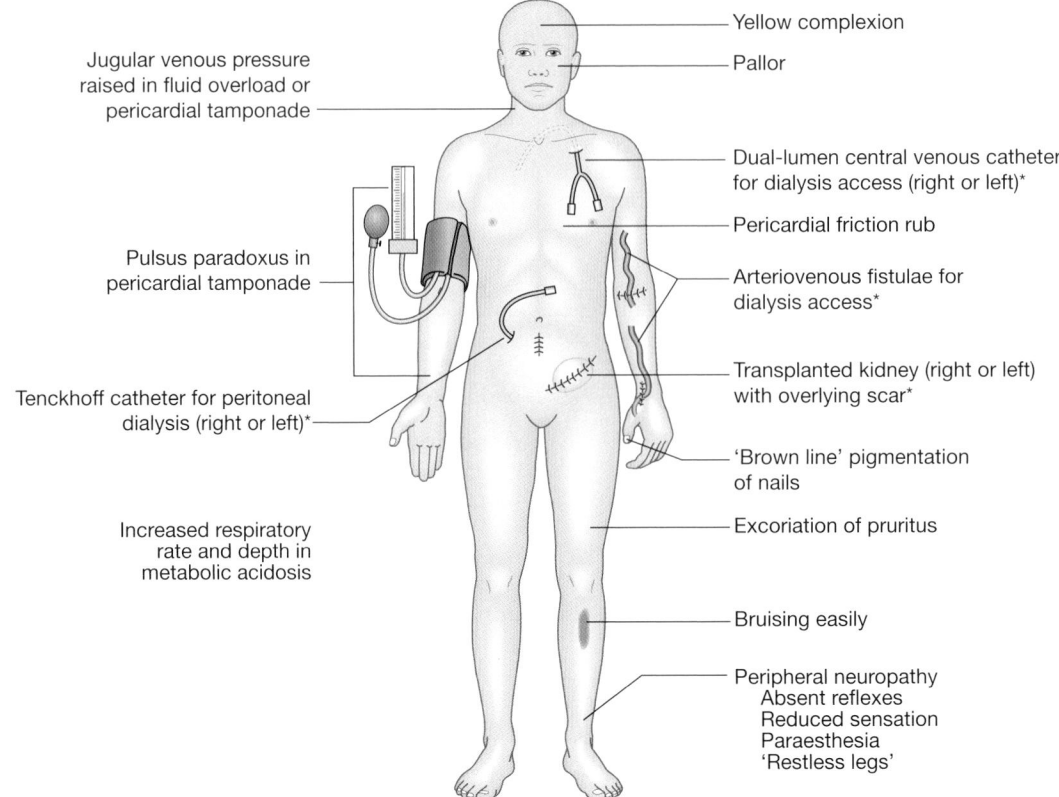

Fig. 17.17 Physical signs in advanced chronic kidney disease. (*Features of renal replacement therapy)

Investigation and management of stages 1–3 CKD

The great majority of patients with CKD stages 1–3 will never develop ESRD—which is fortunate, as they may include 10% of the adult population in developed nations. The large numbers are mainly due to the steep increase in the prevalence of CKD in elderly patients, particularly over the age of 70. However, patients with proteinuria, microalbuminuria or GFR < 50 mL/min/1.73 m^2 are at increased cardiovascular risk.

Recommended investigations in this group are shown in Box 17.30 and management should include:
- blood pressure control: maximum target 130/80 mmHg, reduced to 125/75 mmHg in diabetes mellitus, and anyone with an elevated PCR or ACR
- use of ACE inhibitors or angiotensin receptor blockers (ARBs) in those with proteinuria
- lipid management (pp. 454–456)
- lifestyle advice: smoking, exercise, diet and weight.
Referral to a nephrologist is most appropriate for patients with potentially treatable underlying disease or those who are likely to progress to ESRD:
- young age
- more severe renal damage: in the UK, referral to a nephrologist is recommended at CKD stage 4 (in the absence of other indications)
- deteriorating renal function (e.g. GFR fall > 5 mL/min/1.73 m^2 in 1 year, or > 10 mL/min/1.73 m^2 over 5 years): monitoring can be reduced to annual if disease is stable or very slowly progressive

- proteinuria: PCR > 100 mg/mmol or ACR > 70 mg/mmol has been suggested as a referral threshold, but this should be interpreted with reference to age, comorbidity and other factors
- haematuria: may be a marker for inflammatory nephritis.

Investigation and management of progressive and stage 4+ CKD

Box 17.30 suggests core investigations. The aims of investigation and management are to:
- Identify the underlying renal disease where possible. Additional investigations from Box 17.28 may be relevant, as the cause may be amenable to specific therapy, e.g. immunosuppression in some types of glomerulonephritis.
- Identify reversible factors which are making renal function worse, such as urinary tract obstruction, hypotension due to drug treatment, salt and water depletion, or nephrotoxic medications.
- Prevent further renal damage.
- Limit the adverse effects of the loss of renal function.
- Address any associated cardiovascular risk/disease.
- Institute renal replacement therapy (dialysis, transplantation, pp. 492 and 495) when appropriate.

Retarding the progression of CKD

The rate of deterioration in renal function varies between patients but is relatively constant for an individual patient. A plot of GFR, or of the reciprocal of

17.30 Suggested investigations in chronic kidney disease

Initial tests	Interpretation
Urea and creatinine	To assess stability/progression: compare to previous results
Urinalysis and quantification of proteinuria	Haematuria and proteinuria may indicate cause. Proteinuria indicates risk of progressive CKD requiring preventive ACE inhibitor or ARB therapy
Electrolytes	To identify hyperkalaemia and acidosis
Calcium, phosphate, parathyroid hormone	To assess renal osteodystrophy
Albumin	Low albumin: consider malnutrition, inflammation
Full blood count (± Fe, ferritin, folate, B$_{12}$)	If anaemic, exclude common non-renal explanations then manage as renal anaemia
Lipids, glucose ± HbA1c	Cardiovascular risk high in CKD: treat risk factors aggressively
Renal ultrasound	Only if there are urinary symptoms (to exclude obstruction) or progressive CKD Small kidneys suggest chronicity Asymmetric renal size suggests renovascular or developmental disease
Hepatitis and HIV serology	If dialysis or transplant is planned Hepatitis B vaccination recommended if seronegative
ECG	If patient is > 40 yrs or hyperkalaemic, or there are risk factors for cardiac disease
Other tests	Consider relevant tests from Boxes 17.27 and 17.28, especially if the cause of CKD is unknown

the plasma creatinine concentration against time (Fig. 17.18), predicts when dialysis will be required and detects any unexpected worsening of kidney disease. It can also be used to monitor the success of interventions.

Control of blood pressure

Lowering of blood pressure slows the rate at which renal function declines in CKD, independently of the agent used (Box 17.31). No threshold for this effect has been found; reduction of any level of blood pressure is beneficial. Various target blood pressures have been suggested: for example, 130/80 mmHg for CKD alone, lowered to 125/75 mmHg for those with proteinuria > 1 g/day (PCR > 100 mg/mmol or ACR > 70 mg/mmol). Achieving these targets often requires multiple drugs and may be limited by toxicity or non-compliance. The high incidence of left ventricular hypertrophy, heart failure and occlusive vascular disease in patients with long-standing renal disease also justifies vigorous efforts to control blood pressure.

Proteinuria

There is a clear relationship between the degree of proteinuria and the rate of progression of renal disease, and strong evidence that reducing proteinuria reduces renal risk. ACE inhibitors and ARBs are more effective at reducing proteinuria and retarding the progression of kidney disease than other therapies which lower systemic blood pressure to a similar degree (Box 17.32), even though their effect on glomerular perfusion pressure often causes an immediate reduction in GFR when therapy is initiated (up to 20% reduction is often regarded as acceptable). ACE inhibitors also reduce cardiovascular events and all cause mortality in CKD patients. ACE inhibitors and/or ARBs should be used, if tolerated (check creatinine and potassium), in all patients with incipient or overt diabetic nephropathy or PCR > 50 mg/mmol (ACR > 30 mg/mmol), independently of the presence of hypertension.

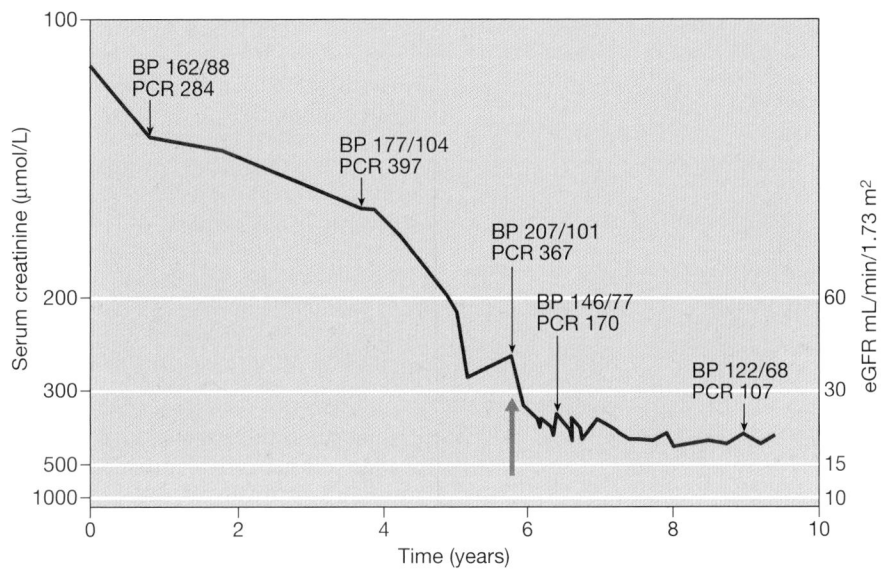

Fig. 17.18 Plot of the reciprocal of serum creatinine concentration against time in a patient with type 1 diabetes mellitus. After approximately 6 years of monitoring (blue arrow) he entered an aggressive treatment programme aimed at optimising blood pressure and glycaemic control. The reduction in blood pressure was accompanied by a fall in proteinuria (protein:creatinine ratio, PCR; mg/mmol) and a stabilisation in renal function.

EBM **17.31 Blood pressure lowering and progression of chronic kidney disease**

'In an analysis of 20 randomised controlled trials, including over 50 000 patients with CKD, the risk of ESRD reduced as BP was lowered. The group with the highest reduction in blood pressure (−6.9 mmHg (95% CI −9.1 to −4.8)) had a relative risk of ESRD of 0.74 (0.59–0.92).'

• Casas JP, et al. Lancet 2005; 366:2026–2033.

EBM **17.32 Renin–angiotensin system blockade in chronic kidney disease**

'ACE inhibitors and ARBs reduce proteinuria and slow the decline in GFR in both diabetic and non-diabetic patients with hypertension, CKD and proteinuria to a greater degree than that seen with blood pressure reduction alone.'

• Scottish Intercollegiate Guidelines Network 103: Diagnosis and management of chronic kidney disease.

For further information: www.sign.ac.uk

Dietary and lifestyle interventions

Although progressive renal disease can be retarded by restricting dietary protein in animals, results are less clear-cut in humans. Low-protein diets are difficult to adhere to and carry a risk of malnutrition. This remains a controversial area but, for most patients living in areas where renal replacement therapy is available, severe protein restriction is not recommended. Dietetic advice should be aimed at preventing excessive consumption of protein and, when approaching ESRD, target an adequate intake of calories to prevent malnutrition.

Smoking cessation also slows the decline in renal function. Exercise and weight loss may reduce proteinuria.

Limiting the adverse effects of CKD

Anaemia

Anaemia is common; it usually correlates with the severity of kidney disease and contributes to many of the non-specific symptoms of CKD. Untreated, haemoglobin can be as low as 50–70 g/L in CKD stage 5. Several mechanisms are implicated, including:

• relative deficiency of erythropoietin
• diminished erythropoiesis due to toxic effects of uraemia on marrow precursor cells
• reduced red cell survival
• increased blood loss due to capillary fragility and poor platelet function
• reduced dietary intake and absorption and utilisation of iron.

In patients with polycystic kidneys, anaemia is often less severe or absent, while in some disorders it appears disproportionately severe for the degree of renal failure. This may be because of the effects of these disorders on the interstitial fibroblasts that secrete erythropoietin.

Recombinant human erythropoietin and other erythropoiesis-stimulating agents (ESAs) are effective in correcting the anaemia of CKD and improve the associated morbidity. However, effects on mortality have not been confirmed and correcting haemoglobin to normal levels may carry some extra risk, including hypertension and thrombosis (e.g. of arteriovenous fistulas used for haemodialysis). The target haemoglobin is usually between 100 and 120 g/L. ESAs are less effective in the presence of iron deficiency, active inflammation or malignancy, or in patients with aluminium overload, which may occur in dialysis.

Fluid and electrolyte balance

Fluid retention is common in advanced CKD. Disproportionate fluid retention in milder CKD, sometimes leading to episodic pulmonary oedema, is particularly associated with renal artery stenosis. Good practice is to limit sodium intake (e.g. 100 mmol/day), for its effects on both fluid balance and blood pressure. Loop diuretics are often also required.

However, some patients with so-called 'salt-wasting' disease may require a high sodium and water intake, including supplements of sodium salts, to prevent fluid depletion and worsening of renal function. This most often occurs in patients with renal cystic disease, obstructive uropathy, reflux nephropathy or other tubulo-interstitial diseases, and is not seen in patients with primary glomerular disease.

If hyperkalaemia occurs, drug therapy should be reviewed, e.g. to avoid potassium-sparing diuretics, ACE inhibitors and ARBs. Correction of acidosis and calcium resonium therapy may be helpful, but limiting potassium intake (e.g. to 70 mmol/day) may be necessary in late CKD.

Acidosis

Declining renal function is associated with metabolic acidosis (p. 443), which is often asymptomatic. Acidosis is associated with increased tissue catabolism and decreased protein synthesis, and may exacerbate bone disease and rate of decline of renal function.

The plasma bicarbonate should be maintained > 22 mmol/L by giving sodium bicarbonate supplements (starting dose of 1 g 8-hourly, increasing as required). The increased sodium intake may induce hypertension or oedema; calcium carbonate (up to 3 g daily) is an alternative that is also used to bind dietary phosphate.

Cardiovascular disease and lipids

CKD is an independent risk factor for occlusive cardiovascular disease. Atherosclerosis is common and may be accelerated by hypertension. Medial vascular calcification, accelerated by high phosphate levels, may develop and is associated with vascular rigidity and occlusion. Left ventricular hypertrophy is frequent in ESRD and may account for many presumed arrhythmic deaths in this group. Pericarditis is common in untreated or inadequately treated ESRD. It may lead to pericardial tamponade and, later, constrictive pericarditis.

Hypercholesterolaemia is almost universal in patients with significant proteinuria, and increased triglyceride levels are also common in patients with CKD. HMG CoA reductase inhibitors (p. 455) achieve substantial reductions in lipids in CKD. In addition to their cardioprotective effect, there is some evidence that control of dyslipidaemia with statins slows the rate of progression of renal disease. Trials to establish the benefits in this patient group are under way.

Renal osteodystrophy

This metabolic bone disease which accompanies CKD consists of a mixture of osteomalacia, hyperparathyroid bone disease (osteitis fibrosa), osteoporosis and osteosclerosis (Fig. 17.19). Osteomalacia (p. 1121) results

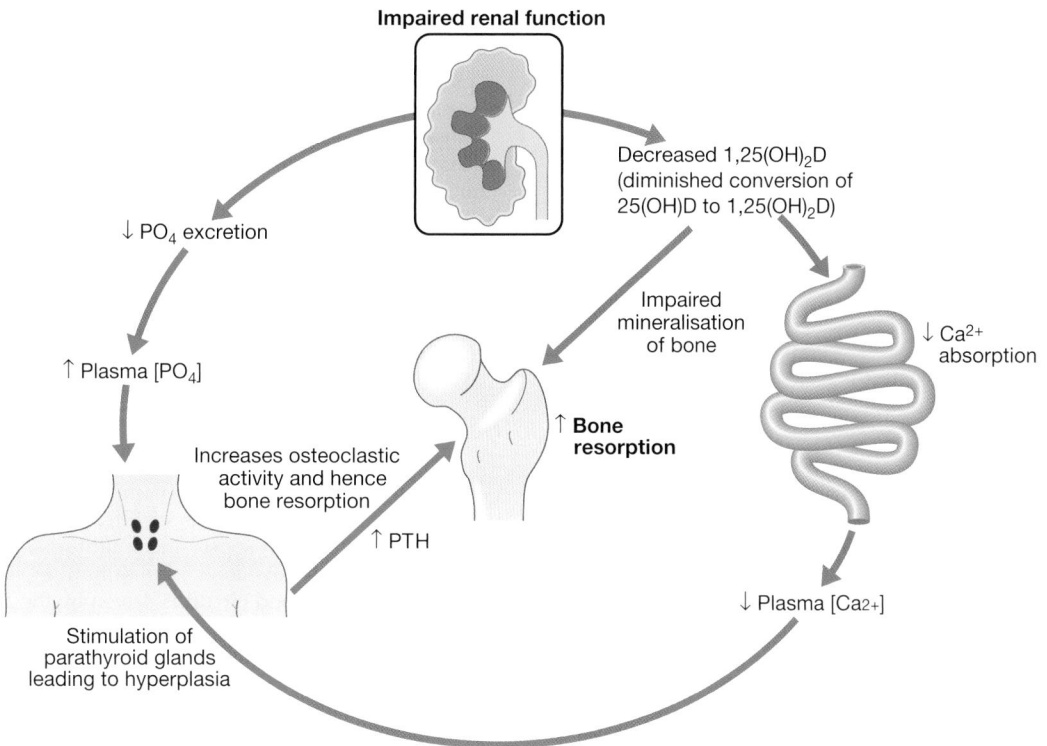

Fig. 17.19 Pathogenesis of renal osteodystrophy. The net result of decreased 1,25(OH)$_2$ cholecalciferol levels and increased parathyroid hormone (PTH) levels in the presence of high [PO$_4$] is bone which exhibits increased osteoclastic activity and increased osteoid as a consequence of decreased mineralisation.

from loss of the renal 1α-hydroxylase enzyme, with failure to convert cholecalciferol (vitamin D) to its active metabolite, 1,25-dihydroxycholecalciferol, and hence diminished intestinal absorption of calcium, hypocalcaemia and reduction in the calcification of osteoid in bone. The parathyroid glands are stimulated by the low plasma calcium, and also by hyperphosphataemia consequent upon reduced urinary phosphate excretion in CKD and poor clearance by conventional haemodialysis. Secondary hyperparathyroidism in the presence of hyperphosphataemia causes osteitis fibrosa. In some patients tertiary (or autonomous) hyperparathyroidism develops, resulting in hypercalcaemia.

Secondary hyperparathyroidism is prevented by giving 1α-hydroxylated vitamin D in patients with hypocalcaemia or high parathyroid hormone (PTH) levels (e.g. more than twice normal). The dose is adjusted to avoid hypercalcaemia. Calcimimetic agents can also reduce PTH via a direct action on the parathyroid glands. In tertiary hyperparathyroidism, parathyroidectomy is sometimes required.

Hyperphosphataemia is controlled by dietary restriction of foods with high phosphate content (milk, cheese, eggs) and the use of phosphate-binding drugs administered with food to prevent absorption (e.g. calcium carbonate, aluminium hydroxide and lanthanum carbonate). Polymer-based phosphate binders are also available.

Other adverse effects

Cellular and humoral immunity are impaired in CKD, with increased susceptibility to infection. Infections are the second most common cause of death in dialysis patients, after cardiovascular disease. Many are staphylococcal infections associated with access devices but some are common infections such as pneumonias.

There is an increased bleeding tendency in CKD which manifests in patients with advanced disease as cutaneous ecchymoses and mucosal bleeds. Platelet function is impaired and bleeding time prolonged. Adequate dialysis treatment partially corrects the bleeding tendency in those with severe uraemia, but dialysis patients have been shown to be at significantly increased risk of complications from anticoagulant therapy.

Generalised myopathy in CKD is due to a combination of poor nutrition, hyperparathyroidism, vitamin D deficiency and disorders of electrolyte metabolism. Muscle cramps are common. The 'restless leg syndrome', in which the patient's legs are jumpy during the night, may be troublesome.

Neuropathy may appear late in the course of CKD but may improve or even resolve once dialysis is established. Sensory neuropathy may cause paraesthesiae. Motor neuropathy may present as foot drop.

A number of hormonal abnormalities may be present. In both sexes there is loss of libido and sexual function, related at least in part to hyperprolactinaemia (p. 788). The half-life of insulin is prolonged in CKD due to reduced tubular metabolism of insulin; insulin requirements may therefore decline in diabetic patients in advanced CKD. However, there is also relative insulin resistance and reduced appetite, so the scale of this effect is unpredictable.

Gastrointestinal manifestations are common at low GFRs. These include anorexia, nausea and vomiting, and a higher incidence of peptic ulcer disease. H_2-receptor antagonists or proton pump inhibitors are used for established peptic ulcer disease in CKD, and as routine prophylaxis in ARF.

Depression is common in patients on or approaching renal replacement therapy, and support should be provided for both them and their relatives.

RENAL REPLACEMENT THERAPY

The facility to replace some functions of the kidney artificially by dialysis first became generally available in the mid-1960s and is now routine in patients with acute or chronic kidney failure. It does not replace the endocrine and metabolic functions of the kidney, but aims to maintain the plasma biochemistry (uraemic toxins, electrolytes and acid–base status) at acceptable levels. Dialysis can also remove fluid from the circulation (ultrafiltration) to maintain euvolaemia.

The original renal replacement therapy (RRT) was haemodialysis, and this is still the most common form of treatment. A variety of other types have been developed, particularly for unstable patients with ARF (Fig. 17.20).

Renal replacement in acute renal failure

The decision to institute RRT is made on an individual basis, taking account of other aspects of the patient's care. Guideline indications are as follows:

- *Hyperkalaemia.* A plasma potassium > 6 mmol/L is hazardous. Elevated plasma potassium can usually be reduced by medical measures in the short term (see Box 16.17, p. 441), and by early restoration of renal function if possible, but dialysis is otherwise often required.
- *Fluid overload and pulmonary oedema.* In patients with continued urine output, this may be controlled by careful fluid balance and use of diuretics, but in oliguric/anuric patients may be an indication for RRT.
- *Metabolic acidosis.* This will often occur together with hyperkalaemia and raise the plasma potassium further.
- *Increased plasma urea and creatinine.* Plasma urea > 30 mmol/L (180 mg/dL) and creatinine > 600 μmol/L (6.8 mg/dL) are undesirable in ARF. At lower levels, if there is progressive biochemical deterioration, and particularly if there is little or no urine output, it may be appropriate to commence dialysis. There is a trend towards earlier institution of dialysis in ARF, although trials of very early dialysis in post-operative or septic patients with oliguria have not shown consistent benefit compared with the more conventional strategy above.
- *Uraemic pericarditis/uraemic encephalopathy.* These are features of severe untreated renal failure; they are uncommon in ARF but are strong indications for RRT.

The principal options for RRT in ARF are haemodialysis, high-volume haemofiltration, or continuous arteriovenous or venovenous haemofiltration. Peritoneal dialysis is less favoured, as it is less efficient and seldom achieves adequate biochemical control in catabolic patients.

Intermittent haemodialysis

This modality offers the best rate of small solute clearance. In previously undialysed patients with ARF and elevated plasma urea, haemodialysis should be started gradually because of the risk of confusion and convulsions due to cerebral oedema (dialysis disequilibrium). Typically, 1 hour of treatment is prescribed initially. Subsequently, patients with ARF who are haemodynamically stable can be treated by 4–5 hours of haemodialysis on alternate days, or 2–3 hours every day if they are severely catabolic. For patients at risk of bleeding, epoprostenol may be used instead of heparin for anticoagulation but can cause hypotension. For short dialyses or patients with abnormal clotting, it may be possible to avoid anticoagulation.

Haemofiltration

This may be either intermittent or continuous, with 1–2 L/hour of filtrate replaced (equivalent to a GFR of 15–30 mL/min); higher rates of filtration may be of benefit in patients with sepsis and multi-organ failure. In continuous, arteriovenous haemofiltration (CAVH) the extracorporeal blood circuit is driven by the arteriovenous pressure difference. Poor filtration rates and clotting of the filter are common and this treatment has fallen out of favour. Continuous venovenous haemofiltration (CVVH, Fig. 17.21) is pump-driven, providing a reliable extracorporeal circulation. Issues concerning anticoagulation are similar to those for haemodialysis, but may be more problematic because longer or continuous anticoagulation is necessary.

Renal replacement in end-stage renal disease (ESRD) (CKD stage 5)

When patients are known to have progressive CKD (see Box 17.3, p. 466) and are under regular clinic review, preparation for RRT should begin at least 12 months before the predicted start date. This involves psychological and social support, assessment of home circumstances and discussion about choice of treatment. The principal decisions required are whether to commence RRT or opt for conservative treatment (see below), the choice between haemodialysis and peritoneal dialysis (Box 17.33), and referral for renal transplantation. In view of the historical high incidence of viral transmission in dialysis units, all patients opting for RRT must be screened in advance for hepatitis B, hepatitis C and HIV, and have hepatitis B vaccine if they are not immune.

The timing of initiation of dialysis is not clear-cut. Typically, it is started when the patient has symptomatic advanced kidney disease but before the development of serious complications, often with a plasma creatinine of 600–800 μmol/L (6.8–9.0 mg/dL) or an eGFR 8–10 mL/min/1.73 m². There is no evidence that early initiation improves survival and the decision to start is usually driven by a combination of patient symptoms and biochemistry.

Of patients starting dialysis in the UK, 77% are treated by haemodialysis and 23% by peritoneal dialysis. Mortality figures in the UK indicate 81% survival at 1 year (87% counted from day 90 of treatment) and 42% at 5 years. Mortality is strongly influenced by age; patients over 75 have an 18% survival at 5 years, whereas patients aged under 35 have an 87% survival at 5 years. Comorbid conditions such

Haemodialysis

There is bidirectional diffusion of solutes between plasma and dialysate across a semipermeable membrane following concentration gradients. The dialysate composition is chosen to achieve a suitable gradient. Fluid is removed by applying negative pressure to the dialysate side (ultrafiltration)

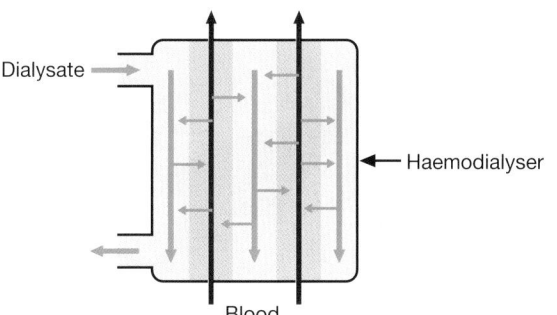

- Typical small solute clearance 160 mL/min
- Used in both acute and chronic renal failure

Haemofiltration

There is filtration of water from plasma to ultrafiltrate across a more porous semipermeable membrane down a pressure gradient with removal of solutes by convection. 'Replacement' fluid of chosen electrolytic composition is added to the blood circuit after the filter. If fluid removal is required, less is replaced than filtered

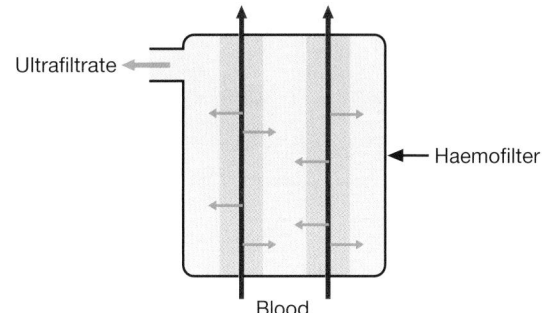

- Typical small solute clearance (2 L/hr exchanges) 33 mL/min
- ? Less circulatory instability than haemodialysis
- Used mostly in acute renal failure

17

- **Access to the circulation** for haemodialysis or filtration is required. Arteriovenous fistulae, temporary or semi-permanent tunnelled central venous lines or arterio-venous shunts (e.g. Scribner shunt) may be used. The extracorporeal circuit requires anticoagulation, typically with heparin

Peritoneal dialysis

This uses peritoneum as a semipermeable dialysis membrane. Solutes move down a concentration gradient, and water down an osmotic gradient achieved by using an osmolar compound (typically glucose) in the dialysis fluid

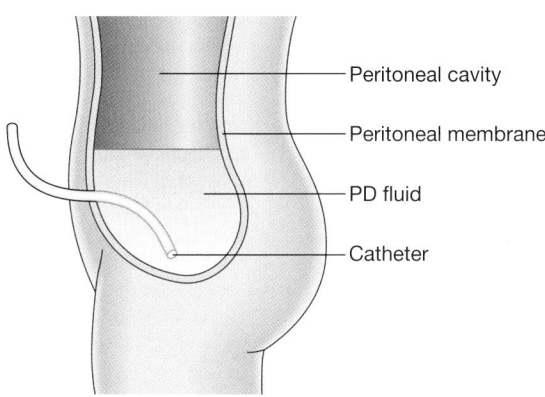

- **Access to the peritoneal cavity** via 'Tenckhoff' catheter
- **Continuous ambulatory peritoneal dialysis** (CAPD): typically 4 exchanges of 2 L of fluid a day 4–6 hrs apart
- **Automated peritoneal dialysis** (APD): uses a machine to perform exchanges overnight (8–10 hrs)
- Used mostly in chronic renal failure (CRF)

Transplantation

A functioning transplant replaces all of the functions of the failed kidneys

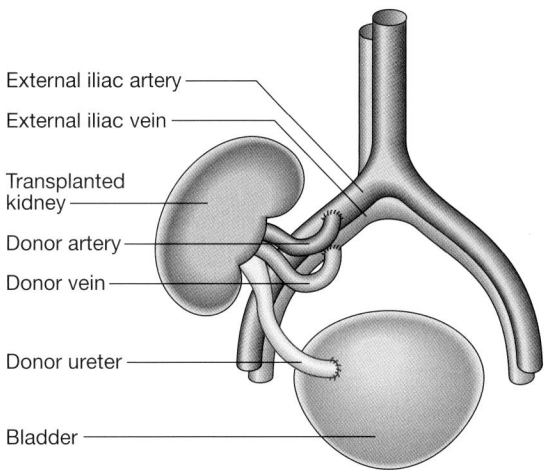

- Successful transplantation extends the life expectancy of patients with end-stage CKD
- Requires long-term use of immunosuppressives with attendant risks

Conservative management

Some patients may elect not to dialyse and can be actively supported to control the symptoms of ESRD

Fig. 17.20 Options for renal replacement therapy.

as diabetes mellitus (30% 5-year survival) and generalised vascular disease (34% 5-year survival) also have a strong influence. However, many patients lead normal and active lives, and patient survival for more than 20 years is commonplace in young patients without extrarenal disease.

Intermittent haemodialysis

This is the standard blood purification therapy in ESRD (Fig. 17.22). Vascular access is required; an arteriovenous fistula should be formed, usually in the forearm, up to a year before dialysis is contemplated, so that the fistula has time to develop. After 4–6 weeks, increased pressure

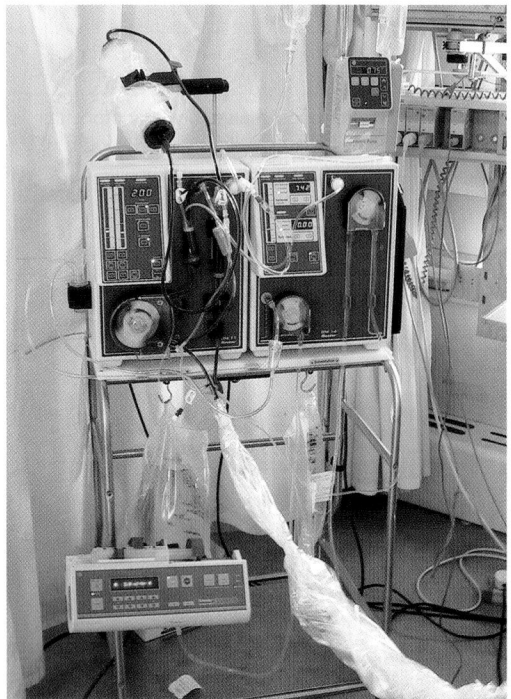

Fig. 17.21 Continuous venovenous haemofiltration (CVVH) on an intensive care unit. In this hypothermic patient the haemofilter and blood lines have been wrapped to reduce heat loss.

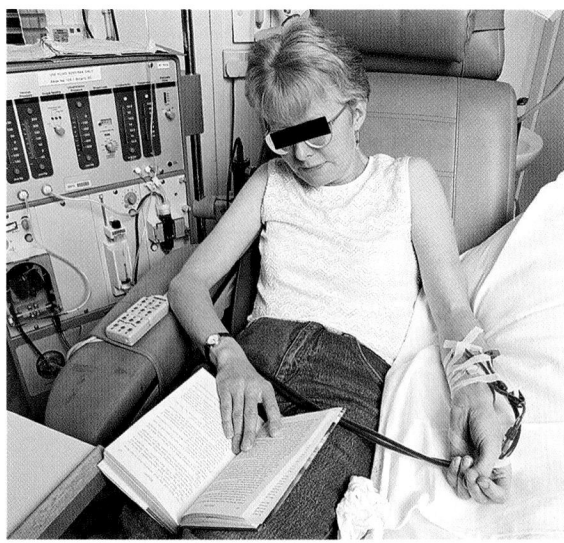

Fig. 17.22 Haemodialysis. A patient receiving haemodialysis through a forearm subcutaneous (Brescia–Cimino) fistula. She subsequently received a live related transplant.

17.33 Comparison of haemodialysis and peritoneal dialysis	
Haemodialysis	**Peritoneal dialysis**
Efficient	Less efficient
4 hrs three times per wk is usually adequate	Four exchanges per day usually required, each taking 30–60 mins (continuous ambulatory peritoneal dialysis) or 8–10 hrs each night (automated peritoneal dialysis)
2–3 days between treatments	A few hours between treatments
Requires visits to hospital (although home treatment possible for some patients)	Performed at home
Requires adequate venous circulation for vascular access	Requires an intact peritoneal cavity without major scarring from previous surgery
Careful compliance with diet and fluid restrictions required between treatments	Diet and fluid less restricted
Fluid removal compressed into treatment periods; may cause symptoms and haemodynamic instability	Slow continuous fluid removal, usually asymptomatic
Infections related to vascular access may occur	Peritonitis and catheter-related infections may occur
Patients are usually dependent on others	Patients can take full responsibility for their treatment

in the vein leading from the fistula causes distension and thickening of the vessel wall (arterialisation). Large-bore needles can then be inserted into the vein to provide access for each haemodialysis treatment. Preservation of arm veins is thus very important in patients with progressive renal disease who may require haemodialysis in the future. If this access is not possible, plastic cannulae in central veins can be used for short-term access.

Haemodialysis is usually carried out for 3–5 hours three times weekly, either at home or in an outpatient dialysis unit. The dialysis 'dose' required is adjusted to achieve a reduction in urea during dialysis (urea reduction ratio) of over 65%. Most patients notice an improvement in symptoms during the first 6 weeks of treatment. Plasma urea and creatinine are lowered by each treatment but do not return to normal. Studies of more frequent (e.g. daily) or longer (e.g. nocturnal) dialysis are under way. These may achieve better fluid balance and electrolyte control. Box 17.34 summarises some of the problems related to haemodialysis.

Haemodiafiltration

This technique uses a large pore membrane and combines the improved middle molecule clearance of haemofiltration with the higher small solute clearance of haemodialysis, but it is more expensive and long-term benefits are not yet established.

Peritoneal dialysis (PD)

Continuous ambulatory peritoneal dialysis (CAPD) involves insertion of a permanent Silastic catheter into the peritoneal cavity. Two litres of sterile, isotonic dialysis fluid are introduced and left in place for approximately 6 hours. Metabolic waste products diffuse from peritoneal capillaries into the dialysis fluid down a concentration gradient. The fluid is then drained and fresh dialysis fluid introduced, in a continuous four-times-daily cycle. The inflow fluid is rendered hyperosmolar by the addition of glucose; this results in net removal of fluid from the patient during each cycle (ultrafiltration).

17.34 Problems with haemodialysis

Problem	Clinical features	Cause	Treatment
Hypotension during dialysis	Sudden ↓BP; often leg cramps; sometimes chest pain	Fluid removal and hypovolaemia	Saline infusion; exclude cardiac ischaemia; quinine may help cramp
Cardiac arrhythmias	↓BP; sometimes chest pain	Potassium and acid–base shifts	Check K+ and arterial blood gases; review dialysis prescription; ?stop dialysis
Haemorrhage	Blood loss (overt or occult); ↓BP	Anticoagulation Venous needle disconnection	Stop dialysis; seek source; consider heparin-free treatment
Air embolism	Circulatory collapse; cardiac arrest	Disconnected or faulty lines and equipment malfunction	Stop dialysis
Dialyser hypersensitivity	Acute circulatory collapse	Allergic reaction to dialysis membrane or sterilisant	Stop dialysis; change to different artificial kidney
Emergencies between treatments Pulmonary oedema Systemic sepsis	Breathlessness Rigors; fever; ↓BP	Fluid overload Usually involves vascular access devices (catheter or fistula)	Ultrafiltration ± dialysis Blood cultures; antibiotics

The patient is mobile and able to undertake normal daily activities.

CAPD is particularly useful in young children, and in elderly patients with cardiovascular instability. Its long-term use may be limited by episodes of bacterial peritonitis and damage to the peritoneal membrane, but patients have been treated successfully for more than 10 years. Box 17.35 summarises some of the problems related to CAPD treatment.

The use of automated peritoneal dialysis (APD) is now widespread. This system is similar to CAPD but uses a mechanical device to perform the fluid exchanges during the night, leaving the patient free, or with only a single exchange to perform, during the day.

Conservative treatment of stage 5 CKD

In older patients with multiple comorbidity, 'conservative' treatment, aimed at limiting the adverse symptomatic effects of ESRD without commencing dialysis, is increasingly viewed as a positive choice (Box 17.36). Current evidence suggests that these patients' survival without dialysis can be similar to equivalent cohorts opting for RRT, but they avoid the hospitalisation and interventions associated with dialysis. Patients are offered full medical, psychological and social support to optimise and sustain their existing renal function and ameliorate the consequences (e.g. erythropoietin treatment for anaemia) for as long as possible, and appropriate palliative care in the terminal phase of their disease. Many of these patients enjoy a good quality of life for several years. It is also appropriate to discontinue dialysis treatment, with the consent of the patient, and to offer conservative therapy and palliative care when quality of life on dialysis is clearly inadequate.

Renal transplantation

Renal transplantation offers the best chance of long-term survival and complete rehabilitation, and is the

17.35 Problems with continuous ambulatory peritoneal dialysis (CAPD)

Problem	Clinical features	Cause	Treatment
CAPD peritonitis	Cloudy drainage fluid; abdominal pain and systemic sepsis are variable	Usually entry of skin contaminants via catheter; bowel organisms less common	Culture of peritoneal dialysis fluid Intraperitoneal antibiotics, e.g. tobramycin, vancomycin Catheter removal sometimes required
Catheter exit site infection	Erythema and pus around exit site	Usually skin organisms	Antibiotics; sometimes surgical drainage
Ultrafiltration failure	Fluid overload	Damage to peritoneal membrane, leading to rapid transport of glucose and loss of osmotic gradient	Replace glucose with synthetic poorly absorbed polymers for some exchanges (e.g. icodextrin)
Peritoneal membrane failure	Inadequate clearance of urea etc.	Scarring/damage to peritoneal membrane	Increase exchange volumes; consider automated peritoneal dialysis or switch to haemodialysis
Sclerosing peritonitis	Intermittent bowel obstruction Malnutrition	Unknown; typically occurs after many years	Switch to haemodialysis (may still progress) Surgery and tamoxifen may be used

17.36 Renal replacement therapy in old age

- **Quality of life**: age itself is not a barrier to good quality of life on RRT.
- **Coexisting cardiovascular disease**: older people are more sensitive to fluid balance changes, predisposing to hypotension during dialysis with rebound hypertension between dialyses. A failing heart cannot cope with fluid overload and pulmonary oedema develops easily.
- **Provision of treatment**: often only hospital-provided haemodialysis is suitable and older patients require more medical and nursing time.
- **Survival on dialysis**: difficult to predict for an individual patient, but old age plus substantial comorbidity are associated with poor median survival.
- **Withdrawal from dialysis**: a common cause of death in older patients with comorbid disease.
- **Transplantation**: relative risks of surgery and immunosuppression, and limited organ availability exclude most older people from transplantation.
- **Conservative therapy**: i.e. without dialysis but with adequate support; may be a popular option for patients at high risk of complications from dialysis, who have a limited prognosis and little hope of functional recovery.

17.37 Contraindications to renal transplantation

Absolute

- Active malignancy: a period of at least 2 yrs of complete remission recommended for most tumours
- Active vasculitis or recent anti-GBM disease
- Severe heart disease
- Severe occlusive aorto-iliac vascular disease

Relative

- Age: while practice varies, transplants are not routinely offered to very young children (< 1 yr) or older people (> 75 yrs)
- High risk of disease recurrence in the transplant kidney
- Disease of the lower urinary tract: in patients with impaired bladder function, an ileal conduit may be considered
- Significant comorbidity

most cost-effective treatment in patients with ESRD. It can restore normal kidney function and correct all the metabolic abnormalities of CKD. All patients should be considered for transplantation unless there are active contraindications (Box 17.37).

Kidney grafts may be taken from a cadaver or from a living donor. As described on pages 93–94, matching of a donor to a specific recipient is strongly influenced by immunological factors, since graft rejection is the major cause of transplant failure. ABO (blood group) compatibility between donor and recipient is required, and the degree of matching for major histocompatibility (MHC) antigens, particularly HLA–DR, influences the incidence of rejection. Further tests pre-transplantation include T- and B-cell cross-matching and tests for antibodies against HLA antigens. Positive tests predict early rejection.

In the transplant operation, the donor vessels are anastomosed to the recipient iliac artery and vein, and the donor ureter to the bladder (see Fig. 17.20; p. 493). Peri-operative problems include:

- *Fluid balance*. Careful matching of input to output is required.
- *Primary graft non-function*. Causes include hypovolaemia, preservation injury/acute tubular necrosis during storage and transfer, other pre-existing renal damage, hyperacute rejection, vascular occlusion and urinary tract obstruction.
- *Sepsis* (risks from operation compounded by uraemia and immunosuppression).

Once the graft begins to function, normal or near-normal biochemistry is usually achieved within days to weeks.

Management after transplantation

All transplant patients require regular life-long follow-up to monitor renal function and immunosuppression. Life-long immunosuppressive therapy (see Box 4.25, p. 94) is required to prevent rejection but it is more intensive in the early post-transplant period when the risk is highest. A common regimen is triple therapy with prednisolone, ciclosporin or tacrolimus, and azathioprine or mycophenolate mofetil. Rapamycin is an alternative that can be introduced later. Antibodies to deplete or modulate specific lymphocyte populations are increasingly used; targeting the lymphocyte IL-2 receptor is particularly effective for preventing rejection. Acute rejection is usually treated by short courses of very high-dose corticosteroids in the first instance, although other more potent therapies, such as antilymphocyte antibodies or plasma exchange, can be used in resistant episodes.

Complications of immunosuppression include infections and malignancy (p. 94). Approximately 50% of white patients develop skin malignancy by 15 years after transplantation.

The prognosis after kidney transplantation has improved significantly. Recent UK statistics for transplants from cadaver donors indicate 96% patient survival and 92% graft survival at 1 year, and 87% patient survival and 82% graft survival at 5 years. Even better figures are obtained with living donor transplantation (88% graft survival at 5 years). Advances in immunosuppression have greatly improved results using genetically unrelated donors such as spouses.

RENAL VASCULAR DISEASES

Diseases which affect renal blood vessels may cause renal ischaemia, leading to acute or chronic kidney disease or secondary hypertension. The rising prevalence of atherosclerosis and diabetes mellitus in ageing populations has made renovascular disease an important cause of ESRD.

Large-vessel disease: renal artery stenosis

Presentations

Hypertension

Renal artery stenosis classically presents as hypertension if it affects a single kidney or as renal failure if it is bilateral. The hypertension is driven by activation of the renin–angiotensin system in response to renal ischaemia. In atherosclerotic renal artery disease, there is usually evidence of vascular disease elsewhere, particularly

17.38 Renal artery stenosis

Renal artery stenosis is more likely if:

- Hypertension is severe, *or* of recent onset, *or* difficult to control
- Kidneys are asymmetrical in size
- Flash pulmonary oedema occurs repeatedly
- There is peripheral vascular disease of lower limbs
- Renal function has deteriorated on ACE inhibitors

in the legs. The selection of hypertensive patients who warrant investigation for secondary hypertension is discussed on page 608. Factors which predict renovascular disease are shown in Box 17.38.

Deterioration of renal function on ACE inhibitors

When renal perfusion pressure drops, the renin–angiotensin–aldosterone system is activated and angiotensin II-mediated glomerular efferent arteriolar vasoconstriction maintains glomerular filtration pressure. ACE inhibitors or ARBs block this physiological response. A drop in GFR of > 20%, or a > 25% rise in creatinine, on ACE inhibitors raises the possibility of renal artery stenosis. This is not a sensitive diagnostic test, however.

Flash pulmonary oedema

Repeated episodes of acute pulmonary oedema associated with severe hypertension, occurring without other obvious cause (e.g. myocardial infarction, dysrhythmia, anaemia, thyrotoxicosis) in patients with normal or only mildly impaired renal and cardiac function, can occur in renal artery stenosis. This presentation is characteristic of bilateral renovascular disease because in unilateral disease salt and water retention are partly corrected by increased 'pressure natriuresis' in the normal kidney.

Acute renal infarction

Sudden occlusion of the renal arteries causes acute loin pain, usually with dipstick haematuria. It may be caused by local atherosclerosis (atheroembolic) or by thromboemboli from a distant source, e.g. mural cardiac thrombus. Bilateral occlusion (as in aortic occlusion—look for absent femoral pulses and reduced lower limb perfusion), or acute occlusion of the artery to a single kidney, will cause acute renal failure. Severe hypertension is common but not universal; presumably, some residual renal perfusion is required to generate renin release.

Aetiology

Reduction of renal blood flow is associated with > 70% narrowing of the artery, and commonly with a dilated region more distally (post-stenotic dilatation).

Atherosclerosis is the most common cause, especially in older patients. The characteristic lesion is an ostial stenosis that is associated with atherosclerosis within the aorta and affecting other major branches, particularly the iliac vessels. Renal impairment is not simply related to the degree of stenosis. The picture is often complicated by small-vessel disease in affected kidneys that may be related to subclinical atheroemboli, hypertension or other disease. As the stenosis becomes more severe, global renal ischaemia leads to shrinkage of the affected kidney and may cause renal failure (ischaemic nephropathy). However, the progression of stenosis is not easily predictable, and many patients die from coronary, cerebral or other vascular disease rather than renal failure.

In younger patients (< 50 years), fibromuscular dysplasia is a more likely cause of renal artery stenosis. This is an uncommon congenital disorder of unknown cause affecting the media ('medial fibroplasia'), which narrows the artery but rarely leads to total occlusion. It may be associated with disease in other arteries; for example, those who have carotid artery dissections are more likely to have this appearance in their renal arteries. It most commonly presents with hypertension in patients aged 15–30 years, and in women more frequently than men. Irregular narrowing ('beading') affects the distal renal artery, sometimes extending into intrarenal branches.

Rarely, large-vessel vasculitis, particularly Takayasu's arteritis (p. 1113), may involve renal arteries. Medium-sized arteries are more typically affected in polyarteritis nodosa (p. 1113).

Investigations

A number of investigations may be abnormal in patients with renovascular disease. Renal function may be impaired and plasma renin activity may be elevated, sometimes with hypokalaemia due to hyperaldosteronism. Ultrasound may reveal a discrepancy in size between the two kidneys. Unfortunately, these simple non-invasive tests are insufficiently sensitive for screening in hypertensive patients and vascular imaging is required to diagnose renovascular disease. Such imaging is usually undertaken only in patients in whom intervention to improve renal perfusion would be contemplated; this is usually limited to young patients and those in whom blood pressure cannot be controlled with antihypertensive agents ('resistant hypertension'), those who have a history of 'flash' pulmonary oedema or accelerated phase ('malignant') hypertension, or those in whom renal function is deteriorating.

CT and MRI angiographic techniques have largely replaced Doppler ultrasound or renal isotope scanning (including 'captopril renography') in diagnosing renal artery stenosis. Conventional renal artery cannulation and arteriography is now usually undertaken for therapeutic rather than diagnostic purposes. CT angiography entails large intravenously administered doses of contrast medium which may be nephrotoxic. MR angiography (Fig. 17.23) is expensive and also carries some risks in patients with severe renal impairment (see Box 17.4, p. 467). Although these techniques at present give good views of the main renal arteries only, these are the vessels affected in atherosclerosis and the most amenable to intervention.

Management

Untreated, atheromatous renal artery stenosis is thought to progress to complete arterial occlusion and loss of kidney function in about 15% of cases. This figure is increased with more severe degrees of stenosis. If the progression is gradual, collateral vessels may develop and some function may be preserved, preventing infarction and loss of kidney structure. Conversely, at least 85% of patients with renal artery stenosis will not develop progressive renal impairment, and indeed in many patients

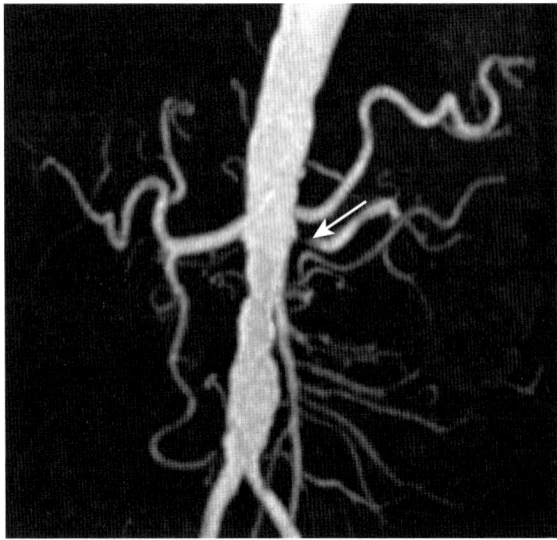

Fig. 17.23 Renal artery stenosis. A magnetic resonance angiogram following injection of contrast. The abdominal aorta is severely irregular and atheromatous. The left renal artery is stenosed (arrow).

the stenosis may be haemodynamically insignificant and not responsible for coexisting essential hypertension. Unfortunately, methods to predict which patients are at risk of progression or will respond to treatment are still imperfect.

Surgical intervention is rarely undertaken now for atherosclerotic disease, as it is associated with high morbidity and mortality. Treatment options are:

- medical management with blood pressure-lowering, low-dose aspirin and lipid-lowering drugs; this should usually have been attempted before angiography is performed.
- angioplasty, with placement of stents in atherosclerotic disease areas to improve primary patency rates and prevent rapid recurrence.

Angioplasty is widely used but there may be substantial risks in patients with atherosclerosis: contrast nephropathy (see Box 17.4, p. 467), renal artery occlusion and renal infarction, and atheroemboli (p. 499) from manipulations in a severely diseased aorta. Small-vessel disease distal to the stenosis may preclude substantial functional recovery. Randomised trials have so far failed to show improved outcome with angioplasty in patients with stable renal function.

In non-atheromatous fibromuscular dysplasia, the renal artery stenosis is much more likely to be the cause of the presentation, and angioplasty has a high chance of success in improving blood pressure and protecting renal function.

Diseases of small intrarenal vessels

A number of conditions are associated with acute damage and occlusion of small blood vessels (arterioles and capillaries) in the kidney (Box 17.39). They may be associated with similar changes elsewhere in the body. A common feature of these syndromes is microangiopathic haemolytic anaemia, in which haemolysis occurs as a consequence of damage incurred to red blood cells during

17.39 Microvascular disorders associated with acute renal damage

- Thrombotic microangiopathy (haemolytic uraemic syndrome and thrombotic thrombocytopenic purpura)
    Associated with verotoxin-producing *E. coli*
    Other (familial, drugs, cancer etc.)
- Disseminated intravascular coagulation
- Malignant hypertension
- Small-vessel vasculitis
- Systemic sclerosis (scleroderma)
- Atheroemboli ('cholesterol' emboli)

passage through the abnormal vessels; fragmented red cells can be seen on a blood film.

Thrombotic microangiopathy: haemolytic uraemic syndrome and thrombotic thrombocytopenic purpura

Haemolytic uraemic syndrome (HUS) and thrombotic thrombocytopenic purpura (TTP) are types of thrombotic microangiopathy. Common features include damage to endothelial cells of the microcirculation, which is followed by cell swelling, platelet adherence and thrombosis. A severe microangiopathy causes a marked reduction in the platelet count and anaemia. Other features of intravascular haemolysis (p. 1023)—raised bilirubin and LDH, decreased haptoglobins—are also present. A reticulocytosis is often seen. The aetiology of the syndromes may be different, although there is substantial overlap. The kidney microcirculation tends to be most affected in HUS, with involvement of other organs (including the brain) in more severe cases. In TTP the brain is commonly affected and involvement of the kidney is usually less severe.

E. coli O157-associated HUS

Thrombotic microangiopathy associated with *E. coli* infection (especially O157 serotypes) is caused by verotoxin-producing organisms (p. 337). Although the bacteria live as commensals in the gut of cattle and other domestic livestock, they can cause haemorrhagic diarrhoea in humans when the infection is contracted from contaminated food products, water or other infected individuals. In a proportion of cases, verotoxin produced by the organisms enters the circulation and binds to specific glycolipid receptors that are expressed on the surface of microvascular endothelial cells. In children, this causes diarrhoea-associated (D+)HUS, although in more severe cases the brain and other organs are also affected. D+HUS is now the most common cause of ARF in children in developed countries. Recovery is good in most patients, often after 5–15 days of dialysis. No specific treatments have been shown to help.

TTP and other HUS

Other causes of thrombotic microangiopathy have a less certain outlook and are more likely to recur (sometimes after renal transplantation). Inherited causes may reflect an abnormality of endothelial cell defence against damage or thrombosis, including deficiency of complement activation inhibitors (associated with familial HUS) or of von Willebrand protease (associated with TTP, p. 1048). The disease may also occur post-partum, in response to certain drugs (especially chemotherapy), after bone marrow transplantation, in malignancy and apparently spontaneously. Plasma exchange using fresh frozen plasma is effective in many of these cases, probably by replacing a deficient substance (e.g. the von Willebrand protease) and sometimes removing an autoantibody.

Disseminated intravascular coagulation

In this condition, consumption of clotting factors and platelets occurs due to uncontrolled thrombosis in the microvasculature (p. 1050). Precipitating conditions include: septic shock, in which bacterial endotoxin directly activates the coagulation cascade; obstetric complications; disseminated cancer; massive transfusion; and other causes of coagulation activation or depletion.

Accelerated phase ('malignant') hypertension

Hypertension is described as being in accelerated phase (p. 608) when it causes acute damage to renal and other arterioles. It is often symptomatic, with headache, impaired vision and, finally, manifestations of renal failure (Fig. 17.24). Severe hypertensive retinopathy with papilloedema is almost always present, usually with some of the features of microangiopathy described above. In the absence of a previous history, it may be difficult to distinguish these patients from those with HUS and hypertension. Patients usually respond to effective control of blood pressure, although renal function is permanently lost in 20% of cases.

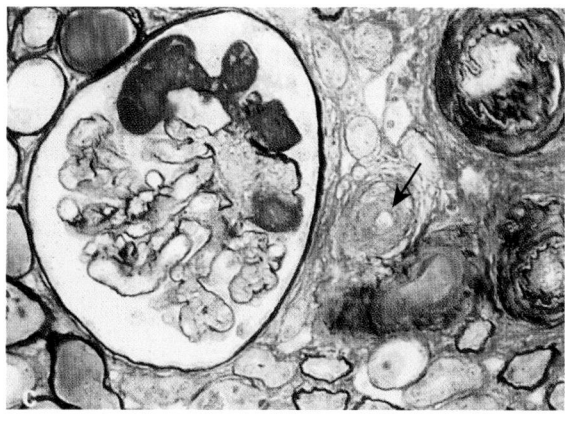

Fig. 17.24 Glomerular capillary thrombosis in malignant hypertension. Similar changes occur in thrombotic microangiopathy. The adjacent arteriole (arrow) shows gross intimal thickening.

Systemic sclerosis (scleroderma)

This connective tissue disease is described on page 1109. Renal involvement is a serious feature, characterised by intimal cell proliferation and luminal narrowing of intrarenal arteries and arterioles. Clinically, it usually presents as 'scleroderma renal crisis', with severe hypertension, microangiopathic features and progressive oliguric renal failure. There is intense intrarenal vasospasm and plasma renin activity is markedly elevated. Use of ACE inhibitors to control the hypertension has improved the 1-year survival from 20% to 75%; however, about 50% of patients continue to require RRT. Onset or acceleration of the syndrome after stopping ACE inhibitors is now well described.

Atheroembolic renal disease ('cholesterol' emboli)

This is caused by showers of cholesterol-containing microemboli, arising in atheromatous plaques in major arteries. It occurs in patients with widespread atheromatous disease, usually after interventions such as surgery or arteriography but sometimes after anticoagulation. There is loss of renal function, haematuria and proteinuria, and sometimes eosinophilia and inflammatory features which may mimic a small-vessel vasculitis. Accompanying signs of microvascular occlusion in the lower limbs (e.g. ischaemic toes, livedo reticularis) are common but not invariable (Fig. 17.25). There is no specific treatment but anticoagulation may be detrimental.

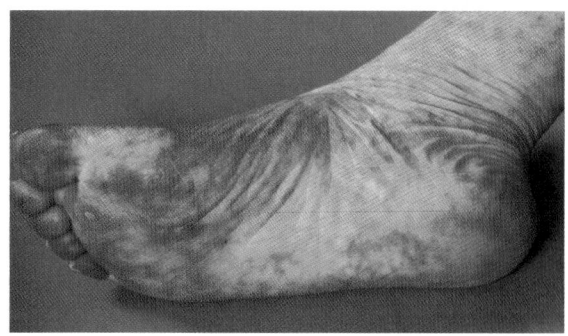

Fig. 17.25 The foot of a patient who suffered extensive atheroembolism following coronary artery stenting.

Small-vessel vasculitis

Renal disease caused by small-vessel vasculitis usually affects the glomeruli, as described in the next section and on page 516.

GLOMERULAR DISEASES

Glomerular diseases account for a significant proportion of acute and chronic kidney disease. Glomerular damage may follow a number of insults: immunological injury, inherited abnormality (e.g. Alport's syndrome, p. 504), metabolic stress (e.g. diabetes mellitus, p. 829), deposition of extraneous materials (e.g. amyloid), or other direct injury to glomerular cells. The cell types of the glomerulus that may be the target of injury are shown in Figure 17.26. The response of the glomerulus to injury and hence the predominant clinical features vary according to the nature of the insult (Fig. 17.27). Glomerular diseases cause some or all of:

- leakage of cells and macromolecules across the glomerular filtration barrier
    proteinuria: characteristic of podocyte diseases or of alteration of architecture by scarring or deposition of foreign material
    haematuria: characteristic of inflammatory and destructive processes
- loss of filtration capacity (GFR)
- hypertension.

Most patients with glomerular disease do not present acutely and are essentially asymptomatic, with abnormalities of blood or urine detected on routine screening, often accompanied by high blood pressure, with or without reduced GFR.

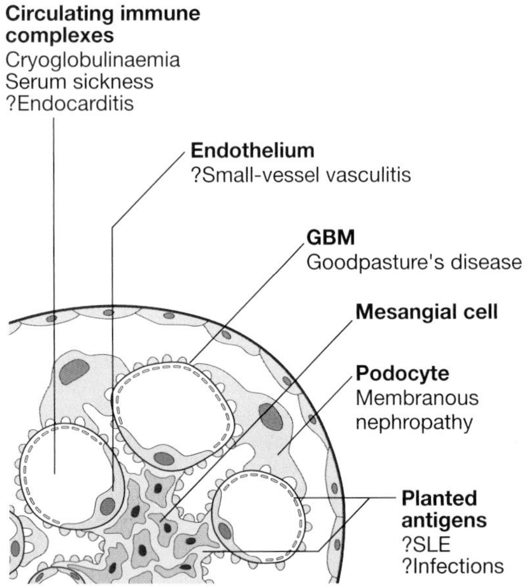

Circulating immune complexes
Cryoglobulinaemia
Serum sickness
?Endocarditis

Endothelium
?Small-vessel vasculitis

GBM
Goodpasture's disease

Mesangial cell

Podocyte
Membranous nephropathy

Planted antigens
?SLE
?Infections

Fig. 17.26 Cells of the glomerulus and targets of immunity and autoimmunity. Antibodies and antigen–antibody (immune) complexes are described according to their site of deposition: subepithelial, between podocyte and GBM; intramembranous, within the GBM; subendothelial, between endothelial cell and GBM; and mesangial, within the mesangial matrix.

Glomerulonephritis

Glomerulonephritis means 'inflammation of glomeruli' and, although inflammation is not apparent in all varieties ('glomerulopathy' is sometimes used to denote this), the name sticks.

Most types of glomerulonephritis seem to be immunologically mediated and several respond to immunosuppressive drugs. Deposition of antibody occurs in many types of glomerulonephritis (Box 17.40) but frequently the presumed mechanisms involve cellular immunity, which is more difficult to investigate. Although deposition of circulating immune complexes was previously thought to be a common mechanism, it now seems that most granular deposits of immunoglobulin are formed 'in situ' by antibodies which complex about glomerular antigens, or about other antigens ('planted' antigens, e.g. viral or bacterial ones) that have localised in glomeruli (see Fig. 17.26).

Classifications of glomerulonephritis are largely histopathological and may appear daunting, but the details are largely a specialist concern. Clinically important types are described in the text. Box 17.40 and Figure 17.29 on pages 502–503 show additional detail and illustrate the major types.

Minimal change nephropathy

Minimal change disease occurs at all ages but accounts for nephrotic syndrome (Box 17.19, p. 479) in most children and about one-quarter of adults. Proteinuria usually remits on high-dose corticosteroid therapy (1 mg/kg prednisolone for 6 weeks), although some patients who respond incompletely or relapse frequently need maintenance corticosteroids, cytotoxic therapy or other agents. Minimal change disease does not progress to CKD; the main problems are those of the nephrotic syndrome and complications of treatment.

Primary focal segmental glomerulosclerosis (FSGS)

FSGS is a histological description (Fig. 17.29B) with many causes. As FSGS is a focal process, abnormal glomeruli

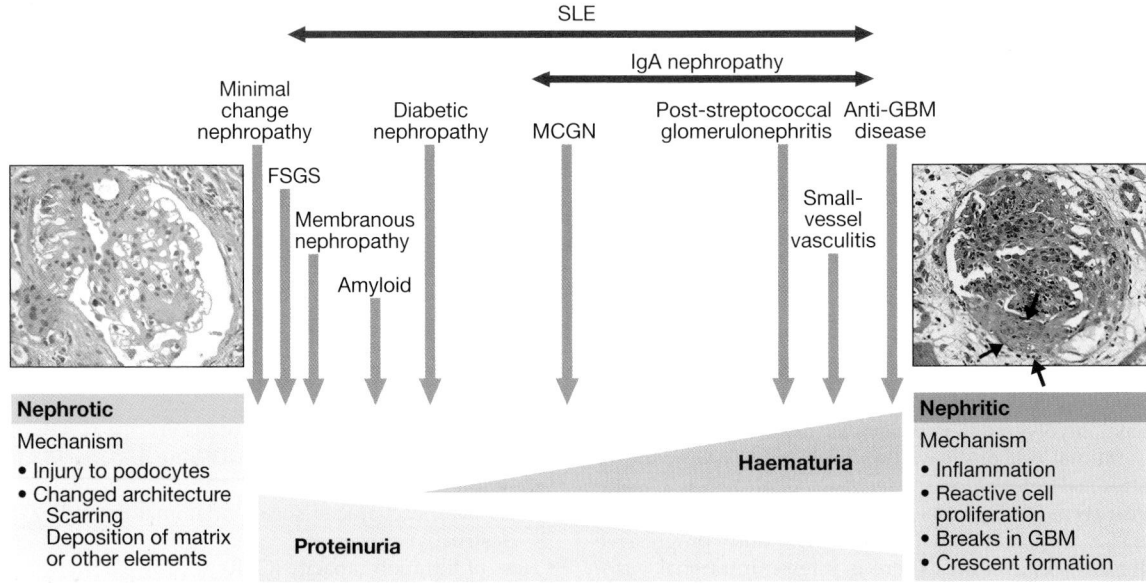

Fig. 17.27 Spectrum of glomerular diseases. At one extreme, specific injury to podocytes, or structural alteration of the glomerulus affecting podocyte function (for example, by scarring or deposition of excess matrix or other material), causes proteinuria and nephrotic syndrome (see Box 17.19, p. 479). The histology to the left shows diabetic nephropathy. At the other end of the spectrum, inflammation leads to cell damage and proliferation, breaks form in the GBM and blood leaks into urine. In its extreme form, with acute sodium retention and hypertension, such disease is labelled nephritic syndrome (FSGS = focal and segmental glomerulosclerosis; MCGN = mesangiocapillary glomerulonephritis). The histology to the right shows a glomerulus with many extra nuclei from proliferating intrinsic cells and influx of inflammatory cells shows crescent formation (arrows) in response to severe post-infectious glomerulonephritis.

may not be seen on renal biopsy if only a few are sampled, leading to an initial diagnosis of minimal change nephropathy. Juxtamedullary glomeruli are more likely to be affected in early disease.

The primary FSGS group that present with idiopathic nephrotic syndrome and no other cause of renal disease typically show little response to corticosteroid treatment and often progress to renal failure. This disease frequently recurs after renal transplantation, and sometimes proteinuria recurs almost immediately. However, a proportion of patients with FSGS do respond to corticosteroids (a good prognostic sign).

In other patients with the histological appearances of FSGS but lesser proteinuria, focal scarring reflects healing of previous focal glomerular injury, such as HUS, cholesterol embolism or vasculitis. In others, it seems to represent particular types of nephropathy: for example, those associated with HIV infection, some podocyte toxins and massive obesity. Associations with numerous other forms of injury and renal disorders are reported. There is no specific treatment for most of these.

Membranous nephropathy

This is the most common cause of nephrotic syndrome in adults. A proportion of cases are associated with known causes (Box 17.40 and Figs 17.29D and F) but most are idiopathic. Of this group, approximately one-third remit spontaneously, one-third remain in a nephrotic state, and one-third show progressive loss of renal function. Short-term treatment with high doses of corticosteroids and alkylating agents (e.g. cyclophosphamide) may improve both the nephrotic syndrome and the long-term prognosis. However, because of the toxicity of these regimens, most nephrologists reserve such treatment for those with severe nephrotic syndrome or deteriorating renal function.

IgA nephropathy and Henoch–Schönlein purpura

IgA nephropathy is the most commonly recognised type of glomerulonephritis and can present in many ways (Figs 17.28 and 17.29G). Haematuria is the earliest sign and is almost universal, proteinuria a later feature, and hypertension very common. There may be severe proteinuria or in some cases progressive loss of renal function. The disease is a common cause of ESRD. A particular hallmark in young adults is acute self-limiting exacerbations, often with gross haematuria, in association with minor respiratory infections. This may be so acute as to resemble acute post-infectious glomerulonephritis, with fluid retention, hypertension and oliguria with dark or red urine. Characteristically, the latency from clinical infection to nephritis is short: a few days or less. Occasionally, IgA nephropathy progresses rapidly and crescent formation may be seen. The response to immunosuppressive therapy is usually poor. The management of less acute disease is largely directed towards the control of blood pressure in an attempt to prevent or retard progressive renal disease.

In children, and occasionally in adults, a systemic vasculitis occurring in response to similar infections is called Henoch–Schönlein purpura. A characteristic petechial rash (cutaneous vasculitis, typically affecting buttocks and lower legs) and abdominal pain (gastrointestinal

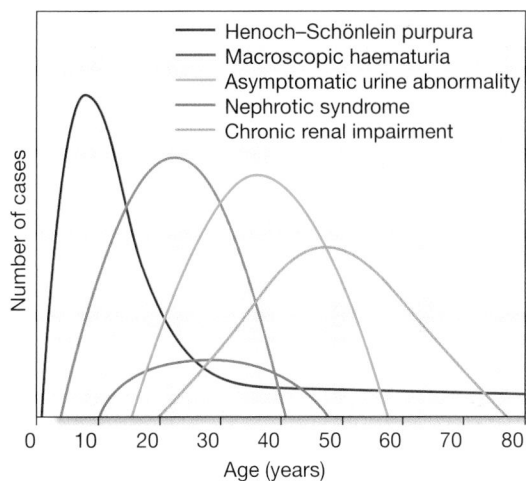

Fig. 17.28 Clinical presentations of IgA nephropathy in relation to age at diagnosis. Henoch–Schönlein purpura is most common in childhood but may occur at any age. Macroscopic haematuria is very uncommon over the age of 40 years. The detection of IgA nephropathy amongst patients with asymptomatic urine abnormality will depend on attitudes to routine urine testing and renal biopsy. It is uncertain whether patients presenting with chronic renal impairment have a disease distinct from that of patients presenting at a younger age with macroscopic haematuria.

vasculitis) usually dominate the clinical picture, with mild glomerulonephritis being indicated by haematuria. When the disease occurs in older children or adults, the glomerulonephritis is usually more prominent. Renal biopsy shows mesangial IgA deposition and appearances indistinguishable from acute IgA nephropathy.

Glomerulonephritis associated with infection

Bacterial infections, usually subacute (typically subacute bacterial endocarditis), may cause a variety of histological patterns of glomerulonephritis, most typically with membranous and mesangiocapillary lesions, and usually with plentiful immunoglobulin deposition and often evidence of complement consumption (low serum C3, Box 17.41). In the developed world, hospital-acquired infections are now a common cause of these syndromes. World-wide, glomerulonephritis occurs more commonly following hepatitis B, hepatitis C, schistosomiasis, leishmaniasis and possibly malaria and other chronic infections. FSGS associated with HIV infection is prevalent in black races. Proving a causative relationship between renal disease and infection in individual cases is difficult. Acute and chronic infections may also cause interstitial renal disease (p. 504).

Acute post-infectious glomerulonephritis

This is most common following infection with certain strains of streptococcus and therefore is often called post-streptococcal nephritis, but it can occur following other infections. It is much more common in children than adults but is now rare in the developed world. The latency is usually about 10 days after a throat infection or longer after skin infection, suggesting an immune mechanism rather than direct infection.

An acute nephritis of varying severity occurs. Sodium retention, hypertension and oedema are particularly

17

17

17.40 Glomerulonephritis: types, associations and causes

Histology	Immune deposits	Pathogenesis	Associations	Comments
Minimal change				
Normal, except on electron microscopy, where fusion of podocyte foot processes is seen (a non-specific finding)	None	Unknown	Atopy HLA–DR7 Drugs	Acute and often severe nephrotic syndrome Good response to corticosteroids Dominant cause of idiopathic nephrotic syndrome in childhood
Focal segmental glomerulosclerosis (FSGS)				
Segmental scars in some glomeruli No acute inflammation Podocyte foot process fusion seen in primary FSGS with nephrotic syndrome	Non-specific trapping in focal scars	Unknown; in some, circulating factors increase glomerular permeability Injury to podocytes may be a common feature	Healing of previous local glomerular injury HIV infection Heroin misuse Morbid obesity	*Primary FSGS* presents as idiopathic nephrotic syndrome but is less responsive to treatment than minimal change; may progress to renal impairment, can recur after transplantation *Secondary FSGS* presents with variable proteinuria and outcome
Focal segmental (necrotising) glomerulonephritis				
Segmental inflammation and/or necrosis in some glomeruli ± crescent formation	Variable according to cause, but typically negative (or 'pauci-immune')	Small-vessel vasculitis	Primary or secondary small-vessel vasculitis	Usually implies presence of systemic disease, and responds to treatment with corticosteroids and cytotoxic agents Check ANCA, ANA
Membranous nephropathy				
Thickening of GBM Progressing to increased matrix deposition and glomerulosclerosis	Granular subepithelial IgG	Antibodies to a podocyte surface antigen, with complement-dependent podocyte injury	HLA–DR3 (for idiopathic) HLA association varies in different populations Drugs Mercury, heavy metals Hepatitis B virus Malignancy	Usually idiopathic; common cause of adult idiopathic nephrotic syndrome One-third progress; may respond to chemotherapy/prednisolone
IgA nephropathy				
Increased mesangial matrix and cells Focal segmental nephritis in acute disease	Mesangial IgA	Unknown	Usually idiopathic Liver disease	Very common disease with range of presentations, but usually including haematuria and hypertension
Mesangiocapillary glomerulonephritis (MCGN) (= membranoproliferative glomerulonephritis, MPGN)				
Type I Mesangial cells interpose between endothelium and GBM	Subendothelial	Deposition of circulating immune complexes or 'planted' antigens	Bacterial infection Hepatitis B virus Cryoglobulinaemia ± hepatitis C virus	Usually proteinuria ± haematuria Most common pattern found in association with subacute bacterial infection No proven treatments
Type II Mesangial cells interpose between endothelium and GBM	Intramembranous dense deposits	Associated with complement consumption caused by autoantibodies	C3 nephritic factor and partial lipodystrophy	Also known as dense deposit disease
Post-infection				
Diffuse proliferation of endothelial and mesangial cells Infiltration by neutrophils and macrophages ± crescent formation	Subendothelial	Immune response to streptococcal infection with presumed cross-reactive epitopes	Streptococcal and other infections	Now rare in developed countries Presents with severe sodium and fluid retention, hypertension, haematuria, oliguria Usually resolves spontaneously
Goodpasture's disease (anti-GBM disease)				
Usually crescentic nephritis	Linear IgG along GBM	Autoantibodies to $\alpha 3$ chain of type IV collagen	HLA–DR15 (previously known as DR2)	Associated with lung haemorrhage but either may occur alone Treat with corticosteroids, cyclophosphamide and plasma exchange
Lupus nephritis				
Almost any histological type	Always positive and often profuse Pattern varies according to type	Some anti-DNA antibodies also bind to glomerular targets	Complement deficiencies Complement consumption	Very variable presentation, sometimes as renal disease alone without systemic features Responds to cytotoxic therapy in addition to prednisolone

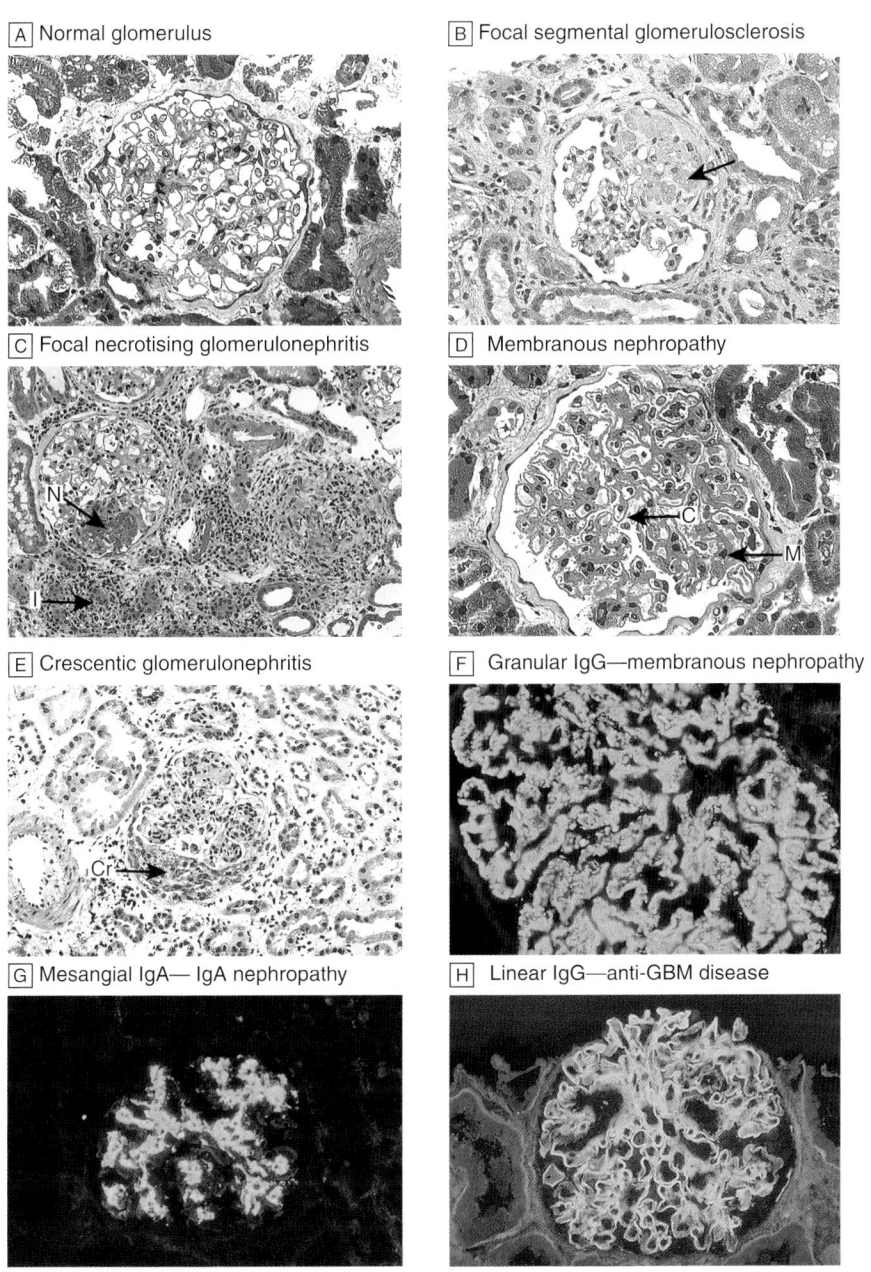

Fig. 17.29 Histopathology of glomerular disease. (A–E light microscopy) A A normal glomerulus. Note the open capillary loops and thinness of their walls—'should look as if you could cut yourself on them'. B Focal segmental glomerulosclerosis. The portion of the glomerulus arrowed shows loss of capillary loops and cells, which are replaced by matrix. C Focal necrotising glomerulonephritis. A portion of the glomerulus (N = focal necrotising lesion) is replaced by bright pink material with some 'nuclear dust'. Neutrophils may be seen elsewhere in the glomerulus. There is surrounding interstitial inflammation (I). This is most commonly associated with small-vessel vasculitis and may progress to crescentic nephritis (see E). D Membranous nephropathy. The capillary loops (C) are thickened (compare with the normal glomerulus) and there is expansion of the mesangial regions by matrix deposition (M). However, there is no gross cellular proliferation or excess of inflammatory cells. E Crescentic glomerulonephritis. The lower part of Bowman's space is occupied by a semicircular formation ('crescent', Cr) of large pale cells, compressing the glomerular tuft. This is usually seen in aggressive inflammatory types of glomerulonephritis. **Antibody deposition in the glomerulus. (F–H direct immunofluorescence)** F Granular deposits of IgG along the basement membrane in a subepithelial pattern, typical of membranous nephropathy. G IgA deposits in the mesangium, as seen in IgA nephropathy. H Ribbon-like linear deposits of anti-GBM antibodies along the GBM in Goodpasture's disease. Glomerular structure is well preserved in all of these examples.

pronounced. There is also reduction of GFR, proteinuria, haematuria and reduced urine volume. Characteristically, this gives the urine a red or smoky appearance. There are low serum concentrations of C3 and C4 (see Box 17.41) and evidence of streptococcal infection (perform antistreptolysin O (ASO) titre, culture of throat swab, and other microbiological sampling if skin infection is suspected).

Renal function begins to improve spontaneously within 10–14 days, and management by fluid and sodium restriction and use of diuretic and hypotensive agents is usually adequate. Remarkably, the renal lesion in almost all children and many adults seems to resolve completely despite the severity of the glomerular inflammation and proliferation seen histologically.

17

> **17.41 Causes of glomerulonephritis associated with low serum complement**
>
> - Post-infection glomerulonephritis
> - Subacute bacterial infection: especially endocarditis
> - SLE
> - Cryoglobulinaemia
> - Mesangiocapillary glomerulonephritis, usually type II

Rapidly progressive (crescentic) glomerulonephritis

This describes an extreme inflammatory nephritis which causes rapid loss of renal function over days to weeks. Renal biopsy shows crescentic lesions often associated with necrotising lesions within the glomerulus (focal segmental (necrotising) glomerulonephritis). It is typically seen in Goodpasture's disease, where there are specific anti-GBM antibodies, and in small-vessel vasculitides (pp. 516 and 1112), but can also be seen in SLE (pp. 517 and 1107) and occasionally IgA and other nephropathies.

Inherited glomerular diseases

Alport's syndrome

A number of uncommon diseases may affect the glomerulus in childhood, but the most important one affecting adults is Alport's syndrome. Most cases arise from a mutation or deletion of the *COL4A5* gene on the X chromosome which encodes type IV collagen, resulting in inheritance as an X-linked recessive disorder (p. 50). Mutations in *COL4A3* or *COL4A4* genes are less common and cause autosomal recessive disease. The accumulation of abnormal collagen results in a progressive degeneration of the GBM (Fig. 17.30). Affected patients progress from haematuria to ESRD in their late teens or twenties. Female carriers of *COL4A5* mutations usually have haematuria but rarely develop significant renal disease. Some other basement membranes containing the same collagen isoforms are similarly affected, notably in the cochlea, so that Alport's syndrome is associated with sensorineural deafness and ocular abnormalities.

No specific treatment is available, but patients with Alport's syndrome are good candidates for RRT, as they are young and usually otherwise healthy. Some of these patients develop an immune response to the normal collagen antigens present in the GBM of the donor kidney, and in a small minority anti-GBM disease develops and destroys the allograft.

Thin GBM disease

In 'thin GBM' disease there is glomerular bleeding, usually only at the microscopic or dipstick level, without associated hypertension, proteinuria or reduction of GFR. The glomeruli appear normal by light microscopy but on electron microscopy the GBM is abnormally thin. This autosomal dominant condition accounts for a large proportion of 'benign familial haematuria' and has an excellent prognosis. Some families may be carriers of autosomal recessive Alport's syndrome but this does not account for all cases.

TUBULO-INTERSTITIAL DISEASES

Acute tubular necrosis is the most common cause of the clinical syndrome of acute renal failure and is described on page 484. Illustrations of this and other tubulo-interstitial pathologies are shown in Figure 17.31.

Interstitial nephritis

A group of inflammatory, inherited and other diseases affect renal tubules and the surrounding interstitium. The clinical presentation is often simply with renal impairment. Proteinuria is generally low level (PCR < 100 mg/mmol) and tubular in type (p. 480). Urine may contain red and white blood cells.

Acute interstitial nephritis (AIN)

Acute inflammation within the tubulo-interstitium is most commonly allergic, particularly to drugs, but other causes include toxins and a variety of systemic diseases and infections (Box 17.42). Deterioration of renal function in drug-induced AIN may be dramatic and resemble rapidly progressive glomerulonephritis.

Diagnosis

A minority of patients with drug-induced AIN have a generalised drug hypersensitivity reaction (e.g. fever, rash, eosinophilia). Dipstick testing of the urine is usually unremarkable, but leucocyturia is common and eosinophils are found in the urine in up to 70% of patients. Many patients are not oliguric despite moderately severe

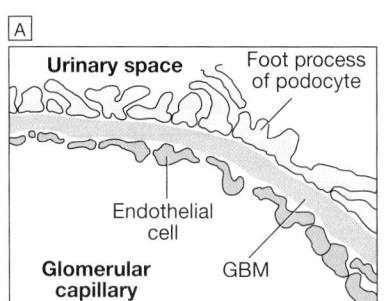
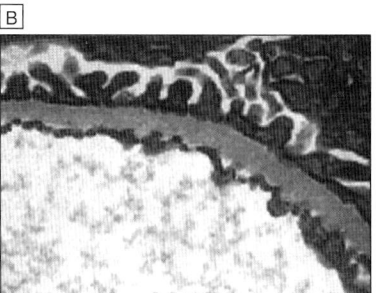
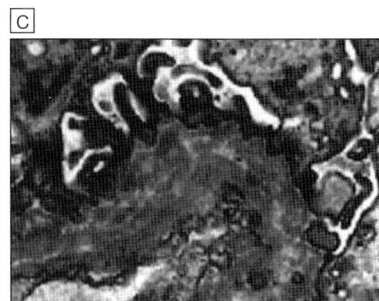

Fig. 17.30 Alport's syndrome. **A** Diagrammatic structure of the normal GBM. **B** The normal GBM (electron micrograph) contains mostly the tissue-specific α3, α4 and α5 chains of type IV collagen. **C** In Alport's syndrome this network is disrupted and replaced by α1 and α2 chains. Although the GBM appears structurally normal in early life, in time thinning appears, progressing to thickening, splitting and degeneration.

In image A labels: Urinary space; Foot process of podocyte; Endothelial cell; GBM; Glomerular capillary

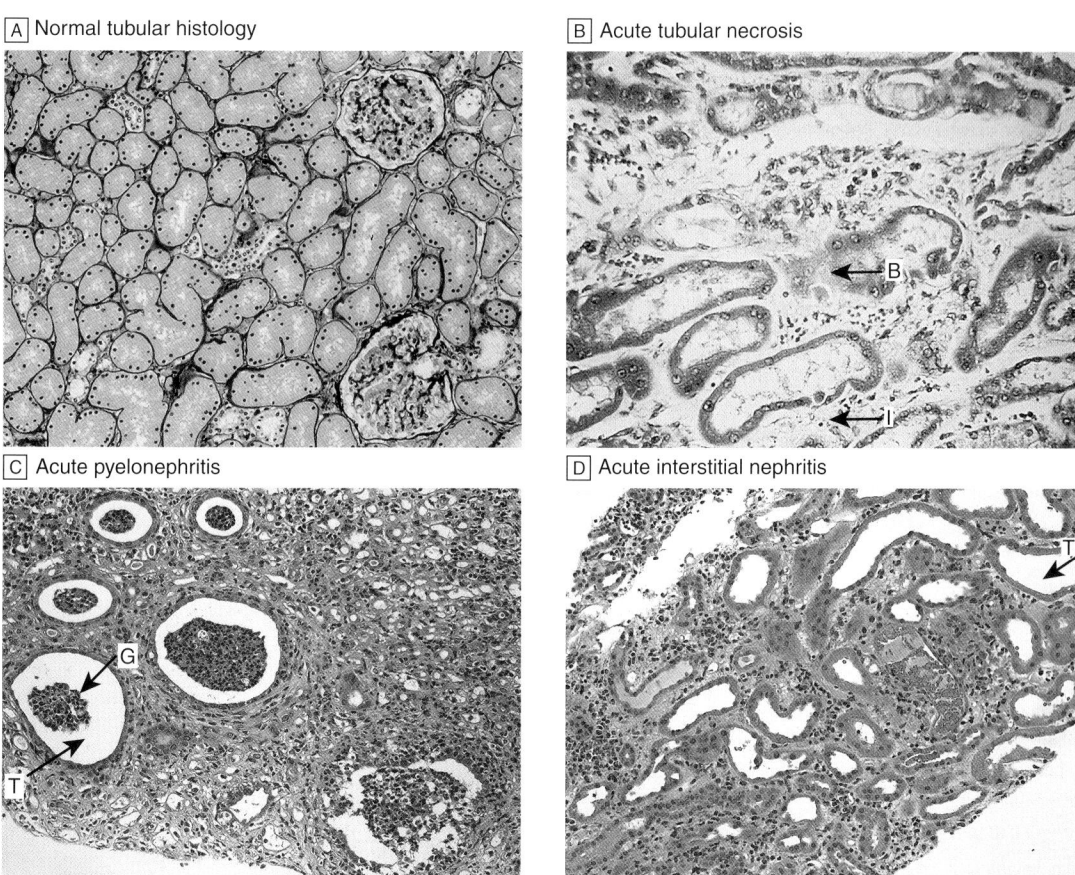

A Normal tubular histology

B Acute tubular necrosis

C Acute pyelonephritis

D Acute interstitial nephritis

Fig. 17.31 Tubular histopathology. **A** Normal tubular histology. The tubules are back to back. Brush borders can be seen on the luminal borders of cells in the proximal tubule. **B** Acute tubular necrosis. There are scattered breaks (B) in tubular basement membranes, swelling and vacuolation of tubular cells, and in places apoptosis and necrosis of tubular cells with shedding of cells into the lumen. During the regenerative phase there is increased tubular mitotic activity. The interstitium (I) is oedematous and infiltrated by inflammatory cells. The glomeruli (not shown) are relatively normal, although there may be endothelial cell swelling and fibrin deposition. **C** Acute bacterial pyelonephritis. A widespread inflammatory infiltrate that includes many neutrophils is seen. Granulocyte casts (G) are forming within some dilated tubules (T). Other tubules are scarcely visible because of the extent of the inflammation and damage. **D** Acute (allergic) interstitial nephritis. In this patient who received an NSAID, an extensive mononuclear cell infiltrate (no neutrophils) involving tubules (T) is seen. This inflammation does not involve the glomeruli (not shown). Sometimes eosinophils are prominent. Transplant rejection looks similar to this.

ARF, and AIN should always be considered in patients with non-oliguric ARF.

Renal biopsy is usually required to confirm the diagnosis (see Fig. 17.31), showing intense inflammation, with polymorphonuclear leucocytes and lymphocytes surrounding tubules and blood vessels and invading tubules (tubulitis), and occasional eosinophils (especially in drug-induced disease). The degree of chronic inflammation in a biopsy is a useful predictor of the eventual outcome for renal function.

Management

Some patients with drug-induced AIN recover following withdrawal of the drug alone, but corticosteroids (e.g. prednisolone 1 mg/kg/day) accelerate recovery and may prevent long-term scarring. Dialysis is sometimes necessary but is usually only short-term. Other specific causes (see Box 17.42) should be treated if possible.

Chronic interstitial nephritis

Aetiology

Chronic interstitial nephritis (CIN) is caused by a heterogeneous group of diseases, summarised in Box 17.43. However, it is quite common for the condition to be diagnosed late and for no aetiology to be apparent.

17.42 Causes of acute interstitial nephritis

Allergic

Many drugs, but particularly
- Penicillins
- NSAIDs
- Proton pump inhibitors
- Mesalazine (delayed)

Immune
- Autoimmune nephritis ± uveitis
- Transplant rejection

Infections
- Acute bacterial pyelonephritis
- Leptospirosis
- Tuberculosis
- Hantavirus

Toxic
- Myeloma light chains
- Mushrooms (*Cortinarius*)

17.43 Causes of chronic interstitial nephritis

Acute interstitial nephritis

• Any of the causes of AIN if persistent (see Box 17.42)

Glomerulonephritis

• Varying degrees of interstitial inflammation occur in association with most types of inflammatory glomerulonephritis

Immune/inflammatory

• Sarcoidosis	• SLE, primary autoimmune
• Sjögren's syndrome	• Chronic transplant rejection

Toxic

• Mushrooms (*Cortinarius*)	• *Aristolochia*
• Lead	• Balkan nephropathy

Drugs

• All drugs causing AIN	• Analgesic nephropathy
• Lithium toxicity	• Ciclosporin, tacrolimus

Infection

• Consequence of severe pyelonephritis

Congenital/developmental

• Vesico-ureteric reflux: is associated; causation not clear
• Renal dysplasias: often associated with reflux
• Inherited: now well recognised but mechanisms unclear
• Other: Wilson's disease, medullary sponge kidney, sickle-cell nephropathy

Metabolic and systemic diseases

• Hypokalaemia, hypercalciuria, hyperoxaluria	• Amyloidosis

Toxic causes of CIN

The combination of interstitial nephritis and tumours of the collecting system is seen in 'Chinese herb nephropathy' (a rapidly progressive syndrome caused by mistaken identity of ingredients in herbal preparations), in analgesic nephropathy, and in Balkan nephropathy (an endemic chronic nephropathy). A plant toxin found in *Aristolochia clematis* is probably responsible for the herb nephropathy and possibly also for Balkan nephropathy. Confusing *Cortinarius* species for wild edible or 'magic' mushrooms causes a devastating irreversible renal tubular toxicity encountered occasionally in Scandinavia and Scotland.

Papillary necrosis and analgesic nephropathy

The renal papillae are at the end of the capillary distribution in the kidney, and may necrose in diabetes mellitus, rarely in infections, in sickle-cell disease and occasionally in other conditions. Necrosed papillae may cause ureteric obstruction and renal colic. Papillary necrosis is difficult to identify other than on pyelography.

Long-term ingestion (years to decades) of certain NSAIDs may cause CIN and renal papillary necrosis. In animals, lesions can be induced with almost any NSAID; however a dramatic fall in the incidence of analgesic nephropathy has been observed which appears to coincide with the withdrawal of phenacetin from compound analgesics.

Clinical and biochemical features

Most patients with CIN present in adult life with CKD, hypertension and small kidneys. CKD is often moderate (stage 3) but, because of tubular dysfunction, electrolyte abnormalities are typically more severe (e.g. hyperkalaemia, acidosis). Urinalysis abnormalities are non-specific. A minority of patients present with salt-losing nephropathy, causing hypotension, polyuria and features of sodium and water depletion (e.g. low blood pressure and jugular venous pressure). Impairment of urine-concentrating ability and sodium conservation places patients with CIN at risk of superimposed ARF with even moderate salt and water depletion during an acute illness.

Hyperkalaemia may be disproportionate in CIN or in diabetic nephropathy because of hyporeninaemic hypoaldosteronism (p. 829). Renal tubular acidosis (p. 444) is seen most often in myeloma, sarcoidosis, cystinosis, amyloidosis and Sjögren's syndrome.

Sickle-cell nephropathy

The longer survival of patients with sickle-cell disease (p. 1028) means that a larger proportion live to develop chronic complications of microvascular occlusion. In the kidney these changes are most pronounced in the medulla, where the vasa recta are the site of sickling because of hypoxia and hypertonicity. Loss of urinary concentrating ability and polyuria are the earliest changes; distal renal tubular acidosis and impaired potassium excretion are typical. Papillary necrosis (as seen in analgesic nephropathy) is very common. A minority of patients develop ESRD. This is managed according to the usual principles, but response to recombinant erythropoietin is poor in the presence of haemoglobinopathy. Patients with sickle trait have an increased incidence of unexplained microscopic haematuria, and occasionally overt papillary necrosis.

Cystic kidney diseases

Polycystic kidney disease

Adult polycystic kidney disease (PKD) is a common condition (prevalence approximately 1:1000) that is inherited as an autosomal dominant trait. Small cysts lined by tubular epithelium develop from infancy or childhood and enlarge slowly and irregularly. Surrounding normal kidney tissue is progressively attenuated. Renal failure is associated with grossly enlarged kidneys (Fig. 17.32).

Mutations in the *PKD1* gene account for 85% of cases and *PKD2* for about 15%. ESRD occurs in approximately 50% of patients with *PKD1* mutations with a mean age of onset of 52 years, but in a minority of patients with *PKD2* mutations with a mean age of onset of 69 years.

Clinical features

Common clinical features are shown in Box 17.44. Affected subjects are usually asymptomatic until later life. After the age of 20 there is often insidious onset of hypertension. One or both kidneys may be palpable and the surface may feel nodular. There is then a gradual reduction in renal function.

About 30% of patients with PKD have hepatic cysts (see Fig. 23.40, p. 967) but disturbance of liver function

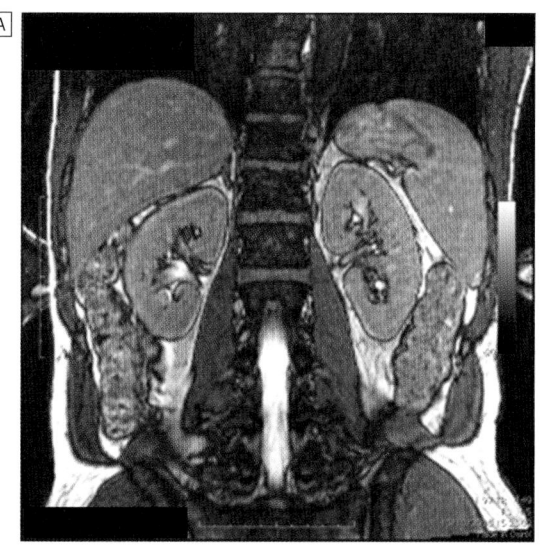 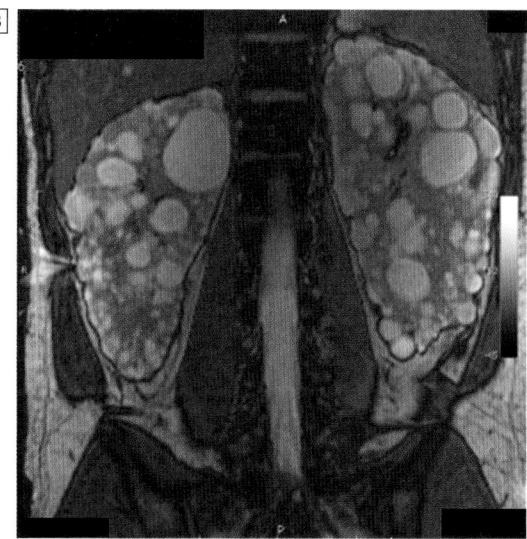

Fig. 17.32 MRI images of kidneys. A Normal kidneys. B Polycystic kidneys; although the kidney enlargement is extreme, this patient had only slightly reduced GFR.

17

> **17.44 Adult polycystic kidney disease: common clinical features**
>
> - Vague discomfort in loin or abdomen due to increasing mass of renal tissue
> - Acute loin pain or renal colic due to haemorrhage into a cyst
> - Hypertension
> - Haematuria (with little or no proteinuria)
> - Urinary tract or cyst infections
> - Renal failure

is rare. Sometimes (almost always in women) this causes massive and symptomatic hepatomegaly, usually concurrent with renal enlargement but occasionally with only minor renal involvement.

Berry aneurysms of cerebral vessels are an associated feature and about 10% of patients have a subarachnoid haemorrhage. This feature appears to be largely restricted to certain families (and presumably specific mutations). Mitral and aortic regurgitation are frequent but rarely severe, and colonic diverticulae and abdominal wall hernias may occur.

PKD is not a pre-malignant condition. The rate of renal malignancy is no different from that of other patients with renal failure.

Investigations and screening

The diagnosis is usually based on family history, clinical findings and ultrasound. Ultrasound demonstrates cysts in approximately 95% of affected patients over the age of 20 but may not detect small developing cysts in younger patients. It is important to identify multiple cysts, not just two or three (see Fig. 17.32). Now that the gene defects responsible for PKD have been identified, it is sometimes possible to make a specific genetic diagnosis, but detecting mutations in the *PKD1* gene is particularly problematic because of its size, the existence of a closely related pseudogene, and the wide variety of mutations that have been described. Linkage analysis (p. 57) may be used to exclude the diagnosis in a young adult with normal renal imaging.

Screening for intracranial aneurysms is not generally indicated. Where non-invasive MR angiography is available, some centres screen patients in families with a history of subarachnoid haemorrhage. However, even then, the yield of screening has been low, and the risk–benefit ratio of intervention in asymptomatic aneurysms in this disease is not known.

Management

Nothing has yet been found to alter the rate of progression of renal failure in human PKD but the first clinical trials of drugs that seem to slow cyst growth are under way. Good control of blood pressure is important because cardiovascular morbidity and mortality are so common in renal disease, but there is no evidence that control of moderate hypertension retards the development of renal failure in PKD, in contrast to the evidence for glomerular diseases.

Patients with PKD are usually good candidates for dialysis and transplantation. Sometimes kidneys are so large that one or both have to be removed to make space for a renal transplant. Otherwise, unless they are a source of pain or infection, they are usually left in situ.

Other cystic diseases

Medullary cystic diseases

Medullary sponge kidney is characterised by cysts confined to papillary collecting ducts. The disease is not inherited and its cause is unknown. Patients usually present as adults with renal stones. These are often recurrent, and preventive measures (p. 511) need to be implemented if so, but the prognosis is generally good. The diagnosis is made by ultrasound or IVU (Fig. 17.33). Contrast medium is seen to fill dilated or cystic tubules, which are sometimes calcified.

Medullary cystic kidney diseases are a heterogenous group of inherited disorders, known as nephronophthisis in children. Small cortical cysts are associated with progressive destruction of the nephron. The childhood variants are characterised by thirst and polyuria due to nephrogenic diabetes insipidus, often with a family

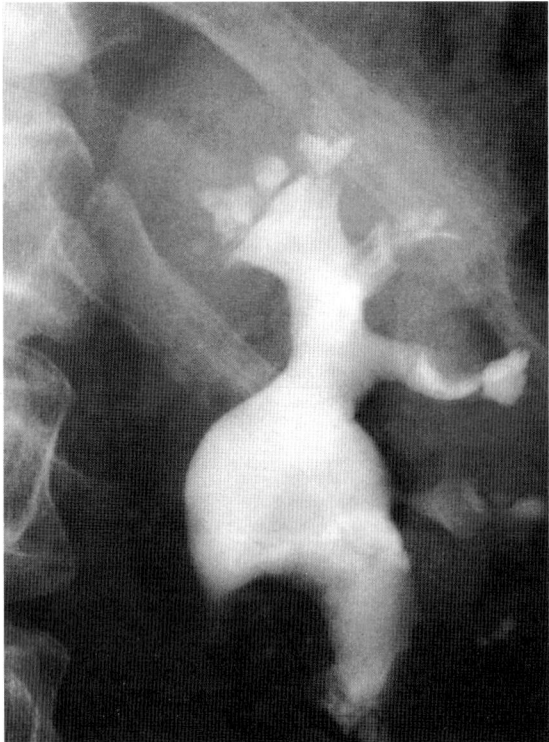

Fig. 17.33 Medullary sponge kidney. Intravenous urogram showing contrast medium filling both the collecting system and cavities arising from collecting ducts, especially within papillae of the upper pole. The cavities have been likened to bunches of grapes. A plain abdominal X-ray may show calcification in the same regions.

history of similar disease. Sometimes, affected patients are 'salt-losing', which aggravates the degree of renal failure. Even when they are treated appropriately, serious renal failure is usual. The genetic basis of these disorders is emerging; several genes involving multiple mechanisms are involved.

Other cystic diseases

A number of other rarer inherited cystic diseases, having some similarities to PKD but distinct genetic causes, are recognised.

Multicystic dysplastic kidneys are often unilateral and are a developmental abnormality found in children. Most of these seem to involute during growth, leaving a solitary kidney in adults.

Acquired cystic kidney disease develops in patients with a very long history of renal failure, usually including many years of dialysis. It is associated with increased erythropoietin production and sometimes with the development of renal cell carcinoma.

Isolated defects of tubular function

An increasing number of disorders are now known to be due to specific defects of transporter molecules or other functions in renal tubular cells. Only the most common are mentioned here.

Renal glycosuria is a benign autosomal recessive defect of tubular reabsorption of glucose, caused by mutations of the sodium/glucose cotransporter *SGLT2*. Glucose appears in the urine in the presence of a normal blood glucose concentration. Targeting of this transporter has been proposed as a treatment for diabetes mellitus.

Cystinuria is a rare condition in which reabsorption of filtered cystine, ornithine, arginine and lysine is defective. It is caused by mutations in the *SLC3A1* amino acid transporter gene. The high concentration of cystine in urine leads to cystine stone formation (pp. 510–511).

Other uncommon tubular disorders include vitamin D-resistant rickets (pp. 112 and 1123), in which reabsorption of filtered phosphate is reduced; nephrogenic diabetes insipidus (p. 792), in which the tubules are resistant to the effects of vasopressin; and Bartter's and Gitelman's syndromes, in which there is sodium-wasting and hypokalaemia (p. 439).

The term 'Fanconi syndrome' is used to describe generalised proximal tubular dysfunction. It is not related to Fanconi anaemia. Notable abnormalities include low blood phosphate and uric acid, the finding of glucose and amino acids in urine, and proximal renal tubular acidosis (p. 444). In addition to the causes of interstitial nephritis described above, some congenital metabolic disorders are associated with Fanconi syndrome, notably Wilson's disease, cystinosis and hereditary fructose intolerance.

Renal tubular acidosis describes the common end-point of a variety of diseases affecting distal (classical or type 1) or proximal (type 2) renal tubular function. These syndromes are described on page 444.

DISEASES OF THE COLLECTING SYSTEM AND URETERS

Congenital abnormalities

Congenital anomalies of the urinary tract (Fig. 17.34) affect more than 10% of infants and, if not immediately lethal, may lead to complications in later life, including obstructive nephropathy and CKD. About 1 in 500 infants are born with only one kidney. Although usually compatible with normal life, this is often associated with other abnormalities.

A ureterocele (see Fig. 17.9, p. 473) occurs behind a pin-hole ureteric orifice when the intramural part of the ureter dilates and bulges into the bladder. It can become very large and cause lower urinary tract obstruction. Incision of the pin-hole opening relieves the obstruction.

Ectopic ureters occur with congenital duplication of one or both kidneys (duplex kidneys). Developmentally, the ureter has two main branches and, if this arrangement persists, the two ureters of the duplex kidneys may drain separately into the bladder. One ureter enters normally on the trigone, while the ectopic ureter (from the upper renal moiety) enters the bladder or, more rarely, the vagina or seminal vesicle. A ureter that is ectopic and drains into the bladder is liable to have an ineffective valve mechanism so that urine passes up the ureter on voiding (vesico-ureteric reflux, see below). Reflux can occur in normally sited ureters if the intramural ureter fails to act as a valve. The management of vesico-ureteric reflux and associated reflux nephropathy is outlined below.

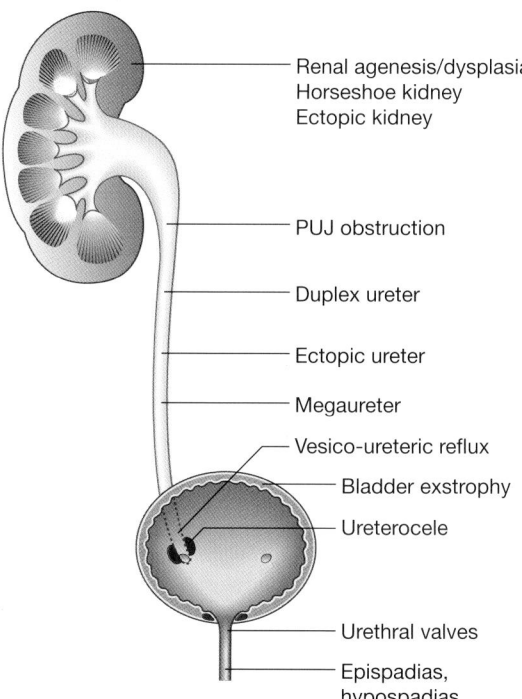

Renal agenesis/dysplasia
Horseshoe kidney
Ectopic kidney

PUJ obstruction

Duplex ureter

Ectopic ureter

Megaureter

Vesico-ureteric reflux

Bladder exstrophy

Ureterocele

Urethral valves

Epispadias,
hypospadias

Fig. 17.34 Congenital abnormalities of the urinary tract.

In primary obstructive megaureter there is dilatation of the ureter in all but its terminal segment without obvious cause and without vesico-ureteric reflux. Radiographic and pressure/flow studies may be needed to determine whether there is obstruction to urine flow. Narrowing of the ureter and reimplantation may be necessary.

Pelviureteric junction obstruction

This causes idiopathic hydronephrosis and results from a functional obstruction at the junction of the ureter and renal pelvis. The aetiology is obscure. The abnormality is likely to be congenital and is often bilateral. It can be seen in very young children but gross hydronephrosis may present at any age.

The common presentation is ill-defined renal pain or ache exacerbated by drinking large volumes of liquid. Rarely, it is asymptomatic. Diagnosis is suspected after ultrasound or IVU, and confirmed with a diuretic renogram. Treatment is surgical excision of the PUJ and reanastomosis (pyeloplasty). This can now be performed laparoscopically. Less invasive alternatives are also possible, including balloon dilatation and endoscopic pyelotomy, but are less effective.

Retroperitoneal fibrosis

Fibrosis of the retroperitoneal connective tissues may encircle and compress the ureter(s), causing obstruction. This fibrosis is most commonly idiopathic, but can represent a reaction to infection, radiation or aortic aneurysm, or be caused by cancer or a drug reaction: to methysergide, for example. Patients usually present with ill-defined symptoms of ureteric obstruction. Typically, there is an acute phase response (high CRP and ESR). IVU or CT shows ureteric obstruction with medial deviation of the ureters. Idiopathic retroperitoneal fibrosis

responds well to corticosteroids and may respond more slowly to tamoxifen, but ureteric stenting is often used to relieve obstruction initially. Failure to respond indicates the need for surgery to relieve obstruction and exclude malignancy.

Reflux nephropathy (chronic pyelonephritis)

This is a chronic interstitial nephritis (p. 505) associated with vesico-ureteric reflux (VUR) in early life, and with the appearance of 'scars' in the kidney, as demonstrated by various imaging techniques. The incidence of reflux nephropathy is not known. About 12% of patients in Europe requiring treatment for ESRD are said to have renal scarring but diagnostic criteria are imprecise.

Pathogenesis

VUR, in which urine refluxes back from the bladder into the ureter, is closely associated with recurrent UTI in childhood, and until recently it was widely assumed that ascending infection is critical in the association of VUR with progressive renal damage. However, antenatal ultrasound has shown that renal scars occur in utero in the absence of infection. Furthermore, epidemiological surveys and controlled trials have found that efforts to reduce progression to ESRD by surgical or other means have not been effective. Reflux diminishes as the child grows and usually disappears. It is often not demonstrable in an adult with a scarred kidney.

Susceptibility to VUR has a genetic component and may be associated with renal dysplasia and other congenital abnormalities of the urinary tract. It can be associated with outflow obstruction, usually caused by urethral valves, but usually occurs in an apparently normal bladder.

Pathology

Abnormalities may be unilateral or bilateral and of any grade of severity. Renal scars are juxtaposed to dilated calyces. Gross scarring of the kidneys, commonly at the poles, is seen, with reduced size and narrowing of the cortex and medulla. In patients who develop heavy proteinuria and hypertension, renal biopsies show glomerulomegaly and focal glomerulosclerosis, probably as a secondary response to reduced nephron number and functional mass.

Clinical features

Usually the renal scarring and dilatation is asymptomatic and the patient presents at any age with hypertension (sometimes severe), proteinuria or features of CKD. There may be no history of overt UTI. However, symptoms arising from the urinary tract may be present and include frequency of micturition, dysuria and aching lumbar pain. Urinary white cells and moderate proteinuria (usually < 1 g/24 hrs) are common but not invariable. There is an increased prevalence of renal calculi.

A number of women first present with hypertension and/or proteinuria in pregnancy. In some families there is a clear inheritance pattern.

Investigations

For detecting renal scars, ultrasound is an insensitive technique, although it will detect major dysplasia and

17

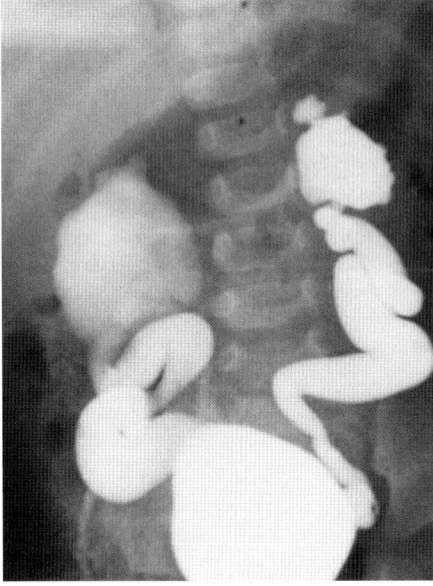

Fig. 17.35 Vesico-ureteric reflux (grade IV) shown by micturating cystogram. The bladder has been filled with contrast medium through a urinary catheter. After micturition there was gross VUR into widely distended ureters and pelvicalyceal systems.

renal dysgenesis, and exclude significant obstruction. Radionuclide DMSA scans are more sensitive (see Fig. 17.7, p. 468). Longitudinal imaging by MRI or CT may be useful.

To investigate VUR, radionuclide techniques can also be used as an alternative to micturating cysto-urethrography (MCUG, when the bladder is filled with contrast media through a urinary catheter and images are taken during and after micturition, Fig. 17.35). However, as surgical intervention for VUR has declined in popularity (see below), these techniques are used less often.

Management

Infection, if present, should be treated (Box 17.45); if recurrent, it should be prevented with prophylactic therapy, as described for UTI (p. 471). If pyelonephrosis develops or unilateral renal infection or pain persists, nephrectomy or other measures may be indicated. Occasionally, hypertension is cured by the removal of a diseased kidney when the disease is predominantly or entirely unilateral.

As most childhood reflux tends to disappear spontaneously and trials have shown small or no benefits from anti-reflux surgery, such intervention is now less common.

EBM **17.45 Prophylactic antibiotics and vesico-ureteric reflux**

'Prophylactic antibiotics reduce recurrences of UTI but there is no evidence that they protect against further renal scarring or dysfunction.'

• Smellie JM, et al. Lancet 2001; 357:1329–1333.

For further information: www.clinicalevidence.org

Prognosis

Children and adults with small or unilateral renal scars have a good prognosis, provided renal growth is normal. With significant unilateral scars there is usually compensatory hypertrophy of the contralateral kidney.

In patients with more severe bilateral disease, prognosis is predicted by the severity of renal dysfunction, hypertension and proteinuria. If the serum creatinine is normal and hypertension and proteinuria are absent, then the long-term prognosis is usually good.

Urinary tract calculi and nephrocalcinosis

Urinary calculi (stones) consist of aggregates of crystals containing small amounts of proteins and glycoprotein. It is surprising that stones and nephrocalcinosis are not more common, since some of the constituents are present in urine in concentrations which exceed their maximum solubility in water. However, urine contains proteins, glycosaminoglycans, pyrophosphate and citrate, which help to keep otherwise insoluble salts in solution.

Different types of stone vary in frequency around the world, probably as a consequence of dietary and environmental factors, but genetic factors may also contribute. In Europe, 80% of renal stones contain crystals of calcium (most commonly as oxalate but also as phosphate). About 15% contain magnesium ammonium phosphate (struvite; these are often associated with infection), and small numbers of pure cystine or uric acid stones are found. Rarely, drugs may form stones (e.g. indinavir, ephedrine). In a North American survey, 12% of men and 5% of women had experienced a renal stone by the age of 70 years. A number of risk factors are known for renal stone formation (Box 17.46). However, in developed countries, most calculi occur in healthy young men in whom investigations reveal no clear predisposing cause.

Urinary concretions vary greatly in size. There may be particles like sand anywhere in the urinary tract, or large round stones in the bladder. In developing countries, bladder stones are common, particularly in children. In

---

i **17.46 Predisposing factors for kidney stones**

Environmental and dietary

• Low urine volumes: high ambient temperatures, low fluid intake
• Diet: high protein, high sodium, low calcium
• High sodium excretion
• High oxalate excretion
• High urate excretion
• Low citrate excretion

Acquired causes

• Hypercalcaemia of any cause (p. 764)
• Ileal disease or resection (increases oxalate absorption and urinary excretion)
• Renal tubular acidosis type I (distal, p. 444)

Congenital and inherited causes

• Familial hypercalciuria
• Medullary sponge kidney
• Cystinuria
• Renal tubular acidosis type I (distal)
• Primary hyperoxaluria

developed countries, the incidence of childhood bladder stones is low; renal stones in adults are more common. Staghorn calculi fill the whole renal pelvis and branch into the calyces (Fig. 17.36); they are usually associated with infection and composed largely of struvite.

Deposits of calcium may be present throughout the renal parenchyma, giving rise to fine calcification within the renal parenchyma (nephrocalcinosis), especially in patients with renal tubular acidosis, hyperparathyroidism, vitamin D intoxication and healed renal tuberculosis. Cortical nephrocalcinosis occurs in areas of cortical necrosis, typically after ARF in pregnancy or other severe ARF.

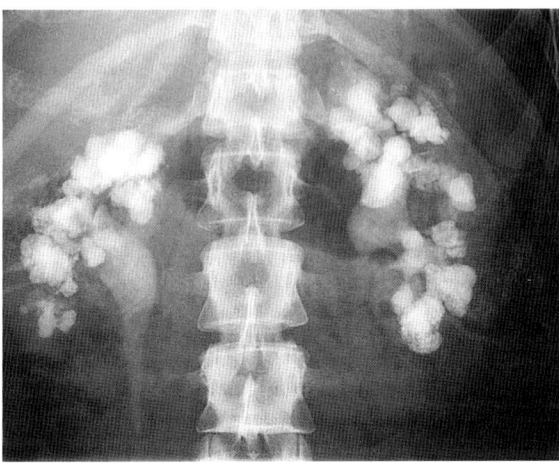

Fig. 17.36 Radio-opaque bilateral staghorn calculi visible during IVU. The intravenous pyelogram demonstrates that, while some dye is being excreted by the right kidney, there is little function on the left.

17.47 Measures to prevent calcium stone formation

Diet

Fluid
- At least 2 L output per day (intake 3–4 L): check with 24-hr urine collections
- Intake distributed throughout the day (especially before bed)

Sodium
- Restrict intake

Protein
- Moderate, not high

Calcium
- Plenty in diet (because calcium forms an insoluble salt with dietary oxalate, lowering oxalate absorption and excretion)
- Avoid supplements away from meals (increase calcium excretion without reducing oxalate excretion)

Oxalate
- Avoid foods that are rich in oxalate (spinach, rhubarb)

N.B. Citrate supplementation is of unproven value

Drugs

Thiazide diuretics
- Reduce calcium excretion
- Valuable in recurrent stone-formers and patients with hypercalciuria

Allopurinol
- If urate excretion high (unproven except for urate stones)

Avoid
- Vitamin D supplements as they increase calcium absorption and excretion
- Vitamin C hypersupplementation as this increases oxalate excretion

17

Indications for intervention
- Obstructive anuria or severe infection (pyonephrosis)
  → Emergency percutaneous nephrostomy only
- Severe pain or solitary kidney
  → Urgent ESWL or surgery
- Pain and failure of the stone to move
  → Elective ESWL or surgery

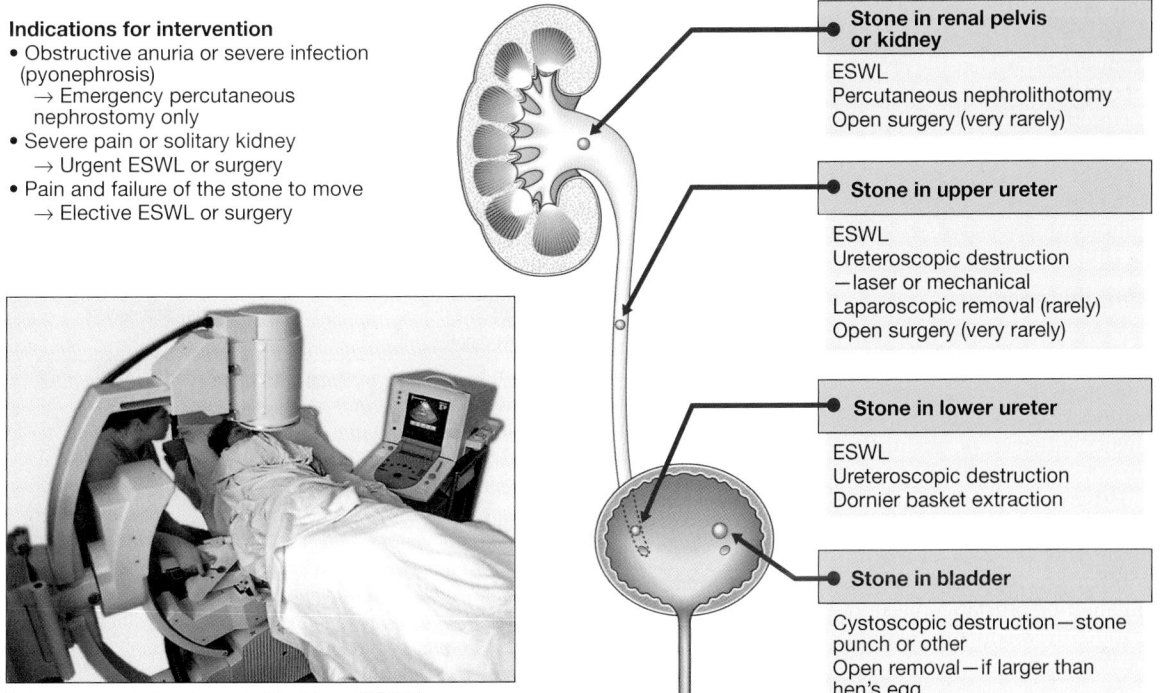

Extracorporeal shock wave lithotripsy (ESWL)

Stone in renal pelvis or kidney
ESWL
Percutaneous nephrolithotomy
Open surgery (very rarely)

Stone in upper ureter
ESWL
Ureteroscopic destruction —laser or mechanical
Laparoscopic removal (rarely)
Open surgery (very rarely)

Stone in lower ureter
ESWL
Ureteroscopic destruction
Dornier basket extraction

Stone in bladder
Cystoscopic destruction—stone punch or other
Open removal—if larger than hen's egg

Fig. 17.37 Surgical options for urinary stones.

Investigations and management

The most common presentation is with renal colic, for which investigations and acute management are described on page 474. Large stones, or stones which do not pass spontaneously through the urinary tract, may require surgical removal and/or fragmentation by extracorporeal shock wave lithotripsy (Fig. 17.37).

Measures to prevent further stone formation are guided by the results of the investigations in Box 17.13 (p. 474). Some general principles apply to almost every patient with calcium-containing stones (Box 17.47). More specific measures apply to some stone types. Urate stones can be prevented by allopurinol, but the role of allopurinol in patients with calcium stones and high urate excretion is uncertain. Stones formed in cystinuria can be reduced by penicillamine therapy. It may also be helpful to attempt to alter urine pH with ammonium chloride (low pH discourages phosphate stone formation) or sodium bicarbonate (high pH discourages urate and cystine stone formation).

DISEASES OF THE LOWER GENITOURINARY TRACT

Several pathologies of the lower urinary tract are discussed elsewhere in this chapter, including infection (pp. 469–472), bladder and urethral dysfunction causing incontinence (p. 476), and urinary tract cancer (p. 515). Testicular tumours are discussed on page 763. Chapter 15 describes infections affecting the genitalia.

DISEASES OF THE PROSTATE GLAND

Benign prostatic hyperplasia

From 40 years of age the prostate increases in volume by $2.4\,cm^3$ per year on average. The process begins in the periurethral (transitional) zone and involves both glandular and stromal tissue to a variable degree. Associated symptoms are common from 60 years of age, and some 50% of men over 80 years will have lower urinary tract symptoms associated with benign prostatic hyperplasia (BPH).

Clinical features

The primary symptoms of BPH are due to the prostate obstructing the urethra; they consist of hesitancy, poor prolonged flow and a sensation of incomplete emptying. Secondary (irritative) symptoms comprising urinary frequency, urgency of micturition and urge incontinence are not specific to BPH.

Patients may present more dramatically with acute urinary retention when they are suddenly unable to micturate and develop a painful distended bladder. This is often precipitated by excessive alcohol intake, constipation or prostatic infection. It is an emergency and requires the bladder to be drained by a catheter to relieve the retention.

In chronic urinary retention the bladder slowly distends due to inadequate emptying over a long period of time. This condition is characterised by pain-free bladder distension which may result in hydroureter, hydronephrosis and renal failure. Patients with chronic retention can also develop acute retention: so-called acute on chronic retention. They require careful management because of their renal failure.

Investigations

Symptoms are scored on the international prostate symptom score (IPSS, Box 17.48), which serves as a valuable starting point for the assessment of urinary problems. Once a baseline value is established, any improvement/deterioration may be assessed on subsequent visits. Flow rates are accurately measured with a flow meter, and prostate volume can be estimated by rectal examination or more accurately by transrectal ultrasound scan (TRUS). Objective assessment of obstruction is only possible by urodynamics (see Fig. 17.11, p. 476). Renal function should be assessed and, if appropriate, obstructive nephropathy identified by ultrasound.

Management

Mild to moderate symptoms can be treated by medication (Boxes 17.49 and 17.50). Alpha-adrenoceptor blockers (e.g. alfuzosin, tamsulosin) reduce the tone of smooth muscle cells in the prostate and bladder neck, thereby reducing the obstruction. 5α-Reductase inhibitors (finasteride and dutasteride) stop the conversion of testosterone to more potent dihydrotestosterone in the prostate and so cause the prostate to shrink. Severe symptoms require surgical removal of some of the obstructing prostate tissue. Transurethral resection of the prostate (TURP) remains the gold standard treatment but enucleation of the prostate by holmium laser appears as effective and has potentially fewer complications. Open surgery is

17.48 How to determine the international prostate symptom score (IPSS) and quality of life scores		
Symptom	**Score**	
1. Straining	Each scored	
2. Weak stream		
3. Intermittency	0	Not at all
4. Incomplete emptying	1	Less than 1 time in 5
	2	Less than half the time
5. Frequency	3	About half the time
6. Urgency	4	More than half the time
7. Nocturia (times per night)	5	Almost always

Total IPSS score
0–7 = mild symptoms
8–19 = moderate symptoms
20–35 = severe symptoms
In addition, consider the quality of life score below

Quality of life	**Score**	
Urinary symptoms	0	Delighted
	1	Pleased
	2	Satisfied
	3	Mixed
	4	Dissatisfied
	5	Unhappy
	6	Terrible

17.49 Treatment for benign prostatic hypertrophy

Medical

- Prostate < 40 cm³: α-adrenoceptor blockers
- Prostate > 40 cm³: 5α-reductase inhibitors

Non-surgical intervention

- Thermotherapy

Surgical

- Transurethral resection of prostate (TURP)
- Holmium laser enucleation
- Open prostatectomy

EBM 17.50 Medical management of benign prostatic hyperplasia

'Oral α-adrenoceptor blockers produce rapid improvement in urinary flow in 60–70% of patients. The 5α-reductase inhibitor, finasteride, causes slow shrinkage of large prostate glands with improvement in symptoms.'

- Clifford GM, et al. Eur Urol 2000; 38:2–19.
- Boyle P, et al. Urology 2001; 58:717–722.

For further information: www.cochrane.org

---

rarely required, except in very large glands (> 100 cm³). Thermotherapy, where the prostate is heated by microwaves of radiofrequency through a urethral catheter, is little better than medication but may have a place in the patient unfit for surgery.

Prostate cancer

Prostatic cancer is common in northern Europe and the USA (particularly in the black population) but rare in China and Japan. In the UK it is the second most common malignancy in males, with a prevalence of 50 per 100 000 population, and is increasing in frequency. It rarely occurs before the age of 50 and has a mean age at presentation of 70 years.

Prostate cancers arise within the peripheral zone of the prostate and almost all are carcinomas. Metastatic spread to pelvic lymph nodes occurs early and metastases to bone, mainly the lumbar spine and pelvis, are common. Prostatic specific antigen (PSA) is a good tumour marker and 40% of patients with a serum PSA > 4.0 ng/mL will have prostate cancer on biopsy. This has led to the introduction of screening programmes, principally in the USA, despite a lack of consensus about their utility.

Clinical features

Most patients present with lower urinary tract symptoms indistinguishable from BPH. Symptoms and signs due to metastases are much less common and include back pain, weight loss, anaemia and obstruction of the ureters. On rectal examination the prostate often feels nodular and stony hard, and the median sulcus may be lost. However, 10–15% of tumours are not palpable.

Whenever possible, the diagnosis is confirmed by needle biopsy, usually aided by TRUS, or by histological examination of tissue removed by endoscopic resection if this is needed to relieve outflow obstruction.

Investigations

Since most patients present with outflow tract obstruction, an ultrasound scan and serum creatinine determination are used to assess the urinary tract. A plain X-ray of the pelvis and lumbar spine (to investigate backache) may show osteosclerotic metastases as the first evidence of prostatic malignancy.

The patient is assessed for distant metastases by a radioisotope bone scan but high levels of serum PSA (> 100 ng/mL) almost always indicate distant bone metastases. PSA is useful for monitoring response to treatment and disease progression.

Management

Tumour confined to the prostate is potentially curable by either radical prostatectomy or radical radiotherapy, and these options should be considered in all patients with more than 10 years' life expectancy. A small focus of tumour found incidentally at TURP does not significantly alter life expectancy and only requires follow-up.

Approximately half of men with prostate cancer will have metastatic disease at the time of diagnosis. Prostatic cancer, like breast cancer, is sensitive to steroid hormones; locally advanced or metastatic prostate cancer is treated by androgen depletion, involving either surgery (orchidectomy) or, more commonly now, androgen-suppressing drugs (Box 17.51). Androgen receptor antagonists such as cyproterone acetate may prevent tumour cell growth. Gonadotrophin-releasing hormone (GnRH) analogues such as goserelin continuously occupy pituitary receptors, preventing them from responding to the GnRH pulses which normally stimulate luteinising hormone (LH) and follicle-stimulating hormone (FSH) release. This initially causes an increase in testosterone before producing a prolonged reduction, and for this reason the initial dose must be covered with an anti-androgen to prevent a tumour flare.

A small proportion of patients fail to respond to endocrine treatment. A larger number respond for a year or two, but then the disease progresses. Chemotherapy with 5-fluorouracil, cyclophosphamide or nitrogen mustard can then be effective. Radiotherapy is useful for localised bone pain. For severe generalised bone pain, hemi-body radiotherapy or [89]strontium may give effective palliation but the basis of treatment remains pain control by analgesia (p. 281).

Prognosis

The life expectancy of a patient with an incidental finding of focal carcinoma of the prostate is normal. With more substantial tumours localised to the prostate, the 10-year survival rate is 60–75%, but if metastases are present this falls to 10%.

EBM 17.51 Hormone manipulation in prostate cancer

'Reducing circulating testosterone levels (either by castration or by medication) results in a 70% initial response rate. Additional androgen blockade produces a small increase in survival but with poorer quality of life.'

- Huggins C, et al. Cancer Res 1941; 1:293–297.
- Schmitt B, et al. Cochrane Library, issue 3, 2005. Oxford: Update Software.

For further information: www.cochrane.org

17

17

Prostatitis

Inflammation of the prostate gland may be acute or chronic. It can be caused by infection with the same bacteria that are associated with UTI (p. 469) or, more commonly, may be 'non-bacterial' (no organisms cultured from urine). Clinical features include frequency, dysuria, perineal or groin pain, difficulty passing urine and, in acute disease, considerable systemic disturbance. The prostate is enlarged and tender. Bacterial prostatitis is confirmed by a positive culture from urine or from urethral discharge obtained after prostatic massage, and the treatment of choice is trimethoprim or a quinolone antibiotic. A 4–6-week course is required (see Box 17.11, p. 471). Non-bacterial prostatitis can be treated with drugs to relax the prostate and bladder neck, such as terodiline or terazosin.

TUMOURS OF THE KIDNEY AND URINARY TRACT

Tumours of the kidney

Tumours of the kidney account for 3% of all malignancies, and a variety of benign, malignant and secondary tumours can occur.

Renal adenocarcinoma

This is by far the most common malignant tumour of the kidney in adults, with a prevalence of 16 cases per 100 000 population. It is twice as common in males as in females. The peak incidence is between 65 and 75 years of age and it is uncommon before 40. The tumour arises from renal tubules. Haemorrhage and necrosis give the cut surface a characteristic mixed golden-yellow and red appearance (Fig. 17.38B). Microscopically, 'clear cell' carcinomas are more common than 'granular cell' tumours. There is early spread of the tumour into the renal pelvis, causing haematuria, and along the renal vein, often extending into the inferior vena cava. Direct invasion

of perinephric tissues is common. Lymphatic spread occurs to para-aortic nodes, while blood-borne metastases (which may be solitary) may develop almost anywhere in the body.

Clinical features

In an increasing number of cases, asymptomatic renal tumours are identified incidentally during imaging investigations carried out for other reasons. Amongst symptomatic patients, about 60% of cases present with haematuria, 40% with loin pain and only 25% with a mass; about 15% have the triad of pain, haematuria and a mass. A remarkable range of systemic effects may be present, including fever, raised ESR, polycythaemia, disorders of coagulation, and abnormalities of plasma proteins and liver function tests. The patient may present with pyrexia of unknown origin or, rarely, with neuropathy. Systemic effects may be due to tumour secretion of products such as renin, erythropoietin, PTH-related peptide and gonadotrophins. The effects disappear when the tumour is removed but may reappear when metastases develop, and so can be used as markers of tumour activity.

Investigations

Ultrasound is often the initial investigation and allows differentiation between solid tumour and simple renal cysts. Contrast-enhanced CT of the abdomen and chest should be performed for staging (see Fig. 17.38A). For tumours < 3 cm in diameter with no evidence of metastatic spread and when the nature of the lesion is uncertain, ultrasound or CT-guided biopsy may be used to avoid nephrectomy for benign disease.

Management and prognosis

Radical nephrectomy that includes the perirenal fascial envelope and ipsilateral para-aortic lymph nodes is performed whenever possible. It should be considered even when metastases are present, as not only do systemic effects often disappear, but also metastases may regress. Solitary metastases tend to remain single for long periods and excision may be worthwhile. Patients at high

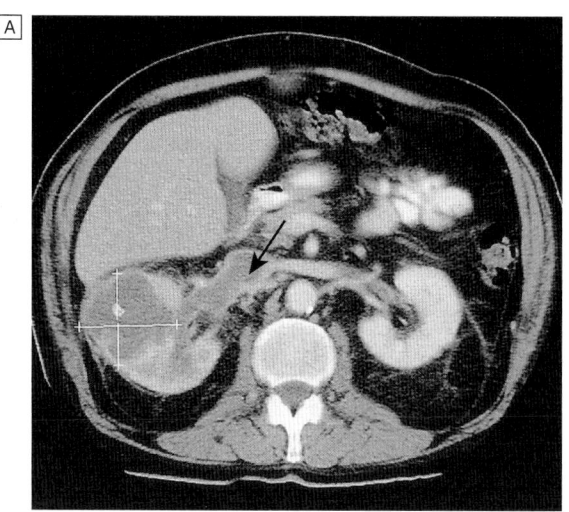
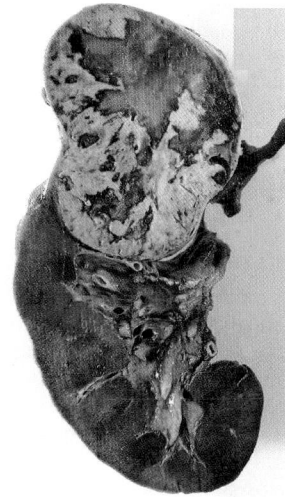

Fig. 17.38 Renal adenocarcinoma. **A** In this CT, the right kidney is expanded by a low-density tumour which fails to take up contrast material. Tumour is shown extending into the renal vein and inferior vena cava (arrow). **B** Pathology specimen showing typical necrosis.

operative or other risk (e.g. single functioning kidney) who have small tumours may be treated percutaneously by radiofrequency ablation or by tissue-sparing surgery or cryoablation.

Renal adenocarcinoma is resistant to most chemo-therapeutic agents, although interferon and interleukin-2 therapy are sometimes beneficial. Two new classes of drug have recently shown promising results: tyrosine kinase inhibitors such as sorafenib and sunitinib; and mTOR (mammalian target of rapamycin) inhibitors such as temsirolimus and everolimus.

Survival studies that antedate the introduction of new chemotherapeutic agents show that if the tumour is confined to the kidney, 5-year survival is 75%, but this falls to 5% when there are distant metastases.

Tumour syndromes

Some uncommon autosomal dominant inherited conditions are associated with multiple renal tumours in adult life. In tuberous sclerosis (p. 1283), replacement of renal tissue by multiple angiomyolipomas (tubers) may occasionally cause renal failure in adults. Other organs affected include the skin (adenoma sebaceum on the face) and brain (causing seizures and mental retardation). The von Hippel–Lindau syndrome (p. 1219) is associated with multiple renal cysts, renal adenomas and renal adenocarcinoma. Other organs affected include the central nervous system (haemangioblastomas) and the adrenals (phaeochromocytoma).

Tumours of the renal pelvis, ureters and bladder

The vast majority of these tumours arise from the urothelium or transitional cell lining. The urothelium is exposed to chemical carcinogens excreted in the urine, such as naphthylamines and benzidine which were extensively used in the chemical and dye industries until their carcinogenic properties were recognised. Almost all tumours are transitional cell carcinomas. Squamous carcinoma may occur in urothelium that has undergone metaplasia, usually following chronic inflammation or irritation due to a stone or schistosomiasis.

The incidence of transitional cell carcinoma in the bladder in the UK is 45 cases per 100 000 population, and is three times more common in men than women. The appearance of a transitional cell tumour ranges from a delicate papillary structure with relatively good prognosis to a solid ulcerating mass in more aggressive disease (Fig. 17.39).

Clinical features and investigations

More than 80% of patients have haematuria, which is usually macroscopic and painless. It should be assumed that such bleeding is from a tumour until proved otherwise (p. 478). A tumour at the lower end of a ureter or a bladder tumour (see Fig. 17.9, p. 473) involving the ureteric orifice may cause obstructive symptoms. Examination is usually unhelpful. Rectal examination detects only very advanced tumours.

Investigation of haematuria is described on page 478. If a suspicious defect is seen on IVU in the ureter or renal pelvis, a retrograde ureteropyelogram is required. Solid invasive tumours are staged by CT of the abdomen, pelvis and chest.

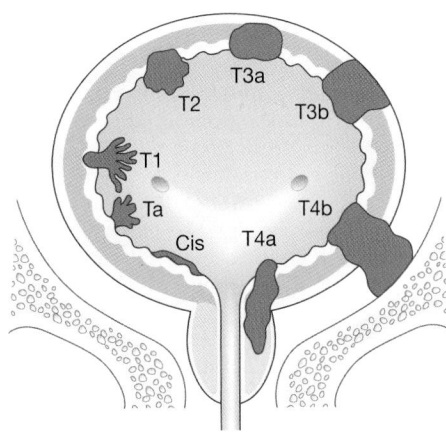

Fig. 17.39 Transitional cell carcinoma of the bladder. Stages are shown from carcinoma in situ (Cis) to invasive tumour progressing beyond the bladder and prostate (T4b). See also Figure 17.9 (p. 473).

Management

Small, large and even multiple superficial bladder tumours can be treated endoscopically by transurethral resection of the tumour(s) (TURT). Intravesical chemotherapy (e.g. epirubicin, mitomycin C) is useful for treating multiple low-grade bladder tumours and for reducing their recurrence rate. Regular 'check' cystoscopies are required and recurrences can usually be controlled by diathermy; only rarely will cystectomy be required for superficial disease.

Untreated patients with carcinoma in situ (Cis) have a high risk of progression to invasive cancer. The tumour responds well to intravesical bacille Calmette–Guérin (BCG) treatment but more aggressive treatment may be needed.

The management of invasive bladder tumours is debated and is largely a matter for specialist urological surgeons, many of whom recommend radical cystectomy with urinary diversion into an incontinent ileal conduit or a continent catheterisable bowel pouch for patients under 70 years of age.

Transitional cell carcinoma of the renal pelvis and ureter is usually treated by nephroureterectomy, but if the tumour is solitary and low-grade it may be treated endoscopically.

Prognosis

The prognosis of bladder tumours depends on tumour stage and grade. The 5-year survival rate varies from 50–60% in those with superficial tumours to 20–30% for those with deep muscle invasion. Overall, about one-third of patients survive for 5 years.

RENAL INVOLVEMENT IN SYSTEMIC CONDITIONS

The kidneys may be directly involved in a number of multisystem diseases or secondarily affected by diseases of other organs. Involvement may be at a pre-renal, renal (glomerular or interstitial) or post-renal level. Many of the diseases are described in other sections of this chapter or in other chapters of the book.

17

Diabetes mellitus

In patients with diabetes, the steady advance from microalbuminuria to dipstick-positive proteinuria, and the progression to frank nephrotic syndrome and renal failure are described on pages 829–831. Few patients require renal biopsy to establish the diagnosis, but atypical features or progression should lead to suspicion that an alternative condition could be present.

Management with ACE inhibitors and other hypotensive agents to slow progression is described on page 830, and has been dramatically effective. In some patients, proteinuria may be eradicated and progression completely halted, even if renal function is abnormal.

Hepatic-renal disease

Severe hepatic dysfunction may cause a haemodynamically mediated type of renal failure, hepatorenal syndrome, described on page 944. It also predisposes the kidney to develop acute renal failure (acute tubular necrosis) in response to relatively minor insults including bleeding and infection. Such patients are often difficult to treat by dialysis and have a poor prognosis. Where treatment is justified—for example, if there is a good chance of recovery or of a liver transplant—very slow or continuous treatments are less likely to precipitate or exacerbate hepatic encephalopathy.

IgA nephropathy (p. 501) is more common in patients with liver disease.

Pulmonary-renal disease

The pulmonary–renal syndrome is a dramatic presentation with renal and respiratory failure that is not explained by excess intravascular fluid or by severe pneumonia; it occurs in Goodpasture's (anti-GBM) disease and small-vessel vasculitis (see below). There are some other uncommon causes of a similar syndrome, including poisoning with the herbicide paraquat.

Malignant diseases

Cancer may affect the kidney in many ways (Box 17.52).

17.52 Renal effects of malignancies

Direct involvement

- Kidney: primary adenocarcinoma (hypernephroma), lymphoma
- Urinary tract: e.g. urothelial tumours, cervical carcinoma

Immune reaction

- Glomerulonephritis: especially membranous nephropathy

Metabolic consequences

- Hypercalcaemia (p. 764)
- Uric acid crystal formation in tubules: usually in tumour lysis syndromes

Remote effects of tumour products

- Light chains in myeloma (p. 1041), amyloidosis (p. 84)
- Antibodies in cryoglobulinaemia (p. 1114)

Tuberculosis of the kidney and urinary tract

Tuberculosis of the kidney is secondary to tuberculosis elsewhere (p. 688) and is the result of blood-borne infection. Initially, lesions develop in the renal cortex; these may ulcerate into the renal pelvis and involve the ureters, bladder, epididymis, seminal vesicles and prostate. Calcification in the kidney and stricture formation in the ureter are typical.

Clinical features may include symptoms of bladder involvement (frequency, dysuria); haematuria (sometimes macroscopic); malaise, fever, night sweats, lassitude, weight loss; loin pain; associated genital disease; and chronic renal failure as a result of urinary tract obstruction or destruction of kidney tissue.

Neutrophils are present in the urine but routine urine culture may be negative ('sterile pyuria'). Special techniques of microscopy and culture may be required to identify tubercle bacilli and are most usefully performed on early morning urine specimens. Bladder involvement should be assessed by cystoscopy. Radiology of the urinary tract and a chest X-ray to look for pulmonary tuberculosis are mandatory. Anti-tuberculous chemotherapy follows standard regimes (p. 693). Surgery to relieve urinary tract obstruction or to remove a very severely infected kidney may be required.

Systemic vasculitis

Medium- to large-vessel vasculitis (e.g. classical polyarteritis nodosa, p. 1113) only causes renal disease when arterial involvement leads to hypertension or renal infarction. In contrast, small-vessel vasculitis (p. 1112) commonly affects the kidneys with rapid and profound impairment of glomerular function.

Small-vessel vasculitis

This causes a focal inflammatory glomerulonephritis, usually with focal necrosis (see Box 17.40, p. 502, and Fig. 17.29, p. 503) and often with crescentic changes. It is usually associated with a systemic illness with acute phase response, weight loss and arthralgia, and characteristically in some patients causes pulmonary haemorrhage, which can be life-threatening. However, in other patients it presents as a kidney-limited disorder, with rapidly deteriorating renal function and crescentic nephritis.

The most important causes of this syndrome, microscopic polyangiitis and Wegener's granulomatosis, are usually associated with antibodies to neutrophil granule enzymes (ANCA, p. 1114); these antibodies are non-specific, however, and cannot be relied upon to make the diagnosis and so biopsy of the affected tissue is usually required. Henoch–Schönlein purpura (pp. 501 and 1114) is associated with IgA nephropathy and ANCA are usually absent. Vasculitis in other organs may give clues to the underlying systemic disorder and its subtype: for example, ear, nose and throat involvement and lung disease in Wegener's granulomatosis, or rash on the buttocks in Henoch–Schönlein purpura.

Treatment of the primary types of small-vessel vasculitis with cyclophosphamide, mycophenolate mofetil or corticosteroids is life-saving (p. 1114). Death from extrarenal manifestations of the disease is prevented and renal function can be salvaged in acute disease, even if the glomerulonephritis is so severe as to cause oliguria. In these circumstances, plasma exchange offers additional benefit.

Vasculitis may also be seen in rheumatoid arthritis, SLE and cryoglobulinaemia, although SLE usually involves the kidney in different ways (see below).

Systemic lupus erythematosus (SLE)

The diverse manifestations of SLE are described on page 1107. Subclinical renal involvement, with low-level haematuria and proteinuria but minimally impaired or normal renal function, is common in SLE. Usually this is due to glomerular disease, although serologically and sometimes clinically overlapping syndromes (e.g. mixed connective tissue disorder, Sjögren's syndrome) may cause interstitial nephritis. As indicated in Box 17.40 (p. 502) and Figure 17.27 (p. 500), SLE can produce almost any histological pattern of glomerular disease and clinical features ranging from florid, rapidly progressive glomerulonephritis to nephrotic syndrome.

Diffuse proliferative lupus nephritis

Typically, patients present with subacute disease and inflammatory features (haematuria, hypertension, variable renal impairment), accompanied by heavy proteinuria that often reaches nephrotic levels. In severely affected patients the most common histological pattern is an inflammatory, diffusely proliferative glomerulonephritis with substantial deposits of immunoglobulins on immunofluorescence. Controlled trials have shown that the risk of ESRD in this type of disease is significantly reduced by cyclophosphamide, often given as regular intravenous pulses, though mycophenolate mofetil appears as effective in short-term studies.

Dialysis and transplantation in SLE

Many patients go into relative remission from SLE once ESRD has developed. This may be because ESRD itself is an immunosuppressed state, as indicated by the higher incidence of bacterial infections in ESRD from all causes. Patients with ESRD caused by SLE are usually good candidates for dialysis and transplantation. Although it may recur in renal allografts, the immunosuppression required to prevent allograft rejection usually controls SLE too.

Pregnancy

Pregnancy has important physiological effects on the renal system. Some diseases are more common in pregnancy, the manifestations of others are modified by the physiological changes of pregnancy, and a few diseases (e.g. pre-eclampsia) are unique to pregnancy.

Physiological adaptations begin in the first few weeks. Peripheral vascular resistance declines, blood volume, cardiac output and GFR increase, and there is usually a reduction in blood pressure and plasma creatinine and urea values in the first trimester. Recordings of baseline blood pressure and urine testing from the first antenatal clinic visit are valuable if problems arise later.

Pregnancy and renal disease

Pyelonephritis is more common during pregnancy, perhaps because of dilatation of the urinary collecting system and ureters, so asymptomatic bacteriuria should be treated (Box 17.53 and p. 472).

Proteinuria caused by glomerular disease is usually exacerbated, and nephrotic syndrome may develop without any alteration in the underlying disease activity in individuals who had only slight proteinuria before pregnancy. This further increases the risk of venous

---

EBM 17.53 **Treatment of asymptomatic bacteriuria in pregnancy**

'Antibiotic therapy for asymptomatic bacteriuria reduces the incidence of pyelonephritis by 75% and pre-term delivery by 40%.'

- Smaill F. (Cochrane Review). Cochrane Library, issue 2, 2007. Oxford: Update Software.

For further information: www.cochrane.org

thromboembolism, which is the leading cause of maternal deaths in developed countries.

Systemic autoimmune diseases are typically relatively quiescent during pregnancy but tend to relapse in the first few weeks and months following delivery. Pre-existing renal disease increases the fetal and maternal risk involved in pregnancy, to a degree dependent on the level of renal function, proteinuria and hypertension. Patients with such diseases who may become pregnant should be aware of the extra associated risks. During pregnancy, therapy should not usually be stopped, but blood pressure targets may be modified (after discussion with the patient) and agents altered to those of proven safety.

Pre-eclampsia and related disorders

Pre-eclampsia is a systemic disorder that occurs in or near the third trimester of pregnancy (Box 17.54). Its aetiology is unknown, although a number of risk factors are described (Box 17.55).

Diagnosis

Pre-eclampsia is traditionally defined by the triad of oedema, proteinuria and hypertension. However, oedema is common in late pregnancy, proteinuria is a late sign and, while hypertension is usually present, it

---

 17.54 **Pre-eclampsia and related diseases in pregnancy**

Clinical syndromes

- Eclampsia: severe hypertension, encephalopathy and fits
- Disseminated intravascular coagulation
- Thrombotic microangiopathy: may also occur post-partum (post-partum haemolytic uraemic syndrome)
- Acute fatty liver of pregnancy
- 'HELLP' syndrome: haemolysis, elevated liver enzymes, low platelets (thrombotic microangiopathy with abnormal liver function)

Clinical signs

- Hypertension
- Proteinuria
- Oedema
- Other evidence of the clinical syndromes listed above

Investigations

- Uric acid levels increased (before renal impairment apparent)
- Platelets decreased
- Reduced GFR (late)
- Fetus small for dates and growing slowly
- Fetal distress (late)

17

17.55 Risk factors for pre-eclampsia

- First pregnancy
- First pregnancy with a new partner or long inter-pregnancy interval
- Pre-eclampsia in previous pregnancies
- Age < 20 yrs or > 35 yrs
- Multiple pregnancy (singleton < twin < triplets etc.)
- Pre-existing hypertension
- Pre-existing renal disease

tinuing the pregnancy for as long as possible may permit delivery of a healthier, more mature baby. Proteinuria and hypertension in the first trimester of pregnancy suggest pre-existing renal disease.

Management

The only effective management for pre-eclampsia is delivery. The role of antiplatelet therapy (low-dose aspirin) remains controversial. Hypertension is a consequence and not the cause of the disorder, and treatment is only justified to lower it from severe and immediately dangerous levels (e.g. > 150–160/100–110 mmHg). Treating lower levels has been shown to confer no benefit and exposes the fetus to additional drugs. If life-threatening complications are not present and the baby is immature, corticosteroids may be given to induce maturation of fetal lungs, and delivery postponed while mother and baby are closely observed. Magnesium sulphate reduces the incidence of eclamptic convulsions.

may be relative, mild or even absent. Furthermore, all these features occur in pre-existing renal disease exacerbated by pregnancy. Distinguishing pre-eclampsia from pre-existing renal disease is important. Pre-eclampsia presents progressively, increasing risks to mother and fetus which can be reversed almost immediately by early delivery. In contrast, in pre-existing renal disease, con-

17.56 Mechanisms and examples of drug-induced renal disease/dysfunction

Mechanism	Drug or toxin	Comments
Haemodynamic	NSAIDs	Especially as a co-factor. Via inhibition of prostaglandin synthesis
	ACE inhibitors	Reduce efferent glomerular arteriolar tone. Toxic in the presence of renal artery stenosis and other conditions of renal hypoperfusion
	Radiographic contrast media	Multifactorial aetiology may include intense vasoconstriction
Acute tubular necrosis	Aminoglycosides, amphotericin	In most examples there is evidence of direct tubular toxicity but haemodynamic and other factors probably contribute
	Paracetamol overdose	May occur with or without serious hepatotoxicity
	Radiographic contrast media	May be secondary to precipitation in tubules. Furosemide is a co-factor
Loss of tubular/ collecting duct function	Lithium	Dose-related, partially reversible loss of concentrating ability
	Cisplatin	
	Aminoglycosides, amphotericin	At lower exposures than cause acute tubular necrosis
Immune (glomerular)	Penicillamine, gold	Membranous nephropathy
	Penicillamine	Crescentic or focal necrotising glomerulonephritis in association with ANCA and systemic small-vessel vasculitis
	NSAIDs	Minimal change nephropathy
Immune (interstitial)	NSAIDs, penicillins, proton pump inhibitors, many others	Acute interstitial nephritis
Chronic interstitial nephritis (alone)	Lithium	As a consequence of acute toxicity. Otherwise controversial
	Ciclosporin, tacrolimus	The major problem with these drugs
Chronic interstitial nephritis (with papillary necrosis)	Various analgesics (p. 506)	
Obstruction (crystal formation)	Aciclovir	Crystals of the drug form in tubules. Aciclovir is now more common than the original example of sulphonamides
	Chemotherapy	Uric acid crystals forming as a consequence of tumour lysis (typically a first-dose effect in haematological malignancy)
Nephrocalcinosis	Oral sodium phosphate containing bowel cleansing agents	Precipitation of calcium phosphate occurring in 1–4% and exacerbated by volume depletion. Usually mild but damage can be irreversible
Retroperitoneal fibrosis	Ergolinic dopamine agonists (e.g. cabergoline), methysergide*, practolol*	Idiopathic is more common (p. 509)

*These drugs are no longer in use in the UK.

Acute renal failure in pregnancy

Maternal acute renal failure may occur in almost any of the pre-eclamptic syndromes. Worldwide, an important cause of acute renal failure is septic abortion, when the uterus becomes infected because of retained products of conception or poor sterility in an often illegally induced abortion. Renal function is usually recoverable, but acute renal failure in pregnancy is particularly prone to progress to cortical necrosis with incomplete or total failure to recover renal function.

DRUGS AND THE KIDNEY

Prescribing in renal disease

Many drugs and drug metabolites are excreted by the kidney so the presence of renal impairment alters the required dose and frequency. This is discussed on page 27.

Drug-induced renal disease

The kidney is susceptible to damage by drugs because it is the route of excretion of many water-soluble compounds, including drugs and their metabolites. Some may reach high concentrations in the renal cortex as a result of proximal tubular transport mechanisms. Others are concentrated in the medulla by the operation of the countercurrent system. The same applies to certain toxins.

Toxic renal damage may occur by a variety of mechanisms (Box 17.56). Very commonly, drugs contribute as one of multiple insults to the development of acute tubular necrosis. Numerically, reactions to NSAIDs and ACE inhibitors are the most important. Haemodynamic renal impairment, acute tubular necrosis and allergic reactions are usually reversible if recognised early enough. However, other types, especially those associated with extensive fibrosis, are less likely to be reversible.

NSAIDs

As described on page 483, NSAIDs impair renal function in individuals in whom prostaglandin-dependent compensatory mechanisms are maintaining renal function (e.g. heart failure, cirrhosis, sepsis and renal impairment of almost any type), and may precipitate ARF in susceptible patients. In addition, idiosyncratic immune reactions may occur; causing minimal change nephrotic syndrome (p. 500) and acute interstitial nephritis (p. 504). Analgesic nephropathy (p. 506) is now a rare complication of long-term use.

ACE inhibitors

These abolish the compensatory angiotensin II-mediated vasoconstriction of the glomerular efferent arteriole that occurs to maintain glomerular perfusion pressure distal to a renal artery stenosis and in renal hypoperfusion (see Fig. 17.1, p. 463). Monitoring of renal function before and after initiation of therapy is essential.

Further information

www.edren.org *Renal Unit, Royal Infirmary of Edinburgh; information about individual diseases, protocols for immediate in-hospital management and a list of educational resources, including key cases; extensive links to other resources.*

www.ndt-educational.org *European Renal Association; gives agreed European Best Practice Guidelines for the management of anaemia, transplantation and haemodialysis.*

www.nephron.com *The links under 'Physicians/ Physicans' resources' are particularly good and include useful urology links; includes an MDRD (Modification of Diet in Renal Disease study) calculator for estimating GFR from serum creatinine; extensive links to other resources.*

www.renal.org *UK Renal Association; link to the current guidelines on the detection, referral and management of chronic kidney disease.*

www.sign.ac.uk *Scottish Intercollegiate Guidelines Network; link to guidelines on the diagnosis and management of chronic kidney disease.*

17

D.E. Newby
N.R. Grubb
A. Bradbury

Cardiovascular disease

18

CLINICAL EXAMINATION OF THE CARDIOVASCULAR SYSTEM

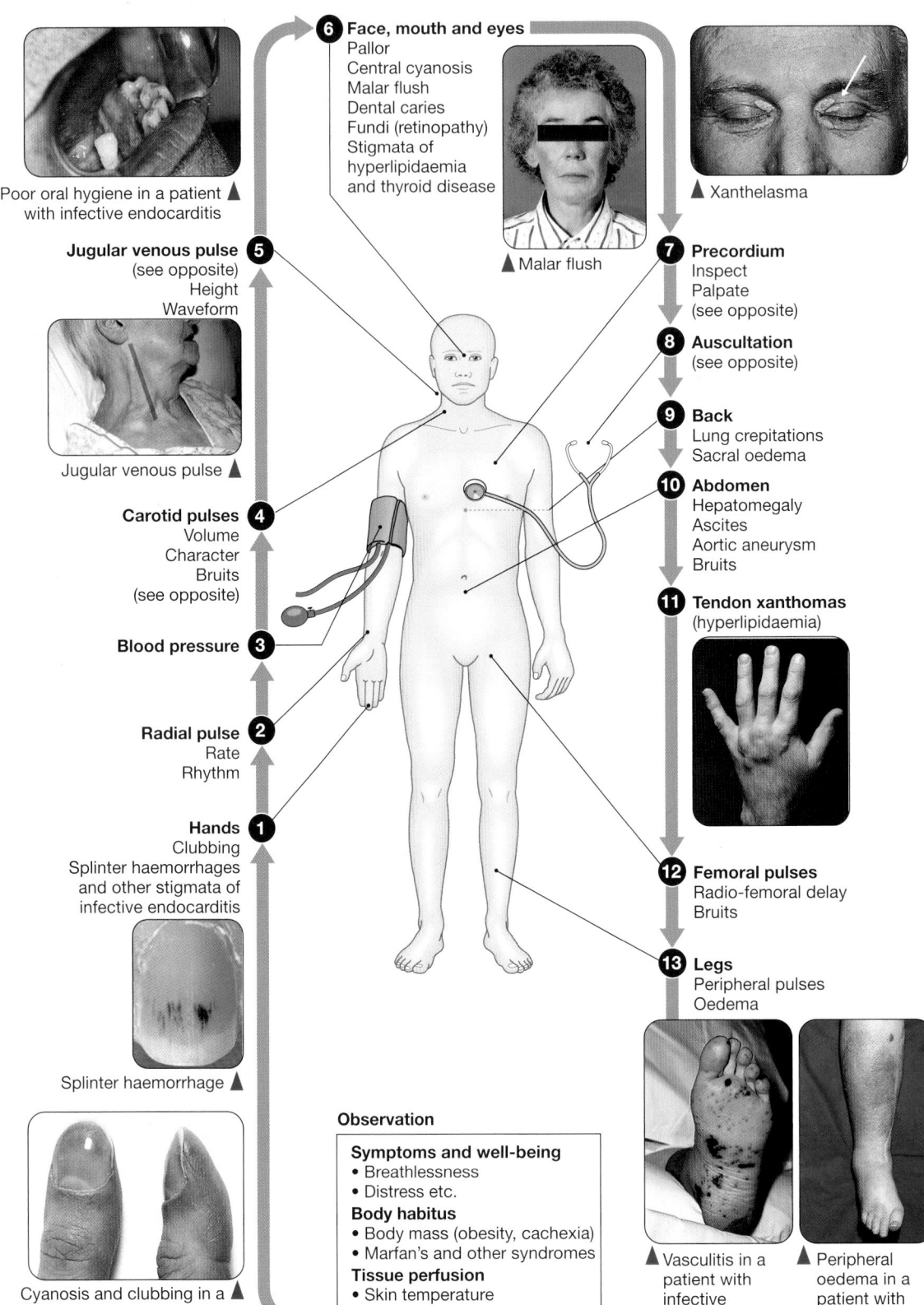

Poor oral hygiene in a patient ▲ with infective endocarditis

6 Face, mouth and eyes
Pallor
Central cyanosis
Malar flush
Dental caries
Fundi (retinopathy)
Stigmata of hyperlipidaemia and thyroid disease

▲ Xanthelasma

▲ Malar flush

Jugular venous pulse 5
(see opposite)
Height
Waveform

Jugular venous pulse ▲

7 Precordium
Inspect
Palpate
(see opposite)

8 Auscultation
(see opposite)

9 Back
Lung crepitations
Sacral oedema

10 Abdomen
Hepatomegaly
Ascites
Aortic aneurysm
Bruits

11 Tendon xanthomas
(hyperlipidaemia)

Carotid pulses 4
Volume
Character
Bruits
(see opposite)

Blood pressure 3

Radial pulse 2
Rate
Rhythm

Hands 1
Clubbing
Splinter haemorrhages
and other stigmata of
infective endocarditis

Splinter haemorrhage ▲

Cyanosis and clubbing in a ▲
patient with complex cyanotic
congenital heart disease

Observation

Symptoms and well-being
• Breathlessness
• Distress etc.
Body habitus
• Body mass (obesity, cachexia)
• Marfan's and other syndromes
Tissue perfusion
• Skin temperature
• Sweating
• Urine output

12 Femoral pulses
Radio-femoral delay
Bruits

13 Legs
Peripheral pulses
Oedema

▲ Vasculitis in a
patient with
infective
endocarditis

▲ Peripheral
oedema in a
patient with
congestive
cardiac failure

4 Examination of the arterial pulse

- The character of the pulse is determined by stroke volume and arterial compliance, and is best assessed by palpating a major artery, such as the carotid or brachial.
- Aortic regurgitation, anaemia, sepsis and other causes of a large stroke volume typically produce a bounding pulse with a high amplitude and wide pulse pressure (panel A).
- Aortic stenosis impedes ventricular emptying and may cause a slow rising, weak and delayed pulse (panel A).
- Normal sinus rhythm produces a pulse that is regular in time and force. Arrhythmias may cause irregularity. Atrial fibrillation produces a pulse that is irregular in time and volume (panel B).

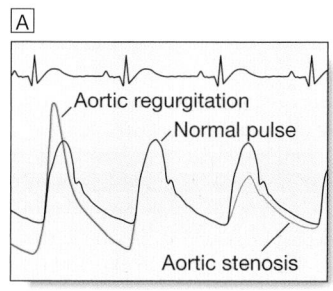

A

Aortic regurgitation
Normal pulse
Aortic stenosis

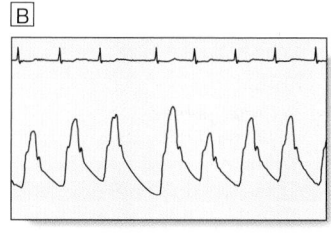

B

5 Examination of the jugular venous pulse

The internal jugular vein, superior vena cava and right atrium are in continuity, so the height of the jugular venous pulsation reflects right atrial pressure. When the patient is placed at 45°, with the head supported and turned a few degrees to the left, the jugular venous pulse (JVP) is visible along the line of the sternocleidomastoid muscle (see opposite).

- The height of the JVP is determined by right atrial pressure and is therefore elevated in right heart failure and reduced in hypovolaemia.
- If the JVP is not easily seen, it may be highlighted by gentle pressure on the abdomen (so-called 'hepato-jugular' reflux).
- In normal sinus rhythm the two venous peaks, the *a* and *v* waves, approximate to atrial and ventricular systole respectively.
- The *x* descent reflects atrial relaxation and apical displacement of the tricuspid valve ring. The *y* descent reflects atrial emptying early in diastole. These signs are subtle.
- Tricuspid regurgitation produces giant *v* waves that coincide with ventricular systole.

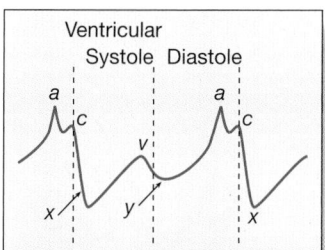

Ventricular
Systole   Diastole

a   *a*
c   *c*
v
x   *y*   *x*

Waveform of the jugular venous pulse.

Features that distinguish venous from arterial pulsation in the neck

- Venous pulse has two peaks in each cardiac cycle (arterial has one).
- The height of the venous pulse varies with respiration (falls on inspiration) and position.
- Abdominal compression causes the venous pulse to rise.
- Venous pulse is not palpable and can be occluded by light pressure.

7 Palpation of the precordium

Technique

- Place fingertips over apex (1) to assess for position and character. Place heel of hand over left sternal edge (2) for a parasternal heave or 'lift'. Assess for the presence of thrills in all areas, including the aortic and pulmonary areas (3).

Common abnormalities of the apex beat

- Volume overload, such as mitral or aortic regurgitation: displaced, forceful
- Pressure overload, such as aortic stenosis, hypertension: discrete, thrusting
- Dyskinetic, such as left ventricular aneurysm: displaced, incoordinate

Other abnormalities

- Palpable S1 (tapping apex beat: mitral stenosis)
- Palpable P2 (severe pulmonary hypertension)
- Left parasternal heave or 'lift' felt by heel of hand (right ventricular hypertrophy)
- Palpable thrill (aortic stenosis)

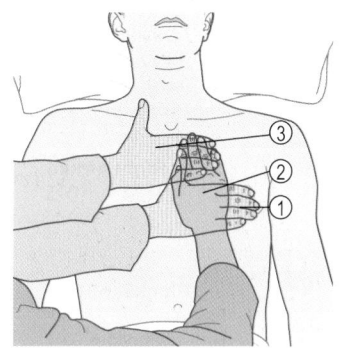

Palpation of the precordium.

8 Auscultation of the heart

- Use the diaphragm to examine at the apex, lower left sternal edge (tricuspid area) and upper left (pulmonary area) and right (aortic area) sternal edges.
- Use the bell to examine low-pitched noises, particularly at the apex for mid-diastolic murmurs.
- Time the sounds and murmurs by feeling the carotid pulse; systolic murmurs are synchronous with the pulse.
- Listen for radiation of systolic murmurs, over the base of the neck (aortic stenosis) and in the axilla (mitral incompetence).
- Listen over the left sternal border with the patient sitting forward (aortic incompetence), then at the apex with the patient rolled on to the left side (mitral stenosis).

The haemodynamic effects of respiration are discussed on page 528.

See pages 557–559 for analysis and interpretation of heart sounds and murmurs.

18

Cardiovascular disease is the most frequent cause of adult death in the Western world; in the UK one-third of men and one-quarter of women will die as a result of ischaemic heart disease. In many developed countries, the incidence of ischaemic heart disease has been falling for the last two or three decades, but it is rising in Eastern Europe and Asia. Cardiovascular disease may thus soon become the leading cause of death on all continents. Strategies for the treatment and prevention of heart disease can be highly effective and have been subjected to rigorous evaluation. The evidence base for the treatment of cardiovascular disease is stronger than for almost any other disease group.

Valvular heart disease is common, but the aetiology varies in different parts of the world. On the Indian subcontinent and in Africa, it is predominantly due to rheumatic fever, whereas calcific aortic valve disease is the most common problem in developed countries.

Prompt recognition of the development of heart disease is limited by two key factors. Firstly, it is often latent; coronary artery disease can proceed to an advanced stage before the patient notices any symptoms. Secondly, the diversity of symptoms attributable to heart disease is limited, so different pathologies may frequently present with the same symptoms.

FUNCTIONAL ANATOMY AND PHYSIOLOGY

Anatomy

The heart acts as two serial pumps that share several electrical and mechanical components. The right heart circulates blood to the lungs where it is oxygenated, and the left heart receives this and circulates it to the rest of the body (Fig. 18.1). The atria are thin-walled structures that act as priming pumps for the ventricles, which provide most of the energy to the circulation. Within the mediastinum, the atria are situated posteriorly and the left atrium (LA) sits anterior to the oesophagus and descending aorta. The interatrial septum separates the two atria. In 20% of adults a patent foramen ovale is found; this communication in the fetal circulation between the right and left atria normally closes at birth (p. 629). The right atrium (RA) receives blood from the superior and inferior venae cavae and the coronary sinus. The LA receives blood from four pulmonary veins, two from each of the left and right lungs. The ventricles are thick-walled structures, adapted to circulating blood through large vascular beds under pressure. The atria and ventricles are separated by the annulus fibrosus, which forms the skeleton for the atrioventricular (AV) valves and which electrically insulates the atria from the ventricles. The right ventricle (RV) is roughly triangular in shape and extends from the annulus fibrosus to near the cardiac apex, which is situated to the left of the midline. Its anterosuperior surface is rounded and convex, and its posterior extent is bounded by the interventricular septum, which bulges into the chamber. Its upper extent is conical, forming the conus arteriosus or outflow tract, from which the pulmonary artery arises. The RV sits anterior to and to the right of the left ventricle (LV). The LV is more conical in shape and in cross-section is nearly circular. It extends from the LA to the apex of the heart. The LV myocardium is normally around 10 mm thick (c.f. RV thickness of 2–3 mm) because it pumps blood at a higher pressure.

The normal heart occupies less than 50% of the transthoracic diameter in the frontal plane, as seen on a chest X-ray. On the patient's left, the cardiac silhouette is formed by the aortic arch, the pulmonary trunk, the left atrial appendage and the LV. On the right, the RA is joined by superior and inferior venae cavae, and

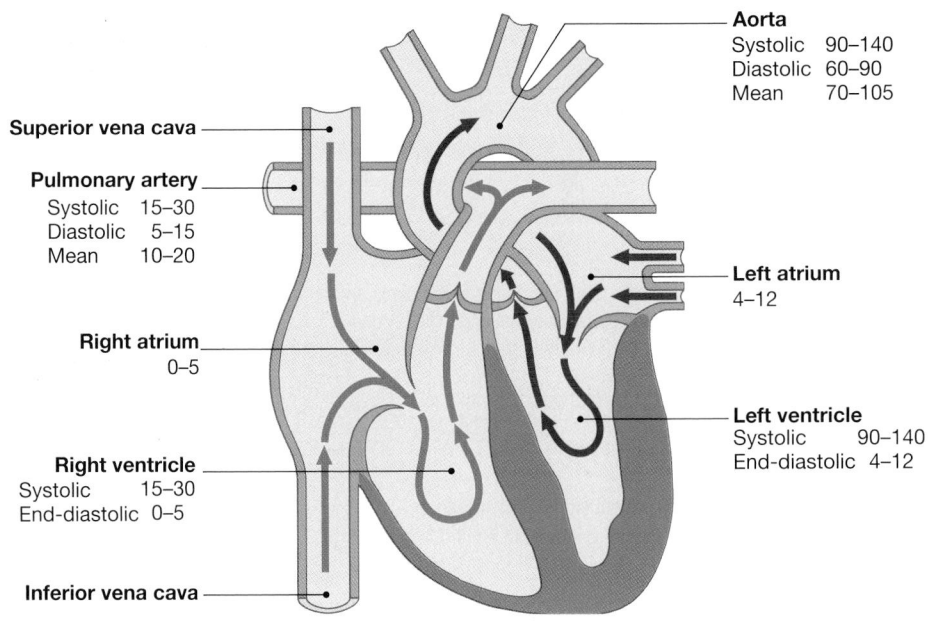

Aorta
Systolic   90–140
Diastolic 60–90
Mean   70–105

Superior vena cava

Pulmonary artery
Systolic   15–30
Diastolic 5–15
Mean   10–20

Left atrium
4–12

Right atrium
0–5

Left ventricle
Systolic   90–140
End-diastolic 4–12

Right ventricle
Systolic   15–30
End-diastolic 0–5

Inferior vena cava

Fig. 18.1 Direction of blood flow through the heart. The blue arrows show deoxygenated blood moving through the right heart to the lungs. The red arrows show oxygenated blood moving from the lungs to the systemic circulation. The normal pressures are shown for each chamber in mmHg.

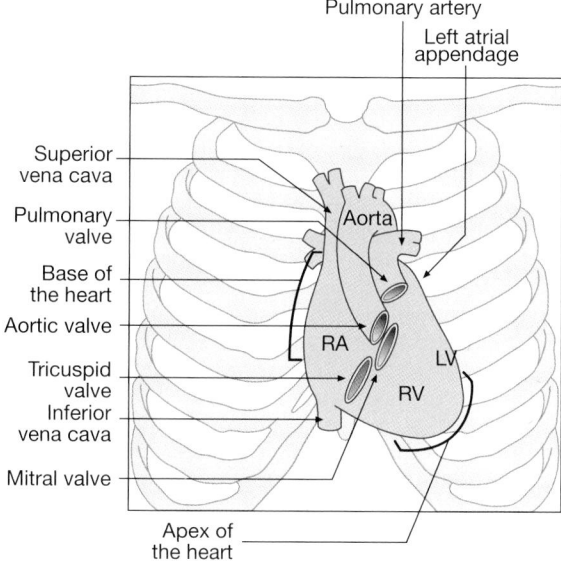

Fig. 18.2 Surface anatomy of the heart. The positions of the major cardiac chambers and heart valves are shown.

the lower right border is made up by the RV (Fig. 18.2). In disease states or congenital cardiac abnormalities, the silhouette may change as a result of hypertrophy or dilatation.

The coronary circulation

The left main and right coronary arteries arise from the left and right coronary sinuses of the aortic root, distal to the aortic valve (Fig. 18.3). Within 2.5 cm of its origin, the left main coronary artery divides into the left anterior descending artery (LAD), which runs in the anterior interventricular groove, and the left circumflex artery (CX), which runs posteriorly in the atrioventricular groove. The LAD gives branches to supply the anterior part of the septum (septal perforators) and the anterior, lateral and apical walls of the LV. The CX gives marginal branches that supply the lateral, posterior and inferior segments

of the LV. The right coronary artery (RCA) runs in the right atrioventricular groove, giving branches that supply the RA, RV and inferoposterior aspects of the LV. The posterior descending artery runs in the posterior interventricular groove and supplies the inferior part of the interventricular septum. This vessel is a branch of the RCA in approximately 90% of people (dominant right system) and is supplied by the CX in the remainder (dominant left system). The coronary anatomy varies greatly from person to person and there are many 'normal variants'.

The RCA supplies the sinoatrial (SA) node in about 60% of individuals and the AV node in about 90%. Proximal occlusion of the RCA therefore often results in sinus bradycardia and may also cause AV nodal block. Abrupt occlusions in the RCA, due to coronary thrombosis, result in infarction of the inferior part of the LV and often the RV. Abrupt occlusion of the LAD or CX causes infarction in the corresponding territory of the LV, and occlusion of the left main coronary artery is usually fatal.

The venous system follows the coronary arteries but drains into the coronary sinus in the atrioventricular groove, and then to the RA. An extensive lymphatic system drains into vessels that travel with the coronary vessels and then into the thoracic duct.

Conducting system of the heart

The SA node is situated at the junction of the superior vena cava and RA (Fig. 18.4). It comprises specialised atrial cells that depolarise at a rate influenced by the autonomic nervous system and by circulating catecholamines. During normal (sinus) rhythm, this depolarisation wave propagates through both atria via sheets of atrial myocytes. The annulus fibrosus forms a conduction barrier between atria and ventricles, and the only pathway through it is the AV node. This is a midline structure, extending from the right side of the interatrial septum, penetrating the annulus fibrosus anteriorly. The AV node conducts relatively slowly, producing a necessary time delay between atrial and ventricular contraction. The His–Purkinje system is comprised of the bundle of His extending from the AV node into the interventricular septum, the right and left bundle branches passing along the ventricular septum and into

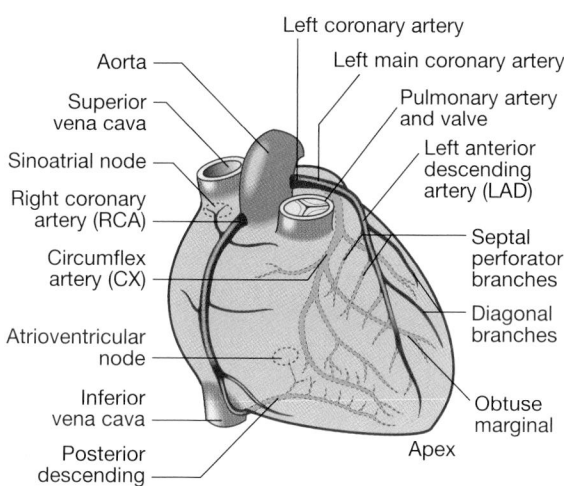

Fig. 18.3 The coronary arteries of the heart. Diagram of the anterior view.

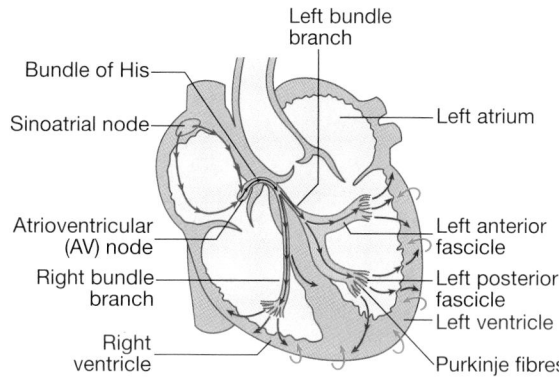

Fig. 18.4 The cardiac conduction system. Depolarisation starts in the sinoatrial node and spreads through the atria (blue arrows), and then through the atrioventricular node (black arrows). Depolarisation then spreads through the bundle of His and the bundle branches to reach the ventricular muscle (red arrows). Repolarisation spreads from epicardium to endocardium (green arrows).

the respective ventricles, the anterior and posterior fascicles of the left bundle branch, and the smaller Purkinje fibres that ramify through the ventricular myocardium. The tissues of the His–Purkinje system conduct very rapidly and allow near-simultaneous depolarisation of the entire ventricular myocardium.

Nerve supply of the heart

The heart is innervated by both sympathetic and parasympathetic fibres. Adrenergic nerves from the cervical sympathetic chain supply muscle fibres in the atria and ventricles and the electrical conducting system. Positive inotropic and chronotropic effects are mediated by β_1-adrenoceptors, whereas β_2-adrenoceptors predominate in vascular smooth muscle and mediate vasodilatation. Parasympathetic pre-ganglionic fibres and sensory fibres reach the heart through the vagus nerves. Cholinergic nerves supply the AV and SA nodes via muscarinic (M2) receptors. Under resting conditions, vagal inhibitory activity predominates and the heart rate is slow. Adrenergic stimulation associated with exercise, emotional stress, fever and so on causes the heart rate to increase. In disease states the nerve supply to the heart may be affected. For example, in heart failure the sympathetic system may be up-regulated, and in diabetes mellitus the nerves themselves may be damaged (autonomic neuropathy, p. 831) so that there is little variation in heart rate.

Physiology

The circulation

The RA receives deoxygenated blood from the superior and inferior venae cavae and discharges blood to the RV, which in turn pumps it into the pulmonary artery. Blood passes through the pulmonary arterial and alveolar capillary bed where it is oxygenated, then drains via four pulmonary veins into the LA. This in turn fills the LV, which delivers blood into the aorta (see Fig. 18.1). During ventricular contraction (systole), the tricuspid valve in the right heart and the mitral valve in the left heart close, and the pulmonary and aortic valves open. In diastole, the pulmonary and aortic valves close, and the two AV valves open. Collectively, these atrial and ventricular events constitute the cardiac cycle of filling and ejection of blood from one heartbeat to the next.

Myocardial contraction

Myocardial cells (myocytes) are about 50–100 μm long; each cell branches and interdigitates with adjacent cells. An intercalated disc permits electrical conduction via gap junctions, and mechanical conduction via the fascia adherens, to adjacent cells. The basic unit of contraction is the sarcomere (2 μm long), which is aligned to those of adjacent myofibrils, giving a striated appearance due to the Z-lines (Fig. 18.5). Actin filaments are attached at

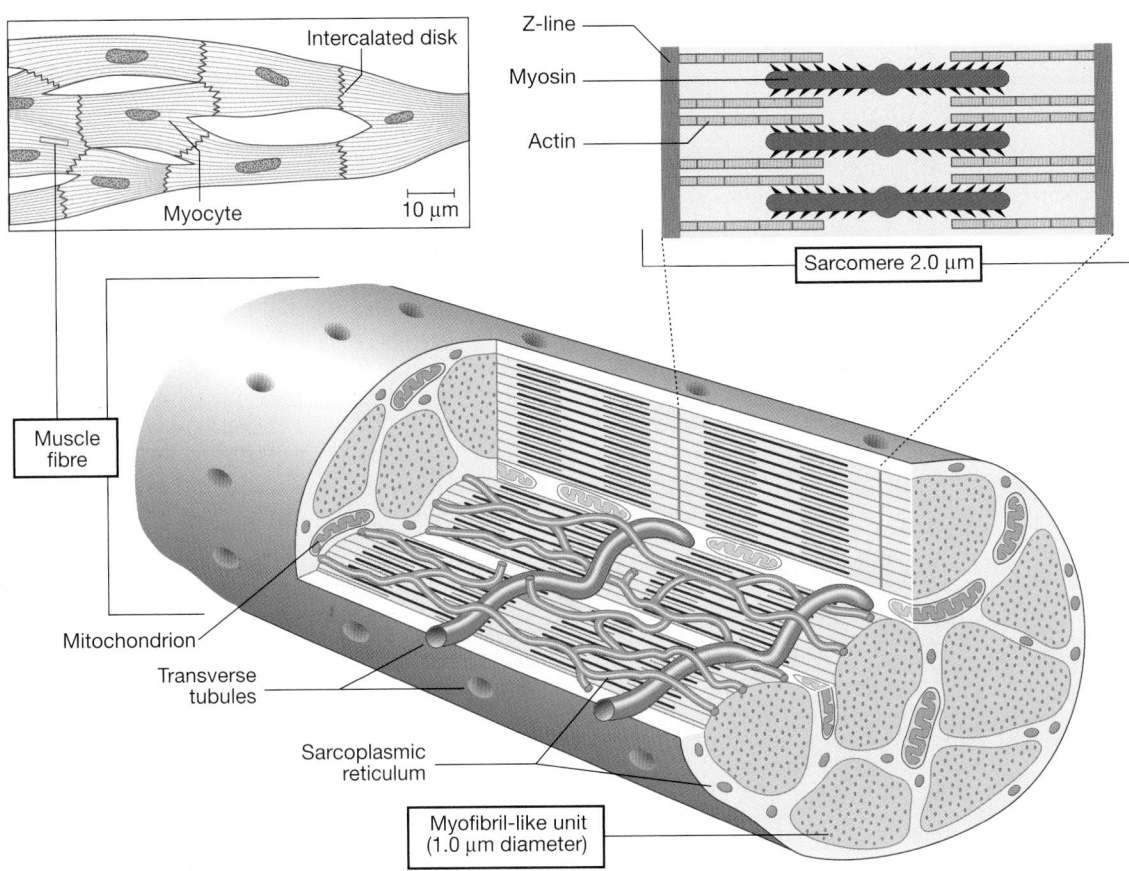

Fig. 18.5 Schematic of myocytes and a muscle fibre. The arrangement of myofibrils, and longitudinal and transverse tubules extending from the sarcoplasmic reticulum are shown. The expanded section shows a schematic of an individual sarcomere with thick filaments composed of myosin and thin filaments composed primarily of actin.

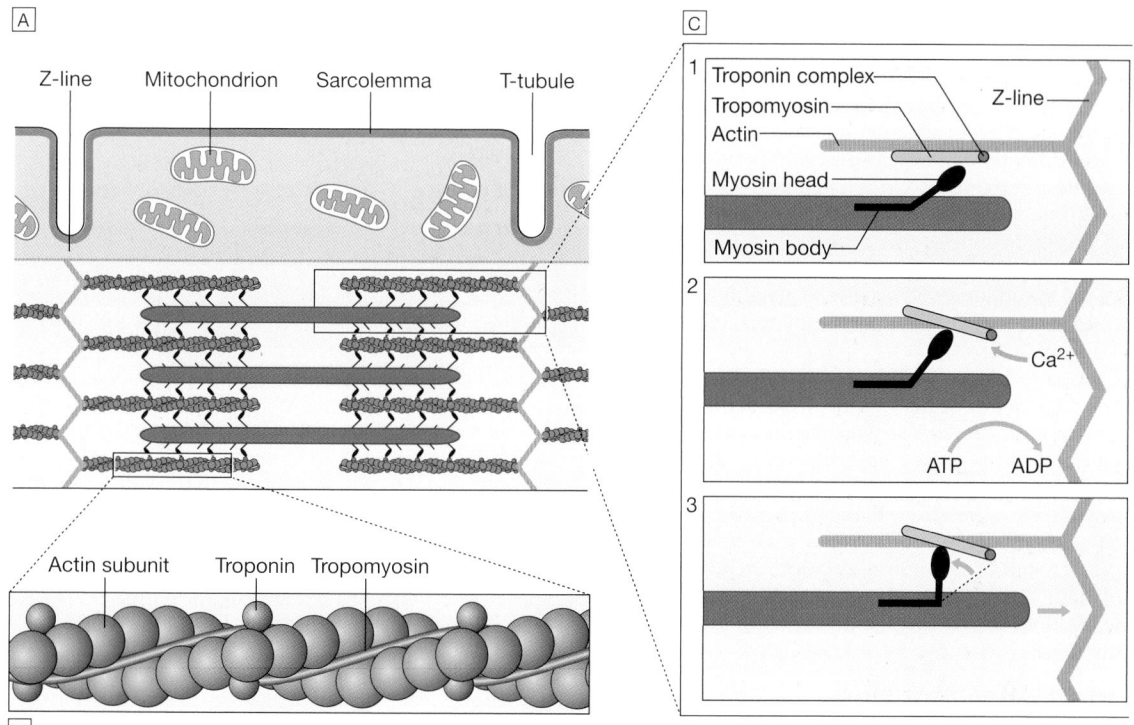

Fig. 18.6 Contraction process within the muscle fibre. **A** Schematic of a sarcomere showing the overlapping of actin and myosin filaments. **B** Enlarged diagram of the structure of an actin filament. **C** The three stages of contraction resulting in shortening of the sarcomere. (1) The actin binding site is blocked by tropomyosin. (2) ATP-dependent release of calcium ions which bind to troponin, displacing tropomyosin. The binding site is exposed. (ADP = adenosine diphosphate; ATP = adenosine triphosphate) (3) Tilting of the angle of attachment of the myosin head, resulting in fibre shortening.

right angles to the Z-lines and interdigitate with thicker parallel myosin filaments. The cross-links between actin and myosin molecules contain myofibrillar ATPase, which breaks down adenosine triphosphate (ATP) to provide the energy for contraction. Two chains of actin molecules form a helical structure, with a second molecule, tropomyosin, in the grooves of the actin helix, and a further molecule complex, troponin, attached to every seventh actin molecule (Fig. 18.6).

During the plateau phase of the action potential, calcium ions enter the cell and are mobilised from the sarcoplasmic reticulum. They bind to troponin and thereby precipitate contraction by shortening of the sarcomere through the interdigitation of the actin and myosin molecules. The force of cardiac muscle contraction, or inotropic state, is regulated by the influx of calcium ions through 'slow calcium channels'. The extent to which the sarcomere can shorten determines stroke volume of the ventricle. It is maximally shortened in response to powerful inotropic drugs or marked exercise. However, the enlargement of the heart seen in heart failure is due to slippage of the myofibrils and adjacent cells rather than lengthening of the sarcomere.

Cardiac output

Cardiac output is the product of stroke volume and heart rate. Stroke volume is the volume of blood ejected in each cardiac cycle (see Fig. 18.36, p. 559), and is dependent upon end-diastolic volume and pressure (preload), myocardial contractility and systolic aortic pressure (afterload). Stretch of cardiac muscle (from increased end-diastolic volume) causes an increase in the force of contraction, producing a greater stroke volume: Starling's Law of the heart (see Fig. 18.22, p. 544).

The contractile state of the myocardium is controlled by neuro-endocrine factors, such as adrenaline (epinephrine), and can be influenced by inotropic drugs and their antagonists. The response to a physiological change or to a drug can be predicted on the basis of its combined influence on preload, afterload and contractility (see Fig. 18.26, p. 548).

Blood flow

Blood passes from the heart through the large central elastic arteries into muscular arteries before encountering the resistance vessels, and ultimately the capillary bed where there is exchange of nutrients, oxygen and waste products of metabolism. The central arteries, such as the aorta, are predominantly composed of elastic tissue with little or no vascular smooth muscle cells. When blood is ejected from the heart, the compliant aorta expands to accommodate the volume of blood before the elastic recoil sustains blood pressure (BP) and flow following cessation of cardiac contraction. This 'Windkessel effect' prevents excessive rises in systolic BP whilst sustaining diastolic BP, thereby reducing cardiac afterload and maintaining coronary perfusion. These benefits are lost with progressive arterial stiffening: a feature of ageing and advanced renal disease.

Passing down the arterial tree, vascular smooth muscle cells progressively play a greater role until the resistance arterioles are encountered. Although all vessels contribute, the resistance vessels (diameter 50–200 µm) provide the greatest contribution to systemic vascular resistance, with small changes in radius having a marked influence on blood flow; resistance is proportional to the fourth power of the radius (Poiseuille's Law). The tone of these resistance vessels is tightly regulated by humoral, neuronal and mechanical factors. Neurogenic constriction operates via α-adrenoceptors on vascular smooth muscle, and dilatation via muscarinic and β$_2$-adrenoceptors. In addition, systemic and locally released vasoactive substances influence tone; vasoconstrictors include noradrenaline (norepinephrine), angiotensin II and endothelin-1, whereas adenosine, bradykinin, prostaglandins and nitric oxide are vasodilators. Resistance to blood flow rises with viscosity and is mainly influenced by red cell concentration (haematocrit).

Coronary blood vessels receive sympathetic and parasympathetic innervation. Stimulation of α-adrenoceptors causes vasoconstriction; stimulation of β$_2$-adrenoceptors causes vasodilatation; the predominant effect of sympathetic stimulation in coronary arteries is vasodilatation. Parasympathetic stimulation also causes modest dilatation of normal coronary arteries. As a result of vascular regulation, an atheromatous narrowing (stenosis) in a coronary artery does not limit flow, even during exercise, until the cross-sectional area of the vessel is reduced by at least 70%.

Endothelial function

The endothelium plays a vital role in the control of vascular homeostasis. It synthesises and releases many vasoactive mediators that cause vasodilatation, including nitric oxide, prostacyclin and endothelium-derived hyperpolarising factor, and vasoconstriction, including endothelin-1 and angiotensin II. A balance exists whereby the release of such factors contributes to the maintenance and regulation of vascular tone and BP. Damage to the endothelium may disrupt this balance and lead to vascular dysfunction, tissue ischaemia and hypertension.

The endothelium also has a major influence on key regulatory steps in the recruitment of inflammatory cells and on the formation and dissolution of thrombus. Once activated, the endothelium expresses surface receptors such as E-selectin, intercellular adhesion molecule type 1 (ICAM-1) and platelet endothelial cell adhesion molecule type 1 (PECAM-1), which mediate rolling, adhesion and migration of inflammatory leucocytes into the subintima. The endothelium also stores and releases the multimeric glycoprotein, von Willebrand factor, which promotes thrombus formation by linking platelet adhesion to denuded surfaces, especially in the arterial vasculature. In contrast, once intravascular thrombus forms, tissue plasminogen activator is rapidly released from a dynamic storage pool within the endothelium to induce fibrinolysis and thrombus dissolution. These processes are critically involved in the development and progression of atherosclerosis, and endothelial function and injury is seen as central to the pathogenesis of many cardiovascular disease states.

Effects of respiration

There is a fall in intrathoracic pressure during inspiration that tends to promote venous flow into the chest, producing an increase in the flow of blood through the right heart. However, a substantial volume of blood is sequestered in the chest as the lungs expand; the increase in the capacitance of the pulmonary vascular bed usually exceeds any increase in the output of the right heart and there is therefore a reduction in the flow of blood into the left heart

18.1 Haemodynamic effects of respiration

	Inspiration	Expiration
Jugular venous pressure	Falls	Rises
Blood pressure	Falls (up to 10 mmHg)	Rises
Heart rate	Accelerates	Slows
Second heart sound	Splits*	Fuses*

*Inspiration prolongs RV ejection, delaying P$_2$, and shortens LV ejection, bringing forward A$_2$; expiration produces the opposite effects.

during inspiration. In contrast, expiration is accompanied by a fall in venous return to the right heart, a reduction in the output of the right heart, a rise in the venous return to the left heart (as blood is squeezed out of the lungs) and an increase in the output of the left heart (Box 18.1).

Pulsus paradoxus

This term is used to describe the exaggerated fall in BP during inspiration that is characteristic of cardiac tamponade (pp. 542 and 639) and severe airways obstruction. In airways obstruction, it is due to accentuation of the change in intrathoracic pressure with respiration. In cardiac tamponade, compression of the right heart prevents the normal increase in flow through the right heart on inspiration, which exaggerates the usual drop in venous return to the left heart and produces a marked fall in BP.

INVESTIGATION OF CARDIOVASCULAR DISEASE

Specific investigations may be required to confirm a diagnosis of cardiac disease. Basic tests, such as electrocardiography, chest X-ray and echocardiography, can be performed in an outpatient clinic or at the bedside. Procedures such as cardiac catheterisation, radionuclide imaging, computed tomography (CT) and magnetic resonance imaging (MRI) require specialised facilities.

Electrocardiogram (ECG)

The ECG is used to assess cardiac rhythm and conduction. It provides information about chamber size and is the main test used to assess for myocardial ischaemia and infarction.

The basis of an ECG recording is that the electrical depolarisation of myocardial tissue produces a small dipole current which can be detected by electrode pairs on the body surface. To produce an ECG, these signals are amplified and either printed or displayed on a monitor (Fig. 18.7). During sinus rhythm, the SA node triggers atrial depolarisation, producing a P wave. Depolarisation proceeds slowly through the AV node, which is too small to produce a depolarisation wave detectable from the body surface. The bundle of His, bundle branches and Purkinje system are then activated, initiating ventricular myocardial depolarisation, which produces the QRS complex. The muscle mass of the ventricles is much larger than that of the atria, so the QRS

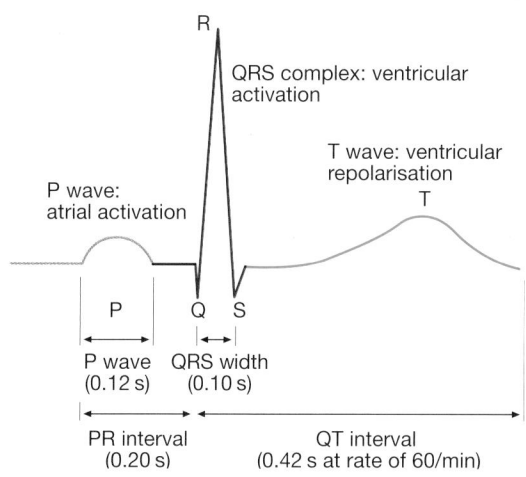

Fig. 18.7 The electrocardiograph. The components correspond to depolarisation and repolarisation, as depicted in Figure 18.4. The upper limit of the normal range for each interval is given in brackets.

In the figure:
- R
- QRS complex: ventricular activation
- T wave: ventricular repolarisation
- T
- P wave: atrial activation
- P Q S
- P wave (0.12 s) QRS width (0.10 s)
- PR interval (0.20 s) QT interval (0.42 s at rate of 60/min)

18.2 How to read a 12-lead ECG: examination sequence

Rhythm strip (lead II)	To determine heart rate and rhythm
Cardiac axis	Normal if QRS complexes +ve in leads I and II
P-wave shape	Tall P waves denote right atrial enlargement (P pulmonale) and notched P waves denote left atrial enlargement (P mitrale)
PR interval	Normal = 0.12–0.20 secs. Prolongation denotes impaired AV nodal conduction. A short PR interval occurs in Wolff–Parkinson–White syndrome (p. 565)
QRS duration	If > 0.12 secs then ventricular conduction is abnormal (left or right bundle branch block)
QRS amplitude	Large QRS complexes occur in slim young patients and in patients with left ventricular hypertrophy
Q waves	May signify previous myocardial infarction (MI)
ST segment	ST elevation may signify MI, pericarditis or left ventricular aneurysm; ST depression may signify myocardial ischaemia or infarction)
T waves	T-wave inversion has many causes, including myocardial ischaemia or infarction, and electrolyte disturbances
QT interval	Normal < 0.42 secs. QT prolongation may occur with congenital long QT syndrome, low K^+, Mg^{2+} or Ca^{2+}, and some drugs (see Box 18.35, p. 568)
ECG conventions	Depolarisation towards electrode: positive deflection
Depolarisation away from electrode: negative deflection
Sensitivity: 10 mm = 1 mV
Paper speed: 25 mm per second
Each large (5 mm) square = 0.2 s
Each small (1 mm) square = 0.04 s
Heart rate = 1500/RR interval (mm) (i.e. 300 ÷ number of large squares between beats)

complex is larger than the P wave. The interval between the onset of the P wave and the onset of the QRS complex is termed the 'PR interval' and largely reflects the duration of AV nodal conduction. Injury to the left or right bundle branch delays ventricular depolarisation, widening the QRS complex. Selective injury of one of the left fascicles (hemiblock, p. 570) affects the electrical axis. Repolarisation is a slower process that spreads from the epicardium to the endocardium. Atrial repolarisation does not cause a detectable signal but ventricular repolarisation produces the T wave. The QT interval represents the total duration of ventricular depolarisation and repolarisation.

The standard 12-lead ECG

The 12-lead ECG (Box 18.2) is generated from ten physical electrodes that are attached to the skin. One electrode is attached to each limb and six electrodes are attached to the chest. In addition the left arm, right arm and left leg electrodes are attached to a central terminal acting as an additional virtual electrode in the centre of the chest (the right leg electrode acts as an earthing electrode). The twelve 'leads' of the ECG refer to recordings made from pairs or sets of these electrodes. They comprise three groups: three dipole limb leads, three augmented voltage limb leads and six unipole chest leads.

Leads I, II and III are the dipole limb leads and refer to recordings obtained from pairs of limb electrodes. Lead I records the signal between the right (-ve) and left (+ve) arms. Lead II records the signal between the right arm (-ve) and left leg (+ve). Lead III records the signal between the left arm (-ve) and left leg (+ve). These three leads thus record electrical activity along three different axes in the frontal plane. Leads aVR, aVL and aVF are the augmented voltage limb leads. These record electrical activity between a limb electrode and a modified central terminal. For example, lead aVL records the signal between the left arm (+ve) and a central (-ve) terminal formed by connecting the right arm and left leg electrodes (Fig. 18.8). Similarly augmented signals are obtained from the right arm (aVR) and left leg (aVF). These leads also record electrical activity in the frontal plane, with each lead 120° apart. Lead

aVF thus examines activity along the axis +90°, and lead aVL along the axis −30° etc.

When depolarisation moves towards a positive electrode, it produces a positive deflection in the ECG; depolarisation in the opposite direction produces a negative deflection. The average vector of ventricular depolarisation is known as the frontal cardiac axis. When the vector is at right angles to a lead, the depolarisation in that lead is equally negative and positive (isoelectric). In Figure 18.8, the QRS complex is isoelectric in aVL, negative in aVR and most strongly positive in lead II; the main vector or axis of depolarisation is therefore 60°. The normal cardiac axis lies between −30° and +90°. Examples of left and right axis deviation are shown in Figures 18.8B and C.

There are six chest leads, V_1–V_6, derived from electrodes placed on the anterior and lateral left side of the chest, over the heart. Each lead records the signal between the corresponding chest electrode (+ve) and the central terminal (−ve). Leads V_1 and V_2 lie approximately over the RV, V_3 and V_4 over the interventricular septum, and V_5 and V_6 over the LV (Fig. 18.9). The LV has the greater muscle mass and contributes the major component of the

18

18

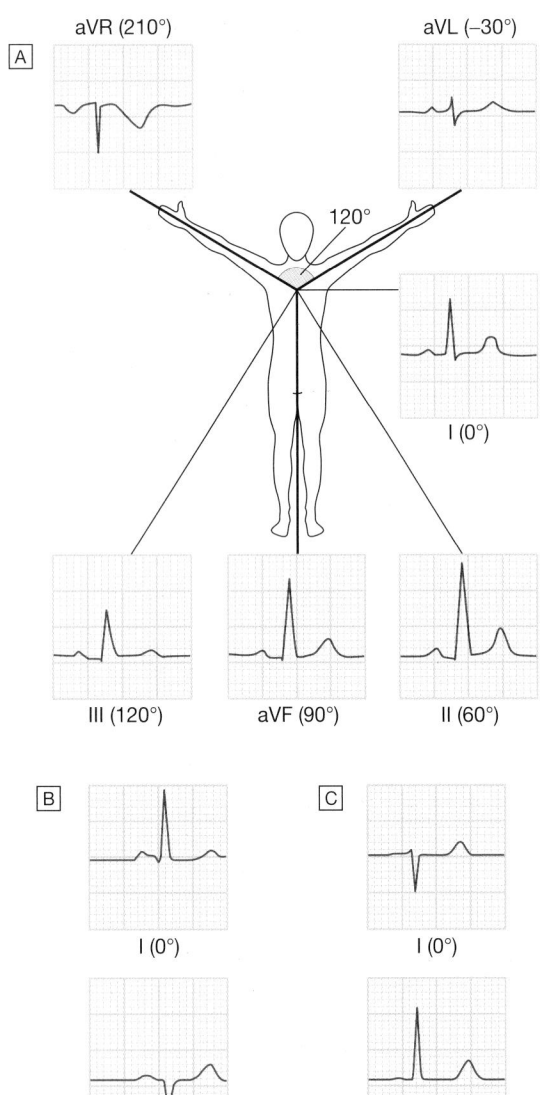

Fig. 18.8 The appearance of the ECG from different leads in the frontal plane. [A] Normal. [B] Left axis deviation, with negative deflection in lead II and positive in lead I. [C] Right axis deviation, with negative deflection in lead I and positive in lead II.

QRS complex. Depolarisation of the interventricular septum occurs first and moves from left to right; this generates a small initial negative deflection in lead V_6 (Q wave) and an initial positive deflection in lead V_1 (R wave). The second phase of depolarisation is activation of the body of the LV, which creates a large positive deflection or R wave in V_6 (with reciprocal changes in V_1). The third and final phase of depolarisation involves the RV and produces a small negative deflection or S wave in V_6.

The ECG in ischaemia and infarction

When an area of the myocardium is ischaemic or undergoing infarction, repolarisation and depolarisation become abnormal relative to the surrounding myocardium. In transmural infarction there is initial ST segment elevation (the current of injury) in the leads facing or overlying the infarct; Q waves (negative deflections)

will then appear as the entire thickness of the myocardial wall becomes electrically neutral relative to the adjacent myocardium. The changes occurring in infarction are described in more detail on page 588, and shown in Figures 18.70–18.74 (pp. 590–591). In myocardial ischaemia, the ECG typically shows ST segment depression and/or T-wave inversion; it is usually the subendocardium that most readily becomes ischaemic. Other conditions, such as left ventricular hypertrophy and electrolyte disturbances, can cause similar ST and T-wave changes.

Exercise (stress) ECG

Exercise electrocardiography is used to detect myocardial ischaemia during physical stress and is helpful in the diagnosis of coronary artery disease. A 12-lead ECG is recorded during exercise on a treadmill or bicycle ergometer. The limb electrodes are placed on the shoulders and hips rather than the wrists and ankles. The Bruce Protocol is the most commonly used protocol for treadmill testing (Box 18.3). BP is recorded and symptoms assessed throughout the test. Common indications for exercise testing are shown in Box 18.4. A test is 'positive' if anginal pain occurs, BP falls or fails to increase, or if there are ST segment shifts of > 1 mm (see Fig. 18.63, p. 583). Exercise testing is useful in confirming the diagnosis in patients with suspected angina, and in such patients has good sensitivity and specificity (see Box 18.4). False negative results can occur in patients with

---

18.3 The Bruce Protocol for exercise tolerance testing

	Speed		
	(mph)	(kph)	Gradient (% incline)
Stage 1*	1.7	2.7	10
Stage 2	2.5	4.0	12
Stage 3	3.4	5.4	14
Stage 4	4.2	6.7	16
Stage 5	5.0	8.0	18

*Each stage lasts for 3 mins.

18.4 Exercise testing

Indications

- To confirm the diagnosis of angina
- To evaluate stable angina
- To assess prognosis following MI
- To assess outcome after coronary revascularisation, e.g. coronary angioplasty
- To diagnose and evaluate the treatment of exercise-induced arrhythmias

High-risk findings

- Low threshold for ischaemia (i.e. within stage 1 or 2 of the Bruce Protocol)
- Fall in BP on exercise
- Widespread, marked or prolonged ischaemic ECG changes
- Exercise-induced arrhythmia

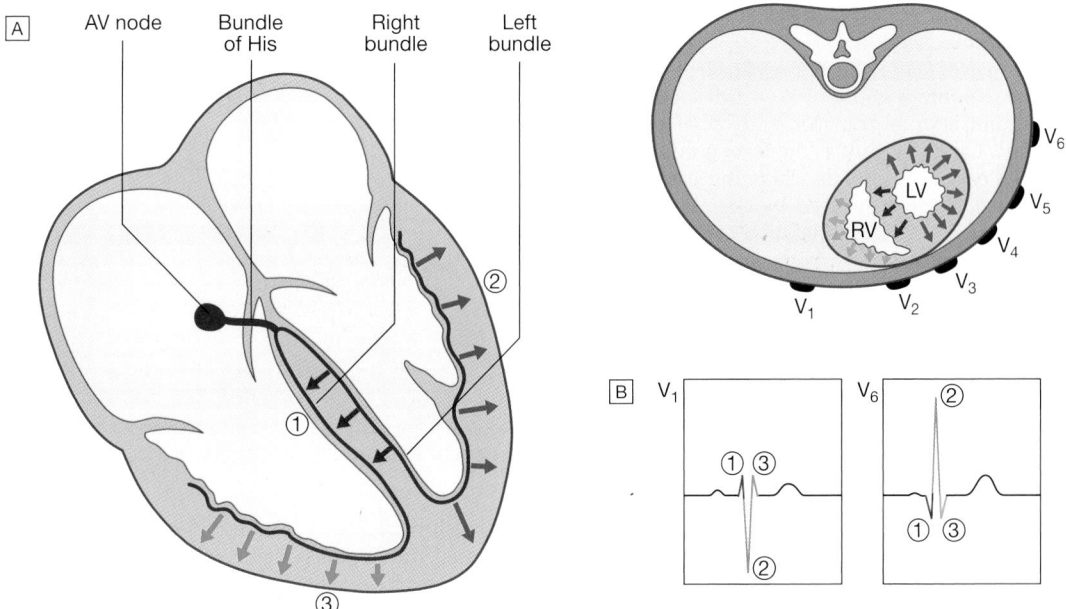

Fig. 18.9 The sequence of activation of the ventricles. [A] Activation of the septum occurs first (red arrows), followed by spreading of the impulse through the LV (blue arrows) and then the RV (green arrows). [B] Normal electrocardiographic complexes from leads V$_1$ and V$_6$.

18

coronary artery disease, and some patients with a positive test will not have coronary disease (false positive). Exercise testing is an unreliable population screening tool because in low-risk individuals (e.g. asymptomatic young or middle-aged women) an abnormal response is more likely to represent a false positive than a true positive test.

Stress testing is contraindicated in the presence of acute coronary syndrome, decompensated heart failure and severe hypertension.

Ambulatory ECG

Continuous (ambulatory) ECG recordings can be obtained using a portable digital recorder. These devices usually provide limb lead ECG recordings only, and can record for between 1 and 7 days. Ambulatory ECG recording is principally used in the investigation of patients with suspected arrhythmia, such as those with intermittent palpitation, dizziness or syncope. For these patients, a 12-lead ECG provides only a snapshot of the cardiac rhythm and is unlikely to detect an intermittent arrhythmia, so a longer period of recording is useful (see Fig. 18.50, p. 569). These devices can also be used to assess rate control in patients with atrial fibrillation, and are sometimes used to detect transient myocardial ischaemia using ST segment analysis. For patients with more infrequent symptoms, small patient-activated ECG recorders can be issued for several weeks until a symptom episode occurs. The patient places the device on the chest to record the rhythm during the episode. With some devices the recording can be transmitted to the hospital via telephone. Implantable 'loop recorders' are small devices that resemble a leadless pacemaker and are implanted subcutaneously. They have a lifespan of 1–3 years and are used to investigate patients with infrequent but potentially serious symptoms, such as syncope.

Cardiac biomarkers

Plasma or serum biomarkers can be measured to assess myocardial dysfunction and ischaemia.

Brain natriuretic peptide

This is a 32 amino acid peptide and is secreted by the LV along with an inactive 76 amino acid N-terminal fragment (NT-proBNP). The latter is diagnostically more useful, as it has a longer half-life. It is elevated principally in conditions associated with left ventricular systolic dysfunction and may aid the diagnosis and assess prognosis and response to therapy in patients with heart failure (p. 543).

Cardiac troponins

Troponin I and troponin T are structural cardiac muscle proteins (see Fig. 18.6, p. 527) that are released during myocyte damage and necrosis, and represent the cornerstone of the diagnosis of acute myocardial infarction (MI, p. 590). However, modern assays are extremely sensitive and can detect very low levels of myocardial damage, so that elevated plasma troponin concentrations are seen in other acute conditions, such as pulmonary embolus, septic shock and acute pulmonary oedema. The diagnosis of MI therefore relies on the patient's clinical presentation (see Box 18.63, p. 588).

Chest X-ray

This is useful for determining the size and shape of the heart, and the state of the pulmonary blood vessels and lung fields. Most information is given by a postero-anterior (PA) projection taken in full inspiration. Anteroposterior (AP) projections are convenient when patient movement is restricted but result in magnification of the cardiac shadow.

An estimate of overall heart size can be made by comparing the maximum width of the cardiac outline with the maximum internal transverse diameter of the thoracic cavity. 'Cardiomegaly' is the term used to describe an enlarged cardiac silhouette where the 'cardiothoracic ratio' is > 0.5. It can be caused by chamber dilatation, especially left ventricular dilatation, or by a pericardial effusion. Artefactual cardiomegaly may be due to a mediastinal mass or pectus excavatum (p. 730), and cannot be reliably assessed from an AP film. Cardiomegaly is not a sensitive indicator of left ventricular systolic dysfunction since the cardiothoracic ratio is normal in many affected patients.

Dilatation of individual cardiac chambers can be recognised by the characteristic alterations to the cardiac silhouette:

- Left atrial dilatation results in prominence of the left atrial appendage, creating the appearance of a straight left heart border, a double cardiac shadow to the right of the sternum, and widening of the angle of the carina (bifurcation of the trachea) as the left main bronchus is pushed upwards (Fig. 18.10).
- Right atrial enlargement projects from the right heart border towards the right lower lung field.
- Left ventricular dilatation causes prominence of the left heart border and enlargement of the cardiac silhouette. Left ventricular hypertrophy produces rounding of the left heart border (Fig. 18.11).
- Right ventricular dilatation increases heart size, displaces the apex upwards and straightens the left heart border.

Lateral or oblique projections may be useful for detecting pericardial calcification in patients with constrictive pericarditis (p. 639) or a calcified thoracic aortic aneurysm, as these abnormalities may be obscured by the spine on the PA view.

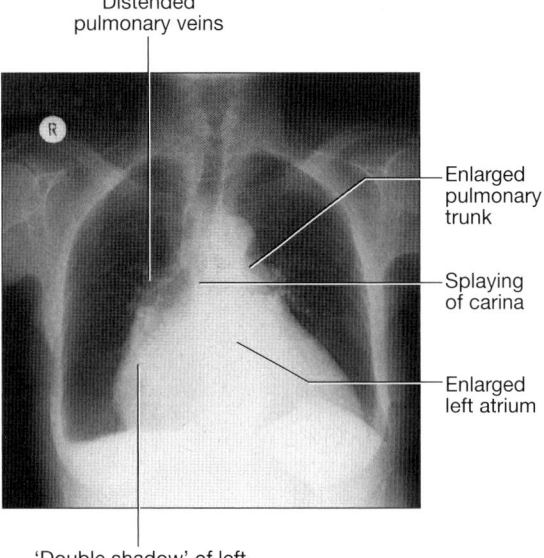

Distended pulmonary veins

Enlarged pulmonary trunk

Splaying of carina

Enlarged left atrium

'Double shadow' of left atrial enlargement

Fig. 18.10 Chest X-ray of a patient with mitral stenosis and regurgitation indicating enlargement of the LA and prominence of the pulmonary artery trunk.

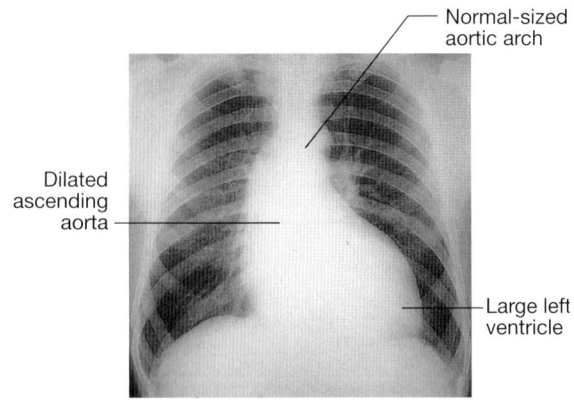

Normal-sized aortic arch

Dilated ascending aorta

Large left ventricle

Fig. 18.11 Chest X-ray of a patient with aortic regurgitation, left ventricular enlargement and dilatation of the ascending aorta.

The lung fields on the chest X-ray may show congestion and oedema in patients with heart failure (see Fig. 18.25, p. 547), and an increase in pulmonary blood flow ('pulmonary plethora') in those with left-to-right shunt. Pleural effusions may also occur in heart failure.

Echocardiography (echo)

Two-dimensional echocardiography

Echocardiography, or cardiac ultrasound, is obtained by placing an ultrasound transducer on the chest wall to image the heart structures as a real-time two-dimensional 'slice'. This permits the rapid assessment of cardiac structure and function. Left ventricular wall thickness and ejection fraction can be estimated from two-dimensional images. Common indications are shown in Box 18.5.

Doppler echocardiography

This depends on the Doppler principle that sound waves reflected from moving objects, such as intracardiac red blood cells, undergo a frequency shift. The speed and direction of the red cells, and thus of blood, can be detected in the heart chambers and great vessels. The greater the frequency shift, the faster the blood is moving. The derived information can be presented either as a plot of blood velocity against time for a particular point in the heart (Fig. 18.12) or as a colour overlay on a two-dimensional real-time echo picture (colour-flow Doppler, Fig. 18.13). Doppler echocardiography can be used to detect valvular regurgitation, where the direction of blood flow is reversed and turbulence is seen, and

18.5 Common indications for echocardiography

- Assessment of left ventricular function
- Diagnosis and quantification of severity of valve disease
- Identification of vegetations in endocarditis
- Identification of structural heart disease in atrial fibrillation, cardiomyopathies or congenital heart disease
- Detection of pericardial effusion
- Identification of structural heart disease or intracardiac thrombus in systemic embolism

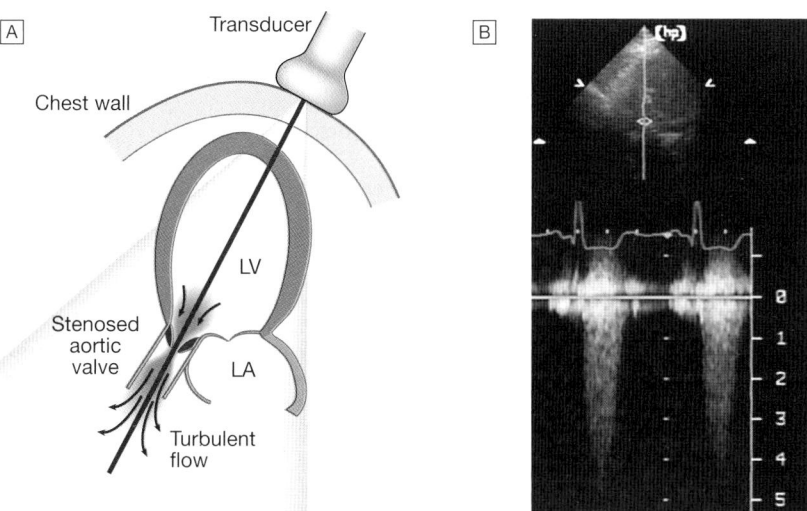

Fig. 18.12 Doppler echocardiography in aortic stenosis. A The aortic valve is imaged and a Doppler beam passed directly through the left ventricular outflow tract and the aorta into the turbulent flow beyond the stenosed valve. B The velocity of the blood cells is recorded to determine the maximum velocity and hence the pressure gradient across the valve. In this example the peak velocity is approximately 450 cm/sec (4.5 m/sec), indicating severe aortic stenosis (peak gradient of 81 mmHg).

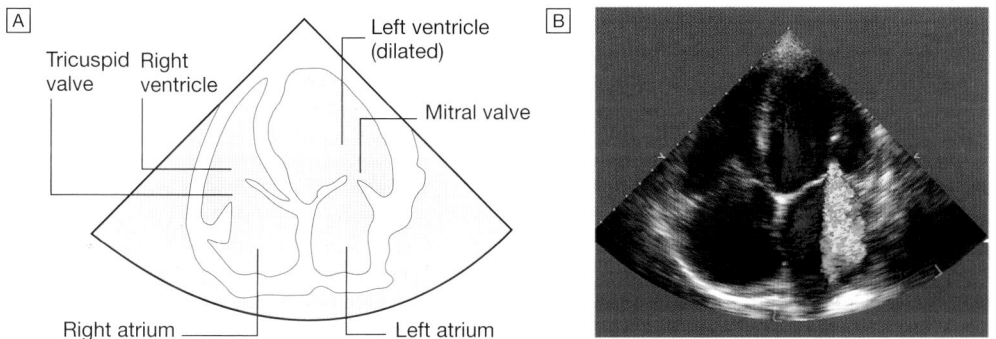

Fig. 18.13 Echocardiographic illustration of the principal cardiac structures in the 'four-chamber' view. A The major chambers and valves. B Colour-flow Doppler has been used to demonstrate mitral regurgitation: a flame-shaped (yellow/blue) turbulent jet into the LA.

is also used to detect the high pressure gradients associated with stenosed valves. For example, the normal resting systolic flow velocity across the aortic valve is approximately 1 m/sec; in the presence of aortic stenosis, this velocity is increased as blood accelerates through the narrow orifice. In severe aortic stenosis the peak aortic velocity may be increased to 5 m/sec (see Fig. 18.12). An estimate of the pressure gradient across a valve or lesion is given by the modified Bernoulli equation:

$$\text{Pressure gradient (mmHg)} = 4 \times (\text{peak velocity in m/sec})^2$$

Advanced techniques include three-dimensional echocardiography, intravascular ultrasound (defines vessel wall abnormalities and guides coronary intervention), intracardiac ultrasound (provides high-resolution images of cardiac structures) and tissue Doppler imaging (quantifies myocardial contractility and diastolic function).

Transoesophageal echocardiography

Transthoracic echocardiography sometimes produces poor images, especially if the patient is overweight or has obstructive airways disease. Some structures are difficult to visualise in transthoracic views, such as the

left atrial appendage, pulmonary veins, thoracic aorta and interatrial septum. Transoesophageal echocardiography (TOE) uses an endoscope-like ultrasound probe which is passed into the oesophagus under light sedation and positioned immediately behind the LA. This produces high-resolution images, which makes the technique particularly valuable for investigating patients with prosthetic (especially mitral) valve dysfunction, congenital abnormalities (e.g. atrial septal defect), aortic dissection, infective endocarditis (vegetations that are too small to be detected by transthoracic echocardiography) and systemic embolism.

Stress echocardiography

Stress echocardiography is used to investigate patients with suspected coronary heart disease who are unsuitable for exercise stress testing, such as those with mobility problems or pre-existing bundle branch block. A two-dimensional echo is performed before and after infusion of a moderate to high dose of an inotrope such as dobutamine. Myocardial segments with poor perfusion become ischaemic and contract poorly under stress, showing as a wall motion abnormality on the scan.

Stress echocardiography is sometimes used to examine myocardial viability in patients with impaired left ventricular function. Low-dose dobutamine can induce contraction in 'hibernating' myocardium; such patients may benefit from bypass surgery or percutaneous coronary intervention.

Computed tomographic (CT) imaging

This is useful for imaging the cardiac chambers, great vessels, pericardium, and mediastinal structures and masses. Multidetector scanners can acquire up to 320 slices per rotation, allowing very high-resolution imaging. CT is often performed using a timed injection of X-ray contrast to produce clear images of blood vessels and associated pathologies. Contrast scans are very useful for imaging the aorta in suspected aortic dissection (see Fig. 18.82, p. 605), and the pulmonary arteries and branches in suspected pulmonary embolism (p. 717).

Multidetector scanning allows non-invasive imaging of the epicardial coronary arteries with a spatial resolution approaching that of conventional coronary arteriography. Coronary artery bypass grafts are also well seen (see Fig. 18.67, p. 587), and in some centres, multidetector scanning is routinely used to assess graft patency. It is likely that CT will supplant invasive coronary angiography for the initial elective assessment of patients with suspected coronary artery disease. Some centres use cardiac CT scans for quantification of coronary artery calcification, which may serve as an index of cardiovascular risk.

Magnetic resonance imaging (MRI)

This requires no ionising radiation and can be used to generate cross-sectional images of the heart, lungs and mediastinal structures. MRI provides better differentiation of soft tissue structures than CT but is poor at demonstrating calcification. MRI scans can be 'gated' to the ECG, allowing the scanner to produce moving images of the heart and mediastinal structures throughout the cardiac cycle. MRI is very useful for imaging the aorta, including suspected dissection (see Fig. 18.81, p. 605), and can define the anatomy of the heart and great vessels in patients with congenital heart disease. It is also useful for detecting infiltrative conditions affecting the heart.

Physiological data can be obtained from the signal returned from moving blood that allows quantification of blood flow across regurgitant or stenotic valves. It is also possible to analyse regional wall motion in patients with suspected coronary disease or cardiomyopathy. The RV is difficult to assess using echocardiography because of its retrosternal position but is readily visualised with MRI.

MRI can also be employed to assess myocardial perfusion and viability. When a contrast agent such as gadolinium is injected, areas of myocardial hypoperfusion can be identified with better spatial resolution than nuclear medicine techniques. Later redistribution of this contrast, so-called delayed enhancement, can be used to identify myocardial scarring and fibrosis. This can help in selecting patients for revascularisation procedures, or in identifying those with myocardial infiltration such as that seen with sarcoid heart disease and right ventricular dysplasia.

Cardiac catheterisation

This involves passage of a preshaped catheter via a vein or artery into the heart under X-ray guidance, which allows the measurement of pressure and oxygen saturation in the cardiac chambers and great vessels, and the performance of angiograms by injecting contrast media into a chamber or blood vessel.

Left heart catheterisation involves accessing the arterial circulation via the radial or femoral artery, to allow catheterisation of the aorta, LV and coronary arteries. Coronary angiography is the most widely performed procedure, in which the left and right coronary arteries are selectively cannulated and imaged, providing information about the extent and severity of coronary stenoses, thrombus and calcification (Fig. 18.14). This permits planning of percutaneous coronary intervention and coronary artery bypass graft surgery. Left ventriculography can be performed during the procedure to determine the size

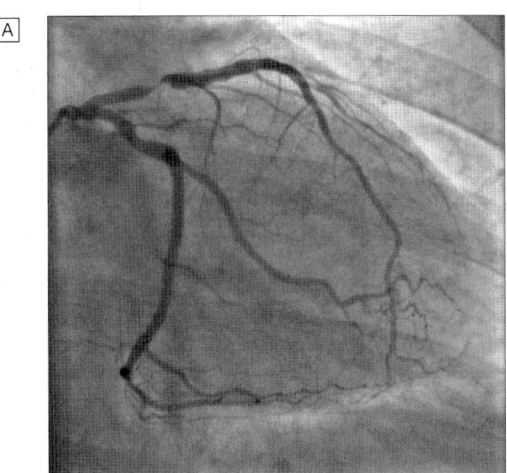

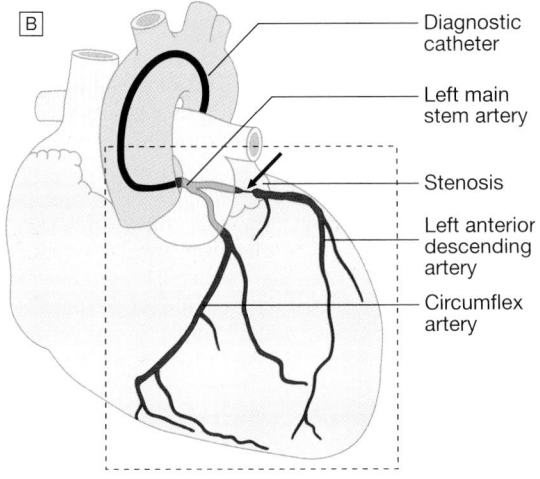

Diagnostic catheter

Left main stem artery

Stenosis

Left anterior descending artery

Circumflex artery

Fig. 18.14 The left anterior descending and circumflex coronary arteries with a stenosis in the left anterior descending vessel. **A** Coronary artery angiogram. **B** Schematic of the vessels and branches.

and function of the LV and to demonstrate mitral regurgitation. Aortography helps define the size of the aortic root and thoracic aorta, and can help quantify aortic regurgitation. Left heart catheterisation can be completed as a day-case procedure and is relatively safe, with serious complications occurring in fewer than 1 in 1000 cases.

Right heart catheterisation is used to assess right heart and pulmonary artery pressures, and to detect intracardiac shunts by measuring oxygen saturations in different chambers. For example, a step up in oxygen saturation from 65% in the RA to 80% in the pulmonary artery is indicative of a large left-to-right shunt that might be due to a ventricular septal defect. Cardiac output can also be measured using thermodilution techniques. Left atrial pressure can be measured directly by puncturing the interatrial septum from the RA with a special catheter. For most purposes, however, a satisfactory approximation to left atrial pressure can be obtained by 'wedging' an end-hole or balloon catheter in a branch of the pulmonary artery. Swan–Ganz balloon catheters are often used to monitor pulmonary 'wedge' pressure as a guide to left heart filling pressure in critically ill patients (p. 190).

Radionuclide imaging

The availability of gamma-emitting radionuclides with a short half-life has made it possible to study cardiac function non-invasively. Two techniques are available.

Blood pool imaging

The isotope is injected intravenously and mixes with the circulating blood. A gamma camera detects the amount of isotope-emitting blood in the heart at different phases of the cardiac cycle, and also the size and 'shape' of the cardiac chambers. By linking the gamma camera to the ECG, information can be collected over multiple cardiac cycles, allowing 'gating' of the systolic and diastolic phases of the cardiac cycle; the left (and right) ventricular ejection fraction (the proportion of blood ejected during each beat) can then be calculated. The reference value for left ventricular ejection fraction depends on the method used but is usually > 60%.

Myocardial perfusion imaging

This technique involves obtaining scintiscans of the myocardium at rest and during stress after the administration of an intravenous radioactive isotope such as ^{99}technetium tetrofosmin (see Fig. 18.64, p. 584). More sophisticated quantitative information is obtained with positron emission tomography (PET), which can be used to assess myocardial metabolism, but this is only available in a few centres.

THERAPEUTIC PROCEDURES

Catheters can be passed into the arterial circulation with X-ray guidance to permit balloon dilatation and/or stenting of diseased arteries (Fig. 18.15, overleaf). Percutaneous coronary intervention (PCI) involves placement of a balloon catheter into one of the coronary arteries via a guide catheter, which is engaged in the coronary ostium. This allows balloon angioplasty and coronary stenting. This technique can also be used to treat stenoses in larger arteries, such as aortic coarctation (p. 631). Balloon valvuloplasty is some-

times used to treat mitral or pulmonary valve stenosis. Patients with congenital heart defects, such as atrial septal defect and patent ductus arteriosus, can have these closed by devices delivered to the heart via a catheter.

Pacemakers are implanted to correct bradycardias or AV block (p. 575). Implantable cardiac defibrillators have similar capabilities to pacemakers and, in addition, can deliver an internal shock to defibrillate the heart if a life-threatening rhythm such as ventricular fibrillation occurs. Cardiac resynchronisation therapy or biventricular pacemakers can improve cardiac function in some patients with heart failure (see Fig. 18.28, p. 550).

Recurrent arrhythmias can be treated by catheter ablation (see Fig. 18.15). Electrode catheters are placed in the heart and can locate re-entry pathways or automatic foci which cause tachycardias. Radiofrequency current is passed through the catheter tip to heat the tissues and cauterise the culprit tissue.

PRESENTING PROBLEMS IN CARDIOVASCULAR DISEASE

18

Cardiovascular disease gives rise to a relatively limited range of symptoms. Differential diagnosis depends on careful analysis of the factors that provoke symptoms, the subtle differences in how they are described by the patient, the clinical findings and appropriate investigations. A close relationship between symptoms and exercise is the hallmark of heart disease. The New York Heart Association (NYHA) functional classification is used to grade disability (Box 18.6).

18.6 New York Heart Association (NYHA) functional classification

- **Class I**   No limitation during ordinary activity
- **Class II**   Slight limitation during ordinary activity
- **Class III** Marked limitation of normal activities without symptoms at rest
- **Class IV**   Unable to undertake physical activity without symptoms; symptoms may be present at rest

Chest pain

Chest pain is a common presentation of cardiac disease but can also be a manifestation of anxiety or disease of the lungs or musculoskeletal or gastrointestinal systems (see Box 18.7 below). Some patients deny 'pain' in favour of 'discomfort' but the significance remains the same.

Characteristics of ischaemic cardiac pain

Several key characteristics help to distinguish cardiac pain from that of other causes (Fig. 18.16). Diagnosis may be difficult and it is helpful to classify pain as possible, probable or definite ischaemic cardiac pain, based on the balance of evidence (Fig. 18.17).
- *Site.* Cardiac pain is typically located in the centre of the chest because of the derivation of the nerve supply to the heart and mediastinum.
- *Radiation.* Ischaemic cardiac pain may radiate to the neck, jaw, and upper or even lower arms. Occasionally, cardiac pain may be experienced only at the sites of radiation or in the back. Pain situated

Balloon dilatations

Coronary angioplasty and stenting

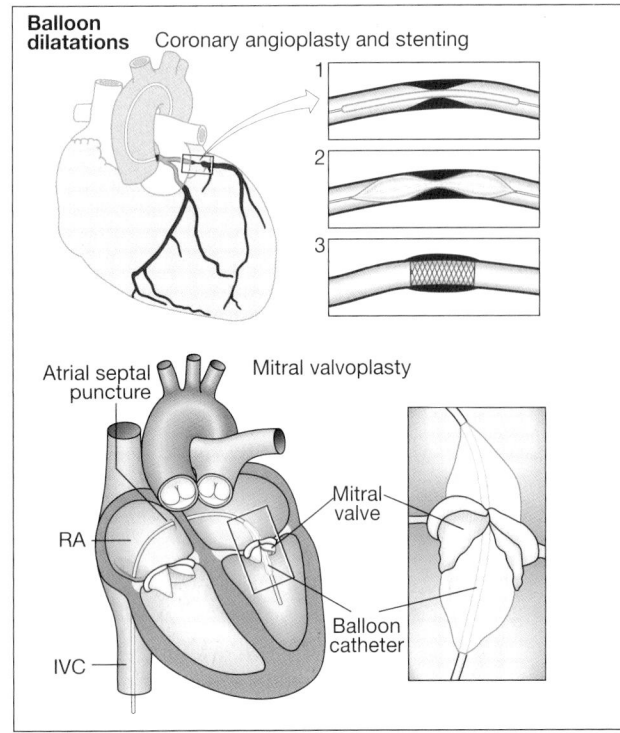

Atrial septal puncture

Mitral valvoplasty

RA

Mitral valve

Balloon catheter

IVC

Closure devices

Atrial septal defect

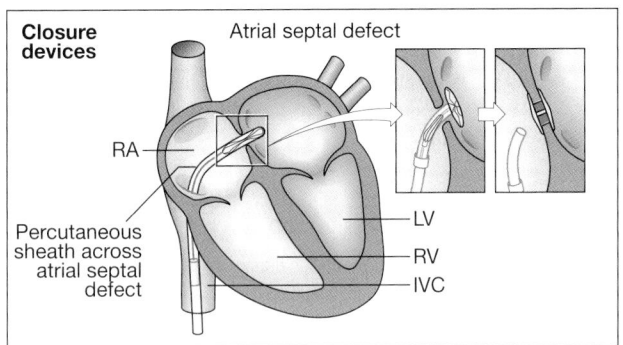

RA

Percutaneous sheath across atrial septal defect

LV

RV

IVC

Radiofrequency ablation

Accessory pathway
(e.g. Wolff–Parkinson–White syndrome)

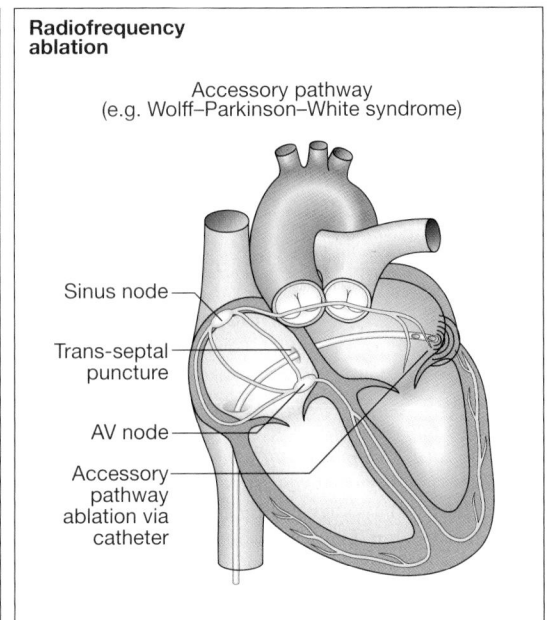

Sinus node

Trans-septal puncture

AV node

Accessory pathway ablation via catheter

Permanent pacemaker

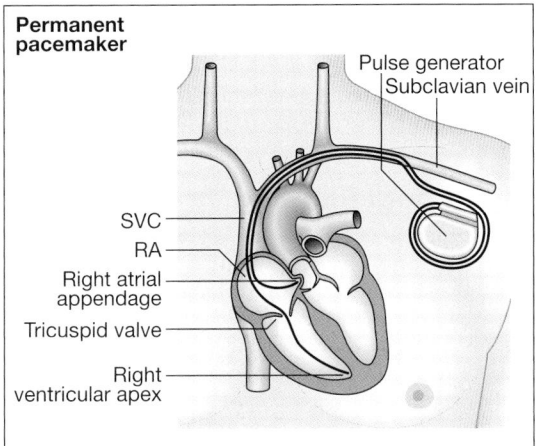

Pulse generator
Subclavian vein

SVC

RA

Right atrial appendage

Tricuspid valve

Right ventricular apex

Fig. 18.15 Percutaneous therapeutic procedures in cardiology. (IVC/SVC = inferior/superior vena cava)

over the left anterior chest and radiating laterally is unlikely to be due to cardiac ischaemia and may have many causes including pleural or lung disorders, musculoskeletal problems and anxiety.

- *Character.* Cardiac pain is typically dull, constricting, choking or 'heavy', and is usually described as squeezing, crushing, burning or aching but not sharp, stabbing, pricking or knife-like. The sensation can be described as breathlessness. Patients often emphasise that it is a discomfort rather than a pain. They typically use characteristic hand gestures (e.g. open hand or clenched fist) when describing ischaemic pain (see Fig. 18.16).
- *Provocation.* Anginal pain occurs during (not after) exertion and is promptly relieved (in less than 5 minutes) by rest. The pain may also be precipitated or exacerbated by emotion but tends to occur more readily during exertion, after a large meal or in a cold wind. In crescendo or unstable angina, similar pain may be precipitated by minimal exertion or at rest. The increase in venous return or preload induced by lying down may also be sufficient to provoke pain in

vulnerable patients (decubitus angina). The pain of MI may be preceded by a period of stable or unstable angina but may occur de novo. In contrast, pleural or pericardial pain is usually described as a 'sharp' or 'catching' sensation that is exacerbated by breathing, coughing or movement. Pain associated with a specific movement (bending, stretching, turning) is likely to be musculoskeletal in origin.

- *Onset.* The pain of MI typically takes several minutes or even longer to develop; similarly, angina builds up gradually in proportion to the intensity of exertion. Pain that occurs after rather than during exertion is usually musculoskeletal or psychological in origin. The pain of aortic dissection, massive pulmonary embolism or pneumothorax is usually very sudden or instantaneous in onset.
- *Associated features.* The pain of MI, massive pulmonary embolism or aortic dissection is often accompanied by autonomic disturbance including sweating, nausea and vomiting. Breathlessness, due to pulmonary congestion arising from transient ischaemic left ventricular dysfunction, is often a prominent and

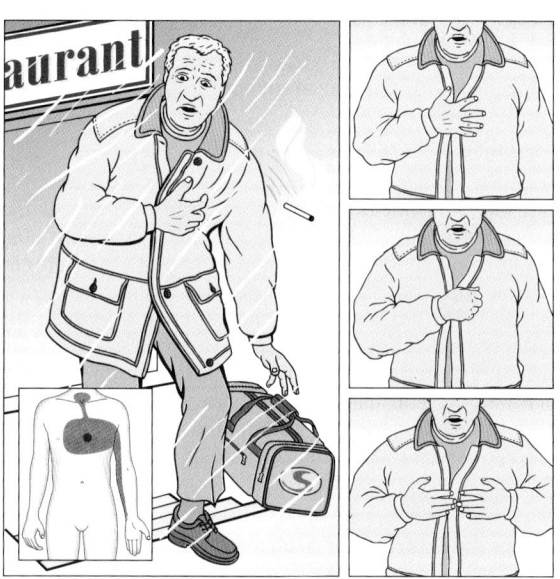

Fig. 18.16 Typical ischaemic cardiac pain. Characteristic hand gestures used to describe cardiac pain. Typical radiation of pain is shown in the schematic.

occasionally the dominant feature of MI or angina (angina equivalent). Breathlessness may also accompany any of the respiratory causes of chest pain and can be associated with cough, wheeze or other respiratory symptoms. Classical gastrointestinal symptoms, such as oesophageal reflux, oesophagitis, peptic ulceration or biliary disease, may indicate non-cardiac chest pain but effort-related 'indigestion' is usually due to heart disease.

Differential diagnosis of chest pain (Box 18.7)
Psychological aspects of chest pain

Emotional distress is a common cause of atypical chest pain. This diagnosis should be considered if there are

18.7 Common causes of chest pain

Anxiety/emotion

Cardiac
- Myocardial ischaemia (angina)
- MI
- Myocarditis
- Pericarditis
- Mitral valve prolapse

Aortic
- Aortic dissection
- Aortic aneurysm

Oesophageal
- Oesophagitis
- Oesophageal spasm
- Mallory–Weiss syndrome

Lungs/pleura
- Bronchospasm
- Pulmonary infarct
- Pneumonia
- Tracheitis
- Pneumothorax
- Pulmonary embolism
- Malignancy
- Tuberculosis
- Connective tissue disorders (rare)

Musculoskeletal
- Osteoarthritis
- Rib fracture/injury
- Costochondritis (Tietze's syndrome)
- Intercostal muscle injury
- Epidemic myalgia (Bornholm disease)

Neurological
- Prolapsed intervertebral disc
- Herpes zoster
- Thoracic outlet syndrome

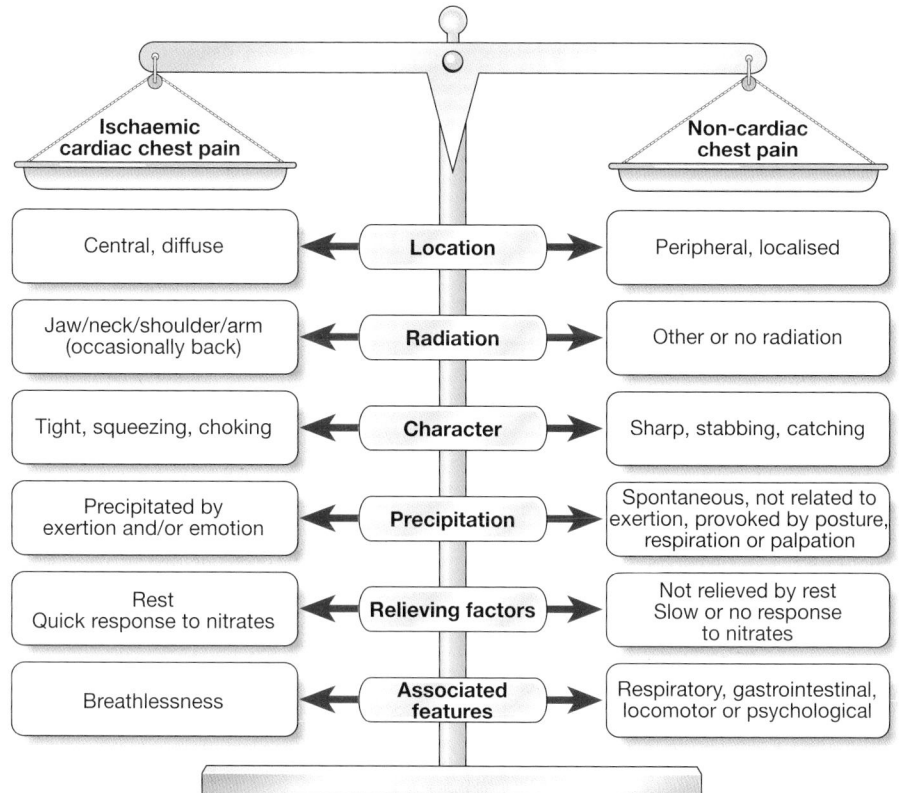

Fig. 18.17 Identifying ischaemic cardiac pain: the 'balance' of evidence.

features of anxiety and the pain lacks a predictable relationship with exercise. However, the prospect of heart disease is a frightening experience, particularly when it has been responsible for the death of a close friend or relative; psychological and organic features therefore often coexist. Anxiety may amplify the effects of organic disease and can create a very confusing picture. Patients who believe they are suffering from heart disease are sometimes afraid to take exercise and this may make it difficult to establish their true effort tolerance; assessment may also be complicated by the impact of physical deconditioning.

Myocarditis and pericarditis

Pain is characteristically felt retrosternally, to the left of the sternum, or in the left or right shoulder, and typically varies in intensity with movement and the phase of respiration. The pain is usually described as 'sharp' and may 'catch' the patient during inspiration, coughing or lying flat; there is occasionally a history of a prodromal viral illness.

Mitral valve prolapse

Sharp left-sided chest pain that is suggestive of a musculoskeletal problem may be a feature of mitral valve prolapse (p. 617).

Aortic dissection

This pain is severe, sharp and tearing, is often felt in or penetrating through to the back, and is typically very abrupt in onset (p. 603). The pain follows the path of the dissection.

Oesophageal pain

This can mimic the pain of angina very closely, is sometimes precipitated by exercise and may be relieved by nitrates. However, it is usually possible to elicit a history relating chest pain to supine posture or eating, drinking or oesophageal reflux. It often radiates to the back.

Bronchospasm

Patients with reversible airways obstruction, such as asthma, may describe exertional chest tightness that is relieved by rest. This may be difficult to distinguish from ischaemic chest tightness. Bronchospasm may be associated with wheeze, atopy and cough (p. 652).

Musculoskeletal chest pain

This is a common problem that is very variable in site and intensity but does not usually fall into any of the patterns described above. The pain may vary with posture or movement of the upper body and is sometimes accompanied by local tenderness over a rib or costal cartilage. There are numerous causes, including arthritis, costochondritis, intercostal muscle injury and Coxsackie viral infection (epidemic myalgia or Bornholm disease). Many minor soft tissue injuries are related to everyday activities such as driving, manual work and sport. The differential diagnosis of peripheral or pleural chest pain is discussed on page 656.

Initial evaluation of suspected cardiac pain

A careful history is crucial in determining whether pain is cardiac or not. Although the physical findings and subsequent investigations may help to confirm the diagnosis, they are of more value in determining the nature and extent of any underlying heart disease, the risk of a serious adverse event, and the best course of management.

Stable angina

Effort-related chest pain is the hallmark of stable angina (Fig. 18.18). The reproducibility, predictability and relationship to physical exertion (and occasionally emotion) of the chest pain are the most important features. The duration of symptoms should be noted because patients with recent-onset angina are at greater risk than those with long-standing and unchanged symptoms.

Physical examination is often normal but may reveal evidence of risk factors (e.g. xanthoma indicating hyperlipidaemia), left ventricular dysfunction (e.g. dyskinetic apex beat, gallop rhythm), other manifestations of arterial disease (e.g. bruits, signs of peripheral vascular disease)

Stable angina	**Unstable angina**
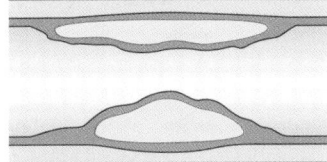	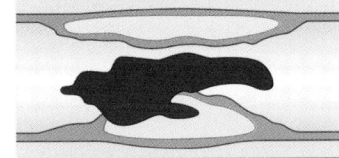

	Stable angina	Unstable angina
Pathophysiology	• Fixed stenosis	• Dynamic stenosis
Clinical features	• Demand-led ischaemia • Related to effort • Predictable • Symptoms over long term	• Supply-led ischaemia • Symptoms at rest • Unpredictable • Symptoms over short term

Risk assessment	• Symptoms on minimal exertion
	• Exercise testing
	   Duration of exercise
	   Degree of ECG changes
	   Abnormal BP response
		• Frequent or nocturnal symptoms
		• ECG changes at rest
		• ECG changes with symptoms
		• Elevation of troponin

Fig. 18.18 Pathophysiology, clinical features and risk assessment of patients with stable or unstable angina.

and unrelated conditions that may exacerbate angina (e.g. anaemia, thyroid disease). Stable angina is usually a symptom of coronary artery disease but may be a manifestation of other forms of heart disease, particularly aortic valve disease and hypertrophic cardiomyopathy. In patients with angina in whom a murmur is found, echocardiography should be performed.

A full blood count, fasting blood glucose, lipids, thyroid function tests and a 12-lead ECG are the most important baseline investigations. Exercise testing may help to confirm the diagnosis and is also used to identify high-risk patients who require further investigation and treatment (p. 530).

Acute coronary syndromes

Prolonged and severe cardiac chest pain may be due to unstable angina (which comprises recent-onset limiting angina, rapidly worsening or crescendo angina, and angina at rest) or acute MI; these are known collectively as the acute coronary syndromes. Although there may be a history of antecedent chronic stable angina, an episode of chest pain at rest is often the first presentation of coronary disease. The diagnosis depends on analysis of the character of the pain and its associated features. Physical examination may reveal signs of important comorbidity, such as peripheral or cerebrovascular disease, autonomic disturbance (such as pallor or sweating) and complications (such as arrhythmia or heart failure).

Patients presenting with symptoms consistent with an acute coronary syndrome require urgent evaluation because there is a high risk of avoidable complications, such as sudden death and MI. Signs of haemodynamic compromise (hypotension, pulmonary oedema), ECG changes (ST segment elevation or depression) and biochemical markers of cardiac damage, such as elevated troponin I or T, are powerful indicators of short-term risk. A 12-lead ECG is mandatory and is the most useful method of initial triage (Fig. 18.19). The release of markers such as creatine kinase, troponin and myoglobin is relatively slow (p. 590) but can help guide immediate management and treatment.

If the diagnosis is unclear, patients with a suspected acute coronary syndrome should be observed in hospital. Repeated ECG recordings are valuable, particularly if obtained during an episode of pain. Plasma troponin concentrations should be measured and, if normal, repeated 12 hours after the onset of symptoms or hospital admission. New ECG changes or an elevated plasma troponin concentration confirm the diagnosis of an acute coronary syndrome. The subsequent management is described on pages 592–595.

If the pain has not recurred 12 hours after the onset of symptoms, plasma troponin concentrations are not elevated and there are no new ECG changes, the patient may be discharged from hospital. At this stage, an exercise test may help to diagnose underlying coronary heart disease but does not reliably exclude the future risk of MI.

Breathlessness (dyspnoea)

Dyspnoea of cardiac origin may vary in severity from an uncomfortable awareness of breathing to a frightening sensation of 'fighting for breath'. The sensation of dyspnoea originates in the cerebral cortex and is described in detail on page 652.

There are several causes of cardiac dyspnoea: acute left heart failure, chronic heart failure, arrhythmia and angina equivalent (Box 18.8). The assessment and treatment of heart failure is described on pages 543–551, and arrhythmias on pages 559–568.

Acute left heart failure

Acute left heart failure may be triggered by a major event such as MI in a previously healthy heart, or by a relatively minor event such as the onset of atrial fibrillation in a diseased heart. An increase in the left ventricular diastolic pressure causes the pressure in the LA, pulmonary veins and pulmonary capillaries to rise. When the hydrostatic pressure of the pulmonary capillaries exceeds the oncotic pressure of plasma (about 25–30 mmHg), fluid moves from the capillaries

18.8 Some causes of dyspnoea

System	Acute dyspnoea	Chronic exertional dyspnoea
Cardiovascular system	*Acute pulmonary oedema	*Chronic congestive cardiac failure Myocardial ischaemia
Respiratory system	*Acute severe asthma *Acute exacerbation of chronic obstructive pulmonary disease *Pneumothorax *Pneumonia *Pulmonary embolus Acute respiratory distress syndrome Inhaled foreign body (especially in a child) Lobar collapse Laryngeal oedema (e.g. anaphylaxis)	*Chronic obstructive pulmonary disease *Chronic asthma Chronic pulmonary thromboembolism Bronchial carcinoma Interstitial lung diseases: sarcoidosis, fibrosing alveolitis, extrinsic allergic alveolitis, pneumoconiosis Lymphatic carcinomatosis (may cause intolerable dyspnoea) Large pleural effusion(s)
Others	Metabolic acidosis (e.g. diabetic ketoacidosis, lactic acidosis, uraemia, overdose of salicylates, ethylene glycol poisoning) Hyperventilation	Severe anaemia Obesity

*Common cause.

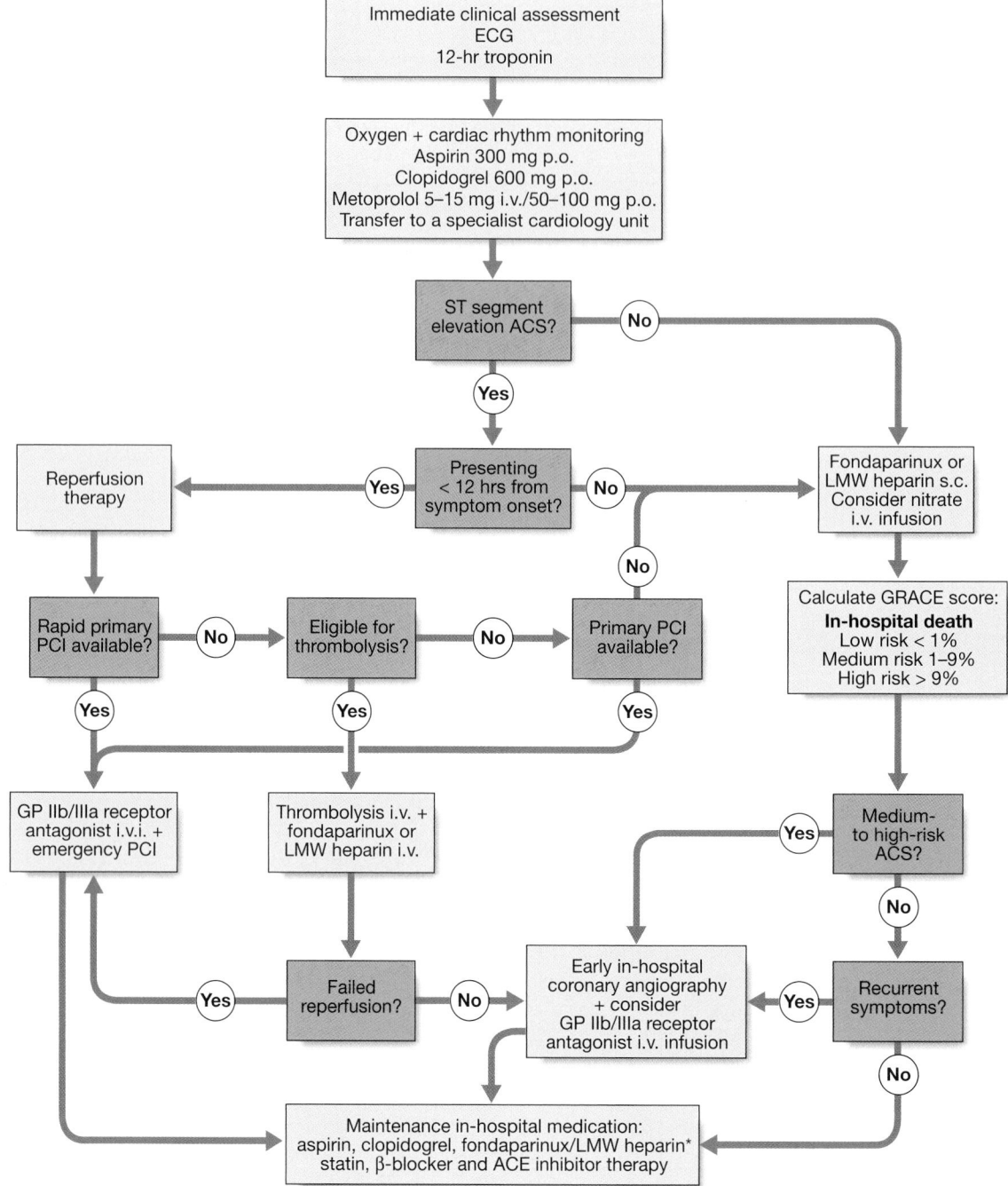

Fig. 18.19 Summary of treatment for acute coronary syndrome (ACS). *Not required following PCI. Amended from SIGN 93. For details of the GRACE score, see Figure 18.69, p. 589. (LMW = low molecular weight; PCI = percutaneous coronary intervention)

into alveoli. This stimulates respiration through a series of autonomic reflexes, producing rapid shallow respiration. Congestion of the bronchial mucosa may cause wheeze (cardiac asthma).

Acute pulmonary oedema is a terrifying experience with the sensation of 'fighting for breath'. Sitting upright or standing may provide some relief by helping to reduce congestion at the apices of the lungs. The patient may be unable to speak and is typically distressed, agitated, sweaty and pale. Respiration is rapid with recruitment of accessory muscles, coughing and wheezing. Sputum may be profuse, frothy and blood-streaked or pink. Extensive

crepitations and rhonchi are usually audible in the chest and there may also be signs of right heart failure.

Chronic heart failure

Chronic heart failure is the most common cardiac cause of chronic dyspnoea. Symptoms may first present on moderate exertion, such as walking up a steep hill, and may be described as a difficulty in 'catching my breath'. As heart failure progresses, the dyspnoea is provoked by less exertion and ultimately the patient may be breathless walking from room to room, washing, dressing or trying to hold a conversation. Other symptoms may include:

- *Orthopnoea.* Lying down increases the venous return to the heart and provokes breathlessness. Patients may prop themselves up with pillows to prevent this.
- *Paroxysmal nocturnal dyspnoea.* In patients with severe heart failure, fluid shifts from the interstitial tissues of the peripheries into the circulation within 1–2 hours of lying down. Pulmonary oedema supervenes, causing the patient to wake and sit upright, profoundly breathless.
- *Cheyne–Stokes respiration.* This cyclical pattern of respiration is due to impaired responsiveness of the respiratory centre to carbon dioxide and occurs in severe left ventricular failure. The pattern of slowly diminishing respiration, leading to apnoea, followed by progressively increasing respiration and hyperventilation, may be accompanied by a sensation of breathlessness and panic during the period of hyperventilation. The Cheyne–Stokes cycle length is a function of the circulation time. The condition can also occur in diffuse cerebral atherosclerosis, stroke or head injury, and may be exaggerated by sleep, barbiturates and opiates.

Arrhythmia

Any arrhythmia may cause breathlessness but usually does so only if the heart is structurally abnormal, such as with the onset of atrial fibrillation in a patient with mitral stenosis.

Angina equivalent

Breathlessness is a common feature of angina. Patients will sometimes describe chest tightness as 'breathlessness'. However, myocardial ischaemia may also induce true breathlessness by provoking transient left ventricular dysfunction or heart failure. When breathlessness is the dominant or sole feature of myocardial ischaemia, it is known as 'angina equivalent'. A history of chest tightness, the close correlation with exercise, and objective evidence of myocardial ischaemia from stress testing may all help to establish the diagnosis.

Acute circulatory failure (cardiogenic shock)

'Shock' is used to describe the clinical syndrome that develops when there is critical impairment of tissue perfusion due to some form of acute circulatory failure. There are numerous causes of shock, described in detail on page 186. The important features and causes (Fig. 18.20) of acute heart failure or cardiogenic shock are described here.

18

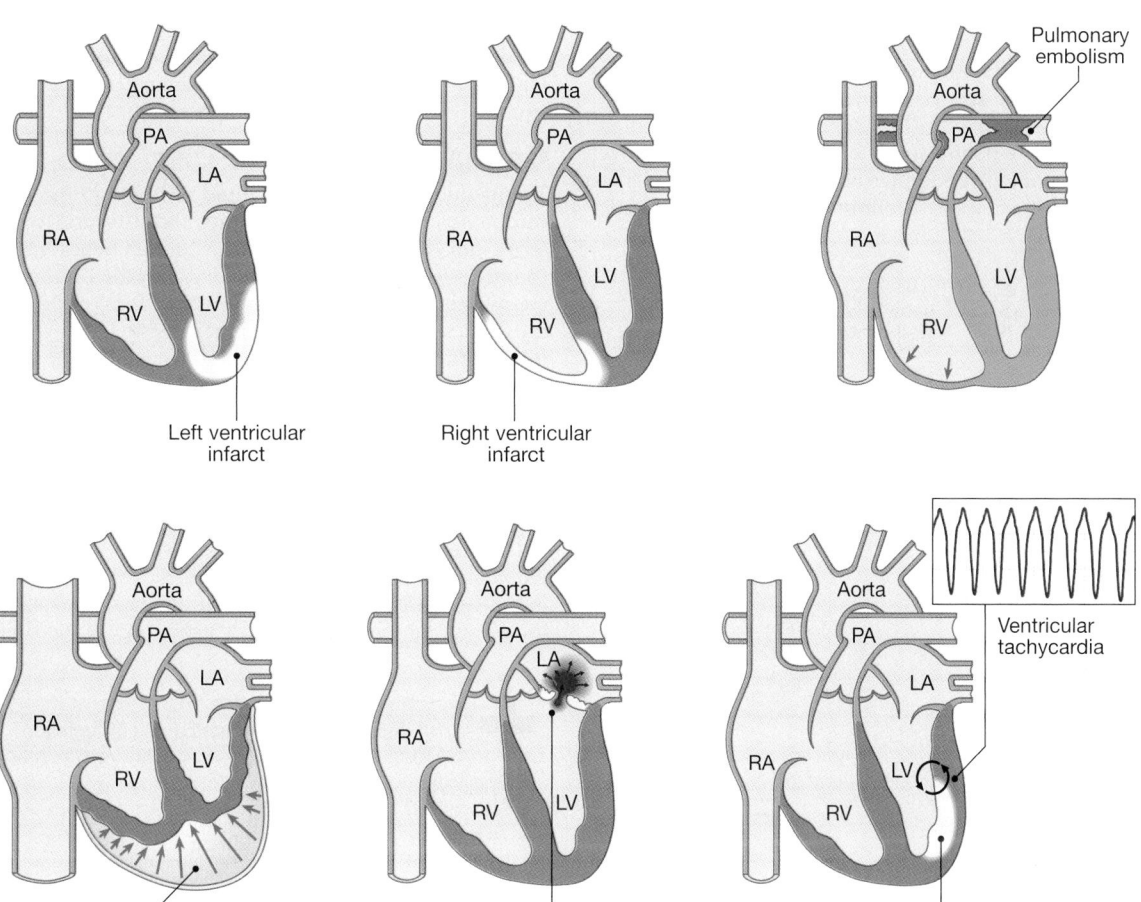

Fig. 18.20 Some common causes of cardiogenic shock.

18

Myocardial infarction

Shock in acute MI is due to left ventricular dysfunction in more than 70% of cases. However, it may also be due to infarction of the RV and a variety of mechanical complications, including tamponade (due to infarction and rupture of the free wall), an acquired ventricular septal defect (due to infarction and rupture of the septum) and acute mitral regurgitation (due to infarction or rupture of the papillary muscles).

Severe myocardial systolic dysfunction causes a fall in cardiac output, BP and coronary perfusion pressure. Diastolic dysfunction causes a rise in left ventricular end-diastolic pressure, pulmonary congestion and oedema, leading to hypoxaemia that worsens myocardial ischaemia. This is further exacerbated by peripheral vasoconstriction. These factors combine to create the 'downward spiral' of cardiogenic shock (Fig. 18.21).

Hypotension, oliguria, confusion and cold clammy peripheries are the manifestations of a low cardiac output, whereas breathlessness, hypoxaemia, cyanosis and inspiratory crackles at the lung bases are typical features of pulmonary oedema. A chest X-ray (see Fig. 18.25, p. 547) may reveal signs of pulmonary congestion when clinical examination is normal. If necessary, a Swan–Ganz catheter can be used to measure the pulmonary artery wedge pressure to guide fluid replacement. The findings can be used to categorise patients with acute MI into four haemodynamic subsets (Box 18.9). Those with cardiogenic shock should be considered for immediate intra-aortic balloon counterpulsation and coronary revascularisation.

The viable myocardium surrounding a fresh infarct may contract poorly for a few days and then recover. This phenomenon is known as myocardial stunning and means that acute heart failure should be treated intensively because overall cardiac function may subsequently improve.

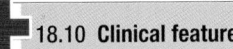

18.9 Acute myocardial infarction: haemodynamic subsets

Cardiac output	Pulmonary oedema	
	No	**Yes**
Normal	Good prognosis and requires no treatment for heart failure	Due to moderate left ventricular dysfunction. Treat with vasodilators and diuretics
Low	Due to right ventricular dysfunction or concomitant hypovolaemia. Give fluid challenge and consider pulmonary artery catheter to guide therapy	Extensive MI and poor prognosis. Consider intra-aortic balloon pump, vasodilators, diuretics and inotropes

Acute massive pulmonary embolism

This may complicate leg or pelvic vein thrombosis and usually presents with sudden collapse. The clinical features and treatment are discussed on page 717. Bedside echocardiography may demonstrate a small underfilled vigorous LV with a dilated RV; it is sometimes possible to see thrombus in the right ventricular outflow tract or main pulmonary artery. CT pulmonary angiography usually provides a definitive diagnosis.

Cardiac tamponade

This is due to a collection of fluid or blood in the pericardial sac, compressing the heart; the effusion may be small and is sometimes < 100 mL. Sudden deterioration (Box 18.10) may be due to bleeding into the pericardial space. Tamponade may complicate any form of pericarditis but can be due to malignant disease. Other causes include trauma and rupture of the free wall of the myocardium following MI.

An ECG may show features of the underlying disease, such as pericarditis or acute MI. When there is a large pericardial effusion, the ECG complexes are small and there may be electrical alternans: a changing axis with alternate beats caused by the heart swinging from side to side in the pericardial fluid. A chest X-ray shows an enlarged globular heart but can look normal. Echocardiography is the best way of confirming the diagnosis and helps to identify the optimum site for aspiration of the fluid.

18.10 Clinical features of pericardial tamponade

- Dyspnoea
- Collapse
- Tachycardia
- Hypotension
- Gross elevation of the JVP
- Soft heart sounds with an early third heart sound
- Pulsus paradoxus (a large fall in BP during inspiration when the pulse may be impalpable)
- Kussmaul's sign (a paradoxical rise in the JVP during inspiration)

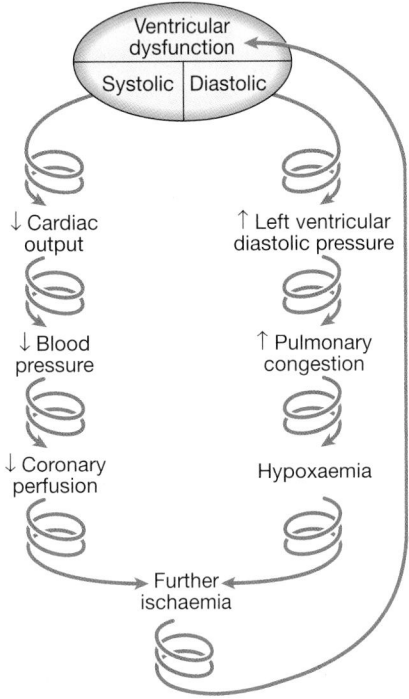

Fig. 18.21 The downward spiral of cardiogenic shock.

Prompt recognition of tamponade is important because the patient usually responds dramatically to percutaneous pericardiocentesis (p. 639) or surgical drainage.

Valvular heart disease

Acute left ventricular failure and shock may be due to the sudden onset of aortic regurgitation, mitral regurgitation or prosthetic valve dysfunction (Box 18.11).

The clinical diagnosis of acute valvular dysfunction is sometimes difficult. Murmurs are often unimpressive because there is usually a tachycardia and a low cardiac output. Transthoracic echocardiography will establish the diagnosis in most cases; however, transoesophageal echocardiography is sometimes required, especially in patients with prosthetic mitral valves.

Patients with acute valve failure usually require cardiac surgery and should be referred for urgent assessment in a cardiac centre.

Aortic dissection may lead to shock by causing aortic regurgitation, coronary dissection, tamponade or blood loss (p. 603).

Management of shock

This is discussed in detail on page 186.

Heart failure

Heart failure describes the clinical syndrome that develops when the heart cannot maintain an adequate cardiac output, or can do so only at the expense of an elevated filling pressure. In mild to moderate forms of heart failure, cardiac output is adequate at rest and only becomes inadequate when the metabolic demand increases during exercise or some other form of stress. In practice, heart failure may be diagnosed whenever a patient with significant heart disease develops the signs or symptoms of a low cardiac output, pulmonary congestion or systemic venous congestion.

Almost all forms of heart disease can lead to heart failure. An accurate aetiological diagnosis (Box 18.12) is important because in some situations a specific remedy may be available.

18

18.11 Causes of acute valve failure

Aortic regurgitation

- Aortic dissection
- Infective endocarditis

Mitral regurgitation

- Papillary muscle rupture due to acute MI
- Infective endocarditis
- Rupture of chordae due to myxomatous degeneration

Prosthetic valve failure

- Mechanical valves: fracture, jamming, thrombosis, dehiscence
- Biological valves: degeneration with cusp tear

18.12 Mechanisms of heart failure

Cause	Examples	Features
Reduced ventricular contractility	MI (segmental dysfunction)	In coronary artery disease, 'akinetic' or 'dyskinetic' segments contract poorly and may impede the function of normal segments by distorting their contraction and relaxation patterns
	Myocarditis/cardiomyopathy (global dysfunction)	Progressive ventricular dilatation
Ventricular outflow obstruction (pressure overload)	Hypertension, aortic stenosis (left heart failure) Pulmonary hypertension, pulmonary valve stenosis (right heart failure)	Initially, concentric ventricular hypertrophy allows the ventricle to maintain a normal output by generating a high systolic pressure. Later, secondary changes in the myocardium and increasing obstruction lead to failure with ventricular dilatation and rapid clinical deterioration
Ventricular inflow obstruction	Mitral stenosis, tricuspid stenosis	Small vigorous ventricle, dilated hypertrophied atrium. Atrial fibrillation is common and often causes marked deterioration because ventricular filling depends heavily on atrial contraction
Ventricular volume overload	Ventricular septal defect Right ventricular volume overload (e.g. atrial septal defect) Increased metabolic demand (high output)	Dilatation and hypertrophy allow the ventricle to generate a high stroke volume and help to maintain a normal cardiac output. However, secondary changes in the myocardium lead to impaired contractility and worsening heart failure
Arrhythmia	Atrial fibrillation	Tachycardia does not allow for adequate filling of the heart, resulting in reduced cardiac output and back pressure
	Tachycardia cardiomyopathy	Incessant tachycardia causes myocardial fatigue
	Complete heart block	Bradycardia limits cardiac output even if stroke volume is normal
Diastolic dysfunction	Constrictive pericarditis	Marked fluid retention and peripheral oedema, ascites, pleural effusions and elevated jugular veins
	Restrictive cardiomyopathy	Bi-atrial enlargement (restrictive filling pattern and high atrial pressures). Atrial fibrillation may cause deterioration
	Left ventricular hypertrophy and fibrosis	Good systolic function but poor diastolic filling
	Cardiac tamponade	Hypotension, elevated jugular veins, pulsus paradoxus, poor urine output

Heart failure is frequently due to coronary artery disease, tends to affect elderly people and often leads to prolonged disability. The prevalence of heart failure rises from 1% in those aged 50–59 years to over 10% in those aged 80–89 years. In the UK, most patients admitted to hospital with heart failure are > 70 years old and remain hospitalised for a week or more.

Although the outlook depends to some extent on the underlying cause of the problem, heart failure carries a very poor prognosis; approximately 50% of patients with severe heart failure due to left ventricular dysfunction will die within 2 years. Many patients die suddenly from malignant ventricular arrhythmias or MI.

Pathophysiology

Cardiac output is a function of the preload (the volume and pressure of blood in the ventricle at the end of diastole), the afterload (the volume and pressure of blood in the ventricle during systole) and myocardial contractility; this is the basis of Starling's Law (Fig. 18.22).

In patients without valvular disease, the primary abnormality is impairment of ventricular function leading to a fall in cardiac output. This activates counter-regulatory neurohumoral mechanisms that in normal physiological circumstances would support cardiac function, but in the setting of impaired ventricular function can lead to a deleterious increase in both afterload and preload (Fig. 18.23). A vicious circle may be established because any additional fall in cardiac output will cause further neurohumoral activation and increasing peripheral vascular resistance.

Stimulation of the renin–angiotensin–aldosterone system leads to vasoconstriction, salt and water retention, and sympathetic nervous system activation. This is mediated by angiotensin II, a potent constrictor of arterioles in both the kidney and the systemic circulation (see Fig. 18.23). Activation of the sympathetic nervous system may initially maintain cardiac output through an increase in myocardial contractility, heart rate and peripheral vasoconstriction. However, prolonged sympathetic stimulation leads to cardiac myocyte apoptosis, hypertrophy and focal myocardial necrosis. Salt and

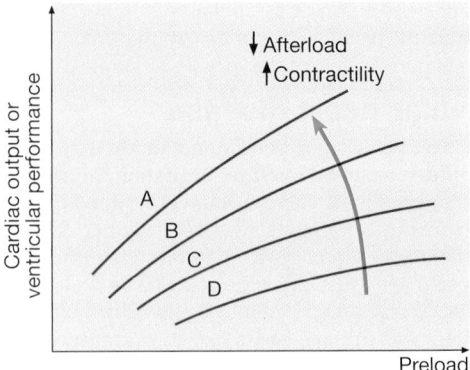

Fig. 18.22 Starling's Law. Normal (A), mild (B), moderate (C) and severe (D) heart failure. Ventricular performance is related to the degree of myocardial stretching. An increase in preload (end-diastolic volume, end-diastolic pressure, filling pressure or atrial pressure) will therefore enhance function; however, overstretching causes marked deterioration. In heart failure the curve moves to the right and becomes flatter. An increase in myocardial contractility or a reduction in afterload will shift the curve upwards and to the left (green arrow).

water retention is promoted by the release of aldosterone, endothelin-1 (a potent vasoconstrictor peptide with marked effects on the renal vasculature) and, in severe heart failure, antidiuretic hormone (ADH). Natriuretic peptides are released from the atria in response to atrial stretch, and act as physiological antagonists to the fluid-conserving effect of aldosterone.

After MI, cardiac contractility is impaired and neurohumoral activation causes hypertrophy of non-infarcted segments, with thinning, dilatation and expansion of the infarcted segment (remodelling; see Fig. 18.77, p. 596). This leads to further deterioration in ventricular function and worsening heart failure.

The onset of pulmonary and peripheral oedema is due to high atrial pressures compounded by salt and water retention caused by impaired renal perfusion and secondary hyperaldosteronism.

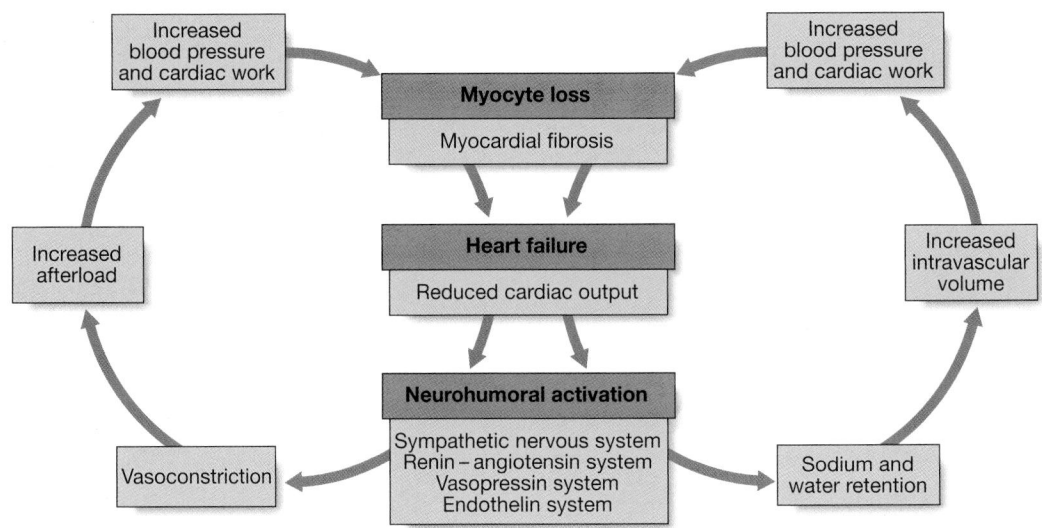

Fig. 18.23 Neurohumoral activation and compensatory mechanisms in heart failure. There is a vicious circle in progressive heart failure.

Types of heart failure

Left, right and biventricular heart failure

The left side of the heart comprises the functional unit of the LA and LV, together with the mitral and aortic valves; the right heart comprises the RA, RV, and tricuspid and pulmonary valves.

- *Left-sided heart failure.* There is a reduction in the left ventricular output and an increase in the left atrial or pulmonary venous pressure. An acute increase in left atrial pressure causes pulmonary congestion or pulmonary oedema; a more gradual increase in left atrial pressure, as occurs with mitral stenosis, leads to reflex pulmonary vasoconstriction, which protects the patient from pulmonary oedema at the cost of increasing pulmonary hypertension.
- *Right-sided heart failure.* There is a reduction in right ventricular output for any given right atrial pressure. Causes of isolated right heart failure include chronic lung disease (cor pulmonale), multiple pulmonary emboli and pulmonary valvular stenosis.
- *Biventricular heart failure.* Failure of the left and right heart may develop because the disease process, such as dilated cardiomyopathy or ischaemic heart disease, affects both ventricles or because disease of the left heart leads to chronic elevation of the left atrial pressure, pulmonary hypertension and right heart failure.

Diastolic and systolic dysfunction

Heart failure may develop as a result of impaired myocardial contraction (systolic dysfunction) but can also be due to poor ventricular filling and high filling pressures caused by abnormal ventricular relaxation (diastolic dysfunction). The latter is caused by a stiff non-compliant ventricle and is commonly found in patients with left ventricular hypertrophy. Systolic and diastolic dysfunction often coexist, particularly in patients with coronary artery disease.

High-output failure

Conditions such as large arteriovenous shunt, beri-beri (p. 126), severe anaemia or thyrotoxicosis can occasionally cause heart failure due to an excessively high cardiac output.

Acute and chronic heart failure

Heart failure may develop suddenly, as in MI, or gradually, as in progressive valvular heart disease. When there is gradual impairment of cardiac function, a variety of compensatory changes may take place.

The term 'compensated heart failure' is sometimes used to describe those with impaired cardiac function in whom adaptive changes have prevented the development of overt heart failure. A minor event, such as an intercurrent infection or development of atrial fibrillation, may precipitate overt or acute heart failure (Box 18.13). Acute left heart failure occurs either de novo or as an acute decompensated episode on a background of chronic heart failure, so-called acute-on-chronic heart failure.

Clinical assessment

Acute left heart failure

Acute de novo left ventricular failure presents with a sudden onset of dyspnoea at rest that rapidly progresses to acute respiratory distress, orthopnoea and prostra-

18.13 Factors that may precipitate or aggravate heart failure in patients with pre-existing heart disease

- Myocardial ischaemia or infarction
- Intercurrent illness, e.g. infection
- Arrhythmia, e.g. atrial fibrillation
- Inappropriate reduction of therapy
- Administration of a drug with negative inotropic properties (e.g. β-blocker) or fluid-retaining properties (e.g. non-steroidal anti-inflammatory drugs (NSAIDs), corticosteroids)
- Pulmonary embolism
- Conditions associated with increased metabolic demand, e.g. pregnancy, thyrotoxicosis, anaemia
- I.v. fluid overload, e.g. post-operative i.v. infusion

tion. The precipitant, such as acute MI, is often apparent from the history.

The patient appears agitated, pale and clammy. The peripheries are cool to the touch and the pulse is rapid. Inappropriate bradycardia or excessive tachycardia should be identified promptly, as this may be the precipitant for the acute episode of heart failure. The BP is usually high because of sympathetic nervous system activation, but may be normal or low if the patient is in cardiogenic shock.

The jugular venous pressure (JVP) is usually elevated, particularly with associated fluid overload or right heart failure. In acute de novo heart failure, there has been no time for ventricular dilatation and the apex is not displaced. Auscultation occasionally identifies the murmur of a catastrophic valvular or septal rupture, or reveals a triple 'gallop' rhythm. Crepitations are heard at the lung bases, consistent with pulmonary oedema.

Acute-on-chronic heart failure will have additional features of long-standing heart failure (see below). Potential precipitants, such as an upper respiratory tract infection or inappropriate cessation of diuretic medication, should be identified.

Chronic heart failure

Patients with chronic heart failure commonly follow a relapsing and remitting course, with periods of stability and episodes of decompensation leading to worsening symptoms that may necessitate hospitalisation. The clinical picture depends on the nature of the underlying heart disease, the type of heart failure that it has evoked, and the neurohumoral changes that have developed (see Box 18.12 and Fig. 18.24).

A low cardiac output causes fatigue, listlessness and a poor effort tolerance; the peripheries are cold and the BP is low. To maintain perfusion of vital organs, blood flow is diverted away from skeletal muscle and this may contribute to fatigue and weakness. Poor renal perfusion leads to oliguria and uraemia.

Pulmonary oedema due to left heart failure presents as described above and with inspiratory crepitations over the lung bases. In contrast, right heart failure produces a high JVP with hepatic congestion and dependent peripheral oedema. In ambulant patients, the oedema affects the ankles, whereas in bed-bound patients it collects around the thighs and sacrum. Ascites or pleural effusion occurs in some cases (see Fig. 18.24). Heart failure is not the only cause of oedema (Box 18.14).

Chronic heart failure is sometimes associated with marked weight loss (cardiac cachexia) caused by a

18

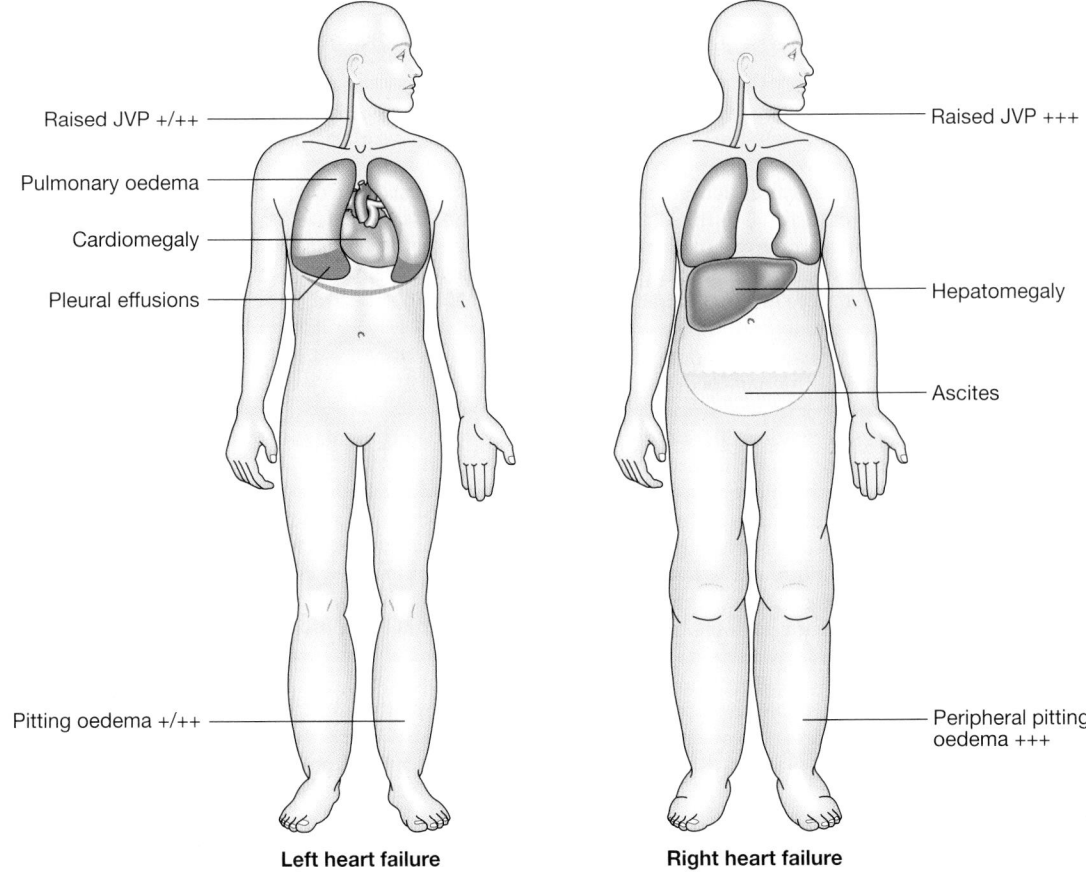

Raised JVP +/++

Pulmonary oedema

Cardiomegaly

Pleural effusions

Pitting oedema +/++

Raised JVP +++

Hepatomegaly

Ascites

Peripheral pitting oedema +++

Left heart failure　　　　**Right heart failure**

Fig. 18.24　Clinical features of left and right heart failure. (JVP = jugular venous pressure)

combination of anorexia and impaired absorption due to gastrointestinal congestion, poor tissue perfusion due to a low cardiac output, and skeletal muscle atrophy due to immobility.

Complications

In advanced heart failure, the following may occur:

- *Renal failure* is caused by poor renal perfusion due to a low cardiac output and may be exacerbated by diuretic therapy, angiotensin-converting enzyme (ACE) inhibitors and angiotensin receptor blockers.
- *Hypokalaemia* may be the result of treatment with potassium-losing diuretics or hyperaldosteronism

18.14　Differential diagnosis of peripheral oedema

- Cardiac failure: right or combined left and right heart failure, pericardial constriction, cardiomyopathy
- Chronic venous insufficiency: varicose veins
- Hypoalbuminaemia: nephrotic syndrome, liver disease, protein-losing enteropathy; often widespread, can affect arms and face
- Drugs:
  Sodium retention: fludrocortisone, NSAIDs
  Increasing capillary permeability: nifedipine, amlodipine
- Idiopathic: women > men
- Chronic lymphatic obstruction

caused by activation of the renin–angiotensin system and impaired aldosterone metabolism due to hepatic congestion. Most of the body's potassium is intracellular and there may be substantial depletion of potassium stores, even when the plasma potassium concentration is in the normal range.

- *Hyperkalaemia* may be due to the effects of drug treatment, particularly the combination of ACE inhibitors and spironolactone (which both promote potassium retention), and renal dysfunction.
- *Hyponatraemia* is a feature of severe heart failure and is a poor prognostic sign. It may be caused by diuretic therapy, inappropriate water retention due to high ADH secretion, or failure of the cell membrane ion pump.
- *Impaired liver function* is caused by hepatic venous congestion and poor arterial perfusion, which frequently cause mild jaundice and abnormal liver function tests; reduced synthesis of clotting factors can make anticoagulant control difficult.
- *Thromboembolism.* Deep vein thrombosis and pulmonary embolism may occur due to the effects of a low cardiac output and enforced immobility, whereas systemic emboli may be related to arrhythmias, atrial flutter or fibrillation, or intracardiac thrombus complicating conditions such as mitral stenosis, MI or left ventricular aneurysm.
- *Atrial and ventricular arrhythmias* are very common and may be related to electrolyte changes (e.g. hypokalaemia, hypomagnesaemia), the underlying

structural heart disease, and the pro-arrhythmic effects of increased circulating catecholamines or drugs. Sudden death occurs in up to 50% of patients with heart failure and is often due to a ventricular arrhythmia. Frequent ventricular ectopic beats and runs of non-sustained ventricular tachycardia are common findings in patients with heart failure and are associated with an adverse prognosis.

Investigations

Serum urea and electrolytes, haemoglobin, thyroid function, ECG and chest X-ray may help to establish the nature and severity of the underlying heart disease and detect any complications. Brain natriuretic peptide (BNP) is elevated in heart failure and is a marker of risk; it is useful in the investigation of patients with breathlessness or peripheral oedema.

Echocardiography is very useful and should be considered in all patients with heart failure in order to:
- determine the aetiology
- detect hitherto unsuspected valvular heart disease, such as occult mitral stenosis, and other conditions that may be amenable to specific remedies
- identify patients who will benefit from long-term therapy with drugs, such as ACE inhibitors (see below).

Chest X-ray

A rise in pulmonary venous pressure from left-sided heart failure first shows on the chest X-ray (Fig. 18.25) as an abnormal distension of the upper lobe pulmonary veins (with the patient in the erect position). The vascularity of the lung fields becomes more prominent, and the right and left pulmonary arteries dilate. Subsequently, interstitial oedema causes thickened interlobular septa and dilated lymphatics. These are evident as horizontal lines in the costophrenic angles (septal or 'Kerley B' lines). More advanced changes due to alveolar oedema cause a hazy opacification spreading from the hilar regions, and pleural effusions.

Management of acute pulmonary oedema

This is urgent:
- Sit the patient up in order to reduce pulmonary congestion.
- Give oxygen (high-flow, high-concentration). Non-invasive positive pressure ventilation (continuous positive airways pressure (CPAP) of 5–10 mmHg) by a tight-fitting facemask results in a more rapid improvement in the patient's clinical state.
- Administer nitrates, such as i.v. glyceryl trinitrate 10–200 µg/min or buccal glyceryl trinitrate 2–5 mg, titrated upwards every 10 minutes, until clinical improvement occurs or systolic BP falls to < 110 mmHg.
- Administer a loop diuretic such as furosemide 50–100 mg i.v.

The patient should initially be kept on strict bed rest with continuous monitoring of cardiac rhythm, BP and pulse oximetry. Intravenous opiates may be cautiously used when patients are in extremis. They reduce sympathetically mediated peripheral vasoconstriction but may cause respiratory depression and exacerbation of hypoxaemia and hypercapnia.

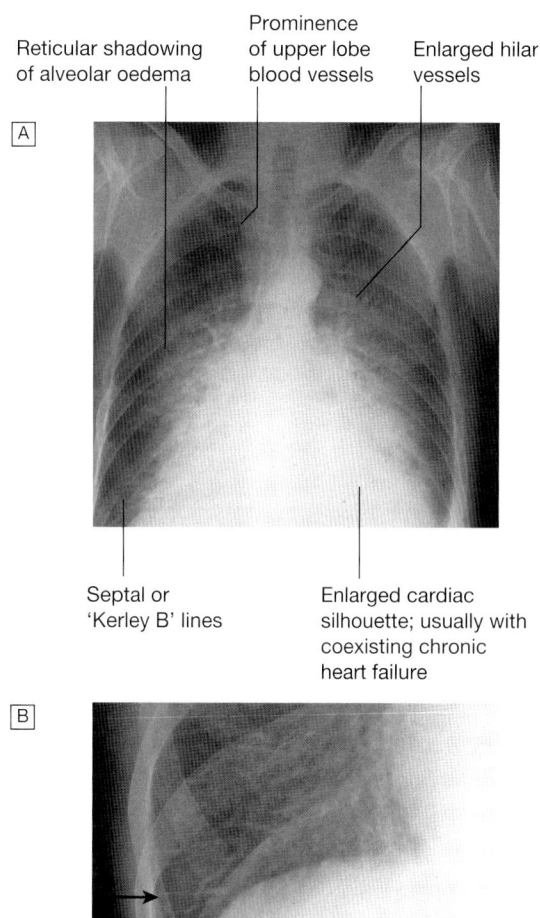

Reticular shadowing of alveolar oedema

Prominence of upper lobe blood vessels

Enlarged hilar vessels

Septal or 'Kerley B' lines

Enlarged cardiac silhouette; usually with coexisting chronic heart failure

Fig. 18.25 Radiological features of heart failure. **A** Chest X-ray of a patient with pulmonary oedema. **B** Enlargement of lung base showing septal or 'Kerley B' lines (arrow).

If these measures prove ineffective, inotropic agents may be required to augment cardiac output, particularly in hypotensive patients. Insertion of an intra-aortic balloon pump can be very beneficial in patients with acute cardiogenic pulmonary oedema, especially when secondary to myocardial ischaemia.

Management of chronic heart failure
General measures

Education of patients and their relatives about the causes and treatment of heart failure can help adherence to a management plan (Box 18.15). Some patients may need to weigh themselves daily and adjust their diuretic therapy accordingly.

In patients with coronary heart disease, secondary preventative measures, such as low-dose aspirin and lipid-lowering therapy, are required (p. 579). However, statins do not appear to be effective in patients with severe heart failure.

Drug therapy

Cardiac function can be improved by increasing contractility, optimising preload or decreasing afterload

18

547

18.15 General measures for the management of heart failure

Education

- Explanation of nature of disease, treatment and self-help strategies

Diet

- Good general nutrition and weight reduction for the obese
- Avoidance of high-salt foods and added salt, especially for patients with severe congestive heart failure

Alcohol

- Moderation or elimination of alcohol consumption. Alcohol-induced cardiomyopathy requires abstinence

Smoking

- Cessation

Exercise

- Regular moderate aerobic exercise within limits of symptoms

Vaccination

- Influenza and pneumococcal vaccination should be considered

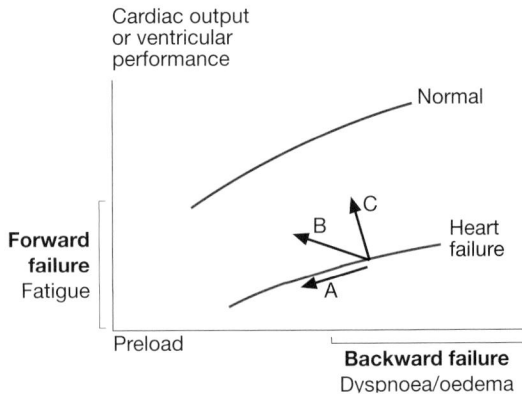

Fig. 18.26 The effect of treatment on ventricular performance curves in heart failure. Diuretics and venodilators (A), angiotensin-converting enzyme (ACE) inhibitors and mixed vasodilators (B), and positive inotropic agents (C).

(see Fig. 18.23). Drugs that reduce preload are appropriate in patients with high end-diastolic filling pressures and evidence of pulmonary or systemic venous congestion. Those that reduce afterload or increase myocardial contractility are more useful in patients with signs and symptoms of a low cardiac output.

Diuretic therapy

In heart failure, diuretics produce an increase in urinary sodium and water excretion, leading to a reduction in blood and plasma volume (p. 433). Diuretic therapy reduces preload and improves pulmonary and systemic venous congestion. It may also reduce afterload and ventricular volume, leading to a fall in wall tension and increased cardiac efficiency.

Although a fall in preload (ventricular filling pressure) tends to reduce cardiac output, the 'Starling curve' in heart failure is flat, so there may be a substantial and beneficial fall in filling pressure with little change in cardiac output (see Figs 18.22 and 18.26). Nevertheless, excessive diuretic therapy may cause an undesirable fall in cardiac output, with a rising serum urea, hypotension and increasing lethargy, especially in patients with a marked diastolic component to their heart failure.

18.16 Congestive cardiac failure in old age

- **Incidence**: rises with age and affects 5–10% of those in their eighties.
- **Common causes**: coronary artery disease, hypertension and calcific degenerative valvular disease.
- **Diastolic dysfunction**: often prominent, particularly in those with a history of hypertension.
- **ACE inhibitors**: improve symptoms and mortality but are more frequently associated with postural hypotension and renal impairment than in younger patients.
- **Loop diuretics**: usually required but may be poorly tolerated in those with urinary incontinence and men with prostate enlargement.

In some patients with severe chronic heart failure, particularly in the presence of chronic renal impairment, oedema may persist despite oral loop diuretics. In such patients an intravenous infusion of furosemide 10 mg/hr may initiate a diuresis. Combining a loop diuretic with a thiazide (e.g. bendroflumethiazide 5 mg daily) or a thiazide-like diuretic (e.g. metolazone 5 mg daily) may prove effective, but this can cause an excessive diuresis.

Aldosterone receptor antagonists, such as spironolactone and eplerenone, are potassium-sparing diuretics that are of particular benefit in patients with heart failure. They may cause hyperkalaemia, particularly when used with an ACE inhibitor. They improve long-term clinical outcome in patients with severe heart failure or heart failure following acute MI.

Vasodilator therapy

These drugs are valuable in chronic heart failure. Venodilators, such as nitrates, reduce preload, and arterial dilators, such as hydralazine, reduce afterload (Fig. 18.26). Their use is limited by pharmacological tolerance and hypotension.

Angiotensin-converting enzyme (ACE) inhibition therapy

This interrupts the vicious circle of neurohumoral activation that is characteristic of moderate and severe heart failure by preventing the conversion of angiotensin I to angiotensin II, thereby preventing salt and water retention, peripheral arterial and venous vasoconstriction, and activation of the sympathetic nervous system (Fig. 18.27). These drugs also prevent the undesirable activation of the renin–angiotensin system caused by diuretic therapy.

Whilst the major benefit of ACE inhibition in heart failure is a reduction in afterload, it also reduces preload and causes a modest rise in the plasma potassium concentrations. Treatment with a combination of a loop diuretic and an ACE inhibitor therefore has many potential advantages.

In moderate and severe heart failure, ACE inhibitors can produce a substantial improvement in effort tolerance and in mortality. They can also improve outcome and prevent the onset of overt heart failure in patients with poor residual left ventricular function following MI (Box 18.17).

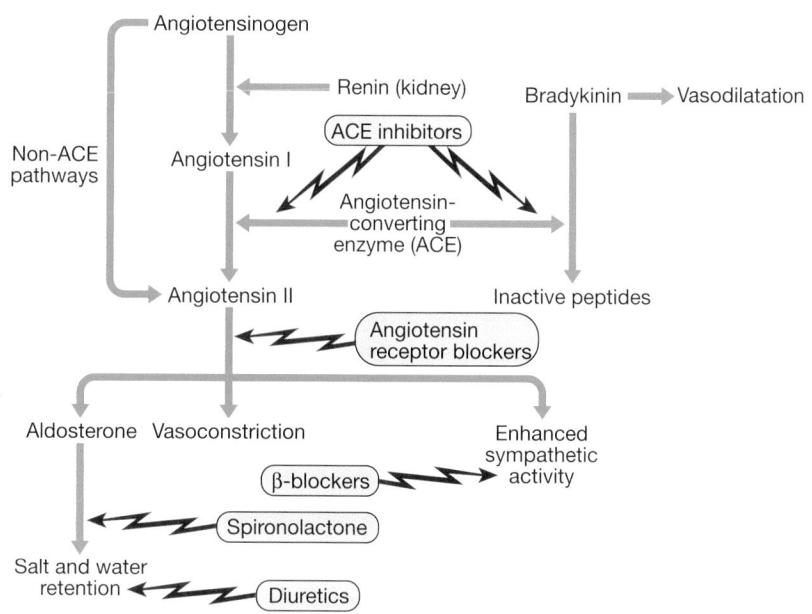

Fig. 18.27 Neurohumoral activation and sites of action of drugs used in the treatment of heart failure.

They can cause symptomatic hypotension and impairment of renal function, especially in patients with bilateral renal artery stenosis or those with pre-existing renal disease. Short-acting ACE inhibitors can cause marked falls in BP, particularly in the elderly or when started in the presence of hypotension, hypovolaemia or hyponatraemia. In stable patients without hypotension (systolic BP > 100 mmHg), ACE inhibitors can usually be safely started in the community. However, in other patients, it is usually advisable to withhold diuretics for 24 hours before starting treatment with a small dose of a long-acting agent, preferably given at night (Box 18.18). Renal function must be monitored and should be checked 1–2 weeks after starting therapy.

Angiotensin receptor blocker (ARB) therapy

These drugs (see Box 18.18) act by blocking the action of angiotensin II on the heart, peripheral vasculature and kidney. In heart failure, they produce beneficial haemodynamic changes that are similar to the effects of ACE inhibitors (see Fig. 18.27) but are generally better tolerated. They have comparable effects on mortality and are a useful alternative for patients who cannot tolerate ACE inhibitors (Box 18.19). Unfortunately, they share all the more serious adverse effects of ACE inhibitors, including renal dysfunction and hyperkalaemia. They may be considered in combination with ACE inhibitors, especially in those with recurrent hospitalisations for heart failure.

Beta-adrenoceptor blocker therapy

Beta-blockade helps to counteract the deleterious effects of enhanced sympathetic stimulation and reduces the risk of arrhythmias and sudden death. When initiated in standard doses, they may precipitate acute-on-chronic heart failure, but when given in small incremental doses (e.g. bisoprolol started at a dose of 1.25 mg daily, and increased gradually over a 12-week period to a target maintenance dose of 10 mg daily), they can increase ejection fraction, improve symptoms, reduce the frequency

---

EBM 18.17 ACE inhibitors and treatment of chronic heart failure

'ACE inhibitors in chronic heart failure due to ventricular dysfunction reduce mortality and readmission rates; average NNT_B for 3 years to prevent one death = 26 and for the combined endpoint of death or readmission = 19.'

- Flather M, et al. Lancet 2000; 355:1575–1581.

For further information: www.sign.ac.uk

18.18 ACE inhibitor and angiotensin receptor blocker (ARB) dosages in heart failure

	Starting dose	Target dose
ACE inhibitors		
Enalapril	2.5 mg 12-hourly	10 mg 12-hourly
Lisinopril	2.5 mg daily	20 mg daily
Ramipril	1.25 mg daily	10 mg daily
Angiotensin receptor blockers		
Losartan	25 mg daily	100 mg daily
Candesartan	4 mg daily	32 mg daily
Valsartan	40 mg daily	160 mg daily

EBM 18.19 ARBs and chronic heart failure

'Compared with ACE inhibitors, ARBs are better tolerated and have similar efficacy in reducing cardiovascular events. ARBs reduce cardiovascular morbidity and mortality in patients with symptomatic heart failure who are intolerant of ACE inhibitors. NNT_B for 5 years to prevent one death or hospitalisation for heart failure = 8. The addition of an ARB to an ACE inhibitor produces further additional benefit. NNT_B for 5 years to prevent one death or hospitalisation for heart failure = 16.'

- Granger CB, et al. Lancet 2003; 362:772–776.
- McMurray JJV, et al. Lancet 2003; 362:767–771.

18

EBM 18.20 β-blockers and treatment of chronic heart failure

'Adding oral β-blockers gradually in small incremental doses to standard therapy including ACE inhibitors in people with heart failure reduces the rate of death or hospital admission. NNT$_B$ for 1 year to prevent one death = 21.'

• Lechat P, et al. Circulation 1998; 98:1184–1191.
• Shibata MC, et al. Eur J Heart Fail 2001; 34:351–357.

For further information: www.escardio.org

of hospitalisation and reduce mortality in patients with chronic heart failure (Box 18.20). Beta-blockers are more effective at reducing mortality than ACE inhibitors: relative risk reduction of 33% versus 20% respectively.

Digoxin

Digoxin (p. 574) can be used to provide rate control in patients with heart failure and atrial fibrillation. In patients with severe heart failure (NYHA class III–IV, see Box 18.6, p. 535), digoxin reduces the likelihood of hospitalisation for heart failure, although it has no effect on long-term survival.

Amiodarone

This is a potent anti-arrhythmic drug (p. 572) that has little negative inotropic effect and may be valuable in patients with poor left ventricular function. It is only effective in the treatment of symptomatic arrhythmias, and should not be used as a preventative agent in asymptomatic patients.

Implantable cardiac defibrillators and resynchronisation therapy

Patients with symptomatic ventricular arrhythmias and heart failure have a very poor prognosis. Irrespective of their response to anti-arrhythmic drug therapy, all should be considered for implantation of a cardiac defibrillator (p. 576). In patients with marked intraventricular conduction delay, prolonged depolarisation may lead to uncoordinated left ventricular contraction. When this is associated with severe symptomatic heart failure, cardiac resynchronisation therapy should be considered. Here, both the LV and RV are paced simultaneously (Fig. 18.28) in an attempt to generate a more coordinated left ventricular contraction and improve cardiac output.

Coronary revascularisation

Coronary artery bypass surgery or percutaneous coronary intervention may improve function in areas of the myocardium that are 'hibernating' because of inadequate blood supply, and can be used to treat carefully selected patients with heart failure and coronary artery disease. If necessary, 'hibernating' myocardium can be identified by stress echocardiography and specialised nuclear or MR imaging.

Heart transplantation

Cardiac transplantation is an established and successful form of treatment for patients with intractable heart failure. Coronary artery disease and dilated cardiomyopathy are the most common indications. The introduction of ciclosporin for immunosuppression (p. 94) has improved survival, which is around 80% at 1 year. The use of trans-

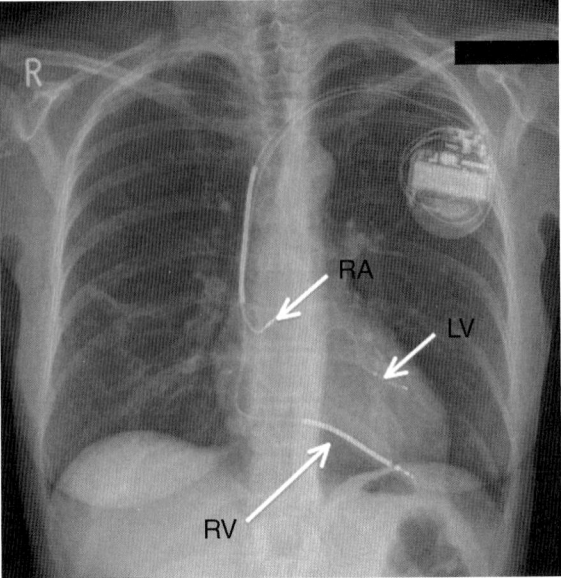

Fig. 18.28 Chest X-ray of a biventricular pacemaker and defibrillator. The right ventricular lead (RV) is in position in the ventricular apex and is used for both pacing and defibrillation. The left ventricular lead (LV) is placed via the coronary sinus and the right atrial lead (RA) is placed in the right atrial appendage; both are used for pacing only.

plantation is limited by the efficacy of modern drug and device therapies, as well as the availability of donor hearts, so it is generally reserved for young patients with severe symptoms despite optimal therapy.

Conventional heart transplantation is contraindicated in patients with pulmonary vascular disease due to long-standing left heart failure, complex congenital heart disease (e.g. Eisenmenger's syndrome) or primary pulmonary hypertension because the RV of the donor heart may fail in the face of high pulmonary vascular resistance. However, heart-lung transplantation can be successful in patients with Eisenmenger's syndrome. Lung transplantation has been used for primary pulmonary hypertension.

Although cardiac transplantation usually produces a dramatic improvement in the recipient's quality of life, serious complications may occur:

• *Rejection.* In spite of routine therapy with ciclosporin A, azathioprine and corticosteroids, episodes of rejection are common and may present with heart failure, arrhythmias or subtle ECG changes; cardiac biopsy is often used to confirm the diagnosis before starting treatment with high-dose corticosteroids.
• *Accelerated atherosclerosis.* Recurrent heart failure is often due to progressive atherosclerosis in the coronary arteries of the donor heart. This is not confined to patients who were transplanted for coronary artery disease and is probably a manifestation of chronic rejection. Angina is rare because the heart has been denervated.
• *Infection.* Opportunistic infection with organisms such as cytomegalovirus or *Aspergillus* remains a major cause of death in transplant recipients.

Ventricular assist devices

Because of the limited supply of donor organs, ventricular assist devices (VADs) have been employed as:

- a bridge to cardiac transplantation
- potential long-term 'destination' therapy
- short-term restoration therapy following a potentially reversible insult such as viral myocarditis.

VADs assist cardiac output by using a roller, centrifugal or pulsatile pump that in some cases is implantable and portable. They withdraw blood through cannulae inserted in the atria or ventricular apex and pump it into the pulmonary artery or aorta. They are designed not only to unload the ventricles but also to provide support to the pulmonary and systemic circulations. Their more widespread application is limited by high complication rates (haemorrhage, systemic embolism, infection, neurological and renal sequelae), although some improvements in survival and quality of life have been demonstrated in patients with severe heart failure.

Hypertension

High BP is a trait as opposed to a specific disease and represents a quantitative rather than a qualitative deviation from the norm. Any definition of hypertension is therefore arbitrary.

Systemic BP rises with age, and the incidence of cardiovascular disease (particularly stroke and coronary artery disease) is closely related to average BP at all ages, even when BP readings are within the so-called 'normal range'. Randomised controlled trials have demonstrated that antihypertensive therapy can reduce the incidence of stroke and, to a lesser extent, coronary artery disease (see Box 18.93, p. 608).

The cardiovascular risks associated with a given BP are dependent upon the combination of risk factors in an individual, such as age, gender, weight, physical activity, smoking, family history, serum cholesterol, diabetes mellitus and pre-existing vascular disease. Effective management of hypertension requires a holistic approach, based on the identification of those at highest cardiovascular risk and the use of multifactorial interventions, targeting not only BP but all modifiable cardiovascular risk factors.

Thus a practical definition of hypertension is 'the level of BP at which the benefits of treatment outweigh the costs and hazards'. The British Hypertension Society classification of hypertension is provided in Box 18.87 (p. 606) and is consistent with those defined by the European Society of Hypertension and the World Health Organization–International Society of Hypertension.

Approach to newly diagnosed hypertension

Hypertension is predominantly an asymptomatic condition and the diagnosis is usually made at routine examination or when a complication arises. A BP check is advisable every 5 years in adults.

The objectives of the initial evaluation of a patient with high BP readings are:

- to obtain accurate and representative measurements of BP
- to identify contributory factors and any underlying cause (secondary hypertension)
- to assess other risk factors and quantify cardiovascular risk
- to detect any complications (target organ damage) that are already present
- to identify comorbidity that may influence the choice of antihypertensive therapy.

These goals are attained by a careful history, clinical examination and some simple investigations. Details of these, along with pathophysiology and management, are discussed on pages 606–612.

Syncope and presyncope

The term 'syncope' refers to sudden loss of consciousness due to reduced cerebral perfusion. 'Presyncope' refers to lightheadedness where the individual thinks he or she may black out. Syncope affects around 20% of the population at some time and accounts for more than 5% of hospital admissions. Dizziness and presyncope are very common in old age (p. 173). Symptoms are disabling, undermine confidence and independence,

18.21 Typical features of cardiac syncope, vasovagal syncope and seizures

	Cardiac syncope	Neuro-cardiogenic syncope	Seizures
Premonitory symptoms	Often none Lightheadedness Palpitation Chest pain Breathlessness	Nausea Lightheadedness Sweating	Confusion Hyperexcitability Olfactory hallucinations 'Aura'
Unconscious period	Extreme 'death-like' pallor	Pallor	Prolonged (> 1 min) unconsciousness Motor seizure activity* Tongue-biting Urinary incontinence
Recovery	Rapid recovery (< 1 min) Flushing	Slow Nausea Lightheadedness	Prolonged confusion (> 5 mins) Headache Focal neurological signs

***N.B.** Cardiac syncope can also cause convulsions by inducing cerebral anoxia.

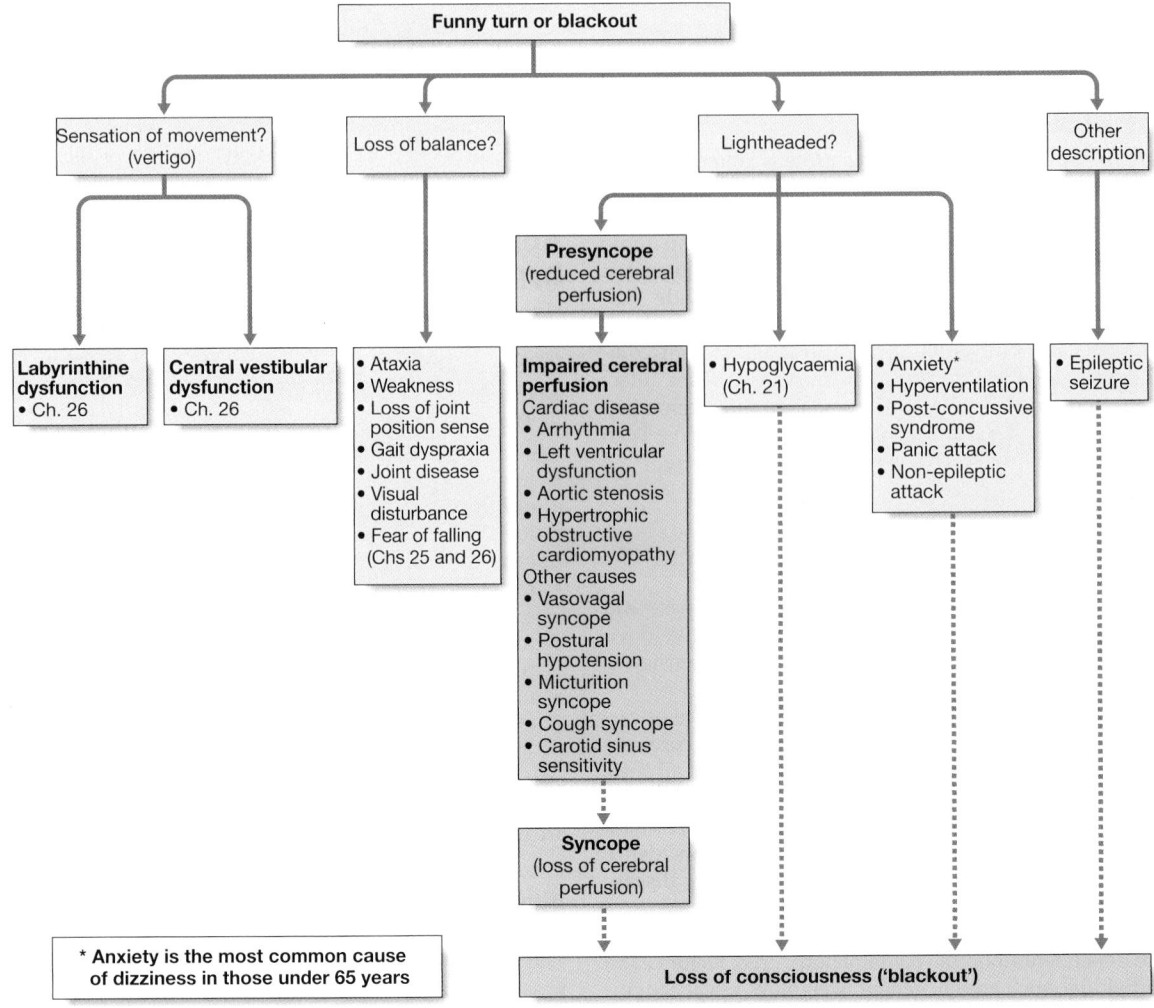

Fig. 18.29 The differential diagnosis of syncope and presyncope.

and can affect an individual's ability to work or to drive. There are several mechanisms that underlie recurrent presyncope or syncope:

- *cardiac syncope* due to mechanical cardiac dysfunction or arrhythmia
- *neurocardiogenic syncope* in which an abnormal autonomic reflex causes bradycardia and/or hypotension.

Blackouts can also be caused by non-cardiac pathology such as epilepsy, cerebrovascular ischaemia or hypoglycaemia (Fig. 18.29).

Differential diagnosis

History-taking, from the patient or a witness, is the key to establishing a diagnosis. Attention should be given to potential triggers (e.g. medication, exertion, posture), the victim's appearance (e.g. colour, seizure activity), the duration of the episode and the speed of recovery (Box 18.21). Cardiac syncope is usually sudden but can be associated with premonitory lightheadedness, palpitation or chest discomfort. The blackout is usually brief and recovery rapid. Neurocardiogenic syncope will often be associated with a situational trigger, and the patient may experience flushing, nausea and malaise for

several minutes afterwards. Patients with seizures do not exhibit pallor, may have abnormal movements, usually take more than 5 minutes to recover and are often confused. A history of rotational vertigo is suggestive of a labyrinthine or vestibular disorder (p. 1149). The pattern and description of the patient's symptoms should indicate the probable mechanism and help to determine subsequent investigations (Fig. 18.30).

Arrhythmia

Lightheadedness may occur with many arrhythmias, but blackouts (Stokes–Adams attacks, p. 570) are usually due to profound bradycardia or malignant ventricular tachyarrhythmias. The 12-lead ECG may show evidence of conducting system disease (e.g. sinus bradycardia, AV block, bundle branch block or axis deviation) which would predispose a patient to bradycardia, but the key to establishing a diagnosis is to obtain an ECG recording *during symptoms*. Since minor rhythm disturbances are common, especially in old age, symptoms must occur at the same time as a recorded arrhythmia before a diagnosis can be made. Ambulatory ECG recordings are helpful only if symptoms occur several times per week. Patient-activated ECG recorders are useful for examining the rhythm in patients with recurrent dizziness, but are not

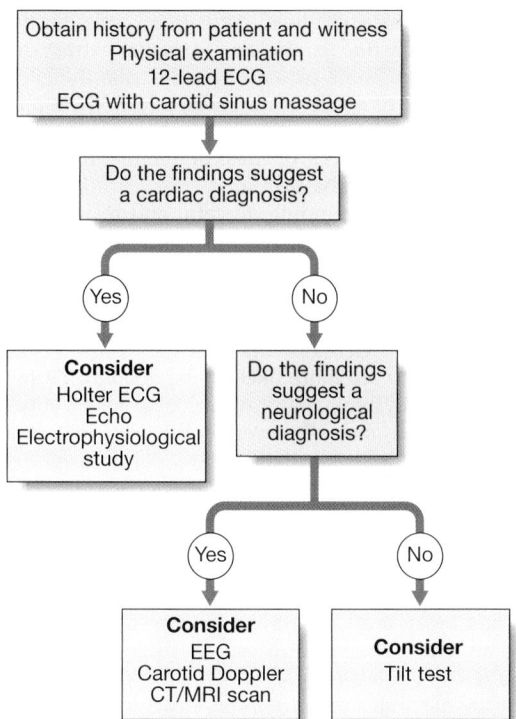

Fig. 18.30 A simple guide to the investigation and diagnosis of recurrent presyncope and syncope.

useful in assessing sudden blackouts. In patients with presyncope or syncope in whom these investigations fail to establish a cause, an implantable 'loop recorder' can be placed subcutaneously in the upper chest. This device continuously records the cardiac rhythm and will activate automatically if extreme bradycardia or tachycardia occurs. The ECG memory can also be frozen by the patient using a hand-held activator. Stored ECGs can be accessed by the implanting centre, using a telemetry device.

Structural heart disease

Severe aortic stenosis, hypertrophic obstructive cardiomyopathy and severe coronary artery disease can cause lightheadedness or syncope on exertion. This is caused by profound hypotension due to a fall in cardiac output, or failure to increase output during exertion, coupled with exercise-induced peripheral vasodilatation. Exertional arrhythmias also occur in these patients.

Neurocardiogenic syncope

This encompasses a family of syndromes in which bradycardia and/or hypotension occur because of a series of abnormal autonomic reflexes. The two main conditions are hypersensitive carotid sinus syndrome (HCSS) and malignant vasovagal syncope.

Situational syncope

This is the collective name given to some variants of neurocardiogenic syncope that occur in the presence of identifiable triggers (e.g. cough syncope, micturition syncope).

Vasovagal syncope

This is normally triggered by a reduction in venous return due to prolonged standing, excessive heat or a large meal. It is mediated by the Bezold–Jarisch reflex, in which there is an initial sympathetic activation that leads to vigorous contraction of the relatively under-filled ventricles. This stimulates ventricular mechano-receptors, producing parasympathetic (vagal) activation and sympathetic withdrawal, and causing bradycardia, vasodilatation or both. Head-up tilt-table testing is a provocation test used to establish the diagnosis, and involves asking the patient to lie on a table that is then tilted to an angle of 60–70° for up to 45 minutes, while the ECG and BP are monitored. A positive test is characterised by bradycardia (cardio-inhibitory response) and/or hypotension (vasodepressor response) associated with typical symptoms. Initial management involves lifestyle modification (salt supplementation and avoiding prolonged standing, dehydration or missing meals). In resistant cases, drug therapy can be used; fludrocortisone, which causes sodium and water retention and expands plasma volume, β-blockers, which inhibit the initial sympathetic activation, disopyramide (a vagolytic agent) or midodrine (a vasoconstrictor α-adrenoceptor agonist) may be helpful. A dual-chamber pacemaker can be useful if symptoms are predominantly due to bradycardia. Patients with a urinary sodium excretion of less than 170 mmol/day may respond to salt loading.

Carotid sinus hypersensitivity

This causes presyncope or syncope because of reflex bradycardia and vasodilatation. Carotid baroreceptors are involved in BP regulation and are activated by increased BP, resulting in a vagal discharge that causes a compensatory drop in BP. In HCSS the baroreceptor is sensitive to external pressure (e.g. during neck movement or if a tight collar is worn), so that pressure over the carotid artery causes an inappropriate and intense vagal discharge. The diagnosis can be established by monitoring the ECG and BP during carotid sinus massage for 6 seconds. This manœuvre should not be attempted in patients with a carotid bruit or with a history of cerebrovascular disease because of the risk of embolic stroke. A positive cardio-inhibitory response is defined as a sinus pause of 3 seconds or more; a positive vasodepressor response is defined as a fall in systolic BP of more than 50 mmHg. Carotid sinus pressure will produce positive findings in about 10% of elderly individuals but less than 25% of these experience spontaneous syncope. Symptoms should not therefore be attributed to HCSS unless they are reproduced by carotid sinus pressure. Dual-chamber pacing usually prevents syncope in patients with the more common cardio-inhibitory response.

Postural hypotension

This is caused by a failure of the normal compensatory mechanisms. Relative hypovolaemia (often due to excessive diuretic therapy), sympathetic degeneration (diabetes mellitus, Parkinson's disease, ageing) and drug therapy (vasodilators, antidepressants) can all cause or aggravate the problem. Treatment is often ineffective; however, withdrawing unnecessary medication and advising the patient to wear graduated elastic stockings and get up slowly may be helpful. Fludrocortisone, which can expand blood volume through sodium and water retention, may be of value.

Palpitation

Palpitation is a very common and sometimes frightening symptom. Patients use the term to describe a wide variety of sensations including an unusually erratic, fast, slow or forceful heart beat, or even chest pain or breathlessness. Initial evaluation should concentrate on determining its likely mechanism, and whether or not there is significant underlying heart disease.

A detailed description of the sensation is essential and patients should be asked to tap out the heart beat they experience, on their chest or a table. A provisional diagnosis can usually be made on the basis of a thorough history (Box 18.22 and Fig. 18.31). It helps to obtain an ECG recording during an episode using an ambulatory monitor or a patient-activated ECG recorder.

✓ 18.22 How to evaluate palpitation

- Is the palpitation continuous or intermittent?
- Is the heart beat regular or irregular?
- What is the approximate heart rate?
- Do symptoms occur in discrete attacks?
    Is the onset abrupt?
    How do attacks terminate?
- Are there any associated symptoms?
    e.g. Chest pain
    Lightheadedness
    Polyuria (a feature of supraventricular tachycardia, p. 564)
- Are there any precipitating factors, e.g. exercise, alcohol?
- Is there a history of structural heart disease, e.g. coronary artery disease, valvular heart disease?

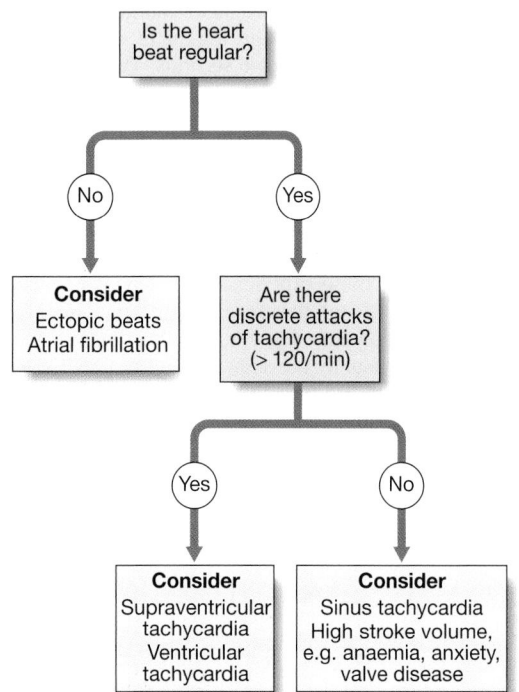

Fig. 18.31 A simple approach to the diagnosis of palpitation.

Recurrent but short-lived bouts of an irregular heart beat are usually due to atrial or ventricular extrasystoles (ectopic beats). Some patients will describe the experience as a 'flip' or a 'jolt' in the chest, while others report dropped or missed beats. Extrasystoles are often more frequent during periods of stress or debility; they can be triggered by alcohol or nicotine.

Episodes of a pounding, forceful and relatively fast (90–120/min) heart beat are a common manifestation of anxiety. They may also reflect a hyperdynamic circulation, such as anaemia, pregnancy and thyrotoxicosis, and can occur in some forms of valve disease (e.g. aortic regurgitation). Discrete bouts of a very rapid (> 120/min) heart beat are more likely to be due to a paroxysmal tachyarrhythmia. Supraventricular and ventricular tachycardias may all present in this way. In contrast, episodes of atrial fibrillation typically present with irregular and usually rapid palpitation.

Palpitation is usually benign and, even if the patient's symptoms are due to an arrhythmia, the outlook is good if there is no underlying structural heart disease. Most cases are due to an awareness of the normal heart beat, a sinus tachycardia or benign extrasystoles, in which case an explanation and reassurance may be all that is required. Palpitation associated with presyncope or syncope may reflect more serious structural or electrical disease and should be investigated promptly.

The diagnosis and management of individual arrhythmias are considered on pages 559–577.

Cardiac arrest and sudden cardiac death

Cardiac arrest describes the sudden and complete loss of cardiac output due to asystole, ventricular tachycardia or ventricular fibrillation, or loss of mechanical cardiac contraction (pulseless electrical activity). The clinical diagnosis is based on the victim being unconscious and pulseless; breathing may take some time to stop completely after cardiac arrest. Death is virtually inevitable unless effective treatment is given promptly.

Sudden cardiac death is usually caused by a catastrophic arrhythmia and accounts for 25–30% of deaths

---

18.23 Common causes of sudden arrhythmic death

Coronary artery disease (85%)

- Myocardial ischaemia
- Acute MI
- Prior MI with myocardial scarring

Structural heart disease (10%)

- Aortic stenosis (p. 619)
- Hypertrophic cardiomyopathy (p. 635)
- Dilated cardiomyopathy (p. 635)
- Arrhythmogenic right ventricular dysplasia (p. 637)
- Congenital heart disease (p. 628)

No structural heart disease (5%)

- Long QT syndrome (p. 567)
- Brugada syndrome (p. 568)
- Wolff–Parkinson–White syndrome (p. 565)
- Adverse drug reactions (torsades de pointes, p. 567)
- Severe electrolyte abnormalities

---

from cardiovascular disease, claiming an estimated 70 000–90 000 lives each year in the UK. Many of these deaths are potentially preventable. Arrhythmias complicate many types of heart disease and can sometimes occur in the absence of recognisable structural abnormalities (Box 18.23). Sudden death less often occurs because of an acute mechanical catastrophe such as cardiac rupture or aortic dissection (pp. 595 and 603).

Coronary artery disease, especially acute MI, is the most common condition leading to cardiac arrest. Ventricular fibrillation or ventricular tachycardia is common in the first few hours of MI and many victims die before medical help is sought. Up to one-third of people developing MI die before reaching hospital, emphasising the importance of educating the public to recognise symptoms and to seek medical help quickly. Acute myocardial ischaemia (in the absence of infarction) can also cause these arrhythmias, although less commonly. Patients with a history of MI may be at risk of sudden arrhythmic death, especially if left ventricular function is impaired or there is ongoing myocardial ischaemia. In these patients, the risk is reduced by the appropriate treatment of heart failure with β-blockers and ACE inhibitors, and by coronary revascularisation, and many require implantation of a cardiac defibrillator (p. 576).

Aetiology of cardiac arrest

Cardiac arrest may be caused by ventricular fibrillation, pulseless ventricular tachycardia, asystole or pulseless electrical activity.

Ventricular fibrillation and pulseless ventricular tachycardia

These are the most common and most easily treatable cardiac arrest rhythms. Ventricular fibrillation produces rapid ineffective uncoordinated movement of the ventricles, which therefore produce no pulse. The ECG (Fig. 18.32) shows rapid, bizarre and irregular ventricular complexes. Ventricular tachycardia (p. 566) can cause

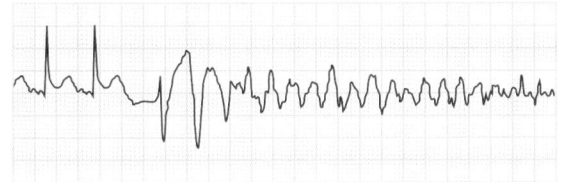

Fig. 18.32 Ventricular fibrillation. A bizarre chaotic rhythm initiated in this case by two ventricular ectopic beats in rapid succession.

cardiac arrest if the ventricular rate is so rapid that effective mechanical contraction and relaxation cannot occur, especially if it occurs in the presence of severe left ventricular impairment. It may degenerate into ventricular fibrillation. Defibrillation will restore cardiac output in more than 80% of patients if delivered immediately. However, the chances of survival fall by at least 10% with each minute's delay, and by more if basic life support is not given (see below); thus provision of these is the key to survival.

Asystole

This occurs when there is no electrical activity within the ventricles and is usually due to failure of the conducting tissue or massive ventricular damage complicating MI. A precordial thump, external cardiac massage, or administration of intravenous atropine or adrenaline (epinephrine) may restore cardiac activity. When due to conducting tissue failure, permanent pacemaker implantation will be required if the individual survives.

Pulseless electrical activity

This occurs when there is no effective cardiac output despite the presence of organised electrical activity. It may be caused by reversible conditions, such as hypovolaemia, cardiac tamponade or tension pneumothorax (see Fig. 18.35 below), but is often due to a catastrophic event such as cardiac rupture or massive pulmonary embolism, and therefore carries an extremely poor prognosis.

Management of cardiac arrest

The Chain of Survival

This term refers to the sequence of events that are necessary to maximise the chances of a cardiac arrest victim surviving (Fig. 18.33). Survival is most likely if all links in the chain are strong, i.e. if the arrest is witnessed, help is called immediately, basic life support is administered by a trained individual, the emergency medical services respond promptly, and defibrillation is achieved within a few minutes. Good training in both basic and advanced life support is essential and should be maintained by regular refresher courses. In recent years, public access defibrillation has been introduced in places of high population density, particularly where traffic congestion may impede the response of emergency services, e.g. railway stations, airports and sports stadia. Designated individuals can respond to a cardiac arrest using basic life support and an automated external defibrillator.

18

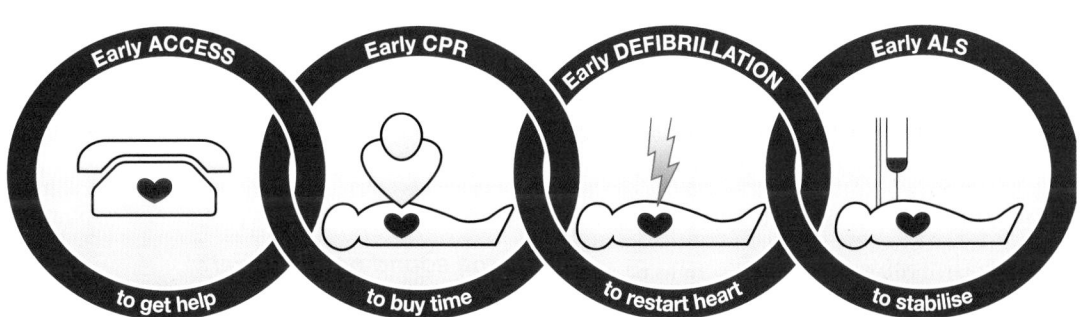

Fig. 18.33 The Chain of Survival in cardiac arrest. (CPR = cardiopulmonary resuscitation; ALS = advanced life support)

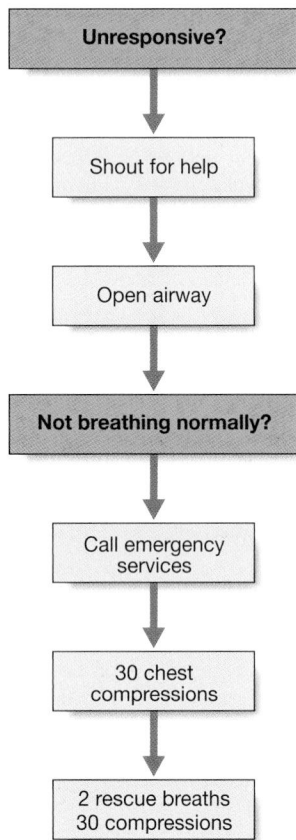

Fig. 18.34 Algorithm for adult basic life support. For further information see www.resus.org.uk.

Basic life support (BLS)

BLS encompasses manœuvres that aim to maintain a low level of circulation until more definitive treatment with advanced life support can be given. Management of the collapsed patient requires prompt assessment and restoration of the airway, maintenance of breathing using rescue breathing ('mouth-to-mouth' breathing) and maintenance of the circulation using chest compressions (Fig. 18.34).

Advanced life support (ALS)

ALS (Fig. 18.35) aims to restore normal cardiac rhythm by defibrillation when the cause of cardiac arrest is due to a tachyarrhythmia, or to restore cardiac output by correcting other reversible causes of cardiac arrest. ALS can also involve administration of intravenous drugs to support the circulation, and endotracheal intubation to ventilate the lungs.

If cardiac arrest is witnessed, a precordial thump may sometimes convert ventricular fibrillation or tachycardia to normal rhythm, but this is futile if cardiac arrest has lasted longer than a few seconds. The priority is to assess the patient's cardiac rhythm by attaching a defibrillator/monitor. Ventricular fibrillation or pulseless ventricular tachycardia is treated with immediate defibrillation. Defibrillation is more likely to be effective if a biphasic shock defibrillator is used, where the polarity of the shock is reversed midway through its delivery. Defibrillation is usually administered using

a 150 Joule biphasic shock, and CPR resumed immediately for 2 minutes without attempting to confirm restoration of a pulse, because restoration of mechanical cardiac output rarely occurs immediately after successful defibrillation. If after 2 minutes a pulse is not restored, a further biphasic shock of 150–200 joules is given. Thereafter, additional biphasic shocks of 150–200 joules are given every 2 minutes after each cycle of cardiopulmonary resuscitation (CPR). During resuscitation, adrenaline (epinephrine, 1 mg i.v.) should be given every 3–5 minutes and consideration given to the use of intravenous amiodarone, especially if ventricular fibrillation or ventricular tachycardia reinitiates after successful defibrillation.

Ventricular fibrillation of low amplitude, or 'fine VF', may mimic asystole. If asystole cannot be confidently diagnosed, the patient should be regarded as having 'fine VF' and defibrillated. If an electrical rhythm is present that would be expected to produce a cardiac output, 'pulseless electrical activity' is present. There are several potentially reversible causes that can be easily remembered as a list of four Hs and four Ts (see Fig. 18.35). Pulseless electrical activity is treated by continuing CPR and adrenaline (epinephrine) administration whilst seeking such causes. Asystole is treated similarly, with the additional support of atropine and sometimes external or transvenous pacing in an attempt to generate an electrical rhythm.

Survivors of cardiac arrest

Patients who survive a cardiac arrest caused by acute MI need no specific treatment beyond that given to those recovering from an uncomplicated infarct, since their prognosis is similar (p. 598). Those with reversible causes, such as exercise-induced ischaemia or aortic stenosis, should have the underlying cause treated if possible. Survivors of ventricular tachycardia or ventricular fibrillation arrest in whom no reversible cause can be identified may be at risk of another episode, and should be considered for an implantable cardiac defibrillator (p. 576) and anti-arrhythmic drug therapy.

Abnormal heart sounds and murmurs

The first clinical manifestation of heart disease may be the discovery of an abnormal sound on auscultation (Box 18.24). This may be incidental—for example, during a routine childhood examination—or may be prompted by symptoms of heart disease. Clinical evaluation is helpful but an echocardiogram is often necessary to confirm the nature of an abnormal heart sound or murmur.

Is the sound cardiac?

Additional heart sounds and murmurs demonstrate a consistent relationship to a specific part of the cardiac cycle but extracardiac sounds (e.g. pleural rub or venous hum) do not. Pericardial friction produces a characteristic scratching or crunching noise, which often has two components corresponding to atrial and ventricular systole, and may vary with posture and respiration.

Is the sound pathological?

Pathological sounds and murmurs are the product of turbulent blood flow or rapid ventricular filling due to abnormal loading conditions. Some added sounds

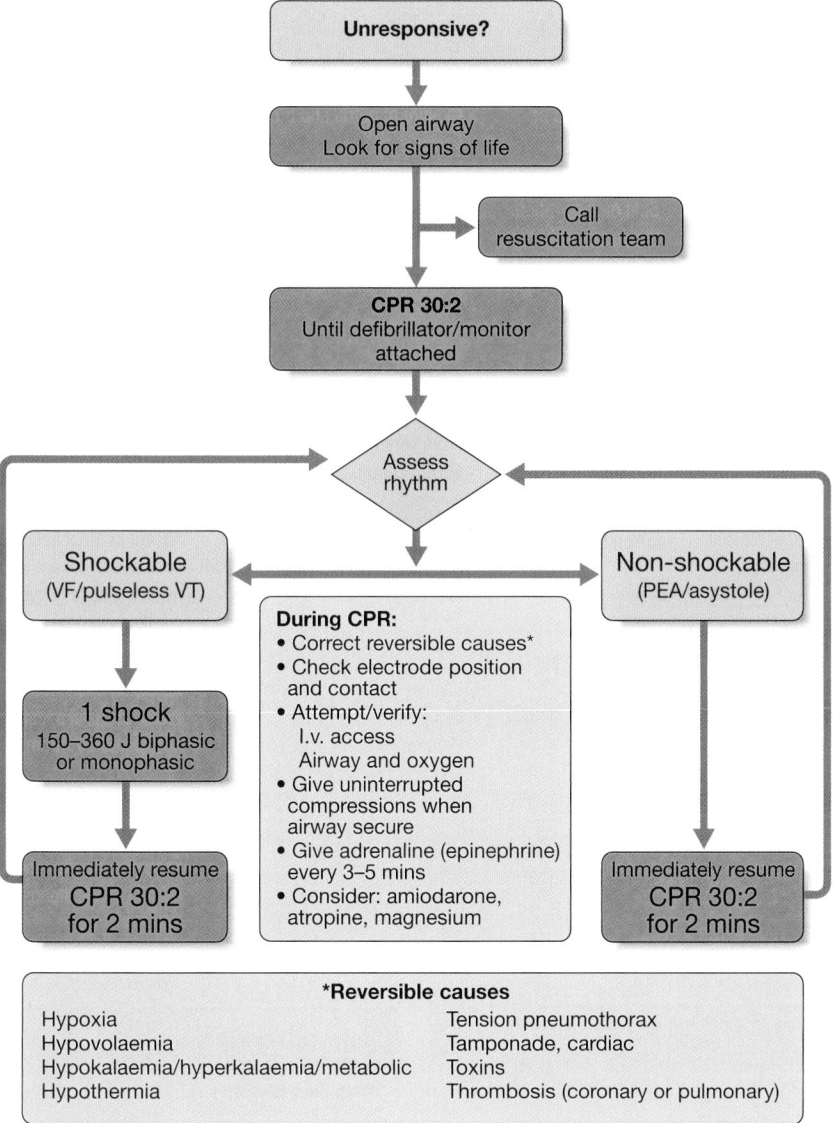

Fig. 18.35 Algorithm for adult advanced life support. For further information see www.resus.org.uk. (CPR = cardiopulmonary resuscitation; PEA = pulseless electrical activity; VF = ventricular fibrillation; VT = pulseless ventricular tachycardia)

18

are physiological but may also occur in pathological conditions; for example, a third sound is common in young people and in pregnancy but is also a feature of heart failure (see Box 18.24). Similarly, a systolic murmur due to turbulence across the right ventricular outflow tract may occur in hyperdynamic states (e.g. anaemia, pregnancy) but may also be due to pulmonary stenosis or an intracardiac shunt leading to volume overload of the RV (e.g. atrial septal defect).

Benign murmurs do not occur in diastole (Box 18.25), and systolic murmurs that radiate or are associated with a thrill are almost always pathological.

Auscultatory evaluation of a heart murmur

Timing, intensity, location, radiation and quality are all useful clues to the origin and nature of a heart murmur (Box 18.26). Radiation of a murmur is determined by the direction of turbulent blood flow and is only detectable when there is a high-velocity jet, such as in

mitral regurgitation (radiation from apex to axilla) or aortic stenosis (radiation from base to neck). Similarly, the pitch and quality of the sound can help to distinguish the murmur, such as the 'blowing' murmur of mitral regurgitation or the 'rasping' murmur of aortic stenosis.

The position of a murmur in relation to the cardiac cycle is crucial and should be assessed by timing it with the heart sounds, carotid pulse and apex beat (Figs 18.36 and 18.37).

Systolic murmurs associated with ventricular outflow tract obstruction

These occur in mid-systole and have a crescendo-decrescendo pattern, reflecting the changing velocity of blood flow (Box 18.27). Pansystolic murmurs maintain a constant intensity and extend from the first heart sound throughout systole (up to and beyond the second heart sound). They occur when blood leaks from a ventricle

557

18.24 Normal and abnormal heart sounds

Sound	Timing	Characteristics	Mechanisms	Variable features
First heart sound (S1)	Onset of systole	Usually single or narrowly split	Closure of mitral and tricuspid valves	Loud: hyperdynamic circulation (anaemia, pregnancy, thyrotoxicosis); mitral stenosis Soft: heart failure; mitral regurgitation
Second heart sound (S2)	End of systole	Split on inspiration Single on expiration (p. 528)	Closure of aortic and pulmonary valve A_2 first P_2 second	Fixed wide splitting with atrial septal defect Wide but variable splitting with delayed right heart emptying (e.g. right bundle branch block) Reversed splitting due to delayed left heart emptying (e.g. left bundle branch block)
Third heart sound (S3)	Early in diastole, just after S2	Low pitch, often heard as 'gallop'	From ventricular wall due to abrupt cessation of rapid filling	Physiological: young people, pregnancy Pathological: heart failure, mitral regurgitation
Fourth heart sound (S4)	End of diastole, just before S1	Low pitch	Ventricular origin (stiff ventricle and augmented atrial contraction) related to atrial filling	Absent in atrial fibrillation A feature of severe left ventricular hypertrophy (e.g. hypertrophic cardiomyopathy)
Systolic clicks	Early or mid-systole	Brief, high-intensity sound	Valvular aortic stenosis Valvular pulmonary stenosis Floppy mitral valve Prosthetic heart sounds from opening and closing of normally functioning mechanical valves	Click may be lost when stenotic valve becomes thickened or calcified Prosthetic clicks lost when valve obstructed by thrombus or vegetations
Opening snap (OS)	Early in diastole	High pitch, brief duration	Opening of stenosed leaflets of mitral valve Prosthetic heart sounds	Moves closer to S2 as mitral stenosis becomes more severe. May be absent in calcific mitral stenosis

18.25 Features of a benign or innocent heart murmur

- Soft
- Mid-systolic
- Heard at left sternal edge
- No radiation
- No other cardiac abnormalities

into a low-pressure chamber at an even or constant velocity. Mitral regurgitation, tricuspid regurgitation and ventricular septal defect are the only causes of a pansystolic murmur. Late systolic murmurs are unusual but may occur in mitral valve prolapse, if the mitral regurgitation is confined to late systole, hypertrophic obstructive cardiomyopathy if dynamic obstruction occurs late in systole.

Mid-diastolic murmurs

These are due to accelerated or turbulent flow across the mitral or tricuspid valves. They are low-pitched noises that are often difficult to hear and should be evaluated with the bell of the stethoscope. A mid-diastolic murmur may be due to mitral stenosis (located at the apex and axilla), tricuspid stenosis (located at the left sternal edge), increased flow across the mitral valve (e.g. the to-and-fro murmur of severe mitral regurgitation) or increased flow across the tricuspid valve (e.g. left-to-right shunt

18.26 How to assess a heart murmur

When does it occur?	Time the murmur using heart sounds, carotid pulse and the apex beat. Is it systolic or diastolic? Does the murmur extend throughout systole or diastole or is it confined to a shorter part of the cardiac cycle?
How loud is it? (intensity)	Grade 1: very soft (only audible in ideal conditions) Grade 2: soft Grade 3: moderate Grade 4: loud with associated thrill Grade 5: very loud Grade 6: heard without stethoscope N.B. Diastolic murmurs are sometimes graded 1–4
Where is it heard best? (location)	Listen over the apex and base of the heart, including the aortic and pulmonary areas
Where does it radiate?	Listen at the neck, axilla or back
What does it sound like? (pitch and quality)	Pitch is determined by flow (high pitch indicates high-velocity flow) Is the intensity constant or variable?

18.27 Features of some common systolic murmurs

Condition	Timing and duration	Quality	Location and radiation	Associated features
Aortic stenosis	Mid-systolic	Loud rasping	Base and left sternal edge, radiating to suprasternal notch and carotids	Single second heart sound Ejection click (in young patients) Slow rising pulse Left ventricular hypertrophy (pressure overload)
Mitral regurgitation	Pansystolic	Blowing	Apex, radiating to axilla	Soft first heart sound Third heart sound Left ventricular hypertrophy (volume overload)
Ventricular septal defect (VSD)	Pansystolic	Harsh	Lower left sternal edge, radiating to whole precordium	Thrill Biventricular hypertrophy
Benign	Mid-systolic	Soft	Left sternal edge, no radiation	No other signs of heart disease

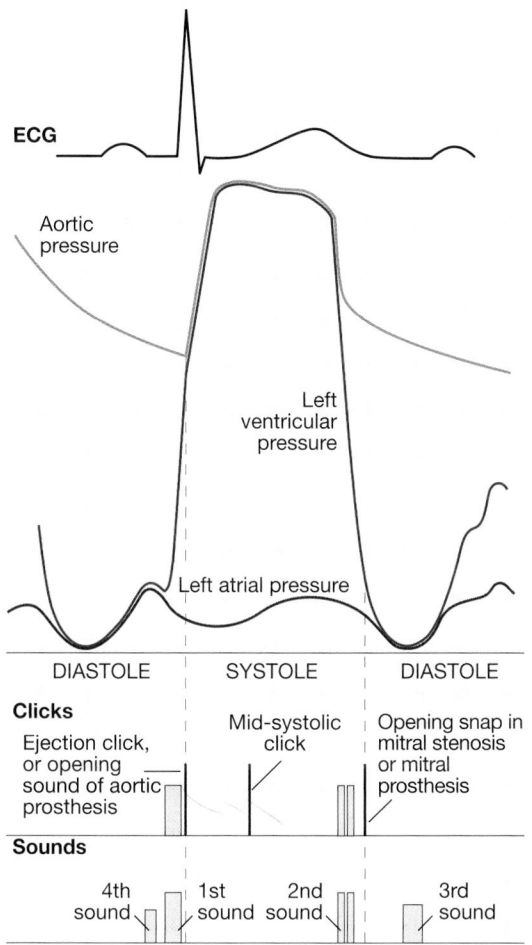

Fig. 18.36 The relationship of the cardiac cycle to the ECG, the left ventricular pressure wave and the position of heart sounds.

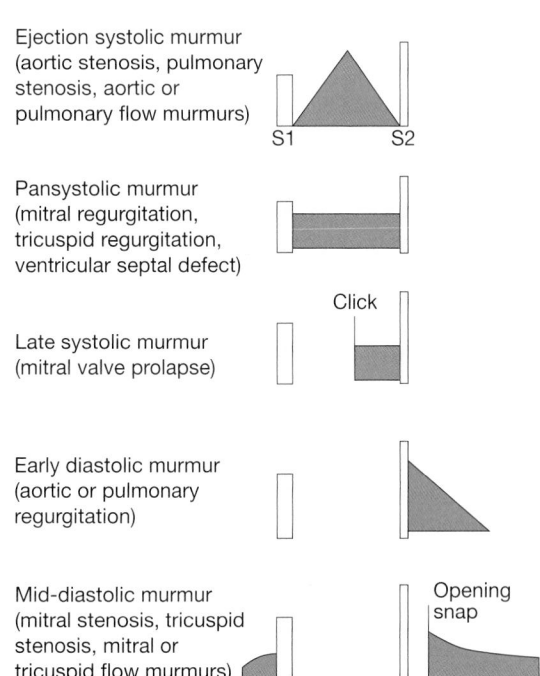

Fig. 18.37 The timing and pattern of cardiac murmurs.

Continuous murmurs

These result from a combination of systolic and diastolic flow (e.g. persistent ductus arteriosus), and must be distinguished from extracardiac noises such as bruits from arterial shunts, venous hums (high rates of venous flow in children) and pericardial friction rubs.

The characteristics of specific valve defects and congenital anomalies are described on pages 612–635.

DISORDERS OF HEART RATE, RHYTHM AND CONDUCTION

The heart beat is normally initiated by an electrical discharge from the sinoatrial (sinus) node. The atria and ventricles then depolarise sequentially as electrical depolarisation passes through specialised conducting tissues (see Fig. 18.4, p. 525). The sinus node acts as a

through a large atrial septal defect). Early diastolic murmurs have a soft, blowing quality with a decrescendo pattern and should be evaluated with the diaphragm of the stethoscope. They are due to regurgitation across the aortic or pulmonary valves and are best heard at the left sternal edge with the patient sitting forwards in held expiration.

pacemaker and its intrinsic rate is regulated by the autonomic nervous system; vagal activity slows the heart rate, and sympathetic activity accelerates it via cardiac sympathetic nerves and circulating catecholamines.

If the sinus rate becomes unduly slow, a lower centre may assume the role of pacemaker. This is known as an escape rhythm and may arise in the AV node or His bundle (junctional rhythm) or the ventricles (idioventricular rhythm).

A cardiac arrhythmia is a disturbance of the electrical rhythm of the heart. Arrhythmias are often a manifestation of structural heart disease but may also occur because of abnormal conduction or depolarisation in an otherwise healthy heart. A heart rate > 100/min is called a tachycardia and a heart rate < 60/min is called a bradycardia.

There are three main mechanisms of tachycardia:

- *Increased automaticity.* The tachycardia is produced by repeated spontaneous depolarisation of an ectopic focus, often in response to catecholamines.
- *Re-entry.* The tachycardia is initiated by an ectopic beat and sustained by a re-entry circuit (Fig. 18.38). Most tachyarrhythmias are due to re-entry.
- *Triggered activity.* This can cause ventricular arrhythmias in patients with coronary heart disease. It is a form of secondary depolarisation arising from an incompletely repolarised cell membrane.

Bradycardia may be due to:

- *Reduced automaticity*, e.g. sinus bradycardia.
- *Blocked or abnormally slow conduction*, e.g. AV block.

An arrhythmia may be 'supraventricular' (sinus, atrial or junctional) or ventricular. Supraventricular rhythms usually produce narrow QRS complexes because the ventricles are depolarised normally through the AV node and bundle of His. In contrast, ventricular rhythms produce broad, bizarre QRS complexes because the ventricles are activated in an abnormal sequence. However, occasionally a supraventricular rhythm can produce broad or wide QRS complexes due to coexisting bundle branch block or the presence of accessory conducting tissue (see below).

Bradycardias tend to cause symptoms that reflect low cardiac output: fatigue, lightheadedness and syncope. Tachycardias cause rapid palpitation, dizziness, chest discomfort or breathlessness. Extreme tachycardias can cause syncope because the heart is unable to contract or relax properly at extreme rates. Extreme bradycardias or tachycardias can precipitate sudden death or cardiac arrest.

Sinus rhythms

Sinus arrhythmia

Phasic alteration of the heart rate during respiration (the sinus rate increases during inspiration and slows during expiration) is a consequence of normal parasympathetic nervous system activity and can be pronounced in children. Absence of this normal variation in heart rate with breathing or with changes in posture may be a feature of autonomic neuropathy (p. 831).

Sinus bradycardia

A sinus rate < 60/min may occur in healthy people at rest and is a common finding in athletes. Some pathological causes are listed in Box 18.28. Asymptomatic sinus bradycardia requires no treatment. Symptomatic acute sinus bradycardia usually responds to intravenous atropine 0.6–1.2 mg. Patients with recurrent or persistent symptomatic sinus bradycardia should be considered for pacemaker implantation.

Sinus tachycardia

This is defined as a sinus rate > 100/min, and is usually due to an increase in sympathetic activity associated with exercise, emotion, pregnancy or pathology (see Box 18.28). Young adults can produce a rapid sinus rate, up to 200/min, during intense exercise.

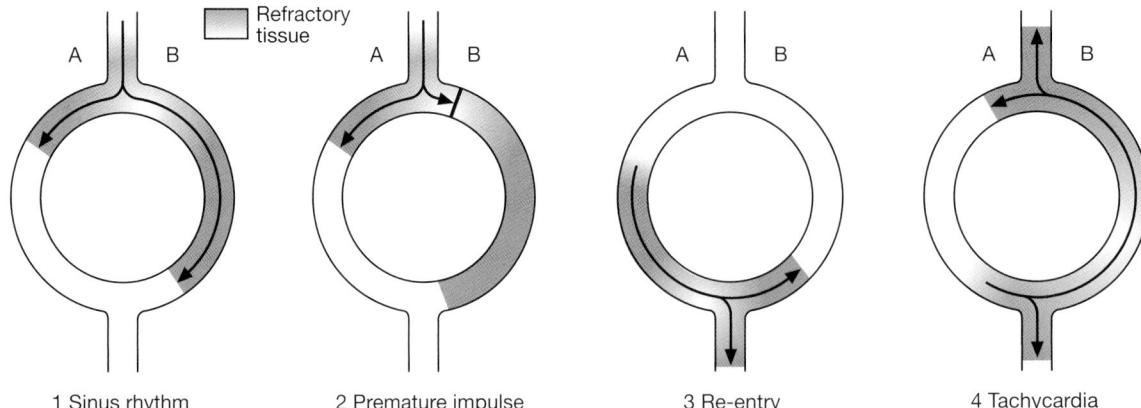

1 Sinus rhythm   2 Premature impulse   3 Re-entry   4 Tachycardia

Fig. 18.38 The mechanism of re-entry. Re-entry can occur when there are two alternative pathways with different conducting properties (e.g. the AV node and an accessory pathway, or an area of normal and an area of ischaemic tissue). Here, pathway A conducts slowly and recovers quickly, while pathway B conducts rapidly and recovers slowly. (1) In sinus rhythm each impulse passes down both pathways before entering a common distal pathway. (2) As the pathways recover at different rates, a premature impulse may find pathway A open and B closed. (3) Pathway B may recover while the premature impulse is travelling selectively down pathway A. The impulse can then travel retrogradely up pathway B, setting up a closed loop or re-entry circuit. (4) This may initiate a tachycardia that continues until the circuit is interrupted by a change in conduction rates or electrical depolarisation.

Atrial tachycardia

Atrial tachycardia may be a manifestation of increased atrial automaticity, sinoatrial disease or digoxin toxicity. It produces a narrow complex tachycardia with abnormal P-wave morphology, sometimes associated with AV block if the atrial rate is rapid. It may respond to β-blockers which reduce automaticity, or class I or III anti-arrhythmic drugs (see Box 18.40, p. 573). The ventricular response in rapid atrial tachycardias may be controlled by AV node-blocking drugs. Catheter ablation (p. 575) can be used to target the ectopic site and should be offered as an alternative to anti-arrhythmic drugs in patients with recurrent atrial tachycardia.

Atrial flutter

Atrial flutter is characterised by a large (macro) re-entry circuit, usually within the RA encircling the tricuspid annulus. The atrial rate is approximately 300/min, and is usually associated with 2:1, 3:1 or 4:1 AV block (with corresponding heart rates of 150, 100 or 75/min). Rarely, in young patients, every beat is conducted, producing a heart rate of 300/min and potentially haemodynamic compromise. The ECG shows saw-toothed flutter waves (Fig. 18.40). When there is regular 2:1 AV block, it may be difficult to identify flutter waves which are buried in the QRS complexes and T waves. Atrial flutter should always be suspected when there is a narrow complex tachycardia of 150/min. Carotid sinus pressure or intravenous adenosine may help to establish the diagnosis by temporarily increasing the degree of AV block and revealing the flutter waves (Fig. 18.41).

18.28 Some pathological causes of sinus bradycardia and tachycardia

Sinus bradycardia

- MI
- Sinus node disease (sick sinus syndrome)
- Hypothermia
- Hypothyroidism
- Cholestatic jaundice
- Raised intracranial pressure
- Drugs, e.g. β-blockers, digoxin, verapamil

Sinus tachycardia

- Anxiety
- Fever
- Anaemia
- Heart failure
- Thyrotoxicosis
- Phaeochromocytoma
- Drugs, e.g. β-agonists (bronchodilators)

Atrial tachyarrhythmias

Atrial ectopic beats (extrasystoles, premature beats)

These usually cause no symptoms but can give the sensation of a missed beat or an abnormally strong beat. The ECG (Fig. 18.39) shows a premature but otherwise normal QRS complex; if visible, the preceding P wave has a different morphology because the atria activate from an abnormal site. In most cases these are of no consequence, although very frequent atrial ectopic beats may herald the onset of atrial fibrillation. Treatment is rarely necessary but β-blockers can be used if symptoms are intrusive.

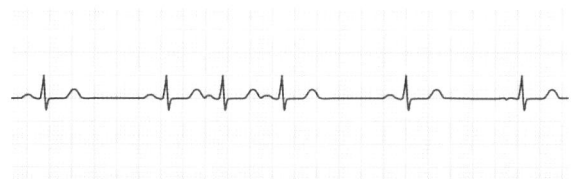

Fig. 18.39 Atrial ectopic beats. The first, second and fifth complexes are normal sinus beats. The third, fourth and sixth complexes are atrial ectopic beats with identical QRS complexes and abnormal (sometimes barely visible) P waves.

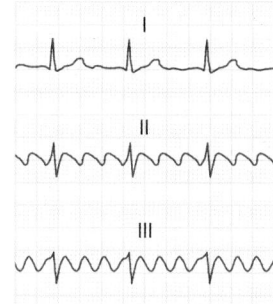

Fig. 18.40 Atrial flutter. Simultaneous recording showing atrial flutter with 3:1 AV block; flutter waves are only visible in leads II and III.

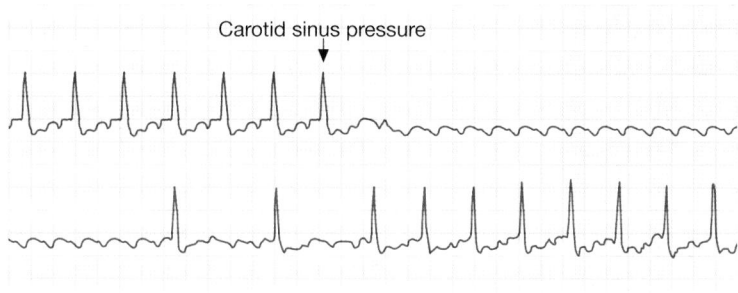

Carotid sinus pressure

Fig. 18.41 Carotid sinus pressure in atrial flutter: continuous trace. The diagnosis of atrial flutter with 2:1 block was established when carotid sinus pressure produced temporary AV block revealing the flutter waves.

18

Management

Digoxin, β-blockers or verapamil can be used to control the ventricular rate (pp. 571–573). However, in many cases it may be preferable to try to restore sinus rhythm by direct current (DC) cardioversion or by using intravenous amiodarone. Beta-blockers or amiodarone can also be used to prevent recurrent episodes of atrial flutter. Although flecainide can also be used for acute treatment or prophylaxis, it should be avoided because there is a risk of slowing the flutter circuit and facilitating 1:1 AV nodal conduction. This can cause a paradoxical tachycardia and haemodynamic compromise. If used, it should always be prescribed along with an AV node-blocking drug, such as a β-blocker. Catheter ablation offers a 90% chance of complete cure and is the treatment of choice for patients with persistent, troublesome symptoms.

Atrial fibrillation

Atrial fibrillation (AF) is the most common sustained cardiac arrhythmia, with an overall prevalence of 0.5% in the adult population of the UK. The prevalence rises with age, affecting 2–5% and 8% of those aged over 70 and 80 years respectively. Atrial fibrillation is a complex arrhythmia characterised by both abnormal automatic firing and the presence of multiple interacting re-entry circuits looping around the atria. Episodes of atrial fibrillation are usually initiated by rapid bursts of ectopic beats arising from conducting tissue in the pulmonary veins or from diseased atrial tissue. AF becomes sustained because of initiation of re-entrant conduction within the atria or sometimes because of continuous ectopic firing (Fig. 18.42). Re-entry is more likely to occur in atria that are enlarged, or in which conduction is slow (as is the case in many forms of heart disease). During episodes of AF, the atria beat rapidly but in an uncoordinated and ineffective manner. The ventricles are activated irregularly at a rate determined by conduction through the AV node. This produces the characteristic 'irregularly irregular' pulse. The ECG (Fig. 18.43) shows normal but irregular QRS complexes; there are no P waves but the baseline may show irregular fibrillation waves.

AF can be classified as paroxysmal (intermittent, self-terminating episodes), persistent (prolonged episodes

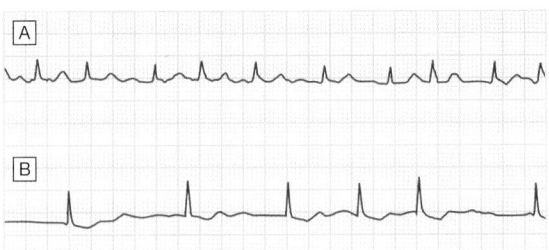

Fig. 18.43 Two examples of atrial fibrillation. The QRS complexes are irregular and there are no P waves. **A** There is usually a fast ventricular rate, e.g. between 120 and 160/min, at the onset of atrial fibrillation. **B** In chronic AF, the ventricular rate may be much slower due to the effects of medication and AV nodal fatigue.

that can be terminated by electrical or chemical cardioversion) or permanent. In patients with AF seen for the first time, it can be difficult to identify which of these is present. Unfortunately for many patients, paroxysmal AF will become permanent as the underlying disease process that predisposes to AF progresses. Electrophysiological changes occur in the atria within a few hours of the onset of AF that tend to maintain fibrillation: electrical remodelling. When AF persists for a period of months, structural remodelling occurs with atrial fibrosis and dilatation that further predispose to AF. Thus early treatment of AF will prevent this and reinitiation of the arrhythmia.

AF may be the first manifestation of many forms of heart disease (Box 18.29), particularly those that are associated with enlargement or dilatation of the atria. Alcohol excess, hyperthyroidism and chronic lung disease are also common causes of AF, although multiple aetiological factors often coexist such as the combination of alcohol, hypertension and coronary disease. About 50% of all patients with paroxysmal AF and 20% of patients with persistent or permanent AF have structurally normal hearts; this is known as 'lone atrial fibrillation'.

AF can cause palpitation, breathlessness and fatigue. In patients with poor ventricular function or valve disease it may precipitate or aggravate cardiac failure because of loss of atrial function and heart rate control. A fall in BP may cause lightheadedness, and chest pain may occur with underlying coronary disease. However, AF is often completely asymptomatic, in which case it is usually discovered as a result of a routine examination or ECG.

AF is associated with significant morbidity and a twofold increase in mortality that are largely attributable to the effects of the underlying heart disease and the risk of cerebral embolism. Careful assessment, risk stratification and therapy can improve the prognosis.

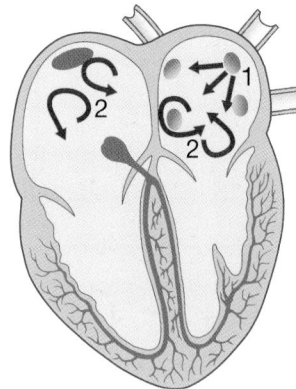

Fig 18.42 Mechanisms of the initiation of atrial fibrillation.
(1) Ectopic beats, often arising from the pulmonary veins, trigger atrial fibrillation. (2) Re-entry within the atria maintains atrial fibrillation, with multiple interacting re-entry circuits operating simultaneously.

18.29 Common causes of atrial fibrillation

- Coronary artery disease (including acute MI)
- Valvular heart disease, especially rheumatic mitral valve disease
- Hypertension
- Sinoatrial disease
- Hyperthyroidism
- Alcohol
- Cardiomyopathy
- Congenital heart disease
- Chest infection
- Pulmonary embolism
- Pericardial disease
- Idiopathic (lone AF)

Management

Assessment of patients with newly diagnosed AF includes a full history, physical examination, 12-lead ECG, echocardiogram and thyroid function tests. Additional investigations such as exercise testing may be needed to determine the nature and extent of any underlying heart disease. Biochemical evidence of hyperthyroidism is found in a small minority of patients with otherwise unexplained AF.

When AF complicates an acute illness (e.g. chest infection, pulmonary embolism), effective treatment of the primary disorder will often restore sinus rhythm. Otherwise, the main objectives are to restore sinus rhythm as soon as possible, prevent recurrent episodes of AF, optimise the heart rate during periods of AF, minimise the risk of thromboembolism and treat any underlying disease.

Paroxysmal atrial fibrillation

Occasional attacks that are well tolerated do not necessarily require treatment. Beta-blockers are normally used as first-line therapy if symptoms are troublesome, and are particularly useful for treating patients with AF associated with ischaemic heart disease, hypertension and cardiac failure. Beta-blockers reduce the ectopic firing that normally initiates AF. Class Ic drugs (see Box 18.40, p. 573), such as propafenone or flecainide, are also effective at preventing episodes but should not be given to patients with coronary disease or left ventricular dysfunction. Flecainide is usually prescribed along with a rate limiting β-blocker because it occasionally precipitates atrial flutter. Amiodarone is the most effective agent for preventing AF but its side-effects restrict its use to patients in whom other measures fail. Digoxin and verapamil are not effective drugs for preventing paroxysms of AF, although they serve to limit the heart rate when AF occurs by blocking the AV node. In patients with AF in whom β-blockers or class Ic drugs are ineffective or cause side-effects, catheter ablation can be considered. Ablation is used to isolate electrically the pulmonary veins from the LA, preventing ectopic triggering of AF. Sometimes ablation is used to create lines of conduction block within the atria to prevent re-entry. Ablation prevents AF in approximately 70% of patients with prior drug-resistant episodes, although drugs may subsequently be needed to maintain sinus rhythm. Ablation for AF is an evolving treatment which is associated with a small risk of embolic stroke or cardiac tamponade. Specialised 'AF suppression' pacemakers have been developed which pace the atria to prevent paroxysms but this has not proved to be as effective as was initially hoped.

Persistent and permanent atrial fibrillation

There are two options for treating persistent AF:
- *rhythm control*: attempting to restore and maintain sinus rhythm
- *rate control*: accepting that AF will be permanent and using treatments to control the ventricular rate and to prevent embolic complications.

Rhythm control. An attempt to restore sinus rhythm is particularly appropriate if the arrhythmia has precipitated troublesome symptoms and there is a modifiable or treatable underlying cause. Electrical cardioversion (p. 574) is initially successful in three-quarters of patients but relapse is frequent (25–50% at 1 month and 70–90% at 1 year). Attempts to restore and maintain

18.30 Atrial fibrillation in old age

- **Prevalence**: rises with age, reaching more than 10% in those > 80 yrs of age.
- **Symptoms**: sometimes asymptomatic but often accompanied by diastolic heart failure.
- **Hyperthyroidism**: AF may be the dominant feature of otherwise silent or occult hyperthyroidism.
- **Cardioversion**: followed by high rates (~70% at 1 yr) of recurrent AF.
- **Stroke**: AF is an important cause of cerebral embolism, found in 15% of all stroke patients and 2–8% of those with transient ischaemic attacks (TIAs).
- **Anticoagulation**: although the risk of thromboembolism rises, the hazards of anticoagulation also rise with age because of increased comorbidity, particularly cognitive impairment and falls.
- **Target INR**: if anticoagulation is recommended in those > 75 yrs, care should be taken to maintain an INR < 3.0 because of the increased risk of intracranial haemorrhage.
- **Aspirin**: a safer alternative if anticoagulation cannot be recommended, but its benefits in reducing the risk of stroke are less significant and consistent than with warfarin.

sinus rhythm are most successful if AF has been present for < 3 months, the patient is young and there is no important structural heart disease.

Immediate DC cardioversion after the administration of intravenous heparin is appropriate if AF has been present for < 48 hours. An attempt to restore sinus rhythm by infusing intravenous flecainide (2 mg/kg over 30 minutes, maximum dose 150 mg) is a safe alternative to electrical cardioversion if there is no underlying structural heart disease. In other situations, DC cardioversion should be deferred until the patient has been established on warfarin, with an international normalised ratio (INR) > 2.0 for a minimum of 4 weeks, and any underlying problems, such as hypertension or alcohol excess, have been eliminated. Anticoagulation should be maintained for at least 3 months following successful cardioversion; if relapse occurs, a second (or third) cardioversion may be appropriate. Concomitant therapy with amiodarone or β-blockers may reduce the risk of recurrence. Catheter ablation is sometimes used to help restore and maintain sinus rhythm in resistant cases, but it is a less effective treatment for persistent AF than for paroxysmal AF.

Rate control. If sinus rhythm cannot be restored, treatment should be directed at maintaining an appropriate heart rate. Digoxin, β-blockers or rate-limiting calcium antagonists such as verapamil or diltiazem (pp. 571–573) will reduce the ventricular rate by increasing the degree of AV block. This alone may produce a striking improvement in overall cardiac function, particularly in patients with mitral stenosis. Beta-blockers and rate-limiting calcium antagonists are often more effective than digoxin at controlling the heart rate during exercise and may have additional benefits in patients with hypertension or structural heart disease. Combination therapy (e.g. digoxin + atenolol) is often advisable.

In exceptional cases, poorly controlled and symptomatic AF can be treated by deliberately inducing complete AV nodal block with catheter ablation; a permanent pacemaker must be implanted beforehand. This is known as the 'pace and ablate' strategy.

18

Prevention of thromboembolism

Loss of atrial contraction and left atrial dilatation cause stasis of blood in the LA and may lead to thrombus formation in the left atrial appendage. This predisposes patients to stroke and other forms of systemic embolism. The annual risk of these events in patients with persistent AF is approximately 5% but it is influenced by many factors (Box 18.31) and may range from less than 1% to 12% (Box 18.32).

Several large randomised trials have shown that treatment with adjusted-dose warfarin (target INR 2.0–3.0) reduces the risk of stroke by about two-thirds, at the cost of an annual risk of bleeding of approximately 1–1.5%, whereas treatment with aspirin reduces the risk of stroke by only one-fifth (Box 18.33). Warfarin is thus indicated for patients with AF who have specific risk factors for stroke. For patients with intermittent AF, the risk of stroke is proportionate to the frequency and duration of AF episodes. Those with frequent, prolonged (> 24 hours) episodes of AF should be considered for warfarin anticoagulation.

An assessment of the risk of embolism helps to define the possible benefits of antithrombotic therapy (see Box 18.31), which must be balanced against its potential hazards. Echocardiography is valuable in risk stratification. Warfarin is indicated in patients at high or very high risk of stroke, unless anticoagulation poses unacceptable risks. Comorbid conditions that may be complicated by bleeding, such as peptic ulcer, uncontrolled hypertension, alcohol misuse, frequent falls, poor drug compliance and potential drug interactions, are all relative contraindications to warfarin. Patients at moderate risk of stroke may be treated with warfarin or aspirin after discussing the balance of risk and benefit with the individual. Young

---

18.31 How to assess risk of thromboembolism in atrial fibrillation: the CHADS score

- Congestive heart failure (1 point)
- Hypertension (1 point)
- Age > 75 (1 point)
- Diabetes mellitus (1 point)
- Stroke or transient ischaemic attack (2 points)

CHADS score	Stroke risk/yr (%)	95% CI
0	1.9	1.2–3.0
1	2.8	2.0–3.8
2	4.0	3.1–5.1
3	5.9	4.6–7.3
4	8.5	6.3–11.1
5	12.5	8.2–17.5
6	18.2	10.5–27.4

Score: 0 = aspirin therapy only, 1 = warfarin or aspirin, ≥ 2 = warfarin

---

18.32 Effect of risk status and treatment on annual risk of stroke in non-rheumatic atrial fibrillation

Risk group	Untreated	Aspirin	Warfarin
Very high	12%	10%	5%
High	6.5%	5%	2.5%
Moderate	4%	3%	1.5%
Low	1.2%	1%	0.5%

N.B. In most studies the annual risk of significant bleeding during warfarin therapy is between 1.0 and 1.5%.

EBM 18.33 **Anticoagulation in atrial fibrillation**

'Anticoagulation with warfarin reduces the risk of ischaemic stroke in non-rheumatic atrial fibrillation by about 62% (absolute risk reduction 2.7% for primary prevention and 8.4% for secondary prevention), while aspirin reduces the risk by only 22% (absolute risk reduction 1.5% for primary prevention and 2.5% for secondary prevention). NNT_B for 1 year (warfarin vs placebo) = 18.'

- Hart RG, et al. Ann Intern Med 1999; 131:492–501.

For further information: www.sign.ac.uk

---

patients (under 65 years) with no evidence of structural heart disease have a very low risk of stroke; they do not require warfarin but may benefit from aspirin.

'Supraventricular' tachycardias

The term 'supraventricular tachycardia' (SVT) is commonly used to describe a range of regular tachycardias that have a similar appearance on an ECG. These are usually associated with a narrow QRS complex and are characterised by a re-entry circuit or automatic focus involving the atria. The term SVT is misleading, as in many cases the ventricles also form part of the re-entry circuit, such as in patients with AV re-entrant tachycardia.

Atrioventricular nodal re-entrant tachycardia (AVNRT)

This is due to re-entry in a circuit involving the AV node and its two right atrial input pathways: a superior 'fast' pathway and an inferior 'slow' pathway (see Fig. 18.45A below). This produces a regular tachycardia with a rate of 120–240/min. It tends to occur in hearts that are otherwise normal and episodes may last from a few seconds to many hours. The patient is usually aware of a fast heart beat and may feel faint or breathless. Polyuria, mainly due to the release of atrial natriuretic peptide, is sometimes a feature, and cardiac pain or heart failure may occur if there is coexisting structural heart disease. The ECG (Fig. 18.44) usually shows a tachycardia with normal QRS complexes but occasionally there may be rate-dependent bundle branch block.

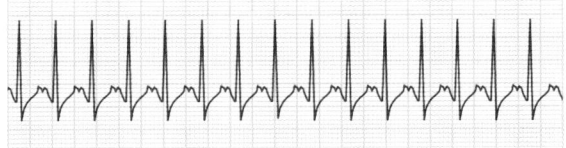

Fig. 18.44 Supraventricular tachycardia. The rate is 180/min and the QRS complexes are normal.

Management

Treatment is not always necessary. However, an episode may be terminated by carotid sinus pressure or other measures that increase vagal tone (e.g. Valsalva manœuvre). Intravenous adenosine or verapamil will restore sinus rhythm in most cases. Suitable alternative drugs include β-blockers or flecainide. In rare cases when there is severe haemodynamic compromise, the tachycardia should be terminated by DC cardioversion (p. 574).

If episodes are frequent or disabling, prophylactic oral therapy with a β-blocker or verapamil may be indicated. Catheter ablation (p. 575) offers a high chance of complete cure and is usually preferable to long-term drug treatment.

Wolff–Parkinson–White syndrome and atrioventricular re-entrant tachycardia

In these conditions, an abnormal band of conducting tissue connects the atria and ventricles. It resembles Purkinje tissue in that it conducts very rapidly, and is known as an accessory pathway. In around half of cases, this pathway only conducts in the retrograde direction (from ventricles to atria) and thus does not alter the appearance of the ECG in sinus rhythm. This is known as a concealed accessory pathway. In the remainder, conduction takes place partly through the AV node and partly through the accessory pathway. Premature activation of ventricular tissue via the pathway produces a short PR interval and a 'slurring' of the QRS complex, called a delta wave (Fig. 18.45B). This is known as a manifest accessory pathway. As the AV node and

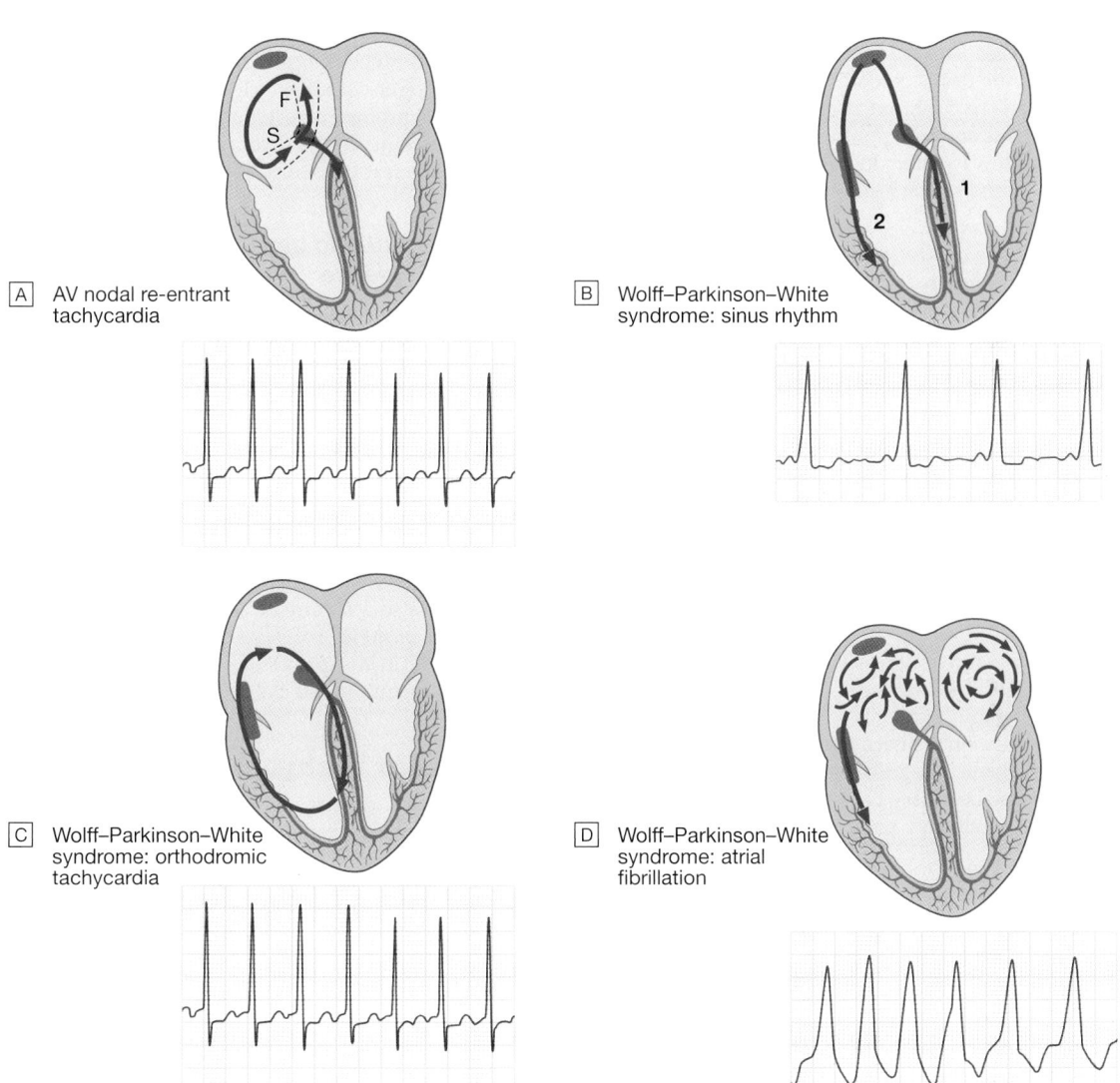

18

A   AV nodal re-entrant tachycardia

B   Wolff–Parkinson–White syndrome: sinus rhythm

C   Wolff–Parkinson–White syndrome: orthodromic tachycardia

D   Wolff–Parkinson–White syndrome: atrial fibrillation

Fig. 18.45 AV nodal re-entrant tachycardia (AVNRT) and Wolff–Parkinson–White (WPW) syndrome. A AV node re-entrant tachycardia. The mechanism of AVNRT occurs via two right atrial AV nodal input pathways: the slow (S) and fast (F) pathways. Antegrade conduction occurs via the slow pathway; the wavefront enters the AV node and passes into the ventricles, at the same time re-entering the atria via the fast pathway.

In WPW syndrome there is a strip of accessory conducting tissue that allows electricity to bypass the AV node and spread from the atria to the ventricles rapidly and without delay. When the ventricles are depolarised through the AV node the ECG is normal, but when the ventricles are depolarised through the accessory conducting tissue the ECG shows a very short PR interval and a broad QRS complex **B** Sinus rhythm. In sinus rhythm the ventricles are depolarised through (1) the AV node and (2) the accessory pathway, producing an ECG with a short PR interval and broadened QRS complexes; the characteristic slurring of the upstroke of the QRS complex is known as a delta wave. The degree of pre-excitation (the proportion of activation passing down the accessory pathway) and therefore the ECG appearances may vary a lot, and at times the ECG can look normal. **C** Orthodromic tachycardia. This is the most common form of tachycardia in WPW. The re-entry circuit passes antegradely through the AV node and retrogradely through the accessory pathway. The ventricles are therefore depolarised in the normal way, producing a narrow-complex tachycardia that is indistinguishable from other forms of SVT. **D** Atrial fibrillation. In this rhythm the ventricles are largely depolarised through the accessory pathway, producing an irregular broad-complex tachycardia which is often more rapid than the example shown.

accessory pathway have different conduction speeds and refractory periods, a re-entry circuit can develop, causing tachycardia (Fig. 18.45C); when this is associated with symptoms, the condition is known as Wolff–Parkinson–White syndrome. The ECG appearance of this tachycardia may be indistinguishable from that of AVNRT (Fig. 18.45A). Carotid sinus pressure or intravenous adenosine can terminate the tachycardia. If atrial fibrillation occurs, it may produce a dangerously rapid ventricular rate because the accessory pathway lacks the rate-limiting properties of the AV node (Fig. 18.45D). This is known as pre-excited atrial fibrillation and may cause collapse, syncope and even death. It should be treated as an emergency, usually with DC cardioversion.

Catheter ablation is first-line treatment in symptomatic patients and is nearly always curative. Prophylactic anti-arrhythmic drugs, such as flecainide, propafenone or amiodarone (p. 573), can also be used. These slow the conduction rate and prolong the refractory period of the accessory pathway. Digoxin and verapamil shorten the refractory period of the accessory pathway and should be avoided.

Ventricular tachyarrhythmias

Ventricular ectopic beats (extrasystoles, premature beats)

QRS complexes in sinus rhythm are normally narrow because the ventricles are activated rapidly and simultaneously via the His–Purkinje system. The complexes of ventricular ectopic beats are premature, broad and bizarre because the ventricles are activated one after the other, rather than simultaneously. The complexes may be unifocal (identical beats arising from a single ectopic focus) or multifocal (varying morphology with multiple foci, Fig. 18.46). 'Couplet' and 'triplet' are terms used to describe two or three successive ectopic beats, whereas a run of alternate sinus and ectopic beats is known as ventricular 'bigeminy'. Ectopic beats produce a low stroke volume because left ventricular contraction occurs before filling is complete. The pulse is therefore irregular, with weak or missed beats (see Fig. 18.46). Patients are usually asymptomatic but may complain of an irregular heart

beat, missed beats or abnormally strong beats (due to the increased output of the post-ectopic sinus beat). The significance of ventricular ectopic beats (VEBs) depends on the presence or absence of underlying heart disease.

Ventricular ectopic beats in otherwise healthy subjects

VEBs are frequently found in healthy people and their prevalence increases with age. Ectopic beats in patients with otherwise normal hearts are more prominent at rest and disappear with exercise. Treatment is not necessary unless the patient is highly symptomatic, in which case β-blockers can be used.

VEBs are sometimes a manifestation of otherwise subclinical heart disease, particularly coronary artery disease. There is no evidence that anti-arrhythmic therapy improves prognosis but the discovery of very frequent VEBs should prompt investigations such as an echocardiogram (looking for structural heart disease) and an exercise stress test (to detect underlying ischaemic heart disease).

Ventricular ectopic beats associated with heart disease

Frequent VEBs often occur during acute MI but need no treatment. Persistent, frequent (> 10/hour) ventricular ectopic beats in patients who have survived the acute phase of MI indicate a poor long-term outcome. Other than β-blockers, anti-arrhythmic drugs do not improve and may even worsen prognosis.

VEBs are common in patients with heart failure, when they are associated with an adverse prognosis, but again the outlook is no better if they are suppressed with anti-arrhythmic drugs. Effective treatment of the heart failure may suppress the ectopic beats.

VEBs are also a feature of digoxin toxicity, are sometimes found in mitral valve prolapse, and may occur as 'escape beats' in the presence of an underlying bradycardia. Treatment should be directed at the underlying condition.

Ventricular tachycardia (VT)

The common causes of VT include acute MI, cardiomyopathy and chronic ischaemic heart disease,

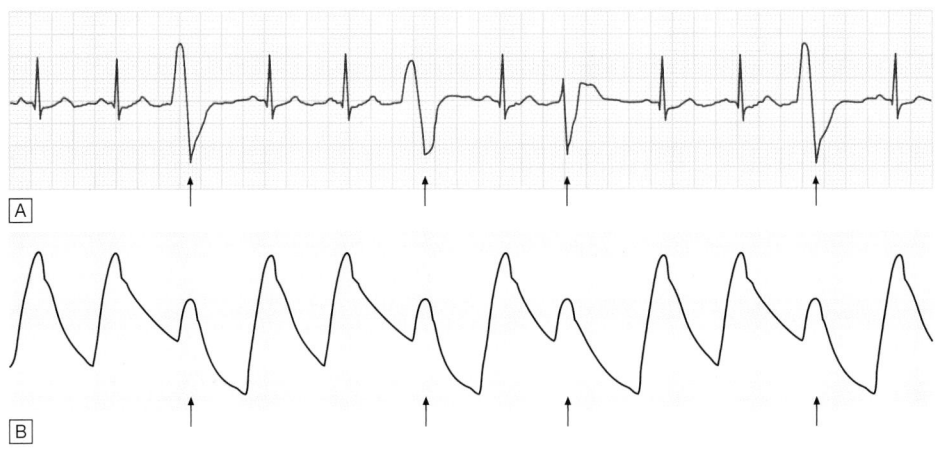

Fig. 18.46 Ventricular ectopic beats. **A** There are broad bizarre QRS complexes (arrows) with no preceding P wave in between normal sinus beats. Their configuration varies, so these are multifocal ectopics. **B** A simultaneous arterial pressure trace is shown. The ectopic beats result in a weaker pulse (arrows), which may be perceived as a 'dropped beat'.

particularly when it is associated with a ventricular aneurysm or poor left ventricular function. In these settings it is serious because it may cause haemodynamic compromise or degenerate into ventricular fibrillation (p. 555). It is caused by abnormal automaticity or triggered activity in ischaemic tissue, or by re-entry within scarred ventricular tissue. Patients may complain of palpitation or symptoms of low cardiac output, such as dizziness, dyspnoea or syncope. The ECG shows tachycardia with broad, abnormal QRS complexes with a rate > 120/min (Fig. 18.47). VT may be difficult to distinguish from SVT with bundle branch block or pre-excitation (WPW syndrome). Features in favour of a diagnosis of VT are listed in Box 18.34. A 12-lead (Fig. 18.48) or intracardiac ECG may help to establish the diagnosis. When there is doubt, it is safer to manage the problem as VT.

Patients recovering from MI sometimes have periods of idioventricular rhythm ('slow' VT) at a rate only slightly above the preceding sinus rate and below 120/min. These episodes often reflect reperfusion of the infarct territory and may be a good sign. They are usually self-limiting and asymptomatic, and do not require treatment. Other forms of VT, if they last for more than a few beats, will require treatment, often as an emergency.

VT occasionally occurs in patients with otherwise healthy hearts ('normal heart VT'), usually because of abnormal automaticity in the right ventricular outflow tract or one of the fascicles of the left bundle branch. The prognosis is good and catheter ablation can be curative.

Management

Prompt action to restore sinus rhythm is required and should usually be followed by prophylactic therapy. Synchronised DC cardioversion is the treatment of choice if systolic BP is < 90 mmHg. If the arrhythmia is well tolerated, intravenous amiodarone may be given as a bolus followed by a continuous infusion (p. 573).

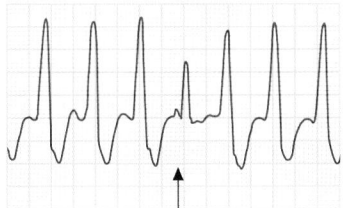

Fig. 18.47 Ventricular tachycardia: fusion beat (arrow). In ventricular tachycardia there is independent atrial and ventricular activity. Occasionally a P wave is conducted to the ventricles through the AV node, producing a normal sinus beat in the middle of the tachycardia (a capture beat); however, more commonly the conducted impulse fuses with an impulse from the tachycardia (a fusion beat). This can only occur when there is AV dissociation and is therefore diagnostic of ventricular tachycardia.

18.34 Features in favour of ventricular tachycardia in the differential diagnosis of broad-complex tachycardia

- History of MI
- AV dissociation (pathognomonic)
- Capture/fusion beats (pathognomonic, see Fig. 18.47)
- Extreme left axis deviation
- Very broad QRS complexes (> 140 ms)
- No response to carotid sinus massage or i.v. adenosine

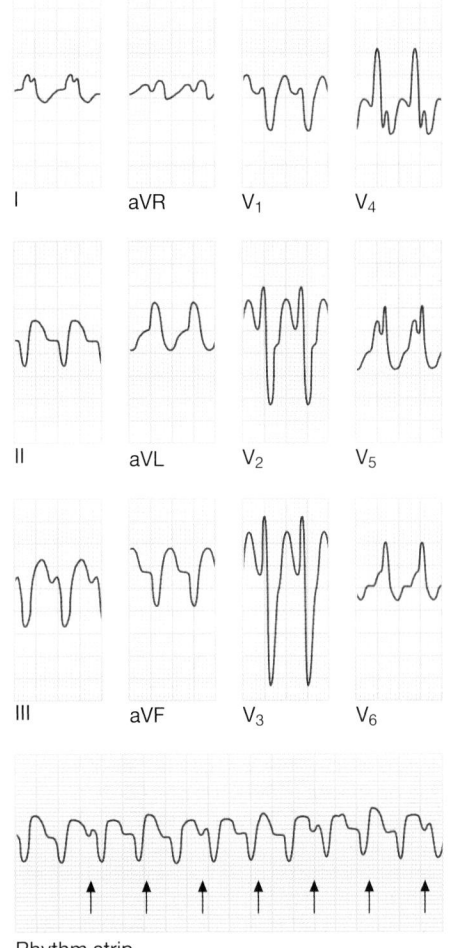

Rhythm strip

Fig. 18.48 Ventricular tachycardia: 12-lead ECG. There are typically very broad QRS complexes and marked left axis deviation. There is also AV dissociation; some P waves are visible and others are buried in the QRS complexes (arrows).

Intravenous lidocaine can be used but may depress left ventricular function, causing hypotension or acute heart failure. Hypokalaemia, hypomagnesaemia, acidosis and hypoxaemia should be corrected.

Beta-blockers are effective at preventing VT by reducing automaticity and by blocking conduction in scar re-entry circuits. Amiodarone can be added if additional control is needed. Class Ic anti-arrhythmic drugs should not be used for prevention of VT in patients with ischaemic heart disease or heart failure because they depress myocardial function and can be pro-arrhythmic (increase the likelihood of a dangerous arrhythmia). In patients at high risk of arrhythmic death (e.g. those with poor left ventricular function, or where VT is associated with haemodynamic compromise), the use of an implantable cardiac defibrillator is recommended (p. 576). Rarely, surgery or catheter ablation can be used to interrupt the arrhythmia focus or circuit.

Torsades de pointes (ventricular tachycardia)

This form of polymorphic VT is a complication of prolonged ventricular repolarisation (prolonged QT interval).

18

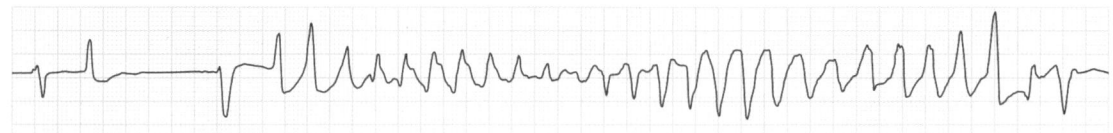

Fig. 18.49 Torsades de pointes. A bradycardia with a long QT interval is followed by polymorphic VT that is triggered by an R on T ectopic.

 18.35 Causes of long QT interval and torsades de pointes

Bradycardia

- Bradycardia compounds other factors that cause torsades de pointes

Electrolyte disturbance

- Hypokalaemia
- Hypomagnesaemia
- Hypocalcaemia

Drugs

- Disopyramide (and other class Ia anti-arrhythmic drugs, p. 573)
- Sotalol, amiodarone (and other class III anti-arrhythmic drugs)
- Amitriptyline (and other tricyclic antidepressants)
- Chlorpromazine (and other phenothiazines)
- Erythromycin (and other macrolides)

… and many more

Congenital syndromes

- LQT1: gene affected *KCNQI:* K$^+$ channel, 30–35%
- LQT2: gene affected *HERG:* K$^+$ channel, 25–30%
- LQT3: gene affected *SCNSA:* Na$^+$ channel, 5–10%
- LQT4–12: rare

The ECG shows rapid irregular complexes that oscillate from an upright to an inverted position and seem to twist around the baseline as the mean QRS axis changes (Fig. 18.49). The arrhythmia is usually non-sustained and repetitive but may degenerate into ventricular fibrillation. During periods of sinus rhythm, the ECG will usually show a prolonged QT interval (> 0.42 s at a rate of 60/min).

Some of the common causes are listed in Box 18.35. The arrhythmia is more common in women and is often triggered by a combination of aetiological factors (e.g. QT-prolonging medications and hypokalaemia). The congenital long QT syndromes are a family of genetic disorders that are characterised by mutations in genes that code for cardiac sodium or potassium channels. Long QT syndrome subtypes have different triggers which are important when counselling patients. Adrenergic stimulation (e.g. exercise) is a common trigger in long QT type 1, and a sudden noise (e.g. an alarm clock) may trigger arrhythmias in long QT type 2. Arrhythmias are more common during sleep in type 3.

Treatment should be directed at the underlying cause. Intravenous magnesium (8 mmol over 15 minutes, then 72 mmol over 24 hours) should be given in all cases. Atrial pacing will usually suppress the arrhythmia through rate-dependent shortening of the QT interval. Intravenous isoprenaline is a reasonable alternative to pacing but should be avoided in patients with the congenital long QT syndromes.

Long-term therapy may not be necessary if the underlying cause can be removed. Beta-blockers are effective at preventing syncope in patients with congenital long QT syndrome. Some patients, particularly those with extreme QT interval prolongation (> 500 ms) or certain high-risk genotypes should be considered for implantation of a defibrillator. Left stellate ganglion block may be of value in patients with resistant arrhythmias.

The Brugada syndrome is a related genetic disorder that may present with polymorphic VT or sudden death. It is characterised by a defect in sodium channel function and an abnormal ECG (right bundle branch block and ST elevation in V$_1$ and V$_2$ but not usually prolongation of the QT interval).

Sinoatrial disease (sick sinus syndrome)

Sinoatrial disease can occur at any age but is most common in older people. The underlying pathology involves fibrosis, degenerative changes or ischaemia of the SA (sinus) node. The condition is characterised by a variety of arrhythmias (Box 18.36) and may present with palpitation, dizzy spells or syncope, due to intermittent tachycardia, bradycardia, or pauses with no atrial or ventricular activity (SA block or sinus arrest) (Fig. 18.50).

A permanent pacemaker may benefit patients with troublesome symptoms due to spontaneous bradycardias, or those with symptomatic bradycardias induced by drugs required to prevent tachyarrhythmias. Atrial pacing may help to prevent episodes of atrial fibrillation. Permanent pacing improves symptoms but not prognosis, and is not indicated in patients who are asymptomatic.

 18.36 Common features of sinoatrial disease

- Sinus bradycardia
- SA block (sinus arrest)
- Paroxysmal atrial tachycardia
- Paroxysmal atrial fibrillation
- AV block

Atrioventricular and bundle branch block

AV block

AV conduction is influenced by autonomic activity. AV block can therefore be intermittent and may only be evident when the conducting tissue is stressed by a rapid atrial rate. Accordingly, atrial tachyarrhythmias are often associated with AV block (see Fig. 18.43, p. 562).

First-degree AV block

In this condition, AV conduction is delayed so the PR interval is prolonged (> 0.20 s; Fig. 18.51). It rarely causes symptoms.

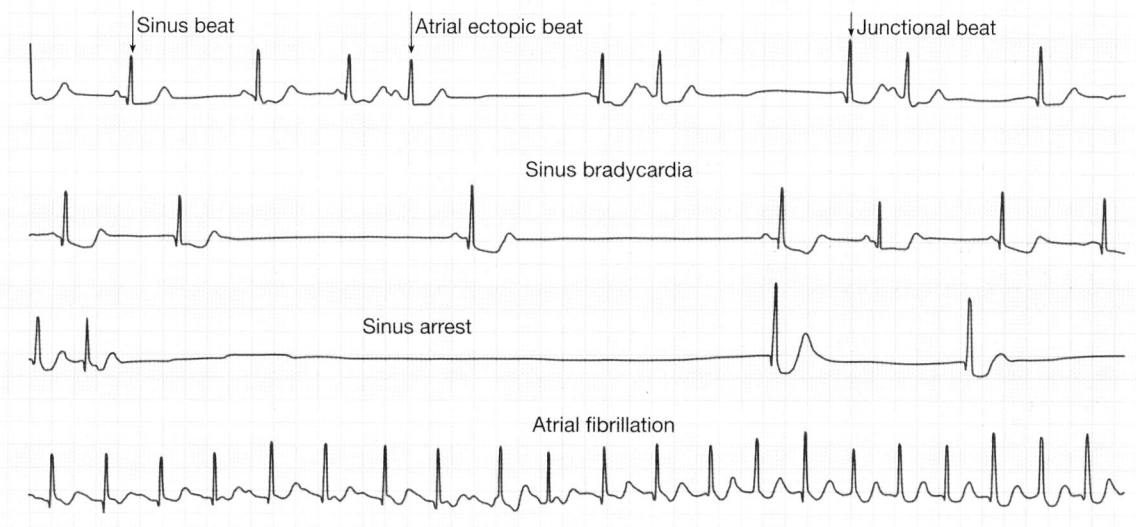

Sinus beat   Atrial ectopic beat   Junctional beat

Sinus bradycardia

Sinus arrest

Atrial fibrillation

Fig. 18.50 Sinoatrial disease (sick sinus syndrome). A continuous rhythm strip from a 24-hour ECG tape recording illustrating periods of sinus rhythm, atrial ectopics, junctional beats, sinus bradycardia, sinus arrest and paroxysmal atrial fibrillation.

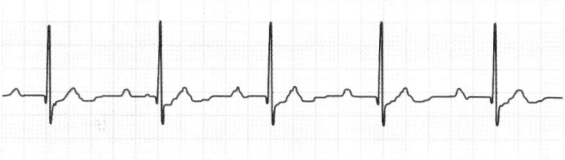

Fig. 18.51 First-degree AV block. The PR interval is prolonged and measures 0.26 s.

Second-degree AV block

In this condition dropped beats occur because some impulses from the atria fail to conduct to the ventricles.

In Mobitz type I second-degree AV block (Fig. 18.52) there is progressive lengthening of successive PR inter-

vals, culminating in a dropped beat. The cycle then repeats itself. This is known as Wenckebach's phenomenon and is usually due to impaired conduction in the AV node itself. The phenomenon may be physiological and is sometimes observed at rest or during sleep in athletic young adults with high vagal tone.

In Mobitz type II second-degree AV block (Fig. 18.53) the PR interval of the conducted impulses remains constant but some P waves are not conducted. This is usually caused by disease of the His–Purkinje system and carries a risk of asystole.

In 2:1 AV block (Fig. 18.54) alternate P waves are conducted, so it is impossible to distinguish between Mobitz type I and type II block.

Third-degree (complete) AV block

When AV conduction fails completely, the atria and ventricles beat independently (AV dissociation, Fig. 18.55).

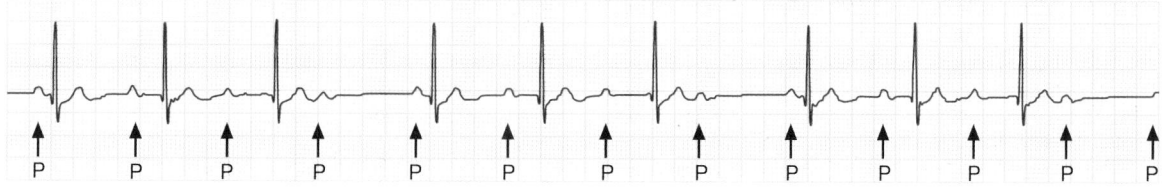

P   P   P   P   P   P   P   P   P   P   P   P   P

Fig. 18.52 Second-degree AV block (Mobitz type I—Wenckebach's phenomenon). The PR interval progressively increases until a P wave is not conducted. The cycle then repeats itself. In this example, conduction is at a ratio of 4:3, leading to groupings of three ventricular complexes in a row.

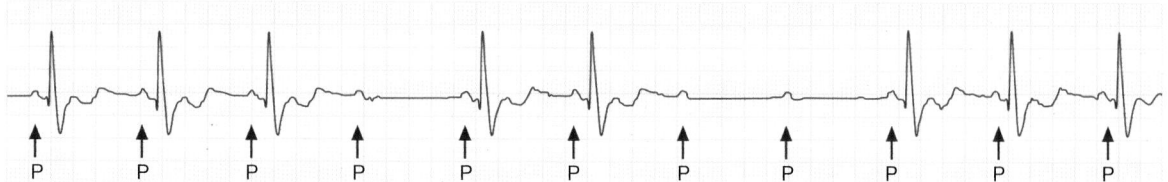

P   P   P   P   P   P   P   P   P   P   P

Fig. 18.53 Second-degree AV block (Mobitz type II). The PR interval of conducted beats is normal but some P waves are not conducted. The constant PR interval distinguishes this from Wenckebach's phenomenon.

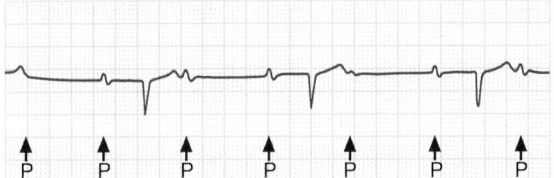

Fig. 18.54 Second-degree AV block with fixed 2:1 block. Alternate P waves are not conducted. This may be due to Mobitz type I or II block.

18.37 Aetiology of complete AV block

Congenital

Acquired
- Idiopathic fibrosis
- MI/ischaemia
- Inflammation
  Acute (e.g. aortic root abscess in infective endocarditis)
  Chronic (e.g. sarcoidosis, p. 708; Chagas disease, p. 354)
- Trauma (e.g. cardiac surgery)
- Drugs (e.g. digoxin, β-blocker)

Ventricular activity is maintained by an escape rhythm arising in the AV node or bundle of His (narrow QRS complexes) or the distal Purkinje tissues (broad QRS complexes). Distal escape rhythms tend to be slower and less reliable.

Complete AV block (Box 18.37) produces a slow (25–50/min), regular pulse that, except in the case of congenital complete AV block, does not vary with exercise. There is usually a compensatory increase in stroke volume producing a large-volume pulse. Cannon waves may be visible in the neck and the intensity of the first heart sound varies due to the loss of AV synchrony.

Stokes–Adams attacks

Episodes of ventricular asystole may complicate complete heart block or Mobitz type II second-degree AV block, or occur in patients with sinoatrial disease (see Fig. 18.50). This may cause recurrent syncope or 'Stokes–Adams' attacks.

A typical episode is characterised by sudden loss of consciousness that occurs without warning and results in collapse. A brief anoxic seizure (due to cerebral ischaemia) may occur if there is prolonged asystole. There is pallor and a death-like appearance during the attack, but when the heart starts beating again there is a characteristic flush. Unlike epilepsy, recovery is rapid. Sinoatrial disease and neurocardiogenic syncope (p. 552) may cause similar symptoms.

Management

AV block complicating acute MI

Acute inferior MI is often complicated by transient AV block because the RCA supplies the AV node. There is usually a reliable escape rhythm and, if the patient remains well, no treatment is required. Symptomatic second- or third-degree AV block may respond to atropine (0.6 mg i.v., repeated as necessary) or, if this fails, a temporary pacemaker. In most cases the AV block will resolve within 7–10 days.

Second- or third-degree AV heart block complicating acute anterior MI indicates extensive ventricular damage involving both bundle branches and carries a poor prognosis. Asystole may ensue and a temporary pacemaker

should be inserted promptly. If the patient presents with asystole, i.v. atropine (3 mg) or i.v. isoprenaline (2 mg in 500 ml 5% dextrose, infused at 10–60 mL/hour) may help to maintain the circulation until a temporary pacing electrode can be inserted. External (transcutaneous) pacing can provide effective temporary rhythm support.

Chronic AV block

Patients with symptomatic bradyarrhythmias associated with AV block should receive a permanent pacemaker (see below). Asymptomatic first-degree or Mobitz type I second-degree AV block (Wenckebach phenomenon) does not require treatment but may be an indication of serious underlying heart disease. A permanent pacemaker is usually indicated in patients with asymptomatic Mobitz type II second- or third-degree AV heart block because of the risk of asystole and sudden death. Pacing improves prognosis.

Bundle branch block and hemiblock

Conduction block in the right or left bundle branch can occur as a result of many pathologies, including ischaemic or hypertensive heart disease or cardiomyopathies (Box 18.38). Depolarisation proceeds

18.38 Common causes of bundle branch block

Right bundle branch block

- Normal variant
- Right ventricular hypertrophy or strain, e.g. pulmonary embolism
- Congenital heart disease, e.g. atrial septal defect
- Coronary artery disease

Left bundle branch block

- Coronary artery disease
- Hypertension
- Aortic valve disease
- Cardiomyopathy

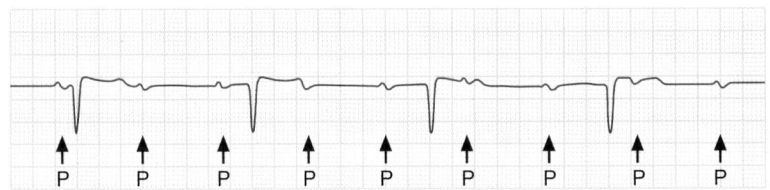

Fig. 18.55 Complete (third-degree) AV block. There is complete dissociation of atrial and ventricular complexes. The atrial rate is 80/min and the ventricular rate is 38/min.

through a slow myocardial route in the affected ventricle rather than through the rapidly conducting Purkinje tissues that constitute the bundle branches. This causes delayed conduction into the LV or RV, broadens the QRS complex (≥ 0.12 s) and produces the characteristic alterations in QRS morphology (Figs 18.56 and 18.57). Right bundle branch block (RBBB) can occur in healthy people but left bundle branch block (LBBB) often signifies important underlying heart disease.

The left bundle branch divides into an anterior and a posterior fascicle. Damage to the conducting tissue at this point (hemiblock) does not broaden the QRS complex but alters the mean direction of ventricular depolarisation (mean QRS axis), causing left axis deviation in left anterior hemiblock and right axis deviation in left posterior hemiblock (see Fig. 18.8, p. 530). The combination of right bundle branch and left anterior or posterior hemiblock is known as bifascicular block.

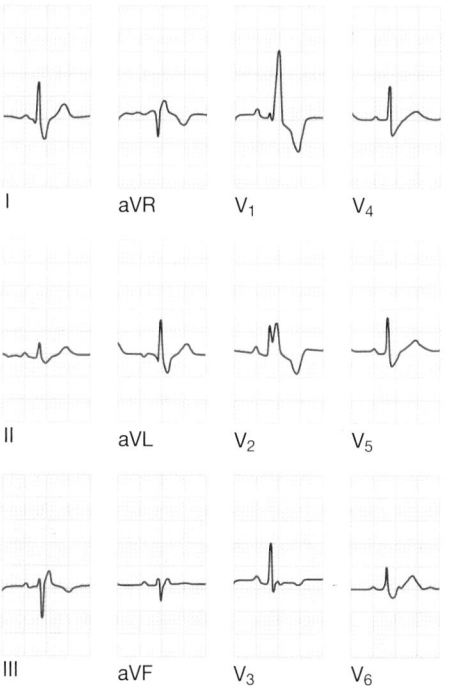

Fig. 18.56 Right bundle branch block. Note the wide QRS complexes with 'M'-shaped configuration in leads V_1 and V_2 and a wide S wave in lead I.

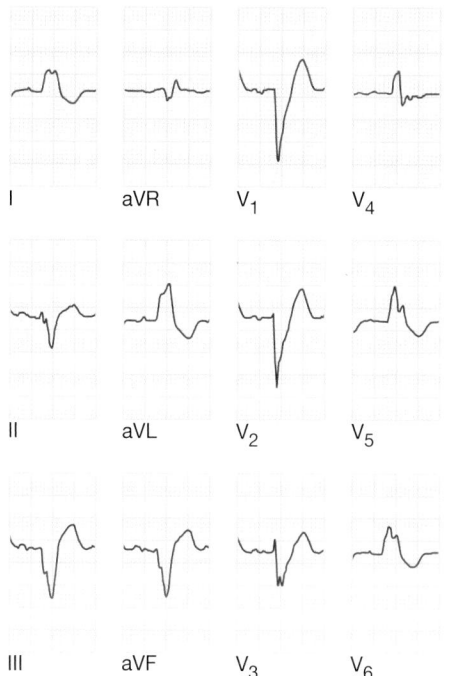

Fig. 18.57 Left bundle branch block. Note the wide QRS complexes with the loss of the Q wave or septal vector in lead I and 'M'-shaped QRS complexes in V_5 and V_6.

Anti-arrhythmic drug therapy

The classification of anti-arrhythmic drugs

These agents may be classified according to their mode or site of action (Box 18.39 and Fig. 18.58). Identification of ion channel subtypes has led to refinement of drug classifications according to the specific mechanisms targeted. The Vaughn Williams classification is a crude system, but is convenient for describing the main mode of action of anti-arrhythmic drugs (Box 18.40) that should be used following guiding principles (Box 18.41). Anti-arrhythmic drugs can also be more accurately categorised by referring to the cardiac ion channels and receptors on which they act.

Class I drugs

Class I drugs act principally by suppressing excitability and slowing conduction in atrial or ventricular muscle. They act by blocking sodium channels, of which there are several types in cardiac tissue. These drugs should generally be avoided in patients with heart failure because they depress myocardial function, and class Ia and Ic drugs are often pro-arrhythmic.

Class Ia drugs

These prolong cardiac action potential duration and increase the tissue refractory period. They are used to prevent both atrial and ventricular arrhythmias.

 18.39 Classification of anti-arrhythmic drugs according to effect on the intracellular action potential

Class I: membrane-stabilising agents (sodium channel blockers)

(a) **Block Na^+ channel and prolong action potential**
• Quinidine, disopyramide
(b) **Block Na^+ channel and shorten action potential**
• Lidocaine, mexiletine
(c) **Block Na^+ channel with no effect on action potential**
• Flecainide, propafenone

Class II: β-adrenoceptor antagonists (β-blockers)

• Atenolol, bisoprolol, metoprolol, l-sotalol

Class III: drugs whose main effect is to prolong the action potential

• Amiodarone, d-sotalol

Class IV: slow calcium channel blockers

• Verapamil, diltiazem

N.B. Some drugs (e.g. digoxin and adenosine) have no place in this classification, while others have properties in more than one class: e.g. amiodarone, which has actions in all four classes.

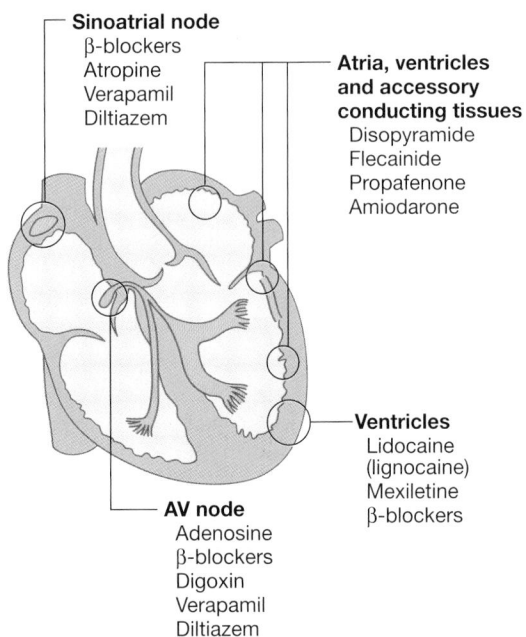

Sinoatrial node
β-blockers
Atropine
Verapamil
Diltiazem

Atria, ventricles and accessory conducting tissues
Disopyramide
Flecainide
Propafenone
Amiodarone

Ventricles
Lidocaine (lignocaine)
Mexiletine
β-blockers

AV node
Adenosine
β-blockers
Digoxin
Verapamil
Diltiazem

Fig. 18.58 Classification of anti-arrhythmic drugs by site of action.

Disopyramide. An effective drug but causes anticholinergic side-effects, such as urinary retention, and can precipitate glaucoma. It can depress myocardial function and should be avoided in cardiac failure.

Quinidine. Now rarely used, as it increases mortality and causes gastrointestinal upset.

Class Ib drugs

These shorten the action potential and tissue refractory period. They act on channels found predominantly in ventricular myocardium so are used to treat or prevent VT and VF.

Lidocaine. Must be given intravenously and has a very short plasma half-life.

Mexiletine. Can be given intravenously or orally, but has many side-effects (see Box 18.40).

Class Ic drugs

These affect the slope of the action potential without altering its duration or refractory period. They are used mainly for prophylaxis of AF but are effective in prophylaxis and treatment of supraventricular or ventricular arrhythmias. They are useful for WPW syndrome because they block conduction in accessory pathways. They should not be used as oral prophylaxis in patients with previous MI because of pro-arrhythmia.

Flecainide. Effective for prevention of atrial fibrillation, and an intravenous infusion may be used for pharmacological cardioversion of atrial fibrillation of less than 24 hours' duration. It should be prescribed along with an AV node-blocking drug, such as a β-blocker, to prevent pro-arrhythmia.

Propafenone. Also has some β-blocker (class II) properties. Important interactions with digoxin, warfarin and cimetidine have been described.

Class II drugs

This group comprises the β-adrenoceptor antagonists (β-blockers). These agents reduce the rate of SA node

depolarisation and cause relative block in the AV node, making them useful for rate control in atrial flutter and AF. They can be used to prevent supraventricular and ventricular tachycardia. They reduce myocardial excitability and reduce risk of arrhythmic death in patients with coronary heart disease and heart failure.

'Non-selective' β-blockers. Act on both β_1 and β_2 receptors. β_2 blockade causes side-effects such as bronchospasm and peripheral vasoconstriction. *Propranolol* is non-selective and is subject to extensive first-pass metabolism in the liver. The effective oral dose is therefore unpredictable and must be titrated after treatment is started with a small dose. Other non-selective drugs include *nadolol* and *carvedilol*.

'Cardioselective' β-blockers. Act mainly on myocardial β_1 receptors and are relatively well tolerated. *Atenolol*, *bisoprolol* and *metoprolol* are all cardioselective β-blockers.

Sotalol. A racemic mixture of two isomers with non-selective β-blocker (mainly l-sotalol) and class III (mainly d-sotalol) activity. It may cause torsades de pointes.

Class III drugs

Class III drugs act by prolonging the plateau phase of the action potential, thus lengthening the refractory period. These drugs are very effective at preventing atrial and ventricular tachyarrhythmias. They cause QT interval prolongation and can predispose to torsades de pointes and VT (p. 566), especially in patients with other predisposing risk factors (see Box 18.35, p. 568).

Amiodarone. The principal drug in this class, although both disopyramide and sotalol have class III activity. Amiodarone is a complex drug that also has class I, II and IV activity. It is probably the most effective drug currently available for controlling paroxysmal AF. It is also used to prevent episodes of recurrent VT, particularly in patients with poor left ventricular function or those with implantable defibrillators (to prevent unnecessary DC shocks). Amiodarone has a very long tissue half-life (25–110 days). An intravenous or oral loading regime is often used to achieve therapeutic tissue concentrations rapidly. The drug's effects may last for weeks or months after treatment has been stopped. Side-effects are common (up to one-third of patients), numerous and potentially serious. Drug interactions are also common (see Box 18.40).

Dronedarone. A related drug that has a short tissue half-life and fewer side effects. It has recently been shown to be effective at preventing episodes of atrial flutter and fibrillation.

Class IV drugs

These block the 'slow calcium channel' which is important for impulse generation and conduction in atrial and nodal tissue, although it is also present in ventricular muscle. Their main indications are prevention of SVT (by blocking the AV node) and rate control in patients with AF.

Verapamil. The most widely used drug in this class. Intravenous verapamil may cause profound bradycardia or hypotension, and should not be used in conjunction with β-blockers.

Diltiazem. Has similar properties.

18.40 The main uses, dosages and side-effects of the most widely used anti-arrhythmic drugs

Drug	Main uses	Route	Dose (adult)	Important side-effects
Class I				
Disopyramide	Prevention and treatment of atrial and ventricular tachyarrhythmias	I.v.	2 mg/kg at 30 mg/min, then 0.4 mg/kg/hr (max 800 mg/day)	Myocardial depression, hypotension, dry mouth, urinary retention
		Oral	300–800 mg daily in divided dosage	
Lidocaine	Treatment and short-term prevention of VT and VF	I.v.	Bolus 50–100 mg, 4 mg/min for 30 mins, then 2 mg/min for 2 hrs, then 1 mg/min for 24 hrs	Myocardial depression, confusion, convulsions
Mexiletine	Prevention and treatment of ventricular tachyarrhythmias	I.v.	Loading dose: 100–250 mg at 25 mg/min, then 250 mg in 1 hr, then 250 mg in 2 hrs Maintenance therapy: 0.5 mg/min	Myocardial depression, GI irritation, confusion, dizziness, tremor, nystagmus, ataxia
		Oral	200–250 mg 8-hourly	
Flecainide	Prevention and treatment of atrial and ventricular tachyarrhythmias	I.v.	2 mg/kg over 10 mins, then 1.5 mg/kg/hr for 1 hr, then 0.1 mg/kg/hr	Myocardial depression, dizziness
		Oral	50–100 mg 12-hourly	
Propafenone	Prevention and treatment of atrial and ventricular tachyarrhythmias	Oral	150 mg 8-hourly for 1 wk, then 300 mg 12-hourly	Myocardial depression, dizziness
Class II				
Atenolol		I.v.	2.5 mg at 1 mg/min repeated at 5-min intervals (max 10 mg)	Myocardial depression, bradycardia, bronchospasm, fatigue, depression, nightmares, cold peripheries
		Oral	25–100 mg daily	
Bisoprolol	Treatment and prevention of SVT and AF Prevention of VEs and exercise-induced VT	Oral	2.5–10 mg daily	
Metoprolol		I.v.	5 mg over 2 mins to a maximum of 15 mg	
		Oral	50–100 mg 8- or 12-hourly	
Sotalol		I.v.	10–20 mg slowly	Sotalol can cause torsades de pointes
		Oral	40–160 mg 12-hourly	
Class III				
Amiodarone	Serious or resistant atrial and ventricular tachyarrhythmias	I.v.	5 mg/kg over 20–120 mins, then up to 15 mg/kg/24 hrs	Photosensitivity, skin discoloration, corneal deposits, thyroid dysfunction, alveolitis, nausea and vomiting, hepatotoxicity, peripheral neuropathy, torsades de pointes; potentiates digoxin and warfarin
		Oral	Initially 600–1200 mg/day, then 100–400 mg daily	
Class IV				
Verapamil	Treatment of SVT, control of AF	I.v.	5–10 mg over 30 secs	Myocardial depression, hypotension, bradycardia, constipation
		Oral	40–120 mg 8-hourly or 240 mg SR daily	
Other				
Atropine	Treatment of bradycardia and/or hypotension due to vagal overactivity	I.v.	0.6–3 mg	Dry mouth, thirst, blurred vision, atrial and ventricular extrasystoles
Adenosine	Treatment of SVT, aid to diagnosis in unidentified tachycardia	I.v.	3 mg over 2 secs, followed if necessary by 6 mg, then 12 mg at intervals of 1–2 mins	Flushing, dyspnoea, chest pain Avoid in asthma
Digoxin	Treatment and prevention of SVT, rate control of AF	I.v.	Loading dose: 0.5–1 mg (total), 0.5 mg over 30 mins, then 0.25–0.5 mg 4- to 8-hourly to maximum total of 1 mg, assessing response before each additional dose	GI disturbance, xanthopsia, arrhythmias (see Box 18.43)
		Oral	0.5 mg 6-hourly for 2 doses, then 0.125–0.25 mg daily	

(AF = atrial fibrillation; SR = sustained-release formulation; SVT = supraventricular tachycardia; VE = ventricular ectopic; VF = ventricular fibrillation; VT = ventricular tachycardia)

18

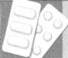

18.41 Anti-arrhythmic drugs: principles of use

Anti-arrhythmic drugs are potentially toxic and should be used carefully according to the following principles:

- Many arrhythmias are benign and do not require specific treatment
- Precipitating or causal factors should be corrected if possible, e.g. excess alcohol or caffeine consumption, myocardial ischaemia, hyperthyroidism, acidosis, hypokalaemia and hypomagnesaemia
- If drug therapy is required, it is best to use as few drugs as possible
- In difficult cases, programmed electrical stimulation (electrophysiological study) may help to identify the optimum therapy
- When managing life-threatening arrhythmias, it is essential to ensure that prophylactic treatment is effective. Ambulatory monitoring and exercise testing may be of value
- Patients on long-term anti-arrhythmic drugs should be reviewed regularly and attempts made to withdraw therapy if the factors which precipitated the arrhythmias are no longer operative
- For patients with recurrent SVT, radiofrequency ablation is often preferable to long-term drug therapy

Other anti-arrhythmic drugs

Atropine sulphate (0.6 mg i.v., repeated if necessary to a maximum of 3 mg). Increases the sinus rate and SA and AV conduction, and is the treatment of choice for severe bradycardia or hypotension due to vagal overactivity. It is used for initial management of symptomatic bradyarrhythmias complicating inferior MI, and in cardiac arrest due to asystole. Repeat dosing may be necessary because the drug disappears rapidly from the circulation after parenteral administration. Side-effects are listed in Box 18.40.

Adenosine. Must be given intravenously. It produces transient AV block lasting a few seconds. Accordingly, it may be used to terminate SVTs when the AV node is part of the re-entry circuit, or to help establish the diagnosis in difficult arrhythmias such as atrial flutter with 2:1 AV block (see Fig. 18.40, p. 561) or broad-complex tachycardia (Boxes 18.40 and 18.42). Adenosine is given as an intravenous bolus, initially 3 mg over 2 seconds (see Box 18.40). If there is no response after 1–2 minutes, 6 mg should be given; if necessary, after another 1–2 minutes, the maximum dose of 12 mg may be given. Patients should be warned that they may experience short-lived and sometimes distressing flushing, breathlessness and chest pain. Adenosine can cause bronchospasm and should be avoided in asthmatics; its effects are greatly potentiated by dipyridamole and inhibited by theophylline and other xanthines.

Digoxin. A purified glycoside from the European foxglove, *Digitalis lanata*, which slows conduction and

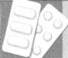

18.42 Response to intravenous adenosine

Arrhythmia	Response
Supraventricular tachycardia	Termination
Atrial fibrillation, atrial flutter	Transient AV block
Ventricular tachycardia	No effect

18.43 Digoxin toxicity

Extracardiac manifestations

- Anorexia, nausea, vomiting
- Diarrhoea
- Altered colour vision (xanthopsia)

Cardiac manifestations

- Bradycardia
- Multiple ventricular ectopics
- Ventricular bigeminy (alternate ventricular ectopics)
- Atrial tachycardia (with variable block)
- VT
- VF

prolongs the refractory period in the AV node. This effect helps to control the ventricular rate in AF and may interrupt SVTs involving the AV node. On the other hand, digoxin tends to shorten refractory periods and enhance excitability and conduction in other parts of the heart (including accessory conduction pathways). It may therefore increase atrial and ventricular ectopic activity and can lead to more complex atrial and ventricular tachyarrhythmias. Digoxin is largely excreted by the kidneys, and the maintenance dose (see Box 18.40) should be reduced in children, older people and those with renal impairment. It is widely distributed and has a long tissue half-life (36 hours), so that effects may persist for several days after the last dose. Measurements of plasma digoxin concentration are useful in demonstrating whether the dose is inadequate or excessive (Box 18.43).

Therapeutic procedures

External defibrillation and cardioversion

The heart can be completely depolarised by passing a sufficiently large electrical current through it from an external source. This will interrupt any arrhythmia and produce a brief period of asystole that is usually followed by the resumption of sinus rhythm. Defibrillators deliver a DC, high-energy, short-duration shock via two metal paddles coated with conducting jelly or a gel pad, positioned over the upper right sternal edge and the apex. Modern units deliver a biphasic shock, during which the shock polarity is reversed mid-shock. This reduces the total shock energy required to depolarise the heart.

Electrical cardioversion

This is the termination of an organised rhythm such as AF or VT with a synchronised shock, usually under general anaesthesia. The shock is delivered immediately after detection of the R wave, because if it is applied during ventricular repolarisation (on the T wave) it may provoke VF. High-energy shocks may cause chest wall pain post-procedure, so if there is no urgency it is appropriate to begin with a lower-amplitude shock (e.g. 50 joules), going on to larger shocks if necessary. Patients with atrial fibrillation or flutter of > 48 hours' duration are at risk of systemic embolism after cardioversion, so it should be ensured that the patient is adequately anticoagulated for at least 4 weeks before and after the procedure.

Defibrillation

This is the delivery of an unsynchronised shock during a cardiac arrest caused by VF. The precise timing of the discharge is not important in this situation. In VF and other emergencies, the energy of the first and second shocks should be 150 joules and thereafter up to 200 joules; there is no need for an anaesthetic as the patient is unconscious.

Catheter ablation

Catheter ablation therapy has become the treatment of choice for many patients with recurrent arrhythmias (see Fig. 18.15, p. 536). A series of catheter electrodes are inserted into the heart via the venous system and are used to record the activation sequence of the heart in sinus rhythm, during tachycardia and after pacing manœuvres. Once the arrhythmia focus or circuit is identified, a steerable catheter is placed into this critical zone (e.g. over an accessory pathway in WPW syndrome) and the culprit tissue is selectively ablated using heat (via radiofrequency current) or sometimes by freezing (cryoablation). The procedure takes approximately 1–3 hours and does not require a general anaesthetic. The patient may experience some discomfort during the ablation itself. Serious complications are rare (< 1%) but include inadvertent complete heart block requiring pacemaker implantation, and cardiac tamponade. For many arrhythmias, radiofrequency ablation is very attractive because it offers the prospect of a lifetime cure, thereby eliminating the need for long-term drug therapy.

The technique has revolutionised the management of many arrhythmias and is now the treatment of choice for AVNRT and AV re-entrant (accessory pathway) tachycardias, when it is curative in > 90% of cases. Focal atrial tachycardias and atrial flutter can also be eliminated by radiofrequency ablation, although some patients subsequently experience episodes of AF. The applications of the technique are expanding and it can now be used to treat some forms of VT. Recently, catheter ablation techniques have been developed to prevent AF. This involves ablation at two sites: the ostia of the pulmonary veins, from which ectopic beats may trigger paroxysms of arrhythmia, and in the LA itself, where re-entry circuits maintain AF once established. This is effective at reducing episodes of AF in around 70–80% of younger patients with structurally normal hearts, and tends to be reserved for patients with drug-resistant AF.

Exceptionally troublesome AF and other refractory atrial tachyarrhythmias can be treated by using radiofrequency ablation to induce complete heart block deliberately; a permanent pacemaker must be implanted as well to achieve proper rate control.

Temporary pacemakers

Temporary pacing involves delivery of an electrical impulse into the heart to initiate tissue depolarisation and to trigger cardiac contraction. This is usually done by inserting a bipolar pacing electrode via the internal jugular, subclavian or femoral vein and positioning it at the apex of the RV, using fluoroscopic imaging. The electrode is connected to an external pacemaker with an adjustable energy output and pacing rate. The threshold is the lowest output that will reliably pace the heart and should be < 1 volt (for pulse width 0.5 ms) at implantation. The generator should be set to deliver an output that is at least twice this figure, and adjusted daily because the threshold tends to rise over time. The ECG of right ventricular pacing is characterised by regular broad QRS complexes with a left bundle branch block pattern. Each complex is immediately preceded by a 'pacing spike' (Fig. 18.59). Nearly all pulse generators are used in the 'demand' mode so that the pacemaker will only operate if the heart rate falls below a preset level. Occasionally temporary atrial or dual-chamber pacing (see below) is used.

Temporary pacing may be indicated in the management of transient AV block and other arrhythmias complicating acute MI or cardiac surgery, to maintain the rhythm in other situations of reversible bradycardia (i.e. due to metabolic disturbance or drug overdose), or as a bridge to permanent pacing. Complications include pneumothorax, brachial plexus or subclavian artery injury, local infection or septicaemia (usually *Staphylococcus aureus*), and pericarditis. Failure of the system may be due to lead displacement or a progressive increase in the threshold (exit block) caused by tissue oedema. Complication rates increase with time and so a temporary pacing system should not be used for more than 7 days.

Transcutaneous pacing is administered by delivering an electrical stimulus through two large adhesive gel pad electrodes placed over the apex and upper right sternal edge, or over the anterior and posterior chest. It is easy and quick to set up, but causes discomfort because it induces forceful pectoral and intercostal muscle contraction. Modern external cardiac defibrillators often incorporate a transcutaneous pacing system that can be used during an emergency until transvenous pacing is established.

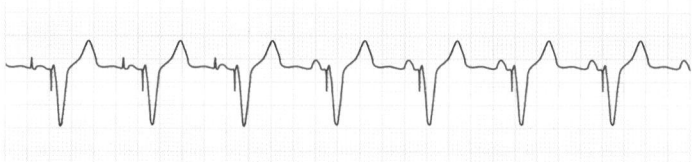

Fig. 18.59 Dual-chamber pacing. The first three beats show atrial and ventricular pacing with narrow pacing spikes in front of each P wave and QRS complex. The last four beats show spontaneous P waves with a different morphology and no pacing spike; the pacemaker senses or tracks these P waves and maintains AV synchrony by pacing the ventricle after an appropriate interval.

18

Permanent pacemakers

Permanent pacemakers are small, flat, metal devices that are implanted under the skin, usually in the pectoral area. They contain a battery, a pulse generator, and programmable electronics that allow adjustment of pacing and memory functions. Pacing electrodes (leads) can be placed via the subclavian or cephalic veins into the RV (usually at the apex), the right atrial appendage or, for AV sequential (dual chamber) pacing, both (see Fig. 18.15, p. 536).

Permanent pacemakers are programmed using an external programmer via a wireless telemetry system. Pacing rate, output, timing and other parameters can be adjusted. This allows the device to be set to the optimum settings to suit the patient's needs. For example, programming can be used to increase output in the face of an unexpected increase in threshold, or to increase the lower rate of the pacemaker in a patient with cardiac failure. Pacemakers store useful diagnostic data about the patient's heart rate trends and the occurrence of tachyarrhythmias, such as VT.

Atrial pacing is appropriate for patients with sinoatrial disease without AV block (the pacemaker acts as an external sinus node). Ventricular pacing is suitable for patients with continuous AF and bradycardia. In dual-chamber pacing, the atrial electrode can be used to detect spontaneous atrial activity and trigger ventricular pacing (see Fig. 18.59), thereby preserving AV synchrony and allowing the ventricular rate to increase together with the sinus node rate during exercise and other forms of stress. Dual-chamber pacing has many advantages over ventricular pacing; these include superior haemodynamics leading to a better effort tolerance, a lower prevalence of atrial arrhythmias in patients with sinoatrial disease, and avoidance of 'pacemaker syndrome' (a fall in BP and dizziness precipitated by loss of AV synchrony).

A code is used to signify the pacing mode (Box 18.44). For example, a system that paces the atrium, senses the atrium and is inhibited if it senses spontaneous activity is designated AAI. Most dual-chamber pacemakers are programmed to a mode termed DDD; here, ventricular pacing is triggered by a sensed sinus P wave and inhibited by a sensed spontaneous QRS complex. A fourth letter, 'R', is added if the pacemaker has a rate response function (e.g. AAIR = atrial demand pacemaker with rate response function). Rate-responsive pacemakers are used in patients who are unable to mount an increase in heart rate during exercise. These devices have a sensor that triggers a rise in heart rate in response to movement or increased respiratory rate. The sensitivity of the sensor is programmable, as is the maximum paced heart rate.

Early complications of permanent pacing include pneumothorax, cardiac tamponade, infection and lead displacement. Late complications include infection (which usually necessitates removing the pacing system), erosion of the generator or lead, chronic pain related to the implant site, and lead fracture due to mechanical fatigue.

Implantable cardiac defibrillators (ICDs)

These devices have all the functions of a permanent pacemaker but can also detect and terminate life-threatening ventricular tachyarrhythmias. ICDs are larger than pacemakers mainly because of the need for a large battery and capacitor to enable cardioversion or defibrillation. ICD leads are similar to pacing leads but have one or two shock coils along the length of the lead, used for delivering defibrillation. ICDs treat ventricular tachyarrhythmias using overdrive pacing, cardioversion or defibrillation. ICD implant procedures have similar complications to pacemaker implants. In addition, patients can be prone to psychological problems and anxiety, particularly if they have experienced repeated shocks from their device.

The evidence-based indications for ICD implantation are shown in Box 18.45. These can be divided into 'secondary prevention' indications, when patients have already had a potentially life-threatening ventricular arrhythmia, and 'primary prevention' indications, when patients are considered to be at significant future risk of arrhythmic death. ICDs may be used prophylactically in selected patients with inherited conditions associated with high risk of sudden cardiac death, such as long QT syndrome (p. 567), hypertrophic cardiomyopathy and arrhythmogenic right ventricular dysplasia (pp. 635–637). ICD treatment is expensive so the indications for which the devices are routinely implanted depend on the health-care resources available.

18.45 Key indications for ICD therapy

Primary prevention

- After MI, if LV ejection fraction < 30%
- Mild to moderate symptomatic heart failure on optimal drug therapy, with LV ejection fraction < 35%

Secondary prevention

- Survivors of VF or VT cardiac arrest not due to transient or reversible cause
- VT with haemodynamic compromise or significant LV impairment (LV ejection fraction < 35%)

Cardiac resynchronisation therapy (CRT)

This is a treatment for selected patients with heart failure who are in sinus rhythm and have left bundle branch block. This conduction defect is associated with left ventricular dys-synchrony (poorly coordinated left ventricular contraction) and can aggravate heart failure in susceptible patients. CRT systems have an additional lead that is placed via the coronary sinus into one of the veins

18.44 International generic pacemaker code

Chamber paced	Chamber sensed	Response to sensing
O = none	O = none	O = none
A = atrium	A = atrium	T = triggered
V = ventricle	V = ventricle	I = inhibited
D = both	D = both	D = both

EBM **18.46 Cardiac resynchronisation therapy (CRT) for heart failure**

'CRT improves symptoms and quality of life, and reduces mortality in patients with moderate to severe symptomatic heart failure who are in sinus rhythm, with left bundle branch block and LV ejection fraction ≤ 35%.'

• Cardiac Resynchronisation-Heart Failure (CARE-HF) Study. Cleland J, et al. N Engl J Med 2005; 352:1539–1549.
• COMPANION Study. Bristow MR, et al. N Engl J Med 2004; 350:2140–2150.

on the epicardial surface of the LV (see Fig. 18.28, p. 550). Simultaneous septal and left ventricular epicardial pacing resynchronises left ventricular contraction. These devices can improve effort tolerance and reduce heart failure symptoms (Box 18.46). Most CRT devices are also defibrillators (CRT-D) because many patients with heart failure are predisposed to ventricular arrhythmias. CRT-pacemakers (CRT-P) are used in patients considered to be at relatively low risk of these arrhythmias.

ATHEROSCLEROSIS

Atherosclerosis can affect any artery in the body. When it occurs in the heart, it may cause angina, MI and sudden death; in the brain, stroke and transient ischaemic attack; and in the limbs, claudication and critical limb ischaemia. Occult coronary artery disease is common in those who present with other forms of atherosclerotic vascular disease, such as intermittent claudication or stroke, and is an important cause of morbidity and mortality in these patients.

Pathophysiology

Atherosclerosis is a progressive inflammatory disorder of the arterial wall that is characterised by focal lipid-rich deposits of atheroma that remain clinically silent until they become large enough to impair tissue perfusion, or until ulceration and disruption of the lesion result in thrombotic occlusion or distal embolisation of the vessel. These mechanisms are common to the entire vascular tree, and the clinical manifestations of atherosclerosis depend upon the site of the lesion and the vulnerability of the organ supplied.

Atherosclerosis begins early in life. Abnormalities of arterial function have been detected among high-risk children and adolescents, such as cigarette smokers and those with familial hyperlipidaemia or hypertension. Early atherosclerotic lesions have been found in the arteries of victims of accidental death in the second and third decades of life. Nevertheless, clinical manifestations often do not appear until the sixth, seventh or eighth decade.

Early atherosclerosis

Fatty streaks tend to occur at sites of altered arterial shear stress, such as bifurcations, and are associated with abnormal endothelial function. They develop when inflammatory cells, predominantly monocytes, bind to receptors expressed by endothelial cells, migrate into the intima, take up oxidised low-density lipoprotein (LDL) particles and become lipid-laden macrophages or foam cells. Extracellular lipid pools appear in the intimal space when these foam cells die and release their contents (Fig. 18.60).

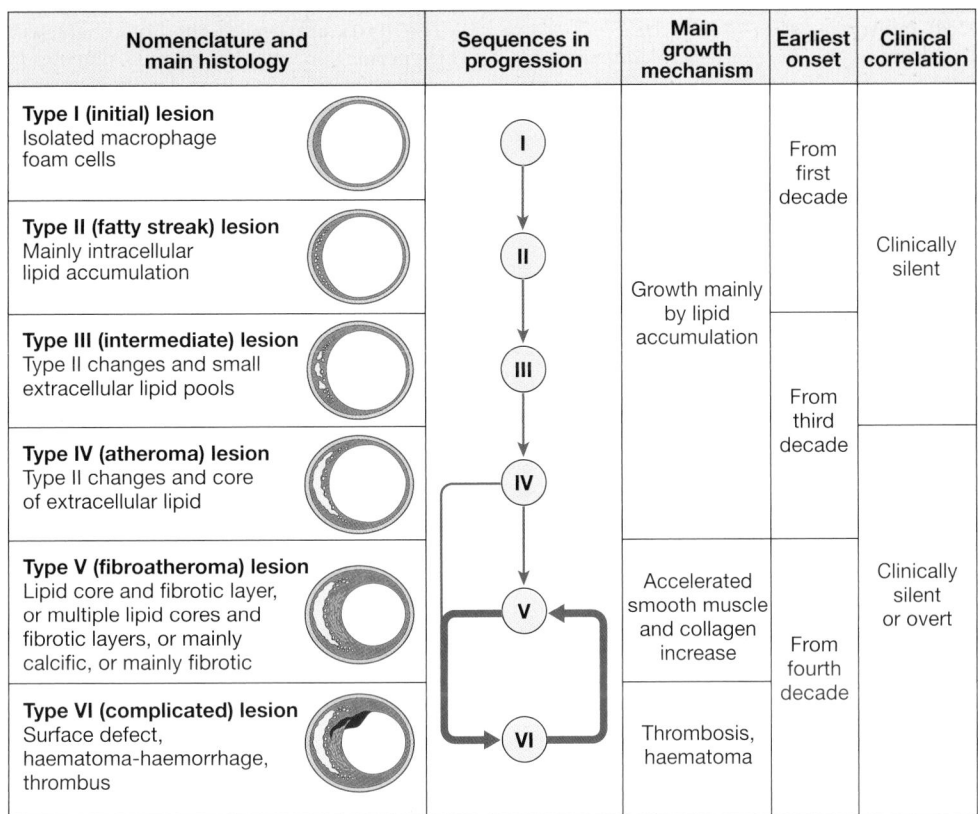

Nomenclature and main histology	Sequences in progression	Main growth mechanism	Earliest onset	Clinical correlation
Type I (initial) lesion Isolated macrophage foam cells	I	Growth mainly by lipid accumulation	From first decade	Clinically silent
Type II (fatty streak) lesion Mainly intracellular lipid accumulation	II			
Type III (intermediate) lesion Type II changes and small extracellular lipid pools	III		From third decade	
Type IV (atheroma) lesion Type II changes and core of extracellular lipid	IV			
Type V (fibroatheroma) lesion Lipid core and fibrotic layer, or multiple lipid cores and fibrotic layers, or mainly calcific, or mainly fibrotic	V	Accelerated smooth muscle and collagen increase	From fourth decade	Clinically silent or overt
Type VI (complicated) lesion Surface defect, haematoma-haemorrhage, thrombus	VI	Thrombosis, haematoma		

Fig. 18.60 **The six stages of atherosclerosis.** American Heart Association classification.

In response to cytokines and growth factors produced by the activated macrophages, smooth muscle cells migrate from the media of the arterial wall into the intima, and change from a contractile to a repair phenotype in an attempt to stabilise the atherosclerotic lesion. If they are successful, the lipid core will be covered by smooth muscle cells and matrix, producing a stable atherosclerotic plaque that will remain asymptomatic until it becomes large enough to obstruct arterial flow.

Advanced atherosclerosis

In an established atherosclerotic plaque, macrophages mediate inflammation and smooth muscle cells promote repair. If inflammation predominates, the plaque becomes active or unstable and may be complicated by ulceration and thrombosis. Cytokines, such as interleukin-1, tumour necrosis factor-alpha, interferon-gamma, platelet-derived growth factors, and matrix metalloproteinases are released by activated macrophages; they cause the intimal smooth muscle cells overlying the plaque to become senescent and collagen cross-struts within the plaque to degrade. This results in thinning of the protective fibrous cap, making the lesion vulnerable to mechanical stress that ultimately causes erosion, fissuring or rupture of the plaque surface (see Fig. 18.60). Any breach in the integrity of the plaque will expose its contents to blood, and trigger platelet aggregation and thrombosis that extend into the atheromatous plaque and the arterial lumen. This type of plaque event may cause partial or complete obstruction at the site of the lesion or distal embolisation resulting in infarction or ischaemia of the affected organ. This common mechanism underlies many of the acute manifestations of atherosclerotic vascular disease, such as acute lower limb ischaemia, MI and stroke.

The number and complexity of arterial plaques increase with age and with risk factors (see below) but the rate of progression of individual plaques is variable. There is a complex and dynamic interaction between mechanical wall stress and atherosclerotic lesions. 'Vulnerable' plaques are characterised by a lipid-rich core, a thin fibrocellular cap and an increase in inflammatory cells that release specific enzymes to degrade matrix proteins. In contrast, stable plaques are typified by a small lipid pool, a thick fibrous cap, calcification and plentiful collagenous cross-struts. Fissuring or rupture tends to occur at sites of maximal mechanical stress, particularly the margins of an eccentric plaque, and may be triggered by a surge in BP, such as during exercise or emotional stress. Surprisingly, plaque events are often subclinical and heal spontaneously, although this may allow thrombus to be incorporated into the lesion, producing plaque growth and further obstruction to flow in the arterial lumen.

Atherosclerosis may induce complex changes in the media that lead to arterial remodelling. Some arterial segments may slowly constrict (negative remodelling) whilst others may gradually enlarge (positive remodelling). These changes are important because they may amplify or minimise the degree to which atheroma encroaches into the arterial lumen.

Risk factors

The role and relative importance of many risk factors for the development of coronary, peripheral and cerebrovascular disease have been defined in experimental animal studies, epidemiological studies and clinical interventional trials. Key factors have emerged but do not explain all the risk, and unknown factors may account for up to 40% of the variation in risk from one person to the next.

The impact of genetic risk is illustrated by twin studies; a monozygotic twin of an affected individual has an eightfold increased risk, and a dizygotic twin a fourfold increased risk of dying from coronary heart disease compared to the general population.

The effect of risk factors is multiplicative rather than additive. People with a combination of risk factors are at greatest risk and so assessment should take account of all identifiable risk factors. It is important to distinguish between relative risk (the proportional increase in risk) and absolute risk (the actual chance of an event). Thus, a man of 35 years with a plasma cholesterol of 7 mmol/L (approximately 170 mg/dL) who smokes 40 cigarettes a day is relatively much more likely to die from coronary disease within the next decade than a non-smoking woman of the same age with a normal cholesterol, but the absolute likelihood of his dying during this time is still small (high relative risk, low absolute risk).

- *Age and sex.* Age is the most powerful independent risk factor for atherosclerosis. Premenopausal women have lower rates of disease than men, although this sex difference disappears after the menopause. However, hormone replacement therapy has no role in the primary or secondary prevention of coronary heart disease, and isolated oestrogen therapy may cause an increased cardiovascular event rate.
- *Family history.* Atherosclerotic vascular disease often runs in families, due to a combination of shared genetic, environmental and lifestyle factors. The most common inherited risk characteristics (hypertension, hyperlipidaemia, diabetes mellitus) are polygenic. A 'positive' family history is present when clinical problems in first-degree relatives occur at relatively young age, such as < 50 years for men and < 55 years for women.
- *Smoking.* This is probably the most important avoidable cause of atherosclerotic vascular disease. There is a strong consistent and dose-linked relationship between cigarette smoking and ischaemic heart disease, especially in younger (< 70 years) individuals.
- *Hypertension* (see below). The incidence of atherosclerosis increases as BP rises, and this excess risk is related to both systolic and diastolic BP as well as pulse pressure. Antihypertensive therapy reduces cardiovascular mortality, stroke and heart failure.
- *Hypercholesterolaemia* (pp. 451–454). Risk rises with increasing serum cholesterol concentrations. Lowering serum total and LDL cholesterol concentrations reduces the risk of cardiovascular events, including death, MI, stroke and coronary revascularisation.
- *Diabetes mellitus.* This is a potent risk factor for all forms of atherosclerosis and is often associated with diffuse disease that is difficult to treat. Insulin resistance (normal glucose homeostasis with high levels of insulin) is associated with obesity and physical inactivity, and is a risk factor for coronary heart disease (p. 802). Glucose intolerance accounts

for a major part of the high incidence of ischaemic heart disease in certain ethnic groups, e.g. South Asians.

- *Haemostatic factors.* Platelet activation and high levels of fibrinogen are associated with an increased risk of coronary thrombosis. Antiphospholipid antibodies are associated with recurrent arterial thromboses (p. 1050).
- *Physical activity.* Physical inactivity roughly doubles the risk of coronary heart disease and is a major risk factor for stroke. Regular exercise (brisk walking, cycling or swimming for 20 minutes two or three times a week) has a protective effect which may be related to increased serum HDL cholesterol concentrations, lower BP, and collateral vessel development.
- *Obesity* (p. 116). Obesity, particularly if central or truncal, is an independent risk factor, although it is often associated with other adverse factors such as hypertension, diabetes mellitus and physical inactivity.
- *Alcohol.* Alcohol consumption is associated with reduced rates of coronary artery disease. Excess alcohol consumption is associated with hypertension and cerebrovascular disease.
- *Other dietary factors.* Diets deficient in fresh fruit, vegetables and polyunsaturated fatty acids are associated with an increased risk of cardiovascular disease. The introduction of a Mediterranean-style diet reduces cardiovascular events. However, dietary supplements, such as vitamin C and E, beta-carotene, folate and fish oils, do not reduce cardiovascular events and, in some cases, have been associated with harm.
- *Personality.* Certain personality traits are associated with an increased risk of coronary disease. Nevertheless, there is little or no evidence to support the popular belief that stress is a major cause of coronary artery disease.
- *Social deprivation.* Health inequalities have a major influence on cardiovascular disease. The impact of established risk factors is amplified in patients who are socially deprived and current guidelines recommend that treatment thresholds should be lowered for them.

Primary prevention

Two complementary strategies can be used to prevent atherosclerosis in apparently healthy but at-risk individuals: population and targeted strategies.

The population strategy aims to modify the risk factors of the whole population through diet and lifestyle advice, on the basis that even a small reduction in smoking or average cholesterol, or modification of exercise and diet will produce worthwhile benefits (Box 18.47). Some risk factors for atheroma, such as obesity and smoking, are also associated with a high risk of other diseases and should be actively discouraged through public health measures. Legislation restricting smoking in public places is associated with reductions in rates of MI.

The targeted strategy aims to identify and treat high-risk individuals who usually have a combination of risk factors and can be identified by using composite scoring systems (Fig. 18.61). It is important to consider the

	18.47 Population advice to prevent coronary disease

- Do not smoke
- Take regular exercise (minimum of 20 mins, three times a week)
- Maintain 'ideal' body weight
- Eat a mixed diet rich in fresh fruit and vegetables
- Aim to get no more than 10% of energy intake from saturated fat

absolute risk of atheromatous cardiovascular disease that an individual is facing before contemplating specific antihypertensive or lipid-lowering therapy because this will help to determine whether the possible benefits of intervention are likely to outweigh the expense, inconvenience and possible side-effects of treatment. For example, a 65-year-old man with an average BP of 150/90 mmHg, who smokes and has diabetes mellitus, a total:HDL cholesterol ratio of 8 and left ventricular hypertrophy on ECG, will have a 10-year risk of CHD of 68% and a 10-year risk of any cardiovascular event of 90%. Lowering his cholesterol will reduce these risks by 30% and lowering his BP will produce a further 20% reduction; both would obviously be worthwhile. Conversely, a 55-year-old woman who has an identical BP, is a non-smoker, does not have diabetes mellitus and has a normal ECG and a total:HDL cholesterol ratio of 6 has a much better outlook, with a predicted CHD risk of 14% and cardiovascular risk of 19% over the next 10 years. Although lowering her cholesterol and BP would also reduce risk by 30% and 20% respectively, the value of either or both treatments would clearly be borderline.

Secondary prevention

Patients who already have evidence of atheromatous vascular disease are at high risk of future cardiovascular events and should be offered treatments and measures to improve their outlook. The energetic correction of modifiable risk factors, particularly smoking, hypertension and hypercholesterolaemia, is particularly important because the absolute risk of further vascular events is high. All patients with coronary heart disease should be given statin therapy irrespective of their serum cholesterol concentration (Box 18.48). BP should be treated to a target of ≤ 140/85 mmHg (p. 609). Aspirin and ACE inhibitors are of benefit in patients with evidence of vascular disease (Boxes 18.49 and 18.50). Beta-blockers benefit patients with a history of MI (see below) or heart failure.

Many clinical events offer an unrivalled opportunity to introduce effective secondary preventive measures; patients who have just survived an MI or undergone bypass surgery are usually keen to help themselves and may be particularly receptive to lifestyle advice, such as dietary modification and smoking cessation.

CORONARY HEART DISEASE

Coronary heart disease (CHD) is the most common form of heart disease and the single most important cause of premature death in Europe, the Baltic states, Russia, North and South America, Australia and New Zealand.

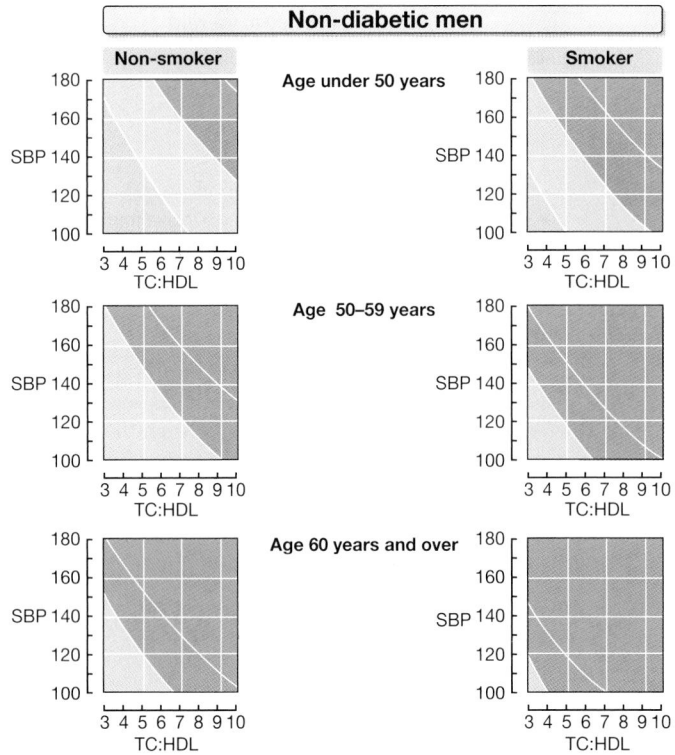

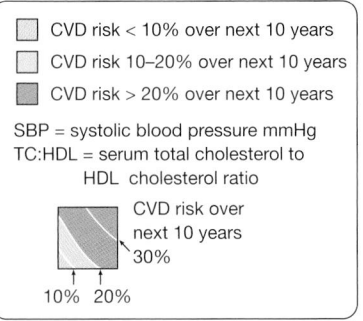

CVD risk < 10% over next 10 years
CVD risk 10–20% over next 10 years
CVD risk > 20% over next 10 years
SBP = systolic blood pressure mmHg
TC:HDL = serum total cholesterol to
HDL cholesterol ratio

CVD risk over
next 10 years
30%
10% 20%

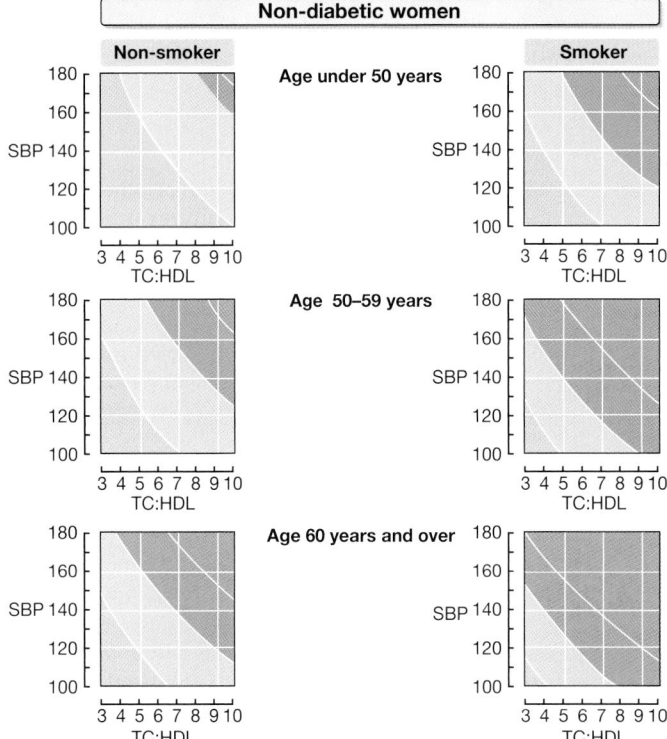

Fig. 18.61 Cardiovascular risk prediction charts. Cardiovascular risk is predicted from the patient's age, sex, smoking habit, BP and cholesterol ratio. The ratio of total to high-density lipoprotein (HDL) cholesterol can be determined in a non-fasting blood sample. Where HDL cholesterol concentration is unknown, it should be assumed to be 1 mmol/L; the lipid scale should be used as total serum cholesterol. Current guidelines suggest initiation of primary prevention in individuals with a 10-year cardiovascular risk ≥ 20%. Patients with diabetes mellitus should be assumed to have a 10-year cardiovascular risk of ≥ 20% and receive secondary prevention therapy.

- To estimate an individual's absolute 10-year risk of developing cardiovascular disease (CVD), choose the panel for the appropriate gender, smoking status and age. Within this, define the level of risk from the point where the coordinates for systolic blood pressure (SBP) and ratio of the total to high-density lipoprotein (HDL)-cholesterol cross.
- Highest-risk individuals (red areas) are those whose 10-year CVD risk exceeds 20%, which is approximately equivalent to a 10-year coronary heart disease risk of > 15%. As a minimum, those with CVD risk > 30% (shown by the line within the red area) should be targeted and treated now. When resources allow, others with a CVD risk > 20% should be targeted progressively.
- The chart also assists in identification of individuals with a moderately high 10-year CVD risk, in the range of 10–20% (orange area) and those in whom it is < 10% (green area).
- Smoking status should reflect lifetime exposure to tobacco. For further information, see www.bhf.org.uk.

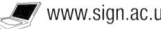

EBM 18.48 **Use of statins in prevention of atherosclerotic disease**

Primary prevention

'In patients *without evidence of coronary disease* but with high serum cholesterol concentrations, cholesterol-lowering with statins does not lower mortality but does prevent coronary events (angina and MI).'

Secondary prevention

'In patients *with established coronary disease* (MI or angina), statin therapy can safely reduce the 5-year incidence of all-cause death as well as major coronary events, coronary revascularisation and stroke. Benefit depends on the overall risk of the study population but the NNT_B for 5 years to prevent one death ranges from 10 to 90.'

• Cholesterol Treatment Trialists' Collaborators. Lancet 2005; 366:1267–1277.

For further information: www.sign.ac.uk

EBM 18.49 **ACE inhibitors and secondary prevention of atherosclerotic disease**

'ACE inhibitor therapy reduces the risk of death, MI and stroke in patients with atherosclerotic vascular disease without apparent left ventricular systolic dysfunction or heart failure. NNT_B to avoid one event over 4 years ranges from 6 to 50, depending upon the level of cardiovascular risk.'

• HOPE trial. N Engl J Med 2000; 342:145–153.
• EUROPA trial. Lancet 2003; 362:782–788.

EBM 18.50 **Aspirin and secondary prevention in atherosclerotic vascular disease**

'In patients with established coronary heart disease, peripheral vascular disease or thrombotic stroke, aspirin is effective in reducing morbidity and mortality (non-fatal MI, stroke and cardiovascular death). In patients at high risk of future vascular events, the overall risk reduction is 22%.'

• Antithrombotic Trialist Collaboration. BMJ 2002; 324:71–86.

For further information: www.clinicalevidence.org

By 2020 it is estimated that it will be the major cause of death in all regions of the world.

In the UK, 1 in 3 men and 1 in 4 women die from CHD, an estimated 330 000 people have a myocardial infarct each year, and approximately 1.3 million people have angina. The death rates from CHD in the UK are amongst the highest in Western Europe (more than 140 000 people) but are falling, particularly in younger age groups; in the last 10 years CHD mortality has fallen by 42% among UK men and women aged 16–64. However, in Eastern Europe and much of Asia, the rates of CHD are rapidly rising.

Disease of the coronary arteries is almost always due to atheroma and its complications, particularly thrombosis (Box 18.51). Occasionally, the coronary arteries are involved in other disorders such as aortitis, polyarteritis and other connective tissue disorders.

 18.51 **Coronary heart disease: clinical manifestations and pathology**

Clinical problem	Pathology
Stable angina	Ischaemia due to fixed atheromatous stenosis of one or more coronary arteries
Unstable angina	Ischaemia caused by dynamic obstruction of a coronary artery due to plaque rupture or erosion with superimposed thrombosis
Myocardial infarction	Myocardial necrosis caused by acute occlusion of a coronary artery due to plaque rupture or erosion with superimposed thrombosis
Heart failure	Myocardial dysfunction due to infarction or ischaemia
Arrhythmia	Altered conduction due to ischaemia or infarction
Sudden death	Ventricular arrhythmia, asystole or massive MI

Stable angina

Angina pectoris is the symptom complex caused by transient myocardial ischaemia and constitutes a clinical syndrome rather than a disease. It may occur whenever there is an imbalance between myocardial oxygen supply and demand (Box 18.52). Coronary atheroma is by far the most common cause of angina, although the symptom may be a manifestation of other forms of heart disease, particularly aortic valve disease and hypertrophic cardiomyopathy.

Clinical features

The history is by far the most important factor in making the diagnosis (pp. 535–539). Stable angina is characterised by central chest pain, discomfort or breathlessness that is precipitated by exertion or other forms of stress (Box 18.53), and is promptly relieved by rest (see Figs 18.17 and 18.18, pp. 537–538). Some patients find that

 18.52 **Factors influencing myocardial oxygen supply and demand**

Oxygen demand: cardiac work

• Heart rate
• BP
• Myocardial contractility
• Left ventricular hypertrophy
• Valve disease, e.g. aortic stenosis

Oxygen supply: coronary blood flow

• Duration of diastole
• Coronary perfusion pressure (aortic diastolic minus coronary sinus or right atrial diastolic pressure)
• Coronary vasomotor tone
• Oxygenation
  Haemoglobin
  Oxygen saturation

N.B. Coronary blood flow occurs mainly in diastole.

18

18.53 Activities precipitating angina

Common

- Physical exertion
- Cold exposure
- Heavy meals
- Intense emotion

Uncommon

- Lying flat (decubitus angina)
- Vivid dreams (nocturnal angina)

18.54 Risk stratification in stable angina

High risk	Low risk
Post-infarct angina	Predictable exertional angina
Poor effort tolerance	Good effort tolerance
Ischaemia at low workload	Ischaemia only at high workload
Left main or three-vessel disease	Single-vessel or two-vessel disease
Poor LV function	Good LV function

N.B. Patients may fall between these categories.

the discomfort comes when they start walking, and that later it does not return despite greater effort ('warm-up angina').

Physical examination is frequently unremarkable but should include a careful search for evidence of valve disease (particularly aortic), important risk factors (e.g. hypertension, diabetes mellitus), left ventricular dysfunction (cardiomegaly, gallop rhythm), other manifestations of arterial disease (carotid bruits, peripheral vascular disease) and unrelated conditions that may exacerbate angina (anaemia, thyrotoxicosis).

Investigations

Resting ECG

The ECG may show evidence of previous MI but is often normal, even in patients with severe coronary artery disease. Occasionally, there is T-wave flattening or inversion in some leads, providing non-specific evidence of myocardial ischaemia or damage. The most convincing ECG evidence of myocardial ischaemia is the demonstration of reversible ST segment depression or elevation, with or without T-wave inversion, at the time the patient is experiencing symptoms (whether spontaneous or induced by exercise testing).

Exercise ECG

An exercise tolerance test (ETT) is usually performed using a standard treadmill or bicycle ergometer protocol (p. 530) while monitoring the patient's ECG, BP and general condition. Planar or down-sloping ST segment depression of ≥ 1 mm is indicative of ischaemia (Fig. 18.62). Up-sloping ST depression is less specific and often occurs in normal individuals.

Exercise testing is also a useful means of assessing the severity of coronary disease and identifying high-risk individuals (Box 18.54). For example, the amount of exercise that can be tolerated and the extent and degree of any ST segment change (Fig. 18.63) provide a useful guide to the likely extent of coronary disease. Exercise testing is not infallible and may produce false positive results in the presence of digoxin therapy, left ventric-

ular hypertrophy, bundle branch block or WPW syndrome. The predictive accuracy of exercise testing is lower in women than men. The test should be classed as inconclusive (rather than negative) if the patient cannot achieve an adequate level of exercise because of locomotor or other non-cardiac problems.

Other forms of stress testing

- *Myocardial perfusion scanning.* This may be helpful in the evaluation of patients with an equivocal or uninterpretable exercise test and those who are unable to exercise (p. 535). It entails obtaining scintiscans of the myocardium at rest and during stress (either exercise testing or pharmacological stress, such as a controlled infusion of dobutamine) after the administration of an intravenous radioactive isotope, such as ^{99}technetium tetrofosmin. Thallium and tetrofosmin are taken up by viable perfused myocardium. A perfusion defect present during stress but not at rest provides evidence of reversible myocardial ischaemia (Fig. 18.64), whereas a persistent perfusion defect seen during both phases of the study is usually indicative of previous MI.
- *Stress echocardiography.* This is an alternative to myocardial perfusion scanning and can achieve similar predictive accuracy. It uses transthoracic echocardiography to identify ischaemic segments of myocardium and areas of infarction (p. 533). The former characteristically exhibit reversible defects in contractility during exercise or pharmacological stress, and the latter do not contract at rest or during stress.

Coronary arteriography

This provides detailed anatomical information about the extent and nature of coronary artery disease (see Fig. 18.14, p. 534), and is usually performed with a view to coronary artery bypass graft (CABG) surgery or percutaneous coronary intervention (PCI, pp. 585–586). In some patients, diagnostic coronary angiography may be indicated when non-invasive tests have failed to establish the cause of atypical chest pain. The procedure is performed under local anaesthesia and requires specialised radiological equipment, cardiac monitoring and an experienced operating team.

Management: general measures

The management of angina pectoris involves:
- a careful assessment of the likely extent and severity of arterial disease

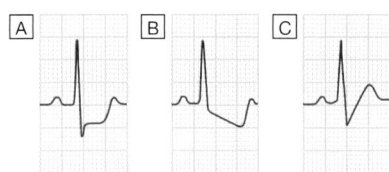

Fig. 18.62 Forms of exercise-induced ST depression. **A** Planar ST depression is usually indicative of myocardial ischaemia. **B** Down-sloping depression also usually indicates myocardial ischaemia. **C** Up-sloping depression may be a normal finding.

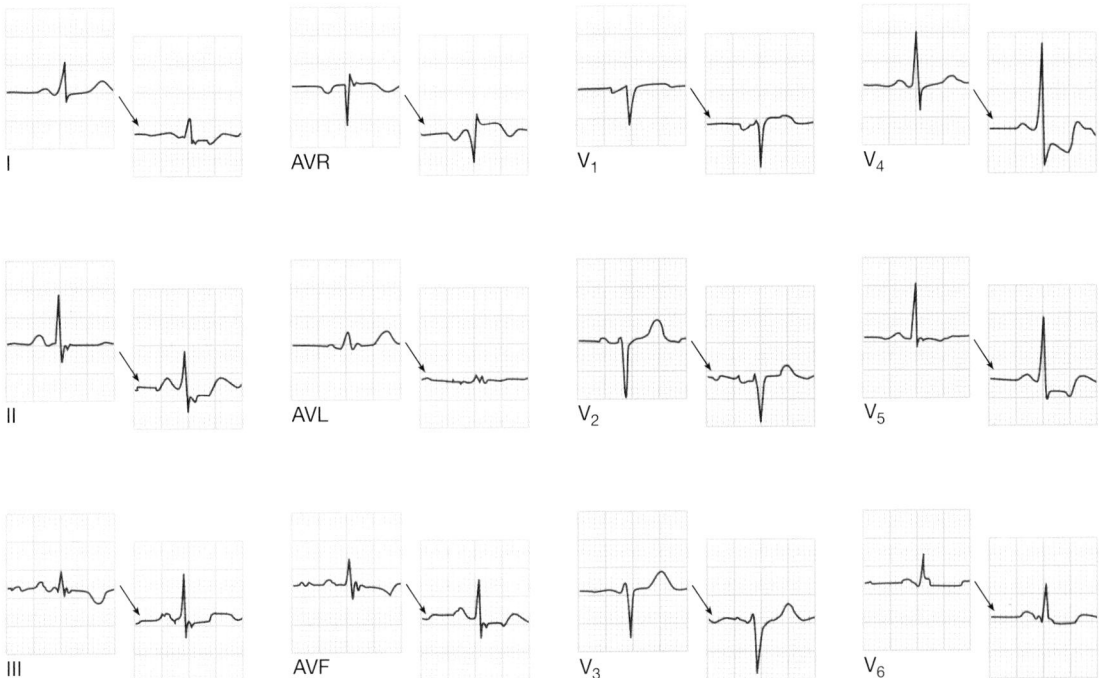

Fig. 18.63 A positive exercise test. The resting 12-lead ECG shows some minor T-wave changes in the inferolateral leads but is otherwise normal. After 3 minutes' exercise on a treadmill there is marked planar ST depression in leads II, V$_4$ and V$_5$ (right offset). Subsequent coronary angiography revealed critical three-vessel coronary artery disease.

- the identification and control of risk factors such as smoking, hypertension and hyperlipidaemia
- the use of measures to control symptoms
- the identification of high-risk patients for treatment to improve life expectancy.

Symptoms alone are a poor guide to the extent of coronary artery disease. Stress testing is therefore advisable in all patients who are potential candidates for revascularisation. An algorithm for the investigation and treatment of patients with stable angina is shown in Figure 18.65.

Management should start with a careful explanation of the problem and a discussion of the potential lifestyle and medical interventions that may relieve symptoms and improve prognosis (Box 18.55). Anxiety and misconceptions often contribute to disability; for example, some patients avoid all forms of exertion because they believe that each attack of angina is a 'mini heart attack' that results in permanent damage. Effective management of these psychological factors can make a huge difference to the patient's quality of life.

---

i **18.55 Advice to patients with stable angina**

- Do not smoke
- Aim for ideal body weight
- Take regular exercise (exercise up to, but not beyond, the point of chest discomfort is beneficial and may promote collateral vessels)
- Avoid severe unaccustomed exertion, and vigorous exercise after a heavy meal or in very cold weather
- Take sublingual nitrate before undertaking exertion that may induce angina

---

Antiplatelet therapy

Low-dose (75 mg) aspirin reduces the risk of adverse events such as MI and should be prescribed for all patients with coronary artery disease indefinitely (see Box 18.50). Clopidogrel (75 mg daily) is an equally effective antiplatelet agent that can be prescribed if aspirin causes troublesome dyspepsia or other side-effects.

Anti-anginal drug treatment

Five groups of drug are used to help relieve or prevent the symptoms of angina: nitrates, β-blockers, calcium antagonists, potassium channel activators and an I$_f$ channel antagonist.

Nitrates

These drugs act directly on vascular smooth muscle to produce venous and arteriolar dilatation. Their beneficial effects are due to a reduction in myocardial oxygen demand (lower preload and afterload) and an increase in myocardial oxygen supply (coronary vasodilatation). Sublingual glyceryl trinitrate (GTN) administered from a metered-dose aerosol (400 µg per spray) or as a tablet (300 or 500 µg) will relieve an attack of angina in 2–3 minutes. Side-effects include headache, symptomatic hypotension and, rarely, syncope.

Patients should be encouraged to use the drug prophylactically before taking exercise that is liable to provoke symptoms. Sublingual GTN has a short duration of action (Box 18.56); however, a variety of alternative nitrate preparations can provide a more prolonged therapeutic effect. GTN can be given transcutaneously as a patch (5–10 mg daily), or as a slow-release buccal tablet (1–5 mg 6-hourly). GTN undergoes extensive first-pass metabolism in the liver and is ineffective when swallowed. Other nitrates such as isosorbide

At rest   During stress

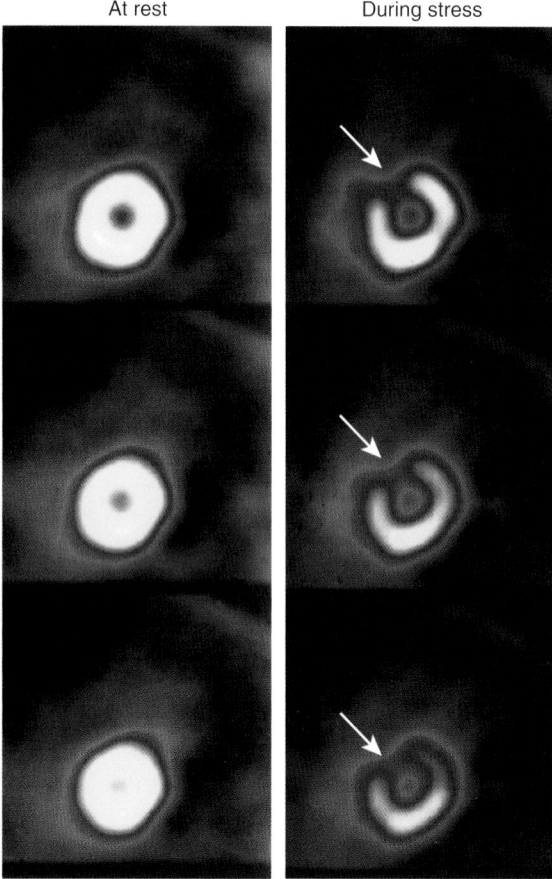

Fig. 18.64 A myocardial perfusion scan showing reversible anterior myocardial ischaemia. The images are cross-sectional tomograms of the LV. The resting scans (left) show even uptake of the [99]technetium-labelled tetrafosmin and look like doughnuts. During stress (e.g. a dobutamine infusion), there is reduced uptake of technetium, particularly along the anterior wall (arrows), and the scans look like crescents (right).

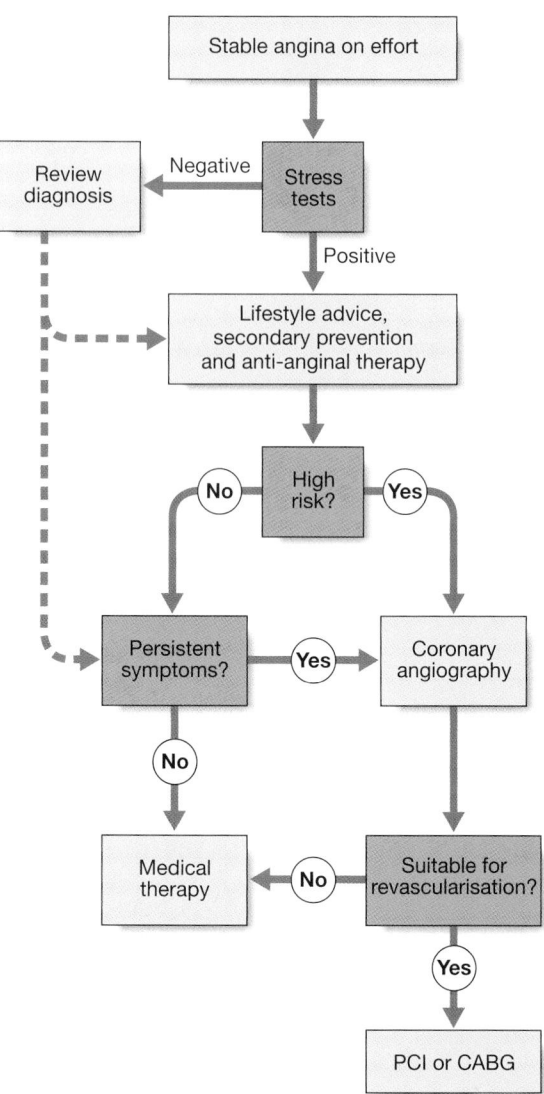

Fig. 18.65 A scheme for the investigation and treatment of stable angina on effort. The selection of percutaneous coronary intervention (PCI) or coronary artery bypass grafting (CABG) depends upon patient choice, coronary artery anatomy and extent of coronary artery disease. In general, left main stem and three-vessel coronary artery disease should be treated by CABG surgery.

dinitrate (10–20 mg 8-hourly) and isosorbide mononitrate (20–60 mg once or twice a day) can be given by mouth. Headache is common but tends to diminish if the patient perseveres with the treatment. Continuous nitrate therapy can cause pharmacological tolerance. This can be avoided by a 6–8-hour nitrate-free period, best achieved at night when the patient is inactive. If nocturnal angina is a predominant symptom, long-acting nitrates can be given at the end of the day.

Beta-blockers

These lower myocardial oxygen demand by reducing heart rate, BP and myocardial contractility, but they may provoke bronchospasm in patients with asthma. The properties and side-effects of β-blockers are discussed on page 597.

In theory, non-selective β-blockers may aggravate coronary vasospasm by blocking the coronary artery β_2-adrenoceptors and so a once-daily cardioselective preparation is used (e.g. slow-release metoprolol 50–200 mg daily, bisoprolol 5–15 mg daily). Beta-blockers should not be withdrawn abruptly because this may have a rebound effect and precipitate dangerous arrhythmias, worsening angina or MI: the β-blocker withdrawal syndrome.

18.56 Duration of action of some nitrate preparations

Preparation	Peak action	Duration of action
Sublingual GTN	4–8 mins	10–30 mins
Buccal GTN	4–10 mins	30–300 mins
Transdermal GTN	1–3 hrs	Up to 24 hrs
Oral isosorbide dinitrate	45–120 mins	2–6 hrs
Oral isosorbide mononitrate	45–120 mins	6–10 hrs

(GTN = glyceryl trinitrate)

Calcium channel antagonists

These drugs inhibit the slow inward current caused by the entry of extracellular calcium through the cell membrane of excitable cells, particularly cardiac and arteriolar smooth muscle, and lower myocardial oxygen demand by reducing BP and myocardial contractility.

Dihydropyridine calcium antagonists, such as nifedipine and nicardipine, often cause a reflex tachycardia. This may be counterproductive and it is best to use them in combination with a β-blocker. In contrast, verapamil and diltiazem are particularly suitable for patients who are not receiving a β-blocker (e.g. those with airways obstruction) because they slow SA node firing, inhibit conduction through the AV node and tend to cause a bradycardia. Calcium channel antagonists reduce myocardial contractility and can aggravate or precipitate heart failure. Other unwanted effects include peripheral oedema, flushing, headache and dizziness (Box 18.57).

Potassium channel activators

These have arterial and venous dilating properties but do not exhibit the tolerance seen with nitrates. Nicorandil (10–30 mg 12-hourly orally) is the only drug in this class currently available for clinical use.

I_f channel antagonist

Ivabradine is the first of this class of drug. It induces bradycardia by modulating ion channels in the sinus node. In contrast to β-blockers and rate-limiting calcium antagonists, it does not have other cardiovascular effects. It appears to be safe to use in patients with heart failure.

Although each of these anti-anginal drugs is superior to placebo in relieving the symptoms of angina, there is little evidence that one group is more effective than another. It is conventional to start therapy with low-dose aspirin, a statin, sublingual GTN and a β-blocker, and then add a calcium channel antagonist or a long-acting nitrate later if needed. The goal is the control of angina with minimum side-effects and the simplest possible drug regimen. There is little evidence that prescribing multiple anti-anginal drugs is of benefit, and revascularisation should be considered if an appropriate combination of two or more drugs fails to achieve an acceptable symptomatic response.

Invasive treatment

Percutaneous coronary intervention (PCI)

This is performed by passing a fine guidewire across a coronary stenosis under radiographic control and using it to position a balloon which is then inflated to dilate the stenosis (see Figs 18.15 (p. 536) and 18.66). A coronary stent is a piece of coated metallic 'scaffolding' that

18.57 Calcium channel antagonists used for the treatment of angina

Drug	Dose	Feature
Nifedipine	5–20 mg 8-hourly*	May cause marked tachycardia
Nicardipine	20–40 mg 8-hourly	May cause less myocardial depression than the other calcium antagonists
Amlodipine	2.5–10 mg daily	Ultra long-acting
Verapamil	40–80 mg 8-hourly*	Commonly causes constipation; useful anti-arrhythmic properties (p. 572)
Diltiazem	60–120 mg 8-hourly*	Similar anti-arrhythmic properties to verapamil

*Once- or twice-daily slow-release preparations are available.

18

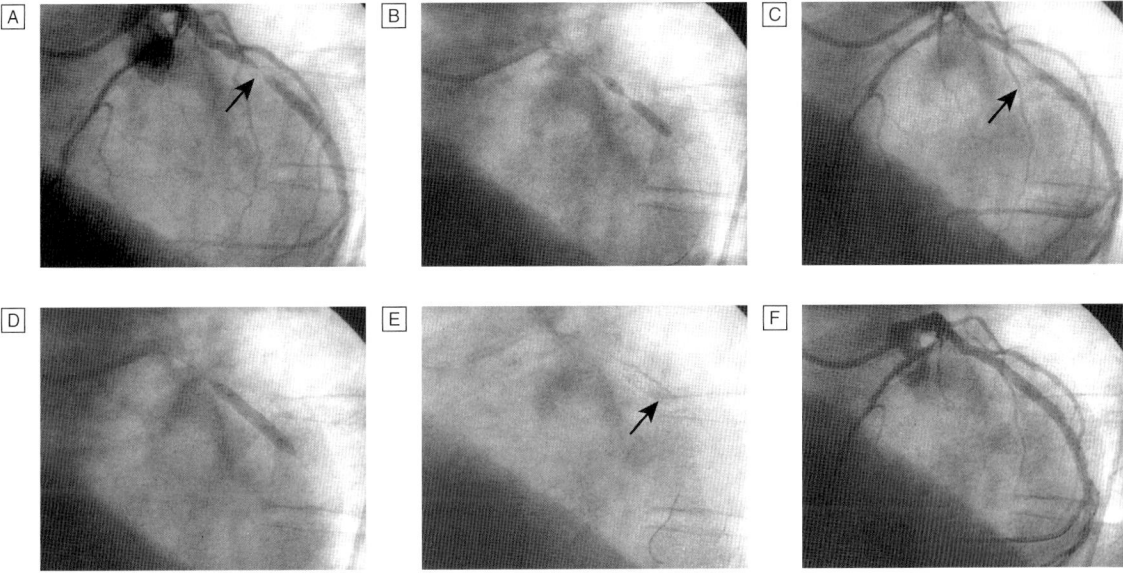

Fig. 18.66 Percutaneous coronary intervention. A sequence of images from a 58-year-old woman with stable angina. **A** Severe stenosis of the circumflex artery (arrow). **B** A balloon has been advanced into the stenosis, over a guidewire, and has been inflated. (Note the waisting caused by the lesion). **C** Residual stenosis and dissection (tramline shadow—arrow) after balloon dilatation. **D** A stent is deployed on a balloon. **E** The stent is visible on plain fluoroscopy (arrow). **F** Angiogram after stenting.

EBM 18.58 **Angioplasty and intracoronary stents in angina**

'In comparison with simple balloon angioplasty, intracoronary stents afford superior acute and long-term clinical and angiographic results with lower rates of restenosis (e.g. 17% vs 40%) and recurrent angina (13% vs 30%). Restenosis rates are reduced even further (< 10%) with drug-eluting stents'

• Stettler C, et al. BMJ 2008; 337:a1331.

For further information: www.nice.org.uk

can be deployed on a balloon and used to maximise and maintain dilatation of a stenosed vessel. The routine use of stents in appropriate vessels reduces both acute complications and the incidence of clinically important restenosis (Box 18.58).

PCI provides an effective symptomatic treatment but definitive evidence that it improves survival in patients with chronic stable angina is lacking. It is mainly used in single or two-vessel disease. Stenoses in bypass grafts can be dilated, as well as those in the native coronary arteries. The technique is often used to provide palliative therapy for patients with recurrent angina after CABG. Coronary surgery is usually the preferred option in patients with three-vessel or left main stem disease, although recent trials have demonstrated that PCI is also feasible in such patients.

The main acute complications of PCI are occlusion of the target vessel or a side branch by thrombus or a loose flap of intima (coronary artery dissection), and consequent myocardial damage. This occurs in about 2–5% of procedures and can often be corrected by deploying a stent; however, emergency CABG is sometimes required. Minor myocardial damage, as indicated by elevation of sensitive intracellular markers (troponins, p. 531), occurs in up to 10% of cases. The main long-term complication of PCI is restenosis (Box 18.59), which occurs in up to one-third of cases. This is due to a combination of elastic recoil and smooth muscle proliferation (neo-intimal hyperplasia) and tends to occur within 3 months. Stenting substantially reduces the risk of restenosis, probably because it allows the operator to achieve more complete dilatation in the first place. Drug-eluting stents can reduce this risk even further by allowing an antiproliferative drug such as sirolimus or paclitaxel to elute slowly from the coating and prevent neo-intimal hyperplasia and in-stent restenosis. There is an increased risk of late stent thrombosis with drug-eluting stents, although the absolute risk is small (< 0.5%). Recurrent angina (affecting up to 15–20% of patients receiving an intracoronary stent at 6 months) may require further PCI or bypass grafting.

EBM 18.59 **Percutaneous coronary intervention vs medical therapy in stable angina**

'PCI is more effective than medical therapy in alleviating angina pectoris and improving exercise tolerance but does not reduce mortality. It carries risks of procedure-related MI, emergency CABG and repeat procedures for restenosis.'

• Weintraub WS, et al. N Engl J Med 2008; 359(7):677–687.

For further information: www.sign.ac.uk

The risk of complications and the likely success of the procedure are closely related to the morphology of the stenoses, the experience of the operator and the presence of important comorbidity, e.g. diabetes, peripheral arterial disease. A good outcome is less likely if the target lesion is complex, long, eccentric or calcified, lies on a bend or within a tortuous vessel, involves a branch or contains acute thrombus.

In combination with aspirin and heparin, adjunctive therapy with potent platelet inhibitors, such as clopidogrel or glycoprotein IIb/IIIa receptor antagonists, improves the outcome of PCI, with lower short- and long-term rates of death and MI.

Coronary artery bypass grafting (CABG)

The internal mammary arteries, radial arteries or reversed segments of the patient's own saphenous vein can be used to bypass coronary artery stenoses (Fig. 18.67). This usually involves major surgery under cardiopulmonary bypass, but in some cases, grafts can be applied to the beating heart: 'off-pump' surgery. The operative mortality is approximately 1.5% but risks are higher in elderly patients, those with poor left ventricular function and those with significant comorbidity, such as renal failure.

Approximately 90% of patients are free of angina 1 year after CABG surgery, but fewer than 60% of patients are asymptomatic after 5 or more years. Early postoperative angina is usually due to graft failure arising from technical problems during the operation, or poor 'run-off' due to disease in the distal native coronary vessels. Late recurrence of angina may be due to progressive disease in the native coronary arteries or graft degeneration. Less than 50% of vein grafts are patent 10 years after surgery. However, arterial grafts have a much better long-term patency rate, with more than 80% of internal mammary artery grafts patent at 10 years. This has led many surgeons to consider total arterial revascularisation during CABG surgery. Aspirin (75–150 mg daily) and clopidogrel (75 mg daily) have both been shown to improve graft patency, and one or other should be prescribed indefinitely if well tolerated. Intensive lipid-lowering therapy slows the progression of disease in the native coronary arteries and bypass grafts, and reduces clinical cardiovascular events. There is substantial excess cardiovascular morbidity and mortality in patients who continue to smoke after bypass grafting. Persistent smokers are twice as likely to die in the 10 years following surgery than those who give up at surgery.

CABG improves survival in symptomatic patients with left main stem stenosis or three-vessel coronary disease (i.e. involving LAD, CX and right coronary arteries, Box 18.60) or two-vessel disease involving the proximal LAD coronary artery. Improvement in survival is most marked in those with impaired left ventricular function or positive stress testing prior to surgery and those who have undergone left internal mammary artery grafting.

Neurological complications are common, with a 1–5% risk of perioperative stroke. Between 30% and 80% of patients develop short-term cognitive impairment that is often mild and typically resolves within 6 months. There are also reports of long-term cognitive decline that may be evident in more than 30% of patients at 5 years. PCI and CABG are compared in Boxes 18.61 and 18.62.

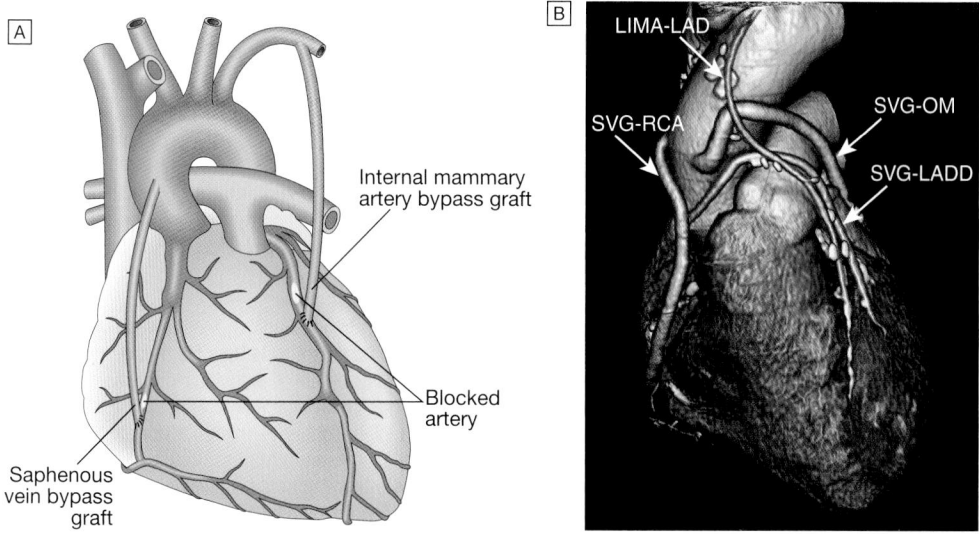

Fig. 18.67 Coronary artery bypass graft surgery. [A] Narrowed or stenosed arteries are bypassed using saphenous vein grafts connected to the aorta, or by utilising the internal mammary artery. [B] Three-dimensional reconstruction of multidetector CT of the heart. The image shows the patent saphenous vein grafts (SVG) to the right coronary artery (RCA), obtuse marginal branch (OM) and diagonal branch (LADD), and left internal mammary artery graft (LIMA) to the left anterior descending (LAD) coronary artery.

18

EBM | 18.60 Coronary artery bypass grafting for stable angina

'CABG is superior to medical treatment for at least 10 years after surgery in terms of survival. Greatest benefit occurs in those with a significant stenosis in the left main coronary artery or those with three-vessel disease and impaired ventricular function.'

- Yusuf S, et al. Lancet 1994; 344:563–570.
- Davies RF, et al. Circulation 1997; 95:2037–2043.

For further information: www.sign.ac.uk

EBM | 18.62 Comparison of PCI and CABG surgery in stable angina

'Systematic reviews and meta-analyses have found similar rates of death and MI, and similar quality of life. PCI is associated with a greater need for repeat procedures, although this has been halved by the introduction of intracoronary stent implantation. For patients with multivessel disease or diabetes, CABG appears to confer better survival rates at 4–5 years.'

- Serruys PW, et al. N Engl J Med 2009; 360:961–972.

For further information: www.sign.ac.uk

18.61 Comparison of PCI and CABG

	PCI	CABG
Death	< 0.5%	< 1.5%
Myocardial infarction*	2%	10%
Hospital stay	12–36 hrs	5–8 days
Return to work	2–5 days	6–12 wks
Recurrent angina	15–20% at 6 mths	10% at 1 yr
Repeat revascularisation	10–20% at 2 yrs	2% at 2 yrs
Neurological complications	Rare	Common (see text)
Other complications	Emergency CABG Vascular damage related to access site	Diffuse myocardial damage Infection (chest, wound) Wound pain

*Defined as CK-MB > 2 × normal, pp. 589–591.

Prognosis

Symptoms are a poor guide to prognosis; nevertheless, the 5-year mortality of patients with severe angina (NYHA class III or IV, p. 535) is nearly double that of patients with mild symptoms. Exercise testing and other forms of stress testing are much more powerful predictors of mortality; for example, in one study, the 4-year mortality of patients with stable angina and a negative exercise test was 1%, compared to more than 20% in those with a strongly positive test.

In general, the prognosis of coronary artery disease is related to the number of diseased vessels and the degree of left ventricular dysfunction. A patient with single-vessel disease and good left ventricular function has an excellent outlook (5-year survival > 90%), whereas a patient with severe left ventricular dysfunction and extensive three-vessel disease has a poor prognosis (5-year survival < 30%) without revascularisation. Spontaneous symptomatic improvement due to the development of collateral vessels is common.

Angina with normal coronary arteries

Approximately 10% of patients who report stable angina on effort will have angiographically normal coronary arteries. Many of these patients are women and the mechanism of their symptoms is often difficult to establish. It is important to review the original diagnosis and explore other potential causes.

Coronary artery spasm

Vasospasm in coronary arteries may coexist with atheroma, especially in unstable angina (see below); in < 1% of cases, vasospasm may occur without angiographically detectable atheroma. This form of angina is sometimes known as variant angina, and may be accompanied by spontaneous and transient ST elevation on the ECG (Prinzmetal's angina). Calcium channel antagonists, nitrates and other coronary vasodilators are the most useful therapeutic agents but may be ineffective.

Syndrome X

The constellation of typical angina on effort, objective evidence of myocardial ischaemia on stress testing, and angiographically normal coronary arteries is sometimes known as syndrome X. This disorder is poorly understood but carries a good prognosis and may respond to treatment with anti-anginal therapy.

Acute coronary syndrome

Acute coronary syndrome is a term that encompasses both unstable angina and MI. Unstable angina is characterised by new-onset or rapidly worsening angina (crescendo angina), angina on minimal exertion or angina at rest in the absence of myocardial damage. In contrast, MI occurs when symptoms occur at rest and there is evidence of myocardial necrosis, as demonstrated by an elevation in cardiac troponin or creatine kinase-MB isoenzyme (Box 18.63).

An acute coronary syndrome may present as a new phenomenon or against a background of chronic stable angina. The culprit lesion is usually a complex ulcerated or fissured atheromatous plaque with adherent platelet-rich thrombus and local coronary artery spasm (see Fig. 18.60, p. 577). This is a dynamic process whereby the degree of obstruction may either increase, leading to complete vessel occlusion, or regress due to the effects of platelet disaggregation and endogenous fibrinolysis. In acute MI, occlusive thrombus is almost always present at

> **18.63 Universal definition of myocardial infarction***
>
> The term 'myocardial infarction' should be used when there is evidence of myocardial necrosis in a clinical setting consistent with myocardial ischaemia, in which case any one of the following meets the diagnosis for MI:
> - Detection of rise and/or fall of cardiac biomarkers (preferably troponin), with at least one value above the 99th percentile of the upper reference limit, together with at least one of the following:
>   Symptoms of ischaemia
>   ECG changes indicative of new ischaemia (new ST-T changes or new left bundle branch block)
>   Development of pathological Q waves
>   Imaging evidence of new loss of viable myocardium or new regional wall motion abnormality
> - Sudden unexpected cardiac death, involving cardiac arrest, often with symptoms suggestive of myocardial ischaemia, and accompanied by presumably new ST elevation or new left bundle branch block, and/or evidence of fresh thrombus by coronary angiography and/or at autopsy, but death occurring before blood samples could be obtained or before the appearance of cardiac biomarkers in the blood
> - Pathological findings of an acute MI
>
> *Further definitions exist for MI during PCI and CABG.
>
> Adapted from Thygesen K, et al. Eur Heart J 2007; 28:2525–2538.

the site of rupture or erosion of an atheromatous plaque. The thrombus may undergo spontaneous lysis over the course of the next few days, although by this time irreversible myocardial damage has occurred. Without treatment, the infarct-related artery remains permanently occluded in 20–30% of patients. The process of infarction progresses over several hours (Fig. 18.68) and most patients present when it is still possible to salvage myocardium and improve outcome.

Clinical features

Pain is the cardinal symptom of an acute coronary syndrome but breathlessness, vomiting, and collapse are common features (Box 18.64). The pain occurs in the same sites as angina but is usually more severe and lasts longer; it is often described as a tightness, heaviness or

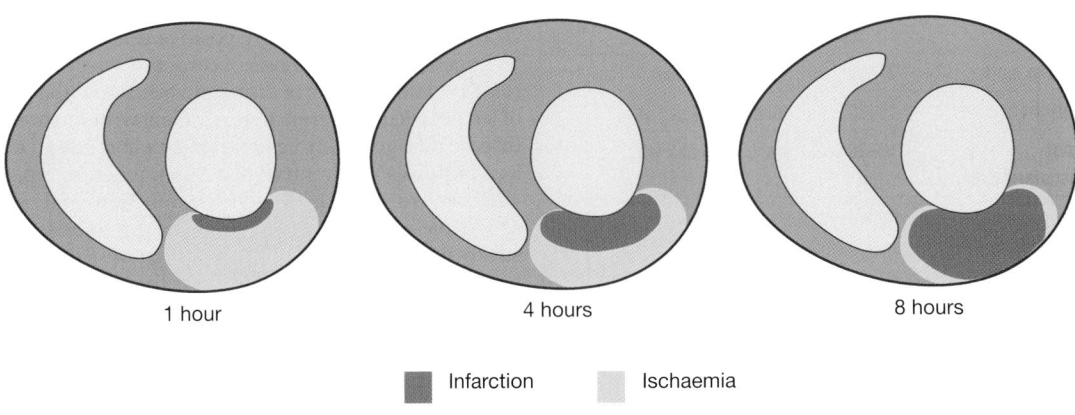

1 hour   4 hours   8 hours

■ Infarction   ■ Ischaemia

Fig. 18.68 The time course of MI. The relative proportion of ischaemic, infarcting and infarcted tissue slowly changes over a period of 12 hours. In the early stages of MI a significant proportion of the myocardium in jeopardy is potentially salvageable.

18.64 Clinical features of acute coronary syndromes

Symptoms

- Prolonged cardiac pain: chest, throat, arms, epigastrium or back
- Anxiety and fear of impending death
- Nausea and vomiting
- Breathlessness
- Collapse/syncope

Physical signs

- Signs of sympathetic activation: pallor, sweating, tachycardia
- Signs of vagal activation: vomiting, bradycardia
- Signs of impaired myocardial function
  Hypotension, oliguria, cold peripheries
  Narrow pulse pressure
  Raised JVP
  Third heart sound
  Quiet first heart sound
  Diffuse apical impulse
  Lung crepitations
- Signs of tissue damage: fever
- Signs of complications: e.g. mitral regurgitation, pericarditis

constriction in the chest. In acute MI, the pain can be excruciating, and the patient's expression and pallor may vividly convey the seriousness of the situation.

Most patients are breathless and in some this is the only symptom. Indeed, MI may pass unrecognised. Painless or 'silent' MI is particularly common in older patients or those with diabetes mellitus. If syncope occurs, it is usually due to an arrhythmia or profound hypotension. Vomiting and sinus bradycardia are often due to vagal stimulation and are particularly common in patients with inferior MI. Nausea and vomiting may also be caused or aggravated by opiates given for pain relief. Sometimes infarction occurs in the absence of physical signs.

Sudden death, from VF or asystole, may occur immediately and often within the first hour. If the patient survives this most critical stage, the liability to dangerous arrhythmias remains, but diminishes as each hour goes by. It is vital that patients know not to delay calling for help if symptoms occur. The development of cardiac failure reflects the extent of myocardial ischaemia and is the major cause of death in those who survive the first few hours.

18

1. Find points for each predictive factor

Killip class	Points	SBP (mmHg)	Points	Heart rate (beats/min)	Points	Age (years)	Points	Serum creatinine level (μmol/L)	Points	Other risk factors	Points
I	0	≤ 80	58	≤ 50	0	≤ 30	0	0–34	1		
II	29	80–99	53	50–69	3	30–39	8	35–70	4	Cardiac arrest at admission	39
III	39	100–119	43	70–89	9	40–49	25	71–105	7		
IV	59	120–139	34	90–109	15	50–59	41	106–140	10	ST-segment deviation	28
		140–159	24	110–149	24	60–69	58	141–176	13		
		160–199	10	150–199	38	70–79	75	177–353	21	Elevated cardiac enzyme levels	14
		≥ 200	0	≥ 200	46	80–89	91	≥ 353	28		
						≥ 90	100				

2. Sum points for all predictive factors

| Killip class | + | SBP | + | Heart rate | + | Age | + | Creatinine level | + | Cardiac arrest at admission | + | ST-segment deviation | + | Elevated cardiac enzyme levels | = | Total points |

3. Look up risk corresponding to total points

Total points	≤ 60	70	80	90	100	110	120	130	140	150	160	170	180	190	200	210	220	230	240	≤ 250
Probability of in-hospital death (%)	≤ 0.2	0.3	0.4	0.6	0.8	1.1	1.6	2.1	2.9	3.9	5.4	7.3	9.8	13	18	23	29	36	44	≤ 52

Examples

A patient has Killip class II, SBP of 99 mmHg, heart rate of 100 beats/min, is 65 years of age, has serum creatinine level of 76 μmol/L, did not have a cardiac arrest at admission but did have ST-segment deviation and elevated enzyme levels. His score would be: 20 + 53 + 15 + 58 + 7 + 0 + 28 + 14 = 195. This gives about a 16% risk of having an in-hospital death.

Similarly, a patient with Killip class I, SPB of 80 mmHg, heart rate of 60 beats/min, is 55 years of age, has a serum creatinine level of 30 μmol/L, and no risk factors would have the following score: 0 + 58 + 3 + 41 + 1 = 103. This gives about a 0.9% risk of having an in-hospital death.

Fig 18.69 Risk stratification in the acute coronary syndrome: the GRACE score. Killip class refers to a categorisation of the severity of heart failure based on easily obtained clinical signs. The main clinical features are as follows: class I = no heart failure; class II = crackles audible halfway up the chest; class III = crackles heard in all the lung fields; class IV = cardiogenic shock. (SBP = systolic blood pressure)

Diagnosis and risk stratification

The differential diagnosis is wide and includes most causes of central chest pain or collapse (pp. 535 and 552). The assessment of acute chest pain depends heavily on an analysis of the character of the pain and its associated features, evaluation of the ECG, and serial measurements of biochemical markers of cardiac damage, such as troponin I and T. A 12-lead ECG is mandatory and defines the initial triage, management and treatment (see Fig. 18.19, p. 540). Patients with ST segment elevation or new bundle branch block require emergency reperfusion therapy (see below). In patients with acute coronary syndrome without ST segment elevation, the ECG may show transient or persistent ST/T wave changes including ST depression and T-wave inversion.

Approximately 12% of patients will die within 1 month and a fifth within 6 months of the index event. The risk markers that are indicative of an adverse prognosis include recurrent ischaemia, extensive ECG changes at rest or during pain, the release of biochemical markers (creatine kinase or troponin), arrhythmias, recurrent ischaemia and haemodynamic complications (e.g. hypotension, mitral regurgitation) during episodes of ischaemia. Risk stratification is important because it guides the use of more complex pharmacological and interventional treatment (Figs 18.69 and 18.19 (p. 540)).

Investigations

Electrocardiography

The ECG is central to confirming the diagnosis but may be difficult to interpret if there is bundle branch block or previous MI. The initial ECG may be normal or non-diagnostic in one-third of cases. Repeated ECGs are important, especially where the diagnosis is uncertain or the patient has recurrent or persistent symptoms.

The earliest ECG change is usually ST-segment deviation. With proximal occlusion of a major coronary artery,

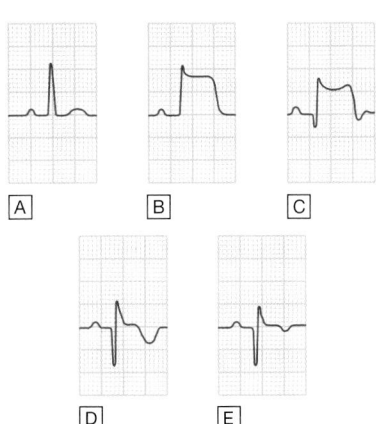

Fig. 18.70 The serial evolution of ECG changes in transmural MI.
A Normal ECG complex. **B** Acute ST elevation ('the current of injury'). **C** Progressive loss of the R wave, developing Q wave, resolution of the ST elevation and terminal T wave inversion. **D** Deep Q wave and T-wave inversion. **E** Old or established infarct pattern; the Q wave tends to persist but the T wave changes become less marked. The rate of evolution is very variable but, in general, stage B appears within minutes, stage C within hours, stage D within days and stage E after several weeks or months. This should be compared with the 12-lead ECGs in Figures 18.71–18.73.

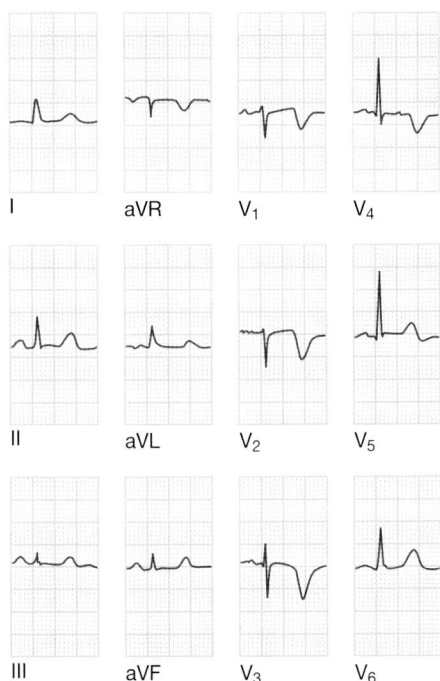

I	aVR	V$_1$	V$_4$
II	aVL	V$_2$	V$_5$
III	aVF	V$_3$	V$_6$

Fig. 18.71 Recent anterior non-ST elevation (subendocardial) MI. There is deep symmetrical T-wave inversion together with a reduction in the height of the R wave in leads V$_1$, V$_2$, V$_3$ and V$_4$.

ST-segment elevation (or new bundle branch block) is seen initially with later diminution in the size of the R wave, and in transmural (full thickness) infarction, development of a Q wave. Subsequently, the T wave becomes inverted because of a change in ventricular repolarisation; this change persists after the ST segment has returned to normal. These sequential features (Fig. 18.70) are sufficiently reliable for the approximate age of the infarct to be deduced.

In non-ST segment elevation acute coronary syndrome, there is partial occlusion of a major vessel or complete occlusion of a minor vessel, causing unstable angina or partial-thickness (subendocardial) MI. This is usually associated with ST-segment depression and T-wave changes. In the presence of infarction, this may be accompanied by some loss of R waves in the absence of Q waves (Fig. 18.71).

The ECG changes are best seen in the leads that 'face' the ischaemic or infarcted area. When there has been anteroseptal infarction, abnormalities are found in one or more leads from V$_1$ to V$_4$, while anterolateral infarction produces changes from V$_4$ to V$_6$, in aVL and in lead I. Inferior infarction is best shown in leads II, III and aVF, while at the same time leads I, aVL and the anterior chest leads may show 'reciprocal' changes of ST depression (Figs 18.72–18.74). Infarction of the posterior wall of the LV does not cause ST elevation or Q waves in the standard leads, but can be diagnosed by the presence of reciprocal changes (ST depression and a tall R wave in leads V$_1$–V$_4$). Some infarctions (especially inferior) also involve the RV. This may be identified by recording from additional leads placed over the right precordium.

Plasma cardiac markers

In unstable angina, there is no detectable rise in cardiac markers or enzymes, and the initial diagnosis is made

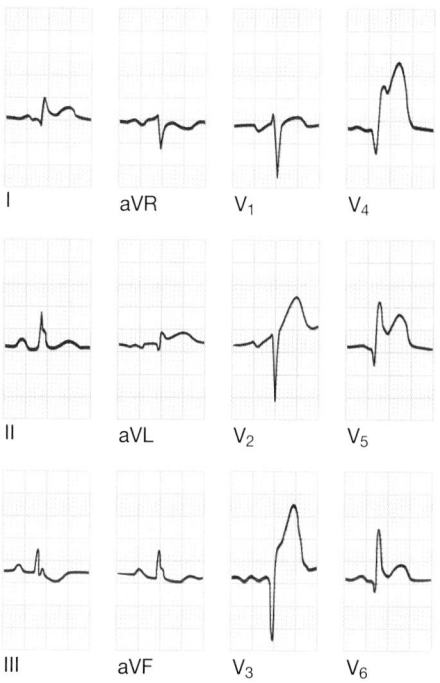

Fig. 18.72 Acute transmural anterior MI. This ECG was recorded from a patient who had developed severe chest pain 6 hours earlier. There is ST elevation in leads I, aVL, V$_2$, V$_3$, V$_4$, V$_5$ and V$_6$, and there are Q waves in leads V$_3$, V$_4$ and V$_5$. Anterior infarcts with prominent changes in leads V$_2$, V$_3$ and V$_4$ are sometimes called 'anteroseptal' infarcts, as opposed to 'anterolateral' infarcts in which the ECG changes are predominantly found in V$_4$, V$_5$ and V$_6$.

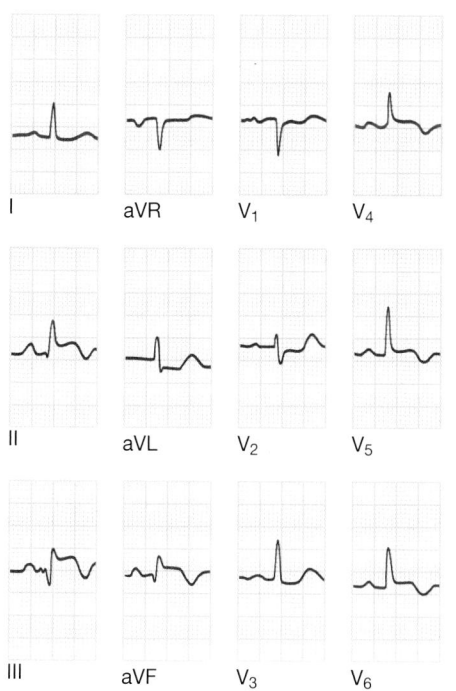

Fig. 18.73 Acute transmural inferolateral MI. This ECG was recorded from a patient who had developed severe chest pain 4 hours earlier. There is ST elevation in the inferior leads II, III and aVF and the lateral leads V$_4$, V$_5$ and V$_6$. There is also 'reciprocal' ST depression in leads aVL and V$_2$.

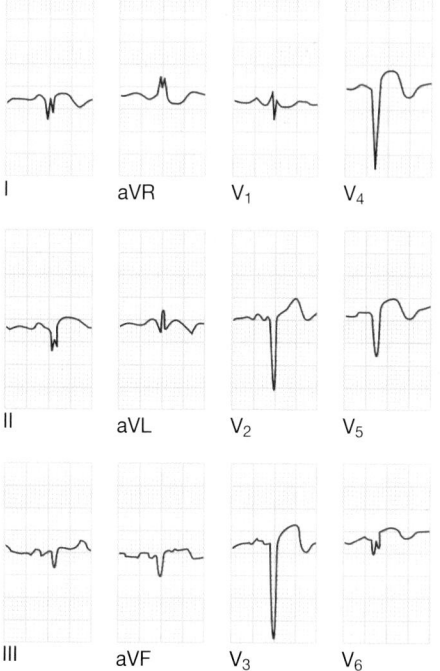

Fig. 18.74 Established anterior and inferior transmural MI. This ECG was recorded from a patient who had presented with an acute anterior infarct 2 days earlier and had been treated for an inferior myocardial infarction 11 months previously. There are Q waves in the inferior leads (II, III and aVF) and Q waves with some residual ST elevation in the anterior leads (I and V$_2$–V$_6$).

from the clinical history and ECG only. In contrast, MI causes a rise in the plasma concentration of enzymes and proteins that are normally concentrated within cardiac cells. These biochemical markers are creatine kinase (CK), a more sensitive and cardiospecific isoform of this enzyme (CK-MB), and the cardiospecific proteins, troponins T and I (p. 531). Admission and serial (usually daily) estimations are helpful because it is the change in plasma concentrations of these markers that confirms the diagnosis of MI (Fig. 18.75 and Box 18.63).

CK starts to rise at 4–6 hours, peaks at about 12 hours and falls to normal within 48–72 hours. CK is also present in skeletal muscle, and a modest rise in CK (but not CK-MB) may sometimes be due to an intramuscular injection, vigorous physical exercise or, particularly in older people, a fall. Defibrillation causes significant release of CK but not CK-MB or troponins. The most sensitive markers of myocardial cell damage are the cardiac troponins T and I, which are released within 4–6 hours and remain elevated for up to 2 weeks.

Other blood tests

A leucocytosis is usual, reaching a peak on the first day. The erythrocyte sedimentation rate (ESR) and C-reactive protein (CRP) are also elevated.

Chest X-ray

This may demonstrate pulmonary oedema that is not evident on clinical examination (see Fig. 18.25, p. 547). The heart size is often normal but there may be cardiomegaly due to pre-existing myocardial damage.

18

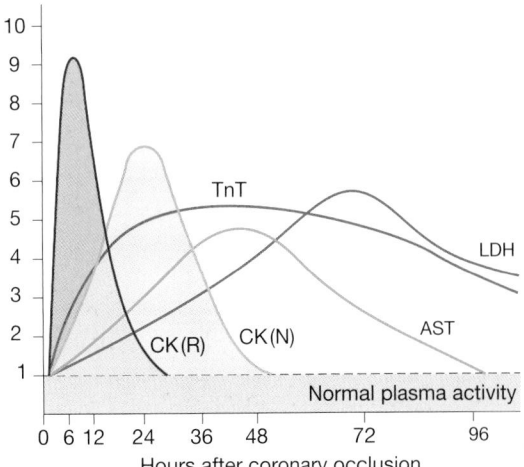

Fig. 18.75 Changes in plasma cardiac marker concentrations after MI. Creatine kinase (CK) and troponin T (TnT) are the first to rise, followed by aspartate aminotransferase (AST) and then lactate (hydroxybutyrate) dehydrogenase (LDH). In patients treated with a thrombolytic agent, reperfusion is usually accompanied by a rapid rise in plasma creatine kinase (curve CK (R)) due to a washout effect; if there is no reperfusion, the rise is less rapid but the area under the curve is often greater (curve CK (N)).

Echocardiography

This is useful for assessing left and right ventricular function and for detecting important complications such as mural thrombus, cardiac rupture, ventricular septal defect, mitral regurgitation and pericardial effusion.

Immediate management: the first 12 hours

Patients should be admitted urgently to hospital because there is a significant risk of death or recurrent myocardial ischaemia during the early unstable phase, and appropriate medical therapy can reduce the incidence of these by at least 60%. The essentials of the immediate in-hospital management of acute coronary syndrome are shown in Figure 18.19 (p. 540).

Patients are usually managed in a dedicated cardiac unit where the necessary expertise, monitoring and resuscitation facilities can be concentrated. If there are no complications, the patient can be mobilised from the second day and discharged from hospital after 3–5 days.

Analgesia

Adequate analgesia is essential not only to relieve distress, but also to lower adrenergic drive and thereby reduce vascular resistance, BP, infarct size and susceptibility to ventricular arrhythmias. Intravenous opiates (initially morphine sulphate 5–10 mg or diamorphine 2.5–5 mg) and antiemetics (initially metoclopramide 10 mg) should be administered and titrated by giving repeated small aliquots until the patient is comfortable. Intramuscular injections should be avoided because the clinical effect may be delayed by poor skeletal muscle perfusion, and a painful haematoma may form following thrombolytic or anti-thrombotic therapy.

Antithrombotic therapy

Antiplatelet therapy

In patients with acute coronary syndrome, oral administration of 75–300 mg aspirin daily improves survival, with a 25% relative risk reduction in mortality. The first tablet (300 mg) should be given orally within the first 12 hours and therapy should be continued indefinitely if there are no side-effects. In combination with aspirin, the early (within 12 hours) use of clopidogrel 600 mg, followed by 150 mg daily for 1 week and 75 mg daily thereafter, confers a further reduction in ischaemic events (Box 18.65). In patients with an acute coronary syndrome with or without ST-segment elevation, ticagrelor (180 mg followed by 90 mg 12-hourly) is more effective than clopidogrel in reducing vascular death, MI or stroke, and all-cause death without affecting overall major bleeding risk.

Glycoprotein IIb/IIIa receptor antagonists, such as tirofiban and abciximab, block the final common pathway of platelet aggregation and are potent inhibitors of platelet-rich thrombus formation. They are of particular benefit in patients with acute coronary syndromes who undergo PCI (Box 18.66), those with recurrent ischaemia and those at particularly high risk, such as patients with diabetes mellitus or an elevated troponin concentration.

Anticoagulants

Anticoagulation reduces the risk of thromboembolic complications, and prevents reinfarction in the absence of reperfusion therapy or after successful thrombolysis (Box 18.67). Anticoagulation can be achieved using unfractionated heparin, fractioned (low molecular weight) heparin or a pentasaccharide. Comparative clinical trials suggest that the pentasaccharides (subcutaneous fondaparinux 2.5 mg daily) have the best safety and efficacy profile, with low molecular weight heparin (subcutaneous enoxaparin 1 mg/kg 12-hourly) being

---

EBM 18.65 Oral antiplatelet agents in acute coronary syndromes

'Aspirin alone (75–325 mg/day) reduces the risk of death, MI and stroke in acute coronary syndromes (NNT_B = 20–25). The addition of clopidogrel (75 mg daily) to aspirin causes a further modest reduction in these events (NNT_B = 45–111).'

• Antithrombotic Trialists Collaboration. BMJ 2002; 324:71–86.
• Clopidogrel in Unstable Angina to prevent Recurrent Events (CURE) trial investigators. N Engl J Med 2001; 345:494–502.

For further information: www.acc.org

EBM 18.66 Intravenous glycoprotein IIb/IIIa inhibitors in acute coronary syndromes

'In patients with acute coronary syndromes, antiplatelet treatment with i.v. glycoprotein IIb/IIIa inhibitors reduces the combined endpoint of death or MI. Most benefit is seen in the context of PCI but there is no convincing evidence of benefit in patients who are treated without revascularisation (NNT_B (death or MI at 30 days) = 100; NNT_B (death, MI or revascularisation at 30 days) = 63).'

• Boersma E, et al. Lancet 2002; 359:189–198.

For further information: www.nice.org.uk

EBM 18.67 **Anticoagulation in acute coronary syndromes**

'Aspirin plus low molecular weight heparin is more effective than aspirin alone in reducing the combined endpoint of death, MI, refractory angina and urgent need for revascularisation. In comparison to low molecular weight heparin, the pentasaccharide, fondaparinux (2.5 mg s.c.), is associated with lower bleeding rates and better overall survival.'

• Antman EM, et al. for the TIMI IIB (Thrombolysis in Myocardial Infarction) and ESSENCE (Efficacy and Safety of Subcutaneous Enoxaparin in Non-Q-wave Coronary Events) Investigators. TIMI IIB-ESSENCE meta-analysis. Circulation 1999; 100:1602–1608.
• Eikelboom JW, et al. Lancet 2000; 355:1936–1942.
• Yusuf S, et al. N Engl J Med 2006; 354:1464–1476.

For further information: www.acc.org

a reasonable alternative. Anticoagulation should be continued for 8 days or until discharge from hospital or coronary revascularisation.

A period of treatment with warfarin should be considered if there is persistent atrial fibrillation or evidence of extensive anterior infarction, or if echocardiography shows mobile mural thrombus, because these patients are at increased risk of systemic thromboembolism.

Anti-anginal therapy

Sublingual glyceryl trinitrate (300–500 µg) is a valuable first-aid measure in unstable angina or threatened infarction, and intravenous nitrates (GTN 0.6–1.2 mg/hour or isosorbide dinitrate 1–2 mg/hour) are useful for the treatment of left ventricular failure and the relief of recurrent or persistent ischaemic pain.

Intravenous β-blockers (e.g. atenolol 5–10 mg or metoprolol 5–15 mg given over 5 mins) relieve pain, reduce arrhythmias and improve short-term mortality in patients who present within 12 hours of the onset of symptoms (see Fig. 18.19). However, they should be avoided if there is heart failure (pulmonary oedema), hypotension (systolic BP < 105 mmHg) or bradycardia (heart rate < 65/min).

18.68 Angina in old age

• **Incidence:** coronary artery disease increases and affects women almost as often as men.
• **Comorbid conditions:** anaemia and thyroid disease are common and may worsen angina.
• **Calcific aortic stenosis:** common and should be sought in all old people with angina.
• **Atypical presentations:** when myocardial ischaemia occurs, age-related changes in myocardial compliance and diastolic relaxation can cause the presentation to be with symptoms of heart failure such as breathlessness, rather than with chest discomfort.
• **Angioplasty and coronary artery bypass surgery:** provide symptomatic relief, although with an increased procedure-related morbidity and mortality. Outcome is determined by the number of diseased vessels, severity of cardiac dysfunction and the number of concomitant diseases, as much as age itself.

A dihydropyridine calcium channel antagonist (e.g. nifedipine or amlodipine) can be added to the β-blocker if there is persistent chest discomfort but may cause an unwanted tachycardia if used alone. Because of their rate-limiting action, verapamil and diltiazem are the calcium channel antagonists of choice if a β-blocker is contraindicated.

Reperfusion therapy

Non-ST segment elevation acute coronary syndrome

Immediate emergency reperfusion therapy has no demonstrable benefit in patients with non-ST segment elevation MI and thrombolytic therapy may be harmful. Selected medium- to high-risk patients do benefit from in-hospital coronary angiography and coronary revascularisation but this does not need to take place in the first 12 hours.

ST segment elevation acute coronary syndrome

Immediate reperfusion therapy restores coronary artery patency, preserves left ventricular function and improves survival. Successful therapy is associated with pain relief, resolution of acute ST elevation and sometimes transient arrhythmias (e.g. idioventricular rhythm).

Primary percutaneous coronary intervention (PCI). This is the treatment of choice for ST segment elevation MI (Figs 18.19 and 18.76). Outcomes are best when it is used in combination with glycoprotein IIb/IIIa receptor antagonists and intracoronary stent implantation. In comparison to thrombolytic therapy, it is associated with a greater reduction in the risk of death, recurrent MI or stroke (Box 18.69). The universal use of primary PCI has been limited by availability of the necessary resources to provide this highly specialised emergency service. Thus, intravenous thrombolytic therapy remains the first-line reperfusion treatment in many hospitals, especially those in rural or remote areas. When primary PCI cannot be achieved within 2 hours of diagnosis, thrombolytic therapy should be administered.

Thrombolysis. The appropriate use of thrombolytic therapy can reduce hospital mortality by 25–50% and this survival advantage is maintained for at least 10 years (Box 18.70). The benefit is greatest in those patients who receive treatment within the first few hours: 'minutes mean muscle'.

Alteplase (human tissue plasminogen activator or tPA) is a genetically engineered drug that is given over 90 minutes (bolus dose of 15 mg, followed by 0.75 mg/kg body weight, but not exceeding 50 mg, over 30 mins and then 0.5 mg/kg body weight, but not exceeding 35 mg, over 60 mins). Its use is associated with better survival rates than other thrombolytic agents, such as streptokinase, but carries a slightly higher risk of intracerebral

EBM 18.69 **Primary PCI in acute ST segment elevation MI**

'Primary PCI is more effective than thrombolysis for the treatment of acute MI. Death, non-fatal reinfarction and stroke are reduced from 14% with thrombolytic therapy to 8% with primary PCI ($NNT_B = 33$ for death and 9 for recurrent ischaemia).'

• Keeley EC, et al. Lancet 2003; 361:13–20.

For further information: www.acc.org; www.sign.ac.uk

18

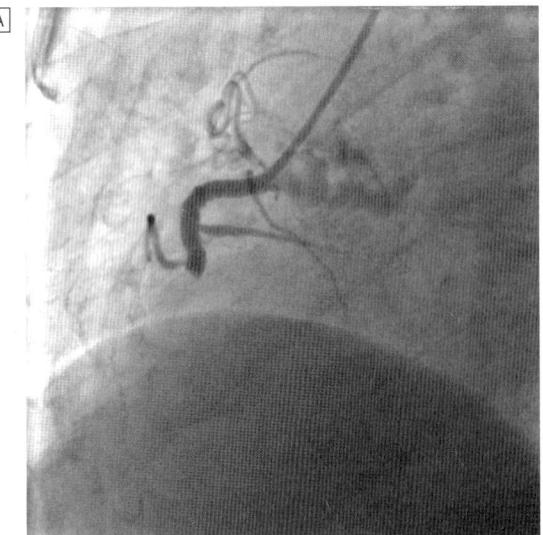

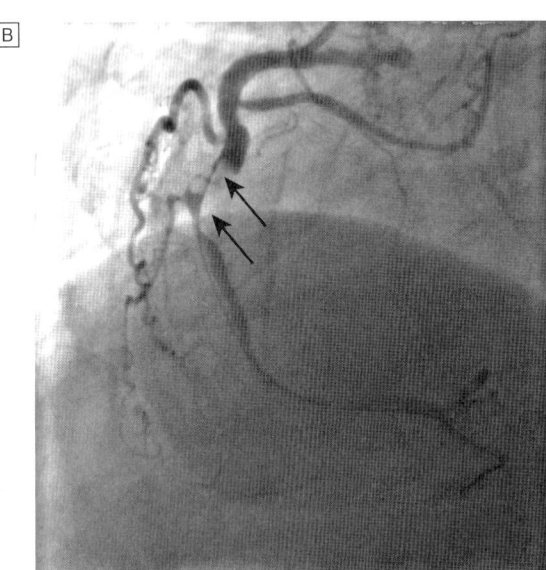

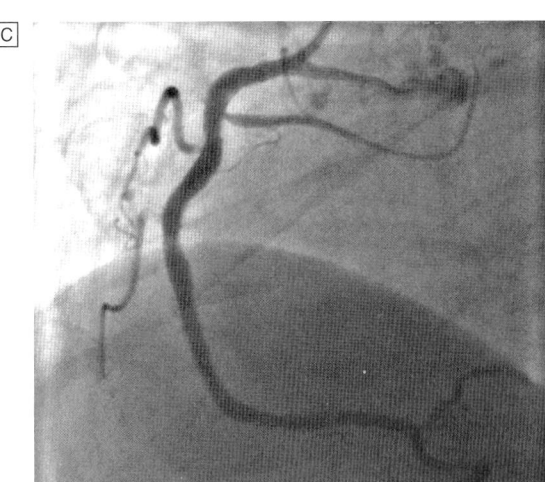

Fig. 18.76 Primary PCI. A Acute right coronary artery occlusion. B Initial angioplasty demonstrates a large thrombus filling defect (arrows). C Complete restoration of normal flow following intracoronary stent insertion.

bleeding (10 per 1000 increased survival, but 1 per 1000 more non-fatal stroke).

Analogues of tPA, such as tenecteplase and reteplase, have a longer plasma half-life than alteplase and can be given as an intravenous bolus. Tenecteplase (TNK) is as effective as alteplase at reducing death and MI whilst conferring similar intracerebral bleeding risks. However, other major bleeding and transfusion risks are lower and the practical advantages of bolus administration may provide opportunities for prompt treatment in the emergency department or in the pre-hospital setting. Reteplase (rPA) is administered as a double bolus and also produces a similar outcome to that achieved with alteplase, although some of the bleeding risks appear slightly higher.

An overview of all the large randomised trials confirms that thrombolytic therapy reduces short-term mortality in patients with MI if it is given within 12 hours of the onset of symptoms and the ECG shows bundle branch block or characteristic ST segment elevation > 1 mm in the limb leads or 2 mm in the chest leads (see Box 18.70). Thrombolysis appears to be of little net benefit and may be harmful in those who present more than 12 hours after the onset of symptoms and in those with a normal ECG or ST depression. In patients with ST elevation or bundle branch block, the absolute benefit of thrombolysis plus aspirin is approximately 50 lives saved per 1000 patients treated within 6 hours and 40 lives saved per 1000 patients treated between 7 and 12 hours after the onset of symptoms. The benefit is greatest for patients treated within the first 2 hours.

The major hazard of thrombolytic therapy is bleeding. Cerebral haemorrhage causes 4 extra strokes per 1000 patients treated and the incidence of other major bleeds is between 0.5% and 1%. Accordingly, the treatment should be withheld if there is a significant risk of serious bleeding (Box 18.71).

EBM | **18.70 Thrombolytic treatment in acute ST segment elevation MI**

'Prompt thrombolytic treatment (within 12 hours, and particularly within 6 hours, of the onset of symptoms) reduces mortality in patients with acute MI and ECG changes of ST elevation or new bundle branch block (NNT$_B$ = 56). Intracranial haemorrhage is more common in people given thrombolysis with one additional stroke for every 250 people treated.'

- Fibrinolytic Therapy Trialists' (FTT) Collaborative Group. Lancet 1994; 343:311–322.
- Collins R. N Engl J Med 1997; 336:847–860.

For further information:  www.escardio.org

---

18.71 Relative contraindications to thrombolytic therapy: potential candidates for primary angioplasty

- Active internal bleeding
- Previous subarachnoid or intracerebral haemorrhage
- Uncontrolled hypertension
- Recent surgery (within 1 mth)
- Recent trauma (including traumatic resuscitation)
- High probability of active peptic ulcer
- Pregnancy

For some patients, thrombolytic therapy is contra-indicated or fails to achieve coronary arterial reperfusion (see Fig. 18.19, p. 540). Early emergency PCI may then be considered, particularly where there is evidence of cardiogenic shock.

Complications of acute coronary syndrome

Complications are seen in all forms of acute coronary syndrome, although the frequency and extent vary with the severity of ischaemia and infarction. Major mechanical and structural complications are only seen with significant, often transmural, MI.

Arrhythmias

Many patients with acute coronary syndrome have some form of arrhythmia (Box 18.72). In the majority of cases this is transient and of no haemodynamic or prognostic importance. Pain relief, rest and the correction of hypokalaemia may help prevent them. Diagnosis and management of arrhythmias are discussed in detail on pages 559–577.

18.72 Common arrhythmias in acute coronary syndrome	
• Ventricular fibrillation	• Atrial fibrillation
• Ventricular tachycardia	• Atrial tachycardia
• Accelerated idioventricular rhythm	• Sinus bradycardia (particularly after inferior MI)
• Ventricular ectopics	• Atrioventricular block

Ventricular fibrillation

This occurs in about 5–10% of patients who reach hospital and is thought to be the major cause of death in those who die before receiving medical attention. Prompt defibrillation will usually restore sinus rhythm and is life-saving. The prognosis of patients with early ventricular fibrillation (within the first 48 hours) who are successfully and promptly resuscitated is identical to that of patients who do not suffer ventricular fibrillation.

Atrial fibrillation

This is common but frequently transient, and usually does not require emergency treatment. However, if the arrhythmia causes a rapid ventricular rate with hypotension or circulatory collapse, prompt cardioversion by immediate synchronised DC shock is essential. In other situations, digoxin or a β-blocker is usually the treatment of choice. Atrial fibrillation (due to acute atrial stretch) is often a feature of impending or overt left ventricular failure, and therapy may be ineffective if heart failure is not recognised and treated appropriately. Anticoagulation is required if atrial fibrillation persists.

Bradycardia

This does not usually require treatment, but if there is hypotension or haemodynamic deterioration, atropine (0.6–1.2 mg i.v.) may be given. AV block complicating inferior infarction is usually temporary and often resolves following reperfusion therapy. If there is clinical deterioration due to second-degree or complete AV block, a temporary pacemaker should be considered. AV block complicating anterior infarction is more serious because asystole may suddenly supervene; a prophylactic temporary pacemaker should be inserted (p. 575).

Ischaemia

Patients who develop recurrent angina at rest or on minimal exertion following an acute coronary syndrome are at high risk and should be considered for prompt coronary angiography with a view to revascularisation. Patients with dynamic ECG changes and ongoing pain should be treated with intravenous glycoprotein IIb/IIIa receptor antagonists. Patients with resistant pain or marked haemodynamic changes should be considered for intra-aortic balloon counterpulsation and emergency coronary revascularisation.

Post-infarct angina occurs in up to 50% of patients treated with thrombolysis. Most patients have a residual stenosis in the infarct-related vessel despite successful thrombolysis, and this may cause angina if there is still viable myocardium downstream. For this reason, all patients who have received successful thrombolysis should be considered for early (within the first 6–24 hours) coronary angiography with a view to coronary revascularisation.

Acute circulatory failure

Acute circulatory failure usually reflects extensive myocardial damage and indicates a bad prognosis. All the other complications of MI are more likely to occur when acute heart failure is present. The assessment and management of heart failure complicating acute MI are discussed in detail on page 542.

Pericarditis

This only occurs following infarction and is particularly common on the second and third days. The patient may recognise that a different pain has developed, even though it is at the same site, and that it is positional and tends to be worse or sometimes only present on inspiration. A pericardial rub may be audible. Opiate-based analgesia should be used. Non-steroidal and steroidal anti-inflammatory drugs may increase the risk of aneurysm formation and myocardial rupture in the early recovery period, and so should be avoided.

The post-MI syndrome (Dressler's syndrome) is characterised by persistent fever, pericarditis and pleurisy, and is probably due to autoimmunity. The symptoms tend to occur a few weeks or even months after the infarct and often subside after a few days; prolonged or severe symptoms may require treatment with high-dose aspirin, NSAIDs or even corticosteroids.

Mechanical complications

Part of the necrotic muscle in a fresh infarct may tear or rupture, with devastating consequences:

- *Rupture of the papillary muscle* can cause acute pulmonary oedema and shock due to the sudden onset of severe mitral regurgitation, which presents with a pansystolic murmur and third heart sound. In the presence of severe valvular regurgitation, the murmur may be quiet or absent. The diagnosis is confirmed by echocardiography and emergency mitral valve replacement may be necessary. Lesser degrees of mitral regurgitation due to papillary muscle dysfunction are common and may be transient.
- *Rupture of the interventricular septum* causes left-to-right shunting through a ventricular septal defect. This usually presents with sudden haemodynamic

18

595

deterioration accompanied by a new loud pansystolic murmur radiating to the right sternal border, but may be difficult to distinguish from acute mitral regurgitation. However, patients with an acquired ventricular septal defect tend to develop right heart failure rather than pulmonary oedema. Doppler echocardiography and right heart catheterisation will confirm the diagnosis. Without prompt surgery, the condition is usually fatal.

- *Rupture of the ventricle* may lead to cardiac tamponade and is usually fatal (p. 542), although it may rarely be possible to support a patient with an incomplete rupture until emergency surgery is performed.

Embolism

Thrombus often forms on the endocardial surface of freshly infarcted myocardium. This can lead to systemic embolism and occasionally causes a stroke or ischaemic limb.

Venous thrombosis and pulmonary embolism may occur but have become less common with the use of prophylactic anticoagulants and early mobilisation.

Impaired ventricular function, remodelling and ventricular aneurysm

Acute transmural MI is often followed by thinning and stretching of the infarcted segment (infarct expansion). This leads to an increase in wall stress with progressive dilatation and hypertrophy of the remaining ventricle (ventricular remodelling, Fig. 18.77). As the ventricle dilates, it becomes less efficient and heart failure may supervene. Infarct expansion occurs over a few days and weeks but ventricular remodelling can take years. ACE

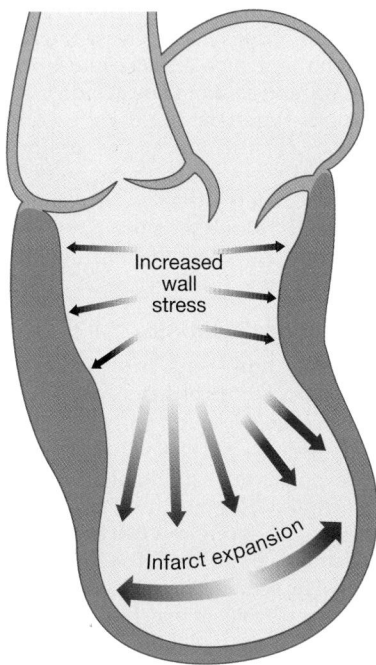

Fig. 18.77 Infarct expansion and ventricular remodelling. Full-thickness MI causes thinning and stretching of the infarcted segment (infarct expansion), which leads to increased wall stress with progressive dilatation and hypertrophy of the remaining ventricle (ventricular remodelling).

inhibitor therapy reduces late ventricular remodelling and can prevent the onset of heart failure (p. 548).

A left ventricular aneurysm develops in approximately 10% of patients with MI and is particularly common when there is persistent occlusion of the infarct-related vessel. Heart failure, ventricular arrhythmias, mural thrombus and systemic embolism are all recognised complications of aneurysm formation. Other clinical features include a paradoxical impulse on the chest wall, persistent ST elevation on the ECG, and sometimes an unusual bulge from the cardiac silhouette on the chest X-ray. Echocardiography is usually diagnostic. Surgical removal of a left ventricular aneurysm carries a high morbidity and mortality but is sometimes necessary.

Later in-hospital management (Box 18.73)
Risk stratification and further investigation

Simple clinical tools can be used to identify medium- to high-risk patients. The GRACE score (see Fig. 18.69, p. 589) is a simple method of calculating early mortality that can help guide which patients should be selected for intensive therapy, and specifically early inpatient coronary angiography.

The prognosis of patients who have survived an acute coronary syndrome is related to the extent of residual myocardial ischaemia, the degree of myocardial damage and the presence of ventricular arrhythmias.

Left ventricular function

The degree of left ventricular dysfunction can be crudely assessed from physical findings (tachycardia, third heart sound, crackles at the lung bases, elevated venous pressure and so on), ECG changes and chest X-ray (size of the heart and presence of pulmonary oedema). However, formal assessment with echocardiography should be undertaken in the early recovery phase.

Ischaemia

Patients with early ischaemia following an acute coronary syndrome should undergo coronary angiography with a view to revascularisation. Low-risk patients without spontaneous ischaemia should undergo an exercise

---

18.73 Late management of MI

Risk stratification and further investigation (see text)

Lifestyle modification
- Cessation of smoking
- Regular exercise
- Diet (weight control, lipid-lowering)

Secondary prevention drug therapy
- Antiplatelet therapy (aspirin and/or clopidogrel)
- β-blocker
- ACE inhibitor/ARB
- Statin
- Additional therapy for control of diabetes and hypertension
- Aldosterone receptor antagonist

Rehabilitation

Devices
- Implantable cardiac defibrillator (high-risk patients)

tolerance test approximately 4 weeks after the acute coronary syndrome. This will help to identify those individuals with residual myocardial ischaemia who require further investigation and may help to boost the confidence of the remainder.

If the exercise test is negative and the patient has a good effort tolerance, the outlook is good, with a 1–4% chance of an adverse event in the next 12 months. In contrast, patients with residual ischaemia in the form of chest pain or ECG changes at low exercise levels are at high risk, with a 15–25% chance of suffering a further ischaemic event in the next 12 months.

Arrhythmias

The presence of ventricular arrhythmias during the convalescent phase of acute coronary syndrome may be a marker of poor ventricular function and may herald sudden death. Although empirical anti-arrhythmic treatment is of no value and even hazardous, selected patients may benefit from electrophysiological testing and specific anti-arrhythmic therapy (including implantable cardiac defibrillators, p. 576).

Recurrent ventricular arrhythmias are sometimes manifestations of myocardial ischaemia or impaired left ventricular function and may respond to appropriate treatment directed at the underlying problem.

Lifestyle and risk factor modification

Smoking

The 5-year mortality of patients who continue to smoke cigarettes is double that of those who quit smoking at the time of their acute coronary syndrome. Giving up smoking is the single most effective contribution a patient can make to his or her future. The success of smoking cessation can be increased by supportive advice and pharmacological therapy (p. 99).

Hyperlipidaemia

The importance of lowering serum cholesterol following acute coronary syndrome has been demonstrated in large-scale randomised clinical trials. Lipids should be measured within 24 hours of presentation because there is often a transient fall in blood cholesterol in the 3 months following infarction. HMG CoA reductase enzyme inhibitors ('statins', p. 455) can produce marked reductions in total (and LDL) cholesterol and reduce the subsequent risk of death, reinfarction, stroke and the need for revascularisation (see Box 18.48, p. 581). Irrespective of serum cholesterol concentrations, all patients should receive statin therapy after acute coronary syndrome, but those with serum LDL cholesterol concentrations > 3.2 mmol/L (~120 mg/dL) benefit from more intensive lipid-lowering, such as atorvastatin 80 mg daily.

Other risk factors

Maintaining an ideal body weight, eating a Mediterranean-style diet, taking regular exercise, and achieving good control of hypertension and diabetes mellitus may all improve the long-term outlook.

Mobilisation and rehabilitation

The necrotic muscle of an acute myocardial infarct takes 4–6 weeks to be replaced with fibrous tissue and it is conventional to restrict physical activities during this period. When there are no complications, the patient can mobilise on the second day, return home in 3–5 days and gradually increase activity with the aim of returning to work in 4–6 weeks. The majority of patients may resume driving after 4–6 weeks, although in most countries vocational driving licence holders (e.g. heavy goods and public service vehicles) require special assessment.

Emotional problems, such as denial, anxiety and depression, are common and must be addressed. Many patients are severely and even permanently incapacitated as a result of the psychological rather than the physical effects of acute coronary syndrome, and all benefit from thoughtful explanation, counselling and reassurance at every stage of the illness. Many patients mistakenly believe that 'stress' was the cause of their heart attack and may restrict their activity inappropriately. The patient's spouse or partner will also require emotional support, information and counselling. Formal rehabilitation programmes based on graded exercise protocols with individual and group counselling are often very successful, and in some cases have been shown to improve the long-term outcome.

Secondary prevention drug therapy

Aspirin and clopidogrel

Low-dose aspirin therapy reduces the risk of further infarction and other vascular events by approximately 25% and should be continued indefinitely if there are no unwanted effects. Clopidogrel should be given in combination with aspirin for at least 3 months. If patients are intolerant of long-term aspirin, clopidogrel is a suitable alternative.

Beta-blockers

Continuous treatment with an oral β-blocker reduces long-term mortality by approximately 25% among the survivors of acute MI (Box 18.74). Unfortunately, a minority of patients do not tolerate β-blockers because of bradycardia, AV block, hypotension or asthma. Patients with heart failure, irreversible chronic obstructive pulmonary disease or peripheral vascular disease derive similar, if not greater secondary preventative benefits from β-blocker therapy if they can tolerate it, so it should be tried. The secondary preventative role of β-blockers in patients with unstable angina is unknown.

ACE inhibitors

Several clinical trials have shown that long-term treatment with an ACE inhibitor (e.g. enalapril 10 mg 12-hourly or ramipril 2.5–5 mg 12-hourly) can counteract ventricular remodelling, prevent the onset of heart failure, improve survival, reduce recurrent MI and avoid rehospitalisation. The benefits are greatest in those with overt heart failure (clinical or radiological) but extend to

18

EBM 18.74 **Beta-blockers in secondary prevention after MI**

'Beta-blockers reduce the risk of overall mortality ($NNT_B = 48$), sudden death ($NNT_B = 63$) and non-fatal reinfarction ($NNT_B = 56$) in patients after MI. The greatest benefit is seen in those at highest risk and about one-quarter of patients suffer adverse events.'

- Freemantle N, et al. Br Med J 1999; 318: 1730–1737.

For further information: www.sign.ac.uk

patients with asymptomatic left ventricular dysfunction and those with preserved left ventricular function. They should therefore be considered in all patients with acute coronary syndrome. Caution must be exercised in hypovolaemic or hypotensive patients because the introduction of an ACE inhibitor may exacerbate hypotension and impair coronary perfusion. In patients intolerant of ACE inhibitor therapy, angiotensin receptor blockers (e.g. valsartan 40–160 mg 12-hourly or candesartan 4–16 mg daily) are suitable alternatives and are better tolerated.

Patients with acute MI and left ventricular dysfunction (ejection fraction < 35%) and either pulmonary oedema or diabetes mellitus further benefit from additional aldosterone receptor antagonism (e.g. eplerenone 25–50 mg daily).

Coronary revascularisation

Most low-risk patients stabilise with aspirin, clopidogrel, anticoagulation and anti-anginal therapy, and can be rapidly mobilised. In the absence of recurrent symptoms, low-risk patients do not benefit from routine coronary angiography. Coronary angiography should be considered with a view to revascularisation in all patients at moderate or high risk, including those who fail to settle on medical therapy, those with extensive ECG changes, those with an elevated plasma troponin and those with severe pre-existing stable angina. This often reveals disease that is amenable to PCI or urgent CABG. In these cases coronary revascularisation is associated with short- and long-term benefits, including reductions in MI and death.

Device therapy

Implantable cardiac defibrillators are of benefit in preventing sudden cardiac death in patients who have severe left ventricular impairment (ejection fraction ≤ 30%) after MI (p. 576).

Prognosis

In almost one-quarter of all cases of MI, death occurs within a few minutes without medical care. Half the deaths occur within 24 hours of the onset of symptoms and about 40% of all affected patients die within the first month. The prognosis of those who survive to reach hospital is much better, with a 28-day survival of more than 85%. Patients with unstable angina have a mortality approximately half those with MI.

Early death is usually due to an arrhythmia and is independent of the extent of MI. However, late outcomes are determined by the extent of myocardial damage and unfavourable features include poor left ventricular function, AV block and persistent ventricular arrhythmias. The prognosis is worse for anterior than for inferior infarcts. Bundle branch block and high cardiac marker levels both indicate extensive myocardial damage. Old age, depression and social isolation are also associated with a higher mortality.

Of those who survive an acute attack, more than 80% live for a further year, about 75% for 5 years, 50% for 10 years and 25% for 20 years.

Cardiac risk of non-cardiac surgery

Non-cardiac surgery, particularly major vascular, abdominal or thoracic surgery, can precipitate serious perioperative cardiac complication such as MI and death in patients with coronary artery and other forms of heart disease. Careful pre-operative cardiac assessment may help to determine the balance of benefit versus risk on an individual basis, and identify measures that minimise the operative risk (Box 18.76).

A hypercoagulable state is part of the normal physiological response to surgery, and may promote coronary thrombosis leading to an acute coronary syndrome in the early post-operative period. Patients with a history of recent PCI or acute coronary syndrome are at greatest risk and, whenever possible, elective non-cardiac surgery should be avoided for 3 months after such an event. Antiplatelet agents, statins and β-blockers reduce the risk of perioperative MI in patients with coronary artery disease and, where possible, should be prescribed throughout the perioperative period.

Careful attention to fluid balance during and after surgery is particularly important in patients with impaired left ventricular function and valvular heart disease because antidiuretic hormone is released as part of the normal physiological response to surgery, and in these circumstances the overzealous administration of intravenous fluids can easily precipitate heart failure. Patients with severe valvular heart disease, particularly aortic stenosis and mitral stenosis, are also at increased risk because they may not be able to increase their cardiac output in response to the stress of surgery.

18.75 Myocardial infarction in old age

- **Atypical presentation**: often with anorexia, fatigue or weakness rather than chest pain.
- **Case fatality**: rises steeply. Hospital mortality exceeds 25% in those > 75 yrs old, which is five times greater than that seen in those aged < 55 yrs.
- **Survival benefit of treatments**: not influenced by age. The absolute benefit of evidence-based treatments may therefore be greatest in older people.
- **Hazards of treatments**: rise with age (e.g. increased risk of intracerebral bleeding after thrombolysis) and are due partly to increased comorbidity.
- **Quality of evidence**: older patients, particularly those with significant comorbidity, were under-represented in many of the randomised controlled clinical trials that helped to establish the treatment of MI. The balance of risk and benefit for many treatments (e.g. thrombolysis, primary percutaneous transluminal coronary angiography) in frail older people is therefore uncertain.

18.76 Major risk factors for cardiac complications of non-cardiac surgery

- Recent (< 6 mths) MI or unstable angina
- Severe coronary artery disease: left main stem or three-vessel disease
- Severe stable angina on effort
- Severe left ventricular dysfunction
- Severe valvular heart disease (especially aortic stenosis)

Atrial fibrillation may be triggered by hypoxia, myocardial ischaemia or heart failure, and is a common postoperative complication in patients with pre-existing heart disease. It usually terminates spontaneously when the precipitating factors have been eliminated, but digoxin or β-blockers can be prescribed to control the heart rate.

VASCULAR DISEASE

Peripheral arterial disease

In developed countries, almost all peripheral arterial disease (PAD) is due to atherosclerosis (pp. 577–579) and so shares common risk factors with coronary artery disease (CAD): namely, smoking, diabetes mellitus, hyperlipidaemia and hypertension. As with CAD, plaque rupture is responsible for the most serious manifestations of PAD, and not infrequently occurs in a plaque that hitherto has been asymptomatic.

Approximately 20% of middle-aged (55–75 years) people in the UK have PAD but only one-quarter of them will have symptoms. The clinical manifestations depend upon the anatomical site, the presence or absence of a collateral supply, the speed of onset and the mechanism of injury (Box 18.77).

Chronic lower limb arterial disease

PAD affects the leg eight times more often than the arm. The lower limb arterial tree comprises the aorto-iliac ('inflow'), femoro-popliteal and infra-popliteal ('outflow') segments. One or more segments may be affected in a variable and asymmetric manner. Lower limb ischaemia presents as two distinct clinical entities: intermittent claudication (IC) and critical limb ischaemia (CLI). The presence and severity of ischaemia can be determined by clinical examination (Box 18.78) and measurement of the ankle-brachial pressure index (ABPI), which is the ratio between the (highest systolic) ankle and brachial blood pressures. In health the ABPI is > 1.0, in IC typically 0.5–0.9 and in CLI usually < 0.5.

Intermittent claudication (IC)

This term describes ischaemic pain affecting the muscles of the leg upon walking. The pain is usually felt in the calf because the disease most commonly affects the superficial femoral artery. However, the pain may be felt in the thigh or buttock if the iliac arteries are involved. Typically, the pain comes on after a reasonably constant 'claudication distance', and rapidly subsides on stopping walking. Resumption of walking leads to a return of the pain. Most patients describe a cyclical pattern of exacerbation and resolution due to the progression of disease and the subsequent development of collaterals.

Approximately 5% of middle-aged men report IC. Provided patients comply with 'best medical therapy' (BMT) (Box 18.79), only 1–2% per year will deteriorate to a point where amputation and/or revascularisation is required. However, the annual mortality rate exceeds 5%, 2–3 times higher than in an equivalent non-claudicant population. This is because IC is nearly always found in association with widespread atherosclerosis, so that most claudicants succumb to MI or stroke. The mainstay of treatment is BMT, including (preferably

---

18.77 Factors influencing the clinical manifestations of peripheral arterial disease

Anatomical site

Cerebral circulation
- TIA, amaurosis fugax, vertebrobasilar insufficiency

Renal arteries
- Hypertension and renal failure

Mesenteric arteries
- Mesenteric angina, acute intestinal ischaemia

Limbs (legs >> arms)
- Intermittent claudication, critical limb ischaemia, acute limb ischaemia

Collateral supply
- In a patient with a complete circle of Willis, occlusion of one carotid artery may be asymptomatic
- In a patient without cross-circulation, stroke is likely

Speed of onset
- Where PAD develops slowly, a collateral supply will develop
- Sudden occlusion of a previously normal artery is likely to cause severe distal ischaemia

Mechanism of injury

Haemodynamic
- Plaque must reduce arterial diameter by 70% ('critical stenosis') to reduce flow and pressure at rest. On exertion (e.g. walking), a much lesser stenosis may become 'critical'. This mechanism tends to have a relatively benign course due to collateralisation

Thrombotic
- Occlusion of a long-standing critical stenosis may be asymptomatic due to collateralisation. However, acute rupture and thrombosis of a non-haemodynamically significant plaque usually has severe consequences

Atheroembolic
- Symptoms depend upon embolic load and size
- Carotid (TIA, amaurosis fugax or stroke) and peripheral arterial (blue toe/finger syndrome) plaque are common examples

Thromboembolic
- Usually secondary to atrial fibrillation
- The clinical consequences are usually dramatic, as the thrombus load is often large and tends to occlude a major, previously healthy, non-collateralised artery suddenly and completely

---

18.78 Clinical features of chronic lower limb ischaemia

- Pulses: diminished or absent
- Bruits: denote turbulent flow but bear no relationship to the severity of the underlying disease
- Reduced skin temperature
- Pallor on elevation and rubor on dependency (Buerger's sign)
- Superficial veins that fill sluggishly and empty ('gutter') upon minimal elevation
- Muscle-wasting
- Skin and nails: dry, thin and brittle
- Loss of hair

18

18.79 Best medical therapy for peripheral arterial disease*

- Smoking cessation
- Regular exercise (30 mins of walking, three times per week)
- Antiplatelet agent (aspirin 75 mg daily or clopidogrel 75 mg daily)
- Reduction of cholesterol (diet + statin therapy)
- Diagnosis and treatment of diabetes mellitus (all should have fasting glucose measured)
- Diagnosis and treatment of frequently associated conditions (e.g. hypertension, anaemia, heart failure)

*All patients with any manifestation of PAD should be considered candidates for BMT.

supervised) exercise therapy. The peripheral vasodilator, cilostazol, has been shown to improve walking distance. Intervention with angioplasty, stenting, endarterectomy or bypass is usually only considered after BMT has been given at least 6 months to effect symptomatic improvement, and then only in patients who are severely disabled or whose livelihood is threatened by their disability.

Critical limb ischaemia (CLI)

This is defined as rest (night) pain, requiring opiate analgesia, and/or tissue loss (ulceration or gangrene), present for more than 2 weeks, in the presence of an ankle BP of < 50 mmHg (Fig. 18.78). Rest pain only, with ankle pressures > 50 mmHg, is known as subcritical limb ischaemia (SCLI). The term severe limb ischaemia (SLI) is used to describe both CLI and SCLI. Whereas IC is usually due to single-segment plaque, SLI is always due to multilevel disease.

Many patients with SLI have not previously sought medical advice for IC, principally because they have other comorbidity that prevents them from walking to a point where claudication pain might develop. In contrast to IC, patients with SLI are at high risk of losing their limb, and sometimes their life, in a matter of weeks or months without surgical bypass or endovascular revascularisation by angioplasty or stenting. However, treatment is difficult because patients have extensive and severe (often bilateral) end-stage disease, are usually elderly and nearly always have significant multisystem comorbidity. Imaging is performed using duplex ultrasonography, MRI or CT with intravenous injection of contrast agents. Intra-arterial digital subtraction angiography (IA-DSA) is usually reserved for those undergoing endovascular revascularisation.

Diabetic vascular disease

Approximately 5–10% of patients with PAD have diabetes but this proportion increases to 30–40% in those with SLI. Diabetes does not cause obstructive microangiopathy at the capillary level, as previously thought, and so is not a contraindication to lower limb revascularisation. Nevertheless, the 'diabetic foot' does pose a number of particular problems (Box 18.80 and p. 833). If the blood supply is adequate, then dead tissue can be excised in the expectation that healing will occur, provided infection is controlled and the foot is protected from pressure. However, if significant ischaemia is also present, the priority is to revascularise the foot if possible. Sadly, many diabetic patients present late with extensive tissue loss, which accounts for the high amputation rate.

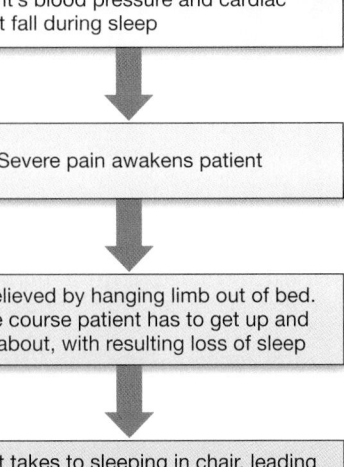

Pain develops, typically in forefoot, about an hour after patient goes to bed because:
- beneficial effects of gravity on perfusion are lost
- patient's blood pressure and cardiac output fall during sleep

↓

Severe pain awakens patient

↓

Pain relieved by hanging limb out of bed. In due course patient has to get up and walk about, with resulting loss of sleep

↓

Patient takes to sleeping in chair, leading to dependent oedema. Interstitial tissue pressure is increased so arterial perfusion is further reduced. Vicious circle of increasing pain and sleep loss

↓

Trivial injury fails to heal, and entry of bacteria leads to infection and increase in metabolic demands of foot. Rapid development of ulcers and gangrene

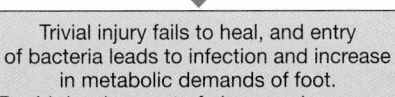

Fig. 18.78 Progressive night pain and the development of tissue loss.

Buerger's disease (thromboangiitis obliterans)

This is an inflammatory obliterative arterial disease that is distinct from atherosclerosis and usually presents in young (20–30 years) male smokers. It is most common in those from the Mediterranean and North Africa. It characteristically affects distal arteries, giving rise to claudication in the feet or rest pain in the fingers or toes. Wrist and ankle pulses are absent but brachial and popliteal are present. Disease also affects the veins, giving rise to superficial thrombophlebitis. It often remits if the patient stops smoking; sympathectomy and prostaglandin infusions may be helpful. Major limb amputation is the most frequent outcome if patients continue to smoke.

Chronic upper limb arterial disease

In the arm, the subclavian artery is the most common site of disease, which may manifest as:
- Arm claudication (rare).
- Atheroembolism (blue finger syndrome). Small emboli lodge in digital arteries and may be confused with Raynaud's phenomenon (see below), but in this case the symptoms are unilateral. Failure to make the diagnosis may eventually lead to amputation.
- Subclavian steal. When the arm is used, blood is 'stolen' from the brain via the vertebral artery.

18.80 Diabetic vascular disease: the 'diabetic foot'

Feature	Difficulty
Arterial calcification	Spuriously high ABPI due to incompressible ankle vessels Inability to clamp arteries for the purposes of bypass surgery Resistant to angioplasty
Immunocompromise	Prone to rapidly spreading cellulitis, gangrene and osteomyelitis
Multisystem arterial disease	Coronary and cerebral arterial disease increase the risks of intervention
Distal disease	Diabetic vascular disease has a predilection for the calf vessels. Although vessels in the foot are often spared, performing a satisfactory bypass or angioplasty to these small vessels is a technical challenge
Sensory neuropathy	Even severe ischaemia and/or tissue loss may be completely painless. Diabetic patients often present late with extensive destruction of the foot. Loss of proprioception leads to abnormal pressure loads and exacerbates joint destruction (Charcot joints)
Motor neuropathy	Weakness of the long and short flexors and extensors leads to abnormal foot architecture, abnormal pressure loads, callus formation and ulceration
Autonomic neuropathy	This leads to a dry foot deficient in sweat that normally lubricates the skin and contains antibacterial substances. Scaling and fissuring create a portal of entry for bacteria. Abnormal blood flow in the bones of the ankle and foot may also contribute to osteopenia and bony collapse

This leads to vertebro-basilar ischaemia, which is characterised by dizziness, cortical blindness and/or collapse. Where possible, subclavian artery disease is treated by means of angioplasty and stenting, as surgery (e.g. carotid-subclavian bypass) can be difficult.

Raynaud's phenomenon and Raynaud's disease

Cold (and emotional) stimuli may trigger vasospasm, leading to the characteristic sequence of digital pallor due to vasospasm, cyanosis due to deoxygenated blood, and rubor due to reactive hyperaemia.

Primary Raynaud's phenomenon (or disease)

This affects 5–10% of young women aged 15–30 years in temperate climates and may be familial. It does not progress to ulceration or infarction, and significant pain is unusual. The underlying cause is unclear. No investigation is necessary. The patient should be reassured and advised to avoid exposure to cold. Long-acting nifedipine may be helpful but sympathectomy is not indicated.

18.81 Atherosclerotic vascular disease in old age

- **Prevalence:** related almost exponentially to age in developed countries, although atherosclerosis is not considered part of the normal ageing process.
- **Statin therapy:** no role in the primary prevention of atherosclerotic disease in those > 75 yrs but reduces cardiovascular events in those with established vascular disease, albeit with no reduction in overall mortality.
- **Presentation in the frail:** frequently with advanced multisystem arterial disease, along with a host of other comorbidities.
- **Intervention in the frail:** in those with extensive disease and limited life expectancy, the risks of surgery may outweigh the benefits, and symptomatic care is all that should be offered.

Secondary Raynaud's phenomenon (or syndrome)

This tends to occur in older people in association with connective tissue disease (most commonly systemic sclerosis or the CREST syndrome, p. 1109), vibration-induced injury (from the use of power tools) and thoracic outlet obstruction (e.g. cervical rib). Unlike primary disease, it is often associated with fixed obstruction of the digital arteries, fingertip ulceration, and necrosis and pain. The fingers must be protected from cold and trauma, infection requires treatment with antibiotics, and surgery should be avoided if possible. Vasoactive drugs have no clear benefit. Sympathectomy helps for a year or two. Prostacyclin infusions are sometimes beneficial.

Acute limb ischaemia

This is most frequently caused by acute thrombotic occlusion of a pre-existing stenotic arterial segment, thrombo-embolism, and trauma which may be iatrogenic. Apart from paralysis (inability to wiggle toes/fingers) and paraesthesia (loss of light touch over the dorsum of the foot/hand), the so-called 'Ps of acute ischaemia' (Box 18.82) are non-specific for ischaemia and/or inconsistently related to its severity. Pain on squeezing the calf indicates muscle infarction and impending irreversible ischaemia.

All patients with suspected acutely ischaemic limbs must be discussed immediately with a vascular surgeon; a few hours can make the difference between death/amputation and complete recovery of limb function.

18.82 Symptoms and signs of acute limb ischaemia

Symptoms/signs	Comment
Pain	May be absent in complete acute ischaemia, and can be present in chronic ischaemia
Pallor	
Pulselessness	
Perishing cold	Unreliable, as the ischaemic limb takes on the ambient temperature
Paraesthesia	Important features of impending irreversible ischaemia
Paralysis	

18.83 Acute limb ischaemia: distinguishing features of embolism and thrombosis in situ		
Clinical features	**Embolism**	**Thrombosis in situ**
Severity	Complete (no collaterals)	Incomplete (collaterals)
Onset	Seconds or minutes	Hours or days
Limb	Leg 3:1 arm	Leg 10:1 arm
Multiple sites	Up to 15%	Rare
Embolic source	Present (usually AF)	Absent
Previous claudication	Absent	Present
Palpation of artery	Soft, tender	Hard, calcified
Bruits	Absent	Present
Contralateral leg pulses	Present	Absent
Diagnosis	Clinical	Angiography
Treatment	Embolectomy, warfarin	Medical, bypass, thrombolysis
Prognosis	Loss of life > loss of limb	Loss of limb > loss of life

If there are no contraindications (for example, acute aortic dissection or trauma, particularly head injury), an intravenous bolus of heparin (3000–5000 U) should be administered to limit propagation of thrombus and protect the collateral circulation. Distinguishing thrombosis from embolism is frequently difficult but is important because treatment and prognosis are different (Box 18.83). Acute limb ischaemia due to thrombosis in situ can usually be treated medically in the first instance with intravenous heparin (target activated partial thromboplastin time (APTT) 2.0–3.0), antiplatelet agents, high-dose statins, intravenous fluids to avoid dehydration, correction of anaemia, oxygen and sometimes prostaglandins such as iloprost. Careful monitoring is required. Embolism will normally result in extensive tissue necrosis within 6 hours unless the limb is revascularised. The indications for thrombolysis, if any, remain controversial. Irreversible ischaemia mandates early amputation or palliative care.

Cerebrovascular disease, renovascular disease and ischaemic gut injury

See pages 1180–1191, 496–499 and 906–907.

Diseases of the aorta

Aneurysm, dissection and aortitis are the main pathologies (Fig. 18.79).

Aortic aneurysm

This is an abnormal dilatation of the aortic lumen; a true aneurysm involves all the layers of the wall, whereas a false aneurysm does not.

Aetiology and types of aneurysm

Non-specific aneurysms

Why some patients develop occlusive vascular disease, some aneurysmal vascular disease and some both in response to atherosclerosis risk factors remains unclear. Unlike occlusive disease, aneurysmal disease tends to run in families and genetic factors are undoubtedly important. The most common site for 'non-specific' aneurysm formation is the infrarenal abdominal aorta. The suprarenal abdominal aorta and a variable length of the descending thoracic aorta may be affected in 10–20% of patients but the ascending aorta is usually spared.

Marfan's syndrome

This disorder of connective tissue is inherited as an autosomal dominant trait and is caused by mutations in the *fibrillin* gene on chromosome 15. Affected systems include the skeleton (arachnodactyly, joint hypermobility, scoliosis, chest deformity and high arched palate), the eyes (dislocation of the lens) and the cardiovascular system (aortic disease and mitral regurgitation). Weakening of the aortic media leads to aortic root dilatation, aortic regurgitation and aortic dissection (see below). Pregnancy is particularly hazardous. Chest X-ray, echocardiography, MRI or CT may detect aortic dilatation at an early stage and can be used to monitor the disease.

Treatment with β-blockers reduces the rate of aortic dilatation and the risk of rupture. Elective replacement of the ascending aorta may be considered in patients with evidence of progressive aortic dilatation but carries a mortality of 5–10%.

Aortitis

Syphilis is a rare cause of aortitis that characteristically produces saccular aneurysms of the ascending aorta containing calcification. Other rare conditions associated with aortitis include Takayasu's disease (p. 1113), Reiter's syndrome (p. 1115), giant cell arteritis and ankylosing spondylitis (pp. 1093–1094).

Thoracic aortic aneurysms

These may produce chest pain, aortic regurgitation, compressive symptoms such as stridor (trachea, bronchus) and hoarseness (recurrent laryngeal nerve), and superior vena cava syndrome (see Fig. 18.79A). If they erode into adjacent structures e.g. aorto-oesophageal fistula, massive bleeding occurs.

Abdominal aortic aneurysms (AAAs)

AAAs are present in 5% of men aged over 60 years and 80% are confined to the infrarenal segment. Men are affected three times more commonly than women. AAA can present in a number of ways (Box 18.84). The usual age at presentation is 65–75 years for elective presentations and 75–85 years for emergency presentations. Ultrasound is the best way of establishing the diagnosis, and of following up patients with asymptomatic aneurysms that are not yet large enough to warrant surgical repair. CT provides more accurate information about the size and extent of the aneurysm, the surrounding structures and whether there is any other intra-abdominal pathology. It is the standard pre-operative investigation but is not suitable for surveillance because of cost and radiation dose.

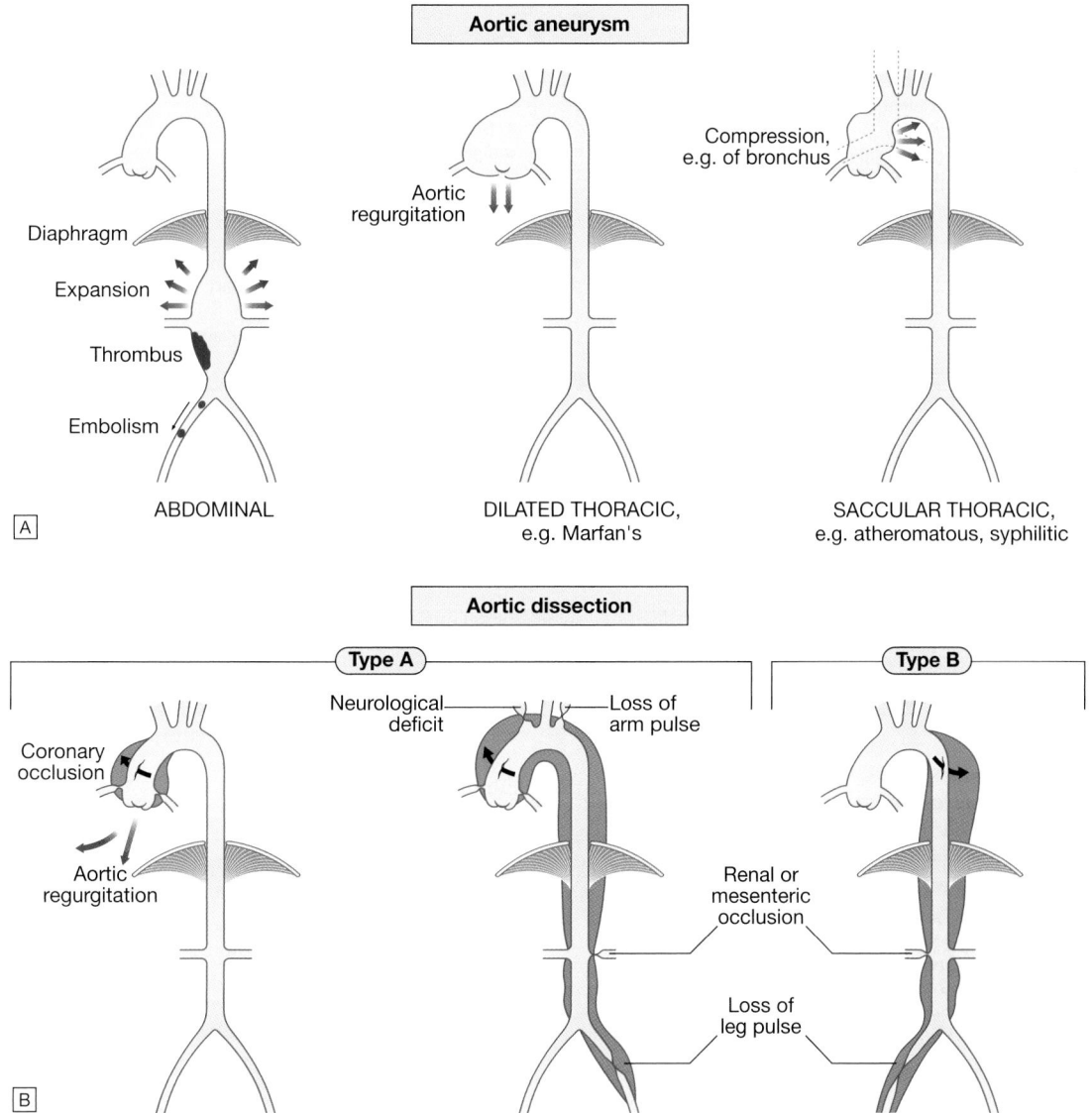

Aortic aneurysm

Diaphragm

Expansion

Thrombus

Embolism

ABDOMINAL

Aortic regurgitation

DILATED THORACIC, e.g. Marfan's

Compression, e.g. of bronchus

SACCULAR THORACIC, e.g. atheromatous, syphilitic

A

Aortic dissection

Type A

Type B

Coronary occlusion

Neurological deficit

Loss of arm pulse

Aortic regurgitation

Renal or mesenteric occlusion

Loss of leg pulse

B

Fig. 18.79 Types of aortic disease and their complications. A Types of aortic aneurysm. B Types of aortic dissection.

Management. Until an asymptomatic AAA has reached a maximum of 5.5 cm in diameter, the risks of surgery generally outweigh the risks of rupture (Box 18.85). All symptomatic AAAs should be considered for repair, not only to rid the patient of symptoms but also because pain often predates rupture. Distal embolisation is a strong indication for repair, regardless of size, because otherwise limb loss is common. Most patients with a ruptured AAA do not survive to reach hospital, but if they do and surgery is thought to be appropriate, there must be no delay in getting them to the operating theatre to clamp the aorta.

Open AAA repair has been the treatment of choice in both the elective and the emergency settings, and entails replacing the aneurysmal segment with a prosthetic (usually Dacron) graft. The 30-day mortality for this procedure is approximately 5–8% for elective asymptomatic AAA, 10–20% for emergency symptomatic AAA and 50% for ruptured AAA. However, patients who survive the operation to leave hospital have a long-term survival which approaches that of the normal population.

Increasingly, endovascular aneurysm repair (EVAR), using a stent-graft introduced via the femoral arteries in the groin, is replacing open surgery. It is cost-effective and likely to become the treatment of choice for infrarenal AAA. It is possible to treat many suprarenal and thoraco-abdominal aneurysms by EVAR too.

Aortic dissection

A breach in the integrity of the aortic wall allows arterial blood to enter the media, which is then split into two layers, creating a 'false lumen' alongside the existing or 'true lumen' (see Fig. 18.79B). The aortic valve may be damaged and the branches of the aorta may be compromised. Typically, the false lumen eventually re-enters the true lumen, creating a double-barrelled aorta, but it may also rupture into the left pleural space or pericardium with fatal consequences.

The primary event is often a spontaneous or iatrogenic tear in the intima of the aorta; multiple tears or entry points are common. Other dissections appear to be triggered by primary haemorrhage in the media of the

18.84 Abdominal aortic aneurysm: common presentations

Incidental

- On physical examination, plain X-ray or, most commonly, abdominal ultrasound
- Even large AAAs can be difficult to feel, so many remain undetected until they rupture
- Studies are currently underway to determine whether screening will reduce the number of deaths from rupture (see Box 18.85)

Pain

- In the central abdomen, back, loin, iliac fossa or groin

Thromboembolic complications

- Thrombus within the aneurysm sac may be a source of emboli to the lower limbs
- Less commonly, the aorta may undergo thrombotic occlusion

Compression

- Surrounding structures such as the duodenum (obstruction and vomiting) and the inferior vena cava (oedema and deep vein thrombosis)

Rupture

- Into the retroperitoneum, the peritoneal cavity or surrounding structures (most commonly the inferior vena cava, leading to an aortocaval fistula)

EBM 18.85 Population screening and prevention of ruptured abdominal aortic aneurysm

'Ultrasound screening for AAA in men aged 65–75 years, with surgical repair of those AAAs that are > 5.5 cm, are rapidly growing or become symptomatic, reduces the community incidence of rupture by ~50% and is cost-effective.'

- MASS Study Group. Lancet 2002; 360:1531–1539.
- MASS Study Group. BMJ 2002; 352:1135.

For further information: www.mrc-bsu.cam.ac.uk

---

aorta that then ruptures through the intima into the true lumen. This form of spontaneous bleeding from the vasa vasorum is sometimes confined to the aortic wall, when it may present as a painful intramural haematoma.

Disease of the aorta and hypertension are the most important aetiological factors but a variety of other conditions may be implicated (Box 18.86). Chronic dissections may lead to aneurysmal dilatation of the aorta, and thoracic aneurysms may be complicated by dissection. It is therefore sometimes difficult to identify the primary pathology.

The peak incidence is in the sixth and seventh decades of life but dissection can occur in younger patients, most commonly in association with Marfan's syndrome, pregnancy or trauma; men are twice as frequently affected as women.

Aortic dissection is classified anatomically and for management purposes into type A and type B (see Fig. 18.79B), involving or sparing the ascending aorta respectively. Type A dissections account for two-thirds of cases and frequently also extend into the descending aorta.

18.86 Factors that may predispose to aortic dissection

- Hypertension (80% of cases)
- Aortic atherosclerosis
- Non-specific aortic aneurysm
- Aortic coarctation (p. 631)
- Collagen disorders (e.g. Marfan's syndrome, Ehlers–Danlos syndrome)
- Fibromuscular dysplasia
- Previous aortic surgery (e.g. CABG, aortic valve replacement)
- Pregnancy (usually third trimester)
- Trauma
- Iatrogenic (e.g. cardiac catheterisation, intra-aortic balloon pumping)

Clinical features

Involvement of the ascending aorta typically gives rise to anterior chest pain, and involvement of the descending aorta to intrascapular pain. The pain is typically described as 'tearing' and very abrupt in onset; collapse is common. Unless there is major haemorrhage, the patient is invariably hypertensive. There may be asymmetry of the brachial, carotid or femoral pulses and signs of aortic regurgitation. Occlusion of aortic branches may cause MI (coronary), stroke (carotid) paraplegia (spinal), mesenteric infarction with an acute abdomen (coeliac and superior mesenteric), renal failure (renal) and acute limb (usually leg) ischaemia.

Investigations

The chest X-ray characteristically shows broadening of the upper mediastinum and distortion of the aortic 'knuckle', but these findings are variable and are absent in 10% of cases. A left-sided pleural effusion is common. The ECG may show left ventricular hypertrophy in patients with hypertension, or rarely changes of acute MI (usually inferior). Doppler echocardiography may show aortic regurgitation, a dilated aortic root and, occasionally, the flap of the dissection. Transoesophageal echocardiography is particularly helpful because transthoracic echocardiography can only image the first 3–4 cm of the ascending aorta (Fig. 18.80). CT and MRI angiography (Figs 18.81 and 18.82) are both highly specific and sensitive.

Management

The early mortality of acute dissection is approximately 1–5% per hour so treatment is urgently required. Initial management comprises pain control and antihypertensive treatment. Type A dissections require emergency surgery to replace the ascending aorta. Type B aneurysms are treated medically unless there is actual or impending external rupture, or vital organ (gut, kidneys) or limb ischaemia, as the morbidity and mortality associated with surgery is very high. The aim of medical management is to maintain a mean arterial pressure (MAP) of 60–75 mmHg to reduce the force of the ejection of blood from the LV. First-line therapy is with β-blockers; the additional α-blocking properties of labetalol make it especially useful. Rate-limiting calcium channel blockers, such as verapamil or diltiazem, are used if β-blockers are contraindicated. Sodium nitroprusside may be considered if these fail to control BP adequately.

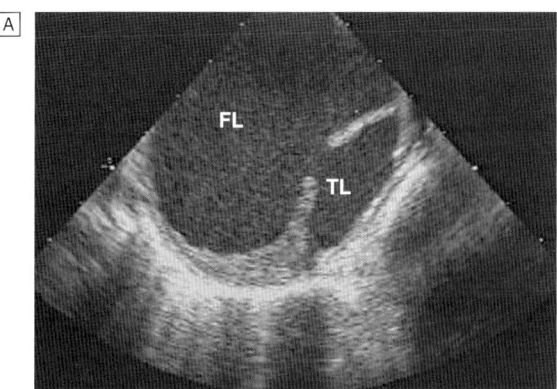

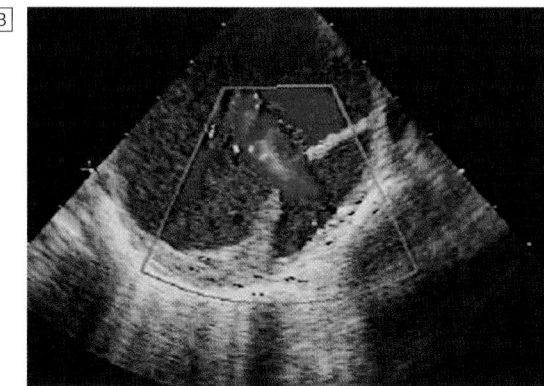

Fig. 18.80 Echocardiograms from a patient with a chronic aortic dissection. A Transoesophageal echocardiogram (FL = false lumen; TL = true lumen). B Colour-flow Doppler shows flow from the larger false lumen into the true lumen, characteristic of chronic disease.

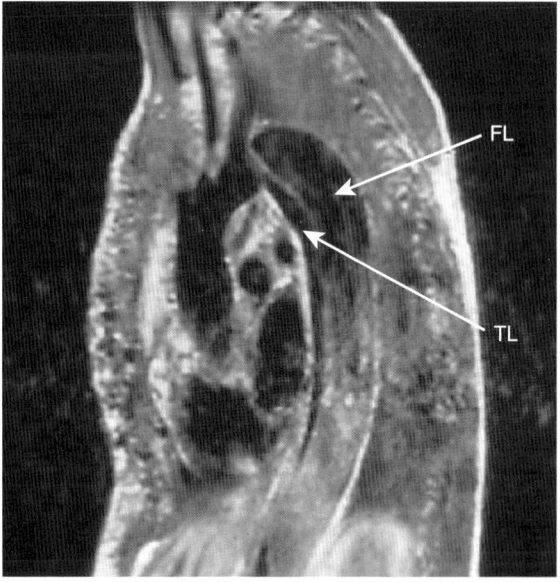

Fig. 18.81 Sagittal view of an MRI scan from a patient with long-standing aortic dissection illustrating a biluminal aorta. There is sluggish flow in the false lumen (FL), accounting for its grey appearance. (TL = true lumen)

Percutaneous or minimal access endoluminal repair is sometimes possible and involves either 'fenestrating' (perforating) the intimal flap so that blood can return from the false to the true lumen (so decompressing the former), or implanting a stent graft placed from the femoral artery (see Fig. 18.82).

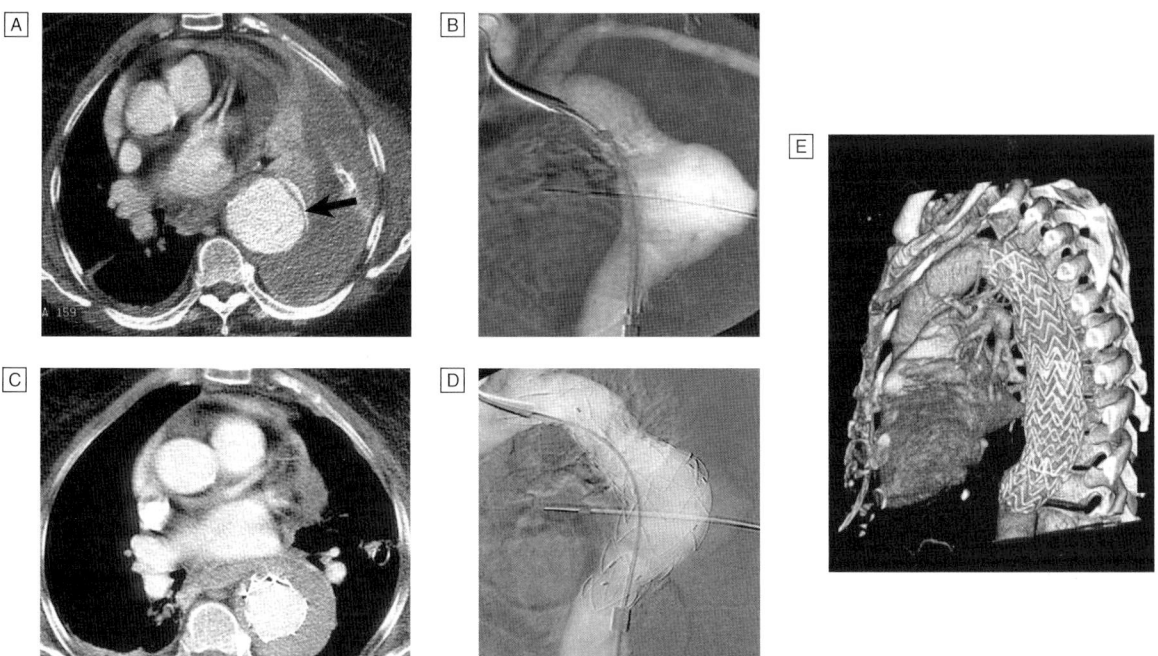

Fig. 18.82 Images from a patient with an acute type B aortic dissection that had ruptured into the left pleural space and was repaired by deploying an endoluminal stent graft. A CT scan illustrating an intimal flap (arrow) in the descending aorta and a large pleural effusion. B Aortogram illustrating aneurysmal dilatation; a stent graft has been introduced from the right femoral artery and is about to be deployed. C CT scan after endoluminal repair. The pleural effusion has been drained but there is a haematoma around the descending aorta. D Aortogram illustrating the stent graft. E Three-dimensional reconstruction of aortic stent graft.

18

Hypertension

Hypertension is a condition in which arterial BP is chronically elevated. BP occurs within a continuous range, so cutoff levels are defined according to their effect on patients' risk. The British Hypertension Society has defined ranges of BP which are normal and those that indicate hypertension (Box 18.87).

Aetiology

In more than 95% of cases, a specific underlying cause of hypertension cannot be found. Such patients are said to have essential hypertension. The pathogenesis of this is not clearly understood. Many factors may contribute to its development, including renal dysfunction, peripheral resistance vessel tone, endothelial dysfunction, autonomic tone, insulin resistance and neurohumoral factors. Hypertension is more common in some ethnic groups, particularly Black Americans and Japanese, and approximately 40–60% is explained by genetic factors. Important environmental factors include a high salt intake, heavy consumption of alcohol, obesity, lack of exercise and impaired intrauterine growth. There is little evidence that 'stress' causes hypertension.

In about 5% of cases, hypertension can be shown to be a consequence of a specific disease or abnormality leading to sodium retention and/or peripheral vasoconstriction (secondary hypertension, Box 18.88).

Measurement of blood pressure

A decision to embark upon antihypertensive therapy effectively commits the patient to life-long treatment, so BP readings must be as accurate as possible.

Measurements should be made to the nearest 2 mmHg, in the sitting position with the arm supported, and repeated after 5 minutes' rest if the first recording is high (Box 18.89). To avoid spuriously high recordings in obese subjects, the cuff should contain a bladder that encompasses at least two-thirds of the circumference of the arm.

Home and ambulatory BP recordings

Exercise, anxiety, discomfort and unfamiliar surroundings can all lead to a transient rise in BP. Sphygmomanometry,

18.88 Causes of secondary hypertension

Alcohol

Obesity

Pregnancy (pre-eclampsia)

Renal disease (Ch. 17)
- Renal vascular disease
- Parenchymal renal disease, particularly glomerulonephritis
- Polycystic kidney disease

Endocrine disease (Ch. 20)
- Phaeochromocytoma
- Cushing's syndrome
- Primary hyperaldosteronism (Conn's syndrome)
- Glucocorticoid-suppressible hyperaldosteronism
- Hyperparathyroidism
- Acromegaly
- Primary hypothyroidism
- Thyrotoxicosis
- Congenital adrenal hyperplasia due to 11-β-hydroxylase or 17α-hydroxylase deficiency
- Liddle's syndrome (p. 439)
- 11-β-hydroxysteroid dehydrogenase deficiency

Drugs
- e.g. Oral contraceptives containing oestrogens, anabolic steroids, corticosteroids, NSAIDs, carbenoxolone, sympathomimetic agents

Coarctation of the aorta (p. 631)

18.89 How to measure blood pressure

- Use a machine that has been validated, well maintained and properly calibrated
- Measure sitting BP routinely, with additional standing BP in elderly and diabetic patients and those with possible postural hypotension
- Remove tight clothing from the arm
- Support the arm at the level of the heart
- Use a cuff of appropriate size (the bladder must encompass > two-thirds of the arm)
- Lower the pressure slowly (2 mmHg per second)
- Read the BP to the nearest 2 mmHg
- Use phase V (disappearance of sounds) to measure diastolic BP
- Take two measurements at each visit

particularly when performed by a doctor, can cause an unrepresentative surge in BP which has been termed 'white coat' hypertension, and as many as 20% of patients with apparent hypertension in the clinic may have a normal BP when it is recorded by automated devices used at home. The risk of cardiovascular disease in these patients is less than that in patients with sustained hypertension but greater than that in normotensive subjects.

A series of automated ambulatory BP measurements obtained over 24 hours or longer provides a better profile than a limited number of clinic readings and correlates

18.87 Definition of hypertension

Category	Systolic BP (mmHg)	Diastolic BP (mmHg)
BP		
Optimal	< 120	< 80
Normal	< 130	85
High normal	130–139	85–89
Hypertension		
Grade 1 (mild)	140–159	90–99
Grade 2 (moderate)	160–179	100–109
Grade 3 (severe)	≥ 180	≥ 110
Isolated systolic hypertension		
Grade 1	140–159	< 90
Grade 2	≥ 160	< 90

more closely with evidence of target organ damage than casual BP measurements. However, treatment thresholds and targets (see Box 18.95, p. 609) must be adjusted downwards because ambulatory BP readings are systematically lower (approximately 12/7 mmHg) than clinic measurements. The average ambulatory daytime (not 24-hour or night-time) BP should be used to guide management decisions.

Patients can measure their own BP at home using a range of commercially available semi-automatic devices. The value of such measurements is less well established and is dependent on the environment and timing of the readings measured. Home or ambulatory BP measurements are particularly helpful in patients with unusually labile BP, those with refractory hypertension, those who may have symptomatic hypotension, and those in whom white coat hypertension is suspected.

History

Family history, lifestyle (exercise, salt intake, smoking habit) and other risk factors should be recorded. A careful history will identify those patients with drug- or alcohol-induced hypertension and may elicit the symptoms of other causes of secondary hypertension such as phaeochromocytoma (paroxysmal headache, palpitation and sweating, p. 779) or complications such as coronary artery disease (e.g. angina, breathlessness).

Examination

Radio-femoral delay (coarctation of the aorta, see Fig. 18.97 (p. 632)), enlarged kidneys (polycystic kidney disease), abdominal bruits (renal artery stenosis) and the characteristic facies and habitus of Cushing's syndrome are all examples of physical signs that may help to identify causes of secondary hypertension (see Box 18.88). Examination may also reveal features of important risk factors such as central obesity and hyperlipidaemia (tendon xanthomas etc.). Most abnormal signs are due to the complications of hypertension.

Non-specific findings may include left ventricular hypertrophy (apical heave), accentuation of the aortic component of the second heart sound, and a fourth heart sound. The optic fundi are often abnormal (see Fig. 18.83 below) and there may be evidence of generalised atheroma or specific complications such as aortic aneurysm or peripheral vascular disease.

Target organ damage

The adverse effects of hypertension on the organs can often be detected clinically.

Blood vessels

In larger arteries (> 1 mm in diameter), the internal elastic lamina is thickened, smooth muscle is hypertrophied and fibrous tissue is deposited. The vessels dilate and become tortuous, and their walls become less compliant. In smaller arteries (< 1 mm), hyaline arteriosclerosis occurs in the wall, the lumen narrows and aneurysms may develop. Widespread atheroma develops and may lead to coronary and cerebrovascular disease, particularly if other risk factors (e.g. smoking, hyperlipidaemia, diabetes) are present.

These structural changes in the vasculature often perpetuate and aggravate hypertension by increasing peripheral

vascular resistance and reducing renal blood flow, thereby activating the renin–angiotensin–aldosterone axis (p. 544).

Hypertension is a major risk factor in the pathogenesis of aortic aneurysm and aortic dissection.

Central nervous system

Stroke is a common complication of hypertension and may be due to cerebral haemorrhage or infarction. Carotid atheroma and transient ischaemic attacks are more common in hypertensive patients. Subarachnoid haemorrhage is also associated with hypertension.

Hypertensive encephalopathy is a rare condition characterised by high BP and neurological symptoms, including transient disturbances of speech or vision, paraesthesiae, disorientation, fits and loss of consciousness. Papilloedema is common. A CT scan of the brain often shows haemorrhage in and around the basal ganglia; however, the neurological deficit is usually reversible if the hypertension is properly controlled.

Retina

The optic fundi reveal a gradation of changes linked to the severity of hypertension; fundoscopy can, therefore, provide an indication of the arteriolar damage occurring elsewhere (Box 18.90).

'Cotton wool' exudates are associated with retinal ischaemia or infarction, and fade in a few weeks (Fig. 18.83A). 'Hard' exudates (small, white, dense deposits of lipid) and microaneurysms ('dot' haemorrhages) are more characteristic of diabetic retinopathy (see Fig. 21.16, p. 827). Hypertension is also associated with central retinal vein thrombosis (Fig. 18.83B).

Heart

The excess cardiac mortality and morbidity associated with hypertension are largely due to a higher incidence of coronary artery disease. High BP places a pressure load on the heart and may lead to left ventricular hypertrophy with a forceful apex beat and fourth heart sound. ECG or echocardiographic evidence of left ventricular hypertrophy is highly predictive of cardiovascular complications and therefore particularly useful in risk assessment.

Atrial fibrillation is common and may be due to diastolic dysfunction caused by left ventricular hypertrophy or the effects of coronary artery disease.

Severe hypertension can cause left ventricular failure in the absence of coronary artery disease, particularly when renal function, and therefore sodium excretion, is impaired.

18.90 Hypertensive retinopathy

- **Grade 1** — Arteriolar thickening, tortuosity and increased reflectiveness ('silver wiring')
- **Grade 2** — Grade 1 plus constriction of veins at arterial crossings ('arteriovenous nipping')
- **Grade 3** — Grade 2 plus evidence of retinal ischaemia (flame-shaped or blot haemorrhages and 'cotton wool' exudates)
- **Grade 4** — Grade 3 plus papilloedema

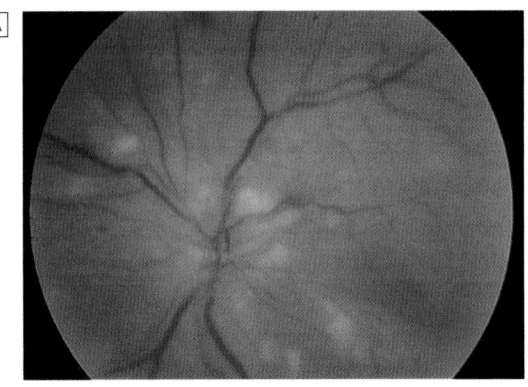
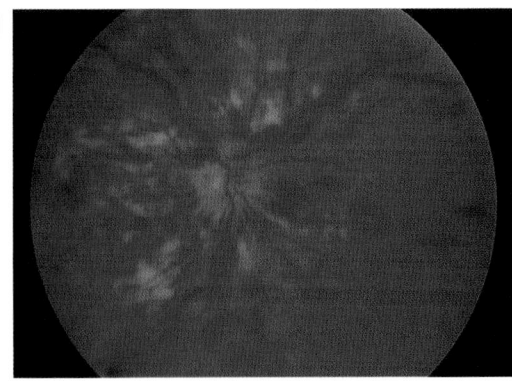

Fig. 18.83 Retinal changes in hypertension. **A** Grade 4 hypertensive retinopathy showing swollen optic disc, retinal haemorrhages and multiple cotton wool spots (infarcts). **B** Central retinal vein thrombosis showing swollen optic disc and widespread fundal haemorrhage, commonly associated with systemic hypertension.

Kidneys

Long-standing hypertension may cause proteinuria and progressive renal failure (p. 482) by damaging the renal vasculature.

'Malignant' or 'accelerated' phase hypertension

This rare condition may complicate hypertension of any aetiology and is characterised by accelerated microvascular damage with necrosis in the walls of small arteries and arterioles ('fibrinoid necrosis') and by intravascular thrombosis. The diagnosis is based on evidence of high BP and rapidly progressive end organ damage, such as retinopathy (grade 3 or 4), renal dysfunction (especially proteinuria) and/or hypertensive encephalopathy (see above). Left ventricular failure may occur and, if this is untreated, death occurs within months.

Investigations

All hypertensive patients should undergo a limited number of investigations (Box 18.91). Additional investigations are appropriate in selected patients (Box 18.92).

Management

Quantification of cardiovascular risk

The sole objective of antihypertensive therapy is to reduce the incidence of adverse cardiovascular events, particularly coronary heart disease, stroke and heart failure. The relative benefit of antihypertensive therapy (approximately 30% reduction in risk of stroke and 20% reduction in risk of coronary heart disease, Box 18.93) is similar in all patient groups, so the absolute benefit of treatment (total number of events prevented) is greatest in those at highest risk. For example, to extrapolate from the Medical Research Council (MRC) Mild Hypertension Trial (1985), 566 young patients would have to be treated with bendroflumethiazide for 1 year to prevent 1 stroke, while in the MRC trial of antihypertensive treatment in the elderly (1992), 1 stroke was prevented for every 286 patients treated for 1 year.

A formal estimate of absolute cardiovascular risk which takes account of all the relevant risk factors may help to determine whether the likely benefits of

18.91 Hypertension: investigation of all patients

- Urinalysis for blood, protein and glucose
- Blood urea, electrolytes and creatinine
    N.B. Hypokalaemic alkalosis may indicate primary hyperaldosteronism but is usually due to diuretic therapy
- Blood glucose
- Serum total and HDL cholesterol
- 12-lead ECG (left ventricular hypertrophy, coronary artery disease)

18.92 Hypertension: investigation of selected patients

- Chest X-ray: to detect cardiomegaly, heart failure, coarctation of the aorta
- Ambulatory BP recording: to assess borderline or 'white coat' hypertension
- Echocardiogram: to detect or quantify left ventricular hypertrophy
- Renal ultrasound: to detect possible renal disease
- Renal angiography: to detect or confirm presence of renal artery stenosis
- Urinary catecholamines: to detect possible phaeochromocytoma (p. 779)
- Urinary cortisol and dexamethasone suppression test: to detect possible Cushing's syndrome (p. 770)
- Plasma renin activity and aldosterone: to detect possible primary aldosteronism (p. 777)

EBM 18.93 Benefit of antihypertensive drug therapy

'Diuretics or β-blockers have been shown to reduce the risk of coronary heart disease by 16%, stroke by 38%, cardiovascular death by 21% and all causes of mortality by 13%. The effects of ACE inhibitors and calcium antagonists are similar. NNT_B varies greatly according to the absolute baseline risk of cardiovascular disease.'

- Blood Pressure Lowering Treatment Trialists' Collaboration. Lancet 2003; 362:1527–1535.

therapy will outweigh its costs and hazards. A variety of risk algorithms are available for this purpose (see Fig. 18.61, p. 580). Most of the excess morbidity and mortality associated with hypertension is attributable to coronary heart disease and many treatment guidelines are therefore based on estimates of the 10-year coronary heart disease risk. Total cardiovascular risk can be estimated by multiplying coronary heart disease risk by 4/3 (i.e. if coronary heart disease risk is 30%, cardiovascular risk is 40%). The value of this approach can be illustrated by comparing the two hypothetical cases on page 579.

Threshold for intervention

Systolic BP and diastolic BP are both powerful predictors of cardiovascular risk. The British Hypertension Society management guidelines therefore utilise both readings, and treatment should be initiated if they exceed the given threshold (Fig. 18.84).

Patients with diabetes or cardiovascular disease are at particularly high risk and the threshold for initiating antihypertensive therapy is therefore lower ($\geq 140/90$ mmHg) in these patient groups. The thresholds for treatment in the elderly are the same as for younger patients (Box 18.94).

Treatment targets

The optimum BP for reduction of major cardiovascular events has been found to be 139/83 mmHg, and even lower in patients with diabetes mellitus. Moreover, reducing BP below this level causes no harm. The targets suggested by the British Hypertension Society (Box 18.95) are ambitious. Primary care strategies have been devised to improve screening and detection of hypertension that, in the past, remained undetected in up to half of affected individuals. Application of new treatment guidelines should help establish patients on appropriate treatment, and allow step-up of treatment if lifestyle modification and first-line drug therapy fail to control patients' BP.

Patients taking antihypertensive therapy require follow-up at 3-monthly intervals to monitor BP, minimise side-effects and reinforce lifestyle advice.

Non-drug therapy

Appropriate lifestyle measures may obviate the need for drug therapy in patients with borderline hypertension, reduce the dose and/or the number of drugs required in patients with established hypertension, and directly reduce cardiovascular risk.

Correcting obesity, reducing alcohol intake, restricting salt intake, taking regular physical exercise and increasing consumption of fruit and vegetables can all lower BP. Moreover, quitting smoking, eating oily fish and adopting a diet that is low in saturated fat may produce further reductions in cardiovascular risk.

Antihypertensive drugs

- *Thiazide and other diuretics.* The mechanism of action of these drugs is incompletely understood and it may take up to a month for the maximum effect to be observed. An appropriate daily dose is 2.5 mg bendroflumethiazide or 0.5 mg cyclopenthiazide. More potent loop diuretics, such as furosemide 40 mg daily or bumetanide 1 mg daily, have few

advantages over thiazides in the treatment of hypertension unless there is substantial renal impairment or they are used in conjunction with an ACE inhibitor.
- *ACE inhibitors* (e.g. enalapril 20 mg daily, ramipril 5–10 mg daily or lisinopril 10–40 mg daily). These inhibit the conversion of angiotensin I to angiotensin II and are usually well tolerated. They should be used with particular care in patients with impaired renal function or renal artery stenosis because they can reduce the filtration pressure in the glomeruli and precipitate renal failure. Electrolytes and creatinine should be checked before and 1–2 weeks after commencing therapy. Side-effects include first-dose hypotension, cough, rash, hyperkalaemia and renal dysfunction.
- *Angiotensin receptor blockers* (e.g. irbesartan 150–300 mg daily, valsartan 40–160 mg daily). These block the angiotensin II type I receptor and have similar effects to ACE inhibitors; however, they do not cause cough and are better tolerated.
- *Calcium channel antagonists.* The dihydropyridines (e.g. amlodipine 5–10 mg daily, nifedipine 30–90 mg daily) are effective and usually well-tolerated antihypertensive drugs that are particularly useful in older people. Side-effects include flushing, palpitations and fluid retention. The rate-limiting calcium channel antagonists (e.g. diltiazem 200–300 mg daily, verapamil 240 mg daily) can be useful when hypertension coexists with angina but they may cause bradycardia. The main side-effect of verapamil is constipation.
- *Beta-blockers.* These are no longer used as first-line antihypertensive therapy, except in patients with another indication for the drug (e.g. angina).

18

18.94 Hypertension in old age

- **Prevalence:** affects more than half of all people over the age of 60 (including isolated systolic hypertension).
- **Risks:** hypertension is the most important risk factor for MI, heart failure and stroke in older people.
- **Benefit of treatment:** absolute benefit from antihypertensives is greatest in older people (at least up to age 80 years).
- **Target BP:** similar to that for younger patients.
- **Tolerance of treatment:** antihypertensives are tolerated as well as in younger patients.
- **Drug of choice:** low-dose thiazides, but in the presence of coexistent disease (e.g. gout, diabetes) other agents may be more appropriate.

18.95 Optimal target blood pressures during antihypertensive treatment: BHS guidelines

	No diabetes	Diabetes
Clinic measurements	< 140/85	< 130/80
Mean day-time ambulatory or home measurement	< 130/80	< 130/75

N.B. Both systolic and diastolic values should be attained.

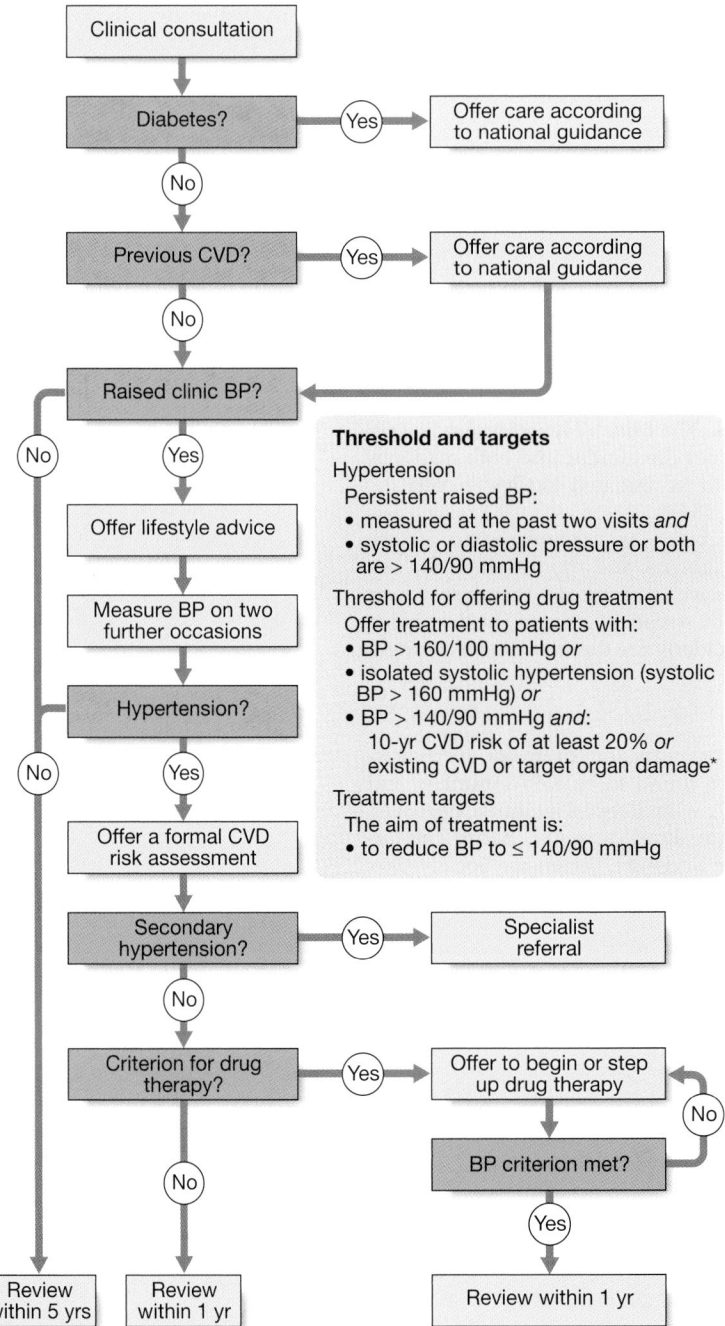

Fig. 18.84 Management of hypertension: British Hypertension Society guidelines. *Assessed with risk chart for cardiovascular disease; see Fig. 18.61. (CVD = cardiovascular disease)

Metoprolol (100–200 mg daily), atenolol (50–100 mg daily) and bisoprolol (5–10 mg daily) preferentially block cardiac β_1-adrenoceptors, as opposed to the β_2-adrenoceptors that mediate vasodilatation and bronchodilatation.

• *Labetalol and carvedilol.* Labetalol (200 mg–2.4 g daily in divided doses) and carvedilol (6.25–25 mg 12-hourly) are combined β- and α-adrenoceptor antagonists which are sometimes more effective than pure β-blockers. Labetalol can be used as an infusion in malignant phase hypertension (see below).

• *Other drugs.* A variety of vasodilators may be used. These include the α_1-adrenoceptor antagonists (α-blockers), such as prazosin (0.5–20 mg daily in divided doses), indoramin (25–100 mg 12-hourly) and doxazosin (1–16 mg daily), and drugs that act directly on vascular smooth muscle, such as hydralazine (25–100 mg 12-hourly) and minoxidil (10–50 mg daily). Side-effects include first-dose and postural hypotension, headache, tachycardia and fluid retention. Minoxidil also causes increased facial hair and is therefore unsuitable for female patients.

Choice of antihypertensive drug

Trials that have compared thiazides, calcium antagonists, ACE inhibitors and angiotensin receptor blockers have not shown consistent differences in outcome, efficacy, side-effects or quality of life. Beta-blockers, which previously featured as first-line therapy in guidelines, have a weaker evidence base (see Box 18.93). The choice of antihypertensive therapy is initially dictated by the patient's age and ethnic background, although cost and convenience will affect the exact drug and preparation used. Response to initial therapy and side-effects dictate subsequent treatment. Comorbid conditions also have an influence on initial drug selection (Box 18.96); for example, a β-blocker might be the most appropriate treatment for a patient with angina. Thiazide diuretics and dihydropyridine calcium channel antagonists are the most suitable drugs for the treatment of high BP in older people.

Although some patients can be satisfactorily treated with a single antihypertensive drug, a combination of drugs is often required to achieve optimal BP control (Fig. 18.85). Combination therapy may be desirable for other reasons; for example, low-dose therapy with two drugs may produce fewer unwanted effects than treatment with the maximum dose of a single drug. Some drug combinations have complementary or synergistic actions; for example, thiazides increase activity of the renin–angiotensin system while ACE inhibitors block it.

Emergency treatment of accelerated phase or malignant hypertension

In accelerated phase hypertension, lowering BP too quickly may compromise tissue perfusion (due to altered autoregulation) and can cause cerebral damage, including occipital blindness, and precipitate coronary or renal insufficiency. Even in the presence of cardiac failure or hypertensive encephalopathy, a controlled reduction to a level of about 150/90 mmHg over a period of 24–48 hours is ideal.

18

18.96 The influence of comorbidity on the choice of antihypertensive drug therapy

Class of drug	Compelling indications	Possible indications	Caution	Compelling contraindications
α-blockers	Benign prostatic hypertrophy	–	Postural hypotension, heart failure[1]	Urinary incontinence
ACE inhibitors	Heart failure Left ventricular dysfunction, post-MI or established coronary heart disease Type 1 diabetic nephropathy Secondary stroke prevention[4]	Chronic renal disease[2] Type 2 diabetic nephropathy	Renal impairment[2] Peripheral vascular disease[3]	Pregnancy Renovascular disease[2]
Angiotensin II receptor blockers	ACE inhibitor intolerance Type 2 diabetic nephropathy Hypertension with left ventricular hypertrophy Heart failure in ACE-intolerant patients, after MI	Left ventricular dysfunction after MI Intolerance of other antihypertensive drugs Proteinuric renal disease, chronic renal disease[2] Heart failure	Renal impairment[2] Peripheral vascular disease[3]	Pregnancy
β-blockers	MI, angina Heart failure[5]		Heart failure[5] Peripheral vascular disease Diabetes (except with coronary heart disease)	Asthma or chronic obstructive pulmonary disease Heart block
Calcium channel blockers (dihydropyridine)	Older patients, isolated systolic hypertension	Angina	–	–
Calcium channel blockers (rate-limiting)	Angina	Older patients	Combination with β-blockade	Atrioventricular block, heart failure
Thiazides or thiazide-like diuretics	Older patients, isolated systolic hypertension, heart failure, secondary stroke prevention	–	–	Gout[6]

[1]In heart failure when used as monotherapy.
[2]ACE inhibitors or angiotensin II receptor blockers may be beneficial in chronic renal failure and those with renovascular disease but should be used with caution, close supervision and specialist advice when there is established and significant renal impairment.
[3]Caution with ACE inhibitors and angiotensin II receptor blockers in peripheral vascular disease because of association with renovascular disease.
[4]In combination with a thiazide or thiazide-like diuretic.
[5]Beta-blockers are used increasingly to treat stable heart failure but may worsen acute heart failure.
[6]Thiazides or thiazide-like diuretics may sometimes be necessary to control BP in people with a history of gout, ideally used in combination with allopurinol.

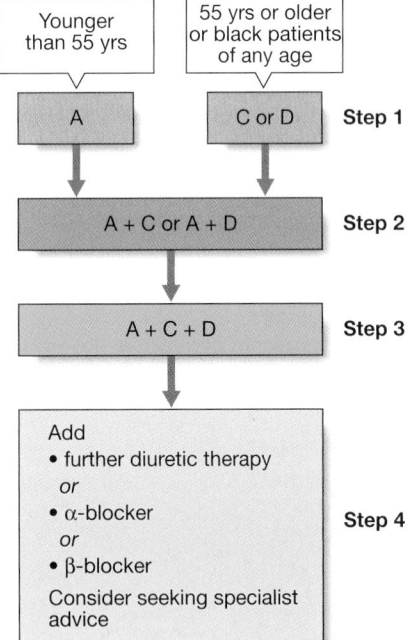

Fig. 18.85 Antihypertensive drug combinations. Black patients are those of African or Caribbean descent, and not mixed-race, Asian or Chinese patients. (A = ACE inhibitor (consider angiotensin II receptor antagonist if ACE-intolerant); C = calcium channel blocker; D = thiazide-type diuretic)

In most patients, it is possible to avoid parenteral therapy and bring BP under control with bed rest and oral drug therapy. Intravenous or intramuscular labetalol (2 mg/min to a maximum of 200 mg), intravenous glyceryl trinitrate (0.6–1.2 mg/hour), intramuscular hydralazine (5 or 10 mg aliquots repeated at half-hourly intervals) and intravenous sodium nitroprusside (0.3–1.0 µg/kg body weight/min) are all effective but require careful supervision, preferably in a high-dependency unit.

Refractory hypertension

The common causes of treatment failure in hypertension are non-adherence to drug therapy, inadequate therapy, and failure to recognise an underlying cause such as renal artery stenosis or phaeochromocytoma; of these, the first is by far the most prevalent. There is no easy solution to compliance problems but simple treatment regimens, attempts to improve rapport with the patient and careful supervision may all help.

Adjuvant drug therapy

- *Aspirin.* Antiplatelet therapy is a powerful means of reducing cardiovascular risk but may cause bleeding, particularly intracerebral haemorrhage, in a small number of patients. The benefits are thought to outweigh the risks in hypertensive patients aged 50 or over who have well-controlled BP and either target organ damage, diabetes or a 10-year coronary heart disease risk of ≥ 15% (or 10-year cardiovascular disease risk of ≥ 20%).
- *Statins.* Treating hyperlipidaemia can produce a substantial reduction in cardiovascular risk. These drugs are strongly indicated in patients who have

established vascular disease, or hypertension with a high (≥ 20% in 10 years) risk of developing cardiovascular disease (p. 579).

DISEASES OF THE HEART VALVES

A diseased valve may be narrowed (stenosed) or may fail to close adequately, and thus permit regurgitation of blood. 'Incompetence' is a less precise term for regurgitation or reflux, and should be avoided. Box 18.97 gives the principal causes of valve disease.

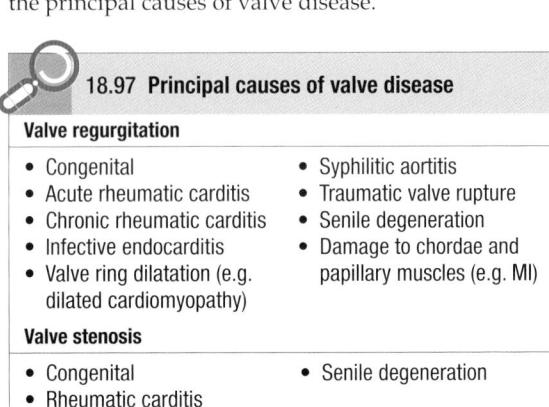

18.97 Principal causes of valve disease

Valve regurgitation

- Congenital
- Acute rheumatic carditis
- Chronic rheumatic carditis
- Infective endocarditis
- Valve ring dilatation (e.g. dilated cardiomyopathy)
- Syphilitic aortitis
- Traumatic valve rupture
- Senile degeneration
- Damage to chordae and papillary muscles (e.g. MI)

Valve stenosis

- Congenital
- Rheumatic carditis
- Senile degeneration

Doppler echocardiography is the most useful technique for assessing valvular heart disease (p. 532) but may also detect minor and even 'physiological' abnormalities, such as trivial mitral regurgitation. Disease of the heart valves may progress with time and selected patients require regular review every 1 or 2 years, to ensure that deterioration is detected before complications such as heart failure ensue. Patients with valvular heart disease are susceptible to bacterial endocarditis, which can be prevented by good dental hygiene. The routine use of antibiotic prophylaxis at times of bacteraemia, such as dental extraction, is no longer recommended.

Rheumatic heart disease

Acute rheumatic fever
Incidence and pathogenesis

Acute rheumatic fever usually affects children (most commonly between 5 and 15 years) or young adults, and has become very rare in Western Europe and North America. However, it remains endemic in parts of Asia, Africa and South America, with an annual incidence in some countries of > 100 per 100 000, and is the most common cause of acquired heart disease in childhood and adolescence.

The condition is triggered by an immune-mediated delayed response to infection with specific strains of group A streptococci, which have antigens that may cross-react with cardiac myosin and sarcolemmal membrane protein. Antibodies produced against the streptococcal antigens cause inflammation in the endocardium, myocardium and pericardium, as well as the joints and skin. Histologically, fibrinoid degeneration is seen in the collagen of connective tissues. Aschoff nodules are pathognomonic and occur only in the heart. They are composed of multinucleated giant cells surrounded by macrophages and T lymphocytes, and are not seen until the subacute or chronic phases of rheumatic carditis.

Clinical features

Acute rheumatic fever is a multisystem disorder that usually presents with fever, anorexia, lethargy and joint pain, 2–3 weeks after an episode of streptococcal pharyngitis. There may, however, be no history of sore throat. Arthritis occurs in approximately 75% of patients. Other features include rashes, carditis and neurological changes (Fig. 18.86). The diagnosis, made using the revised Jones criteria (Box 18.98), is based upon two or more major manifestations, or one major and two or more minor manifestations, along with evidence of preceding streptococcal infection. Only about 25% of patients will have a positive culture for group A streptococcus at the time of diagnosis because there is a latent period between infection and presentation. Serological evidence of recent streptococcal infection with a raised antistreptolysin O (ASO) antibody titre is helpful. A presumptive diagnosis of acute rheumatic fever can be made without evidence of preceding streptococcal infection in cases of isolated chorea or pancarditis, if other causes for these have been excluded. In cases of established rheumatic heart disease or prior rheumatic fever, a diagnosis of acute rheumatic fever can be made based only on the presence of

i	**18.98** Jones criteria for the diagnosis of rheumatic fever

Major manifestations

• Carditis	• Erythema marginatum
• Polyarthritis	• Subcutaneous nodules
• Chorea	

Minor manifestations

• Fever	• Raised ESR or CRP
• Arthralgia	• Leucocytosis
• Previous rheumatic fever	• First-degree AV block

Plus

- Supporting evidence of preceding streptococcal infection: recent scarlet fever, raised antistreptolysin O or other streptococcal antibody titre, positive throat culture

N.B. Evidence of recent streptococcal infection is particularly important if there is only one major manifestation.

multiple minor criteria and evidence of preceding group A streptococcal pharyngitis.

Carditis

A 'pancarditis' involves the endocardium, myocardium and pericardium to varying degrees. Its incidence declines with increasing age, ranging from 90% at 3 years to around 30% in adolescence. It may manifest as breathlessness (due to heart failure or pericardial effusion), palpitations or chest pain (usually due to pericarditis or pancarditis). Other features include tachycardia, cardiac enlargement and new or changed cardiac murmurs. A soft systolic murmur due to mitral regurgitation is very common. A soft mid-diastolic murmur (the Carey Coombs murmur) is typically due to valvulitis, with nodules forming on the mitral valve leaflets. Aortic regurgitation occurs in about 50% of cases but the tricuspid and pulmonary valves are rarely involved. Pericarditis may cause chest pain, a pericardial friction rub and precordial tenderness. Cardiac failure may be due to myocardial dysfunction or valvular regurgitation. ECG changes commonly include ST and T wave changes. Conduction defects sometimes occur and may cause syncope.

Arthritis

This is the most common major manifestation and tends to occur early when streptococcal antibody titres are high. An acute painful asymmetric and migratory inflammation of the large joints typically affects the knees, ankles, elbows and wrists. The joints are involved in quick succession and are usually red, swollen and tender for between a day and 4 weeks. The pain characteristically responds to aspirin; if not, the diagnosis is in doubt.

Skin lesions

Erythema marginatum occurs in < 5% of patients. The lesions start as red macules (blotches) that fade in the centre but remain red at the edges and occur mainly on the trunk and proximal extremities but not the face. The resulting red rings or 'margins' may coalesce or overlap (see Fig. 18.86). Subcutaneous nodules occur in 5–7% of patients. They are small (0.5–2.0 cm), firm and painless, and are best felt over extensor surfaces of bone or tendons. They typically appear more than 3 weeks after

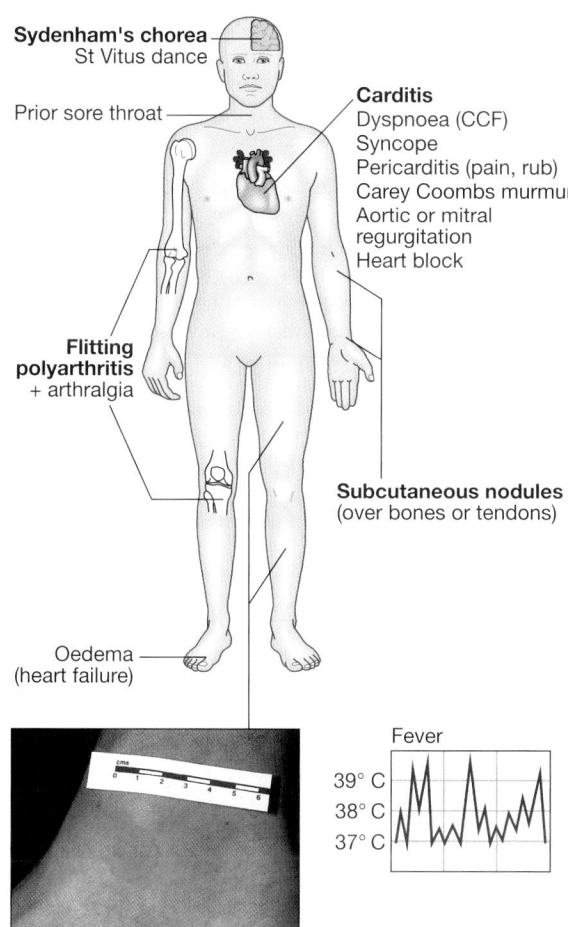

Sydenham's chorea
St Vitus dance

Prior sore throat

Carditis
Dyspnoea (CCF)
Syncope
Pericarditis (pain, rub)
Carey Coombs murmur
Aortic or mitral regurgitation
Heart block

Flitting polyarthritis
+ arthralgia

Subcutaneous nodules
(over bones or tendons)

Oedema
(heart failure)

Fever
39° C
38° C
37° C

Erythema marginatum

Fig. 18.86 Clinical features of rheumatic fever. Bold labels indicate Jones major criteria. (CCF = congestive cardiac failure)

18

the onset of other manifestations and therefore help to confirm rather than make the diagnosis.

Other systemic manifestations are rare but include pleurisy, pleural effusion and pneumonia.

Sydenham's chorea (St Vitus dance)

This is a late neurological manifestation that appears at least 3 months after the episode of acute rheumatic fever, when all the other signs may have disappeared. It occurs in up to one-third of cases and is more common in females. Emotional lability may be the first feature and is typically followed by purposeless involuntary choreiform movements of the hands, feet or face. Speech may be explosive and halting. Spontaneous recovery usually occurs within a few months. Approximately one-quarter of affected patients will go on to develop chronic rheumatic valve disease.

Investigations

The ESR and CRP are useful for monitoring progress of the disease (Box 18.99). Positive throat swab cultures are obtained in only 10–25% of cases. ASO titres are normal in one-fifth of adult cases of rheumatic fever and most cases of chorea. Echocardiography typically shows mitral regurgitation with dilatation of the mitral annulus and prolapse of the anterior mitral leaflet, and may also show aortic regurgitation and pericardial effusion.

18.99 Investigations in acute rheumatic fever

Evidence of a systemic illness (non-specific)

- Leucocytosis, raised ESR and CRP

Evidence of preceding streptococcal infection (specific)

- Throat swab culture: group A β-haemolytic streptococci (also from family members and contacts)
- Antistreptolysin O antibodies (ASO titres): rising titres, or levels of > 200 U (adults) or > 300 U (children)

Evidence of carditis

- Chest X-ray: cardiomegaly; pulmonary congestion
- ECG: first- and rarely second-degree AV block; features of pericarditis; T-wave inversion; reduction in QRS voltages
- Echocardiography: cardiac dilatation and valve abnormalities

Management of the acute attack

A single dose of benzyl penicillin 1.2 million U i.m. or oral phenoxymethylpenicillin 250 mg 6-hourly for 10 days should be given on diagnosis to eliminate any residual streptococcal infection. If the patient is penicillin-allergic, erythromycin or a cephalosporin can be used. Treatment is then directed towards limiting cardiac damage and relieving symptoms.

Bed rest and supportive therapy

Bed rest is important, as it lessens joint pain and reduces cardiac workload. The duration should be guided by symptoms along with temperature, leucocyte count and ESR, and should be continued until these have settled. Patients can then return to normal physical activity but strenuous exercise should be avoided in those who have had carditis.

Cardiac failure should be treated as necessary. Some patients, particularly those in early adolescence, develop a fulminant form of the disease with severe mitral regurgitation and sometimes concomitant aortic regurgitation. If heart failure in these cases does not respond to medical treatment, valve replacement may be necessary and is often associated with a dramatic decline in rheumatic activity. AV block is seldom progressive and pacemaker insertion rarely needed.

Aspirin

This will usually relieve the symptoms of arthritis rapidly and a response within 24 hours helps to confirm the diagnosis. A reasonable starting dose is 60 mg/kg body weight/day, divided into six doses. In adults, 100 mg/kg per day may be needed up to the limits of tolerance or a maximum of 8 g per day. Mild toxic effects include nausea, tinnitus and deafness; vomiting, tachypnoea and acidosis are more serious. Aspirin should be continued until the ESR has fallen and then gradually tailed off.

Corticosteroids

These produce more rapid symptomatic relief than aspirin and are indicated in cases with carditis or severe arthritis. There is no evidence that long-term steroids are beneficial. Prednisolone, 1.0–2.0 mg/kg per day in divided doses, should be continued until the ESR is normal then tailed off.

Secondary prevention

Patients are susceptible to further attacks of rheumatic fever if another streptococcal infection occurs, and long-term prophylaxis with penicillin should be given as benzathine penicillin 1.2 million U i.m. monthly (if compliance is in doubt) or oral phenoxymethylpenicillin 250 mg 12-hourly. Sulfadiazine or erythromycin may be used if the patient is allergic to penicillin; sulphonamides prevent infection but are not effective in the eradication of group A streptococci. Further attacks of rheumatic fever are unusual after the age of 21, when treatment may be stopped. However, it should be extended if an attack has occurred in the last 5 years, or if the patient lives in an area of high prevalence or has an occupation (e.g. teaching) with high exposure to streptococcal infection. In those with residual heart disease, prophylaxis should continue until 10 years after the last episode or 40 years of age, whichever is longer. Long-term antibiotic prophylaxis prevents another attack of acute rheumatic fever but does not protect against infective endocarditis.

Chronic rheumatic heart disease

Chronic valvular heart disease develops in at least half of those affected by rheumatic fever with carditis. Two-thirds of cases occur in women. Some episodes of rheumatic fever pass unrecognised and it is only possible to elicit a history of rheumatic fever or chorea in about half of all patients with chronic rheumatic heart disease.

The mitral valve is affected in more than 90% of cases; the aortic valve is the next most frequently affected, followed by the tricuspid and then the pulmonary valve. Isolated mitral stenosis accounts for about 25% of all cases of rheumatic heart disease, and an additional 40% have mixed mitral stenosis and regurgitation. Valve disease may be symptomatic during fulminant forms of acute rheumatic fever but may remain asymptomatic for many years.

Pathology

The main pathological process in chronic rheumatic heart disease is progressive fibrosis. The heart valves are predominantly affected but involvement of the pericardium and myocardium may contribute to heart failure and conduction disorders. Fusion of the mitral valve commissures and shortening of the chordae tendineae may lead to mitral stenosis with or without regurgitation. Similar changes in the aortic and tricuspid valves produce distortion and rigidity of the cusps, leading to stenosis and regurgitation. Once a valve has been damaged, the altered haemodynamic stresses perpetuate and extend the damage, even in the absence of a continuing rheumatic process.

Mitral valve disease

Mitral stenosis

Aetiology and pathophysiology

Mitral stenosis is almost always rheumatic in origin, although in older people it can be caused by heavy calcification of the mitral valve apparatus. There is also a rare form of congenital mitral stenosis.

In rheumatic mitral stenosis, the mitral valve orifice is slowly diminished by progressive fibrosis, calcification of the valve leaflets, and fusion of the cusps and subvalvular apparatus. The flow of blood from LA to LV is restricted and left atrial pressure rises, leading to pulmonary venous congestion and breathlessness. There is dilatation and hypertrophy of the LA, and left ventricular filling becomes more dependent on left atrial contraction.

Any increase in heart rate shortens diastole when the mitral valve is open and produces a further rise in left atrial pressure. Situations that demand an increase in cardiac output also increase left atrial pressure, so exercise and pregnancy are poorly tolerated.

The mitral valve orifice is normally about $5\,cm^2$ in diastole and may be reduced to $1\,cm^2$ in severe mitral stenosis. Patients usually remain asymptomatic until the stenosis is $< 2\,cm^2$. Reduced lung compliance, due to chronic pulmonary venous congestion, contributes to breathlessness and a low cardiac output may cause fatigue.

Atrial fibrillation due to progressive dilatation of the LA is very common. Its onset often precipitates pulmonary oedema because the accompanying tachycardia and loss of atrial contraction lead to marked haemodynamic deterioration with a rapid rise in left atrial pressure. In contrast, a more gradual rise in left atrial pressure tends to cause an increase in pulmonary vascular resistance, which leads to pulmonary hypertension that may protect the patient from pulmonary oedema. Pulmonary hypertension leads to right ventricular hypertrophy and dilatation, tricuspid regurgitation and right heart failure.

Fewer than 20% of patients remain in sinus rhythm; many of these have a small fibrotic LA and severe pulmonary hypertension.

Clinical features

Effort-related dyspnoea is usually the dominant symptom (Box 18.100). Exercise tolerance typically diminishes very slowly over many years and patients often do not appreciate the extent of their disability.

18.100 Clinical features (and their causes) in mitral stenosis

Symptoms

- Breathlessness (pulmonary congestion)
- Fatigue (low cardiac output)
- Oedema, ascites (right heart failure)
- Palpitation (atrial fibrillation)
- Haemoptysis (pulmonary congestion, pulmonary embolism)
- Cough (pulmonary congestion)
- Chest pain (pulmonary hypertension)
- Thromboembolic complications (e.g. stroke, ischaemic limb)

Signs

- Atrial fibrillation
- Mitral facies
- Auscultation
    Loud first heart sound, opening snap
    Mid-diastolic murmur
- Crepitations, pulmonary oedema, effusions (raised pulmonary capillary pressure)
- RV heave, loud P_2 (pulmonary hypertension)

18

Eventually symptoms occur at rest. Acute pulmonary oedema or pulmonary hypertension can lead to haemoptysis. All patients with mitral stenosis, and particularly those with atrial fibrillation, are at risk from left atrial thrombosis and systemic thromboembolism. Prior to the advent of anticoagulant therapy, emboli caused one-quarter of all deaths.

The physical signs of mitral stenosis are often found before symptoms develop and their recognition is of particular importance in pregnancy. The forces that open and close the mitral valve increase as left atrial pressure rises. The first heart sound (S1) is therefore loud and can be palpable (tapping apex beat). An opening snap may be audible and moves closer to the second sound (S2) as the stenosis becomes more severe and left atrial pressure rises. However, the first heart sound and opening snap may be inaudible if the valve is heavily calcified.

Turbulent flow produces the characteristic low-pitched mid-diastolic murmur and sometimes a thrill (Fig. 18.87). The murmur is accentuated by exercise and during atrial systole (pre-systolic accentuation). Early in the disease, a pre-systolic murmur may be the only auscultatory abnormality, but in patients with symptoms the murmur extends from the opening snap to the first heart sound. Coexisting mitral regurgitation causes a pansystolic murmur that radiates towards the axilla.

Pulmonary hypertension may ultimately lead to right ventricular hypertrophy and dilatation with secondary tricuspid regurgitation, which causes a systolic murmur and giant 'v waves' in the venous pulse.

Investigations

The ECG may show either atrial fibrillation or bifid P waves (P mitrale) associated with left atrial hypertrophy (Box 18.101). A typical chest X-ray is shown in Figure 18.10 (p. 532). Doppler echocardiography provides the definitive evaluation of mitral stenosis (see Fig. 18.87). Cardiac catheterisation is used in the assessment of coexisting conditions.

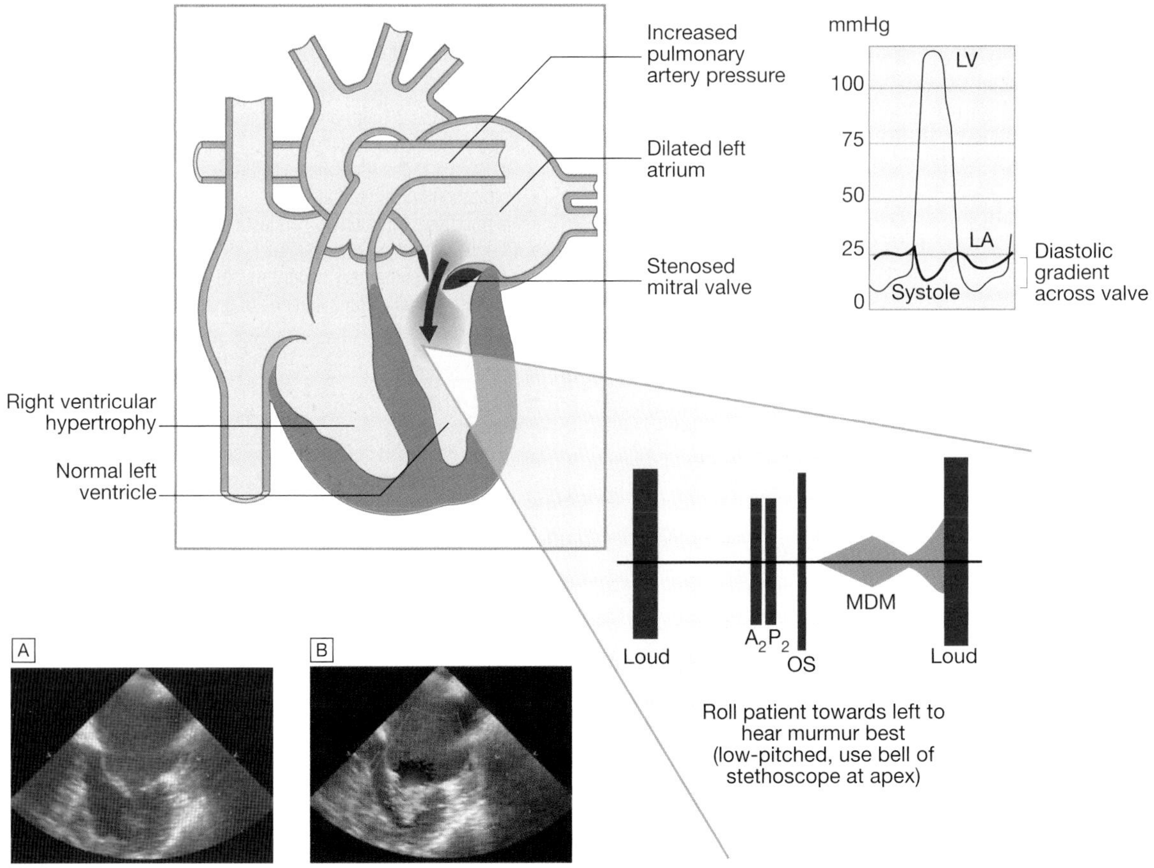

Increased
pulmonary
artery pressure

Dilated left
atrium

Stenosed
mitral valve

Right ventricular
hypertrophy

Normal left
ventricle

mmHg

Diastolic
gradient
across valve

Systole

MDM

A₂P₂
OS

Loud

Loud

Roll patient towards left to
hear murmur best
(low-pitched, use bell of
stethoscope at apex)

Fig. 18.87 Mitral stenosis: murmur and the diastolic pressure gradient between LA and LV. (Mean gradient is reflected by the area between LA and LV in diastole.) The first heart sound is loud, and there is an opening snap (OS) and mid-diastolic murmur (MDM) with pre-systolic accentuation. **A** Echocardiogram showing reduced opening of the mitral valve in diastole. **B** Colour Doppler showing turbulent flow.

18.101 Investigations in mitral stenosis

ECG

- P mitrale or atrial fibrillation
- Right ventricular hypertrophy: tall R waves in V_1–V_3

Chest X-ray

- Enlarged LA and appendage
- Signs of pulmonary venous congestion

Echo

- Thickened immobile cusps
- Reduced valve area
- Reduced rate of diastolic filling of LV
- Enlarged LA

Doppler

- Pressure gradient across mitral valve
- Pulmonary artery pressure
- Left ventricular function

Cardiac catheterisation

- Coronary artery disease
- Mitral stenosis and regurgitation
- Pulmonary artery pressure

Management

Patients with minor symptoms should be treated medically. Intervention by balloon valvuloplasty, mitral valvotomy or mitral valve replacement should be considered if the patient remains symptomatic despite medical treatment or if pulmonary hypertension develops.

Medical management

This consists of anticoagulation to reduce the risk of systemic embolism, ventricular rate control (digoxin, β-blockers or rate-limiting calcium antagonists) in atrial fibrillation, and diuretic therapy to control pulmonary congestion. Antibiotic prophylaxis against infective endocarditis is no longer routinely recommended.

Mitral balloon valvuloplasty and valve replacement

Valvuloplasty is the treatment of choice if specific criteria are fulfilled (Box 18.102 and Fig. 18.15, p. 536), although surgical closed or open mitral valvotomy are acceptable alternatives. Patients who have undergone mitral valvuloplasty or valvotomy should be followed up at 1–2-yearly intervals because restenosis may occur. Clinical symptoms and signs are a guide to the severity of mitral restenosis but Doppler echocardiography provides a more accurate assessment.

18.102 Criteria for mitral valvuloplasty*

- Significant symptoms
- Isolated mitral stenosis
- No (or trivial) mitral regurgitation
- Mobile, non-calcified valve/subvalve apparatus on echo
- LA free of thrombus

*For comprehensive guidelines on valvular heart disease see www.acc.org.

18.103 Causes of mitral regurgitation

- Mitral valve prolapse
- Dilatation of the LV and mitral valve ring (e.g. coronary artery disease, cardiomyopathy)
- Damage to valve cusps and chordae (e.g. rheumatic heart disease, endocarditis)
- Ischaemia or infarction of the papillary muscle
- MI

Valve replacement is indicated if there is substantial mitral reflux or if the valve is rigid and calcified (p. 628).

Mitral regurgitation

Aetiology and pathophysiology

Rheumatic disease is the principal cause in countries where rheumatic fever is common but elsewhere, including in the UK, other causes are more important (Box 18.103). Mitral regurgitation may also follow mitral valvotomy or valvuloplasty.

Chronic mitral regurgitation causes gradual dilatation of the LA with little increase in pressure and therefore relatively few symptoms. Nevertheless, the LV dilates slowly and the left ventricular diastolic and left atrial pressures gradually increase as a result of chronic volume overload of the LV. In contrast, acute mitral regurgitation causes a rapid rise in left atrial pressure (because left atrial compliance is normal) and marked symptomatic deterioration.

Mitral valve prolapse

This is also known as 'floppy' mitral valve and is one of the more common causes of mild mitral regurgitation (Fig. 18.88). It is caused by congenital anomalies or degenerative myxomatous changes, and is sometimes a feature of connective tissue disorders such as Marfan's syndrome (p. 602).

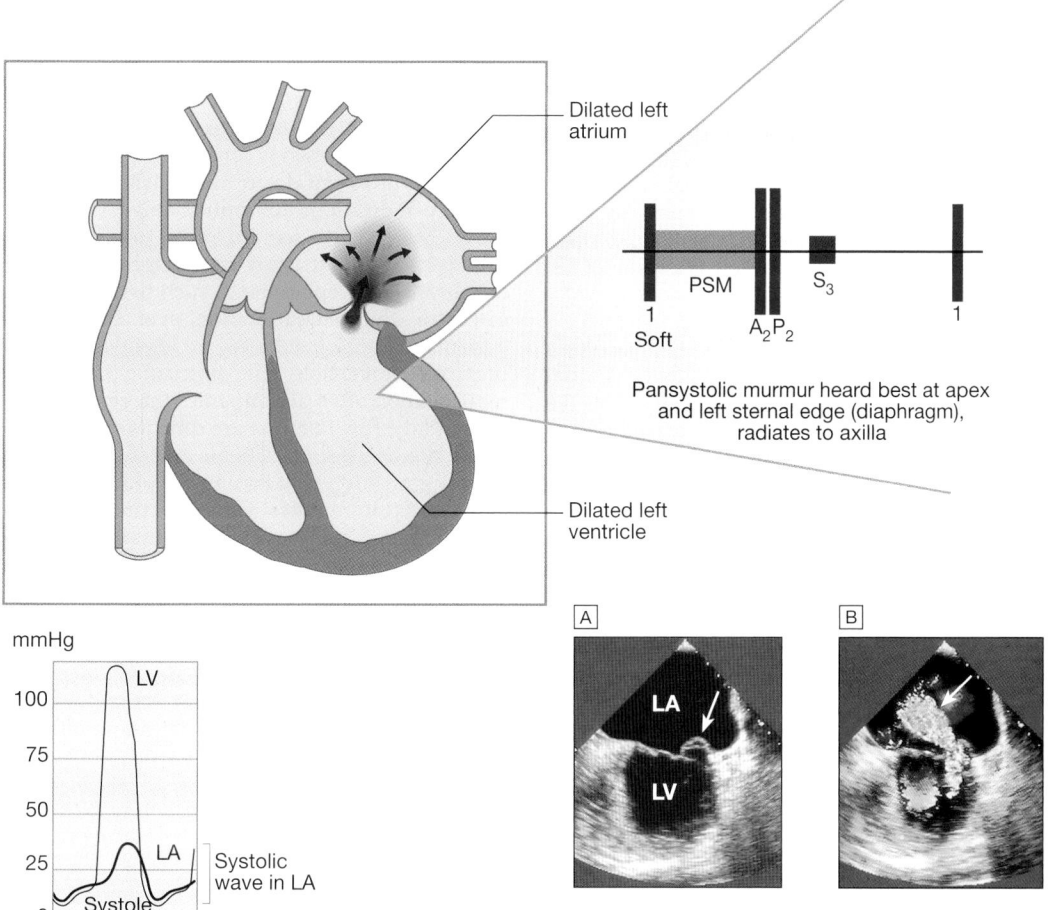

Fig. 18.88 Mitral regurgitation: murmur and systolic wave in left atrial pressure. The first sound is normal or soft and merges with a pansystolic murmur (PSM) extending to the second heart sound. A third heart sound occurs with severe regurgitation. **A** A transoesophageal echocardiogram shows mitral valve prolapse, with one leaflet bulging towards the LA (arrow). **B** This results in a jet of mitral regurgitation on colour Doppler (arrow).

In its mildest forms, the valve remains competent but bulges back into the atrium during systole, causing a midsystolic click but no murmur. In the presence of a regurgitant valve, the click is followed by a late systolic murmur which lengthens as the regurgitation becomes more severe. A click is not always audible and the physical signs may vary with both posture and respiration. Progressive elongation of the chordae tendineae leads to increasing mitral regurgitation, and if chordal rupture occurs, regurgitation suddenly becomes severe. This is rare before the fifth or sixth decade of life.

Mitral valve prolapse is associated with a variety of typically benign arrhythmias, atypical chest pain and a very small risk of embolic stroke or TIA. Nevertheless, the overall long-term prognosis is good.

Other causes of mitral regurgitation

Mitral valve function depends on the chordae tendineae and their papillary muscles; dilatation of the LV distorts the geometry of these and may cause mitral regurgitation (see Box 18.103). Dilated cardiomyopathy and heart failure from coronary artery disease are common causes of so-called 'functional' mitral regurgitation. Endocarditis is an important cause of acute mitral regurgitation.

Clinical features

Symptoms depend on how suddenly the regurgitation develops (Box 18.104). Chronic mitral regurgitation produces a symptom complex that is similar to that of mitral stenosis but sudden-onset mitral regurgitation usually presents with acute pulmonary oedema.

The regurgitant jet causes an apical systolic murmur (see Fig. 18.88) which radiates into the axilla and may be accompanied by a thrill. Increased forward flow through the mitral valve causes a loud third heart sound and even a short mid-diastolic murmur. The apex beat feels active and rocking due to left ventricular volume overload and is usually displaced to the left as a result of left ventricular dilatation.

Investigations

Atrial fibrillation is common, as a consequence of atrial dilatation. At cardiac catheterisation (Box 18.105), the severity of mitral regurgitation can be assessed by left ventriculography and by the size of the v (systolic) waves in the left atrial or pulmonary artery wedge pressure trace.

18.104 Clinical features (and their causes) in mitral regurgitation

Symptoms

- Dyspnoea (pulmonary venous congestion)
- Fatigue (low cardiac output)
- Palpitation (atrial fibrillation, increased stroke volume)
- Oedema, ascites (right heart failure)

Signs

- Atrial fibrillation/flutter
- Cardiomegaly: displaced hyperdynamic apex beat
- Apical pansystolic murmur ± thrill
- Soft S1, apical S3
- Signs of pulmonary venous congestion (crepitations, pulmonary oedema, effusions)
- Signs of pulmonary hypertension and right heart failure

18.105 Investigations in mitral regurgitation

ECG

- Left atrial hypertrophy (if not in AF)
- Left ventricular hypertrophy

Chest X-ray

- Enlarged LA
- Enlarged LV
- Pulmonary venous congestion
- Pulmonary oedema (if acute)

Echo

- Dilated LA, LV
- Dynamic LV (unless myocardial dysfunction predominates)
- Structural abnormalities of mitral valve (e.g. prolapse)

Doppler

- Detects and quantifies regurgitation

Cardiac catheterisation

- Dilated LA, dilated LV, mitral regurgitation
- Pulmonary hypertension
- Coexisting coronary artery disease

Management

Mitral regurgitation of moderate severity can be treated medically (Box 18.106). In all patients with mitral regurgitation, high afterload may worsen the degree of regurgitation and hypertension should be treated with vasodilators such as ACE inhibitors. Patients should be reviewed at regular intervals because worsening symptoms, progressive cardiomegaly or echocardiographic evidence of deteriorating left ventricular function are indications for mitral valve replacement or repair. Mitral valve repair is used to treat mitral valve prolapse and offers many advantages when compared to mitral valve replacement, such that it is now advocated for severe regurgitation, even in asymptomatic patients, because results are excellent and early repair prevents irreversible left ventricular damage. Mitral regurgitation often accompanies the ventricular dilatation and dysfunction that are concomitants of coronary artery disease. If such patients are to undergo coronary bypass graft surgery, it is common practice to repair the valve and restore mitral valve function by inserting an annuloplasty ring to overcome annular dilatation and to bring the valve leaflets closer together. It can be difficult, however, to determine whether it is the ventricular dilatation or the mitral regurgitation that is the predominant problem. If ventricular dilatation is the underlying cause of mitral regurgitation, then mitral valve repair or replacement may actually worsen ventricular function, as the ventricle can no longer empty into the low-pressure LA.

18.106 Medical management of mitral regurgitation

- Diuretics
- Vasodilators, e.g. ACE inhibitors
- Digoxin if atrial fibrillation is present
- Anticoagulants if atrial fibrillation is present

Aortic valve disease

Aortic stenosis

Aetiology and pathophysiology

The likely aetiology depends on the age of the patient (Box 18.107). In congenital aortic stenosis, obstruction is present from birth or becomes apparent in infancy. With bicuspid aortic valves, obstruction may take years to develop as the valve becomes fibrotic and calcified. The aortic valve is the second most frequently affected by rheumatic fever, and commonly both the aortic and mitral valves are involved. In older people, a structurally normal tricuspid aortic valve may be affected by fibrosis and calcification, in a process that is histologically similar to that of atherosclerosis affecting the arterial wall. Haemodynamically significant stenosis develops slowly, typically occurring at 30–60 years in those with rheumatic disease, 50–60 in those with bicuspid aortic valves and 70–90 in those with degenerative calcific disease.

Cardiac output is initially maintained at the cost of a steadily increasing pressure gradient across the aortic valve. The LV becomes increasingly hypertrophied and coronary blood flow may then be inadequate; patients may therefore develop angina, even in the absence of concomitant coronary disease. The fixed outflow obstruction limits the increase in cardiac output required on exercise. Eventually, the LV can no longer overcome the outflow tract obstruction and pulmonary oedema supervenes. In contrast to mitral stenosis, which tends to progress very slowly, patients with aortic stenosis typically remain asymptomatic for many years but deteriorate rapidly when symptoms develop, and death usually ensues within 3–5 years of these.

18.107 Causes of aortic stenosis

Infants, children, adolescents

- Congenital aortic stenosis
- Congenital subvalvular aortic stenosis
- Congenital supravalvular aortic stenosis

Young adults to middle-aged

- Calcification and fibrosis of congenitally bicuspid aortic valve
- Rheumatic aortic stenosis

Middle-aged to elderly

- Senile degenerative aortic stenosis
- Calcification of bicuspid valve
- Rheumatic aortic stenosis

Clinical features

Aortic stenosis is commonly picked up in asymptomatic patients at routine clinical examination but the three cardinal symptoms are angina, breathlessness and syncope (Box 18.108). Angina arises because of the increased demands of the hypertrophied LV working against the high-pressure outflow tract obstruction, leading to a mismatch between oxygen demand and supply, but may also be due to coexisting coronary artery disease, especially in old age when it affects over 50% of patients. Exertional breathlessness suggests cardiac decompensation as a consequence of the excessive pressure overload

18.108 Clinical features of aortic stenosis

Symptoms

- Mild or moderate stenosis: usually asymptomatic
- Exertional dyspnoea
- Angina
- Exertional syncope
- Sudden death
- Episodes of acute pulmonary oedema

Signs

- Ejection systolic murmur
- Slow-rising carotid pulse
- Narrow pulse pressure
- Thrusting apex beat (LV pressure overload)
- Signs of pulmonary venous congestion (e.g. crepitations)

placed on the LV. Syncope usually occurs on exertion when cardiac output fails to rise to meet demand, leading to a fall in BP.

The characteristic clinical signs of severe aortic stenosis are shown in Box 18.108. A harsh ejection systolic murmur radiates to the neck, with a soft second heart sound, particularly in those with calcific valves. The murmur is often likened to a saw cutting wood and may (especially in older patients) have a musical quality like the 'mew' of a seagull (Fig. 18.89). The severity of aortic stenosis may be difficult to gauge clinically, as older patients with a non-compliant 'stiff' arterial system may have an apparently normal carotid upstroke in the presence of severe aortic stenosis. Milder degrees of stenosis may be difficult to distinguish from aortic sclerosis in which the valve is thickened or calcified but not obstructed. A careful examination should be made for other valve lesions, particularly in rheumatic heart disease when there is frequently concomitant mitral valve disease.

Investigations

In advanced cases, ECG features of hypertrophy (Box 18.109) are often gross (Fig. 18.90), and down-sloping ST segments and T inversion ('strain pattern') are seen in leads reflecting the LV. Nevertheless, especially in old age, the ECG can be normal despite severe stenosis. Echocardigraphy demonstrates restricted valve opening (Fig. 18.91) and Doppler assessment permits calculation of the systolic gradient across the aortic valve, from which the severity of stenosis can be assessed (see Fig. 18.12, p. 533). In patients with an impaired left ventricle, velocities across the aortic valve may be diminished because of a reduced stroke volume, while in those in whom aortic regurgitation is present, velocities are increased because of an increased stroke volume. In these circumstances, aortic valve area calculated from Doppler measurements is a more accurate assessment of severity. CT and MRI are useful in assessing the degree of valve calcification and stenosis respectively but are rarely necessary.

Management

Irrespective of the severity of valve stenosis, patients with asymptomatic aortic stenosis have a good immediate prognosis and conservative management is appropriate. Such patients should be kept under review, as the development of angina, syncope, symptoms of low cardiac output or heart failure has a poor prognosis and is an

18

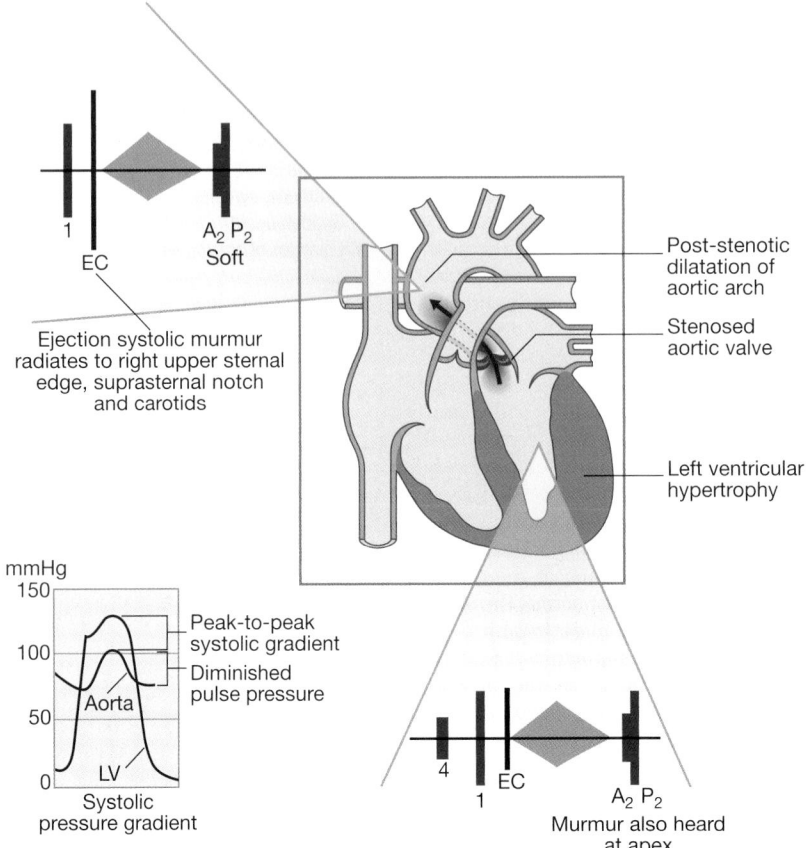

Fig. 18.89 Aortic stenosis. Pressure traces show the systolic gradient between LV and aorta. The 'diamond-shaped' murmur is heard best with the diaphragm in the aortic outflow and also at the apex. An ejection click (EC) may be present in young patients with a bicuspid aortic valve but not in older patients with calcified valves. Aortic stenosis may lead to left ventricular hypertrophy with a fourth sound at the apex and post-stenotic dilatation of the aortic arch. Figure 18.12 (p. 533) shows the typical Doppler signal with aortic stenosis.

indication for prompt surgery. In practice, patients with moderate or severe stenosis are evaluated every 1–2 years with Doppler echocardiography to detect progression in severity; this is more rapid in older patients with heavily calcified valves.

Patients with symptomatic severe aortic stenosis should have prompt aortic valve replacement. Old age is not a contraindication to valve replacement and results are very good in experienced centres, even for those in their eighties (Box 18.110). Delay exposes the patient to the risk of sudden death or irreversible

---

18.109 Investigations in aortic stenosis

ECG

- Left ventricular hypertrophy (usually)
- Left bundle branch block

Chest X-ray

- May be normal; sometimes enlarged LV and dilated ascending aorta on PA view, calcified valve on lateral view

Echo

- Calcified valve with restricted opening, hypertrophied LV (see Fig. 18.91)

Doppler

- Measurement of severity of stenosis
- Detection of associated aortic regurgitation

Cardiac catheterisation

- Mainly to identify associated coronary artery disease
- May be used to measure gradient between LV and aorta

18.110 Aortic stenosis in old age

- **Incidence:** the most common form of valve disease affecting the very old.
- **Symptoms:** a common cause of syncope, angina and heart failure in the very old.
- **Signs:** because of increasing stiffening in the central arteries, low pulse pressure and a slow rising pulse may not be present.
- **Surgery:** can be successful in those aged 80 or more in the absence of comorbidity, but with a higher operative mortality. The prognosis without surgery is poor once symptoms have developed.
- **Valve replacement type:** a biological valve is often preferable to a mechanical, because this obviates the need for anticoagulation, and the durability of biological valves usually exceeds the patient's anticipated life expectancy.

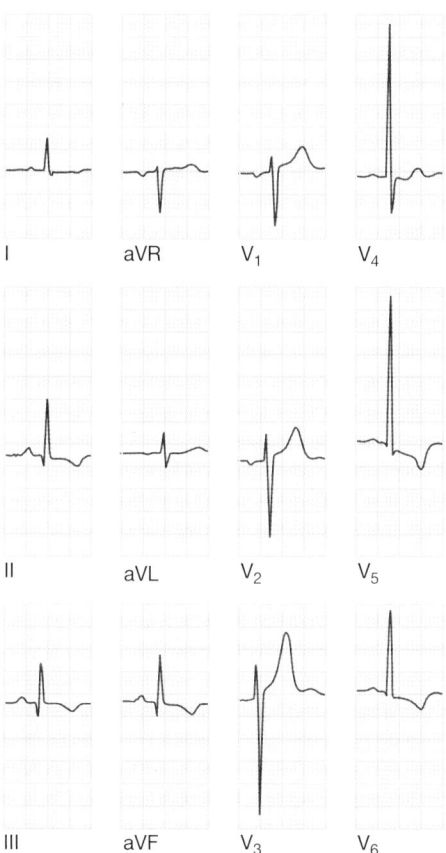

Fig. 18.90 Left ventricular hypertrophy. QRS complexes in limb leads have increased amplitude with a very large R wave in V_5 and S wave in V_2. There is ST depression and T-wave inversion in leads II, III, AVF, V_5 and V_6: a 'left ventricular strain' pattern.

deterioration in ventricular function. Some patients with severe aortic stenosis deny symptoms, and if this could be due to a sedentary lifestyle, a careful exercise test may reveal symptoms on modest exertion. Aortic balloon valvuloplasty is useful in congenital aortic stenosis but is of no value in older patients with calcific aortic stenosis.

Anticoagulants are only required in patients who have atrial fibrillation or those who have had a valve replacement with a mechanical prosthesis.

Aortic regurgitation

Aetiology and pathophysiology

This condition is due to disease of the aortic valve cusps or dilatation of the aortic root (Box 18.111). The LV dilates and hypertrophies to compensate for the regurgitation. The stroke volume of the LV may eventually be doubled or trebled, and the major arteries are then conspicuously pulsatile. As the disease progresses, left ventricular diastolic pressure rises and breathlessness develops.

Clinical features

Until the onset of breathlessness, the only symptom may be an awareness of the heart beat (Box 18.112), particularly when lying on the left side, which results from the increased stroke volume. Paroxysmal nocturnal dyspnoea is sometimes the first symptom, and peripheral oedema or angina may occur. The characteristic murmur

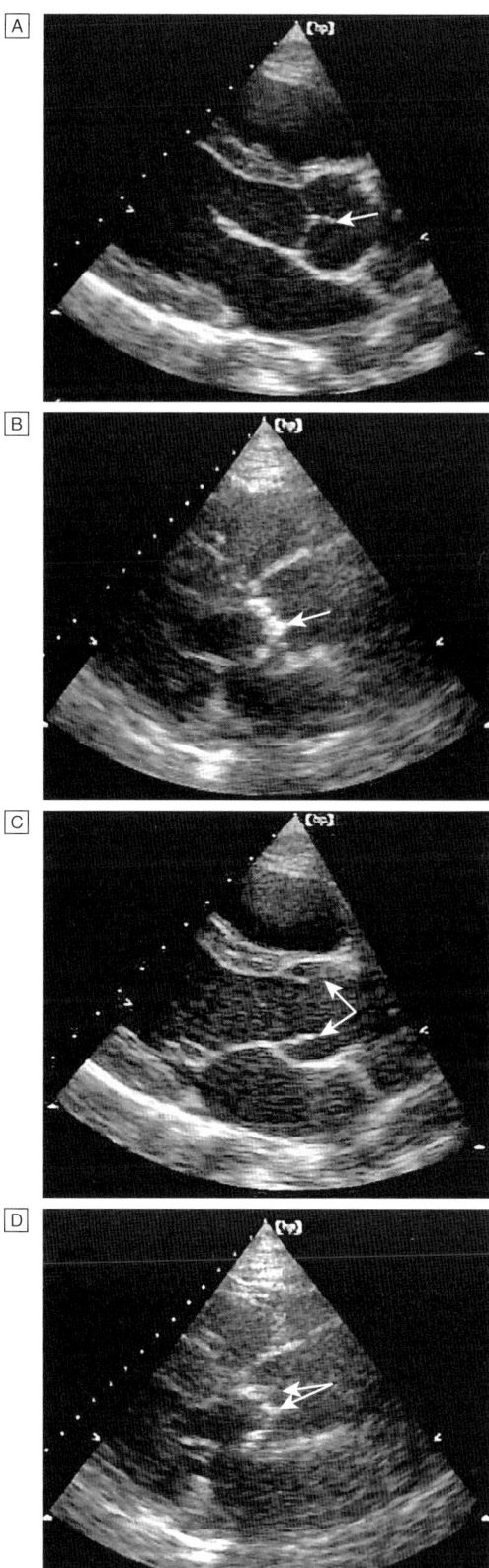

Fig. 18.91 Two-dimensional echocardiogram comparing a normal subject with a patient with calcific aortic stenosis. **A** Normal subject in diastole; the aortic leaflets are closed and thin, and a point of coaptation is seen (arrow). **B** Calcific aortic stenosis in diastole; the aortic leaflets are thick and calcified (arrow). **C** Normal in systole; the aortic leaflets are open (arrows). **D** Calcific aortic stenosis in systole; the thickened leaflets have barely moved (arrows).

18

18.111 Causes of aortic regurgitation

Congenital

- Bicuspid valve or disproportionate cusps

Acquired

- Rheumatic disease
- Infective endocarditis
- Trauma
- Aortic dilatation (Marfan's syndrome, aneurysm, dissection, syphilis, ankylosing spondylitis)

18.112 Clinical features of aortic regurgitation (AR)

Symptoms

Mild to moderate AR

- Often asymptomatic
- Awareness of heart beat, 'palpitations'

Severe AR

- Breathlessness
- Angina

Signs

Pulses

- Large-volume or 'collapsing' pulse
- Low diastolic and increased pulse pressure
- Bounding peripheral pulses
- Capillary pulsation in nail beds: Quincke's sign
- Femoral bruit ('pistol shot'): Duroziez's sign
- Head nodding with pulse: de Musset's sign

Murmurs

- Early diastolic murmur
- Systolic murmur (increased stroke volume)
- Austin Flint murmur (soft mid-diastolic)

Other signs

- Displaced, heaving apex beat (volume overload)
- Presystolic impulse
- Fourth heart sound
- Crepitations (pulmonary venous congestion)

is best heard to the left of the sternum during held expiration (Fig. 18.92); a thrill is rare. A systolic murmur due to the increased stroke volume is common and does not necessarily indicate stenosis. The regurgitant jet causes fluttering of the mitral valve and, if severe, causes partial closure of the anterior mitral leaflet leading to functional mitral stenosis and a soft mid-diastolic (Austin Flint) murmur.

In acute severe regurgitation (e.g. perforation of aortic cusp in endocarditis) there may be no time for compensatory left ventricular hypertrophy and dilatation to develop and the features of heart failure may predominate. In this situation, the classical signs of aortic regurgitation may be masked by tachycardia and an abrupt rise in left ventricular end-diastolic pressure; thus, the pulse pressure may be near normal and the diastolic murmur may be short or even absent.

Investigations

Regurgitation is detected by Doppler echocardiography (Box 18.113). In severe acute aortic regurgitation, the rapid rise in left ventricular diastolic pressure may cause premature mitral valve closure. Cardiac catheterisation and aortography can help in assessing the severity of regurgitation, and dilatation of the aorta and the presence of coexisting coronary artery disease. MRI is useful in assessing the degree and extent of aortic dilatation.

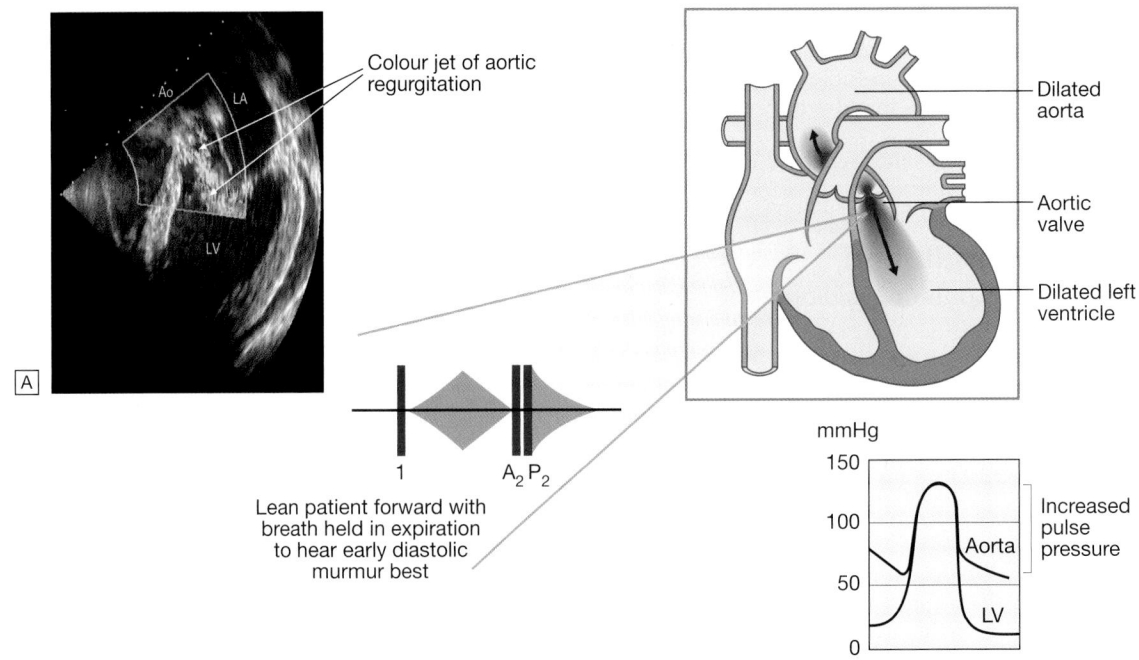

Fig. 18.92 Aortic regurgitation. The early diastolic murmur is best heard at the left sternal edge and may be accompanied by an ejection systolic murmur ('to and fro' murmur). The aortic arch and LV may become dilated. **A** Doppler echocardiogram with the regurgitant jet (arrows).

18.113 Investigations in aortic regurgitation

ECG

• Initially normal, later left ventricular hypertrophy and T-wave inversion

Chest X-ray

• Cardiac dilatation, maybe aortic dilatation
• Features of left heart failure

Echo

• Dilated LV
• Hyperdynamic LV
• Fluttering anterior mitral leaflet
• Doppler detects reflux

Cardiac catheterisation (may not be required)

• Dilated LV
• Aortic regurgitation
• Dilated aortic root

Management

Treatment may be required for underlying conditions such as endocarditis or syphilis. Aortic valve replacement is indicated if aortic regurgitation causes symptoms, and this may need to be combined with aortic root replacement and coronary bypass surgery. Those with chronic aortic regurgitation can remain asymptomatic for many years because compensatory ventricular dilatation and hypertrophy occur, but should be advised to report the development of any symptoms of breathlessness or angina. Asymptomatic patients should also be followed up annually with echocardiography for evidence of increasing ventricular size. If this occurs or if the end-systolic dimension increases to ≥ 55 mm, then aortic valve replacement should be undertaken. Systolic BP should be controlled with vasodilating drugs such as nifedipine or ACE inhibitors. There is conflicting evidence regarding the need for aortic valve replacement in asymptomatic patients with severe aortic regurgitation. When aortic root dilatation is the cause of aortic regurgitation (e.g. Marfan's syndrome), aortic root replacement is usually necessary.

Tricuspid valve disease

Tricuspid stenosis

Aetiology

Tricuspid stenosis is usually rheumatic in origin and is seldom seen in developed countries. Tricuspid disease occurs in fewer than 5% of patients with rheumatic heart disease and nearly always in association with mitral and aortic valve disease. Tricuspid stenosis and regurgitation are also features of the carcinoid syndrome (p. 782).

Clinical features and investigations

Although the symptoms of mitral and aortic valve disease predominate, tricuspid stenosis may cause symptoms of right heart failure, including hepatic discomfort and peripheral oedema.

The main clinical feature is a raised JVP with a prominent *a* wave, and a slow *y* descent due to the loss of normal rapid right ventricular filling (p. 523). There is also a mid-diastolic murmur best heard at the lower left or right sternal edge. This is generally higher-pitched than the murmur of mitral stenosis and is increased by inspiration. Right heart failure causes hepatomegaly with presystolic pulsation (large *a* wave), ascites and peripheral oedema. On Doppler echocardiography, the valve has similar appearances to those of rheumatic mitral stenosis.

Management

In patients who require surgery to other valves, either the tricuspid valve is replaced or valvotomy is performed at the time of surgery. Balloon valvuloplasty can be used to treat rare cases of isolated tricuspid stenosis.

Tricuspid regurgitation

Aetiology, clinical features and investigations

Tricuspid regurgitation is common, and is most frequently 'functional' as a result of right ventricular dilatation (Box 18.114).

Symptoms are usually non-specific, with tiredness related to reduced forward flow, and oedema and hepatic enlargement due to venous congestion. The most prominent sign is a 'giant' *v* wave in the jugular venous pulse (a *cv* wave replaces the normal *x* descent). Other features include a pansystolic murmur at the left sternal edge and a pulsatile liver. Echocardiography may reveal dilatation of the RV. If the valve has been affected by rheumatic disease, the leaflets will appear thickened, and in endocarditis vegetations may be seen. Ebstein's anomaly (see Box 18.125, p. 634) is a congenital abnormality in which the tricuspid valve is displaced towards the right ventricular apex, with consequent enlargement of the RA. It is commonly associated with tricuspid regurgitation.

Management

Tricuspid regurgitation due to right ventricular dilatation often improves when the cause of right ventricular overload is corrected, with diuretic and vasodilator treatment of congestive cardiac failure. Patients with a normal pulmonary artery pressure tolerate isolated tricuspid reflux well, and valves damaged by endocarditis do not usually need to be replaced. Patients undergoing mitral valve replacement who have tricuspid regurgitation due to marked dilatation of the tricuspid annulus benefit from repair of the valve with an annuloplasty ring to bring the leaflets closer together. Those with rheumatic damage may require tricuspid valve replacement.

18.114 Causes of tricuspid regurgitation

Primary

• Rheumatic heart disease
• Endocarditis, particularly in injection drug-users
• Ebstein's congenital anomaly (see Box 18.125, p. 634)

Secondary

• Right ventricular dilatation due to chronic left heart failure ('functional tricuspid regurgitation')
• Right ventricular infarction
• Pulmonary hypertension (e.g. cor pulmonale)

18

Pulmonary valve disease

Pulmonary stenosis

This can occur in the carcinoid syndrome but is usually congenital, in which case it may be isolated or associated with other abnormalities such as Fallot's tetralogy (p. 633).

The principal finding on examination is an ejection systolic murmur, loudest at the left upper sternum and radiating towards the left shoulder. There may be a thrill, best felt when the patient leans forward and breathes out. The murmur is often preceded by an ejection sound (click). Delay in right ventricular ejection may cause wide splitting of the second heart sound. Severe pulmonary stenosis is characterised by a loud harsh murmur, an inaudible pulmonary closure sound (P_2), an increased right ventricular heave, prominent *a* waves in the jugular pulse, ECG evidence of right ventricular hypertrophy, and post-stenotic dilatation in the pulmonary artery on the chest X-ray. Doppler echocardiography is the definitive investigation.

Mild to moderate isolated pulmonary stenosis is relatively common and does not usually progress or require treatment. Severe pulmonary stenosis (resting gradient > 50 mmHg with a normal cardiac output) is treated by percutaneous pulmonary balloon valvuloplasty or, if this is not available, by surgical valvotomy. Long-term results are very good. Post-operative pulmonary regurgitation is common but benign.

Pulmonary regurgitation

This is rare in isolation and is usually associated with pulmonary artery dilatation due to pulmonary hypertension. It may complicate mitral stenosis, producing an early diastolic decrescendo murmur at the left sternal edge that is difficult to distinguish from aortic regurgitation (Graham Steell murmur). The pulmonary hypertension may be secondary to other disease of the left side of the heart, primary pulmonary vascular disease or Eisenmenger's syndrome (p. 630). Trivial pulmonary regurgitation is a frequent finding in normal individuals and has no clinical significance.

Infective endocarditis

This is due to microbial infection of a heart valve (native or prosthetic), the lining of a cardiac chamber or blood vessel, or a congenital anomaly (e.g. septal defect). The causative organism is usually a bacterium, but may be a rickettsia, chlamydia or fungus.

Pathophysiology

Infective endocarditis typically occurs at sites of pre-existing endocardial damage, but infection with particularly virulent or aggressive organisms (e.g. *Staphylococcus aureus*) can cause endocarditis in a previously normal heart; staphylococcal endocarditis of the tricuspid valve is a common complication of intravenous drug misuse. Many acquired and congenital cardiac lesions are vulnerable to endocarditis, particularly areas of endocardial damage caused by a high-pressure jet of blood, such as ventricular septal defect, mitral regurgitation and aortic regurgitation, many of which are haemodynamically insignificant. In contrast,

the risk of endocarditis at the site of haemodynamically important low-pressure lesions, such as a large atrial septal defect, is minimal.

Infection tends to occur at sites of endothelial damage because they attract deposits of platelets and fibrin that are vulnerable to colonisation by blood-borne organisms. The avascular valve tissue and presence of fibrin and platelet aggregates help to protect proliferating organisms from host defence mechanisms. When the infection is established, vegetations composed of organisms, fibrin and platelets grow and may become large enough to cause obstruction or embolism. Adjacent tissues are destroyed and abscesses may form. Valve regurgitation may develop or increase if the affected valve is damaged by tissue distortion, cusp perforation or disruption of chordae. Extracardiac manifestations such as vasculitis and skin lesions are due to emboli or immune complex deposition. Mycotic aneurysms may develop in arteries at the site of infected emboli. At autopsy, infarction of the spleen and kidneys, and sometimes an immune glomerulonephritis are found.

Microbiology

Over three-quarters of cases are due to streptococci or staphylococci. The *viridans* group of streptococci (*Strep. mitis*, *Strep. sanguis*) are commensals in the upper respiratory tract that may enter the blood stream on chewing or teeth-brushing, or at the time of dental treatment, and are common causes of subacute endocarditis (Box 18.115). Other organisms, including *Enterococcus faecalis*, *E. faecium* and *Strep. bovis*, may enter the blood from the bowel or urinary tract. *Strep. milleri* and *Strep. bovis* endocarditis is associated with large-bowel neoplasms.

Staph. aureus has now overtaken streptococci as the most common cause of acute endocarditis. It originates from skin infections, abscesses or vascular access sites (e.g. intravenous and central lines), or from intravenous

18.115 Microbiology of infective endocarditis

Pathogen	Of native valve (n = 280)	In i.v. drug users (n = 87)	Of prosthetic valve Early (n = 15)	Of prosthetic valve Late (n = 72)
Staphylococci	124 (44%)	60 (69%)	10 (67%)	33 (46%)
Staph. aureus	106 (38%)	60 (69%)	3 (20%)	15 (21%)
Coagulase-negative	18 (6%)	0	7 (47%)	18 (25%)
Streptococci	86 (31%)	7 (8%)	0	25 (35%)
Oral	59 (21%)	3 (3%)	0	19 (26%)
Others (non-enterococcal)	27 (10%)	4 (5%)	0	6 (8%)
***Enterococcus* spp.**	21 (8%)	2 (2%)	1 (7%)	5 (7%)
HACEK group	12 (4%)	0	0	1 (1%)
Polymicrobial	6 (2%)	8 (9%)	0	1 (1%)
Other bacteria	12 (4%)	4 (5%)	0	2 (3%)
Fungi	3 (1%)	2 (2%)	0	0
Negative blood culture	16 (6%)	4 (5%)	4 (27%)	5 (7%)

Adapted from Moreillon P, Que YA. Lancet 2004; 363:139–149.

drug misuse. It is a highly virulent and invasive organism, usually producing florid vegetations, rapid valve destruction and abscess formation. Other causes of acute endocarditis include *Strep. pneumoniae* and *Strep. pyogenes*.

Post-operative endocarditis after cardiac surgery may affect native or prosthetic heart valves or other prosthetic materials. The most common organism is a coagulase-negative staphylococcus (*Staph. epidermidis*), a normal skin commensal. There is frequently a history of post-operative wound infection with the same organism. *Staph. epidermidis* occasionally causes endocarditis in patients who have not had cardiac surgery, and its presence in blood cultures may be erroneously dismissed as contamination. Another coagulase-negative staphylococcus, *Staph. lugdenensis*, causes a rapidly destructive acute endocarditis that is associated with previously normal valves and multiple emboli. Unless accurately identified, it may also be overlooked as a contaminant.

In Q fever endocarditis due to *Coxiella burnetii*, the patient often has a history of contact with farm animals. The aortic valve is usually affected and there may be hepatic complications and purpura. Life-long antibiotic therapy may be required.

Gram-negative bacteria of the so-called HACEK group (*Haemophilus* spp., *Actinobacillus actinomycetemcomitans*, *Cardiobacterium hominis*, *Eikenella* spp. and *Kingella kingae*) are slow-growing fastidious organisms that are only revealed after prolonged culture and may be resistant to penicillin.

Brucella is associated with a history of contact with goats or cattle and often affects the aortic valve.

Yeasts and fungi (*Candida*, *Aspergillus*) may attack previously normal or prosthetic valves, particularly in immunocompromised patients or those with indwelling intravenous lines. Abscesses and emboli are common, therapy is difficult (surgery is often required) and mortality is high. Concomitant bacterial infection may be present.

Incidence

The incidence of infective endocarditis in community-based studies ranges from 5 to 15 cases per 100 000 per annum. More than 50% of affected patients are over 60 years of age (Box 18.116). In a large British study, the underlying condition was rheumatic heart disease in 24% of patients, congenital heart disease in 19%, and some other cardiac abnormality (e.g. calcified aortic valve, floppy mitral valve) in 25%. The remaining 32% were not thought to have a pre-existing cardiac abnormality.

Clinical features

Endocarditis occurs as either an acute or a more insidious 'subacute' form. However, there is considerable overlap because the clinical pattern is influenced not only by the organism, but also by the site of infection, prior antibiotic therapy and the presence of a valve or shunt prosthesis. The subacute form may abruptly develop acute life-threatening complications such as valve disruption or emboli.

Subacute endocarditis

This should be suspected when a patient with congenital or valvular heart disease develops a persistent fever, complains of unusual tiredness, night sweats or weight loss, or develops new signs of valve dysfunction or heart failure. Less often, it presents as an embolic stroke or peripheral arterial embolism. Other features (Fig. 18.93) include purpura and petechial haemorrhages in the skin and mucous membranes, and splinter haemorrhages under the fingernails or toe nails. Osler's nodes are painful tender swellings at the fingertips that are probably the product of vasculitis; they are rare. Digital clubbing is a late sign. The spleen is frequently palpable; in *Coxiella* infections the spleen and the liver may be considerably enlarged. Microscopic haematuria is common. The finding of any of these features in a patient with persistent fever or malaise is an indication for re-examination to detect hitherto unrecognised heart disease.

Acute endocarditis

This presents as a severe febrile illness with prominent and changing heart murmurs and petechiae. Clinical stigmata of chronic endocarditis are usually absent. Embolic events are common, and cardiac or renal failure may develop rapidly. Abscesses may be detected on echocardiography. Partially treated acute endocarditis behaves like subacute endocarditis.

Post-operative endocarditis

This may present as an unexplained fever in a patient who has had heart valve surgery. The infection usually affects the valve ring and may resemble subacute or acute endocarditis, depending on the virulence of the organism. Morbidity and mortality are high and redo surgery is often required. The range of organisms is similar to that seen in native valve disease, but when endocarditis occurs during the first few weeks after surgery, it is usually due to infection with a coagulase-negative staphylococcus that was introduced during the perioperative period. A clinical diagnosis of endocarditis can be made on the presence of two major, one major and three minor, or five minor criteria (Box 18.117).

Investigations

Blood culture is the crucial investigation because it may identify the infection and guide antibiotic therapy. Three to six sets of blood cultures should be taken prior to commencing therapy and should not wait for episodes of pyrexia. The first two specimens will detect bacteraemia in 90% of culture-positive cases. Aseptic technique is essential and the risk of contaminants should be minimised by sampling from different venepuncture sites. An in-dwelling line should not be used to take cultures. Aerobic and anaerobic cultures are required.

Echocardiography is key for detecting and following the progress of vegetations, for assessing valve damage and for detecting abscess formation. Vegetations as

18.116 Endocarditis in old age

- **Symptoms and signs:** may be non-specific, e.g. confusion, weight loss, malaise and weakness, and the diagnosis may not be suspected.
- **Common causative organisms:** often enterococci (from the urinary tract) and *Strep. bovis* (from a colonic source).
- **Morbidity and mortality:** much higher.

18

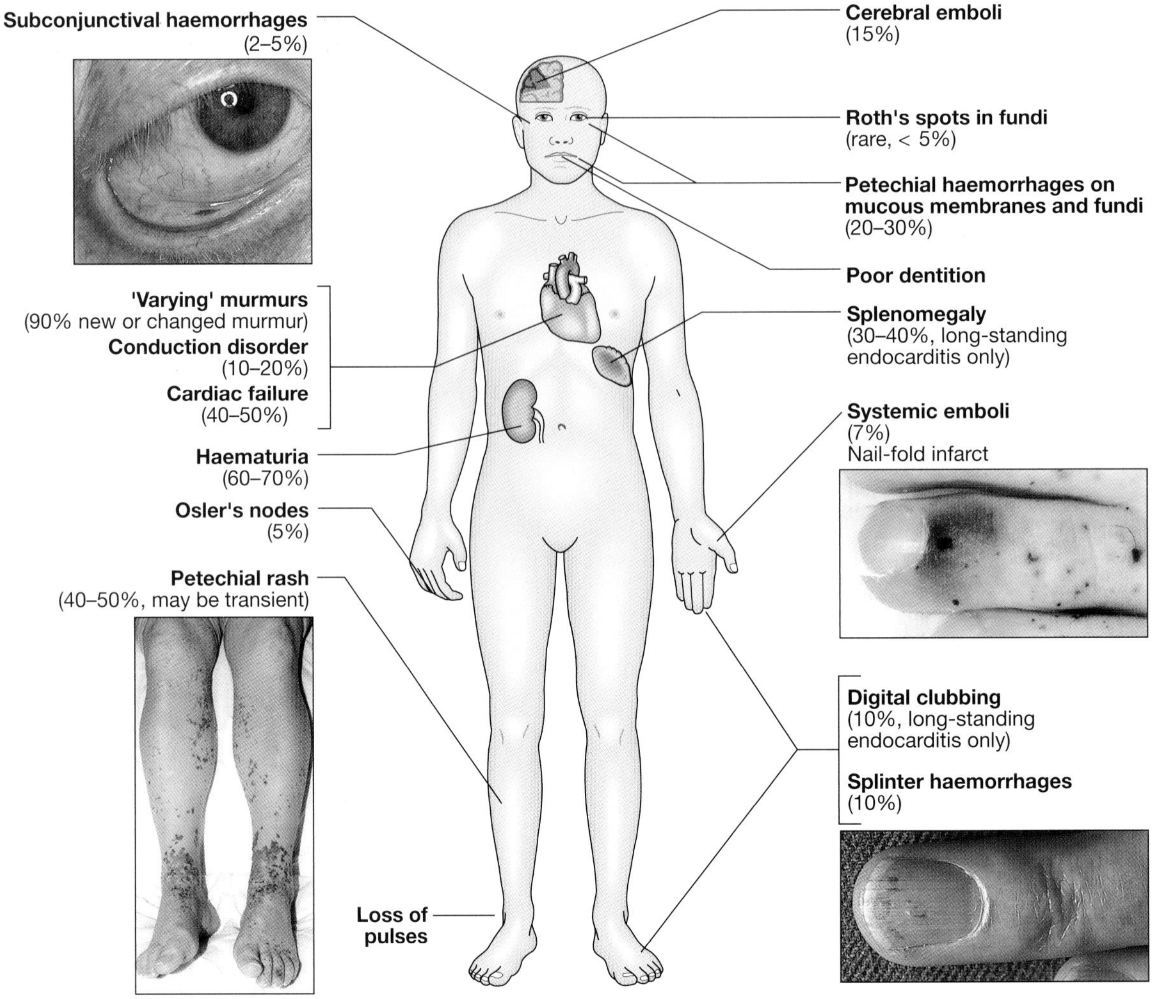

Subconjunctival haemorrhages
(2–5%)

Cerebral emboli
(15%)

Roth's spots in fundi
(rare, < 5%)

Petechial haemorrhages on
mucous membranes and fundi
(20–30%)

Poor dentition

Splenomegaly
(30–40%, long-standing
endocarditis only)

'Varying' murmurs
(90% new or changed murmur)
Conduction disorder
(10–20%)
Cardiac failure
(40–50%)

Haematuria
(60–70%)

Osler's nodes
(5%)

Systemic emboli
(7%)
Nail-fold infarct

Digital clubbing
(10%, long-standing
endocarditis only)

Splinter haemorrhages
(10%)

Petechial rash
(40–50%, may be transient)

Loss of
pulses

Fig. 18.93 Clinical features which may be present in endocarditis.

18.117 Diagnosis of infective endocarditis (modified Duke criteria)

Major criteria

- Positive blood culture
  Typical organism from two cultures
  Persistent positive blood cultures taken > 12 hrs apart
  Three or more positive cultures taken over > 1 hr
- Endocardial involvement
  Positive echocardiographic findings of vegetations
  New valvular regurgitation

Minor criteria

- Predisposing valvular or cardiac abnormality
- Intravenous drug misuse
- Pyrexia ≥ 38 °C
- Embolic phenomenon
- Vasculitic phenomenon
- Blood cultures suggestive: organism grown but not achieving major criteria
- Suggestive echocardiographic findings

Definite endocarditis = two major, or one major and three minor, or five minor

Possible endocarditis = one major and one minor, or three minor

---

small as 2–4 mm can be detected by transthoracic echocardiography, and even smaller ones (1–1.5 mm) can be visualised by transoesophageal echocardiography, which is particularly valuable for identifying abscess formation and investigating patients with prosthetic heart valves. Vegetations may be difficult to distinguish in the presence of an abnormal valve; the sensitivity of transthoracic echo is approximately 65% but that of transoesophageal echo is more than 90%. Failure to detect vegetations does not exclude the diagnosis.

Elevation of the ESR, a normocytic normochromic anaemia, and leucocytosis are common but not invariable. Measurement of serum CRP is more reliable than the ESR in monitoring progress. Proteinuria may occur and microscopic haematuria is usually present.

The ECG may show the development of AV block (due to aortic root abscess formation) and occasionally infarction due to emboli. The chest X-ray may show evidence of cardiac failure and cardiomegaly.

Management

The case fatality of bacterial endocarditis is approximately 20% and even higher in those with prosthetic valve endocarditis and those infected with antibiotic-resistant organisms. A multidisciplinary approach with cooperation between the physician, surgeon and bacteriologist increases the chance of a successful outcome. Any source of infection should be removed as soon as possible; for example, a tooth with an apical abscess should be extracted.

Empirical treatment depends on the mode of presentation, the suspected organism, and whether the patient has a prosthetic valve or penicillin allergy (Box 18.118). If the presentation is acute, flucloxacillin and gentamicin are recommended, while for a subacute or indolent presentation, benzyl penicillin and gentamicin are preferred. In those with penicillin allergy, a prosthetic valve or suspected meticillin-resistant *Staph. aureus* (MRSA) infection, triple therapy with vancomycin, gentamicin and oral rifampicin should be considered. Following identification of the causal organism, determination of the minimum inhibitory concentration (MIC) for the organism is essential to guide antibiotic therapy.

A 2-week treatment regimen may be sufficient for fully sensitive strains of *Strep. viridans* and *Strep. bovis*, provided specific conditions are met (Box 18.119). For the empirical treatment of bacterial endocarditis, penicillin plus gentamicin is the regimen of choice for most patients; however, when staphylococcal infection is suspected, vancomycin plus gentamicin is recommended.

Cardiac surgery (débridement of infected material and valve replacement) is advisable in a substantial proportion of patients, particularly those with *Staph. aureus* and fungal infections (Box 18.120). Antimicrobial therapy must be started before surgery.

18.119 Conditions to be met for the short-course treatment of *Strep. viridans* and *Strep. bovis* endocarditis

- Native valve infection
- MIC ≤ 0.1 mg/L
- No adverse prognostic factors (e.g. heart failure, aortic regurgitation, conduction defect)
- No evidence of thromboembolic disease
- No vegetations > 5 mm diameter
- Clinical response within 7 days

18.120 Indications for cardiac surgery in infective endocarditis

- Heart failure due to valve damage
- Failure of antibiotic therapy (persistent or uncontrolled infection)
- Large vegetations on left-sided heart valves with evidence or 'high risk' of systemic emboli
- Abscess formation

N.B. Patients with prosthetic valve endocarditis or fungal endocarditis often require cardiac surgery.

Prevention

Until recently, antibiotic prophylaxis was routinely given to people at risk of infective endocarditis undergoing interventional procedures. However, as this has not been proven to be effective and the link between episodes of infective endocarditis and interventional

18

18.118 Antimicrobial treatment of common causative organisms in infective endocarditis

Organism	Antimicrobial	Dose	Native valve	Prosthetic valve
			Duration	
Viridans* streptococci and *Strep. bovis				
MIC ≤ 0.1 mg/L	Benzyl penicillin i.v.	1.2 g 4-hourly	4 wks[1]	6 wks
	and gentamicin i.v.	1 mg/kg 8–12-hourly	2 wks	2 wks
MIC > 0.1 to < 0.5 mg/L	Benzyl penicillin i.v.	1.2 g 4-hourly	4 wks	6 wks
	and gentamicin i.v.	1 mg/kg 8–12-hourly	2 wks	4–6 wks
MIC ≥ 0.5 mg/L	Benzyl penicillin i.v.	1.2 g 4-hourly	4 wks	6 wks
	and gentamicin i.v.	1 mg/kg 8–12-hourly	4 wks	4–6 wks
Enterococci				
Ampicillin-sensitive	Ampicillin i.v.	2 g 4-hourly	4 wks	6 wks
	and gentamicin i.v.[2]	1 mg/kg 8–12-hourly	4 wks	6 wks
Ampicillin-resistant	Vancomycin i.v.	1 g 12-hourly	4 wk	6 wks
	and gentamicin i.v.[2]	1 mg/kg 8–12-hourly	4 wks	6 wks
Staphylococci				
Penicillin-sensitive	Benzyl penicillin i.v.	1.2 g 4-hourly	4 wks	6 wks
Penicillin-resistant Meticillin-sensitive	Flucloxacillin i.v.	2 g 4-hourly (< 85 kg 6-hourly)	4 wks	6 wks[3]
Penicillin-resistant Meticillin-resistant	Vancomycin i.v. and gentamicin i.v.	1 g 12-hourly 1 mg/kg 8-hourly	4 wks 4 wks	6 wks[3] 6 wks[3]

[1]When conditions in Box 18.119 are met, 2 wks of benzyl penicillin.
[2]In high-level gentamicin resistance, consider streptomycin.
[3]Consider additional rifampicin 300–600 mg 12-hourly orally for 2 wks.
(MIC = minimum inhibitory concentration)

18

procedures has not been demonstrated, antibiotic prophylaxis is no longer offered routinely for defined interventional procedures.

Valve replacement surgery

Diseased heart valves can be replaced with mechanical or biological prostheses. The three most commonly used types of mechanical prosthesis are the ball and cage, tilting single disc and tilting bi-leaflet valves. All generate prosthetic sounds or clicks on auscultation. Pig or allograft valves mounted on a supporting stent are the most commonly used biological valves. They generate normal heart sounds. All prosthetic valves used in the aortic position produce a systolic flow murmur.

All mechanical valves require long-term anticoagulation because they can cause systemic thromboembolism or may develop valve thrombosis or obstruction (Box 18.121); the prosthetic clicks may become inaudible if the valve malfunctions. Biological valves have the advantage of not requiring anticoagulants to maintain proper function; however, many patients undergoing valve replacement surgery, especially mitral valve replacement, will have atrial fibrillation that requires anticoagulation anyway. Biological valves are less durable than mechanical valves and may degenerate 7 or more years after implantation, particularly when used in the mitral position. They are more durable in the aortic position and in older patients, so are particularly appropriate for patients over 65 undergoing aortic valve replacement.

Symptoms or signs of unexplained heart failure in a patient with a prosthetic heart valve may be due to valve dysfunction, and urgent assessment is required. Biological valve dysfunction is usually associated with the development of a regurgitant murmur.

18.121 Prosthetic heart valves: optimal anticoagulant control

Mechanical valves	Target INR
Ball and cage (e.g. Starr–Edwards) Tilting disc (e.g. Bjork–Shiley)	3.5
Bi-leaflet (e.g. St Jude)	3.0
Biological valves with atrial fibrillation	2.5

CONGENITAL HEART DISEASE

Congenital heart disease usually manifests in childhood but may pass unrecognised and not present until adult life. Defects that are well tolerated, such as atrial septal defect, may cause no symptoms until adult life or may be detected incidentally on routine examination or chest X-ray. Congenital defects that were previously fatal in childhood can now be corrected, or at least partially, so that survival to adult life is the norm. Such patients remain well for many years but subsequently re-present in later life with related problems such as arrhythmia or ventricular dysfunction (Box 18.122).

18.122 Presentation of congenital heart disease throughout life

Birth and neonatal period

- Cyanosis
- Heart failure

Infancy and childhood

- Cyanosis
- Heart failure
- Arrhythmia
- Murmur
- Failure to thrive

Adolescence and adulthood

- Heart failure
- Murmur
- Arrhythmia
- Cyanosis due to shunt reversal (Eisenmenger's syndrome)
- Hypertension (coarctation)
- Late consequences of previous cardiac surgery, e.g. arrhythmia, heart failure

The fetal circulation

Understanding the fetal circulation helps clarify how some forms of congenital heart disease occur. The fetus has only a small flow of blood through the lungs, as it does not breathe in utero. The fetal circulation allows oxygenated blood from the placenta to pass directly to the left side of the heart through the foramen ovale without having to flow through the lungs (Fig. 18.94).

Congenital defects may arise if the changes from fetal circulation to the extrauterine circulation are not properly completed. Atrial septal defects occur at the site of the foramen ovale. A patent ductus arteriosus may remain if it fails to close after birth. Failure of the aorta to develop at the point of the aortic isthmus and where the ductus arteriosus attaches can lead to narrowing or coarctation of the aorta.

In fetal development, the heart develops as a single tube which folds back on itself and then divides into two separate circulations. Failure of septation can lead to some forms of atrial and ventricular septal defect. Failure of alignment of the great vessels with the ventricles contributes to transposition of the great arteries, tetralogy of Fallot and truncus arteriosus.

Aetiology and incidence

The incidence of haemodynamically significant congenital cardiac abnormalities is about 0.8% of live births (Box 18.123). Maternal infection or exposure to drugs or toxins may cause congenital heart disease. Maternal rubella infection is associated with persistent ductus arteriosus, pulmonary valvular and/or artery stenosis, and atrial septal defect. Maternal alcohol misuse is associated with septal defects, and maternal lupus erythematosus with congenital complete heart block. Genetic or chromosomal abnormalities such as Down's syndrome may cause septal defects, and gene defects have also been identified as causing specific abnormalities, such as Marfan's syndrome (p. 602) and DiGeorge's (deletion in chromosome 22q) syndrome.

Clinical features

Symptoms may be absent, or the child may be breathless or fail to attain normal growth and development. Some defects are not compatible with extrauterine life, or only for a short time. Clinical signs vary with the anatomical lesion. Murmurs, thrills or signs of cardiomegaly

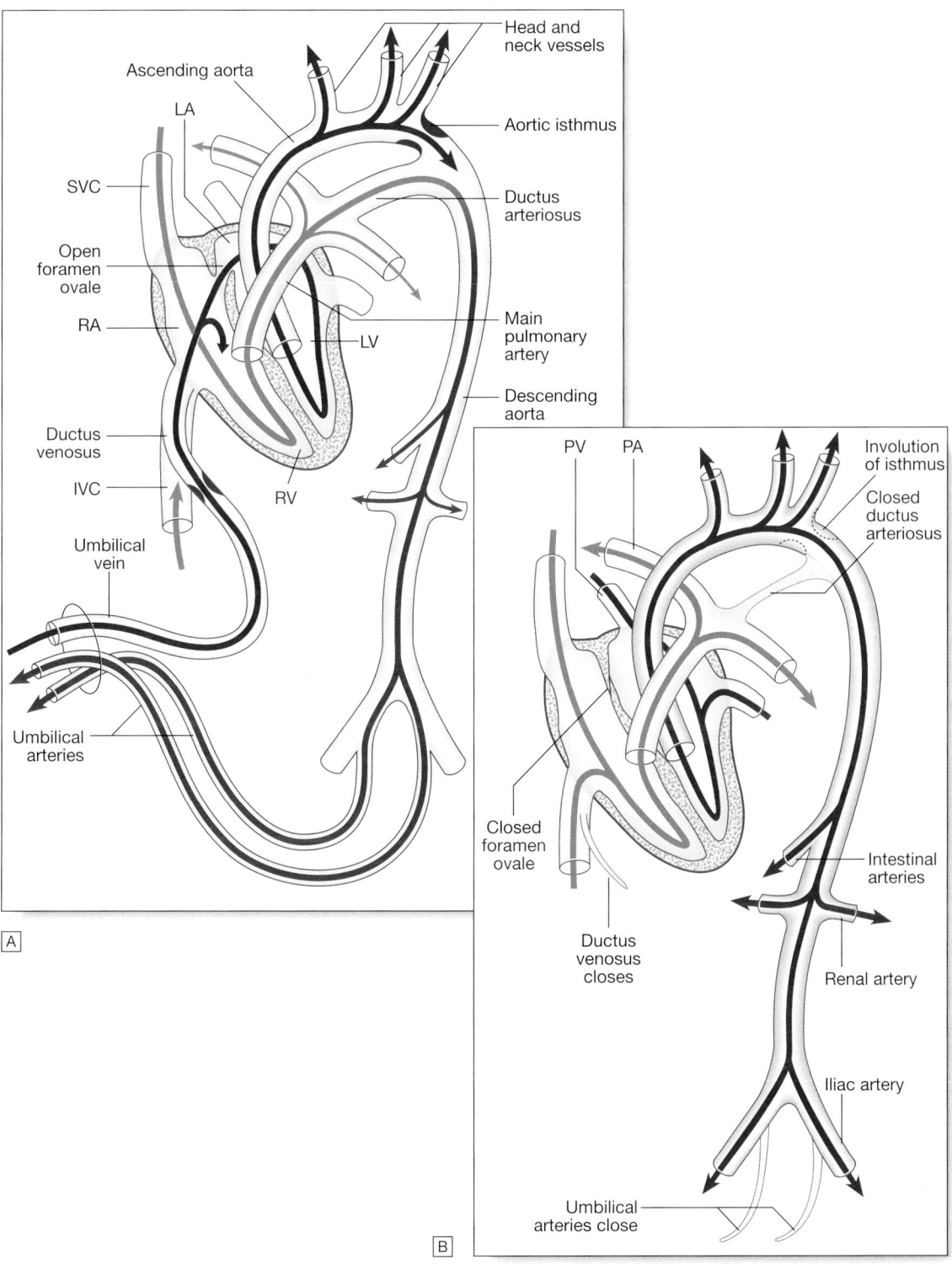

Fig. 18.94 Changes in the circulation at birth. **A** In the fetus, oxygenated blood comes through the umbilical vein where it enters the inferior vena cava via the ductus venosus (red). The oxygenated blood streams from the RA through the open foramen ovale to the LA and via the LV into the aorta. Venous blood from the superior vena cava (blue) crosses under the main blood stream into the RA and then, partly mixed with oxygenated blood (purple), into the RV and pulmonary artery. The pulmonary vasculature has a high resistance and so little blood passes to the lungs; most blood passes through the ductus arteriosus to the descending aorta. The aortic isthmus is a constriction in the aorta that lies in the aortic arch before the junction with the ductus arteriosus and limits the flow of oxygen-rich blood to the descending aorta. This configuration means that less oxygen-rich blood is supplied to organ systems that take up their function mainly after birth, e.g. the kidneys and intestinal tract. **B** At birth, the lungs expand with air and pulmonary vascular resistance falls, so that blood now flows to the lungs and back to the LA. The left atrial pressure rises above right atrial pressure and the flap valve of the foramen ovale closes. The umbilical arteries and the ductus venosus close. In the next few days, the ductus arteriosus closes under the influence of hormonal changes (particularly prostaglandins) and the aortic isthmus expands.

18.123 Incidence and relative frequency of congenital cardiac malformations

Lesion	% of all CHD defects
Ventricular septal defect	30
Atrial septal defect	10
Patent ductus arteriosus	10
Pulmonary stenosis	7
Coarctation of aorta	7
Aortic stenosis	6
Tetralogy of Fallot	6
Complete transposition of great arteries	4
Others	20

may be present. In coarctation of the aorta, radio-femoral delay may be noted (Fig. 18.95) and some female patients have the features of Turner's syndrome (p. 761). Features of other congenital conditions such as Marfan's syndrome or Down's syndrome may also be apparent. Cerebrovascular accidents and cerebral abscesses may complicate severe cyanotic congenital disease.

Early diagnosis is important because many types of congenital heart disease are amenable to surgical treatment, but this opportunity is lost if secondary changes such as pulmonary vascular damage occur.

Central cyanosis and digital clubbing

Central cyanosis of cardiac origin occurs when desaturated blood enters the systemic circulation without passing through the lungs (i.e. a right-to-left shunt). In the neonate, the most common cause is transposition of the great arteries, in which the aorta arises from the RV and the pulmonary artery from the LV. In older children, cyanosis is usually the consequence of a ventricular septal defect combined with severe pulmonary stenosis (tetralogy of Fallot) or with pulmonary vascular disease (Eisenmenger's syndrome). Prolonged cyanosis is associated with finger and toe clubbing (p. 522).

Growth retardation and learning difficulties

These may occur with large left-to-right shunts at ventricular or great arterial level, and also with other defects, especially if they form part of a genetic syndrome.

Major intellectual impairment is uncommon in children with isolated congenital heart disease; however, minor learning difficulties can occur and may complicate cardiac surgery if cerebral perfusion is compromised.

Syncope

In the presence of increased pulmonary vascular resistance or severe left or right ventricular outflow obstruction, exercise may provoke syncope as systemic vascular resistance falls but pulmonary vascular resistance rises, worsening right-to-left shunting and cerebral oxygenation. Syncope can also occur because of associated arrhythmias.

Pulmonary hypertension and Eisenmenger's syndrome

Persistently raised pulmonary flow (e.g. with left-to-right shunt) causes increased pulmonary resistance followed by pulmonary hypertension. Progressive changes, including obliteration of distal vessels, occur and are irreversible. Central cyanosis appears and digital clubbing develops. The chest X-ray shows enlarged central pulmonary arteries and peripheral 'pruning' of the pulmonary vessels. The ECG shows right ventricular hypertrophy. If severe pulmonary hypertension develops, a left-to-right shunt may reverse, resulting in right-to-left shunt and marked cyanosis (Eisenmenger's syndrome), which may be more apparent in the feet and toes than in the upper part of the body: differential cyanosis. This is more common with large ventricular septal defects or persistent ductus arteriosus than with atrial septal defects. Patients with Eisenmenger's syndrome are at particular risk from abrupt changes in afterload that exacerbate right-to-left shunting, such as vasodilatation, anaesthesia and pregnancy.

Pregnancy

During pregnancy, there is a 50% increase in plasma volume, a 40% increase in whole blood volume and a similar increase in cardiac output, so problems may arise in women with congenital heart disease (Box 18.124). However, many with palliated or untreated disease will tolerate pregnancy well. Pregnancy is particularly hazardous in the presence of conditions associated with cyanosis or severe pulmonary hypertension; maternal mortality in patients with Eisenmenger's syndrome is more than 50%.

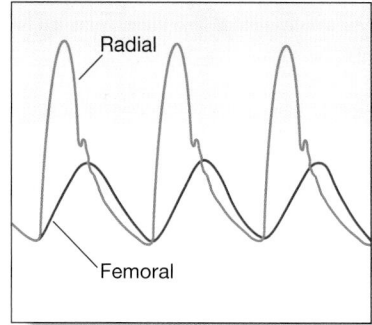

Fig. 18.95 Radio-femoral delay. The difference in pulse pressures is shown.

18.124 Pregnancy in women with congenital heart disease

- **Obstructive lesions** (e.g. severe aortic stenosis): poorly tolerated and associated with significant maternal morbidity and mortality.
- **Cyanotic conditions** (e.g. Eisenmenger's syndrome): especially poorly tolerated and pregnancy should be avoided.
- **Surgically corrected disease:** patients often tolerate pregnancy well.
- **Children of patients with congenital heart disease:** 2–5 % will be born with cardiac abnormalities, especially if the mother is affected.

Persistent ductus arteriosus

Aetiology

During fetal life, before the lungs begin to function, most of the blood from the pulmonary artery passes through the ductus arteriosus into the aorta (see Fig. 18.94). Normally, the ductus closes soon after birth but sometimes fails to do so. Persistence of the ductus is associated with other abnormalities and is more common in females.

Since the pressure in the aorta is higher than that in the pulmonary artery, there will be a continuous arteriovenous shunt, the volume of which depends on the size of the ductus. As much as 50% of the left ventricular output is recirculated through the lungs, with a consequent increase in the work of the heart (Fig. 18.96).

Clinical features

With small shunts there may be no symptoms for years, but when the ductus is large, growth and development may be retarded. Usually there is no disability in infancy but cardiac failure may eventually ensue, dyspnoea being the first symptom. A continuous 'machinery' murmur is heard with late systolic accentuation, maximal in the second left intercostal space below the clavicle (see Fig. 18.96). It is frequently accompanied by a thrill. Pulses are increased in volume.

A large left-to-right shunt in infancy may cause a considerable rise in pulmonary artery pressure, and sometimes this leads to progressive pulmonary vascular damage. Enlargement of the pulmonary artery may be detected radiologically. The ECG is usually normal.

Persistent ductus with reversed shunting

If pulmonary vascular resistance increases, pulmonary artery pressure may rise until it equals or exceeds aortic pressure. The shunt through the defect may then reverse, causing Eisenmenger's syndrome. The murmur becomes quieter, may be confined to systole or may disappear. The ECG shows evidence of right ventricular hypertrophy.

Management

A patent ductus is closed at cardiac catheterisation with an implantable occlusive device. Closure should be undertaken in infancy if the shunt is significant and pulmonary resistance not elevated, but this may be delayed until later childhood in those with smaller shunts, for whom closure remains advisable to reduce the risk of endocarditis.

Pharmacological treatment in the neonatal period

When the ductus is structurally intact, a prostaglandin synthetase inhibitor (indometacin or ibuprofen) may be used in the first week of life to induce closure. However, in the presence of a congenital defect with impaired lung perfusion (e.g. severe pulmonary stenosis and left-to-right shunt through the ductus), it may be advisable to improve oxygenation by keeping the ductus open with prostaglandin treatment. Unfortunately, these treatments do not work if the ductus is intrinsically abnormal.

Coarctation of the aorta

Aetiology

Narrowing of the aorta occurs in the region where the ductus arteriosus joins the aorta, i.e. at the isthmus just below the origin of the left subclavian artery (see Fig. 18.94). The condition is twice as common in males and occurs in 1 in 4000 children. It is associated with other abnormalities, most frequently bicuspid aortic valve and 'berry' aneurysms of the cerebral circulation (p. 1145). Acquired coarctation of the aorta is rare but may follow trauma or occur as a complication of a progressive arteritis (Takayasu's disease, p. 1113).

Clinical features and investigations

Aortic coarctation is an important cause of cardiac failure in the newborn, but symptoms are often absent when it is detected in older children or adults. Headaches may occur from hypertension proximal to the coarctation, and occasionally weakness or cramps in the legs may result from decreased circulation in the lower part of the body. The BP is raised in the upper body but normal or low in the legs. The femoral pulses are weak, and delayed in comparison with the radial pulse (see Fig. 18.95). A systolic murmur is usually heard posteriorly, over the coarctation. There may also be an ejection click and systolic murmur in the aortic area due to a bicuspid aortic valve. As a result of the aortic narrowing, collaterals form and mainly involve the periscapular, internal mammary and intercostal arteries, and may result in localised bruits.

Chest X-ray in early childhood is often normal but later may show changes in the contour of the aorta (indentation of the descending aorta, '3 sign') and notching of the under-surfaces of the ribs from collaterals. MRI is ideal for demonstrating the lesion (Fig. 18.97). The ECG may show left ventricular hypertrophy.

Management

In untreated cases, death may occur from left ventricular failure, dissection of the aorta or cerebral haemorrhage.

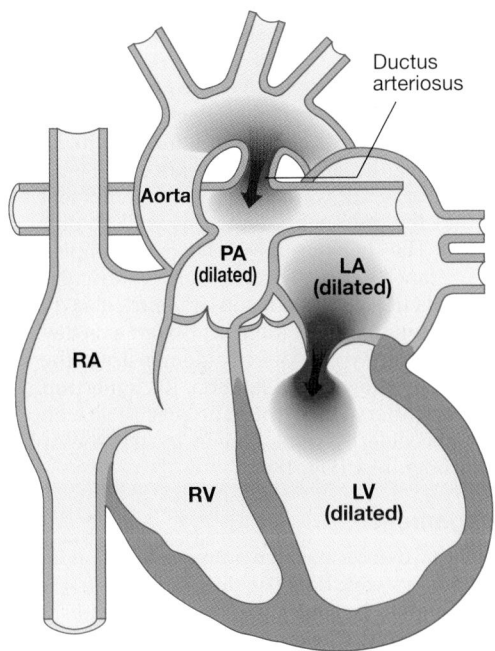

Fig. 18.96 Persistent ductus arteriosus. There is a connection between the aorta and the pulmonary artery with left-to-right shunting.

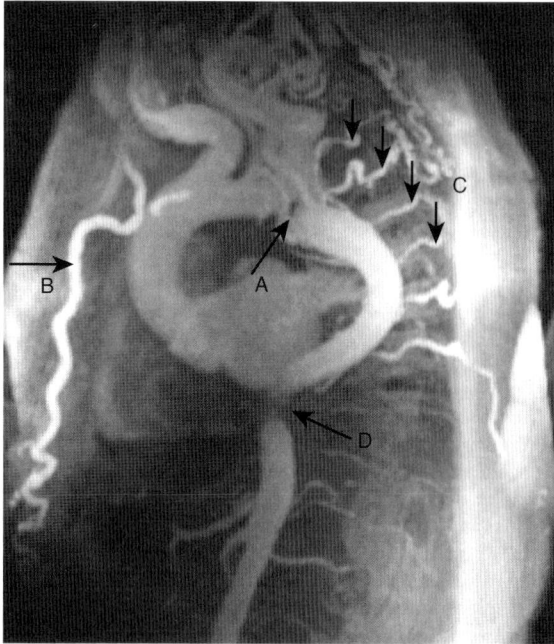

Fig. 18.97 MRI scan of coarctation of the aorta. The aorta is severely narrowed just beyond the arch at the start of the descending aorta (arrow A). Extensive collaterals have developed with a large internal mammary artery shown (arrow B), and several intercostal arteries (arrows C). Unusually, in this case there is also a coarctation of the abdominal aorta (arrow D).

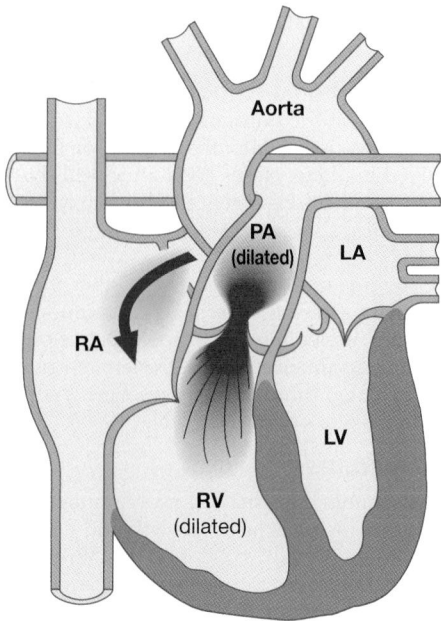

Fig. 18.98 Atrial septal defect. Blood flows across the atrial septum (arrow) from left to right. The murmur is produced by increased flow velocity across the pulmonary valve, as a result of left-to-right shunting and a large stroke volume. The density of shading is proportional to velocity of blood flow.

Surgical correction is advisable in all but the mildest cases. If this is carried out sufficiently early in childhood, persistent hypertension can be avoided. Patients repaired in late childhood or adult life often remain hypertensive or develop recurrent hypertension later on. Recurrence of stenosis may occur as the child grows and this may be managed by balloon dilatation, which can also be used as the primary treatment in some cases. Coexistent bicuspid aortic valve, which occurs in over 50% of cases, may lead to progressive aortic stenosis or regurgitation, and also requires long-term follow-up.

Atrial septal defect

Aetiology

Atrial septal defect is one of the most common congenital heart defects and occurs twice as frequently in females. Most are 'ostium secundum' defects, involving the fossa ovalis that in utero was the foramen ovale (see Fig. 18.94). 'Ostium primum' defects result from a defect in the atrioventricular septum and are associated with a 'cleft mitral valve' (split anterior leaflet).

Since the normal RV is more compliant than the LV, a large volume of blood shunts through the defect from the LA to the RA, and then to the RV and pulmonary arteries (Fig. 18.98). As a result there is gradual enlargement of the right side of the heart and of the pulmonary arteries. Pulmonary hypertension and shunt reversal sometimes complicate atrial septal defect, but are less common and tend to occur later in life than with other types of left-to-right shunt.

Clinical features and investigations

Most children are asymptomatic for many years and the condition is often detected at routine clinical examination or following a chest X-ray. Dyspnoea, chest infections, cardiac failure and arrhythmias, especially atrial fibrillation, are other possible manifestations. The characteristic physical signs are the result of the volume overload of the RV:

- wide fixed splitting of the second heart sound: wide because of delay in right ventricular ejection (increased stroke volume and right bundle branch block) and fixed because the septal defect equalises left and right atrial pressures throughout the respiratory cycle
- a systolic flow murmur over the pulmonary valve.

In children with a large shunt, there may be a diastolic flow murmur over the tricuspid valve. Unlike a mitral flow murmur, this is usually high-pitched.

The chest X-ray typically shows enlargement of the heart and the pulmonary artery, as well as pulmonary plethora. The ECG usually shows incomplete right bundle branch block because right ventricular depolarisation is delayed as a result of ventricular dilatation (with a 'primum' defect there is also left axis deviation). Echocardiography can directly demonstrate the defect and typically shows RV dilatation, RV hypertrophy and pulmonary artery dilatation. The precise size and location of the defect can be shown by transoesophageal echocardiography (Fig. 18.99).

Management

Atrial septal defects in which pulmonary flow is increased 50% above systemic flow (i.e. flow ratio of 1.5:1) are often large enough to be clinically recognisable and should be closed surgically. Closure can also be accomplished at cardiac catheterisation using implantable closure devices (see Fig. 18.15, p. 536). The long-term prognosis thereafter is excellent unless pulmonary hypertension has

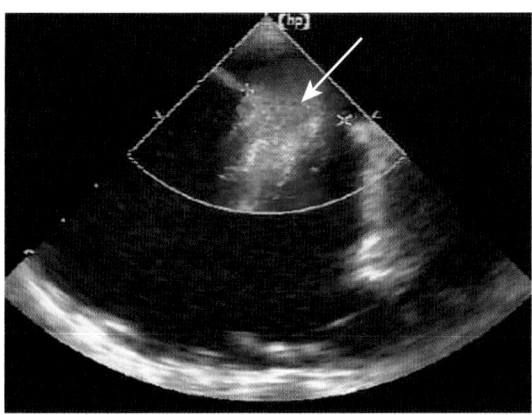

Fig. 18.99 Transoesophageal echocardiogram of an atrial septal defect (ASD). The defect is clearly seen (arrow) between the LA above and RA below. Doppler colour-flow imaging shows flow (blue) across the defect.

developed. Severe pulmonary hypertension and shunt reversal are both contraindications to surgery.

Ventricular septal defect

Aetiology

Congenital ventricular septal defect occurs as a result of incomplete septation of the ventricles. Embryologically, the interventricular septum has a membranous and a muscular portion, and the latter is further divided into inflow, trabecular and outflow portions. Most congenital defects are 'perimembranous', i.e. at the junction of the membranous and muscular portions.

Ventricular septal defects are the most common congenital cardiac defect, occurring once in 500 live births. The defect may be isolated or part of complex congenital heart disease. Acquired ventricular septal defect may result from rupture as a complication of acute MI, or rarely from trauma.

Clinical features

Flow from the high-pressure LV to the low-pressure RV during systole produces a pansystolic murmur usually heard best at the left sternal edge but radiating all over the precordium (Fig. 18.100). A small defect often produces a loud murmur (maladie de Roger) in the absence of other haemodynamic disturbance. Conversely, a large defect produces a softer murmur, particularly if pressure in the RV is elevated. This may be found immediately after birth, while pulmonary vascular resistance remains high, or when the shunt is reversed in Eisenmenger's syndrome.

Congenital ventricular septal defect may present as cardiac failure in infants, as a murmur with only minor haemodynamic disturbance in older children or adults, or rarely as Eisenmenger's syndrome. In a proportion of infants, the murmur gets quieter or disappears due to spontaneous closure of the defect.

If cardiac failure complicates a large defect, it is usually absent in the immediate postnatal period and only becomes apparent in the first 4–6 weeks of life. In addition to the murmur, there is prominent parasternal pulsation, tachypnoea and indrawing of the lower ribs on inspiration. The chest X-ray shows pulmonary plethora and the ECG shows bilateral ventricular hypertrophy.

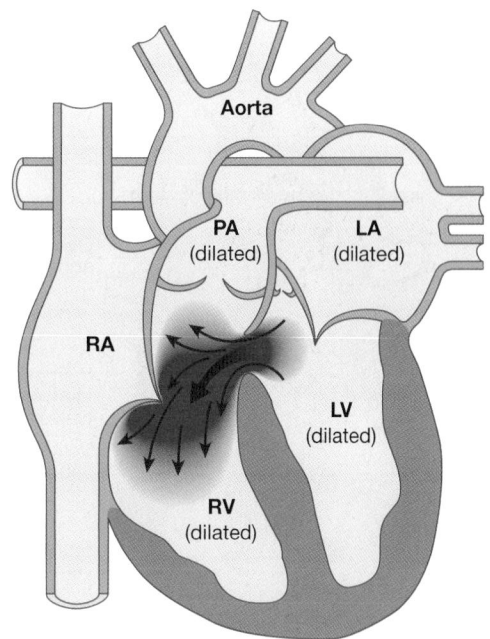

Fig. 18.100 Ventricular septal defect. In this example a large left-to-right shunt (arrows) has resulted in chamber enlargement.

Management and prognosis

Small ventricular septal defects require no specific treatment. Cardiac failure in infancy is initially treated medically with digoxin and diuretics. Persisting failure is an indication for surgical repair of the defect. Percutaneous closure devices are under development.

Doppler echocardiography helps to predict the small septal defects that are likely to close spontaneously. Eisenmenger's syndrome is avoided by monitoring for signs of rising pulmonary resistance (serial ECG and echocardiography) and carrying out surgical repair when appropriate. Surgical closure is contraindicated in fully developed Eisenmenger's syndrome when heart-lung transplantation may be the only effective treatment.

Except in Eisenmenger's syndrome, long-term prognosis is very good in congenital ventricular septal defect. Many patients with Eisenmenger's syndrome die in the second or third decade of life, but a few survive to the fifth decade without transplantation.

Tetralogy of Fallot

The RV outflow obstruction is most often subvalvular (infundibular) but may be valvular, supravalvular or a combination of these (Fig. 18.101). The ventricular septal defect is usually large and similar in aperture to the aortic orifice. The combination results in elevated right ventricular pressure and right-to-left shunting of cyanotic blood across the ventricular septal defect.

Aetiology

The embryological cause is abnormal development of the bulbar septum which separates the ascending aorta from the pulmonary artery, and which normally aligns and fuses with the outflow part of the interventricular septum. The defect occurs in about 1 in 2000 births and is the most common cause of cyanosis in infancy after the first year of life.

18

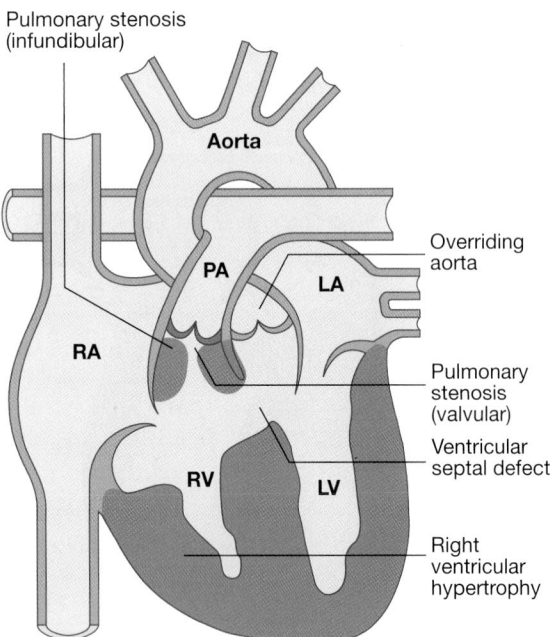

Pulmonary stenosis
(infundibular)

Aorta

PA

RA

LA

Overriding
aorta

Pulmonary
stenosis
(valvular)

Ventricular
septal defect

RV

LV

Right
ventricular
hypertrophy

Fig. 18.101 Tetralogy of Fallot. The tetralogy comprises (1) pulmonary stenosis, (2) overriding of the ventricular septal defect by the aorta, (3) a ventricular septal defect and (4) right ventricular hypertrophy.

Clinical features

Children are usually cyanosed but this may not be the case in the neonate because it is only when right ventricular pressure rises to equal or exceed left ventricular pressure that a large right-to-left shunt develops. The subvalvular component of the RV outflow obstruction is dynamic and may increase suddenly under adrenergic stimulation. The affected child suddenly becomes increasingly cyanosed, often after feeding or a crying attack, and may become apnoeic and unconscious. These attacks are called 'Fallot's spells'. In older children, Fallot's spells are uncommon but cyanosis becomes increasingly apparent, with stunting of growth, digital clubbing and polycythaemia. Some children characteristically obtain relief by squatting after exertion, which increases the afterload of the left heart and reduces the right-to-left shunting: Fallot's sign. The natural history before the development of surgical correction was variable but most patients died in infancy or childhood.

On examination the most characteristic feature is the combination of cyanosis with a loud ejection systolic murmur in the pulmonary area (as for pulmonary stenosis). However, cyanosis may be absent in the newborn or in patients with only mild right ventricular outflow obstruction ('acyanotic tetralogy of Fallot').

Investigations and management

The ECG shows right ventricular hypertrophy and the chest X-ray shows an abnormally small pulmonary artery and a 'boot-shaped' heart. Echocardiography is diagnostic and demonstrates that the aorta is not continuous with the anterior ventricular septum.

The definitive management is total correction of the defect by surgical relief of the pulmonary stenosis and closure of the ventricular septal defect. Primary surgical correction may be undertaken prior to age 5. If the pulmonary arteries are too hypoplastic then palliative treatment in the

form of a Blalock–Taussig shunt may be performed, with an anastomosis created between the pulmonary artery and subclavian artery. This improves pulmonary blood flow and pulmonary artery development, and may facilitate definitive correction at a later stage.

The prognosis after total correction is good, especially if the operation is performed in childhood. Follow-up is needed to identify residual shunting, recurrent pulmonary stenosis and rhythm disorders.

Other causes of cyanotic congenital heart disease

Other causes of cyanotic congenital heart disease occur (Box 18.125) and echocardiography is usually the definitive diagnostic procedure, supplemented if necessary by cardiac catheterisation.

Adult congenital heart disease

There are increasing numbers of children who have had surgical correction of congenital defects and who may have further cardiological problems as adults. Those who have undergone correction of coarctation of the aorta may develop hypertension in adult life. Those with transposition of the great arteries who have had a 'Mustard' repair, where blood is redirected at atrial level leaving the RV connected to the aorta, may develop right ventricular failure in adult life. The RV is unsuited for function at systemic pressures and may begin to dilate and fail when patients are in their twenties or thirties.

Those who have had surgery involving the atria may develop atrial arrhythmias, and those who have ventricular scars may develop ventricular arrhythmias and need consideration for implantation of an ICD device. Such patients require careful follow-up from the

18.125 Other causes of cyanotic congenital heart disease	
Defect	**Features**
Tricuspid atresia	Absent tricuspid orifice, hypoplastic RV, RA to LA shunt, ventricular septal defect shunt, other anomalies
	Surgical correction may be possible
Transposition of the great vessels	Aorta arises from the morphological RV, pulmonary artery from LV
	Shunt via atria, ductus and possibly ventricular septal defect
	Palliation by balloon atrial septostomy/enlargement
	Surgical correction possible
Pulmonary atresia	Pulmonary valve atretic and pulmonary artery hypoplastic
	RA to LA shunt, pulmonary flow via ductus
	Palliation by balloon atrial septostomy
	Surgical correction may be possible
Ebstein's anomaly	Tricuspid valve is dysplastic and displaced into RV, RV 'atrialised'
	Tricuspid regurgitation and RA to LA shunt
	Wide spectrum of severity
	Arrhythmias
	Surgical repair possible but significant risks

teenage years throughout adult life so that problems can be identified early and appropriate medical or surgical treatment instituted. The management of these adult or 'grown-up' congenital heart disease patients has developed as a cardiological subspecialty.

DISEASES OF THE MYOCARDIUM

Although the myocardium is involved in most types of heart disease, the terms 'myocarditis' and 'cardiomyopathy' are usually reserved for conditions that primarily affect the heart muscle.

Myocarditis

This is an acute inflammatory condition that can have an infectious, toxic or autoimmune aetiology. Myocarditis can complicate many infections in which inflammation may be due directly to infection of the myocardium or the effects of circulating toxins. Viral infections are the most common causes, such as Coxsackie (35 cases per 1000 infections) and influenza A and B (25 cases per 1000 infections) viruses. Myocarditis may occur several weeks after the initial viral symptoms and susceptibility is increased by corticosteroid treatment, immunosuppression, radiation, previous myocardial damage and exercise. Some bacterial and protozoal infections may be complicated by myocarditis; for example, approximately 5% of patients with Lyme disease (*Borrelia burgdorferi*, p. 329) develop myopericarditis, which is often associated with AV block. Toxic aetiologies include drugs, which may directly injure the myocardium (e.g. cocaine, lithium and anticancer drugs such as doxorubicin) or which may cause a hypersensitivity reaction and associated myocarditis (e.g. penicillins and sulphonamides), lead and carbon monoxide. Occasionally, autoimmune conditions such as systemic lupus erythematosus and rheumatoid arthritis are associated with myocarditis.

The clinical picture ranges from a symptomless disorder, sometimes recognised by the presence of an inappropriate tachycardia or abnormal ECG, to fulminant heart failure. Myocarditis may be heralded by an influenza-like illness. ECG changes are common but non-specific. Biochemical markers of myocardial injury (e.g. troponin I and T, creatine kinase) are elevated in proportion to the extent of damage. Echocardiography may reveal left ventricular dysfunction that is sometimes regional (due to focal myocarditis), and if the diagnosis is uncertain it can be confirmed by endomyocardial biopsy.

In most patients, the disease is self-limiting and the immediate prognosis is excellent. However, death may occur due to a ventricular arrhythmia or rapidly progressive heart failure. Myocarditis has been reported as a cause of sudden and unexpected death in young athletes. There is strong evidence that some forms of myocarditis may lead to chronic low-grade myocarditis or dilated cardiomyopathy (see below); for example, in Chagas disease (p. 354) the patient frequently recovers from the acute infection but goes on to develop a chronic dilated cardiomyopathy 10 or 20 years later.

Specific antimicrobial therapy may be used if a causative organism has been identified; however, this is rare and in most cases only supportive therapy is available. Treatment for cardiac failure or arrhythmias may be required and patients should be advised to avoid intense physical exertion because there is some evidence that this can induce potentially fatal ventricular arrhythmias. There is no evidence for any benefit from treatment with corticosteroids and immunosuppressive agents.

Cardiomyopathy

The aetiology of most intrinsic disorders of the myocardium has not been elucidated and a functional classification is used (Fig. 18.102).

Dilated cardiomyopathy

This is characterised by dilatation and impaired contraction of the LV (and sometimes the RV); left ventricular mass is increased but wall thickness is normal or reduced (see Fig. 18.102). Histological changes are variable but include myofibrillary loss, interstitial fibrosis and T-cell infiltrates. The differential diagnosis includes coronary artery disease and some specific disorders of heart muscle (see below), and a diagnosis of dilated cardiomyopathy should only be made when these have been excluded.

The pathogenesis is not clear but dilated cardiomyopathy probably encompasses a heterogenous group of conditions. Alcohol is an important aetiological factor in a significant proportion of patients. At least 25% of cases are inherited as an autosomal dominant trait and a variety of single gene mutations have been identified. Most of these mutations affect proteins in the cytoskeleton of the myocyte (e.g. dystrophin, lamin A and C, emerin and metavinculin) and many are associated with minor skeletal muscle abnormalities. Most of the X-linked inherited skeletal muscular dystrophies (e.g. Becker and Duchenne, p. 1233) are associated with cardiomyopathy. Finally, a late autoimmune reaction to viral myocarditis is thought to be the main aetiological factor in a substantial subgroup of patients with dilated cardiomyopathy; a similar mechanism is thought to be responsible for the heart muscle disease that occurs in up to 10% of patients with advanced HIV infection.

In North America and Europe, symptomatic dilated cardiomyopathy has an incidence of 20 per 100 000 and a prevalence of 38 per 100 000. Men are affected more than twice as often as women. Most patients present with heart failure or are found to have the condition during routine investigation. Arrhythmia, thromboembolism and sudden death are common and may occur at any stage; sporadic chest pain is a surprisingly frequent symptom. The ECG usually shows non-specific changes but echocardiography is useful in establishing the diagnosis. Treatment is aimed at controlling the resulting heart failure. Although some patients remain well for many years, the prognosis is variable and cardiac transplantation may be indicated. Patients with dilated cardiomyopathy and moderate or severe heart failure may be at risk of sudden arrhythmic death. This risk is substantially reduced by rigorous medical therapy with β-blockers and angiotensin receptor antagonists. Some patients may be considered for implantation of a cardiac defibrillator and/or cardiac resynchronisation therapy (p. 576).

Hypertrophic cardiomyopathy

This is the most common form of cardiomyopathy, with a prevalence of approximately 100 per 100 000 and is char-

18

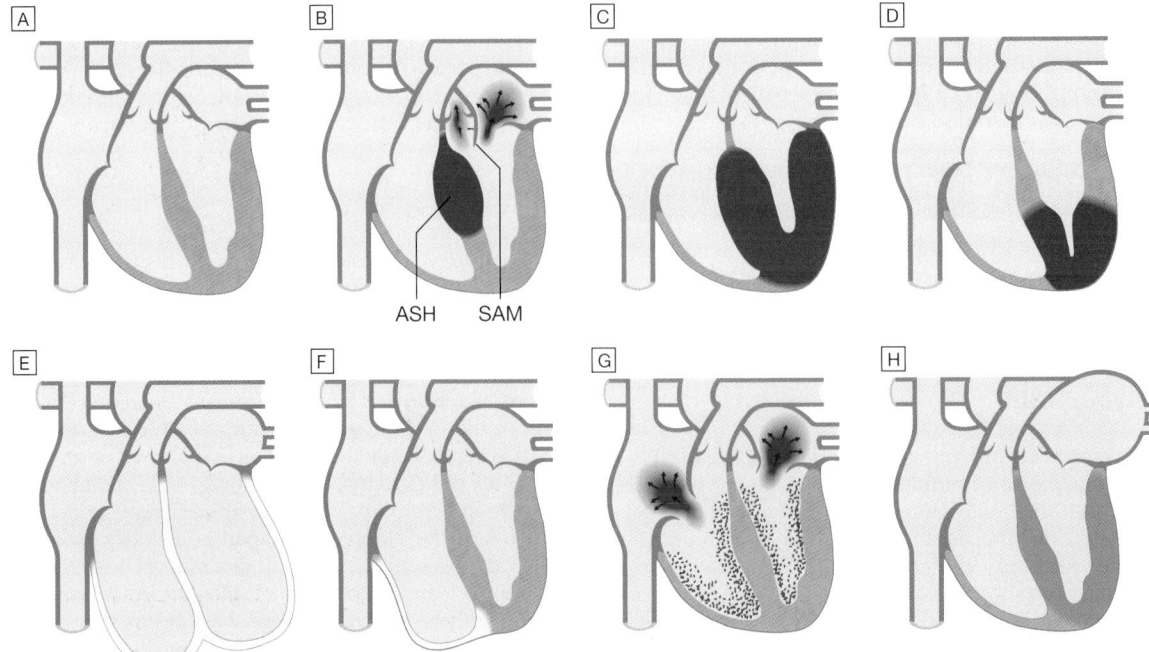

Fig. 18.102 Types of cardiomyopathy. A Normal. B Hypertrophic cardiomyopathy: asymmetric septal hypertrophy (ASH) with systolic anterior motion of the mitral valve (SAM), causing mitral reflux and dynamic left ventricular outflow tract obstruction. C Hypertrophic cardiomyopathy: concentric hypertrophy. D Hypertrophic cardiomyopathy: apical hypertrophy. E Dilated cardiomyopathy. F Arrhythmogenic right ventricular cardiomyopathy. G Obliterative cardiomyopathy. H Restrictive cardiomyopathy.

acterised by inappropriate and elaborate left ventricular hypertrophy with malalignment of the myocardial fibres. The hypertrophy may be generalised or confined largely to the interventricular septum (asymmetric septal hypertrophy, see Fig. 18.102) or other regions (e.g. apical hypertrophic cardiomyopathy, a variant which is common in the Far East).

Heart failure may develop because the stiff non-compliant ventricles impede diastolic filling. Septal hypertrophy may also cause dynamic left ventricular outflow tract obstruction (hypertrophic obstructive cardiomyopathy, or HOCM) and mitral regurgitation due to abnormal systolic anterior motion of the anterior mitral valve leaflet. Effort-related symptoms (angina and breathlessness), arrhythmia and sudden death are the dominant clinical problems.

The condition is a genetic disorder, usually with autosomal dominant transmission, a high degree of penetrance and variable expression. In most patients, it appears to be due to a single point mutation in one of the genes that encode sarcomeric contractile proteins. There are three common groups of mutation with different phenotypes. Beta-myosin heavy chain mutations are associated with elaborate ventricular hypertrophy. Troponin mutations are associated with little, and sometimes even no hypertrophy but marked myocardial fibre disarray, an abnormal vascular response (e.g. exercise-induced hypotension) and a high risk of sudden death. Myosin-binding protein C mutations tend to present late in life and are often associated with hypertension and arrhythmia.

Symptoms and signs are similar to those of aortic stenosis, except that in hypertrophic cardiomyopathy the character of the arterial pulse is jerky (Box 18.126).

> **18.126 Clinical features of hypertrophic cardiomyopathy**
>
> **Symptoms**
>
> - Angina on effort
> - Dyspnoea on effort
> - Syncope on effort
> - Sudden death
>
> **Signs**
>
> - Jerky pulse*
> - Palpable left ventricular hypertrophy
> - Double impulse at the apex (palpable fourth heart sound due to left atrial hypertrophy)
> - Midsystolic murmur at the base*
> - Pansystolic murmur (due to mitral regurgitation) at the apex
>
> *Signs of left ventricular outflow tract obstruction may be augmented by standing up (reduced venous return), inotropes and vasodilators (e.g. sublingual nitrate).

The ECG is abnormal and shows features of left ventricular hypertrophy with a wide variety of often bizarre abnormalities (e.g. pseudo-infarct pattern, deep T-wave inversion). Echocardiography is diagnostic, although the diagnosis may be difficult when another cause of left ventricular hypertrophy is present (e.g. physical training—athletes' heart, hypertension) but the degree of hypertrophy is greater than expected. Genetic testing may facilitate diagnosis.

The natural history is variable but clinical deterioration is often slow. The annual mortality from sudden death is 2–3% among adults and 4–6% in children and adolescents (Box 18.127). Sudden death typically occurs

18.127 Risk factors for sudden death in hypertrophic cardiomyopathy

- A history of previous cardiac arrest or sustained ventricular tachycardia
- Recurrent syncope
- An adverse genotype and/or family history
- Exercise-induced hypotension
- Non-sustained ventricular tachycardia on ambulatory ECG monitoring
- Marked increase in left ventricular wall thickness

during or just after vigorous physical activity; indeed, hypertrophic cardiomyopathy is the most common cause of sudden death in young athletes. Ventricular arrhythmias are thought to be responsible for many of these deaths.

Beta-blockers, rate-limiting calcium antagonists (e.g. verapamil) and disopyramide can help to relieve symptoms and sometimes prevent syncopal attacks; however, there is no pharmacological treatment that is definitely known to improve prognosis. Arrhythmias are common and often respond to treatment with amiodarone. Outflow tract obstruction can be improved by partial surgical resection (myectomy) or by iatrogenic infarction of the basal septum (septal ablation) using a catheter-delivered alcohol solution. An ICD should be considered in patients with clinical risk factors for sudden death (see Box 18.127). Digoxin and vasodilators may increase outflow tract obstruction and should be avoided.

Arrhythmogenic right ventricular cardiomyopathy

In this condition, patches of the right ventricular myocardium are replaced with fibrous and fatty tissue (see Fig. 18.102). It is inherited as an autosomal dominant trait and has a prevalence of approximately 10 per 100 000. The dominant clinical problems are ventricular arrhythmias, sudden death and right-sided cardiac failure. The ECG typically shows a slightly broadened QRS complex and inverted T waves in the right precordial leads. MRI is a useful diagnostic tool and is often used to screen the first-degree relatives of affected individuals. Patients at high risk of sudden death can be offered an ICD.

Obliterative cardiomyopathy

This disease involves the endocardium of one or both ventricles and is characterised by thrombosis and elaborate fibrosis with gradual obliteration of the ventricular cavities (e.g. endomyocardial fibroelastosis, see Fig. 18.102). The mitral and tricuspid valves become regurgitant. Heart failure and pulmonary and systemic embolism are prominent features. It can sometimes be associated with eosinophilia (e.g. eosinophilic leukaemia, Churg–Strauss syndrome, p. 1114). In tropical countries, the disease can be responsible for up to 10% of cardiac deaths. Mortality is high at 50% at 2 years. Anticoagulation and antiplatelet therapy are usually advisable, and diuretics may help symptoms of heart failure. Surgery (tricuspid and/or mitral valve replacement with decortication of the endocardium) may be helpful in selected cases.

Restrictive cardiomyopathy

In this rare condition, ventricular filling is impaired because the ventricles are 'stiff' (see Fig. 18.102). This leads to high atrial pressures with atrial hypertrophy, dilatation and later atrial fibrillation. Amyloidosis is the most common cause of restrictive cardiomyopathy in the UK, although other forms of infiltration (e.g. glycogen storage diseases), idiopathic perimyocyte fibrosis and a familial form of restrictive cardiomyopathy do occur. Diagnosis can be very difficult and requires complex Doppler echocardiography, CT or MRI, and endomyocardial biopsy. Treatment is symptomatic but the prognosis is usually poor and transplantation may be indicated.

Specific diseases of heart muscle

Many forms of specific heart muscle disease produce a clinical picture that is indistinguishable from dilated cardiomyopathy (e.g. connective tissue disorders, sarcoidosis, haemochromatosis, alcoholic heart muscle disease, Box 18.128). In contrast, amyloidosis and eosinophilic heart disease produce symptoms and signs similar to those found in restrictive or obliterative cardiomyopathy, whereas the heart disease associated with Friedreich's ataxia (p. 1203) can mimic hypertrophic cardiomyopathy.

Treatment and prognosis are determined by the underlying disorder. Abstention from alcohol may lead to a dramatic improvement in patients with alcoholic heart muscle disease.

18.128 Specific diseases of heart muscle

Infections
- Viral, e.g. Coxsackie A and B, influenza, HIV
- Bacterial, e.g. diphtheria, *Borrelia burgdorferi*
- Protozoal, e.g. trypanosomiasis

Endocrine and metabolic disorders
- Diabetes, hypo- and hyperthyroidism, acromegaly, carcinoid syndrome, phaeochromocytoma, inherited storage diseases

Connective tissue diseases
- Systemic sclerosis, systemic lupus erythematosus, polyarteritis nodosa

Infiltrative disorders
- Haemochromatosis, haemosiderosis, sarcoidosis, amyloidosis

Toxins
- Doxorubicin, alcohol, cocaine, irradiation

Neuromuscular disorders
- Dystrophia myotonica, Friedreich's ataxia

Cardiac tumours

Primary cardiac tumours are rare (< 0.2% of autopsies) but the heart and mediastinum may be the site of metastases. Most primary tumours are benign (75%) and, of these, the majority are myxomas. The remainder are fibromas, lipomas, fibroelastomas and haemangiomas.

Atrial myxoma

Myxomas most commonly arise in the LA as single or multiple polypoid tumours, attached by a pedicle to the interatrial septum. They are usually gelatinous but may be solid and even calcified, with superimposed thrombus.

On examination the first heart sound is usually loud, and there may be a murmur of mitral regurgitation with a variable diastolic sound (tumour 'plop') due to prolapse of the mass through the mitral valve. The tumour can be detected incidentally on echocardiography, or following investigation of pyrexia, syncope, arrhythmias or emboli. Occasionally, the condition presents with malaise and features suggestive of a connective tissue disorder, including a raised ESR.

Treatment is by surgical excision. If the pedicle is removed, fewer than 5% of tumours recur.

DISEASES OF THE PERICARDIUM

The normal pericardial sac contains about 50 mL of fluid, similar to lymph, which lubricates the surface of the heart. The pericardium limits distension of the heart, contributes to the haemodynamic interdependence of the ventricles, and acts as a barrier to infection. Nevertheless, congenital absence of the pericardium does not appear to result in significant clinical or functional limitations.

Acute pericarditis

Aetiology

Pericardial inflammation may be due to a number of pathologies (Box 18.129) but sometimes remains unexplained. Pericarditis and myocarditis often coexist, and all forms of pericarditis may produce a pericardial effusion (see below) that, depending on the aetiology, may be fibrinous, serous, haemorrhagic or purulent.

A fibrinous exudate may eventually lead to varying degrees of adhesion formation, whereas serous pericarditis often produces a large effusion of turbid, straw-coloured fluid with a high protein content.

A haemorrhagic effusion is often due to malignant disease, particularly carcinoma of the breast or bronchus, and lymphoma.

Purulent pericarditis is rare and may occur as a complication of septicaemia, by direct spread from an intrathoracic infection, or from a penetrating injury.

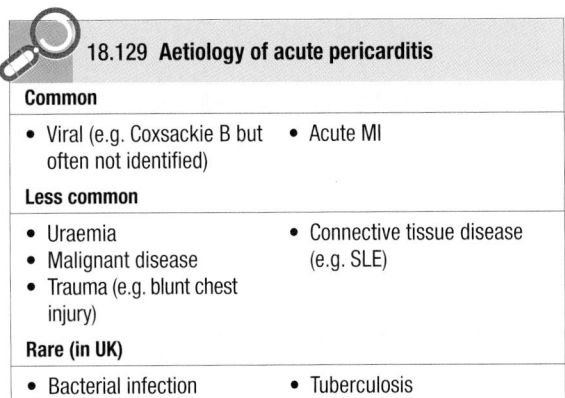

18.129 Aetiology of acute pericarditis	
Common	
• Viral (e.g. Coxsackie B but often not identified)	• Acute MI
Less common	
• Uraemia • Malignant disease • Trauma (e.g. blunt chest injury)	• Connective tissue disease (e.g. SLE)
Rare (in UK)	
• Bacterial infection • Rheumatic fever	• Tuberculosis

Clinical features

The characteristic pain of pericarditis is retrosternal, radiates to the shoulders and neck, and is typically aggravated by deep breathing, movement, a change of position, exercise and swallowing. A low-grade fever is common.

A pericardial friction rub is a high-pitched superficial scratching or crunching noise produced by movement of the inflamed pericardium and is diagnostic of pericarditis; it is usually heard in systole but may also be audible in diastole and frequently has a 'to-and-fro' quality.

Investigations and management

The ECG shows ST elevation with upward concavity (Fig. 18.103) over the affected area, which may be widespread. PR interval depression is a very specific indicator of acute pericarditis. Later, there may be T-wave inversion, particularly if there is a degree of myocarditis.

The pain is usually relieved by aspirin (600 mg 4-hourly) but a more potent anti-inflammatory agent such as indometacin (25 mg 8-hourly) may be required. Corticosteroids may suppress symptoms but there is no evidence that they accelerate cure.

In viral pericarditis, recovery usually occurs within a few days or weeks but there may be recurrences (chronic relapsing pericarditis). Purulent pericarditis requires treatment with antimicrobial therapy, pericardiocentesis and, if necessary, surgical drainage.

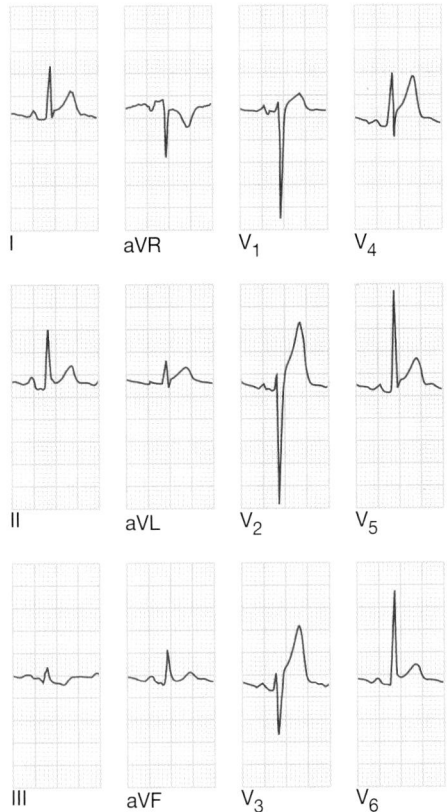

Fig. 18.103 ECG in viral pericarditis. Widespread ST elevation (leads I, II, aVL and V$_1$–V$_6$) is shown. The upward concave shape of the ST segments (see leads II and V$_6$) and the unusual distribution of changes (involving anterior and inferior leads) help to distinguish pericarditis from acute MI.

Pericardial effusion

If a pericardial effusion develops, there is sometimes a sensation of retrosternal oppression. An effusion is difficult to detect clinically. The heart sounds may become quieter, although a pericardial friction is not always abolished.

The QRS voltages on the ECG are often reduced in the presence of a large effusion. The QRS complexes may alternate in amplitude due to a to-and-fro motion of the heart within the fluid-filled pericardial sac (electrical alternans). Serial chest X-rays may show a rapid increase in the size of the cardiac shadow over days or even hours, and when there is a large effusion the heart often has a globular or pear-shaped appearance. Echocardiography is the definitive investigation (Fig. 18.104).

Cardiac tamponade

This term is used to describe acute heart failure due to compression of the heart by a large or rapidly developing effusion and is described in detail on page 542. Typical physical findings are of a markedly raised jugular venous pulse, hypotension, pulsus paradoxus (p. 528) and oliguria. Atypical presentations may occur when the effusion is loculated as a result of previous pericarditis or cardiac surgery.

Pericardial aspiration

Aspiration of a pericardial effusion is indicated for diagnostic purposes or for the treatment of cardiac tamponade. A needle is inserted under echocardiographic guidance medial to the cardiac apex or below the xiphoid process, directing upwards towards the left shoulder. The route of choice will depend on the experience of the operator, the shape of the patient and the position of the effusion. A few millilitres of fluid aspirated through the needle may be sufficient for diagnostic purposes but a drain is needed for symptom relief.

Complications of pericardiocentesis include arrhythmias, damage to a coronary artery, and bleeding with exacerbation of tamponade as a result of injury to the RV. When tamponade is due to cardiac rupture or aortic dissection, pericardial aspiration may precipitate further potentially fatal bleeding and in these situations emergency surgery is the treatment of choice. A viscous, loculated or recurrent effusion may also require formal surgical drainage.

Tuberculous pericarditis

Tuberculous pericarditis may complicate pulmonary tuberculosis but may also be the first manifestation of the infection. In Africa, a tuberculous pericardial effusion is a common feature of AIDS (p. 396).

The condition typically presents with chronic malaise, weight loss and a low-grade fever. An effusion usually develops and the pericardium may become thick and unyielding, leading to pericardial constriction or tamponade. An associated pleural effusion is often present.

The diagnosis may be confirmed by aspiration of the fluid and direct examination or culture for tubercle bacilli. Treatment requires specific antituberculous chemotherapy (p. 693); in addition, a 3-month course of prednisolone (initial dose 60 mg a day, tapering down rapidly) improves outcome.

Chronic constrictive pericarditis

Constrictive pericarditis is due to progressive thickening, fibrosis and calcification of the pericardium. In effect, the heart is encased in a solid shell and cannot fill properly. The calcification may extend into the myocardium, so there may also be impaired myocardial contraction. The condition often follows an attack of tuberculous pericarditis but can also complicate haemopericardium, viral pericarditis, rheumatoid arthritis and purulent pericarditis. It is often impossible to identify the original insult.

Clinical features and management

The symptoms and signs of systemic venous congestion are the hallmarks of constrictive pericarditis. Atrial fibrillation is common and there is often dramatic ascites and hepatomegaly (Box 18.130). Breathlessness is not a prominent symptom because the lungs are seldom congested.

The condition is sometimes overlooked but should be suspected in any patient with unexplained right heart failure and a small heart. A chest X-ray, which may show pericardial calcification (Fig. 18.105), and

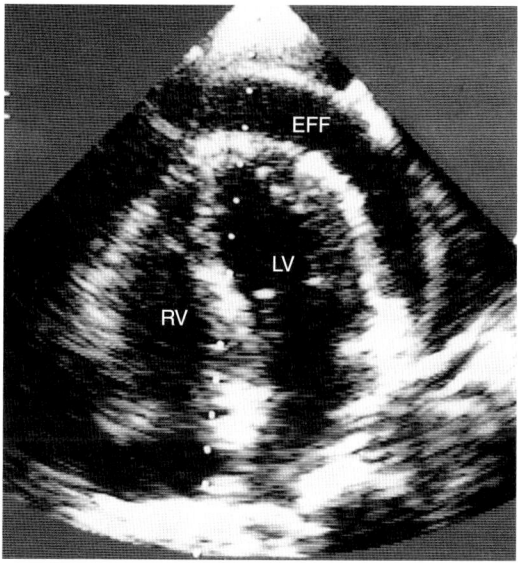
Fig. 18.104 **Pericardial effusion (EFF).** Echocardiogram (apical view).

18.130 Clinical features of constrictive pericarditis

- Fatigue
- Rapid, low-volume pulse
- Elevated JVP with a rapid *y* descent
- Kussmaul's sign (a paradoxical rise in the JVP during inspiration)
- Loud early third heart sound or 'pericardial knock'
- Hepatomegaly
- Ascites
- Peripheral oedema
- Pulsus paradoxus (excessive fall in BP during inspiration): present in some cases

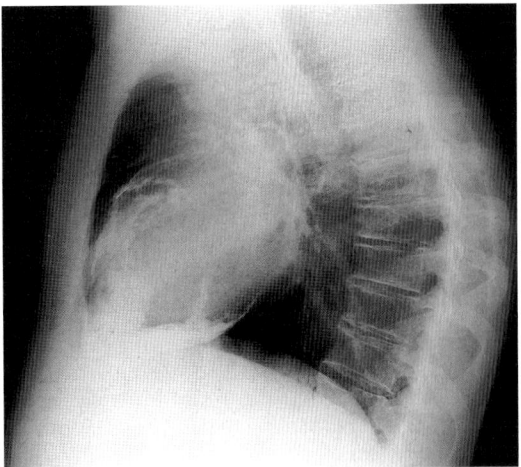

Fig. 18.105 Lateral chest X-ray from a patient with severe heart failure due to chronic constrictive pericarditis. There is heavy calcification of the pericardium.

echocardiography often help to establish the diagnosis. CT and MRI are also useful techniques for imaging the pericardium.

Constrictive pericarditis is often difficult to distinguish from restrictive cardiomyopathy and the final diagnosis may depend on complex echo-Doppler studies and cardiac catheterisation. Surgical resection of the diseased pericardium can lead to a dramatic improvement but carries a high morbidity with disappointing results in up to 50% of patients.

Further information

www.acc.org *American College of Cardiology (ACC): free access to guidelines for the evaluation and management of many cardiac conditions.*

www.americanheart.org *American Heart Association (AHA): free access to all the ACC/AHA/ESC guidelines, AHA scientific statements and fact sheets for patients.*

www.escardio.org *European Society of Cardiology (ESC): free access to guidelines for the diagnosis and management of many cardiac conditions, and to educational modules.*

www.nice.org.uk *Reviews of the evidence base for a number of cardiological treatments and procedures.*

www.sign.ac.uk *Evidence-based guidelines on the management of most common cardiac conditions.*

P.T. Reid
J.A. Innes

Respiratory disease

19

CLINICAL EXAMINATION OF THE RESPIRATORY SYSTEM

Thorax 6 – 9
(see opposite)

Inspection 6
Deformity
(e.g. pectus excavatum)
Scars
Intercostal indrawing
Symmetry of expansion
Hyperinflation
Paradoxical rib movement
(low flat diaphragm)

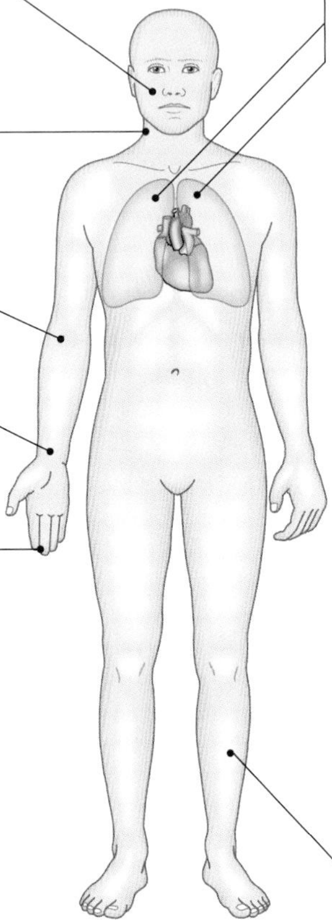

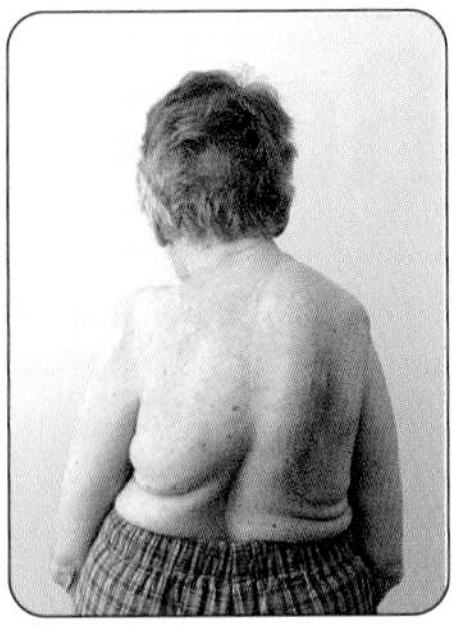

▲ Idiopathic kyphoscoliosis

Face, mouth and eyes 5
Pursed lips
Central cyanosis
Anaemia
Horner's syndrome
(Ch. 26)

Jugular venous pulse 4
Elevated
Pulsatile

Blood pressure 3
Arterial paradox

Radial pulse 2
Rate
Rhythm

Hands 1
Digital clubbing
Tar staining
Peripheral cyanosis
Signs of occupation
CO_2 retention flap

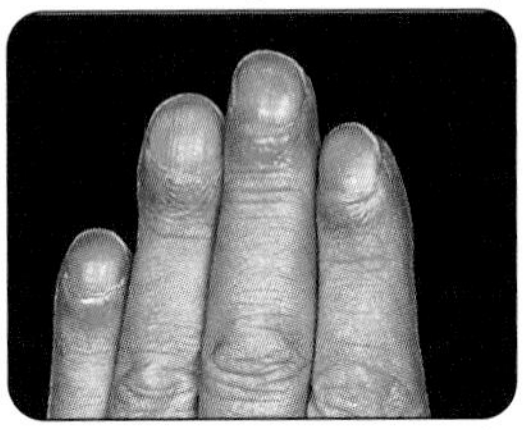

Finger clubbing ▲

7 Palpation
From the front:
Trachea central
Cricosternal distance
Cardiac apex displaced
Expansion
From behind:
Cervical lymphadenopathy
Expansion

8 Percussion
Resonant or dull
'Stony dull' (effusion)

9 Auscultation
Breath sounds:
normal, bronchial, louder or softer
Added sounds:
wheezes, crackles, rubs
Spoken voice (vocal resonance):
absent (effusion), increased
(consolidation)
Whispered voice:
whispering pectoriloquy

10 Leg oedema
Cor pulmonale
Venous thrombosis

Observation

- Respiratory rate
- Cachexia, fever, rash
- Sputum (see below)
- Fetor

- Locale
  Oxygen delivery (mask, cannulae)
  Nebulisers
  Inhalers

Sputum

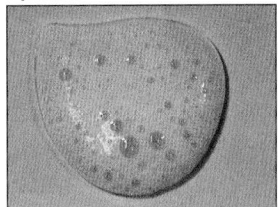

▲ Serous/frothy/pink
Pulmonary oedema

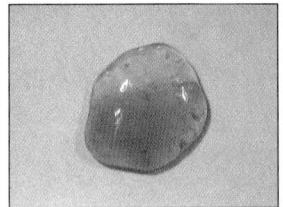

▲ Mucopurulent
Bronchial or pneumonic
infection

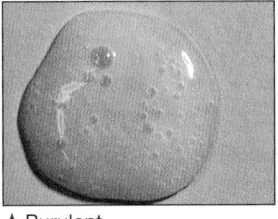

▲ Purulent
Bronchial or pneumonic
infection

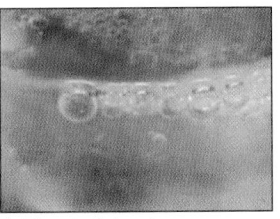

▲ Blood-stained
Cancer, tuberculosis,
bronchiectasis,
pulmonary embolism

Chronic obstructive pulmonary disease

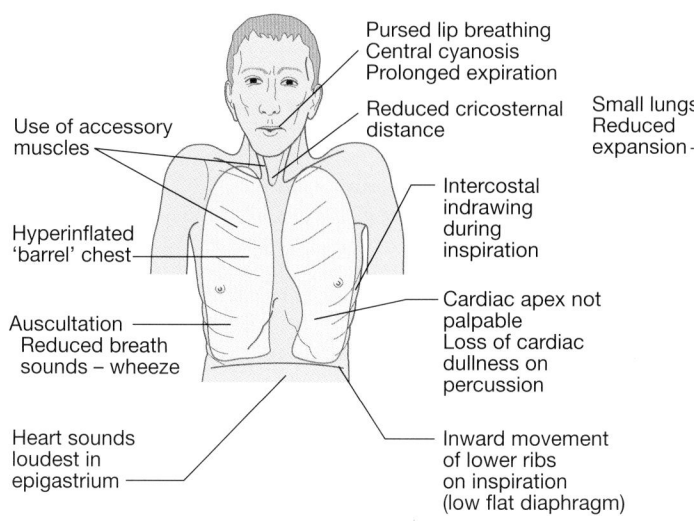

Pursed lip breathing
Central cyanosis
Prolonged expiration

Reduced cricosternal distance

Use of accessory muscles

Intercostal indrawing during inspiration

Hyperinflated 'barrel' chest

Auscultation
Reduced breath sounds – wheeze

Cardiac apex not palpable
Loss of cardiac dullness on percussion

Heart sounds loudest in epigastrium

Inward movement of lower ribs on inspiration (low flat diaphragm)

Also: raised JVP, peripheral oedema if cor pulmonale

Pulmonary fibrosis

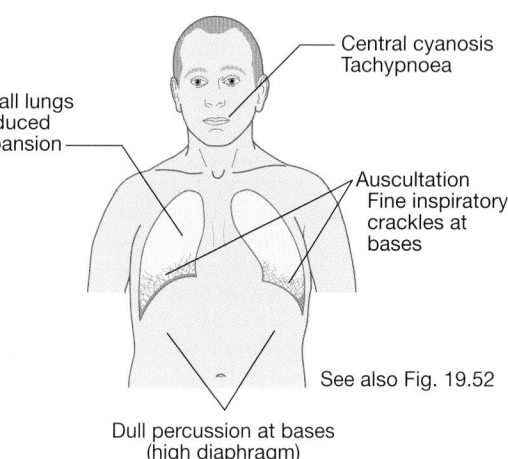

Central cyanosis
Tachypnoea

Small lungs
Reduced expansion

Auscultation
Fine inspiratory crackles at bases

See also Fig. 19.52

Dull percussion at bases (high diaphragm)

Also: finger clubbing common in idiopathic pulmonary fibrosis; raised JVP and peripheral oedema if cor pulmonale

Right middle lobe pneumonia

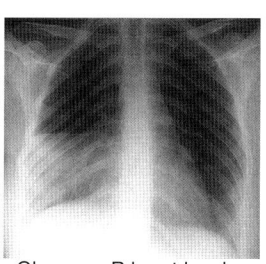

Obscures R heart border on X-ray

Inspection
 Tachypnoea
 Central cyanosis (if severe)
Palpation
 ↓Expansion on R
Percussion
 Dull R mid-zone and axilla
Auscultation
 Bronchial breath sounds and ↑vocal resonance over consolidation and whispering pectoriloquy
 Pleural rub if pleurisy

Right upper lobe collapse

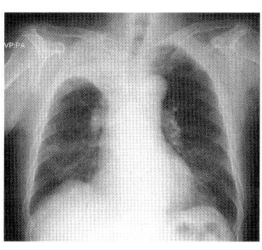

Inspection
 ↓Volume R upper zone
Palpation
 Trachea deviated to R
 ↓Expansion R upper zone
Percussion
 Dull R upper zone
Auscultation
 ↓Breath sounds with central obstruction

X-ray
 Deviated trachea (to R)
 Elevated horizontal fissure
 ↓Volume R hemithorax
 Central (hilar) mass may be seen

Right pneumothorax

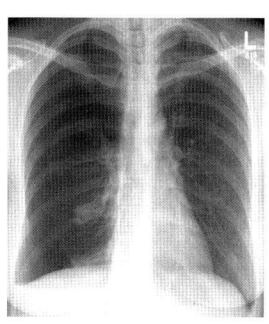

Inspection
 Tachypnoea (pain, deflation reflex)
Palpation
 ↓Expansion R side
Percussion
 Resonant or hyper-resonant on R
Auscultation
 Absent breath sounds on R

Tension pneumothorax also causes
 Deviation of trachea to opposite side
 Tachycardia and hypotension

Large right pleural effusion

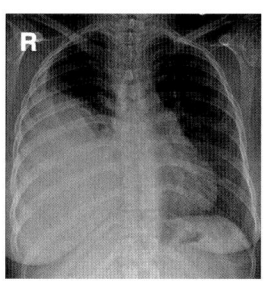

Inspection
 Tachypnoea
Palpation
 ↓Expansion on R
 Trachea and apex may be moved to L
Percussion
 Stony dull
 R mid- and lower zones
Auscultation
 Absent breath sounds and vocal resonance R base
 Crackles above effusion

19

Respiratory disease is responsible for a major burden of morbidity and untimely death, and conditions such as tuberculosis, pandemic influenza and pneumonia are the most important conditions in world health terms. In addition, the increasing prevalence of allergy, asthma and chronic obstructive pulmonary disease (COPD) contribute to the overall burden of chronic disease in the community. By 2025, the number of cigarette smokers world-wide is anticipated to increase to 1.5 billion, ensuring a growing burden of tobacco-related respiratory conditions.

The approach to respiratory disease embraces the basic medical sciences and covers a breadth of pathologies, including infectious, inflammatory, neoplastic and degenerative processes. The practice of respiratory medicine thus requires the collaboration of a range of disciplines. Recent advances have improved the lives of many patients with obstructive lung disease, cystic fibrosis, obstructive sleep apnoea and pulmonary hypertension, but the outlook remains poor for lung and other respiratory cancers, and for some of the fibrosing lung conditions.

FUNCTIONAL ANATOMY AND PHYSIOLOGY

The lungs occupy the upper two-thirds of the bony thorax, bounded medially by the spine, the heart and the mediastinum and inferiorly by the diaphragm. During breathing, free movement of the lung surface relative to the chest wall is facilitated by sliding contact between the parietal and visceral pleura, which cover the inner surface of the chest wall and the lung respectively, and are normally in close apposition. Inspiration involves downward contraction of the dome-shaped diaphragm (innervated by the phrenic nerves originating from C3, 4 and 5) and upward, outward movement of the ribs on the costovertebral joints, caused by contraction of the external intercostal muscles (innervated by the corresponding intercostal nerves originating from the thoracic spinal cord). Expiration is largely passive, driven by elastic recoil of the lungs. The control of this 'respiratory cycle' is described below.

The conducting airways from the nose to the alveoli connect the external environment with the extensive, thin and vulnerable alveolar surface. As air is inhaled through the upper airways, it is filtered in the nose, heated to body temperature and fully saturated with water vapour; partial recovery of this heat and moisture occurs on expiration. Total airway cross-section is smallest in the glottis and trachea, which means that airflow is rapid here and the airway is particularly vulnerable to obstruction by foreign bodies and tumours. Normal breath sounds originate mainly from the rapid turbulent airflow in the larynx and in these central airways.

The multitude of small airways within the lung parenchyma have a very large combined cross-sectional area (over 300 cm^2 in the third-generation respiratory bronchioles), resulting in very slow flow rates. Airflow is normally silent here, and gas transport occurs largely by diffusion in the final generations. Major bronchial and pulmonary divisions are shown in Figure 19.1.

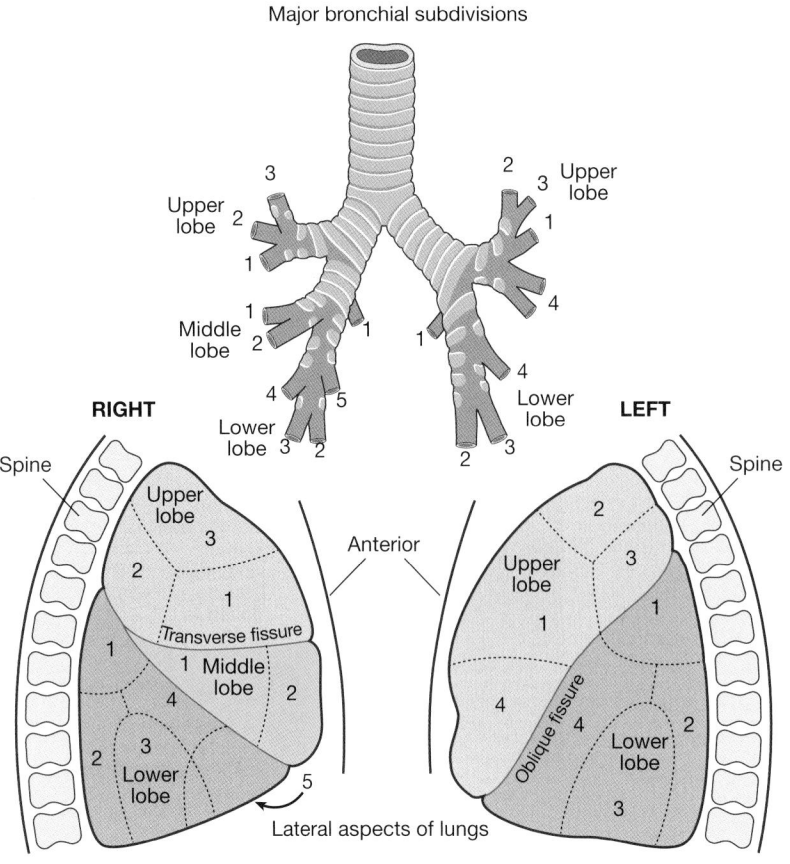

Major bronchial subdivisions

Fig. 19.1 The major bronchial divisions and the fissures, lobes and segments of the lungs. The angle of the oblique fissure means that the left upper lobe is largely anterior to the lower lobe. On the right, the transverse fissure separates the upper from the anteriorly placed middle lobe, which is matched by the lingular segment on the left side. The site of a lobe determines whether physical signs are mainly anterior or posterior. Each lobe is composed of two or more bronchopulmonary segments which are supplied by the main branches of each lobar bronchus. *Bronchopulmonary segments:* **Right**—*Upper lobe*: (1) Anterior, (2) Posterior, (3) Apical. Middle lobe: (1) Lateral, (2) Medial. *Lower lobe*: (1) Apical, (2) Posterior basal, (3) Lateral basal, (4) Anterior basal, (5) Medial basal. **Left**—*Upper lobe*: (1) Anterior, (2) Apical, (3) Posterior, (4) Lingular. *Lower lobe*: (1) Apical, (2) Posterior basal, (3) Lateral basal, (4) Anterior basal.

The acinus is the gas exchange unit of the lung (Fig. 19.2) and comprises branching respiratory bronchioles and clusters of alveoli. The filtered, moistened and heated air makes close contact here with the blood in the pulmonary capillaries (gas-to-blood distance < 0.4 μm), and oxygen uptake and CO_2 excretion occur. The alveoli are lined with flattened epithelial cells (type I pneumocytes) and a few, more cuboidal, type II pneumocytes. The latter produce surfactant, which is a mixture of phospholipids that reduces surface tension and counteracts the tendency of alveoli to collapse. Type II pneumocytes can also divide to reconstitute type I pneumocytes after lung injury.

Lung mechanics

Healthy lung parenchyma contains a fine network of elastin and collagen fibres within the alveolar walls (see Fig. 19.2). At the end of a tidal breath out, the inward elastic recoil of the lungs (resulting from stretch of the elastin fibres and surface tension in the alveolar lining fluid) is balanced by resistance of the chest wall to inward distortion, resulting in a negative pleural pressure. The arrangement of fibres results in the lung being easily distended (elastin) at physiological lung volumes, but increasingly stiff (collagen) as full inflation is approached. The elastic forces are distributed evenly throughout the parenchyma, maintaining airway patency by radial traction on small airway walls. Even in health, however, these airways narrow during exhalation because they are surrounded by alveoli at higher pressure. Airway collapse is prevented by radial elastic traction, so in health the minimum lung volume achievable is limited by the capacity of the respiratory muscles to distort the chest wall inwards. In emphysema, loss of alveolar walls leaves the small airways unsupported and collapsible, resulting in expiratory air trapping and hyperinflation (p. 672).

Control of breathing

The respiratory motor neurons in the medulla oblongata discharge rhythmically and are the origin of the respiratory cycle. These neurons receive information on the state of the respiratory system from multiple inputs in health and in disease (see Fig. 19.9, p. 653):

- Central chemoreceptors in the ventrolateral medulla sense the pH of the cerebrospinal fluid (CSF) and are indirectly stimulated by a rise in arterial PCO_2.
- The carotid bodies sense hypoxaemia but are mainly activated by arterial PO_2 values below 8 KPa (60 mmHg).
- Muscle spindles in the respiratory muscles sense changes in mechanical load.
- Vagal sensory fibres from the lung may be stimulated by stretch or by various disease processes in the interstitium.
- Cortical influences can override the automatic control of breathing.

19

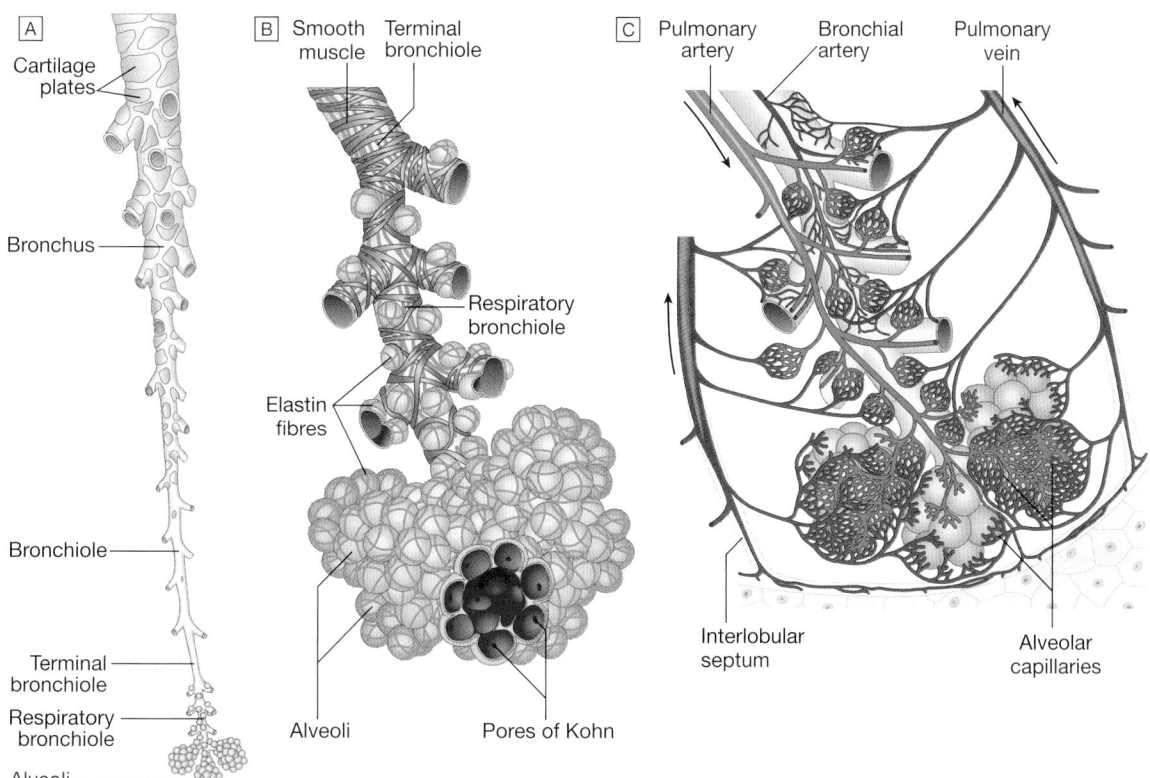

Fig. 19.2 Functional anatomy of the lung. **A** The tapering, branching bronchus is armoured against compression by plates of cartilage. The more distal bronchioles are collapsible, but held patent by surrounding elastic tissue. **B** The unit of lung supplied by a terminal bronchiole is called an acinus. The bronchiolar wall contains smooth muscle and elastin fibres. The latter also run through the alveolar walls. Gas exchange occurs in the alveoli, which are connected to each other by the pores of Kohn. **C** Vascular anatomy of an acinus. Both the pulmonary artery (carrying desaturated blood) and the bronchial artery (systemic supply to airway tissue) run along the bronchus. The venous drainage to the left atrium follows the interlobular septa.

19

Ventilation/perfusion matching and the pulmonary circulation

To achieve optimal gas exchange within the lungs, the regional distribution of ventilation and perfusion must be matched. Gravity determines the distribution of ventilation and blood flow in the lungs, with most of both going to the dependent zones. Within each lung, hypoxia constricts pulmonary arterioles and airway CO_2 dilates bronchi, helping to maintain good matching of ventilation and perfusion within pulmonary segments. Lung disease may create regions of relative underventilation or underperfusion, which disturb this physiological matching of regional ventilation and perfusion, causing respiratory failure (pp. 660–662). In addition to causing ventilation–perfusion mismatch, diseases that destroy or thicken the alveolar capillary membrane (e.g. emphysema or fibrosis) can impair gas diffusion directly.

The pulmonary circulation in health operates at low pressure (approximately 24/9 mmHg), and can accommodate large increases in flow without much rise in pressure, e.g. during exercise. Pulmonary hypertension occurs when pulmonary vessels are destroyed by emphysema, obstructed by thrombus or involved in interstitial inflammation or fibrosis. The right ventricle responds by hypertrophy, with right axis deviation and P pulmonale on the ECG. Pulmonary hypertension with hypoxia and hypercapnia is associated with generalised salt and water retention ('cor pulmonale'), with elevation of the jugular venous pressure (JVP) and peripheral oedema. This is thought to result mainly from a failure of the hypoxic and hypercapnic kidney to excrete sufficient salt and water.

Lung defences

Upper airway defences

Large airborne particles are trapped by nasal hairs, and smaller particles settling on the mucosa are cleared towards the oropharynx by the columnar ciliated epithelium which covers the turbinates and septum (Fig. 19.3). During cough, expiratory muscle effort against a closed glottis results in high intrathoracic pressure, which is then released explosively. The flexible posterior tracheal wall is pushed inwards by the high surrounding pressure, reducing tracheal cross-section and maximising

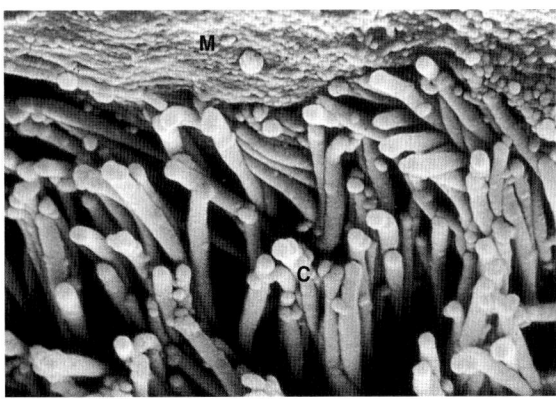

Fig. 19.3 The mucociliary escalator. Scanning electron micrograph of the respiratory epithelium showing large numbers of cilia (C) overlaid by the mucus 'raft' (M).

19.1 Respiratory function in old age

- **Reserve capacity:** a significant reduction in function can occur with ageing with only minimal effect on normal breathing, although the ability to combat acute intercurrent disease is reduced.
- **Decline in FEV_1:** the FEV_1/FVC (forced expiratory volume/forced vital capacity) ratio falls by around 0.2% per year from 70% at the age of 40–45 years, due to a decline in elastic recoil in the small airways with age. Smoking accelerates this decline threefold on average. Symptoms usually only occur when FEV_1 drops below 50% of predicted.
- **Increasing ventilation–perfusion mismatch:** the reduction in elastic recoil causes a tendency for the small airways to collapse during expiration, particularly in dependent areas of the lungs, thus reducing ventilation.
- **Reduced ventilatory responses to hypoxia and hypercapnia:** older people may be less tachypnoeic for any given fall in PaO_2 or rise in $PaCO_2$.
- **Impaired defences against infection:** due to reduced numbers of glandular epithelial cells which lead to a reduction in protective mucus.
- **Decline in maximum oxygen uptake:** due to a combination of changes in muscle, and the respiratory and cardiovascular systems. This leads to a reduction in cardiorespiratory reserve and exercise capacity.
- **Loss of chest wall compliance:** due to reduced intervertebral disc spaces and ossification of the costal cartilages; respiratory muscle strength and endurance also decline. These changes only become important in the presence of other respiratory disease.

---

the airspeed to achieve effective expectoration. The larynx also acts as a sphincter protecting the airway during swallowing and vomiting.

Lower airway defences

The sterility, structure and function of the lower airways are maintained by close cooperation between the innate and adaptive immune responses (pp. 70–76).

The innate response in the lungs is characterised by a number of non-specific defence mechanisms. Inhaled particulate matter is trapped in airway mucus and cleared by the mucociliary escalator. Cigarette smoke increases mucus secretion but reduces mucociliary clearance and predisposes towards lower respiratory tract infections, including pneumonia. Defective mucociliary transport is also a feature of several rare diseases, including Kartagener's syndrome, Young's syndrome and ciliary dysmotility syndrome, which are characterised by repeated sino-pulmonary infections and bronchiectasis.

Airway secretions contain an array of antimicrobial peptides (such as defensins, immunoglobulin A (IgA) and lysozyme), antiproteinases and antioxidants. Many of these assist with the opsonisation and killing of bacteria, and the regulation of the powerful proteolytic enzymes secreted by inflammatory cells. In particular, α_1-antiproteinase (A1Pi) regulates neutrophil elastase, and deficiency of this may be associated with premature emphysema.

Macrophages engulf microbes, organic dusts and other particulate matter. They are unable to digest inorganic agents such as asbestos or silica, which result in their death and the release of powerful proteolytic enzymes that cause parenchymal damage. Neutrophil numbers in the airway are low, but the pulmonary circulation contains a marginated pool that may be recruited rapidly in response to bacterial infection. This may explain the prominence of lung injury in sepsis syndromes and trauma.

Adaptive immunity is characterised by the specificity of the response and the development of memory. Lung dendritic cells facilitate antigen presentation to T- and B-lymphocytes.

INVESTIGATION OF RESPIRATORY DISEASE

A detailed history, thorough examination and basic haematological and biochemical tests usually suggest the likely diagnosis and key differentials. However, a number of further investigations are usually required to confirm the diagnosis and/or monitor disease activity.

Imaging

The 'plain' chest X-ray

This is performed on the majority of patients suspected of having chest disease. A postero-anterior (PA) film provides information on the lung fields, heart, mediastinum, vascular structures and the thoracic cage (Fig. 19.4). Additional information may be obtained from a lateral film, particularly if pathology is suspected behind the heart shadow or deep in the diaphragmatic sulci. An approach to interpreting the chest X-ray is given in Box 19.2, and common abnormalities in Box 19.3.

19.2 **How to interpret a chest X-ray**	
Name, date, orientation	Films are postero-anterior (PA) unless marked AP to denote antero-posterior
Lung fields	Equal translucency? Check horizontal fissure from right hilum to sixth rib at the anterior axillary line Masses? Consolidation? Cavitation?
Lung apices	Check behind the clavicles Masses? Consolidation? Cavitation?
Trachea	Central? (Midway between the clavicular heads) Paratracheal mass? Goitre?
Heart	Normal shape? Cardiothoracic ratio (should be < half the intrathoracic diameter) Retrocardiac mass?
Hila	Left should be higher than right Shape? (Should be concave laterally; if convex, consider mass or lymphadenopathy) Density?
Diaphragms	Right should be higher than left Hyperinflation? No more than 10 ribs should be visible posteriorly above the diaphragm)
Costophrenic angles	Acute and well-defined? (Pleural fluid or thickening, if not)
Soft tissues	Breast shadows in females Chest wall for masses or subcutaneous emphysema
Bones	Ribs, vertebrae, scapulae and clavicles Any fracture visible at bone margins or lucencies?

19

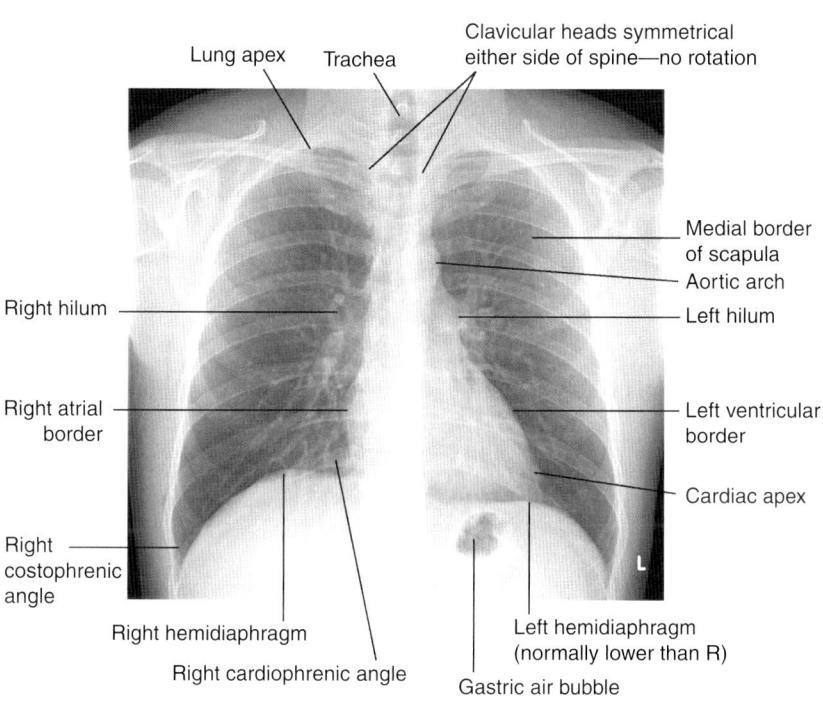

Fig. 19.4 The normal chest X-ray.

Labels on figure:
Lung apex — Trachea — Clavicular heads symmetrical either side of spine—no rotation
Right hilum
Right atrial border
Right costophrenic angle
Right hemidiaphragm
Right cardiophrenic angle
Medial border of scapula
Aortic arch
Left hilum
Left ventricular border
Cardiac apex
Left hemidiaphragm (normally lower than R)
Gastric air bubble

Fig. 19.4 The normal chest X-ray. Note lung markings consist of branching and tapering lines radiating out from the hila; where airways and vessels turn towards the film they can appear as open or filled circles (see upper pole of right hilum). The scapulae may overlie the lung fields; trace the edge of bony structures to avoid mistaking them for pleural or pulmonary shadows. To check for hyperinflation, count the ribs; if more than 10 are visible posteriorly above the diaphragm, the lungs are hyperinflated.

19.3 Common chest X-ray abnormalities

Pulmonary and pleural shadowing

- **Consolidation:** infection, infarction, inflammation, and rarely bronchoalveolar cell carcinoma
- **Lobar collapse:** mucus plugging, tumour, compression by lymph nodes
- **Solitary nodule:** see pages 657–658
- **Multiple nodules:** miliary tuberculosis (TB), dust inhalation, metastatic malignancy, healed varicella pneumonia, rheumatoid disease
- **Ring shadows, tramlines and tubular shadows:** bronchiectasis
- **Cavitating lesions:** tumour, abscess, infarct, pneumonia (*Staphylococcus/Klebsiella*), Wegener's granulomatosis
- **Reticular, nodular and reticulonodular shadows:** diffuse parenchymal lung disease, infection
- **Pleural abnormalities:** fluid, plaques, tumour

Increased translucency

- Bullae
- Pneumothorax
- Oligaemia

Hilar abnormalities

- **Unilateral hilar enlargement:** TB, bronchial carcinoma, lymphoma
- **Bilateral hilar enlargement:** sarcoid, lymphoma, TB, silicosis

Other abnormalities

- Hiatus hernia
- Surgical emphysema

Increased shadowing may represent accumulation of fluid, lobar collapse or consolidation. Uncomplicated consolidation should not change the position of the mediastinum and the presence of an air bronchogram means that proximal bronchi are patent. Collapse (implying obstruction of the proximal bronchus) is accompanied by loss of volume and displacement of the mediastinum towards the affected side (see Fig. 19.43, p. 700).

The presence of ring shadows (diseased bronchi seen end-on), tramline shadows (diseased bronchi side-on) or tubular shadows (bronchi filled with secretions) suggests bronchiectasis. The presence of pleural fluid is suggested by a dense basal shadow which, in the erect patient, ascends towards the axilla. In large pulmonary embolism, relative oligaemia may cause a lung field to appear abnormally dark.

Computed tomography (CT)

CT provides detailed images of the pulmonary parenchyma, mediastinum, pleura and bony structures (Figs 19.5 and 19.57, p. 714) The displayed range of densities can be adjusted to highlight different structures such as the lung parenchyma, the mediastinal vascular structures or bone. Sophisticated software facilitates three-dimensional reconstruction of the thorax and virtual bronchoscopy.

CT is superior to chest radiography in determining the position and size of a pulmonary lesion and whether calcification or cavitation is present. It is now routinely used in the assessment of patients with suspected lung cancer and facilitates guided percutaneous

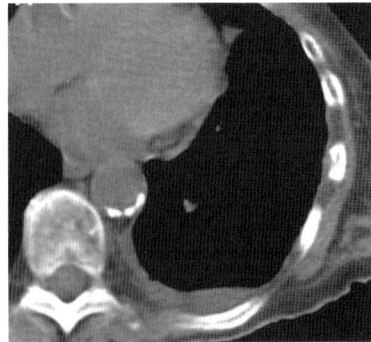

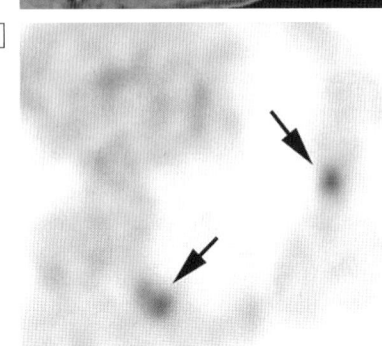

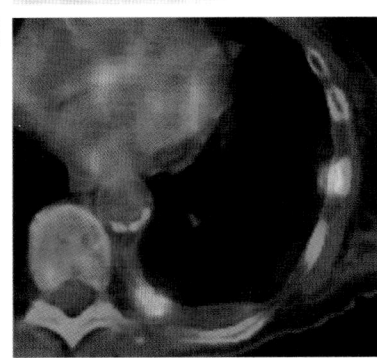

Fig. 19.5 CT and positron emission tomography (PET) combined to reveal intrathoracic metastases. In a patient with lung cancer, CT **A** shows some posterior pleural thickening. PET scanning **B** reveals FDG uptake in two pleural lesions (arrows), highlighted in yellow in the combined PET/CT image **C** .

needle biopsy. Information on tumour stage may be gained by examining the mediastinum, liver and adrenal glands.

High-resolution CT (HRCT) uses thin sections to provide detailed images of the pulmonary parenchyma and is particularly useful in assessing diffuse parenchymal lung disease, identifying bronchiectasis (see Fig. 19.28, p. 677), and assessing the type and extent of emphysema.

CT pulmonary angiography (CTPA) is used increasingly in the diagnosis of pulmonary thromboembolism (see Fig. 19.60, p. 719), when it may either confirm the suspected embolism or highlight an alternative diagnosis.

Ultrasound

Ultrasound is sensitive at detecting pleural fluid and may also be employed to direct and improve the diagnostic yield from pleural biopsy. It is also used to investigate the anatomy of an empyema cavity to facilitate directed drainage, and to guide needle biopsy of superficial lymph node or chest wall masses. Endobronchial ultrasound is now possible using specialised bronchoscopes, and is used for imaging and sampling peribronchial lymph nodes.

Ventilation–perfusion imaging

In this technique, the lungs are imaged using a gamma camera that is able to distinguish two isotopes, inhaled ^{133}Xe (yielding ventilation images) and injected macroaggregates of ^{99m}Tc-albumin (yielding perfusion images). Pulmonary emboli appear as perfusion defects with preserved ventilation. However, the utility of this technique is limited in patients with underlying lung disease, in whom up to 70% of scans may be indeterminate. It is increasingly being replaced by CTPA.

Positron emission tomography (PET)

PET scanners exploit the avid ability of malignant tissue to absorb and metabolise glucose. The radiotracer ^{18}F-fluorodeoxyglucose (FDG) is administered and rapidly taken up by malignant tissue. It is then phosphorylated but cannot be metabolised further, becoming 'trapped' in the cell. PET is useful in the investigation of pulmonary nodules, and in staging mediastinal lymph nodes and distal metastatic disease in patients with lung cancer. The negative predictive value is high; however, the positive predictive value is poor. Co-registration of PET and CT (PET-CT) enhances localisation and characterisation of metabolically active deposits (see Fig. 19.5C).

Pulmonary angiography

Images taken with contrast medium in the main pulmonary artery are rarely used, particularly now that CTPA is widely available. Right heart catheterisation remains useful in the investigation of patients with pulmonary hypertension, providing information on pulmonary and right heart pressures.

Endoscopic examination

Laryngoscopy

The larynx may be inspected indirectly with a mirror or directly with a laryngoscope. Fibreoptic instruments allow a magnified view to be obtained.

Bronchoscopy

The trachea and larger bronchi may be inspected using either a flexible or a rigid bronchoscope. Flexible bronchoscopy may be performed under local anaesthesia with sedation on an outpatient basis. Structural changes, such as distortion or obstruction, can be seen. Abnormal tissue in the bronchial lumen or wall can be biopsied, and bronchial brushings, washings or aspirates can be taken for cytological or bacteriological examination. Small biopsy specimens of lung tissue, taken by forceps passed through the bronchial wall (transbronchial biopsies), may reveal sarcoid granulomas or malignant diseases and may be helpful in diagnosing certain bronchocentric disorders (e.g. hypersensitivity pneumonitis, cryptogenic organising pneumonia), but are generally too small to be of diagnostic value in other diffuse parenchymal pulmonary disease (p. 705). Transbronchial needle aspiration (TBNA) may be used to sample mediastinal lymph nodes and in the staging of lung cancer.

Rigid bronchoscopy requires general anaesthesia and is reserved for specific situations such as massive haemoptysis or removal of foreign bodies (see Fig. 19.8, p. 652). Endobronchial laser therapy and endobronchial stenting may be performed more easily with rigid bronchoscopy.

Assessment of the mediastinum

Lymph nodes down to the main carina can be sampled using a mediastinoscope passed through a small incision at the suprasternal notch under general anaesthetic. This procedure is particularly useful in lung cancer as a means of determining whether nodal disease is present. Endobronchial ultrasound (EBUS) using a specialised bronchoscope allows directed needle aspiration from peribronchial nodes but is not yet widely available. Lymph nodes in the lower mediastinum may be biopsied via the oesophagus using endoscopic ultrasound (EUS), an oesophageal endoscope equipped with an ultrasound transducer and biopsy needle.

Investigation of pleural disease

The traditional method of pleural biopsy using an Abram's needle is largely being replaced by the use of core biopsy guided by either ultrasound or CT. Thoracoscopy, which involves the insertion of an endoscope through the chest wall, facilitates biopsy under direct vision and is practised by many surgeons and an increasing number of physicians.

Skin tests

The tuberculin test (pp. 694–695) may be of value in the diagnosis of tuberculosis. Skin hypersensitivity tests are useful in the investigation of allergic diseases (p. 88).

Immunological and serological tests

The presence of pneumococcal antigen (revealed by counter-immunoelectrophoresis) in sputum, blood or urine may be of diagnostic importance in pneumonia. Exfoliated cells colonised by influenza A virus can be detected by fluorescent antibody techniques. In blood, high or rising antibody titres to specific organisms (such as *Legionella*, *Mycoplasma*, *Chlamydia* or viruses) may eventually clinch a diagnosis suspected on clinical grounds. Precipitating antibodies may be found as a reaction to fungi such as *Aspergillus* (p. 697) or to antigens involved in hypersensitivity pneumonitis (p. 710).

Microbiological investigations

Sputum, pleural fluid, throat swabs, blood and bronchial washings and aspirates can be examined for bacteria, fungi and viruses. In some cases, as when *Mycobacterium tuberculosis* is isolated, the information is diagnostically conclusive, but in others the findings must be interpreted in conjunction with the results of clinical and radiological examination.

Induced sputum

The use of hypertonic saline to induce expectoration of sputum is useful in facilitating the collection of specimens for microbiology, particularly in patients in whom

19

more invasive procedures such as bronchoscopy are not possible. The technique also allows assessment of the inflammatory cell constituency of the airway, which is a useful research tool in many conditions including asthma, COPD and interstitial lung disease.

Histopathological and cytological examination

Histopathological examination of biopsy material obtained from pleura, lymph node or lung often allows a 'tissue diagnosis' to be made. This is of particular importance in suspected malignancy or in elucidating the pathological changes in interstitial lung disease. Important causative organisms, such as *M. tuberculosis*, *Pneumocystis jirovecii* or fungi, may be identified in bronchial washings, brushings or transbronchial biopsies.

Cytological examination of exfoliated cells in sputum, pleural fluid or bronchial brushings and washings, or of fine needle aspirates from lymph nodes or pulmonary lesions can support a diagnosis of malignancy, but if this is indeterminate a tissue biopsy is necessary. Cellular patterns in bronchial lavage fluid may help to distinguish pulmonary changes due to sarcoidosis (p. 708) from those caused by idiopathic pulmonary fibrosis (p. 707) or hypersensitivity pneumonitis (p. 710).

Respiratory function testing

Respiratory function tests are used to aid diagnosis, assess functional impairment, and monitor treatment or progression of disease. Airway narrowing, lung volume and gas exchange capacity are quantified and compared with normal values adjusted for age, gender, height and ethnic origin. Typical laboratory traces are illustrated in Figure 19.6.

Forced expiratory volume (FEV$_1$) and forced vital capacity (FVC)

In diseases characterised by airway narrowing (e.g. asthma, bronchitis and emphysema), maximum expiratory flow is limited by dynamic compression of small intrathoracic airways, some of which close completely during expiration, limiting the volume which can be expired (obstructive defect). Hyperinflation of the chest results, and can become extreme if elastic recoil is also lost due to parenchymal destruction, as in emphysema. In contrast, diseases which cause interstitial inflammation and/or fibrosis lead to progressive loss of lung volume (restrictive defect) with normal expiratory flow rates.

Airway narrowing is assessed by asking patients to blow out as hard and as fast as they can into a peak flow meter or a spirometer. Peak flow meters are

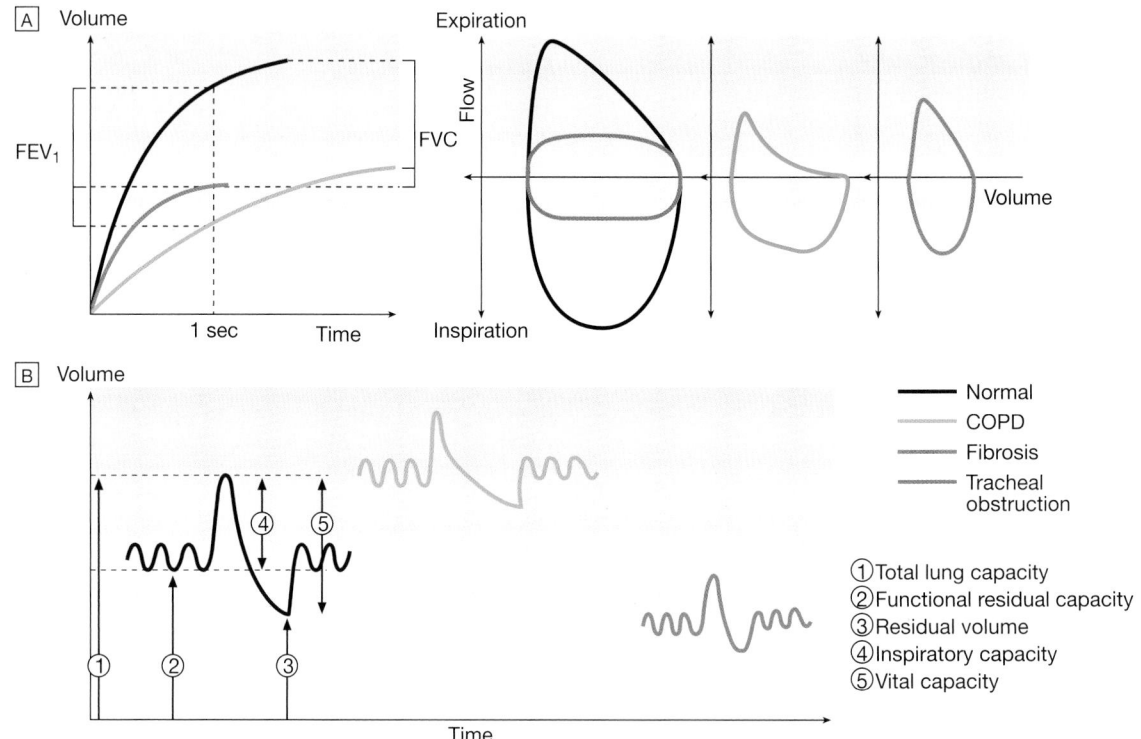

Fig. 19.6 Respiratory function tests in health and disease. [A] Volume/time traces from forced expiration in a normal subject, a patient with COPD and a patient with fibrosis. COPD causes slow, prolonged and limited exhalation. In fibrosis, forced expiration results in rapid expulsion of a reduced forced vital capacity (FVC). Forced expiratory volume (FEV$_1$) is reduced in both diseases but is disproportionately reduced compared to FVC in COPD. [B] The same data plotted as flow/volume loops. In COPD, collapse of intrathoracic airways limits flow, particularly during mid- and late expiration. The blue trace illustrates large airway obstruction, which particularly limits peak flow rates. [C] Lung volume measurement. Volume/time graphs during quiet breathing with a single maximal breath in and out. COPD causes hyperinflation with increased residual volume. Fibrosis causes a proportional reduction in all lung volumes.

cheap and convenient for home monitoring of peak expiratory flow (PEF) in the detection and monitoring of asthma, but values are effort-dependent. The FEV₁ and FVC are obtained from a maximal forced expiration into a spirometer. FEV_1 is disproportionately reduced in airflow obstruction, resulting in FEV_1/FVC ratios of less than 70%. When airflow obstruction is seen, spirometry should be repeated following inhaled short-acting β_2-adrenoceptor agonists (e.g. salbutamol); reversibility to normal is suggestive of asthma (p. 665).

Flow/volume loops

To distinguish large airway narrowing (e.g. tracheal stenosis or compression) from small airway narrowing, flow/volume loops are recorded using spirometry. These display flow as it relates to lung volume (rather than time) during maximum expiration and inspiration, and the pattern of flow reveals the site of airflow obstruction (see Fig. 19.6).

Lung volumes

Tidal volume and vital capacity (VC) can be measured by spirometry. Total lung capacity (TLC) can be measured by asking the patient to rebreathe an inert non-absorbed gas (usually helium) and recording the dilution of test gas by lung gas. This measures the volume of intrathoracic gas which mixes quickly with tidal breaths. Alternatively, lung volume may be measured by body plethysmography, which determines the pressure/volume relationship of the thorax. This method measures total intrathoracic gas volume, including poorly ventilated areas such as bullae.

Transfer factor

To measure the capacity of the lungs to exchange gas, patients inhale a test mixture of 0.3% carbon monoxide, which is avidly bound to haemoglobin in pulmonary capillaries. After a short breath-hold, the rate of disappearance of CO into the circulation is calculated from a sample of expirate, and expressed as the TL_{CO} or carbon monoxide transfer factor. Helium is also included in the test breath to allow calculation of the volume of lung examined by the test breath. Transfer factor expressed per unit lung volume is termed K_{CO}. Common respiratory function abnormalities are summarised in Box 19.4.

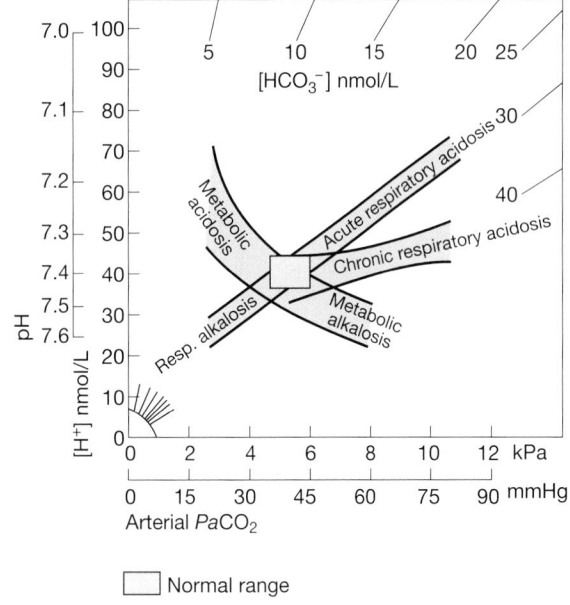

Fig. 19.7 Changes in blood [H⁺], *Pa*CO₂ and plasma [HCO₃⁻] in acid–base disorders. The rectangle indicates limits of normal reference ranges for [H⁺] and *Pa*CO₂. The bands represent 95% confidence limits of single disturbances in human blood in vivo. When the point obtained by plotting [H⁺] against *Pa*CO₂ does not fall within one of the labelled bands, compensation is incomplete or a mixed disorder is present.

Arterial blood gases and oximetry

The measurement of hydrogen ion concentration, PaO_2 and $PaCO_2$, and derived bicarbonate concentration in an arterial blood sample is essential in assessing the degree and type of respiratory failure and for measuring acid–base status. This is discussed in detail on pages 660 and 442. Interpretation of results is made easier by blood gas diagrams (Fig. 19.7), which indicate whether any acidosis or alkalosis is due to acute or chronic respiratory derangements of $PaCO_2$, or to metabolic causes. Pulse oximeters with finger or ear probes allow non-invasive continuous assessment of oxygen saturation in patients, in order to assess hypoxaemia and its response to therapy. They measure the difference in absorbance of light by oxygenated and deoxygenated blood to calculate its oxygen saturation (SaO₂).

Exercise tests

Resting measurements are sometimes unhelpful in early disease or in patients complaining only of exercise-induced symptoms. Exercise testing with spirometry before and after can be helpful in demonstrating exercise-induced asthma. Walk tests include the self-paced 6-minute walk and the externally paced incremental 'shuttle' test, where patients walk at increasing pace between two cones 10 m apart. These provide simple, repeatable assessments of disability and response to treatment. Cardiopulmonary bicycle or treadmill exercise testing with measurement of metabolic gas exchange, ventilation and cardiac responses is useful for quantifying exercise limitation and for detecting occult cardiovascular or respiratory limitation in the breathless patient.

19.4 How to interpret respiratory function abnormalities

	Asthma	Chronic bronchitis	Emphysema	Pulmonary fibrosis
FEV₁	↓↓	↓↓	↓↓	↓
VC	↓	↓	↓	↓↓
FEV₁/VC	↓	↓	↓	→/↑
TL_CO	→	→	↓↓	↓↓
K_CO	→/↑	→	↓	–/↓
TLC	→/↑	↑	↑↑	↓
RV	→/↑	↑	↑↑	↓

(RV = residual volume; see text for other abbreviations)

19

Cough

Cough is the most frequent symptom of respiratory disease. It is caused by stimulation of sensory nerves in the mucosa of the pharynx, larynx, trachea and bronchi. Acute sensitisation of the normal cough reflex occurs in a number of conditions, and it is typically induced by changes in air temperature or exposure to irritants such as cigarette smoke or perfumes. The characteristics of cough originating at various levels of the respiratory tract are detailed in Box 19.5.

The explosive quality of a normal cough is lost in patients with respiratory muscle paralysis or vocal cord palsy. Paralysis of a single vocal cord gives rise to a prolonged, low-pitched, inefficient 'bovine' cough accompanied by hoarseness. Coexistence of an inspiratory noise (stridor) indicates partial obstruction of a major airway (e.g. laryngeal oedema, tracheal tumour, scarring, compression or inhaled foreign body) and requires urgent investigation and treatment. Sputum production is common in patients with acute or chronic cough, and its nature and appearance can provide clues to the aetiology (p. 642).

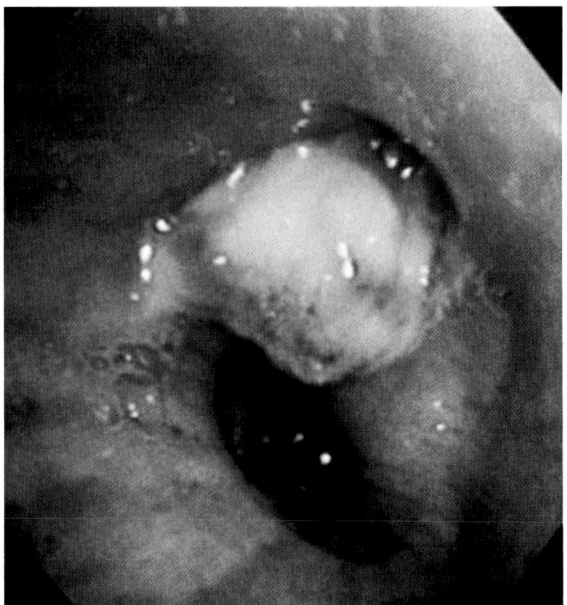

Fig. 19.8 Bronchoscopic appearance of inhaled foreign body (tooth) with a covering mucous film.

Causes of cough

Acute transient cough is most commonly caused by viral lower respiratory tract infection, post-nasal drip resulting from rhinitis or sinusitis, aspiration of a foreign body or throat-clearing secondary to laryngitis or pharyngitis. When it occurs in the context of more serious diseases such as pneumonia, aspiration, congestive heart failure or pulmonary embolism, it is usually easy to diagnose from other clinical features.

Patients with chronic cough present more of a diagnostic challenge, especially when physical examination, chest X-ray and lung function studies are normal. In this context, it is most often explained by cough-variant asthma (where cough may be the principal or exclusive clinical manifestation), post-nasal drip secondary to nasal or sinus disease, or gastro-oesophageal reflux with aspiration. Diagnosis of the latter may require ambulatory pH monitoring or a prolonged trial of anti-reflux therapy (p. 863). Between 10 and 15% of patients (particularly women) taking angiotensin-converting enzyme (ACE) inhibitors develop a drug-induced chronic cough. *Bordetella pertussis* infection in adults (p. 681) can also result in protracted cough and should be suspected in those in close contact with children. While most patients with a bronchogenic carcinoma have an abnormal chest X-ray on presentation, fibreoptic bronchoscopy or thoracic CT is advisable in most adults (especially smokers) with otherwise unexplained cough of recent onset, as this may reveal a small endobronchial tumour or unexpected foreign body (Fig. 19.8). In a small percentage of patients, dry cough may be the presenting feature of interstitial lung disease.

Breathlessness

Breathlessness or dyspnoea can be defined as the feeling of an uncomfortable need to breathe. It is unusual

19.5 **Cough**		
Origin	**Common causes**	**Clinical features**
Pharynx	Post-nasal drip	History of chronic rhinitis
Larynx	Laryngitis, tumour, whooping cough, croup	Voice or swallowing altered, harsh or painful cough. Paroxysms of cough, often associated with stridor
Trachea	Tracheitis	Raw retrosternal pain with cough
Bronchi	Bronchitis (acute) and COPD	Dry or productive, worse in mornings
	Asthma	Usually dry, worse at night
	Eosinophilic bronchitis	Features similar to asthma but no airway hyper-reactivity (AHR)
	Bronchial carcinoma	Persistent (often with haemoptysis)
Lung parenchyma	Tuberculosis	Productive, often with haemoptysis
	Pneumonia	Dry initially, productive later
	Bronchiectasis	Productive, changes in posture induce sputum production
	Pulmonary oedema	Often at night (may be productive of pink, frothy sputum)
	Interstitial fibrosis	Dry, irritant and distressing
Drug side-effect	ACE inhibitors	Dry cough

among sensations in having no defined receptors, no localised representation in the brain, and multiple causes both in health (e.g. exercise) and in diseases of the lungs, heart or muscles.

Pathophysiology

Stimuli to breathing resulting from disease processes are summarised in Figure 19.9. Respiratory diseases can stimulate breathing and dyspnoea by:

- stimulating intrapulmonary sensory nerves (e.g. pneumothorax, interstitial inflammation and pulmonary embolus)
- increasing the mechanical load on the respiratory muscles (e.g. airflow obstruction or pulmonary fibrosis)
- causing hypoxia, hypercapnia or acidosis, stimulating chemoreceptors.

In cardiac failure, pulmonary congestion reduces lung compliance and can also obstruct the small airways. In addition, during exercise, reduced cardiac output limits oxygen supply to the skeletal muscles, causing early lactic acidaemia and further stimulating breathing via the central chemoreceptors.

Breathlessness and the effects of treatment can be quantified using a symptom scale. Patients tend to report breathlessness in proportion to the sum of the above stimuli to breathe. Individual patients differ greatly in the intensity of breathlessness reported for a given set of circumstances, but breathlessness scores during exercise within individuals are reproducible, and can be used to monitor the effects of therapy.

Differential diagnosis

Patients with breathlessness present either with chronic exertional breathlessness or as an emergency with acute breathlessness with prominent symptoms even at rest, and the causes are most easily classified accordingly (Box 19.6).

Chronic exertional breathlessness

The cause of breathlessness is often apparent from a careful clinical history. Key questions include:

How is your breathing at rest and overnight?

In COPD, there is a fixed, structural limit to maximum ventilation, and a tendency for progressive hyperinflation during exercise. Breathlessness is mainly apparent during mobilisation, and patients usually report minimal symptoms at rest and overnight. In contrast, patients with significant asthma are often woken from their sleep by breathlessness with chest tightness and wheeze.

Orthopnoea, however, is common in COPD as well as in heart disease, because airflow obstruction is made worse by cranial displacement of the diaphragm by the abdominal contents when recumbent, so many patients

19

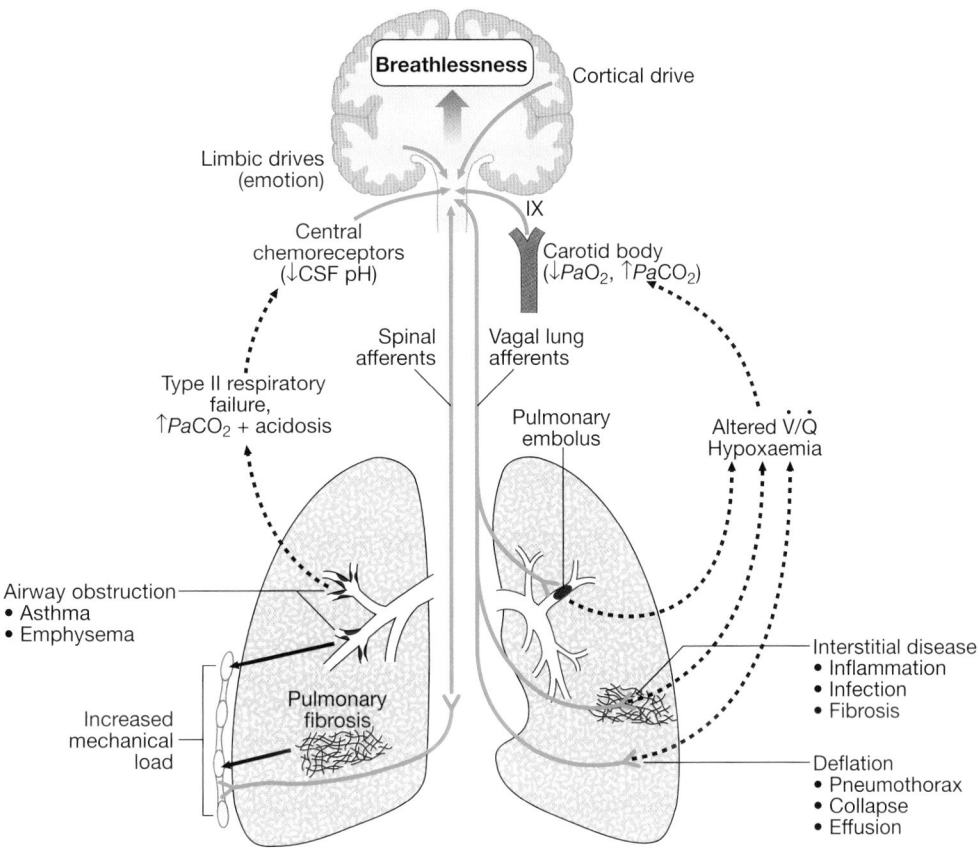

Fig. 19.9 Respiratory stimuli contributing to breathlessness. Mechanisms by which disease can stimulate the respiratory motor neurons in the medulla. Breathlessness is usually felt in proportion to the sum of these stimuli.

19

19.6 Causes of breathlessness

System	Acute dyspnoea	Chronic exertional dyspnoea
Cardiovascular	*Acute pulmonary oedema (p. 540)	Chronic heart failure (p. 540) Myocardial ischaemia (angina equivalent) (p. 541)
Respiratory	*Acute severe asthma *Acute exacerbation of COPD *Pneumothorax *Pneumonia *Pulmonary embolus Acute respiratory distress syndrome (ARDS) Inhaled foreign body (especially in the child) Lobar collapse Laryngeal oedema (e.g. anaphylaxis)	*COPD *Chronic asthma Bronchial carcinoma Interstitial lung disease (sarcoidosis, fibrosing alveolitis, extrinsic allergic alveolitis, pneumoconiosis) Chronic pulmonary thromboembolism Lymphatic carcinomatosis (may cause intolerable breathlessness) Large pleural effusion(s)
Others	Metabolic acidosis (e.g. diabetic ketoacidosis, lactic acidosis, uraemia, overdose of salicylates, ethylene glycol poisoning) Psychogenic hyperventilation (anxiety or panic-related)	Severe anaemia Obesity Deconditioning

*Denotes a common cause.

choose to sleep propped up. It may thus not be a useful differentiating symptom, unless there is a clear history of previous angina or infarction to suggest cardiac disease.

How much can you do on a good day?

Noting 'breathless on exertion' is not enough; the approximate distance the patient can walk on the level should be documented, along with capacity to climb inclines or stairs. Variability within and between days is a hallmark of asthma; in mild asthma the patient may be free of symptoms and signs when well. Gradual, progressive loss of exercise capacity over months and years with consistent disability over days is typical of COPD. When asthma is suspected, the degree of variability is best documented by home peak flow monitoring.

Relentless, progressive breathlessness that is also present at rest, often accompanied by a dry cough, suggests interstitial fibrosis. Impaired left ventricular function can also cause chronic exertional breathlessness, cough and wheeze. A history of angina, hypertension or myocardial infarction may be useful in implicating a cardiac cause. The suspicion of cardiac impairment may be confirmed by a displaced apex beat, a raised JVP and cardiac murmurs (although these signs can occur in severe cor pulmonale). The chest X-ray may show cardiomegaly and an electrocardiogram (ECG) and echocardiogram may provide evidence of left ventricular disease. Measurement of arterial blood gases may be of value, since in the absence of an intracardiac shunt or pulmonary oedema the PaO_2 in cardiac disease is normal and the $PaCO_2$ is low or normal.

Did you have breathing problems in childhood or at school?

When present, a history of childhood wheeze increases the likelihood of asthma, although this history may be absent in late-onset asthma. Similarly, a history of atopic allergy increases the likelihood of asthma.

Do you have other symptoms along with your breathlessness?

Digital or perioral paraesthesiae and a feeling that 'I cannot get a deep enough breath in' are typical features of psychogenic hyperventilation, but this cannot be diagnosed until investigations have excluded other potential causes of breathlessness. Additional symptoms include lightheadedness, central chest discomfort or even carpopedal spasm due to acute respiratory alkalosis. These alarming symptoms may provoke further anxiety and exacerbate hyperventilation. Psychogenic breathlessness rarely disturbs sleep, frequently occurs at rest, may be provoked by stressful situations and may even be relieved by exercise. The Nijmegen questionnaire can be used to enumerate some of the typical symptoms of hyperventilation (Box 19.7). Arterial blood gases show normal PO_2, low PCO_2 and alkalosis.

Pleuritic chest pain in a patient with chronic breathlessness, particularly if it occurs in more than one site over time, should raise suspicion of thromboembolic disease. Thromboembolism may occasionally present as chronic breathlessness with no other specific features, and should always be considered before a diagnosis of psychogenic hyperventilation is made.

Morning headache is an important symptom in patients with breathlessness, as it may signal the onset of carbon dioxide retention and respiratory failure. This

19.7 Factors suggesting psychogenic hyperventilation

- 'Inability to take a deep breath'
- Frequent sighing/erratic ventilation at rest
- Short breath-holding time in the absence of severe respiratory disease
- Difficulty in performing/inconsistent spirometry manoeuvres
- High score (over 26) on Nijmegen questionnaire
- Induction of symptoms during submaximal hyperventilation
- Resting end-tidal $CO_2 < 4.5\%$
- Associated digital paraesthesiae

is particularly significant in patients with musculoskeletal disease impairing respiratory function (e.g. kyphoscoliosis or muscular dystrophy).

Acute severe breathlessness

This is one of the most common and dramatic medical emergencies. Although there are a number of possible causes, the history and a rapid but careful examination will usually suggest a diagnosis which can be confirmed by routine investigations, including chest X-ray, ECG and arterial blood gases. Specific features that aid the diagnosis of the important causes are shown in Box 19.8.

History

It is important to establish the rate of onset and severity of the breathlessness and whether associated cardiovascular symptoms (chest pain, palpitations, sweating and nausea) or respiratory symptoms (cough, wheeze, haemoptysis, stridor—Fig. 19.10) are present. A previous history of repeated episodes of left ventricular failure, asthma or exacerbations of COPD is valuable. In the severely ill patient it may be necessary to obtain the history from accompanying relatives or carers. In children, the possibility of inhalation of a foreign body (see Fig. 19.8) or acute epiglottitis (p. 681) should always be considered.

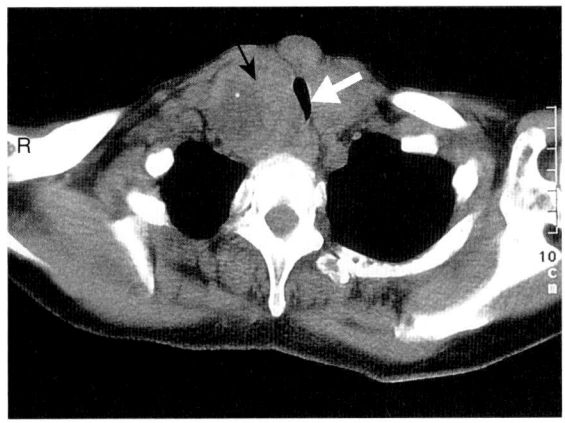

Fig. 19.10 CT showing retrosternal multinodular goitre (small arrow) causing acute severe breathlessness and stridor due to tracheal compression (large arrow).

Clinical assessment

The following should be assessed and documented immediately:
- level of consciousness
- degree of central cyanosis
- evidence of anaphylaxis (urticaria or angioedema)

19

19.8 Differential diagnosis of acute breathlessness

Condition	History	Signs	CXR	ABG	ECG
Pulmonary oedema	Chest pain, palpitations, orthopnoea, cardiac history*	Central cyanosis, ↑JVP, sweating, cool extremities, basal crepitations*	Cardiomegaly, oedema/pleural effusions*	↓PaO_2 ↓$PaCO_2$	Sinus tachycardia, ischaemia*, arrhythmia
Massive pulmonary embolus	Risk factors, chest pain, pleurisy, syncope*, dizziness*	Central cyanosis, ↑JVP*, absence of signs in the lung*, shock (tachycardia, hypotension)	Often normal Prominent hilar vessels, oligaemic lung fields*	↓PaO_2 ↓$PaCO_2$	Sinus tachycardia, RBBB, $S_1Q_3T_3$ pattern ↓T (V_1–V_4)
Acute severe asthma	History of asthma, asthma medications, wheeze*	Tachycardia, pulsus paradoxus, cyanosis (late), JVP →*, ↓peak flow, wheeze*	Hyperinflation only (unless complicated by pneumothorax)*	↓PaO_2 ↓$PaCO_2$ (↑$PaCO_2$ in extremis)	Sinus tachycardia (bradycardia in extremis)
Acute exacerbation of COPD	Previous episodes*, smoker. If in type II respiratory failure may be drowsy	Cyanosis, hyperinflation*, signs of CO_2 retention (flapping tremor, bounding pulses)*	Hyperinflation*, bullae, complicating pneumothorax	↓ or ⇓PaO_2 ↑$PaCO_2$ in type II failure ± ↑H+, ↑HCO_3 in chronic type II failure	Normal, or signs of right ventricular strain
Pneumonia	Prodromal illness*, fever*, rigors*, pleurisy*	Fever, confusion, pleural rub*, consolidation*, cyanosis (if severe)	Pneumonic consolidation*	↓PaO_2 ↓$PaCO_2$ (↑ in extremis)	Tachycardia
Metabolic acidosis	Evidence of diabetes mellitus or renal disease, aspirin or ethylene glycol overdose	Fetor (ketones), hyperventilation without heart or lung signs*, dehydration*, air hunger	Normal	PaO_2 normal ⇓$PaCO_2$, ↑H+	
Psychogenic	Previous episodes, digital or peri-oral dysaesthesia	No cyanosis, no heart or lung signs, carpopedal spasm	Normal	PaO_2 normal* ⇓$PaCO_2$, ↓H+*	

*Denotes a valuable discriminatory feature. (RBBB = right bundle branch block)

- patency of the upper airway
- ability to speak (in single words or sentences)
- cardiovascular status (heart rate and rhythm, blood pressure and degree of peripheral perfusion).

Pulmonary oedema is suggested by pink frothy sputum and bi-basal crackles, asthma or COPD by wheeze and prolonged expiration, pneumothorax by a silent resonant hemithorax, and pulmonary embolus by severe breathlessness with normal breath sounds. The peak expiratory flow should be measured whenever possible. Leg swelling may suggest cardiac failure or, if asymmetrical, venous thrombosis. Arterial blood gases, chest X-ray and an ECG should be obtained to confirm the clinical diagnosis, and high concentrations of oxygen given pending results. Urgent endotracheal intubation (p. 196) may become necessary if the conscious level declines or if severe respiratory acidosis is present.

Chest pain

Chest pain is a frequent manifestation of both cardiac and respiratory disease, and is considered in detail on page 535. Pleural or chest wall involvement by lung disease gives rise to sharp, peripheral pain which is exacerbated by deep breathing or coughing (Box 19.9). Central chest pain suggests heart disease but also occurs with tumours affecting the mediastinum, oesophageal disease (pp. 863–870) or disease of the thoracic aorta (p. 602). Massive pulmonary embolus may cause ischaemic cardiac pain as well as severe breathlessness. Tracheitis produces raw upper retrosternal pain, exacerbated by the accompanying cough. Musculoskeletal chest wall pain is usually exacerbated by movement and associated with local tenderness.

Haemoptysis

Coughing up blood, irrespective of the amount, is an alarming symptom and patients nearly always seek medical advice. A history should be taken to establish that it is true haemoptysis and not haematemesis, or gum or nose bleeding. Haemoptysis must always be assumed to have a serious cause until this is excluded (Box 19.10).

Many episodes of haemoptysis remain unexplained even after full investigation, and are likely to be caused by simple bronchial infection. A history of repeated small haemoptysis, or blood-streaking of sputum, is highly suggestive of bronchial carcinoma. Fever, night sweats and weight loss suggest tuberculosis. Pneumococcal pneumonia often causes 'rusty'-coloured sputum but can cause frank haemoptysis, as can all suppurative pneumonic infections including lung abscess (p. 686). Bronchiectasis (p. 676) and intracavitary mycetoma (p. 698) can cause catastrophic bronchial haemorrhage, and in these patients there may be a history of previous tuberculosis or pneumonia in early life. Finally, pulmonary thromboembolism is a common cause of haemoptysis and should always be considered.

19.9 Differential diagnosis of chest pain

Central

Cardiac
- Myocardial ischaemia (angina)
- Myocardial infarction
- Myocarditis
- Pericarditis
- Mitral valve prolapse syndrome

Aortic
- Aortic dissection
- Aortic aneurysm

Oesophageal
- Oesophagitis
- Oesophageal spasm
- Mallory–Weiss syndrome

Massive pulmonary embolus

Mediastinal
- Tracheitis
- Malignancy

Anxiety/emotion[1]

Peripheral

Lungs/pleura
- Pulmonary infarct
- Pneumonia
- Pneumothorax
- Malignancy
- Tuberculosis
- Connective tissue disorders

Musculoskeletal[2]
- Osteoarthritis
- Rib fracture/injury
- Costochondritis (Tietze's syndrome)
- Intercostal muscle injury
- Epidemic myalgia (Bornholm disease)

Neurological
- Prolapsed intervertebral disc
- Herpes zoster
- Thoracic outlet syndrome

[1]May also cause peripheral chest pain.
[2]Can sometimes cause central chest pain.

19.10 Causes of haemoptysis

Bronchial disease
- Carcinoma*
- Bronchiectasis*
- Acute bronchitis*
- Bronchial adenoma
- Foreign body

Parenchymal disease
- Tuberculosis*
- Suppurative pneumonia
- Lung abscess
- Parasites (e.g. hydatid disease, flukes)
- Trauma
- Actinomycosis
- Mycetoma

Lung vascular disease
- Pulmonary infarction*
- Goodpasture's syndrome (p. 502)
- Polyarteritis nodosa
- Idiopathic pulmonary haemosiderosis

Cardiovascular disease
- Acute left ventricular failure*
- Mitral stenosis
- Aortic aneurysm

Blood disorders
- Leukaemia
- Haemophilia
- Anticoagulants

*More common causes.

Physical examination may reveal additional clues. Finger clubbing suggests bronchial carcinoma or bronchiectasis; other signs of malignancy, such as cachexia, hepatomegaly and lymphadenopathy, should also be sought. Fever, pleural rub or signs of consolidation occur in pneumonia or pulmonary infarction; a minority of patients with pulmonary infarction also have unilateral leg swelling or pain suggestive of deep venous thrombosis. Rashes, haematuria and digital infarcts suggest an underlying systemic disease such as a vasculitis, which may be associated with haemoptysis.

Management

In severe acute haemoptysis, the patient should be nursed upright (or on the side of the bleeding if this is known), and given high-flow oxygen and appropriate haemodynamic resuscitation. Bronchoscopy in the acute phase is difficult and often merely shows blood throughout the bronchial tree. If radiology shows an obvious central cause, then rigid bronchoscopy under general anaesthesia may allow intervention to stop bleeding; however, the source often cannot be visualised. Intubation with a divided endotracheal tube may allow protected ventilation of the unaffected lung to stabilise the patient. Bronchial arteriography and embolisation (Fig. 19.11), or even emergency pulmonary surgery, can be life-saving in the acute situation.

In the vast majority of cases, however, the haemoptysis itself is not life-threatening and a logical sequence of investigations should be followed:

- chest X-ray, which may give evidence of a localised lesion including pulmonary infarction, tumour (malignant or benign), pneumonia, mycetoma or tuberculosis

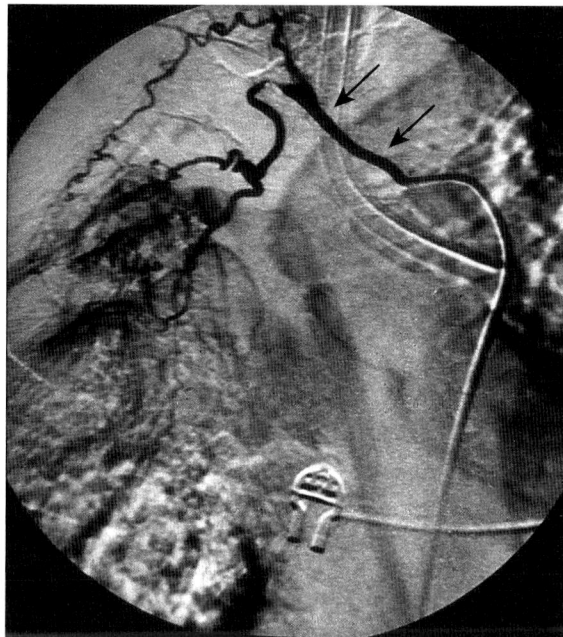

Fig. 19.11 Bronchial artery angiography. An angiography catheter has been passed via the femoral artery and aorta into an abnormally dilated right bronchial artery (arrows). Contrast is seen flowing into the lung. This patient had post-tuberculous bronchiectasis affecting the right upper lobe and presented with massive haemoptysis. Bronchial artery embolisation was successfully performed.

- full blood count and clotting screen
- bronchoscopy after acute bleeding has settled, which may reveal a central bronchial carcinoma (not visible on the chest X-ray) and permit biopsy and tissue diagnosis
- CTPA, which may reveal underlying pulmonary thromboembolic disease or alternative causes of haemoptysis not seen on the chest X-ray (e.g. pulmonary arteriovenous malformation or small or hidden tumours).

Incidental pulmonary nodule on imaging

A pulmonary nodule may be defined as a round opacity which is at least moderately well marginated and no greater than 3 cm in diameter. The increased use of imaging, particularly volumetric thin slice CT, has increased the number of pulmonary nodules reported, with non-calcified pulmonary nodules (NCN) seen in around two-thirds of thoracic CT studies performed in smokers over the age of 50 years. The majority are benign; however, the differential diagnosis is extensive (Box 19.11) and includes early malignant disease that may be treatable.

The problem is most satisfactorily resolved if it can be shown that the lesion was present on old films and has remained unchanged over 2 years of follow-up; however, if there are no previous films, or if previous films are normal, further assessment is required. Factors to take into account are the status of the patient and the characteristics of the nodule (Box 19.12). Whenever bacterial infection is a differential diagnosis, an antibiotic should be given during the period in which the investigations are being performed; the patient should then undergo a repeat X-ray to see whether there has been a reduction in size of the opacity. Tuberculous, fungal and hydatid disease may have to be considered, depending on the clinical context.

PET (p. 649) is useful in selected patients. In a patient older than 60 years a positive ^{18}FDG-PET scan equates to a probability of malignancy of 90%; if negative, the probability of malignancy is less than 5%. However, it is unreliable when the size of the lesion is below 1 cm and false negatives may be seen with carcinoid and bronchoalveolar cell carcinomas.

Percutaneous needle biopsy under CT guidance allows tissue to be obtained with few complications,

19.11 Causes of pulmonary nodules

Common causes

- Bronchial carcinoma
- Single metastasis
- Localised pneumonia
- Lung abscess
- Tuberculoma
- Pulmonary infarct

Uncommon causes

- Benign tumours
- Lymphoma
- Arteriovenous malformation
- Hydatid cyst (p. 375)
- Bronchogenic cyst
- Rheumatoid nodule
- Pulmonary sequestration
- Pulmonary haematoma
- Wegener's granuloma
- 'Pseudotumour'—fluid collection in a fissure
- Aspergilloma (usually surrounded by air 'halo')

19

i 19.12 Clinical and radiographic features distinguishing benign from malignant nodules*

Risk status of patient

Age	Increasing age increases likelihood of malignancy. Lung cancer is uncommon under the age of 40 and rare under 35
Smoking history	Risk of malignancy increases in proportion to duration and amount smoked
History of malignancy	Risk of malignancy increased by history of lung cancer in a first-degree relative, and by exposure to asbestos, silica, uranium and radon

Characteristics of nodule

Size	Greater probability of malignancy with increasing size. Nearly all nodules > 3 cm are malignant; less than 1% of very small (< 4 mm) nodules are malignant, even in smokers; 10–20% in the 8 mm range will prove cancerous
Margin	Usually smooth in benign lesions; malignant lesions have a spiculated margin
Density	Most cancerous lesions are solid, but most solid lesions are non-cancerous. A partly solid lesion or one with air lucencies is more likely to be malignant than a solid lesion. Ground glass lesions with malignant potential grow very slowly and require longer follow-up
Calcification or fat	These favour benign disease, although CT may detect calcification in some malignant lesions. A laminated or central deposition of calcification is typical of a granuloma, while a 'popcorn' pattern is suggestive of a hamartoma. Fat content is consistent with a hamartoma or a lipoid granuloma
Location	70% of lung cancers occur in the upper lobes and the right lung is more commonly affected than the left lung. Benign lesions are equally distributed throughout upper and lower lobes
Contrast enhancement	Lack of contrast enhancement (< 15 HU) has a high negative predictive value for malignancy, but is non-specific with a poor positive predictive value. Not useful in lesions < 8 mm in diameter
Lymphadenopathy	Hilar or mediastinal adenopathy favours a malignant process and is important for staging

*Linear or sheet-like lung opacities are unlikely to represent neoplasms and do not require follow-up, and some nodular opacities may be judged sufficiently typical of scarring that follow-up is not warranted.
Adapted from Fleischer Society Statement Radiology 2005; 237:395–400.

e.g. pneumothorax and haemorrhage. Bronchoscopy is usually unrewarding, as the lesion is often beyond the vision of the operator and as the diagnostic yield from blind washings is low. If the lesion has a high probability of malignancy and the patient is fit for surgery, resection may be considered.

Serial imaging of an indeterminate lesion can be very helpful (Box 19.13). The doubling times of tumours are characterised; however, the limits of reproducibility in measurement on most CT scanners require an increase in diameter of at least 1.7 mm or an increase in volume of at least 25%. These changes may be difficult to measure, and may be more accurately assessed by specially adapted computer programs, particularly those that facilitate three-dimensional reconstruction of nodules.

Finally, in considering further imaging, account should be taken not only of the risks of further radiation exposure to the patient (greater in younger than in older individuals), but also of the fact that further scans may detect new nodules so that investigation may need to start all over again.

Pleural effusion

The accumulation of serous fluid within the pleural space is termed pleural effusion. The accumulation of frank pus is termed empyema (p. 725), that of blood is haemothorax, and that of chyle is chylothorax. In general, pleural fluid accumulates as a result of either increased hydrostatic pressure or decreased osmotic pressure ('transudative effusion', as seen in cardiac, liver or renal failure), or from increased microvascular pressure due to disease of the pleural surface itself or injury

19.13 Recommendations for follow-up of incidental nodules smaller than 8 mm[1]

Nodule size (mm)[2]	Low-risk patient[3]	High-risk patient[4]
≤ 4	No follow-up needed[5]	Follow-up CT at 12 months; if unchanged, no further follow-up
4–6	Follow-up at 12 months; if unchanged, no further follow-up	Initial follow-up CT at 6–12 months, then at 18–24 months if no change
6–8	Initial follow-up CT at 6–12 months then at 18–24 months if no change	Initial follow-up CT at 3–6 months, then at 9–12 months if no change
> 8	Follow-up CT at around 3, 9 and 24 months, dynamic contrast-enhanced CT, PET and/or biopsy	As for low-risk patient

[1]Excludes patients known to have or suspected of having malignant disease, younger patients, and patients with unexplained fever.
[2]Average of length and width.
[3]Minimal or absent history of smoking and of other known risk factors.
[4]History of smoking or of other known risk factors.
[5]Very low risk of malignancy (< 1%). Non-solid (ground glass) or partly solid nodules may require longer follow-up to exclude indolent adenocarcinoma.

in the adjacent lung ('exudative effusion'). The cause of the majority of pleural effusions (Boxes 19.14 and 19.15) can be identified through a thorough history, examination and relevant investigations.

19.14 Causes of pleural effusion

Common causes

- Pneumonia ('para-pneumonic effusion')
- Tuberculosis
- Pulmonary infarction*
- Malignant disease

- Cardiac failure*
- Subdiaphragmatic disorders (subphrenic abscess, pancreatitis etc.)

Uncommon causes

- Hypoproteinaemia* (nephrotic syndrome, liver failure, malnutrition)
- Connective tissue diseases* (particularly systemic lupus erythematosus (SLE) and rheumatoid arthritis)
- Acute rheumatic fever
- Post-myocardial infarction syndrome

- Meigs' syndrome (ovarian tumour plus pleural effusion)
- Myxoedema*
- Uraemia*
- Asbestos-related benign pleural effusion

*May cause bilateral effusions.

Clinical assessment

Symptoms (pain on inspiration and coughing) and signs of pleurisy (a pleural rub) often precede the development of an effusion, especially in patients with underlying pneumonia, pulmonary infarction or connective tissue disease. However, the onset may be insidious. Breathlessness is the only symptom related to the effusion itself, and its severity depends on the size and rate of accumulation. The physical signs are detailed on page 643.

Investigations

Imaging

The classical appearance of pleural fluid on the erect PA chest film is of a curved shadow at the lung base, blunting the costophrenic angle and ascending towards the axilla (p. 643). Fluid appears to track up the lateral chest wall. In fact, fluid surrounds the whole lung at this level, but casts a radiological shadow only where the X-ray beam passes tangentially across the fluid against the lateral chest wall. Around 200 mL of fluid is required to be detectable on a PA chest X-ray, but smaller effusions can be identified by ultrasound or CT. Previous scarring or adhesions in the pleural space can cause localised effusions. Pleural fluid localised below the lower lobe ('subpulmonary effusion') simulates an elevated hemidiaphragm. Fluid localised within an oblique fissure may produce a rounded opacity, simulating a tumour.

Ultrasonography is more accurate than plain chest radiography for determining the volume of pleural fluid and frequently provides additional helpful information. Visualisation of fluid facilitates skin marking to indicate a site for safe needle aspiration and guides pleural biopsy, increasing diagnostic yield. The presence of loculation may suggest an evolving empyema or resolving haemothorax. The technique may also distinguish pleural fluid from pleural thickening. CT displays pleural abnormalities more readily than either plain radiography or ultrasound, and may distinguish benign from malignant pleural disease.

Pleural aspiration and biopsy

In some clinical settings (e.g. left ventricular failure) it should not be necessary to sample fluid unless atypical

19.15 Pleural effusion: main causes and features

Cause	Appearance of fluid	Type of fluid	Predominant cells in fluid	Other diagnostic features
Tuberculosis	Serous, usually amber-coloured	Exudate	Lymphocytes (occasionally polymorphs)	Positive tuberculin test Isolation of *M. tuberculosis* from pleural fluid (20%) Positive pleural biopsy (80%)
Malignant disease	Serous, often blood-stained	Exudate	Serosal cells and lymphocytes Often clumps of malignant cells	Positive pleural biopsy (40%) Evidence of malignant disease elsewhere
Cardiac failure	Serous, straw-coloured	Transudate	Few serosal cells	Other evidence of left ventricular failure Response to diuretics
Pulmonary infarction	Serous or blood-stained	Exudate (rarely transudate)	Red blood cells Eosinophils	Evidence of pulmonary infarction Source of embolism Factors predisposing to venous thrombosis
Rheumatoid disease	Serous Turbid if chronic	Exudate	Lymphocytes (occasionally polymorphs)	Rheumatoid arthritis; rheumatoid factor and anti-CCP antibodies Cholesterol in chronic effusion; very low glucose in pleural fluid
SLE	Serous	Exudate	Lymphocytes and serosal cells	Other manifestations of SLE Antinuclear factor or anti-DNA in serum
Acute pancreatitis	Serous or blood-stained	Exudate	No cells predominate	High amylase in pleural fluid (greater than in serum)
Obstruction of thoracic duct	Milky	Chyle	None	Chylomicrons

19

19.16 Light's criteria for distinguishing pleural transudate from exudate

Pleural fluid is an exudate if one or more of the following criteria are met:
- Pleural fluid protein:serum protein ratio > 0.5
- Pleural fluid LDH:serum LDH ratio > 0.6
- Pleural fluid LDH > two-thirds of the upper limit of normal serum LDH

(LDH = lactate dehydrogenase)

features are present (such as a unilateral effusion); appropriate treatment should be administered and the effusion re-evaluated. However, in most other circumstances, sampling is necessary to establish a diagnosis. Simple aspiration provides information on the colour and texture of fluid and on appearance alone may immediately suggest an empyema or chylothorax. The presence of blood is consistent with pulmonary infarction or malignancy, but may represent a traumatic tap. Biochemical analysis allows differentiation of transudates from exudates (Box 19.16) and Gram stain may indicate parapneumonic effusion. Cytological examination is essential, as the predominant cell type provides useful information. A low pH suggests infection but may also be seen in rheumatoid arthritis, ruptured oesophagus or advanced malignancy.

Combining pleural aspiration with biopsy increases the diagnostic yield, particularly when guided by either ultrasound or CT. The best results are obtained from video-assisted thoracoscopy, allowing the operator to visualise the pleura and guide the biopsy directly.

Management

Therapeutic aspiration may be required to palliate breathlessness, but removing more than 1.5 L in one episode is inadvisable as there is a small risk of re-expansion pulmonary oedema. An effusion should never be drained to dryness before establishing a diagnosis, as further biopsy may be precluded until further fluid accumulates. Treatment of the underlying cause — for example, heart failure, pneumonia, pulmonary embolism or subphrenic abscess — will often be followed by resolution of the effusion. The management of pleural effusion in association with pneumonia, tuberculosis and malignancy is discussed in the relevant sections.

Respiratory failure

The term respiratory failure is used when pulmonary gas exchange fails to maintain normal arterial oxygen and carbon dioxide levels. Its classification into types I and II relates to the absence or presence of hypercapnia (raised $PaCO_2$).

Pathophysiology

When disease impairs ventilation of part of a lung (e.g. in asthma or pneumonia), perfusion of that underventilated region results in hypoxic and CO_2-laden blood entering the pulmonary veins. Increased ventilation of neighbouring regions of normal lung can increase their CO_2 excretion, correcting arterial CO_2 to normal, but cannot augment their oxygen uptake because the haemoglobin flowing through these normal regions is already fully saturated. Admixture of blood from the underventilated and normal regions thus results in hypoxia with normocapnia, which is called 'type I respiratory failure'. Diseases causing this abnormality include any that impair ventilation locally, with sparing of other regions (Box 19.17).

Arterial hypoxia with hypercapnia (type II respiratory failure) is seen if there is severe generalised ventilation–perfusion mismatch (insufficient normal lung to correct $PaCO_2$) or a disease which reduces total ventilation. The latter category includes not just diseases of the lung but also disorders affecting any part of the neuromuscular mechanism of ventilation (see Box 19.17).

Management of acute respiratory failure

Prompt diagnosis and management of the underlying cause is crucial to the management of patients with acute respiratory failure. In type I respiratory failure, high concentrations of oxygen (40–60% by mask) will usually relieve hypoxia by increasing the alveolar PO_2 in poorly ventilated lung units. Occasionally, however (e.g. severe pneumonia affecting several lobes), mechanical ventilation may be needed to relieve hypoxia. Patients who

19.17 How to interpret blood gas abnormalities in respiratory failure

	Type I		Type II	
	Hypoxia (PaO_2 < 8.0 kPa (60 mmHg))		Hypoxia (PaO_2 < 8.0 kPa (60 mmHg))	
	Normal or low $PaCO_2$ (< 6.6 kPa (50 mmHg))		Raised $PaCO_2$ (> 6.6 kPa (50 mmHg))	
	Acute	Chronic	Acute	Chronic
H⁺	→ or ↑	→	↑	→ or ↑
Bicarbonate	→	→	→	↑
Causes	Acute asthma	Emphysema	Acute severe asthma	COPD
	Pulmonary oedema	Lung fibrosis	Acute exacerbation COPD	Sleep apnoea
	Pneumonia	Lymphangitis	Upper airway obstruction	Kyphoscoliosis
	Lobar collapse	carcinomatosa	Acute neuropathies/paralysis	Myopathies/muscular
	Pneumothorax	Right-to-left shunts	Narcotic drugs	dystrophy
	Pulmonary embolus	Brain-stem lesion	Primary alveolar hypoventilation	Ankylosing spondylitis
	ARDS		Flail chest injury	

need high concentrations of oxygen for more than a few hours should receive humidified oxygen.

Acute type II respiratory failure is an emergency, which requires immediate intervention. It is useful to distinguish between patients with high ventilatory drive (rapid respiratory rate and accessory muscle recruitment) who cannot move sufficient air, and those with reduced or inadequate respiratory effort. In the former situation, particularly if inspiratory stridor is present, acute upper airway obstruction from foreign body inhalation or laryngeal obstruction (angioedema, carcinoma or vocal cord paralysis) must be considered, as the Heimlich manœuvre (p. 724), immediate intubation or emergency tracheostomy may be life-saving.

More commonly, however, the problem is in the lungs, with severe generalised bronchial obstruction from COPD or asthma, ARDS arising from a variety of insults (p. 187), or occasionally tension pneumothorax. In all such cases, high-concentration (e.g. 60%) oxygen should be administered pending a rapid examination of the respiratory system and measurement of arterial blood gases. Patients with the trachea deviated away from a silent and resonant hemithorax are likely to have tension pneumothorax, and air should be aspirated from the pleural space and a chest drain inserted as soon as possible. Patients with generalised wheeze, scanty breath sounds bilaterally or a history of asthma or COPD should be treated with nebulised salbutamol 2.5 mg plus oxygen, repeated until bronchospasm is relieved. Failure to respond to initial treatment, declining conscious level or worsening respiratory acidosis ($H^+ > 50$ nmol/L, $PaCO_2 > 6.6$ kPa (50 mmHg)) on blood gases are all indications that supported ventilation is required (p. 196).

A small percentage of patients with severe chronic COPD and type II respiratory failure develop abnormal tolerance to raised $PaCO_2$ and may become dependent on hypoxic drive to breathe. In these patients only, lower concentrations of oxygen (24–28% by Venturi mask) should be used to avoid precipitating worsening respiratory depression (see below). In all cases, regular monitoring of arterial blood gases is important to assess progress.

Patients with acute type II respiratory failure who have reduced drive or conscious level may be suffering from sedative poisoning, CO_2 narcosis or a primary failure of neurological drive (e.g. following intracerebral haemorrhage or head injury). History from an accompanying person may be invaluable, and reversal of specific drugs with (for example) opiate antagonists is occasionally successful, but should not delay intubation and supported mechanical ventilation in appropriate cases.

Chronic and 'acute on chronic' type II respiratory failure

The most common cause of chronic type II respiratory failure is severe COPD. Although CO_2 may be persistently raised, there is no persisting acidaemia because the kidneys retain bicarbonate, correcting arterial pH to normal. This 'compensated' pattern, which may also occur in chronic neuromuscular disease or kyphoscoliosis, is maintained until there is a further pulmonary insult (see Box 19.17), such as an exacerbation of COPD which precipitates an episode of 'acute on chronic' respiratory failure, with acidaemia and initial respiratory distress followed by drowsiness and eventu-

ally coma. Because these patients have lost their chemosensitivity to elevated $PaCO_2$, they may paradoxically depend on hypoxia for respiratory drive, and are at risk of respiratory depression if given high concentrations of oxygen—for example, during ambulance transfers or in emergency departments. Moreover, in contrast to acute severe asthma, a patient with 'acute on chronic' type II respiratory failure due to COPD may not feel overtly distressed despite being critically ill with severe hypoxaemia, hypercapnia and acidaemia. While the physical signs of CO_2 retention (confusion, flapping tremor, bounding pulses etc.) can be helpful if present, they may not be, so arterial blood gases are mandatory in the assessment of initial severity and response to treatment.

Management

The principal aim of treatment in acute on chronic type II respiratory failure is to achieve a safe PaO_2 (> 7.0 kPa (52 mmHg)) without increasing $PaCO_2$ and acidosis, while identifying and treating the precipitating condition. In this patient group it is not necessary to achieve a normal PaO_2; even a small increase will often have a greatly beneficial effect on tissue oxygen delivery since the PaO_2 values of these patients are often on the steep part of the oxygen saturation curve (p. 181). The risks of worsening hypercapnia and coma must be balanced against those of severe hypoxaemia, which include potentially fatal arrhythmias or severe cerebral complications. Immediate treatment is shown in Box 19.18. Patients who are conscious, with adequate respiratory

19.18 Assessment and management of 'acute on chronic' type II respiratory failure

Initial assessment

Patient may not appear distressed despite being critically ill
- Conscious level (response to commands, ability to cough)
- CO_2 retention (warm periphery, bounding pulses, flapping tremor)
- Airways obstruction (wheeze, prolonged expiration, hyperinflation, intercostal indrawing, pursed lips)
- Cor pulmonale (peripheral oedema, raised JVP, hepatomegaly, ascites)
- Background functional status and quality of life
- Signs of precipitating cause (see Box 19.17)

Investigations
- Arterial blood gases (severity of hypoxaemia, hypercapnia, acidaemia, bicarbonate)
- Chest X-ray

Management
- Maintenance of airway
- Treatment of specific precipitating cause
- Frequent physiotherapy ± pharyngeal suction
- Nebulised bronchodilators
- Controlled oxygen therapy
    Start with 24% Venturi mask
    Aim for a $PaO_2 > 7$ kPa (52 mmHg) (a $PaO_2 < 5$ (37 mmHg) is dangerous)
- Antibiotics
- Diuretics

Progress
- If $PaCO_2$ continues to rise or patient cannot achieve a safe PaO_2 without severe hypercapnia and acidaemia, mechanical ventilatory support may be required

drive, may benefit from non-invasive ventilation (NIV), which has been shown to reduce the need for intubation and shorten hospital stay. Patients who are drowsy, with low respiratory drive, require an urgent decision regarding the appropriateness of intubation and ventilation, which is likely to be the only effective treatment, although weaning off the ventilator may be difficult in severe disease. This decision is difficult, and useful factors to consider include patient and family wishes, presence of a potentially remediable precipitating condition, prior functional capacity and quality of life. The various types of non-invasive (via a face or nasal mask) or invasive (via an endotracheal tube) ventilation are detailed on pages 194–197.

Doxapram (1.5–4 mg/min by slow intravenous infusion) is a respiratory stimulant that is occasionally used in patients with acute on chronic type II respiratory failure and low respiratory drive. It causes unacceptable distress due to increased dyspnoea in those with preserved drive, and should not be used as a substitute for intubation and mechanical ventilation in suitable patients with CO_2 narcosis, as it provides only minor and transient improvements in arterial blood gases.

Home ventilation for chronic respiratory failure

NIV has proved to be of great value in the long-term treatment of respiratory failure due to skeletal deformity, neuromuscular disease and central alveolar hypoventilation. These conditions often present subacutely, with a very gradual onset of type II respiratory failure. Morning headache (due to elevated $PaCO_2$) and fatigue are common symptoms but in many cases the diagnosis is only revealed by sleep studies or blood gas analysis. In the initial stages, ventilation is insufficient for metabolic needs only during sleep, when ventilatory drive declines physiologically. Over time, however, CO_2 retention becomes chronic, with renal compensation of acidosis. Treatment by home-based NIV overnight is often sufficient to restore the daytime PCO_2 to normal, and to relieve fatigue and headache. In advanced muscle disease (e.g. muscular dystrophies), daytime NIV may also be required.

Lung transplantation

Lung transplantation is now an established treatment for carefully selected patients with advanced lung disease unresponsive to medical treatment (Box 19.19). Single-lung transplantation may be used for selected patients with advanced emphysema or lung fibrosis, but is contraindicated in patients with chronic bilateral pulmonary infection, such as cystic fibrosis and bronchiectasis, because the transplanted lung is vulnerable to cross-infection. In these cases bilateral lung transplantation is the standard procedure. Combined heart-lung transplantation is still occasionally needed for patients with advanced congenital heart disease such as Eisenmenger's syndrome and is preferred by some surgeons for the treatment of primary pulmonary hypertension unresponsive to medical therapy.

The prognosis following lung transplantation is improving steadily with modern immunosuppressive drugs (over 60% 5-year survival in some UK centres); however, chronic rejection resulting in obliterative bronchiolitis continues to afflict some recipients. While corticosteroids continue to be used in the short-term management of acute rejection, maintenance treatment to prevent chronic rejection depends on drugs which inhibit cell-mediated immunity specifically, such as ciclosporin, mycophenolate and tacrolimus (p. 93). The major factor limiting the availability of lung transplantation is the shortage of donor lungs. To improve donor availability, techniques to preserve the lungs after cardiac arrest are being developed, and living donor lobar transplantation is performed in some cases.

OBSTRUCTIVE PULMONARY DISEASES

Asthma

There is no universally agreed definition of asthma. Descriptions of the condition focus on clinical, physiological and pathological characteristics stressing the central role of both chronic airway inflammation and increased airway hyper-responsiveness. Typical symptoms include wheeze, cough, chest tightness and dyspnoea which are accompanied by the presence of airflow obstruction that is variable over short periods of time, or is reversible with treatment.

Epidemiology

The prevalence of asthma increased steadily over the latter part of the last century, first in the developed and then in the developing world (Fig. 19.12). Current estimates suggest that asthma affects 300 million people world-wide and an additional 100 million persons will be diagnosed by 2025. The socio-economic impact is enormous, particularly when poor control leads to days lost from school or work, unscheduled health-care visits and hospital admissions.

Although the development, course of disease and response to treatment are influenced by genetic determinants, the rapid rise in the prevalence of asthma implies that environmental factors are critically important in terms of its expression. To date, studies have explored the potential role of microbial exposure, diet, vitamins, breastfeeding, air pollution and obesity, but no clear consensus has emerged (Fig. 19.13).

Pathophysiology

Airway hyper-reactivity (AHR) — the tendency for airways to contract too easily and too much in response to triggers that have little or no effect in normal individuals — is integral to the diagnosis of asthma

19.19 Indications for lung transplantation

Parenchymal lung disease

- Cystic fibrosis
- Emphysema
- Pulmonary fibrosis
- Langerhans cell histiocytosis
- Lymphangioleiomyomatosis
- Obliterative bronchiolitis

Pulmonary vascular disease

- Primary pulmonary hypertension
- Thromboembolic pulmonary hypertension
- Veno-occlusive disease
- Eisenmenger's syndrome (p. 630)

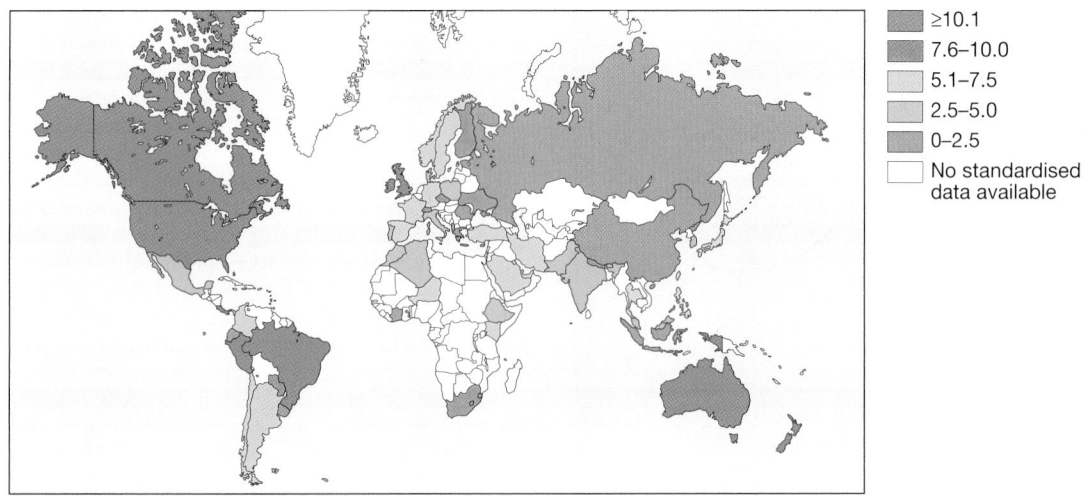

Fig. 19.12 World map showing the prevalence of clinical asthma (proportion of population (%)). Data drawn from the European Community Respiratory Health Study (ECRHS) and the International Study of Asthma and Allergies in Childhood (ISAAC).

Legend:
- ≥10.1
- 7.6–10.0
- 5.1–7.5
- 2.5–5.0
- 0–2.5
- No standardised data available

19

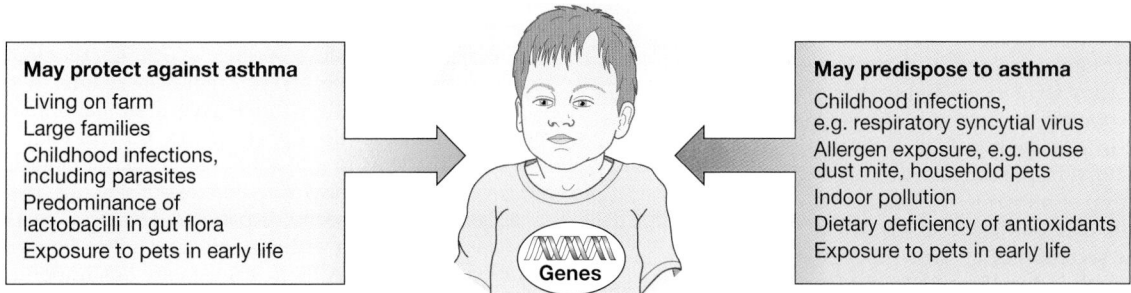

May protect against asthma

Living on farm
Large families
Childhood infections, including parasites
Predominance of lactobacilli in gut flora
Exposure to pets in early life

May predispose to asthma

Childhood infections, e.g. respiratory syncytial virus
Allergen exposure, e.g. house dust mite, household pets
Indoor pollution
Dietary deficiency of antioxidants
Exposure to pets in early life

Fig. 19.13 Factors implicated in the development of, or protection from, asthma.

and appears to be related, although not exclusively so, to airway inflammation (Fig. 19.14). Other factors likely to be important include the degree of airway narrowing and the influence of neurogenic mechanisms.

With increasing severity and chronicity of the disease, remodelling of the airway occurs, leading to fibrosis of the airway wall, fixed narrowing of the airway and a reduced response to bronchodilator medication.

The relationship between atopy (a propensity to produce IgE) and asthma is well established, and in many individuals there is clear relationship between sensitisation (demonstration of skin prick reactivity or elevated serum specific IgE) and allergen exposure. Inhalation of an allergen into the airway is followed by a two-phase bronchoconstrictor response with both an early and a late-phase response (Fig. 19.15). Common examples include house dust mites, pets such as cats and dogs, pests such as cockroaches, and fungi (particularly *Aspergillus*: allergic bronchopulmonary aspergillosis, p. 697). Allergic mechanisms are also implicated in some cases of occupational asthma (see below).

In aspirin-sensitive asthma, symptoms follow the ingestion of salicylates. These inhibit the cyclo-oxygenase,

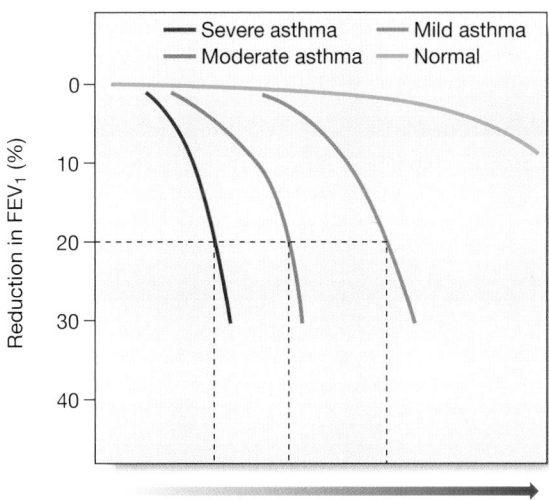

Fig. 19.14 Airway hyper-reactivity in asthma. This is demonstrated by bronchial challenge tests by the administration of sequentially increasing concentrations of either histamine, methacholine or mannitol. The reactivity of the airways is expressed as the concentration or dose of either chemical required to produce a certain decrease (usually 20%) in the FEV_1 (PC_{20} or PD_{20} respectively).

663

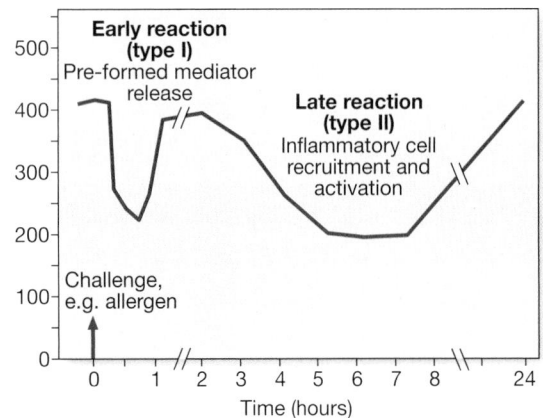

Fig. 19.15 Changes in peak flow following allergen challenge.
A similar biphasic response is observed following a variety of different
challenges. Occasionally an individual will develop an isolated late response
with no early reaction.

which leads to shunting of arachidonic acid metabolism
through the lipoxygenase pathway, resulting in the production of the cysteinyl leukotrienes. In exercise-induced
asthma, hyperventilation results in water loss from the
pericellular lining fluid of the respiratory mucosa, which
in turn triggers mediator release. Heat loss from the
respiratory mucosa may also be important.

In persistent asthma, a chronic and complex inflammatory response ensues, which is characterised by an
influx of numerous inflammatory cells, the transformation and participation of airway structural cells, and
the secretion of an array of cytokines, chemokines and
growth factors. Smooth muscle hypertrophy and hyperplasia, thickening of the basement membrane, mucous
plugging and epithelial damage result. Examination of
the inflammatory cell profile in induced sputum samples demonstrates that, although asthma is predominantly characterised by airway eosinophilia, in some
patients neutrophilic inflammation predominates, and
in others, scant inflammation is observed: so-called
'pauci-granulocytic' asthma.

Clinical features

Typical symptoms include recurrent episodes of wheeze,
chest tightness, breathlessness and cough. Not uncommonly, asthma is mistaken for a cold or chest infection
that is failing to resolve (e.g. after more than 10 days).
Classical precipitants include exercise, particularly in
cold weather, exposure to airborne allergens or pollutants, and viral upper respiratory tract infections.
Wheeze apart, there is often little to find on examination. An inspection for nasal polyps and eczema should
be performed. Rarely, a vasculitic rash may be present
in Churg–Strauss syndrome (p. 1114).

Patients with mild intermittent asthma are usually
asymptomatic between exacerbations. Patients with
persistent asthma report on-going breathlessness and
wheeze, but variability is usually present with symptoms fluctuating over the course of one day, from day to
day, or from month to month.

Asthma characteristically displays a diurnal pattern, with symptoms and lung function being worse in
the early morning. Particularly when poorly controlled,

symptoms such as cough and wheeze disturb sleep
and have led to the use of the term 'nocturnal asthma'.
Cough may be the dominant symptom in some patients,
and the lack of wheeze or breathlessness may lead to
a delay in reaching the diagnosis of so-called 'cough-
variant asthma'.

Although the aetiology of asthma is often elusive,
an attempt should be made to identify any agents that
may contribute to the appearance or aggravation of
the condition. With regard to potential allergens, particular enquiry should be made into exposure to a pet
cat, guinea pig, rabbit or horse, pest infestation, or
mould growth following water damage to a home or
building.

In some circumstances, the appearance of asthma is
triggered by medications. For example, β-adrenoceptor
antagonists (β-blockers), even when administered topically as eye drops, may induce bronchospasm, and aspirin and other non-steroidal anti-inflammatory drugs
(NSAIDs) may also induce wheeze as above. The classical
aspirin-sensitive patient is female and presents in middle
age with asthma, rhinosinusitis and nasal polyps. Aspirin-
sensitive patients may also report symptoms following
alcohol (in particular white wine) and foods containing
salicylates. Other medications implicated include the oral
contraceptive pill, cholinergic agents and prostaglandin
F2α. Betel nuts contain aceroline, which is structurally
similar to methacholine, and can aggravate asthma.

Some patients with asthma have a similar inflammatory response in the upper airway. Careful enquiry
should be made as to a history of sinusitis, sinus headache, a blocked or runny nose, and loss of sense of smell.

An important minority of patients develop a particularly severe form of asthma; this appears to be more
common in women. Allergic triggers are less important
and airway neutrophilia predominates.

Diagnosis

The diagnosis of asthma is predominantly clinical and
based on a characteristic history. Supportive evidence
is provided by the demonstration of variable airflow
obstruction, preferably by using spirometry (Box 19.20).
The measurement of FEV_1 and VC identify the obstructive nature of the ventilatory defect, define its severity,
and provide the basis of bronchodilator reversibility (Fig.
19.16). If spirometry is not available, a peak flow meter
may be used. Patients should be instructed to record peak
flow readings after rising in the morning and before retiring in the evening. A diurnal variation in PEF (the lowest
values typically being recorded in the morning) of more
than 20% is considered diagnostic and the magnitude of
variability provides some indication of disease severity

19.20 Making a diagnosis of asthma

Compatible clinical history *plus either/or*:
- $FEV_1 \geq 15\%^*$ (and 200 mL) increase following administration
  of a bronchodilator/trial of corticosteroids
- > 20% diurnal variation on $\geq$ 3 days in a week for 2 weeks
  on PEF diary
- $FEV_1 \geq 15\%$ decrease after 6 mins of exercise

*Global Initiative for Asthma (GINA) definition accepts an increased FEV_1
12%.

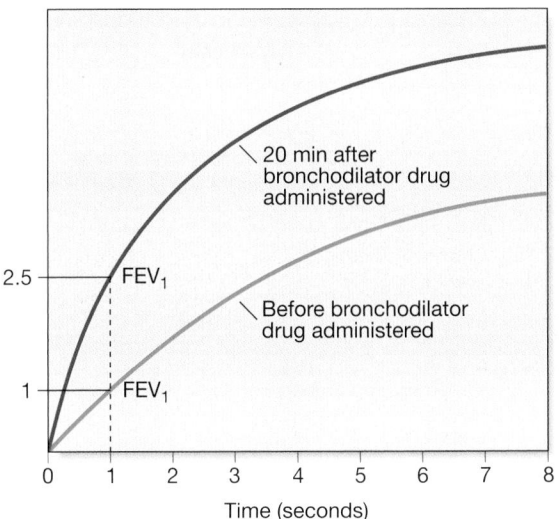

Fig. 19.16 **Reversibility test.** Forced expiratory manœuvres before and 20 minutes after inhalation of a β_2-adrenoceptor agonist. Note the increase in FEV_1 from 1.0 to 2.5 L.

(Fig. 19.17). A trial of corticosteroids (e.g. 30 mg daily for 2 weeks) may be useful in documenting improvement in either FEV_1 or PEF to establish the diagnosis.

It is not uncommon for patients whose symptoms are suggestive of asthma to have normal lung function. In these circumstances, the demonstration of AHR by challenge tests may be useful to confirm the diagnosis (see Fig. 19.14). AHR is sensitive but non-specific; it therefore has a high negative predictive value but positive results may be seen in other conditions such as COPD,

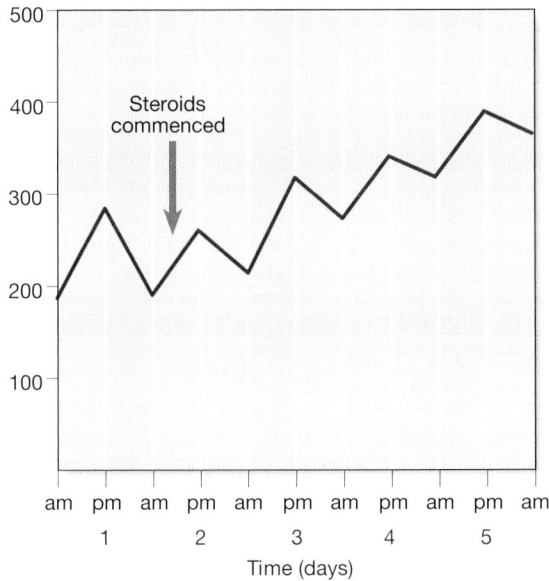

Fig. 19.17 **Serial recordings of peak expiratory flow (PEF) in a patient with asthma.** Note the sharp overnight fall (morning dip) and subsequent rise during the day. In this example corticosteroids have been commenced, followed by a subsequent improvement in PEF rate and loss of morning dipping.

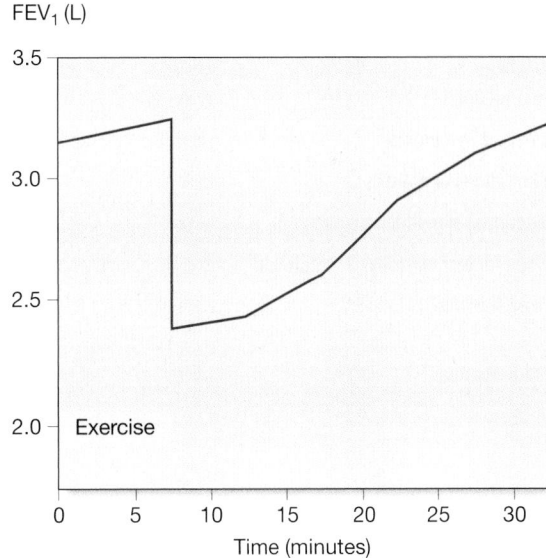

Fig. 19.18 **Exercise-induced asthma.** Serial recordings of FEV_1 in a patient with bronchial asthma before and after 6 minutes of strenuous exercise. Note initial slight rise on completion of exercise, followed by sudden fall and gradual recovery. Adequate warm-up exercise or pre-treatment with a β_2-adrenoceptor agonist, nedocromil sodium or a leukotriene antagonist (e.g. montelukast sodium) can protect against exercise-induced symptoms.

bronchiectasis and CF. Challenge tests using adenosine may improve specificity. When symptoms are predominantly related to exercise, an exercise challenge may be followed by a drop in lung function (Fig. 19.18).

Other useful investigations

- *Measurement of allergic status.* The presence of atopy may be demonstrated by skin prick tests. Similar information may be provided by the measurement of total and allergen-specific IgE. A full blood picture may show peripheral blood eosinophilia.
- *Radiological examination.* Chest X-ray appearances are often normal or show hyperinflation of lung fields. Lobar collapse may be seen if mucus occludes a large bronchus, and if accompanied by the presence of flitting infiltrates, may suggest that asthma has been complicated by allergic bronchopulmonary aspergillosis (p. 697). An HRCT scan may be useful to detect bronchiectasis.
- *Assessment of eosinophilic airway inflammation.* An induced sputum differential eosinophil count of greater than 2% or exhaled breath nitric oxide concentration (FE_{NO}) may support the diagnosis but is non-specific.

Management

Setting goals

Asthma is a chronic condition but effective treatment is available for the majority of patients. The goal of management should be to obtain and sustain complete control (Box 19.21). However, goals may have to be modified according to the circumstances and the patient. Unfortunately, surveys consistently demonstrate that the majority of asthmatics report suboptimal control, perhaps reflecting poor expectations of patients and their clinicians.

19.21 Levels of asthma control*			
Characteristic	Controlled	Partly controlled (any present in any week)	Uncontrolled
Daytime symptoms	None (2 or less/week)	More than twice/week	
Limitations of activities	None	Any	
Nocturnal symptoms/awakening	None	Any	3 or more features of partly controlled asthma present in any week
Need for rescue/'reliever' treatment	None (2 or less/week)	More than twice/week	
Lung function (PEF or FEV$_1$)	Normal	< 80% predicted or personal best (if known) on any day	
Exacerbation	None	One or more/year	1 in any week

*Based on GINA guidelines.

Whenever possible, patients should be encouraged to take responsibility for managing their own disease. Time should be taken to encourage an understanding of the nature of the condition, the relationship between symptoms and inflammation, the importance of key symptoms such as nocturnal waking, the different types of medication, and, if appropriate, the use of PEF to guide management decisions. A variety of tools/questionnaires have been validated to assist in assessing asthma control. Written action plans may be helpful in developing self-management skills.

Avoidance of aggravating factors

This is particularly important in the management of occupational asthma, but may also be relevant to atopic patients where removing or reducing exposure to relevant antigens, e.g. a pet animal, may effect improvement. House dust mite exposure may be minimised by replacing carpets with floorboards and using mite-impermeable bedding, although improvements in asthma control following such measures have been difficult to demonstrate. Many patients are sensitised to several ubiquitous aeroallergens, making avoidance strategies largely impractical. Measures to reduce fungal exposure and eliminate cockroaches may be applicable in specific circumstances, and medications known to precipitate or aggravate asthma should be avoided. Smoking cessation (p. 99) is particularly important, as smoking not only encourages sensitisation but also induces a relative corticosteroid resistance in the airway.

A stepwise approach to the management of asthma (Fig. 19.19)

Step 1: Occasional use of inhaled short-acting β$_2$-adrenoreceptor agonist bronchodilators

For patients with mild intermittent asthma (symptoms less than once a week for 3 months and fewer than two nocturnal episodes/month), it is usually sufficient to prescribe an inhaled short-acting β$_2$-agonist (salbutamol or terbutaline), to be used on an as-required basis. However, many patients (and their physicians) underestimate the severity of asthma and these patients require careful supervision. A history of a severe exacerbation should lead to a step up in treatment.

A variety of different inhaled devices are available and choice should be guided by patient preference and competence in using the device. The metered-dose inhaler remains the most widely prescribed (Fig. 19.20).

Step 2: Introduction of regular 'preventer' therapy

Regular anti-inflammatory therapy (preferably inhaled corticosteroids (ICS) such as beclometasone, budesonide, fluticasone or ciclesonide) should be started in addition to inhaled β$_2$-agonists taken on an as-required basis in any patient who:

- has experienced an exacerbation of asthma in the last 2 years (Box 19.22)
- uses inhaled β$_2$-agonists three times a week or more
- reports symptoms three times a week or more
- is awakened by asthma one night per week.

For adults, a reasonable starting dose is 400 μg beclometasone dipropionate (BDP) or equivalent per day, although higher doses may be required in smokers. Alternative but much less effective preventive agents include chromones, leukotriene receptor antagonists, and theophyllines.

Step 3: Add-on therapy

If a patient remains poorly controlled despite regular use of ICS, a thorough review should be undertaken focusing on adherence, inhaler technique and on-going exposure to modifiable aggravating factors. A further increase in the dose of ICS may benefit some patients, but in general, add-on therapy should be considered in adults taking 800 μg/day BDP (or equivalent).

Long-acting β$_2$-agonists (LABAs), such as salmeterol and formoterol, with a duration of action of at least 12 hours, represent the first choice of add-on therapy. They have consistently been demonstrated to improve asthma control and reduce the frequency and severity of exacerbations when compared to increasing the dose of ICS alone. Fixed combination inhalers of ICS and LABAs have been developed; these are more convenient, increase compliance, and prevent patients using a LABA as monotherapy (which may be accompanied by an increased risk of life-threatening attacks or asthma death). The onset of action of formoterol is similar to that of salbutamol, such that, in carefully selected patients, a fixed combination of

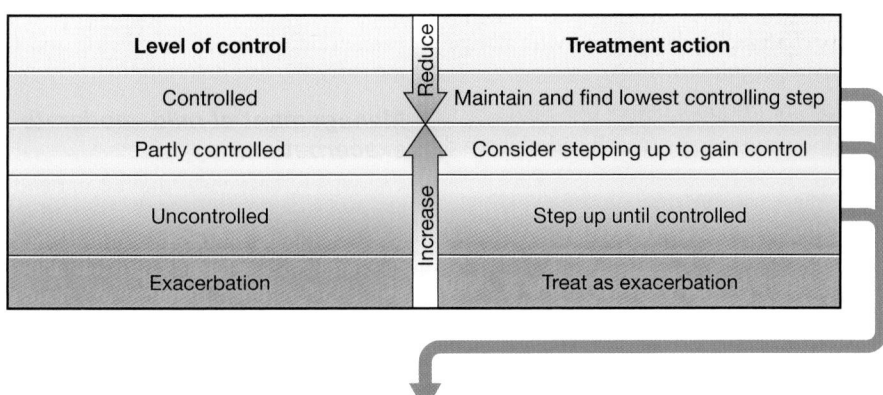

Level of control	Reduce / Increase	Treatment action
Controlled	Reduce	Maintain and find lowest controlling step
Partly controlled		Consider stepping up to gain control
Uncontrolled	Increase	Step up until controlled
Exacerbation		Treat as exacerbation

	Reduce ◄ Treatment steps ► Increase				
	Step 1	Step 2	Step 3	Step 4	Step 5
	Asthma education				
	Environmental control				
	As needed rapid-acting β₂-agonist				
		Select one	Select one	Add one or more	Add one or both
Controller options	Low-dose ICS	Low-dose ICS *plus* long-acting β₂-agonist	Medium- *or* high-dose ICS *plus* long-acting β₂-agonist	Oral glucocorticosteroid (lowest dose)
	Leukotriene modifier*	Medium- *or* high-dose ICS	Leukotriene modifier	Anti-IgE treatment
		Low-dose ICS *plus* leukotriene modifier	Sustained-release theophylline	
		Low-dose ICS *plus* sustained-release theophylline		

Fig. 19.19 Management approach based on asthma control. For children older than 5 years, adolescents and adults. (ICS = inhaled corticosteroid) *Receptor antagonist or synthesis inhibitors.

budesonide and formoterol may be contemplated for use as both rescue and maintenance therapy.

Oral leukotriene receptor antagonists (e.g. montelukast 10 mg daily) are generally less effective than LABA as add-on therapy but may facilitate a reduction in the dose of ICS and control exacerbations. Oral theophyllines may be considered in some patients but their unpredictable metabolism, propensity for drug interactions and prominent side-effect profile limit their widespread use.

Step 4: Poor control on moderate dose of inhaled steroid and add-on therapy: addition of a fourth drug

In adults, the dose of ICS may be increased to 2000 μg BDP/budesonide (or equivalent) daily. A nasal corticosteroid preparation should be used in patients with prominent upper airway symptoms. Oral therapy with leukotriene receptor antagonists, theophyllines or a slow-release β₂-agonist may be considered. If the trial of add-on

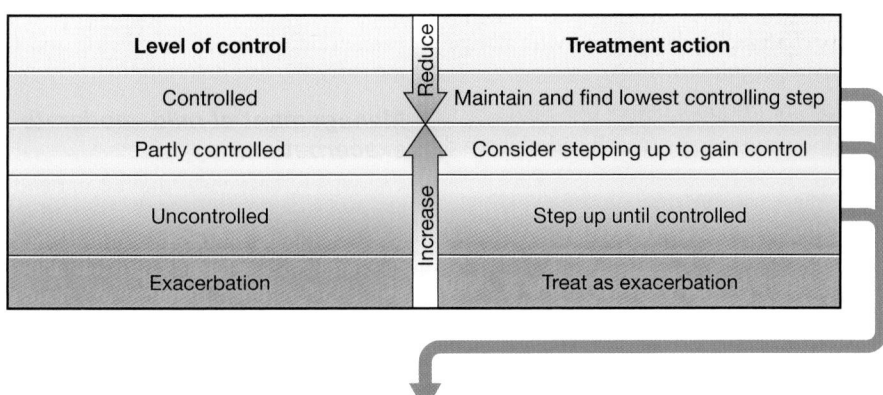

- Remove the cap and shake the inhaler

- Breathe out gently and place the mouthpiece into the mouth

- Incline the head backwards to minimise oropharyngeal deposition

- Simultaneously, begin a slow deep inspiration, depress the cannister and continue to inhale

- Hold the breath for 10 seconds

Fig. 19.20 How to use a metered-dose inhaler.

EBM 19.22 Inhaled corticosteroids and asthma

'Regular therapy with low-dose budesonide reduces the risk of severe exacerbations in patients with mild persistent asthma.'

• Pauwels RA, et al. Lancet 2003; 361:1066–1067.

therapy is ineffective, it should be discontinued. Oral itraconazole should be contemplated in patients with allergic bronchopulmonary aspergillosis (ABPA).

Step 5: Continuous or frequent use of oral steroids

At this stage prednisolone therapy (usually administered as a single daily dose in the morning) should be prescribed in the lowest amount necessary to control symptoms. Patients on long-term oral corticosteroids (> 3 months) or receiving more than three or four courses per year will be at risk of systemic side-effects (p. 770). Osteoporosis can be prevented in this group of patients by using bisphosphonates (p. 1119). Steroid-sparing therapies such as methotrexate, ciclosporin or oral gold may be considered. New therapies, such as omalizumab, a monoclonal antibody directed against IgE, may prove helpful in atopic patients.

Step-down therapy

Once asthma control is established, the dose of inhaled (or oral) corticosteroid should be titrated to the lowest dose at which effective control of asthma is maintained. Decreasing the dose of ICS by around 25–50% every 3 months is a reasonable strategy for most patients.

Asthma in pregnancy

The management of asthma in pregnancy is described in Box 19.23.

19.23 Asthma in pregnancy

- **Unpredictable clinical course:** one-third worsen, one-third remain stable and one-third improve.
- **Labour and delivery:** 90% have no symptoms.
- **Safety data:** good for β_2-agonists, inhaled steroids, theophyllines, oral prednisolone, and chromones.
- **Oral leukotriene receptor antagonists:** no evidence that these harm the fetus and they should not be stopped in women who have previously demonstrated significant improvement in asthma control prior to pregnancy.
- **Steroids:** women on maintenance prednisolone > 7.5 mg/day should receive hydrocortisone 100 mg 6–8-hourly during labour.
- **Prostaglandin F2α:** may induce bronchospasm and should be used with extreme caution.
- **Breastfeeding:** use medications as normal.
- **Uncontrolled asthma represents the greatest danger to the fetus:** Associated with maternal (hyperemesis, hypertension, pre-eclampsia, vaginal haemorrhage, complicated labour) and fetal (intrauterine growth restriction and low birth weight, preterm birth, increased perinatal mortality, neonatal hypoxia) complications.

Exacerbations of asthma

The course of asthma may be punctuated by exacerbations characterised by increased symptoms, deterioration in lung function, and an increase in airway inflammation. Exacerbations are most commonly precipitated by viral infections, but moulds (*Alternaria* and *Cladosporium*), pollens (particularly following thunderstorms) and air pollution are also implicated. Most attacks are characterised by a gradual deterioration over several hours to days but some appear to occur with little or no warning: so-called brittle asthma. An

important minority of patients appear to have a blunted perception of airway narrowing and fail to appreciate the early signs of deterioration.

Management of mild–moderate exacerbations

The widely held view that an impending exacerbation may be avoided by doubling the dose of ICS has failed to be validated by recent studies. Short courses of 'rescue' oral corticosteroids (prednisolone 30–60 mg daily) are therefore often required to regain control of symptoms. Tapering of the dose to withdraw treatment is not necessary unless given for more than 3 weeks.

Indications for 'rescue' courses include:

- symptoms and PEF progressively worsening day by day
- fall of PEF below 60% of the patient's personal best recording
- onset or worsening of sleep disturbance by asthma
- persistence of morning symptoms until midday
- progressively diminishing response to an inhaled bronchodilator
- symptoms severe enough to require treatment with nebulised or injected bronchodilators.

Management of acute severe asthma

Initial assessment

Box 19.24 lists the features requiring immediate assessment in acute asthma. Measurement of PEF is mandatory unless the patient is too ill to cooperate, and is most easily interpreted when expressed as a percentage of the predicted normal or of the previous best value obtained on optimal treatment (Fig. 19.21). Arterial blood gas analysis is essential to determine the $PaCO_2$, a normal or elevated level being particularly dangerous. A chest X-ray is not immediately necessary unless pneumothorax is suspected.

19.24 Immediate assessment of acute severe asthma

Acute severe asthma

- PEF 33–50% predicted (< 200 L/min)
- Respiratory rate $\geq$ 25/min
- Heart rate $\geq$ 110/min
- Inability to complete sentences in 1 breath

Life-threatening features

- PEF < 33% predicted (< 100 L/min)
- SpO_2 < 92% or PaO_2 < 8 kPa (60 mmHg) (especially if being treated with oxygen)
- Normal or raised $PaCO_2$
- Silent chest
- Cyanosis
- Feeble respiratory effort
- Bradycardia or arrhythmias
- Hypotension
- Exhaustion
- Confusion
- Coma

Near-fatal asthma

- Raised $PaCO_2$ and/or requiring mechanical ventilation with raised inflation pressures

---

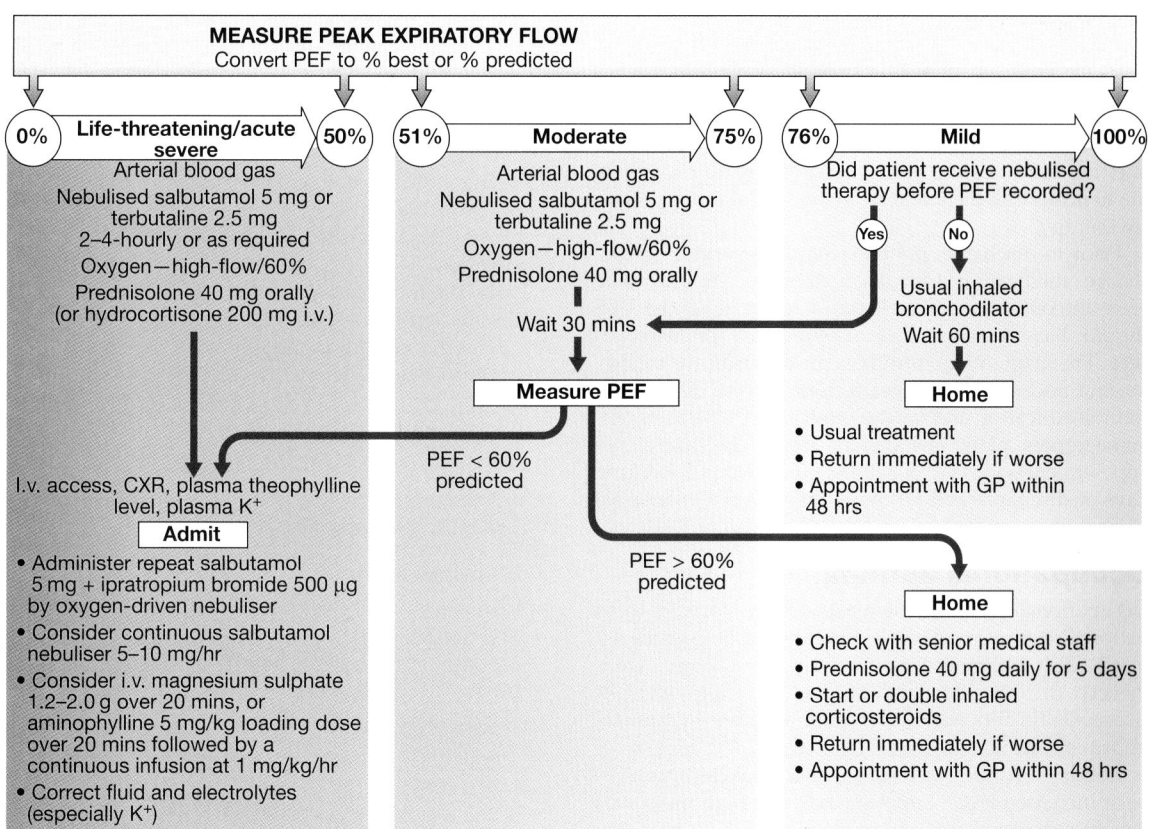

Fig. 19.21 Immediate treatment of patients with acute severe asthma.

Treatment

- *Oxygen.* High concentrations of oxygen (humidified if possible) should be administered to maintain the oxygen saturation above 92% in adults. The presence of a high $PaCO_2$ should not be taken as an indication to reduce oxygen concentration but as a warning sign of a severe or life-threatening attack. Failure to achieve appropriate oxygenation is an indication for assisted ventilation.
- *High doses of inhaled bronchodilators.* Short-acting β_2-agonists are the agent of first choice. In hospital they are most conveniently administered via a nebuliser driven by oxygen but delivery of multiple doses of salbutamol via a metered-dose inhaler through a spacer device provides equivalent bronchodilatation and may be used in primary care. Ipratropium bromide should be added to salbutamol in patients with acute severe or life-threatening attacks.
- *Systemic corticosteroids.* Systemic corticosteroids reduce the inflammatory response and hasten the resolution of exacerbations. They should be administered to all patients experiencing an acute severe attack. They can usually be administered orally as prednisolone, but intravenous hydrocortisone may be given in patients who are vomiting or unable to swallow.
- *Intravenous fluids.* There are no controlled trials to support the use of intravenous fluids but many patients are dehydrated due to high insensible water loss and probably benefit from these. Potassium supplements may be necessary because repeated doses of salbutamol can lower serum potassium.

Subsequent management

If patients fail to improve, a number of further options may be considered. Intravenous magnesium may provide additional bronchodilatation in some patients whose presenting PEF is < 30% predicted. Some patients benefit from the use of intravenous aminophylline but careful monitoring is required. The potential for intravenous leukotriene receptor antagonists remains under investigation.

Monitoring of treatment

PEF should be recorded every 15–30 minutes and then every 4–6 hours. Pulse oximetry should ensure that SaO_2 remains > 92%, but repeat arterial blood gases are necessary if the initial $PaCO_2$ measurements were normal or raised, the PaO_2 was < 8 kPa (60 mmHg) or the patient deteriorates. Box 19.25 lists the indications for endotracheal intubation and intermittent positive pressure ventilation.

> **19.25 Indications for assisted ventilation in acute severe asthma**
>
> - Coma
> - Respiratory arrest
> - Deterioration of arterial blood gas tensions despite optimal therapy
>   - PaO_2 < 8 kPa (60 mmHg) and falling
>   - $PaCO_2$ > 6 kPa (45 mmHg) and rising
>   - pH low and falling (H^+ high and rising)
> - Exhaustion, confusion, drowsiness

19

Prognosis

The outcome from acute severe asthma is generally good. Death is fortunately rare but a considerable number of deaths occur in young people and many are preventable. Failure to recognise the severity of an attack, on the part of either the assessing physician or the patient, contribute to undertreatment and delay in delivering appropriate therapy.

Prior to discharge, patients should be stable on discharge medication (nebulised therapy should have been discontinued for at least 24 hours) and the PEF should have reached 75% of predicted or personal best. The acute attack provides an opportunity to look for and address any trigger factors, for the delivery of asthma education and for the provision of a written self-management plan. The patient should be offered an appointment with a GP or asthma nurse within 2 working days of discharge and follow-up at a specialist hospital clinic within a month.

Occupational asthma

Occupational asthma is the most common form of occupational respiratory disorder and should be considered in all adult asthmatics, particularly if symptoms commenced during a particular period of employment. It is especially important to enquire whether symptoms improve during time away from work, e.g. weekends or holidays. Atopic individuals and smokers appear to be at increased risk. Numerous low and high molecular weight substances have been implicated. The most frequently reported causative agents commonly affecting workers are shown in Box 19.26.

The diagnosis of occupational asthma can be particularly difficult and requires specialist assessment. The patient should be instructed to perform 2-hourly peak flow recording which can be analysed by a computer-based programme such as Occupational Asthma System (OASYS) (Fig. 19.22). Skin prick tests or the measurement of specific IgE may confirm sensitivity to the suspected agent. Bronchial provocation tests with the suspected agent may be necessary, but require highly specialist laboratories.

Early diagnosis and removal from exposure often results in significant improvement and may occasionally cure the condition. Recognition also has important medico-legal implications and should prompt a

19.26 Occupational asthma	
Most frequently reported causative agents	
• Isocyanates	• Animals
• Flour and grain dust	• Aldehydes
• Colophony and fluxes	• Wood dust
• Latex	
Workers most commonly reported to occupational asthma schemes	
• Paint sprayers	• Animal handlers
• Bakers and pastry-makers	• Welders
• Nurses	• Food processing workers
• Chemical workers	• Timber workers

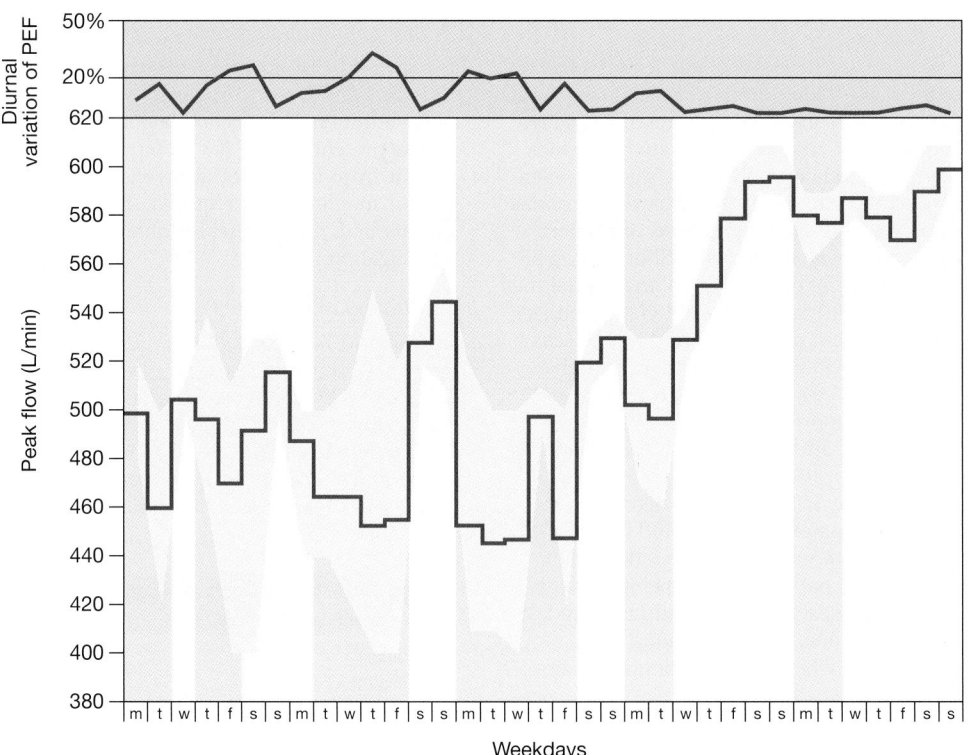

Fig. 19.22 Peak flow readings in occupational asthma. Subjects with suspected occupational asthma are asked to perform 2-hourly serial peak flows at, and away from, work. The maximum, mean and minimum values are plotted daily. Days at work are indicated by the shaded areas. The diurnal variation is displayed at the top. In this example, a period away from work is followed by a marked improvement in peak flow readings and a reduction in diurnal variation.

workplace visit to identify and rectify exposure, and to trigger screening of other employees who may also have developed the disease.

Byssinosis

Byssinosis occurs as a result of exposure to cotton brack (dried leaf and plant debris) in cotton and flax mills. An acute form of the disease occurs in about one-third of individuals on first exposure to cotton dust and is characterised by an acute bronchiolitis with symptoms and signs of airflow obstruction. Many of those affected may give up such work at this stage. Chronic byssinosis, unlike occupational asthma, usually develops after 20–30 years' exposure. The condition is more common in smokers. Typical symptoms include chest tightness or breathlessness accompanied by a drop in lung function; classically, these are most severe on the first day of the working week ('Monday fever') or following a period away from work. As the week progresses, symptoms improve and the fall in lung function becomes less dramatic (across-shift variation). Affected workers should be offered alternative employment. Continued exposure leads to the development of persistent symptoms and a progressive decline in FEV_1.

Chronic obstructive pulmonary disease (COPD)

COPD is defined as a preventable and treatable lung disease with some significant extrapulmonary effects that may contribute to the severity in individual patients. The pulmonary component is characterised by airflow limitation that is not fully reversible. The airflow limitation is usually progressive and associated with an abnormal inflammatory response of the lung to noxious particles or gases. Related diagnoses include chronic bronchitis (cough and sputum on most days for at least 3 consecutive months for at least 2 successive years) and emphysema (abnormal permanent enlargement of the airspaces distal to the terminal bronchioles, accompanied by destruction of their walls and without obvious fibrosis). Extrapulmonary manifestations include impaired nutrition, weight loss and skeletal muscle dysfunction (Fig. 19.23).

Epidemiology

Prevalence is directly related to the prevalence of tobacco smoking and, in low- and middle-income countries, the use of biomass fuels. Current estimates suggest that 80 million people world-wide suffer from moderate to severe disease. In 2005, COPD contributed to more than 3 million deaths (5% of deaths globally), but by 2020 it is forecast to represent the third most important cause of death world-wide. The anticipated rise in morbidity and mortality from COPD will be greatest in Asian and African countries as a result of their increasing tobacco consumption.

Aetiology

Risk factors are shown in Box 19.27. Cigarette smoking represents the most significant risk factor for COPD and relates to both the amount and the duration of smoking. It is unusual to develop COPD with less than 10 pack years (1 pack year = 20 cigarettes/day/year) and not all smokers develop the condition, suggesting that individual susceptibility factors are important.

19

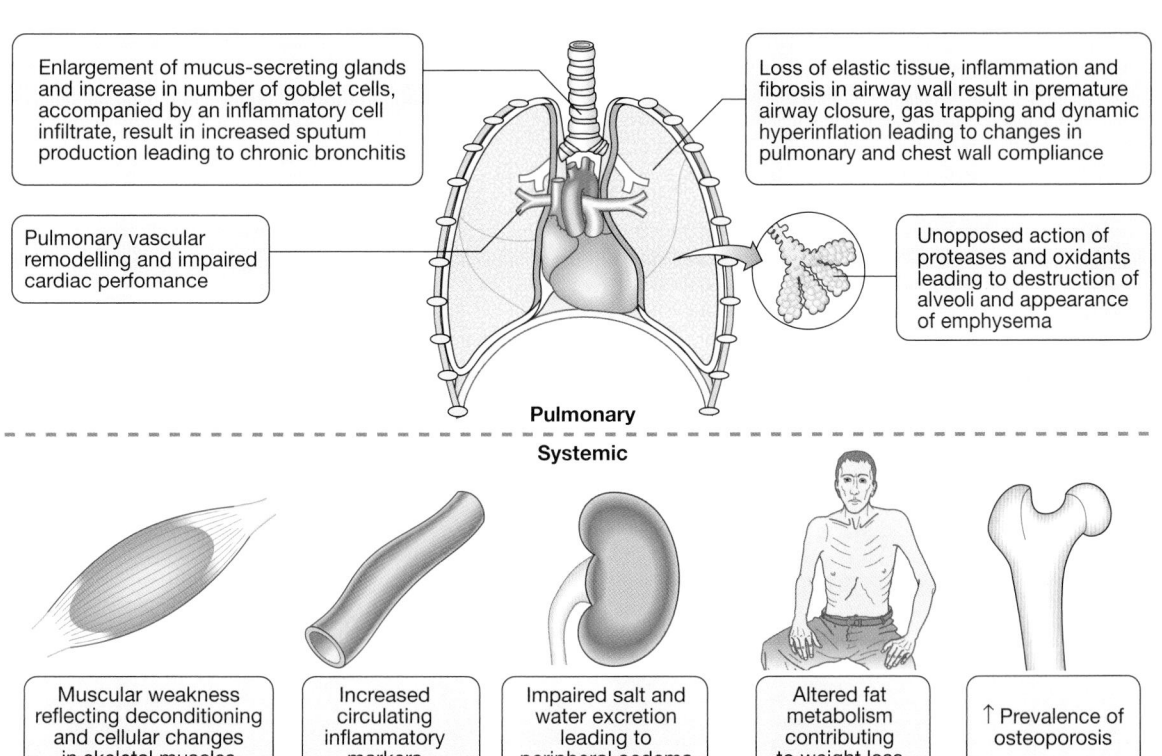

Enlargement of mucus-secreting glands and increase in number of goblet cells, accompanied by an inflammatory cell infiltrate, result in increased sputum production leading to chronic bronchitis

Loss of elastic tissue, inflammation and fibrosis in airway wall result in premature airway closure, gas trapping and dynamic hyperinflation leading to changes in pulmonary and chest wall compliance

Pulmonary vascular remodelling and impaired cardiac perfomance

Unopposed action of proteases and oxidants leading to destruction of alveoli and appearance of emphysema

Pulmonary

Systemic

Muscular weakness reflecting deconditioning and cellular changes in skeletal muscles

Increased circulating inflammatory markers

Impaired salt and water excretion leading to peripheral oedema

Altered fat metabolism contributing to weight loss

↑ Prevalence of osteoporosis

Fig. 19.23 The pulmonary and systemic features of COPD.

19.27 Risk factors for development of COPD

Exposures

- Tobacco smoke: accounts for 95% of cases in UK
- Biomass solid fuel fires: wood, animal dung, crop residues and coal lead to high levels of indoor air pollution
- Occupation: coal miners and those who work with cadmium
- Outdoor and indoor air pollution
- Low birth weight: may reduce maximally attained lung function in young adult life
- Lung growth: childhood infections or maternal smoking may affect growth of lung during childhood, resulting in a lower maximally attained lung function in adult life
- Infections: recurrent infection may accelerate decline in FEV_1; persistence of adenovirus in lung tissue may alter local inflammatory response predisposing to lung damage; HIV infection is associated with emphysema
- Low socioeconomic status
- Nutrition: role as independent risk factor unclear
- Cannabis smoking

Host factors

- Genetic factors: α_1-antiproteinase deficiency; other COPD susceptibility genes are likely to be identified
- Airway hyper-reactivity

Pathophysiology

COPD has both pulmonary and systemic components (Fig. 19.23).

The changes in pulmonary and chest wall compliance mean that collapse of intrathoracic airways during expiration is exacerbated, during exercise as the time available for expiration shortens, resulting in dynamic hyperinflation. Increased $\dot{V}/\dot{Q}$ mismatch increases the dead space volume and wasted ventilation. Flattening of the diaphragmatic muscles and an increasingly horizontal alignment of the intercostal muscles place the respiratory muscles at a mechanical disadvantage. The work of breathing is therefore markedly increased, first on exercise but, as the disease advances, at rest too.

Emphysema (Fig. 19.24) may be classified by the pattern of the enlarged airspaces: centriacinar, panacinar and periacinar. Bullae form in some individuals. This results in impaired gas exchange and respiratory failure.

Clinical features

COPD should be suspected in any patient over the age of 40 years who presents with symptoms of chronic bronchitis and/or breathlessness. Depending on the presentation, important differential diagnoses include chronic asthma, tuberculosis, bronchiectasis and congestive cardiac failure.

Cough and associated sputum production are usually the first symptoms, often referred to as a 'smoker's cough'. Haemoptysis may complicate exacerbations of COPD but should not be attributed to COPD without thorough investigation.

Breathlessness usually brings about the first presentation to medical attention. The level should be quantified for future reference by documenting the exercise the patient can manage before stopping; the modified Medical Research Council (MRC) dyspnoea scale may also be useful (Box 19.28). In advanced disease, enquiry should be made as to the presence of oedema (which may be seen for the first time during an exacerbation) and morning headaches, which may suggest hypercapnia.

Physical signs (pp. 642–643) are non-specific, correlate poorly with lung function, and are seldom obvious until the disease is advanced. Breath sounds are typically quiet; crackles may accompany infection but if persistent raise the possibility of bronchiectasis. Finger clubbing is not a feature of COPD and should trigger further investigation for lung cancer, bronchiectasis or fibrosis. The presence of

19.28 Modified MRC dyspnoea scale

Grade	Degree of breathlessness related to activities
0	No breathlessness except with strenuous exercise
1	Breathlessness when hurrying on the level or walking up a slight hill
2	Walks slower than contemporaries on level ground because of breathlessness or has to stop for breath when walking at own pace
3	Stops for breath after walking about 100 m or after a few minutes on level ground
4	Too breathless to leave the house, or breathless when dressing or undressing

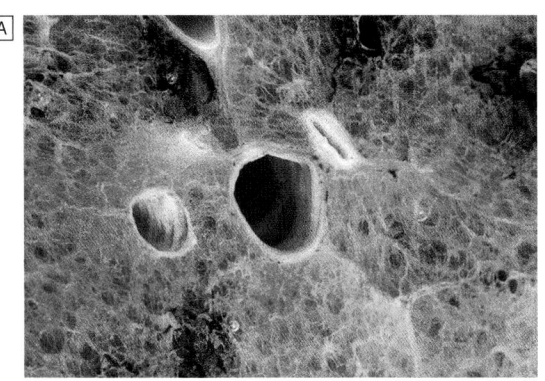
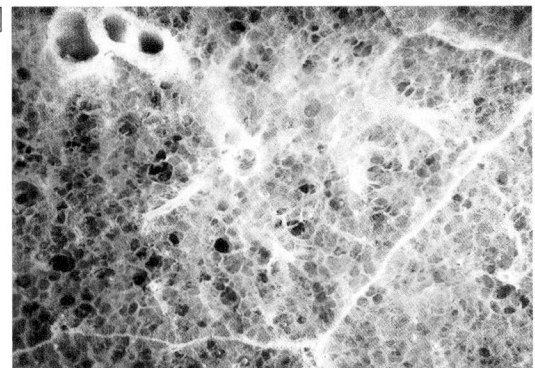

Fig. 19.24 The pathology of emphysema. [A] Normal lung. [B] Emphysematous lung showing gross loss of the normal surface area available for gas exchange.

pitting oedema should be documented but the frequently used term 'cor pulmonale' is actually a misnomer, as the right heart seldom 'fails' in COPD and the occurrence of oedema usually relates to failure of salt and water excretion by the hypoxic, hypercapnic kidney. The body mass index (BMI) is of prognostic significance and should be recorded.

Two classical phenotypes have been described: 'pink puffers' and 'blue bloaters'. The former are typically thin and breathless, and maintain a normal $PaCO_2$ until the late stage of disease. The latter develop (or tolerate) hypercapnia earlier and may develop oedema and secondary polycythaemia. In practice, these phenotypes often overlap.

Investigations

Although there are no reliable radiographic signs that correlate with the severity of airflow limitation, a chest X-ray is essential to identify alternative diagnoses such as cardiac failure, other complications of smoking such as lung cancer, and the presence of bullae. A full blood count is useful to exclude anaemia or document polycythaemia, and in younger patients with predominantly basal emphysema, α_1-antiproteinase should be assayed.

The diagnosis requires objective demonstration of airflow obstruction by spirometry and is established when the post-bronchodilator FEV_1 is less than 80% of the predicted value and accompanied by $FEV_1/FVC < 70\%$. An $FEV_1/FVC < 70\%$ with an FEV_1 of 80% or more suggests the presence of mild disease, although this may be a normal finding in older patients. The severity of COPD may be defined according to the post-bronchodilator FEV_1 as a percentage of the predicted value for the patient's age (Box 19.29). A low peak flow is consistent with COPD but is non-specific, does not discriminate between obstructive and restrictive disorders, and may underestimate the severity of airflow limitation.

Measurement of lung volumes provides an assessment of hyperinflation. This is generally performed using the helium dilution technique (p. 650); however, in patients with severe COPD, and in particular large bullae, body plethysmography is preferred because the use of helium may underestimate lung volumes. The presence of emphysema is suggested by a low gas transfer factor (p. 650). Exercise tests provide an objective assessment of exercise tolerance and a baseline on which to judge the response to bronchodilator therapy or rehabilitation programmes; they may also be valuable when assessing prognosis. Pulse oximetry may

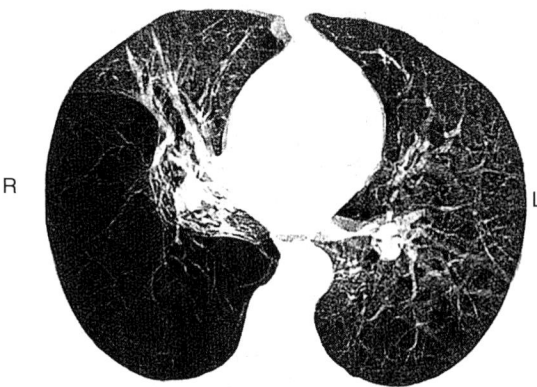

Fig. 19.25 Gross emphysema. HRCT showing emphysema most evident in the right lower lobe.

> **EBM** 19.30 **Smoking cessation and COPD**
>
> 'Sustained smoking cessation in mild to moderate COPD is accompanied by a reduced decline in FEV_1 compared to persistent smokers.'
>
> • Anthonisen NR, et al. Am J Respir Crit Care Med 2002; 166:675–679.

prompt referral for a domiciliary oxygen assessment if less than 93%.

Health status questionnaires provide valuable clinical information but are currently too cumbersome for day-to-day practice.

HRCT is likely to play an increasing role in the assessment of COPD, as it allows the detection, characterisation and quantification of emphysema (Fig. 19.25) and is more sensitive than a chest X-ray at detecting bullae.

Management

The management of COPD (Fig. 19.26) has been the subject of unjustified pessimism. It is usually possible to improve breathlessness, reduce the frequency and severity of exacerbations, and improve health status and the prognosis.

Smoking cessation

Every attempt should be made to highlight the role of smoking in the development and progress of COPD, advising and assisting the patient toward smoking cessation (p. 99). Reducing the number of cigarettes smoked each day has little impact on the course and prognosis of COPD, but complete cessation is accompanied by an improvement in lung function and deceleration in the rate of FEV_1 decline (Fig. 19.27 and Box 19.30). In regions where the indoor burning of biomass fuels is important, the introduction of non-smoking cooking devices or the use of alternative fuels should be encouraged.

Bronchodilators

Bronchodilator therapy is central to the management of breathlessness. The inhaled route is preferred and a number of different agents delivered by a variety of devices are available. Choice should be informed by patient preference and inhaler assessment. Short-acting bronchodilators, such as the β_2-agonists salbutamol and terbutaline, or the anticholinergic, ipratropium bromide,

Stage	Severity	FEV_1
I	Mild	$FEV_1/FVC < 0.70$ $FEV_1 \geq 80\%$ predicted
II	Moderate	$FEV_1/FVC < 0.70$ $50\% \leq FEV_1 < 80\%$ predicted
III	Severe	$FEV_1/FVC < 0.70$ $30\% \leq FEV_1 < 50\%$ predicted
IV	Very severe	$FEV_1/FVC < 0.70$ $FEV_1 < 30\%$ predicted or $FEV_1 < 50\%$ predicted plus chronic respiratory failure

19.29 Spirometric classification of COPD severity based on post-bronchodilator FEV_1

19

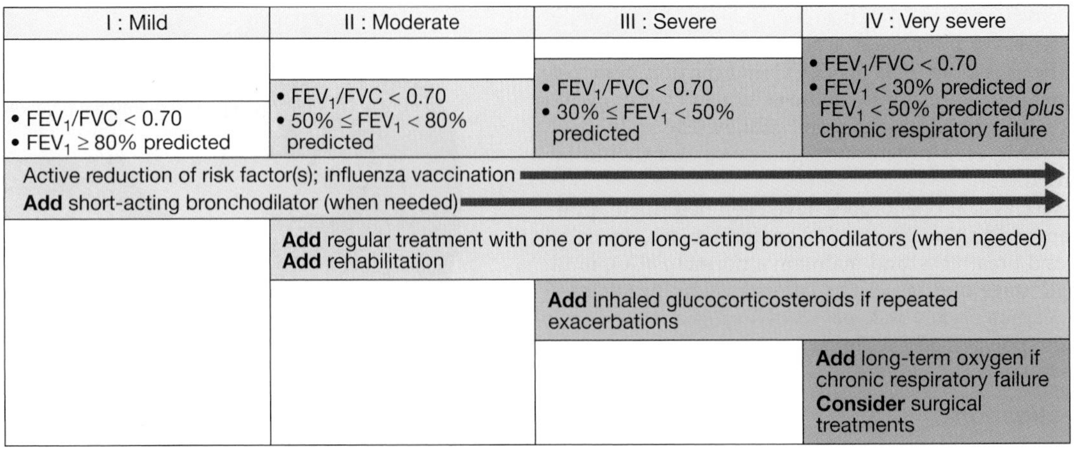

I : Mild	II : Moderate	III : Severe	IV : Very severe
			• FEV$_1$/FVC < 0.70 • FEV$_1$ < 30% predicted *or* FEV$_1$ < 50% predicted *plus* chronic respiratory failure
• FEV$_1$/FVC < 0.70 • FEV$_1$ ≥ 80% predicted	• FEV$_1$/FVC < 0.70 • 50% ≤ FEV$_1$ < 80% predicted	• FEV$_1$/FVC < 0.70 • 30% ≤ FEV$_1$ < 50% predicted	
Active reduction of risk factor(s); influenza vaccination ━━━━━━━━━━━━━━▶			
Add short-acting bronchodilator (when needed) ━━━━━━━━━━━━━━▶			
	Add regular treatment with one or more long-acting bronchodilators (when needed) **Add** rehabilitation		
		Add inhaled glucocorticosteroids if repeated exacerbations	
			Add long-term oxygen if chronic respiratory failure **Consider** surgical treatments

Fig. 19.26 Global Initiative for Chronic Obstructive Lung Disease (GOLD) guidelines for treatment of COPD. Post-bronchodilator FEV$_1$ is recommended for the diagnosis and assessment of severity of COPD.

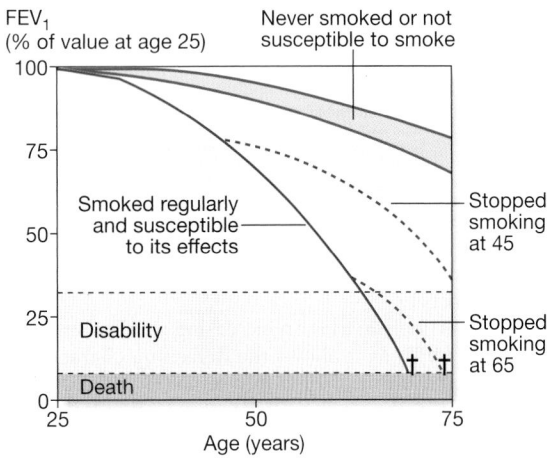

Fig. 19.27 Model of annual decline in FEV$_1$ with accelerated decline in susceptible smokers. When smoking is stopped, subsequent loss is similar to that in healthy non-smokers.

may be used for patients with mild disease. Longer-acting bronchodilators, such as the β$_2$-agonists salmeterol and formoterol, or the anticholinergic tiotropium bromide, are more appropriate for patients with moderate to severe disease. Significant improvements in breathlessness may be reported despite minimal changes in FEV$_1$, probably reflecting improvements in lung emptying that reduce dynamic hyperinflation and ease the work of breathing.

Oral bronchodilator therapy may be contemplated in patients who cannot use inhaled devices efficiently. Theophylline preparations improve breathlessness and quality of life, but their use has been limited by side-effects, unpredictable metabolism and drug interactions. Bambuterol, a pro-drug of terbutaline, is used on occasion. Orally active highly selective phosphodiesterase inhibitors are currently under development.

Corticosteroids

Inhaled corticosteroids (ICS) reduce the frequency and severity of exacerbations; they are currently recommended in patients with severe disease (FEV$_1$ < 50%)

who report two or more exacerbations requiring antibiotics or oral steroids per year. Regular use is associated with a small improvement in FEV$_1$, but they do not alter the natural history of the FEV$_1$ decline. It is more usual to prescribe a fixed combination of an ICS with a LABA.

Oral corticosteroids are useful during exacerbations but maintenance therapy contributes to osteoporosis and impaired skeletal muscle function and should be avoided. Oral corticosteroid trials assist in the diagnosis of asthma but do not predict response to inhaled steroids in COPD.

Pulmonary rehabilitation

Exercise should be encouraged at all stages and patients should be reassured that breathlessness, whilst distressing, is not dangerous. Multidisciplinary programmes that incorporate physical training, disease education and nutritional counselling reduce symptoms, improve health status and enhance confidence. Most programmes include 2–3 sessions per week, last between 6 and 12 weeks, and are accompanied by demonstrable and sustained improvements in exercise tolerance and health status.

Oxygen therapy

Long-term domiciliary oxygen therapy (LTOT) has been shown to be of significant benefit in specific patients (Boxes 19.31 and 19.32). It is most conveniently provided by an oxygen concentrator and patients should be instructed to use oxygen for a minimum of 15 hours/day; greater benefits are seen in patients who receive > 20 hours/day. The aim of therapy is to increase the PaO_2 to at least 8 kPa (60 mmHg) or SaO_2 to at least 90%. Ambulatory oxygen therapy should be considered in

---

EBM **19.31 Long-term domiciliary oxygen therapy (LTOT)**

'Long-term home oxygen therapy improves survival in selected patients with COPD complicated by severe hypoxaemia (arterial PaO_2 less than 8.0 kPa (55 mmHg)).'

• Cranston JM, et al. (Cochrane Review). Cochrane Library, issue 4, 2005. Oxford: Update Software.

For further information: ✎ www.brit-thoracic.org.uk

19.32 Prescription of long-term oxygen therapy (LTOT) in COPD

Arterial blood gases measured in clinically stable patients on optimal medical therapy on at least two occasions 3 weeks apart:
- $PaO_2 < 7.3$ kPa (55 mmHg) irrespective of $PaCO_2$ and $FEV_1 < 1.5$ L
- PaO_2 7.3–8 kPa (55–60 mmHg) plus pulmonary hypertension, peripheral oedema or nocturnal hypoxaemia
- patient stopped smoking.

Use at least 15 hours/day at 2–4 L/min to achieve a $PaO_2 > 8$ kPa (60 mmHg) without unacceptable rise in $PaCO_2$.

---

patients who desaturate on exercise and show objective improvement in exercise capacity and/or dyspnoea with oxygen. Oxygen flow rates should be adjusted to maintain SaO_2 above 90%.

Surgical intervention

Some patients with COPD may benefit from surgical intervention. Young patients in whom large bullae compress surrounding normal lung tissue, who otherwise have minimal airflow limitation and a lack of generalised emphysema, may be considered for bullectomy. Patients with predominantly upper lobe emphysema, with preserved gas transference and no evidence of pulmonary hypertension, may benefit from lung volume reduction surgery (LVRS), in which peripheral emphysematous lung tissue is resected with the aim of reducing hyperinflation and decreasing the work of breathing may lead to improvements in FEV_1, lung volumes, exercise tolerance and quality of life. Both bullectomy and LVRS can be performed thorascopically, minimising morbidity, and endoscopic techniques for lung volume reduction are also under development. Lung transplantation may benefit carefully selected patients with advanced disease but is limited by shortage of donor organs.

Other measures

Patients with COPD should be offered an annual influenza vaccination and, as appropriate, pneumococcal vaccination. Obesity, poor nutrition, depression and social isolation should be identified and, if possible, improved. Mucolytic therapy such as acetylcysteine, or antioxidant agents are occasionally used but with limited evidence.

Palliative care

Addressing end-of-life needs is an important, yet often ignored aspect of care in advanced disease. Morphine preparations may be used for palliation of breathlessness in advanced disease and benzodiazepines in low dose may reduce anxiety. Decisions regarding resuscitation should be addressed in advance of critical illness.

Prognosis

COPD has a variable natural history but is usually progressive. The prognosis is inversely related to age and directly related to the post-bronchodilator FEV_1. Additional poor prognostic indicators include weight loss and pulmonary hypertension. A recent study has suggested that a composite score (BODE index) comprising the body mass index (B), the degree of airflow obstruction (O), a measurement of dyspnoea (D) and exercise capacity (E), may assist in predicting death from respiratory and other causes (Box 19.33). Respiratory failure, cardiac disease and lung cancer represent common modes of death.

19.33 Calculation of the BODE index

Variable	Points on BODE index			
	0	1	2	3
FEV_1	≥ 65	50–64	36–49	≤ 35
Distance walked in 6 min (m)	≥ 350	250–349	150–249	≤ 149
MRC dyspnoea scale*	0–1	2	3	4
Body mass index	> 21	≤ 21		

A patient with a BODE score of 0–2 has a mortality rate of around 10% at 52 months, whereas a patient with a BODE score of 7–10 has a mortality rate of around 80% at 52 months.

*See Box 19.28.

Acute exacerbations of COPD

Acute exacerbations of COPD are characterised by an increase in symptoms and deterioration in lung function and health status. They become more frequent as the disease progresses and are usually triggered by bacteria, viruses or a change in air quality. They may be accompanied by the development of respiratory failure and/or fluid retention and represent an important cause of death.

Many patients can be managed at home with the use of increased bronchodilator therapy, a short course of oral corticosteroids, and if appropriate, antibiotics. The presence of cyanosis, peripheral oedema or an alteration in consciousness should prompt referral to hospital. In other patients, consideration of comorbidity and social circumstances may influence decisions regarding hospital admission.

19.34 Obstructive pulmonary disease in old age

- **Asthma:** may appear de novo in old age so airflow obstruction should not always be assumed to be due to COPD.
- **PEF recordings:** older people with poor vision have difficulty reading PEF meters.
- **Perception of bronchoconstriction:** impaired by age, so an older patient's description of symptoms may not be a reliable indicator of severity.
- **Stopping smoking:** the benefits on the rate of loss of lung function decline with age but remain valuable up to the age of 80.
- **Metered-dose inhalers:** many older people cannot use these because of difficulty coordinating and triggering the device. Even mild cognitive impairment virtually precludes their use. Frequent demonstration and reinstruction in the use of all devices are required.
- **Mortality rates for acute asthma:** higher in old age, partly because patients underestimate the severity of bronchoconstriction and also develop a lower degree of tachycardia and pulsus paradoxus for the same degree of bronchoconstriction.
- **Treatment decisions:** advanced age in itself is not a barrier to intensive care or mechanical ventilation in an acute episode of asthma or COPD, but this decision may be difficult and should be shared with the patient (if possible), the relatives and the GP.

19

19

Oxygen therapy

In patients with an exacerbation of severe COPD, high concentrations of oxygen may cause respiratory depression and worsening acidosis (pp. 661–662). Controlled oxygen at 24% or 28% should be used with the aim of maintaining a PaO_2 > 8 kPa (60 mmHg) (or an SaO_2 > 90%) without worsening acidosis.

Bronchodilators

Nebulised short-acting β_2-agonists combined with an anticholinergic agent (e.g. salbutamol with ipratropium) should be administered. With careful supervision, it is usually safe to drive nebulisers with oxygen, but if concern exists regarding oxygen sensitivity, nebulisers may be driven by compressed air and supplemental oxygen delivered by nasal cannula.

Corticosteroids

Oral prednisolone reduces symptoms and improves lung function. Currently, doses of 30 mg for 10 days are recommended but shorter courses may be acceptable. Prophylaxis against osteoporosis should be considered in patients who receive repeated courses of steroids (p. 770).

Antibiotic therapy

The role of bacteria in exacerbations remains controversial and there is little evidence for the routine administration of antibiotics. They are currently recommended for patients reporting an increase in sputum purulence, sputum volume or breathlessness. In most cases, simple regimens are advised, such as an aminopenicillin or a macrolide. Co-amoxiclav is only required in regions where β-lactamase-producing organisms are known to be common.

Non-invasive ventilation

If, despite the above measures, the patient remains tachypnoeic and acidotic (H⁺ ≥ 45/pH < 7.35), then NIV should be commenced (p. 196). Several studies have demonstrated its benefit (Box 19.35). It is not useful in patients who cannot protect their airway. Mechanical ventilation may be contemplated in those with a reversible cause for deterioration (e.g. pneumonia), or when no prior history of respiratory failure has been noted.

Additional therapy

Exacerbations may be accompanied by the development of peripheral oedema; this usually responds to diuretics. There has been a vogue for using an infusion of intravenous aminophylline but evidence for benefit is limited and there are risks of inducing arrhythmias and drug interactions. The use of the respiratory stimulant doxapram has been largely superseded by the develop-

ment of NIV, but it may be useful for a limited period in selected patients with a low respiratory rate.

Discharge

Discharge from hospital may be planned once the patient is clinically stable on his or her usual maintenance medication. The provision of a nurse-led 'hospital at home' team providing short-term nebuliser loan improves discharge rates and provides additional support for the patient.

Bronchiectasis

Bronchiectasis means abnormal dilatation of the bronchi. Chronic suppurative airway infection with sputum production, progressive scarring and lung damage are present, whatever the cause.

Aetiology and pathogenesis

Bronchiectasis may result from a congenital defect affecting airway ion transport or ciliary function, such as cystic fibrosis (p. 678), or be acquired secondary to damage to the airways by a destructive infection, inhaled toxin or foreign body. The result is chronic inflammation and infection in airways. Box 19.36 shows the common causes, of which tuberculosis is the most common world-wide.

Localised bronchiectasis may occur due to the accumulation of pus beyond an obstructing bronchial lesion, such as enlarged tuberculous hilar lymph nodes, a bronchial tumour or an inhaled foreign body (e.g. an aspirated peanut).

Pathology

The bronchiectatic cavities may be lined by granulation tissue, squamous epithelium or normal ciliated epithelium. There may also be inflammatory changes in the deeper layers of the bronchial wall and hypertrophy of the bronchial arteries. Chronic inflammatory and fibrotic changes are usually found in the surrounding lung tissue, resulting in progressive destruction of the normal lung architecture in advanced cases.

19.36 Causes of bronchiectasis

Congenital

- Cystic fibrosis
- Ciliary dysfunction syndromes
  Primary ciliary dyskinesia (immotile cilia syndrome)
  Kartagener's syndrome (sinusitis and transposition of the viscera)
- Primary hypogammaglobulinaemia (p. 881)

Acquired: children

- Pneumonia (complicating whooping cough or measles)
- Primary TB
- Inhaled foreign body

Acquired: adults

- Suppurative pneumonia
- Pulmonary TB
- Allergic bronchopulmonary aspergillosis complicating asthma (p. 696)
- Bronchial tumours

EBM **19.35 Non-invasive ventilation in COPD exacerbations**

'Non-invasive ventilation is safe and effective in patients with an acute exacerbation of COPD complicated by mild to moderate respiratory acidosis and should be considered early in the course of respiratory failure to reduce the need for endotracheal intubation, treatment failure and mortality.'

• Ram FS, et al. (Cochrane Review). Cochrane Library, issue 3, 2004. Oxford: Update Software.

Clinical features

The symptoms of bronchiectasis are summarised in Box 19.37.

Physical signs in the chest may be unilateral or bilateral. If the bronchiectatic airways do not contain secretions and there is no associated lobar collapse, there are no abnormal physical signs. When there are large amounts of sputum in the bronchiectatic spaces, numerous coarse crackles may be heard over the affected areas. Collapse with retained secretions blocking a proximal bronchus may lead to locally diminished breath sounds, while advanced disease may lead to scarring and overlying bronchial breathing. Acute haemoptysis is an important complication of bronchiectasis; management is covered on page 657.

19.37 Symptoms of bronchiectasis

Cough

- Chronic productive cough due to accumulation of pus in dilated bronchi; usually worse in mornings and often brought on by changes of posture. Sputum often copious and persistently purulent in advanced disease. Halitosis is a common accompanying feature

Pneumonia and pleurisy

- Due to inflammatory changes in lung and pleura surrounding dilated bronchi when spread of infection occurs: fever, malaise and increased cough and sputum volume, which may be associated with pleurisy. Recurrent pleurisy in the same site often occurs in bronchiectasis

Haemoptysis

- Can be slight or massive and is often recurrent. Usually associated with purulent sputum or an increase in sputum purulence. Can, however, be the only symptom in so-called 'dry bronchiectasis'

Poor general health

- When disease is extensive and sputum persistently purulent, there may be associated weight loss, anorexia, lassitude, low-grade fever, and failure to thrive in children. In these patients, digital clubbing is common

Investigations

Bacteriological and mycological examination of sputum

In addition to common respiratory pathogens, sputum culture may reveal *Pseudomonas aeruginosa*, fungi such as *Aspergillus* and various mycobacteria. Frequent cultures are necessary to ensure appropriate treatment of resistant organisms.

Radiological examination

Bronchiectasis, unless very gross, is not usually apparent on a chest X-ray. In advanced disease, thickened airway walls, cystic bronchiectatic spaces, and associated areas of pneumonic consolidation or collapse may be visible. CT is much more sensitive, and shows thickened dilated airways (Fig. 19.28).

Assessment of ciliary function

A screening test can be performed in patients suspected of having a ciliary dysfunction syndrome by measuring the time taken for a small pellet of saccharin placed in

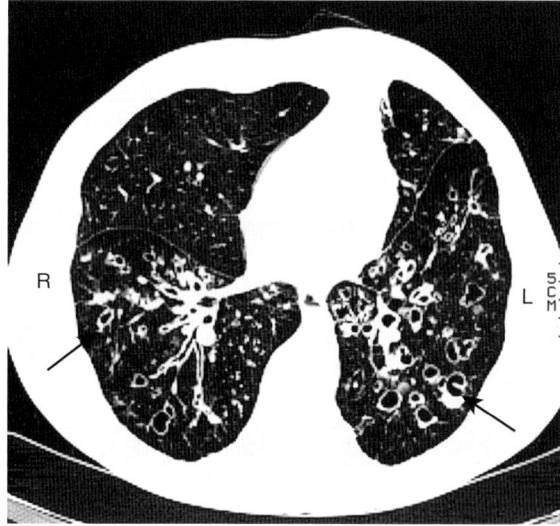

Fig. 19.28 CT of bronchiectasis. This scan shows extensive dilatation of the bronchi with thickened walls (arrows) in both lower lobes.

the anterior chamber of the nose to reach the pharynx, when the patient can taste it. This time should not exceed 20 minutes but is greatly prolonged in patients with ciliary dysfunction. Ciliary beat frequency may also be assessed using biopsies taken from the nose. Structural abnormalities of cilia can be detected by electron microscopy.

Management

In patients with airflow obstruction, inhaled bronchodilators and corticosteroids should be used to enhance airway patency.

Physiotherapy

Patients should be instructed on how to perform regular daily physiotherapy to assist the drainage of excess bronchial secretions. Efficiently executed, this is of great value both in reducing the amount of cough and sputum and in preventing recurrent episodes of bronchopulmonary infection. Patients should adopt a position in which the lobe to be drained is uppermost. Deep breathing followed by forced expiratory manœuvres (the 'active cycle of breathing' technique) is of help in moving secretions in the dilated bronchi towards the trachea, from which they can be cleared by vigorous coughing. 'Percussion' of the chest wall with cupped hands may help to dislodge sputum, but does not suit all patients. Devices which increase airway pressure, either by a constant amount (positive expiratory pressure mask) or in an oscillatory manner (flutter valve), aid sputum clearance in some patients, and a variety of techniques should be tried to find one that suits the individual. The optimum duration and frequency of physiotherapy depend on the amount of sputum, but 5–10 minutes once or twice daily is a minimum for most patients.

Antibiotic therapy

For most patients with bronchiectasis, the appropriate antibiotics are the same as those used in COPD (p. 676); however, in general, larger doses and longer courses are required, while resolution of symptoms is often incomplete. When secondary infection occurs with staphylococci and Gram-negative bacilli, in particular

Pseudomonas species, antibiotic therapy becomes more challenging and should be guided by the microbiological sensitivities. For *Pseudomonas*, oral ciprofloxacin (250–750 mg 12-hourly) or ceftazidime by intravenous injection or infusion (1–2 g 8-hourly) may be required. Haemoptysis in bronchiectasis often responds to treating the underlying infection, although in severe cases percutaneous embolisation of the bronchial circulation by an interventional radiologist may be necessary.

Surgical treatment

Excision of bronchiectatic areas is only indicated in a small proportion of cases. These are usually young patients in whom the bronchiectasis is unilateral and confined to a single lobe or segment on CT. Unfortunately, many of the patients in whom medical treatment proves unsuccessful are also unsuitable for surgery because of either extensive bronchiectasis or coexisting chronic lung disease. In progressive forms of bronchiectasis, resection of destroyed areas of lung which are acting as a reservoir of infection should only be considered as a last resort.

Prognosis

The disease is progressive when associated with ciliary dysfunction and cystic fibrosis, and eventually causes respiratory failure. In other patients the prognosis can be relatively good if physiotherapy is performed regularly and antibiotics are used aggressively.

Prevention

As bronchiectasis commonly starts in childhood following measles, whooping cough or a primary tuberculous infection, it is essential that these conditions receive adequate prophylaxis and treatment. The early recognition and treatment of bronchial obstruction is also important.

Cystic fibrosis

Genetics, pathogenesis and epidemiology

Cystic fibrosis (CF) is the most common fatal genetic disease in Caucasians, with autosomal recessive inheritance, a carrier rate of 1 in 25 and an incidence of about 1 in 2500 live births (pp. 45 and 50). CF is the result of mutations affecting a gene on the long arm of chromosome 7 which codes for a chloride channel known as cystic fibrosis transmembrane conductance regulator (*CFTR*), that influences salt and water movement across epithelial cell membranes. The most common *CFTR* mutation in northern European and American populations is Δ*F508*, but over one thousand mutations of this gene have now been identified. The genetic defect causes increased sodium and chloride content in sweat and increased resorption of sodium and water from respiratory epithelium (Fig. 19.29). Relative dehydration of the airway epithelium is thought to predispose to chronic bacterial infection and ciliary dysfunction, leading to bronchiectasis. The gene defect also causes disorders in the gut epithelium, pancreas, liver and reproductive tract (see below).

In the 1960s, few patients with CF survived childhood, yet with aggressive treatment of airway infection and nutritional support, life expectancy has improved dramatically, such that there are now more adults than children with CF in many developed countries. Until recently, the diagnosis was most commonly made from the clinical picture (bowel obstruction, failure to thrive, steatorrhoea and/or chest symptoms in a young child) supported by sweat electrolyte testing and genotyping. Patients with unusual phenotypes were commonly missed, however, and late diagnosis led to poorer outcomes. Neonatal screening for CF using immunoreactive trypsin and genetic testing of newborn blood samples is now routine in the UK, and should reduce delayed diagnosis and

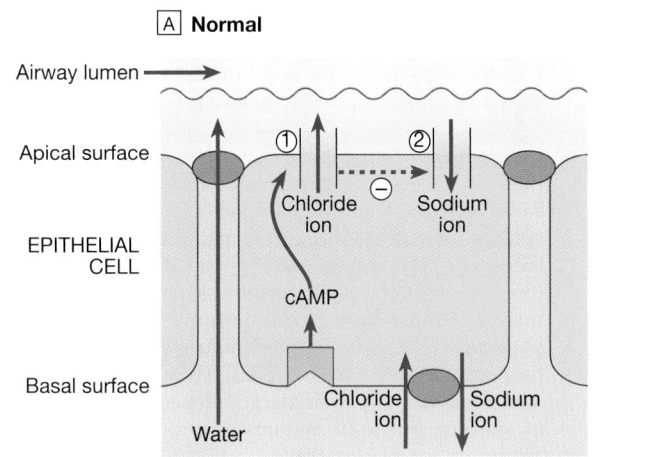
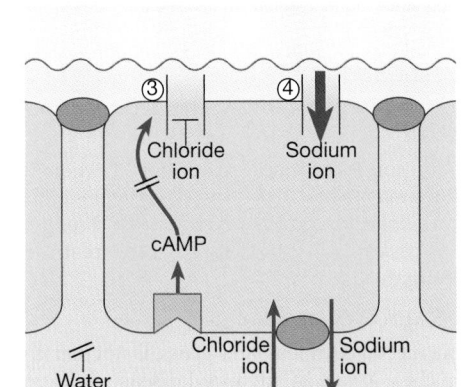

A │ **Normal**

Airway lumen →

Apostrophe surface

Chloride ion ① ② Sodium ion

cAMP

EPITHELIAL CELL

Basal surface

Water Chloride ion Sodium ion

B │ **Cystic fibrosis**

③ Chloride ion ④ Sodium ion

cAMP

Water Chloride ion Sodium ion

β₂-adrenoceptor

Fig. 19.29 Cystic fibrosis: basic defect in the pulmonary epithelium. A The CF gene codes for a chloride channel (1) in the apical (luminal) membrane of epithelial cells in the conducting airways. This is normally controlled by cyclic adenosine monophosphate (cAMP) and indirectly by β-adrenoceptor stimulation, and is one of several apical ion channels which control the quantity and solute content of airway-lining fluid. Normal channels appear to inhibit the adjacent epithelial sodium channels (2). B In CF, one of many CF gene defects causes absence or defective function of this chloride channel (3). This leads to reduced chloride secretion and loss of inhibition of sodium channels with excessive sodium resorption (4) and dehydration of the airway lining. The resulting abnormal airway-lining fluid predisposes to infection by mechanisms still to be fully explained

improve outcomes. Prenatal screening by amniocentesis may be offered to those known to be at high risk.

Clinical features

The lungs are macroscopically normal at birth, but bronchiolar inflammation and infections usually lead to bronchiectasis in childhood. At this stage, the lungs are most commonly infected with *Staphylococcus aureus*; however, many patients become colonised with *Pseudomonas aeruginosa* by the time they reach adulthood. Recurrent exacerbations of bronchiectasis, initially in the upper lobes but subsequently throughout both lungs, cause progressive lung damage resulting ultimately in death from respiratory failure. Other clinical manifestations are shown in Box 19.38. Most men with CF are infertile due to failure of development of the vas deferens, but microsurgical sperm aspiration and in vitro fertilisation are now possible. Genotype is a poor predictor of disease severity in individuals; even siblings with matching genotypes may have quite different phenotypes. This suggests that other 'modifier genes', as yet unidentified, influence clinical outcome.

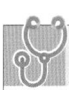

19.38 **Complications of cystic fibrosis**	
Respiratory	
• Infective exacerbations of bronchiectasis • Spontaneous pneumothorax • Haemoptysis • Nasal polyps	• Respiratory failure • Cor pulmonale • Lobar collapse due to secretions
Gastrointestinal	
• Malabsorption and steatorrhoea • Distal intestinal obstruction syndrome	• Biliary cirrhosis and portal hypertension • Gallstones
Others	
• Diabetes (25% of adults) • Delayed puberty • Male infertility • Stress incontinence due to repeated forced cough	• Psychosocial problems • Osteoporosis • Arthropathy • Cutaneous vasculitis

Management

Treatment of CF lung disease

The management of CF lung disease is that of severe bronchiectasis. All patients with CF who produce sputum should perform regular chest physiotherapy, and should do so more frequently during exacerbations. While infections with *Staph. aureus* can often be managed with oral antibiotics, intravenous treatment (often self-administered at home through a subcutaneous vascular port) is usually needed for *Pseudomonas* species. Regular nebulised antibiotic therapy (colomycin or tobramycin) is used between exacerbations in an attempt to suppress chronic *Pseudomonas* infection.

Unfortunately, the bronchi of many CF patients eventually become colonised with pathogens which are resistant to most antibiotics. Resistant strains of *P. aeruginosa*, *Stenotrophomonas maltophilia* and *Burkholderia cepacia* are the main culprits, and may require prolonged treatment with unusual combinations of antibiotics. *Aspergillus* and

19.39 **Treatments that may reduce chest exacerbations and/or improve lung function in CF**	
Therapy	**Patients treated**
Nebulised recombinant human DNase 2.5 mg daily	Age ≥ 5, FVC > 40% predicted
Nebulised tobramycin 300 mg 12-hourly, given in alternate months	Patients colonised with *Pseudomonas aeruginosa*
Regular oral azithromycin 500 mg three times/week	Patients colonised with *Pseudomonas aeruginosa*

'atypical mycobacteria' are also frequently found in the sputum of CF patients, but in most cases these behave as benign 'colonisers' of the bronchiectatic airways and do not require specific therapy. Some patients have coexistent asthma, which is treated with inhaled bronchodilators and corticosteroids; allergic bronchopulmonary aspergillosis (p. 696) also occurs occasionally in CF.

Three maintenance treatments have been shown to cause modest rises in lung function and/or to reduce the frequency of chest exacerbations in CF patients (Box 19.39). Individual responses are variable and should be carefully monitored to avoid burdening patients with treatments that prove ineffective.

For advanced CF lung disease, home oxygen and NIV may be necessary to treat respiratory failure. Ultimately, lung transplantation can produce dramatic improvements but is limited by donor organ availability.

Treatment of non-respiratory manifestations of CF

There is a clear link between good nutrition and prognosis in CF. Malabsorption is treated with oral pancreatic enzyme supplements and vitamins. The increased calorie requirements of CF patients are met by supplemental feeding, including nasogastric or gastrostomy tube feeding if required. Diabetes eventually appears in over 25% of patients and often requires insulin therapy. Osteoporosis secondary to malabsorption and chronic ill health should be sought and treated (p. 1116).

Somatic gene therapy

The discovery of the CF gene and the fact that the lethal defect is located in the respiratory epithelium (which is accessible by inhaled therapy) presents an exciting opportunity for gene therapy. Manufactured normal CF gene can be 'packaged' within a viral or liposome vector and delivered to the respiratory epithelium to correct the genetic defect. Initial trials in the nasal and bronchial epithelium have shown some effect, and further trials of nebulised bronchial delivery are planned. Improved gene transfer efficiency is needed before this will become a practical clinical treatment.

INFECTIONS OF THE RESPIRATORY SYSTEM

Infections of the upper and lower respiratory tract are a major cause of morbidity and mortality throughout the world; patients at the extremes of age, and those with pre-existing lung disease or immune suppression are at particular risk.

19

19

Upper respiratory tract infection

The causes, clinical features, complications and management of the common and most important upper respiratory tract infections are summarised in Boxes 19.40 and 19.41. The vast majority of these illnesses are caused by viruses (Box 19.40), of which acute coryza (common cold) is by far the most common. Immunity is short-lived and virus-specific. Bacterial infection is the usual cause of acute tonsillitis, otitis media and epiglottitis.

Acute epiglottis represents a medical emergency because of the risk of asphyxia, requiring prompt diagnosis and treatment, but those with other upper respiratory tract infections recover rapidly and specific investigation is rarely warranted. Viruses can be isolated from exfoliated cells collected on throat swabs, and may be identified retrospectively by serological tests. Throat swabs may also be helpful if streptococcal pharyngitis is suspected, and a blood film and serological testing (p. 316) will identify infectious mononucleosis. X-rays of the sinuses may be required if an underlying chronic sinusitis is suspected.

19.40 Respiratory infections caused by viruses

Clinical syndrome	Usual cause (other causes in parentheses)
Epidemic influenza	Influenza A and B
'Influenza-like' illness	Adenoviruses, rhinoviruses (enteroviruses)
Pharyngitis	Adenoviruses (enteroviruses, parainfluenza viruses, influenza A and B in partially immune)
Common cold (coryza)	Rhinoviruses (coronaviruses, enteroviruses, adenoviruses, respiratory syncytial virus)
'Feverish' cold	Rhinoviruses, enteroviruses (influenza A and B, parainfluenza viruses, respiratory syncytial virus)
Croup	Parainfluenza 1, 2, 3 (rhinoviruses, enteroviruses)
Bronchitis	Rhinoviruses, adenoviruses (influenza A and B)
Bronchiolitis	Respiratory syncytial virus (parainfluenza 3)
Pneumonia	Influenza A and B, chickenpox (respiratory syncytial virus, parainfluenza, measles and adenoviruses)

Pneumonia

Pneumonia is defined as an acute respiratory illness associated with recently developed radiological pulmonary shadowing which may be segmental, lobar or multilobar. The context in which pneumonia develops is highly suggestive of the likely organism(s) involved;

therefore, pneumonias are usually classified as community- or hospital-acquired, or those occurring in immunocompromised hosts. 'Lobar pneumonia' is a radiological and pathological term referring to homogeneous consolidation of one or more lung lobes, often with associated pleural inflammation; bronchopneumonia refers to more patchy alveolar consolidation associated with bronchial and bronchiolar inflammation often affecting both lower lobes.

Community-acquired pneumonia (CAP)

UK figures suggest that an estimated 5–11/1000 adults suffer from CAP each year, accounting for around 5–12% of all lower respiratory tract infections. The incidence varies with age, being much higher in the very young and very old, in whom the mortality rates are also much higher. World-wide, CAP continues to kill more children than any other illness.

Most cases are spread by droplet infection and occur in previously healthy individuals but several factors may impair the effectiveness of local defences and predispose to CAP (Box 19.42). *Strep. pneumoniae* (Fig. 19.30) remains the most common infecting agent, and thereafter, the likelihood that other organisms may be involved depends on the age of the patient and the clinical context. Viral infections are an important cause of CAP in children, and their contribution to adult CAP is increasingly recognised. The common causative organisms are shown in Box 19.43.

Clinical features

Pneumonia usually presents as an acute illness in which systemic features such as fever, rigors, shivering and vomiting predominate (see Box 19.43). The appetite is usually lost and headache is common. Pulmonary symptoms include breathlessness and cough, which at first is characteristically short, painful and dry, but later accompanied by the expectoration of mucopurulent sputum. Rust-coloured sputum may be seen in patients with *Strep. pneumoniae* infection, and the occasional patient may report haemoptysis. Pleuritic chest pain may be a presenting feature and on occasion may be referred to the shoulder or anterior abdominal wall. Upper abdominal tenderness is sometimes apparent in patients with lower lobe pneumonia or if there is associated hepatitis. Less typical presentations may be seen at the extremes of

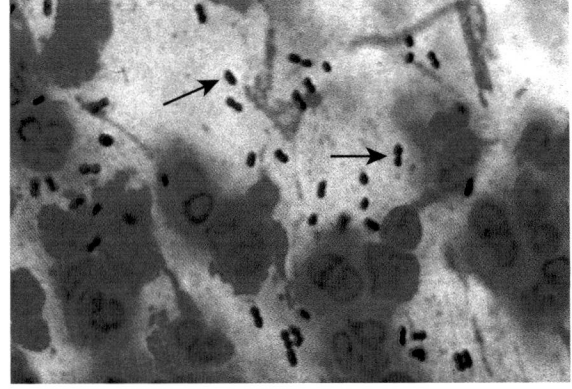

Fig. 19.30 Gram stain of sputum showing Gram-positive diplococci characteristic of *Strep. pneumoniae* (arrows).

19.41 Common upper respiratory tract infections

Infection	Clinical features	Complications	Management
Acute coryza (common cold)	Rapid onset. Sneezing. Sore throat. Watery nasal discharge. Cough (Similar features in nasal allergy)	Sinusitis, bronchitis, pneumonia. Hearing impairment, otitis media due to blockage of Eustachian tubes	Treatment not usually required. Paracetamol 0.5–1 g 4–6-hourly. Nasal decongestant. Antibiotics not necessary if uncomplicated
Acute pharyngitis	More severe sore throat. Hoarse voice or loss of voice with pain on speaking. Painful and unproductive cough. Stridor in children, caused by inflammatory oedema leading to partial obstruction of a small larynx	Rare. Chronic laryngitis, tracheitis, bronchitis or pneumonia	Rest voice. Paracetamol 0.5–1 g 4–6-hourly for relief of discomfort and pyrexia. Steam inhalations may help. Antibiotics not necessary if uncomplicated
Sinusitis	Fever. Severe unilateral pain over maxillary or other sinus. Purulent nasal discharge. Commonly viral, but bacterial (e.g. *Strep. pneumoniae, H. influenzae*) likely if persists 7–10 days	CNS or orbital spread of infection	Steam inhalation and nasal decongestants. Co-amoxiclav if bacterial cause suspected.
Acute laryngo-tracheobronchitis (croup)*	Sudden paroxysms of cough accompanied by stridor and breathlessness. Contraction of accessory muscles and indrawing of intercostal spaces. Cyanosis and asphyxia in small children	Death from asphyxia. Superinfection with bacteria, especially *Strep. pneumoniae* and *Staph. aureus*. Viscid secretions may occlude bronchi	Steam inhalations and humidified air/high concentrations of oxygen. Endotracheal intubation or tracheostomy may be required to relieve laryngeal obstruction and allow clearing of bronchial secretions. Intravenous co-amoxiclav or erythromycin for serious illness. Maintain adequate hydration
Acute epiglottitis	Mostly affects young children. Fever and sore throat, progressing to stridor and dysphagia caused by swelling of epiglottis and surrounding structures. Due to *H. influenzae* type b	Death from asphyxia, which may be precipitated by attempts to examine the throat—*avoid using a tongue depressor or any instrument* unless facilities for endotracheal intubation or tracheostomy are immediately available	I.v. co-amoxiclav or chloramphenicol therapy essential. Urgent endotracheal intubation or tracheostomy may be necessary. Routine immunisation has reduced incidence in the UK
Acute bronchitis and tracheitis	Often follows acute coryza. Initial dry, painful cough with retrosternal discomfort in tracheitis. Chest tightness, wheeze and breathlessness if bronchitis develops. Sputum is initially scanty or mucoid, then becomes mucopurulent, more copious and, in tracheitis, often blood-stained. Acute bronchitis may be associated with a pyrexia of 38–39°C. Spontaneous recovery occurs over a few days	Bronchopneumonia. Exacerbation of asthma or COPD which, if severe, may result in type II respiratory failure	Specific treatment rarely necessary in previously healthy individuals. Amoxicillin 250 mg 8-hourly should be given to those developing bronchopneumonia. Cough may be eased by pholcodine 5–10 mg 6–8-hourly. In COPD and asthma, aggressive treatment of exacerbations may be required (pp. 675 and 668)
Influenza	Range from mild to rapidly fatal. Sudden onset of pyrexia with generalised aching, headache, anorexia, nausea and vomiting, and harsh unproductive cough. Most recover within 3–5 days, but may be followed by 'post-viral syndrome' with debility that persists for weeks. During epidemics, diagnosis is usually obvious. Sporadic cases diagnosed by virus isolation, fluorescent antibody techniques or serological tests for specific antibodies	Tracheitis, bronchitis, bronchiolitis and bronchopneumonia. Secondary bacterial invasion by *Strep. pneumoniae, H. influenzae* and *Staph. aureus* may occur. Rarely, toxic cardiomyopathy (may cause sudden death), encephalitis, demyelinating encephalopathy and peripheral neuropathy	Bed rest. Paracetamol 0.5–1 g 4–6-hourly. Pholcodine 5–10 mg 6–8-hourly for cough. Specific treatment for pneumonia may be necessary. Antiviral agents (e.g. zanamivir) reduce the rate of viral replication and may be effective when used as an adjunct to vaccination. Antiviral resistance is a potential problem

*Whooping cough (caused by *Bordetella pertussis*) is often considered a disease of non-immunised children but it also occurs in sporadic 'epidemics' in middle life when immunisation effectiveness has waned. After a short febrile tracheobronchitis (which is responsive to antibiotics), severe episodic paroxysmal coughing bouts, associated with laryngospasm and post-tussive vomiting, often lead to intercostal muscle tears or fractured ribs, and may persist for many weeks.

19

19.42 Factors that predispose to pneumonia

- Cigarette smoking
- Upper respiratory tract infections
- Alcohol
- Corticosteroid therapy
- Old age
- Recent influenza infection
- Pre-existing lung disease
- HIV
- Indoor air pollution

age. Clinical signs reflect the nature of the inflammatory response. Proteinaceous fluid and inflammatory cells congest the airspaces, leading to consolidation of lung tissue (which takes on the appearance of liver on a cut surface: phases of red, then grey hepatisation). This improves the conductivity of sound to the chest wall and the clinician may hear bronchial breathing and whispering pectoriloquy (p. 642). Crackles are often also detected.

Investigations

The objectives are to exclude other conditions that mimic pneumonia (Box 19.44), assess the severity, and identify the development of complications.

A chest X-ray usually provides confirmation of the diagnosis. In lobar pneumonia, a homogeneous opacity localised to the affected lobe or segment usually appears within 12–18 hours of the onset of the illness (Fig. 19.31). Radiological examination is helpful if a complication such as parapneumonic effusion, intrapulmonary abscess formation or empyema is suspected.

Many cases of CAP can be managed successfully without identification of the organism, particularly if there are no features indicating severe disease. A full range of microbiological tests should be performed on patients with severe CAP (Box 19.45). The identification of *Legionella pneumophila* has important public health

19.43 Common clinical features of community-acquired pneumonia (CAP)

Organism	Clinical features
Streptococcus pneumoniae	Most common cause. Affects all age groups, particularly young to middle-aged. Characteristically rapid onset, high fever and pleuritic chest pain; may be accompanied by herpes labialis and 'rusty' sputum. Bacteraemia more common in women and those with diabetes or COPD
Mycoplasma pneumoniae	Children and young adults. Epidemics occur every 3–4 years, usually in autumn. Rare complications include haemolytic anaemia, Stevens–Johnson syndrome, erythema nodosum, myocarditis, pericarditis, meningoencephalitis, Guillain–Barré syndrome
Legionella pneumophila	Middle to old age. Local epidemics around contaminated source, e.g. cooling systems in hotels, hospitals. Person-to-person spread unusual. Some features more common, e.g. headache, confusion, malaise, myalgia, high fever and vomiting and diarrhoea. Laboratory abnormalities include hyponatraemia, elevated liver enzymes, hypoalbuminaemia and elevated creatine kinase. Smoking, corticosteroids, diabetes, chronic kidney disease increase risk
Chlamydia pneumoniae	Young to middle-aged. Large-scale epidemics or sporadic; often mild, self-limiting disease. Headaches and a longer duration of symptoms before hospital admission. Usually diagnosed on serology
Haemophilus influenzae	More common in old age and those with underlying lung disease (COPD, bronchiectasis)
Staphylococcus aureus	Associated with debilitating illness and often preceded by influenza. Radiographic features include multilobar shadowing, cavitation, pneumatocoeles and abscesses. Dissemination to other organs may cause osteomyelitis, endocarditis or brain abscesses. Mortality up to 30%
Chlamydia psittaci	Consider in those in contact with birds, especially recently imported and exotic. Malaise, low-grade fever, protracted illness, hepatosplenomegaly and occasionally headache with meningism
***Coxiella burnetii* (Q fever, 'querry' fever)**	Consider in workers in dairy farms, abattoirs and hide factories (as amniotic fluid and placenta carry high risk). Risk of infection increases with age and male sex. Acute illness characterised by severe headache, high fever, hepatitis, myalgia, conjunctivitis. Chronic disease causes endocarditis, hepatomegaly
***Klebsiella pneumoniae* (Freidländer's bacillus)**	More common in men, alcoholics, diabetics, elderly, hospitalised patients, and those with poor dental hygiene. Predilection for upper lobes and particularly liable to suppurate and form abscesses. May progress to pulmonary gangrene
Actinomyces israelii	Mouth commensal. Cervicofacial, abdominal or pulmonary infection, empyema, chest wall sinuses, pus with sulphur granules
Primary viral pneumonias	
Influenza, parainfluenza, measles	May cause pneumonia commonly complicated by secondary bacterial infection
Herpes simplex	May cause tracheobronchitis or pneumonia in the immunosuppressed
Varicella	May cause severe pneumonia. Heals with small nodules that calcify and become visible on chest X-ray
Adenovirus	Pneumonia reported in malnourished children and immunocompromised adults
Cytomegalovirus (CMV)	Pneumonia may be a major problem in transplant recipients (particularly bone marrow) and those with AIDS
Coronavirus (Urbani SARS-associated coronavirus)	SARS (severe acute respiratory distress syndrome) should be suspected if a high fever (> 38°C), malaise, muscle aches, a dry cough and breathlessness follow within 10 days of travel to an area affected by an epidemic

19.44 Differential diagnosis of pneumonia

- Pulmonary infarction
- Pulmonary/pleural TB
- Pulmonary oedema (can be unilateral)
- Pulmonary eosinophilia (p. 715)
- Malignancy: bronchoalveolar cell carcinoma
- Rare disorders: cryptogenic organising pneumonia/ bronchiolitis obliterans organising pneumonia (COP/BOOP)

19.45 Microbiological investigations in patients with CAP

All patients

- Sputum: direct smear by Gram (see Fig. 19.30) and Ziehl–Neelsen stains. Culture and antimicrobial sensitivity testing
- Blood culture: frequently positive in pneumococcal pneumonia
- Serology: acute and convalescent titres for *Mycoplasma*, *Chlamydia*, *Legionella*, and viral infections. Pneumococcal antigen detection in serum or urine
- PCR: *Mycoplasma* can be detected from swab of oropharynx

Severe community-acquired pneumonia

The above tests *plus* consider:
- Tracheal aspirate, induced sputum, bronchoalveolar lavage, protected brush specimen or percutaneous needle aspiration. Direct fluorescent antibody stain for *Legionella* and viruses
- Serology: *Legionella* antigen in urine. Pneumococcal antigen in sputum and blood. Immediate IgM for *Mycoplasma*
- Cold agglutinins: positive in 50% of patients with *Mycoplasma*

Selected patients

- Throat/nasopharyngeal swabs: helpful in children or during influenza epidemic
- Pleural fluid: should always be sampled when present in more than trivial amounts, preferably with ultrasound guidance

implications and requires notification. In patients who do not respond to initial therapy, microbiological results may allow its appropriate modification. Microbiology also provides useful epidemiological information.

Pulse oximetry provides a non-invasive method of measuring arterial oxygen saturation (SaO_2) and monitoring response to oxygen therapy. An arterial blood gas is important in those with $SaO_2 < 93\%$ or with features of severe pneumonia, to identify ventilatory failure or acidosis.

The white cell count may be normal or only marginally raised in pneumonia caused by atypical organisms, whereas a neutrophil leucocytosis of more than $15 \times 10^9/L$ favours a bacterial aetiology. A very high ($> 20 \times 10^9/l$) or low ($< 4 \times 10^9/l$) white cell count may be seen in severe pneumonia. Urea and electrolytes and liver function tests should also be checked. The C-reactive protein (CRP) is typically elevated.

Assessment of disease severity

This is best assessed by an experienced clinician; however, the CURB-65 scoring system helps guide antibiotic and admission policies, and gives useful prognostic information (Fig. 19.32).

Management

The most important aspects of management include oxygenation, fluid balance and antibiotic therapy. In severe or prolonged illness, nutritional support may be required.

Oxygen

Oxygen should be administered to all patients with tachypnoea, hypoxaemia, hypotension or acidosis with the aim of maintaining the $PaO_2 \geq 8$ kPa (60 mmHg) or $SaO_2 \geq 92\%$. High concentrations ($\geq 35\%$), preferably humidified, should be used in all patients who do not have hypercapnia associated with COPD. Assisted ventilation should be considered at an early stage in those who remain hypoxaemic despite adequate oxygen therapy. NIV (p. 194) may have a limited role but early recourse to mechanical ventilation is often more appropriate (Box 19.46).

19

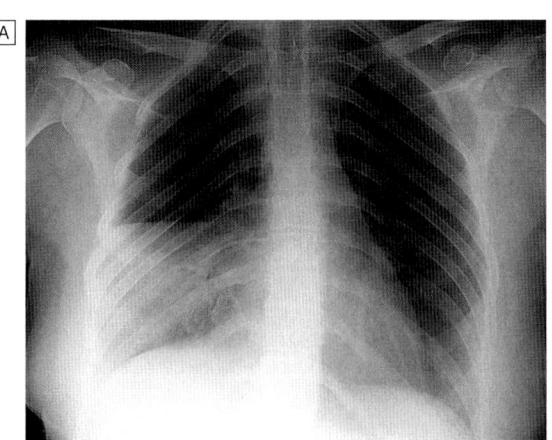
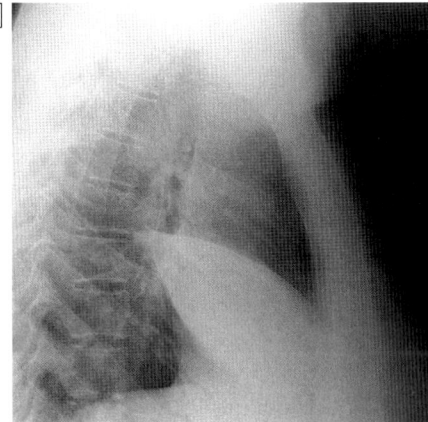

Fig. 19.31 Pneumonia of the right middle lobe. **A** PA view: consolidation in the right middle lobe with characteristic opacification beneath the horizontal fissure and loss of normal contrast between the right heart border and lung. **B** Lateral view: consolidation confined to the anteriorly situated middle lobe.

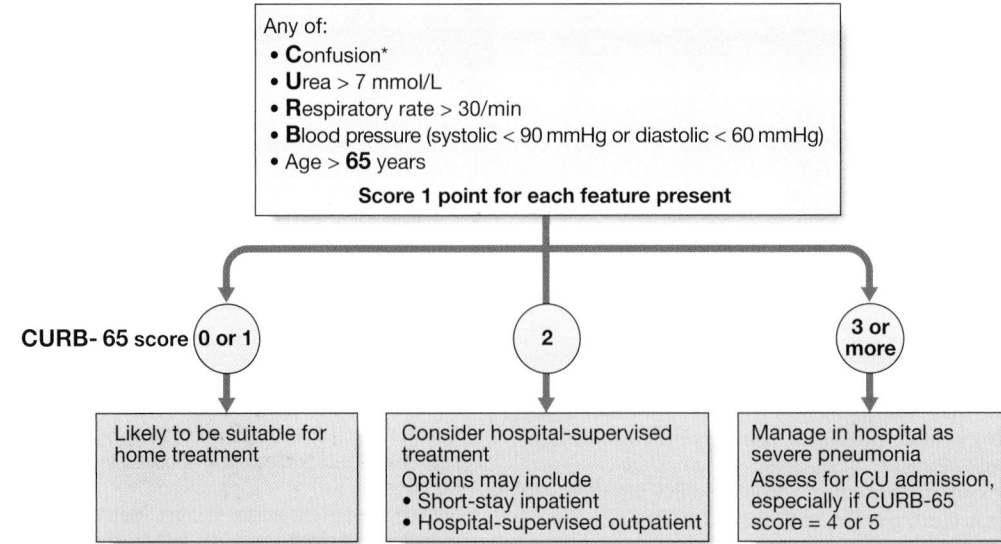

Any of:
- **C**onfusion*
- **U**rea > 7 mmol/L
- **R**espiratory rate > 30/min
- **B**lood pressure (systolic < 90 mmHg or diastolic < 60 mmHg)
- Age > **65** years

Score 1 point for each feature present

CURB- 65 score (0 or 1) (2) (3 or more)

| Likely to be suitable for home treatment | Consider hospital-supervised treatment
Options may include
• Short-stay inpatient
• Hospital-supervised outpatient | Manage in hospital as severe pneumonia
Assess for ICU admission, especially if CURB-65 score = 4 or 5 |

Fig. 19.32 Hospital CURB-65. *Defined as a Mental Test Score of 8 or less, or new disorientation in person, place or time. (A urea of 7 mmol/L ≅ 20 mg/dL.)

19.46 Indications for referral to ITU

- CURB score 4–5 failing to respond rapidly to initial management
- Persisting hypoxia ($PaO_2 < 8$ kPa (60 mmHg)) despite high concentrations of oxygen
- Progressive hypercapnia
- Severe acidosis
- Circulatory shock
- Reduced conscious level

Fluid balance

Intravenous fluids should be considered in those with severe illness, in older patients and in those with vomiting. Otherwise, an adequate oral intake of fluid should be encouraged. Inotropic support may be required in patients with circulatory shock (p. 193).

Antibiotic treatment

Prompt administration of antibiotics improves outcome. The initial choice of antibiotic is guided by clinical context, severity assessment, local knowledge of antibiotic resistance patterns, and at times epidemiological information, e.g. during a mycoplasma epidemic (Box 19.47). In most patients with uncomplicated pneumonia a 7–10-day course is adequate, although treatment is usually required for longer in patients with *Legionella*, staphylococcal or *Klebsiella* pneumonia. Oral antibiotics are usually adequate unless the patient has severe illness, impaired consciousness, loss of swallowing reflex or malabsorption.

Treatment of pleural pain

It is important to relieve pleural pain, in order to allow the patient to breathe normally and cough efficiently. For the majority, simple analgesia with paracetamol, co-codamol or NSAIDs is sufficient. In some patients, opiates may be required but these must be used with extreme caution in patients with poor respiratory function.

Physiotherapy

Physiotherapy may be helpful to assist expectoration in patients who suppress cough because of pleural pain or when mucus plugging leads to bronchial collapse.

Prognosis

Most patients respond promptly to antibiotic therapy. However, fever may persist for several days and the chest X-ray often takes several weeks or even months to resolve, especially in old age. Delayed recovery suggests either that a complication has occurred (Box 19.48) or that the diagnosis is incorrect (see Box 19.44). Alternatively, the pneumonia may be secondary to a proximal bron-

19.47 Antibiotic treatment for CAP*

Uncomplicated CAP

- Amoxicillin 500 mg 8-hourly orally

If patient is allergic to penicillin
- Clarithromycin 500 mg 12-hourly orally *or* Erythromycin 500 mg 6-hourly orally

If *Staphylococcus* is cultured or suspected
- Flucloxacillin 1–2 g 6-hourly i.v. *plus*
- Clarithromycin 500 mg 12-hourly i.v.

If *Mycoplasma* or *Legionella* is suspected
- Clarithromycin 500 mg 12-hourly orally or i.v. *or* Erythromycin 500 mg 6-hourly orally or i.v. *plus*
- Rifampicin 600 mg 12-hourly i.v. in severe cases

Severe CAP

- Clarithromycin 500 mg 12-hourly i.v. *or* Erythromycin 500 mg 6-hourly i.v. *plus*
- Co-amoxiclav 1.2 g 8-hourly i.v. *or* Ceftriaxone 1–2 g daily i.v. *or* Cefuroxime 1.5 g 8-hourly i.v. *or* Amoxicillin 1 g 6-hourly i.v. *plus* flucloxacillin 2 g 6-hourly i.v.

*Adapted from British Thoracic Society Guidelines.

19.48 Complications of pneumonia

- Para-pneumonic effusion—common
- Empyema (p. 725)
- Retention of sputum causing lobar collapse
- DVT and pulmonary embolism
- Pneumothorax, particularly with *Staph. aureus*
- Suppurative pneumonia/lung abscess
- ARDS, renal failure, multi-organ failure
- Ectopic abscess formation (*Staph. aureus*)
- Hepatitis, pericarditis, myocarditis, meningoencephalitis
- Pyrexia due to drug hypersensitivity

chial obstruction or recurrent aspiration. The mortality rate in adults managed at home is very low (< 1%); hospital death rates are typically between 5 and 10%, but may be as high as 50% in severe illness.

Discharge and follow-up

The decision to discharge a patient depends on home circumstances and the likelihood of complications. A chest X-ray need not be repeated before discharge in those making a satisfactory clinical recovery. Clinical review should be arranged around 6 weeks later and a chest X-ray obtained if there are persistent symptoms, physical signs or reasons to suspect underlying malignancy.

Prevention

The risk of further pneumonia is increased by smoking, so current smokers should be advised to stop. Influenza and pneumococcal vaccination should be considered in selected patients (Box 19.49 and p. 146). Because of the mode of spread (see Box 19.43), *Legionella pneumophila* has important public health implications and usually requires notification to the appropriate health authority. In developing countries, tackling malnourishment and indoor air pollution, and encouraging immunisation against measles, pertussis and *Haemophilus influenzae* type b are particularly important in children.

EBM   19.49 Influenza and pneumococcal vaccines in old age

'Influenza vaccine reduces the risk of influenza and death in elderly people.'

'Polysaccharide pneumococcal vaccines do not appear to reduce the incidence of pneumonia or death but may reduce the incidence of invasive pneumococcal disease.'

- Andrew R, et al. (Cochrane Review). Cochrane Library, issue 4, 2003. Oxford: Update Software.

Hospital-acquired pneumonia

Hospital-acquired or nosocomial pneumonia refers to a new episode of pneumonia occurring at least 2 days after admission to hospital. It is the second most common hospital-acquired infection (HAI) and the leading cause of HAI-associated death. Older people are particularly at risk, as are patients in intensive care units, especially when mechanically ventilated, in which case the term ventilator-associated pneumonia (VAP) is applied. Health care-associated pneumonia (HCAP) refers to the development of pneumonia in a person who has spent at least

2 days in hospital within the last 90 days, attended a haemodialysis unit, received intravenous antibiotics, or been resident in a nursing home or other long-term care facility.

Aetiology

When HAP occurs within 4–5 days of admission (early-onset), the organisms involved are similar to those involved in CAP; however, late-onset HAP is more often attributable to Gram-negative bacteria (e.g. *Escherichia*, *Pseudomonas* and *Klebsiella* species), *Staph. aureus* (including meticillin-resistant *Staph. aureus* (MRSA)) and anaerobes. The factors predisposing to the development of HAP are listed in Box 19.50.

19.50 Factors predisposing to hospital-acquired pneumonia

Reduced host defences against bacteria

- Reduced immune defences (e.g. corticosteroid treatment, diabetes, malignancy)
- Reduced cough reflex (e.g. post-operative)
- Disordered mucociliary clearance (e.g. anaesthetic agents)
- Bulbar or vocal cord palsy

Aspiration of nasopharyngeal or gastric secretions

- Immobility or reduced conscious level
- Vomiting, dysphagia, achalasia or severe reflux
- Nasogastric intubation

Bacteria introduced into lower respiratory tract

- Endotracheal intubation/tracheostomy
- Infected ventilators/nebulisers/bronchoscopes
- Dental or sinus infection

Bacteraemia

- Abdominal sepsis
- I.v. cannula infection
- Infected emboli

Clinical features and investigations

Universally agreed diagnostic criteria are lacking; however, HAP should be considered in any hospitalised or ventilated patient who develops purulent sputum (or endotracheal secretions), new radiological infiltrates, an otherwise unexplained increase in oxygen requirement, a core temperature > 38.3°C, and a leucocytosis or leucopenia. Circulating biomarkers may assist with the diagnosis but are currently non-specific. Appropriate investigations are similar to those outlined for CAP, although whenever possible, microbiological confirmation should be sought. In mechanically ventilated patients, bronchoscopy-directed protected brush specimens or bronchoalveolar lavage (BAL) may be performed. Endotracheal aspirates are easy to obtain but less reliable.

Management

The choice of empirical antibiotic therapy should be based on local knowledge of pathogens and drug resistance patterns, and variables such as length of hospital stay, recent antibiotics and comorbidity. Adequate Gram-negative cover is usually provided by:

- a third-generation cephalosporin (e.g. cefotaxime) with an aminoglycoside (e.g. gentamicin)

19

- meropenem or
- a monocyclic β-lactam (e.g. aztreonam) and flucloxacillin.

MRSA is treated with intravenous vancomycin, but when appropriate, oral therapy may be considered with doxycycline, rifampicin or linezolid.

The nature and severity of most HAPs dictate that these antibiotics are all given intravenously, at least initially. Physiotherapy is important in those who are immobile or old. Adequate oxygen therapy, fluid support and monitoring are essential.

Prevention

Despite appropriate management, the mortality from HAP is high at approximately 30%, emphasising the importance of prevention. Good hygiene is paramount, including both hand washing and equipment. Steps should be taken to minimise the chances of aspiration and limit the use of stress ulcer prophylaxis with proton pump inhibitors. Oral antiseptic (chlorhexidine 2%) may be used to decontaminate the upper airway and some intensive care units use selective decontamination of the digestive tract when the anticipated requirement for ventilation will exceed 48 hours.

Suppurative pneumonia, aspiration pneumonia and pulmonary abscess

These conditions are considered together, as their aetiology and clinical features overlap. Suppurative pneumonia is characterised by destruction of the lung parenchyma by the inflammatory process and, although microabscess formation is a characteristic histological feature, 'pulmonary abscess' is usually taken to refer to lesions in which there is a large localised collection of pus, or a cavity lined by chronic inflammatory tissue, from which pus has escaped by rupture into a bronchus.

Suppurative pneumonia and pulmonary abscess often develop after the inhalation of septic material dur-

ing operations on the nose, mouth or throat, under general anaesthesia, or of vomitus during anaesthesia or coma, particularly if oral hygiene is poor. Additional risk factors for aspiration pneumonia include bulbar or vocal cord palsy, stroke, achalasia or oesophageal reflux, and alcoholism. Aspiration tends to localise to dependent areas of the lung such as the apical segment of the lower lobe in a supine patient. Suppurative pneumonia and abscess may also complicate local bronchial obstruction from a neoplasm or foreign body.

Infections are usually due to a mixture of anaerobes and aerobes in common with the typical flora encountered in the mouth and upper respiratory tract, and isolates of *Bacteroides melaninogenicus*, *Fusobacterium necrophorum*, anaerobic or microaerophilic cocci, and *Bacteroides fragilis* may be identified. When suppurative pneumonia or pulmonary abscess occurs in a previously healthy lung, the most likely infecting organisms are *Staph. aureus* or *Klebsiella pneumoniae*.

Bacterial infection of a pulmonary infarct or a collapsed lobe may also produce a suppurative pneumonia or lung abscess. The organism(s) isolated from the sputum include *Strep. pneumoniae*, *Staph. aureus*, *Strep. pyogenes*, *H. influenzae* and, in some cases, anaerobic bacteria. In many cases, however, no pathogen can be isolated, particularly when antibiotics have been given.

Recently, cases of community-acquired MRSA (CA-MRSA) have been reported. This organism is distinct from MRSA but produces the toxin Panton–Valentine leukocidin, which causes a rapidly progressive severe necrotising pneumonia.

Lemierre's syndrome is a rare cause of pulmonary abscesses. The usual causative agent is the anaerobe, *Fusobacterium necrophorum*. It typically commences as a sore throat, painful swollen neck, fever, rigor, haemoptysis and dyspnoea, and bacterial spread into the jugular veins leads to thrombosis and metastatic spread of the organisms.

Injecting drug-users are at particular risk of developing haematogenous lung abscess, often in association with endocarditis affecting the pulmonary and tricuspid valves.

The clinical features of a suppurative pneumonia are summarised in Box 19.52. A non-infective form of aspiration pneumonia — exogenous lipid pneumonia — may follow the aspiration of animal, vegetable or mineral oils.

Investigations

Radiological features of suppurative pneumonia include homogeneous lobar or segmental opacity consistent with consolidation or collapse. Abscesses are characterised by cavitation and fluid level. Occasionally, a pre-existing emphysematous bulla becomes infected and appears as a cavity containing an air-fluid level. Sputum and blood should be sent for culture.

Management

Oral treatment with amoxicillin 500 mg 6-hourly is effective in many patients. Aspiration pneumonia can be treated with co-amoxiclav 1.2 g 8-hourly. If an anaerobic bacterial infection is suspected (e.g. from fetor of the sputum), oral metronidazole 400 mg 8-hourly should be added. Further modification of antibiotics should be informed by clinical response and the microbiological

---

19.51 Respiratory infection in old age

- **Increased risk of and from respiratory infection:** because of reduced immune responses, increased closing volumes, reduced respiratory muscle strength and endurance, altered mucus layer, poor nutritional status and the increased prevalence of chronic lung disease.
- **Predisposing factors:** other medical conditions may predispose to infection, e.g. swallowing difficulties due to stroke increase the risk of aspiration pneumonia.
- **Atypical presentation:** older patients often present with, for example, confusion, rather than breathlessness or cough.
- **Mortality:** the vast majority of deaths from pneumonia in developed countries occur in older people.
- **Influenza:** has a much higher complication rate, morbidity and mortality. Vaccination significantly reduces morbidity and mortality in old age but uptake is poor.
- **Tuberculosis:** most cases in old age represent reactivation of previous, often unrecognised disease and may be precipitated by steroid therapy, diabetes mellitus and the factors above. Cryptic miliary TB is an occasional alternative presentation. Older people more commonly suffer adverse effects from antituberculous chemotherapy and require close monitoring.

19.52 Clinical features of suppurative pneumonia

Symptoms

- Cough productive of large amounts of sputum which is sometimes fetid and blood-stained
- Pleural pain common
- Sudden expectoration of copious amounts of foul sputum occurs if abscess ruptures into a bronchus

Clinical signs

- High remittent pyrexia
- Profound systemic upset
- Digital clubbing may develop quickly (10–14 days)
- Chest examination usually reveals signs of consolidation; signs of cavitation rarely found
- Pleural rub common
- Rapid deterioration in general health with marked weight loss can occur if disease not adequately treated

19.53 Causes of immune suppression-associated lung infection

	Causes	Infecting organisms
Defective phagocytic function	Acute leukaemia Cytotoxic drugs Agranulocytosis	Gram-positive bacteria, including *Staph. aureus* Gram-negative bacteria Fungi, e.g. *Candida albicans* and *Aspergillus fumigatus*
Defects in cell-mediated immunity	Immunosuppressive drugs Cytotoxic chemotherapy Lymphoma Thymic aplasia	Viruses Cytomegalovirus Herpesvirus Adenovirus Influenza Fungi *Pneumocystis jirovecii* (formerly *carinii*) *Candida albicans* *Aspergillus fumigatus*
Defects in antibody production	Multiple myeloma Chronic lymphocytic leukaemia	*Haemophilus influenzae* *Mycoplasma pneumoniae*

results. CA-MRSA is usually susceptible to a variety of oral non-β-lactam antibiotics, such as trimethoprim/sulfamethoxazole, clindamycin, tetracyclines and linezolid. Parenteral therapy with vancomycin or daptomycin can also be considered. *Fusobacterium necrophorum* is highly susceptible to β-lactam antibiotics and to metronidazole, clindamycin and third-generation cephalosporins. Prolonged treatment for 4–6 weeks may be required in some patients with lung abscess.

Physiotherapy is of great value, especially when suppuration is present in the lower lobes or when a large abscess cavity has formed. In most patients, there is a good response to treatment, and although residual fibrosis and bronchiectasis are common sequelae, these seldom give rise to serious morbidity. Surgery should be contemplated if no improvement occurs despite optimal medical therapy. Removal or treatment of any obstructing endobronchial lesion is essential.

Pneumonia in the immunocompromised patient

Patients immunocompromised by drugs or disease (particularly HIV; pp. 395–397) are at high risk of pulmonary infection. The majority of infections are caused by the same pathogens that cause pneumonia in non-immunocompromised individuals, but in patients with more profound immunosuppression, unusual organisms, or those normally considered to be of low virulence or non-pathogenic, may become 'opportunistic' pathogens (Box 19.53). In addition to the more common agents, the possibility of Gram-negative bacteria, especially *Pseudomonas aeruginosa*, viral agents, fungi, mycobacteria, and less common organisms such as *Nocardia asteroides*, must be considered. Infection is often due to more than one organism.

Clinical features

These typically include fever, cough and breathlessness, but are less specific with more profound degrees of immunosuppression. In general, the onset of symptoms tends to be less rapid when caused by opportunistic organisms such as *Pneumocystis jirovecii* and in mycobacterial infections, than with bacterial infections

(p. 395). In *P. jirovecii* pneumonia, symptoms of cough and breathlessness can be present several days or weeks before the onset of systemic symptoms or the appearance of radiographic abnormality. The clinical features of invasive pulmonary aspergillosis are described on page 697.

Diagnosis

The approach to investigation is informed by the clinical context and severity of the illness. Invasive investigations such as bronchoscopy, BAL, transbronchial biopsy or surgical lung biopsy are often impractical, as many patients are too ill to undergo these safely. However, 'induced sputum' (p. 649) may offer a relatively safe method of obtaining microbiological samples. HRCT is useful in differentiating the likely cause:

- Focal unilateral airspace opacification favours bacterial infection, mycobacteria or nocardia.
- Bilateral opacification favours *P. jirovecii* pneumonia, fungi, viruses and unusual bacteria, e.g. nocardia.
- Cavitation may be seen with *N. asteroides*, mycobacteria and fungi.
- The presence of a 'halo sign' may suggest *Aspergillus* (see Fig. 19.40, p. 696).
- Pleural effusions suggest a pyogenic bacterial infection and are uncommon in *P. jirovecii* pneumonia.

Management

In theory, treatment should be based on an established aetiological diagnosis; in practice, the causative agent is frequently unknown and broad-spectrum antibiotic therapy is required, such as:

- a third-generation cephalosporin, or a quinolone, plus an antistaphylococcal antibiotic, *or*
- an antipseudomonal penicillin plus an aminoglycoside.

Thereafter treatment may be tailored according to the results of investigations and the clinical response.

19

Depending on the clinical context and response to treatment, antifungal or antiviral therapies may be added. The management of *P. jirovecii* infection is detailed on page 395 and of invasive aspergillosis on page 697.

Mechanical ventilation increases the risk of nosocomial pneumonia and is associated with a greater mortality rate. It may be avoided by the early use of NIV. The delivery of NIV via a hood (p. 194) is as effective as a face mask and allows the patient to expectorate, communicate and feed.

Tuberculosis

Epidemiology

Tuberculosis (TB) is caused by infection with *Mycobacterium tuberculosis* (MTB), which is part of a complex of organisms including *M. bovis* (reservoir cattle) and *M. africanum* (reservoir human). The impact of TB on world health is significant; in 2006, there were an estimated 9.2 million new cases, 14.4 million prevalent cases and 1.5 million deaths attributable to TB. Furthermore, it is estimated that around one-third of the world's population has latent TB. The majority of cases occur in the world's poorest nations, who struggle to cover the costs associated with management and control programmes (Fig. 19.33). The resurgence of TB has been largely driven in Africa by HIV disease, and in the former Soviet Union and Baltic states by lack of appropriate health care exacerbated by social and political upheaval.

Pathology and pathogenesis

M. bovis infection arises from drinking non-sterilised milk from infected cows. *M. tuberculosis* is spread by the inhalation of aerosolised droplet nuclei from other infected patients. Once inhaled, the organisms lodge in the alveoli and initiate the recruitment of macrophages and lymphocytes. Macrophages undergo transformation into epithelioid and Langhans cells which aggregate with the lymphocytes to form the classical tuberculous granuloma (Fig. 19.34). Numerous granulomas aggregate to form a primary lesion or 'Ghon focus'

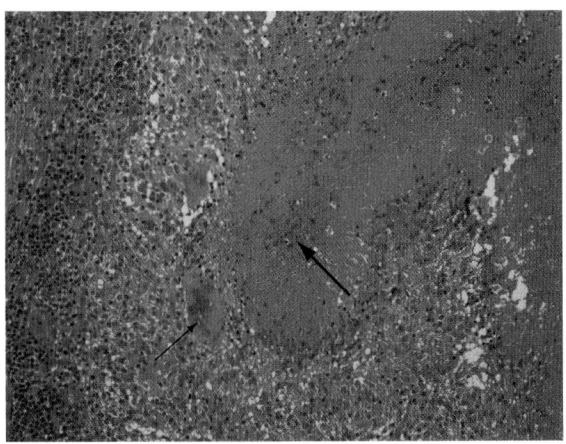

Fig. 19.34 Tuberculous granuloma. The normal lung tissue is lost and replaced by a mass of fibrous tissue with granulomatous inflammation characterised by the presence of large numbers of macrophages and multinucleate giant cells (small arrow). The central area of this focus of granulomatous inflammation shows caseous degeneration (large arrow).

(a pale yellow, caseous nodule, usually a few mm to 1–2 cm in diameter), which is characteristically situated in the periphery of the lung. Spread of organisms to the hilar lymph nodes is followed by a similar pathological reaction; the combination of a primary lesion and regional lymph nodes is referred to as the 'primary complex of Ranke'. Reparative processes encase the primary complex in a fibrous capsule limiting the spread of bacilli: so-called latent TB. If no further complications ensue, this lesion eventually calcifies and is clearly seen on a chest X-ray. However, lymphatic or haematogenous spread may occur before immunity is established, seeding secondary foci in other organs including lymph nodes, serous membranes, meninges, bones, liver, kidneys and lungs, which may lie dormant for years. The only clue that infection has occurred may be the appearance of a cell-mediated, delayed-type hypersensitivity reaction to tuberculin, demonstrated by tuberculin skin testing. If these reparative processes fail, primary progressive disease ensues (Fig. 19.35). The estimated

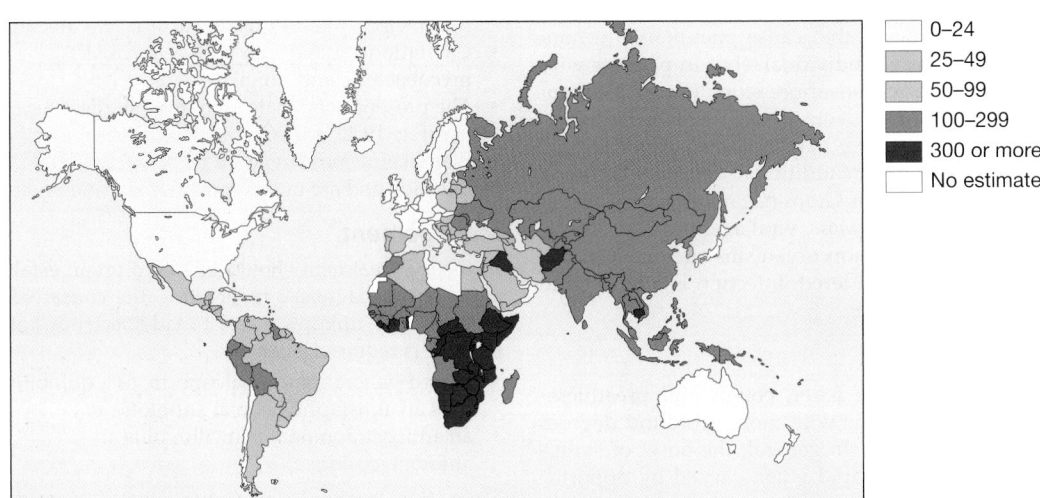

0–24
25–49
50–99
100–299
300 or more
No estimate

Fig. 19.33 World-wide incidence of tuberculosis. Estimated new cases (all forms) per 100 000 population (WHO).

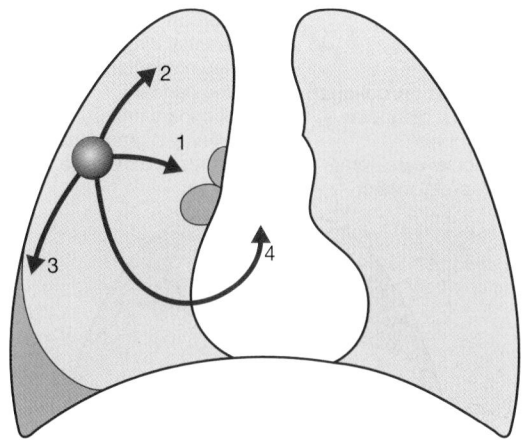

Fig. 19.35 Primary pulmonary TB. (1) Spread from the primary focus to hilar and mediastinal lymph glands to form the 'primary complex', which in most cases heals spontaneously. (2) Direct extension of the primary focus—progressive pulmonary TB. (3) Spread to the pleura—tuberculous pleurisy and pleural effusion. (4) Blood-borne spread: *few bacilli*—pulmonary, skeletal, renal, genitourinary infection often months or years later; *massive spread*—miliary TB and meningitis.

lifetime risk of developing disease after primary infection is 10%, with roughly half of this risk occurring in the first 2 years after infection. Box 19.54 lists factors predisposing to TB and Box 19.55 shows the timetable of disease progression.

Clinical features: pulmonary disease

Primary pulmonary TB

Primary TB refers to the infection of a previously uninfected (tuberculin-negative) individual. A few patients develop a self-limiting febrile illness but clinical disease only occurs if there is a hypersensitivity reaction or progressive infection (Box 19.56). Progressive primary dis-

19.54 Factors increasing the risk of TB

Patient-related

- Age (children > young adults < elderly)
- First-generation immigrants from high-prevalence countries
- Close contacts of patients with smear-positive pulmonary TB
- Overcrowding (prisons, collective dormitories); homelessness (doss houses and hostels)
- Chest radiographic evidence of self-healed TB
- Primary infection < 1 year previously
- Smoking: cigarettes and bidis (Indian cigarettes made of tobacco wrapped in temburini leaves)

Associated diseases

- Immunosuppression: HIV, anti-TNF therapy, high-dose corticosteroids, cytotoxic agents
- Malignancy (especially lymphoma and leukaemia)
- Type 1 diabetes mellitus
- Chronic renal failure
- Silicosis
- Gastrointestinal disease associated with malnutrition (gastrectomy, jejuno-ileal bypass, cancer of the pancreas, malabsorption)
- Deficiency of vitamin D or A
- Recent measles: increases risk of child contracting TB

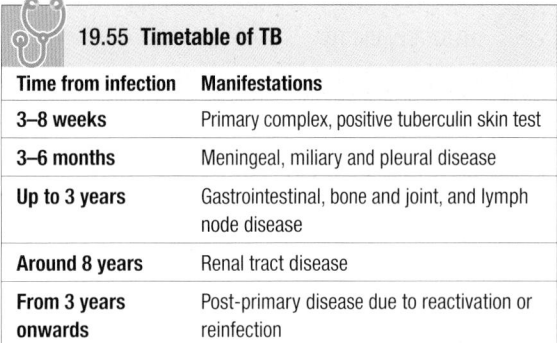

19.55 Timetable of TB

Time from infection	Manifestations
3–8 weeks	Primary complex, positive tuberculin skin test
3–6 months	Meningeal, miliary and pleural disease
Up to 3 years	Gastrointestinal, bone and joint, and lymph node disease
Around 8 years	Renal tract disease
From 3 years onwards	Post-primary disease due to reactivation or reinfection

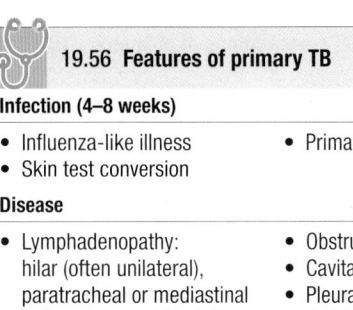

19.56 Features of primary TB

Infection (4–8 weeks)

- Influenza-like illness
- Skin test conversion
- Primary complex

Disease

- Lymphadenopathy: hilar (often unilateral), paratracheal or mediastinal
- Collapse (especially right middle lobe)
- Consolidation (especially right middle lobe)
- Obstructive emphysema
- Cavitation (rare)
- Pleural effusion
- Endobronchial
- Miliary
- Meningitis
- Pericarditis

Hypersensitivity

- Erythema nodosum
- Phlyctenular conjunctivitis
- Dactylitis

ease may appear during the course of the initial illness or after a latent period of weeks or months.

Miliary TB

Blood-borne dissemination gives rise to miliary TB, which may present acutely but more frequently is characterised by 2–3 weeks of fever, night sweats, anorexia, weight loss and a dry cough. Hepatosplenomegaly may develop and the presence of a headache may indicate coexistent tuberculous meningitis. Auscultation of the chest is frequently normal, although with more advanced disease widespread crackles are evident. Fundoscopy may show choroidal tubercles. The classical appearances on chest X-ray are of fine 1–2 mm lesions ('millet seed') distributed throughout the lung fields, although occasionally the appearances are coarser. Anaemia and leucopenia reflect bone marrow involvement. 'Cryptic' miliary TB is an unusual presentation sometimes seen in old age (Box 19.57).

Post-primary pulmonary TB

Post-primary disease refers to exogenous ('new' infection) or endogenous (reactivation of a dormant primary lesion) infection in a person who has been sensitised by earlier exposure. It is most frequently pulmonary and characteristically occurs in the apex of an upper lobe where the oxygen tension favours survival of the strictly aerobic organism. The onset is usually insidious, developing slowly over several weeks. Systemic symptoms include fever, night sweats, malaise, and loss of appetite

19

19.57 Cryptic TB

- Age over 60 years
- Intermittent low-grade pyrexia of unknown origin
- Unexplained weight loss, general debility (hepatosplenomegaly in 25–50%)
- Normal chest X-ray
- Blood dyscrasias; leukaemoid reaction, pancytopenia
- Negative tuberculin skin test
- Confirmation by biopsy (granulomas and/or acid-fast bacilli demonstrated) of liver or bone marrow

19.58 Clinical presentations of pulmonary TB

- Chronic cough, often with haemoptysis
- Pyrexia of unknown origin
- Unresolved pneumonia
- Exudative pleural effusion
- Asymptomatic (diagnosis on chest X-ray)
- Weight loss, general debility
- Spontaneous pneumothorax

and weight, and are accompanied by progressive pulmonary symptoms (Box 19.58). Very occasionally, this form of TB may present with one of the complications listed in Box 19.59. Radiological changes include ill-defined opacification in one or both of the upper lobes, and as progression occurs, consolidation, collapse and cavitation develop to varying degrees (Fig. 19.36). It is often difficult to distinguish active from quiescent disease on radiological criteria alone, but the presence of a miliary pattern or cavitation favours active disease. In extensive disease, collapse may be marked and result in significant displacement of the trachea and mediastinum. Occasionally, a caseous lymph node may drain into an adjoining bronchus resulting in tuberculous pneumonia.

Clinical features: extrapulmonary disease

Extrapulmonary tuberculosis (Fig. 19.37) accounts for about 20% of cases in those who are HIV-negative but is more prevalent in HIV-positive individuals.

19.59 Chronic complications of pulmonary TB

Pulmonary

• Massive haemoptysis	• Aspergilloma
• Cor pulmonale	• Lung/pleural calcification
• Fibrosis/emphysema	• Obstructive airways disease
• Atypical mycobacterial infection	• Bronchiectasis
	• Bronchopleural fistula

Non-pulmonary

• Empyema necessitans	• Anorectal disease*
• Laryngitis	• Amyloidosis
• Enteritis*	• Poncet's polyarthritis

*From swallowed sputum.

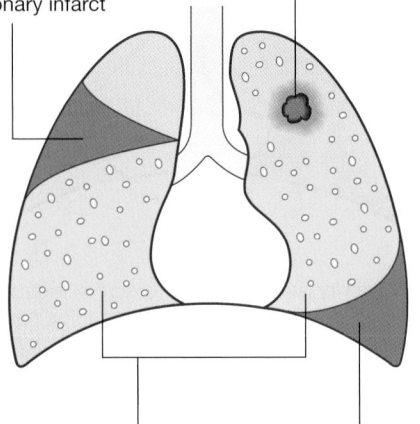

Consolidation/collapse
Differential diagnosis
- Pneumonia
- Bronchial carcinoma
- Pulmonary infarct

Cavitation
Differential diagnosis
- Pneumonia/lung abscess
- Lung cancer
- Pulmonary infarct
- Wegener's granulomatosis
- Progressive massive fibrosis

'Miliary' diffuse shadowing
Differential diagnosis
- Sarcoidosis
- Malignancy
- Pneumoconiosis
- Infection (e.g. histoplasmosis infection)

Pleural effusion/empyema
Differential diagnosis
- Bacterial pneumonia
- Pulmonary thromboembolism (pulmonary infarct)
- Carcinoma
- Connective tissue disorder

Fig. 19.36 Chest X-ray: major manifestations and differential diagnosis of pulmonary TB. Less common manifestations include pneumothorax, ARDS (p. 187), cor pulmonale and localised emphysema.

Lymphadenitis

Lymph nodes are the most common extrapulmonary site of disease. Cervical and mediastinal glands are affected most frequently, followed by axillary and inguinal; more than one region may be involved. Disease may represent primary infection, spread from contiguous sites or reactivation. Supraclavicular lymphadenopathy is often the result of spread from mediastinal disease. The nodes are usually painless and initially mobile but become matted together with time. When caseation and liquefaction occur, the swelling becomes fluctuant and may discharge through the skin with the formation of a 'collar-stud' abscess and sinus formation. Approximately half of cases fail to show any constitutional features such as fevers or night sweats. The tuberculin test is usually strongly positive. During or after treatment, paradoxical enlargement, development of new nodes and suppuration may all occur but without evidence of continued infection; rarely, surgical excision is necessary. In non-immigrant children in the UK, most mycobacterial lymphadenitis is caused by opportunistic mycobacteria, especially of the *M. avium* complex.

Gastrointestinal disease

TB can affect any part of the bowel and patients may present with a wide range of symptoms and signs (see Fig. 19.37). Upper gastrointestinal tract involvement is rare and is usually an unexpected histological finding in an endoscopic or laparotomy specimen. Ileocaecal disease accounts for approximately half of abdominal TB

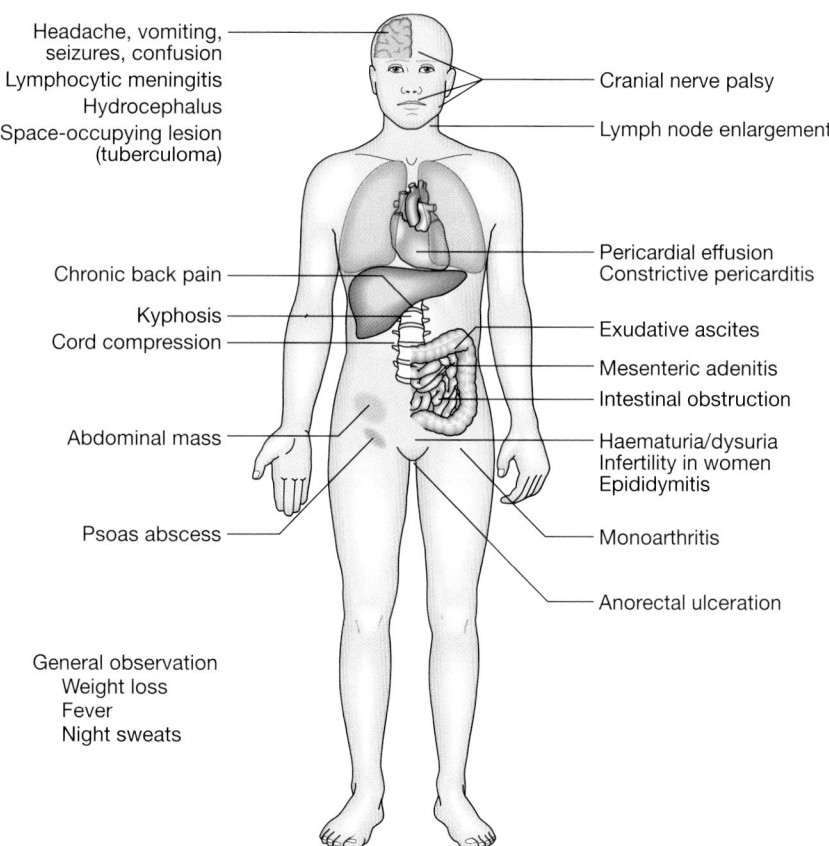

Headache, vomiting,
seizures, confusion
Lymphocytic meningitis
Hydrocephalus
Space-occupying lesion
(tuberculoma)

Cranial nerve palsy

Lymph node enlargement

Chronic back pain

Pericardial effusion
Constrictive pericarditis

Kyphosis

Exudative ascites

Cord compression

Mesenteric adenitis

Intestinal obstruction

Abdominal mass

Haematuria/dysuria
Infertility in women
Epididymitis

Psoas abscess

Monoarthritis

Anorectal ulceration

General observation
Weight loss
Fever
Night sweats

Fig. 19.37 Systemic presentations of extrapulmonary TB.

cases. Fever, night sweats, anorexia and weight loss are usually prominent and a right iliac fossa mass may be palpable. Up to 30% of cases present with an acute abdomen. Ultrasound or CT may reveal thickened bowel wall, abdominal lymphadenopathy, mesenteric thickening or ascites. Barium enema and small bowel enema reveal narrowing, shortening and distortion of the bowel with caecal involvement predominating. Diagnosis rests on obtaining histology by either colonoscopy or mini-laparotomy. The main differential diagnosis is Crohn's disease (p. 895). Tuberculous peritonitis is characterised by abdominal distension, pain and constitutional symptoms. The ascitic fluid is exudative and cellular with a predominance of lymphocytes. Laparoscopy reveals multiple white 'tubercles' over the peritoneal and omental surfaces. Low-grade hepatic dysfunction is common in miliary disease when biopsy reveals granulomas. Occasionally, patients may be frankly icteric with a mixed hepatic/cholestatic picture.

Pericardial disease

Disease occurs in two forms: pericardial effusion and constrictive pericarditis (p. 639). Fever and night sweats are rarely prominent and the presentation is usually insidious with breathlessness and abdominal swelling. Coexistent pulmonary disease is very rare, with the exception of pleural effusion. Pulsus paradoxus, a raised JVP, hepatomegaly, prominent ascites and peripheral oedema are common to both types. Pericardial effusion is associated with increased pericardial dullness and a

globular enlarged heart on chest X-ray. Constriction is associated with a raised JVP, an early third heart sound and, occasionally, atrial fibrillation; pericardial calcification occurs in around 25% of cases. Diagnosis is on clinical, radiological and echocardiographic grounds (p. 639). The effusion is frequently blood-stained. Open pericardial biopsy can be performed where there is diagnostic uncertainty. The addition of corticosteroids to antituberculosis treatment has been shown to be beneficial for both forms of pericardial disease.

Central nervous system disease

Meningeal disease represents the most important form of central nervous system TB (see Fig. 19.37). Unrecognised and untreated, it is rapidly fatal. Even when appropriate treatment is prescribed, mortality rates of 30% have been reported and survivors may be left with neurological sequelae. Clinical features, investigations and management are described on page 1208.

Bone and joint disease

The spine is the most common site for bony TB (Pott's disease), which usually presents with chronic back pain and typically involves the lower thoracic and lumbar spine (see Fig. 19.37). The infection starts as a discitis and then spreads along the spinal ligaments to involve the adjacent anterior vertebral bodies, causing angulation of the vertebrae with subsequent kyphosis. Paravertebral and psoas abscess formation is common and the disease may present with a large (cold) abscess in the inguinal region. CT and/or MRI are valuable in gauging the extent of disease, the amount of cord compression, and the site for needle biopsy or open exploration if required. The major differential diagnosis is malignancy, which tends to affect the vertebral body and leave the disc intact. Important complications include spinal instability or cord compression.

TB can affect any joint, but most frequently involves the hip or knee. Presentation is usually insidious with pain and swelling; fever and night sweats are uncommon. Radiological changes are often non-specific, but as disease progresses, reduction in joint space and erosions appear. Poncet's arthropathy refers to an immunologically mediated polyarthritis that usually resolves within 2 months of starting treatment.

Genitourinary disease

Fever and night sweats are rare with renal tract TB and patients are often only mildly symptomatic for many years. Haematuria, frequency and dysuria are often present, with sterile pyuria found on urine microscopy and culture. In women, infertility from endometritis, or pelvic pain and swelling from salpingitis or a tubo-ovarian abscess occur occasionally. In men, genitourinary TB may present as epididymitis or prostatitis.

Diagnosis

The presence of an otherwise unexplained cough for more than 2–3 weeks, particularly in an area where TB is highly prevalent, or typical chest X-ray changes should prompt further investigation (Box 19.60). Direct microscopy of sputum is the most important first step. The probability of detecting acid-fast bacilli is proportional

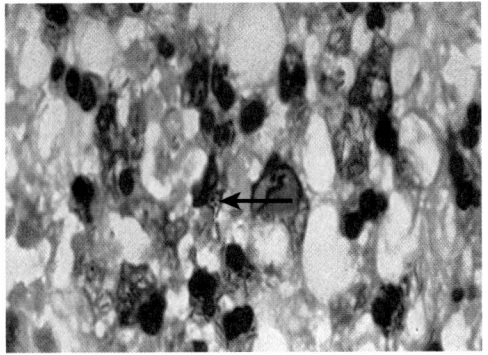

Fig. 19.38 Positive Ziehl–Neelsen stain. Mycobacteria retain the red carbol fuschin stain despite washing with acid and alcohol.

to the bacillary burden in the sputum (typically positive when 5000–10 000 organisms are present). By virtue of their substantial lipid-rich wall, tuberculous bacilli are difficult to stain. The most effective techniques are the Ziehl–Neelsen and rhodamine–auramine (Fig. 19.38) stains. The latter causes the tuberculous bacilli to fluoresce against a dark background and is easier to use when numerous specimens need to be examined; however, it is more complex and expensive, limiting applicability in resource-poor regions.

A positive smear is sufficient for the presumptive diagnosis of TB but definitive diagnosis requires culture. Smear-negative sputum should also be cultured, as only 10–100 viable organisms are required for sputum to be culture-positive. A diagnosis of smear-negative TB may be made in advance of culture if the chest X-ray appearances are typical of TB and there is no response to a broad-spectrum antibiotic.

MTB grows slowly and may take between 4 and 6 weeks to appear on solid medium such as Löwenstein–Jensen or Middlebrook. Faster growth (1–3 weeks) occurs in liquid media such as the radioactive BACTEC system or the non-radiometric mycobacteria growth indicator tube (MGIT). The BACTEC method is commonly used in developed nations and detects mycobacterial growth by measuring the liberation of $^{14}CO_2$, following metabolism of ^{14}C-labelled substrate present in the medium. New strategies for the rapid confirmation of TB at low cost are being developed; these include the nucleic acid amplification test (NAT), designed to amplify nucleic acid regions specific to MTB such as IS6110, and the MPB64 skin patch test, in which immunogenic antigen detects active but not latent TB, and has the potential to provide a simple, non-invasive test which does not require a laboratory or highly skilled personnel.

Drug sensitivity testing is particularly important in those with a previous history of TB, treatment failure or chronic disease, those who are resident in or have visited an area of high prevalence of resistance, or those who are HIV-positive. The detection of rifampicin resistance, using molecular tools to test for the presence of the *rpo* gene currently associated with around 95% of rifampicin-resistant cases, is important as the drug forms the cornerstone of 6-month chemotherapy. Rapid tests for other forms of drug resistance are under development. If a cluster of cases suggests a common source, confirmation may be sought by fingerprinting of isolates

---

19.60 Diagnosis of TB

Specimens required

Pulmonary
- Sputum* (induced with nebulised hypertonic saline if not expectorating)
- Bronchoscopy with washings or BAL
- Gastric washing* (mainly used for children)

Extrapulmonary
- Fluid examination (cerebrospinal, ascitic, pleural, pericardial, joint): yield classically very low
- Tissue biopsy (from affected site); also bone marrow/liver may be diagnostic in patients with disseminated disease

Diagnostic tests
- Circumstantial (ESR, CRP, anaemia etc.)
- Tuberculin skin test (low sensitivity/specificity; useful only in primary or deep-seated infection)
- Stain
   Ziehl–Neelsen
   Auramine fluorescence
- Nucleic acid amplification
- Culture
   Solid media (Löwenstein–Jensen, Middlebrook)
   Liquid media (e.g. BACTEC or MGIT)
- Response to empirical antituberculous drugs (usually seen after 5–10 days)

*At least 2 but preferably 3, including an early morning sample.
(MGIT = mycobacteria growth indicator tube)

with restriction-fragment length polymorphism (RFLP) or DNA amplification.

The diagnosis of extrapulmonary TB can be more challenging. There are generally fewer organisms (particularly in meningeal or pleural fluid), so culture or histopathological examination of tissue is more important. In the presence of HIV, however, examination of sputum may still be useful, as subclinical pulmonary disease is common.

Management

Chemotherapy

A variety of highly effective short-course regimens are available; choice depends on local health resources and infrastructure (Box 19.61). They are based on the principle of an initial intensive phase (which rapidly reduces the bacterial population), followed by a continuation phase to destroy any remaining bacteria. Treatment should be commenced immediately in any patient who is smear-positive, or who is smear-negative but with typical chest X-ray changes and no response to standard antibiotics.

Quadruple therapy has become standard in the UK, although ethambutol may be omitted under certain circumstances. Fixed-dose tablets combining two or three drugs are generally favoured: for example, Rifater (rifampicin, isoniazid and pyrazinamide) daily for 2 months, followed by 4 months of Rifinah (rifampicin and isoniazid). Streptomycin is rarely used in the UK, but is an important component of short-course treatment regimens in developing nations. Six months of therapy is appropriate for all patients with new-onset, uncomplicated pulmonary disease. However, 9–12 months of therapy should be considered if the patient is HIV-positive, or if drug intolerance occurs and a second-line agent is substituted. Meningitis should be treated for a minimum of 12 months. Pyridoxine should be prescribed in pregnant women and malnourished patients to reduce the risk of peripheral neuropathy with isoniazid. Where drug resistance is not anticipated, patients can be assumed to be non-infectious after 2 weeks of appropriate therapy.

Most patients can be treated at home. Admission to a hospital unit with appropriate isolation facilities should be considered where there is uncertainty about the diagnosis, intolerance of medication, questionable compliance, adverse social conditions or a significant risk of multidrug-resistant TB (MDR-TB: culture-positive after 2 months on treatment, or contact with known MDR-TB).

In choosing a suitable drug regimen, underlying comorbidity (renal and hepatic dysfunction, eye disease, peripheral neuropathy and HIV status), as well as the potential for drug interactions, must be considered. Baseline liver function and regular monitoring are important for patients treated with standard therapy including rifampicin, isoniazid and pyrazinamide, as all of these agents are potentially hepatotoxic. Mild asymptomatic increases in transaminases are common but serious liver damage is rare. Patients treated with rifampicin should be advised that their urine, tears and other secretions will develop a bright orange/red coloration, and women taking the oral contraceptive pill must be warned that its efficacy will be reduced and alternative contraception may be necessary. Ethambutol should be used with caution in patients with renal failure, with appropriate dose reduction and monitoring of drug levels. Adverse drug reactions occur in about 10% of patients, but are significantly more common in the presence of HIV co-infection (Box 19.62).

Corticosteroids reduce inflammation and limit tissue damage, and are currently recommended when treating pericardial or meningeal disease, and in children with endobronchial disease. They may confer benefit in TB of the ureter, pleural effusions and extensive pulmonary disease, and can suppress hypersensitivity drug reactions. Surgery is still occasionally required (e.g. for massive haemoptysis, loculated empyema, constrictive pericarditis, lymph node suppuration, spinal disease with cord compression), but usually only after a full course of antituberculosis treatment.

19.61 Treatment of TB (World Health Organization recommendations)

	Category of TB	Initial phase*	Continuation phase
1	New cases of smear-positive pulmonary TB Severe extrapulmonary TB Severe smear-negative pulmonary TB Severe concomitant HIV disease	2 months $H_3R_3Z_3E_3$ or 2 months $H_3R_3Z_3S_3$ 2 months HRZE or 2 months HRZS	4 months H_3R_3 4 months HR 6 months HE[†]
2[§]	Previously treated smear-positive pulmonary TB Relapse Treatment failure Treatment after default	2 months $H_3R_3Z_3E_3$ or 1 month $H_3R_3Z_3E$ 2 months HRZES or 1 month HRZE	5 months $H_3R_3E_3$ 5 months HRE
3[‡]	New cases of smear-negative pulmonary TB Less severe extrapulmonary TB	2 months $H_3R_3Z_3E_3$ 2 months HRZE	4 months H_3R_3 4 months HR 6 months HE[†]

*The subscript after the letter refers to the number of doses per week; daily has no subscript. (H = isoniazid; R = rifampicin; Z = pyrazinamide; E = ethambutol; S = streptomycin)
[†]A continuation phase of 6 months HE has a higher failure and relapse rate than a continuation phase of 4 months of HR but can be used for mobile patients and those with a limited access to health services; the HE regimen can also be used concomitantly with anti-retroviral treatment of HIV-infected patients.
[§]Treatment should be guided by sensitivity testing.
[‡]Ethambutol may be omitted in the initial phase of category 3 patients if disease is non-cavitary, smear-negative pulmonary TB, or if patients are known to have a drug-susceptible organism, or for young children with primary TB.

19.62 Main adverse reactions of first-line antituberculous drugs

	Isoniazid	Rifampicin	Pyrazinamide	Streptomycin	Ethambutol
Mode of action	Cell wall synthesis	DNA transcription	Unknown	Protein synthesis	Cell wall synthesis
Major adverse reactions	Peripheral neuropathy[1] Hepatitis[2] Rash	Febrile reactions Hepatitis Rash Gastrointestinal disturbance	Hepatitis Gastrointestinal disturbance Hyperuricaemia	8th nerve damage Rash	Retrobulbar neuritis[3] Arthralgia
Less common adverse reactions	Lupoid reactions Seizures Psychoses	Interstitial nephritis Thrombocytopenia Haemolytic anaemia	Rash Photosensitisation Gout	Nephrotoxicity Agranulocytosis	Peripheral neuropathy Rash

[1] The risk of peripheral neuropathy may be reduced by prescribing pyridoxine.
[2] Hepatitis is more common in patients with a slow acetylator status and in alcoholics.
[3] Reduced visual acuity and colour vision may be reported with higher doses and are usually reversible.

The effectiveness of therapy for pulmonary TB may be judged by a further sputum smear at 2 months and at 5 months. A positive sputum smear at 5 months defines treatment failure. Extrapulmonary TB must be assessed clinically or radiographically as appropriate.

Control and prevention

The WHO is committed to reducing the incidence of TB by 2015. Important components of this goal include supporting the development of laboratory and health-care services to improve detection and treatment of active and latent TB.

Detection of latent TB

Contact tracing is a legal requirement in many countries. It has the potential to identify the probable index case, other cases infected by the same index patient (with or without evidence of disease), and close contacts who should receive BCG vaccination (see below) or chemotherapy. Approximately 10–20% of close contacts of patients with smear-positive pulmonary TB and 2–5% of those with smear-negative, culture-positive disease have evidence of TB infection.

Cases are commonly identified using the tuberculin skin test (Box 19.63 and Fig. 19.39). An otherwise asymptomatic contact with a positive tuberculin skin test but a normal chest X-ray may be treated with chemoprophylaxis to prevent infection progressing to clinical disease. Chemoprophylaxis is also recommended for children aged less than 16 years identified during contact tracing to have a strongly positive tuberculin test, children aged less than 2 years in close contact with smear-positive pulmonary disease, those in whom recent tuberculin conversion has been confirmed, and babies of mothers with pulmonary TB. It should also be considered for HIV-infected close contacts of a patient with smear-positive disease. Rifampicin plus isoniazid for 3 months or isoniazid for 6 months is effective.

Tuberculin skin testing may be associated with false-positive reactions in those who have had a BCG vaccination and in areas where exposure to non-tuberculous mycobacteria is high. These limitations may be overcome by employing interferon-gamma release assays (IGRAs). These tests measure the release of IFN-γ from sensitised T cells in response to antigens such as early secreted

19.63 Skin testing in TB: tests using purified protein derivative (PPD)

Heaf test

- Read at 3–7 days
- Multipuncture method
  Grade 1: 4–6 papules
  Grade 2: Confluent papules forming ring
  Grade 3: Central induration
  Grade 4: > 10 mm induration

Mantoux test

- Read at 2–4 days
- Using 10 tuberculin units
  Positive when induration 5–14 mm (equivalent to Heaf grade 2) and > 15 mm (Heaf grade 3–4)

False negatives

- Severe TB (25% of cases negative)
- Newborn and elderly
- HIV (if CD4 count < 200 cells/mL)
- Malnutrition
- Recent infection (e.g. measles) or immunisation
- Immunosuppressive drugs
- Malignancy
- Sarcoidosis

antigenic target (ESAT)-6 or culture filtrate protein (CFP)-10 that are encoded by genes specific to the MTB and are not shared with BCG or opportunistic mycobacteria. The greater specificity of these tests, combined with the logistical convenience of one blood test, as opposed to two visits for skin testing, suggests that IGRAs will replace the tuberculin skin test in low-incidence, high-income countries.

Directly observed therapy (DOT)

Poor adherence to therapy is a major factor in prolonged infectious illness, risk of relapse and the emergence of drug resistance. DOT involves the supervised administration of therapy thrice weekly and improves adherence. It has become an important control strategy in resource-poor nations. In the UK, it is currently only recommended for patients thought unlikely to be adherent to therapy: those who are homeless, alcohol or drug users, drifters, those with serious mental illness and those with a history of non-compliance.

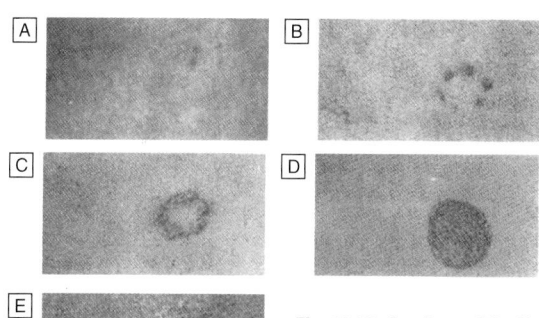

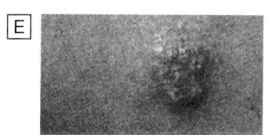

Fig. 19.39 Gradings of the Heaf test response. A Negative. B Grade 1. C Grade 2. D Grade 3. E Grade 4.

TB and HIV/AIDS

The close links between HIV and TB, particularly in sub-Saharan Africa, and the potential for both diseases to overwhelm health-care funding in resource-poor nations have been recognised with the promotion of programmes that link detection and treatment of TB with detection and treatment of HIV. It is recommended that all patients with TB should be counselled and tested for HIV disease. Mortality is high and TB is a leading cause of death in HIV patients. Full discussion of its presentation and management is given on pages 396–397.

Drug-resistant TB

Drug-resistant TB is defined by the presence of resistance to any first-line agent. Multidrug-resistant (MDR) TB is defined by resistance to at least rifampicin and isoniazid, with or without other drug resistance. Extensively drug-resistant (XDR) TB is defined by resistance to at least rifampicin and isoniazid, in addition to any quinolone and at least one injectable second-line agent. The prevalence of MDR-TB is rising, particularly in the former Soviet Union, Central Asia and Africa. It is more common in those with a prior history of TB, particularly if treatment has been inadequate, and those with HIV infection (Box 19.64). Diagnosis is challenging, especially in developing countries, and although cure may be possible, it requires prolonged treatment with less effective, more toxic and more expensive therapies. Mortality rate from MDR-TB is high and that from XDR-TB higher still.

Vaccines

BCG (the Calmette–Guérin bacillus), a live attenuated vaccine derived from *M. bovis*, is the most established TB vaccine. It is administered by intradermal injection and is highly immunogenic. BCG appears to be effective in preventing disseminated disease, including tuberculous meningitis, in children, but its efficacy in adults is incon-

sistent and new vaccines are urgently needed. Current vaccination policies vary world-wide according to incidence and health-care resources, but usually target children and other high-risk individuals. BCG is very safe with the occasional complication of local abscess formation. It should not be administered to those who are immunocompromised (e.g. by HIV) or pregnant.

Prognosis

Following successful completion of chemotherapy, cure should be anticipated in the majority of patients. There is a small (< 5%) and unavoidable risk of relapse, which usually occurs within 5 months and has the same drug susceptibility. In the absence of treatment, a patient with smear-positive TB will remain infectious for an average of 2 years; in 1 year, 25% of untreated cases will die. Death is more likely in those who are smear-positive and those who smoke. A few patients die unexpectedly soon after commencing therapy and it is possible that some have subclinical hypoadrenalism that is unmasked by a rifampicin-induced increase in steroid metabolism. HIV-positive patients have higher mortality rates and a modestly increased risk of relapse.

Opportunistic mycobacterial infection

Other species of environmental mycobacteria (termed 'atypical') may cause human disease (Box 19.65). The sites commonly involved are the lungs, lymph nodes, skin and soft tissues. The most widely recognised *M. avium* complex (MAC) is well described in severe HIV disease (CD4 count < 50 cells/mL; p. 396); however, several others (including MAC) colonise and/or infect apparently immunocompetent patients with chronic lung diseases such as COPD, bronchiectasis, pneumoconiosis, old TB, or cystic fibrosis. The clinical presentation varies from a relatively indolent course in some, to an aggressive course characterised by cavitatory or nodular disease in others. Radiological appearances may be similar to classical TB, but in patients with bronchiectasis, opportunistic infection may present

19.64 Factors contributing to emergence of drug-resistant TB

- Drug shortages
- Poor-quality drugs
- Lack of appropriate supervision
- Transmission of drug-resistant strains
- Prior anti-tuberculosis treatment
- Treatment failure (smear-positive at 5 months)

19.65 Site-specific opportunistic mycobacterial disease

Pulmonary	
• *M. xenopi*	• *M. malmoense*
• *M. kansasii*	• MAC

Lymph node	
• MAC	• *M. fortuitum*
• *M. malmoense*	• *M. chelonei*

Soft tissue/skin	
• *M. leprae*	• *M. marinum*
• *M. ulcerans* (prevalent in Africa, northern Australia and South-east Asia)	• *M. fortuitum*
	• *M. chelonei*

Disseminated	
• MAC (HIV-associated)	• *M. fortuitum*
• *M. haemophilum*	• *M. chelonei*
• *M. genavense*	• BCG

(MAC = Mycobacterium avium complex—M. scrofulaceum, M. intracellulare and M. avium) with lower zone nodules. The most commonly reported organisms include *M. kansasii, M. malmoense, M. xenopi* and *M. abscessus,* but geographical variation is marked. *M. abscessus* and *M. fortuitum* grow rapidly, but the majority grow slowly. More rapid discriminating systems are under development, including DNA probes, high-performance liquid chromatography (HPLC), PCR restriction enzyme analysis (PRA) and 16S rRNA gene sequence analysis. With the exception of *M. kansasii,* drug sensitivity testing is usually unhelpful in predicting treatment response. There is no requirement for notification as the organisms are not normally communicable.

Respiratory diseases caused by fungi

The majority of fungi encountered by humans are harmless saprophytes, but in certain circumstances (Box 19.66) some species may infect human tissue, promoting damaging allergic reactions or producing toxins. 'Mycosis' is the term used to describe disease caused by fungal infection.

Aspergillus spp

Most cases of bronchopulmonary aspergillosis are caused by *Aspergillus fumigatus,* but other members of the genus (*A. terreus, A. flavus* and *A. niger*) occasionally cause disease. The conditions associated with *Aspergillus* species are listed in Box 19.67.

Allergic bronchopulmonary aspergillosis (ABPA)

ABPA is a hypersensitivity reaction to germinating fungal spores, which may complicate asthma and cystic fibrosis. It is a recognised cause of pulmonary eosinophilia (p. 715). The prevalence of ABPA is approximately 1–2% in asthma and 5–10% in CF. A variety of HLA antigens convey either an increased or a decreased risk of developing the condition, suggesting that genetic susceptibility is important.

> **19.66 Factors predisposing to fungal disease**
>
> **Systemic factors**
>
> - Metabolic disorders: diabetes mellitus
> - Chronic alcoholism
> - HIV and AIDS
> - Corticosteroids and other immunosuppressant medication
> - Radiotherapy
>
> **Local factors**
>
> - Tissue damage by suppuration or necrosis
> - Alteration of normal bacterial flora by antibiotic therapy

> **19.67 Classification of bronchopulmonary aspergillosis**
>
> - Allergic bronchopulmonary aspergillosis (asthmatic pulmonary eosinophilia)
> - Extrinsic allergic alveolitis (*Aspergillus clavatus*)
> - Intracavitary aspergilloma
> - Invasive pulmonary aspergillosis
> - Chronic and subacute pulmonary aspergillosis

> **19.68 Features of allergic bronchopulmonary aspergillosis**
>
> - Asthma (in the majority of cases)
> - Proximal bronchiectasis (inner two-thirds of chest CT field)
> - Positive skin test to an extract of *A. fumigatus*
> - Elevated total serum IgE > 417 KU/L or 1000 ng/mL
> - Elevated serum IgE (*A. fumigatus*) or IgG (*A. fumigatus*)
> - Peripheral blood eosinophilia > 0.5×10^9/L
> - Presence or history of chest X-ray abnormalities
> - Fungal hyphae of *A. fumigatus* on microscopic examination of sputum

Clinical features and investigations

Clinical features depend on the stage of disease. Common early manifestations include fever, breathlessness, cough productive of bronchial casts and worsening of asthmatic symptoms. The appearance of radiographic infiltrates may cause ABPA to be mistaken for pneumonia, but the diagnosis may also be suggested by abnormalities such as segmented or lobar collapse on chest X-rays of patients whose asthmatic symptoms are stable. Diagnostic features are shown in Box 19.68. If bronchiectasis develops, its symptoms and complications often overshadow those of asthma.

Management

ABPA is generally an indication for regular low-dose oral corticosteroids (prednisolone 7.5–10 mg daily) to suppress the immunopathological responses and prevent progress to tissue damage. In some patients, itraconazole (400 mg/day) allows a reduction in oral steroids; a 4-month trial is usually recommended to assess its efficacy. The use of specific anti-IgE monoclonal antibodies is under consideration. Exacerbations, particularly when associated with new chest X-ray changes, should be treated promptly with prednisolone 40–60 mg daily and physiotherapy. If persistent lobar collapse occurs, bronchoscopy (usually under general anaesthetic) should be performed to remove impacted mucus and ensure prompt reinflation.

Aspergilloma

Inhaled *Aspergillus* may lodge and germinate in areas of damaged lung tissue forming a fungal ball or aspergilloma. The upper lobes are most frequently involved, and fungal balls readily form in tuberculous cavities (Fig. 19.40). Less common causes include damage from a lung abscess cavity, a bronchiectatic space, pulmonary infarct,

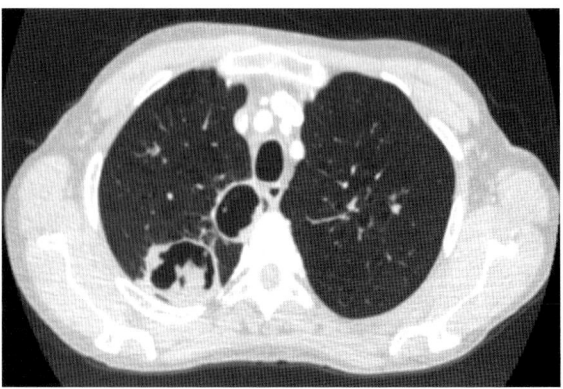

Fig. 19.40 CT of aspergilloma in the left upper lobe. The rounded fungal ball is separated from the wall of the cavity by a 'halo' of air.

sarcoid, ankylosing spondylitis or a cavitated tumour. The presence of multiple aspergilloma cavities in a diseased area of lung has been termed 'complex aspergilloma' (see below).

Clinical features and diagnosis

Simple aspergillomas are often asymptomatic, and are identified incidentally on chest X-ray. However, they may cause recurrent haemoptysis which can be severe and life-threatening.

The fungal ball produces a tumour-like opacity on X-ray, but can be distinguished from a carcinoma by the presence of a crescent of air between the fungal ball and the upper wall of the cavity. HRCT is more sensitive (see Fig. 19.40). Elevated serum precipitins to *A. fumigatus* are found in virtually all patients. Sputum microscopy typically demonstrates scanty hyphal fragments, and is usually positive on culture. Less than half exhibit skin hypersensitivity to extracts of *A. fumigatus*. Rarely, other filamentous fungi can cause intracavitary mycetoma and are identified by culture; antibody tests are unavailable.

Management

Asymptomatic cases do not require treatment. Specific antifungal therapy is of no value and steroids may predispose to invasion. Aspergillomas complicated by haemoptysis should be excised surgically. In those unfit for surgery, palliative procedures range from local instillation of amphotericin B to bronchial artery embolisation. The latter has also been used to control haemoptysis as a prelude to definitive surgery.

Invasive pulmonary aspergillosis (IPA)

IPA is most commonly a complication of profound neutropenia caused by drugs (especially immunosuppressants) and/or disease (Box 19.69).

Clinical features and diagnosis

Acute IPA causes a severe necrotising pneumonia, and must be considered in any immunocompromised patient who develops fever, new respiratory symptoms (particularly pleural pain or haemoptysis) or a pleural rub. Invasion of pulmonary vessels causes thrombosis and infarction, and systemic spread may occur to the brain, heart, kidneys and other organs. Tracheobronchial aspergillosis complicates lung transplant and presents with large airway invasion, fungal plaques and ulceration.

HRCT characteristically shows macronodules (usually ≥ 1 cm), which may be surrounded by a 'halo' of low attenuation if captured early (< 5 days). Culture or histopathological evidence of *Aspergillus* in diseased tissue gives a definitive diagnosis, but the majority of patients are too ill for invasive tests such as bronchoscopy or lung biopsy. Other investigations include detection of *Aspergillus* cell wall components (galactomannan and β-1,3-glucan) in blood or BAL fluid, and *Aspergillus* DNA by PCR. Diagnosis is most often inferred from a combination of features (Box 19.70).

Management and prevention

IPA carries a high mortality rate, especially if treatment is delayed. The treatment of choice is voriconazole. Second-line agents include lipid-associated amphotericin, caspofungin or posaconazole. Response is assessed both clinically and radiologically. Recovery is dependent on immune reconstitution, which may be accompanied by enlargement and/or cavitation of pulmonary nodules.

Patients at risk of *Aspergillus* (and other fungal infections) should be nursed in rooms with high-efficiency particulate air (HEPA) filters and laminar airflow. In

19.70 Criteria for the diagnosis of probable invasive pulmonary aspergillosis[1]

Host factors

- Recent history of neutropenia ($< 0.5 \times 10^9$/L for ≥ 10 days) temporally related to the onset of fungal disease
- Recipient of allogeneic stem cell transplant
- Prolonged use of corticosteroids (average minimum 0.3 mg/kg/day prednisolone or equivalent) for > 3 weeks (excludes ABPA)
- Treatment with other recognised T-cell immune suppressants such as ciclosporin, TNF-α blockers, specific monoclonal antibodies (e.g. alemtuzumab) or nucleoside analogues during the last 90 days
- Inherited severe immune deficiency, e.g. chronic granulomatous disease or severe combined immune deficiency (p. 79)

Clinical criteria[2]

- The presence of one of the following three imaging signs on CT:
    1. Dense, well-circumscribed lesion(s) with or without a halo sign
    2. Air crescent sign
    3. Cavity

Tracheobronchitis

- Tracheobronchial ulceration, nodule, pseudomembrane, plaque or eschar seen on bronchoscopy

Mycological criteria

- Mould in sputum, BAL fluid or bronchial brush, indicated by one of the following:
    1. Recovery of fungal elements indicating a mould of *Aspergillus*
    2. Recovery by culture of a mould of *Aspergillus*
- Indirect tests (detection of antigen or cell wall constituents)
    1. Galactomannan antigen in plasma, serum or BAL fluid
    2. β-1,3-glucan detected in serum (detects other species of fungi as well as *Aspergillus*)[3]

[1]Adapted from European Organisation for Research and Treatment of Cancer/Mycoses Study Group.
[2]Must be consistent with the mycological findings, if any, and temporally related to current episode.
[3]May be useful as a preliminary screening tool for invasive aspergillosis.

19.69 Risk factors for invasive aspergillosis

- Neutropenia: risk related to duration and degree
- Solid organ or allogenic stem cell transplantation
- Prolonged high dose corticosteroid therapy
- Leukaemia and other haematological malignancies
- Cytotoxic chemotherapy
- Advanced HIV disease
- Severe COPD
- Critically ill patients on intensive care units
- Chronic granulomatous disease

areas with high spore counts, patients may be advised to wear a mask if venturing outside their hospital room. Posaconazole (200 mg 8-hourly) or itraconazole (200 mg/day) may be prescribed for primary prophylaxis, and patients with a history of definite or probable IPA should be considered for secondary prophylaxis before further immunosuppression.

Chronic and subacute pulmonary aspergillosis

Chronic pulmonary aspergillosis (CPA) is an indolent, non-invasive complication of chronic lung disease such as COPD, tuberculosis/non-tuberculous mycobacterial disease or fibrotic conditions; it may be associated with malnutrition, diabetes or liver disease, and co-infection with non-tuberculous mycobacteria. CPA may mimic TB, resulting in its delayed diagnosis. Features include cough (with or without haemoptysis), weight loss, anorexia and fatigue over months or years, with associated fever, night sweats, and an elevated CRP and ESR. Radiological features include thick-walled cavities (predominantly apical), pulmonary infiltrates, pleural thickening and, later, fibrosis. The terms chronic necrotising (CNPA), cavitary ('complex aspergilloma') and fibrosing pulmonary aspergillosis have been applied, depending on predominant features. There is overlap between CNPA, 'subacute' and 'semi-invasive' aspergillosis. Subacute aspergillosis/CNPA is an increasingly recognised complication in patients in intensive care, especially in the presence of pre-existing COPD. Diagnosis is achieved by a combination of radiological examination, histopathology, isolation of the fungus in sputum and detection of *Aspergillus* IgG in serum. Disease is usually treated with prolonged/indefinite courses of itraconazole or voriconazole, but cure is unusual. The most frequent pattern is chronic relapse/remission with gradual, inexorable deterioration. Surgical intervention is fraught with complications and should be avoided.

Other fungal infections
Pulmonary mucormycosis and endemic mycoses

Mucormycosis (p. 379) may present with a pulmonary syndrome indistinguishable clinically from acute IPA. Diagnosis relies on histopathology (where available) and/or culture of the organism from diseased tissue. The principles of treatment are as for other forms of mucormycosis: correction of predisposing factors, antifungal therapy with high-dose lipid-amphotericin B or posaconazole, and surgical débridement.

Histoplasmosis, coccidioidomycosis, blastomycosis and cryptococcosis

These are discussed on pages 379–381.

TUMOURS OF THE BRONCHUS AND LUNG

Lung cancer is the most common cause of death from cancer world-wide, causing 1.4 million deaths per year. Tobacco use is the major preventable cause; however,

> **19.71 The burden of lung cancer**
>
> - Strikes 900 000 men and 330 000 women each year
> - Accounts for 18% of all cancer deaths
> - More than a threefold increase in deaths since 1950
> - Rates rising in women: female lung cancer deaths outnumber male in some Nordic countries
> - Has overtaken breast cancer in several countries, making it the most common cause of cancer death in men and women

just as tobacco use and cancer rates are falling in some developed countries, both smoking and lung cancer are rising in Eastern Europe and in many developing countries (Box 19.71). The great majority of tumours in the lung are primary bronchial carcinomas, and in contrast to many other tumours, the prognosis remains poor, with fewer than 30% of patients surviving at 1 year and 6–8 % at 5 years. Carcinomas of many other organs, as well as osteogenic and other sarcomas, may cause metastatic pulmonary deposits.

Primary tumours of the lung

Aetiology

Cigarette smoking is by far the most important cause of lung cancer. It is thought to be directly responsible for at least 90% of lung carcinomas, the risk being proportional to the amount smoked and to the tar content of cigarettes. The death rate from the disease in heavy smokers is 40 times that in non-smokers. Risk falls slowly after smoking cessation, but remains above that in non-smokers for many years. It is estimated that 1 in 2 smokers dies from a smoking-related disease, about half in middle age. The effect of 'passive' smoking is more difficult to quantify but is currently thought to be a factor in 5% of all lung cancer deaths. Exposure to naturally occurring radon is another risk. The incidence of lung cancer is slightly higher in urban than in rural dwellers, which may reflect differences in atmospheric pollution (including tobacco smoke) or occupation, since a number of industrial materials (e.g. asbestos, silica, beryllium, cadmium and chromium) are associated with lung cancer. In recent years, the strong link between smoking and ill health has led many Western governments to legislate against smoking in public places, and smoking prevalence and some smoking-related diseases are already declining in these countries (pp. 98–99).

Bronchial carcinoma

The incidence of bronchial carcinoma increased dramatically during the 20th century as a direct result of the tobacco epidemic (Fig. 19.41). In women, smoking prevalence and deaths from lung cancer continue to increase, and more women now die of lung cancer than breast cancer in the USA and the UK.

Pathology

Bronchial carcinomas arise from the bronchial epithelium or mucous glands. The common cell types are listed in Box 19.72. When the tumour occurs in a large bronchus, symptoms arise early, but tumours originating in a peripheral bronchus can grow very large

Males

Rate per 100 000

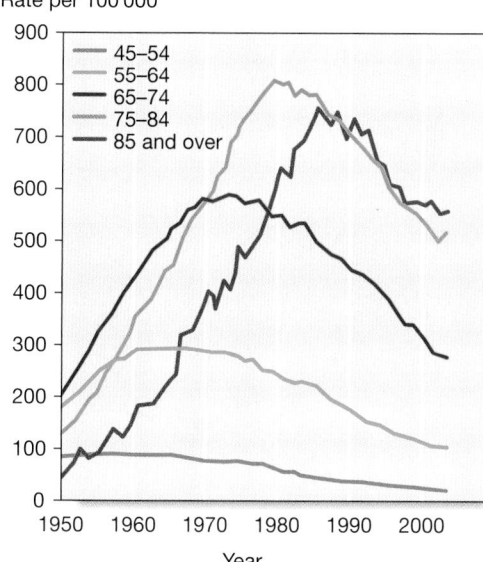

Females

Rate per 100 000

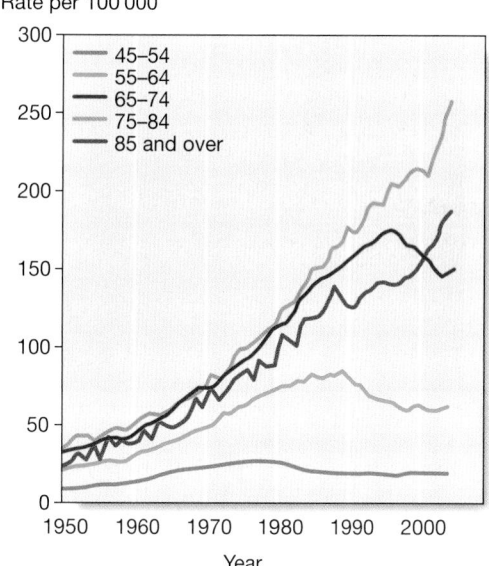

Fig. 19.41 Mortality trends from lung cancer in England and Wales, 1950–2004 by age and year of death. A Males. B Females. Note the decline in mortality from lung cancer in men towards the end of this period, reflecting a change in smoking habit.

19.72 Common cell types in bronchial carcinoma

Cell type	%
Squamous	35
Adenocarcinoma	30
Small-cell	20
Large-cell	15

without producing symptoms, resulting in delayed diagnosis. Peripheral squamous tumours may undergo central necrosis and cavitation, and may resemble a lung abscess on X-ray (Fig. 19.42). Bronchial carcinoma may involve the pleura either directly or by lymphatic spread and may extend into the chest wall, invading the intercostal nerves or the brachial plexus and causing pain. Lymphatic spread to mediastinal and supraclavicular lymph nodes frequently occurs prior to diagnosis. Blood-borne metastases occur most commonly in liver, bone, brain, adrenals and skin. Even a small primary tumour may cause widespread metastatic deposits and this is a particular characteristic of small-cell lung cancers.

Clinical features

Lung cancer presents in many different ways, reflecting local, metastatic or paraneoplastic tumour effects.

- *Cough.* The most common early symptom, cough is often dry; however, secondary infection may cause purulent sputum. A change in the character of a smoker's cough, particularly if associated with other new symptoms, should always raise suspicion of bronchial carcinoma.
- *Haemoptysis.* This is common, especially with central bronchial tumours. Although it frequently

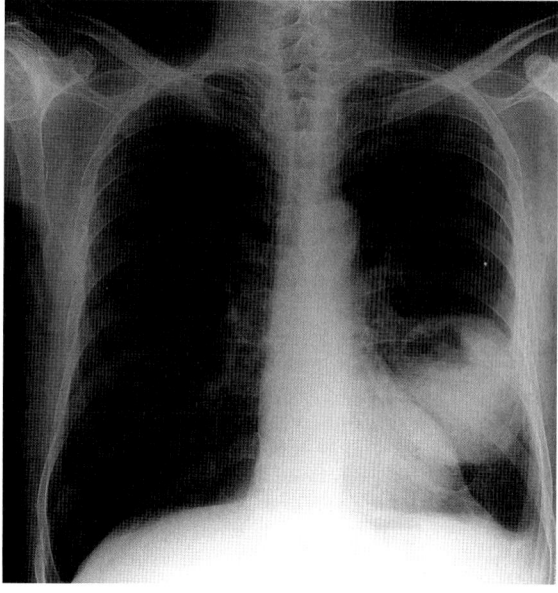

Fig. 19.42 Large cavitated bronchial carcinoma in left lower lobe.

accompanies bronchitic infection and may be benign, haemoptysis in a smoker should always be investigated to exclude a bronchial carcinoma. Occasionally, central tumours invade large vessels, causing sudden massive haemoptysis which may be fatal.
- *Bronchial obstruction.* This is another common presentation, and the clinical and radiological manifestations (Figs 19.43 and 19.44; Box 19.73) depend on the site and extent of the obstruction, any secondary infection, and the extent of coexisting lung disease. Complete obstruction causes collapse

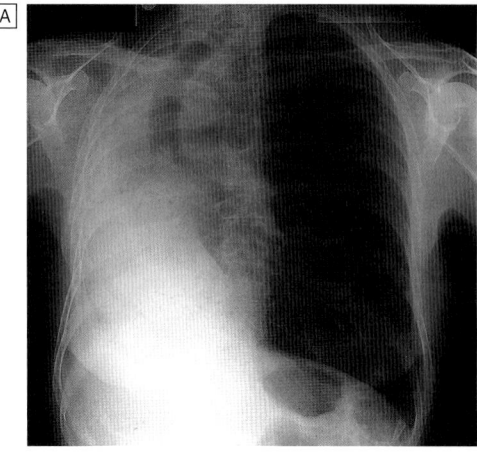

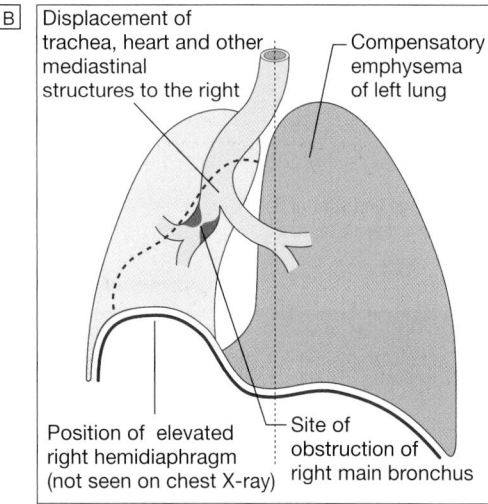

Fig. 19.43 Collapse of the right lung: effects on neighbouring structures. A Chest X-ray. B Abnormalities highlighted.

of a lobe or lung, with breathlessness, mediastinal displacement and dullness to percussion with reduced breath sounds. Partial bronchial obstruction may cause a monophonic, unilateral wheeze that fails to clear with coughing and may also impair the drainage of secretions sufficiently to cause pneumonia or lung abscess as a presenting problem. Pneumonia that recurs at the same site or responds slowly to treatment, particularly in a smoker, should always suggest an underlying bronchial carcinoma. Stridor (a harsh inspiratory noise) occurs when the lower trachea, carina or main bronchi are narrowed by the primary tumour or by compression from malignant enlargement of the subcarinal and paratracheal lymph nodes.

- *Breathlessness.* This may be caused by collapse or pneumonia, or by tumour causing a large pleural effusion or compressing a phrenic nerve causing diaphragmatic paralysis.
- *Pain and nerve entrapment.* Pleural pain usually indicates malignant pleural invasion, although it can occur with distal infection. Intercostal nerve involvement causes pain in the distribution of a thoracic dermatome. Carcinoma in the lung apex may cause Horner's syndrome (ipsilateral partial

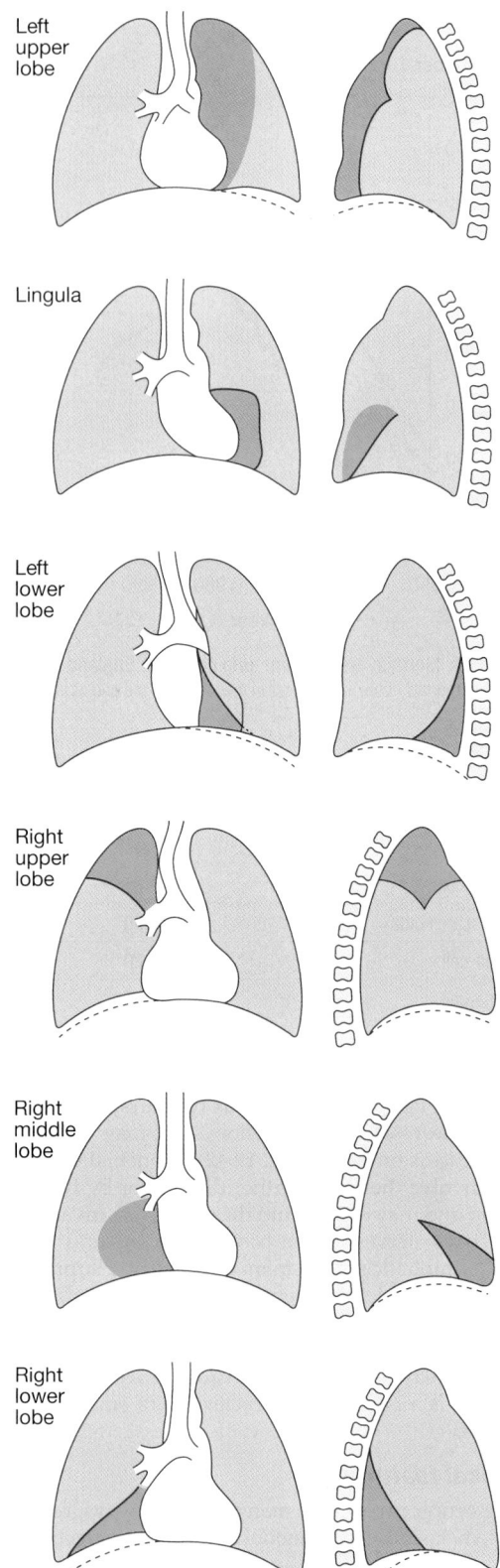

Fig. 19.44 Radiological features of lobar collapse caused by bronchial obstruction. The dotted line in the drawings represents the normal position of the diaphragm.

19.73 Causes of large bronchus obstruction

Common

- Bronchial carcinoma or adenoma
- Enlarged tracheobronchial lymph nodes (malignant or tuberculous)
- Inhaled foreign bodies (especially right lung and in children)
- Bronchial casts or plugs consisting of inspissated mucus or blood clot (especially asthma, cystic fibrosis, haemoptysis, debility)
- Collections of mucus or mucopus retained in the bronchi as a result of ineffective expectoration (especially post-operative following abdominal surgery)

Rare

- Aortic aneurysm
- Giant left atrium
- Pericardial effusion
- Congenital bronchial atresia
- Fibrous bronchial stricture (e.g. following TB or bronchial surgery/lung transplant)

19.74 Non-metastatic extrapulmonary manifestations of bronchial carcinoma

Endocrine (Ch. 20)

- Inappropriate antidiuretic hormone secretion causing hyponatraemia
- Ectopic adrenocorticotrophic hormone secretion
- Hypercalcaemia due to secretion of parathyroid hormone-related peptides
- Carcinoid syndrome (p. 887)
- Gynaecomastia

Neurological (Ch. 26)

- Polyneuropathy
- Myelopathy
- Cerebellar degeneration
- Myasthenia (Lambert–Eaton syndrome, p. 1219)

Other

- Digital clubbing
- Hypertrophic pulmonary osteoarthropathy
- Nephrotic syndrome
- Polymyositis and dermatomyositis
- Eosinophilia

19

ptosis, enophthalmos, miosis and hypohidrosis of the face – p. 1166) due to involvement of the sympathetic chain at or above the stellate ganglion. Pancoast's syndrome (pain in the shoulder and inner aspect of the arm, sometimes with small muscle wasting in the hand) indicates malignant destruction of the T1 and C8 roots in lower part of the brachial plexus by an apical lung tumour.

- *Mediastinal spread.* Involvement of the oesophagus may cause dysphagia. If the pericardium is invaded, arrhythmia or pericardial effusion may occur. Superior vena cava obstruction by malignant nodes causes suffusion and swelling of the neck and face, conjunctival oedema, headache and dilated veins on the chest wall, and is most commonly due to bronchial carcinoma. Involvement of the left recurrent laryngeal nerve by tumours at the left hilum causes vocal cord paralysis, voice alteration and a 'bovine' cough (lacking the normal explosive character). Supraclavicular lymph nodes may be palpably enlarged; if so, a needle aspirate may provide a simple means of cytological diagnosis.
- *Metastatic spread.* This may lead to focal neurological defects, epileptic seizures, personality change, jaundice, bone pain or skin nodules. Lassitude, anorexia and weight loss usually indicate metastatic spread.
- *Digital clubbing.* Overgrowth of the soft tissue of the terminal phalanx leading to increased nail curvature is often seen (p. 642). This may be associated with hypertrophic pulmonary osteoarthropathy (HPOA), characterised by periostitis of the long bones, most commonly the distal tibia, fibula, radius and ulna. This causes pain and tenderness over the affected bones and often pitting oedema over the anterior aspect of the shin. X-rays reveal subperiosteal new bone formation. While most frequently associated with bronchial carcinoma, HPOA can occur with other tumours.
- *Non-metastatic extrapulmonary effects* (Box 19.74). Syndrome of inappropriate antidiuretic hormone secretion (SIADH, p. 436) and ectopic

adrenocorticotrophic hormone secretion (p. 774) are usually associated with small-cell lung cancer. Hypercalcaemia is usually caused by squamous cell carcinoma. Associated neurological syndromes may occur with any type of bronchial carcinoma.

Investigations

The main aims of investigation are to confirm the diagnosis, establish the histological cell type and define the extent of the disease.

Imaging

The features of bronchial carcinoma on plain X-rays are illustrated in Figures 19.44 and 19.45 and Box 19.75. CT is usually performed early, as it may reveal mediastinal or metastatic spread, and helps to direct histological sampling procedures. Imaging also indicates whether a tumour is likely to be accessible by bronchoscopy.

Histological characterisation

Around three-quarters of primary lung tumours can be visualised and sampled directly by biopsy and brushing using a flexible bronchoscope. Bronchoscopy also allows an assessment of operability, from the proximity of central tumours to the main carina (Fig. 19.46).

For tumours which are too peripheral to be accessible by bronchoscope, the yield of 'blind' bronchoscopic washings and brushings from the radiologically affected area is low, and percutaneous needle biopsy under CT or ultrasound guidance is a more reliable way to obtain a histological diagnosis. There is a small risk of iatrogenic pneumothorax, which may preclude the procedure if there is extensive coexisting COPD in the remaining lung. In patients who are not fit enough for invasive investigation, at least three sputum samples should be obtained for cytology, which may confirm the diagnosis non-invasively (Fig. 19.47).

In patients with pleural effusions, pleural aspiration and biopsy is the preferred investigation. Where facilities exist, thoracoscopy increases yield by allowing targeted biopsies under direct vision. In patients with

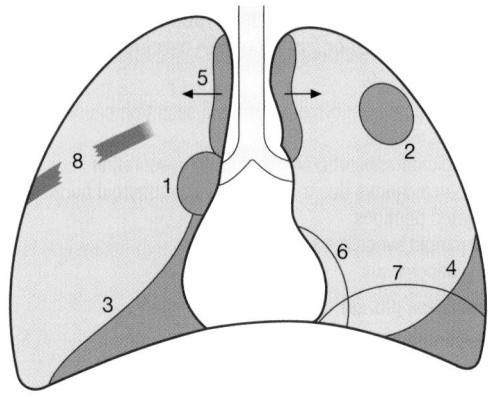

Fig. 19.45 Common radiological presentations of bronchial carcinoma.

19.75 Common radiological presentations of bronchial carcinoma

① Unilateral hilar enlargement

- Central tumour. Hilar glandular involvement. However, a peripheral tumour in the apical segment of a lower lobe can look like an enlarged hilar shadow on the PA X-ray

② Peripheral pulmonary opacity (p. 657)

- Usually irregular but well circumscribed, and may contain irregular cavitation. Can be very large

③ Lung, lobe or segmental collapse

- Usually caused by tumour within the bronchus leading to occlusion. Lung collapse may be due to compression of the main bronchus by enlarged lymph glands

④ Pleural effusion

- Usually indicates tumour invasion of pleural space; very rarely, a manifestation of infection in collapsed lung tissue distal to a bronchial carcinoma

⑤-⑦ Broadening of mediastinum, enlarged cardiac shadow, elevation of a hemidiaphragm

- Paratracheal lymphadenopathy may cause widening of the upper mediastinum. A malignant pericardial effusion will cause enlargement of the cardiac shadow. If a raised hemidiaphragm is caused by phrenic nerve palsy, screening will show it to move paradoxically upwards when patient sniffs

⑧ Rib destruction

- Direct invasion of the chest wall or blood-borne metastatic spread can cause osteolytic lesions of the ribs

metastatic disease, the diagnosis can often be confirmed by needle aspiration or biopsy of affected lymph nodes, skin lesions, liver or bone marrow.

Staging to guide treatment

The propensity of small-cell lung cancer to metastasise early dictates that patients with this tumour type are usually not suitable for surgical intervention. In patients with other cell types, subsequent investigations should focus on determining whether the tumour is operable, because complete resection may be curative. While CT may show obvious spread of disease, for many patients the results are equivocal and further investiga-

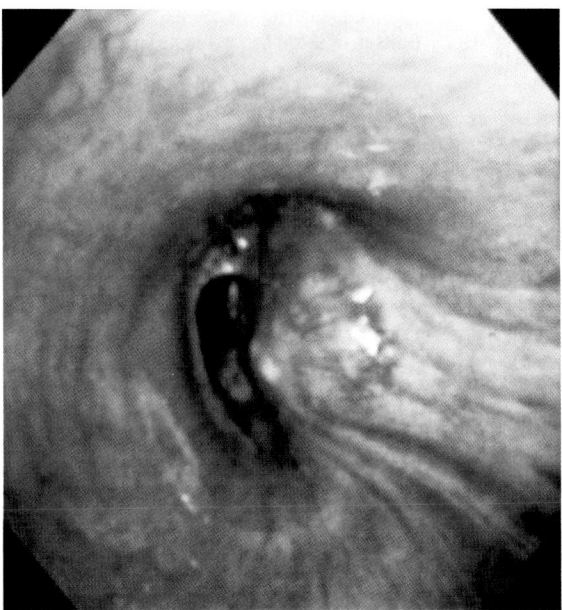

Fig. 19.46 Bronchoscopic view of a bronchogenic carcinoma. There is distortion of mucosal folds, partial occlusion of the airway lumen and abnormal tumour tissue.

tion is required before deciding whether curative surgery is feasible. Enlarged upper mediastinal nodes may be sampled by using a bronchoscope equipped with endobronchial ultrasound (EBUS) or by mediastinoscopy. Nodes in the lower mediastinum can be sampled through the oesophageal wall using endoscopic ultrasound. Combined CT and PET imaging (see Fig. 19.5, p. 648) is used increasingly to detect metabolically active tumour metastases. Head CT, radionuclide bone scanning, liver ultrasound and bone marrow biopsy are generally reserved for patients with clinical, haematological or biochemical evidence of tumour spread to such sites.

Finally, detailed physiological testing is required to ensure that the patient's respiratory and cardiac function is sufficient to allow surgical treatment (Box 19.76).

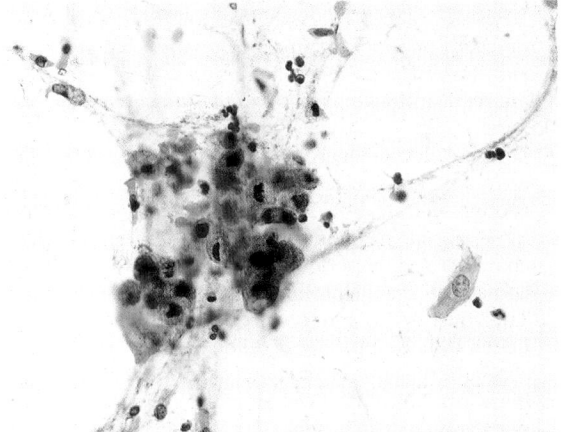

Fig. 19.47 Sputum sample showing a cluster of carcinoma cells. There is keratinisation, showing orangeophilia of the cytoplasm, and non-keratinised forms are also seen. The nuclei are large and 'coal-black' in density. These are the features of squamous cell bronchogenic carcinoma.

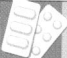

19.76 Contraindications to surgical resection in bronchial carcinoma

- Distant metastasis (M1)
- Invasion of central mediastinal structures including heart, great vessels, trachea and oesophagus (T4)
- Malignant pleural effusion (T4)
- Contralateral mediastinal nodes (N3)
- $FEV_1 < 0.8$ L
- Severe or unstable cardiac or other medical condition

N.B. In otherwise fit individuals, direct extension of tumour into the chest wall, diaphragm, mediastinal pleura or pericardium or to within 2 cm of the main carina does not exclude surgery. Though surgically resectable, patients with N2 (ipsilateral mediastinal) nodes may require neoadjuvant or adjuvant therapy.

Management

Surgical resection carries the best hope of long-term survival; however, some patients treated with radical radiotherapy and chemotherapy also achieve prolonged remission or cure. Unfortunately, in over 75% of cases, treatment with curative intent is not possible, or is inappropriate due to extensive spread or comorbidity. Such patients can only be offered palliative therapy and best supportive care. Radiotherapy, and in some cases chemotherapy, can relieve distressing symptoms.

Surgical treatment

Accurate pre-operative staging, coupled with improvements in surgical and post-operative care, now offers 5-year survival rates of over 75% in stage I disease (N0, tumour confined within visceral pleura) and 55% in stage II disease, which includes resection in patients with ipsilateral peribronchial or hilar node involvement.

Radiotherapy

While much less effective than surgery, radical radiotherapy can offer long-term survival in selected patients with localised disease in whom comorbidity precludes surgery. Continuous hyper-fractionated accelerated radiotherapy (CHART), in which a similar total dose is given in smaller but more frequent fractions, may offer better survival prospects than conventional schedules. The greatest value of radiotherapy, however, is in the palliation of distressing complications such as superior vena cava obstruction, recurrent haemoptysis, and pain caused by chest wall invasion or by skeletal metastatic deposits. Obstruction of the trachea and main bronchi can also be relieved temporarily. Radiotherapy can be used in conjunction with chemotherapy in the treatment of small-cell carcinoma, and is particularly efficient at preventing the development of brain metastases in patients who have had a complete response to chemotherapy (p. 272).

Chemotherapy

The treatment of small-cell carcinoma with combinations of cytotoxic drugs, sometimes in combination with radiotherapy, can increase the median survival from 3 months to well over a year. Combination chemotherapy leads to better outcomes than single-agent treatment. In particular, oral etoposide leads to more toxicity and worse survival than standard combination chemotherapy. Regular cycles of therapy, including combinations of i.v. cyclophosphamide, doxorubicin and vincristine or i.v. cisplatin and etoposide, are commonly used. Nausea and vomiting are common side-effects and are best treated with $5\text{-}HT_3$ receptor antagonists (p. 285).

The use of combinations of chemotherapeutic drugs requires considerable skill and should be overseen by teams of expert clinicians and nurses. In general, chemotherapy is less effective in non-small-cell bronchial cancers. However, studies in such patients using platinum-based chemotherapy regimens have shown a 30% response rate associated with a small increase in survival.

Neoadjuvant and adjuvant chemotherapy

In non-small-cell carcinoma, there is some evidence that chemotherapy given before surgery may increase survival and can effectively 'down-stage' disease with limited nodal spread. Post-operative chemotherapy is now proven to improve survival rates when operative samples show nodal involvement by tumour.

Laser therapy and stenting

Palliation of symptoms caused by major airway obstruction can be achieved in selected patients using bronchoscopic laser treatment to clear tumour tissue and allow re-aeration of collapsed lung. The best results are achieved in tumours of the main bronchi. Endobronchial stents can be used to maintain airway patency in the face of extrinsic compression by malignant nodes.

General aspects of management

The best outcomes are obtained when lung cancer is managed in specialist centres by multidisciplinary teams including oncologists, thoracic surgeons, respiratory physicians and specialist nurses; effective communication, pain relief and attention to diet are important. Lung tumours can cause clinically significant depression and anxiety, and these may need specific therapy. The management of non-metastatic endocrine manifestations is described in Chapter 20. When a malignant pleural effusion is present, an attempt should be made to drain the pleural cavity using an intercostal drain; provided the lung fully re-expands, pleurodesis with a sclerosing agent such as talc should be performed.

Prognosis

The overall prognosis in bronchial carcinoma is very poor, with around 70% of patients dying within a year of diagnosis and only 6–8% of patients surviving 5 years after diagnosis. The best prognosis is with well-differentiated squamous cell tumours that have not metastasised and are amenable to surgical resection. The clinical features and prognosis of some less common benign and malignant lung tumours are given in Box 19.77.

Secondary tumours of the lung

Blood-borne metastatic deposits in the lungs may be derived from many primary tumours, in particular the breast, kidney, uterus, ovary, testes and thyroid. The secondary deposits are usually multiple and bilateral. Often there are no respiratory symptoms and the diagnosis is made on radiological examination. Breathlessness may occur if a considerable amount of lung tissue has been replaced by metastatic tumour. Endobronchial deposits are uncommon but can cause haemoptysis and lobar collapse.

19

ℹ

19.77 Rare types of lung tumour

Tumour	Status	Histology	Typical presentation	Prognosis
Adenosquamous carcinoma	Malignant	Tumours with areas of unequivocal squamous and adeno-differentiation	Peripheral or central lung mass	Stage-dependent
Carcinoid tumour (p. 887)	Low-grade malignant	Neuroendocrine differentiation	Bronchial obstruction, cough	95% 5-year survival with resection
Bronchial gland adenoma	Benign	Salivary gland differentiation	Tracheobronchial irritation/obstruction	Local resection curative
Bronchial gland carcinoma	Low-grade malignant	Salivary gland differentiation	Tracheobronchial irritation/obstruction	Local recurrence occurs
Hamartoma	Benign	Mesenchymal cells, cartilage	Peripheral lung nodule	Local resection curative
Bronchoalveolar carcinoma	Malignant	Tumour cells line alveolar spaces	Alveolar shadowing, productive cough	Variable, worse if multifocal

Lymphangitic spread of carcinoma in the lung

Lymphatic infiltration may develop in patients with carcinoma of the breast, stomach, bowel, pancreas or bronchus. This grave condition causes severe and rapidly progressive breathlessness associated with marked hypoxaemia. The chest X-ray shows diffuse pulmonary shadowing radiating from the hilar regions, often associated with septal lines, and CT scans show characteristic polygonal thickened interlobular septa. Palliation of breathlessness with opiates may help (p. 285).

Tumours of the mediastinum

The mediastinum can be divided into four major compartments with reference to the lateral chest X-ray (Fig. 19.48):

- superior mediastinum: above a line drawn between the lower border of the 4th thoracic vertebra and the upper end of the body of the sternum
- anterior mediastinum: in front of the heart

- middle mediastinum: between the anterior and posterior compartments
- posterior mediastinum: behind the heart.

A variety of conditions can present radiologically as a mediastinal mass (Box 19.78).

Benign tumours and cysts arising within the mediastinum are frequently diagnosed when radiological examination of the chest is undertaken for some other reason. In general, they do not invade vital structures but may cause symptoms by compressing the trachea or occasionally the superior vena cava. A dermoid cyst may very occasionally rupture into a bronchus.

Malignant mediastinal tumours are distinguished by their power to invade as well as compress surrounding structures. As a result, even a small malignant tumour can produce symptoms, although more commonly the tumour has attained a considerable size before this happens (Box 19.79). The most common cause is mediastinal lymph node metastases from bronchogenic carcinoma, but lymphomas, leukaemia, malignant thymic tumours and germ-cell tumours can cause similar features. Aortic and innominate aneurysms have destructive features resembling those of malignant mediastinal tumours.

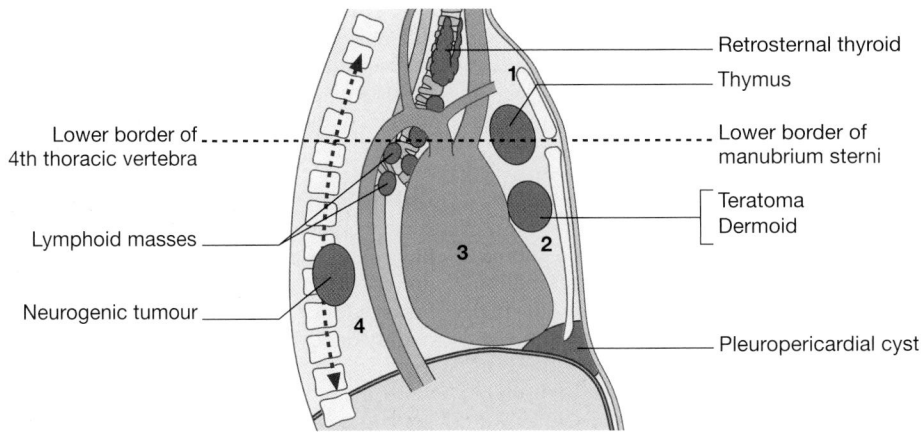

Fig. 19.48 The divisions of the mediastinum. (1) Superior mediastinum. (2) Anterior mediastinum. (3) Middle mediastinum. (4) Posterior mediastinum. Sites of the more common mediastinal tumours are also illustrated.

19.78 Causes of a mediastinal mass

Superior mediastinum

- Retrosternal goitre
- Persistent left superior vena cava
- Prominent left subclavian artery
- Thymic tumour
- Dermoid cyst
- Lymphoma
- Aortic aneurysm

Anterior mediastinum

- Retrosternal goitre
- Dermoid cyst
- Thymic tumour
- Lymphoma
- Aortic aneurysm
- Germ cell tumour
- Pericardial cyst
- Hiatus hernia through the diaphragmatic foramen of Morgagni

Posterior mediastinum

- Neurogenic tumour
- Paravertebral abscess
- Oesophageal lesion
- Aortic aneurysm
- Foregut duplication

Middle mediastinum

- Bronchial carcinoma
- Lymphoma
- Sarcoidosis
- Bronchogenic cyst
- Hiatus hernia

19.79 Clinical presentations with malignant invasion of the structures of the mediastinum

Trachea and main bronchi

- Stridor, breathlessness, cough, pulmonary collapse

Oesophagus

- Dysphagia, oesophageal displacement or obstruction on barium swallow examination

Phrenic nerve

- Diaphragmatic paralysis

Left recurrent laryngeal nerve

- Paralysis of left vocal cord giving rise to hoarseness and 'bovine' cough

Sympathetic trunk

- Horner's syndrome

Superior vena cava

- SVC obstruction results in non-pulsatile distension of neck veins, subconjunctival oedema, and oedema and cyanosis of head, neck, hands and arms. Dilated anastomotic veins on chest wall

Pericardium

- Pericarditis and/or pericardial effusion

Investigations

Radiological examination

A benign mediastinal tumour generally appears as a sharply circumscribed opacity situated in the mediastinum but encroaching on one or both lung fields (Fig. 19.49). CT (or MRI) is the investigation of choice for mediastinal tumours (e.g. see Fig. 20.12B, p. 750). A malignant mediastinal tumour seldom has a clearly defined margin and often presents as a general broadening of the mediastinal shadow.

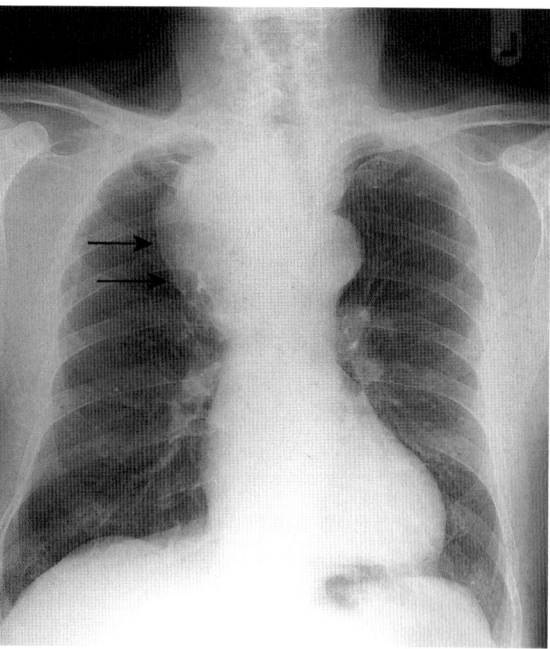

Fig. 19.49 Large mass (intrathoracic goitre—arrows) extending from right upper mediastinum.

Endoscopic investigation

Bronchoscopy may reveal a primary bronchial carcinoma causing mediastinal tumour by secondary lymphatic spread. EBUS may be used to image and guide sampling of peribronchial masses. The posterior mediastinum can be imaged via the oesophagus using EUS, which also facilitates needle biopsies of tumours or lymph node masses (p. 650).

Surgical exploration

Mediastinoscopy under general anaesthetic can be used to visualise and biopsy masses in the superior and anterior mediastinum; however, surgical exploration of the chest with removal of part or all of the tumour is often required to obtain a histological diagnosis.

Management

Benign mediastinal tumours should be removed surgically because most produce symptoms sooner or later. Some of them, particularly cysts, may become infected, while others, especially neural tumours, have the potential to undergo malignant transformation. The operative mortality is low provided there is no relative contraindication to surgical treatment, such as coexisting cardiovascular disease, COPD or extreme age.

INTERSTITIAL AND INFILTRATIVE PULMONARY DISEASES

Diffuse parenchymal lung disease

The diffuse parenchymal lung diseases (DPLDs) are a heterogeneous group of conditions affecting the pulmonary interstitium and/or alveolar lumen. The presentation and natural history of these may differ widely, but they are frequently considered collectively as they

19

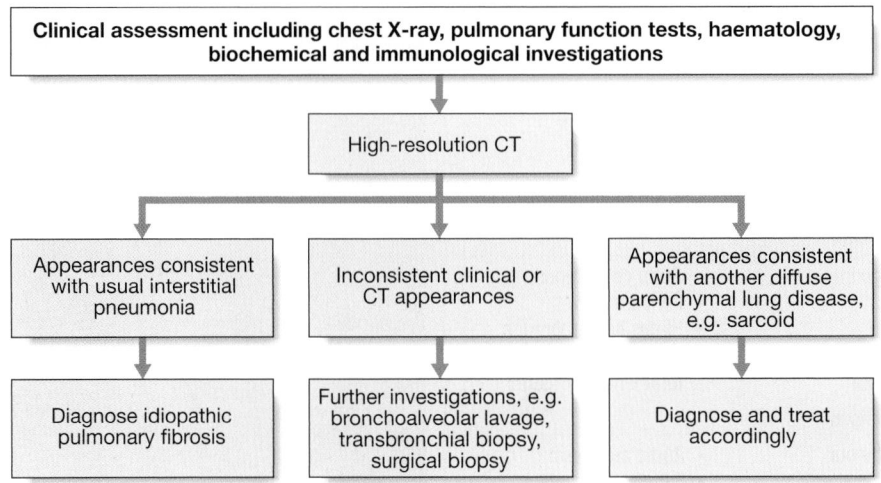

Fig. 19.50 Algorithm for the investigation of patients with interstitial lung disease following initial clinical and chest X-ray examination.

share similar symptoms, physical signs, pulmonary function abnormalities and radiological changes. HRCT has become the critical first step in the investigation of DPLD, indicating the diagnosis or directing further investigation (Fig. 19.50). The classification of DPLD is shown in Figure 19.51. A range of conditions may mimic interstitial lung disease (Box 19.80).

Idiopathic interstitial pneumonias

The idiopathic interstitial pneumonias (IIPs) are characterised by varying patterns of inflammation and fibrosis in the lung parenchyma, and comprise a number of clinicopathological entities that are sufficiently different from one another to be considered as separate diseases

> **i** **19.80 Conditions which mimic interstitial lung diseases**
>
> **Infection**
> - Viral pneumonia
> - *Pneumocystis jirovecii*
> - *Mycoplasma pneumoniae*
> - TB
> - Parasites, e.g. filariasis
> - Fungal infection
>
> **Malignancy**
> - Leukaemia and lymphoma
> - Lymphatic carcinomatosis
> - Multiple metastases
> - Bronchoalveolar carcinoma
>
> **Pulmonary oedema**
>
> **Aspiration pneumonitis**

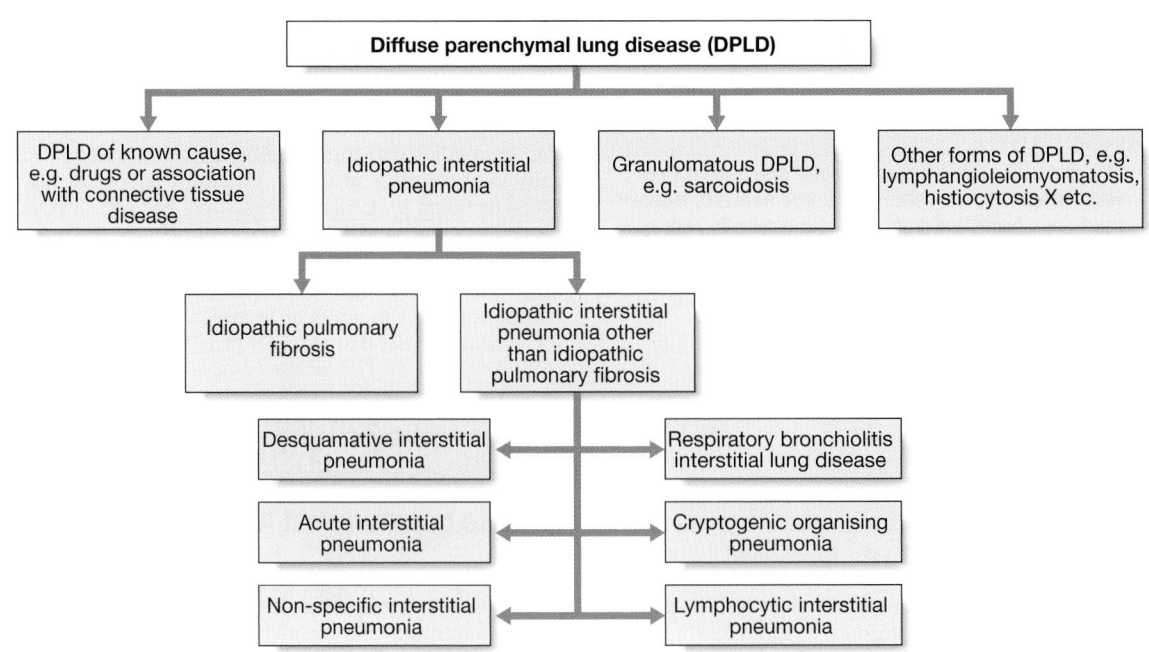

Fig. 19.51 Classification of diffuse parenchymal lung disease (see Box 19.81).

19.81 Differential diagnoses of the interstitial pneumonias

Clinical diagnosis	Notes
Usual interstitial pneumonia (UIP)	Idiopathic pulmonary fibrosis
Non-specific interstitial pneumonia (NSIP)	See page 708
Respiratory bronchiolitis-interstitial lung disease	More common in men and smokers. Usually presents in those aged 40–60. Smoking cessation may lead to improvement. Natural history unclear
Acute interstitial pneumonia	Often preceded by viral upper respiratory tract infection. Severe exertional dyspnoea, widespread pneumonic consolidation and diffuse alveolar damage on biopsy. Prognosis is often poor
Desquamative interstitial pneumonia (DIP)	More common in men and smokers. Presents in those aged 40–60. Insidious onset of dyspnoea. Clubbing in 50%. Biopsy shows increased macrophages in the alveolar space, septal thickening and type II pneumocyte hyperplasia. Prognosis is generally good
Cryptogenic organising pneumonia ('bronchiolitis obliterans organising pneumonia'—BOOP)	Presents as clinical and radiological pneumonia. Systemic features and markedly raised ESR common. Finger clubbing is absent. Biopsy shows a florid proliferation of immature collagen (Masson bodies) and fibrous tissue. Response to corticosteroids is classically excellent
Lymphocytic interstitial pneumonia (LIP)	More common in women, slow onset over years. Investigate for associations with connective tissue disease or HIV. Unclear whether corticosteroids helpful

19

(Box 19.81). The most common and important of these is idiopathic pulmonary fibrosis (IPF), which accounts for over 85% of new cases.

Idiopathic pulmonary fibrosis

Idiopathic pulmonary fibrosis refers to a specific form of DPLD characterised by pathological (or HRCT) evidence of 'usual interstitial pneumonia' (UIP). The histological features are suggestive of repeated episodes of focal damage to the alveolar epithelium consistent with an autoimmune process, but the aetiology remains elusive; putative factors include viruses (e.g. Epstein–Barr virus), occupational dusts (metal or wood), drugs (antidepressants) or chronic gastro-oesophageal reflux. Familial cases are rare but genetic factors that control the inflammatory and fibrotic response are likely to be important. There is a strong association with cigarette smoking.

Clinical features

IPF is uncommon before the age of 50 years. It usually presents with insidiously progressive breathlessness and a non-productive cough. Constitutional symptoms are unusual. Clinical findings include finger clubbing and the presence of bi-basal fine late inspiratory crackles likened to the unfastening of Velcro. The natural history is usually one of steady decline, but some patients are prone to exacerbations which are accompanied by an acute deterioration in breathlessness, disturbed gas exchange, and new ground glass changes or consolidation on HRCT. In advanced disease, central cyanosis is detectable and patients may develop features of right heart failure.

Investigations (Box 19.82)

There is no circulating marker for IPF. Non-specific findings include hypergammaglobulinaemia, positive rheumatoid factor or antinuclear factor (p. 1063), and an elevated LDH which may reflect active pneumonitis. Pulmonary function tests classically show a restric-

tive defect with reduced lung volumes and gas transfer. However, lung volumes may be paradoxically preserved in patients with concomitant emphysema. Dynamic tests are useful to document exercise tolerance and demonstrate exercise-induced arterial hypoxaemia, but as IPF advances, arterial hypoxaemia and hypocapnia are

19.82 Investigations in DPLD

Laboratory investigations

- Full blood count: lymphopenia in sarcoid; eosinophilia in pulmonary eosinophilias and drug reactions; neutrophilia in hypersensitivity pneumonitis
- Ca^{2+}: may be elevated in sarcoid
- Lactate dehydrogenase (LDH): may provide non-specific indicator of disease activity in DPLD
- Serum ACE: non-specific indicator of disease activity in sarcoid
- ESR and CRP may be non-specifically raised
- Autoimmune screen, rheumatoid factor and anti-CCP antibodies may suggest connective tissue disease

Radiology

- Chest X-ray
- HRCT

Pulmonary function

- Spirometry, lung volumes, gas transfer, exercise tests

Bronchoscopy

- Bronchoalveolar lavage: infection, differential cell counts
- Bronchial biopsy may be useful in sarcoid

Lung biopsy (in selected cases)

- Transbronchial biopsy useful in sarcoid and differential of malignancy or infection
- Video-assisted thoracoscopy (VATS)

Others

- Liver biopsy may be useful in sarcoidosis
- Urinary calcium excretion may be useful in sarcoidosis

present at rest. Virtually all patients have an abnormal chest X-ray at presentation with lower zone bi-basal reticular and reticulonodular opacities. A 'honeycomb' appearance may be seen in advanced disease but is non-specific (Fig. 19.52A). HRCT typically demonstrates a patchy, predominantly peripheral, subpleural and basal reticular pattern with subpleural cysts (honeycombing) and/or traction bronchiectasis (Fig. 19.52B). A lung biopsy is not usually required in those with typical clinical features and HRCT appearances, particularly if other known causes of interstitial lung disease have been excluded, but should be considered in cases of diagnostic uncertainty or with atypical features.

Management

Treatment is challenging. Prednisolone therapy (0.5 mg/kg) combined with azathioprine (2–3 mg/kg) is advocated for patients who are highly symptomatic or have rapidly progressive disease, have a predominantly 'ground glass' appearance on CT or a sustained fall of > 15% in their FVC or gas transfer over a 3–6-month period. However, response rates are notoriously poor, side-effects are guaranteed, and there is little evidence that this therapy impacts on the natural history of the disease. If objective evidence of improvement can be demonstrated, the prednisolone dose may be gradually reduced to a maintenance dose of 10–12.5 mg daily. The potential of therapies such as warfarin, N-acetyl-cysteine, IFN-γ1b, pirfenidone, bosentan or etanercept is being explored but cannot be recommended outside clinical trials at present. Lung transplantation should be considered in young patients with advanced disease. Oxygen may be provided for palliation of breathlessness but opiates may be required for relief of severe dyspnoea. The optimum treatment for acute exacerbations is unknown.

Prognosis

A median survival of 3 years is widely quoted; however, the rate of disease progression varies considerably from death within a few months to survival with minimal symptoms for many years. Serial lung function testing may provide useful prognostic information, with relative preservation of lung function suggesting longer survival and desaturation on exercise heralding a poorer prognosis. The finding of high numbers of fibroblastic foci on biopsy suggests a more rapid deterioration. IPF is associated with an increased risk of carcinoma of the lung.

Non-specific interstitial pneumonia

The clinical picture of fibrotic NSIP is similar to that of IPF, although patients tend to be women and younger in age. The aetiology is unknown but recognised associations occur with connective tissue disease, certain drugs and chronic hypersensitivity pneumonitis. HRCT findings are less specific than with IPF and lung biopsy may be required. NSIP is more likely to respond to immunosuppressive therapy than IPF; accordingly, the prognosis is significantly better, particularly in the cellular form of the condition, and the 5-year mortality rate is typically less than 15%.

Sarcoidosis

Sarcoidosis is a multisystem granulomatous disorder of unknown aetiology that is characterised by the presence of non-caseating granulomas (Fig. 19.53). The condition is more frequently described in colder parts of northern Europe. It also appears to be more common and more severe in those from a West Indian or Asian background; Eskimos, Arabs and Chinese are rarely affected. The tendency for sarcoid to present in the spring and summer has led to speculation as to the role of infective agents,

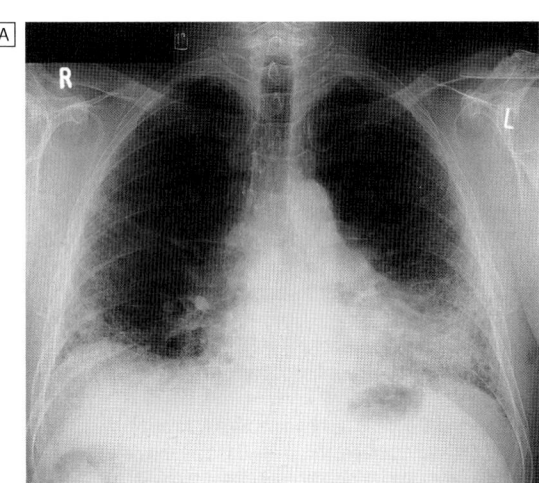

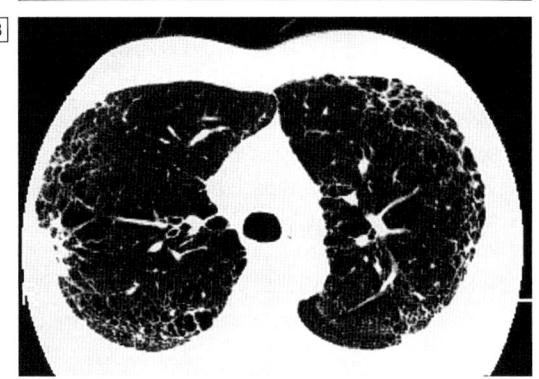

Fig. 19.52 Idiopathic pulmonary fibrosis. **A** Chest X-ray showing bilateral, predominantly lower zone and peripheral coarse reticulonodular shadowing and small lungs. **B** The CT scan shows honeycombing and scarring which is most marked peripherally.

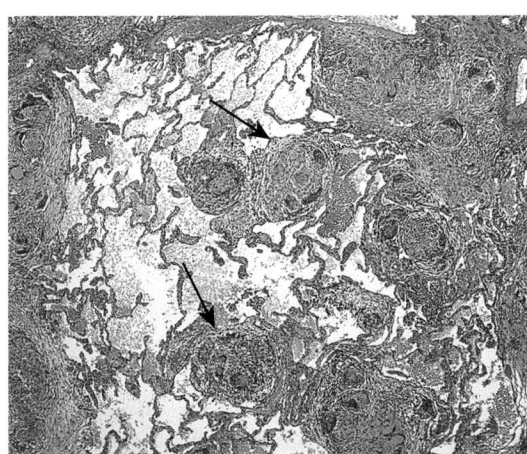

Fig. 19.53 Sarcoidosis of the lung. Histology showing non-caseating granulomas (arrows).

including mycobacteria, propionibacteria and viruses, but the cause remains elusive. Genetic susceptibility is supported by familial clustering; a range of class II HLA alleles confer protection from or susceptibility to the condition. Sarcoidosis occurs less frequently in smokers.

Clinical features

Sarcoidosis is considered with other DPLD as over 90% of cases affect the lungs, but the condition can affect almost any organ (Fig. 19.54 and Box 19.83). Löfgren's syndrome — an acute illness characterised by erythema nodosum, peripheral arthropathy, uveitis, bilateral hilar lymphadenopathy (BHL), lethargy and occasionally fever — is often seen in young adults. Alternatively, BHL may be detected in an otherwise asymptomatic individual undergoing a chest X-ray for other purposes. Pulmonary disease may also present in a more insidious manner with cough, exertional breathlessness and radiographic infiltrates; chest auscultation is often surprisingly unremarkable. Fibrosis occurs in around 20% of cases of pulmonary sarcoidosis and may cause a silent loss of lung function. Pleural disease is uncommon and finger clubbing is not a feature. Complications such as bronchiectasis, aspergilloma, pneumothorax, pulmonary hypertension and cor pulmonale have been reported but are rare.

19.83 Presentation of sarcoidosis

- Asymptomatic: abnormal routine chest X-ray (~30%) or abnormal liver function tests
- Respiratory and constitutional symptoms (20–30%)
- Erythema nodosum and arthralgia (20–30%)
- Ocular symptoms (5–10%)
- Skin sarcoid (including lupus pernio) (5%)
- Superficial lymphadenopathy (5%)
- Other (1%), e.g. hypercalcaemia, diabetes insipidus, cranial nerve palsies, cardiac arrhythmias, nephrocalcinosis

Investigations

Lymphopenia is characteristic and liver function tests may be mildly deranged. Hypercalcaemia may be present (reflecting increased formation of calcitriol — 1,25-dihydroxyvitamin D_3 — by alveolar macrophages), particularly if the patient has been exposed to strong sunlight. Hypercalciuria may also be seen and may lead to nephrocalcinosis. Serum angiotensin-converting enzyme (ACE) is a non-specific marker of disease activity and can assist in monitoring the clinical course. Chest radiography has been used to stage sarcoid (Box 19.84).

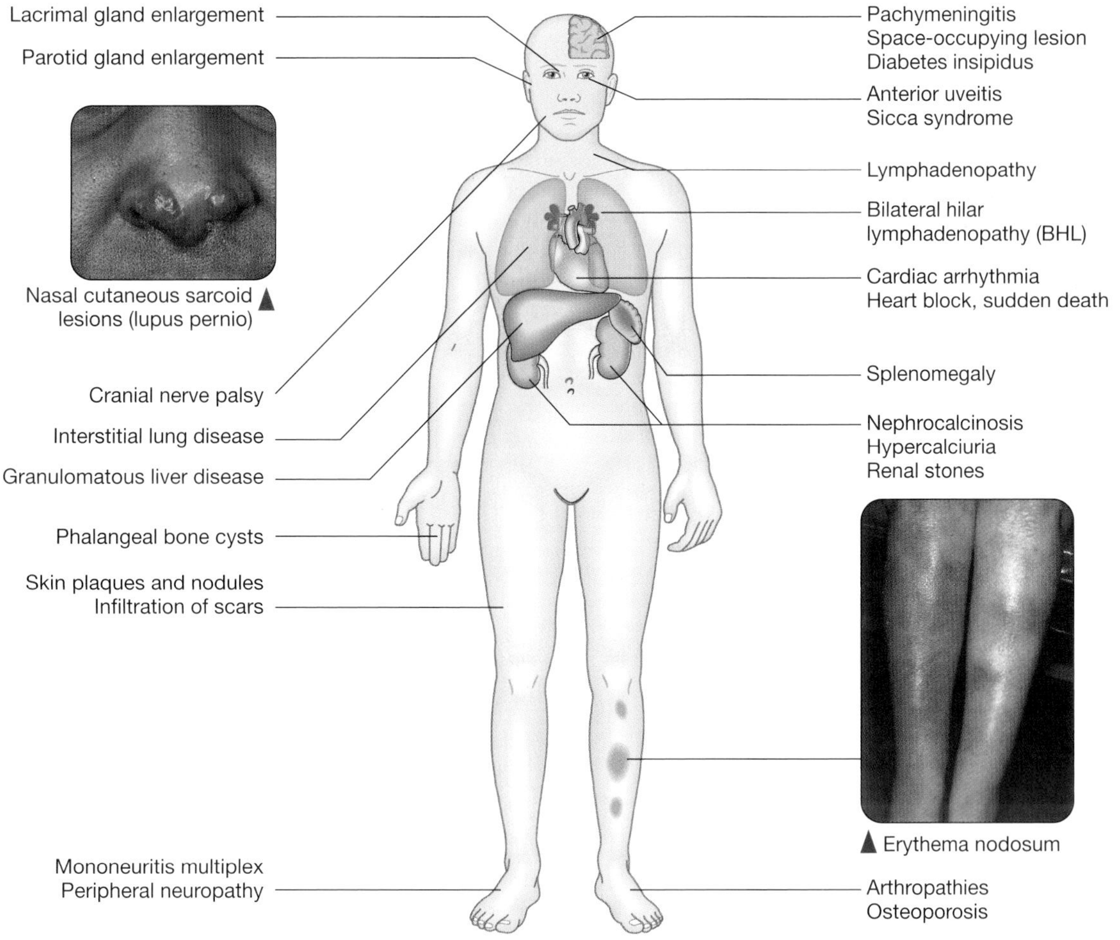

19

Lacrimal gland enlargement
Parotid gland enlargement
Nasal cutaneous sarcoid lesions (lupus pernio) ▲
Cranial nerve palsy
Interstitial lung disease
Granulomatous liver disease
Phalangeal bone cysts
Skin plaques and nodules Infiltration of scars
Mononeuritis multiplex Peripheral neuropathy

Pachymeningitis Space-occupying lesion Diabetes insipidus
Anterior uveitis Sicca syndrome
Lymphadenopathy
Bilateral hilar lymphadenopathy (BHL)
Cardiac arrhythmia Heart block, sudden death
Splenomegaly
Nephrocalcinosis Hypercalciuria Renal stones
▲ Erythema nodosum
Arthropathies Osteoporosis

Fig. 19.54 Possible systemic involvement in sarcoidosis.

19.84 Chest X-ray changes in sarcoidosis

Stage I: BHL (usually symmetrical); paratracheal nodes often enlarged

- Often asymptomatic, but may be associated with erythema nodosum and arthralgia. The majority of cases resolve spontaneously within 1 year

Stage II: BHL and parenchymal infiltrates

- Patients may present with breathlessness or cough. The majority of cases resolve spontaneously

Stage III: parenchymal infiltrates without BHL

- Disease less likely to resolve spontaneously

Stage IV: pulmonary fibrosis

- Can cause progression to ventilatory failure, pulmonary hypertension and cor pulmonale

In patients with pulmonary infiltrates, pulmonary function testing may show a restrictive defect accompanied by impaired gas exchange. Exercise tests may reveal oxygen desaturation. Transbronchial (and bronchial) biopsies show non-caseating granulomas (see Fig. 19.53) and the mucosa may have a 'cobblestone' appearance at bronchoscopy. The BAL fluid typically contains an increased CD4:CD8 T-cell ratio. Characteristic HRCT appearances include reticulonodular opacities that follow a perilymphatic distribution centred on bronchovascular bundles and the subpleural areas.

The occurrence of erythema nodosum with BHL on chest X-ray is often sufficient for a confident diagnosis, without recourse to a tissue biopsy. Similarly, a typical presentation with classical HRCT features may also be accepted. However, in other instances the diagnosis should be confirmed by histological examination of the involved organ. The presence of anergy (e.g. to tuberculin skin tests) may support the diagnosis.

Management

Patients who present with acute illness and erythema nodosum should receive NSAIDs and, if symptoms are severe, a short course of corticosteroids. The majority of patients enjoy spontaneous remission and so if there is no evidence of organ damage, systemic corticosteroid therapy can be withheld for 6 months. However, prednisolone (at a starting dose of 20–40 mg/day) should be commenced immediately in the presence of hypercalcaemia, pulmonary impairment, renal impairment and uveitis (Box 19.85). Topical steroids may be useful in cases of mild uveitis, and inhaled corticosteroids have been used to shorten the duration of systemic corticosteroid use in asymptomatic parenchymal sarcoid. Patients should be

EBM 19.85 Systemic corticosteroids in pulmonary sarcoidosis

'Oral glucocorticoids administered for 6–24 months improve chest X-ray appearances and symptoms but there is little evidence of an improvement in lung function and there are no data from follow-up beyond 2 years.'

- Paramathayan NS, et al. (Cochrane Review). Cochrane Library, issue 2, 2005. Oxford: Update Software.

warned that strong sunlight may precipitate hypercalcaemia and endanger renal function.

Features suggesting a less favourable outlook include age > 40 years, Afro-Caribbean ethnicity, persistent symptoms for more than 6 months, the involvement of more than three organs, lupus pernio and a stage III/IV chest X-ray. In patients with severe disease methotrexate (10–20 mg/week), azathioprine (50–150 mg/day) and specific TNF-α inhibitors (p. 1080) have been effective. Chloroquine, hydroxychloroquine and low-dose thalidomide may be useful in cutaneous sarcoid with limited pulmonary involvement. Selected patients may be referred for consideration of single lung transplantation. The overall mortality is low (1–5%) and usually reflects cardiac involvement or pulmonary fibrosis.

Lung diseases due to organic dusts

A wide range of organic agents may cause respiratory disorders (Box 19.86). Disease results from a local immune response to animal proteins (e.g. bird fancier's lung) or fungal antigens in mouldy vegetable matter. Hypersensitivity pneumonitis is the most common of these conditions.

Hypersensitivity pneumonitis (HP)

Hypersensitivity pneumonitis (also called extrinsic allergic alveolitis) results from the inhalation of a wide variety of organic antigens which give rise to a diffuse immune complex reaction in the walls of the alveoli and bronchioles. Common causes include farm worker's lung and bird fancier's lung.

Pathogenesis and pathology

The pathology of HP is consistent with both type III and type IV immunological mechanisms (p. 86). Precipitating IgG antibodies may be detected in the serum and a type III Arthus reaction is believed to occur in the lung, where the precipitation of immune complexes results in

19.86 Examples of lung diseases caused by organic dusts

Disorder	Source	Antigen/agent
Farmer's lung*	Mouldy hay, straw, grain	*Micropolyspora faeni* *Aspergillus fumigatus*
Bird fancier's lung*	Avian excreta, proteins and feathers	Avian serum proteins
Malt worker's lung*	Mouldy maltings	*Aspergillus clavatus*
Byssinosis (p. 671)	Textile industries	Cotton, flax, hemp dust
Inhalation ('humidifier') fever	Contamination of air conditioning	Thermophilic actinomycetes
Cheese worker's lung*	Mouldy cheese	*Aspergillus clavatus* *Penicillium casei*
Maple bark stripper's lung*	Bark from stored maple	*Cryptostroma corticale*

*Denotes lung disease presenting as hypersensitivity pneumonitis.

activation of complement and an inflammatory response in the alveolar walls, characterised by the influx of mononuclear cells and foamy histiocytes. The presence of poorly formed non-caseating granulomas in the alveolar walls suggests that type IV responses are also important. The distribution of the inflammatory infiltrate is predominantly peribronchiolar, which helps to distinguish the appearances from non-specific or lymphocytic interstitial pneumonias which display a more diffuse distribution. Chronic forms of the disease may be accompanied by fibrosis. For reasons that remain uncertain, there is a lower incidence of HP in smokers compared to non-smokers.

Clinical features

The acute form of the disease should be suspected when anyone who is exposed to organic dust complains, within a few hours of re-exposure to the same dust, of influenza-like symptoms such as headache, myalgia, malaise, pyrexia, dry cough and breathlessness. Chest auscultation reveals widespread end-inspiratory crackles and squeaks. In cases attributable to chronic low-level exposure (as may be the case with an indoor pet bird), the presentation is more often insidious and established fibrosis may be present by the time the disease is recognised. If unchecked, HP may progress to cause severe respiratory disability, hypoxaemia, pulmonary hypertension, cor pulmonale and eventually death.

Investigations

The classical chest X-ray shows upper zone diffuse micronodular shadowing. HRCT is more sensitive and the appearances may provide information on the stage of disease. Acute forms are characterised by ground glass shadowing and areas of consolidation superimposed on small centrilobar nodular opacities; the distribution is typically bilateral with upper and middle lobe predominance. In more chronic disease, features of fibrosis such as volume loss, linear opacities and architectural distortion appear. Pulmonary function tests show a restrictive ventilatory defect with reduced lung volumes and impaired gas transfer, dynamic tests may detect oxygen desaturation and, in more advanced disease, type I respiratory failure is present at rest.

Diagnosis

The diagnosis of HP is usually based on the characteristic clinical and radiological features, together with the identification of a potential source of antigen at the patient's home or place of work (Box 19.87). It may be supported by a positive precipitin test or by more sensitive serological tests based on the enzyme-linked immunosorbent assay (ELISA) technique. However, the great majority of farmers with positive precipitins do not have farmer's lung, and up to 15% of pigeon breeders may have positive serum precipitins yet remain healthy.

Where HP is suspected but the cause is not readily apparent, a visit to the patient's home or workplace should be arranged. Occasionally, such as when an agent not previously recognised as causing HP is suspected, provocation testing may be necessary to prove the diagnosis; inhalation of the relevant antigen is followed by pyrexia and a reduction in VC and gas transfer factor after 3–6 hours, if positive. BAL fluid usually shows an increase in the number of $CD8^+$ T lymphocytes. Transbronchial biopsy can occasionally provide sufficient tissue for a confident diagnosis, but open lung biopsy may be necessary.

Management

Whenever possible, the patient should cease exposure to the inciting agent. However, in some cases this may be difficult to achieve, because of either implications for livelihood (e.g. farmers) or addiction to hobbies (e.g. pigeon breeders). Dust masks with appropriate filters may minimise exposure and may be combined with methods of reducing levels of antigen (e.g. drying hay before storage). In acute cases prednisolone should be given for 3–4 weeks, starting with an oral dose of 40 mg per day. Severely hypoxaemic patients may require high-concentration oxygen therapy initially. Most patients recover completely, but the development of interstitial fibrosis is usually accompanied by permanent disability.

Inhalation ('humidifier') fever

Inhalation fever shares similarities with HP. It occurs as a result of contaminated humidifiers or air-conditioning units that release a fine spray of microorganisms into the atmosphere. The illness is characterised by self-limiting fever and breathlessness; permanent sequelae are unusual. An identical syndrome can also develop after disturbing an accumulation of mouldy hay, compost or mulch. So-called 'hot tub lung' appears to be attributable to *M. avium*. Outbreaks of HP in workers using metalworking fluids appear linked to *Acinetobacter* or *Ochrobactrum*.

Lung diseases due to inorganic dusts

In certain occupations, the inhalation of inorganic dusts, fumes or other noxious substances leads to specific pathological changes in the lungs. Industrial inorganic gases and fumes can cause acute respiratory diseases including pulmonary oedema and asthma (Box 19.88). In general, prolonged exposure to inorganic dusts (Box 19.89) leads to diffuse pulmonary fibrosis (the pneumoconioses), although beryllium causes an interstitial granulomatous disease similar to sarcoidosis. The pathological result depends largely on the inflammatory and fibrotic responses: silica is highly fibrogenic whereas iron and tin are almost inert. The most important types of pneumoconiosis are coal worker's pneumoconiosis, silicosis and asbestosis. In many types, a long period of dust

19.87 Predictive factors in the identification of hypersensitivity pneumonitis

- Exposure to a known offending antigen
- Positive precipitating antibodies to offending antigen
- Recurrent episodes of symptoms
- Inspiratory crackles on examination
- Symptoms occurring 4–8 hours after exposure
- Weight loss

19.88 Lung diseases caused by inorganic gases and fumes

Cause	Occupation	Disease
Irritant gases (chlorine, ammonia, phosgene, nitrogen dioxide)	Various (industrial accidents)	Acute lung injury ARDS
Cadmium	Welding and electroplating	COPD
Isocyanates (e.g. epoxy resins, paints)	Plastic, paints; manufacture of epoxy resins and adhesives	Bronchial asthma Eosinophilic pneumonia

19.89 Lung diseases caused by exposure to inorganic dusts

Cause	Occupation	Description	Characteristic pathological features
Coal dust	Coal mining	Coal worker's pneumoconiosis	Focal and interstitial fibrosis, centrilobular emphysema, progressive massive fibrosis
Silica	Mining, quarrying, stone dressing, metal grinding, pottery, boiler scaling	Silicosis	
Asbestos	Demolition, ship breaking, manufacture of fireproof insulating materials, pipe and boiler lagging	Asbestos-related disease	Pleural plaques Diffuse pleural thickening Acute benign pleurisy Carcinoma of lung Interstitial fibrosis Mesothelioma
Iron oxide	Arc welding	Siderosis	Mineral deposition only
Tin oxide	Tin mining	Stannosis	Tin-laden macrophages
Beryllium	Aircraft, atomic energy and electronics industries	Berylliosis	Granulomas, interstitial fibrosis

exposure is required before radiological changes appear, and these may precede clinical symptoms. A detailed occupational history is essential not only to avoid missing a case of occupational lung disease, but also to allow appropriate advice to be given to the patient, and if relevant, the employer and legal advisors. Many countries encourage the registration of cases of occupational lung disease.

Coal worker's pneumoconiosis

Simple coal worker's pneumoconiosis (SCWP) follows prolonged inhalation of coal dust. Dust-laden alveolar macrophages aggregate to form macules in or near the centre of the secondary pulmonary lobule and a fibrotic reaction ensues, resulting in the appearance of scattered discrete fibrotic lesions. Classification is based on the size and extent of radiographic nodularity.

SCWP is asymptomatic, does not impair lung function, and once exposure ceases will seldom progress. In some cases, SCWP may be 'complicated' by an additional pathology such as progressive massive fibrosis (PMF) or Caplan's syndrome. PMF refers to the formation of large dense masses (mainly in the upper lobes); cavitation may occur, raising important differential diagnoses such as lung cancer, tuberculosis and Wegener's granulomatosis. In contrast to SCWP, PMF is usually associated with cough, sputum that may be black (melanoptysis), and breathlessness. It may progress after coal dust exposure ceases and in extreme cases leads to respiratory failure and right ventricular failure. Caplan's syndrome describes the coexistence of rheumatoid arthritis and pneumoconiosis, with rounded fibrotic nodules 0.5–5 cm in diameter. They show pathological features similar to a rheumatoid nodule including central necrosis, palisading histiocytes, and a peripheral rim of lymphocytes and plasma cells. This syndrome may also occur in other types of pneumoconiosis.

Silicosis

Silicosis results from the inhalation of crystalline or free silica, usually in the form of quartz, by workers cutting, grinding and polishing stone. The clinical presentation reflects the intensity of exposure. Classic silicosis is most common and usually manifests after 10–20 years of continuous silica exposure, during which time the patient remains asymptomatic. Accelerated silicosis is associated with a much shorter duration of dust exposure (typically 5–10 years), may present as early as 1 year of exposure, and as the name suggests, follows a more aggressive course. Typical symptoms include cough, with sputum and breathlessness. Very rarely, intense exposure to very fine crystalline silica dust can cause a more acute disease: silicoproteinosis, similar to alveolar proteinosis (Box 19.94, p. 717).

Radiological features are similar to those of SCWP, with multiple well-circumscribed 3–5 mm nodular opacities predominantly in the mid- and upper zones. As the disease progresses, PMF may develop (Fig. 19.55). Enlargement of the hilar glands with an 'eggshell' pattern of calcification is said to be characteristic, but is uncommon and non-specific.

Silica is highly fibrogenic and the disease is usually progressive, even when exposure ceases. The disease is associated with an increased risk of tuberculosis (silicotuberculosis), lung cancer and COPD; associations with renal and connective tissue disease have also been described.

Asbestosis

The main types of the fibrous mineral asbestos are chrysotile (white asbestos), which accounts for 90% of the world's production, crocidolite (blue asbestos) and amosite (brown asbestos). By virtue of their aerodynamic shape, airborne asbestos fibres can penetrate deep within the lung parenchyma, then lodge in small airways where their inert mineral structure confounds the attempts of pulmonary macrophages to clear them. In the lung, pulmonary fibrosis and bronchial carcinoma

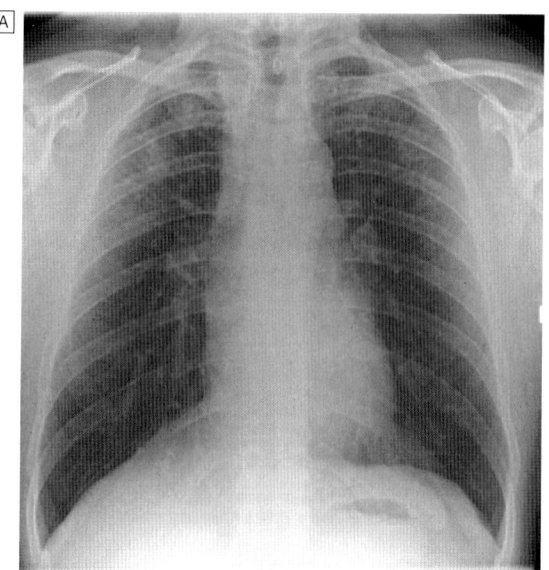

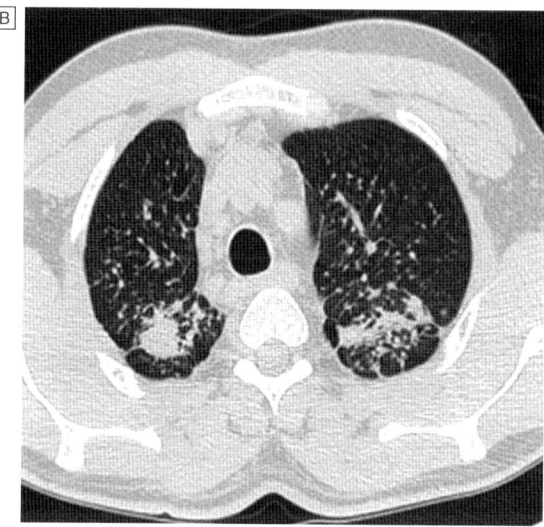

Fig. 19.55 Silicosis. [A] A chest X-ray from a patient with silicosis showing the presence of small rounded nodules predominantly seen in the upper zones. [B] HRCT from the same patient demonstrating conglomeration of nodules with posterior bias.

are the most serious consequences. Exposure occurs in a variety of occupations and is a recognised risk factor for several respiratory diseases (Fig. 19.56). Asbestos-related pleural disease is described on page 728.

Asbestosis is a diffuse interstitial fibrosis of the lungs. The risk of development and severity of the disease increase in relation to the amount of dust inhaled, although individual susceptibility appears to be important. Patients usually present with exertional breathlessness and fine, late inspiratory crackles over the lower zones. Digital clubbing (reported in 40% of patients) is an adverse prognostic feature. The chest X-ray shows bi-basal reticulonodular shadowing and asbestos-related pleural disease is usually (but not invariably) present. HRCT is more sensitive than plain radiography and typically shows bi-basal, subpleural, dot-like opacities, curvilinear subpleural lines, ground glass opacification and interlobular septal thickening. In more advanced disease, honeycombing may be present. Pulmonary function tests typically show a restrictive defect with decreased lung volumes and reduced gas transfer factor.

The diagnosis is usually established by a history of substantial asbestos exposure with the clinical, radiological and pulmonary function abnormalities described above. Asbestos bodies may be identified in sputum or BAL and confirm asbestos exposure. Lung biopsy is rarely necessary but may be required to exclude other causes of interstitial lung disease. Asbestos fibre counts may be performed on lung biopsy material.

Management

No specific treatment is available and asbestosis is usually slowly progressive. In advanced cases, respiratory failure and cor pulmonale may develop. About 40% of patients (who usually smoke) develop carcinoma of the lung and 10% may develop mesothelioma (p. 729). Patients should be provided with appropriate legal advice if asbestos exposure occurred as a result of negligent exposure.

Berylliosis

The presence of cough, progressive breathlessness, night sweats and arthralgia in a worker exposed to dusts, fumes or vapours containing beryllium should

19

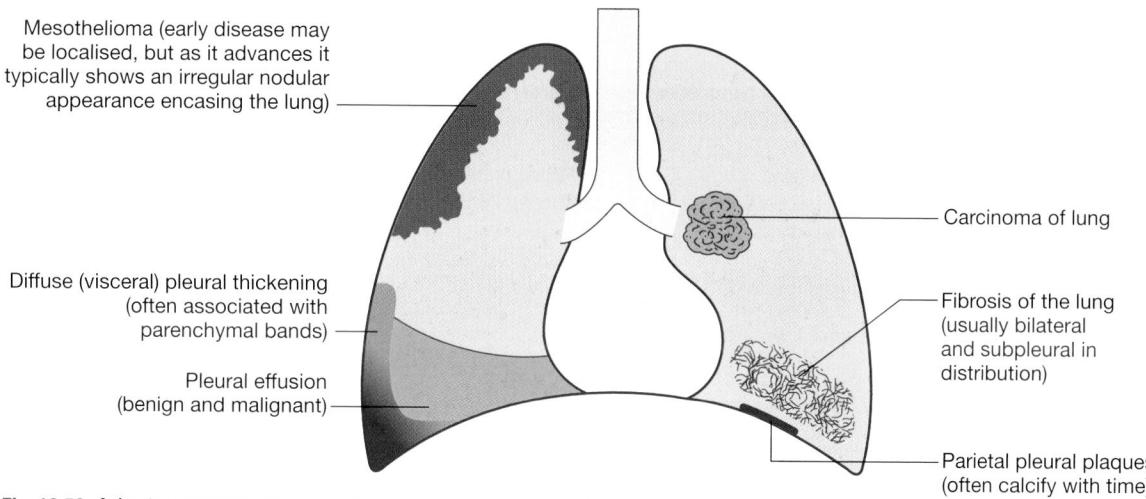

Mesothelioma (early disease may be localised, but as it advances it typically shows an irregular nodular appearance encasing the lung)

Diffuse (visceral) pleural thickening (often associated with parenchymal bands)

Pleural effusion (benign and malignant)

Carcinoma of lung

Fibrosis of the lung (usually bilateral and subpleural in distribution)

Parietal pleural plaques (often calcify with time)

Fig. 19.56 Asbestos exposure. The range of possible effects on the respiratory tract.

raise suspicions of chronic berylliosis. The radiographic appearances are similar in type and distribution to sarcoid and biopsy shows sarcoid-like granulomas.

Lung diseases due to systemic inflammatory disease

Acute respiratory distress syndrome

See page 187.

Respiratory involvement in connective tissue disorders

Pulmonary complications of connective tissue disease are common, affecting the airways, the alveoli, the pulmonary vasculature, the diaphragm and chest wall muscles, and the chest wall itself. In some instances, pulmonary disease may precede the appearance of the connective tissue disorder (Box 19.90). Indirect associations between connective tissue disorders and respiratory complications include those due to disease in other organs, e.g. thrombocytopenia causing haemoptysis, pulmonary toxic effects of drugs used to treat the connective tissue disorder (e.g. gold and methotrexate), and secondary infection due to the disease itself, neutropenia or immunosuppressive drug regimens.

Rheumatoid arthritis

Pulmonary involvement is important, accounting for around 10–20% of the mortality associated with the condition (p. 1088). The majority of cases occur within 5 years of the rheumatological diagnosis but pulmonary manifestations may precede joint involvement in 10–20%. Pulmonary fibrosis is the most common pulmonary manifestation. All forms of interstitial disease have been described but NSIP (see Box 19.81, p. 708) is probably the most common.

Pleural effusion is common, especially in men with seropositive disease. Effusions are usually small and unilateral but can be large and bilateral. Most resolve spontaneously. Biochemical testing reveals an exudate with markedly reduced glucose levels and raised LDH. Effusions that fail to resolve spontaneously may respond to a short course of oral prednisolone (30–40 mg daily) but some become chronic.

Rheumatoid pulmonary nodules are usually asymptomatic and detected incidentally on imaging. They are usually multiple and subpleural in site (Fig. 19.57). Solitary nodules can mimic primary bronchial carcinoma and, when multiple, the differential diagnoses include pulmonary metastatic disease. Cavitation raises the possibility of tuberculosis and predisposes to pneumothorax. The combination of rheumatoid nodules and pneumoconiosis is known as Caplan's syndrome (p. 712).

Bronchitis and bronchiectasis are both more common in rheumatoid arthritis. Rarely, the potentially fatal condition called obliterative bronchiolitis may develop. Bacterial lower respiratory tract infections are frequent. Treatments given for rheumatoid arthritis may also be relevant; corticosteroid therapy predisposes to infections, methotrexate may cause pulmonary fibrosis, and anti-TNF therapy may precipitate the reactivation of tuberculosis.

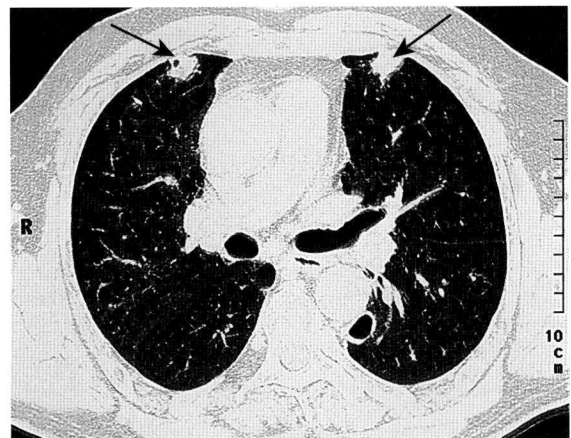

Fig. 19.57 Rheumatoid (necrobiotic) nodules. Thoracic CT just below the level of the main carina showing the typical appearance of peripheral, pleural-based nodules. The nodule in the left lower lobe shows characteristic cavitation.

19.90 Respiratory complications of connective tissue disorders

Disorder	Airways	Parenchyma	Pleura	Diaphragm and chest wall
Rheumatoid arthritis	Bronchitis, obliterative bronchiolitis, bronchiectasis, crico-arytenoid arthritis, stridor	Pulmonary fibrosis, nodules, upper lobe fibrosis, infections	Pleurisy, effusion, pneumothorax	Poor healing of intercostal drain sites
Systemic lupus erythematosus	–	Pulmonary fibrosis, 'vasculitic' infarcts	Pleurisy, effusion	Diaphragmatic weakness (shrinking lungs)
Systemic sclerosis	Bronchiectasis	Pulmonary fibrosis, aspiration pneumonia	–	Cutaneous thoracic restriction (hidebound chest)
Dermatomyositis/ polymyositis	Bronchial carcinoma	Pulmonary fibrosis	–	Intercostal and diaphragmatic myopathy
Rheumatic fever	–	Pneumonia	Pleurisy, effusion	–

Systemic lupus erythematosus (SLE)

Pleuropulmonary involvement is more common in SLE (p. 1107) than in any other connective tissue disorder and may be a presenting problem, when it is sometimes attributed incorrectly to infection or pulmonary embolism. Up to two-thirds of patients have repeated episodes of pleurisy, with or without effusions. Effusions may be bilateral and may also involve the pericardium.

The most serious manifestation of lupus is an acute alveolitis that may be associated with diffuse alveolar haemorrhage. This condition is life-threatening and requires immunosuppression.

Pulmonary fibrosis is a relatively uncommon manifestation. Some patients present with exertional dyspnoea and orthopnoea but without overt signs of pulmonary fibrosis. The chest X-ray reveals elevated diaphragms, and pulmonary function testing shows reduced lung volumes. This condition has been described as 'shrinking lungs' and attributed to diaphragmatic myopathy.

SLE patients with antiphospholipid antibodies are at increased risk of venous and pulmonary thromboembolism and these patients require life-long anticoagulation.

Systemic sclerosis

Most patients with systemic sclerosis (p. 1109) eventually develop diffuse pulmonary fibrosis; at necropsy more than 90% have evidence of lung fibrosis. In some patients, it is indolent, but when progressive, as in IPF, the median survival time is around 4 years. Pulmonary fibrosis is rare in the CREST variant of progressive systemic sclerosis but pulmonary hypertension is an important complication.

Other pulmonary complications include recurrent aspiration pneumonias secondary to oesophageal disease. Rarely, sclerosis of the skin of the chest wall may be so extensive and cicatrising as to restrict chest wall movement: the so-called 'hidebound chest'.

Pulmonary eosinophilia and vasculitides

Pulmonary eosinophilia refers to the association of radiographic (usually pneumonic) abnormalities and peripheral blood eosinophilia. The term encompasses a group of disorders of different aetiology (Box 19.91). Eosinophils are the predominant cell recovered in sputum or BAL and their products are likely to be the prime mediators of tissue damage.

Acute eosinophilic pneumonia

Acute eosinophilic pneumonia is an acute febrile illness of less than 5 days' duration, characterised by diffuse pulmonary infiltrates and hypoxic respiratory failure. The pathology is usually that of diffuse alveolar damage. Diagnosis is confirmed by BAL, which characteristically demonstrates > 25% eosinophils. The condition is usually idiopathic but drug reactions should be considered. Corticosteroids invariably induce prompt and complete resolution.

Chronic eosinophilic pneumonia

Chronic eosinophilic pneumonia typically presents in an insidious manner with malaise, fever, weight loss, breathlessness and unproductive cough. It is more common in middle-aged females. The classical chest X-ray appearance has been likened to the photographic negative of pulmonary oedema with bilateral, peripheral and predominantly upper lobe parenchymal shadowing. The peripheral blood eosinophil count is almost always very high, and the ESR and total serum IgE are elevated. BAL reveals a high proportion of eosinophils in the lavage fluid. Response to prednisolone (20–40 mg daily) is usually dramatic. Prednisolone can usually be withdrawn after a few weeks without relapse, but long-term low-dose therapy is occasionally necessary.

Tropical pulmonary eosinophilia

Tropical pulmonary eosinophilia occurs as a result of a mosquito-borne filarial infection with *Wuchereria bancrofti* or *Brugia malayi*. The condition presents with

19

19.92 Interstitial lung disease in old age

- **Idiopathic pulmonary fibrosis:** the most common interstitial lung disease, with a worse prognosis.
- **Chronic aspiration pneumonitis:** must always be considered in elderly patients presenting with bilateral basal shadowing on a chest X-ray.
- **Wegener's granulomatosis:** a rare condition but more common in old age. Renal involvement is more common at presentation and upper respiratory problems are fewer.
- **Asbestosis:** symptoms may only appear in old age because of the prolonged latent period between exposure and disease.
- **Drug-induced interstitial lung disease:** more common, presumably because of the increased chance of exposure to multiple drugs.
- **Rarer interstitial disease:** sarcoidosis, idiopathic pulmonary haemosiderosis, alveolar proteinosis and eosinophilic pneumonia rarely present.
- **Increased dyspnoea:** coexistent muscle weakness, chest wall deformity (e.g. thoracic kyphosis) and deconditioning may all exacerbate dyspnoea associated with interstitial lung disease.
- **Surgical lung biopsy:** often inappropriate in the very frail. A diagnosis therefore frequently depends on clinical and HRCT findings alone.

19.91 Pulmonary eosinophilia

Extrinsic (cause known)

- Helminths: e.g. *Ascaris, Toxocara, Filaria*
- Drugs: nitrofurantoin, para-aminosalicylic acid (PAS), sulfasalazine, imipramine, chlorpropamide, phenylbutazone
- Fungi: e.g. *Aspergillus fumigatus* causing allergic bronchopulmonary aspergillosis (p. 696)

Intrinsic (cause unknown)

- Cryptogenic eosinophilic pneumonia
- Churg–Strauss syndrome (diagnosed on the basis of four or more of the following features: asthma, peripheral blood eosinophilia > 1.5 × 10⁹/L (or > 10% of a total white cell count), mononeuropathy or polyneuropathy, pulmonary infiltrates, paranasal sinus disease or eosinophilic vasculitis on biopsy of an affected site)
- Hypereosinophilic syndrome
- Polyarteritis nodosa (p. 1113; rare)

fever, weight loss, dyspnoea and asthma-like symptoms. Peripheral blood eosinophilia is marked, as is the elevation of total IgE. High antifilarial antibody titres are seen. The diagnosis may be confirmed by a response to treatment with diethylcarbamazine (6 mg/kg/day for 3 weeks). Important differential diagnoses include infection with *Strongyloides stercoralis* (p. 365), *Ascaris* ('larva migrans', p. 365) and other hookworm infestation (p. 364).

Wegener's granulomatosis

Wegener's granulomatosis is a rare vasculitic and granulomatous condition (p. 1113). The lung is commonly involved in systemic forms of the condition but a limited pulmonary form may also occur. Respiratory symptoms include cough, haemoptysis and chest pain. Associated upper respiratory tract manifestations include nasal discharge and crusting, and otitis media. Fever, weight loss and anaemia are common. Radiological features include multiple nodules and cavitation which may resemble primary or metastatic carcinoma, or a pulmonary abscess. Tissue biopsy confirms the distinctive pattern of necrotising granulomas and necrotising vasculitis. Other respiratory complications include tracheal subglottic stenosis and saddle nose deformity. The differential diagnoses include mycobacterial and fungal infection and other forms of pulmonary vasculitis (p. 1112), including polyarteritis nodosa (pulmonary infarction), microscopic polyangiitis, Churg–Strauss syndrome, necrotising sarcoid, bronchocentric granulomatosis, lymphomatoid granulomatosis and cavitating tumours.

Goodpasture's syndrome

This describes the association of pulmonary haemorrhage and glomerulonephritis, in which IgG antibodies bind to the glomerular or alveolar basement membranes (see Box 17.40, p. 502). Pulmonary disease usually precedes renal involvement and includes radiographic infiltrates and hypoxia with or without haemoptysis. It occurs more commonly in men and almost exclusively in smokers.

19.93 Drug-induced respiratory disease

Non-cardiogenic pulmonary oedema (ARDS)

- Hydrochlorothiazide
- Thrombolytics (streptokinase)
- I.v. β-adrenoceptor agonists (e.g. for premature labour)
- Aspirin and opiates (in overdose)

Non-eosinophilic alveolitis

- Amiodarone, flecainide, gold, nitrofurantoin, cytotoxic agents—especially bleomycin, busulfan, mitomycin C, methotrexate, sulfasalazine

Pulmonary eosinophilia

- Antimicrobials (nitrofurantoin, penicillin, tetracyclines, sulphonamides, nalidixic acid)
- Antirheumatic agents (gold, aspirin, penicillamine, naproxen)
- Cytotoxic drugs (bleomycin, methotrexate, procarbazine)
- Psychotropic drugs (chlorpromazine, dosulepin, imipramine)
- Anticonvulsants (carbamazepine, phenytoin)
- Others (sulfasalazine, nadolol)

Pleural disease

- Bromocriptine, amiodarone, methotrexate, methysergide
- Induction of SLE—phenytoin, hydralazine, isoniazid

Asthma

- Pharmacological mechanisms (β-blockers, cholinergic agonists, aspirin and NSAIDs)
- Idiosyncratic reactions (tamoxifen, dipyridamole)

Lung diseases due to irradiation and drugs

Radiotherapy

Targeting radiotherapy to certain tumours is inevitably accompanied by irradiation of normal lung tissue. Although delivered in divided doses, the effects are cumulative. Acute radiation pneumonitis is typically seen within 6–12 weeks and presents with cough and dyspnoea. This may resolve spontaneously but responds to corticosteroid treatment. Chronic interstitial fibrosis may present several months later with symptoms of exertional dyspnoea and cough. Changes are often confined to the area irradiated but may be bilateral. Established post-irradiation fibrosis does not usually respond to corticosteroid treatment. The pulmonary effects of radiation (p. 272) are exacerbated by treatment with cytotoxic drugs, and the phenomenon of 'recall pneumonitis' describes the appearance of radiation injury in a previously irradiated area when chemotherapy follows radiotherapy. If the patient survives, there are long-term risks of lung cancer.

Drugs

Drugs may cause a number of parenchymal reactions, including ARDS, eosinophilic reactions and diffuse interstitial inflammation/scarring (Box 19.93). Drugs can also cause other lung disorders, including asthma, haemorrhage (e.g. anticoagulants, penicillamine) and occasionally pleural effusions and pleural thickening. An ARDS-like syndrome of acute non-cardiogenic pulmonary oedema may present with dramatic onset of breathlessness, severe hypoxaemia and signs of alveolar oedema on the chest X-ray.

Pulmonary fibrosis may occur in response to a variety of drugs, but is seen most frequently with bleomycin, methotrexate, amiodarone and nitrofurantoin. The pathogenesis of drug-induced eosinophilic pulmonary reactions may be an immune reaction similar to that in hypersensitivity pneumonitis, which specifically attracts large numbers of eosinophils into the lungs. Patients usually present with breathlessness, cough and fever. The chest X-ray characteristically shows patchy shadowing. Most cases resolve completely on withdrawal of the drug, but if the reaction is severe, rapid resolution can be obtained with corticosteroids.

Rare interstitial lung diseases

See Box 19.94.

i 19.94 Rare interstitial lung diseases

Disease	Presentation	Chest X-ray	Course
Idiopathic pulmonary haemosiderosis	Haemoptysis, breathlessness, anaemia	Bilateral infiltrates often perihilar Diffuse pulmonary fibrosis	Rapidly progressive in children Slow progression or remission in adults Death from massive pulmonary haemorrhage or cor pulmonale and respiratory failure
Alveolar proteinosis	Breathlessness and cough Occasionally fever, chest pain and haemoptysis	Diffuse bilateral shadowing, often more pronounced in the hilar regions Air bronchogram	Spontaneous remission in one-third Whole-lung lavage or granulocyte macrophage-colony stimulating factor (GM-CSF) therapy may be effective
Langerhans cell histiocytosis (histiocytosis X)	Breathlessness, cough, pneumothorax	Diffuse interstitial shadowing progressing to honeycombing	Course unpredictable but may progress to respiratory failure Smoking cessation may be followed by significant improvement Poor response to immunosuppressive treatment
Neurofibromatosis	Breathlessness and cough in a patient with multiple organ involvement with neurofibromas including skin	Bilateral reticulonodular shadowing of diffuse interstitial fibrosis	Slow progression to death from respiratory failure Poor response to corticosteroid therapy
Alveolar microlithiasis	May be asymptomatic Breathlessness and cough	Diffuse calcified micronodular shadowing more pronounced in the lower zones	Slowly progressive to cor pulmonale and respiratory failure May stabilise in some
Lymphangioleiomyomatosis	Haemoptysis, breathlessness, pneumothorax and chylous effusion in females	Diffuse bilateral shadowing CT shows characteristic thin-walled cysts with well-defined walls throughout both lungs	Progressive to death within 10 years Oestrogen ablation and progesterone therapy of doubtful value Consider lung transplantation
Pulmonary tuberous sclerosis	Very similar to lymphangioleiomyomatosis except occasionally occurs in men		

19

PULMONARY VASCULAR DISEASE

Venous thromboembolism (VTE)

Deep venous thrombosis (DVT, p. 1004) and pulmonary embolism (PE) can be considered under this heading. The majority (79%) of pulmonary emboli arise from the propagation of lower limb DVT. Rare causes include septic emboli (from endocarditis affecting the tricuspid or pulmonary valves), tumour (especially choriocarcinoma), fat, air, amniotic fluid and placenta.

The incidence of VTE in the community is unknown; it occurs in approximately 1% of all patients admitted to hospital and accounts for around 5% of in-hospital deaths. It is a common mode of death in patients with cancer, stroke and pregnancy.

Clinical features

VTE can be difficult to diagnose. It may be helpful to consider the following:

- Is the clinical presentation consistent with PE?
- Does the patient have risk factors for PE?
- Are there any alternative diagnoses that can explain the patient's presentation?

Presentation varies depending on the number, size and distribution of emboli, and the underlying cardiorespiratory reserve (Box 19.95). A recognised risk factor is present in between 80% and 90% of patients (Box 19.96). The presence of one or more risk factors may multiply the risk.

Investigations

Chest radiography

A variety of non-specific appearances have been described (Fig. 19.58) but the chest X-ray is most useful in excluding key differential diagnoses, e.g. pneumonia or pneumothorax. Normal appearances in an acutely breathless and hypoxaemic patient should raise the suspicion of PE, as should bilateral changes in a patient presenting with unilateral pleuritic chest pain.

Electrocardiography

The ECG is often normal but is useful in excluding other important differential diagnoses such as acute myocardial infarction and pericarditis. The most common abnormalities in PE include sinus tachycardia and anterior T-wave inversion but are non-specific; larger emboli may cause right heart strain revealed by an $S_1Q_3T_3$ pattern, ST-segment and T-wave changes, or the appearance of right bundle branch block.

Arterial blood gases

Arterial blood gases typically show a reduced PaO_2, a normal or low $PaCO_2$, and an increased alveolar–arterial oxygen gradient, but may be normal in a significant minority. A metabolic acidosis may be seen in acute massive PE with cardiovascular collapse.

D-dimer and other circulating markers

D-dimer is a specific degradation product released into the circulation when cross-linked fibrin undergoes

717

i 19.95 Features of pulmonary thromboemboli

	Acute massive PE	Acute small/medium PE	Chronic PE
Pathophysiology	Major haemodynamic effects: ↓cardiac output; acute right heart failure	Occlusion of segmental pulmonary artery → infarction ± effusion	Chronic occlusion of pulmonary microvasculature, right heart failure
Symptoms	Faintness or collapse, crushing central chest pain, apprehension, severe dyspnoea	Pleuritic chest pain, restricted breathing, haemoptysis	Exertional dyspnoea. Late symptoms of pulmonary hypertension or right heart failure
Signs	Major circulatory collapse: tachycardia, hypotension, ↑JVP, right ventricular gallop rhythm, loud P_2, severe cyanosis, ↓urinary output	Tachycardia, pleural rub, raised hemidiaphragm, crackles, effusion (often blood-stained), low-grade fever	May be minimal early in disease. Later: RV heave, loud P_2. Terminal: signs of right heart failure
Chest X-ray	Usually normal. May be subtle oligaemia	Pleuropulmonary opacities, pleural effusion, linear shadows, raised hemidiaphragm	Enlarged pulmonary artery trunk, enlarged heart, prominent RV
ECG	$S_1Q_3T_3$ anterior T-wave inversion, right bundle branch block (RBBB)	Sinus tachycardia	RV hypertrophy and strain
Arterial blood gases	Markedly abnormal with ↓PaO_2 and ↓$PaCO_2$. Metabolic acidosis	May be normal or ↓PaO_2 or ↓$PaCO_2$	Exertional ↓PaO_2 or desaturation on formal exercise testing
Alternative diagnoses	Myocardial infarction, pericardial tamponade, aortic dissection	Pneumonia, pneumothorax, musculoskeletal chest pain	Other causes of pulmonary hypertension

🔍 19.96 Risk factors for venous thromboembolism

Surgery

- Major abdominal/pelvic surgery
- Hip/knee surgery
- Post-operative intensive care

Obstetrics

- Pregnancy/puerperium

Cardiorespiratory disease

- COPD
- Congestive cardiac failure
- Other disabling disease

Lower limb problems

- Fracture
- Varicose veins
- Stroke/spinal cord injury

Malignant disease

- Abdominal/pelvic
- Advanced/metastatic
- Concurrent chemotherapy

Miscellaneous

- Increasing age
- Previous proven VTE
- Immobility
- Thrombotic disorders (Ch. 24)
- Trauma

endogenous fibrinolysis (p. 992). An elevated D-dimer is of limited value, as it occurs in a number of conditions including PE, myocardial infarction, pneumonia and sepsis. However, low D-dimer levels (< 500 ng/mL measured by ELISA), particularly where clinical risk is low, have a high negative predictive value and further investigation is unnecessary (Fig. 19.59). The D-dimer result should be disregarded in high-risk patients, as further investigation is mandatory even if it is normal. Other circulating markers that reflect right ventricular micro-infarction, such as troponin I and brain natriuretic peptide, are under investigation.

Imaging

A range of imaging techniques can be used to confirm suspected PE. The choice depends on the clinical probability of VTE, the condition of the patient, local availability, risks from iodinated contrast medium, radiation exposure and the associated costs.

CT pulmonary angiography (CTPA, Fig. 19.60) is the most commonly sought first-line diagnostic test. It has the advantage of visualising the distribution and extent of the emboli, or highlighting alternative diagnoses such as consolidation, pneumothorax or aortic dissection. The sensitivity of CT may be increased by simultaneous visualisation of the femoral and popliteal veins. As contrast may be nephrotoxic, care should be taken in patients with renal impairment and the use of iodinated contrast media should be avoided in those with a history of allergy to it.

Ventilation–perfusion scanning is less commonly used, as its utility is limited in patients with pre-existing chronic cardiopulmonary pathology and the scan is most frequently regarded as indeterminate. It is most useful in patients without significant cardiopulmonary disease and a normal chest X-ray; interpretation should be informed by clinical probability.

Colour Doppler ultrasound of the leg veins remains the investigation of choice in patients with suspected DVT, but may also be applied to patients in whom PE is suspected, particularly if there are clinical signs in a limb, as many will have identifiable proximal thrombus in the leg veins.

Echocardiography

Bedside echocardiography is extremely helpful in the differential diagnosis and assessment of acute circulatory collapse (p. 541). Acute dilatation of the right heart

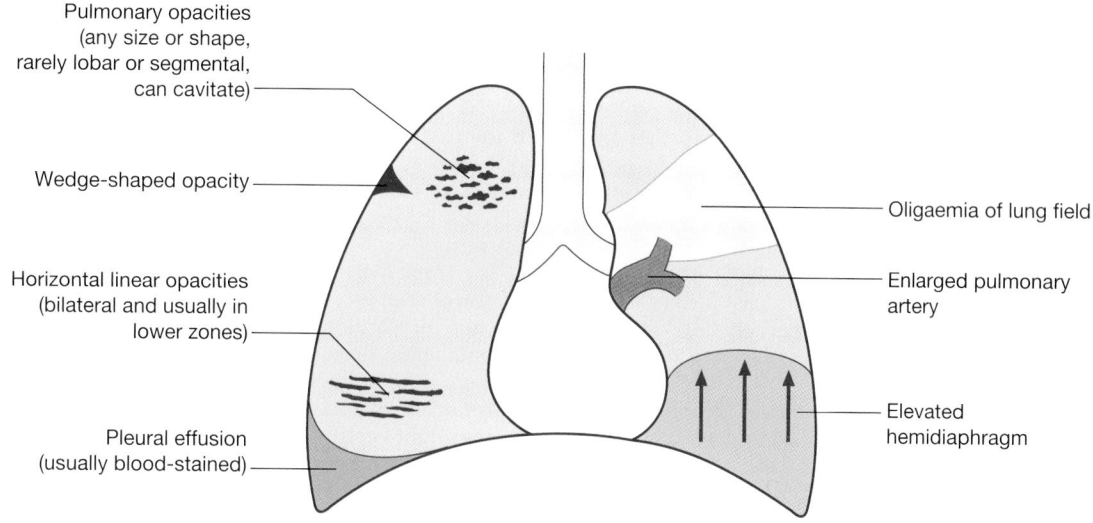

Fig. 19.58 **Features of pulmonary thromboembolism/infarction on chest X-ray.**

Pulmonary opacities
(any size or shape,
rarely lobar or segmental,
can cavitate)

Wedge-shaped opacity

Horizontal linear opacities
(bilateral and usually in
lower zones)

Pleural effusion
(usually blood-stained)

Oligaemia of lung field

Enlarged pulmonary
artery

Elevated
hemidiaphragm

is usually present in massive PE, and thrombus (embolism in transit) may be visible. Alternative diagnoses, including left ventricular failure, aortic dissection and pericardial tamponade, can also be established.

Pulmonary angiography

Conventional pulmonary angiography has been largely superseded by CTPA but may still be used in selected settings or for delivering catheter-based therapies.

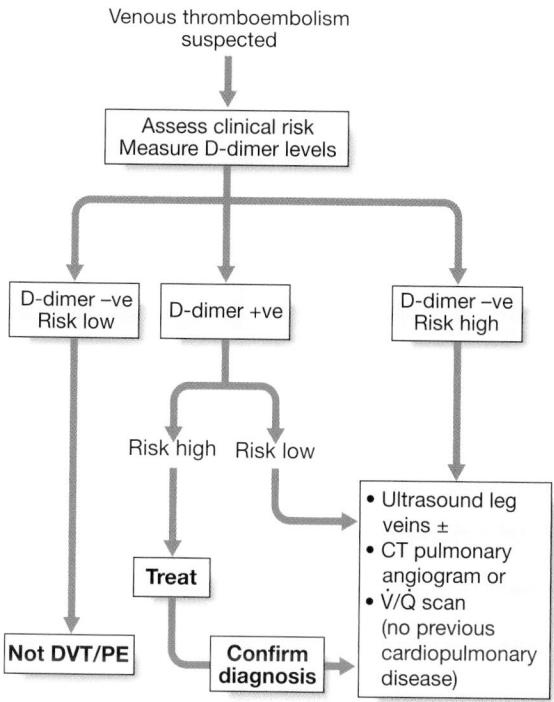

Fig. 19.59 **Algorithm for the investigation of patients with suspected pulmonary thromboembolism.** Clinical risk is based on the presence of risk factors for VTE and the probability of another diagnosis.

Venous thromboembolism
suspected

Assess clinical risk
Measure D-dimer levels

D-dimer –ve
Risk low

D-dimer +ve

D-dimer –ve
Risk high

Risk high   Risk low

Treat

Not DVT/PE

**Confirm
diagnosis**

• Ultrasound leg
  veins ±
• CT pulmonary
  angiogram or
• V̇/Q̇ scan
  (no previous
  cardiopulmonary
  disease)

Management

General measures

Prompt recognition and treatment are potentially life-saving. Oxygen should be given to all hypoxaemic patients at a concentration necessary to maintain arterial oxygen saturation above 90%. Circulatory shock should be treated with intravenous fluids or plasma expander, but inotropic agents are of limited value, as the hypoxic dilated right ventricle is near maximally stimulated by endogenous catecholamines. Diuretics and vasodilators should also be avoided, as they will reduce cardiac output. Opiates may be necessary to relieve pain and distress but should be used with caution in the hypotensive patient. Resuscitation by external cardiac massage may be successful in the moribund patient by dislodging and breaking up a large central embolus.

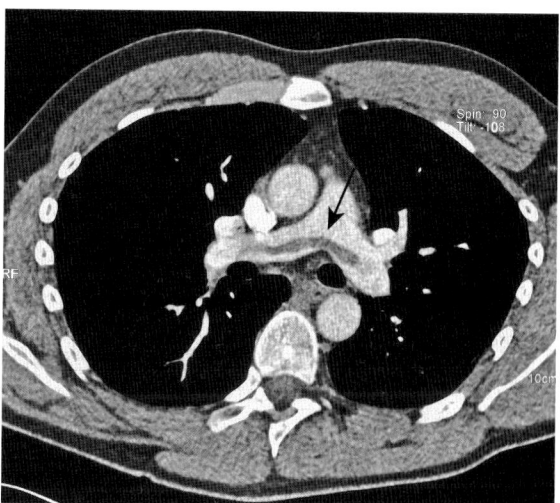

Fig. 19.60 **CT pulmonary angiogram.** The arrow points to a saddle embolism in the bifurcation of the pulmonary artery.

19

Anticoagulation

Anticoagulation should be commenced immediately in patients with a high or intermediate probability, but may be safely withheld in patients with low clinical probability pending investigation. Heparin reduces further propagation of clot, the risk of further emboli, and lowers mortality. It is most easily administered as subcutaneous low molecular weight heparin. The dose is based on the patient's weight and there is usually no requirement to monitor tests of coagulation (p. 1005). The duration of LMWH treatment should be at least 5 days, during which time oral warfarin is commenced. LMWH should not be discontinued until the international normalised ratio (INR) is greater than 2.

Patients with a persistent prothrombotic risk or a history of previous emboli should be anticoagulated for life, whereas those with an identifiable and reversible risk factor usually require only 3 months of therapy. If the condition is idiopathic or risk factors are weak, anticoagulation for 6 months is recommended, although the appropriate duration is unclear. Long-term, low-intensity warfarin therapy (target INR 1.5–2.0) appears to be associated with reduced risk of bleeding and may prevent recurrent thromboembolism (p. 1005). The role of D-dimer and right heart function in decision-making on duration of anticoagulation is currently being examined.

Thrombolytic therapy

Thrombolysis is indicated in any patient presenting with acute massive PE accompanied by cardiogenic shock. In the absence of shock, the benefits are less clear but it may be considered in patients presenting with right ventricular dilatation and hypokinesis or severe hypoxaemia. Patients must be screened carefully for haemorrhagic risk, as there is a high risk of intracranial haemorrhage. Surgical pulmonary embolectomy may be considered in selected patients but carries a high mortality risk.

Caval filters

A patient in whom anticoagulation is contraindicated, who has suffered massive haemorrhage on anticoagulation, or recurrent VTE despite anticoagulation, should be considered for an inferior vena caval filter. The introduction of retrievable caval filters has been useful in patients with temporary risk factors.

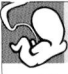

19.97 VTE and pregnancy

- **Maternal mortality:** VTE is the leading cause.
- **CTPA:** may be performed safely with fetal shielding (0.01–0.06 mGy). It is important to consider the risk of radiation to breast tissue (particularly if family history of breast carcinoma) and the risk of iodinated contrast media to mother and fetus (neonatal hypothyroidism).
- **V̇/Q̇ scanning:** greater radiation dose to fetus (0.11–0.22 mGy) but less to maternal breast tissue.
- **In utero radiation exposure:** estimated incidence of childhood malignancy is about 1 in 16 000 per mGy.
- **Warfarin:** teratogenic, so VTE should be treated with LMWH during pregnancy.

Prognosis

Patients who have suffered symptomatic VTE carry an increased risk of further events, particularly if a persisting risk factor is present. The risk of recurrence is highest in the first 6–12 months after the initial event, and by follow-up at 10 years just under one-third of patients may have suffered a further event. Risks of recurrent VTE are lowest in those with temporary or reversible risk factors.

The immediate mortality is greatest in those with echocardiographic evidence of right ventricular dysfunction or cardiogenic shock. The vast majority of patients attain normal right heart function by 3 weeks but persisting pulmonary hypertension may be present in around 4% of patients by 2 years. A minority progress to overt right ventricular failure.

Pulmonary hypertension

Pulmonary hypertension (PH) is defined as a mean pulmonary artery pressure > 25 mmHg at rest or 30 mmHg with exercise. Pulmonary arterial hypertension (PAH) also requires the presence of a pulmonary capillary wedge pressure ≤ 15 mmHg and a pulmonary vascular resistance ≥ 240 dynes/s/cm⁵. The causes of pulmonary hypertension by site of pathology are listed in Box 19.98.

19.98 Classification of pulmonary hypertension

Pulmonary arterial hypertension

- Primary pulmonary hypertension: sporadic and familial
- Related to: connective tissue disease (limited cutaneous systemic sclerosis), congenital systemic to pulmonary shunts, portal hypertension, HIV infection, exposure to various drugs or toxins, and persistent pulmonary hypertension of the newborn

Pulmonary venous hypertension

- Left-sided atrial or ventricular heart disease
- Left-sided valvular heart disease
- Pulmonary veno-occlusive disease
- Pulmonary capillary haemangiomatosis

Pulmonary hypertension associated with disorders of the respiratory system and/or hypoxaemia

- COPD
- DPLD
- Sleep-disordered breathing
- Alveolar hypoventilation disorders
- Chronic exposure to high altitude
- Neonatal lung disease
- Alveolar capillary dysplasia
- Severe kyphoscoliosis

Pulmonary hypertension caused by chronic thromboembolic disease

- Thromboembolic obstruction of the proximal pulmonary arteries
- In situ thrombosis
- Sickle cell disease

Miscellaneous

- Inflammatory conditions
- Extrinsic compression of central pulmonary veins

Further classification is based on the degree of functional disturbance according to the New York Heart Association (NYHA) grades I–IV. Although respiratory failure due to intrinsic pulmonary disease is the most common cause of pulmonary hypertension, severe pulmonary hypertension may occur as a primary disorder, as a complication of connective tissue disease (e.g. systemic sclerosis), or as a result of chronic thromboembolic events.

Primary pulmonary hypertension (PPH) is a rare but important disease that affects young people, predominantly women, aged between 20 and 30 years. Familial disease is rarer still, but is known to be associated with mutations in the gene encoding type II bone morphogenetic protein receptor (BMPR2), a member of the TGF-β superfamily. Mutations in this gene have been identified in some patients with sporadic pulmonary hypertension.

Pathological features include hypertrophy of both the media and intima of the vessel wall, and a clonal expansion of endothelial cells which take the appearance of plexiform lesions. There is marked narrowing of the vessel lumen and this together with the frequently observed in situ thrombosis leads to an increase in pulmonary vascular resistance and pulmonary hypertension.

Clinical features

Pulmonary hypertension presents insidiously and is often diagnosed late. Typical symptoms include breathlessness, chest pain, fatigue, palpitation and syncope. Important signs include elevation of the JVP (with a prominent 'a' wave if in sinus rhythm), a parasternal heave (RV hypertrophy), accentuation of the pulmonary component of the second heart sound and a right ventricular third heart sound.

Investigations

Pulmonary hypertension may be suspected if an ECG show a right ventricular 'strain' pattern or a chest X-ray shows enlarged pulmonary arteries, peripheral pruning and right ventricle enlargement. Confirmation is by transthoracic echocardiography; Doppler assessment of the tricuspid regurgitant jet provides a non-invasive estimate of the pulmonary artery pressure. Further assessment should be undertaken in specialist centres that can perform right heart catheterisation to assess pulmonary haemodynamics and measure vasodilator responsiveness, to guide further therapy.

Management

Pulmonary hypertension is incurable but new treatments have delivered significant improvements in exercise performance, symptoms and prognosis. All patients should be anticoagulated with warfarin, and oxygen, diuretics and digoxin prescribed as appropriate. Specific treatment options include high-dose calcium channel blockers, prostaglandins such as epoprostenol (prostacyclin) or iloprost therapy, the PDE5 inhibitor sildenafil, and the oral endothelin antagonist bosentan. Selected patients can be referred for heart-lung transplantation, and pulmonary thromboendarterectomy may be contemplated in those with chronic proximal pulmonary thromboembolic disease. Atrial septostomy (the creation of a right to left shunt) decompresses the right ventricle and improves haemodynamic performance at the expense of shunting and hypoxaemia.

19.99 Thromboembolic disease in old age

- **Risk:** rises by a factor of 2.5 over the age of 60 years.
- **Prophylaxis for VTE:** should be considered in all older patients who are immobile as a result of acute illness, except when this is due to acute stroke.
- **Association with cancer:** the prevalence of cancer among those with DVT increases with age but the relative risk of malignancy with DVT falls; therefore intensive investigation is not justified if initial assessment reveals no evidence of an underlying neoplasm.
- **Warfarin:** older patients are more sensitive to the anticoagulant effects of warfarin, partly due to the concurrent use of other drugs and the presence of other pathology. Life-threatening or fatal bleeds on warfarin are significantly more common in those aged over 80 years.
- **Chronic immobility:** long-term anticoagulant therapy is not required as there is no associated increase in thromboembolism.

DISEASES OF THE UPPER AIRWAY

19

Diseases of the nasopharynx

Allergic rhinitis

This is a disorder in which there are episodes of nasal congestion, watery nasal discharge and sneezing. It may be seasonal or perennial.

Aetiology

Allergic rhinitis is due to an immediate hypersensitivity reaction in the nasal mucosa. Seasonal antigens include pollens from grasses, flowers, weeds or trees. Grass pollen is responsible for hay fever, the most common type of seasonal allergic rhinitis in northern Europe, which is at its peak between May and July. This is, however, a world-wide problem, which may be aggravated during harvest seasons.

Perennial allergic rhinitis may be a specific reaction to antigens derived from house dust, fungal spores or animal dander, but similar symptoms can be caused by physical or chemical irritants—for example, pungent odours or fumes, including strong perfumes, cold air and dry atmospheres. The term 'vasomotor rhinitis' is often used in this context, as the term 'allergic' is a misnomer.

Clinical features

In the seasonal type, there are frequent sudden attacks of sneezing, with profuse watery nasal discharge and nasal obstruction. These attacks last for a few hours and are often accompanied by smarting and watering of the eyes and conjunctival infection. In perennial rhinitis, the symptoms are similar but more continuous and generally less severe. Skin hypersensitivity tests with the relevant antigen are usually positive in seasonal allergic rhinitis, but are less useful in perennial rhinitis.

Prevention

In those sensitised to house dust, simple measures such as thorough dust removal from the bed area, leaving a window open and renewing old pillows are often helpful. Avoidance of pollen and antigens from domestic pets, however desirable and beneficial, is usually impractical.

Management

The following medications, singly or in combination, are usually effective in both seasonal and perennial allergic rhinitis:

- an antihistamine such as loratadine
- sodium cromoglicate nasal spray
- nasal steroid spray, e.g. beclometasone dipropionate, fluticasone, mometasone or budesonide.

In patients whose symptoms are very severe and seriously interfering with school, business or social activities, systemic corticosteroids are occasionally indicated, but side-effects limit their usefulness. Vasomotor rhinitis is often difficult to treat, but may respond to ipratropium bromide, administered into each nostril 6–8-hourly.

Sleep-disordered breathing

A variety of respiratory disorders affect sleep or are affected by sleep. Cough and wheeze disturbing sleep are characteristic of asthma, while the hypoventilation that accompanies normal sleep can precipitate respiratory failure in patients with disordered ventilation due to kyphoscoliosis, diaphragmatic palsy or muscle disease (e.g. muscular dystrophy).

In contrast, a small but important group of disorders cause problems only during sleep. Patients with these may have normal lungs and daytime respiratory function, but during sleep have either abnormalities of ventilatory drive (central sleep apnoea) or upper airway obstruction (obstructive sleep apnoea). Of these, the obstructive sleep apnoea/hypopnoea syndrome is by far the most common and important. When this coexists with COPD, severe respiratory failure can result even if the COPD is mild.

The sleep apnoea/hypopnoea syndrome

It is now recognised that 2–4% of the middle-aged population suffer from recurrent upper airway obstruction during sleep. The ensuing sleep fragmentation causes daytime sleepiness, especially in monotonous situations, resulting in a threefold increased risk of road traffic accidents and a ninefold increased risk of single-vehicle accidents.

Aetiology

Sleep apnoea results from recurrent occlusion of the pharynx during sleep, usually at the level of the soft palate. Inspiration results in negative pressure within the pharynx. During wakefulness, upper airway dilating muscles, including palatoglossus and genioglossus, contract actively during inspiration to preserve airway patency. During sleep, muscle tone declines, impairing the ability of these muscles to maintain pharyngeal patency. In a minority of people, a combination of an anatomically narrow palatopharynx and underactivity of the dilating muscles during sleep results in inspiratory airway obstruction. Incomplete obstruction causes turbulent flow, resulting in snoring (around 40% of middle-aged men and 20% of middle-aged women snore). More severe obstruction triggers increased inspiratory effort and transiently wakes the patient, allowing the dilating muscles to re-open the airway. These awakenings are so brief that patients have no recollection of them. After a series of loud deep breaths that may wake their bed partner, the patient rapidly returns to sleep, snores and becomes apnoeic once more. This cycle of apnoea and awakening may repeat itself many hundreds of times per night and results in severe sleep fragmentation and secondary variations in blood pressure, which may predispose over time to sustained hypertension, coronary events and stroke.

Predisposing factors to the sleep apnoea/hypopnoea syndrome include being male, which doubles the risk probably due to a testosterone effect on the upper airway, and obesity, found in about half of patients, because parapharyngeal fat deposits tend to narrow the pharynx. Nasal obstruction or a recessed mandible can further exacerbate the problem. Acromegaly and hypothyroidism also predispose by causing submucosal infiltration and narrowing of the upper airway. Sleep apnoea is often familial, and in these families the maxilla and mandible are back-set, narrowing the upper airway. Alcohol and sedatives predispose to snoring and apnoea by relaxing the upper airway dilating muscles.

Clinical features

Excessive daytime sleepiness is the principal symptom and snoring is virtually universal. The patient usually feels that he or she has been asleep all night but wakes unrefreshed. Bed partners report loud snoring in all body positions and will often have noticed multiple breathing pauses (apnoeas). Difficulty with concentration, impaired cognitive function and work performance, depression, irritability and nocturia are other features.

Investigations

Provided that the sleepiness does not result from inadequate time in bed or from shift work and so on, any person who repeatedly falls asleep during the day when not in bed, who complains that his or her work is impaired by sleepiness, or who is a habitual snorer with multiple witnessed apnoeas should be referred to a respiratory specialist for a sleep assessment. A more quantitative assessment of daytime sleepiness can be obtained by questionnaire (Box 19.100).

Overnight studies of breathing, oxygenation and sleep quality are diagnostic (Fig. 19.61) but the appropriate level of investigations depends on local resources and the probability of the diagnosis. The current threshold for diagnosing the sleep apnoea/hypopnoea syndrome is 15 apnoeas/hypopnoeas per hour of sleep, where an apnoea is a 10-second or longer breathing pause and a hypopnoea a 10-second or longer 50% reduction in breathing.

Differential diagnosis

Several other conditions can cause daytime sleepiness but can usually be excluded by a careful history (Box 19.101). Narcolepsy is a rare cause of sleepiness, occurring in 0.05% of the population (p. 1179). Idiopathic hypersomnolence occurs in younger individuals and is characterised by long nocturnal sleeps.

19.100 Epworth sleepiness scale

How likely are you to doze off or fall asleep in the situations described below? Use the following scale to choose the most appropriate number for each situation:

0 = would never doze
1 = slight chance of dozing
2 = moderate chance of dozing
3 = high chance of dozing

- Sitting and reading
- Watching TV
- Sitting, inactive in a public place (e.g. a theatre or a meeting)
- As a passenger in a car for an hour without a break
- Lying down to rest in the afternoon when circumstances permit
- Sitting and talking to someone
- Sitting quietly after a lunch without alcohol
- In a car, while stopped for a few minutes in the traffic

Normal subjects average 5.9 (SD 2.2) and patients with severe obstructive sleep apnoea average 16.0 (SD 4.4).

19.101 Differential diagnosis of persistent sleepiness

Lack of sleep

- Inadequate time in bed
- Extraneous sleep disruption (e.g. babies/children)
- Shift work
- Excessive caffeine intake
- Physical illness (e.g. pain)

Sleep disruption

- Sleep apnoea/hypopnoea syndrome
- Periodic limb movement disorder (recurrent limb movements during non-REM sleep, frequent nocturnal awakenings)

Sleepiness with relatively normal sleep

- Narcolepsy
- Idiopathic hypersomnolence (rare)
- Neurological lesions (e.g. hypothalamic or upper brain-stem infarcts or tumours)
- Drugs

Psychological/psychiatric

- Depression

Management

The major hazard to patients and those around them is traffic accidents, so all drivers must be advised not to drive until treatment has relieved their sleepiness. In a minority, relief of nasal obstruction or the avoidance of alcohol may prevent obstruction. Advice to obese patients to lose weight is often unheeded, and the majority of patients need to use continuous positive airway pressure (CPAP) delivered by a nasal mask every night to splint the upper airway open. When CPAP is tolerated, the effect is often dramatic (see Fig. 19.61), with relief of somnolence and improved daytime performance, quality of life and survival. Unfortunately, 30–50% of patients do not tolerate CPAP. Mandibular advancement devices worn within the mouth are an alternative that is effective in some patients. There is no evidence that palatal surgery is of benefit.

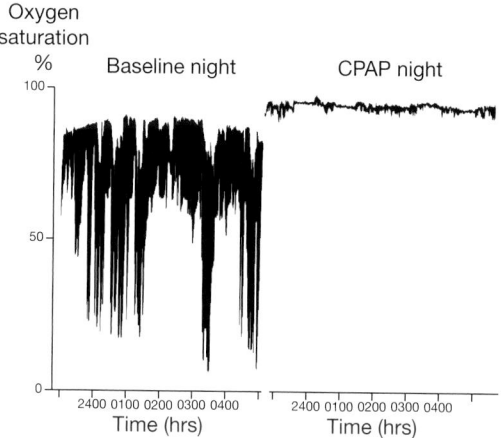

Fig. 19.61 Sleep apnoea/hypopnoea syndrome: overnight oxygen saturation trace. The left-hand panel shows the trace of a 46-year-old patient when he slept without continuous positive airway pressure (CPAP) and had 53 apnoeas plus hypopnoeas/hour, 55 brief awakenings/hour and marked oxygen desaturation. The right-hand panel shows the effect of CPAP of 10 cm H_2O delivered through a tight-fitting nasal mask, which abolished his breathing irregularity and awakenings, and improved his oxygenation.

Laryngeal disorders

Acute infections are described in Box 19.41 (p. 681). Other disorders of the larynx include chronic laryngitis, laryngeal tuberculosis, laryngeal paralysis and laryngeal obstruction. Tumours of the larynx are relatively common, particularly in smokers. For further details, the reader should refer to an otolaryngology text.

Chronic laryngitis

The common causes are listed in Box 19.102. The chief symptoms are hoarseness or loss of voice (aphonia). There is irritation of the throat and a spasmodic cough. The disease pursues a chronic course, frequently uninfluenced by treatment, and the voice may become permanently impaired. The causes of chronic hoarseness are listed in Box 19.103.

In some patients a chest X-ray may bring to light an unsuspected bronchial carcinoma or pulmonary tuberculosis. If no such abnormality is found,

19.102 Causes of chronic laryngitis

- Repeated attacks of acute laryngitis
- Excessive use of the voice, especially in dusty atmospheres
- Heavy tobacco smoking
- Mouth-breathing from nasal obstruction
- Chronic infection of nasal sinuses

19.103 Causes of chronic hoarseness

If hoarseness persists for more than a few days, consider:
- Adverse effect of inhaled corticosteroid treatment
- TB
- Laryngeal paralysis
- Tumour of the larynx

19

laryngoscopy should be performed, usually by a specialist in otolaryngology.

Management

When no specific treatable cause is found, the voice must be rested completely. This is particularly important in public speakers and singers. Smoking should be avoided. Some benefit may be obtained from frequent inhalations of medicated steam.

Laryngeal paralysis

Interruption of the motor nerve supply of the larynx is nearly always unilateral and, because of the intrathoracic course of the left recurrent laryngeal nerve, usually left-sided. One or both recurrent laryngeal nerves may be damaged at thyroidectomy, by carcinoma of the thyroid or by anterior neck injury. Rarely, the vagal trunk itself is involved by tumour, aneurysm or trauma.

Clinical features

* *Hoarseness* always accompanies laryngeal paralysis, whatever its cause. Paralysis of organic origin is seldom reversible, but when only one vocal cord is affected, hoarseness may improve or even disappear after a few weeks, as the normal cord compensates by crossing the midline to approximate with the paralysed cord on phonation.
* *'Bovine cough'* is a characteristic feature of organic laryngeal paralysis, and has a cow-like quality which lacks the explosive quality of normal coughing because the cords fail to close the glottis. Sputum clearance may also be impaired. A normal cough in patients with partial loss of voice or aphonia virtually excludes laryngeal paralysis.
* *Stridor* is occasionally present but seldom severe, except when laryngeal paralysis is bilateral.

Diagnosis and management

Laryngoscopy is necessary to establish the diagnosis of laryngeal paralysis with certainty. The paralysed cord lies in the so-called 'cadaveric' position, midway between abduction and adduction.

The cause of laryngeal paralysis should be treated if possible. In unilateral paralysis, persistent dysphonia may be improved by the injection of Teflon into the affected vocal cord. In bilateral organic paralysis, tracheal intubation, tracheostomy or plastic surgery on the larynx may be necessary.

Psychogenic hoarseness and aphonia

Psychogenic causes of hoarseness or complete loss of voice may be suggested by associated symptoms in the history (p. 238). However, laryngoscopy may be necessary to exclude a physical cause of the abnormality. In psychogenic aphonia, only the voluntary movement of adduction of the vocal cords is seen to be impaired. Speech therapy may be helpful.

Laryngeal obstruction

Laryngeal obstruction is more liable to occur in children than in adults because of the smaller size of the glottis. Important causes are given in Box 19.104.

19.104 Causes of laryngeal obstruction

* Inflammatory or allergic oedema, or exudate
* Spasm of laryngeal muscles
* Inhaled foreign body
* Inhaled blood clot or vomitus in an unconscious patient
* Tumours of the larynx
* Bilateral vocal cord paralysis
* Fixation of both cords in rheumatoid disease

Clinical features

Sudden complete laryngeal obstruction by a foreign body produces the clinical picture of acute asphyxia: violent but ineffective inspiratory efforts with indrawing of the intercostal spaces and the unsupported lower ribs, accompanied by cyanosis. Unrelieved, the condition progresses rapidly to coma and death within a few minutes. When, as in most cases, the obstruction is incomplete at first, the main clinical features are progressive breathlessness accompanied by stridor and cyanosis. Urgent treatment to prevent complete obstruction is needed.

Management

Transient laryngeal obstruction due to exudate and spasm, which may occur with acute pharyngitis in children (p. 681) and with whooping cough, is potentially dangerous but can usually be relieved by steam inhalation. Laryngeal obstruction from all other causes carries a high mortality and demands prompt treatment.

Relief of obstruction

When a foreign body causes laryngeal obstruction in children, it can often be dislodged by turning the patient head downwards and squeezing the chest vigorously. In adults, a sudden forceful compression of the upper abdomen (Heimlich manœuvre) may be effective. Otherwise, the cause of the obstruction should be investigated by direct laryngoscopy, which may also permit the removal of an unsuspected foreign body or the insertion of a tube past the obstruction into the trachea. Tracheostomy must be performed without delay if these procedures fail to relieve obstruction, but except in dire emergencies this should be performed in theatre by a surgeon.

Treatment of the cause

In diphtheria, antitoxin should be administered, and for other infections the appropriate antibiotic should be given. In angioedema, complete laryngeal occlusion can usually be prevented by treatment with adrenaline (epinephrine) 0.5–1 mg (0.5–1 mL of 1:1000) i.m., chlorphenamine maleate (10–20 mg by slow i.v. injection) and intravenous hydrocortisone sodium succinate (200 mg).

Tracheal disorders

Acute tracheitis

See Box 19.41 (p. 681).

Tracheal obstruction

External compression by enlarged mediastinal lymph nodes containing metastatic deposits, usually from a bronchial carcinoma, is a more frequent cause of tracheal obstruction than the uncommon primary benign or malignant tumours. The trachea may also be compressed by a retrosternal goitre (see Fig. 19.10, p. 655). Rare causes include an aneurysm of the aortic arch and (in children) tuberculous mediastinal lymph nodes. Tracheal stenosis is an occasional complication of tracheostomy, prolonged intubation, Wegener's granulomatosis (p. 1113) or trauma.

Clinical features and management

Stridor can be detected in every patient with severe tracheal narrowing. Bronchoscopic examination of the trachea should be undertaken without delay to determine the site, degree and nature of the obstruction.

Localised tumours of the trachea can be resected, but reconstruction after resection may be technically difficult. Endobronchial laser therapy, bronchoscopically placed tracheal stents, chemotherapy and radiotherapy are alternatives to surgery. The choice of treatment depends upon the nature of the tumour and the general health of the patient. Benign tracheal strictures can sometimes be dilated but may require resection.

Tracheo-oesophageal fistula

This may be present in newborn infants as a congenital abnormality. In adults, it is usually due to malignant lesions in the mediastinum, such as carcinoma or lymphoma, eroding both the trachea and oesophagus to produce a communication between them. Swallowed liquids enter the trachea and bronchi through the fistula and provoke coughing.

Surgical closure of a congenital fistula, if undertaken promptly, is usually successful. There is usually no curative treatment for malignant fistulae, and death from overwhelming pulmonary infection rapidly supervenes.

DISEASES OF THE PLEURA, DIAPHRAGM AND CHEST WALL

Diseases of the pleura

Pleurisy

Pleurisy is not a diagnosis but a term used to describe pleuritic pain resulting from any one of a number of disease processes involving the pleura. Pleurisy is a common feature of pulmonary infection and infarction; it may also occur in malignancy.

Clinical features

Sharp pain that is aggravated by deep breathing or coughing is characteristic. On examination, rib movement is restricted and a pleural rub may be present. Sometimes this is only audible in deep inspiration or near the pericardium (pleuro-pericardial rub). The other clinical features depend on the cause. Loss of a pleural rub and diminution in the chest pain may indicate either recovery or the development of a pleural effusion.

Every patient should have a chest X-ray, but if normal, this does not exclude a pulmonary cause of pleurisy. A preceding history of cough, purulent sputum and pyrexia is presumptive evidence of a pulmonary infection which may not have been severe enough to produce a radiographic abnormality, or which may have resolved before the chest X-ray was taken.

Management

The primary cause of pleurisy must be treated. The symptomatic treatment of pleural pain is described on page 684.

Pleural effusion

See page 658.

Empyema

This is a collection of pus in the pleural space. The pus may be as thin as serous fluid or so thick that it is impossible to aspirate even through a wide-bore needle. Microscopically, neutrophil leucocytes are present in large numbers. The causative organism may or may not be isolated from the pus. An empyema may involve the whole pleural space or only part of it ('loculated' or 'encysted' empyema) and is usually unilateral.

Aetiology

Empyema is always secondary to infection in a neighbouring structure, usually the lung, most commonly due to the bacterial pneumonias and tuberculosis. Over 40% of patients with community-acquired pneumonia develop an associated pleural effusion ('parapneumonic' effusion) and about 15% of these become secondarily infected. Other causes are infection of a haemothorax following trauma or surgery, oesophageal rupture and rupture of a subphrenic abscess through the diaphragm. Despite the widespread availability of antibiotics effective against pneumonia, empyema remains a significant cause of morbidity and mortality even in developed countries. This reflects delays in the diagnosis or in the instigation of appropriate therapy.

Pathology

Both layers of pleura are covered with a thick, shaggy inflammatory exudate. The pus in the pleural space is often under considerable pressure, and if the condition is not adequately treated, pus may rupture into a bronchus causing a bronchopleural fistula and pyopneumothorax, or track through the chest wall with the formation of a subcutaneous abscess or sinus, so-called empyema necessitans.

An empyema will only heal if infection is eradicated and the empyema space is obliterated, allowing apposition of the visceral and parietal pleural layers. This can only occur if re-expansion of the compressed lung is secured at an early stage by removal of all the pus from the pleural space. Successful re-expansion and resolution will not occur if:

- the visceral pleura becomes grossly thickened and rigid due to delayed treatment or inadequate drainage of the infected pleural fluid
- the pleural layers are kept apart by air entering the pleura through a bronchopleural fistula

19

- there is underlying disease in the lung, such as bronchiectasis, bronchial carcinoma or pulmonary TB preventing re-expansion.

In these circumstances an empyema tends to become chronic, and healing will only occur with surgical intervention.

Clinical features

An empyema should be suspected in patients with pulmonary infection if there is persisting or recurrent pyrexia despite treatment with a suitable antibiotic. In other cases the illness associated with the primary infection may be so slight that it passes unrecognised and the first definite clinical features are due to the empyema itself. Once an empyema has developed, systemic features are prominent (Box 19.105).

19.105 Clinical features of empyema
Systemic features
• Pyrexia, usually high and remittent
• Rigors, sweating, malaise and weight loss
• Polymorphonuclear leucocytosis, high CRP
Local features
• Pleural pain; breathlessness; cough and sputum usually because of underlying lung disease; copious purulent sputum if empyema ruptures into a bronchus (bronchopleural fistula)
• Clinical signs of pleural effusion

Investigations

Radiological examination

The appearances may be indistinguishable from those of pleural effusion. When air is present in addition to pus (pyopneumothorax), a horizontal 'fluid level' marks the air/liquid interface. Ultrasound shows the position of the fluid, the extent of pleural thickening and whether fluid is in a single collection or multiloculated by fibrin and debris. Sometimes, pleural adhesions confine the empyema to form a 'D'-shaped shadow against the inside of the chest wall. CT gives information on the pleura, the underlying lung parenchyma and patency of the major bronchi.

Aspiration of fluid

Ultrasound or CT is used to identify the optimal site to undertake aspiration, which is best performed using a wide-bore needle. If the fluid is thick and turbid pus, empyema is confirmed. Other features suggesting empyema are a fluid glucose < 3.3 mmol/L (60 mg/dL), LDH > 1000 U/L or a fluid pH < 7.0 (H^+ >100 nmol/L). However, pH measurement should be avoided if pus is thick, as it damages blood gas machines. The pus is frequently sterile on culture if antibiotics have already been given. The distinction between tuberculous and non-tuberculous disease can be difficult and often requires pleural biopsy, histology and culture.

Management

Treatment of non-tuberculous empyema

When the patient is acutely ill and the pus is sufficiently thin, a wide-bore intercostal tube should be inserted into the most dependent part of the empyema space (using ultrasound or CT guidance in difficult cases) and connected to an underwater-seal drain system. If the initial aspirate reveals turbid fluid or frank pus, or if loculations are seen on ultrasound, the tube should be put on suction (−5 to −10 cm H_2O) and flushed regularly with 20 mL normal saline. Trials have failed to show any benefit from intrapleural fibrinolytic therapy in empyema. An antibiotic directed against the organism causing the empyema should be given for 2–4 weeks. Empirical antibiotic treatment (e.g. intravenous co-amoxiclav or cefuroxime with metronidazole) should be used if the organism is unknown.

An empyema can often be aborted if these measures are started early. If, however, the intercostal tube is not providing adequate drainage—e.g. when the pus is thick or loculated, surgical intervention is required. The empyema cavity is cleared of pus and adhesions, and a wide-bore tube inserted to allow optimal drainage. Surgical 'decortication' of the lung may also be required if gross thickening of the visceral pleura is preventing re-expansion of the lung.

Treatment of tuberculous empyema

Antituberculosis chemotherapy must be started immediately (p. 693) and the pus in the pleural space aspirated through a wide-bore needle until it ceases to reaccumulate. Intercostal tube drainage is often required. In many patients, no other treatment is necessary but surgery is occasionally required to ablate a residual empyema space. Fibrothorax, with restriction and encasement of the lung in thickened, often calcified pleura is a late complication.

Spontaneous pneumothorax

Pneumothorax is the presence of air in the pleural space, which can either occur spontaneously, or result from iatrogenic injury or trauma to the lung or chest wall (Box 19.106). Primary spontaneous pneumothorax occurs in patients with no history of lung disease in whom smoking, tall stature and the presence of apical subpleural blebs are additional risk factors. Secondary pneumothorax affects patients with pre-existing lung disease and is associated with higher mortality rates (Fig. 19.62).

Clinical features

The most common symptoms are sudden-onset unilateral pleuritic chest pain or breathlessness. In those with

19.106 Classification of pneumothorax
Spontaneous
Primary
• No evidence of overt lung disease. Air escapes from the lung into the pleural space through rupture of a small subpleural emphysematous bulla or pleural bleb, or the pulmonary end of a pleural adhesion
Secondary
• Underlying lung disease, most commonly COPD and TB; also seen in asthma, lung abscess, pulmonary infarcts, bronchogenic carcinoma, all forms of fibrotic and cystic lung disease
Traumatic
• Iatrogenic (e.g. following thoracic surgery or biopsy) or chest wall injury

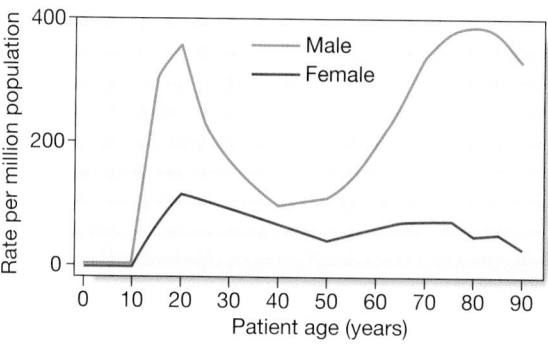

Fig. 19.62 Bimodal age distribution for hospital admissions for pneumothorax in England. The incidence of primary spontaneous pneumothorax peaks in males aged 15–30. Secondary spontaneous pneumothorax occurs mainly in males > 55 years.

underlying chest disease, breathlessness can be severe and may not resolve spontaneously. In patients with a small pneumothorax, physical examination may be normal. A larger pneumothorax (> 15% of the hemithorax) results in decreased or absent breath sounds (p. 643). The combination of absent breath sounds and resonant percussion note is diagnostic of pneumothorax.

Occasionally, the communication between the airway and the pleural space acts as a one-way valve, allowing air to enter the pleural space during inspiration but not to escape on expiration. Large amounts of trapped air accumulate progressively in the pleural space and the intrapleural pressure rises to well above atmospheric levels. This is a tension pneumothorax. The pressure causes mediastinal displacement towards the opposite side, with compression of the opposite normal lung and impairment of systemic venous return, causing cardiovascular compromise (Fig. 19.63C). Clinically, the findings are rapidly progressive breathlessness associated with a marked tachycardia, hypotension, cyanosis and tracheal displacement away from the side of the silent hemithorax. Occasionally, tension pneumothorax may occur without mediastinal shift, if malignant disease or scarring has splinted the mediastinum.

Where the communication between the airway and the pleural space seals off as the lung deflates and does not re-open, the pneumothorax is referred to as 'closed' (Fig. 19.63A). In such circumstances the mean pleural pressure remains negative, spontaneous reabsorption of air and re-expansion of the lung occur over a few days or weeks, and infection is uncommon. This contrasts with an 'open' pneumothorax, where the communication fails to seal and air continues to pass freely between the bronchial tree and pleural space (Fig. 19.63B). An example of the latter is a bronchopleural fistula, which, if large, can also facilitate the transmission of infection from the airways into the pleural space, leading to empyema. An open pneumothorax is commonly seen following rupture of an emphysematous bulla, tuberculous cavity or lung abscess into the pleural space.

Investigations

The chest X-ray shows the sharply defined edge of the deflated lung with complete translucency (no lung markings) between this and the chest wall (p. 643). Care must be taken to differentiate between a large pre-existing emphysematous bulla and a pneumothorax to avoid misdirected attempts at aspiration. Where doubt exists, CT is useful in distinguishing bullae from pleural air. X-rays also show the extent of any mediastinal displacement and reveal any pleural fluid or underlying pulmonary disease.

Management

Primary pneumothorax in which the lung edge is less than 2 cm from the chest wall and the patient is not breathless normally resolves without intervention. In young patients presenting with a moderate or large spontaneous primary pneumothorax, percutaneous needle aspiration of air is a simple and well-tolerated alternative to intercostal tube drainage, with a 60–80% chance of avoiding the need for a chest drain (Fig. 19.64). In patients with significant underlying chronic lung disease, however, secondary pneumothorax may cause respiratory distress. In these patients, the success rate of aspiration is much lower, and intercostal tube drainage and inpatient observation are usually required, particularly in those over 50 years old and those with respiratory compromise.

When needed, intercostal drains are inserted in the 4th, 5th or 6th intercostal space in the mid-axillary line, connected to an underwater seal or one-way Heimlich

19

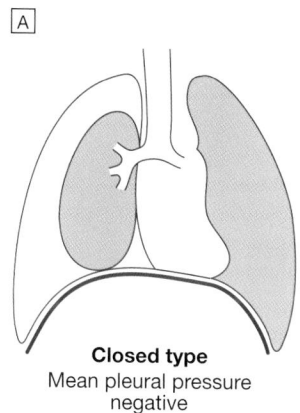

Closed type
Mean pleural pressure
negative

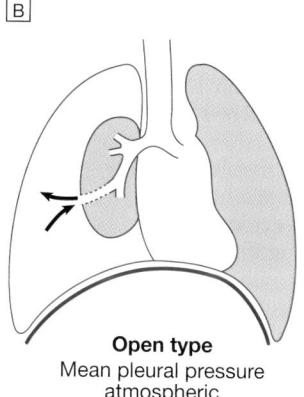

Open type
Mean pleural pressure
atmospheric

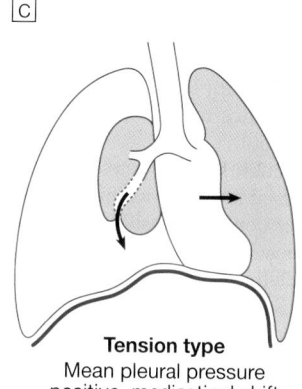

Tension type
Mean pleural pressure
positive, mediastinal shift
to opposite side

Fig. 19.63 Types of spontaneous pneumothorax. A Closed type. B Open type. C Tension (valvular) type.

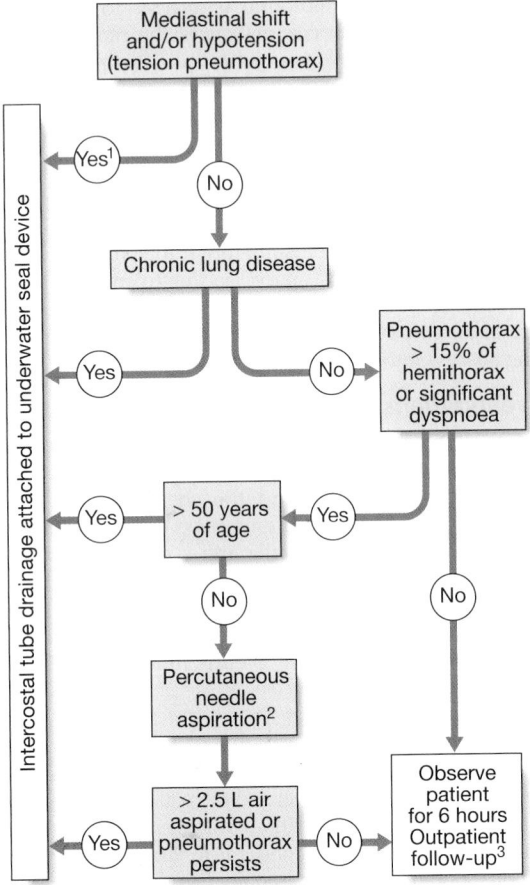

Fig. 19.64 Management of spontaneous pneumothorax.
(1) Immediate decompression is required prior to insertion of intercostal drain. (2) Aspirate in the 2nd intercostal space anteriorly in the mid-clavicular line using a 16 F cannula; discontinue if resistance is felt, the patient coughs excessively, or > 2.5 L of air are removed. (3) Beware: the post-aspiration chest X-ray is not a reliable indicator of whether a pleural leak remains, and all patients should be told to attend again immediately in the event of deterioration.

valve, and secured firmly to the chest wall. Clamping of an intercostal drain is potentially dangerous and rarely indicated. The drain should be removed 24 hours after the lung has fully reinflated and bubbling stopped. Continued bubbling after 5–7 days is an indication for surgery. If bubbling in the drainage bottle stops before full reinflation, the tube is either blocked, kinked or displaced. Supplemental oxygen may speed resolution as it accelerates the rate at which nitrogen is reabsorbed by the pleura.

Patients with a closed pneumothorax should be advised not to fly as the trapped gas expands at altitude. After complete resolution, there is no clear evidence to indicate how long patients should avoid flying, although guidelines suggest that a wait of 1–2 weeks, with confirmation of full inflation prior to flight, is prudent. Patients should also be advised to stop smoking and informed about the risks of a recurrent pneumothorax.

Recurrent spontaneous pneumothorax

After primary spontaneous pneumothorax, recurrence occurs within a year of either aspiration or tube

drainage in approximately 25% of patients, and should prompt definitive treatment. Surgical pleurodesis is recommended in all patients following a second pneumothorax and should be considered following the first episode of secondary pneumothorax if low respiratory reserve makes recurrence hazardous. Pleurodesis can be achieved by pleural abrasion or parietal pleurectomy at thoracotomy or thoracoscopy.

Asbestos-related pleural disease

Asbestos-related lung disease is described on page 712. In the pleura, the chronic tissue reaction may take a variety of clinical and radiological forms.

Benign pleural plaques

Pleural plaques are discrete raised areas situated on the pleura, chest wall, diaphragm, pericardium or mediastinum. They are strongly associated with asbestos exposure but do not usually cause any impairment of lung function and do not contribute to disability. Pleural plaques gradually calcify with time, making them more obvious on radiological imaging (Fig. 19.65).

Benign pleural effusion

Benign asbestos pleurisy occurs in around 20% of asbestos workers, usually within 10 years of exposure but sometimes much later. They present with features of pleurisy including pleural pain, fever and leucocytosis. The pleural liquid may be blood-stained, and differentiation of this benign condition from a malignant effusion caused by mesothelioma can be difficult. The disease is self-limiting but may cause diffuse pleural fibrosis.

Diffuse pleural fibrosis

This involves the visceral pleura, and if sufficiently extensive it may restrict chest expansion and cause breathlessness. Typical appearances on chest X-ray include thickening of the pleura along the chest wall and obliteration of the costophrenic angles (which is uncommon with pleural plaques). Early manifestations may be detected on CT, including the appearance of parenchymal bands. On occasion, shrinkage of the pleura

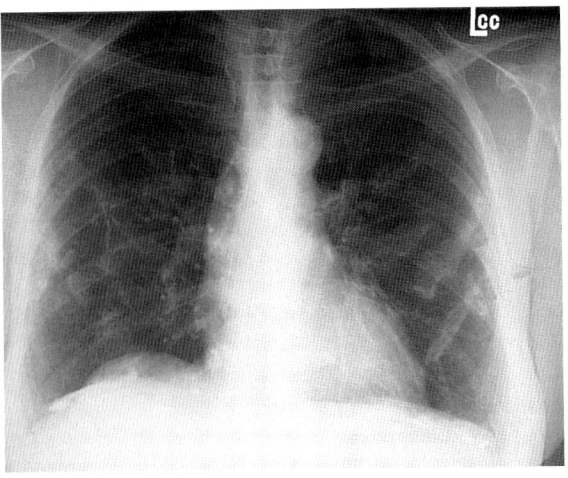

Fig. 19.65 Asbestos-related benign pleural plaques. Chest X-ray showing extensive calcified pleural plaques ('candle wax' appearance), particularly marked on the diaphragm and lateral pleural surfaces.

results in 'round atelectasis', which has the appearance of a mass adjacent to the pleura. This may cause confusion with a tumour.

Mesothelioma

Mesothelioma is a malignant tumour affecting the pleura (pleural mesothelioma) or, less commonly, the peritoneum (peritoneal mesothelioma). Although all fibre types are implicated, crocidolite (p. 712) appears to be the most potent cause. A time lag of 20 years or more between asbestos exposure and the development of mesothelioma is typical. In the UK, the incidence of mesothelioma has increased markedly over the past 20 years and is predicted to peak between 2011 and 2015.

The condition most frequently presents with chest pain or breathlessness from a pleural effusion. Histological diagnosis is difficult and generous (often surgical) pleural biopsies are needed, although tumour may invade along the surgical track following biopsy. The main differential diagnosis is adenocarcinoma and differentiation is aided by the characteristic immuno-histochemistry profile. The prognosis is poor (usually in the order of 12–18 months), although small survival advantages have been reported following the use of chemotherapy. Radiotherapy may be helpful in preventing tumour growth through previous chest drain or biopsy sites. Highly selected patients may be considered for radical surgery; but in general, a palliative approach is all that is possible.

19.107 Pleural disease in old age

- **Spontaneous pneumothorax:** invariably associated with underlying lung disease in old age and has a significant mortality. Surgical or chemical pleurodesis is advised in all such patients.
- **Rib fracture:** common cause of pleural-type pain; may be spontaneous (due to coughing), traumatic or pathological. Underlying osteomalacia may contribute to poor healing, especially in the housebound with no exposure to sunlight.
- **Tuberculosis:** should always be considered and actively excluded in any elderly patient presenting with a unilateral pleural effusion.
- **Mesothelioma:** more common in older than younger people due to a long latency between asbestos exposure (often > 20 years) and the development of disease.
- **Analgesia:** frail older people are particularly sensitive to the respiratory depressant effects of opiate-based analgesia and careful monitoring is required when using these agents for pleural pain.

Diseases of the diaphragm

Congenital disorders

Diaphragmatic hernias

Congenital defects of the diaphragm can allow herniation of abdominal viscera. Posteriorly situated hernias through the foramen of Bochdalek are more common than anterior hernias through the foramen of Morgagni.

Eventration of the diaphragm

Abnormal elevation or bulging of one hemidiaphragm, more often the left, results from total or partial absence of muscular development of the septum transversum. Most eventrations are asymptomatic and are detected by chance on X-ray in adult life, but severe respiratory distress can be caused in infancy if the diaphragmatic muscular defect is extensive.

Acquired disorders

Diaphragmatic paralysis

Phrenic nerve damage leading to paralysis of a hemidiaphragm may be idiopathic but is most often due to bronchial carcinoma (Box 19.108). It may also be damaged by disease of cervical vertebrae, tumours of the cervical cord, shingles, trauma including road traffic and birth injuries, surgery, and stretching of the nerve by mediastinal masses and aortic aneurysms. Paralysis of one hemidiaphragm results in loss of approximately 20% of ventilatory capacity, but is not usually noticed by otherwise healthy individuals. The diagnosis is suggested by elevation of the hemidiaphragm on chest X-ray and is confirmed by using ultrasound screening to demonstrate paradoxical upward movement of the paralysed hemidiaphragm on sniffing.

Bilateral diaphragmatic weakness occurs in peripheral neuropathies of any type including Guillain–Barré syndrome (p. 1229), in disorders affecting the anterior horn cells, e.g. poliomyelitis (p. 1210), in muscular dystrophies and in connective tissue disorders such as SLE and polymyositis (pp. 1107 and 1111).

Other acquired diaphragmatic disorders

Hiatus hernia is common (p. 864). Diaphragmatic rupture is usually caused by a crush injury and may not be detected until years later. Respiratory disorders that cause pulmonary hyperinflation, e.g. emphysema, and those which result in small stiff lungs, e.g. diffuse pulmonary fibrosis, decrease diaphragmatic efficiency and predispose to fatigue. Severe skeletal deformity, such as kyphosis, causes gross distortion of diaphragmatic muscle configuration and mechanical disadvantage.

19.108 Causes of elevation of a hemidiaphragm

- Phrenic nerve paralysis
- Eventration of the diaphragm
- Decrease in volume of one lung (e.g. lobectomy, unilateral pulmonary fibrosis)
- Severe pleuritic pain
- Pulmonary infarction
- Subphrenic abscess
- Large volume of gas in the stomach or colon
- Large tumours or cysts of the liver

Deformities of the chest wall

Thoracic kyphoscoliosis

Abnormalities of alignment of the dorsal spine and their consequent effects on thoracic shape may be caused by:

19

- congenital abnormality
- vertebral disease, including tuberculosis, osteoporosis and ankylosing spondylitis
- trauma
- neuromuscular disease such as poliomyelitis.

Simple kyphosis (increased anteroposterior curvature) causes less pulmonary embarrassment than kyphoscoliosis (anteroposterior and lateral curvature). Kyphoscoliosis, if severe, restricts and distorts expansion of the chest wall, causing ventilation–perfusion mismatch in the lungs and impaired diaphragmatic function. Patients with severe deformity may develop type II respiratory failure (initially manifest during sleep), pulmonary hypertension and right ventricular failure. They can often be successfully treated with non-invasive ventilatory support (p. 194).

Pectus excavatum

Pectus excavatum (funnel chest) is an idiopathic condition in which the body of the sternum, usually only the lower end, is curved inwards. The heart is displaced to the left and may be compressed between the sternum and the vertebral column; however, only rarely is there associated disturbance of cardiac function. The deformity may restrict chest expansion and reduce vital capacity. Operative correction is rarely performed, and only for cosmetic reasons.

Pectus carinatum

Pectus carinatum (pigeon chest) is frequently caused by severe asthma during childhood. Very occasionally, this deformity can be produced by rickets or be idiopathic.

Further information

www.agius.com *A useful website with information on health, work and the environment.*

www.brit-thoracic.org.uk *Website of the British Thoracic Society with access to guidelines on a range of respiratory conditions.*

www.ersnet.org *European Respiratory Society provides information on education and research, and patient information.*

www.ginasthma.com *Global Initiative for Asthma website with a comprehensive overview of asthma.*

www.goldcopd.com *Global Initiative for Chronic Obstructive Lung Disease website containing a comprehensive overview of COPD.*

www.thoracic.org *American Thoracic Society provides information on education and research, and patient information.*

www.who.int *World Health Organization. Tuberculosis: a manual for medical students. WHO/CDS/TB/99.272.*

M.W.J. Strachan
B.R. Walker

Endocrine disease

20

CLINICAL EXAMINATION IN ENDOCRINE DISEASE

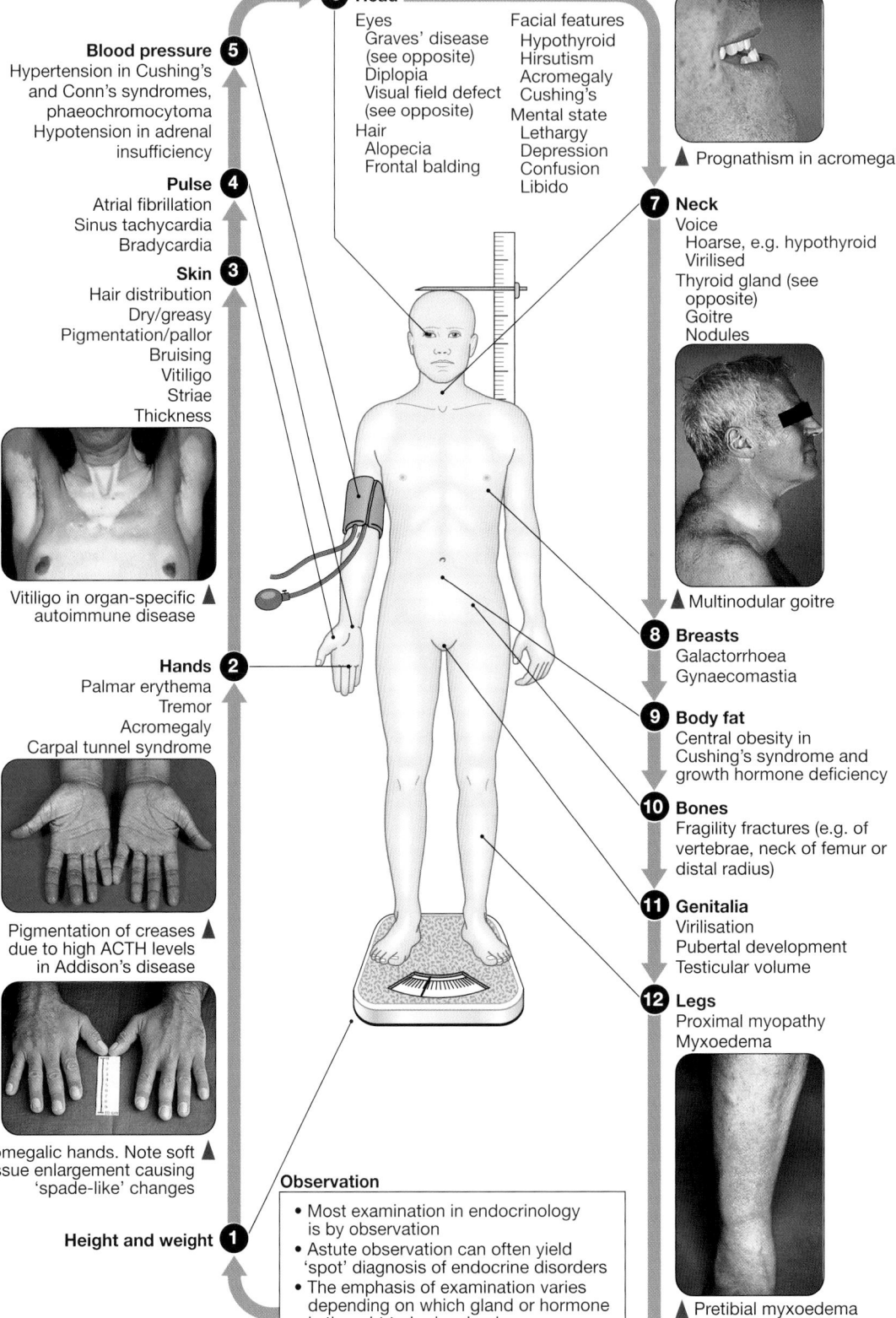

Blood pressure ⑤
Hypertension in Cushing's and Conn's syndromes, phaeochromocytoma
Hypotension in adrenal insufficiency

Pulse ④
Atrial fibrillation
Sinus tachycardia
Bradycardia

Skin ③
Hair distribution
Dry/greasy
Pigmentation/pallor
Bruising
Vitiligo
Striae
Thickness

Vitiligo in organ-specific ▲ autoimmune disease

Hands ②
Palmar erythema
Tremor
Acromegaly
Carpal tunnel syndrome

Pigmentation of creases ▲ due to high ACTH levels in Addison's disease

Acromegalic hands. Note soft ▲ tissue enlargement causing 'spade-like' changes

Height and weight ①

⑥ **Head**
Eyes
  Graves' disease
  (see opposite)
  Diplopia
  Visual field defect
  (see opposite)
Hair
  Alopecia
  Frontal balding
Facial features
  Hypothyroid
  Hirsutism
  Acromegaly
  Cushing's
Mental state
  Lethargy
  Depression
  Confusion
  Libido

▲ Prognathism in acromegaly

⑦ **Neck**
Voice
  Hoarse, e.g. hypothyroid
  Virilised
Thyroid gland (see opposite)
  Goitre
  Nodules

▲ Multinodular goitre

⑧ **Breasts**
Galactorrhoea
Gynaecomastia

⑨ **Body fat**
Central obesity in Cushing's syndrome and growth hormone deficiency

⑩ **Bones**
Fragility fractures (e.g. of vertebrae, neck of femur or distal radius)

⑪ **Genitalia**
Virilisation
Pubertal development
Testicular volume

⑫ **Legs**
Proximal myopathy
Myxoedema

▲ Pretibial myxoedema in Graves' disease

Observation

- Most examination in endocrinology is by observation
- Astute observation can often yield 'spot' diagnosis of endocrine disorders
- The emphasis of examination varies depending on which gland or hormone is thought to be involved

Endocrine disease causes clinical syndromes with symptoms and signs involving many organ systems, reflecting the diverse effects of hormone deficiency and excess. The emphasis of the clinical examination depends on the gland or hormone that is thought to be abnormal. Diabetes mellitus (Ch. 21) and thyroid disease are the most common endocrine diseases.

⑥ Examination of the visual fields by confrontation

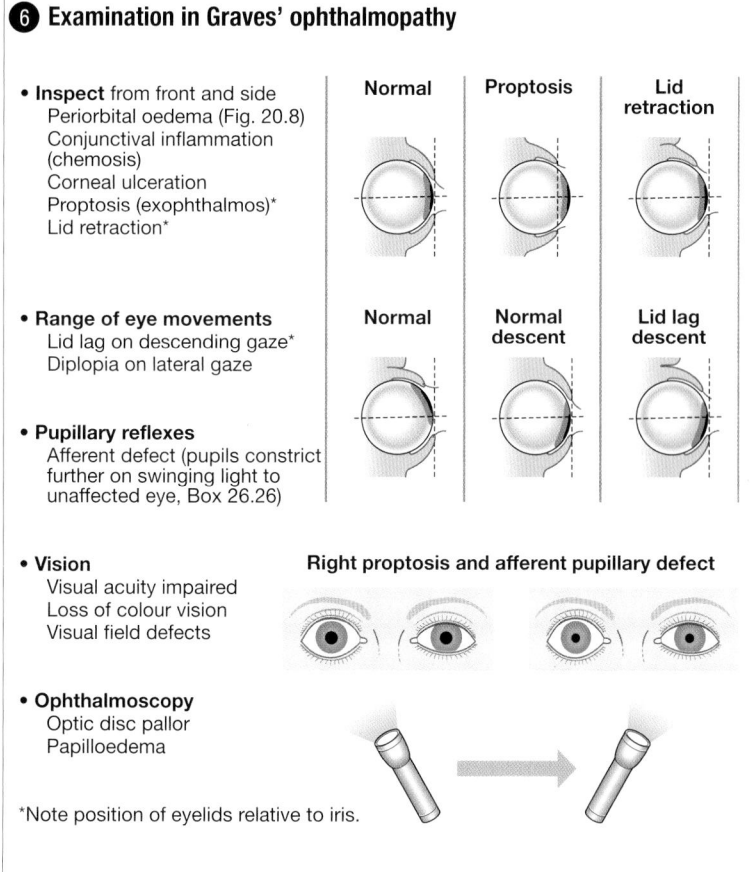

- Sit opposite patient
- You and patient cover opposite eyes
- Bring red pin (or wiggling finger) slowly into view from extreme of your vision, as shown
- Ask patient to say 'now' when it comes into view
- Continue to move pin into centre of vision and ask patient to tell you if it disappears
- Repeat in each of four quadrants
- Repeat in other eye

A bitemporal hemianopia is the classical finding in pituitary macroadenomas (p. 787)

⑥ Examination in Graves' ophthalmopathy

- **Inspect** from front and side
  Periorbital oedema (Fig. 20.8)
  Conjunctival inflammation (chemosis)
  Corneal ulceration
  Proptosis (exophthalmos)*
  Lid retraction*

| Normal | Proptosis | Lid retraction |

- **Range of eye movements**
  Lid lag on descending gaze*
  Diplopia on lateral gaze

| Normal | Normal descent | Lid lag descent |

- **Pupillary reflexes**
  Afferent defect (pupils constrict further on swinging light to unaffected eye, Box 26.26)

- **Vision**
  Visual acuity impaired
  Loss of colour vision
  Visual field defects

Right proptosis and afferent pupillary defect

- **Ophthalmoscopy**
  Optic disc pallor
  Papilloedema

*Note position of eyelids relative to iris.

⑦ Examination of the thyroid gland

- **Inspect** from front to side

- **Palpate** from behind
  Thyroid moves on swallowing
  Cervical lymph nodes
  Tracheal deviation

- **Auscultate** for bruit
  Ask patient to hold breath
  If present, check for radiating murmur

- **Percuss** for retrosternal thyroid

- Consider systemic signs of thyroid dysfunction (Box 20.7) incl. tremor, palmar erythema, warm peripheries, tachycardia, lid lag

- Consider signs of Graves' disease incl. ophthalmopathy, pretibial myxoedema

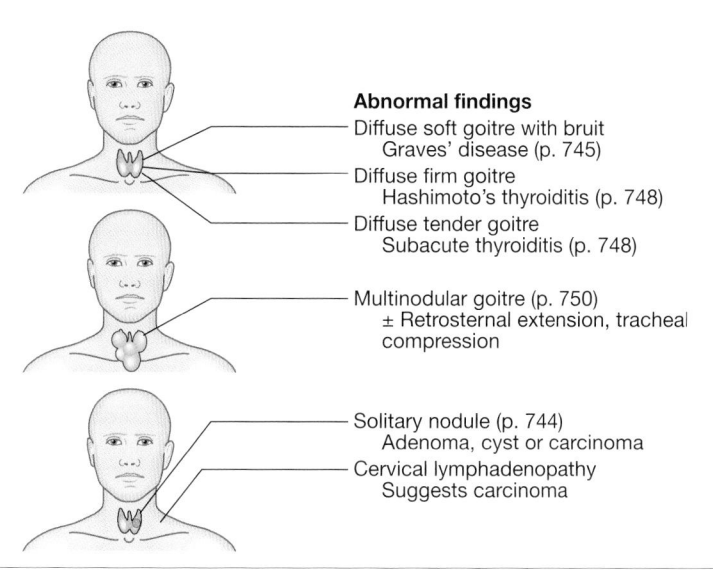

Abnormal findings
Diffuse soft goitre with bruit
  Graves' disease (p. 745)
Diffuse firm goitre
  Hashimoto's thyroiditis (p. 748)
Diffuse tender goitre
  Subacute thyroiditis (p. 748)

Multinodular goitre (p. 750)
  ± Retrosternal extension, tracheal compression

Solitary nodule (p. 744)
  Adenoma, cyst or carcinoma
Cervical lymphadenopathy
  Suggests carcinoma

Endocrinology concerns the synthesis, secretion and action of hormones. These are chemical messengers released from endocrine glands that coordinate the activities of many different cells. Endocrine diseases can therefore affect multiple organs and systems. This chapter describes the principles of endocrinology before dealing with the function and diseases of each gland in turn.

Some endocrine diseases are common, particularly those of the thyroid gland, reproductive system and β cells of the pancreas (Ch. 21). For example, thyroid dysfunction occurs in more than 10% of the population in areas with iodine deficiency, such as the Himalayas, and 4% of women aged 20–50 years in the UK. Some endocrine diseases are becoming more common in association with emerging diseases; HIV infection is associated in particular with adrenal insufficiency. Less common endocrine syndromes are described later in the chapter.

Few endocrine therapies have been evaluated by randomised controlled trials, in part because hormone replacement therapy (for example, with thyroxine) has obvious clinical benefits and placebo-controlled trials would be unethical, and in part because many endocrine diseases are rare, making trials difficult to perform. Recommendations for 'evidence-based medicine' are, therefore, relatively scarce. They relate mainly to use of therapy that is 'optional' and/or recently available, such as oestrogen replacement in post-menopausal women and growth hormone replacement.

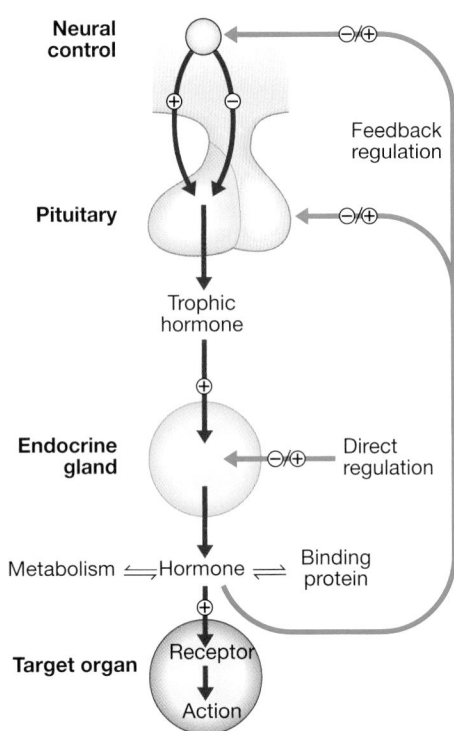

Fig. 20.1 An archetypal endocrine axis. Regulation by negative feedback and direct control is shown along with the equilibrium between active circulating free hormone and bound or metabolised hormone.

AN OVERVIEW OF ENDOCRINOLOGY

Functional anatomy and physiology

Some endocrine glands, such as the parathyroids and pancreas, respond directly to metabolic signals, but most are controlled by hormones released from the pituitary gland. Anterior pituitary hormone secretion is controlled in turn by substances produced in the hypothalamus and released into portal blood which drains directly down the pituitary stalk (Fig. 20.1). Posterior pituitary hormones are synthesised in the hypothalamus and transported down nerve axons to be released from the posterior pituitary. Hormone release in the hypothalamus and pituitary is regulated by numerous stimuli and through feedback control by hormones produced by the target glands (thyroid, adrenal cortex and gonads). These integrated endocrine systems are called 'axes', and are listed in Figure 20.2.

A wide variety of molecules act as hormones. Peptides (e.g. insulin), glycoproteins (e.g. thyroid-stimulating hormone, TSH) and amines (e.g. noradrenaline/norepinephrine) act on specific cell surface receptors which signal through G-proteins and/or enzymes on the cytosolic side of the plasma membrane. Other hormones (e.g. steroids, triiodothyronine and vitamin D) bind to specific intracellular receptors, which in turn bind to response elements on DNA to regulate gene transcription (p. 41).

The classical model of endocrine function involves hormones which are synthesised in endocrine glands, are released into the circulation, and act at sites distant from those of secretion (as in Fig. 20.1). However, additional levels of regulation are now recognised. Many other organs secrete hormones or contribute to the peripheral metabolism and activation of prohormones. A notable example is the production of oestrogens from adrenal androgens in adipose tissue by the enzyme aromatase. Some hormones such as neurotransmitters act in a paracrine fashion to affect adjacent cells or act in an autocrine way to affect behaviour of the cell that produces the hormone.

Endocrine pathology

For each endocrine axis or major gland, diseases can be classified as shown in Box 20.1. Pathology arising within the gland is often called 'primary' disease (e.g. primary hypothyroidism in Hashimoto's thyroiditis), while abnormal stimulation of the gland is often called 'secondary' disease (for example, secondary hypothyroidism in patients with a pituitary tumour and TSH deficiency). Two types of endocrine disease affect multiple glands (p. 794): organ-specific autoimmune diseases (which are common) and multiple endocrine neoplasia (MEN) syndromes (which are rare).

Investigation of endocrine disease

Biochemical investigations play a central role in endocrinology. Most hormones can be measured in blood, but the circumstances in which the sample is taken are often crucial, especially for hormones with pulsatile secretion such as growth hormone; diurnal variation such as cortisol; or monthly variation such as oestrogen or progesterone. Other investigations such as imaging and biopsy are

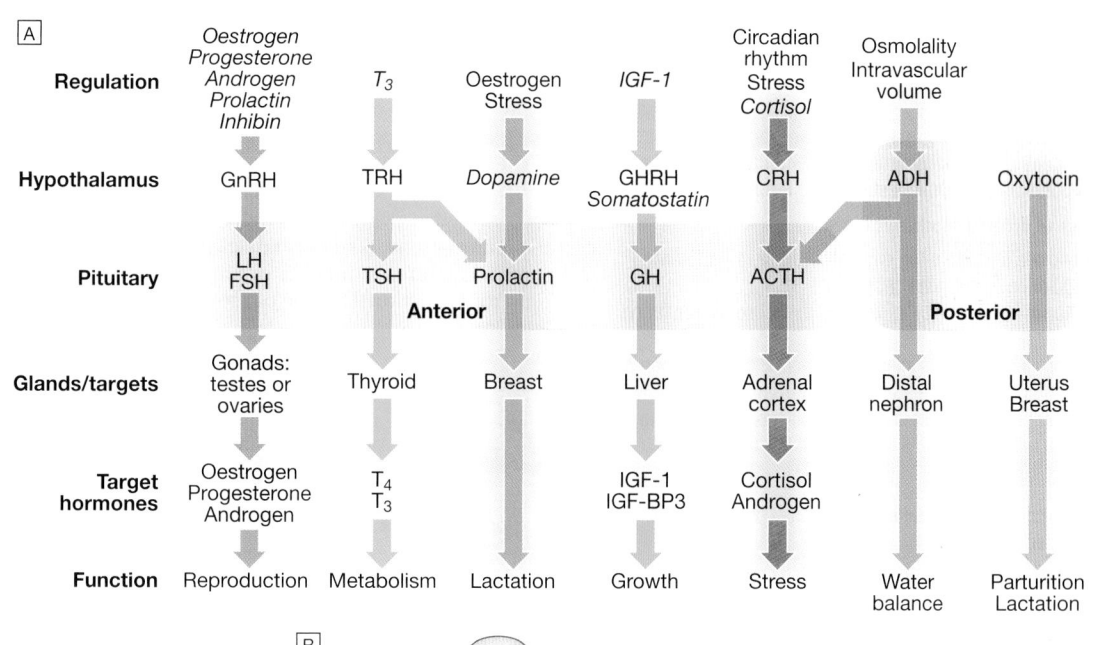

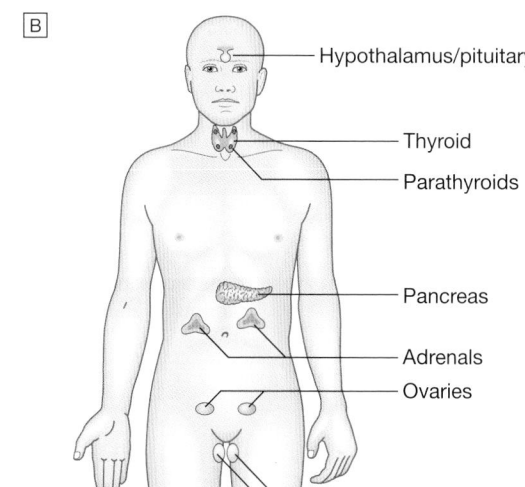

Fig. 20.2 The principal endocrine 'axes' and glands. **A** Endocrine axes. Some major endocrine glands are not controlled by the pituitary. These include the parathyroid glands (regulated by calcium concentrations, p. 764), the adrenal zona glomerulosa (regulated by the renin–angiotensin system, p. 769) and the endocrine pancreas (Ch. 21). Italics show negative regulation. (ACTH = adrenocorticotrophic hormone; ADH = antidiuretic hormone, arginine vasopressin; CRH = corticotrophin-releasing hormone; FSH = follicle-stimulating hormone; GH = growth hormone; GHRH = growth hormone-releasing hormone; GnRH = gonadotrophin-releasing hormone; IGF-1 = insulin-like growth factor-1; IGF-BP3 = IGF-binding protein-3; LH = luteinising hormone; T_3 = triiodothyronine; T_4 = thyroxine; TRH = thyrotrophin-releasing hormone; TSH = thyroid-stimulating hormone) **B** Endocrine glands.

20.1 Classification of endocrine disease

Hormone excess
- Primary gland over-production
- Secondary to excess trophic substance

Hormone deficiency
- Primary gland failure
- Secondary to deficient trophic hormone

Hormone hypersensitivity
- Failure of inactivation of hormone
- Target organ over-activity/hypersensitivity

Hormone resistance
- Failure of activation of hormone
- Target organ resistance

Non-functioning tumours

usually reserved for patients who present with a tumour. The principles of investigation are shown in Box 20.2. The choice of test is often pragmatic, taking local access to reliable sampling facilities and laboratory measurements into account.

Presenting problems in endocrine disease

Endocrine diseases present in many different ways and to clinicians in many different disciplines. Classical syndromes are described in relation to individual glands in the following sections. Often, however, the presentation is with non-specific symptoms (Box 20.3) or with asymptomatic biochemical abnormalities. In addition, endocrine

20.2 Principles of endocrine investigation

Timing of measurement

- Release of many hormones is rhythmical (pulsatile, circadian or monthly), so random measurement may be invalid and sequential or dynamic tests may be required

Choice of dynamic biochemical tests

- Abnormalities are often characterised by loss of normal regulation of hormone secretion
- If hormone deficiency is suspected, choose a stimulation test
- If hormone excess is suspected, choose a suppression test
- The more tests there are to choose from, the less likely it is that any single test is infallible, so avoid interpreting one result in isolation

Imaging

- Secretory cells also take up substrates, which can be labelled
- Most endocrine glands have a high prevalence of 'incidentalomas', so do not scan unless the biochemistry confirms endocrine dysfunction or the primary problem is a tumour

Biopsy

- Many endocrine tumours are difficult to classify histologically (e.g. adrenal carcinoma and adenoma)

---

diseases are encountered in the differential diagnosis of common complaints discussed in other chapters of this book, including electrolyte abnormalities (Ch. 16), hypertension (Ch. 18), obesity (Ch. 5) and osteoporosis (Ch. 25). Although diseases of the adrenal glands, hypothalamus and pituitary are relatively rare, their diagnosis often relies on astute clinical observation in a patient with non-specific complaints, so it is important that clinicians are familiar with their key features.

20.3 Examples of non-specific presentations of endocrine disease

Symptom	Most likely endocrine disorder(s)
Lethargy and depression	Hypothyroidism, diabetes mellitus, hyperparathyroidism, hypogonadism, adrenal insufficiency, Cushing's syndrome
Weight gain	Hypothyroidism, Cushing's syndrome
Weight loss	Thyrotoxicosis, adrenal insufficiency, diabetes mellitus
Polyuria and polydipsia	Diabetes mellitus, diabetes insipidus, hyperparathyroidism, hypokalaemia (Conn's syndrome)
Heat intolerance	Thyrotoxicosis, menopause
Palpitations	Thyrotoxicosis, phaeochromocytoma
Headache	Acromegaly, pituitary tumour, phaeochromocytoma
Muscle weakness (usually proximal)	Thyrotoxicosis, Cushing's syndrome, hypokalaemia (e.g. Conn's syndrome), hyperparathyroidism, hypogonadism
Coarsening of features	Acromegaly, hypothyroidism

THE THYROID GLAND

Diseases of the thyroid predominantly affect females and are common, occurring in about 5% of the population. The thyroid axis is involved in the regulation of cellular differentiation and metabolism in virtually all nucleated cells, so that disorders of thyroid function have diverse manifestations. Structural diseases of the thyroid gland, such as goitre, commonly occur in patients with normal thyroid function. Disease of the thyroid are summarised in Box 20.4.

20.4 Classification of thyroid disease

	Primary	Secondary
Hormone excess	Graves' disease Multinodular goitre Adenoma Subacute thyroiditis	Pituitary TSHoma
Hormone deficiency	Hashimoto's thyroiditis Atrophic hypothyroidism	Hypopituitarism
Hormone hypersensitivity	–	
Hormone resistance	Thyroid hormone resistance syndrome 5'-monodeiodinase deficiency	
Non-functioning tumours	Differentiated carcinoma Medullary carcinoma Lymphoma	

Functional anatomy, physiology and investigations

Thyroid physiology is illustrated in Figure 20.3. The para-follicular C cells secrete calcitonin, which is of no apparent physiological significance in humans. The follicular epithelial cells synthesise thyroid hormones by incorporating iodine into the amino acid tyrosine on the surface of thyroglobulin (Tg), a protein secreted into the colloid of the follicle. Iodide is a key substrate for thyroid hormone synthesis; a dietary intake in excess of 100 µg/day is required to maintain thyroid function in adults. The thyroid secretes predominantly thyroxine (T_4) and only a small amount of triiodothyronine (T_3); approximately 85% of T_3 in blood is produced from T_4 by a family of monodeiodinase enzymes which are active in many tissues including liver, muscle, heart and kidney. T_4 can be regarded as a pro-hormone, since it has a longer half-life in blood than T_3 (approximately 1 week compared with approximately 18 hours), and binds and activates thyroid hormone receptors less effectively than T_3. T_4 can also be converted to the inactive metabolite, reverse T_3.

T_3 and T_4 circulate in plasma almost entirely (> 99%) bound to transport proteins, mainly thyroxine-binding globulin (TBG). It is the unbound or free hormones which diffuse into tissues and exert diverse metabolic

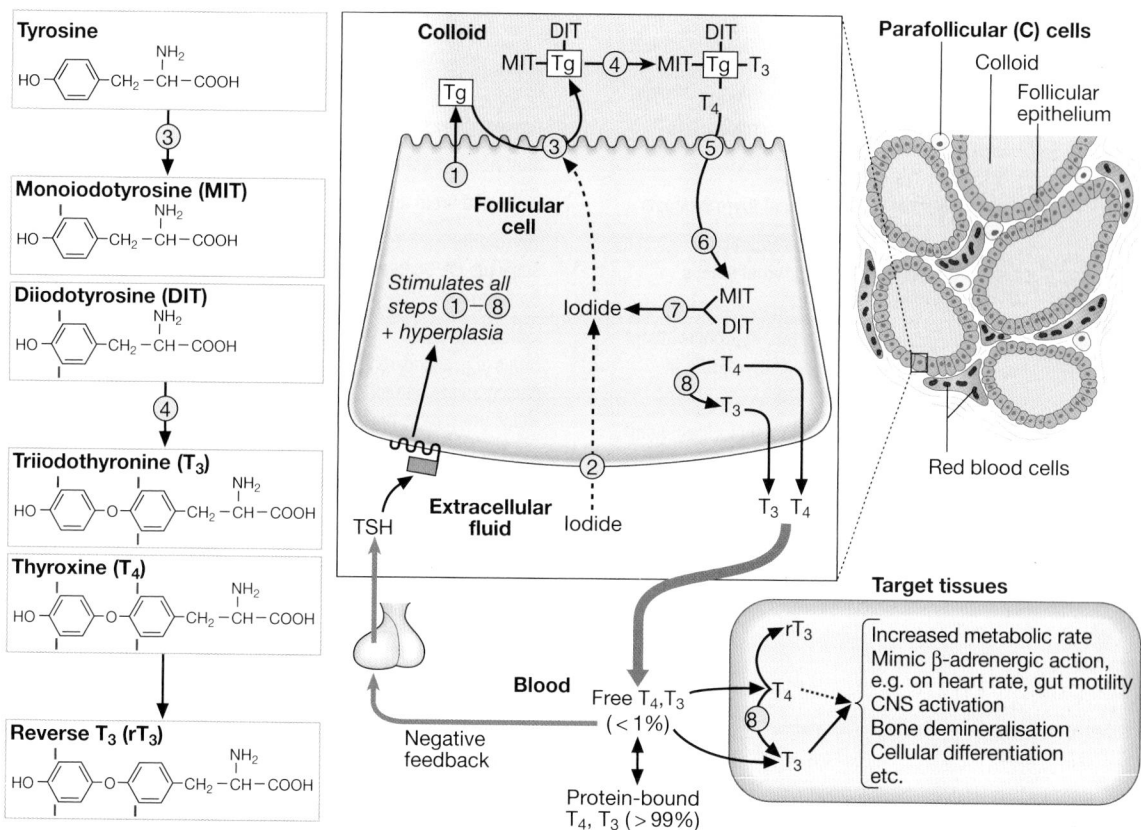

Fig. 20.3 Structure and function of the thyroid gland. (1) Thyroglobulin (Tg) is synthesised and secreted into the colloid of the follicle. (2) Inorganic iodide (I^-) is actively transported into the follicular cell ('trapping'). (3) Iodide is transported on to the colloidal surface by a transporter (pendrin, defective in Pendred's syndrome) and 'organified' by the thyroid peroxidase enzyme, which incorporates it into the amino acid tyrosine on the surface of Tg to form monoiodotyrosine (MIT) and diiodotyrosine (DIT). (4) Iodinated tyrosines couple to form T_3 and T_4. (5) Tg is endocytosed. (6) Tg is cleaved by proteolysis to free the iodinated tyrosine and thyroid hormones. (7) Iodinated tyrosine is dehalogenated to recycle the iodide. (8) T_4 is converted to T_3 by 5'-monodeiodinase.

20

actions. Some laboratories use assays which measure total T_4 and T_3 in plasma but it is increasingly common to measure free T_4 and free T_3. The advantage of the free hormone measurements is that they are not influenced by changes in the concentration of binding proteins; in pregnancy, for example, TBG levels are increased and total T_3 and T_4 may be raised, but free thyroid hormone levels are normal.

Production of T_3 and T_4 in the thyroid is stimulated by thyrotrophin (thyroid-stimulating hormone, TSH), a glycoprotein released from the thyrotroph cells of the anterior pituitary in response to the hypothalamic tripeptide, thyrotrophin-releasing hormone (TRH). A circadian rhythm of TSH secretion can be demonstrated with a peak at 0100 hrs and trough at 1100 hrs, but the variation is small so that thyroid function can be assessed reliably from a single blood sample taken at any time of day and does not usually require any dynamic stimulation or suppression tests. There is a negative feedback of thyroid hormones on the hypothalamus and pituitary such that in thyrotoxicosis, when plasma concentrations of T_3 and T_4 are raised, TSH secretion is suppressed. Conversely, in hypothyroidism due to disease of the thyroid gland, low T_3 and T_4 are associated with high circulating TSH levels. The anterior pituitary is very sensitive to minor changes in thyroid hormone levels within the normal range. Although the reference range for free T_4 is 9–21

pmol/L (700–1632 pg/dL), a rise or fall of 5 pmol/L in an individual in whom the level is usually 15 pmol/L would be associated on the one hand with undetectable TSH, and on the other hand with a raised TSH. For this reason, TSH is usually regarded as the most useful investigation of thyroid function. However, interpretation of TSH values without considering thyroid hormone levels may be misleading in patients with pituitary disease (see Box 20.56, p. 784). Moreover, TSH may take several weeks to 'catch up' with T_4 and T_3 levels, for example, when prolonged suppression of TSH in thyrotoxicosis is relieved by antithyroid therapy. Common patterns of abnormal thyroid function test results and their interpretation are shown in Box 20.5.

Other modalities commonly employed in the investigation of thyroid disease include measurement of antibodies against the TSH receptor or other thyroid antigens (see Box 20.8, p. 740), radioisotope imaging, fine needle aspiration biopsy and ultrasound. Their use is described below.

Presenting problems in thyroid disease

The most common presentations are hyperthyroidism (thyrotoxicosis), hypothyroidism and enlargement of the thyroid (goitre). Widespread availability of thyroid

20.5 How to interpret thyroid function test results

TSH	T$_4$	T$_3$	Most likely interpretation(s)
U.D.	Raised	Raised	**Primary thyrotoxicosis**
U.D.	Normal[1]	Raised	**Primary T$_3$-toxicosis**
U.D.	Normal[1]	Normal[1]	**Subclinical thyrotoxicosis**
U.D.	Raised	Low, normal or raised[2]	**Sick euthyroidism/ non-thyroidal illness**
U.D.	Low	Low	**Secondary hypothyroidism[5] Transient thyroiditis in evolution**
Normal	Low	Low[3]	**Secondary hypothyroidism[5]**
Mildly elevated 5–20 mU/L	Low	Low[3]	**Primary hypothyroidism Secondary hypothyroidism[5]**
Elevated > 20 mU/L	Low	Low[3]	**Primary hypothyroidism**
Mildly elevated 5–20 mU/L	Normal[4]	Normal[3]	**Subclinical hypothyroidism**
Elevated 20–500 mU/L	Normal	Normal	**Artefact** Endogenous IgG antibodies which interfere with TSH assay
Elevated	Raised	Raised	**Non-compliance with T$_4$ replacement**—recent 'loading' dose **Secondary thyrotoxicosis[5] Thyroid hormone resistance**

[1]Usually upper part of reference range.
[2]Depending on the assay system.
[3]T$_3$ is not a sensitive indicator of hypothyroidism and should not be requested.
[4]Usually lower part of normal range.
[5]I.e. secondary to pituitary or hypothalamic disease. Note that TSH assays may report detectable TSH.
(U.D. = undetectable)

20.6 Causes of thyrotoxicosis and their relative frequencies

Cause	Frequency[1] (%)
Graves' disease	76
Multinodular goitre	14
Solitary thyroid adenoma	5
Thyroiditis	
Subacute (de Quervain's)[2]	3
Post-partum[2]	0.5
Iodide-induced	
Drugs (e.g. amiodarone)[2]	1
Radiographic contrast media[2]	–
Iodine prophylaxis programme[2]	–
Extrathyroidal source of thyroid hormone	
Factitious thyrotoxicosis[2]	0.2
Struma ovarii[2,3]	–
TSH-induced	
TSH-secreting pituitary adenoma	0.2
Choriocarcinoma and hydatidiform mole[4]	–
Follicular carcinoma ± metastases	0.1

[1]In a series of 2087 patients presenting to the Royal Infirmary of Edinburgh, over a 10-year period.
[2]Characterised by negligible radio-isotope uptake.
[3]i.e. Ovarian teratoma containing thyroid tissue.
[4]Human chorionic gonadotrophin has thyroid-stimulating activity.

goitre of Graves' disease from the irregular enlargement of a multinodular goitre. All causes of thyrotoxicosis can cause lid retraction and lid lag, due to potentiation of sympathetic innervation of the levator palpebrae muscles, but only Graves' disease causes other features of ophthalmopathy, including periorbital oedema, conjunctival irritation, exophthalmos and diplopia. Pretibial myxoedema (p. 733) and the rare thyroid acropachy (a periosteal hypertrophy indistinguishable from finger clubbing) are also specific to Graves' disease.

Investigations

The first-line investigations are serum T$_3$, T$_4$ and TSH. If abnormal values are found, the tests should be repeated and the abnormality confirmed in view of the likely need for prolonged medical treatment or destructive therapy. In most patients serum T$_3$ and T$_4$ are both elevated but T$_4$ is in the upper part of the normal range and T$_3$ raised (T$_3$ toxicosis) in about 5%. Serum TSH is undetectable in primary thyrotoxicosis but values can be raised in the very rare syndrome of secondary thyrotoxicosis caused by a TSH-producing pituitary adenoma. When biochemical thyrotoxicosis has been confirmed, further investigations should be undertaken to determine the underlying cause, including measurement of TSH receptor antibodies (TRAb, elevated in Graves' disease, Box 20.8) and isotope scanning, as shown in Figure 20.4. Other non-specific abnormalities are common (Box 20.9). An ECG may demonstrate sinus tachycardia or atrial fibrillation.

Radio-iodine uptake tests measure the proportion of isotope which is trapped in the whole gland, but have been largely superseded by [99m]technetium scintigraphy scans which also indicate trapping, are quicker to

function tests has led to the increasingly frequent identification of patients with abnormal results who are either asymptomatic or have non-specific complaints such as tiredness and weight gain.

Thyrotoxicosis

Thyrotoxicosis describes a constellation of clinical features arising from elevated circulating levels of thyroid hormone. The most common causes are Graves' disease, multinodular goitre and autonomously functioning thyroid nodules (toxic adenoma) (Box 20.6). Thyroiditis is more common in parts of the world where relevant viral infections occur, such as North America.

Clinical assessment

The clinical manifestations of thyrotoxicosis are shown in Box 20.7 and an approach to differential diagnosis is given in Figure 20.4. The most common symptoms are weight loss with a normal or increased appetite, heat intolerance, palpitations, tremor and irritability. Tachycardia, palmar erythema and lid lag are common signs. Not all patients have a palpable goitre, but experienced clinicians can discriminate the diffuse soft

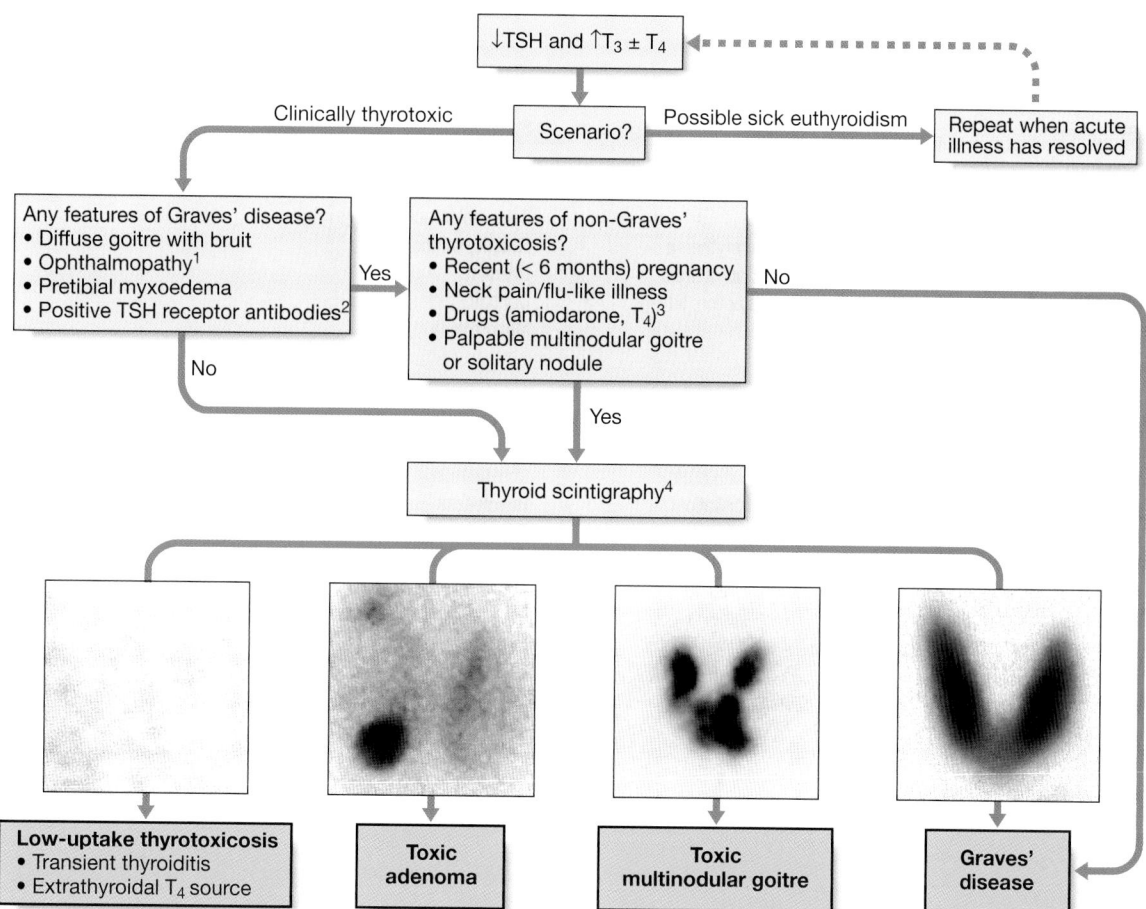

Fig. 20.4 Establishing the differential diagnosis in thyrotoxicosis. (1) Graves' ophthalmopathy refers to clinical features of exophthalmos and periorbital and conjunctival oedema, not simply the lid lag and lid retraction which can occur in all forms of thyrotoxicosis. (2) TSH receptor antibodies are very rare in patients without autoimmune thyroid disease, but only occur in 80–95% of patients with Graves' disease; a positive test is therefore confirmatory, but a negative test does not exclude Graves' disease. Other thyroid antibodies (e.g. anti-peroxidase and anti-thyroglobulin antibodies) are unhelpful in the differential diagnosis since they occur frequently in the population and are found with several of the disorders which cause thyrotoxicosis. (3) Scintigraphy is not necessary in most cases of drug-induced thyrotoxicosis. (4) ^{99m}Technetium pertechnetate scans of patients with thyrotoxicosis. In low-uptake thyrotoxicosis, most commonly due to a viral, post-partum or iodine-induced thyroiditis, there is negligible isotope detected in the region of the thyroid, although uptake is apparent in nearby salivary glands (not shown here). In a toxic adenoma there is lack of uptake of isotope by the rest of the thyroid gland due to suppression of serum TSH. In multinodular goitre there is relatively low, patchy uptake within the nodules; such an appearance is not always associated with a palpable thyroid. In Graves' disease there is diffuse uptake of isotope.

perform with a lower dose of radioactivity, and provide a higher-resolution image. In low-uptake thyrotoxicosis, the cause is usually a transient thyroiditis (p. 748). Occasionally, patients induce 'factitious thyrotoxicosis' by consuming excessive amounts of a thyroid hormone preparation, most often levothyroxine. The exogenous thyroxine suppresses pituitary TSH secretion and hence iodine uptake, serum thyroglobulin and release of endogenous thyroid hormones. The T_4:T_3 ratio (typically 30:1 in conventional thyrotoxicosis) is increased to above 70:1 because circulating T_3 in factitious thyrotoxicosis is derived exclusively from the peripheral monodeiodination of T_4 and not from thyroid secretion. The combination of negligible iodine uptake, high T_4:T_3 ratio and a low or undetectable thyroglobulin is diagnostic.

Management

Definitive treatment of thyrotoxicosis depends on the underlying cause and may include antithyroid drugs, radioactive iodine or surgery. A non-selective β-adrenoceptor antagonist (β-blocker), such as propranolol (160 mg daily) or nadolol (40–80 mg daily), will alleviate but not abolish symptoms in most patients within 24–48 hours. Beta-blockers should not be used for long-term treatment of thyrotoxicosis, but are extremely useful in the short term, whilst patients are awaiting hospital consultation or following ^{131}I therapy.

Atrial fibrillation in thyrotoxicosis

Atrial fibrillation occurs in about 10% of patients with thyrotoxicosis. The incidence increases with age so that almost half of all males with thyrotoxicosis over the age of 60 are affected (Fig. 20.5). Moreover, subclinical thyrotoxicosis (p. 744) is a risk factor for atrial fibrillation. Characteristically, the ventricular rate is little influenced by digoxin, but responds to the addition of a β-blocker. Thromboembolic vascular complications are particularly common in thyrotoxic atrial fibrillation so that anticoagulation with warfarin is required,

20.7 Clinical features of thyroid dysfunction

Thyrotoxicosis		Hypothyroidism	
Symptoms	**Signs**	**Symptoms**	**Signs**
Common			
Weight loss despite normal or increased appetite	Weight loss	Weight gain	Weight gain
Heat intolerance	Tremor	Cold intolerance	
Palpitations	Palmar erythema	Fatigue, somnolence	
Dyspnoea	Sinus tachycardia	Dry skin	
Irritability, emotional lability	Lid retraction, lid lag	Dry hair	
Fatigue		Menorrhagia	
Sweating			
Tremor			
Less common			
Osteoporosis (fracture, loss of height)	Goitre with bruit[1]	Constipation	Hoarse voice
Diarrhoea, steatorrhoea	Atrial fibrillation[2]	Hoarseness	Facial features:
Angina	Systolic hypertension/ increased pulse pressure	Carpal tunnel syndrome	Purplish lips
Ankle swelling		Alopecia	Malar flush
Anxiety, psychosis	Cardiac failure[2]	Aches and pains	Periorbital oedema/myxoedema
Muscle weakness	Hyper-reflexia	Muscle stiffness	Loss of lateral eyebrows
Periodic paralysis (predominantly in Chinese)	Ill-sustained clonus	Deafness	Anaemia
Pruritus	Proximal myopathy	Depression	Carotenaemia
Alopecia	Bulbar myopathy[2]	Infertility	Erythema ab igne (Granny's tartan)
Amenorrhoea/oligomenorrhoea			Bradycardia
Infertility, spontaneous abortion			Hypertension
Loss of libido, impotence			Delayed relaxation of tendon reflexes
Excessive lacrimation			Dermal myxoedema
Rare			
Vomiting	Lymphadenopathy	Psychosis (myxoedema madness)	Ileus
Apathy	Spider naevi		Ascites
Anorexia	Onycholysis	Galactorrhoea	Pericardial and pleural effusions
Exacerbation of asthma	Pigmentation	Impotence	Cerebellar ataxia
	Gynaecomastia		Myotonia

[1]In Graves' disease only.
[2]Features found particularly in elderly patients.

20.8 Prevalence of thyroid autoantibodies (%)

	Antibodies to:		
	Thyroid peroxidase[1]	**Thyroglobulin**	**TSH receptor[2]**
Normal population	8–27	5–20	0
Graves' disease	50–80	50–70	80–95
Autoimmune hypothyroidism	90–100	80–90	10–20
Multinodular goitre	~30–40	~30–40	0
Transient thyroiditis	~30–40	~30–40	0

[1]Thyroid peroxidase (TPO) antibodies are the principal component of what was previously measured as thyroid 'microsomal' antibodies.
[2]TSH receptor antibodies (TRAb) can be agonists (stimulatory, causing Graves' thyrotoxicosis) or antagonists ('blocking', causing hypothyroidism).

20.9 Non-specific laboratory abnormalities in thyroid dysfunction*

Thyrotoxicosis

- Serum enzymes
  Raised alanine aminotransferase, γ-glutamyl transferase (GGT), and alkaline phosphatase from liver and bone
- Raised bilirubin
- Mild hypercalcaemia
- Glycosuria
  Associated diabetes mellitus
  'Lag storage' glycosuria

Hypothyroidism

- Serum enzymes
  Raised creatine kinase, aspartate aminotransferase, lactate dehydrogenase (LDH)
- Hypercholesterolaemia
- Anaemia
  Normochromic normocytic or macrocytic
- Hyponatraemia

*These abnormalities are not useful in differential diagnosis, so the tests should be avoided and any further investigation undertaken only if abnormalities persist when the patient is euthyroid.

unless contraindicated. Once thyroid hormone and TSH concentrations have been returned to normal, atrial fibrillation will spontaneously revert to sinus rhythm in about 50% of patients, but cardioversion may be required in the remainder.

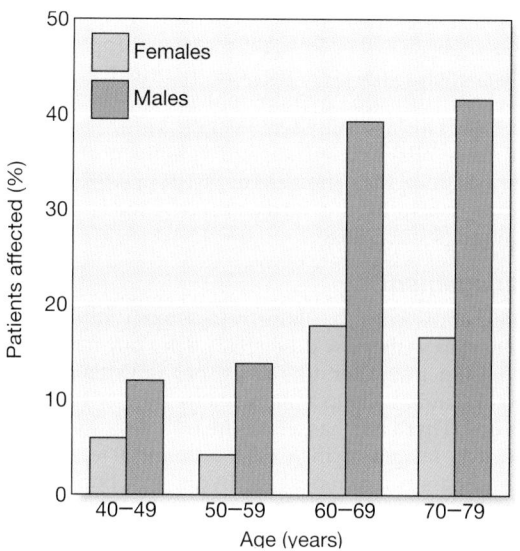

Fig. 20.5 Age-related incidence of atrial fibrillation in patients with thyrotoxicosis.

Thyrotoxic crisis ('thyroid storm')

This is a rare but life-threatening complication of thyrotoxicosis. The most prominent signs are fever, agitation, confusion, tachycardia or atrial fibrillation and, in the older patient, cardiac failure. It is a medical emergency, which has a mortality of 10% despite early recognition and treatment. Thyrotoxic crisis is most commonly precipitated by infection in a patient with previously unrecognised or inadequately treated thyrotoxicosis. It may also develop shortly after subtotal thyroidectomy in an ill-prepared patient or within a few days of ^{131}I therapy when acute irradiation damage may lead to a transient rise in serum thyroid hormone levels.

Patients should be rehydrated and given a broad-spectrum antibiotic and propranolol, either orally (80 mg 6-hourly) or intravenously (1–5 mg 6-hourly). Sodium ipodate (500 mg per day orally) will restore serum T_3 levels to normal in 48–72 hours. This is a radiographic contrast medium which not only inhibits the release of thyroid hormones, but also reduces the conversion of T_4 to T_3 and is, therefore, more effective than potassium iodide or Lugol's solution. Dexamethasone (2 mg 6-hourly) and amiodarone have similar effects. Oral carbimazole 40–60 mg daily (p. 746) should be given to inhibit the synthesis of new thyroid hormone. If the patient is unconscious or uncooperative, carbimazole can be administered rectally with good effect, but no preparation is available for parenteral use. After 10–14 days the patient can usually be maintained on carbimazole alone.

Thyrotoxicosis and pregnancy

Thyrotoxicosis during pregnancy is usually due to Graves' disease and its treatment is described on pages 745–747. Thyrotoxicosis within the first 6 months after pregnancy may be due to post-partum thyroiditis, which is described on page 747. See also Box 20.19 (p. 753).

Hypothyroidism

Hypothyroidism is a common condition with various causes (Box 20.10), but autoimmune disease (Hashimoto's thyroiditis) and thyroid failure following ^{131}I or surgical

---

20.10 Causes of hypothyroidism

Causes	Anti-TPO antibodies[1]	Goitre[2]
Autoimmune		
Hashimoto's thyroiditis	++	±
Spontaneous atrophic hypothyroidism	−	−
Graves' disease with TSH receptor-blocking antibodies	+	±
Iatrogenic		
Radioactive iodine ablation	+	±
Thyroidectomy	+	−
Drugs		
Carbimazole, methimazole, propylthiouracil	+	±
Amiodarone	+	±
Lithium	−	±
Transient thyroiditis		
Subacute (de Quervain's) thyroiditis	+	±
Post-partum thyroiditis	+	±
Iodine deficiency, e.g. in mountainous regions	−	++
Congenital		
Dyshormonogenesis	−	++
Thyroid aplasia	−	−
Infiltrative		
Amyloidosis, Riedel's thyroiditis, sarcoidosis etc.	+	++
Secondary hypothyroidism		
TSH deficiency	−	−

[1] As shown in Box 20.8, thyroid autoantibodies are common in the healthy population, so might be present in anyone. ++ high titre; + more likely to be detected than in the healthy population; − not especially likely.
[2] Goitre: − absent; ± may be present; ++ characteristic.

---

treatment of thyrotoxicosis account for over 90% of cases, except in areas where iodine deficiency is endemic. Women are affected approximately six times more frequently than men.

Clinical assessment

The clinical presentation depends on the duration and severity of the hypothyroidism. Those in whom complete thyroid failure has developed insidiously over months or years may present with many of the clinical features listed in Box 20.7. A consequence of prolonged hypothyroidism is the infiltration of many body tissues by the mucopolysaccharides, hyaluronic acid and chondroitin sulphate, resulting in a low-pitched voice, poor hearing, slurred speech due to a large tongue, and compression of the median nerve at the wrist (carpal tunnel syndrome). Infiltration of the dermis gives rise to non-pitting oedema (myxoedema) which is most marked in the skin of the hands, feet and eyelids. The resultant periorbital puffiness is often striking and, when combined with facial pallor due to vasoconstriction and anaemia, or a lemon-yellow tint to the skin due to carotenaemia, purplish lips and malar flush, the clinical diagnosis is simple. Most cases of hypothyroidism are not clinically obvious, however, and a high index of suspicion needs to be maintained so that the diagnosis is

20

not overlooked in the middle-aged woman complaining of non-specific symptoms such as tiredness, weight gain, depression or carpal tunnel syndrome.

The key discriminatory features in the history and examination are highlighted in Figure 20.6. Care must be taken to identify patients with transient hypothyroidism, in whom life-long thyroxine therapy is inappropriate. This is often observed during the first 6 months after subtotal thyroidectomy or ^{131}I treatment of Graves' disease, in the post-thyrotoxic phase of subacute thyroiditis and in post-partum thyroiditis. In these conditions thyroxine treatment is not always necessary as the patient may be asymptomatic during the short period of thyroid failure.

Investigations

In the vast majority of cases hypothyroidism results from an intrinsic disorder of the thyroid gland (primary hypothyroidism). In this situation serum T_4 is low and TSH is elevated, usually in excess of 20 mU/L. Measurements of serum T_3 are unhelpful since they do not discriminate reliably between euthyroidism and hypothyroidism. The rare condition of secondary hypothyroidism is caused by failure of TSH secretion in a patient with hypothalamic or anterior pituitary disease.

This is characterised by a low serum T_4 but TSH may be low, normal or even slightly elevated (pp. 784–785). Other non-specific abnormalities are shown in Box 20.9. In severe prolonged hypothyroidism, the electrocardiogram (ECG) classically demonstrates sinus bradycardia with low-voltage complexes and ST segment and T wave abnormalities. Measurement of thyroid peroxidase antibodies is helpful, but further investigations are rarely required (see Fig. 20.6).

Management

Treatment is with thyroxine replacement. It is customary to start with a low dose of 50 µg per day for 3 weeks, increasing thereafter to 100 µg per day for a further 3 weeks and finally to a maintenance dose of 100–150 µg per day. Thyroxine has a half-life of 7 days so it should always be taken as a single daily dose and at least 6 weeks should pass before repeating thyroid function tests and adjusting the dose, usually in increments of 25 µg per day. Patients feel better within 2–3 weeks. Reduction in weight and periorbital puffiness occurs quickly, but the restoration of skin and hair texture and resolution of any effusions may take 3–6 months. As illustrated in Figure 20.6, most patients do not require specialist review but will require life-long thyroxine therapy.

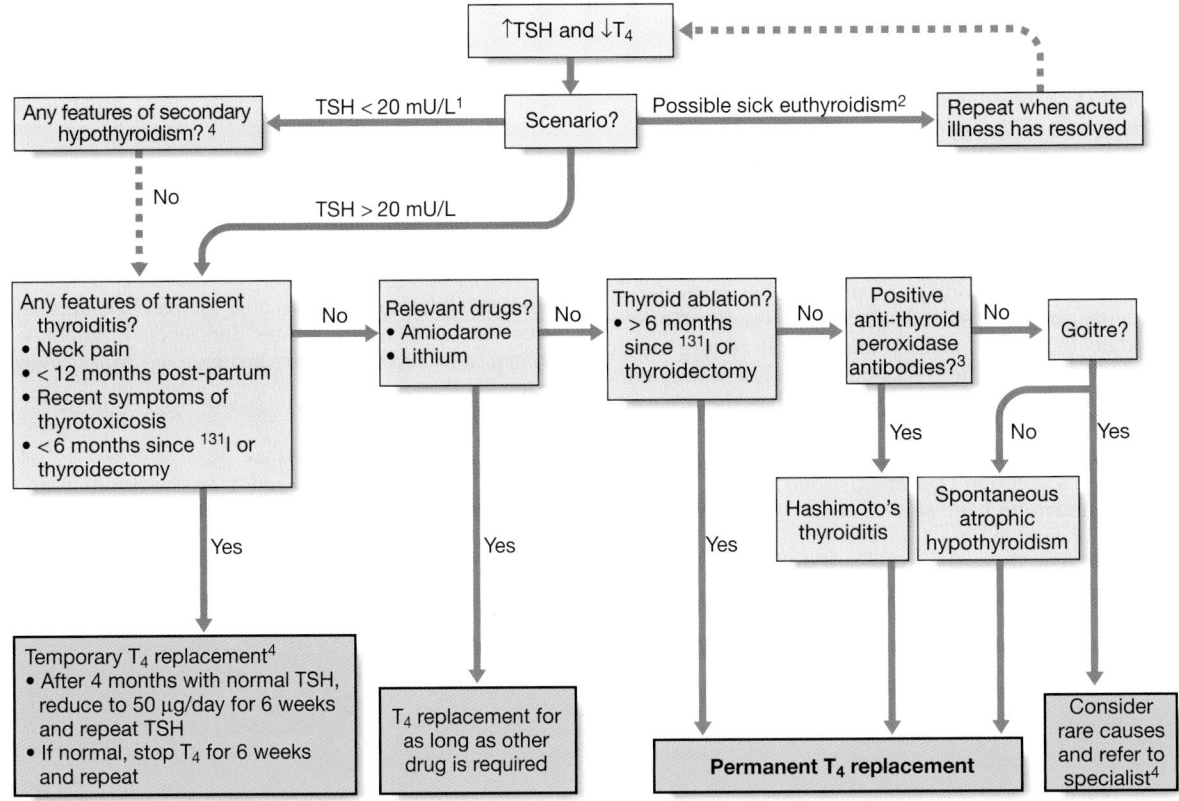

Fig. 20.6 An approach to adults with suspected primary hypothyroidism. This scheme ignores congenital causes of hypothyroidism (see Box 20.10) such as thyroid aplasia and dyshormonogenesis (associated with nerve deafness in Pendred's syndrome), which are usually diagnosed in childhood. (1) Immunoreactive TSH may be detected at normal or even modestly elevated levels in patients with pituitary failure; unless T_4 is only marginally low then TSH should be > 20 mU/L to confirm the diagnosis of primary hypothyroidism. (2) The usual abnormality in sick euthyroidism is a low TSH, but any pattern can occur. (3) Thyroid peroxidase antibodies are highly sensitive, but not very specific for autoimmune thyroid disease (see Boxes 20.8 and 20.10). (4) Specialist advice is most appropriate where indicated. Secondary hypothyroidism is rare, but is suggested by deficiency of pituitary hormones or by clinical features of pituitary tumour such as headache or visual field defect (p. 787). Rare causes of hypothyroidism with goitre include dyshormonogenesis and infiltration of the thyroid (see Box 20.10).

The dose of thyroxine should be adjusted to maintain serum TSH within the reference range. To achieve this, serum T$_4$ often needs to be in the upper part of the normal range or even slightly raised, because the T$_3$ required for receptor activation is derived exclusively from conversion of T$_4$ within the target tissues, without the usual contribution from thyroid secretion. Some physicians advocate combined replacement with T$_4$ and T$_3$ but this approach remains controversial and no ideal preparation exists (Box 20.11). Some patients remain symptomatic despite normalisation of TSH and may wish to take extra thyroxine which suppresses TSH values. However, there is evidence that suppressed TSH is a risk factor for osteoporosis and atrial fibrillation (p. 744; subclinical thyrotoxicosis), so this approach cannot be recommended.

It is important to measure thyroid function every 1–2 years once the dose of thyroxine is stabilised. This encourages patient compliance with therapy and allows adjustment for variable underlying thyroid activity and other changes in thyroxine requirements (Box 20.12).

EBM **20.11 Therapy with T$_3$ in addition to T$_4$ in hypothyroidism**

'One RCT showed that combined T$_3$ + T$_4$ has beneficial effects on neuropsychological tests compared with T$_4$ alone. However, these findings were not replicated in more recent RCTs, no satisfactory combined synthetic preparation is available and the potency of animal thyroid extract is too variable.'

• Bunevicius R, et al. N Engl J Med 1999; 340:420–429.
• Clyde PW, et al. JAMA 2003; 290:2952–2958.
• Sawha AM, et al. J Clin Endocrine Metab 2004; 88:4551–4555.

For further information: www.british-thyroid-association.org

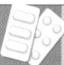 **Box 20.12 Situations in which an adjustment of the dose of levothyroxine may be necessary**

Increased dose required

Use of other medication
• Increase T$_4$ clearance
  Phenobarbital
  Phenytoin
  Carbamazepine
  Rifampicin
  Sertraline*
  Chloroquine*
• Interfere with intestinal T$_4$ absorption
  Colestyramine
  Sucralfate
  Aluminium hydroxide
  Ferrous sulphate
  Dietary fibre supplements
  Calcium carbonate

Pregnancy or oestrogen therapy
• Increases concentration of serum thyroxine-binding globulin

After surgical or ^{131}I ablation of Graves' disease
• Reduces thyroidal secretion with time

Malabsorption, e.g. coeliac disease

Decreased dose required

Ageing
• Decreases T$_4$ clearance

Graves' disease developing in patient with long-standing primary hypothyroidism
• Switch from production of blocking to stimulating TSH receptor antibodies

*Mechanism not fully established.

In some poorly compliant patients, thyroxine is taken diligently or even in excess for a few days prior to a clinic visit, resulting in the seemingly anomalous combination of a high serum T$_4$ and high TSH (see Box 20.5, p. 738).

Thyroxine replacement in ischaemic heart disease

Hypothyroidism and ischaemic heart disease are common conditions which often occur together. Although angina may remain unchanged in severity or paradoxically disappear with restoration of metabolic rate, exacerbation of myocardial ischaemia, infarction and sudden death are recognised complications of thyroxine replacement, even using doses as low as 25 µg per day. In patients with known ischaemic heart disease, thyroid hormone replacement should be introduced at low dose and increased very slowly under specialist supervision. It has been suggested that T$_3$ has an advantage over T$_4$, since T$_3$ has a shorter half-life and any adverse effect will reverse more quickly, but the more distinct peak in hormone levels after each dose of T$_3$ is a disadvantage. Coronary artery surgery or angioplasty is required in the minority of patients with angina who cannot tolerate full thyroxine replacement therapy despite maximal anti-anginal therapy.

Hypothyroidism in pregnancy

Most pregnant women with primary hypothyroidism require an increase in the dose of thyroxine of approximately 50 µg daily to maintain normal TSH levels. This may reflect increased metabolism of thyroxine by the placenta and increased serum thyroxine-binding globulin during pregnancy, resulting in an increase in the total thyroid hormone pool to maintain the same free T$_4$ and T$_3$ concentrations. Recent research suggests that inadequate maternal T$_4$ therapy is associated with impaired cognitive development in their offspring. Serum TSH and free T$_4$ should be measured during each trimester and the dose of thyroxine adjusted to maintain a normal TSH. See also Box 20.19 (p. 753).

Myxoedema coma

This is a rare presentation of hypothyroidism in which there is a depressed level of consciousness, usually in an elderly patient who appears myxoedematous. Body temperature may be as low as 25°C, convulsions are not uncommon and cerebrospinal fluid (CSF) pressure and protein content are raised. The mortality rate is 50% and survival depends upon early recognition and treatment of hypothyroidism and other factors contributing to the altered consciousness level, such as phenothiazines, cardiac failure, pneumonia, dilutional hyponatraemia and respiratory failure.

Myxoedema coma is a medical emergency and treatment must begin before biochemical confirmation of the diagnosis. Suspected cases should be treated with an intravenous injection of 20 µg triiodothyronine followed by further injections of 20 µg 8-hourly until there is sustained clinical improvement. In survivors there is a rise in body temperature within 24 hours and, after 48–72 hours, it is usually possible to switch patients on to oral thyroxine in a dose of 50 µg daily. Unless it is apparent that the patient has primary hypothyroidism, the thyroid failure should also be assumed to be secondary to hypothalamic or pituitary disease and treatment given with hydrocortisone 100 mg i.m. 8-hourly, pending the results of T$_4$, TSH and cortisol measurement (p. 784).

20

Other measures include slow rewarming (p. 102), cautious use of intravenous fluids, broad-spectrum antibiotics and high-flow oxygen. Occasionally, assisted ventilation may be necessary.

Asymptomatic abnormal thyroid function tests

One of the most common problems in medical practice is how to manage patients with abnormal thyroid function tests who have no obvious signs or symptoms of thyroid disease. These can be divided into three categories.

Subclinical thyrotoxicosis

Serum TSH is undetectable, and serum T_3 and T_4 are at the upper end of the reference range. This combination is most often found in older patients with multinodular goitre. These patients are at increased risk of atrial fibrillation and osteoporosis, and hence the consensus view is that they have mild thyrotoxicosis and require therapy, usually with [131]I. Otherwise, annual review is essential as the conversion rate to overt thyrotoxicosis with elevated T_4 and/or T_3 concentrations is 5% each year.

Subclinical hypothyroidism

Serum TSH is raised, and serum T_3 and T_4 concentrations are at the lower end of the reference range. This may persist for many years, although there is a risk of progression to overt thyroid failure, particularly if antibodies to thyroid peroxidase are present or if the TSH rises above 10 mU/L. In patients with non-specific symptoms, a trial of thyroxine therapy may be appropriate. In those with positive autoantibodies or TSH > 10 mU/L it is better to treat the thyroid failure early rather than risk loss to follow-up and subsequent presentation with profound hypothyroidism. Thyroxine should be given in a dose sufficient to restore the serum TSH concentration to normal.

Non-thyroidal illness ('sick euthyroidism')

This typically presents with a low serum TSH, raised T_4 and normal or low T_3, in a patient with systemic illness who does not have clinical evidence of thyroid disease. These abnormalities are caused by decreased peripheral conversion of T_4 to T_3, altered levels of binding proteins and their affinity for thyroid hormones, and often reduced secretion of TSH. During convalescence, serum TSH concentrations may increase to levels found in primary hypothyroidism. Because thyroid function tests are difficult to interpret in patients with non-thyroidal illness it is wise to avoid performing thyroid function tests unless there is clinical evidence of concomitant thyroid disease. If an abnormal result is found, treatment should only be given with specialist advice and the diagnosis should be re-evaluated after recovery.

Thyroid enlargement

Palpable thyroid enlargement is common, affecting about 5% of the population, but only a minority seek medical attention, often because a friend or relative has noticed a lump in the neck. Multinodular goitres and solitary nodules sometimes present with acute painful enlargement due to haemorrhage into a nodule. There are numerous causes of thyroid enlargement (Box 20.13), ranging from the soft diffuse goitre of puberty and youth, to the multinodular goitre of middle age and beyond, and the

20.13 Causes of thyroid enlargement

Diffuse goitre
- Simple goitre[1] (p. 750)
- Hashimoto's thyroiditis[1] (p. 748)
- Graves' disease (p. 745)
- Drugs
    Iodine, amiodarone (p. 749), lithium
- Iodine deficiency (endemic goitre)[1] (p. 749)
- Suppurative thyroiditis[2]
- Transient thyroiditis[2] (p. 748)
- Dyshormonogenesis[1] (p. 752)
- Infiltrative
    Amyloidosis, sarcoidosis etc
- Riedel's thyroiditis[2] (p. 752)

Multinodular goitre (p. 750)

Solitary nodule
- Simple cyst
- Colloid nodule
- Follicular adenoma (p. 751)
- Papillary carcinoma (p. 751)
- Follicular carcinoma (p. 751)
- Medullary cell carcinoma (p. 752)
- Anaplastic carcinoma
- Lymphoma
- Metastasis

[1]Goitre likely to shrink with thyroxine therapy.
[2]Usually tender.

solitary nodule which can present at any age. Whereas diffuse and multinodular goitre are almost invariably benign, there is a 1:20 chance of malignancy in the truly solitary lesion.

Palpation of the neck (including the thyroid gland and any lymph nodes, p. 732) will allow discrimination of the following distinct groups of patients. Thyroid function tests should always be performed.

Diffuse goitre

In the absence of thyrotoxicosis or hypothyroidism a diffuse goitre rarely needs further investigation or treatment unless it is very large and causing cosmetic symptoms or compression of other local structures (resulting in stridor or dysphagia). The presence of autoantibodies may support the diagnosis of Graves' disease or Hashimoto's thyroiditis, while their absence in a younger patient suggests a simple goitre. Thyroxine therapy is sometimes justified in an attempt to shrink the goitre.

Multinodular goitre

This condition is described on page 750. It is usually necessary to confirm the clinical diagnosis using ^{99m}Tc scintigraphy (see Fig. 20.4, p. 739) or ultrasonography. Sometimes one of the nodules is much larger than any other (a 'dominant' nodule); if such a nodule is 'cold' on isotope scanning, it may be investigated in the same way as a truly solitary nodule since the risk of malignancy is not negligible in such lesions.

Solitary thyroid nodule

It is important to determine whether the nodule is benign or malignant. It is rarely possible to make this distinction on clinical grounds alone, although the presence of cervical lymphadenopathy increases the likelihood of malignancy. However, a solitary nodule presenting in childhood or adolescence, particularly if there is a past history of head and neck irradiation, or one presenting in the elderly should heighten suspicion of a primary thyroid malignancy (pp. 751–752). Very occasionally, a secondary deposit from a renal, breast or lung carcinoma presents as a painful, rapidly growing solitary thyroid nodule.

Investigations

Serum T_3, T_4 and TSH should be measured in all patients with a solitary thyroid nodule. The finding of undetectable TSH is very suggestive of a benign autonomously functioning thyroid follicular adenoma, but this diagnosis can only be confirmed by thyroid isotope scanning (see Fig. 20.4, p. 739).

For euthyroid patients, the most useful investigation is fine needle aspiration of the nodule. This can be performed in the outpatient clinic using a standard 21-gauge needle and a 20 mL syringe, usually making several passes through different parts of the lesion. Aspiration may be therapeutic in the small proportion of patients in whom the swelling is a cyst, although recurrence on more than one occasion is an indication for surgery. Cytological examination can differentiate benign (80%) from definitely malignant or indeterminate nodules (20%), of which 25–50% are confirmed as cancer at surgery. The advantage of fine needle aspiration over isotope scanning is that a much higher proportion of patients avoid surgery; isotope scanning identifies suspicious 'cold nodules', but most of these are benign. The limitations of fine needle aspiration are that it cannot differentiate between follicular adenoma and carcinoma and that in 10–20% of cases an inadequate specimen is obtained. Ultrasound-guided needle aspiration can be helpful in increasing the quality of specimens.

Management

Solitary nodules with a solid component in which cytology either is inconclusive or shows malignant cells are treated by surgical excision. Those in which malignancy is confirmed by formal histology are then treated as described on page 751. Benign lesions are sometimes excised, if they are growing, but the majority of patients can be reassured.

Autoimmune thyroid disease

Thyroid diseases are amongst the most prevalent antibody-mediated autoimmune diseases and are associated with other organ-specific autoimmunity (Ch. 4 and p. 794). Autoantibodies may produce inflammation and destruction of thyroid tissue resulting in hypothyroidism, goitre (in Hashimoto's thyroiditis) or sometimes even transient thyrotoxicosis ('Hashitoxicosis'), or they may stimulate the TSH receptor to cause thyrotoxicosis (in Graves' disease). There is overlap between these conditions, since some patients have multiple autoantibodies.

Graves' disease

Graves' disease can occur at any age but is unusual before puberty and most commonly affects women aged 30–50 years. The most common manifestation is thyrotoxicosis with or without a diffuse goitre. The clinical features and differential diagnosis are described on pages 738–740. Graves' disease also causes ophthalmopathy and rarely pretibial myxoedema (p. 732). These extrathyroidal features usually occur in thyrotoxic patients, but can occur in the absence of thyroid dysfunction.

Graves' thyrotoxicosis

Pathophysiology

The thyrotoxicosis results from the production of IgG antibodies directed against the TSH receptor on the thyroid follicular cell, which stimulate thyroid hormone production and proliferation of follicular cells, leading to goitre in the majority of patients. These antibodies are termed thyroid-stimulating immunoglobulins or TSH receptor antibodies (TRAb) and can be detected in the serum of 80–95% of patients with Graves' disease. The concentration of TRAb in the serum is presumed to fluctuate to account for the natural history of Graves' thyrotoxicosis (Fig. 20.7). The thyroid failure seen in some patients may result from the presence of blocking antibodies against the TSH receptor, and from tissue destruction by cytotoxic antibodies and cell-mediated immunity.

There is an association of Graves' disease with HLA-B8, DR3 and DR2 and with inability to secrete the water-soluble glycoprotein form of the ABO blood group antigens. There is 50% concordance for thyrotoxicosis between monozygotic twins, but only 5% concordance between dizygotic twins.

A suggested trigger for the development of thyrotoxicosis in genetically susceptible individuals may be infection with viruses or bacteria. Certain strains of the gut organisms *Escherichia coli* and *Yersinia enterocolitica* possess cell membrane TSH receptors; antibodies to these microbial antigens may cross-react with the TSH receptors on the host thyroid follicular cell. In regions of iodine deficiency (p. 749), iodine supplementation can precipitate thyrotoxicosis, but only in those with pre-existing subclinical Graves' disease. Smoking is weakly associated with Graves' thyrotoxicosis, but strongly linked with the development of ophthalmopathy.

Management

Symptoms of thyrotoxicosis respond to β-blockade (p. 739), but definitive treatment requires control of thyroid hormone secretion. The different options are compared in Box 20.14. For patients under 40 years of age most clinicians adopt the empirical approach of prescribing a course of carbimazole and recommending surgery if relapse occurs, while ^{131}I is employed as first- or second-line treatment in those aged over 40. A number of observational studies have linked therapeutic ^{131}I with increased incidence of some malignancies, particularly of the thyroid and gastrointestinal tract, but the results have been inconsistent; the association may be with Graves' disease rather than its therapy, and the magnitude of the effect, if any, is small. Experience from the Chernobyl disaster suggests that younger people are more sensitive to radiation-induced thyroid cancer. In many centres, however, ^{131}I is used more extensively, even in young patients.

Antithyroid drugs. The most commonly used are carbimazole and its active metabolite, methimazole (not available in the UK). Propylthiouracil is equally effective. These drugs reduce the synthesis of new thyroid hormones by inhibiting the iodination of tyrosine (see Fig. 20.3, p. 737). Carbimazole also has an immunosuppressive action, leading to a reduction in serum TRAb concentrations, but this is not enough to influence the natural history of the thyrotoxicosis significantly.

20

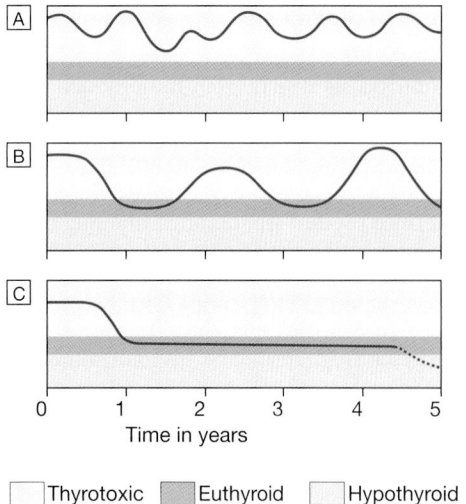

Fig. 20.7 **Natural history of the thyrotoxicosis of Graves' disease.** A and B The majority (60%) of patients have either prolonged periods of thyrotoxicosis of fluctuating severity, or periods of alternating relapse and remission. C It is the minority who experience a single short-lived episode followed by prolonged remission and, in some cases, by the eventual onset of hypothyroidism.

Antithyroid drugs should be introduced at high doses (carbimazole 40–60 mg daily or prophylthiouracil 400–600 mg daily). Usually this results in subjective improvement within 10–14 days and renders the patient clinically and biochemically euthyroid at 3–4 weeks. At this point the dose can be reduced and titrated to maintain T_4 and TSH within their reference range. In most patients carbimazole is continued at 5–20 mg/day for 12–18 months in the hope that remission will occur. Thyrotoxicosis relapses in at least 50% of cases, usually within 2 years of stopping treatment. Rarely, T_4 and TSH levels fluctuate between those of thyrotoxicosis and hypothyroid-ism at successive review appointments, despite good drug compliance, presumably due to rapidly changing concentrations of TRAb. In these patients satisfactory control can be achieved by blocking thyroid hormone synthesis with carbimazole 30–40 mg daily and adding thyroxine 100–150 µg daily as replacement therapy.

Antithyroid drugs can have adverse effects. The most common is a rash. Agranulocytosis is a rare but potentially serious complication which cannot be predicted by routine measurement of white blood cell count but which is reversible on stopping treatment. Patients should be warned to stop the drug and seek medical advice immediately should a severe sore throat or fever develop whilst on treatment. If side-effects do develop, another member of the group can be substituted as cross-sensitivity between the antithyroid drugs is unusual.

Subtotal thyroidectomy. Patients should be rendered euthyroid with antithyroid drugs before operation. Potassium iodide, 60 mg 8-hourly orally, is often added for 2 weeks before surgery to inhibit thyroid hormone release and reduce the size and vascularity of the gland, making surgery technically easier. Complications of surgery are rare. One year after surgery, 80% of patients are euthyroid, 15% are permanently hypothyroid and 5% remain thyrotoxic. Thyroid failure within 6 months of operation may be temporary. Long-term follow-up of patients treated surgically is necessary, as the late development of hypothyroidism and recurrence of thyrotoxicosis are well recognised.

Radioactive iodine. [131]I is administered orally as a single dose, and is trapped and organified in the thyroid (see Fig. 20.3, p. 737). Although ^{131}I decays within a few weeks, it has long-lasting inhibitory effects on survival and replication of follicular cells. The variable radio-iodine uptake and radiosensitivity of the gland means that the choice of dose is empirical; in most centres approximately 400 MBq (10 mCi) is given orally. This regimen is effective in 75% of patients within

---

20.14 Comparison of treatments for the thyrotoxicosis of Graves' disease

Management	Common indications	Contraindications	Disadvantages/complications
Antithyroid drugs (carbimazole, propylthiouracil)	First episode in patients < 40 yrs	Breastfeeding (propylthiouracil suitable)	Hypersensitivity rash 2% Agranulocytosis 0.2% > 50% relapse rate usually within 2 years of stopping drug
Subtotal thyroidectomy	Large goitre Poor drug compliance, especially in young patients Recurrent thyrotoxicosis after course of antithyroid drugs in young patients	Previous thyroid surgery Dependence upon voice, e.g. opera singer, lecturer[1]	Hypothyroidism (~25%) Transient hypocalcaemia (10%) Permanent hypoparathyroidism (1%) Recurrent laryngeal nerve palsy[1] (1%)
Radio-iodine	Patients > 40 yrs[2] Recurrence following surgery irrespective of age Other serious comorbidity	Pregnancy or planned pregnancy within 6 months of treatment Active Graves' ophthalmopathy[3]	Hypothyroidism, ~40% in first year, 80% after 15 years Most likely treatment to result in exacerbation of ophthalmopathy[3]

[1]It is not only vocal cord palsy due to recurrent laryngeal nerve damage which alters the voice following thyroid surgery; the superior laryngeal nerves are frequently transected and result in minor changes in voice quality.
[2]In many institutions, ^{131}I is used more liberally and prescribed for much younger patients.
[3]The extent to which radio-iodine exacerbates ophthalmopathy is controversial and practice varies; some use prednisolone for 4 months to reduce this risk (see Box 20.15).

EBM 20.15 **Effects of ¹³¹I and prednisolone in Graves' ophthalmopathy**

'The deterioration of ophthalmopathy, which occurs in some patients following ¹³¹I therapy, can be prevented by a 3-month course of oral prednisolone.'

• Bartalena L, et al. N Engl J Med 1989; 321:1349–1352.

For further information: www.rcplondon.ac.uk

4–12 weeks. During the lag period, symptoms can be controlled by a β-blocker or, in more severe cases, by carbimazole. However, carbimazole reduces the efficacy of ¹³¹I therapy because it prevents organification of ¹³¹I in the gland, and so should be avoided until 48 hours after radio-iodine administration. If thyrotoxicosis persists after 6 months, a further dose of ¹³¹I can be given. The disadvantage of ¹³¹I treatment is that the majority of patients eventually develop hypothyroidism. ¹³¹I is usually avoided in patients with Graves' ophthalmopathy and evidence of active orbital inflammation, and used only with caution in those with 'burnt out' eye disease (Box 20.15). In women of reproductive age, pregnancy must be excluded before administration of ¹³¹I and avoided for 6 months thereafter; men are also advised against fathering children for 6 months.

Thyrotoxicosis in pregnancy

The coexistence of pregnancy and thyrotoxicosis is unusual, as anovulatory cycles are common in thyrotoxic patients and autoimmune disease tends to remit during pregnancy, when the maternal immune response is suppressed. Thyroid function tests must be interpreted in the knowledge that thyroid-binding globulin, and hence total T_4 and T_3 levels, are increased in pregnancy and that TSH normal ranges may be lower (see Box 20.19, p. 753); a fully suppressed TSH with elevated free thyroid hormone levels indicates thyrotoxicosis. The thyrotoxicosis is almost always caused by Graves' disease. Both mother and fetus must be considered, since maternal thyroid hormones, TRAb and antithyroid drugs can all cross the placenta to some degree, exposing the fetus to the risks of thyrotoxicosis, iatrogenic hypothyroidism and goitre.

Thyrotoxicosis should be treated with antithyroid drugs which cross the placenta and also treat the fetus, whose thyroid gland is exposed to the action of maternal TRAb. Propylthiouracil may be preferable to carbimazole since the latter might be associated with a skin defect in the child, known as aplasia cutis. In order to avoid fetal hypothyroidism and goitre, it is important to use the smallest dose of antithyroid drug (optimally less than 150 mg propylthiouracil per day) that will maintain maternal (and presumably fetal) free T_4, T_3 and TSH within their respective normal ranges. Frequent review of mother and fetus (using ultrasonography and heart rate monitoring) is important. TRAb levels can be measured in the third trimester to predict the likelihood of neonatal thyrotoxicosis. When TRAb levels are not elevated, the antithyroid drug can be discontinued 4 weeks before the expected date of delivery to minimise the risk of fetal hypothyroidism at the time of maximum brain development. After delivery, if antithyroid drug is required and the patient wishes to breastfeed, then propylthiouracil is the drug of choice, as it is excreted in the milk to a much lesser extent than carbimazole.

If subtotal thyroidectomy is necessary because of poor drug compliance or drug hypersensitivity, it is most safely performed in the second trimester. Radioactive iodine is absolutely contraindicated, as it invariably induces fetal hypothyroidism.

Graves' ophthalmopathy

This condition is immunologically mediated, but the autoantigen has not been identified. Within the orbit (and the dermis) there is cytokine-mediated proliferation of fibroblasts which secrete hydrophilic glycosaminoglycans. The resulting increase in interstitial fluid content, combined with a chronic inflammatory cell infiltrate, causes marked swelling and ultimately fibrosis of the extraocular muscles (Fig. 20.8) and a rise in retrobulbar pressure. The eye is displaced forwards (proptosis, exophthalmos; see p. 733) and in severe cases there is optic nerve compression.

Ophthalmopathy, like thyrotoxicosis (see Fig. 20.7), typically follows an episodic course and it is helpful to distinguish patients with active inflammation (periorbital oedema and conjunctival inflammation with changing orbital signs) from those in whom the inflammation has 'burnt out'. Eye disease is detectable in up to 50% of thyrotoxic patients at presentation, but active ocular inflammation may occur before or after thyrotoxic episodes (exophthalmic Graves' disease). It is more common in cigarette smokers and is exacerbated by poor control of thyroid function, especially hypothyroidism.

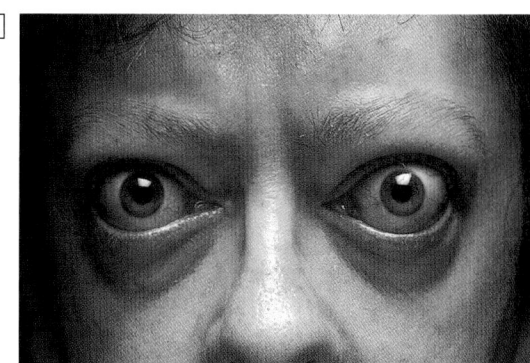
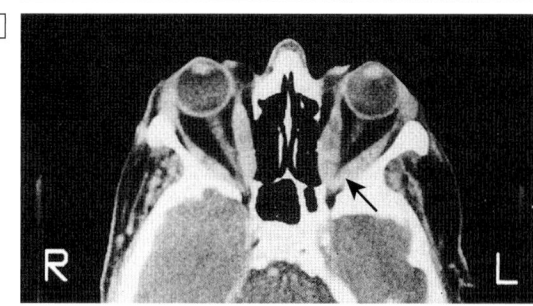

Fig. 20.8 Graves' disease. **A** Bilateral ophthalmopathy in a 42-year-old man. The main symptoms were diplopia in all directions of gaze and reduced visual acuity in the left eye. The periorbital swelling is due to retrobulbar fat prolapsing into the eyelids, and increased interstitial fluid as a result of raised intraorbital pressure. **B** Transverse CT of the orbits, showing the enlarged extraocular muscles. This is most obvious at the apex of the left orbit (arrow), where compression of the optic nerve caused reduced visual acuity.

The most frequent presenting symptoms are related to increased exposure of the cornea, resulting from proptosis and lid retraction. There may be excessive lacrimation made worse by wind and bright light, a 'gritty' sensation in the eye, and pain due to conjunctivitis or corneal ulceration. In addition, there may be reduction of visual acuity and/or visual fields as a consequence of corneal oedema or optic nerve compression. Other signs of optic nerve compression include reduced colour vision and a relative afferent pupillary defect (pp. 733 and 1163). If the extraocular muscles are involved and do not act in concert, diplopia results.

The majority of patients require no treatment other than reassurance. Methylcellulose eye drops and gel counter the gritty discomfort of dry eyes, and tinted glasses or side shields attached to spectacle frames reduce the excessive lacrimation triggered by sun or wind. Severe inflammatory episodes are treated with glucocorticoids (e.g. daily oral prednisolone or pulsed i.v. methylprednisolone) and sometimes orbital irradiation. Loss of visual acuity is an indication for urgent surgical decompression of the orbit. In 'burnt out' disease, surgery to the eyelids and/or ocular muscles may improve conjunctival exposure, cosmetic appearance and diplopia.

Pretibial myxoedema

This infiltrative dermopathy occurs in fewer than 10% of patients with Graves' disease and has similar pathological features as occur in the orbit. It takes the form of raised pink-coloured or purplish plaques on the anterior aspect of the leg, extending on to the dorsum of the foot (p. 732). The lesions may be itchy and the skin may have a 'peau d'orange' appearance with growth of coarse hair; less commonly, the face and arms are affected. Treatment is rarely required, but in severe cases topical glucocorticoids may be helpful.

Hashimoto's thyroiditis

Hashimoto's thyroiditis is characterised by destructive lymphoid infiltration of the thyroid, ultimately leading to a varying degree of fibrosis and thyroid enlargement. There is an increased risk of thyroid lymphoma (p. 752), although this is exceedingly rare. The nomenclature of autoimmune hypothyroidism is confusing. Some authorities reserve the term 'Hashimoto's thyroiditis' for patients with positive anti-thyroid peroxidase autoantibodies and a firm goitre who may or may not be hypothyroid, and use the term 'spontaneous atrophic hypothyroidism' for hypothyroid patients without a goitre in whom TSH receptor-blocking antibodies may be more important than anti-peroxidase antibodies. However, these syndromes can both be considered as variants of the same underlying disease process.

Hashimoto's thyroiditis increases in incidence with age and affects approximately 3.5 per 1000 women and 0.8 per 1000 men each year. Many present with a small or moderately sized diffuse goitre, which is characteristically firm or rubbery in consistency. The goitre may be soft, however, and impossible to differentiate from simple goitre (p. 750) by palpation alone. Around 25% of patients are hypothyroid at presentation. In the remainder, serum T_4 is normal and TSH normal or raised, but these patients are at risk of developing overt hypothyroidism in future years. Anti-thyroid peroxidase antibodies are present in the serum in more than 90% of patients with Hashimoto's thyroiditis. In those under the age of 20 years, antinuclear factor (ANF) may also be positive.

Thyroxine therapy is indicated as treatment for hypothyroidism (p. 742), and also to shrink an associated goitre. In this context, the dose of thyroxine should be sufficient to suppress serum TSH to low but detectable levels.

Transient thyroiditis

Subacute (de Quervain's) thyroiditis

In its classical painful form, subacute thyroiditis is a transient inflammation of the thyroid gland occurring after infection with Coxsackie, mumps or adenoviruses. There is pain in the region of the thyroid that may radiate to the angle of the jaw and the ears, and is made worse by swallowing, coughing and movement of the neck. The thyroid is usually palpably enlarged and tender. Systemic upset is common. Affected patients are usually females aged 20–40 years. Painless transient thyroiditis can also occur after viral infection and in patients with underlying autoimmune disease. The condition can also be precipitated by drugs, including interferon-α and lithium.

Irrespective of the clinical presentation, inflammation in the thyroid gland occurs and is associated with release of colloid and stored thyroid hormones, but also with damage to follicular cells and impaired synthesis of new thyroid hormones. As a result, T_4 and T_3 levels are raised for 4–6 weeks until the preformed colloid is depleted. Thereafter, there is usually a period of hypothyroidism of variable severity before the follicular cells recover and normal thyroid function is restored within 4–6 months (Fig. 20.9). In the thyrotoxic phase, the iodine uptake is low, because the damaged follicular cells are unable to trap iodine and because TSH secretion is suppressed. Low-titre thyroid autoantibodies appear transiently in the serum, and the erythrocyte sedimentation rate (ESR) is usually raised. High-titre autoantibodies suggest an underlying autoimmune pathology and greater risk of recurrence and ultimate progression to hypothyroidism.

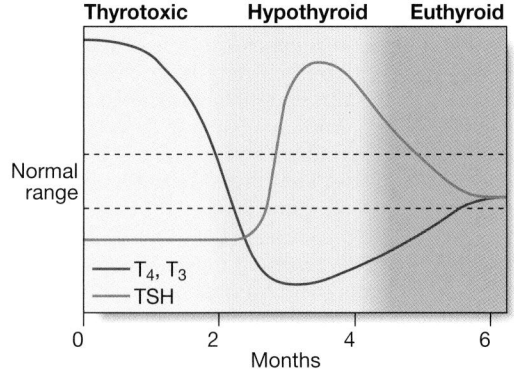

Fig. 20.9 Thyroid function tests in an episode of transient thyroiditis. This pattern might be observed in classical subacute (de Quervain's) thyroiditis, painless thyroiditis or post-partum thyroiditis. The duration of each phase varies between patients. Note that the lower limit of detection of TSH is close to the lower limit of the normal range.

The pain and systemic upset usually respond to simple measures such as non-steroidal anti-inflammatory drugs (NSAIDs). Occasionally, however, it may be necessary to prescribe prednisolone 40 mg daily for 3–4 weeks. The thyrotoxicosis is mild and treatment with a β-blocker is usually adequate. Antithyroid drugs are of no benefit because thyroid hormone synthesis is impaired rather than enhanced. Careful monitoring of thyroid function and symptoms is required so that thyroxine can be prescribed temporarily in the hypothyroid phase. Care must be taken to identify patients presenting with hypothyroidism who are in the later stages of a transient thyroiditis, since they are unlikely to require life-long thyroxine therapy (see Fig. 20.6, p. 742).

Post-partum thyroiditis

The maternal immune response, which is modified during pregnancy to allow survival of the fetus, is enhanced after delivery and may unmask previously unrecognised subclinical autoimmune thyroid disease. Surveys have shown that transient biochemical disturbances of thyroid function occur in 5–10% of women within 6 months of delivery (see Box 20.19, p. 753). Those affected are likely to have anti-thyroid peroxidase antibodies in the serum in early pregnancy. Symptoms of thyroid dysfunction are rare and there is no association between postnatal depression and abnormal thyroid function tests. However, symptomatic thyrotoxicosis presenting for the first time within 12 months of childbirth is likely to be due to post-partum thyroiditis and the diagnosis is confirmed by a negligible radioisotope uptake. The clinical course and treatment are similar to painless subacute thyroiditis (see above). Post-partum thyroiditis tends to recur after subsequent pregnancies and eventually patients progress over a period of years to permanent hypothyroidism.

Iodine-associated thyroid disease

Iodine deficiency

Thyroid enlargement is extremely common in certain mountainous parts of the world, such as the Andes, the Himalayas and central Africa, where there is dietary iodine deficiency (endemic goitre). Most patients are euthyroid with normal or raised TSH levels, although hypothyroidism can occur with severe iodine deficiency. Iodine supplementation programmes have abolished this condition in most developed countries.

Iodine-induced thyroid dysfunction

Iodine has complex effects on thyroid function. Very high concentrations of iodine inhibit thyroid hormone release and this forms the rationale for iodine treatment of thyroid storm (p. 741) and prior to subtotal thyroidectomy (p. 746). Iodine administration initially enhances, but then inhibits, iodination of tyrosine and thyroid hormone synthesis (see Fig. 20.3, p. 737). The resulting effect of iodine on thyroid function varies according to whether the patient has an iodine-deficient diet or underlying thyroid disease. In iodine-deficient parts of the world, transient thyrotoxicosis may be precipitated by prophylactic iodinisation programmes. In iodine-sufficient areas, thyrotoxicosis can be precipitated by radiographic contrast medium or expectorants in individuals who have underlying thyroid disease predisposing to thyrotoxicosis, such as multinodular goitre or Graves' disease in remission. Induction of thyrotoxicosis by iodine is called the Jod–Basedow effect. Chronic excess iodine administration can, however, result in hypothyroidism. Increased iodine within the thyroid gland down-regulates iodine trapping, so that uptake is low in all circumstances.

Amiodarone

The anti-arrhythmic agent amiodarone has a structure that is analogous to T_4 (Fig. 20.10) and contains huge amounts of iodine; a 200 mg dose contains 75 mg iodine, compared with a daily dietary requirement of just 125 μg. Amiodarone also has a cytotoxic effect on thyroid follicular cells and inhibits conversion of T_4 to T_3. Most patients receiving amiodarone have normal thyroid function, but up to 20% develop hypothyroidism or thyrotoxicosis and so thyroid function should be monitored regularly. The ratio of T_4:T_3 is elevated and TSH provides the best indicator of thyroid function.

The thyrotoxicosis can be classified as either:

- type I: a Jod–Basedow effect in patients with underlying thyroid disease, *or*
- type II: thyroiditis due to cytotoxicity, resulting in a transient thyrotoxicosis.

These patterns can overlap and can be difficult to distinguish clinically, as iodine uptake is low in both. There is no widely accepted management algorithm, although the iodine excess renders the gland completely resistant to radioiodine. Antithyroid drugs may be effective in patients with the type I form, but are ineffective in type II thyrotoxicosis. Prednisolone is beneficial in the type II form. A pragmatic approach is to commence combination therapy with an antithyroid drug and glucocorticoid in patients with significant thyrotoxicosis. A rapid response (within 1–2 weeks) usually indicates a type II picture and permits withdrawal of the antithyroid therapy; a slower response suggests a type I picture, when antithyroid drugs may be continued and prednisolone withdrawn. Potassium perchlorate can also be used to inhibit iodine trapping in the thyroid. If the cardiac state allows, amiodarone should be discontinued, but it has a long half-life (50–60 days) so its effects are long-lasting. To minimise the risk of type I thyrotoxicosis, thyroid function should be measured in all patients prior to

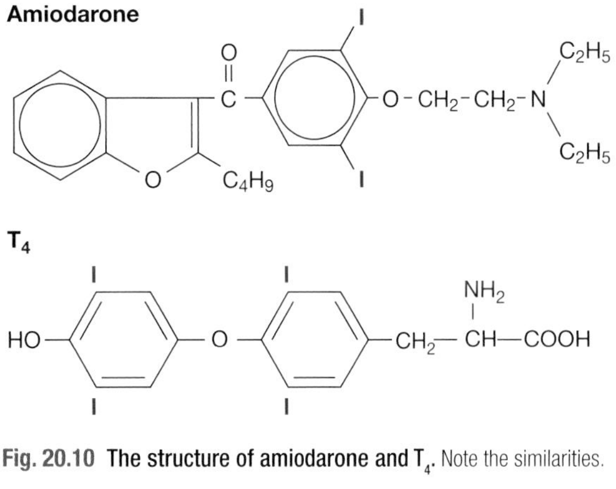

Fig. 20.10 The structure of amiodarone and T_4. Note the similarities.

commencement of amiodarone therapy, and amiodarone avoided if TSH is suppressed.

Hypothyroidism should be treated with thyroxine, which can be given while amiodarone is continued.

Simple and multinodular goitre

These terms describe diffuse or multinodular enlargement of the thyroid, which occurs sporadically and is of unknown aetiology.

Simple diffuse goitre

This form of goitre usually presents between the ages of 15 and 25 years, often during pregnancy, and tends to be noticed, not by the patient, but by friends and relatives. Occasionally, there is a tight sensation in the neck, particularly when swallowing. The goitre is soft and symmetrical and the thyroid is enlarged to two or three times its normal size. There is no tenderness, lymphadenopathy or overlying bruit. Concentrations of T_3, T_4 and TSH are normal and no thyroid autoantibodies are detected in the serum. No treatment is necessary and in most cases the goitre regresses. In some, however, the unknown stimulus to thyroid enlargement persists and, as a result of recurrent episodes of hyperplasia and involution during the following 10–20 years, the gland becomes multinodular with areas of autonomous function.

Multinodular goitre

The natural history is shown in Figure 20.11. Patients with thyroid enlargement in the absence of thyroid dysfunction or positive autoantibodies (i.e. with 'simple goitre', see above) as young adults may progress to develop nodules. These nodules grow at varying rates and secrete thyroid hormone 'autonomously', thereby suppressing TSH-dependent growth and function in the rest of the gland. Ultimately, complete suppression of TSH occurs in about 25% of cases, with T_4 and T_3 levels often within the normal range (subclinical thyrotoxicosis, p. 744) but sometimes elevated (toxic multinodular goitre, Fig. 20.4, p. 739). Opinions differ as to whether

Age (in years)	15–25	35–55	> 55
Goitre	Diffuse	Nodular	Nodular
Tracheal compression/ deviation	No	Minimal	Yes
T_3, T_4	Normal	Normal	Raised
TSH	Normal	Normal or undetectable	Undetectable

Fig. 20.11 Natural history of simple goitre.

the nodules represent multiple adenomas or focal hyperplasia. There are reports that the prevalence of foci of thyroid cancer is increased in multinodular goitres, but for practical purposes patients can be reassured that it is a benign condition and malignancy need only be considered in patients with a large 'dominant' nodule that is 'cold' (i.e. does not take up radioisotope, p. 744).

Clinical features and investigations

Multinodular goitre is usually diagnosed in patients presenting with thyrotoxicosis, a large goitre with or without tracheal compression, or sudden painful swelling caused by haemorrhage into a nodule or cyst. The goitre is nodular or lobulated on palpation and may extend retrosternally; however, not all multinodular goitres causing thyrotoxicosis are easily palpable. Very large goitres may cause mediastinal compression with stridor (Fig. 20.12), dysphagia and obstruction of the superior vena cava. Hoarseness due to recurrent laryngeal nerve palsy can occur, but is far more suggestive of thyroid carcinoma.

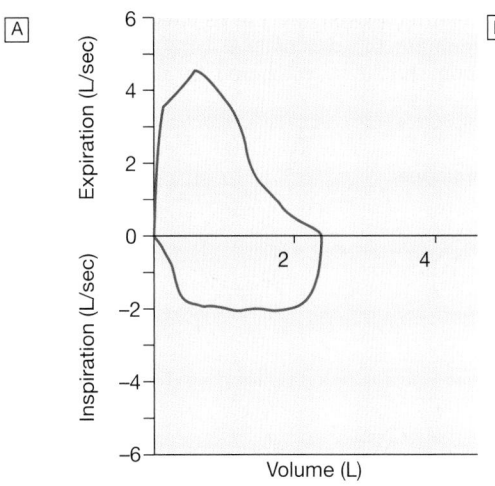

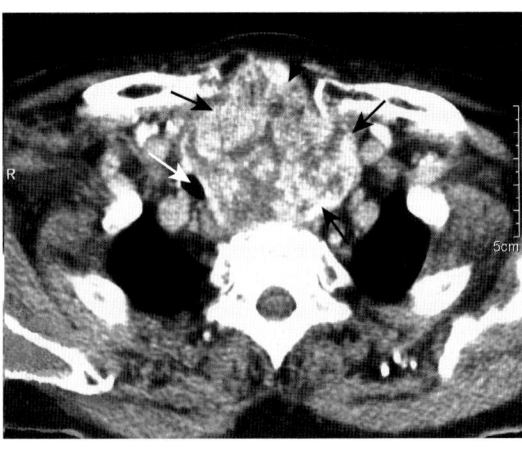

Fig. 20.12 Multinodular goitre with retrosternal extension and tracheal compression. **A** A flow-volume loop (p. 650) showing a square-shaped inspiratory curve indicating extrathoracic airflow obstruction. **B** A CT scan of the upper mediastinum showing a large retrosternal goitre (black arrows) with marked deviation and compression of the trachea (white arrow).

The diagnosis can be confirmed by a radioisotope thyroid scan (see Fig. 20.4, p. 739) and/or ultrasonography. In patients with large goitres a flow-volume loop is a good screening test for significant tracheal compression (see Fig. 20.12). If intervention is contemplated, a CT or MRI of the thoracic inlet should be performed to quantify the degree of tracheal displacement or compression and the extent of retrosternal extension. In those with a 'dominant', 'cold' nodule, fine needle aspiration is indicated to exclude thyroid cancer.

Management

If the goitre is small, no treatment is necessary but annual thyroid function testing should be arranged, as the natural history is progression to a toxic multinodular goitre. Partial thyroidectomy is indicated for large goitres which cause mediastinal compression or which are cosmetically unattractive. [131]I can result in a significant reduction in thyroid size and may be of value in elderly patients (Box 20.16). Unfortunately, recurrence 10–20 years later is not uncommon. Thyroxine therapy is of no benefit in shrinking multinodular goitres and may simply aggravate any associated thyrotoxicosis.

In toxic multinodular goitre treatment is usually with [131]I. The iodine uptake is lower than in Graves' disease so a higher dose may be administered (up to 800 Mbq (approximately 20 mCi)) and hypothyroidism is less common. In thyrotoxic patients with a large goitre, partial thyroidectomy may be indicated. Long-term treatment with antithyroid drugs is not usually employed, as relapse is invariable after drug withdrawal.

Asymptomatic patients with subclinical thyrotoxicosis (p. 744) are increasingly being treated with ^{131}I on the grounds that a suppressed TSH is a risk factor for atrial fibrillation and, particularly in post-menopausal women, osteoporosis.

EBM | **20.16 Medical therapy to shrink non-toxic multinodular goitre**

'[131]I, but not thyroxine therapy, reduces thyroid volume in patients with large multinodular goitres and normal thyroid function.'

- Wesche MFT, et al. J Clin Endocrinol Metab 2001; 86:998–1005.

For further information: 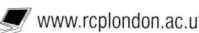 www.rcplondon.ac.uk

---

Thyroid neoplasia

Patients with thyroid tumours usually present with a solitary nodule (p. 744). Most are benign and a few of these, called 'toxic adenomas', secrete excess thyroid hormones. Primary thyroid malignancy is rare, accounting for less than 1% of all carcinomas, and has an incidence of 25 per million per annum. As shown in Box 20.17, it can be classified according to the cell type of origin. With the exception of medullary carcinoma, thyroid cancer is more common in females.

Toxic adenoma

The presence of a toxic solitary nodule is the cause of less than 5% of all cases of thyrotoxicosis. The nodule is a follicular adenoma, which autonomously secretes excess

i | **20.17 Malignant thyroid tumours**

Type of tumour	Frequency (%)	Age at presentation (years)	20-year survival (%)
Follicular cells			
Differentiated carcinoma			
Papillary	70	20–40	95
Follicular	10	40–60	60
Undifferentiated carcinoma			
Anaplastic	5	> 60	< 1
Parafollicular C cells			
Medullary carcinoma	5–10	> 40*	50
Lymphocytes			
Lymphoma	5–10	> 60	10

*Patients with medullary carcinoma as part of MEN type 2 (p. 793) may present in childhood.

thyroid hormones and inhibits endogenous TSH secretion with subsequent atrophy of the rest of the thyroid gland. The adenoma is usually greater than 3 cm in diameter.

Most patients are female and over 40 years of age. Although many nodules are palpable, the diagnosis can be made with certainty only by isotope scanning (see Fig. 20.4, p. 739). The thyrotoxicosis is usually mild and in almost 50% of patients the plasma T_3 alone is elevated (T_3 thyrotoxicosis). [131]I (400–800 MBq (10–20 mCi)) is highly effective and is an ideal treatment since the atrophic cells surrounding the nodule do not take up iodine and so receive little or no radiation. For this reason, permanent hypothyroidism is unusual. A surgical hemithyroidectomy is an alternative.

Differentiated carcinoma

Papillary carcinoma

This is the most common of the malignant thyroid tumours and accounts for 90% of irradiation-induced thyroid cancer. It may be multifocal and spread is to regional lymph nodes. Some patients present with cervical lymphadenopathy and no apparent thyroid enlargement; in such instances, the primary lesion may be less than 10 mm in diameter.

Follicular carcinoma

This is always a single encapsulated lesion. Spread to cervical lymph nodes is rare. Metastases are blood-borne and are most often found in bone, lungs and brain.

Management

This is usually by total thyroidectomy followed by a large dose of [131]I (3700 MBq (approximately 100 mCi)) in order to ablate any remaining thyroid tissue, normal or malignant. Thereafter, long-term treatment with thyroxine in a dose sufficient to suppress TSH (usually 150–200 µg daily) is important, as there is evidence that growth of differentiated thyroid carcinomas is TSH-dependent. Follow-up is by measurement of serum thyroglobulin, which should be undetectable in patients whose normal thyroid has been ablated and who are taking a suppressive dose of thyroxine. Detectable thyroglobulin is suggestive of tumour recurrence or metastases, which may be localised

20

by whole-body scanning with ^{131}I and may respond to further radio-iodine therapy. For meaningful results, isotope scanning requires serum TSH concentrations to be elevated (> 20 mU/L). In the past this was achieved by stopping thyroxine for 4–6 weeks, inducing symptomatic hypothyroidism. The availability of recombinant human TSH now allows measurement of stimulated thyroglobulin and radio-iodine uptake without the need to stop thyroxine therapy.

Prognosis

Most patients have an excellent prognosis when treated appropriately. Those under 50 years of age with papillary carcinoma have a near-normal life expectancy if the tumour is less than 2 cm in diameter, confined to the thyroid and cervical nodes, and of low-grade malignancy histologically. Even for patients with distant metastases at presentation, the 10-year survival is approximately 40%.

Anaplastic carcinoma and lymphoma

These two conditions are difficult to distinguish clinically but are distinct cytologically and histologically. Patients are usually elderly women in whom there is rapid thyroid enlargement over 2–3 months. The goitre is hard and symmetrical. There is usually stridor due to tracheal compression and hoarseness due to recurrent laryngeal nerve palsy. There is no effective treatment of anaplastic carcinoma, although radiotherapy may afford temporary relief of mediastinal compression. The prognosis for lymphoma, which may arise from pre-existing Hashimoto's thyroiditis, is better (p. 1037). External irradiation often produces dramatic goitre shrinkage and, when combined with chemotherapy, may result in survival for 5 years or more.

Medullary carcinoma

This tumour arises from the parafollicular C cells of the thyroid. In addition to calcitonin, the tumour may secrete 5-hydroxytryptamine (5-HT, serotonin), various peptides of the tachykinin family, ACTH and prostaglandins. As a consequence, carcinoid syndrome (p. 782) and Cushing's syndrome (p. 770) may occur.

Patients usually present in middle age with a firm thyroid mass. Cervical lymphadenopathy is common, but distant metastases are rare initially. Serum calcitonin levels are raised and are useful in monitoring response to treatment. Despite the very high levels of calcitonin found in some patients, hypocalcaemia is extremely rare.

Treatment is by total thyroidectomy with removal of affected cervical nodes. Since the C cells do not concentrate iodine, there is no role for ^{131}I therapy. Prognosis is very variable, some patients surviving 20 years or more and others less than 1 year.

Medullary carcinoma of the thyroid may occur sporadically, or in families as part of the MEN type 2 syndrome (p. 793).

Riedel's thyroiditis

This is not a form of thyroid cancer, but the presentation is similar and the differentiation can usually only be made by thyroid biopsy. It is an exceptionally rare condition of unknown aetiology in which there is extensive infiltration of the thyroid and surrounding structures with fibrous tissue. There may be associated

20.18 The thyroid gland in old age

Thyrotoxicosis

- **Causes**: commonly due to multinodular goitre.
- **Clinical features**: apathy, anorexia, proximal myopathy, atrial fibrillation and cardiac failure predominate.
- **Non-thyroidal illness**: thyroid function tests are performed more frequently in the elderly, but interpretation may be altered by intercurrent illness.

Hypothyroidism

- **Clinical features**: non-specific features such as physical and mental slowing are often attributed to increasing age and the diagnosis is delayed.
- **Myxoedema coma** (p. 743): more likely in the elderly.
- **Thyroxine dose**: to avoid exacerbating latent or established heart disease, the starting dose should be 25 μg daily. Thyroxine requirements fall with increasing age and few patients need > 100 μg daily.
- **Other medication** (see Box 20.12, p. 743): may interfere with absorption or metabolism of thyroxine, necessitating an increase in dose.

mediastinal and retroperitoneal fibrosis. Presentation is with a slow-growing goitre which is irregular and stony-hard. There is usually tracheal and oesophageal compression necessitating partial thyroidectomy. Other recognised complications include recurrent laryngeal nerve palsy, hypoparathyroidism and eventually hypothyroidism.

Congenital thyroid disease

Early treatment with thyroxine is essential to prevent irreversible brain damage in children with congenital hypothyroidism. Routine screening of TSH levels in blood spot samples obtained 5–7 days after birth (as part of the Guthrie test) has revealed an incidence of approximately 1 in 3000, resulting from thyroid agenesis, ectopic or hypoplastic glands, or dyshormonogenesis. Congenital hypothyroidism is thus six times more common than phenylketonuria. It is now possible to start thyroid replacement therapy within 2 weeks of birth. Developmental assessment of infants treated at this early stage has revealed no differences between cases and controls in most children.

Dyshormonogenesis

Several autosomal recessive defects in thyroid hormone synthesis have been described; the most common results from deficiency of the intrathyroidal peroxidase enzyme. Homozygous individuals present with congenital hypothyroidism; heterozygotes present in the first two decades of life with goitre, normal thyroid hormone levels and a raised TSH. The combination of dyshormonogenetic goitre and nerve deafness is known as Pendred's syndrome and is due to mutations in pendrin, the protein which transports iodide to the luminal surface of the follicular cell (see Fig. 20.3, p. 737).

Thyroid hormone resistance

This is a rare disorder in which the pituitary and hypothalamus are resistant to feedback suppression of TSH by T_3, sometimes due to mutations in the

20.19 Thyroid disease in pregnancy

Normal pregnancy

- **Trimester-specific normal ranges:** should be used to interpret thyroid function test results in pregnancy. In the first trimester, TSH is lower and free free T_4 and T_3 higher, in part due to thyroid stimulation by human chorionic gonadotrophin (hCG). In later pregnancy, free T_4 and T_3 are lower. Binding globulin levels are induced by oestrogen, so total T_4 and T_3 levels are invariably high.
- **Iodine requirements:** increased in pregnancy. The World Health Organization (WHO) recommends minimum intake of 200 µg/day.
- **Screening of thyroid function and autoantibodies:** not recommended for every woman, but should be performed in first trimester in those with a personal or family history of thyroid disease, goitre, other autoimmune disease including type 1 diabetes, or when there is clinical suspicion of thyroid dysfunction.

Thyrotoxicosis

- **Hyperemesis gravidarum:** associated with thyrotoxic biochemistry, sometimes requiring antithyroid drugs.
- **Subclinical thyrotoxicosis:** not usually treated, to avoid fetal hypothyroidism.
- **Anti-thyroid drugs:** propylthiouracil is first choice.

Hypothyroidism

- **Preterm labour and impaired cognitive development in the offspring:** may be associated with even subclinical hypothyroidism.
- **Thyroxine replacement therapy dose requirements:** increase by 30–50% from early in pregnancy. Monitoring to maintain TSH results within the trimester-specific reference range is recommended in early pregnancy and at least once in each trimester.

Post-partum thyroiditis

- **Screening:** not recommended for every woman, but thyroid function should be tested 4–6 weeks post-partum in those with a personal history of thyroid disease, goitre or other autoimmune disease including type 1 diabetes, those known to have positive anti-thyroid peroxidase antibodies, or when there is clinical suspicion of thyroid dysfunction.

thyroid hormone receptor β or due to defects in monodeiodinase activity. The result is high levels of TSH, T_4 and T_3, often with a moderate goitre which may not be noted until adulthood. Thyroid hormone signalling is highly complex and involves different isozymes of both monodeiodinases and thyroid hormone receptors in different tissues. For that reason, other tissues may or may not share the resistance to thyroid hormone and there may be features of thyrotoxicosis (e.g. tachycardia). This condition can be difficult to distinguish from an equally rare TSH-producing pituitary tumour (see Box 20.5, p. 738); administration of TRH results in elevation of TSH in thyroid hormone resistance and not in TSHoma, but an MRI scan of the pituitary may be necessary to exclude a macroadenoma.

THE REPRODUCTIVE SYSTEM

Clinical practice in reproductive medicine is shared between several specialties, including gynaecology, urology, paediatrics, psychiatry and endocrinology. The following section is focused on disorders managed by endocrinologists.

Functional anatomy, physiology and investigations

The physiology of male and female reproductive function is illustrated in Figures 20.13 and 20.14 respectively. Pathways for synthesis of sex steroids are shown in Figure 20.20 (p. 770).

The male

In the male, the testis subserves two principal functions: synthesis of testosterone by the interstitial Leydig cells under the control of luteinising hormone (LH), and spermatogenesis by Sertoli cells under the control of follicle-stimulating hormone (FSH) (but also requiring adequate testosterone). Negative feedback suppression of LH is mediated principally by testosterone, while secretion of another hormone by the testis, inhibin, suppresses FSH. The axis can be assessed easily by a random blood sample for testosterone, LH and FSH. If testosterone is marginally low, it may be worth repeating sampling in the morning, when values are somewhat higher. Testosterone is largely

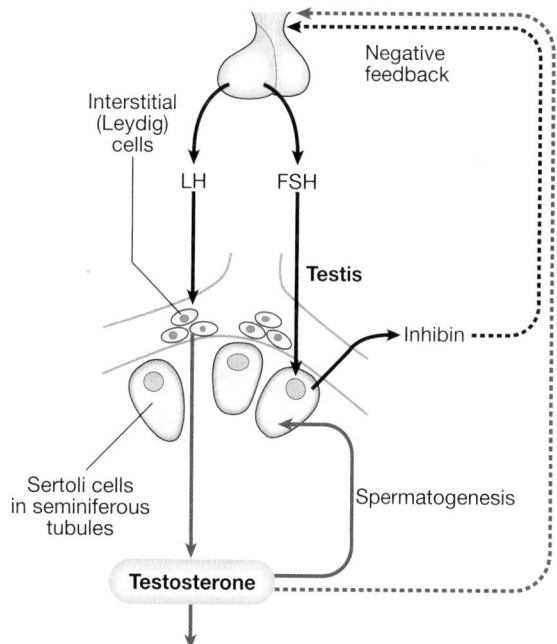

Fig. 20.13 Male reproductive physiology.

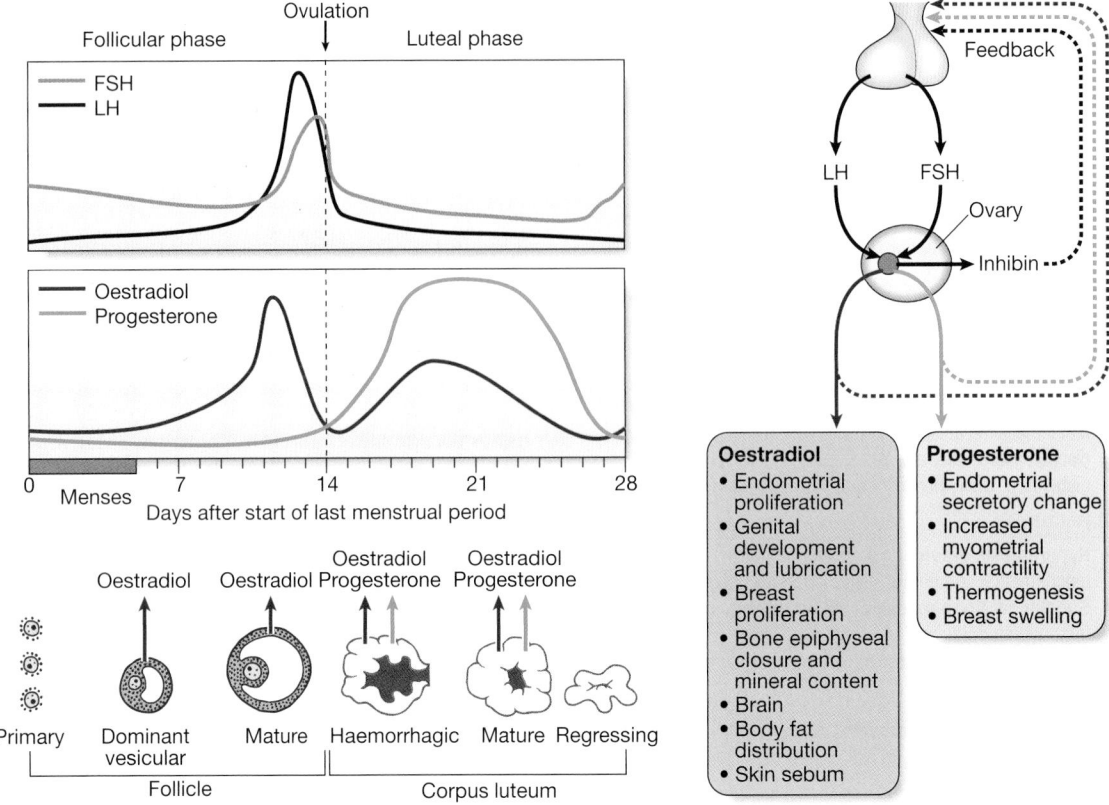

Fig. 20.14 Female reproductive physiology and the normal menstrual cycle.

bound in plasma to sex hormone-binding globulin, and this can also be measured to calculate the 'free androgen index' or the 'bioavailable' testosterone. Testicular function can also be tested by semen analysis.

There is no equivalent of the menopause in men, although testosterone concentrations decline slowly from the fourth decade onwards.

The female

In the female, physiology is complicated by variations in function during the normal menstrual cycle. FSH stimulates growth and development of ovarian follicles during the first 14 days after the menses. This leads to a gradual increase in oestradiol production from granulosa cells, which initially suppresses FSH secretion (negative feedback) but then, above a certain level, stimulates an increase in both the frequency and amplitude of gonadotrophin-releasing hormone (GnRH) pulses, resulting in a marked increase in LH secretion (positive feedback). The mid-cycle 'surge' of LH induces ovulation. After release of the ovum the follicle differentiates into a corpus luteum which secretes progesterone. Withdrawal of progesterone results in menstrual bleeding. Circulating levels of oestrogen and progesterone in pre-menopausal women are, therefore, critically dependent on the time of the cycle. The most useful 'test' of ovarian function is a careful menstrual history. In addition, ovulation can be confirmed by measuring plasma progesterone levels during the luteal phase ('day 21 progesterone') or by tracking changes in oestrogen and progesterone metabolites in urine specimens collected at weekly intervals.

Cessation of menstruation (the menopause) occurs at an average age of approximately 50 years in developed countries. In the 5 years before, there is a gradual increase in the number of anovulatory cycles and this is referred to as the climacteric. Oestrogen and inhibin secretion falls and negative feedback results in increased pituitary secretion of LH and FSH (typically to levels > 30 U/L (3.3 μg/L)).

The pathophysiology of male and female reproductive dysfunction is summarised in Box 20.20.

Presenting problems in reproductive disease

Delayed puberty

Puberty is considered to be delayed if the onset of the physical features of sexual maturation has not occurred by a chronological age that is 2.5 standard deviations above the national average. In the UK this is by the age of 14 in boys and 13 in girls. Genetic factors have a major influence in determining the timing of the onset of puberty, such that the age of menarche (the onset of menstruation) is often comparable within sibling and mother–daughter pairs and within ethnic groups. However, because there is also a threshold for body weight that acts as a trigger for normal puberty, the onset of puberty can be influenced by other factors including nutritional status and chronic illness (p. 107).

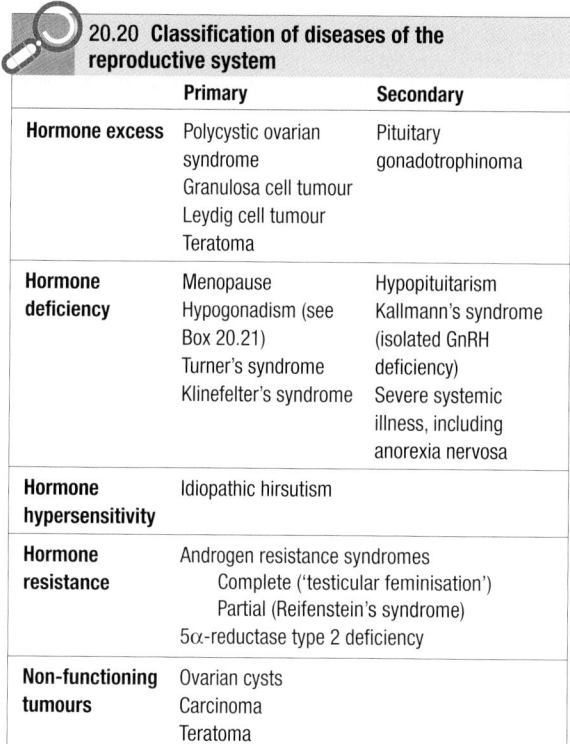

20.20 Classification of diseases of the reproductive system

	Primary	Secondary
Hormone excess	Polycystic ovarian syndrome Granulosa cell tumour Leydig cell tumour Teratoma	Pituitary gonadotrophinoma
Hormone deficiency	Menopause Hypogonadism (see Box 20.21) Turner's syndrome Klinefelter's syndrome	Hypopituitarism Kallmann's syndrome (isolated GnRH deficiency) Severe systemic illness, including anorexia nervosa
Hormone hypersensitivity	Idiopathic hirsutism	

Hormone resistance	Androgen resistance syndromes
	    Complete ('testicular feminisation')
	    Partial (Reifenstein's syndrome)
	5α-reductase type 2 deficiency	

Non-functioning tumours	Ovarian cysts Carcinoma Teratoma Seminoma	

20.21 Causes of delayed puberty and hypogonadism

Constitutional delay

Hypogonadotrophic hypogonadism
- Structural hypothalamic/pituitary disease (see Box 20.57)
- Functional gonadotrophin deficiency
    Chronic systemic illness (e.g. asthma, malabsorption, coeliac disease, cystic fibrosis, renal failure)
    Psychological stress
    Anorexia nervosa
    Excessive physical exercise
    Hyperprolactinaemia
    Other endocrine disease (e.g. Cushing's syndrome, primary hypothyroidism)
- Isolated gonadotrophin deficiency (Kallmann's syndrome)

Hypergonadotrophic hypogonadism
- Acquired gonadal damage
    Chemotherapy/radiotherapy to gonads
    Trauma/surgery to gonads
    Autoimmune gonadal failure
    Mumps orchitis
    Tuberculosis
    Haemochromatosis
- Developmental/congenital gonadal disorders
    Steroid biosynthetic defects
    Anorchidism/cryptorchidism in males
    Klinefelter's syndrome (47XXY, male phenotype)
    Turner's syndrome (45XO, female phenotype)

20

Clinical assessment

The differential diagnosis is shown in Box 20.21. The key issue is to determine whether the delay in puberty is simply because the 'clock is running slow' (constitutional delay of puberty) or because there is pathology in the hypothalamus/pituitary (hypogonadotrophic hypogonadism) or the gonads (hypergonadotrophic hypogonadism). A general history and physical examination should be performed with particular reference to previous or current medical disorders, social circumstances and family history. Body proportions, sense of smell and pubertal stage should be carefully documented and, in boys, the presence or absence of testes in the scrotum noted. Current weight and height may be plotted on centile charts along with parental heights. Previous growth measurements in childhood, which can usually be obtained from health records, are extremely useful. Children with constitutional delay have usually always been small, but have maintained a normal growth velocity that is appropriate for bone age. Poor linear growth, with 'crossing of the centiles', is more likely to be associated with acquired disease.

Constitutional delay of puberty

This is the most common cause of delayed puberty. Affected children are healthy and have usually been more than 2 standard deviations below the mean height for their age throughout childhood. There is often a history of delayed puberty in siblings or parents. 'Bone age' can be estimated by X-rays of epiphyses, usually in the wrist and hand; in constitutional delay, bone age is lower than chronological age. Constitutional delay of puberty should be considered as a normal variant as puberty will commence

spontaneously. However, affected children can experience significant psychological distress because of their lack of physical development, particularly when compared with their peers.

Hypogonadotrophic hypogonadism

This may be due to structural, inflammatory or infiltrative disorders of the pituitary and/or hypothalamus (see Box 20.57, p. 786). In such circumstances, other pituitary hormones, such as growth hormone, are also likely to be deficient.

'Functional' gonadotrophin deficiency is caused by a variety of factors, including low body weight, chronic systemic illness (as a consequence of the disease itself or secondary malnutrition), endocrine disorders and profound psychosocial stress.

Isolated gonadotrophin deficiency is usually due to a genetic abnormality that affects the synthesis of either GnRH or gonadotrophins. The most common form is Kallmann's syndrome, in which there is primary GnRH deficiency and, in most affected individuals, agenesis or hypoplasia of the olfactory bulbs resulting in anosmia or hyposmia. If isolated gonadotrophin deficiency is left untreated, the epiphyses fail to fuse, resulting in tall stature with disproportionately long arms and legs relative to trunk height (eunuchoid habitus).

Cryptorchidism (undescended testes) and gynaecomastia are commonly observed in all forms of hypogonadotrophic hypogonadism.

Hypergonadotrophic hypogonadism

Hypergonadotrophic hypogonadism associated with delayed puberty is usually due to Klinefelter's syndrome in boys and Turner's syndrome in girls (p. 761). Other causes of primary gonadal failure are shown in Box 20.21.

Investigations

Key measurements are LH and FSH, testosterone (in boys) and oestradiol (in girls). Chromosome analysis is performed if gonadotrophin concentrations are elevated. If gonadotrophin concentrations are low, then the differential diagnosis lies between constitutional delay and hypogonadotrophic hypogonadism. A plain X-ray of the wrist and hand may be compared with a set of standard films to obtain a bone age. Full blood count, renal function, liver function, thyroid function and coeliac disease autoantibodies (p. 879) should be measured, but further tests may be unnecessary if the blood tests are normal and the child has all the clinical features of constitutional delay. If hypogonadotrophic hypogonadism is suspected, neuroimaging and further investigations will be required (p. 784).

Management

Puberty can be induced using low doses of oral oestrogen in girls (e.g. ethinylestradiol 2 µg daily) or testosterone in boys (e.g. depot testosterone ester injections 50 mg i.m. each month). Higher doses carry a risk of early fusion of epiphyses. This therapy should be given in a specialist clinic where the progress of puberty and growth can be carefully monitored. In children with constitutional delay, this 'priming' therapy can be discontinued when endogenous puberty is established, usually in less than a year. In children with hypogonadism, the underlying cause should be treated and reversed if possible. If hypogonadism is permanent, then sex hormone doses are gradually increased during puberty and full adult replacement doses given when development is complete.

Amenorrhoea

Primary amenorrhoea describes the condition of a female patient who has never menstruated; this usually occurs as a manifestation of delayed puberty, but may also be a consequence of anatomical defects of the female reproductive system, such as endometrial hypoplasia or vaginal agenesis. Secondary amenorrhoea describes the cessation of menstruation. The causes of this common presentation are shown in Box 20.22. In non-pregnant women, secondary amenorrhoea is almost invariably a consequence of either ovarian or hypothalamic/pituitary dysfunction. Premature ovarian failure (premature menopause) is defined, arbitrarily, as occurring before 40 years of age. Rarely, endometrial adhesions (Asherman's syndrome) can form after uterine curettage, surgery or infection, e.g. with tuberculosis or schistosomiasis, preventing endometrial proliferation and shedding.

Clinical assessment

The underlying cause can often be suspected from associated clinical features and the patient's age. Hypothalamic/pituitary disease and premature ovarian failure result in oestrogen deficiency, which causes a variety of symptoms usually associated with the menopause (Box 20.23). If there is weight loss, then this may be primary, as in anorexia nervosa (p. 249), or secondary to underlying disease such as tuberculosis or malabsorption. Weight gain may suggest hypothyroidism, Cushing's syndrome or, very rarely, a hypothalamic lesion. Hirsutism, obesity and long-standing irregular periods suggest the polycystic ovarian syndrome (PCOS, p. 760). The presence of other autoimmune disease raises the possibility of autoimmune premature ovarian failure. The breasts should be examined for galactorrhoea and a vaginal examination should be performed, particularly if disease of the uterus is suspected.

Investigations

Pregnancy should be excluded in women of reproductive age by measuring human chorionic gonadotrophin (hCG) in a sample of urine. Serum LH, FSH, oestradiol, prolactin, testosterone, T_4 and TSH should be measured, and in the absence of a menstrual cycle, can be taken at any time. Investigation of hyperprolactinaemia is described on page 789. High concentrations of LH and FSH with low or low normal oestradiol suggest primary ovarian failure. Ovarian autoantibodies may be positive when there is an underlying autoimmune aetiology, and a karyotype should be performed in younger women to exclude mosaic Turner's syndrome. Elevated LH, prolactin and testosterone levels with normal oestradiol are common in PCOS. Low levels of LH, FSH and oestradiol suggest hypothalamic or pituitary disease.

There is some overlap in gonadotrophin and oestrogen concentrations between women with hypogonadotrophic hypogonadism and PCOS. If there is doubt as to the underlying cause of secondary amenorrhoea, then the response to 5 days of treatment with an oral progestogen (e.g. medroxyprogesterone acetate 10 mg 12-hourly) can be assessed. In women with PCOS, the progestogen will cause maturation of the endometrium and menstruation

20.22 Causes of secondary amenorrhoea

Physiological
- Pregnancy
- Menopause

Hypogonadotrophic hypogonadism (see Box 20.21)

Ovarian dysfunction
- Hypergonadotrophic hypogonadism (see Box 20.21)
- Polycystic ovarian syndrome
- Androgen-secreting tumours

Uterine dysfunction
- Asherman's syndrome

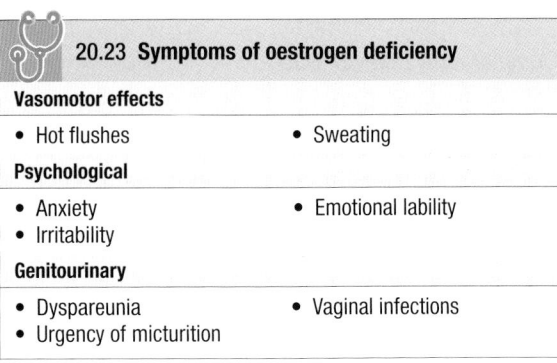

20.23 Symptoms of oestrogen deficiency

Vasomotor effects	
• Hot flushes	• Sweating

Psychological	
• Anxiety	• Emotional lability
• Irritability	

Genitourinary	
• Dyspareunia	• Vaginal infections
• Urgency of micturition	

will occur a few days after the progestogen is stopped. In women with hypogonadotrophic hypogonadism, menstruation does not occur following progestogen withdrawal because the endometrium is atrophic as a result of oestrogen deficiency. If doubt persists in distinguishing oestrogen deficiency from a uterine abnormality, the capacity for menstruation can be tested with 1 month of treatment with cyclical oestrogen and progestogen (usually administered as a combined oral contraceptive pill).

Assessment of bone mineral density by dual energy X-ray absorptiometry (DEXA, p. 1118) may be appropriate in patients with low androgen and oestrogen levels.

Management

Where possible, the underlying cause should be treated. For example, women with functional amenorrhoea due to excessive exercise and low weight should be encouraged to reduce their exercise and regain some weight. The management of structural pituitary and hypothalamic disease is described on page 788 and PCOS on page 761.

In oestrogen-deficient women, replacement therapy may be necessary to treat symptoms and/or to prevent osteoporosis. Women who have had a hysterectomy can be treated with oestrogen alone, but those with a uterus should be treated with combined oestrogen/progestogen therapy, since unopposed oestrogen increases the risk of endometrial cancer. Cyclical hormone replacement therapy (HRT) regimens typically involve giving oestrogen on days 1–21 and progestogen on days 14–21 of the cycle and this can be conveniently administered as the oral contraceptive pill. If oestrogenic side-effects (fluid retention, weight gain, hypertension and thrombosis) are a concern, then lower-dose oral or transdermal HRT may be more appropriate.

The timing of the discontinuation of oestrogen replacement therapy is still a matter of debate. In post-menopausal women HRT has been shown to relieve menopausal symptoms and to prevent osteoporotic fractures, but is associated with adverse effects, which are related to the duration of therapy and to the patient's age (Box 20.24). In patients with premature menopause HRT should be continued up to the age of 50 years but

---

EBM 20.24 Hormone replacement therapy (HRT) in post-menopausal women

'Administering HRT for 5 years to 10 000 women aged 50–79 years prevents 5 hip fractures and 6 cases of colorectal cancer, while inducing 8 extra cases of breast cancer, 8 of pulmonary embolism, 7 of coronary heart disease and 8 of stroke. The risks increase with age.'

• Writing Group for the Women's Health Initiative Investigators. JAMA 2002; 288:321–333.

---

only continued beyond this age if there are continued symptoms of oestrogen deficiency on discontinuation.

Management of infertility in oestrogen-deficient women is described on page 758.

Male hypogonadism

The clinical features of both hypo- and hypergonadotrophic hypogonadism include loss of libido, lethargy with muscle weakness, and decreased frequency of shaving. Patients may also present with gynaecomastia, infertility, delayed puberty and/or anaemia of chronic disease. The causes of hypogonadism are listed in Box 20.21.

Investigations

Male hypogonadism is confirmed by demonstrating a low serum testosterone level. The distinction between hypo- and hypergonadotrophic hypogonadism is by measurement of random LH and FSH. Patients with hypogonadotrophic hypogonadism should be investigated as described for pituitary disease on pages 784–785. Patients with hypergonadotrophic hypogonadism should have the testes examined for cryptorchidism or atrophy and a karyotype performed (to identify Klinefelter's syndrome).

Management

Testosterone replacement is indicated in hypogonadal men to prevent osteoporosis and to restore muscle power and libido. Routes of testosterone administration are shown in Box 20.25. First-pass hepatic metabolism of testosterone is highly efficient so bioavailability of ingested preparations is poor. Doses of systemic

20

20.25 Options for androgen replacement therapy

Route of administration	Preparation	Dose	Frequency	Comments
Intramuscular	Testosterone enantate	50–250 mg	Every 3–4 wks	Produces peaks and troughs of testosterone levels which are outside the physiological range and may be symptomatic
Intramuscular	Testosterone undecanoate	1000 mg	Every 3 mths	Smoother profile than testosterone enantate, less frequent injections
Subcutaneous	Testosterone pellets	600–800 mg	Every 4–6 mths	Smoother profile than testosterone enantate, but implantation causes scarring and infection
Transdermal	Testosterone patch	5–10 mg	Daily	Stable testosterone levels, but high incidence of skin hypersensitivity
Transdermal	Testosterone gel	50–100 mg	Daily	Stable testosterone levels; transfer of gel can occur following skin-to-skin contact with another person
Oral	Testosterone undecanoate	40–120 mg	12-hourly	Very variable testosterone levels; risk of hepatotoxicity

testosterone can be titrated against symptoms; circulating testosterone levels may provide only a rough guide to dosage because they may be highly variable (see Box 20.25). Testosterone therapy can aggravate prostatic carcinoma; prostate-specific antigen (PSA) should be measured before commencing testosterone therapy in men older than 50 years and monitored annually thereafter. Haemoglobin concentration should also be monitored in older men as androgen replacement can cause polycythaemia. Testosterone replacement inhibits spermatogenesis; treatment for fertility is described below.

Infertility

Infertility affects around 1 in 7 couples of reproductive age, often causing substantial psychological distress. The main causes are listed in Box 20.26. In women, infertility may result from anovulation or from abnormalities of the reproductive tract that prevent fertilisation or embryonic implantation, most commonly damaged fallopian tubes from previous infection. In men, infertility may result from impaired sperm quality (e.g. reduced motility) or number. Azoospermia or oligospermia is usually idiopathic, but may be a consequence of hypogonadism (see Box 20.21). Microdeletions of the Y chromosome are increasingly recognised as a cause of severely abnormal spermatogenesis. In many couples, more than one factor causing subfertility is present, and in a substantial proportion no cause can be identified.

20.26 Causes of infertility

Female factor (35–40%)

Ovulatory dysfunction
- Polycystic ovarian syndrome
- Hypogonadotrophic hypogonadism (see Box 20.21)
- Hypergonadotrophic hypogonadism (see Box 20.21)

Tubular dysfunction
- Pelvic inflammatory disease (chlamydia, gonorrhoea)
- Endometriosis
- Previous sterilisation
- Previous pelvic or abdominal surgery

Cervical and/or uterine dysfunction
- Congenital abnormalities
- Fibroids
- Asherman's syndrome
- Treatment for cervical carcinoma

Male factor (35–40%)

Reduced sperm quality or production
- Y chromosome microdeletions
- Varicocoele
- Hypogonadotrophic hypogonadism (see Box 20.21)
- Hypergonadotrophic hypogonadism (see Box 20.21)

Tubular dysfunction
- Varicocoele
- Congenital abnormality of vas deferens/epididymis
- Previous vasectomy
- Previous sexually transmitted infection (chlamydia, gonorrhoea)

Unexplained or mixed factor (20–35%)

Clinical assessment

A history of previous pregnancies, relevant infections and surgery is important in both men and women. A sexual history must be explored sensitively as some couples have intercourse infrequently or only when they consider the woman to be ovulating, and psychosexual difficulties are common. Irregular and/or infrequent menstrual periods are an indicator of anovulatory cycles in the woman, in which case causes such as PCOS should be considered. In men, the testes should be examined to confirm that both are in the scrotum and to identify any structural abnormality, such as small size, absent vas deferens or the presence of a varicocoele.

Investigations

Investigations are generally performed after a couple has failed to conceive despite unprotected intercourse for 12 months, unless there is an obvious abnormality (e.g. amenorrhoea). Investigations are guided by the history and examination; for example, if the male partner already has a child then the focus may, at least initially, be on the woman, but otherwise both partners need to be investigated. The male partner should provide at least two fresh semen samples, over an interval of several weeks, for analysis of sperm count and quality. Home testing for ovulation (either by commercial urine dipstick kits, temperature measurement, or assessment of cervical mucus) is not recommended as the information provided is often counterbalanced by increased anxiety if interpretation is inconclusive. In women with regular periods, ovulation can be confirmed by an elevated serum progesterone concentration on day 21 of the menstrual cycle. In women with irregular periods, such as in PCOS, weekly urine samples can be collected over several months to detect any peaks in progesterone metabolites which indicate ovulation. Transvaginal ultrasound can be used to assess uterine and ovarian anatomy. Tubal patency may be examined at laparoscopy or by hysterosalpingography (HSG; a radio-opaque medium is injected into the uterus and should normally outline the fallopian tubes). In vitro assessments of sperm survival in cervical mucus may be ascertained in cases of unexplained infertility but are rarely helpful.

Management

Couples should be advised to have regular sexual intercourse, ideally every 2–3 days throughout the menstrual cycle. It is not uncommon for 'spontaneous' pregnancies to occur in couples undergoing investigations for infertility or with identified causes of male or female subfertility.

In women with anovulatory cycles secondary to PCOS (p. 760), anti-oestrogen therapy with clomifene or tamoxifen blocks negative feedback of oestrogen on the hypothalamus/pituitary and encourages gonadotrophin secretion and thus ovulation. In women with gonadotrophin deficiency or in whom anti-oestrogen therapy is unsuccessful, ovulation may be induced by direct stimulation of the ovary by daily injection of FSH and an injection of hCG to induce follicular rupture at the appropriate time. In hypothalamic disease, pulsatile GnRH therapy with a portable infusion pump can be used to stimulate pituitary gonadotrophin secretion (note that non-pulsatile administration of GnRH or its analogues paradoxically suppresses LH and FSH secretion). Whatever method of ovulation induction is employed, monitoring of response is essential to avoid multiple ovulation. For clomifene, ultrasound monitoring is recommended for at least the first cycle. During gonadotrophin therapy, closer monitoring of follicular growth by transvaginal ultrasonography and blood oestradiol levels is mandatory. 'Ovarian hyperstimulation syndrome' is characterised by grossly enlarged ovaries and capillary leak with circulatory shock, pleural effusions and ascites. Anovulatory women who fail to respond to ovulation induction or who have primary ovarian failure may wish to consider using donated eggs or embryos, surrogacy and adoption.

Surgery to restore fallopian tube patency can be effective, but in vitro fertilisation (IVF) is normally recommended. IVF is widely used for many causes of infertility and in unexplained cases of prolonged (> 3 years) infertility. The success of IVF depends on age, with low success rates in women over 40 years.

Men with hypogonadotrophic hypogonadism who wish fertility are usually given injections of hCG several times a week (recombinant FSH may also be required in men with hypogonadism of pre-pubertal origin); it may take up to 2 years to achieve satisfactory sperm counts. Surgery is rarely an option in primary testicular disease, but removal of a varicocoele can improve semen quality. Extraction of sperm from the epididymis for IVF, and intracytoplasmic sperm injection (ICSI, when single spermatozoa are injected into each oöcyte), are being used increasingly in men with oligospermia or poor sperm quality who have primary testicular disease. Azoospermic men may opt to use donated sperm, but this is now in short supply.

Gynaecomastia

Gynaecomastia is the presence of glandular breast tissue in males. Normal breast development in women is oestrogen-dependent, while androgens oppose this effect. Gynaecomastia results from an imbalance between androgen and oestrogen activity, which may reflect androgen deficiency or oestrogen excess. Causes are listed in Box 20.27. The most common are physiological: for example, in the newborn baby (due to maternal and placental oestrogens), in pubertal boys (in whom oestradiol concentrations reach adult levels before testosterone) and in elderly men (due to decreasing testosterone concentrations). Prolactin excess alone does not cause gynaecomastia (p. 789).

20.27 Causes of gynaecomastia

Idiopathic

Physiological

Drug-induced
- Cimetidine
- Digoxin
- Anti-androgens (cyproterone acetate, spironolactone)
- Some exogenous anabolic steroids (diethylstilbestrol)

Hypogonadism (see Box 20.21)

Androgen resistance syndromes

Oestrogen excess
- Liver failure (impaired steroid metabolism)
- Oestrogen-secreting tumour (for example, of testis)
- hCG-secreting tumour (for example, of testis or lung)

Clinical assessment

A drug history is important. Gynaecomastia is often asymmetrical and palpation may allow breast tissue to be distinguished from the prominent adipose tissue around the nipple that is often observed in obesity. Features of hypogonadism should be sought (see above) and the testes examined for evidence of cryptorchidism, atrophy or a tumour.

Investigations

If a clinical distinction between gynaecomastia and adipose tissue cannot be made, then ultrasonography or mammography is required. A random blood sample should be taken for testosterone, LH, FSH, oestradiol, prolactin and hCG. Elevated oestrogen concentrations are found in testicular tumours and hCG-producing neoplasms.

Management

An adolescent with gynaecomastia who is progressing normally through puberty may be reassured that the gynaecomastia will usually resolve once development is complete. If puberty does not proceed in a harmonious manner, then there may be an underlying abnormality that requires investigation (p. 754). Gynaecomastia may cause significant psychological distress, especially in adolescent boys, and surgical excision may be justified for cosmetic reasons. Androgen replacement will usually improve gynaecomastia in hypogonadal males and any other identifiable underlying cause should be addressed if possible. The anti-oestrogen tamoxifen may also be effective in reducing the size of the breast tissue.

Hirsutism

Hirsutism refers to the excessive growth of thick terminal hair in an androgen-dependent distribution in women (upper lip, chin, chest, back, lower abdomen, thigh, forearm) and is one of the most common presentations of endocrine disease. It should be distinguished from hypertrichosis, which is generalised excessive growth of vellus hair. The aetiology of androgen excess is shown in Box 20.28.

Clinical assessment

The severity of hirsutism is subjective. Some women suffer profound embarrassment from a degree of hair growth which others would not consider remarkable. Important observations are a drug and menstrual history, calculation of body mass index, measurement of blood pressure, examination for virilisation (clitoromegaly, deep voice, male-pattern balding, breast atrophy), and associated features including acne vulgaris or Cushing's syndrome (p. 770). Hirsutism of recent onset associated with virilisation is suggestive of an androgen-secreting tumour, but this is rare.

Investigations

A random blood sample should be taken for testosterone, prolactin, LH and FSH. If there are clinical features of Cushing's syndrome, an overnight 1 mg dexamethasone suppression test should be performed (p. 772).

If testosterone levels are elevated above twice the upper limit of the normal female range, especially if this is associated with low LH and FSH, then causes other than idiopathic hirsutism and PCOS are more

20.28 **Causes of hirsutism**

Cause	Clinical features	Investigation findings	Treatment
Idiopathic	Often familial Mediterranean or Asian background	Normal	Cosmetic measures Anti-androgens
Polycystic ovarian syndrome (see Box 20.29)	Obesity Oligomenorrhoea or secondary amenorrhoea Infertility	LH:FSH ratio > 2.5:1 Minor elevation of androgens* Mild hyperprolactinaemia	Weight loss Cosmetic measures Anti-androgens (Metformin, glitazones may be useful)
Congenital adrenal hyperplasia (95% 21-hydroxylase deficiency)	Pigmentation History of salt-wasting in childhood, ambiguous genitalia, or adrenal crisis when stressed Jewish background	Elevated androgens* which suppress with dexamethasone Abnormal rise in 17OH-progesterone with ACTH	Glucocorticoid replacement administered in reverse rhythm to suppress early morning ACTH
Exogenous androgen administration	Athletes Virilisation	Low LH and FSH Analysis of urinary androgens may detect drug of misuse	Stop steroid misuse
Androgen-secreting tumour of ovary or adrenal cortex	Rapid onset Virilisation: clitoromegaly, deep voice, balding, breast atrophy	High androgens* which do not suppress with dexamethasone or oestrogen Low LH and FSH CT or MRI usually demonstrates a tumour	Surgical excision
Cushing's syndrome	Clinical features of Cushing's syndrome (p. 771)	Normal or mild elevation of adrenal androgens* See investigations (p. 772)	Treat the cause (p. 773)

*e.g. Serum testosterone levels in women: < 2 nmol/L (< 58 ng/dL) is normal; 2–5 nmol/L (58–144 ng/dL) is minor elevation; > 5 nmol/L (> 144 ng/dL) is high and requires further investigation.

likely, and the source of the androgen excess should be established. Congenital adrenal hyperplasia due to 21-hydroxylase deficiency is diagnosed by a short ACTH stimulation test with measurement of 17OH-progesterone (p. 780). In patients with androgen-secreting tumours, serum testosterone does not suppress following dexamethasone (either as an overnight or a 48-hour low-dose suppression test) or oestrogen (30 µg daily for 7 days). The tumour should then be sought by CT or MRI of the adrenals and ovaries.

Management

This depends on the cause (see Box 20.28). Options for the treatment of PCOS and idiopathic hirsutism are similar and are described below.

Polycystic ovarian syndrome (PCOS)

PCOS describes a constellation of clinical and biochemical features (Box 20.29) for which the primary cause remains uncertain. PCOS often affects several family members and is aggravated by obesity. Women with PCOS vary in the severity and combination of features that they manifest; the diagnosis is usually made during investigation of patients presenting with hirsutism (p. 759) or amenorrhoea/oligomenorrhoea (p. 756) with or without infertility (p. 758). There is no universally accepted definition, but it has been recommended that PCOS requires the presence of two of the following three features:

- menstrual irregularity
- clinical or biochemical androgen excess
- multiple cysts in the ovaries (most readily detected by transvaginal ultrasound; Fig. 20.15).

Women with PCOS are at increased risk of glucose intolerance and some authorities recommend screening for type 2 diabetes and other cardiovascular risk factors associated with the metabolic syndrome (p. 802).

20.29 **Features of polycystic ovarian syndrome**

Mechanisms*	Manifestations
Pituitary dysfunction	High serum LH High serum prolactin
Anovulatory menstrual cycles	Oligomenorrhoea Secondary amenorrhoea Cystic ovaries Infertility
Androgen excess	Hirsutism Acne
Obesity	Hyperglycaemia Elevated oestrogens
Insulin resistance	Dyslipidaemia Hypertension

* These mechanisms are interrelated; it is not known which, if any, is primary. PCOS probably represents the common endpoint of several different pathologies.

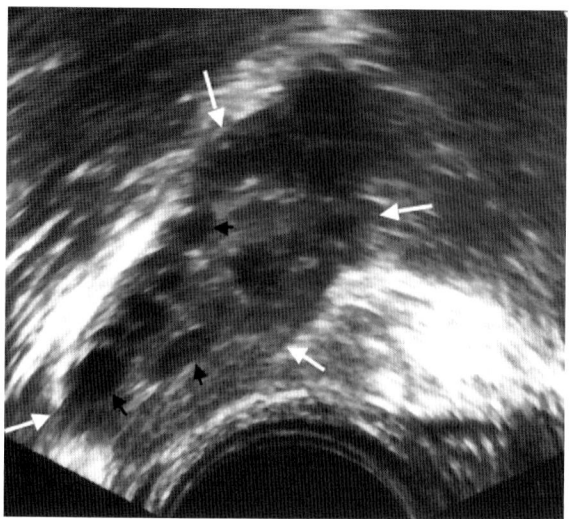

Fig. 20.15 Polycystic ovary. A transvaginal ultrasound scan showing multiple cysts (some indicated by black arrows) in the ovary (highlighted by white arrows) of a woman with PCOS.

Management

This depends on the clinical problem, but all overweight women with PCOS should be encouraged to lose weight as this may improve the clinical manifestations (especially menstrual irregularity) and reduce the risk of type 2 diabetes.

Menstrual irregularity and infertility

Most women with PCOS have oligomenorrhoea, with irregular, heavy menstrual periods. This may not require treatment unless fertility is desired. Metformin (p. 820), by reducing insulin resistance, may restore regular ovulatory cycles in overweight women, although it is less effective than clomifene (p. 758) at restoring fertility as measured by successful pregnancy (Box 20.30). Thiazolidinediones (p. 821) also enhance insulin sensitivity and restore menstrual regularity in PCOS, but are contraindicated in women planning pregnancy.

In women who have very few periods each year or are amenorrhoeic, the high oestrogen concentrations associated with PCOS can cause endometrial hyperplasia. Progestogens can be administered on a cyclical basis to induce regular shedding of the endometrium and a withdrawal bleed, or a progestogen-impregnated intrauterine coil can be fitted.

Hirsutism

For hirsutism, most patients will have used cosmetic measures such as shaving, bleaching and waxing before

---

EBM 20.30 **Treatment of infertility in women with PCOS**

'In one RCT, 626 infertile women with PCOS were randomised to receive clomifene, metformin or combination therapy. After 6 months, the live birth rates were 22.5%, 7.2% and 26.8% respectively. Multiple births occurred in 6% of women receiving clomifene and none receiving metformin.'

• RS Legro, et al. New Engl J Med 2008; 356:551–566.

---

consulting a doctor. Electrolysis and laser treatment are effective for small areas, e.g. upper lip and chest hair, but are expensive. Eflornithine cream inhibits ornithine decarboxylase in hair follicles and may reduce hair growth when applied daily to affected areas of the face.

If these conservative measures are unsuccessful, then anti-androgen therapy may be employed (Box 20.31). The life cycle of each hair follicle is at least 3 months and so no improvement is likely before this time, when previous follicles have all shed their hair and replacement hair growth has been suppressed. Metformin and thiazolidinediones are less effective at treating hirsutism than at restoring menstrual regularity. Unless the patient has lost weight, the hirsutism will return if therapy is discontinued. The patient should be aware that prolonged exposure to some of these agents may not be desirable and that they should be discontinued in advance of pregnancy.

Turner's syndrome

Turner's syndrome affects approximately 1 in 2500 females. The syndrome is classically associated with a 45XO karyotype, but other cytogenetic abnormalities may be responsible, including mosaic forms (e.g. 45XO/46XX or 45XO/46XY) and partial deletions of an X chromosome.

Clinical features

These are shown in Figure 20.16.

Individuals with Turner's syndrome invariably have short stature from an early age and this is often the initial presenting symptom. It is probably due to haploinsufficiency of the *SHOX* gene, one copy of which is found on both the X and Y chromosomes, which encodes a protein that is predominantly found in bone fibroblasts.

The genital tract and external genitalia in Turner's syndrome are female in character, since this is the default developmental outcome in the absence of testes. Ovarian tissue develops normally until the third month of gestation, but thereafter there is gonadal dysgenesis with accelerated degeneration of oöcytes and increased ovarian stromal fibrosis, resulting in 'streak ovaries'. The inability of the ovarian tissue to produce oestrogen results in loss of negative feedback and elevation of FSH and LH concentrations.

There is a wide variation in the spectrum of associated somatic abnormalities. The severity of the phenotype is, in part, related to the underlying cytogenetic abnormality. Mosaic individuals may have only mild short stature and may enter puberty spontaneously before developing gonadal failure.

Diagnosis and management

The diagnosis of Turner's syndrome can be confirmed by karyotype analysis. Short stature, although not directly due to growth hormone deficiency, responds to high doses of growth hormone. Prophylactic gonadectomy is recommended for individuals with 45XO/46XY mosaicism because there is an increased risk of gonadoblastoma. Pubertal development is induced with oestrogen therapy, but will result in

20

20.31 Anti-androgen therapy

Mechanism of action	Drug	Dose	Hazards
Androgen receptor antagonists	Cyproterone acetate	2, 50 or 100 mg on days 1–11 of 28-day cycle with ethinylestradiol 30 µg on days 1–21	Hepatic dysfunction Feminisation of male fetus Progesterone receptor agonist Dysfunctional uterine bleeding
	Spironolactone	100–200 mg daily	Electrolyte disturbance
	Flutamide	Not recommended	Hepatic dysfunction
5α-reductase inhibitors (prevent conversion of testosterone to active dihydrotestosterone)	Finasteride	5 mg daily	Limited clinical experience; possibly less efficacious than other treatments
Suppress ovarian steroid production and elevate sex hormone-binding globulin	Oestrogen	See combination with cyproterone acetate above *or* Conventional oestrogen-containing contraceptive	Venous thromboembolism Hypertension Weight gain Dyslipidaemia Increased breast and endometrial carcinoma
Suppress adrenal androgen production	Exogenous glucocorticoid to suppress ACTH	e.g. Hydrocortisone 5 mg on waking and dexamethasone 0.5 mg at bedtime	Cushing's syndrome

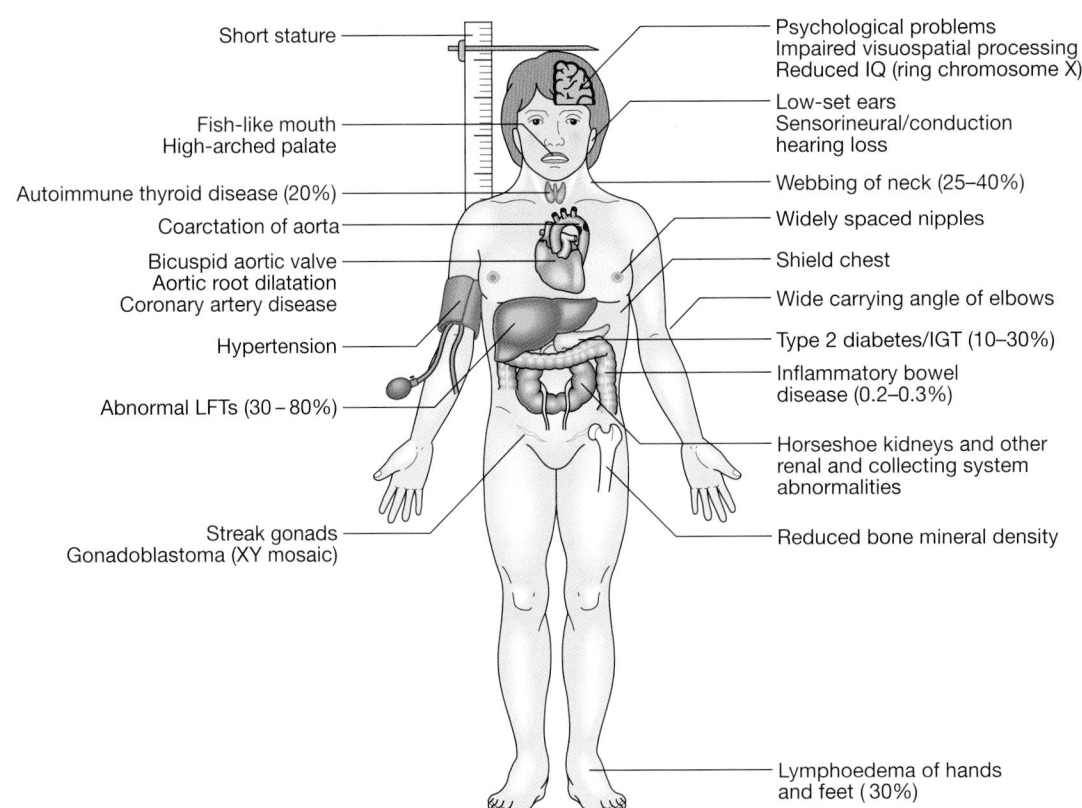

Fig. 20.16 Clinical features of Turner's syndrome (45XO). (IGT = impaired glucose tolerance)

fusion of the epiphyses and cessation of growth. Therefore, the timing of pubertal induction needs to be carefully planned. Adults with Turner's syndrome require long-term oestrogen replacement therapy and should be monitored periodically for the development of aortic root dilatation, hearing loss and other somatic complications.

Klinefelter's syndrome

Klinefelter's syndrome affects approximately 1 in 1000 males and is usually associated with a 47XXY karyotype. However, other cytogenetic variants may be responsible, especially 46XY/47XXY mosaicism. The principal pathological abnormality is dysgenesis of the seminiferous tubules. This is evident from infancy (and possibly even in utero) and progresses with age. By adolescence, hyalinisation and fibrosis are present within the seminiferous tubules and Leydig cell function is impaired, resulting in hypogonadism.

Clinical features

The diagnosis is typically made in adolescents who have presented with gynaecomastia and failure to progress normally through puberty. Affected individuals usually have small, firm testes. Tall stature is apparent from early childhood, reflecting characteristically long leg length associated with 47XXY, and may be exacerbated by androgen deficiency with lack of epiphyseal closure in puberty. Other clinical features may include learning difficulties and behavioural disorders, as well as an increased risk of breast cancer and type 2 diabetes in later life. The spectrum of clinical features is wide and some individuals, especially those with 46XY/47XXY mosaicism, may pass through puberty normally and be identified only when undergoing investigation for infertility.

Diagnosis and management

Klinefelter's syndrome is suggested by the typical phenotype in a patient with hypergonadotrophic hypogonadism and can be confirmed by karyotype analysis. Individuals with clinical and biochemical evidence of androgen deficiency require androgen replacement (see Box 20.25, p. 757).

Testicular tumours

Testicular tumours are uncommon, with a prevalence of 5 cases per 100 000 population. They occur mainly in young men between the age of 20 and 40 years. They often secrete α-fetoprotein (AFP) and β-human chorionic gonadotrophin (β-hCG), which are useful biochemical markers for both diagnosis and prognosis. Seminoma and teratoma account for 85% of all tumours of the testis. Leydig cell tumours are less common.

Seminomas arise from seminiferous tubules and represent a relatively low-grade malignancy. Metastases occur mainly via the lymphatics and may involve the lungs.

Teratomas arise from primitive germinal cells and tend to occur at a younger age than seminomas. They may contain cartilage, bone, muscle, fat and a variety of

20.32 Gonadal function in old age

- **Post-menopausal osteoporosis**: a major public health issue due to the high incidence of associated fragility fractures, especially of hip.
- **Hormone replacement therapy**: should only be prescribed above the age of 50 for the short-term relief of symptoms of oestrogen deficiency.
- **Sexual activity**: many older people remain sexually active.
- **'Male menopause'**: does not occur, although testosterone concentrations do fall with age. Testosterone therapy in mildly hypogonadal men may be of benefit for body composition, muscle and bone. Large randomised trials are required to determine whether benefits outweigh potentially harmful effects on the prostate and the cardiovascular system.
- **Androgens in older women**: hirsutism and balding occur. In the rare patients in whom androgen levels are elevated this may be pathological, e.g. from an ovarian tumour.

other tissues, and are classified according to the degree of differentiation. Well-differentiated tumours are the least aggressive; at the other extreme, trophoblastic teratoma is highly malignant. Occasionally, teratoma and seminoma occur together.

Leydig cell tumours are usually small and benign, but secrete oestrogens leading to presentation with gynaecomastia (p. 759).

Clinical features and investigations

The common presentation is incidental discovery of a painless testicular lump, although some patients complain of a testicular ache.

All suspicious scrotal lumps should be imaged by ultrasound. Serum levels of AFP and β-hCG are elevated in extensive disease. Oestradiol may be elevated, suppressing LH, FSH and testosterone. Accurate staging is based on CT of the lungs, liver and retroperitoneal area.

Management and prognosis

The primary treatment is surgical orchidectomy. Subsequent treatment depends on the histological type and stage. Radiotherapy is the treatment of choice for early-stage seminoma. Teratoma confined to the testes may be managed conservatively, but more advanced cancers are treated with chemotherapy, usually the combination of bleomycin, etoposide and cisplatin. Follow-up is by CT and assessment of AFP and β-hCG. Retroperitoneal lymph node dissection is now only performed for residual or recurrent nodal masses.

The 5-year survival rate for patients with seminoma is 90–95%. For teratomas the 5-year survival varies between 60% and 95%, depending on tumour type, stage and volume.

THE PARATHYROID GLANDS

Parathyroid hormone (PTH) plays a key role in the regulation of calcium and phosphate homeostasis and vitamin D metabolism, as shown in Figure 20.17. The consequences of altered function of this axis in gut and

20

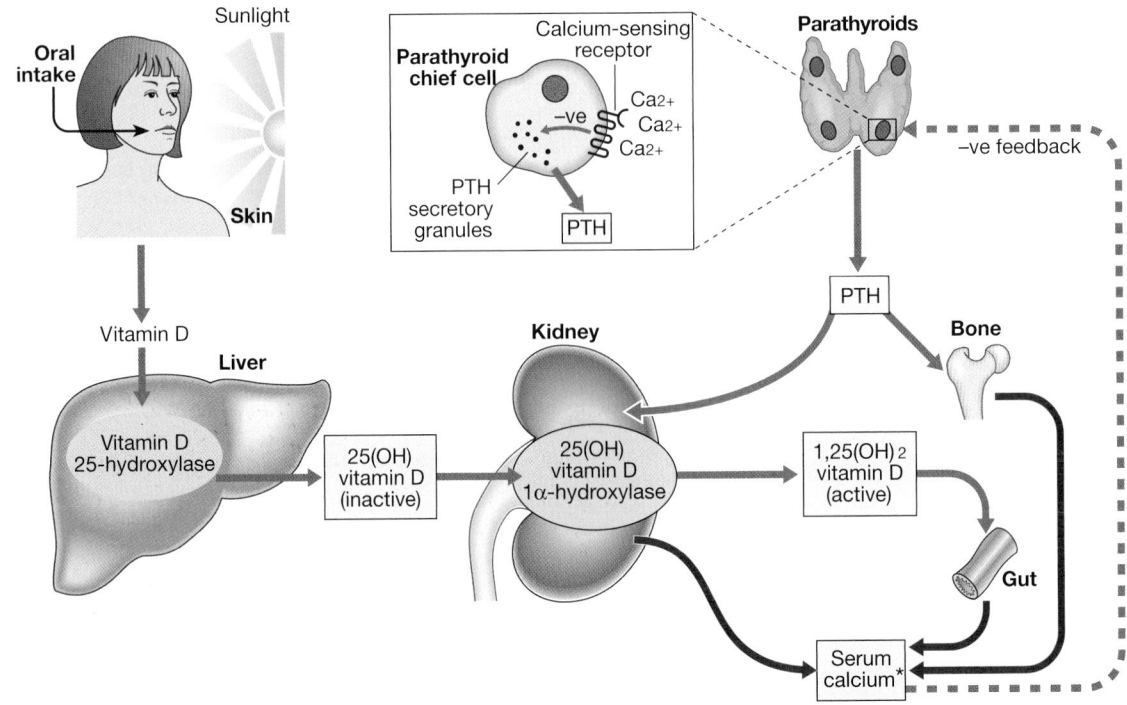

Fig. 20.17 Outline of calcium homeostasis showing interactions between parathyroid hormone (PTH), vitamin D and calcium. *Calcium in serum exists as 50% ionised (Ca^{2+}), 10% non-ionised or complexed with organic ions such as citrate and phosphate, and 40% protein-bound, mainly to albumin. It is the ionised calcium concentration which regulates PTH production.

renal disease are covered in Chapters 22 and 17, respectively. Other metabolic bone diseases are explored in Chapter 25. Here, the investigation of hypercalcaemia and hypocalcaemia and disorders of the parathyroid glands are discussed.

Functional anatomy, physiology and investigations

The four parathyroid glands lie behind the lobes of the thyroid. The parathyroid chief cells respond directly to changes in calcium concentrations via a G-protein-coupled cell surface receptor (the calcium-sensing receptor) located on the cell surface (see Fig. 20.17). When serum ionised calcium levels fall, PTH secretion rises. PTH is a single-chain polypeptide of 84 amino acids. It acts on the renal tubules to promote reabsorption of calcium and reduce reabsorption of phosphate, and on the skeleton to increase osteoclastic bone resorption and bone formation. PTH also promotes conversion of 25-hydroxycholecalciferol to the active metabolite 1,25-dihydroxycholecalciferol; the 1,25-dihydroxycholecalciferol, in turn, enhances calcium absorption from the gut.

More than 99% of total body calcium is in bone. Prolonged exposure of bone to high levels of PTH is associated increased osteoclastic activity and new bone formation, but the net effect is to cause bone loss with mobilisation of calcium into the extracellular fluid. In contrast, pulsatile release of PTH causes net bone gain, an effect that is exploited therapeutically in the treatment of osteoporosis (p. 1116).

The differential diagnosis of disorders of calcium metabolism usually requires measurement of calcium phosphate, alkaline phosphatase, renal function and sometimes 25(OH)D and PTH. Although the parathyroid glands detect and respond to ionised calcium levels, most clinical laboratories only measure total serum calcium levels and about 50% of total calcium is bound to organic ions, such as citrate or phosphate, and to proteins, especially albumin. Accordingly, if the serum albumin level is reduced, total calcium concentrations should be 'corrected' by adjusting the value for calcium upwards by 0.1 mmol/L (0.4 mg/dL) for each 5 g/L reduction in albumin below 40 g/L.

Calcitonin is secreted from the parafollicular C cells of the thyroid gland. Although calcitonin is a useful tumour marker in medullary carcinoma of thyroid (p. 752) and can be administered therapeutically in Paget's disease of bone (p. 1124), its release from the thyroid is of no clinical relevance to calcium homeostasis in humans.

Disorders of the parathyroid glands are summarised in Box 20.33.

Presenting problems in parathyroid disease

Hypercalcaemia

Hypercalcaemia is one of the most common biochemical abnormalities and is often detected during routine biochemical analysis in asymptomatic patients. However, it can present with chronic symptoms as described below, and occasionally as an acute emergency with severe hypercalcaemia and dehydration.

Box 20.33 Classification of diseases of the parathyroid glands

	Primary	Secondary
Hormone excess	Primary hyperpara-thyroidism 　Parathyroid adenoma 　Parathyroid carcinoma[1] 　Parathyroid hyperplasia[2] Tertiary hyperparathyroidism 　Following prolonged secondary hyperparathyroidism	Secondary hyperparathyroidism 　Chronic kidney disease 　Malabsorption 　Vitamin D deficiency
Hormone deficiency	Hypoparathyroidism 　Post-surgical 　Autoimmune 　Inherited	
Hormone hypersensitivity	Autosomal dominant hypercalciuric hypocalcaemia (activating mutation in CASR)	
Hormone resistance	Pseudohypoparathyroidism Familial hypocalciuric hypercalcaemia (inactivating mutation in CASR)	
Non-functioning tumours	Parathyroid carcinoma[1]	

[1]Parathyroid carcinomas may or may not produce PTH.
[2]In multiple endocrine neoplasia (MEN) syndromes (p.793).
(CASR = calcium-sensing receptor)

Causes of hypercalcaemia are listed in Box 20.34. Of these, primary hyperparathyroidism and malignant hypercalcaemia are by far the most common. Familial hypocalciuric hypercalcaemia (FHH) is a rare but important cause. Lithium may cause hyperparathyroidism by reducing the sensitivity of the calcium-sensing receptor.

Clinical assessment

Symptoms and signs of hypercalcaemia include polyuria and polydipsia, renal colic, lethargy, anorexia, nausea, dyspepsia and peptic ulceration, constipation, depression, drowsiness and impaired cognition. Patients with

20.34 Causes of hypercalcaemia

With normal or elevated (i.e. inappropriate) PTH levels

- Primary or tertiary hyperparathyroidism
- Lithium-induced hyperparathyroidism
- Familial hypocalciuric hypercalcaemia

With low (i.e. suppressed) PTH levels

- Malignancy (e.g. lung, breast, renal, ovarian, colonic and thyroid carcinoma, lymphoma, multiple myeloma)
- Elevated 1,25(OH)$_2$ vitamin D (vitamin D intoxication, sarcoidosis, HIV, other granulomatous disease)
- Thyrotoxicosis
- Paget's disease with immobilisation
- Milk-alkali syndrome
- Thiazide diuretics
- Glucocorticoid deficiency

malignant hypercalcaemia can have a rapid onset of symptoms and may have clinical features that help to localise the tumour.

The classic symptoms are described by the adage 'bones, stones and abdominal groans'. However, about 50% of patients with primary hyperparathyroidism are asymptomatic and many have non-specific symptoms. In others, symptoms may go unrecognised until patients present with renal calculi (5% of first stone formers and 15% of recurrent stone formers have primary hyperparathyroidism; p. 766). Hypertension is common in hyperparathyroidism. Parathyroid tumours are almost never palpable.

A family history of hypercalcaemia raises the possibility of FHH or MEN (p. 793).

Investigations

The most discriminant investigation is measurement of PTH. If PTH levels are detectable or elevated in the presence of hypercalcaemia then primary hyperparathyroidism is the most likely diagnosis. High plasma phosphate and alkaline phosphatase accompanied by renal impairment suggest tertiary hyperparathyroidism. Hypercalcaemia may cause nephrocalcinosis and renal tubular impairment, resulting in hyperuricaemia and hyperchloraemia.

Patients with FHH can present with a similar biochemical picture to primary hyperparathyroidism but typically have low urinary calcium excretion (a ratio of urinary calcium clearance to creatinine clearance of < 0.01). The diagnosis of FHH can be confirmed by screening family members for hypercalcaemia and/or a mutation in the gene encoding the calcium-sensing receptor.

If PTH is low and no other cause is apparent, then malignancy with or without bony metastases is likely. PTH-related peptide, which is often responsible for the hypercalcaemia associated with malignancy, is not detected by PTH assays, but can be measured by a specific assay (although this is not usually necessary). Unless the source is obvious, the patient should be screened for malignancy with a chest X-ray, myeloma screen (p. 1041) and CT as appropriate.

Management

Treatment of severe hypercalcaemia and primary hyperparathyroidism is described on pages 269 and 767, respectively. FHH does not require any specific intervention.

Hypocalcaemia

Aetiology

Hypocalcaemia is much less common than hypercalcaemia. The differential diagnosis is shown in Box 20.35. The most common cause of hypocalcaemia is a low serum albumin with normal ionised calcium concentration. Conversely, ionised calcium may be low in the face of normal total serum calcium in patients with alkalosis: for example, as a result of hyperventilation.

Hypocalcaemia may also develop as a result of magnesium depletion and should be considered in patients with malabsorption, on diuretic therapy or with a history of alcohol excess. Magnesium deficiency causes hypocalcaemia by impairing the ability of the parathyroid glands to secrete PTH (resulting in PTH concentrations that are low or inappropriately in

20

20.35 Differential diagnosis of hypocalcaemia

	Total serum calcium	Ionised serum calcium	Serum phosphate	Serum PTH	Comments
Hypoalbuminaemia	↓	↔	↔	↔	Adjust calcium upwards by 0.1 mmol/L (0.4 mg/dL) for every 5 g/L reduction in albumin below 40 g/L
Alkalosis Respiratory, e.g. hyperventilation Metabolic, e.g. Conn's syndrome	↔	↓	↔	↔ or ↑	Chapter 16
Vitamin D deficiency	↓	↓	↓	↑	Chapter 25
Chronic renal failure	↓	↓	↑	↑	Due to impaired vitamin D hydroxylation Serum creatinine ↑
Hypoparathyroidism	↓	↓	↑	↓	See text
Pseudohypoparathyroidism	↓	↓	↑	↑	Characteristic phenotype (see text)
Acute pancreatitis	↓	↓	↔ or ↓	↑	Usually clinically obvious Serum amylase ↑
Hypomagnesaemia	↓	↓	Variable	↓ or ↔	Treatment of hypomagnesaemia may correct hypocalcaemia

(↑ = levels increased; ↓ = levels reduced; ↔ = levels normal)

the normal range) and may also impair the actions of PTH on bone and kidney.

Clinical assessment

Mild hypocalcaemia is often asymptomatic but, with more profound reductions in serum calcium, tetany can occur. This is characterised by muscle spasms due to increased excitability of peripheral nerves.

Children are more liable to develop tetany than adults and present with a characteristic triad of carpopedal spasm, stridor and convulsions, although one or more of these may be found independently of the others. In carpopedal spasm, the hands adopt a characteristic position with flexion of the metacarpophalangeal joints of the fingers and adduction of the thumb ('main d'accoucheur'). Pedal spasm can also occur but is less frequent. Stridor is caused by spasm of the glottis. Adults can also develop carpopedal spasm in association with tingling of the hands and feet and around the mouth, but stridor and fits are rare.

Latent tetany may be detected by eliciting Trousseau's sign; inflation of a sphygmomanometer cuff on the upper arm to more than the systolic blood pressure is followed by carpal spasm within 3 minutes. Less specific is Chvostek's sign, in which tapping over the branches of the facial nerve as they emerge from the parotid gland produces twitching of the facial muscles.

Hypocalcaemia can cause papilloedema and prolongation of the ECG QT interval, which may predispose to ventricular arrhythmias. Prolonged hypocalcaemia and hyperphosphataemia (as in hypoparathyroidism) may cause calcification of the basal ganglia, grand mal epilepsy, psychosis and cataracts. Hypocalcaemia associated with hypophosphataemia, as in vitamin D deficiency, causes rickets in children and osteomalacia in adults (p. 1121).

20.36 Management of severe hypocalcaemia

Immediate management

- 10–20 mL 10% calcium gluconate i.v. over 10–20 minutes
- Continuous i.v. infusion may be required for several hours (equivalent of 10 mL 10% calcium gluconate/hr)
- Cardiac monitoring is recommended

If associated hypomagnesaemia

- 50 mmol magnesium chloride i.v. over 24 hours
- Most parenteral magnesium will be excreted in the urine, so further doses may be required to replenish body stores

Management

Emergency management of hypocalcaemia associated with tetany is described in Box 20.36. Treatment of chronic hypocalcaemia is described on page 768.

Primary hyperparathyroidism

Primary hyperparathyroidism is caused by autonomous secretion of PTH, usually by a single parathyroid adenoma which can vary in diameter from a few millimetres to several centimetres. It should be distinguished from secondary hyperparathyroidism, in which there is a physiological increase in PTH secretion to compensate for prolonged hypocalcaemia (such as in vitamin D deficiency, p. 1121), and tertiary hyperparathyroidism, in which continuous stimulation of the parathyroids over a prolonged period of time results in adenoma formation and autonomous PTH secretion (Box 20.37). This is most commonly seen in individuals with advanced chronic kidney disease (p. 487).

20.37 Hyperparathyroidism

Type	Serum calcium	PTH
Primary	Raised	Not suppressed
Single adenoma (90%)		
Multiple adenomas (4%)		
Nodular hyperplasia (5%)		
Carcinoma (1%)		
Secondary	Low	Raised
Chronic renal failure		
Malabsorption		
Osteomalacia and rickets		
Tertiary	Raised	Not suppressed

The prevalence of primary hyperparathyroidism is about 1 in 800 and it is 2–3 times more common in women than men; 90% of patients are over 50 years of age. It also occurs in the familial MEN syndromes (p. 793), when hyperplasia or multiple adenomas of all four parathyroid glands rather than a solitary adenoma are more likely.

Clinical and radiological features

The clinical presentation of primary hyperparathyroidism is described on page 765. Parathyroid bone disease is now rare due to earlier diagnosis and treatment. Osteitis fibrosa results from increased bone resorption by osteoclasts with fibrous replacement in the lacunae. This may present as bone pain and tenderness, fracture and deformity. Chondrocalcinosis can occur due to deposition of calcium pyrophosphate crystals within articular cartilage. It typically affects the menisci at the knees and can result in secondary degenerative arthritis or predispose to attacks of acute pseudogout (p. 1101). Skeletal X-rays are usually normal in mild primary hyperparathyroidism, but in patients with advanced disease characteristic changes are observed. In the early stages there is demineralisation, with subperiosteal erosions and terminal resorption in the phalanges. A 'pepper-pot' appearance may be seen on lateral X-rays of the skull. Reduced bone mineral density, resulting in either osteopenia or osteoporosis, is now the most common skeletal manifestation of hyperparathyroidism. This is usually not evident radiographically and requires assessment by DEXA (p. 1118).

In nephrocalcinosis, scattered opacities may be visible within the renal outline. There may be soft tissue calcification in arterial walls, soft tissues of the hands and the cornea.

Investigations

The diagnosis can be confirmed by finding a raised PTH level in the presence of hypercalcaemia, provided that FHH is excluded (p. 768). Parathyroid scanning by ^{99m}Tc-sestamibi scintigraphy (Fig. 20.18) or ultrasound examination can be performed prior to surgery, in an attempt to localise an adenoma and allow a targeted resection. However, negative imaging does not exclude the diagnosis.

Management

The treatment of choice for primary hyperparathyroidism is surgery, with excision of a solitary parathyroid adenoma or hyperplastic glands. Experienced surgeons will identify solitary tumours in more than 90% of cases. Patients with parathyroid bone disease run a significant risk of developing hypocalcaemia post-operatively and in such patients treatment with active vitamin D metabolites and calcium supplements should be commenced in the immediate post-operative period. Often therapy can be gradually withdrawn after 2–3 weeks as the bone remineralises and the residual parathyroid tissue recovers.

Surgery is usually indicated for individuals aged less than 50 years, and in those with significant hypercalcaemia (corrected serum calcium > 2.85 mmol/L (> 11.4 mg/dL)), clear-cut symptoms or documented complications (such as peptic ulceration, renal stones, renal impairment or osteoporosis). However, a large number of patients have only vague symptoms or are asymptomatic and for these individuals surgery has no clear advantage over conservative treatment. They should be reviewed every 6–12 months to assess symptoms, serum calcium levels and renal function, and undergo DEXA scans periodically. They should be encouraged to maintain a high oral fluid intake to avoid renal stones.

Occasionally, primary hyperparathyroidism presents with severe life-threatening hypercalcaemia. This is often due to dehydration and should be managed medically with intravenous fluids and bisphosphonates, as described on page 269. If this is not effective, then urgent parathyroidectomy should be considered.

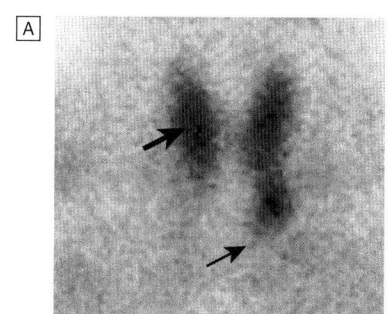 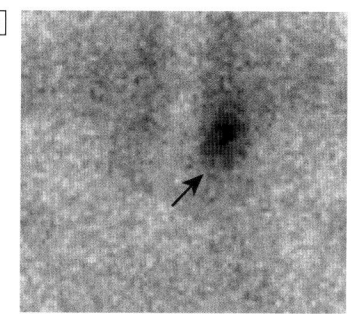

Fig. 20.18 ^{99m}Tc-sestamibi scan of a patient with primary hyperparathyroidism secondary to a parathyroid adenoma. **A** After 1 hour, there is uptake in the thyroid gland (thick arrow) and the enlarged left inferior parathyroid gland (thin arrow). **B** After 3 hours, uptake is evident only in the parathyroid.

Cinacalcet is a calcimimetic which enhances the sensitivity of the calcium-sensing receptor and is licensed for tertiary hyperparathyroidism and as a treatment for patients with primary hyperparathyroidism who are unwilling to have surgery or are medically unfit.

Familial hypocalciuric hypercalcaemia

This autosomal dominant disorder is caused by an inactivating mutation in one of the alleles of the calcium-sensing receptor gene, which reduces the ability of the parathyroid gland to 'sense' ionised calcium concentrations. As a result, higher than normal calcium levels are required to suppress PTH secretion. The typical presentation is with mild hypercalcaemia with PTH concentrations that are 'inappropriately' at the upper end of the normal range or are slightly elevated. Calcium-sensing receptors in the renal tubules are also affected and this leads to increased renal tubular reabsorption of calcium and hypocalciuria. The hypercalcaemia of FHH is always asymptomatic and complications do not occur. The main risk of FHH is being subjected to an unnecessary (and ineffective) parathyroidectomy if misdiagnosed as having primary hyperparathyroidism. Testing of family members for hypercalcaemia is helpful in confirming the diagnosis and it is also possible to perform genetic testing. No treatment is necessary.

Hypoparathyroidism

The most common cause of hypoparathyroidism is damage to the parathyroid glands (or their blood supply) during thyroid surgery, although this complication is only permanent in 1% of thyroidectomies. Transient hypocalcaemia develops in 10% of patients 12–36 hours following subtotal thyroidectomy for Graves' disease. Rarely, hypoparathyroidism can occur as a result of infiltration of the glands, e.g. in haemochromatosis (p. 959) and Wilson's disease (p. 960).

There are a number of rare congenital or inherited forms of hypoparathyroidism. One form is associated with autoimmune polyendocrine syndrome type 1 (p. 794) and another with DiGeorge syndrome (p. 53). Autosomal dominant hypoparathyroidism (ADH) is the mirror image of familial hypocalciuric hypercalcaemia (see above) in that an activating mutation in the calcium-sensing receptor results in hypocalcaemia, hypercalciuria and PTH concentrations that are 'inappropriately' low.

Pseudohypoparathyroidism

In this disorder, the individual is functionally hypoparathyroid, but instead of PTH deficiency there is tissue resistance to the effects of PTH, such that PTH concentrations are markedly elevated. The PTH receptor itself is normal, but there are defective post-receptor mechanisms due to mutations at the *GNAS1* locus. There are several subtypes, but in the most common form (type 1a) features include short stature, short 4th metacarpals and metatarsals, rounded face, obesity and subcutaneous calcification (Albright's hereditary osteodystrophy, AHO).

The term 'pseudo-pseudohypoparathyroidism' is used to describe patients with AHO in whom serum calcium and PTH concentrations are normal. The inheritance

20.38 The parathyroid glands in old age

- **Osteoporosis**: always exclude osteomalacia and hyperparathyroidism by checking vitamin D and calcium concentrations.
- **Primary hyperparathyroidism**: more common with ageing. Older people can often be observed without surgical intervention.
- **Hypercalcaemia**: may cause confusion.
- **Vitamin D deficiency**: common because of poor diet and limited exposure to the sun.

of these disorders is an example of genetic imprinting (p. 49); inheritance of the defective allele from a mother with pseudohypoparathyroidism results in pseudohypoparathyroidism in the offspring, but inheritance from the father results in pseudo-pseudohypoparathyroidism.

Management of hypoparathyroidism

Persistent hypoparathyroidism and pseudohypoparathyroidism are treated with oral calcium salts and vitamin D analogues, either 1α-hydroxycholecalciferol (alfacalcidol) or 1,25-dihydroxycholecalciferol (calcitriol). This therapy needs careful monitoring because of the risks of iatrogenic hypercalcaemia, hypercalciuria and nephrocalcinosis. Recombinant PTH is available as subcutaneous injection therapy for osteoporosis (p. 1116) and, although not currently licensed, has been used in hypoparathyroidism (but not in pseudohypoparathyroidism). It is much more expensive than calcium and vitamin D analogue therapy, but has the advantage that it is less likely to cause hypercalciuria. ADH usually does not require therapy.

THE ADRENAL GLANDS

The adrenals comprise several separate endocrine glands within a single anatomical structure. The adrenal medulla is an extension of the sympathetic nervous system which secretes catecholamines into capillaries rather than synapses. Most of the adrenal cortex is made up of cells which secrete cortisol and adrenal androgens, and form part of the hypothalamic–pituitary–adrenal (HPA) axis. The small outer glomerulosa of the cortex secretes aldosterone under the control of the renin–angiotensin system. These functions are important in the integrated control of cardiovascular, metabolic and immune responses to stress.

There is increasing evidence that subtle alterations in adrenal function contribute to the pathogenesis of common diseases such as hypertension, obesity and type 2 diabetes mellitus. However, classical syndromes of adrenal hormone deficiency and excess are relatively rare.

Functional anatomy and physiology

Adrenal anatomy and function are shown in Figure 20.19. Histologically, the cortex is divided into three zones, but these function as two units (zona glomerulosa and zonae fasciculata/reticularis) which produce corticosteroids in response to humoral stimuli. Pathways for the biosynthesis of corticosteroids are shown in Figure 20.20.

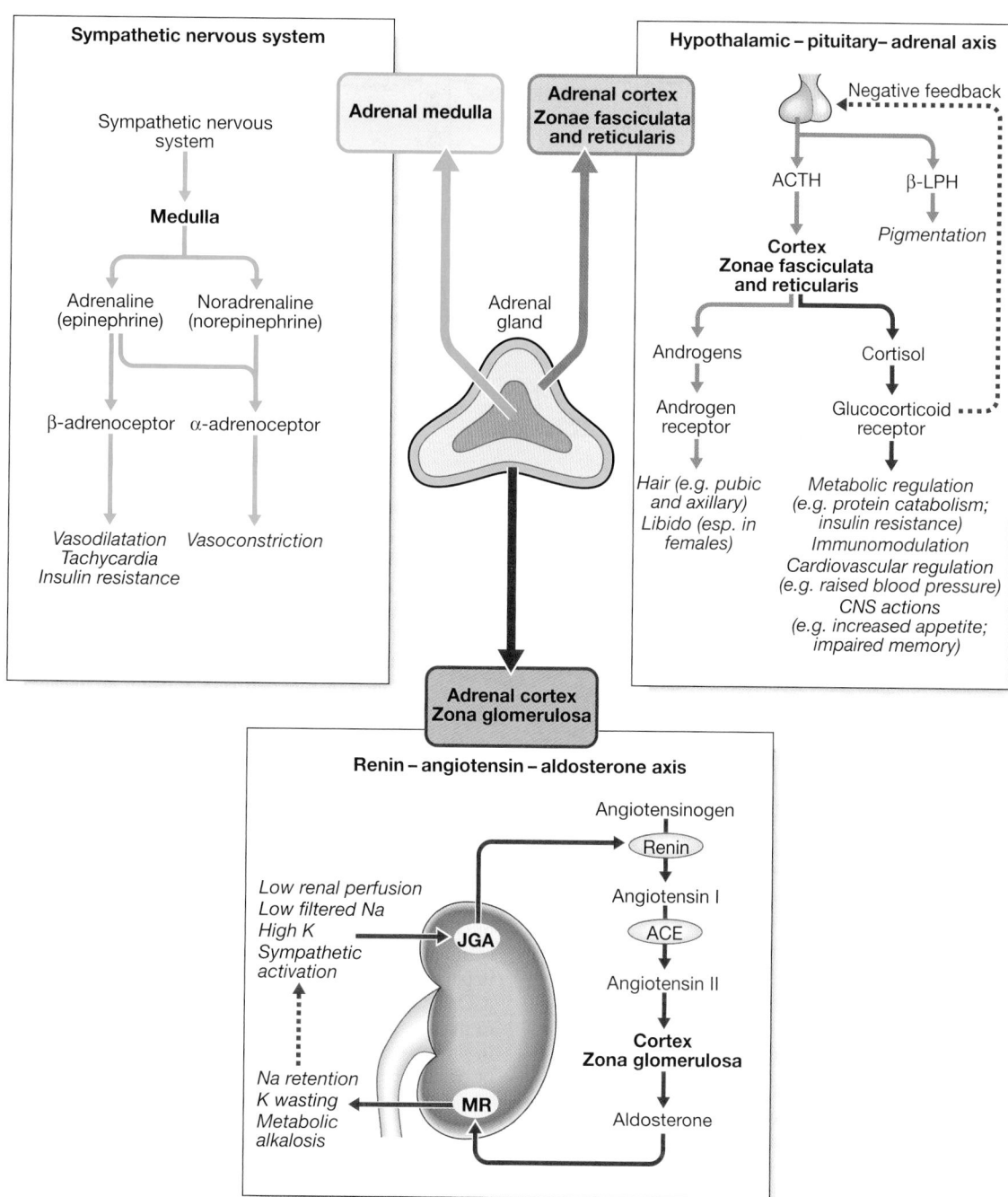

Fig. 20.19 Structure and function of the adrenal glands. (ACE = angiotensin-converting enzyme; JGA = juxtaglomerular apparatus; MR = mineralocorticoid receptor; β-LPH = β-lipotrophic hormone, a fragment of the ACTH precursor peptide pro-opiomelanocortin which contains melanocyte-stimulating hormone activity)

20

Investigation of adrenal function is described under specific diseases below. The different types of adrenal disease are shown in Box 20.39.

Glucocorticoids

Cortisol is the major glucocorticoid in humans. Levels are highest in the morning on waking and lowest in the middle of the night. Cortisol rises dramatically during stress, including any illness. This elevation protects key metabolic functions (such as the maintenance of cerebral glucose supply during starvation) and inhibits poten-

tially damaging inflammatory responses to infection and injury. The clinical importance of cortisol deficiency is, therefore, most obvious at times of stress.

More than 95% of circulating cortisol is bound to protein, principally cortisol-binding globulin. It is the free fraction which is biologically active. Cortisol regulates cell function by binding to glucocorticoid receptors which regulate the transcription of many genes. It can also activate mineralocorticoid receptors, but it does not normally do so because most cells containing mineralocorticoid receptors also express an enzyme,

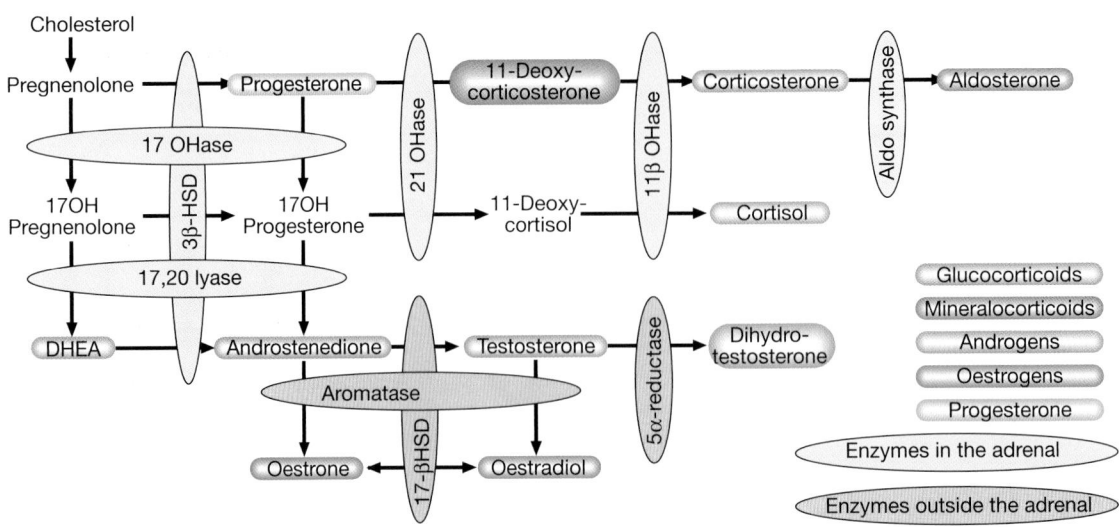

Fig. 20.20 The major pathways of synthesis of steroid hormones. (DHEA = dehydroepiandrosterone; OHase = hydroxylase; HSD = hydroxysteroid dehydrogenase)

20.39 Classification of diseases of the adrenal glands

	Primary	Secondary
Hormone excess	Non-ACTH-dependent Cushing's syndrome (see Box 20.40)	ACTH-dependent Cushing's syndrome
	Primary hyperaldosteronism (see Box 20.49, p. 777)	Secondary hyperaldosteronism
	Phaeochromocytoma	
Hormone deficiency	Addison's disease (see Box 20.44, p. 775)	Hypopituitarism
	Congenital adrenal hyperplasia	
Hormone hypersensitivity	11β-hydroxysteroid dehydrogenase type 2 deficiency	
	Liddle's syndrome	
Hormone resistance	Pseudohypoaldosteronism	
	Glucocorticoid resistance syndrome	
Non-functioning tumours	Adenoma	
	Carcinoma (usually functioning)	
	Metastatic tumours	

11β-hydroxysteroid dehydrogenase type 2 (11β-HSD2), which converts cortisol to its inactive metabolite, cortisone. Loss of the protection of mineralocorticoid receptors by inhibition of 11β-HSD2 (e.g. by liquorice or as a result of an inherited enzyme defect) results in cortisol acting like aldosterone as a potent sodium-retaining steroid (see Box 20.49, p. 777).

Mineralocorticoids

Aldosterone is the most important mineralocorticoid. It binds to mineralocorticoid receptors in the kidney and causes sodium retention and increased excretion of potas-

sium and protons (Ch. 16). The principal stimulus to aldosterone secretion is angiotensin II, a peptide produced by activation of the renin–angiotensin system (see Fig. 20.19). Renin activity in the juxtaglomerular apparatus of the kidney is stimulated by low perfusion pressure in the afferent arteriole, low sodium filtration leading to low sodium concentrations at the macula densa, or increased sympathetic nerve activity. As a result, renin activity is increased in hypovolaemia and renal artery stenosis, and is approximately doubled when standing up from a recumbent position.

Catecholamines

In humans, only a small proportion of circulating noradrenaline (norepinephrine) is derived from the adrenal medulla; much more is released from sympathetic nerve endings. Conversion of noradrenaline to adrenaline (epinephrine) is catalysed by catechol-o-methyltransferase (COMT), which is induced by glucocorticoids. Blood flow in the adrenal is centripetal so that the medulla is bathed in high concentrations of cortisol and is the major source of circulating adrenaline. However, after surgical removal of the adrenal medullae, there appear to be no clinical consequences attributable to deficiency of circulating catecholamines.

Adrenal androgens

Adrenal androgens are secreted in response to ACTH and are the most abundant steroids in the blood stream. They are probably important in the initiation of puberty (the adrenarche). The adrenals are also the major source of androgens in adult females and may be important in female libido.

Presenting problems in adrenal disease

Cushing's syndrome

Cushing's syndrome is caused by excessive activation of glucocorticoid receptors. By far the most common cause is iatrogenic, due to prolonged administration of synthetic glucocorticoids such as prednisolone. Non-iatrogenic Cushing's syndrome is rare and is often a 'spot diagnosis' made by an astute clinician.

Aetiology

The causes are shown in Box 20.40. Amongst endogenous causes, pituitary-dependent cortisol excess (by convention, called Cushing's disease) accounts for approximately 80% of cases. Both Cushing's disease and cortisol-secreting adrenal tumours are four times more common in women than men. In contrast, ectopic ACTH syndrome (often due to a small-cell carcinoma of the bronchus) is more common in men.

Clinical assessment

The diverse manifestations of glucocorticoid excess are shown in Figure 20.21. Many of these are not specific to Cushing's syndrome and, because spontaneous Cushing's syndrome is rare, the positive predictive value of any one feature alone is low. Moreover, some common disorders can be confused with Cushing's syndrome because they are associated with alterations in cortisol secretion: for example, obesity and depression (see Box 20.40). Features which favour Cushing's syndrome in an obese patient are bruising, myopathy and hypertension. Any clinical suspicion of cortisol excess is best resolved by further investigation.

It is vital to exclude iatrogenic causes in all patients with Cushing's syndrome since even inhaled or topical glucocorticoids can induce the syndrome in susceptible individuals. A careful drug history must therefore be taken before embarking on complex investigations.

Some clinical features are more common in ectopic ACTH syndrome. Unlike pituitary tumours secreting ACTH, ectopic tumours have no residual negative feedback sensitivity to cortisol, and both ACTH and cortisol levels are usually higher than with other causes. Very

20.40 Classification of Cushing's syndrome

ACTH-dependent

- Pituitary adenoma secreting ACTH (Cushing's disease)
- Ectopic ACTH syndrome (bronchial carcinoid, small-cell lung carcinoma, other neuro-endocrine tumour)
- Iatrogenic (ACTH therapy)

Non-ACTH-dependent

- Iatrogenic (chronic glucocorticoid therapy)
- Adrenal adenoma
- Adrenal carcinoma

Pseudo-Cushing's syndrome*

- Alcohol excess (biochemical and clinical features)
- Major depressive illness (biochemical features only, some clinical overlap)
- Primary obesity (mild biochemical features, some clinical overlap)

*Cortisol excess as part of another illness.

20

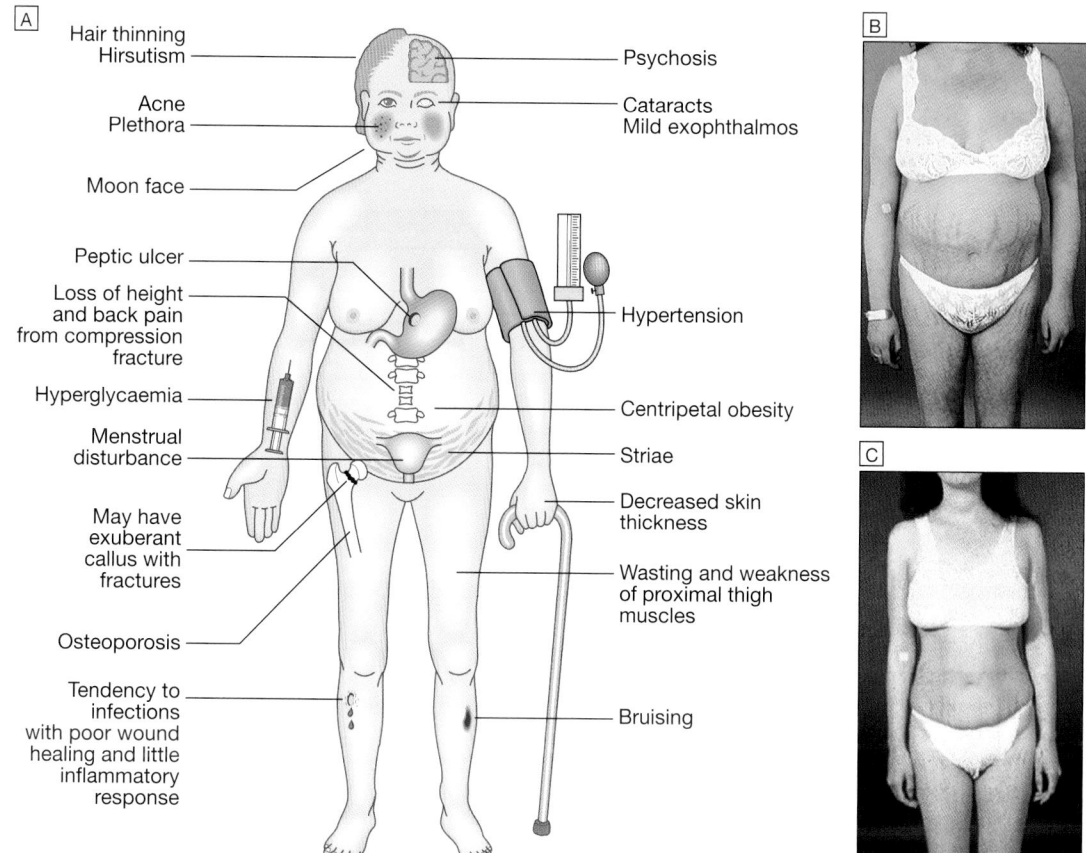

Fig. 20.21 Cushing's syndrome. **A** Clinical features common to all causes. **B** A patient with Cushing's disease before treatment. **C** The same patient 1 year after the successful removal of an ACTH-secreting pituitary microadenoma by trans-sphenoidal surgery.

high ACTH levels are associated with marked pigmentation. Very high cortisol levels overcome the barrier of 11β-HSD2 in the kidney (p. 770) and cause hypokalaemic alkalosis. Hypokalaemia aggravates both myopathy and hyperglycaemia (by inhibiting insulin secretion). When the tumour secreting ACTH is malignant, then the onset is usually rapid and may be associated with cachexia. For these reasons, the classical features of Cushing's syndrome are less common in ectopic ACTH syndrome, and if present suggest that a less aggressive tumour (e.g. bronchial carcinoid) is responsible.

In Cushing's disease, the pituitary tumour is usually a microadenoma (< 10 mm in diameter); hence other features of a pituitary macroadenoma (hypopituitarism, visual failure or disconnection hyperprolactinaemia, p. 784) are rare.

Investigations

The large number of tests available for Cushing's syndrome reflects the limited specificity and sensitivity of each test in isolation. Several tests are usually combined to establish the diagnosis. It is useful to divide investigations into those which establish whether the patient has Cushing's syndrome, and those which are used subsequently to define the cause.

A recommended sequence of investigations is shown in Figure 20.22 and the interpretation of these tests is shown in Box 20.41. Some additional tests are useful in all cases of Cushing's syndrome, including plasma electrolytes, glucose, glycosylated haemoglobin and bone mineral density measurement.

In iatrogenic Cushing's syndrome, cortisol levels are low unless the patient is taking a corticosteroid (such as prednisolone) which cross-reacts in immunoassays with cortisol.

Establishing the presence of Cushing's syndrome

Cushing's syndrome is confirmed by the demonstration of increased secretion of cortisol (measured in plasma

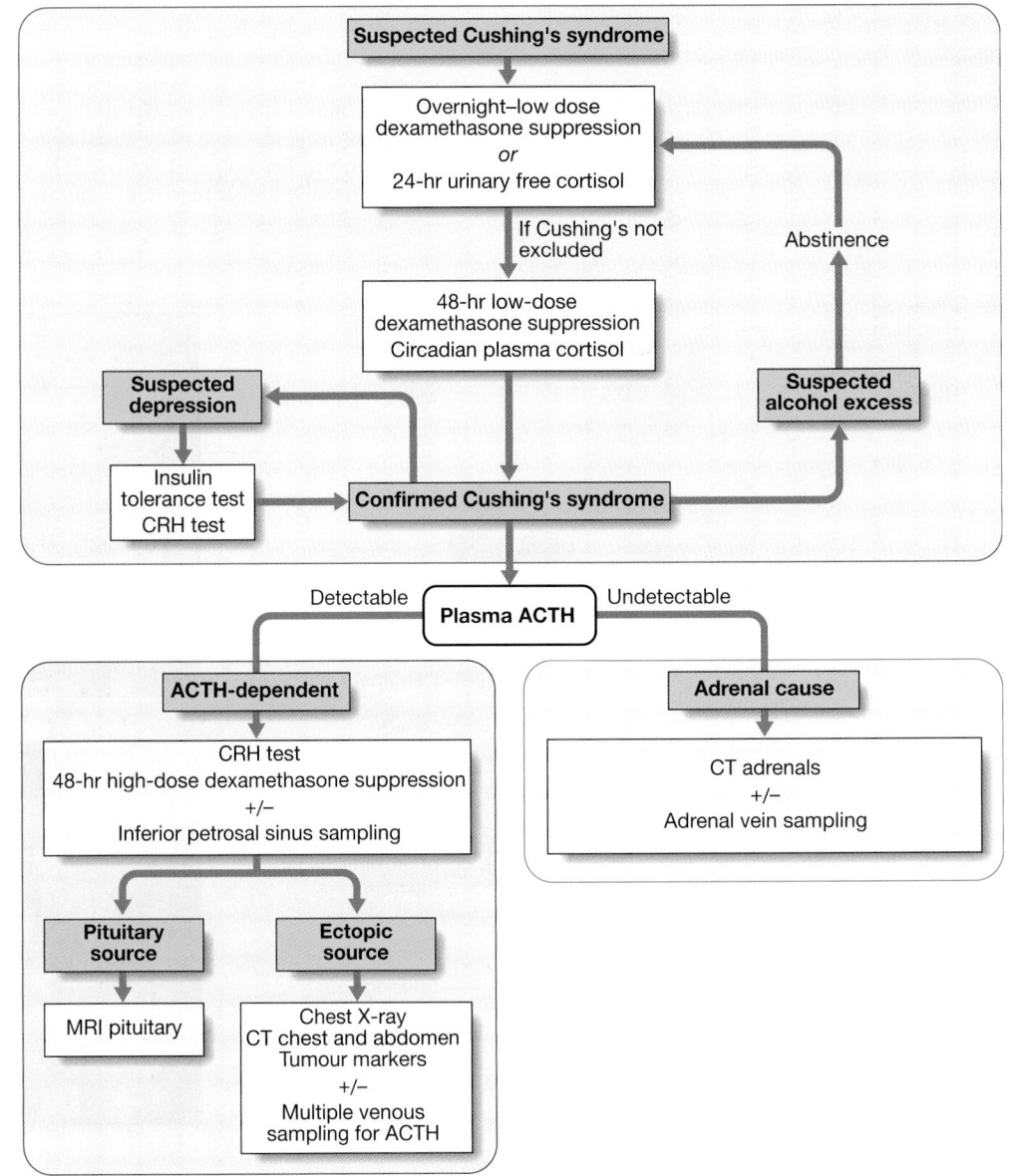

Fig. 20.22 Sequence of investigations in suspected spontaneous Cushing's syndrome. (CRH = corticotrophin-releasing hormone)

20.41 Tests for Cushing's syndrome

Test	Protocol	Interpretation
Urine free cortisol	24-hr timed collection (some centres use overnight collections corrected for creatinine)	Normal range depends on assay
Overnight dexamethasone suppression test	1 mg orally at midnight; measure plasma cortisol at 0800–0900 hrs	Plasma cortisol < 60 nmol/L (< 2.2 µg/dL) excludes Cushing's
Diurnal rhythm of plasma cortisol	Sample for cortisol at 0900 hrs and at 2300 hrs (requires acclimatisation to ward for at least 48 hrs)	Evening level > 75% of morning level in Cushing's
Low-dose dexamethasone suppression test	0.5 mg 6-hourly for 48 hrs; sample 24-hr urine cortisol during second day and 0900-hr plasma cortisol after 48 hrs	Urine cortisol < 100 nmol/day (36 µg/day) or plasma cortisol < 60 nmol/L (< 2.2 µg/dL) excludes Cushing's
Insulin tolerance test	Box 20.59, page 786	Peak plasma cortisol > 120% of baseline excludes Cushing's
High-dose dexamethasone suppression test	2 mg 6-hourly for 48 hrs; sample 24-hr urine cortisol at baseline and during second day	Urine cortisol < 50% of basal suggests pituitary-dependent disease; > 50% of basal suggests ectopic ACTH syndrome
Corticotrophin-releasing hormone test	100 µg ovine CRH i.v. and monitor plasma ACTH and cortisol for 2 hrs	Peak plasma cortisol > 120% and/or ACTH > 150% of basal values suggests pituitary-dependent disease; lesser responses suggest ectopic ACTH syndrome
Inferior petrosal sinus sampling	Catheters placed in both inferior petrosal sinuses and simultaneous sampling from these and peripheral blood for ACTH; may be repeated 10 minutes after peripheral CRH injection	ACTH concentration in either petrosal sinus > 200% peripheral ACTH suggests pituitary-dependent disease; < 150% suggests ectopic ACTH syndrome

20

or urine) that fails to suppress with relatively low doses of oral dexamethasone (see Box 20.41). Loss of diurnal variation, with elevated evening plasma cortisol, is also characteristic of Cushing's syndrome, but samples are awkward to obtain. Plasma cortisol levels are highly variable in healthy subjects and random measurement of daytime plasma cortisol is of no value in supporting or refuting the diagnosis.

Dexamethasone is used for suppression testing because, unlike prednisolone, it does not cross-react in radioimmunoassays for cortisol. The hypothalamic–pituitary–adrenal axis may 'escape' from suppression by dexamethasone if a more potent influence, such as psychological stress, supervenes.

In the rare cyclical Cushing's syndrome there is episodic excessive secretion of cortisol. If there is a strong clinical suspicion of Cushing's syndrome but initial screening tests are normal, then weekly 24-hour urine cortisol measurements for up to 3 months are sometimes justified.

Determining the underlying cause

Once the presence of Cushing's syndrome is confirmed, measurement of plasma ACTH is the key to establishing the differential diagnosis. In the presence of excess cortisol secretion, an undetectable ACTH indicates an adrenal tumour, while any detectable ACTH suggest a pituitary cause or ectopic ACTH. Tests to discriminate pituitary from ectopic sources of ACTH rely on the fact that pituitary tumours, but not ectopic tumours, retain some features of normal regulation of ACTH secretion. Thus, in pituitary-dependent Cushing's disease, ACTH secretion is suppressed by high-dose dexamethasone and ACTH is stimulated by corticotrophin-releasing hormone (CRH).

Techniques for localisation of tumours secreting ACTH or cortisol are listed in Figure 20.22. MRI detects around 70% of pituitary microadenomas secreting ACTH. Inferior petrosal sinus sampling with measurement of ACTH may be helpful in confirming Cushing's disease if the MRI does not show a microadenoma. CT or MRI detects most adrenal tumours; adrenal carcinomas are usually large (> 5 cm) and have other features of malignancy (p. 777).

Management

Untreated Cushing's syndrome has a 50% 5-year mortality. Most patients are treated surgically with medical therapy given for a few weeks prior to operation. A number of drugs are used to inhibit corticosteroid biosynthesis, including metyrapone and ketoconazole. The dose of these agents is best titrated against 24-hour urine free cortisol.

Cushing's disease

Trans-sphenoidal surgery with selective removal of the adenoma is the treatment of choice. Experienced surgeons can identify microadenomas which were not detected by MRI and cure about 80% of patients. If the operation is unsuccessful, then bilateral adrenalectomy is an alternative.

If bilateral adrenalectomy is used in patients with pituitary-dependent Cushing's syndrome, then there is a risk that the pituitary tumour will grow in the absence of the negative feedback suppression previously provided by elevated cortisol levels. This can result in Nelson's syndrome, with an aggressive pituitary macroadenoma and very high ACTH levels causing pigmentation. Nelson's syndrome can be prevented by pituitary irradiation.

Adrenal tumours

Adrenal adenomas are removed by laparoscopy or a loin incision. Surgery offers the only prospect of cure for adreno-cortical carcinomas, but in general prognosis is poor with high rates of recurrence even in patients with localised disease at presentation. Although often used, there is little evidence that radiotherapy, chemotherapy or the adreno-lytic drug mitotane improves recurrence rates or survival.

Ectopic ACTH syndrome

Localised tumours such as bronchial carcinoid should be removed surgically. In patients with incurable malignancy it is important to reduce the severity of the Cushing's syndrome using medical therapy (see above) or, if appropriate, bilateral adrenalectomy.

Therapeutic use of glucocorticoids

The remarkable anti-inflammatory properties of gluco-corticoids have led to their use in a wide variety of clinical conditions, but the hazards are significant. Equivalent doses of commonly used glucocorticoids are listed in Box 20.42. Topical preparations (dermal, rectal and inhaled) can also be absorbed into the systemic circulation. Although this rarely occurs to a sufficient degree to produce clinical features of Cushing's syndrome, it can result in significant suppression of endogenous ACTH and cortisol secretion.

20.42 Equivalent doses of glucocorticoids

- Hydrocortisone: 20 mg
- Cortisone acetate: 25 mg
- Prednisolone: 5 mg
- Dexamethasone: 0.5 mg

Side-effects of glucocorticoids

The clinical features of glucocorticoid excess are illustrated in Figure 20.21 (p. 771). Adverse effects are related to dose, duration of therapy, and pre-existing conditions that might be worsened by corticosteroid therapy, such as diabetes mellitus or osteoporosis. Osteoporosis is a particularly important problem because, for a given bone mineral density, the fracture risk is greater in glucocorticoid-treated patients than in post-menopausal osteoporosis. Therefore, when systemic glucocorticoids are prescribed and the anticipated duration of steroid therapy is more than 3 months, bone-protective therapy should be considered, as detailed on page 1081. Rapid changes in glucocorticoid levels can also lead to marked mood disturbance, either depression or mania, and insomnia.

The anti-inflammatory effect of glucocorticoids may mask signs of disease. For example, perforation of a viscus may be masked and the patient may show no febrile response to an infection. Although there is debate about whether or not corticosteroids increase the risk of peptic ulcer when used alone, they act synergistically with NSAIDs, including aspirin, to increase the risk of serious gastrointestinal adverse effects. Latent tuberculosis may be reactivated and patients on corticosteroids should be advised to avoid contact with varicella zoster virus if they are not immune.

20.43 Advice to patients on glucocorticoid replacement therapy

Intercurrent stress

- Febrile illness: double dose of hydrocortisone

Surgery

- Minor operation: hydrocortisone 100 mg i.m. with pre-medication
- Major operation: hydrocortisone 100 mg 6-hourly for 24 hours, then 50 mg i.m. 6-hourly until ready to take tablets

Vomiting

- Patients must have parenteral hydrocortisone if unable to take it by mouth

Steroid card

- Patient should carry this at all times. It should give information regarding diagnosis, steroid, dose and doctor

Bracelet

- Patients should be encouraged to buy one of these and have it engraved with the diagnosis and a reference number for a central database

---

Management of glucocorticoid withdrawal

All glucocorticoid therapy, even if inhaled or applied topically, can suppress the HPA axis. In practice, this is only likely to result in a crisis due to adrenal insufficiency on withdrawal of treatment if glucocorticoids have been administered orally or systemically for longer than 3 weeks, if repeated courses have been prescribed within the previous year, or if the dose is higher than the equivalent of 7.5 mg prednisolone per day. In these circumstances, the drug, when it is no longer required for the underlying condition, must be withdrawn slowly at a rate dictated by the duration of treatment. If glucocorticoid therapy has been prolonged, then it may take many months for the HPA axis to recover. All patients must be advised to avoid sudden drug withdrawal. They should be issued with a steroid card and/or wear an engraved bracelet (Box 20.43).

Recovery of the HPA axis is aided if there is no exogenous glucocorticoid present during the nocturnal surge in ACTH secretion. This can be achieved by giving glucocorticoid in the morning. Giving ACTH to stimulate adrenal recovery is of no value as the pituitary remains suppressed.

In patients who have received glucocorticoids for longer than a few weeks, it is often valuable to confirm that the HPA axis is recovering during glucocorticoid withdrawal. Once the dose of glucocorticoid is reduced to a minimum (e.g. 4 mg prednisolone or 0.5 mg dexamethasone per day), then measure plasma cortisol at 0900 hrs before the next dose. If this is detectable, then perform an ACTH stimulation test (see Box 20.46) to confirm that glucocorticoids can be withdrawn completely. Even once glucocorticoids have been successfully withdrawn, short-term replacement therapy is often advised during significant intercurrent illness occurring in subsequent months, as the HPA axis may not be able to respond fully to severe stress.

Adrenal insufficiency

Adrenal insufficiency results from inadequate secretion of cortisol and/or aldosterone. It is potentially fatal

20.44 Causes of adrenocortical insufficiency

Secondary (↓ACTH)

- Withdrawal of suppressive glucocorticoid therapy
- Hypothalamic or pituitary disease

Primary (↑ACTH)

Addison's disease

Common causes
- Autoimmune
  Sporadic
  Polyglandular syndromes
  (p. 794)
- Tuberculosis
- HIV/AIDS
- Metastatic carcinoma
- Bilateral adrenalectomy

Rare causes
- Lymphoma
- Intra-adrenal haemorrhage (Waterhouse–Friderichsen syndrome following meningococcal septicaemia)
- Amyloidosis
- Haemochromatosis

Corticosteroid biosynthetic enzyme defects
- Congenital adrenal hyperplasias
- Drugs
  Metyrapone, ketoconazole, etomidate

coid or mineralocorticoid deficiency may come first, but eventually all patients fail to secrete both classes of corticosteroid.

Patients may present with chronic features and/or in acute circulatory shock. With a chronic presentation, initial symptoms are often misdiagnosed as chronic fatigue syndrome or depression. Adrenocortical insufficiency should also be considered in patients with hyponatraemia, even in the absence of symptoms (p. 435).

Features of an acute adrenal crisis include circulatory shock with severe hypotension, hyponatraemia, hyperkalaemia and, in some instances, hypoglycaemia and hypercalcaemia. Muscle cramps, nausea, vomiting, diarrhoea and unexplained fever may be present. The crisis is often precipitated by intercurrent disease, surgery or infection.

Vitiligo occurs in 10–20% of patients with autoimmune Addison's disease (p. 732).

Investigations

In patients presenting with chronic illness, investigations should be performed before any treatment. In patients with suspected acute adrenal crisis, treatment should not be delayed pending results. A random blood sample should be stored for measurement of cortisol. It may be appropriate to spend 30 minutes performing a short ACTH stimulation test (Box 20.46) before administering hydrocortisone, but investigations may need to be delayed until after recovery.

Assessment of glucocorticoids

Random plasma cortisol is usually low in patients with adrenal insufficiency, but it may be within the normal range, yet inappropriately low for a seriously ill patient. Random measurement of plasma cortisol cannot therefore be used to confirm or refute the diagnosis, unless the value is high (> 460 nmol/L (> 17 µg/dL)).

and notoriously variable in its presentation. A high index of suspicion is therefore required in patients with unexplained fatigue, hyponatraemia or hypotension. Causes are shown in Box 20.44. The most common is ACTH deficiency (secondary adrenocortical failure), usually because of inappropriate withdrawal of chronic glucocorticoid therapy or a pituitary tumour (p. 785). Congenital adrenal hyperplasias and Addison's disease (primary adrenocortical failure) are rare.

Clinical assessment

The clinical features of adrenal insufficiency are shown in Box 20.45. In Addison's disease, either glucocorti-

20

20.45 Clinical and biochemical features of adrenal insufficiency

	Glucocorticoid insufficiency	Mineralocorticoid insufficiency	ACTH excess	Adrenal androgen insufficiency
Withdrawal of exogenous glucocorticoid	+	−	−	+
Hypopituitarism	+	−	−	+
Addison's disease	+	+	+	+
Congenital adrenal hyperplasia (21 OHase deficiency)	+	+	+	−
Clinical features	Weight loss Malaise Weakness Anorexia Nausea Vomiting Diarrhoea or constipation Postural hypotension Shock Hypoglycaemia Hyponatraemia (dilutional) Hypercalcaemia	Hypotension Shock Hyponatraemia (depletional) Hyperkalaemia	Pigmentation of: Sun-exposed areas Pressure areas, (e.g. elbows, knees) Palmar creases, knuckles Mucous membranes Conjunctivae Recent scars	Decreased body hair and loss of libido, especially in female

20.46 How and when to do an ACTH stimulation test

Use

- Diagnosis of primary or secondary adrenal insufficiency
- Assessment of HPA axis in patients taking suppressive glucocorticoid therapy
- Relies on ACTH-dependent adrenal atrophy in secondary adrenal insufficiency, so may not detect acute ACTH deficiency (e.g. in pituitary apoplexy, p. 787)

Dose

- 250 µg ACTH$_{1-24}$ (Synacthen) by i.m. injection at any time of day

Blood samples

- 0 and 30 mins for plasma cortisol
- 0 mins also for ACTH (on ice) if Addison's disease is being considered (i.e. patient not known to have pituitary disease or to be taking exogenous glucocorticoids)

Results

- Normal subjects plasma cortisol > 460 nmol/L (~17 µg/dL)* either at baseline or at 30 mins
- Incremental change in cortisol is not a criterion

*The exact cortisol concentration depends on the cortisol assay being used.

More useful is the short ACTH stimulation test (also called the tetracosactrin or short Synacthen test) described in Box 20.46. Cortisol levels fail to increase in response to exogenous ACTH in patients with primary or secondary adrenal insufficiency. These can be distinguished by measurement of ACTH (which is low in ACTH deficiency and high in Addison's disease). If an ACTH assay is unavailable, then a long ACTH stimulation test can be used (1 mg depot ACTH i.m. daily for 3 days); in secondary adrenal insufficiency there is a progressive increase in plasma cortisol with repeated ACTH administration, whereas in Addison's disease, cortisol remains less than 700 nmol/L (25.4 µg/dL) at 8 hours after the last injection.

In a patient who is already receiving glucocorticoids, the short ACTH stimulation test can be performed first thing in the morning, more than 12 hours after the last dose of glucocorticoid, or the treatment can be changed to a synthetic steroid such as dexamethasone (0.75 mg daily), which does not cross-react in the plasma cortisol immunoassay.

Assessment of mineralocorticoids

Mineralocorticoid secretion in patients with suspected Addison's disease cannot be adequately assessed by electrolyte measurements since hyponatraemia occurs in both aldosterone and cortisol deficiency (see Box 20.45 and p. 435). Hyperkalaemia is common, but not universal, in aldosterone deficiency. Plasma renin activity and aldosterone should be measured in the supine position. In mineralocorticoid deficiency, plasma renin activity is high, with plasma aldosterone being either low or in the lower part of the normal range.

Assessment of adrenal androgens

This is not necessary in men because testosterone from the testes is the principal androgen. In women, dehydroepiandrosterone (DHEA) and androstenedione may be measured in a random specimen of blood, though levels are highest in the morning.

Other tests to establish the cause

Patients with unexplained secondary adrenocortical insufficiency should be investigated as described on page 785. In patients with elevated ACTH, further tests are required to establish the cause of Addison's disease. In those who have autoimmune adrenal failure, antibodies can often be measured against steroid-secreting cells (adrenal and gonad), thyroid antigens, pancreatic β cells and gastric parietal cells. Thyroid function tests, full blood count (to screen for pernicious anaemia), plasma calcium, glucose and tests of gonadal function (p. 753) should be performed. Other causes of adrenocortical disease are usually obvious clinically, particularly if health is not fully restored by corticosteroid replacement therapy. Tuberculosis causes adrenal calcification, visible on plain X-ray or ultrasound scan. A chest X-ray and early morning urine for culture should also be taken. An HIV test should be performed if risk factors for infection are present (p. 385). Imaging of the adrenals by CT or MRI to identify metastatic malignancy may also be appropriate.

Management

Patients with adrenocortical insufficiency always need glucocorticoid replacement therapy and usually, but not always, mineralocorticoid. Adrenal androgen replacement for women is controversial. Other treatments depend on the underlying cause. The emergency management of adrenal crisis is described in Box 20.47.

Glucocorticoid replacement

Hydrocortisone (cortisol) is the drug of choice. In someone who is not critically ill, hydrocortisone should be given by mouth, 15 mg on waking and 5 mg at around 1800 hrs. The dose may need to be adjusted for the individual patient but this is subjective. Excess weight gain usually indicates over-replacement, whilst persistent lethargy or hyperpigmentation may be due to an inadequate dose. Measurement of plasma cortisol levels is

20.47 Management of adrenal crisis

Correct volume depletion

- I.v. saline as required to normalise BP and pulse
- In severe hyponatraemia (< 125 mmol/L) avoid increases of plasma Na >10 mmol/L/day to prevent pontine demyelination (p. 435)
- Fludrocortisone is not required during the acute phase of treatment

Replace glucocorticoids

- I.v. hydrocortisone succinate 100 mg stat
- Continue parenteral hydrocortisone (50–100 mg i.m. 6-hourly) until the patient is well enough for reliable oral therapy

Correct other metabolic abnormalities

- Acute hypoglycaemia: i.v. 10% glucose
- Hyperkalaemia: should respond to volume replacement, but occasionally requires specific therapy (Box 16.17, p. 441)

Identify and treat underlying cause

- Consider acute precipitant, e.g. infection
- Consider adrenal or pituitary pathology (see Box 20.44)

unhelpful, because the dynamic interaction between cortisol and glucocorticoid receptors is not predicted by measurements such as the maximum or minimum plasma cortisol level after each dose. Advice to patients dependent on glucocorticoid replacement is given in Box 20.43. These are physiological replacement doses which should not cause Cushingoid side-effects.

Mineralocorticoid replacement

Fludrocortisone (9α-fluoro-hydrocortisone) is administered in a dose 0.05–0.1 mg daily and adequacy of replacement may be assessed objectively by measurement of blood pressure, plasma electrolytes and plasma renin activity.

Androgen replacement

DHEA (approximately 50 mg/day) is sometimes given to women with primary adrenal insufficiency. Some trials have suggested that DHEA increases libido and sense of well-being, but complications include acne and hirsutism.

Incidental adrenal mass

It is not uncommon for a mass in the adrenal gland to be identified on a CT or MRI scan of the abdomen that has been performed for another indication. Such lesions are known as adrenal 'incidentalomas'. They are present in up to 10% of adults and the prevalence increases with age.

Eighty-five per cent of adrenal incidentalomas are non-functioning adrenal adenomas. The remainder includes functional tumours of the adrenal cortex (secreting cortisol, aldosterone or androgens), phaeochromocytomas, primary and secondary carcinomas, hamartomas and other rare disorders including granulomatous infiltrations.

Clinical assessment and investigations

There are two key questions to be resolved: is the lesion secreting hormones, and is it benign or malignant?

Patients with an adrenal incidentaloma are usually asymptomatic. However, clinical signs and symptoms of excess glucocorticoids (p. 771), mineralocorticoids (see below), catecholamines (p. 779) and, in women, androgens (p. 759) should be sought. Investigations should include a 24-hour urine collection for metanephrines and urine free cortisol and, in women, measurement of serum testosterone, DHEA and androstenedione concentrations. Patients with hypertension should be investigated for mineralocorticoid excess as described below.

CT and MRI are equally effective in assessing the malignant potential of an adrenal mass, using the following parameters:

- *Size.* The larger the lesion, the greater the malignant potential. Around 90% of adrenocortical carcinomas are > 4 cm in diameter, but specificity is poor since only approximately 25% of such lesions are malignant.
- *Configuration.* Homogeneous and smooth lesions are more likely to be benign. The presence of metastatic lesions elsewhere increases the risk of malignancy, but as many as two-thirds of adrenal incidentalomas in patients with cancer are benign.

20.48 Glucocorticoids in old age

- **Adrenocortical insufficiency**: often insidious and difficult to spot.
- **Glucocorticoid therapy**: especially hazardous in older people, who are already relatively immunocompromised and susceptible to osteoporosis, diabetes, hypertension and other complications.
- **'Physiological' glucocorticoid replacement therapy**: increased risk of adrenal crisis, because compliance may be poor and there is a greater incidence of intercurrent illness. Patient and carer education with regular reinforcement of principles described in Box 20.43 is crucial.

- *Presence of lipid.* Adenomas are usually lipid-rich, resulting in an attenuation of < 10 Hounsfield Units (HU) on an unenhanced CT and in signal dropout on chemical shift MRI.
- *Enhancement.* Benign lesions demonstrate rapid washout of contrast, whereas malignant lesions tend to retain contrast.

Histology in a sample obtained by CT-guided biopsy is not useful in distinguishing an adrenal adenoma from an adrenal carcinoma, although it is occasionally helpful in confirming adrenal metastases from other cancers.

Management

Functional lesions and tumours > 5 cm in diameter should be removed by laparoscopic adrenalectomy. In patients with radiologically benign, non-functioning lesions < 5 cm in diameter, surgery is only required if serial imaging suggests tumour growth.

Primary hyperaldosteronism

Estimates of the prevalence of primary hyperaldosteronism vary according to the screening tests employed,

20.49 Causes of mineralocorticoid excess

With renin high and aldosterone high (secondary hyperaldosteronism)

- Inadequate renal perfusion, e.g. diuretic therapy, cardiac failure, liver failure, nephrotic syndrome, renal artery stenosis
- Renin-secreting renal tumour (very rare)

With renin low and aldosterone high (primary hyperaldosteronism)

- Adrenal adenoma secreting aldosterone (Conn's syndrome)
- Idiopathic bilateral adrenal hyperplasia
- Glucocorticoid-suppressible hyperaldosteronism (rare)

With renin low and aldosterone low (non-aldosterone-dependent activation of mineralocorticoid pathway)

- Ectopic ACTH syndrome
- Liquorice misuse (inhibition of 11β-HSD2)
- Liddle's syndrome
- 11-deoxycorticosterone-secreting adrenal tumour
- Rare forms of congenital adrenal hyperplasia and 11β-HSD2 deficiency

20

but it may occur in as many as 10% of people with hypertension. Indications to test for mineralocorticoid excess in hypertensive patients include hypokalaemia (including hypokalaemia induced by thiazide diuretics), poor control of blood pressure with conventional therapy, a family history of early-onset hypertension, or presentation at a young age.

Causes of excessive activation of mineralocorticoid receptors are shown in Box 20.49. It is important to differentiate primary hyperaldosteronism, caused by an intrinsic abnormality of the adrenal glands resulting in aldosterone excess, from secondary hyperaldosteronism, which is usually a consequence of enhanced activity of renin in response to inadequate renal perfusion and hypotension. Most individuals with primary hyperaldosteronism have bilateral adrenal hyperplasia (idiopathic hyperaldosteronism), while only a minority have an aldosterone-producing adenoma (APA; Conn's syndrome). Glucocorticoid-suppressible hyperaldosteronism is a rare autosomal dominant condition in which aldosterone is secreted 'ectopically' from the adrenal fasciculata/reticularis in response to ACTH. Rarely, the mineralocorticoid receptor pathway in the distal nephron is activated, even though aldosterone concentrations are low.

Clinical features

Individuals with primary hyperaldosteronism are usually asymptomatic, but they may have features of sodium retention or potassium loss. Sodium retention may cause oedema, while hypokalaemia may causes muscle weakness (or even paralysis, especially in Chinese), polyuria (secondary to renal tubular damage which produces nephrogenic diabetes insipidus) and occasionally tetany (because of associated metabolic alkalosis and low ionised calcium). Blood pressure is elevated but accelerated phase hypertension is rare.

Investigations

Biochemical

Routine bloods may show a hypokalaemic alkalosis. Sodium is usually at the upper end of the normal range in primary hyperaldosteronism, but is characteristically low in secondary hyperaldosteronism (because low plasma volume stimulates ADH release and high angiotensin II levels stimulate thirst). The key measurements are plasma renin and aldosterone (see Box 20.49). In many centres, the aldosterone:renin ratio (ARR) is employed as a screening test for primary hyperaldosteronism in hypertensive patients. Almost all antihypertensive drugs interfere with this ratio (β-blockers inhibit, whilst thiazide diuretics stimulate renin secretion). Thus, individuals with an elevated ARR require further testing after stopping interfering antihypertensive drugs for at least 2 weeks. If necessary, antihypertensive agents that have minimal effects on the renin–angiotensin system, such as calcium antagonists and α-blockers, may be substituted. Oral potassium supplementation may also be required, as hypokalaemia itself suppresses renin activity. If, on repeat testing, renin activity is low and aldosterone concentrations are elevated, then further investigation under specialist supervision may include suppression tests (sodium loading) and/or stimulation tests (captopril or furosemide administration) to differentiate angiotensin II-dependent aldosterone secretion in idiopathic hyperplasia from autonomous aldosterone

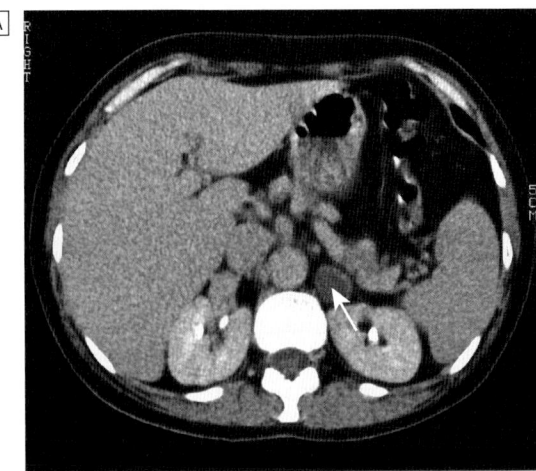

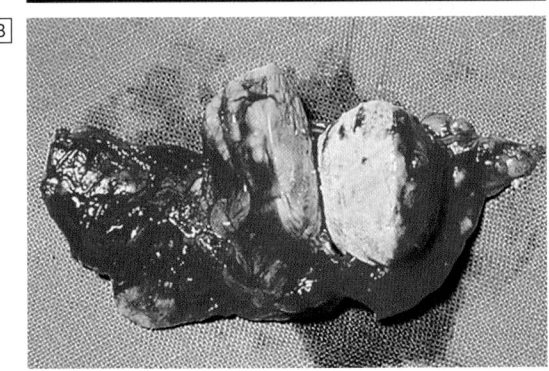

Fig. 20.23 Aldosterone-producing adenoma causing Conn's syndrome. **A** CT scan of left adrenal adenoma (arrow). **B** The tumour is 'canary yellow' because of intracellular lipid accumulation.

secretion typical of an aldosterone-producing adenoma (APA).

Imaging and localisation

Imaging with CT or MRI will identify most APAs (Fig. 20.23), but it is important to recognise the risk of false positives (non-functioning adrenal adenomas are common) and false negatives (imaging may have insufficient resolution to identify adenomas with diameter < 0.5 cm). If the imaging is inconclusive and there is an intention to proceed with surgery on the basis of strong biochemical evidence of an APA, then adrenal vein catheterisation with measurement of aldosterone (and cortisol to confirm positioning of the catheters) is required.

Management

Mineralocorticoid receptor antagonists are valuable in treating both hypokalaemia and hypertension in all forms of mineralocorticoid excess. Up to 20% of males develop gynaecomastia on spironolactone. Eplerenone or amiloride (10–40 mg/day), which blocks the epithelial sodium channel regulated by aldosterone, is an alternative.

In patients with an APA, medical therapy is usually given for a few weeks to normalise whole-body electrolyte balance before unilateral adrenalectomy. Laparoscopic surgery cures the biochemical abnormality but hypertension remains in as many as 70% of cases, probably because of irreversible damage to the systemic microcirculation.

Phaeochromocytoma and paraganglioma

These are rare neuro-endocrine tumours that may secrete catecholamines (adrenaline/epinephrine, noradrenaline/norepinephrine) and are responsible for less than 0.1% of cases of hypertension. Approximately 80% of these tumours occur in the adrenal medulla (phaeochromocytomas), while 20% arise elsewhere in the body in sympathetic ganglia (paragangliomas). Most are benign but approximately 15% show malignant features. Around 25% of phaeochromocytomas are associated with inherited disorders, including neurofibromatosis (p. 1218), von Hippel–Lindau syndrome (p. 1219) and MEN type 2 (p. 793). Paragangliomas are particularly associated with mutations in the succinate dehydrogenase B, C and D genes.

Clinical features

These depend on the pattern of catecholamine secretion and are listed in Box 20.50.

Some patients present with a complication of hypertension, such as stroke, myocardial infarction, left ventricular failure, hypertensive retinopathy or accelerated phase hypertension. The apparent paradox of postural

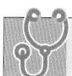

20.50 Clinical features of phaeochromocytoma

- Hypertension (usually paroxysmal; often postural drop of blood pressure)
- Paroxysms of:
  Pallor (occasionally flushing)
  Palpitations
  Sweating
  Headache
  Anxiety (fear of death—angor animi)
- Abdominal pain, vomiting
- Constipation
- Weight loss
- Glucose intolerance

hypotension between episodes is explained by 'pressure natriuresis' during hypertensive episodes so that intravascular volume is reduced. There may also be features of the familial syndromes associated with phaeochromocytoma.

Investigations

Excessive secretion of catecholamines can be confirmed by measuring metabolites in plasma and/or urine (metanephrine and normetanephrine). There is a high 'false positive' rate as misleading metanephrine concentrations may be seen in stressed patients (during acute illness or following vigorous exercise or severe pain) and following ingestion of some drugs such as tricyclic antidepressants. For this reason, a repeat sample should usually be requested if elevated levels are found, although as a rule the higher the concentration of metanephrines, the more likely the diagnosis of phaeochromocytoma/paraganglioma. Serum chromogranin A is often elevated and may be a useful tumour marker in patients with non-secretory tumours and/or metastatic disease. Genetic testing should be considered in individuals with other features of a genetic syndrome, with a family history of phaeochromocytoma/paraganglioma and in those presenting under the age of 50 years.

Localisation

Phaeochromocytomas are usually identified by abdominal CT or MRI (Fig. 20.24). Localisation of paragangliomas may be more difficult. Scintigraphy using meta-iodobenzyl guanidine (MIBG) can be useful, particularly if combined with CT. ^{18}F-deoxyglucose PET is a sensitive but not specific test, and is not universally available.

Management

Medical therapy is required to prepare the patient for surgery, preferably for a minimum of 6 weeks to allow restoration of normal plasma volume. The most useful drug in the face of very high circulating catecholamines is the α-blocker phenoxybenzamine (10–20 mg orally 6–8-hourly) because it is a non-competitive antagonist, unlike prazosin or doxazosin. If α-blockade produces a marked tachycardia, then a β-blocker (e.g. propranolol) or combined α- and β-antagonist (e.g. labetalol) can be

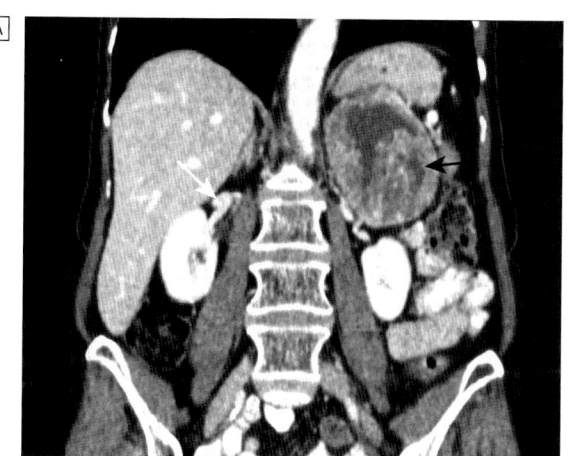
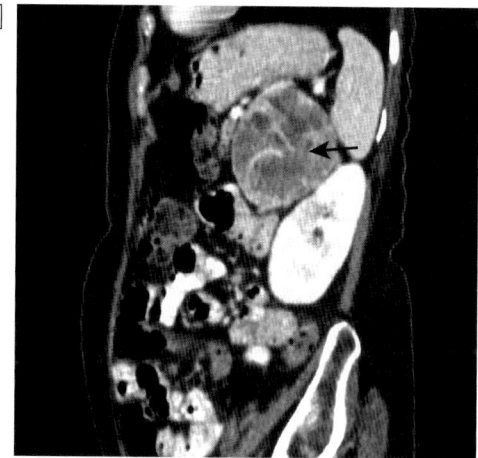

Fig. 20.24 CT scan of abdomen showing large left adrenal phaeochromocytoma. **A** Coronal view. **B** Sagittal view. The normal right adrenal (white arrow) contrasts with the large heterogeneous phaeochromocytoma arising from the left adrenal gland (black arrows).

20

added. On no account should the β-antagonist be given before the α-antagonist, as it may cause a paradoxical rise in blood pressure due to unopposed α-mediated vasoconstriction.

During surgery sodium nitroprusside and the short-acting α-antagonist phentolamine are useful in controlling hypertensive episodes which may result from anaesthetic induction or tumour mobilisation. Post-operative hypotension may occur and require volume expansion and, very occasionally, noradrenaline (norepinephrine) infusion. This is uncommon if the patient has been prepared adequately with phenoxybenzamine.

Metastatic tumours may behave in an aggressive or a very indolent fashion. Management options include debulking surgery, radionuclide therapy with ^{131}I-MIBG, chemotherapy and (chemo)embolisation of hepatic metastases.

Congenital adrenal hyperplasia

Pathophysiology and clinical features

Inherited defects in enzymes of the cortisol biosynthetic pathway (see Fig. 20.20, p. 770) result in insufficiency of hormones 'distal' to the block, with impaired negative feedback and increased ACTH secretion. ACTH then stimulates the production of steroids 'proximal' to the enzyme block. This produces adrenal hyperplasia and a combination of clinical features that depend on the severity and site of the defect in biosynthesis. All of these enzyme abnormalities are inherited as autosomal recessive traits.

The most common enzyme defect is 21-hydroxylase deficiency. This results in impaired synthesis of cortisol and aldosterone and accumulation of 17OH-progesterone, which is then diverted to form adrenal androgens. In about one-third of cases this defect is severe and presents in infancy with features of glucocorticoid and mineralocorticoid deficiency (see Box 20.45, p. 775) and androgen excess (i.e. ambiguous genitalia in girls). In the other two-thirds, mineralocorticoid secretion is adequate, but there may be features of cortisol insufficiency and/or ACTH and androgen excess, including precocious pseudopuberty, which is distinguished from 'true' precocious puberty by low gonadotrophins. Sometimes the mildest enzyme defects are not apparent until adult life, when females may present with amenorrhoea and/or hirsutism (p. 759). This is called 'non-classical' or 'late-onset' congenital adrenal hyperplasia.

Defects of all the other enzymes in Figure 20.20 (p. 770) are rare. Both 17-hydroxylase and 11β-hydroxylase deficiency may produce hypertension due to excess production of 11-deoxycorticosterone, which has mineralocorticoid activity.

Investigations

Circulating 17OH-progesterone levels are raised in 21-hydroxylase deficiency, but this may only be demonstrated after ACTH administration in late-onset cases. To avoid salt-wasting crises in infancy, 17OH-progesterone can be routinely measured in heel prick blood spot samples taken from all infants in the first week of life. Assessment is otherwise as described for adrenal insufficiency on page 775.

In siblings of affected children, antenatal genetic diagnosis can be made by amniocentesis or chorionic villus sampling. This allows prevention of virilisation of affected female fetuses by administration of dexamethasone to the mother.

Management

The aim is to replace deficient corticosteroids and to suppress ACTH-driven adrenal androgen production. In contrast to glucocorticoid replacement therapy in other forms of cortisol deficiency (p. 776), it is usual to give 'reverse' treatment. This involves giving a larger dose of a long-acting synthetic glucocorticoid just before going to bed to suppress the early morning ACTH peak, and a smaller dose in the morning. A careful balance is required between adequate suppression of adrenal androgen excess and excessive glucocorticoid replacement resulting in features of Cushing's syndrome. In children, growth velocity is an important measurement, since either under- or over-replacement with glucocorticoids suppresses growth. In adults, clinical features (menstrual cycle, hirsutism, weight gain, blood pressure) and biochemical profiles (plasma renin activity, 17OH-progesterone and testosterone levels) provide a guide.

Women with late-onset 21-hydroxylase deficiency may not require corticosteroid replacement. If hirsutism is the main problem, anti-androgen therapy may be just as effective (p. 762).

THE ENDOCRINE PANCREAS AND GASTROINTESTINAL TRACT

A series of hormones are secreted from cells distributed throughout the gastrointestinal tract and pancreas. Functional anatomy and physiology are described in Chapters 21 and 22. Diseases associated with abnormalities of these hormones are listed in Box 20.51. Most are rare, with the exception of diabetes mellitus (Ch. 21).

20.51 Classification of endocrine diseases of the pancreas and gastrointestinal tract

	Primary	Secondary
Hormone excess	Insulinoma Gastrinoma (Zollinger–Ellison syndrome) Carcinoid syndrome (secretion of 5-HT) Glucagonoma VIPoma Somatostatinoma	Hypergastrinaemia of achlorhydria Hyperinsulinaemia after bariatric surgery
Hormone deficiency	Diabetes mellitus	
Hormone hypersensitivity	Rare, e.g. pseudoacromegaly	
Hormone resistance	Insulin resistance syndromes (e.g. type 2 diabetes mellitus, lipodystrophy, leprechaunism)	
Non-functioning tumours	Pancreatic carcinoma Pancreatic neuro-endocrine tumour	

Presenting problems in endocrine pancreas disease

Spontaneous hypoglycaemia

Hypoglycaemia most commonly occurs as a side-effect of treatment with insulin or sulphonylurea drugs in people with diabetes mellitus. In non-diabetic individuals, symptomatic hypoglycaemia is rare, but it is not uncommon to detect venous blood glucose concentrations below 3.0 mmol/L in asymptomatic patients. For this reason, and because the symptoms of hypoglycaemia are non-specific, a hypoglycaemic disorder should only be diagnosed if all three conditions of Whipple's triad are met (Fig. 20.25). There is no specific blood glucose concentration at which spontaneous hypoglycaemia can be said to occur, although the lower the blood glucose concentration, the more likely it is to have pathological significance.

Clinical assessment

The clinical features of hypoglycaemia are described in the section on insulin-induced hypoglycaemia on page 812. Individuals with chronic spontaneous hypoglycaemia often have attenuated autonomic responses, and may present with a wide variety of features of neuroglycopenia, including odd behaviour and convulsions. The symptoms are usually episodic and relieved by consumption of carbohydrate. Symptoms occurring while fasting (such as before breakfast) or following exercise are much more likely to be representative of pathological hypoglycaemia than those which develop after food (post-prandial or 'reactive' symptoms). Hypoglycaemia should be considered in all comatose patients, even if there is an apparently obvious cause, such as hemiplegic stroke or alcohol intoxication.

Investigations

Does the patient have a hypoglycaemic disorder?

Patients who present acutely with confusion, coma or convulsions should be tested for hypoglycaemia at the bedside with a capillary blood sample and an automated meter. While this is sufficient to exclude hypoglycaemia, blood glucose meters are relatively inaccurate in the hypoglycaemic range and the diagnosis should always be confirmed by a laboratory-based glucose measurement. At the same time, a sample should be taken for later measurement, if necessary, of alcohol, insulin, C-peptide and sulphonylurea levels. Taking these samples during an acute presentation prevents subsequent unnecessary dynamic tests and is of medico-legal importance in cases where poisoning is suspected.

Patients who attend the outpatient clinic with episodic symptoms suggestive of hypoglycaemia present a more challenging problem. The main diagnostic test is the prolonged (72-hour) fast. If symptoms of hypoglycaemia develop during the fast, then blood samples should be taken to confirm hypoglycaemia and for later measurement of insulin and C-peptide. Hypoglycaemia is then corrected with oral or intravenous glucose and Whipple's triad completed by confirmation of the resolution of symptoms. The absence of clinical and biochemical evidence of hypoglycaemia during a prolonged fast effectively excludes the diagnosis of a hypoglycaemic disorder.

What is the cause of the hypoglycaemia?

In the acute setting, the underlying diagnosis is often obvious. In non-diabetic individuals, alcohol excess is the most common cause of hypoglycaemia in the UK, but other drugs, for example salicylates, quinine and pentamidine, may also be implicated. Hypoglycaemia is one of many metabolic derangements which occur in patients with hepatic failure, renal failure, sepsis or malaria.

Hypoglycaemia in the absence of insulin, or any insulin-like factor, in the blood indicates impaired gluconeogenesis and/or availability of glucose from glycogen in the liver. Hypoglycaemia associated with high insulin and low C-peptide concentrations is indicative of administration of exogenous insulin, either factitiously or feloniously. Adults with high insulin and C-peptide concentrations during an episode of hypoglycaemia are most likely to have an insulinoma, but sulphonylurea ingestion should also be considered (particularly in

20

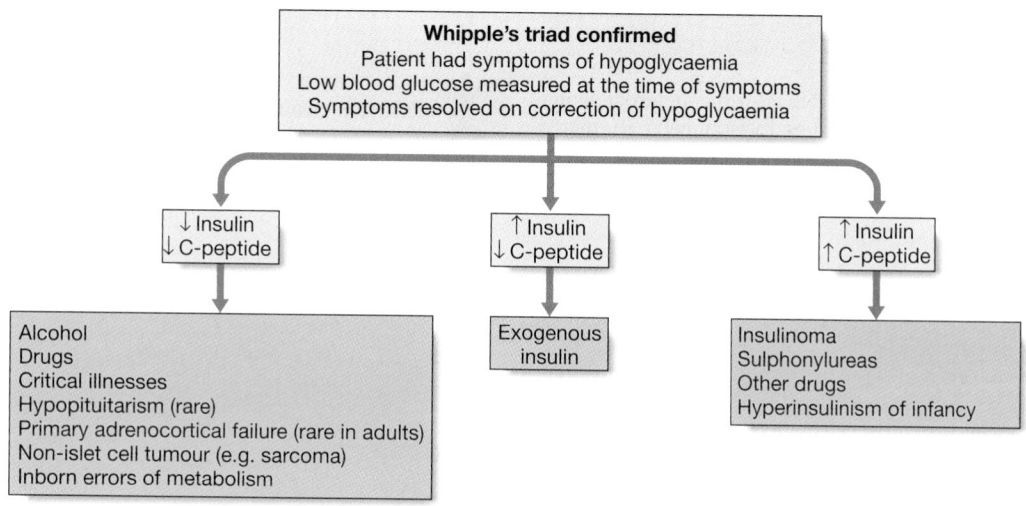

Whipple's triad confirmed
Patient had symptoms of hypoglycaemia
Low blood glucose measured at the time of symptoms
Symptoms resolved on correction of hypoglycaemia

↓ Insulin
↓ C-peptide

↑ Insulin
↓ C-peptide

↑ Insulin
↑ C-peptide

Alcohol
Drugs
Critical illnesses
Hypopituitarism (rare)
Primary adrenocortical failure (rare in adults)
Non-islet cell tumour (e.g. sarcoma)
Inborn errors of metabolism

Exogenous insulin

Insulinoma
Sulphonylureas
Other drugs
Hyperinsulinism of infancy

Fig. 20.25 Differential diagnosis of spontaneous hypoglycaemia. Measurement of insulin and C-peptide concentrations during an episode is helpful in determining the underlying cause.

individuals with access to such medication, such as health-care professionals or family members of someone with type 2 diabetes). Insulinomas in the pancreas are usually small (< 5 mm diameter), but can usually be identified by CT, MRI or ultrasound (endoscopic or laparoscopic). Imaging should include the liver since around 10% of insulinomas are malignant. Rarely, large non-pancreatic tumours, such as sarcomas, may cause recurrent hypoglycaemia because of their ability to produce excess insulin-like growth factor-2.

Management

Treatment of acute hypoglycaemia should be initiated as soon as laboratory blood samples have been taken, and should *not* be deferred until the formal laboratory confirmation is obtained. Intravenous dextrose (5% or 10%) is effective in the short term in the obtunded patient, and should be followed on recovery with oral unrefined carbohydrate (starch). Continuous dextrose infusion may be necessary, especially in sulphonylurea poisoning. Intramuscular glucagon (1 mg) stimulates hepatic glucose release, but is ineffective in patients with depleted glycogen reserves such as alcohol excess, liver disease.

Chronic recurrent hypoglycaemia in insulin-secreting tumours can be treated by regular consumption of oral carbohydrate combined with agents that inhibit insulin secretion (diazoxide or somatostatin analogues). Insulinomas are resected when benign, providing the individual is fit enough to undergo surgery. Metastatic malignant insulinomas are incurable and are managed along the same lines as other metastatic neuro-endocrine tumours (see below).

20.52 Spontaneous hypoglycaemia in old age

- **Presentation**: may present with focal neurological abnormality. Blood glucose should be checked in all patients with acute neurological symptoms and signs, especially stroke, as these will reverse with early treatment of hypoglycaemia.

Gastroenteropancreatic neuro-endocrine tumours

Neuro-endocrine tumours (NETs) are a heterogeneous group derived from neuro-endocrine cells in many organs, including the gastrointestinal tract, lung, adrenals (phaeochromocytoma, p. 779) and thyroid (medullary carcinoma, p. 752). Most NETs occur sporadically, but a proportion are associated with genetic cancer syndromes such as MEN 1, MEN 2 and neurofibromatosis type 1 (pp. 793 and 1218). NETs may secrete hormones into the circulation.

Gastroenteropancreatic NETs arise in organs that are derived embryologically from the gastrointestinal tract. Most commonly they occur in the small bowel, but they can also arise elsewhere in the bowel, pancreas, thymus and bronchi. The term 'carcinoid' is often used when referring to non-pancreatic gastroenteropancreatic NETs, because when initially described they were thought to behave in an indolent fashion compared with conventional cancers. It is now recognised that there is a wide spectrum of malignant potential for all NETs; some are benign (most insulinomas and appendiceal carcinoid tumours) while others have an aggressive clinical course with widespread metastases (small cell carcinoma of the lung). The majority of gastroenteropancreatic NETs behave in an intermediate manner with relatively slow growth, but a propensity to invade and metastasise to remote organs, especially the liver.

Clinical features

Gastroenteropancreatic NETs usually present with local mass effects, such as small bowel obstruction, appendicitis, and pain from hepatic metastases. Thymic and bronchial carcinoids occasionally present with ectopic ACTH syndrome (p. 771). Pancreatic NETs can also cause hormone excess (Box 20.53) but most are non-functional. The classic 'carcinoid syndrome' (Box 20.54) occurs when vasoactive hormones, such as serotonin (5-HT), reach the systemic circulation. In the case of gastrointestinal carcinoids, this invariably means that the tumour has metastasised to the liver, as hormones secreted by the primary tumour into the portal vein are metabolised and inactivated in the liver.

Investigations

A combination of imaging with ultrasound, CT, MRI and/or radiolabelled somatostatin analogue (Fig. 20.26) will usually identify the primary tumour and allow staging, which is crucial for determining prognosis. Biopsy of the primary tumour or a metastatic deposit is required to confirm the histological type. NETs demonstrate immunohistochemical staining for the proteins chromogranin A and synaptophysin, and the histological grade may also provide prognostic information.

Carcinoid syndrome is confirmed by measuring elevated concentrations of 5-hydroxyindoleacetic acid (5-HIAA), a metabolite of serotonin, in a 24-hour urine collection. False positives can occur, particularly if the individual has been eating certain foods, such as avocado and pineapple. Chromogranin A and synaptophysin can be measured in a fasting blood sample, along with the hormones listed in Box 20.53; these can be useful as tumour markers.

20.53 Pancreatic neuro-endocrine tumours

Tumour	Hormone	Effects
Gastrinoma	Gastrin	Peptic ulcer and steatorrhoea (Zollinger–Ellison syndrome)
Insulinoma	Insulin	Recurrent hypoglycaemia (see above)
VIPoma	Vasoactive intestinal peptide (VIP)	Watery diarrhoea and hypokalaemia
Glucagonoma	Glucagon	Diabetes mellitus, necrolytic migratory erythema
Somatostatinoma	Somatostatin	Diabetes mellitus and steatorrhoea

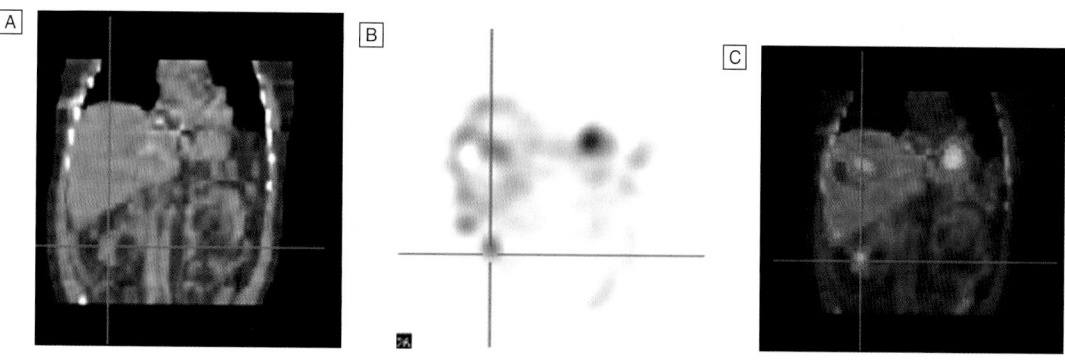

Fig. 20.26 Octreotide scintigraphy in a metastatic neuro-endocrine tumour. [A] Coronal CT scan showing hepatomegaly and a mass inferior to the liver (at the intersection of the horizontal and vertical red lines). [B] Octreotide scintogram showing patches of increased uptake in the upper abdomen. [C] When the octreotide and CT scans are superimposed, it shows that the areas of increased uptake are in hepatic metastases and in the tissue mass which may be lymph nodes or a primary tumour.

20.54 Clinical features of the carcinoid syndrome

- Episodic flushing, wheezing and diarrhoea
- Facial telangiectasia
- Cardiac involvement (tricuspid regurgitation, pulmonary stenosis, right ventricular endocardial plaques) leading to heart failure

Management

Treatment of solitary tumours is by surgical resection. If metastatic or multifocal primary disease is present, then surgery is usually not indicated, unless there is, for example, gastrointestinal obstruction. Diazoxide may reduce insulin secretion in insulinomas and high doses of proton pump inhibitors suppress acid production in gastrinomas. Somatostatin analogues are effective in reducing the symptoms of carcinoid syndrome and of excess glucagon and vasoactive intestinal peptide (VIP) production. The slow-growing nature of NETs means that conventional cancer therapies, such as chemotherapy and radiotherapy, have a limited role. Other treatments, such as interferon, targeted radionuclide therapy with ^{131}I-MIBG and radiolabelled somatostatin analogues (which may be taken up by NET metastases), and resection/embolisation of hepatic metastases, may have a role in the palliation of symptoms, but there is little evidence that they prolong life.

THE HYPOTHALAMUS AND THE PITUITARY GLAND

Diseases of the hypothalamus and pituitary are rare, with an annual incidence of approximately 1:50 000. The pituitary plays a central role in several major endocrine axes, so that investigation and treatment invariably involve several other glands.

Functional anatomy, physiology and investigations

The anatomical relationships of the pituitary are shown in Figure 20.27 and its numerous functions are shown in Figure 20.2 (p. 735). The pituitary gland is enclosed in the sella turcica and bridged over by a fold of dura mater called the diaphragma sellae, with the sphenoidal air sinuses below and the optic chiasm above. The cavernous sinuses are lateral to the pituitary fossa and contain the 3rd, 4th and 6th cranial nerves and the internal carotid arteries. The gland is composed of two lobes, anterior and posterior, and is connected to the hypothalamus by the infundibular stalk, which has portal vessels carrying blood from the median eminence of the hypothalamus to the anterior lobe and nerve fibres to the posterior lobe.

Diseases of the hypothalamus and pituitary are classified in Box 20.55. By far the most common disorder is an adenoma of the anterior pituitary gland.

20.55 Classification of diseases of the pituitary and hypothalamus

	Primary	Secondary
Hormone excess		
Anterior pituitary	Prolactinoma	Disconnection
	Acromegaly	hyperprolactinaemia
	Cushing's disease	
	Rare TSH-, LH-	
	and FSH-secreting	
	adenomas	
Hypothalamus and	Syndrome of	
posterior pituitary	inappropriate	
	antidiuretic hormone	
	(SIADH; p. 436)	
Hormone deficiency		
Anterior pituitary	Hypopituitarism	GnRH deficiency
Hypothalamus and	Cranial diabetes	(Kallmann's
posterior pituitary	insipidus	syndrome)
Hormone resistance	Growth hormone	
	resistance (Laron	
	dwarfism)	
	Nephrogenic diabetes	
	insipidus	
Non-functioning tumours	Pituitary adenoma	
	Craniopharyngioma	
	Metastatic tumours	

20

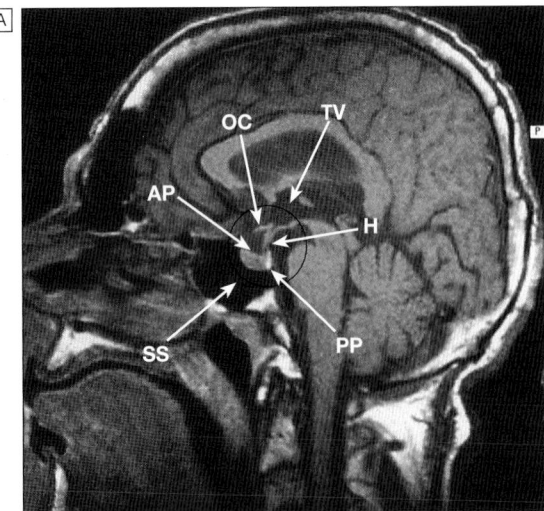

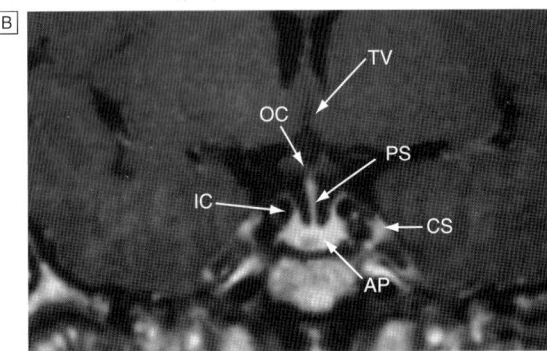

Fig. 20.27 Anatomical relationships of the normal pituitary gland and hypothalamus. See also Figure 20.2 (p. 735). **A** Sagittal MRI. **B** Coronal MRI. (AP = anterior pituitary; CS = cavernous sinus; H = hypothalamus; IC = internal carotid artery; OC = optic chiasm; PP = posterior pituitary; PS = pituitary stalk; SS = sphenoid sinus; TV = third ventricle)

Investigation of patients with pituitary disease

Although pituitary disease presents with diverse clinical manifestations (see below), the approach to investigation is similar in all cases (Box 20.56).

The approach to testing for hormone deficiency is outlined in Box 20.56. Details are given in the sections on individual glands elsewhere in this chapter. This approach has generally superseded the potentially hazardous 'combined pituitary function test', which involves simultaneous administration of thyrotrophin-releasing hormone (TRH), gonadotrophin-releasing hormone (GnRH) and insulin (to induce hypoglycaemic stress and stimulate ACTH and growth hormone secretion).

Tests for hormone excess vary according to the hormone in question. For example, prolactin is not secreted in pulsatile fashion, although it rises with significant psychological stress. Assuming that the patient was not distressed by venepuncture, a random measurement of serum prolactin is sufficient to diagnose hyperprolactinaemia. In contrast, growth hormone is secreted in a pulsatile fashion. A high random level does not confirm acromegaly; the diagnosis is only confirmed by failure of growth hormone to be suppressed (by the insulin-induced rise in insulin-like growth factor-1) during an oral glucose tolerance test. Similarly, in suspected ACTH-dependent Cushing's disease (p. 772), random measurement of plasma cortisol is unreliable and the diagnosis is usually made by a dexamethasone suppression test.

The most common local complication of a large pituitary tumour is compression of the optic pathway. The resulting visual field defect can be documented using a Goldman's perimetry chart.

MRI reveals 'abnormalities' of the pituitary gland in as many as 10% of 'healthy' middle-aged people. It should therefore be performed only if there is a clear biochemical abnormality or in a patient who presents with clinical features of pituitary tumour (see below). A pituitary tumour may be classified as either a macroadenoma (> 10 mm diameter) or a microadenoma (< 10 mm diameter). Microadenomas are not associated with hypopituitarism or compression of local structures and are only treated if they are secreting excess hormones.

Surgical biopsy is usually only performed as part of a therapeutic operation. Conventional histology identifies tumours as chromophobe (usually non-functioning), acidophil (typically prolactin- or growth hormone-

---

20.56 How to investigate patients with suspected pituitary hypothalamic disease

Identify pituitary hormone deficiency

ACTH deficiency
- Short ACTH stimulation test (see Box 20.46, p. 776)
- Insulin tolerance test (see Box 20.59, p. 786): only if uncertainty in interpretation of short ACTH stimulation test (e.g. acute presentation)

LH/FSH deficiency
- In the male, measure random serum testosterone, LH and FSH
- In the pre-menopausal female, ask if menses are regular
- In the post-menopausal female, measure random serum LH and FSH (which would normally be > 30 mU/L)

TSH deficiency
- Measure random serum T_4
- Note that TSH is often detectable in secondary hypothyroidism, due to inactive TSH isoforms in the blood

Growth hormone deficiency
Only investigate if growth hormone replacement therapy is being contemplated; p. 787
- Measure immediately after exercise
- Consider other stimulatory tests (Box 20.58, p. 786)

Cranial diabetes insipidus
Only investigate if patient complains of polyuria/polydipsia, which may be masked by ACTH or TSH deficiency
- Exclude other causes of polyuria with blood glucose, potassium and calcium measurements
- Water deprivation test (see Box 20.64, p. 793) or 5% saline infusion test

Identify hormone excess
- Measure random serum prolactin
- Investigate for acromegaly (glucose tolerance test) or Cushing's syndrome (p. 772) if there are clinical features

Establish the anatomy and diagnosis
- Consider visual field testing
- Image the pituitary and hypothalamus by MRI or CT

secreting) or basophil (typically ACTH-secreting); immunohistochemistry may confirm their secretory capacity but is poorly predictive of growth potential of the tumour.

Presenting problems in hypothalamic and pituitary disease

The clinical features of pituitary disease are shown in Figure 20.28. Younger women with pituitary disease most commonly present with secondary amenorrhoea (p. 756) or galactorrhoea (in hyperprolactinaemia). Postmenopausal women and men of any age are less likely to report symptoms of hypogonadism and so are more likely to present late with larger tumours causing visual field defects. Nowadays, many patients present with the incidental finding of a pituitary tumour on a CT or MRI scan.

Hypopituitarism

Hypopituitarism describes combined deficiency of any of the anterior pituitary hormones. The clinical presentation is variable and depends on the underlying lesion and the pattern of resulting hormone deficiency. The most common cause is a pituitary macroadenoma but other causes are listed in Box 20.57.

Clinical assessment

The presentation is highly variable. With progressive lesions of the pituitary there is a characteristic sequence of loss of pituitary hormone secretion. Growth hormone secretion is often the earliest to be lost. In adults, this produces lethargy, muscle weakness and increased fat mass, but these features are not obvious in isolation. Next, gonadotrophin (LH and FSH) secretion becomes impaired with, in the male, loss of libido and, in the female, oligomenorrhoea or amenorrhoea. Later, in the male there may be gynaecomastia and decreased frequency of shaving. In both sexes axillary and pubic hair eventually become sparse or even absent and the skin becomes characteristically finer and wrinkled. Chronic anaemia may also occur. The next hormone to be lost is usually ACTH, resulting in symptoms of cortisol insufficiency. In contrast to primary adrenal insufficiency (p. 774), angiotensin II-dependent zona glomerulosa function is not lost and hence aldosterone secretion maintains normal plasma potassium. However, there may be postural hypotension and a dilutional hyponatraemia for three reasons:

- Failure of vasoconstriction in the absence of cortisol results in pooling of blood in the legs on standing.
- Antidiuretic hormone (ADH) release is enhanced by hypotension and cortisol deficiency.
- Cortisol is required for normal water excretion by the kidney.

In contrast to the pigmentation of Addison's disease, a striking degree of pallor is usually present, principally because of lack of stimulation of melanocytes by β-lipotrophic hormone (β-LPH, a fragment of the ACTH precursor peptide) in the skin. Finally, TSH secretion is lost with consequent secondary hypothyroidism. This contributes further to apathy and cold intolerance. In contrast to primary hypothyroidism, frank myxoedema is rare, presumably because the thyroid retains some autonomous function. The onset of all of the above symptoms is notoriously insidious. However, patients sometimes

20

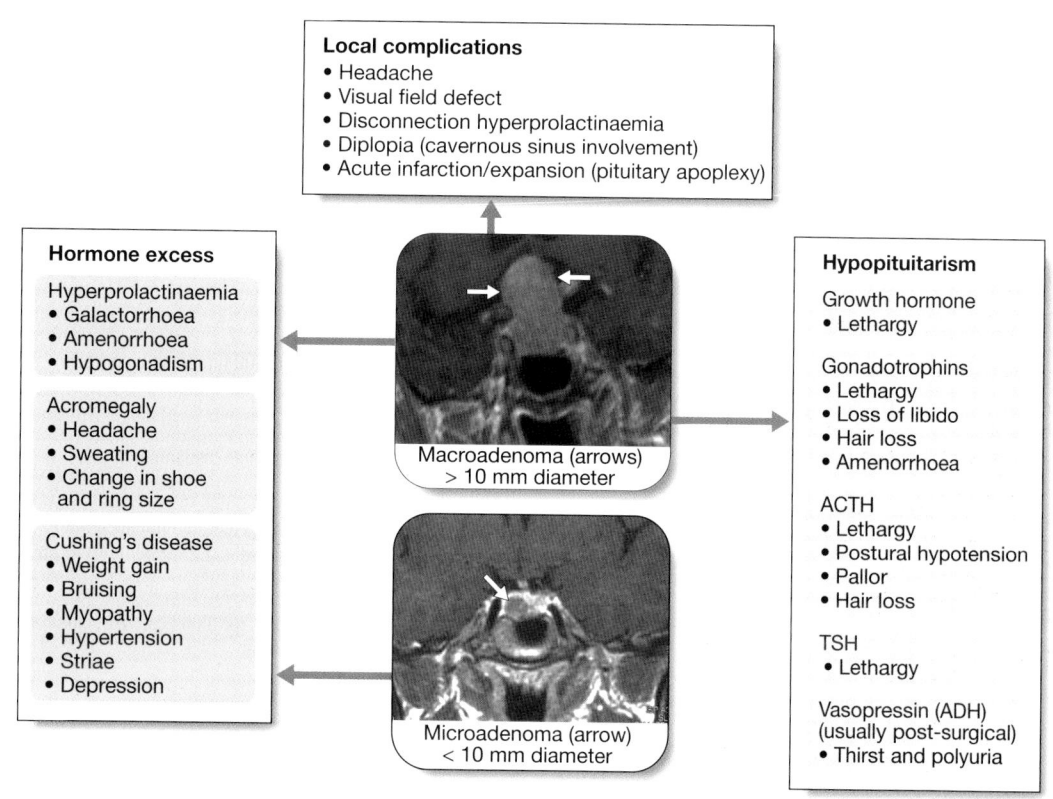

Local complications
- Headache
- Visual field defect
- Disconnection hyperprolactinaemia
- Diplopia (cavernous sinus involvement)
- Acute infarction/expansion (pituitary apoplexy)

Hormone excess

Hyperprolactinaemia
- Galactorrhoea
- Amenorrhoea
- Hypogonadism

Acromegaly
- Headache
- Sweating
- Change in shoe and ring size

Cushing's disease
- Weight gain
- Bruising
- Myopathy
- Hypertension
- Striae
- Depression

Macroadenoma (arrows)
> 10 mm diameter

Microadenoma (arrow)
< 10 mm diameter

Hypopituitarism

Growth hormone
- Lethargy

Gonadotrophins
- Lethargy
- Loss of libido
- Hair loss
- Amenorrhoea

ACTH
- Lethargy
- Postural hypotension
- Pallor
- Hair loss

TSH
- Lethargy

Vasopressin (ADH)
(usually post-surgical)
- Thirst and polyuria

Fig. 20.28 Common symptoms and signs to consider in a patient with suspected pituitary disease.

20.57 Causes of anterior pituitary hormone deficiency

Structural

- Primary pituitary tumour
  - Adenoma*
  - Carcinoma (exceptionally rare)
- Craniopharyngioma*
- Meningioma*
- Secondary tumour (including leukaemia and lymphoma)

- Chordoma
- Germinoma (pinealoma)
- Arachnoid cyst
- Rathke's cleft cyst
- Langerhans cell histiocytosis
- Haemorrhage (apoplexy)

Inflammatory/infiltrative

- Sarcoidosis
- Lymphocytic hypophysitis
- Haemochromatosis

- Infections, e.g. pituitary abscess, TB, syphilis, encephalitis

Congenital deficiencies

- GnRH (Kallmann's syndrome)*—gonadotrophin-releasing hormone
- GHRH*—growth hormone-releasing hormone

- TRH—thyrotrophin-releasing hormone
- CRH—corticotrophin-releasing hormone

Functional*

- Chronic systemic illness
- Anorexia nervosa

- Excessive exercise

Other

- Head injury*
- (Para-)sellar surgery*
- (Para-)sellar radiotherapy*

- Post-partum necrosis (Sheehan's syndrome)

*The most common causes of pituitary hormone deficiency.

present acutely unwell with glucocorticoid deficiency. This may be precipitated by a mild infection or injury, or may occur secondary to pituitary apoplexy (p. 787).

Other features of pituitary disease may be present (see Fig. 20.28).

Investigations

The strategy for investigation of pituitary disease is described in Box 20.56. In acutely unwell patients, the priority is to diagnose and treat cortisol deficiency (p. 774). Other tests can be undertaken later. Specific dynamic tests for diagnosing hormone deficiency are described in Boxes 20.46 (p. 776) and 20.58. More specialised biochemical tests, such as insulin tolerance tests (Box 20.59), GnRH and TRH tests, are rarely required. All patients with biochemical evidence of pituitary hormone deficiency should have an MRI or CT scan to identify pituitary or hypothalamic tumours. If a tumour is not identified, then further investigations are indicated to exclude infectious or infiltrative causes.

Management

Treatment of acutely ill patients is similar to that described for adrenocortical insufficiency on page 776, except that sodium depletion is not an important component to correct. Chronic hormone replacement therapies are described below. Once the cause of hypopituitarism is established, specific treatment—of a pituitary macroadenoma, for example (see below)—may be required.

Cortisol replacement

Hydrocortisone should be given if there is ACTH deficiency. Suitable doses are described in the section on adrenal disease on page 46. Mineralocorticoid replacement is not required.

Thyroid hormone replacement

Thyroxine 100–150 µg once daily should be given as described on page 742. Unlike in primary hypothyroidism, measuring TSH is not helpful in adjusting the replacement dose because patients with hypopituitarism often secrete glycoproteins which are measured in the TSH assays but are not bioactive. The aim is to maintain serum T_4 in the upper part of the reference

20.58 Tests of growth hormone secretion

GH levels are commonly undetectable, so a choice from the range of 'stimulation' tests is required*:

- 1 hour after going to sleep
- Frequent sampling during sleep
- Post-exercise
- Insulin-induced hypoglycaemia
- Arginine (may be combined with GHRH)
- Glucagon
- Clonidine

*In pre-pubertal patients, priming with sex steroid is required before 'stimulation' tests are performed.

20.59 How and when to do an insulin tolerance test

Use

- Assessment of the HPA axis
- Assessment of growth hormone deficiency
- Indicated when there is doubt after other tests in Box 20.56
- Usually performed in specialist centres, especially in children
- I.v. glucose and hydrocortisone must be available for resuscitation

Contraindications

- Ischaemic heart disease
- Epilepsy
- Severe hypopituitarism (0800 hrs plasma cortisol < 180 nmol/L (6.6 µg/dL))

Dose

- 0.15 U/kg body weight soluble insulin i.v.

Aim

- To produce adequate hypoglycaemia (tachycardia and sweating with blood glucose < 2.2 mmol/L (40 mg/dL))

Blood samples

- 0, 30, 45, 60, 90, 120 mins for blood glucose, plasma cortisol and growth hormone

Results

- Normal subjects GH > 6.7 µg/L (20 mU/L)*
- Normal subjects cortisol > 550 nmol/L (~20.2 µg/dL)*

*The precise cut-off figure for a satisfactory cortisol and GH response depends on the assay used and so varies between centres.

range. It is dangerous to give thyroid replacement to patients with adrenal insufficiency without first giving glucocorticoid therapy, since this may precipitate adrenal crisis.

Sex hormone replacement

This is indicated if there is gonadotrophin deficiency in men of any age and in women under the age of 50 to restore normal sexual function and to prevent osteoporosis (p. 1116).

Growth hormone replacement

Growth hormone (GH) is administered by daily subcutaneous self-injection to children and adolescents with GH deficiency and, until recently, was discontinued once the epiphyses had fused. However, although hypopituitary adults receiving 'full' replacement with hydrocortisone, thyroxine and sex steroids are usually much improved by these therapies, some individuals remain lethargic and unwell compared with a healthy population. Some of these patients feel better, and have objective improvements in their fat:muscle mass ratios and other metabolic parameters, if they are also given GH replacement. GH therapy may also help young adults to achieve a higher peak bone mineral density. The principal side-effect is sodium retention, manifest as peripheral oedema or carpal tunnel syndrome. For this reason, GH replacement should be started at a low dose, with monitoring of the response by measurement of serum insulin-like growth factor-1 (IGF-1) levels.

Pituitary tumour

Pituitary tumours produce a variety of mass effects, depending on their size and location, but also present as incidental findings on CT or MRI, or with hypopituitarism, as described above. A wide variety of disorders can present as mass lesions in or around the pituitary gland (see Box 20.57). Most intrasellar tumours are pituitary macroadenomas (most commonly non-functioning adenomas, Fig. 20.28), whereas the majority of suprasellar masses are craniopharyngiomas (see Fig. 20.32, p. 792). The most common cause of a parasellar mass is a meningioma.

Clinical assessment

Clinical features are shown in Figure 20.28. A common but non-specific presentation is with headache, which may be the consequence of stretching of the diaphragma sellae. Compression of the neural connections between the retina and occipital cortex may lead to a visual field defect. Although the classical abnormalities associated with compression of the optic chiasm are bitemporal hemianopia (see Fig. 20.29) or upper quadrantanopia, any type of visual field defect can result from suprasellar extension of a tumour because it may compress the optic nerve (unilateral loss of acuity or scotoma) or the optic tract (homonymous hemianopia). Optic atrophy may be apparent on ophthalmoscopy. Lateral extension of a sellar mass into the cavernous sinus with subsequent compression of the 3rd, 4th or 6th cranial nerves may cause diplopia and strabismus.

Occasionally, pituitary tumours infarct or there is bleeding into cystic lesions. This is termed 'pituitary apoplexy' and may result in sudden expansion with local compression symptoms and acute-onset

hypopituitarism. Non-haemorrhagic infarction can also occur in a normal pituitary gland; predisposing factors include obstetric haemorrhage (Sheehan's syndrome), diabetes mellitus and raised intracranial pressure.

Investigations

Patients suspected of having a pituitary tumour should undergo MRI or CT. Whilst some lesions have distinctive neuroradiological features, definitive diagnosis often requires biopsy which is usually done at the same time as operative treatment to resect or debulk a tumour that is compressing the optic chiasm. All patients with (para-) sellar space-occupying lesions should have pituitary function assessed as described in Box 20.56 (p. 784).

Management

Modalities of treatment of common pituitary and hypothalamic tumours are shown in Box 20.60. Associated hypopituitarism should be treated as described above.

Urgent treatment is required if there is evidence of pressure on visual pathways. The chances of recovery of a visual field defect are proportional to the duration of symptoms, with full recovery unlikely if the defect has been present for longer than 4 months. It is crucial that serum prolactin is measured before emergency surgery is performed. If the prolactin is > 5000 mU/L, then the lesion may be a macroprolactinoma and a therapeutic trial of a dopamine agonist for just a few days may successfully shrink the lesion and make surgery unnecessary (see Fig. 20.29).

Most operations on the pituitary are performed using the trans-sphenoidal approach via the nostrils, while transfrontal surgery via a craniotomy is reserved for suprasellar tumours. It is uncommon to be able to resect large lesions completely, particularly if there is lateral extension into the cavernous sinuses. All operations on the pituitary carry a risk of damaging normal endocrine function; this risk increases with the size of the primary lesion.

Pituitary function (see Box 20.56, p. 784) should be retested 4–6 weeks following surgery, primarily to detect the development of any new hormone deficits. Rarely, the surgical treatment of a sellar lesion can result in recovery of hormone secretion that was deficient pre-operatively.

Following surgery, imaging should be repeated, usually after a few months and, if there is any residual mass and the histology confirms a radiosensitive tumour, external radiotherapy may be given to reduce the risk of recurrence. Radiotherapy is not useful in patients requiring urgent therapy because it takes many months or years to be effective and there is a risk of acute swelling of the mass. Radiotherapy carries a life-long risk of hypopituitarism (50–70% in the first 10 years) and annual pituitary function tests are obligatory. There is also concern that radiotherapy might impair cognitive function, cause vascular changes and even induce primary brain tumours, but these side-effects have not been quantified reliably and are likely to be rare.

Non-functioning tumours should be followed up by repeated imaging at intervals that depend on the size of the lesion and on whether or not radiotherapy has been administered. For smaller lesions that are not causing mass effects, therapeutic surgery may not be indicated and the lesion may simply be monitored by serial

20.60 Therapeutic modalities for hypothalamic and pituitary tumours

	Surgery	Radiotherapy	Medical	Comment
Non-functioning pituitary macroadenoma	1st line	2nd line	–	
Prolactinoma	2nd line	2nd line	1st line Dopamine agonists	Dopamine agonists usually cause macroadenomas to shrink
Acromegaly	1st line	2nd line	2nd line Somatostatin analogues Dopamine agonists GH receptor antagonists	Medical therapy does not reliably cause macroadenomas to shrink Radiotherapy and medical therapy are used in combination for inoperable tumours
Cushing's disease	1st line	2nd line	–	Radiotherapy is used in children and to prevent Nelson's syndrome
Craniopharyngioma	1st line	2nd line	–	

neuroimaging without a clear-cut diagnosis having been established.

Hyperprolactinaemia/galactorrhoea

Hyperprolactinaemia is a common abnormality which usually presents with hypogonadism and/or galactorrhoea (lactation in the absence of breastfeeding). Since prolactin stimulates milk secretion but not breast development, galactorrhoea rarely occurs in men and only does so if gynaecomastia has been induced by hypogonadism (p. 759). The differential diagnosis of hyperprolactinaemia is shown in Box 20.61. Many drugs, especially dopamine antagonists, elevate prolactin concentrations. Pituitary tumours can cause hyperprolactinaemia by directly secreting prolactin (prolactinomas, see below), or by compressing the infundibular stalk and thus interrupting the tonic inhibitory effect of hypothalamic dopamine on prolactin secretion ('disconnection' hyperprolactinaemia).

Prolactin usually circulates as a free (monomeric) hormone in plasma, but in some individuals prolactin becomes bound to an IgG antibody. This complex is known as macroprolactin and such patients have macroprolactinaemia (not to be confused with macroprolactinoma, a prolactin-secreting pituitary tumour > 1 cm in diameter). Since macroprolactin cannot cross blood vessel walls to reach prolactin receptors in target tissues it is of no pathological significance. Some commercial prolactin assays do not distinguish prolactin from macroprolactin and so macroprolactinaemia is a cause of spurious hyperprolactinaemia. Identification of macroprolactin requires gel filtration chromatography or polyethylene glycol precipitation techniques and one of these tests should be performed in all patients with hyperprolactinaemia, if the prolactin assay is known to cross-react.

Clinical assessment

In women, in addition to galactorrhoea, hypogonadism associated with hyperprolactinaemia causes secondary amenorrhoea and anovulation with infertility (p. 756). Important points in the history include drug use, recent pregnancy and menstrual history. The quantity of milk produced is variable, and it may be observed

20.61 Causes of hyperprolactinaemia

Physiological

- Stress (e.g. post-seizure)
- Pregnancy
- Lactation
- Nipple stimulation
- Sleep
- Coitus
- Exercise
- Baby crying

Drug-induced

Dopamine antagonists
- Antipsychotics (phenothiazines and butyrophenones)
- Antidepressants
- Antiemetics (e.g. metoclopramide, domperidone)

Dopamine-depleting drugs
- Reserpine
- Methyldopa

Oestrogens
- Oral contraceptive pill

Pathological

Common
- Disconnection hyperprolactinaemia (e.g. non-functioning pituitary macroadenoma)
- Prolactinoma (usually microadenoma)
- Primary hypothyroidism
- Polycystic ovarian syndrome
- Macroprolactinaemia

Uncommon
- Hypothalamic disease
- Renal failure
- Pituitary tumour secreting prolactin and growth hormone

Rare
- Chest wall reflex (e.g. post-herpes zoster)
- Ectopic source

only by manual expression. In men there is decreased libido, reduced shaving frequency and lethargy (p. 757). Unilateral galactorrhoea may be confused with nipple discharge, and careful breast examination to exclude malignancy or fibrocystic disease is important. Further assessment should address the features in Figure 20.28 (p. 785).

Investigations

Pregnancy should first be excluded before further investigations are performed in women of child-bearing potential. The upper limit of normal for many assays of serum prolactin is approximately 500 mU/L (14 ng/mL). In non-pregnant and non-lactating patients, monomeric prolactin concentrations of 500–1000 mU/L are likely to be induced by stress or drugs, and a repeat measurement is indicated. Levels between 1000 and 5000 mU/L are likely to be due to either drugs, a microprolactinoma or 'disconnection' hyperprolactinaemia. Levels above 5000 mU/L are highly suggestive of a macroprolactinoma.

Patients with prolactin excess should have tests of gonadal function (p. 753), and T_4 and TSH measured to exclude primary hypothyroidism causing TRH-induced prolactin excess. Unless the prolactin falls after withdrawal of relevant drug therapy, a serum prolactin of > 1000 mU/L is an indication for MRI or CT scan of the hypothalamus and pituitary. Patients with a macroadenoma also need tests for hypopituitarism (see Box 20.56).

Management

If possible, the underlying cause should be corrected (for example, cessation of offending drugs and giving thyroxine replacement in primary hypothyroidism). If this is not possible, then in almost all cases of hyperprolactinaemia, dopamine agonist therapy (see Box 20.62) will normalise prolactin levels with return of gonadal function. If gonadal function does not return despite effective lowering of prolactin, then there may be associated gonadotrophin deficiency or, in the female, the onset of the menopause. Troublesome physiological galactorrhoea can also be treated with dopamine agonists. Management of prolactinomas is described below.

Prolactinoma

Most prolactinomas in pre-menopausal women are microadenomas because the symptoms of prolactin excess usually result in early presentation. In men and post-menopausal women, however, the presentation is often much more insidious and due to mass effects rather than hyperprolactinaemia, with the result that these tumours are almost invariably macroadenomas at the time of diagnosis. Prolactin-secreting cells of the anterior pituitary share a common lineage with growth hormone-secreting cells, so occasionally prolactinomas can secrete excess growth hormone and cause acromegaly. In prolactinomas there is a relationship between prolactin concentration and tumour size: the higher the level, the bigger the tumour. Some macroprolactinomas can elevate prolactin concentrations > 100 000 mU/L. The investigation of prolactinomas is the same as for other pituitary tumours (see above).

Management

As shown in Box 20.60, several therapeutic modalities can be employed in the management of prolactinomas.

Medical

Dopamine agonist drugs are first-line therapy for the majority of patients (Box 20.62). They usually reduce serum prolactin concentrations and cause significant tumour shrinkage (Fig. 20.29). It is possible to withdraw dopamine agonist therapy without recurrence of hyperprolactinaemia after a few years of treatment in some patients with a microadenoma. Also, after the menopause, suppression of prolactin is only required in microadenomas if galactorrhoea is troublesome, since hypogonadism is then physiological and tumour growth unlikely. In patients with macroadenomas, drugs can only be withdrawn after curative surgery or radiotherapy and under close supervision.

Ergot-derived dopamine agonists (bromocriptine and cabergoline) can bind to 5-HT$_{2B}$ receptors in the heart and elsewhere and have been associated with fibrotic reactions, particularly tricuspid valve regurgitation, in

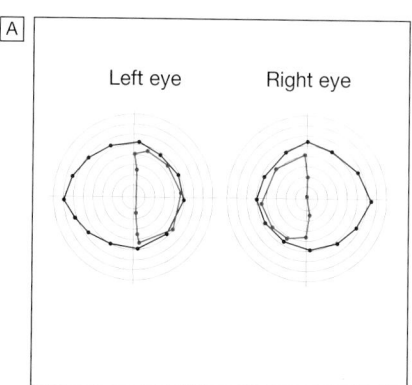

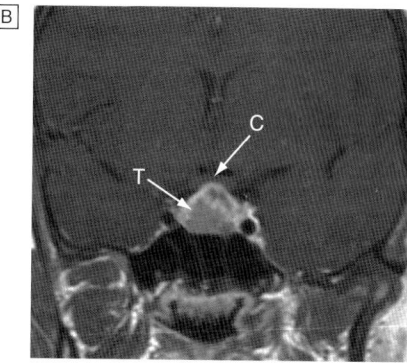

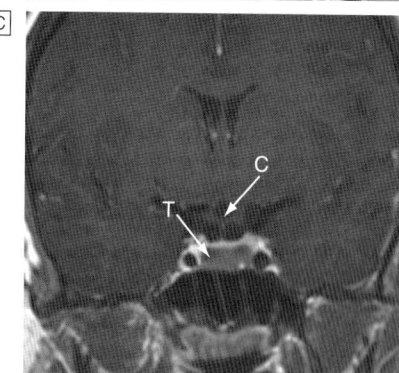

Fig. 20.29 Visual field defect in a patient with a macroprolactinoma and shrinkage of tumour following treatment with a dopamine agonist. [A] Goldmann visual field chart showing normal visual fields (black) and bitemporal hemianopia (red) in a patient with hyperprolactinaemia. [B] MRI scan showing a pituitary macroadenoma (T) compressing the optic chiasm (C). [C] MRI scan of the same tumour following treatment with a dopamine agonist. The macroadenoma, which was a prolactinoma, has decreased in size substantially and is no longer compressing the optic chiasm.

20

20.62	Dopamine agonist therapy: drugs used to treat prolactinomas		
	Oral dose*	**Advantages**	**Disadvantages**
Bromocriptine	2.5–15 mg/day 8–12-hourly	Available for parenteral use Short half-life; useful in treating infertility Proven long-term efficacy	Ergotamine-like side-effects (nausea, headache, postural hypotension, constipation) Frequent dosing so poor compliance Rare reports of fibrotic reactions in various tissues
Cabergoline	250–1000 µg/week 2 doses/week	Long-acting, so missed doses less important Reported to have fewer ergotamine-like side-effects	Limited data on safety in pregnancy Associated with cardiac valvular fibrosis in Parkinson's disease
Quinagolide	50–150 µg/day Once daily	A non-ergot with few side-effects in patients intolerant of the above	Untested in pregnancy

*Tolerance develops for the side-effects. All of these agents, especially bromocriptine, must be introduced at low dose and increased slowly. If several doses of bromocriptine are missed, the process must start again.

patients with Parkinson's disease and, less commonly, prolactinoma. At the relatively low doses used in prolactinomas it is uncertain whether systematic screening for cardiac fibrosis is required, but if dopamine agonist therapy is prolonged many authorities recommend periodic screening by echocardiography or use of non-ergot agents (quinagolide).

Surgery and radiotherapy

Surgical decompression is usually only necessary when a macroprolactinoma has failed to shrink sufficiently with dopamine agonist therapy and this may be because the tumour has a significant cystic component. Surgery may also be performed in patients who are intolerant of dopamine agonists. Microadenomas can be removed selectively by trans-sphenoidal surgery with a cure rate of about 80%; the cure rate for surgery in macroadenomas is substantially lower.

External irradiation may be required for some macroadenomas to prevent regrowth if dopamine agonists are stopped.

Pregnancy

Hyperprolactinaemia often presents with infertility, so dopamine agonist therapy may be followed by pregnancy. Patients with microadenomas should be advised to withdraw dopamine agonist therapy as soon as pregnancy is confirmed. In contrast, macroprolactinomas may enlarge rapidly under oestrogen stimulation and these patients should continue dopamine agonist therapy and need measurement of prolactin levels and visual fields during pregnancy. All patients should be advised to report headache or visual disturbance promptly.

Acromegaly

Acromegaly is caused by growth hormone (GH) secretion from a pituitary tumour, usually a macroadenoma.

Clinical features

If GH hypersecretion occurs before puberty then the presentation is with gigantism. More commonly, GH excess occurs in adult life and presents with acromegaly. If hypersecretion starts in adolescence and persists into adult life, then the two conditions may be combined. The clinical features are shown in Figure 20.30.

The most common complaints are headache and sweating. Additional features include those of any pituitary tumour (see Fig. 20.28, p. 785).

Investigations

The clinical diagnosis must be confirmed by measuring GH levels during an oral glucose tolerance test (Fig. 20.31). In normal subjects, plasma GH suppresses to below 0.5 µg/L (approximately 2 mU/L). In acromegaly, GH does not suppress and in about 50% of patients there is a paradoxical rise. The rest of pituitary function should be investigated as described in Box 20.56 (p. 784). Prolactin concentrations are elevated in about 30% of patients due to co-secretion of prolactin from the tumour.

The diagnosis of acromegaly is more difficult in patients with insulin deficiency, either type 1 or long-standing type 2 diabetes mellitus. GH may fail to suppress following a glucose load in these patients because inadequate insulin secretion results in failure of glucose to stimulate IGF-1 from the liver. It is IGF-1 that, in turn, suppresses GH secretion. This is important because acromegaly can cause diabetes mellitus by exacerbating insulin resistance. However, measuring IGF-1 usually resolves matters; in diabetic patients without acromegaly, IGF-1 concentrations are low, while in acromegalic patients IGF-1 levels are high.

Additional tests in acromegaly may include screening for colonic neoplasms with colonoscopy.

Management

This is summarised in Box 20.60.

Surgical

Trans-sphenoidal surgery is usually the first line of treatment and may result in cure of GH excess, especially in patients with microadenomas. More often, surgery serves to debulk the tumour and further second-line therapy is required, according to post-operative imaging and glucose tolerance test results.

Radiotherapy

External radiotherapy is usually employed as second-line treatment if acromegaly persists after surgery, to stop tumour growth and lower GH levels. However, GH levels fall slowly (over many years) and there is a risk of hypopituitarism.

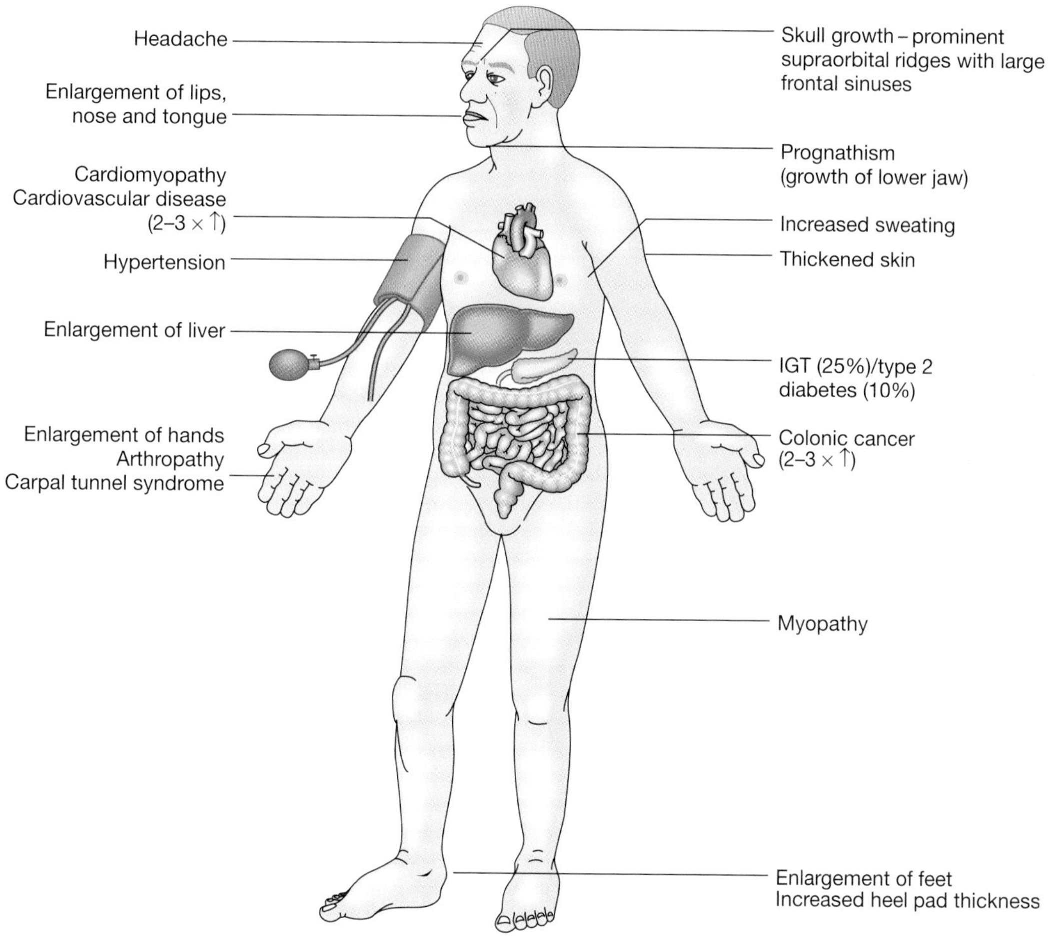

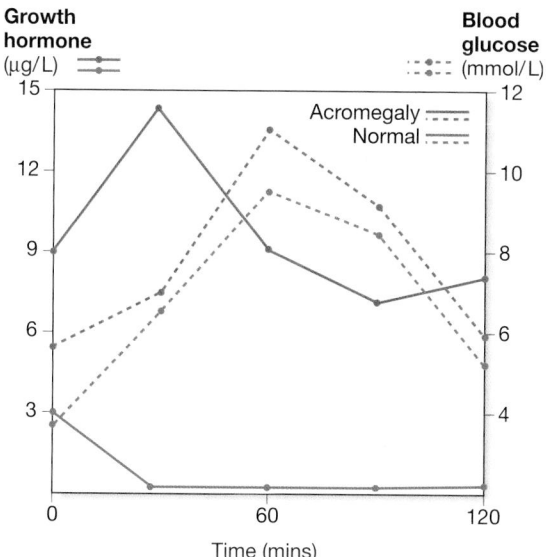

Headache
Enlargement of lips, nose and tongue
Cardiomyopathy
Cardiovascular disease (2–3 × ↑)
Hypertension
Enlargement of liver
Enlargement of hands
Arthropathy
Carpal tunnel syndrome
Skull growth – prominent supraorbital ridges with large frontal sinuses
Prognathism (growth of lower jaw)
Increased sweating
Thickened skin
IGT (25%)/type 2 diabetes (10%)
Colonic cancer (2–3 × ↑)
Myopathy
Enlargement of feet
Increased heel pad thickness

Fig. 20.30 Clinical features of acromegaly. (IGT = impaired glucose tolerance)

Growth hormone (μg/L)
Blood glucose (mmol/L)
15
12
9
6
3
12
10
8
6
4
Acromegaly
Normal
0
60
120
Time (mins)

Fig. 20.31 Oral glucose tolerance tests in a normal subject and a patient with acromegaly with measurement of blood glucose and plasma growth hormone. Note the suppression of growth hormone secretion to < 0.5 μg/L in the normal subject, and failure to suppress (sometimes accompanied by paradoxical elevation) in acromegaly. Glucose tolerance may also be impaired in acromegaly. (To convert GH in μg/L to mU/L multiply by 3. To convert glucose in mmol/L to mg/dL multiply by 18.)

Medical

In patients with persisting acromegaly after surgery, medical therapy is usually employed to lower GH levels to < 1.5 μg/L (approximately < 5 mU/L) and to normalise IGF-1 concentrations. Medical therapy may be discontinued after several years in patients who have received radiotherapy. Somatostatin analogues (such as octreotide or lanreotide) can be administered as slow-release injections every few weeks. Somatostatin analogues can also be used as primary therapy for acromegaly either as an alternative or in advance of surgery, given evidence that they can induce modest tumour shrinkage in a proportion of patients. Dopamine agonists are less potent in lowering GH but may be helpful, especially in patients with associated prolactin excess. Pegvisomant is a peptide GH receptor antagonist which is administered by daily self-injection and may be indicated in some patients whose GH and IGF-1 concentrations fail to suppress sufficiently following somatostatin analogue therapy.

Craniopharyngioma

Craniopharyngiomas are benign tumours that develop in cell rests of Rathke's pouch, and may be located within the sella turcica, or commonly in the suprasellar

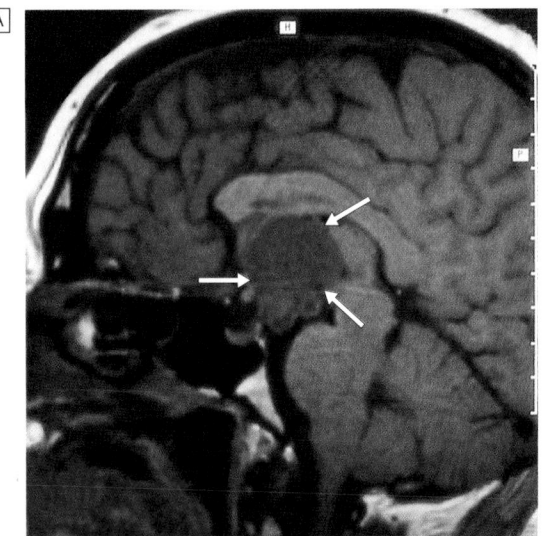

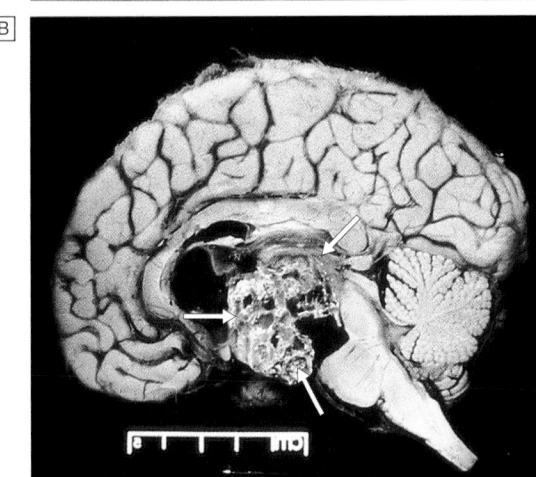

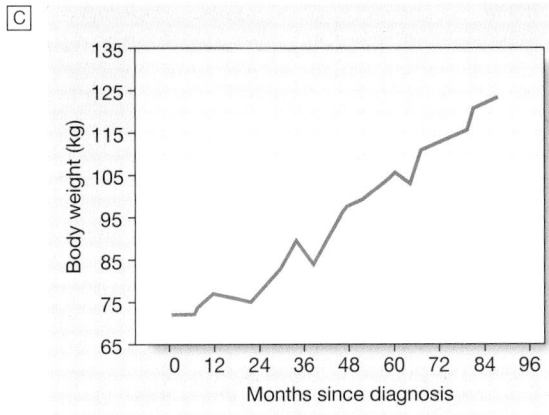

Fig 20.32 Craniopharyngioma. **A** This developmental tumour characteristically presents in younger patients; it is often cystic and calcified, as shown in this MRI scan (arrows). **B** Pathology specimen. **C** Hypothalamic damage is manifest as diabetes insipidus and loss of satiety, leading to relentless weight gain, as in this young woman following successful surgical resection and irradiation of her craniopharyngioma.

space. They are often cystic with a solid component that may or may not be calcified (Fig. 20.32). In young people, they are diagnosed more commonly than pituitary adenomas. They may present with pressure effects on adjacent structures, hypopituitarism and/or cranial diabetes insipidus. In addition, other clinical features that are directly related to hypothalamic damage may also occur. These include hyperphagia and obesity (see Fig. 20.32C), loss of the sensation of thirst and disturbance of temperature regulation.

Craniopharyngiomas can rarely be reached by the trans-sphenoidal route and so surgery may involve a craniotomy, with a relatively high risk of hypothalamic damage and other complications. If the tumour has a large cystic component it may be safer to place in the cyst cavity a drain which is attached to a subcutaneous access device, rather than attempt a resection. Whatever form it takes, surgery is unlikely to be curative and radiotherapy is usually given, although there is uncertainty about its efficacy. Unfortunately, craniopharyngiomas often recur, requiring repeated surgery. They often cause considerable morbidity, usually from hypothalamic obesity, water balance problems and/or visual failure.

Diabetes insipidus

This uncommon disorder is characterised by the persistent excretion of excessive quantities of dilute urine and by thirst. Diabetes insipidus is classified into two types:

- cranial diabetes insipidus, in which there is deficient production of ADH by the hypothalamus
- nephrogenic diabetes insipidus, in which the renal tubules are unresponsive to ADH.

The underlying causes are listed in Box 20.63.

20.63 Causes of diabetes insipidus

Cranial

Structural hypothalamic or high stalk lesion
- See Box 20.57

Idiopathic

Genetic defect
- Dominant (AVP gene mutation)
- Recessive (DIDMOAD syndrome—association of diabetes insipidus with diabetes mellitus, optic atrophy, deafness)

Nephrogenic

Genetic defect
- V2 receptor mutation
- Aquaporin-2 mutation
- Cystinosis

Metabolic abnormality
- Hypokalaemia
- Hypercalcaemia

Drug therapy
- Lithium
- Demeclocycline

Poisoning
- Heavy metals

Chronic kidney disease
- Polycystic kidney disease
- Sickle-cell anaemia
- Infiltrative disease

Clinical features

The most marked symptoms are polyuria and polydipsia. The patient may pass 5–20 L or more of urine in 24 hours. This is of low specific gravity and osmolality. If the patient has an intact thirst mechanism, is conscious and has access to oral fluids, then he or she can maintain adequate fluid intake. However, in an unconscious patient or a patient with damage to the hypothalamic thirst centre, diabetes insipidus is potentially lethal. If there is associated cortisol deficiency, then diabetes insipidus may not be manifest until glucocorticoid replacement therapy is given. The most common differential diagnosis is primary polydipsia, caused by drinking excessive amounts of fluid in the absence of a defect in ADH or thirst control.

Investigations

Diabetes insipidus can be confirmed if serum ADH is undetectable or the urine is not maximally concentrated (i.e. is < 600 mOsm/kg) in the presence of increased plasma osmolality (i.e. > 300 mOsm/kg). Sometimes, the diagnosis can be confirmed or refuted by random simultaneous samples of blood and urine, but more often a dynamic test is required. The water deprivation test described in Box 20.64 is widely used, but an alternative is to infuse hypertonic (5%) saline and measure ADH secretion in response to increasing plasma osmolality. Thirst can also be assessed during these tests on a visual analogue scale. Anterior pituitary function and suprasellar anatomy should be assessed in patients with cranial diabetes insipidus as indicated in Box 20.56 (p. 784).

20.64 How and when to do a water deprivation test

Use

- To establish a diagnosis of diabetes insipidus, and differentiate cranial from nephrogenic causes

Protocol

- No coffee, tea or smoking on the test day
- Free fluids until 0730 hrs on the morning of the test, but discourage patients from 'stocking up' with extra fluid in anticipation of fluid deprivation
- No fluids from 0730 hrs
- Attend at 0830 hrs for body weight, plasma and urine osmolality
- Record body weight, urine volume, urine and plasma osmolality and thirst score on a visual analogue scale every 2 hrs for up to 8 hrs
- Stop the test if the patient loses 3% of body weight
- If plasma osmolality reaches > 300 mOsm/kg and urine osmolality < 600 mOsm/kg, then administer DDAVP (see text) 2 μg i.m.

Interpretation

- Diabetes insipidus is confirmed by a plasma osmolality > 300 mOsm/kg with a urine osmolality < 600 mOsm/kg
- Cranial diabetes insipidus is confirmed if urine osmolality rises by at least 50% after DDAVP
- Nephrogenic diabetes insipidus is confirmed if DDAVP does not concentrate the urine
- Primary polydipsia is suggested by low plasma osmolality at the start of the test

---

20.65 The pituitary and hypothalamus in old age

- **Late presentation**: often with large tumours causing visual disturbance, because early symptoms such as amenorrhoea and sexual dysfunction do not occur or are not recognised.
- **Coincidentally discovered pituitary tumours**: may not require surgical intervention if the visual apparatus is not involved, because of slow growth. Radiotherapy alone is sometimes employed simply to prevent further growth.
- **Hyperprolactinaemia**: less impact in post-menopausal women who are already 'physiologically' hypogonadal. Macroprolactinomas, however, require treatment because of their potential to cause mass effects.

In primary polydipsia, the urine may be excessively dilute because of chronic diuresis which 'washes out' the solute gradient across the loop of Henle, but plasma osmolality is low rather than high. DDAVP (see below) should not be administered to patients with primary polydipsia, since it will prevent excretion of water and risks severe water intoxication if the patient continues to drink fluid to excess.

In nephrogenic diabetes insipidus appropriate further tests include plasma electrolytes, calcium and investigation of the renal tract (Chs 16 and 17).

Management

Treatment of cranial diabetes insipidus is with desamino-des-aspartate-arginine vasopressin (desmopressin, DDAVP), an analogue of ADH which has a longer half-life. DDAVP is usually administered intranasally. An oral formulation is also available but bioavailability is low and rather unpredictable. In sick patients, DDAVP should be given by intramuscular injection. The dose of DDAVP should be adjusted on the basis of serum sodium concentrations and/or osmolality. The principal hazard should be excessive treatment resulting in water intoxication and hyponatraemia. Conversely, inadequate treatment results in thirst and polyuria. The ideal dose prevents nocturia but allows a degree of polyuria from time to time before the next dose (e.g. DDAVP nasal dose 5 μg in the morning and 10 μg at night).

The polyuria in nephrogenic diabetes insipidus is improved by thiazide diuretics (e.g. bendroflumethiazide 5–10 mg/day), amiloride (5–10 mg/day) and NSAIDs (e.g. indometacin 15 mg 8-hourly), although the last of these carries a risk of reducing glomerular filtration rate.

DISEASES AFFECTING MULTIPLE ENDOCRINE GLANDS

Multiple endocrine neoplasia (MEN)

These rare autosomal dominant syndromes are characterised by hyperplasia and formation of adenomas or malignant tumours in multiple glands. They fall into two groups, as shown in Box 20.66. Some other genetic diseases also have an increased risk of endocrine tumours; for example, phaeochromocytoma is associated with von Hippel–Lindau syndrome (p. 1219) and neurofibromatosis type 1 (p. 1218).

20.66 Multiple endocrine neoplasia (MEN) syndromes

MEN 1 (Wermer's syndrome)

- Primary hyperparathyroidism
- Pituitary tumours
- Pancreatic neuro-endocrine tumours (insulinoma, gastrinoma)

MEN 2 (Sipple's syndrome)

- Primary hyperparathyroidism
- Medullary carcinoma of thyroid
- Phaeochromocytoma

In addition, in MEN 2b syndrome there are phenotypic changes (including marfanoid habitus, skeletal abnormalities, abnormal dental enamel, multiple mucosal neuromas)

20.67 Autoimmune polyendocrine syndromes (APS)*

Type 1 (APECED)

- Addison's disease
- Hypoparathyroidism
- Type 1 diabetes
- Primary hypothyroidism
- Chronic mucocutaneous candidiasis
- Nail dystrophy
- Dental enamel hypoplasia

Type 2 (Schmidt's syndrome)

- Addison's disease
- Primary hypothyroidism
- Graves' disease
- Pernicious anaemia
- Primary hypogonadism
- Type 1 diabetes
- Vitiligo
- Coeliac disease
- Myasthenia gravis

*In both types of APS, the precise pattern of disease varies between affected individuals.

MEN syndromes should be considered in all patients with two or more endocrine tumours and in patients with solitary tumours who report other endocrine tumours in their family. MEN 1 results from inactivating mutations in *MENIN*, a tumour suppressor gene on chromosome 11, whereas MEN 2 is caused by mutations in the *RET* proto-oncogene on chromosome 10. This causes constitutive activation of the membrane-associated tyrosine kinase RET, which controls the development of cells that migrate from the neural crest. Different mutations causing loss of function of the RET kinase are associated with Hirschsprung's disease (p. 914). Genetic testing can be performed on relatives of affected individuals, after appropriate counselling (p. 64).

Individuals who carry mutations associated with MEN should be entered into a surveillance programme. In MEN 1, this typically involves annual history, examination and measurements of serum calcium, gastrointestinal hormones (see Box 20.53, p. 782) and prolactin; MRI of the pituitary is performed at less frequent intervals. In individuals with MEN 2, annual history, examination and measurement of serum calcium and urinary catecholamine metabolites should be performed. Because the penetrance of medullary carcinoma of the thyroid is 100% in individuals with a *RET* mutation, prophylactic thyroidectomy should be performed in early childhood.

Autoimmune polyendocrine syndromes (APS)

Two distinct autoimmune polyendocrine syndromes are known: APS types 1 and 2.

The most common is APS type 2 (Schmidt's syndrome) which typically presents in women between the ages of 20 and 60. It is usually defined as the occurrence in the same individual of two or more autoimmune endocrine disorders, some of which are listed in Box 20.67. The mode of inheritance is autosomal dominant with incomplete penetrance and there is a strong association with HLA-DR3 and CTLA-4. APS type 2 may be further subdivided, depending on the precise combination of endocrine disorders observed, but this is of limited value.

APS type 1, which is also termed autoimmune polyendocrinopathy-candidiasis-ectodermal dystrophy (APECED), is much rarer and is inherited in an autosomal recessive fashion. It is caused by mutations in the autoimmune regulator gene (*AIRE*). *AIRE* is responsible for the presentation of self-antigens to thymocytes in utero, which is essential for the deletion of thymocyte clones that react against self-antigens and hence for the development of immune tolerance (Ch. 4). The most common clinical features are described in Box 20.67, although the pattern of presentation is variable and other autoimmune disorders are often observed.

Further information

www.british-thyroid-association.org *British Thyroid Association: provider of guidelines, e.g. for use of thyroid function tests.*

www.endocrinology.org *British Society for Endocrinology: useful online education resources and links to patient-support group.*

www.endo-society.org *American Endocrine Society: provider of clinical practice guidelines.*

www.pituitary.org.uk *Pituitary Foundation: an excellent resource for patient and general practitioner leaflets and further information.*

B.M. Frier
M. Fisher

Diabetes mellitus

21

CLINICAL EXAMINATION OF THE PATIENT WITH DIABETES

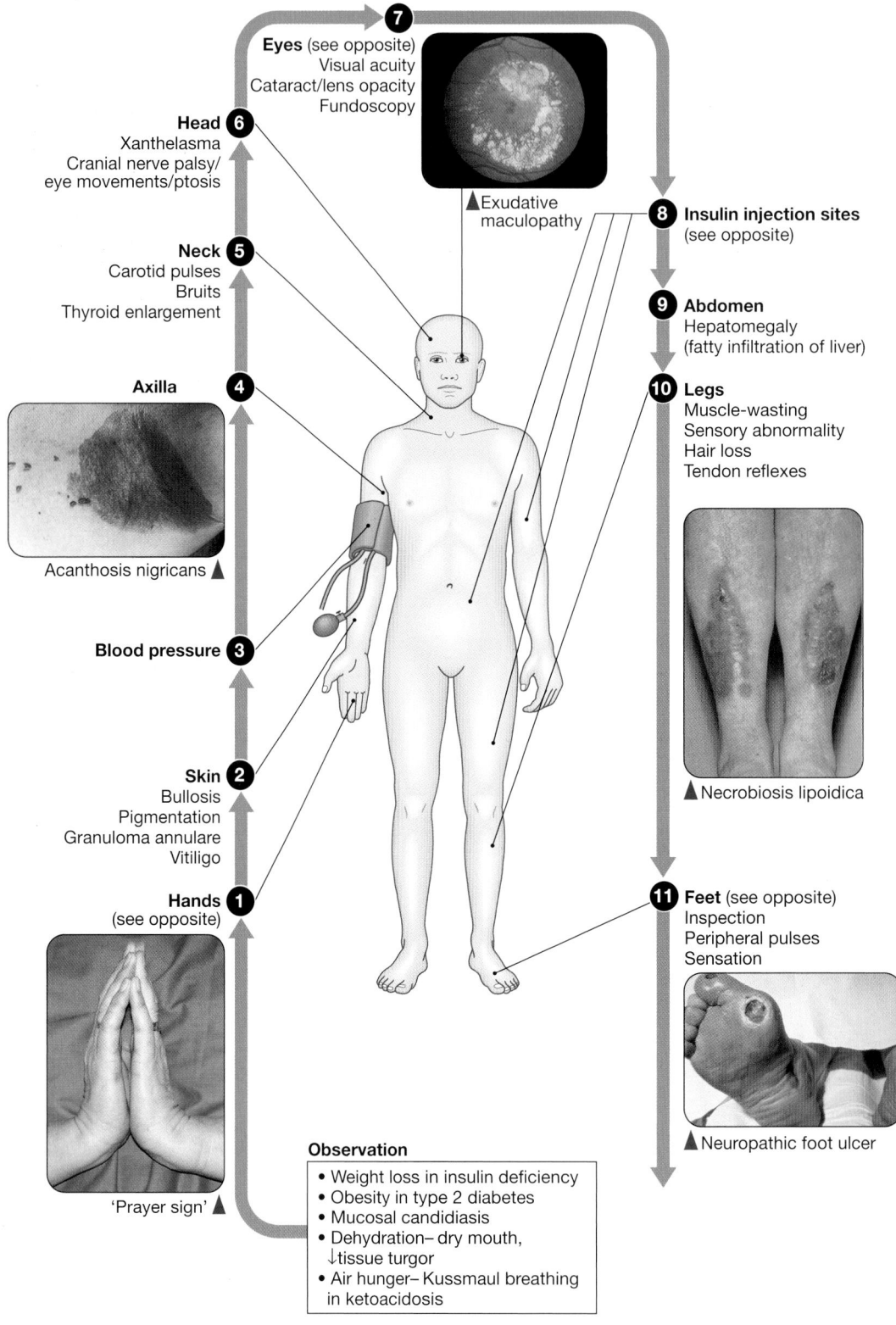

7 Eyes (see opposite)
Visual acuity
Cataract/lens opacity
Fundoscopy

▲Exudative maculopathy

Head 6
Xanthelasma
Cranial nerve palsy/
eye movements/ptosis

8 Insulin injection sites
(see opposite)

Neck 5
Carotid pulses
Bruits
Thyroid enlargement

9 Abdomen
Hepatomegaly
(fatty infiltration of liver)

Axilla 4

10 Legs
Muscle-wasting
Sensory abnormality
Hair loss
Tendon reflexes

Acanthosis nigricans ▲

Blood pressure 3

▲ Necrobiosis lipoidica

Skin 2
Bullosis
Pigmentation
Granuloma annulare
Vitiligo

Hands 1
(see opposite)

11 Feet (see opposite)
Inspection
Peripheral pulses
Sensation

▲Neuropathic foot ulcer

'Prayer sign' ▲

Observation

- Weight loss in insulin deficiency
- Obesity in type 2 diabetes
- Mucosal candidiasis
- Dehydration– dry mouth,
  ↓tissue turgor
- Air hunger– Kussmaul breathing
  in ketoacidosis

Diabetes can affect every system in the body. In routine clinical practice, examination of the patient with diabetes is focused on **1** hands, **3** blood pressure, **7** eyes, **8** insulin injection sites and **11** feet.

7 Examination of the eyes

Visual acuity

- Distance vision using Snellen chart at 6 metres
- Near vision using standard reading chart

Impaired visual acuity may indicate diabetic eye disease, including maculopathy, and serial decline suggests development or deterioration

Lens opacification

- Look for the red reflex using the ophthalmoscope held 30 cm from the eye

Fundal examination

- Dilate pupils with a mydriatic (e.g. tropicamide) and examine with ophthalmoscope in a darkened room
- Note features of diabetic retinopathy (p. 826), including photocoagulation scars from previous laser treatment

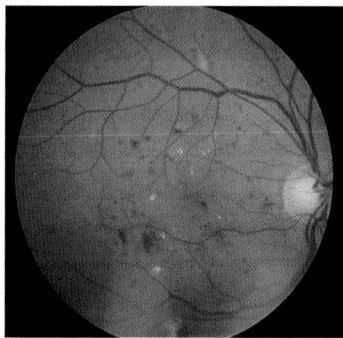

Background retinopathy.

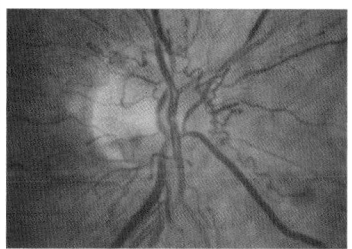

Proliferative retinopathy.

1 Examination of the hands

Several abnormalities are more common in diabetes:
- Limited joint mobility ('cheiroarthropathy') causes painless stiffness in the hands, and occasionally affects the wrists and shoulders. The inability to extend (to 180°) the metacarpophalangeal or interphalangeal joints of at least one finger bilaterally can be demonstrated in the 'prayer sign'
- Dupuytren's contracture (p. 1070) causes nodules or thickening of the skin and knuckle pads
- Carpal tunnel syndrome (p. 1228) presents with wrist pain radiating into the hand
- Trigger finger (flexor tenosynovitis)
- Muscle-wasting/sensory changes may be present as features of a peripheral sensorimotor neuropathy, although this is more common in the lower limbs

8 Insulin injection sites

Main areas used

- Anterior abdominal wall
- Upper thighs/buttocks
- Upper outer arms

Inspection

- Bruising
- Lumps (lipodystrophy)
- Subcutaneous fat deposition (lipohypertrophy)
- Subcutaneous fat loss (lipoatrophy; associated with injection of unpurified animal insulins—now rare)
- Erythema, infection (rare)

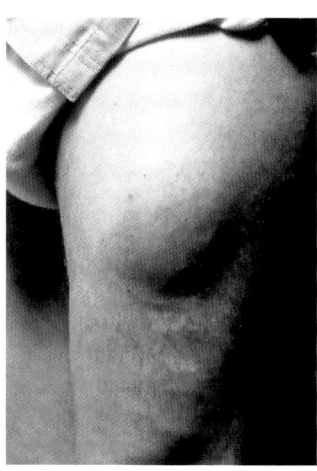

Lipohypertrophy.

11 Examination of the feet

Inspection

- Look for evidence of callus formation on weight-bearing areas, clawing of the toes (a feature of neuropathy), loss of the plantar arch, discoloration of the skin (ischaemia), localised infection and the presence of ulcers
- Deformity may be present, especially in Charcot neuroarthropathy
- Fungal infection may affect skin between toes, and nails

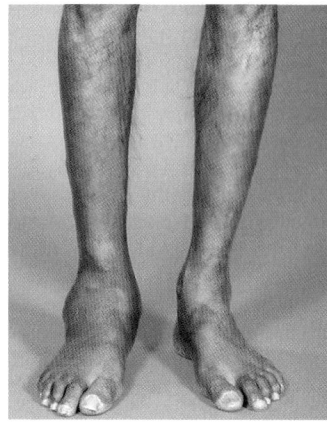

Charcot neuroarthropathy.

Circulation

- Peripheral pulses, skin temperature and capillary refill may be abnormal

Sensation

- Abnormal in stocking distribution in typical peripheral sensorimotor neuropathy
- Light touch: use monofilaments
- Vibration sense: use 128 Hz tuning fork over big toe/malleoli
- Pin-prick: use pin
- Pain: pressure over Achilles tendon
- Proprioception: test position of big toe

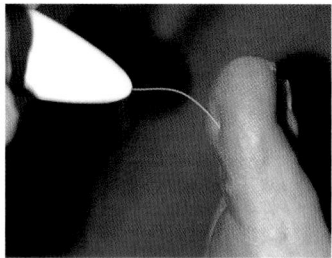

Monofilaments.

Reflexes

- Loss of ankle reflexes in typical sensorimotor neuropathy
- Test plantar and ankle reflexes

Diabetes mellitus is a clinical syndrome characterised by hyperglycaemia caused by absolute or relative deficiency of insulin. Hyperglycaemia has many causes (see Box 21.7, p. 804) but is most commonly due to type 1 or type 2 diabetes. Lack of insulin affects the metabolism of carbohydrate, protein and fat, and can cause significant disturbance of water and electrolyte homeostasis; death may result from acute metabolic decompensation. Long-standing metabolic derangement is associated with functional and structural changes in many organs, particularly those of the vascular system, which lead to the clinical 'complications' of diabetes. These characteristically affect the eye, the kidney and the nervous system.

The distribution of blood glucose concentration in populations is unimodal, with no clear division between people with normal and abnormal values. Hyperglycaemia represents an independent risk factor for disease of both small and large blood vessels. Diagnostic criteria for diabetes (pp. 805–806) have been selected to identify those who have a degree of hyperglycaemia which, if untreated, is associated with a significant risk of microvascular disease, and in particular diabetic retinopathy. Less severe hyperglycaemia is called 'impaired glucose tolerance'. This is not associated with substantial risk of microvascular disease, but is associated with increased risk of large vessel disease (e.g. atheroma leading to myocardial infarction) and with a greater risk of developing diabetes in future. The implication of these criteria is that there is no such thing as 'mild' diabetes not requiring effective treatment.

The incidences of both type 1 and type 2 diabetes are rising; it is estimated that, in the year 2000, 171 million people had diabetes, and this is expected to double by 2030 (Fig. 21.1). This global pandemic principally involves type 2 diabetes and is associated with greater longevity, obesity, unsatisfactory diet, sedentary lifestyle and increasing urbanisation. Many cases of type 2 diabetes remain undetected. However, the prevalence of both types of diabetes varies considerably around the world, and is related to differences in genetic and environmental factors. The prevalence of known diabetes in

21.1 The current cost of diabetes in the UK

- 10–30% reduction in life expectancy
- Most common cause of blindness in age group 20–65 years
- 1000 patients per annum reach end-stage renal failure
- Lower limb amputation rate increased 25-fold
- Use of hospital beds increased sixfold
- 7% of total National Health Service budget

the UK is around 4%, but is higher in the Middle and Far East (e.g. > 12% in urban areas of the Indian subcontinent). A pronounced rise in the prevalence of type 2 diabetes occurs in migrant populations to industrialised countries, as in Asian and Afro-Caribbean immigrants to the UK. Type 2 diabetes is now being observed in children and adolescents, particularly in some ethnic groups, such as Hispanics and Afro-Americans.

Type 1 diabetes is more common in Caucasian populations, and in northern Europe its prevalence in children has doubled in the last 20 years, with a particular increase in children under 5 years of age.

Diabetes is a major burden upon health-care facilities in all countries. Estimated costs in the UK are shown in Box 21.1.

FUNCTIONAL ANATOMY AND PHYSIOLOGY

Normal glucose and fat metabolism

Blood glucose is tightly regulated and maintained within a narrow range. A balance is preserved between the entry of glucose into the circulation from the liver, supplemented by intestinal absorption after meals, and glucose uptake by peripheral tissues, particularly skeletal muscle. A continuous supply of glucose is essential for the brain, which cannot oxidise free fatty acids and relies upon glucose as its principal metabolic fuel.

When intestinal glucose absorption declines between meals, hepatic glucose output is increased in response to low insulin levels and increased levels of the counter-regulatory hormones, glucagon and epinephrine (adrenaline). The liver produces glucose by gluconeogenesis and glycogen breakdown. The main substrates for gluconeogenesis are glycerol and amino acids, as shown in Figure 21.2.

After meals, blood insulin levels rise. Insulin is an anabolic hormone with profound effects on the metabolism of carbohydrate, fat and protein (Box 21.2). Insulin is secreted from pancreatic β cells into the portal circulation, with a brisk increase in response to a rise in blood glucose (Fig. 21.3). A number of other factors can augment insulin release, including amino acids and hormones, such as glucagon-like peptide 1 (GLP-1), released from the gut following food intake (p. 822). Insulin lowers blood glucose by suppressing hepatic glucose production and stimulating glucose uptake in skeletal muscle and fat, mediated by the glucose transporter, GLUT 4.

Adipocytes (and the liver) synthesise triglyceride from non-esterified ('free') fatty acids (FFAs) and glycerol. Insulin stimulates lipogenesis and inhibits lipolysis,

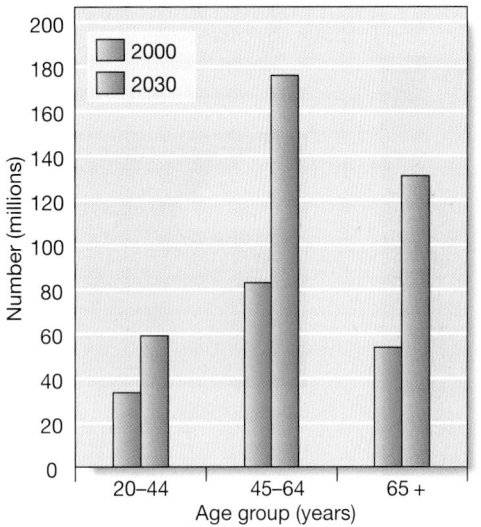

Fig. 21.1 World-wide estimated number of adults with diabetes by age group and year.

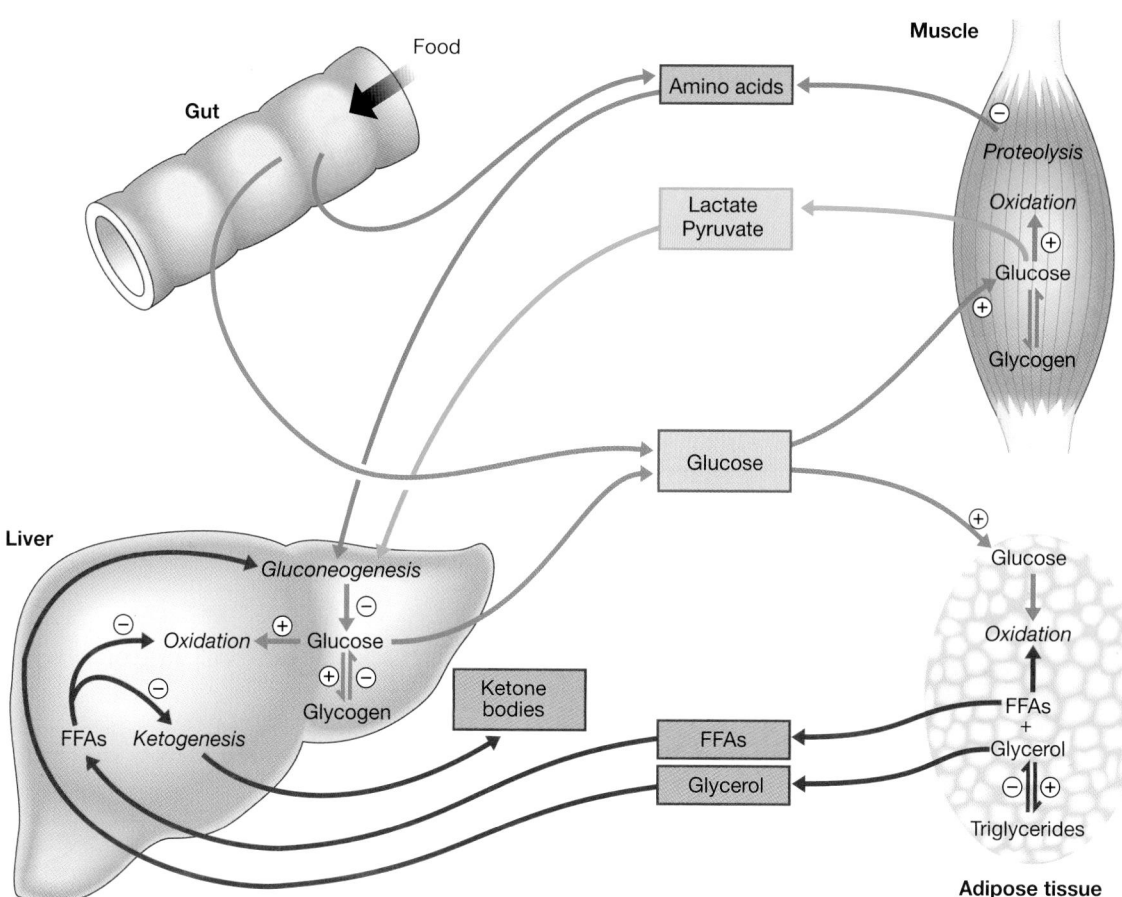

Fig. 21.2 Major metabolic pathways of fuel metabolism and the actions of insulin. $\oplus$ indicates stimulation and $\ominus$ indicates suppression by insulin. In response to a rise in blood glucose, e.g. after a meal, insulin is released, suppressing gluconeogenesis and promoting glycogen synthesis and storage. Insulin promotes the peripheral uptake of glucose, particularly in skeletal muscle, and encourages storage (as muscle glycogen). It also promotes protein synthesis and lipogenesis, and suppresses lipolysis. The release of intermediate metabolites, including amino acids (glutamine, alanine), 3-carbon intermediates in oxidation (lactate, pyruvate) and free fatty acids (FFAs), is controlled by insulin. In the absence of insulin, e.g. during fasting, these processes are reversed and favour gluconeogenesis in liver from glycogen, glycerol, amino acids and other 3-carbon precursors.

21

21.2 Metabolic actions of insulin

Increase (anabolic effects)	Decrease (anticatabolic effects)
Carbohydrate metabolism	
Glucose transport (muscle, adipose tissue)	Gluconeogenesis
	Glycogenolysis
Glucose phosphorylation	
Glycogenesis	
Glycolysis	
Pyruvate dehydrogenase activity	
Pentose phosphate shunt	
Lipid metabolism	
Triglyceride synthesis	Lipolysis
Fatty acid synthesis (liver)	Lipoprotein lipase (muscle)
Lipoprotein lipase activity (adipose tissue)	Ketogenesis
	Fatty acid oxidation (liver)
Protein metabolism	
Amino acid transport	Protein degradation
Protein synthesis	

promoting triglyceride accumulation. Lipolysis is stimulated by catecholamines and liberates FFAs which can be oxidised by many tissues. Their partial oxidation in the liver provides energy to drive gluconeogenesis and also produces ketone bodies (acetoacetate, which can be reduced to 3-hydroxybutyrate or decarboxylated to acetone) which are generated in hepatocyte mitochondria. Ketone bodies are organic acids which, when formed in small amounts, are oxidised and utilised as metabolic fuel. However, the rate of utilisation of ketone bodies by peripheral tissues is limited, and when the rate of production by the liver exceeds their removal, hyperketonaemia results. This occurs physiologically during starvation, when low insulin levels and high catecholamine levels increase lipolysis and delivery of FFAs to the liver.

Aetiology and pathogenesis of diabetes

In both of the common types of diabetes, environmental factors interact with genetic susceptibility to determine which people develop the clinical syndrome,

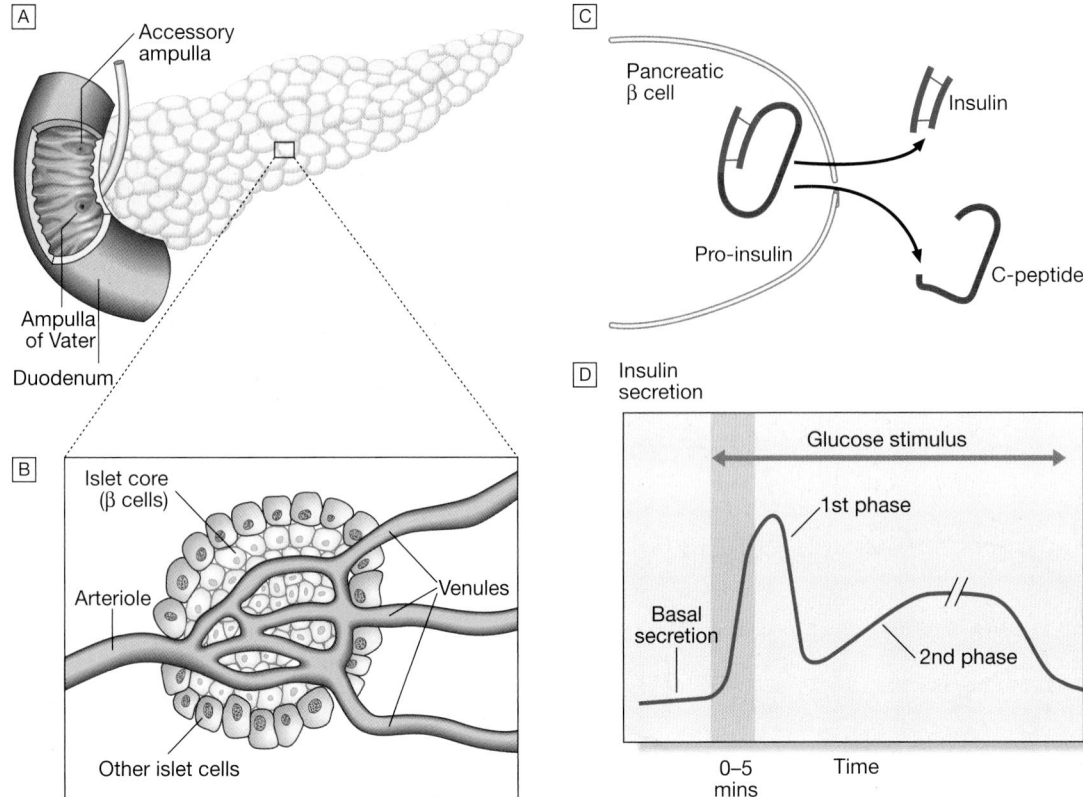

Fig. 21.3 Pancreatic structure and endocrine function. [A] The normal adult pancreas contains about 1 million islets which are scattered throughout the exocrine parenchyma. Histology is shown in Figure 21.4. [B] The core of each islet consists of β cells that produce insulin, and is surrounded by a cortex of endocrine cells that produce other hormones including glucagon (α cells), somatostatin (δ cells) and pancreatic polypeptide (PP cells). [C] Pro-insulin in the pancreatic β cell is cleaved to release insulin and equimolar amounts of inert C-peptide (connecting peptide). Measurement of C-peptide can be used to assess endogenous insulin secretory capacity. [D] An acute first phase of insulin secretion occurs in response to an elevated blood glucose, followed by a sustained second phase.

and the timing of its onset. However, the underlying genes, precipitating environmental factors and pathophysiology differ substantially between type 1 and type 2 diabetes. Type 1 diabetes was previously termed 'insulin-dependent diabetes mellitus' (IDDM) and is invariably associated with profound insulin deficiency requiring replacement therapy. Type 2 diabetes was previously termed 'non-insulin-dependent diabetes mellitus' (NIDDM) because patients retain the capacity to secrete some insulin but exhibit impaired sensitivity to insulin (insulin resistance) and initially can usually be treated without insulin replacement therapy. However, 20% or more of patients with type 2 diabetes will ultimately develop profound insulin deficiency requiring replacement therapy so that IDDM and NIDDM were misnomers.

Type 1 diabetes

Pathology

Type 1 diabetes is a T cell-mediated autoimmune disease (p. 85) involving destruction of the insulin-secreting β cells in the pancreatic islets which takes place over many years. Hyperglycaemia accompanied by the classical symptoms of diabetes occurs only when 70–90% of β cells have been destroyed.

The pathology in the pre-diabetic pancreas in type 1 diabetes is characterised by:

- 'insulitis' (Fig. 21.4): infiltration of the islets with mononuclear cells containing activated macrophages, helper cytotoxic and suppressor T lymphocytes, natural killer cells and B lymphocytes
- initial patchiness of this lesion with, until a very late stage, lobules containing heavily infiltrated islets seen adjacent to unaffected lobules
- β-cell specificity of the destructive process, with the glucagon and other hormone-secreting cells in the islet remaining intact.

Islet cell antibodies can be detected before the clinical development of type 1 diabetes, but have a variable predictive value as a marker of disease, and disappear with increasing duration of diabetes (see Fig. 21.4). These antibodies are generally not suitable for screening or diagnostic purposes. However, glutamic acid decarboxylase (GAD) antibodies may have a role in identifying late-onset type 1 diabetes in middle-aged people (latent autoimmune diabetes in adults, LADA) in whom type 2 diabetes might otherwise be presumed.

Type 1 diabetes is associated with other autoimmune disorders (Ch. 4), including thyroid disease (p. 736), coeliac disease (p. 879), Addison's disease (p. 775), pernicious anaemia (p. 1021) and vitiligo (p. 1253).

Genetic predisposition

Genetic factors account for about one-third of the susceptibility to type 1 diabetes, the inheritance of which

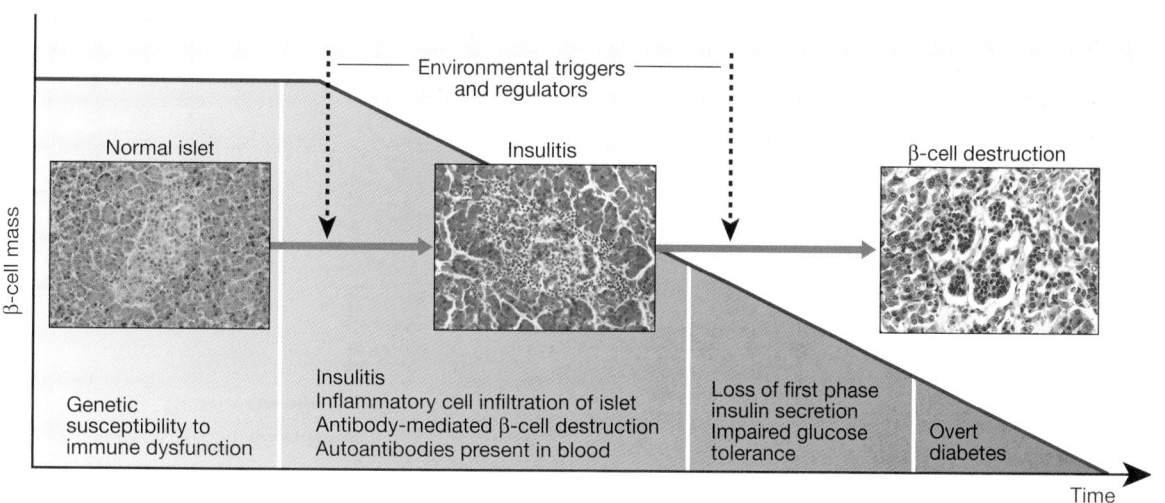

Fig. 21.4 Pathogenesis of type 1 diabetes. Proposed sequence of events in the development of type 1 diabetes. Environmental triggers are described in the text.

21.3 Risk of developing type 1 diabetes in an individual who has a first-degree relative with type 1 diabetes	
Relative with type 1 diabetes	% overall risk
Identical twin	35
Non-identical twin	20
HLA-identical sibling	16
Non-HLA-identical sibling	3
Father	9
Mother	3
Both parents	Up to 30

is polygenic (Box 21.3). Over 20 different regions of the human genome show some linkage with type 1 diabetes but most interest has focused on the human leucocyte antigen (HLA) region within the major histocompatibility complex on the short arm of chromosome 6; this locus is designated IDDM 1. The HLA haplotypes *DR3* and/or *DR4* are associated with increased susceptibility to type 1 diabetes in Caucasians and are in 'linkage disequilibrium', i.e. they tend to be transmitted together, with the neighbouring alleles of the *HLA-DQA1* and *DQB1* genes. The latter may be the main determinants of the genetic susceptibility, since these HLA class II genes code for proteins on the surface of cells which present foreign and self antigens to T lymphocytes (p. 85). Candidate gene and genome-wide association studies have also implicated other genes in type 1 diabetes, e.g. *CD25*, *PTPN22*, *IL2RA*, which are involved in immune recognition of pancreatic islet antigens, T cell development and immune regulation. The genes associated with type 1 diabetes overlap with those for other autoimmune disorders such as coeliac disease and thyroid disease, consistent with clustering of these conditions in individuals or families.

Environmental factors

Although genetic susceptibility appears to be a prerequisite for type 1 diabetes, the concordance rate between monozygotic twins is less than 40% (see Box 21.3), and environmental factors have an important role in promoting clinical expression of the disease. Although

hypotheses abound, the nature of these environmental factors is uncertain.

One proposal is that reduced exposure to microorganisms in early childhood limits maturation of the immune system and increases susceptibility to autoimmune disease (the 'hygiene hypothesis'). Another is that viral infection in the pancreas alters β cells' immunogenicity; several viruses have been implicated, including mumps, Coxsackie B4, retroviruses, rubella (in utero), cytomegalovirus and Epstein–Barr virus. Stress may precipitate type 1 diabetes by stimulating the secretion of counter-regulatory hormones and possibly by modulating immune activity. Dietary factors may also be important. Various nitrosamines (found in smoked and cured meats) and coffee have been proposed as potentially diabetogenic toxins. Bovine serum albumin (BSA), a major constituent of cow's milk, has been implicated, since children who are given cow's milk early in infancy are more likely to develop type 1 diabetes than those who are breastfed. BSA may cross the neonatal gut and raise antibodies which cross-react with a heat-shock protein expressed by β cells.

Metabolic disturbances in type 1 diabetes

Patients with type 1 diabetes present when progressive β-cell destruction has crossed a threshold at which adequate insulin secretion and normal blood glucose levels can no longer be sustained. Above a certain level, high glucose levels may be toxic to the remaining β cells so that profound insulin deficiency rapidly ensues. Severe insulin deficiency is associated with the metabolic sequelae shown in Figure 21.5. Hyperglycaemia leads to glycosuria and dehydration, which in turn induces secondary hyperaldosteronism (p. 433). Unrestrained lipolysis and proteolysis result in weight loss, increased gluconeogenesis and ketogenesis. Ketoacidosis occurs when generation of ketone bodies exceeds the capacity for their metabolism. Elevated blood H^+ ions drive K^+ out of the intracellular compartment, while secondary hyperaldosteronism encourages urinary loss of K^+. Thus patients usually present with a short history (typically a few weeks) of hyperglycaemic symptoms (thirst, polyuria, nocturia and fatigue), infections and weight loss, and may have developed ketoacidosis (p. 809).

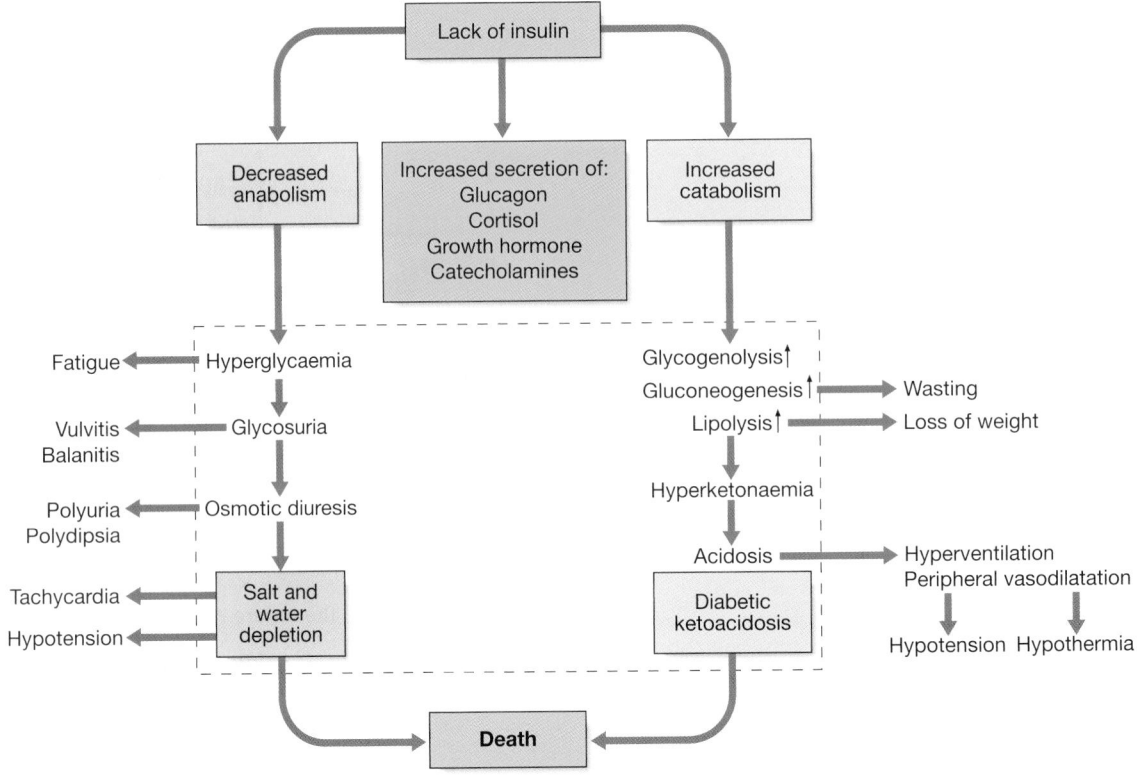

Fig. 21.5 Pathophysiological basis of the symptoms and signs of uncontrolled diabetes mellitus.

Type 2 diabetes

Pathology

Type 2 diabetes is a more complex condition than type 1 diabetes because there is a combination of resistance to the actions of insulin in liver and muscle together with impaired pancreatic β-cell function leading to 'relative' insulin deficiency. The natural history is shown in Figure 21.6. Insulin resistance appears to come first, and leads to elevated insulin secretion in order to maintain normal blood glucose levels. However, in susceptible individuals the pancreatic β cells are unable to sustain the increased demand for insulin and a slowly progressive insulin deficiency develops.

Insulin resistance

Type 2 diabetes, or its antecedent impaired glucose tolerance, is often associated with other disorders, particularly central (visceral) obesity, hypertension and dyslipidaemia (characterised by elevated levels of small dense low-density lipoprotein (LDL) cholesterol and triglycerides, and a low level of high-density lipoprotein (HDL) cholesterol) (Box 21.4). It has been suggested that coexistence of this cluster of conditions, all of which predispose to cardiovascular disease, is a specific entity (the 'insulin resistance syndrome' or 'metabolic syndrome'), with insulin resistance being the primary defect and the presence of obesity being a powerful amplifier of the insulin resistance.

The primary cause of insulin resistance remains unclear. Intra-abdominal 'central' adipose tissue is metabolically active, and releases large quantities of FFAs which may induce insulin resistance because they

compete with glucose as a fuel supply for oxidation in peripheral tissues such as muscle. In addition, adipose tissue releases a number of hormones (including a variety of peptides, called 'adipokines' because they are structurally similar to immunological 'cytokines') which act on specific receptors to influence sensitivity to insulin in other tissues. Because visceral adipose tissue drains into the portal vein, central obesity may have a particularly potent influence on insulin sensitivity in the liver, and thereby adversely affect gluconeogenesis and hepatic lipid metabolism.

Physical activity is another important determinant of insulin sensitivity. Inactivity is associated with down-regulation of insulin-sensitive kinases and may promote accumulation of FFAs within skeletal muscle. Sedentary

21.4 Features of the insulin resistance (metabolic) syndrome*

- Hyperinsulinaemia
- Type 2 diabetes or impaired glucose tolerance
- Hypertension
- Low HDL cholesterol; elevated triglycerides
- Central (visceral) obesity
- Microalbuminuria
- Increased fibrinogen
- Increased plasminogen activator inhibitor-1
- Increased C-reactive protein (CRP)
- Elevated plasma uric acid

*This constellation of features has also been called Reaven's syndrome and syndrome X. It describes the co-segregation in the population of a group of risk factors for atherosclerosis, manifested by macrovascular disease (coronary, cerebral, peripheral) and an excess mortality. It is not a discrete clinical disorder. Additional associations include polycystic ovary syndrome (p. 760) and non-alcoholic fatty liver disease (NAFLD, p. 956).

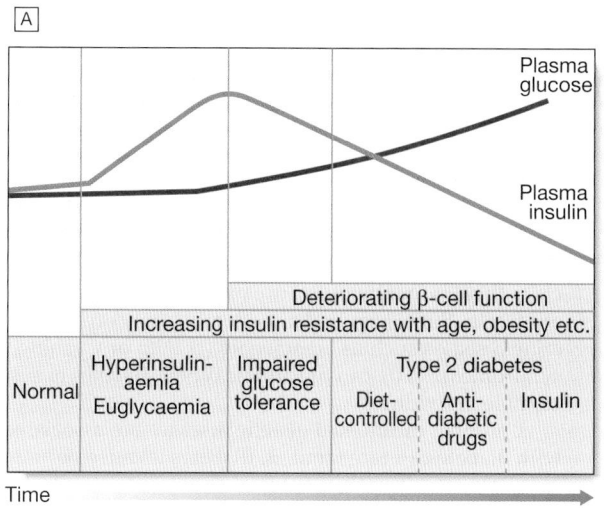

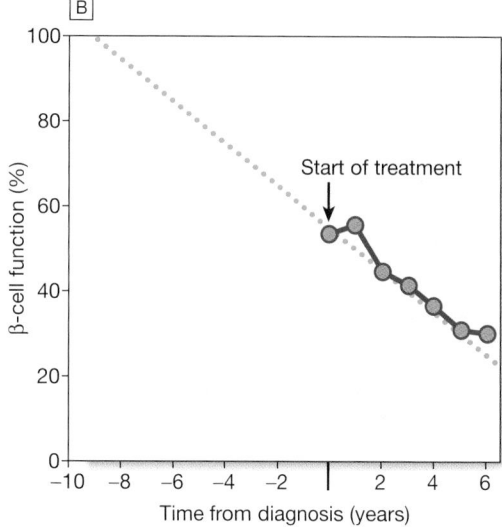

Fig. 21.6 Natural history of type 2 diabetes. **A** In the early stage of the disorder the response to progressive insulin resistance is an increase in insulin secretion by the pancreatic cells, causing hyperinsulinaemia. Eventually the β cells are unable to compensate adequately and blood glucose rises, producing hyperglycaemia. With further β-cell failure (type 2 diabetes) glycaemic control deteriorates and treatment requirements escalate. **B** Progressive pancreatic β-cell failure in patients in the United Kingdom Prospective Diabetes Study (UKPDS). β-cell function was estimated using the homeostasis model assessment (HOMA) and was already < 50% at the time of diagnosis. Thereafter, long-term increments in fasting plasma glucose were accompanied by progressive β-cell dysfunction. By extrapolating the slope of this progression, it appears that pancreatic dysfunction may have been developing for many years before diagnosis of diabetes.

people are therefore more insulin-resistant than active people with the same degree of obesity. Moreover, physical activity allows non-insulin-dependent glucose uptake into muscle, reducing the 'demand' on the pancreatic β cells to produce insulin.

Additional disorders have been associated more recently with insulin resistance. Deposition of fat in the liver is a common association with central obesity and is exacerbated by insulin resistance and/or deficiency. Many patients with type 2 diabetes have evidence of fatty infiltration of the liver (non-alcoholic fatty liver disease (NAFLD), p. 956). This condition may improve with effective treatment of the diabetes and dyslipidaemia, but despite this a few patients progress to non-alcoholic steatohepatitis (NASH) (p. 957) and cirrhosis.

Pancreatic β-cell failure

In the early stages of type 2 diabetes, reduction in the total mass of pancreatic islet tissue is modest. At the time of diagnosis, around 50% of β-cell function has been lost and this declines progressively with time (see Fig. 21.6B). Some pathological changes are typical of type 2 diabetes, the most consistent of which is deposition of amyloid. In addition, elevated plasma glucose and FFAs exert toxic effects on pancreatic β cells to impair insulin secretion. However, while β-cell numbers are reduced, α-cell mass is unchanged and glucagon secretion is increased, which may contribute to the hyperglycaemia.

Genetic predisposition

Genetic factors are important in type 2 diabetes, as shown by marked differences in susceptibility in different ethnic groups and by studies in monozygotic twins where concordance rates for type 2 diabetes approach 100%. However, many genes are involved and the chance of developing diabetes is also influenced very powerfully by environmental factors (Box 21.5). Genome-wide association studies have identified over 20 genes or gene

i 21.5 Risk of developing type 2 diabetes for siblings of probands with type 2 diabetes

Age at onset of type 2 diabetes in proband	Age-corrected risk of type 2 diabetes for siblings (%)
25–44	53
45–54	37
55–64	38
65–80	31

regions that are associated with type 2 diabetes, each exerting a small effect. The largest effect is seen with variation in *TCF7L2*; the 10% of the population with two copies of the risk variant for this gene have a nearly two-fold increase in risk of developing type 2 diabetes. Most of the genes known to contribute to risk of type 2 diabetes are involved in β-cell function or in regulation of cell cycling and turnover, suggesting that altered regulation of β-cell mass is a primary predisposing factor.

Environmental and other risk factors
Diet and obesity

Epidemiological studies show that type 2 diabetes is associated with overeating, especially when combined with obesity and underactivity. Middle-aged people with diabetes eat significantly more and are fatter and less active than their non-diabetic siblings. The risk of developing type 2 diabetes increases tenfold in people with a body mass index (BMI) > 30 kg/m² (p. 115). However, although the majority of patients with type 2 diabetes are obese, only a minority of obese people develop diabetes. Obesity probably acts as a diabetogenic factor (through increasing resistance to the action of insulin) only in those who are genetically predisposed both to insulin resistance and to β-cell failure.

In addition to the effect of total calorie content on obesity, the constituents of the diet and the style of eating may be important. Sweet foods rich in refined carbohydrate consumed frequently may increase the demand for insulin secretion, while high-fat foods may increase FFAs and exacerbate insulin resistance.

Age

Type 2 diabetes is more common in the middle-aged and elderly (Box 21.6). In the UK, it affects 10% of the population over 65, and over 70% of all cases of diabetes occur after the age of 50 years.

21.6 Diagnosis of diabetes mellitus in old age

- **Prevalence**: increases with age, affecting ~10% of people over 65 years. Half of these people are undiagnosed. Impaired β-cell function and exaggerated insulin resistance with ageing both contribute.
- **Glycosuria**: the renal threshold for glucose rises with age, so glycosuria may not develop until the blood glucose concentration is markedly raised.
- **Pancreatic carcinoma**: may present in old age with the development of diabetes, in association with weight loss and diminished appetite.

Pregnancy

During normal pregnancy, insulin sensitivity is reduced through the action of placental hormones and this affects glucose tolerance. The insulin-secreting cells of the pancreatic islets may be unable to meet this increased demand in women genetically predisposed to develop diabetes. The term 'gestational diabetes' refers to hyperglycaemia occurring for the first time during pregnancy (p. 815). Repeated pregnancy increases the likelihood of developing irreversible diabetes, particularly in obese women; 80% of women with gestational diabetes ultimately develop permanent diabetes.

Metabolic disturbances in type 2 diabetes

Patients with type 2 diabetes have a slow onset of 'relative' insulin deficiency. Relatively small amounts of insulin are required to suppress lipolysis, and some glucose uptake is maintained in muscle, so that, in contrast with type 1 diabetes, lipolysis and proteolysis are not unrestrained and weight loss and ketoacidosis seldom occur. The severity of the classical 'osmotic' symptoms of polyuria and polydipsia is related to the degree of glycosuria. In type 2 diabetes, hyperglycaemia develops slowly over months or years and there is a rise in the renal threshold for glucose (the capacity of renal tubules to reabsorb glucose from the glomerular filtrate), so that glycosuria is limited and osmotic symptoms are usually mild. This is one reason that many cases of type 2 diabetes are discovered coincidentally and a large number are undetected. Thus, patients are often asymptomatic and usually present with a long history (typically many months) of fatigue, with or without osmotic symptoms.

In some patients with type 2 diabetes, presentation is late and pancreatic β-cell failure has reached an advanced stage of insulin deficiency (see type 1 diabetes, p. 801). These patients may present with weight loss but ketoacidosis is uncommon.

Intercurrent illness, e.g. with infections, increases the production of counter-regulatory hormones such as cortisol, growth hormone and catecholamines. This can precipitate an acute exacerbation of insulin resistance and insulin deficiency, and result in more severe hyperglycaemia and dehydration (see hyperosmolar non-ketotic coma, p. 812).

Other forms of diabetes

Other causes of diabetes are shown in Box 21.7. In most cases there is an obvious cause of destruction of pancreatic β cells. Some acquired disorders, notably other endocrine diseases such as acromegaly (p. 790) or Cushing's syndrome (p. 770), can precipitate type 2 diabetes in susceptible individuals.

A number of unusual genetic diseases are associated with diabetes. In rare families, diabetes is caused by single gene defects with autosomal dominant inheritance. These subtypes constitute less than 5% of all cases of diabetes and typically present as 'maturity-onset diabetes of the young' (MODY), i.e. non-insulin-requiring diabetes presenting before the age of 25 years (Box 21.8).

21.7 Aetiological classification of diabetes mellitus

Type 1 diabetes
- Immune-mediated
- Idiopathic

Type 2 diabetes

Other specific types
- Genetic defects of β-cell function (see Box 21.8)
- Genetic defects of insulin action (e.g. leprechaunism, lipodystrophies)
- Pancreatic disease (e.g. pancreatitis, pancreatectomy, neoplastic disease, cystic fibrosis, haemochromatosis, fibrocalculous pancreatopathy)
- Excess endogenous production of hormonal antagonists to insulin (e.g. growth hormone—acromegaly; glucocorticoids—Cushing's syndrome; glucagon—glucagonoma; catecholamines—phaeochromocytoma; thyroid hormones—thyrotoxicosis)
- Drug-induced (e.g. corticosteroids, thiazide diuretics, phenytoin)
- Viral infections (e.g. congenital rubella, mumps, Coxsackie virus B)
- Uncommon forms of immune-mediated diabetes
- Associated with genetic syndromes (e.g. Down's syndrome; Klinefelter's syndrome; Turner's syndrome; DIDMOAD (Wolfram's syndrome) —diabetes insipidus, diabetes mellitus, optic atrophy, nerve deafness; Friedreich's ataxia; myotonic dystrophy)

Gestational diabetes

INVESTIGATIONS

Urine testing

Glucose

Testing the urine for glucose with dipsticks is a common screening procedure for detecting diabetes. If pos-

21.8 Monogenic diabetes mellitus: maturity onset diabetes of the young (MODY)

Functional defect	Main type*	Gene mutated*
β-cell glucose sensing	MODY2	*GCK*

The set point for basal insulin release is altered, causing a high fasting glucose, but sufficient insulin is released after meals. As a result the HbA_{1c} is often normal and microvascular complications are rare. Treatment is only rarely required

β-cell transcriptional regulation	MODY3	*HNF-1α*
	MODY5	*HNF-1β*
	MODY1	*HNF-4α*

Diabetes develops during adolescence/early adulthood and can be managed with diet and tablets for many years, but ultimately insulin treatment is required. The HNF-1α and 4α forms respond particularly well to sulphonylurea drugs. All types are associated with microvascular complications. HNF-1β mutations also cause renal cysts and renal failure

*Other gene mutations have been found in rare cases. For further information, see http://projects.exeter.ac.uk/diabetesgenes/mody/

sible, testing should be performed on urine passed 1–2 hours after a meal to maximise sensitivity. Glycosuria always warrants further assessment by blood testing (see below). The greatest disadvantage of urinary glucose measurement is the individual variation in renal threshold for glucose. The most common cause of glycosuria is a low renal threshold, which is common during pregnancy and in young people; 'renal glycosuria' is a benign condition unrelated to diabetes. Some drugs may interfere with urine glucose tests.

Ketones

Ketone bodies can be identified by the nitroprusside reaction, which measures acetoacetate, using either tablets or dipsticks. Ketonuria may be found in normal people who have been fasting or exercising strenuously for long periods, who have been vomiting repeatedly, or who have been eating a diet high in fat and low in carbohydrate. Ketonuria is therefore not pathognomonic of diabetes but, if associated with glycosuria, the diagnosis of diabetes is highly likely. In diabetic ketoacidosis (p. 809), ketones can also be detected in plasma using dipsticks.

Protein

Standard dipstick testing for albumin detects urinary albumin at concentrations > 300 mg/L, but smaller amounts (microalbuminuria, Box 17.21, p. 480) can only be measured using specific albumin dipsticks or by quantitative biochemical laboratory measurement. Microalbuminuria or proteinuria, in the absence of urinary tract infection, is an important indicator of the development of diabetic nephropathy and/or increased risk of macrovascular disease (see Box 21.44, p. 830).

Blood testing

Glucose

Laboratory glucose testing in blood relies upon an enzymatic reaction (glucose oxidase) and is cheap, usually automated and highly reliable. However, variation in blood glucose depends on whether the patient has eaten recently, so it is important to consider the circumstances in which the blood sample was taken.

Blood glucose can also be measured with colorimetric or other testing sticks, which are often read with a portable electronic meter. These are used for capillary (fingerprick) testing to monitor diabetes treatment (p. 808). To make the diagnosis of diabetes, the blood glucose concentration should be estimated using an accurate laboratory method rather than a portable technique.

Glucose concentrations are lower in venous than in arterial or capillary (fingerprick) blood. Whole blood glucose concentrations are lower than plasma concentrations because red blood cells contain relatively little glucose. In general, venous plasma values are the most reliable for diagnostic purposes (Boxes 21.9 and 21.10).

Glycated haemoglobin

Glycated haemoglobin provides an accurate and objective measure of glycaemic control over a period of weeks to months. This allows assessment of glycaemic control by repeated measurements every few months in patients with known diabetes, but current assays may not be sufficiently sensitive to make a diagnosis of diabetes and are usually within the normal range in patients with impaired glucose tolerance.

In diabetes, the slow non-enzymatic covalent attachment of glucose to haemoglobin (glycation) increases the amount in the HbA_1 (HbA_{1c}) fraction relative to non-glycated adult haemoglobin (HbA_0). These fractions can be separated by chromatography; laboratories may report glycated haemoglobin as total glycated haemoglobin (GHb), HbA_1 or HbA_{1c}. In most countries HbA_{1c} is the preferred measurement. The rate of formation of HbA_{1c} is directly proportional to the ambient blood glucose concentration; a rise of 1% in HbA_{1c} corresponds to an approximate average increase of 2 mmol/L (36 mg/dL) in blood glucose. Although HbA_{1c} concentration reflects the integrated blood glucose control over the lifespan of the erythrocyte (120 days), half of the erythrocytes are replaced in 60 days and HbA_{1c} is most sensitive to changes in glycaemic control occurring in the month before measurement.

Various assay methods are used to measure HbA_{1c}, but most laboratories have been reporting HbA_{1c} values (as %) aligned with the reference range that was used in the Diabetes Control and Complications Trial (DCCT). To allow world-wide comparisons of HbA_{1c} values, the International Federation of Clinical Chemistry and Laboratory Medicine (IFCC) has developed a standard method; IFCC-standardised HbA_{1c} values are reported in mmol/mol. The equivalent of typical DCCT HbA_{1c} targets of 6.5% and 7.5% (p. 809) are 48 and 59 mmol/mol using the IFCC assay. In some countries, including the USA, DCCT-aligned HbA_{1c} is reported along with the estimated average blood glucose value (eAG) that is represented by the HbA_{1c} measurement. However, the clinical applicability of this eAG measurement is uncertain.

HbA_{1c} estimates may be erroneously diminished in anaemia or during pregnancy, and may be difficult to interpret with some assay methods in patients who have uraemia or a haemoglobinopathy.

21

21.9 Diagnosis of diabetes[1]

Patient complains of symptoms suggesting diabetes

- Test urine for glucose and ketones
- Measure random or fasting venous blood glucose. Diagnosis confirmed by[2]:
    Fasting plasma glucose ≥ 7.0 mmol/L (126 mg/dL)
    Random plasma glucose ≥ 11.1 mmol/L (200 mg/dL)

Indications for oral glucose tolerance test (see Box 21.10)

- Fasting plasma glucose 6.1–7.0 mmol/L (110–126 mg/dL)
- Random plasma glucose 7.8–11.0 mmol/L (140–198 mg/dL)

[1]The use of HbA$_{1c}$ for diagnosis is uncertain.
[2]In asymptomatic patients two samples are required to confirm diabetes.

21.10 How to perform an oral glucose tolerance test (OGTT)

Preparation before the test

- Unrestricted carbohydrate diet for 3 days
- Fasted overnight for at least 8 hrs
- Rest for 30 mins
- Remain seated for the duration of the test, with no smoking

Sampling

- Plasma glucose is measured before and 2 hrs after a 75 g oral glucose drink

Interpretation (venous plasma glucose)

	Fasting	2 hrs after glucose load
Fasting hyperglycaemia	6.1–6.9 mmol/L (110–125 mg/dL)	< 7.8 mmol/L (< 140 mg/dL)
Impaired glucose tolerance	< 7.0 mmol/L (< 126 mg/dL)	7.8–11.0 mmol/L (140–199 mg/dL)
Diabetes	≥ 7.0 mmol/L (≥ 126 mg/dL)	≥ 11.1 mmol/L (≥ 200 mg/dL)

PRESENTING PROBLEMS IN DIABETES MELLITUS

Newly discovered hyperglycaemia

Hyperglycaemia is a very common biochemical abnormality. It is frequently detected on routine biochemical analysis of asymptomatic patients, following routine dipstick testing of urine showing glycosuria, or during severe illness ('stress hyperglycaemia'). Alternatively, hyperglycaemia may present with the chronic symptoms described in Box 21.11. Occasionally, patients present as an emergency with acute metabolic decompensation (see below). The key goals are to establish whether the patient has diabetes, what type of diabetes it is and how it should be treated.

Establishing the diagnosis of diabetes

When diabetes is suspected, the diagnosis may be confirmed by a random plasma glucose concentration greater than 11.0 mmol/L (199 mg/dL) (see Box 21.9). When random plasma glucose values are elevated but are not diagnostic of diabetes, glucose tolerance is usually assessed either by a fasting plasma glucose estimation or by an oral glucose tolerance test (OGTT) (see Box 21.10).

21.11 Symptoms of hyperglycaemia

- Thirst, dry mouth
- Polyuria
- Nocturia
- Tiredness, fatigue, lethargy
- Noticeable change in weight (usually weight loss)
- Blurring of vision
- Pruritus vulvae, balanitis (genital candidiasis)
- Nausea; headache
- Hyperphagia; predilection for sweet foods
- Mood change, irritability, difficulty in concentrating, apathy

The diagnostic criteria for diabetes mellitus (and normality) recommended by the World Health Organization (WHO) in 2000 are shown in Boxes 21.9 and 21.10, and Figure 21.7. The values are based on the threshold for risk of developing vascular disease. Patients who do not meet the criteria for diabetes may have 'impaired glucose tolerance' (IGT, Box 21.10 and Fig. 21.7) or 'fasting hyperglycaemia' (sometimes called 'impaired fasting glucose', when the fasting glucose is between 6.1 and 6.9 mmol/L (110–125 mg/dL)). These patients have increased risks of progression to frank diabetes with time and of macrovascular atheromatous disease. Lowering the cut-off defining impaired fasting glucose to 5.6 mmol/L has been proposed; this would triple the prevalence of this condition.

In some people, an abnormal blood glucose result is observed under conditions which impose a burden on the pancreatic β cells, e.g. during pregnancy, infection, myocardial infarction or other severe stress, or during treatment with diabetogenic drugs such as corticosteroids. This 'stress hyperglycaemia' usually disappears after the acute illness has resolved. However, blood glucose should be remeasured and an OGTT will often show persistence of impaired glucose tolerance.

The diagnostic criteria for diabetes in pregnancy are more stringent than those recommended for non-pregnant subjects. Pregnant women with abnormal glucose tolerance should be referred urgently to a specialist unit for full evaluation.

When a diagnosis of diabetes is confirmed, other investigations should include plasma urea, creatinine and electrolytes, lipids, liver and thyroid function tests, and urine testing for ketones, protein or microalbuminuria.

Clinical assessment and classification

Hyperglycaemia causes a wide variety of symptoms (see Box 21.11). The clinical features of the two main types of diabetes are compared in Box 21.12. The classical symptoms of thirst, polyuria, nocturia and rapid weight loss are prominent in type 1 diabetes, but are often absent in patients with type 2 diabetes, many of whom are asymptomatic or have non-specific complaints such as chronic fatigue and malaise. Uncontrolled diabetes is associated with an increased susceptibility to infection and patients may present with skin sepsis (boils) or genital candidiasis, and complain of pruritus vulvae or balanitis. A history of pancreatic disease (see Box 21.7, p. 804), particularly in patients with a history of alcohol excess, makes insulin deficiency more likely, although such patients may develop incidental classical type 2 diabetes.

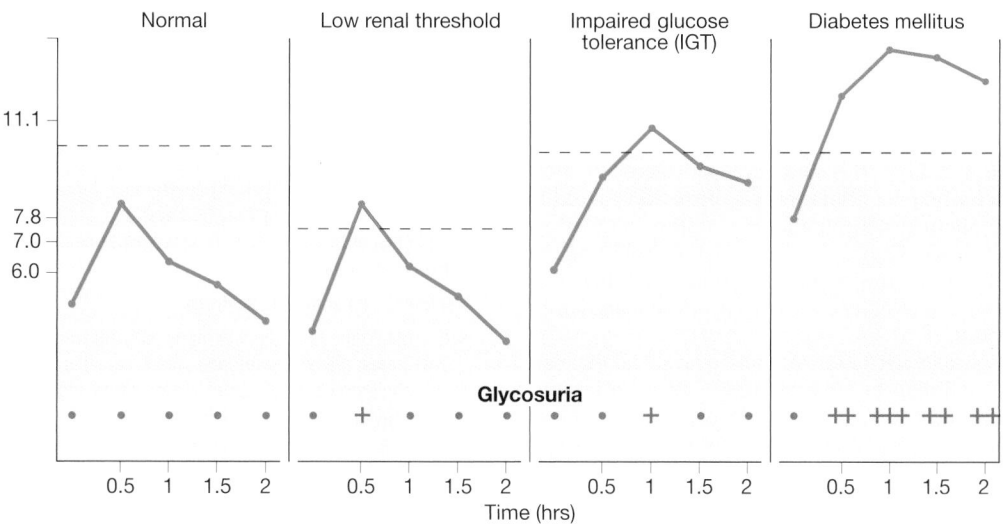

Plasma glucose (mmol/L)

Fig. 21.7 **Glucose tolerance tests: venous plasma glucose after 75 g glucose by mouth.** The dotted lines indicate the 'renal threshold', i.e. the blood glucose concentration above which glycosuria occurs. (To convert glucose in mmol/L to mg/dL, multiply by 18.)

i	21.12 **Comparative features of type 1 and type 2 diabetes**	
	Type 1	**Type 2**
Typical age at onset	< 40 yrs	> 50 yrs
Duration of symptoms	Weeks	Months to years
Body weight	Normal or low	Obese
Ketonuria	Yes	No
Rapid death without treatment with insulin	Yes	No
Autoantibodies	Yes	No
Diabetic complications at diagnosis	No	25%
Family history of diabetes	Uncommon	Common
Other autoimmune disease	Common	Uncommon

While the distinction between type 1 and type 2 diabetes is usually obvious, overlap occurs particularly in age at onset, duration of symptoms and family history. A few young people have a form of diabetes designated 'maturity-onset diabetes of the young' (MODY; see Box 21.8, p. 805); they usually have a remarkably strong family history of early-onset diabetes. Classical type 2 diabetes is developing increasingly in obese sedentary young people, including children. Some middle-aged and elderly people present with typical autoimmune type 1 diabetes. Others with apparent type 2 diabetes have evidence of autoimmune activity against pancreatic β cells, and may have a slowly evolving variant of type 1 diabetes (latent autoimmune diabetes in adults (LADA)). Some patients with type 2 diabetes have advanced pancreatic β-cell failure at the time of presentation and require treatment with insulin. For these reasons, the definitive diagnosis of the type of diabetes may sometimes be unclear until the natural history or responsiveness to different therapies becomes apparent with time.

The physical signs in patients with type 2 diabetes at diagnosis depend on the mode of presentation. In Western populations more than 80% are overweight, and the obesity is often central (truncal or abdominal). Obesity is much less evident in Asians. Hypertension is present in at least 50% of patients with type 2 diabetes. Although dyslipidaemia is also common, skin lesions such as xanthelasma and eruptive xanthomas are rare. An increasing number of patients now present with non-alcoholic fatty liver disease, usually identified by their elevated blood transaminase values, but they may also have non-tender hepatomegaly.

Management

The methods of treatment of diabetes are: dietary/lifestyle modification, oral anti-diabetic drugs and injected therapies. These are described in detail on pages 818–824. In patients with suspected type 1 diabetes, urgent treatment with insulin is required and prompt referral to a specialist is usually needed. In patients with suspected type 2 diabetes, the first line of therapy involves advice about dietary and lifestyle modification. Oral anti-diabetic drugs are added in those who do not achieve glycaemic targets as a result, or who have severe symptomatic hyperglycaemia at diagnosis and a high HbA_{1c}.

In parallel with treatment of hyperglycaemia, other risk factors for complications of diabetes need to be addressed, including treatment of hypertension (p. 606) and dyslipidaemia (p. 454), and advice on smoking cessation (p. 98).

Educating patients

It is essential that people with diabetes understand their disorder and learn to handle all aspects of their management as comprehensively and quickly as possible. Ideally, this can be achieved by a multidisciplinary team (doctor, dietitian, specialist nurse and podiatrist) in the outpatient setting. However, patients commencing insulin need daily advice at first and admission to hospital may sometimes be necessary.

21

Those requiring insulin need to learn how to measure doses of insulin accurately with an insulin syringe or pen device, how to inject, and how to adjust the dose on the basis of blood glucose values and in relation to factors such as exercise, illness and episodic hypoglycaemia. They must therefore acquire a working knowledge of diabetes, be familiar with the symptoms of hypoglycaemia (Box 21.21, p. 812), and have ready access to medical advice when the need arises. Information should be provided about driving (national statutory regulations and practical safety measures, Box 21.13). Providing this education is time-consuming but essential if patients are to undertake normal activities safely while maintaining good control.

It is a sensible precaution for those who are taking insulin or oral anti-diabetic medications to carry a card stating their name and address, the fact that they have diabetes, the nature and dose of any insulin or other drugs they may be taking, and the contact details of their family doctor and any specialist diabetes clinic that they attend.

Self-assessment of glycaemic control

Urine testing to assess blood glucose control has major limitations, particularly in people with type 1 diabetes, but also in those with type 2 diabetes in whom a raised renal threshold for glucose may mask persistent hyperglycaemia. Negative urine tests fail to distinguish between normal and low blood glucose levels, which is a serious disadvantage since the aim of treatment is a normal blood glucose level while avoiding hypoglycaemia. However, semi-quantitative urine glucose testing with visually read strips is very cheap and may suffice for many people with type 2 diabetes treated with diet alone or in those taking oral therapy who have stable glycaemic control.

Many patients (particularly those treated with insulin) should be taught to perform capillary blood glucose measurements using blood glucose test strips, read either visually or with a glucose meter (Box 21.14). The principal advantage of self-monitoring of blood glucose is that information is available immediately and permits

21.14 Blood glucose (BG) testing and diabetes

Treatment with insulin

- Regular BG monitoring should be performed by all patients to adjust the insulin dose and detect hypoglycaemia
- Daily pre-prandial and bedtime measurements are usually recommended
- Target BG levels are typically 5–8 mmol/L (~90–144 mg/dL), although target ranges may be lower (e.g. in gestational diabetes) or higher (e.g. in impaired awareness of hypoglycaemia)

Treatment with anti-diabetic drugs

- BG monitoring is optional in many patients with stable type 2 diabetes; patient preference usually decides
- BG monitoring is most useful in patients taking sulphonylureas (risk of hypoglycaemia), during intercurrent illness and prescription of corticosteroids, and during changes in therapy
- BG is usually measured before breakfast (typical target 4–7 mmol/L (~72–126 mg/dL)) and 2 hrs after food (typical target 4–10 mmol/L (~72–180 mg/dL))

the well-informed and motivated patient to make appropriate adjustments in treatment (particularly in insulin dose) on a day-to-day basis. Thus changes in routine can be accommodated, ketoacidosis avoided, compliance with diet encouraged and near-normal metabolism achieved while avoiding frequent and disabling hypoglycaemia. Blood glucose monitoring involves a significant cost and may not be justified in many patients with type 2 diabetes. Single random blood glucose estimations obtained at routine clinic visits are of limited value and profiles measured in hospital may be unrepresentative of normal circumstances. Continuous blood glucose monitoring methodology is available but is costly and not yet applicable to routine monitoring.

Advice to patients with IGT

These patients have an increased risk both of progression to type 2 diabetes and of developing macrovascular disease. There is evidence that the lifestyle advice recommended for patients with type 2 diabetes will reduce the risk of progression in IGT. Patients with IGT should be monitored annually by measurement of fasting blood glucose. Other cardiovascular risk factors should be treated aggressively.

Long-term supervision of diabetes

Diabetes is a complex disorder which progresses in severity with time, so people with diabetes should be seen at regular intervals for the remainder of their lives, either at a specialist diabetic clinic or in primary care where facilities are available and staff are trained in diabetes care. A checklist for follow-up visits is given in Box 21.15. The frequency of visits is very variable, ranging from weekly during pregnancy to annually in the case of patients with well-controlled type 2 diabetes.

Therapeutic goals

The aims of treatment are to relieve the symptoms of hyperglycaemia and to achieve as near normal

21.13 Diabetes and driving

- Licensing regulations vary considerably between countries. In the UK, diabetes requiring insulin therapy or any complication that could affect driving should be declared to the Driver and Vehicle Licensing Agency; ordinary driving licences are 'period-restricted' for insulin-treated drivers, and vocational licences (large goods vehicles and public service vehicles) are generally refused unless very strict criteria can be met
- The main risk to driving performance is hypoglycaemia. Visual impairment and other complications may occasionally cause problems
- Insulin-treated diabetic drivers should be advised to:
  Check blood glucose before driving and 2-hourly during long journeys
  Keep an accessible supply of fast-acting carbohydrate in the vehicle
  Take regular snacks or meals during long journeys
  Stop driving if hypoglycaemia develops
  Refrain from driving until at least 45 mins after treatment of hypoglycaemia (delayed recovery of cognitive function)
  Carry identification in case of injury

21.15 How to review a patient in the diabetes clinic

Body weight and BMI

Urinalysis
- Analyse fasting specimen for glucose, ketones, albumin (both macro- and microalbuminuria)

Biochemistry
- Lipid profile and renal, liver and thyroid function

Glycaemic control
- Glycated haemoglobin (HbA$_{1c}$)
- Inspection of home blood glucose monitoring record

Hypoglycaemic episodes
- Number and cause of severe (requiring assistance for treatment) events and frequency of mild (self-treated) episodes
- Time of day when 'hypos' are experienced
- Nature and intensity of symptoms
- Ability to identify onset (awareness)

Blood pressure

Smoking

Eye examination
- Visual acuities (near and distance)
- Ophthalmoscopy (with pupils dilated) or digital photography

Lower limbs and feet
- Peripheral pulses
- Tendon reflexes
- Perception of vibration sensation, light touch and proprioception
- Callus indicating pressure areas
- Nails
- Deformity
- Ulceration
- Need for podiatry

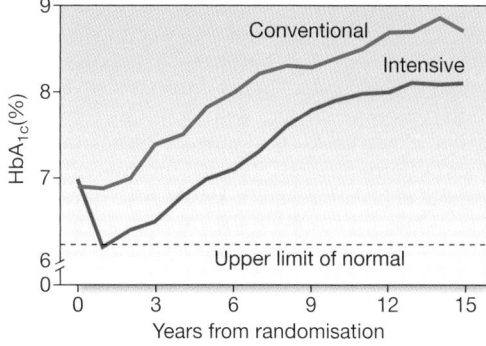

Fig. 21.8 Time course of changes in HbA$_{1c}$ during the United Kingdom Prospective Diabetes Study (UKPDS). In the UKPDS there was loss of glycaemic control with time in patients receiving monotherapy, independently of their randomisation to conventional or intensive glycaemic control, consistent with progressive decline in β-cell function (see Fig. 21.6, p. 803).

4 mmol/L should be avoided. The importance of routinely measuring post-prandial glucose is debatable, and multiple daily measurements (> 4/day) are seldom practical or tolerated.

In people with type 2 diabetes, treatment of coexisting hypertension and dyslipidaemia is usually required. This can be determined by assessment of cardiovascular risk and targets are adjusted to individual circumstances. The target for blood pressure is usually < 140/80 mmHg. The target levels for lipids are usually a total cholesterol < 5.0 mmol/L (approximately 190 mg/dL) and LDL cholesterol < 3.0 mmol/L (approximately 115 mg/dL). Similar targets would be appropriate in type 1 diabetes, with modification depending on age and the presence of microalbuminuria.

Diabetic ketoacidosis

Ketoacidosis is a major medical emergency and remains a serious cause of morbidity, principally in people with type 1 diabetes. A significant number of newly diagnosed diabetic patients present in ketoacidosis. In established diabetes a common course of events is that patients develop an intercurrent infection, lose their appetite, and either stop or reduce their dose of insulin in the mistaken belief that under these circumstances less insulin is required. Any form of stress, particularly that produced by infection, may precipitate severe ketoacidosis, even in patients with type 2 diabetes. No obvious precipitating cause can be found in many cases.

The average mortality in developed countries is 5–10% and is higher in the elderly. Although some deaths from ketoacidosis are associated with severe medical conditions such as acute myocardial infarction or septicaemia, others are the consequence of delays in diagnosis and management errors.

Pathogenesis

A clear understanding of the biochemical basis and pathophysiology of diabetic ketoacidosis is essential for its efficient treatment. The cardinal biochemical features are:
- hyperglycaemia
- hyperketonaemia
- metabolic acidosis.

metabolism as is practicable, while avoiding hypoglycaemia and therapeutic side-effects. The nearer the body weight approaches the ideal level and the closer the blood glucose is kept to normal, the more the total metabolic profile is improved and the lower the incidence of vascular disease and of specific diabetic complications. Excellent glycaemic control may also slow the progression of pancreatic β-cell failure.

The recommended target HbA$_{1c}$ is 7% or less, to minimise the risk of vascular complications. However, this may be difficult to achieve and to maintain, particularly with increasing duration of diabetes. Type 2 diabetes progresses in severity with time, with evidence of a gradual rise in HbA$_{1c}$ despite escalation in treatment (Fig. 21.8). Strict glycaemic control in type 1 diabetes increases the risk of hypoglycaemia. Glycaemic targets should therefore be appropriate to the age and physical condition of the patient; strict control may be inappropriate in the very young, the elderly, people with several comorbidities or cancer, and those with advanced diabetic complications or cardiovascular disease. Blood glucose targets depend similarly on individual requirements, but fasting blood glucose values below 6 mmol/L (108 mg/dL) are desirable in type 2 diabetes. Preprandial values between 5 and 8 mmol/L would be ideal in patients with type 1 diabetes, in whom values below

21

The hyperglycaemia causes a profound osmotic diuresis leading to dehydration and electrolyte loss, particularly of sodium and potassium. Potassium loss is exacerbated by secondary hyperaldosteronism as a result of reduced renal perfusion. Ketosis results from insulin deficiency, exacerbated by elevated catecholamines and other stress hormones, resulting in unrestrained lipolysis and supply of FFAs for hepatic ketogenesis (see Fig. 21.5, p. 802). When this exceeds the capacity to metabolise acidic ketones, these accumulate in blood. The resulting metabolic acidosis forces hydrogen ions into cells, displacing potassium ions.

The average loss of fluid and electrolytes in moderately severe diabetic ketoacidosis in an adult is shown in Box 21.16. About half the deficit of total body water is derived from the intracellular compartment and occurs comparatively early in the development of acidosis with relatively few clinical features; the remainder represents loss of extracellular fluid sustained largely in the later stages, when marked contraction of the size of the extracellular space occurs, with haemoconcentration, a decreased blood volume, and finally a fall in blood pressure with associated renal ischaemia and oliguria.

21.16 Average loss of fluid and electrolytes in adult diabetic ketoacidosis of moderate severity	
• Water: 6 L	3 L extracellular
• Sodium: 500 mmol	—replace with saline
• Chloride: 400 mmol	3 L intracellular
• Potassium: 350 mmol	—replace with dextrose

Every patient in diabetic ketoacidosis is potassium-depleted, but the plasma concentration of potassium gives very little indication of the total body deficit. Plasma potassium may even be raised initially due to disproportionate loss of water, catabolism of protein and glycogen, and displacement of potassium from the intracellular compartment by H⁺ ions. However, soon after insulin treatment is started there is likely to be a precipitous fall in the plasma potassium due to dilution of extracellular potassium by administration of intravenous fluids, the movement of potassium into cells induced by insulin, and the continuing renal loss of potassium.

The magnitude of the hyperglycaemia does not correlate with the severity of the metabolic acidosis; moderate elevation of blood glucose may be associated with life-threatening ketoacidosis. In some cases, hyperglycaemia predominates and acidosis is minimal, with patients presenting in a hyperosmolar state (p. 812).

Clinical assessment

The clinical features of ketoacidosis are listed in Box 21.17. In the fulminating case the striking features are those of salt and water depletion, with loss of skin turgor, furred tongue and cracked lips, tachycardia, hypotension and reduced intra-ocular pressure. Breathing may be deep and sighing, the breath is usually fetid, and the sickly-sweet smell of acetone may be apparent. Mental apathy, confusion or a reduced conscious level may be present. The state of consciousness is very variable in patients with diabetic ketoacidosis; coma is uncommon. A patient with dangerous ketoacidosis requiring urgent

21.17 Clinical features of diabetic ketoacidosis	
Symptoms	
• Polyuria, thirst	• Leg cramps
• Weight loss	• Blurred vision
• Weakness	• Abdominal pain
• Nausea, vomiting	
Signs	
• Dehydration	• Air hunger (Kussmaul breathing)
• Hypotension (postural or supine)	• Smell of acetone
• Cold extremities/peripheral cyanosis	• Hypothermia
• Tachycardia	• Confusion, drowsiness, coma (10%)

treatment may walk into the consulting room. For this reason the term 'diabetic ketoacidosis' is to be preferred to 'diabetic coma', which implies that there is no urgency until unconsciousness supervenes. In fact, it is imperative that energetic treatment is started at the earliest possible stage.

Abdominal pain is sometimes a feature of diabetic ketoacidosis, particularly in children. Serum amylase may be elevated but rarely indicates coexisting pancreatitis. In infected patients, pyrexia may not be present initially because of vasodilatation secondary to acidosis.

Investigations

The following are important but should not delay the institution of intravenous fluid and insulin replacement:
- *Venous blood*: for urea and electrolytes, glucose, bicarbonate.
- *Arterial blood gases* to assess the severity of acidosis. (The severity of ketoacidosis can be assessed rapidly by measuring the venous plasma bicarbonate; less than 12 mmol/L indicates severe acidosis. The hydrogen ion concentration gives a more precise measure but requires arterial blood.)
- *Urinalysis for ketones*. (A meter is available to quantify ketones in plasma, and a test strip can be used as a semi-quantitative guide to the plasma concentration of acetoacetate and acetone.)
- *ECG*.
- *Infection screen*: full blood count, blood and urine culture, C-reactive protein, chest X-ray. Although leucocytosis invariably occurs, this represents a stress response and does not necessarily indicate infection.

Management

Diabetic ketoacidosis is a medical emergency which should be treated in hospital, preferably in a high-dependency area. Regular clinical and biochemical review is essential, particularly during the first 24 hours of treatment (Box 21.18). Guidelines for the management of ketoacidosis are shown in Box 21.19.

The principal components of treatment are:
- the administration of short-acting (soluble) insulin
- fluid replacement
- potassium replacement
- the administration of antibiotics if infection is present.

21.18 Monitoring in diabetic ketoacidosis[1]

Laboratory	Baseline	1 hr	2 hr	3 hr	6 hr	12 hr	24 hr
Glucose[2]	✓	✓	✓	✓	✓	✓	✓
Urea, electrolytes	✓	✓	✓	✓	✓	✓	✓
Creatinine	✓				✓	✓	✓
Bicarbonate	✓	✓	✓	✓	✓	✓	✓
Blood gases	(✓)		✓[3]		✓[3]		

[1]The following should be monitored hourly: pulse, blood pressure, respiratory rate, urine output, capillary blood glucose.
[2] A capillary blood glucose measurement of > 17 mmol/L (approximately 300 mg/dL) using a meter or visually read glucose strips can be very misleading since the actual blood glucose concentration is often considerably higher when measured precisely in the laboratory; therefore an accurate measurement should be made at an early stage.
[3] If no clinical improvement. Blood gases at baseline are not necessary if plasma bicarbonate is > 15 mmol/L.

21.19 Management of diabetic ketoacidosis

Fluid replacement

- 0.9% saline (NaCl) i.v.
    - 1 L over 30 mins
    - 1 L over 1 hr
    - 1 L over 2 hrs
    - 1 L over next 2–4 hrs
- When blood glucose < 15 mmol/L (270 mg/dL)
    - Switch to 5% dextrose, 1 L 8-hourly
    - If still dehydrated, continue 0.9% saline and add 5% dextrose, 1 L per 12 hrs
- Typical requirement is 6 L in first 24 hrs but avoid fluid overload in elderly patients
- Subsequent fluid requirement should be based on clinical response including urine output

Insulin

- 50 U soluble insulin in 50 mL 0.9% saline i.v. via infusion pump
    - 6 U/hr initially
    - 3 U/hr when blood glucose < 15 mmol/L (270 mg/dL)
    - 2 U/hr if blood glucose < 10 mmol/L (180 mg/dL)
- Check blood glucose hourly initially; if no reduction in first hour, rate of insulin infusion should be increased
- Aim for fall in blood glucose of 3–6 mmol/L (approximately 55–110 mg/dL) per hour

Potassium

- None in first L of i.v fluid unless plasma potassium < 3.0 mmol/L
- When < 3.5 mmol/L, give 20 mmol/hr
- When plasma potassium is 3.5–5.0 mmol/L, give 10 mmol/hr

Additional procedures

- Catheterisation if no urine passed after 3 hrs
- Nasogastric tube to keep stomach empty in unconscious or semiconscious patients, or if vomiting is protracted
- Central venous line if cardiovascular system compromised, to allow fluid replacement to be adjusted accurately
- Plasma expander if systolic BP is < 90 mmHg or does not rise with i.v. saline
- Antibiotic if infection demonstrated or suspected
- ECG monitoring in severe cases

Insulin

If an intravenous infusion of insulin (see Box 21.19) is not possible, soluble insulin can be given by intramuscular injection (loading dose of 10–20 U followed by 5 U hourly) or, alternatively, a fast-acting insulin analogue can be given hourly by subcutaneous injection (initially 0.3 U/kg body weight, then 0.1 U/kg hourly). The blood glucose concentration should fall by 3–6 mmol/L (approximately 55–110 mg/dL) per hour. A more rapid fall in blood glucose should be avoided, as hypoglycaemia can be precipitated and the serious complication of cerebral oedema may develop, particularly in children. If blood glucose does not fall within 1 hour of commencing treatment, the dose of insulin should be increased until a satisfactory response is obtained. Ketosis, dehydration, acidaemia, infection and stress combine to produce severe insulin resistance in some cases but most will respond to a low-dose insulin regimen. When the blood glucose concentration has fallen to 10–15 mmol/L (180–270 mg/dL) the dose of insulin should be reduced to 1–4 U hourly. The half-life of intravenous insulin is short (2.5 mins) so the insulin infusion should not be interrupted.

Restoration of the usual insulin regimen, by subcutaneous injection, should not be instituted until the patient is able to eat and drink normally. 'Sliding scales' of subcutaneous insulin administration (in which insulin is prescribed according to blood glucose levels immediately before injection) should not be used.

Fluid replacement

Intravenous fluid replacement is required since, even when the patient is able to swallow, fluids given by mouth may be poorly absorbed. The extracellular fluid deficit should be replenished by infusing isotonic saline (0.9% NaCl). Early and rapid rehydration is essential; otherwise the administered insulin will not reach the poorly perfused tissues. If the plasma sodium is greater than 155 mmol/L, 0.45% saline may be given initially.

The intracellular water deficit must be replaced by using 5% or 10% dextrose and not by more saline. Dextrose is best given when the blood glucose concentration approaches normal. An accurate record of fluid balance must be maintained.

Potassium

As the plasma potassium is often high at presentation, treatment with intravenous potassium chloride should be started cautiously (see Box 21.19) and carefully monitored. Sufficient should be given to maintain a normal plasma concentration and large amounts may be required (100–300 mmol in the first 24 hours). Cardiac rhythm should be monitored in severe cases because of the risk of electrolyte-induced cardiac arrhythmia.

Bicarbonate

In patients who are severely acidotic ($[H^+] > 100$ nmol/L, pH < 7.0) the infusion of sodium bicarbonate (300 mL 1.26% over 30 mins into a large vein) should be considered, with the simultaneous administration of potassium. Its use is controversial, however, and should only be considered in exceptional circumstances. Complete correction of the acidosis should not be attempted.

21

811

21.20 **Complications of diabetic ketoacidosis**

- Cerebral oedema
  - May be caused by very rapid reduction of blood glucose, use of hypotonic fluids and/or bicarbonate
  - High mortality
  - Treat with mannitol, oxygen
- Acute respiratory distress syndrome (p. 187)
- Thromboembolism
- Disseminated intravascular coagulation (rare)
- Acute circulatory failure

Antibiotics

Infections must be carefully sought and vigorously treated since it may not be possible to abolish ketosis until they are controlled. The management of diabetic ketoacidosis may be complicated by the development of other conditions (Box 21.20) which require active therapy.

Non-ketotic hyperosmolar diabetic coma

This condition is characterised by severe hyperglycaemia (> 50 mmol/L (900 mg/dL)) without significant hyperketonaemia or acidosis. Severe dehydration and pre-renal uraemia are common. It usually affects elderly patients, many with previously undiagnosed type 2 diabetes. Mortality is high (40%). Treatment differs from ketoacidosis in two main respects. Firstly, these patients are usually relatively sensitive to insulin and approximately half the dose of insulin recommended for the treatment of ketoacidosis should usually be employed (3 U/hr). Secondly, the plasma osmolality should be measured or, less accurately, calculated using the following formula based on plasma values in mmol/L:

$$\text{Plasma osmolality} = 2[Na^+] + 2[K^+] + [\text{glucose}] + [\text{urea}]$$

The normal value is 280–290 mmol/kg and the conscious level is depressed when it is high (> 340 mmol/kg). The patient should be given 0.45% saline until the osmolality approaches normal, when isotonic (0.9%) saline should be substituted. The rate of fluid replacement should be adjusted on the basis of the central venous pressure, and plasma sodium concentration checked frequently. Thromboembolic complications are common, and prophylactic subcutaneous low molecular weight heparin is recommended.

Lactic acidosis

In coma due to lactic acidosis the patient is likely to be taking metformin for type 2 diabetes and is very ill and overbreathing but not as profoundly dehydrated as is usual in coma due to ketoacidosis. The patient's breath does not smell of acetone, and ketonuria is mild or even absent, yet plasma bicarbonate is reduced and the anion gap and H^+ are increased (p. 441). The diagnosis is confirmed by a high (usually > 5.0 mmol/L) concentration of lactic acid in the blood. Treatment is with intravenous sodium bicarbonate sufficient to reduce H^+ below 60 nmol/L (pH 7.2), along with insulin and glucose.

Despite energetic treatment, the mortality in this condition is over 50%. Sodium dichloroacetate may be given to lower blood lactate.

Hypoglycaemia

When hypoglycaemia (blood glucose < 3.5 mmol/L (63 mg/dL)) occurs in a person with diabetes it is a result of treatment and not a manifestation of the disease itself. It occurs often in those treated with insulin, occasionally in those taking oral insulin secretagogues such as a sulphonylurea drug, and rarely with other anti-diabetic drugs. When hypoglycaemia develops in non-diabetic people, it is called 'spontaneous' hypoglycaemia, the causes and investigation of which are described on page 781. The risk of hypoglycaemia is the most important single factor limiting the attainment of near-normal glycaemia; fear of severe hypoglycaemia is common among patients and their relatives.

Clinical assessment

Symptoms of hypoglycaemia (Box 21.21) comprise two main groups: those related to acute activation of the autonomic nervous system and those secondary to glucose deprivation of the brain (neuroglycopenia). Symptoms of hypoglycaemia are idiosyncratic and differ with age. The ability to recognise their onset is an important aspect of the initial education of diabetic patients treated with insulin. The severity of hypoglycaemia is defined by ability to self-treat; 'mild' episodes are self-treated, while 'severe' require assistance for recovery.

Circumstances of hypoglycaemia

Nocturnal hypoglycaemia in patients with type 1 diabetes is probably common and under-recognised. As hypoglycaemia does not usually waken a person who is asleep and the usual warning symptoms are not perceived, it is often undetected. However, on direct questioning, patients may admit to poor quality of sleep, morning headaches, 'hangover', chronic fatigue and vivid dreams or nightmares. Sometimes a partner may observe profuse sweating, restlessness, twitching or even

21.21 **Most common symptoms of hypoglycaemia**	
Autonomic	
- Sweating	- Hunger
- Trembling	- Anxiety
- Pounding heart	
Neuroglycopenic	
- Confusion	- Inability to concentrate
- Drowsiness	- Incoordination
- Speech difficulty	- Irritability, anger
Non-specific	
- Nausea	- Headache
- Tiredness	

N.B. Symptoms differ with age; children exhibit behavioural changes (such as naughtiness or irritability), while elderly people experience more prominent neurological symptoms such as visual disturbance and ataxia.

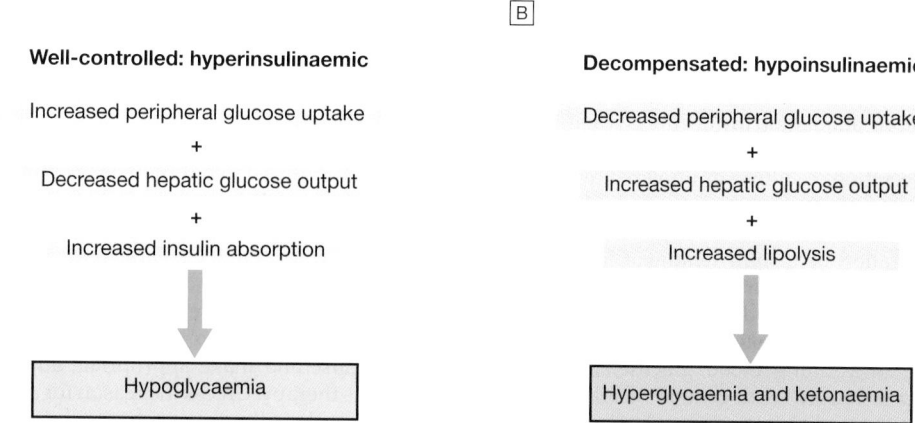

Fig. 21.9 The potential effects of exercise in diabetic patients being treated with insulin. **A** Well-controlled hyperinsulinaemic patients. **B** Decompensated hypoinsulinaemic patients.

21

seizures. The only reliable way to identify this problem is to measure the blood glucose during the night.

Exercise-induced hypoglycaemia (Fig. 21.9) occurs in people with well-controlled, insulin-treated diabetes because of hyperinsulinaemia and the absence of the capacity to suppress secretion of endogenous insulin, a key factor in the normal adaptation to exercise.

Risk factors and causes of hypoglycaemia in patients taking insulin or sulphonylurea drugs are listed in Box 21.22. Severe hypoglycaemia can have serious morbidity (Box 21.23) and has a recognised mortality of up to 4% in insulin-treated patients. The unrecognised mortality

21.22 Hypoglycaemia: common causes and risk factors

Causes of hypoglycaemia

- Missed, delayed or inadequate meal
- Unexpected or unusual exercise
- Alcohol
- Errors in oral anti-diabetic agent(s) or insulin dose/schedule/administration
- Poorly designed insulin regimen, particularly if predisposing to nocturnal hyperinsulinaemia
- Lipohypertrophy at injection sites causing variable insulin absorption
- Gastroparesis due to autonomic neuropathy
- Malabsorption, e.g. coeliac disease
- Unrecognised other endocrine disorder, e.g. Addison's disease
- Factitious (deliberately induced)
- Breastfeeding by diabetic mother

Risk factors for severe hypoglycaemia

- Strict glycaemic control
- Impaired awareness of hypoglycaemia
- Age (very young and elderly)
- Increasing duration of diabetes
- Sleep
- C-peptide negativity (indicating complete insulin deficiency)
- History of previous severe hypoglycaemia
- Renal impairment
- Genetic, e.g. angiotensin-converting enzyme (ACE) genotype

21.23 Morbidity of severe hypoglycaemia in diabetic patients

CNS

- Impaired cognitive function
- Coma
- Convulsions
- Intellectual decline
- Transient ischaemic attack, stroke
- Brain damage (rare)
- Focal neurological lesions (rare)

Heart

- Cardiac arrhythmias
- Myocardial ischaemia

Eye

- Vitreous haemorrhage
- ? Worsening of retinopathy

Other

- Accidents (including road traffic accidents) with injury
- Hypothermia

may be higher. Occasionally, sudden death occurs during sleep in otherwise healthy young patients with type 1 diabetes ('dead-in-bed syndrome'); hypoglycaemia-induced cardiac arrhythmia has been implicated. Severe hypoglycaemia is very disruptive and impinges on many aspects of the patient's life, including employment, driving (see Box 21.13, p. 808), travel, sport and personal relationships.

Awareness of hypoglycaemia

In most instances patients have no difficulty in recognising the symptoms of hypoglycaemia and can take appropriate remedial action. In certain circumstances (e.g. during sleep, lying supine or when distracted by other activities) warning symptoms are not always perceived, so that appropriate action is not taken and neuroglycopenia with reduced consciousness ensues.

If short-acting insulin is administered to a non-diabetic person, symptoms of hypoglycaemia are usually experienced when the venous or capillary blood glucose falls to 2.5–3.0 mmol/L (45–54 mg/dL). In diabetic patients who are chronically hyperglycaemic the same symptoms may develop at a higher blood glucose level. Conversely, patients who have strict glycaemic control (HbA$_{1c}$ within the non-diabetic range) may not experience any symptoms even when the blood glucose is well below 2.5 mmol/L. In patients exposed to frequent hypoglycaemia, cerebral adaptation lowers the glycaemic thresholds for the onset of symptoms and counter-regulatory hormonal secretion, resulting in impaired awareness of hypoglycaemia. The prevalence of impaired perception of the onset of symptoms of hypoglycaemia increases with the duration of insulin treatment, and it affects around 20–25% of people with type 1 diabetes and < 10% with insulin-treated type 2 diabetes.

Counter-regulatory responses may also be impaired. In response to a falling blood glucose, there is normally suppression of endogenous insulin secretion (absent in type 1 diabetes) and a brisk secretion of counter-regulatory hormones, such as glucagon and epinephrine (adrenaline), which antagonise the blood glucose-lowering effect of insulin. Hypoglycaemia-induced secretion of glucagon becomes impaired in most people within 5 years of developing type 1 diabetes and many also develop a defective adrenaline response to hypoglycaemia so that glucose recovery may be seriously compromised. Both autonomic neuropathy and impaired central activation of counter-regulation following exposure to recurrent hypoglycaemia may contribute. Counter-regulatory deficiency is closely associated with impaired awareness of hypoglycaemia, and has been described as 'hypoglycaemia-associated autonomic failure'.

Management

Acute treatment of hypoglycaemia

Treatment of acute hypoglycaemia depends on its severity and on whether the patient is conscious and able to swallow (Box 21.24). Oral carbohydrate usually suffices if hypoglycaemia is recognised early. If parenteral therapy is required, then as soon as the patient is able to swallow, glucose should be given orally. Full recovery may not occur immediately and reversal of cognitive impairment may not be complete until 60 minutes after normoglycaemia is restored. Further, when hypoglycaemia has occurred in a patient treated with a long- or intermediate-acting insulin or a long-acting sulphonylurea, such as glibenclamide, the possibility of recurrence should be anticipated; to prevent this, infusion of 10% dextrose, titrated to the patient's blood glucose, may be necessary.

If the patient fails to regain consciousness after blood glucose is restored to normal, then cerebral oedema and other causes of impaired consciousness, such as alcohol intoxication, a post-ictal state or cerebral haemorrhage, should be considered. Cerebral oedema has a high mortality and morbidity, and requires urgent treatment with mannitol and high-dose oxygen.

Following recovery, it is important to try to identify a cause and make appropriate adjustments to the patient's therapy. Unless the reason for a hypoglycaemic episode is clear, the patient should reduce the next dose of insulin by 10–20% and seek medical advice about further adjustments in dose.

The management of self-poisoning with oral anti-diabetic agents is given on page 214.

Prevention of hypoglycaemia

Patient education on the potential causes and risks of inducing hypoglycaemia and on its treatment, including the need to have an accessible supply of glucose (and glucagon) and to perform regular blood glucose monitoring, is fundamental to the prevention of this potentially dangerous side-effect of treatment. If strenuous or protracted exercise is anticipated, the preceding dose of insulin should be reduced (the degree of reduction varying widely between individuals but often being substantial) and extra carbohydrate ingested. Advice for during travel is shown in Box 21.25.

Relatives and friends also need to be familiar with the symptoms and signs of hypoglycaemia and should be instructed as to how this should be managed (including how to inject glucagon).

Unfortunately, many insulin regimens in current use produce inappropriate nocturnal hyperinsulinaemia. With a basal-bolus regimen (pp. 822–823) the times of maximum risk of hypoglycaemia are between 2300 and 0200 hrs and between 0500 and 0700 hrs. When an intermediate-acting insulin such as isophane (pp. 822–823) is taken before the main evening meal between 1700 and 1900 hrs, its peak action will coincide with the period of maximum sensitivity to insulin, namely 2300–0200 hrs. Short-acting insulin administered before a late evening meal (after 2000 hrs) can cause hypoglycaemia after retiring to bed. To reduce the risk of nocturnal

---

21.24 Emergency treatment of hypoglycaemia

Mild (self-treated)

- Oral fast-acting carbohydrate (10–15 g) is taken as glucose drink or tablets or confectionery
- This should be followed with a snack containing complex carbohydrate

Severe (external help required)

- If patient is semiconscious or unconscious, parenteral treatment is required:
    I.v. 75 mL 20% dextrose (=15 g; give 0.2 g/kg in children)*
    or
    I.m. glucagon (1 mg; 0.5 mg in children)
- If patient is conscious and able to swallow:
    Give oral refined glucose as drink or sweets (=25 g)
    or
    Apply glucose gel or jam or honey to buccal mucosa

*Use of 50% dextrose is no longer recommended.

21.25 Measures for avoidance and treatment of hypoglycaemia during travel

- Carry a supply of fast-acting carbohydrate (non-perishable, in suitable containers)
    Screwtop plastic bottles for glucose drinks
    Packets of powdered glucose (for use in hot, humid climates)
    Confectionery (foil-wrapped in hot climates)
- Companions should carry additional oral carbohydrate, and glucagon
- Perform frequent blood glucose testing (carry spare meter, visually read strips)
- Use fast-acting insulin analogues for long-distance air travel

hypoglycaemia, administration of the evening dose of depot intermediate-acting insulin can be deferred until bedtime (after 2300 hrs) or a fast-acting insulin analogue used for the evening meal. A long-acting insulin analogue should be taken with breakfast instead of at bedtime, so that its action is then waning during the night. It is a sensible precaution for patients to measure their blood glucose before they retire to bed and to eat a carbohydrate snack if the reading is less than 6.0 mmol/L (approximately 110 mg/dL).

In patients with impaired awareness of hypoglycaemia the risk of severe hypoglycaemia is greatly increased. The usual therapeutic goals need to be modified and frequent self-monitoring of blood glucose is mandatory. Therapy-induced impaired awareness of hypoglycaemia is usually reversible if glycaemic control is relaxed and hypoglycaemia avoided completely.

Diabetes in pregnancy

Maternal glucose metabolism changes during normal pregnancy to meet the nutritional demands of the developing fetus. Pregnant women develop marked insulin resistance, particularly in the second half of pregnancy. Fasting plasma glucose decreases slightly, while postprandial blood glucose may be increased. The renal threshold for glycosuria (p. 805) is reduced in pregnancy.

Gestational diabetes

Gestational diabetes is defined as diabetes with first onset or recognition during pregnancy. While this definition will include a small number of women with pre-existing (and previously clinically undetected) type 1 or type 2 diabetes, the majority of women can expect to return to normal glucose tolerance immediately after pregnancy. Risk factors for gestational diabetes are shown in Box 21.26.

Controversy surrounds the precise glucose levels at which gestational diabetes should be diagnosed and the most appropriate screening method for its detection. A number of factors have led to this difficulty. Firstly, a continuous relationship exists between maternal blood glucose and risk of adverse perinatal outcomes, with no easily definable 'threshold' of increased risk. Secondly, labelling a woman as having gestational diabetes may increase certain adverse outcomes such as caesarean section as doctors respond to a perceived increased risk. Finally, the risk of gestational diabetes and adverse outcomes varies widely between populations due to differing prevalences of underlying risk factors (see Box 21.26); this variation affects the sensitivity and specificity of screening programmes (p. 5). Screening practice varies between countries, although the WHO suggests that all women who meet the criteria for impaired glucose tolerance or diabetes after a 75 g OGTT (see Box 21.10, p. 806) should be classified as having gestational diabetes.

Implications for the mother

Gestational diabetes is managed where possible by dietary modification, particularly by reducing consumption of refined carbohydrates (see Box 21.26). Blood glucose is monitored closely and insulin is introduced if glycaemic control is unsatisfactory. In certain cases metformin or glibenclamide (the only sulphonylurea that

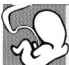

21.26 Diabetes in pregnancy

Gestational diabetes

- **Glucose metabolism**: insulin resistance occurs in normal pregnancy, particularly in the second half. Gestational diabetes develops when the pancreas is unable to secrete sufficient insulin to compensate for the insulin resistance.
- **Risk factors**: include obesity, ethnicity (South Asian, black, Hispanic, Native American), family history of type 2 diabetes, previous glucose abnormalities during pregnancy and previous macrosomia.
- **Treatment**: strict glycaemic control is required, if possible by dietary modification, particularly reducing consumption of refined carbohydrates. Metformin can be useful. Insulin is often required.
- **Monitoring**: as below for established diabetes in pregnancy, except for items marked *.
- **Inadequate control**: risks increasing fetal size and perinatal morbidity.

Pregnancy in women with established diabetes

- **Glucose metabolism**: insulin doses must be increased substantially to overcome physiological insulin resistance.
- **Pre-conception preparation**: strict glycaemic control very early in pregnancy prevents fetal malformations. Pregnancy should be planned: folic acid supplementation is introduced before conception and patients with type 2 diabetes should usually be converted to insulin therapy. If possible, use basal-bolus insulin regimens.
- **Monitoring**:
  Frequent self-monitoring of blood glucose, including post-prandial measurements, plus HbA$_{1c}$.
  Maintain strict glycaemic control, i.e. HbA$_{1c}$ close to the non-diabetic range. Do not strive for normoglycaemia at the expense of hypoglycaemia.
  Check blood glucose periodically during the night.
  Check overnight sample of urine for ketones regularly; increase intake of carbohydrate and dose of insulin to eliminate ketonuria.
  Microalbuminuria* and retinal screening* should be performed on three occasions during the pregnancy.
  Regular monitoring of fetal size, and screening for fetal abnormalities*.
- **Inadequate control**: early risks are congenital malformations and later risks are increased fetal size, neonatal hypoglycaemia and increased perinatal morbidity.

does not cross the placenta) is used. Other oral hypoglycaemic drugs are not used in pregnancy.

Gestational diabetes is associated with an increased risk of later development of type 2 diabetes in the mother. The risk is as high as 50% at 5 years in certain ethnic groups such as Hispanic women in the USA but is lower in Caucasian populations. Women with gestational diabetes should have glucose tolerance re-assessed after pregnancy (generally at 6 weeks post-partum or later). If post-partum glucose tolerance has returned to normal (fasting glucose < 6.1 mmol/L (110 mg/dL) and 2 hour glucose < 7.8 mmol/L (140 mg/dL)) advice on lifestyle changes should be given to minimise the long-term risk of developing type 2 diabetes. When glucose intolerance persists after pregnancy in a patient with a strong family history of diabetes, the presence of one of the rare autosomal dominant forms of diabetes (MODY, p. 805) should be considered.

21

815

Implications for the fetus

A clear relationship exists between maternal blood glucose and perinatal morbidity for the baby. Maternal glucose crosses the placenta and is an important fuel for the developing fetus. An elevated maternal blood glucose promotes fetal insulin production and hence stimulates fetal growth (macrosomia), which may complicate labour and delivery, resulting in a higher caesarean section rate. Fetal hyperinsulinaemia may also result in neonatal hypoglycaemia. Reduction of maternal blood glucose by insulin therapy can reduce fetal growth.

Pregnancy in women with established diabetes

Historically, pregnancy in patients with type 1 diabetes was associated with a very high incidence of morbidity for mother and child. In the 1940s and 1950s perinatal mortality rates were of the order of 40–50% and maternal mortality could be as high as 5%. Dramatic improvements in these outcomes for mother and child have been driven by the introduction of home monitoring of blood glucose, dietetic advice, modern intensive regimens for insulin delivery using either multiple injections or infusion pumps, improved obstetrical management and the support of a multidisciplinary team.

Type 2 diabetes in pregnancy used to be rare, but the increased prevalence of obesity and the emergence of type 2 diabetes in younger patients have increased its occurrence in women of reproductive age in most populations. The risk of complications and adverse outcomes in women with type 2 diabetes appears to be as high as those for women with type 1 diabetes.

Maternal hyperglycaemia early in pregnancy (during the first 6 weeks of development) has teratogenic effects. These include cardiac, renal and skeletal malformations, of which the caudal regression syndrome is the most characteristic. All women with diabetes should, if possible, be offered pre-pregnancy counselling and encouraged to achieve excellent glycaemic control before becoming pregnant (see Box 21.26). Later in pregnancy maternal hyperglycaemia is associated with macrosomia and neonatal hypoglycaemia, as described above for gestational diabetes.

Ideally, mothers should attempt to maintain near-normal glycaemia while avoiding hypoglycaemia in advance of conception and throughout all of pregnancy (see Box 21.26), but this is often difficult to achieve. Pregnancy is also associated with an increased potential for ketosis, particularly, but not exclusively, in women with type 1 diabetes. Ketoacidosis during pregnancy is dangerous for the mother and is associated with a high rate (10–35%) of fetal mortality.

Pregnancy is also associated with a worsening of diabetic complications, most notably retinopathy and nephropathy, so careful monitoring of eyes and kidneys is required throughout pregnancy.

While the outlook for mother and child has been vastly improved, pregnancy outcomes are still not equivalent to those of non-diabetic mothers. Perinatal mortality rates remain 3–4 times those of the non-diabetic population (at around 30–40 per 1000 pregnancies) and the rate of congenital malformation is increased 5–6-fold.

Hyperglycaemia in acute myocardial infarction

Hyperglycaemia is often found in patients who have sustained an acute myocardial infarction. In some, this represents stress hyperglycaemia (p. 806), some have previously undiagnosed diabetes, and many have established diabetes. Many patients with stress hyperglycaemia will have impaired glucose tolerance on a subsequent glucose tolerance test. There is much that can be done to reduce mortality from myocardial infarction in those with diabetes (Box 21.27). Hyperglycaemia should be treated with insulin and, in patients with type 2 diabetes, oral anti-diabetic drugs should be stopped in the peri-infarct period. Studies have suggested that good glycaemic control using insulin therapy for type 2 diabetes in patients with acute myocardial infarction may reduce their long-term mortality from coronary heart disease.

21.27 Treatments to reduce mortality from myocardial infarction in people with diabetes
Primary prevention of myocardial infarction
• Strict glycaemic control
• Aggressive control of hypertension
• Cholesterol reduction with a statin
Immediate measures in acute myocardial infarction
• Primary angioplasty or thrombolysis/fibrinolysis
• Aspirin and clopidogrel
• ACE inhibitor
• β-blocker
• ? Intravenous insulin
Secondary prevention of myocardial infarction
• Aspirin
• β-blocker
• ACE inhibitor
• Cholesterol reduction with high-dose statin
• Intensive subcutaneous insulin or anti-diabetic medication

Surgery and diabetes

Surgery, whether performed electively or in an emergency, causes catabolic stress and secretion of counter-regulatory hormones both in normal and in diabetic subjects. This results in increased glycogenolysis, gluconeogenesis, lipolysis, proteolysis and insulin resistance. In the non-diabetic person these metabolic effects lead to a secondary increase in the secretion of insulin, which exerts a restraining and controlling influence. In diabetic patients either there is absolute deficiency of insulin (type 1 diabetes) or insulin secretion is delayed and impaired (type 2 diabetes), so that in untreated or poorly controlled diabetes the uptake of metabolic substrate is significantly reduced, catabolism is increased and ultimately metabolic decompensation in the form of diabetic ketoacidosis may develop in both types of diabetes. Starvation exacerbates this process by increasing lipolysis. In addition, hyperglycaemia impairs phagocytic function (leading to reduced resistance to infection) and wound healing.

Thus surgery must be carefully planned and managed in the diabetic patient, with particular emphasis on good metabolic control and avoidance of hypoglycaemia, which is especially dangerous in the unconscious or semiconscious patient.

Pre-operative assessment

Careful pre-operative assessment is mandatory (Box 21.28). Much of this can be done as an outpatient but, if cardiovascular or renal function is impaired, there are signs of neuropathy (particularly autonomic), diabetic control is poor or alterations need to be made to the patient's usual treatment, then admission to hospital some days before operation is required.

21.28 How to assess diabetic patients pre-operatively

- Assess cardiovascular and renal function
- Check for features of neuropathy, particularly autonomic
- Assess glycaemic control
  Measure HbA$_{1c}$
  Monitor pre-prandial and bedtime blood glucose
- Review treatment of diabetes
  Modify insulin regimen if necessary; use intermediate and short-acting insulins
  Stop metformin and long-acting sulphonylureas; replace with insulin if necessary

---

Perioperative management

The management of diabetic patients undergoing surgery requiring general anaesthesia is summarised in Figure 21.10. Post-operatively, a glucose/insulin/potassium infusion should be continued until the patient's intake of food is adequate, when the normal insulin or tablet regimen can be resumed. If the intravenous infusion has to be continued for more than 24 hours, plasma electrolytes and urea should be measured and urinary ketones checked daily. If the infusion is prolonged, the concentration of potassium may require adjustment, and if dilutional hyponatraemia occurs, a parallel saline infusion may be necessary. If fluids need to be restricted, e.g. in patients with cardiovascular or renal disease, the rate of infusion can be halved by using a 20% dextrose solution and doubling the concentration of insulin and potassium. The insulin requirement is likely to be higher than that indicated in Figure 21.10 in patients with hepatic disease, obesity or sepsis and in those being treated with corticosteroids or undergoing cardiopulmonary bypass surgery.

Surgical emergencies

If the patient is significantly hyperglycaemic and/or ketoacidotic, this should be corrected first with an intravenous infusion of saline and/or dextrose plus insulin, 6 U/hour, with potassium as required. Subsequent treatment is as described in Figure 21.10.

Diabetes management if emergency surgery is required in a patient with well-controlled insulin-treated

21

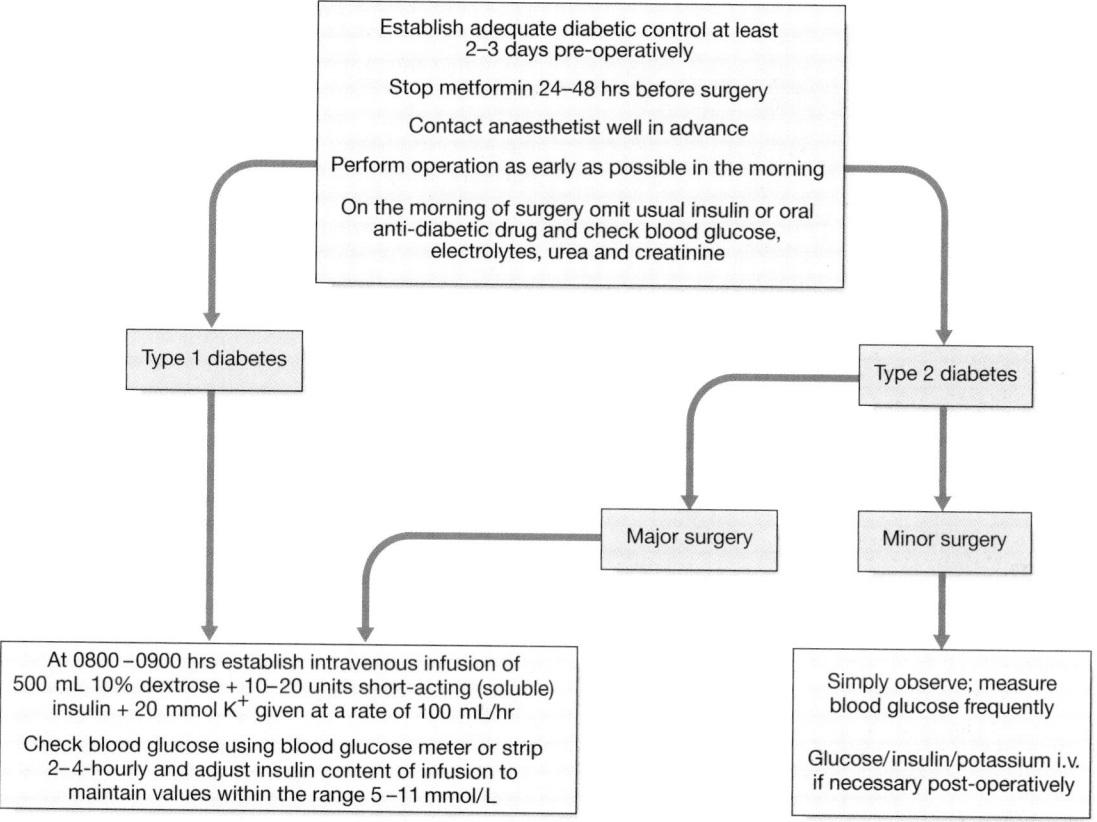

Fig. 21.10 Management of diabetic patients undergoing surgery and general anaesthesia. (Glucose of 5–11 mmol/L ≅ 90–199 mg/dL.)

diabetes depends on when the last subcutaneous injection of insulin was given. If this was recent, an infusion of dextrose alone may be sufficient, but frequent monitoring is essential.

Children, adolescents and young adults with diabetes

Children and teenagers generally have type 1 diabetes, but more cases of type 2 diabetes in obese children are now appearing, and the possibility of a diagnosis of MODY (p. 805) should also be considered. The management of diabetes in children and adolescents presents particular challenges which should be addressed in specialised paediatric clinics. Insulin therapy and diet require modification to accommodate the physiological changes associated with growth and puberty and the physical and emotional challenges of adolescence. Adherence to prescribed treatment may be erratic, and glycaemic control often deteriorates during adolescence.

Wide fluctuations in blood glucose and frequent metabolic emergencies occur in a few adolescents and young adults, but use of the term 'brittle diabetes' should be discouraged, as this is not considered to be a pathological entity. The problem (mostly affecting young women) is usually associated with persistent manipulation of therapy (stopping insulin or taking excessive doses) to induce recurrent diabetic ketoacidosis or severe hypoglycaemia requiring hospital admission. This attention-seeking behaviour may be a manifestation of psychological disturbance (p. 251).

Complications of diabetes

Patients with long-standing diabetes are at risk of developing a variety of complications of the disorder (Box 21.29). Moreover, as many as 25% of people with type 2 diabetes have evidence of diabetic complications at the time of initial diagnosis. Thus, diabetes may be first suspected when a patient visits an optometrist or podiatrist, or presents with hypertension or a vascular event such as an acute myocardial infarction or stroke. Blood glucose should therefore be checked in all patients presenting with such pathology. The detailed investigation and management of diabetic complications are described on pages 824–834.

MANAGEMENT OF DIABETES

In new cases of diabetes, adequate glycaemic control can be obtained by diet and lifestyle advice alone in approximately 50%, 20–30% will need oral anti-diabetic medication, and 20–30% will require insulin. Regardless of aetiology, the choice of treatment is determined by the adequacy of residual β-cell function. However, this cannot be determined easily by measurement of circulating plasma insulin concentration because a level which is adequate in one patient may be inadequate in another, depending upon sensitivity to insulin. Consideration of the features in Box 21.12 (p. 807), and in particular the age and weight of the patient at diagnosis, usually indicate the type of treatment required. However, in each individual the regimen adopted is effectively a therapeutic trial and should be reviewed regularly.

The ideal management for diabetes would allow the person to lead a completely normal life, to remain not only symptom-free but in good health, to achieve a normal metabolic state and to escape the long-term complications of diabetes. This is achievable to a variable degree. Setting individual goals for each patient is discussed on page 809.

Patients whose glycaemic control deteriorates after a period of satisfactory control are not a homogeneous group; they include some with late-onset type 1 diabetes who develop an absolute deficiency of insulin, some with type 2 diabetes whose β-cell failure is advanced, and others who are not adhering to the recommended diet. The most common precipitant of deteriorating glycaemic control is decreasing care with diet, usually associated with weight gain. Weight loss suggests worsening β-cell function. During continuing follow-up many patients will require combinations of anti-diabetic drugs to obtain satisfactory glycaemic control.

Diet and lifestyle

The importance of lifestyle changes such as undertaking regular physical activity, observing a healthy diet and reducing alcohol consumption should not be underestimated in improving glycaemic control, but many people, particularly the middle-aged and elderly, find

---

21.29 Complications of diabetes

Microvascular/neuropathic

Retinopathy, cataract
- Impaired vision

Nephropathy
- Renal failure

Peripheral neuropathy
- Sensory loss
- Pain
- Motor weakness

Autonomic neuropathy
- Gastrointestinal problems (gastroparesis; altered bowel habit)
- Postural hypotension

Foot disease
- Ulceration
- Arthropathy

Macrovascular

Coronary circulation
- Myocardial ischaemia/infarction

Cerebral circulation
- Transient ischaemic attack
- Stroke

Peripheral circulation
- Claudication
- Ischaemia

21.30 Aims of dietary management

- Achieve good glycaemic control
- Reduce hyperglycaemia and avoid hypoglycaemia
- Assist with weight management:
    Weight maintenance for type 1 diabetes and non-obese type 2 diabetes
    Weight loss for overweight and obese type 2 diabetes
- Reduce the risk of micro- and macrovascular complications
- Ensure adequate nutritional intake
- Avoid 'atherogenic' diets or those that aggravate complications, e.g. high protein intake in nephropathy

them difficult to sustain. Patients should also be encouraged to stop smoking.

Dietary measures are required in the treatment of all people with diabetes. The aims are shown in Box 21.30. People with diabetes should have access to dietitians at diagnosis, review and at times of treatment change. Nutritional advice should be tailored to individuals and take account of their age and lifestyle. Structured education programmes are available for both common types of diabetes.

Composition of the diet

Recommended dietary composition is summarised in Box 21.31 (see also p. 107). Consumption of fruit and vegetables should be encouraged as components of a healthy diet.

Carbohydrate

Traditionally, people with diabetes, especially type 1 diabetes, have been advised to maintain a regular intake of carbohydrate in meals throughout the day. The development of modern insulin regimens, particularly using insulin analogues or continuous subcutaneous insulin infusion (CSII), has allowed greater flexibility in the timing and choice of carbohydrate intake. It is now possible to match the amount of carbohydrate in a meal with a dose of short-acting insulin using methods such as DAFNE (dose adjustment for normal eating), although this is demanding and requires extensive patient education. This approach enables motivated individuals with type 1 diabetes to achieve and maintain good glycaemic control, while avoiding post-prandial hyper- and hypoglycaemia.

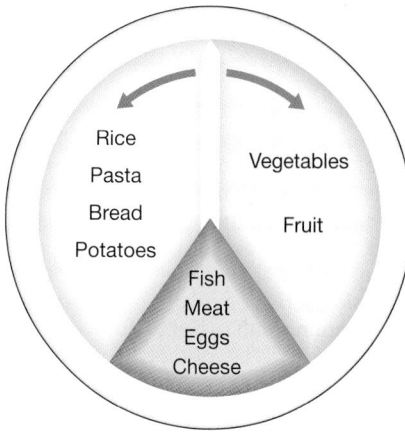

Fig. 21.11 A 'plate model' for meal planning. The plate is divided into three sections. The smallest section (one-fifth of total area) is for the meat, fish, eggs or cheese, and the remainder divided in roughly equal proportions between the staple food (rice, pasta, potatoes, bread etc.) and vegetables or fruit.

For people with type 2 diabetes, limitation of refined carbohydrate and restriction of total caloric intake is important, and a 'plate model' (Fig. 21.11) can provide a simple visual aid to show the proportions of carbohydrate and other food groups for selection at mealtimes.

Both the amount and source of carbohydrate determine post-prandial glucose (p. 109). The glycaemic index (GI) of a carbohydrate-containing food is a measure of the change in blood glucose following its ingestion. Different foods can be ranked by their effect on post-prandial glycaemia. Consumption of foods with a low GI is encouraged because they produce a slow, gradual rise in blood glucose. Examples include starchy foods such as basmati rice, spaghetti, porridge, noodles, granary bread, and beans and lentils. However, different methods of food processing and preparation can influence the GI of foods, as can the ripeness of some foods and differences in strains of rice. In addition, GI is limited to assessing the effect of consuming types of carbohydrate, and does not address the total amount consumed.

Fat

The intake of total fat should be restricted to less than 35% of energy intake, with less than 10% as saturated fat, and 10–20% from monounsaturated fat through consumption of oils and spreads made from olive, rapeseed or groundnut oils (see Box 21.31). The influence of dietary fats on plasma lipid profile and cardiovascular disease is discussed on page 110.

Diabetic foods and sweeteners

Low-calorie and sugar-free drinks are useful for patients with diabetes. These drinks usually contain non-nutritive sweeteners. Many 'diabetic foods' contain sorbitol, are expensive and high in calories, and may cause gastrointestinal side-effects. As a result, these foods are not recommended as part of the diabetic diet.

Salt

People with diabetes should follow the advice given to the general population: namely, to reduce sodium intake to no more than 6 g daily.

21.31 Recommended composition of diet for people with diabetes

Dietary constituent	Percentage of energy intake
Carbohydrate	45–60%
Sucrose	Up to 10%
Fat (total)	< 35%
n-6 Polyunsaturated	< 10%
n-3 Polyunsaturated	Eat 1 portion (140 g) oily fish once or twice weekly
Monounsaturated	10–20%
Saturated	< 10%
Protein	10–15% (do not exceed 1 g/kg body weight)
Fruit/vegetables	5 portions daily

21

Weight management

In patients with diabetes, weight management is a key factor, as a high percentage of people with type 2 diabetes are overweight or obese, and many anti-diabetic drugs including insulin encourage weight gain. Obesity, particularly central obesity with increased waist circumference, also predicts insulin resistance and cardiovascular risk.

Management of obesity is described on pages 118–121. Weight loss can be achieved through a reduction in energy intake and an increase in energy expenditure through physical activity. Some people find group motivation in a slimming club to be helpful when attempting to lose weight and this is appropriate for most patients with type 2 diabetes. Patients on oral anti-diabetic drugs, and especially those on insulin, may need to adjust their therapy when changing their diet.

Exercise

Diabetic patients should be strongly encouraged to take regular physical activity, in the form of walking, gardening, swimming or cycling, for approximately 30 minutes daily, as this improves insulin sensitivity and the lipid profile and lowers blood pressure.

Alcohol

Alcohol can be consumed in moderation unless there is a coexisting medical problem that requires abstinence. As alcohol suppresses gluconeogenesis, it can precipitate or protract hypoglycaemia, particularly in patients taking insulin or sulphonylureas. In the UK the weekly recommended limits are a maximum of 14 U for women and 21 U for men, a unit being defined as half a pint of beer/lager, a measure of spirits or a small glass of wine. Drinks containing alcohol can be a substantial (and often overlooked) source of calories and total intake may have to be reduced to assist weight reduction.

Anti-diabetic drugs

Various drugs are effective in reducing hyperglycaemia in patients with type 2 diabetes (Fig. 21.12). Although their mechanisms of action are different, most depend upon a supply of endogenous insulin and therefore have little hypoglycaemic effect in patients with type 1 diabetes. Metformin and sulphonylureas have been the mainstay of treatment for many years and have the strongest evidence of preventing complications of diabetes. However, newer agents include the α-glucosidase inhibitors, the thiazolidinediones and the dipeptidyl peptidase 4 inhibitors. These drugs may be used as monotherapy or in combinations as dual or triple therapy, but adherence to prescribed medication is best when few drugs are used, preferably with once-daily administration. The effects of these drugs are compared in Box 21.32.

Biguanides

Metformin is the only biguanide available. Its long-term benefits were shown in the UKPDS (p. 826), and it is now widely used as first-line therapy for type 2 diabetes, irrespective of body weight. Metformin is also used increasingly as an adjunct to insulin therapy in obese patients with type 1 diabetes. However, it is less well tolerated than sulphonylureas because of a higher incidence of side-effects, particularly gastrointestinal symptoms.

Mechanism of action

The mechanism of action of metformin has not been precisely defined. It has no hypoglycaemic effect in non-diabetic individuals, but in diabetes, insulin sensitivity and peripheral glucose uptake are increased, possibly through inhibition of mitochondrial respiration and activation of AMP-regulated kinase (AMPK) in muscle. There is some evidence that it also impairs glucose absorption by the gut and inhibits hepatic gluconeogenesis. Although secretion of some endogenous insulin is mandatory for its glucose-lowering action, it does not increase insulin secretion and seldom causes hypoglycaemia.

Indications for use

Administration of metformin is not associated with a rise in body weight and it may be beneficial for the overweight or obese patient. In addition, as the glucose-lowering effect of metformin is synergistic with that of sulphonylureas, the two can be combined when either alone has proved inadequate. It can also be given in combination with most other anti-diabetic medications. Metformin is given with food, usually starting with

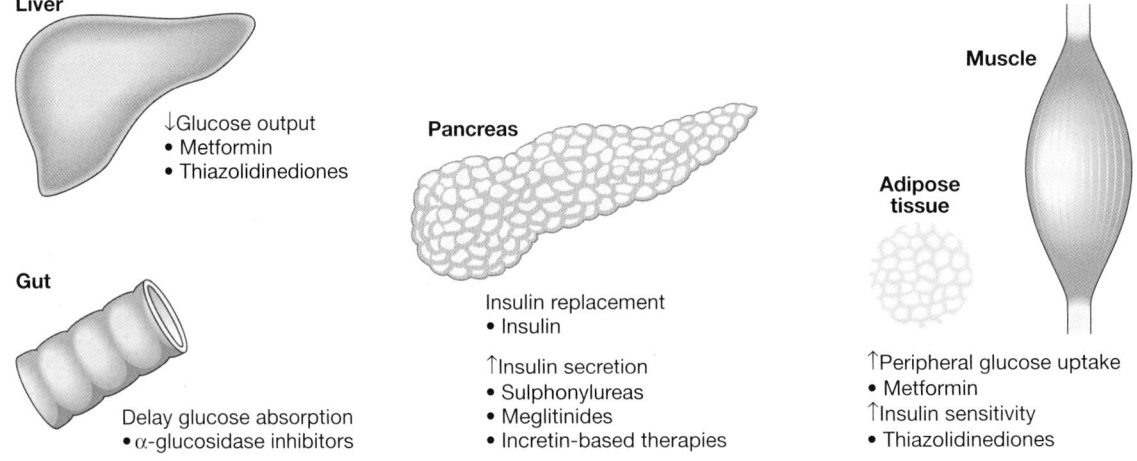

Fig. 21.12 Principal modes and sites of action of pharmacological treatments for type 2 diabetes.

21.32 Effects of anti-diabetic drugs used in the treatment of type 2 diabetes

	Insulin	Sulphonylureas and meglitinides	Metformin	Acarbose	Thiazolidinediones	Incretin-based therapies
Reduce basal glycaemia	Yes	Yes	Yes	Slightly	Yes	Yes
Reduce post-prandial glycaemia	Yes	Yes	Yes	Yes	Yes	Yes
Raise plasma insulin	Yes	Yes	No	No	No	Yes
Increase body weight	Yes	Yes	No	No	Yes	No
Improve lipid profile	Yes	No	Slightly	Slightly	Variably	Yes
Risk of hypoglycaemia	Yes	Yes	No	No	No	No
Tolerability	Good	Good	Moderate	Moderate	Good	Moderate

500 mg 12-hourly, gradually increased as required to a maximum of 1 g 8-hourly.

Metformin can increase susceptibility to lactic acidosis. Its use is contraindicated in patients with impaired renal or hepatic function and in those who drink alcohol in excess in whom the risk of lactic acidosis is significantly increased. It should be discontinued, at least temporarily, if any other serious medical condition develops, especially one causing severe shock or hypoxaemia. In such circumstances, treatment with insulin should be substituted.

Sulphonylureas

Mechanism of action

Sulphonylureas are 'insulin secretagogues' that act through a specific receptor which is linked to a K^+ channel on the surface of pancreatic β cells. K^+ transport triggers insulin secretion.

Indications for use

Sulphonylureas are valuable in the treatment of non-obese patients with type 2 diabetes who fail to respond to dietary measures alone. Although sulphonylureas will lower the blood glucose concentration of obese patients with type 2 diabetes, such patients should be treated energetically in the first instance by dietary measures with or without metformin, since treatment with sulphonylureas is often associated with an increase in weight which will exacerbate insulin resistance.

The main differences between the individual compounds lie in their potency, duration of action and cost. Tolbutamide, the mildest of the first-generation sulphonylureas, is very well tolerated. Its duration of action is relatively short, it is usually administered 8- or 12-hourly, and it is a useful drug in the elderly in whom the risk and the consequences of inducing hypoglycaemia are greater. Chlorpropamide has a biological half-life of about 36 hours and is taken once daily, but may cause severe and prolonged hypoglycaemia and is rarely used.

Of the second-generation sulphonylureas, gliclazide and glipizide cause few side-effects, but glibenclamide is prone to induce severe hypoglycaemia and should be avoided in the elderly. Newer long-acting preparations such as glimepiride and a modified-release form of gliclazide can be administered once daily with no apparent increased risk of hypoglycaemia. The dose-response of all sulphonylureas is steepest at low doses; little additional hypoglycaemic benefit is obtained when the dose is increased to maximal levels. Several drugs can potentiate the hypoglycaemic effect of sulphonylureas by displacing them from their plasma protein-binding sites, e.g. salicylates, phenylbutazone and antifungal agents.

Meglitinides

These insulin secretagogues are called prandial glucose regulators. Repaglinide directly stimulates endogenous insulin secretion through the sulphonylurea receptor and is taken immediately before food. It is less likely to cause hypoglycaemia than sulphonylureas. Nateglinide has a similar mode of action, restores first-phase insulin secretion, and can be prescribed with metformin.

Alpha-glucosidase inhibitors

The α-glucosidase inhibitors delay carbohydrate absorption in the gut by selectively inhibiting disaccharidases. Acarbose and miglitol are available and are taken with each meal. Both lower post-prandial blood glucose and modestly improve overall glycaemic control. They can be combined with a sulphonylurea. The main side-effects are flatulence, abdominal bloating and diarrhoea. They are used widely in the Far East but infrequently in the UK.

Thiazolidinediones

Mechanism of action

These drugs (also called TZD drugs, 'glitazones' or PPARγ agonists) bind and activate peroxisome proliferator-activated receptor-γ, a nuclear receptor present mainly in adipose tissue that regulates the expression of several genes involved in metabolism. TZDs enhance the actions of endogenous insulin, partly directly (in the adipose cells) and partly indirectly (by altering release of 'adipokines' such as adiponectin and resistin which alter insulin sensitivity in the liver). Plasma insulin concentrations are not increased and hypoglycaemia does not occur.

21

Indications for use

Pioglitazone or rosiglitazone are usually prescribed as second-line therapy with metformin, or as third-line therapy in combination with sulphonylurea and metformin (known as 'triple therapy'). However, their use as monotherapy and in combination with insulin is increasing.

TZDs are most likely to be effective in patients with pronounced insulin resistance (e.g. in abdominal obesity) and redistribute fat away from the abdominal stores and into subcutaneous depots. However, body weight and total body fat are increased by TZDs.

A clinical study and meta-analysis have shown that pioglitazone reduces myocardial infarctions and strokes, so may benefit patients with cardiovascular disease. However, rosiglitazone may slightly increase acute ischaemic events, so should be avoided in patients with coronary heart disease.

TZDs have significant side-effects. The first drug of this class, troglitazone, had to be withdrawn because of hepatotoxicity and newer TZDs are avoided in patients with liver dysfunction, but it appears that this effect was specific to troglitazone. An important side-effect of all TZDs is sodium and fluid retention, which is aggravated if they are combined with insulin. TZDs must be avoided in patients with cardiac failure. They also increase upper limb fractures, mainly in women.

Incretin-based therapies

The secretion of insulin in response to a rise in blood glucose is greater when glucose is given by mouth than by intravenous infusion. In part this is caused by secretion of gut hormones, or incretins, which potentiate glucose-induced insulin secretion. Glucagon-like peptide (GLP-1) is an incretin hormone which stimulates insulin secretion in a glucose-dependent manner; thus hypoglycaemia does not occur. In addition, GLP-1 suppresses glucagon secretion, delays gastric emptying, reduces appetite and encourages weight loss.

As GLP-1 is rapidly degraded by the enzyme, dipeptidyl peptidase 4, inhibitors of this enzyme can be used to prolong its biological effect. The DPP-4 inhibitors or gliptins (sitagliptin, vildagliptin and saxagliptin) are oral agents which act in this manner. They are weight-neutral and have few side-effects.

Synthetic GLP-1 receptor antagonists with longer therapeutic action include exenatide (synthetic exendin-4) and liraglutide but, although they have the advantage of inducing weight loss in most patients, they have to be given daily by subcutaneous injection and may cause nausea. Pancreatitis is a rare complication of treatment with exenatide. Long-acting GLP-1 receptor antagonists are being evaluated, which will be administered once weekly.

Incretin-based therapies are most useful in obese patients and can be used in combination with other oral anti-diabetic agents.

Insulin therapy

Manufacture and formulation

Insulin was discovered in 1921 and transformed the management of type 1 diabetes, until then a fatal disorder. Until the 1980s insulin was obtained by extraction and purification from pancreata of cows and pigs

21.33 Duration of action (in hours) of insulin preparations

Insulin	Onset	Peak	Duration
Rapid-acting (insulin analogues: lispro, aspart, glulisine)	< 0.5	0.5–2.5	3–4.5
Short-acting (soluble (regular))	0.5–1	1–4	4–8
Intermediate-acting (isophane (NPH), lente)	1–3	3–8	7–14
Long-acting (bovine ultralente)	2–4	6–12	12–30
Long-acting (insulin analogues: glargine, detemir)	1–2	None	18–24

(bovine and porcine insulins), and some patients still prefer to use animal insulins. Recombinant DNA technology enabled large-scale production of human insulin. More recently, the amino acid sequence of insulin has been altered to produce analogues of insulin, which differ in their rate of absorption from the site of injection.

The duration of action of short-acting, unmodified insulin ('soluble' or 'regular' insulin), which is a clear solution, can be extended by the addition of protamine and zinc at neutral pH (isophane or NPH insulin) or excess zinc ions (lente insulins). These modified 'depot' insulins are cloudy preparations. Pre-mixed formulations containing short-acting and isophane insulins in various proportions are available. The pharmacokinetics of these various insulins are shown in Box 21.33.

In most countries, the insulin concentration in available formulations has been standardised at 100 U/mL.

Subcutaneous multiple dose insulin therapy

In most patients, insulin is injected subcutaneously several times a day into the anterior abdominal wall, upper arms, outer thighs and buttocks (Box 21.34). Accidental intramuscular injection often occurs in children and thin adults. The rate of absorption of insulin may be influenced by many factors other than the insulin formulation, including the site, depth and volume of injection, skin temperature (warming), local massage and exercise. Absorption is delayed from areas of lipohypertrophy at injection sites (p. 797), which results from the local trophic action of insulin, so repeated injection at the same site should be avoided. Other routes of administration (intravenous and intraperitoneal) are reserved for specific circumstances.

Insulin can be administered using a disposable plastic syringe with a fine needle (which can be reused several times) in preference to the traditional glass syringe

21.34 How to inject insulin subcutaneously

- Needle sited at right angle to the skin
- Subcutaneous (not intramuscular) injection
- Delivery devices: glass syringe (requires re-sterilisation), plastic syringe (disposable), pen device, infusion pump

and metal needle which require repeated sterilisation. Pen injectors with insulin in cartridge form are popular and convenient and are also available as pre-loaded disposable pens.

Short-acting insulin has to be injected at least 30 minutes before a meal to allow adequate time for absorption. Many patients find this inconvenient and ignore this requirement. However, the rapidly absorbed fast-acting insulin analogues can be administered immediately before, during or even after meals, and their peak action coincides more closely with the post-prandial rise in blood glucose (see Box 21.33).

Once absorbed into the blood, insulin has a half-life of a few minutes. It is removed mainly by the liver and also the kidneys; plasma insulin concentrations are elevated in patients with liver disease or renal failure. The rate of clearance is also affected by binding to insulin antibodies (associated with the use of animal insulins).

The complications of insulin therapy are listed in Box 21.35; the most important of these is hypoglycaemia (p. 812). A common problem is fasting hyperglycaemia ('the dawn phenomenon') associated with the normal circadian rhythm and causing release of counter-regulatory hormones during the later part of the night, which antagonise insulin action before wakening.

21.35 Side-effects of insulin therapy

- Hypoglycaemia
- Weight gain
- Peripheral oedema (insulin treatment causes salt and water retention in the short term)
- Insulin antibodies (animal insulins)
- Local allergy (rare)
- Lipodystrophy at injection sites

Insulin dosing regimens

The choice of regimen depends on the desired degree of glycaemic control, the severity of underlying insulin deficiency, the patient's lifestyle, and his or her ability to adjust the insulin dose. The time-action profile of different insulin regimens, compared to the secretory pattern of insulin in the non-diabetic state, is shown in Figure 21.13. Most people require two or more injections of insulin daily. Once-daily injections rarely achieve satisfactory glycaemic control and are reserved either for some elderly patients or for those who retain substantial endogenous insulin secretion and have a low insulin requirement.

Twice-daily administration of a short-acting and intermediate-acting insulin (usually soluble and isophane insulins), given in combination before breakfast and the evening meal, is the simplest regimen and is still used commonly. Individual doses vary considerably but usually two-thirds of the total daily requirement of insulin is given in the morning in a ratio of 1:2, short-:intermediate-acting insulins. The remaining third is given in the evening, and doses are adjusted according to blood glucose measurements. Several pre-mixed formulations are available containing different proportions of soluble and isophane insulins (e.g. 30:70 and 50:50). These are useful for patients who have difficulty mix-

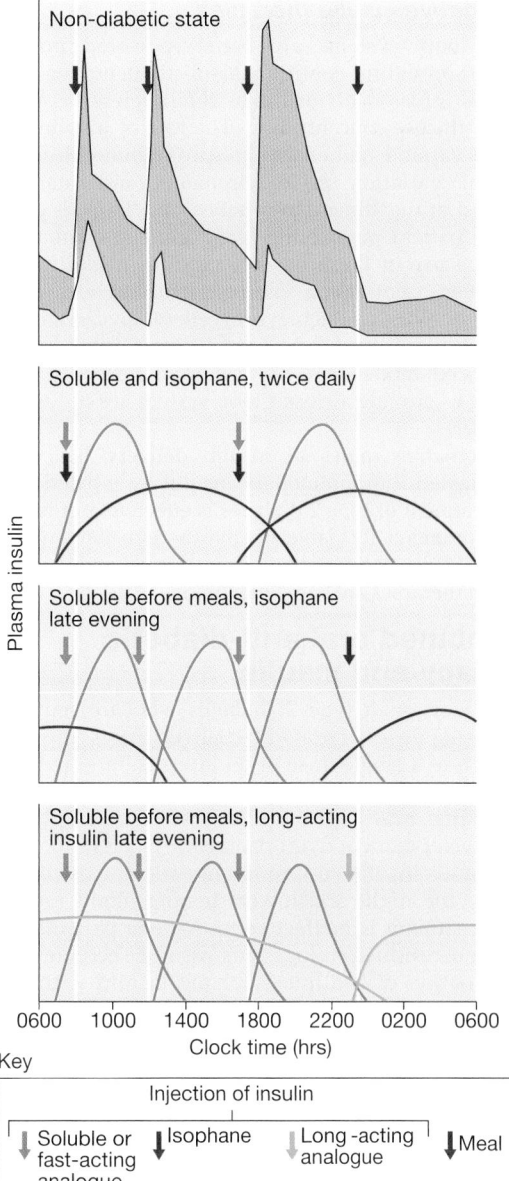

Fig. 21.13 Profiles of plasma insulin associated with different insulin regimens. The schematic profiles are compared with the insulin responses (mean ± standard deviation) observed in non-diabetic adults, shown in the top panel (shaded area). These are theoretical patterns of plasma insulin and may differ considerably in magnitude and duration of action between individuals.

ing insulins, but are inflexible as the individual components cannot be adjusted independently, and require to be resuspended by shaking the vial several times before administration.

Multiple injection regimens are popular, with short-acting insulin being taken before each meal (usually by en injector), and intermediate- or long-acting insulin being injected once or twice daily (basal-bolus regimen). This type of regimen allows greater freedom of timing of meals and more variable day-to-day physical activity, but snacks may have to be taken between meals to prevent hypoglycaemia.

Alternative insulin therapies

'Open-loop' systems are battery-powered portable pumps providing continuous subcutaneous or intra-venous infusion of insulin without reference to the blood glucose concentration. The rate of insulin infusion is variable and can be pre-programmed to match diurnal variation in requirements and manually boosted at mealtimes. In practice, the 'loop' is closed by the patient performing blood glucose estimations, and the use of these devices requires a high degree of patient motivation. These increasingly sophisticated systems can achieve excellent glycaemic control but widespread therapeutic use is limited by cost. Advanced models linked to a miniaturised glucose sensor to provide a closed loop system are not widely available.

Alternative routes of insulin delivery have been investigated. Intrapulmonary insulin by inhalation for the treatment of type 2 diabetes is effective, but has not been commercially viable and may be associated with an increased risk of lung cancer. Transdermal and even oral insulin therapies are being explored.

Combined oral anti-diabetic therapy and insulin

In patients with type 2 diabetes who are requiring increasing doses of oral anti-diabetic drugs, the introduction of a single dose of an intermediate- (e.g. isophane) or long-acting insulin analogue, administered at bedtime, may improve glycaemic control and delay the development of overt pancreatic β-cell failure. The exogenous insulin suppresses hepatic glucose output during the night and lowers fasting blood glucose. This treatment is ineffective in diabetic patients who have no residual endogenous insulin secretion. The combination of bedtime isophane insulin with metformin is the regimen least likely to promote weight gain.

Transplantation

Whole pancreas transplantation is carried out in a small number of patients with diabetes each year, but it presents problems relating to the exocrine pancreatic secretions and long-term immunosuppression is necessary. While results are steadily improving, they remain less favourable than for renal transplantation. At present the procedure is usually undertaken only in patients with end-stage renal failure who require a combined pancreas/kidney transplantation in whom diabetes control is particularly difficult, e.g. because of recurrent hypoglycaemia.

Transplantation of isolated pancreatic islets (usually into the liver via the portal vein) has been achieved safely in an increasing number of centres around the world. Progress is being made towards meeting the needs of supply, purification and storage of islets, but the problems of transplant rejection, and of destruction by the patient's autoantibodies against β cells, remain. Nevertheless, the development of methods of inducing tolerance to transplanted islets and the potential use of stem cells means that this may still prove the most promising approach in the long term.

LONG-TERM COMPLICATIONS OF DIABETES

The long-term results of treatment of diabetes are disappointing in many patients. Although a few diabetic patients die from acute metabolic complications (ketoacidosis and hypoglycaemia), the major problem is the excess mortality and serious morbidity suffered as a result of the long-term complications of diabetes (see Box 21.29, p. 818). The factors associated with these are listed in Box 21.36.

As shown in Box 21.37, excess mortality in diabetes is caused mainly by large blood vessel disease, particularly myocardial infarction and stroke. Macrovascular disease also causes substantial morbidity from myocardial infarction, stroke, angina, cardiac failure and intermittent claudication. The pathological changes associated with atherosclerosis in diabetic patients are similar to those seen in the non-diabetic population but they occur earlier in life and are more extensive and severe. Diabetes amplifies the effects of the other major cardiovascular risk factors: smoking, hypertension and dyslipidaemia (Fig. 21.14). Moreover, patients with type 2 diabetes are more likely to have additional cardiovascular risk factors, which co-segregate in the metabolic (insulin resistance) syndrome (see Box 21.4, p. 802).

Disease of small blood vessels is a specific complication of diabetes and is termed diabetic microangiopathy. It contributes to mortality through renal failure caused by diabetic nephropathy, and is responsible for substantial morbidity and disability: for example, blindness

21.36 Factors associated with increased mortality and morbidity in people with diabetes

- Duration of diabetes
- Early age at onset of disease
- High glycated haemoglobin (HbA_{1c})
- Raised blood pressure
- Proteinuria; microalbuminuria
- Dyslipidaemia
- Obesity

21.37 Mortality in diabetes

Risk versus non-diabetic controls (mortality ratio)

• Overall	2.6
• Coronary heart disease	
Cerebrovascular disease	2.8
Peripheral vascular disease	
• All other causes, including renal failure	2.7

Causes of death in diabetes (approximate proportion)

• Cardiovascular disease	70%
• Renal failure	10%
• Cancer	10%
• Infections	6%
• Diabetic ketoacidosis	1%
• Other	3%

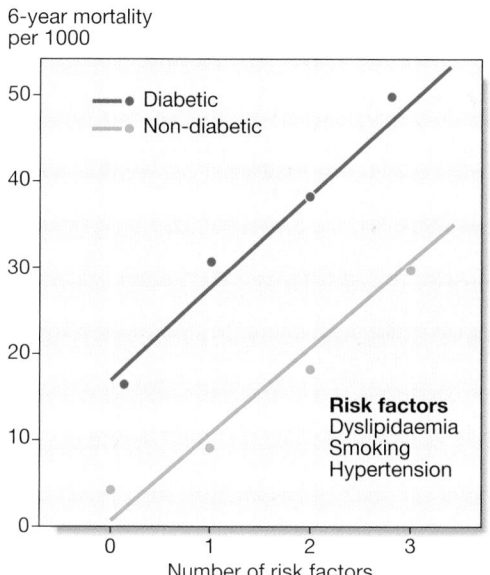

6-year mortality
per 1000

Fig. 21.14 Diabetes mellitus as a risk factor for coronary heart disease (CHD). Three major factors—smoking, hypertension and dyslipidaemia—are associated with risk of CHD in the general population. The presence of diabetes mellitus produces an increment in risk in addition to these conventional factors (p. 580).

from diabetic retinopathy, difficulty in walking, chronic ulceration of the feet from peripheral neuropathy, and bowel and bladder dysfunction from autonomic neuropathy. Positive correlations exist between the duration and degree of sustained hyperglycaemia, however caused and at whatever age it develops, and the risk of microvascular disease.

Pathophysiology

The histopathological hallmark of diabetic microangiopathy is thickening of the capillary basement membrane, with associated increased vascular permeability throughout the body. The development of the characteristic clinical syndromes of diabetic retinopathy, nephropathy, neuropathy and accelerated atherosclerosis is thought to result from the local response to the generalised vascular injury. For example, in the wall of large vessels, increased permeability of arterial endothelium, particularly when combined with hyperinsulinaemia and hypertension, may increase the deposition of atherogenic lipoproteins.

The mechanisms linking hyperglycaemia to these pathological changes are, however, poorly characterised. Functional abnormalities found in long-standing, poorly controlled diabetes include endothelial dysfunction, haemodynamic disturbances, haemorrheological and coagulation abnormalities, microvascular hypertension and increased capillary permeability. Some of the numerous biochemical abnormalities are shown in Figure 21.15. It is thought that increased metabolism of glucose to sorbitol via the polyol pathway is of central importance in pathogenesis, since haemodynamic, vascular permeability and structural changes in capillaries are preventable in diabetic animals by treatment with a variety of structurally different aldose-reductase inhibitors which inhibit this process.

Preventing diabetes complications
Glycaemic control

The possibility of reversing early microvascular disease by improving metabolic control has been examined in several prospective randomised controlled clinical trials involving patients with early background retinopathy and minimal proteinuria. None of these

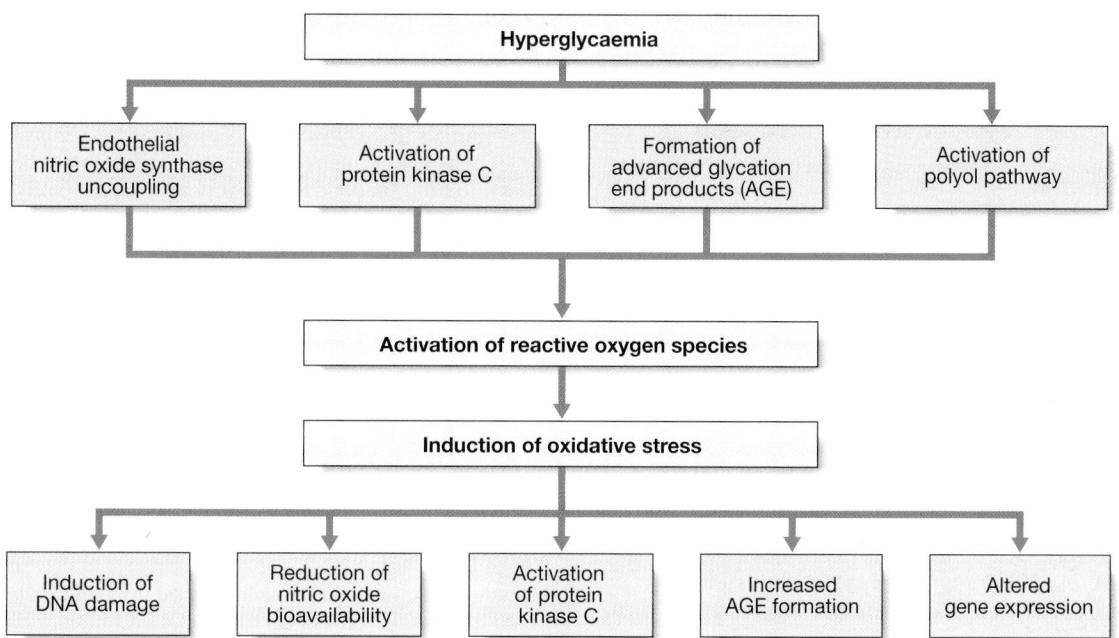

Fig. 21.15 The roles of hyperglycaemia-induced accumulation of reactive oxygen species and oxidative stress in causation of diabetic vascular complications. The induction of oxidative stress causes haemodynamic changes and endothelial and vascular dysfunction, leading to vascular damage.

studies produced any evidence of reversal of either retinopathy or nephropathy, and in some cases retinopathy worsened abruptly soon after control was improved. Despite this, in the long term the rate of progression of both retinopathy and nephropathy was reduced by maintaining good glycaemic control. These studies stimulated a search for markers of early reversible retinal, renal and neural dysfunction, and shifted the emphasis in the management of diabetes to primary prevention of complications.

The Diabetes Control and Complications Trial (DCCT) was a large study that lasted 9 years in type 1 diabetic patients. There was a 60% overall reduction in the risk of developing diabetic complications in those on intensive therapy with strict glycaemic control (mean HbA_{1c} around 7%), compared with those on conventional therapy (mean HbA_{1c} around 9%, Box 21.38). No single factor other than glycaemic control had a significant effect on outcome. A large study of patients with type 2 diabetes, the UK Prospective Diabetes Study (UKPDS), also showed that the frequency of diabetic complications is lower and progression is slower with good glycaemic control and effective treatment of hypertension, irrespective of the type of therapy used (Box 21.39). These landmark trials demonstrated that diabetic complications are preventable and that the aim of treatment should be 'near-normal' glycaemia.

However, in the patients with strict glycaemic control in the DCCT, weight gain was common and severe hypoglycaemic episodes occurred three times more often. Although there was no detectable increase in deaths, major macrovascular events or neurological/cognitive defects, this increased risk of hypoglycaemia may alter

---

21.40 Diabetes management in old age

- **Glycaemic control**: the optimal target for glycaemic control in older people has yet to be determined. Strict glycaemic control should be avoided in very frail patients.
- **Cognitive and affective function**: may benefit from improving glycaemic control.
- **Hypoglycaemia**: older people have reduced symptomatic awareness of hypoglycaemia and limited knowledge of symptoms, and are at greater risk of, and from, hypoglycaemia.
- **Mortality**: the mortality rate of older people with diabetes is more than double that of age-matched non-diabetic people, largely because of increased deaths from cardiovascular disease.

---

the risk:benefit ratio of good control in certain patients. Thus less intensive treatment may be indicated in:

- those with impaired awareness of hypoglycaemia
- those with severe macrovascular disease (particularly if they have a past history of myocardial infarction or cerebrovascular accident)
- those at the extremes of life (very young children and the frail elderly, Box 21.40).

Control of other risk factors

Randomised controlled trials have shown that aggressive management of blood pressure minimises the microvascular and macrovascular complications of diabetes. ACE inhibitors are valuable in improving outcome in heart disease and in preventing diabetic nephropathy (p. 829). The management of dyslipidaemia with a statin limits macrovascular disease in people with diabetes. This often results in the necessary use of multiple medications, which augments the problem of adherence to therapy by patients.

Other approaches

There are new approaches to preventing diabetic complications which have been effective in animal models. Aldose-reductase inhibitors have been disappointing in clinical trials. Aminoguanidine, an inhibitor of the formation of advanced glycation end-products, prevents damage to the retina, kidney, nerve and artery in diabetic animals. It has low toxicity and may be applicable for human use. Protein kinase C inhibitors have been shown to limit diabetic retinopathy and nephropathy in humans and are undergoing clinical trials.

Diabetic retinopathy

Diabetic retinopathy is one of the commonest causes of blindness in adults between 30 and 65 years of age in developed countries. Retinal photocoagulation is an effective treatment, particularly if it is given at a relatively early stage when the patient is usually symptomless. Expert annual examination of the fundi is therefore mandatory in all diabetic patients.

Pathogenesis

Hyperglycaemia increases retinal blood flow and metabolism and has direct effects on retinal endothelial cells and pericyte loss, which impairs vascular autoregulation. The resulting uncontrolled blood flow initially dilates capillaries but also increases production of vasoactive substances and endothelial cell proliferation,

---

EBM **21.38 Glycaemic control in type 1 diabetes**

'In patients with type 1 diabetes, strict glycaemic control (mean HbA_{1c} 7%) reduced the development of retinopathy and other microvascular complications by 76% compared with conventional therapy (mean HbA_{1c} 9%). On longer-term follow-up strict glycaemic control also reduced cardiovascular events, including myocardial infarction, stroke and death from cardiovascular disease.'

- Diabetes Control and Complications Trial Research Group. N Engl J Med 1993; 329:977–986.
- Diabetes Control and Complications Trial/Epidemiology of Diabetes Interventions and Complications (DCCT/EDIC) Study Research Group. N Engl J Med 2005; 353:2643–2653.

For further information: 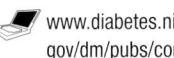 www.diabetes.niddk.nih. gov/dm/pubs/control/

EBM **21.39 Glycaemic control in type 2 diabetes**

'In patients with type 2 diabetes, intensive glycaemic control (mean HbA_{1c} 7%) with oral anti-diabetic drugs or insulin reduced the development of microvascular complications, particularly retinopathy, by 25% compared with conventional treatment (mean HbA_{1c} 8%). On longer-term follow-up there was a significant reduction in myocardial infarction and all-cause mortality.'

- UKPDS Group. Lancet 1998; 352:837–853, 854–865.
- Holman RR, et al. N Engl J Med 2008; 359:1577–1589.

For further information: www.dtu.ox.ac.uk

resulting in capillary closure. This causes chronic retinal hypoxia and stimulates production of growth factors, including vascular endothelial growth factor (VEGF), which plays a major role in stimulating the deleterious changes of endothelial cell growth (causing new vessel formation) and increased vascular permeability (causing retinal leakage and exudation).

Clinical features

These are listed in Box 21.41. They occur in varying combinations in different patients and are used to classify the severity of retinopathy and assess the need for specialist referral, as shown in Box 21.42.

21.41 Clinical features of diabetic retinopathy

- Microaneurysms
- Retinal haemorrhages (dot and blot)
- Exudates
- Cotton wool spots
- Venous changes
- Neovascularisation (retina and iris)
- Pre-retinal/subhyaloid haemorrhage
- Vitreous haemorrhage
- Fibrosis/gliosis

Microaneurysms

In most cases these are the earliest clinical abnormality detected. They appear as tiny, discrete, circular, dark red dots near to, but apparently separate from, the retinal vessels (Fig. 21.16A). They look like tiny haemorrhages but they are in fact minute aneurysms arising mainly from the venous end of capillaries. They may give rise to retinal leakage of plasma constituents.

Haemorrhages

These most characteristically occur in the deeper layers of the retina and hence are round and regular in shape and described as 'blot' haemorrhages (see Fig. 21.16A). The smaller ones may be difficult to differentiate from microaneurysms and the two are often grouped together as 'dots and blots'. Superficial flame-shaped haemorrhages in the nerve fibre layer may also occur, particularly if the patient is hypertensive.

Exudates

These are characteristic of diabetic retinopathy. They vary in size from tiny specks to large confluent patches and tend to occur particularly in the perimacular area (Fig. 21.16B). They result from leakage of plasma from abnormal retinal capillaries and overlie areas of neuronal degeneration. The terms 'hard' exudates and 'soft' exudates (i.e. cotton wool spots) are no longer recommended.

Cotton wool spots

These are similar to retinal changes that occur in hypertension, and also occur particularly within five disc diameters of the optic disc (Fig. 21.16E). They represent arteriolar occlusions causing retinal ischaemia and, if numerous, may represent pre-proliferative diabetic retinopathy; they are most often seen in rapidly advancing retinopathy or in association with uncontrolled hypertension.

21

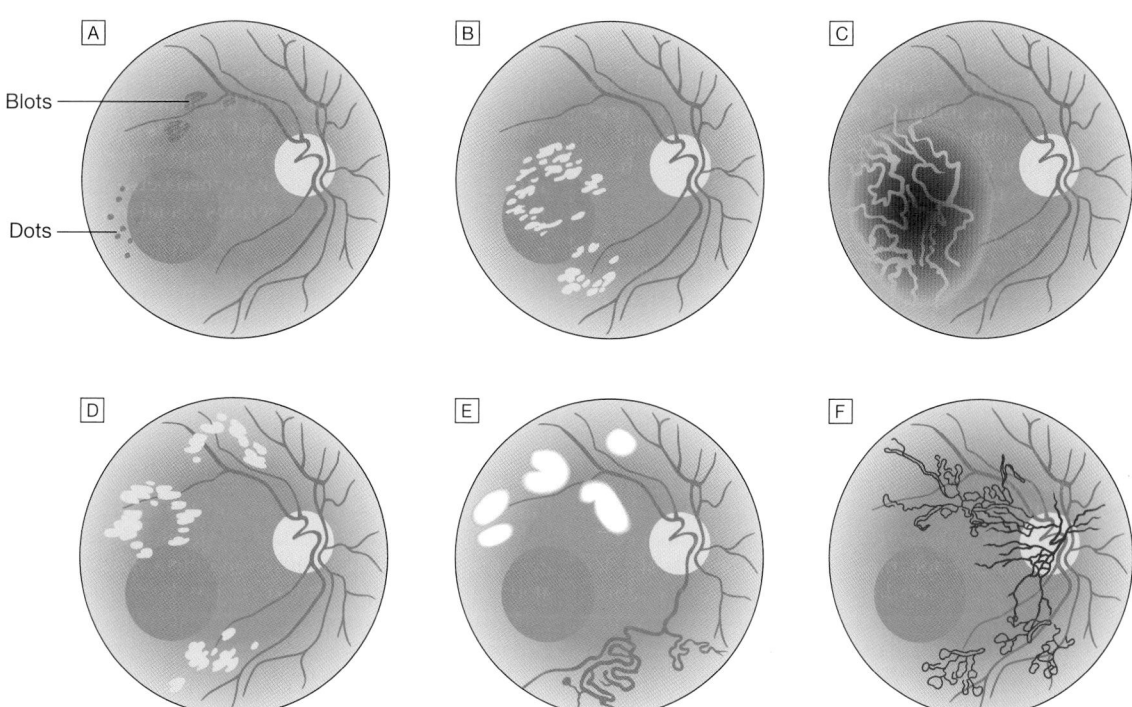

Fig. 21.16 Diagrammatic representation of diabetic eye disease. **A** Background diabetic retinopathy showing microaneurysms and blot haemorrhages. **B** Background retinopathy showing exudates. **C** Maculopathy showing oedema. **D** Maculopathy with exudates. **E** Pre-proliferative retinopathy showing venous changes and cotton wool spots. **F** Proliferative retinopathy showing neovascularisation.

21

Type of retinopathy	Prognosis	Action required
Non-proliferative 'background' retinopathy without maculopathy		
Venous dilatation	No immediate threat to vision	Maximise control of blood glucose, lipids and blood pressure
Peripheral		Give advice to stop smoking and reduce intake of alcohol
Microaneurysms		On first appearance inform diabetes team and carers
Blot haemorrhages		Observe carefully, i.e. fundoscopy with dilated pupils every 6–12 mths
Exudates		Refer for specialist opinion if rate of progression increases significantly
Maculopathy		
Macula	Sight-threatening	Refer for specialist opinion
Exudation		Medical review of risk factors, glycaemic control, blood pressure and
Haemorrhage		lipid levels
Ischaemia		
Oedema		
Pre-proliferative retinopathy		
Venous loops and beading	Sight-threatening	Refer for specialist opinion
Clusters/sheets of microaneurysms and		At this stage rapid lowering of the blood glucose may result in abrupt
small blot haemorrhages and/or large		worsening of retinopathy with the appearance of cotton wool spots and
retinal haemorrhages		an increased number of haemorrhages; it may be safer to lower the
Intra-retinal microvascular		blood glucose gradually over a period of months
abnormalities		
Multiple cotton wool spots		
Macular oedema with reduced visual		
acuity		
Perimacular exudates ± retinal		
haemorrhages of any size		
Proliferative retinopathy		
Pre-retinal haemorrhage	Sight-threatening	Urgent review and treatment by specialist is mandatory
Neovascularisation		
Fibrosis		
Exudative maculopathy		

Intra-retinal microvascular abnormalities

Intra-retinal microvascular abnormalities (IRMA) are dilated, tortuous capillaries which develop in severe pre-proliferative retinopathy. They represent the remaining patent capillaries in an area of ischaemic retina where most have been occluded.

Venous changes

These include venous dilatation (an early feature probably representing increased blood flow), 'beading' (sausage-like changes in calibre) and increased tortuosity, sometimes in the form of 'oxbow lakes' or loops. These latter changes indicate widespread non-perfusion of capillaries and are a feature of severe pre-proliferative retinopathy.

Neovascularisation

New vessel formation may arise from the venous circulation either on the optic disc (NVD) or elsewhere in the retina (NVE), in response to widespread retinal ischaemia. The earliest appearance is that of fine tufts of delicate vessels forming arcades on the surface of the retina (Fig. 21.16F). As they grow, they may extend forwards on to the posterior surface of the vitreous. They are fragile and leaky, and are liable to rupture during vitreous movement, causing a pre-retinal ('subhyaloid') or a vitreous haemorrhage. New vessels may be symptomless until haemorrhage occurs, when there may be sudden visual loss. Serous products leaking from these new vessels stimulate a connective tissue reaction, called gliosis and fibrosis. This first appears as a white, cloudy haze among the network of new vessels. As it extends, the new vessels may be obliterated and the surrounding retina is covered by a dense white sheet. By this stage, haemorrhage is less common but retinal detachment can occur through traction on adhesions formed between the vitreous and the retina, causing serious visual impairment.

Rubeosis iridis

Proliferative retinopathy and severe ocular ischaemia may be accompanied by the development of new vessels on the anterior surface of the iris: 'rubeosis iridis'. These vessels may obstruct the drainage angle of the eye and the outflow of aqueous fluid, causing secondary glaucoma.

Loss of visual acuity

Microaneurysms, abnormalities of the veins, and small blot haemorrhages and exudates situated in the periphery will not interfere with vision unless they are associated with oedema and thickening in the macular area.

Macular oedema should be suspected if there is impairment of visual acuity, even if this is associated with only mild peripheral non-proliferative retinopathy and no other obvious pathology. Macular oedema can only be confirmed or excluded on slit lamp retinal biomicroscopy. If macular changes are observed by direct ophthalmoscopy or retinal photography, referable maculopathy should be suspected.

Sudden visual loss occurs with vitreous haemorrhage or retinal detachment. In pre-proliferative and proliferative retinopathy, whether or not visual acuity is impaired, prompt laser treatment is important to reduce the risk of haemorrhage, fibrosis/gliosis and severe irreversible visual impairment.

Prevention

Glycaemic, blood pressure and lipid profile control

Risk factors for retinopathy include early onset and long duration of diabetes, hypertension, poor glycaemic control, pregnancy, use of the oral contraceptive pill, smoking, excessive alcohol consumption and evidence of microangiopathy elsewhere, particularly neuropathy and nephropathy. Good glycaemic control, particularly in the early years following the development of diabetes, reduces the risk of developing retinopathy.

Hyperglycaemia promotes retinal hyperperfusion, so a rapid reduction in blood glucose may cause an initial deterioration of retinopathy by causing relative ischaemia. Improvement in glycaemic control should therefore be effected gradually. The rate of progression of retinopathy is significantly slower in intensively treated patients than in matched control subjects after a 12–18-month period.

Blood pressure lowering is of proven benefit in hypertensive patients, and there may be specific benefit from angiotensin II receptor antagonists. While the effect of statins in retinopathy is limited, clinical trials have suggested that fibrate treatment may reduce the requirement for laser therapy in type 2 diabetes.

Screening

Annual screening for retinopathy is essential in all diabetic patients as the disease is asymptomatic in the early stages, when treatment is most effective. Screening is particularly important in those with risk factors. It should be undertaken by trained personnel in an organised and audited programme. The preferred method is a digital photographic system for retinal imaging, with prompt referral of patients with sight-threatening retinopathy to an ophthalmologist for examination with slit lamp biomicroscopy. If direct ophthalmoscopy is used, the pupils should be dilated for adequate examination. Unfortunately, many people with diabetes receive no regular supervision and do not attend for eye screening.

Management

Severe retinopathy is treated with retinal photocoagulation (laser treatment), which has been shown to reduce severe visual loss by 85% (50% in patients with maculopathy). Photocoagulation is used:
- to treat leaking microaneurysms and areas of retinal thickening in the macular area, and to reduce macular oedema (focal laser)
- to destroy areas of retinal ischaemia and hence lower intra-ocular levels of VEGF which play a major role in the development of neovascularisation
- to reduce the risk of recurrent haemorrhage by inducing gliosis and fibrosis of new vessels (pan-retinal photocoagulation (PRP)).

Argon laser photocoagulation is the usual method used for PRP and focal treatment. This simple procedure can be carried out under topical anaesthesia. Patients should be reviewed regularly to look for further development of new vessels and/or maculopathy. Extensive

bilateral photocoagulation can cause significant visual field loss, which may interfere with driving ability and reduce night vision.

Vitrectomy may be used in selected cases with advanced diabetic eye disease where visual loss has been caused by recurrent vitreous haemorrhage that has failed to clear or by retinal detachment resulting from retinitis proliferans (extensive glial/fibrous tissue on the retina). Rubeosis iridis is a severe complication requiring early and extensive PRP.

Other causes of visual loss in people with diabetes

Around 50% of visual loss in people with type 2 diabetes results from causes other than diabetic retinopathy. These include cataract, age-related macular degeneration, retinal vein occlusion, retinal arterial occlusion, non-arteritic ischaemic optic neuropathy and glaucoma. Some of these conditions are to be expected in this group as they relate to cardiovascular risk factors (e.g. hypertension, hyperlipidaemia and smoking), all of which are prevalent in people with type 2 diabetes.

Cataract

Cataract is a permanent lens opacity and is a common cause of visual deterioration in the elderly. The lens thickens and opacifies with age; with diabetes, the increased metabolic insult to the lens causes these changes to accelerate and occur prematurely. A rare type of 'snow-flake' cataract occurs in young patients with poorly controlled diabetes. This does not usually affect vision but tends to make fundal examination difficult.

The indications for cataract extraction are similar to those for the non-diabetic population and depend on the degree of visual impairment. An additional indication in diabetes is when adequate assessment of the fundus, or laser treatment to the retina, is prevented. The usual method of extraction is by phakoemulsification, with implantation of an intra-ocular lens.

Diabetic nephropathy

Diabetic nephropathy is an important cause of morbidity and mortality, and is now among the most common causes of end-stage renal failure (ESRF) in developed countries. As it is found with other microvascular and macrovascular complications, management is frequently difficult. The benefits of prevention are substantial.

About 30% of patients with type 1 diabetes have developed diabetic nephropathy 20 years after diagnosis, but the risk after this time falls to less than 1% per year, and from the outset the risk is not equal in all patients (Box 21.43). Epidemiological data have indicated that the overall

21.43 Risk factors for developing diabetic nephropathy

- Poor control of blood glucose
- Long duration of diabetes
- Presence of other microvascular complications
- Ethnicity (e.g. Asian races, Pima Indians)
- Pre-existing hypertension
- Family history of diabetic nephropathy
- Family history of hypertension

21

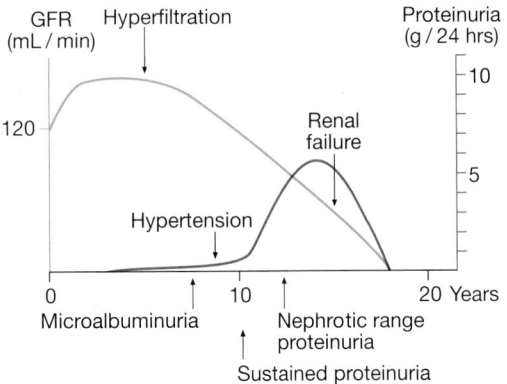

Fig. 21.17 Natural history of diabetic nephropathy. In the first few years of type 1 diabetes mellitus there is hyperfiltration which declines fairly steadily to return to a normal value at approximately 10 years (blue line). In susceptible patients (about 30%), after about 10 years there is sustained proteinuria and by approximately 14 years it has reached the nephrotic range (red line). Renal function continues to decline, with the end stage being reached at approximately 16 years.

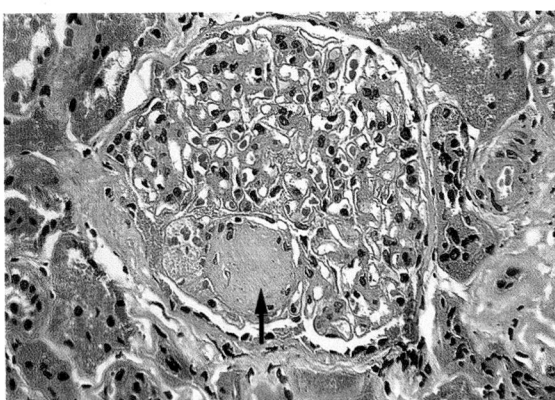

Fig. 21.18 Nodular diabetic glomerulosclerosis. There is thickening of basement membranes and mesangial expansion, and a Kimmelstiel–Wilson nodule (arrow).

incidence is declining as standards of glycaemic and blood pressure control have improved.

The pattern of progression of renal abnormalities in diabetes is shown schematically in Figure 21.17. Pathologically, the first changes coincide with the onset of microalbuminuria and include thickening of the glomerular basement membrane and accumulation of matrix material in the mesangium. Subsequently, nodular deposits (Fig. 21.18) are characteristic, and glomerulosclerosis worsens as heavy proteinuria develops, until glomeruli are progressively lost and renal function deteriorates.

Diagnosis and screening

Microalbuminuria (Box 21.44) is an important indicator of the risk of developing overt diabetic nephropathy, although it is also found in other conditions (p. 481). Microalbuminuria is therefore most reliable as an indicator of incipient diabetic nephropathy within the first 10 years of type 1 diabetes, when the majority of patients with microalbuminuria will progress to overt nephropathy within a further 10 years. It is a less reliable predictor of nephropathy in older patients with type 2 diabetes, in whom it may be accounted for by other

21.44 Screening for microalbuminuria (MA)

- Identifies incipient nephropathy in type 1 and type 2 diabetes; independent predictor of macrovascular disease in type 2 diabetes
- Risk factors include increased blood pressure, poor glycaemic control, smoking
- Random urine sample can estimate urinary albumin:creatinine ratio (MA values 3–30 mg/mmol (27–270 µg/mg)); normal range (mg/mmol) differs in males (< 2.5) and females (< 3.5)
- If possible, confirm MA with a timed collection of urine (overnight or 24 hrs) to quantify the albumin excretion rate (AER) (MA values 20–200 µg/min or 30–300 mg/24 hrs)

Who to screen

- Patients with type 1 diabetes annually from 5 yrs after diagnosis
- Patients with type 2 diabetes annually from time of diagnosis

Abnormal results

- Exclude recent (24 hrs) vigorous exercise, fever, heart failure, urine infection, prostatitis, menstruation
- Confirm observation twice within 3–6 mths
- Look for blood pressure above target levels

diseases, although it is a potentially useful marker of an increased risk of macrovascular disease. Nevertheless, progressively increasing albuminuria, or albuminuria accompanied by hypertension, is most likely to be due to early diabetic nephropathy.

Management

If there is evidence of incipient nephropathy, vigorous efforts should be made to reduce the risk of progression and of cardiovascular disease by:
- improved control of blood glucose
- aggressive reduction of blood pressure
- aggressive cardiovascular risk factor reduction (Box 21.45).

In type 1 diabetes ACE inhibitors have been shown to provide greater benefit than equal blood pressure reduction achieved with other drugs (p. 609), and subsequent studies have shown similar benefits from angiotensin II receptor blockers in patients with type 2 diabetes. There may be particular problems with the use of either in diabetic nephropathy because of hyperkalaemia (p. 440) and renal artery stenosis (p. 496). Non-dihydropyridine calcium antagonists (diltiazem, verapamil) may be suitable alternatives.

Diabetic control becomes difficult as renal impairment progresses. Treatment with metformin should be withdrawn when creatinine is higher than 150 µmol/L

EBM 21.45 Multi-risk factor intervention in type 2 diabetes

'In type 2 patients with microalbuminuria, intensive treatment (including control of glycaemia and hypertension, with use of ACE inhibitors, statins and aspirin) reduced the risk of cardiovascular disease by 53%, of nephropathy by 61%, and of retinopathy by 58% compared with conventional treatment. On longer-term follow-up there was a reduction in total mortality and death from cardiovascular causes.'

- Gaede P, et al. N Engl J Med 2003; 348:383–393.
- Gaede P, et al. N Engl J Med 2008; 358:580–591.

(1.7 mg/dL), as the risk of lactic acidosis is increased. Long-acting sulphonylureas should be replaced by short-acting agents that are metabolised rather than excreted.

Renal replacement therapy (p. 492) may benefit diabetic patients at an earlier stage than other patients with ESRF, although it may carry additional difficulties. Renal transplantation can dramatically improve the life of many, and any recurrence of diabetic nephropathy in the allograft is usually too slow to be a serious problem, but associated macrovascular and microvascular disease elsewhere may still progress. Pancreatic transplantation (generally carried out at the same time as renal transplantation) can produce insulin independence and slow or reverse microvascular disease, but the supply of organs is very limited and this is available to few. For further information on management, see Chapter 17.

Diabetic neuropathy

This is a relatively early and common complication affecting approximately 30% of diabetic patients. Although in a few patients it can cause severe disability, it is symptomless in the majority. Like retinopathy, it occurs secondary to metabolic disturbance, and prevalence is related to the duration of diabetes and the degree of metabolic control. Although there is some evidence that the central nervous system is affected in long-term diabetes, the clinical impact of diabetes is mainly manifest in the peripheral nervous system.

The main pathological features are listed in Box 21.46. They can occur in motor, sensory and autonomic nerves.

Various classifications of diabetic neuropathy have been proposed. One is shown in Box 21.47, but motor, sensory and autonomic nerves may be involved in varying combinations so that clinically mixed syndromes usually occur.

21.46 Diabetic neuropathy: histopathology

- Axonal degeneration of both myelinated and unmyelinated fibres
  Early: axon shrinkage
  Later: axonal fragmentation; regeneration
- Thickening of Schwann cell basal lamina
- Patchy, segmental demyelination
- Thickening of basement membrane and microthrombi in intraneural capillaries

21.47 Classification of diabetic neuropathy

Somatic

- Polyneuropathy
  Symmetrical, mainly sensory and distal
  Asymmetrical, mainly motor and proximal (including amyotrophy)
- Mononeuropathy (including mononeuritis multiplex)

Visceral (autonomic)

- Cardiovascular
- Gastrointestinal
- Genitourinary
- Sudomotor
- Vasomotor
- Pupillary

Clinical features

Symmetrical sensory polyneuropathy

This is frequently asymptomatic. The most common clinical signs are diminished perception of vibration sensation distally, 'glove-and-stocking' impairment of all other modalities of sensation, and loss of tendon reflexes in the lower limbs. In symptomatic patients, sensory abnormalities are predominant. Symptoms include paraesthesiae in the feet (and, rarely, in the hands), pain in the lower limbs (dull, aching and/or lancinating, worse at night, and mainly felt on the anterior aspect of the legs), burning sensations in the soles of the feet, cutaneous hyperaesthesia and an abnormal gait (commonly wide-based), often associated with a sense of numbness in the feet. Muscle weakness and wasting develop only in advanced cases, but subclinical motor nerve dysfunction is common. The toes may be clawed with wasting of the interosseous muscles, which results in increased pressure on the plantar aspects of the metatarsal heads with the development of callus skin at these and other pressure points. Electrophysiological tests (p. 1141) demonstrate slowing of both motor and sensory conduction, and tests of vibration sensitivity and thermal thresholds are abnormal.

A diffuse small-fibre neuropathy causes altered perception of pain and temperature, and is associated with symptomatic autonomic neuropathy; characteristic features include foot ulcers and Charcot neuroarthropathy.

Asymmetrical motor diabetic neuropathy

Sometimes called diabetic amyotrophy, this presents as severe and progressive weakness and wasting of the proximal muscles of the lower (and occasionally the upper) limbs. It is commonly accompanied by severe pain, mainly felt on the anterior aspect of the leg, and hyperaesthesia and paraesthesiae. Sometimes there may also be marked loss of weight ('neuropathic cachexia'). The patient may look extremely ill and be unable to get out of bed. Tendon reflexes may be absent on the affected side(s). Sometimes there are extensor plantar responses and the cerebrospinal fluid protein is often raised. This condition is thought to involve acute infarction of the lower motor neurons of the lumbosacral plexus. Other lesions involving this plexus, such as neoplasms and lumbar disc disease, must be excluded. Although recovery usually occurs within 12 months, some deficits become permanent. Management is mainly supportive.

Mononeuropathy

Either motor or sensory function can be affected within a single peripheral or cranial nerve. Unlike the gradual progression of distal symmetrical and autonomic neuropathies, mononeuropathies are severe and of rapid onset but they eventually recover. The nerves most commonly affected are the 3rd and 6th cranial nerves (resulting in diplopia), and the femoral and sciatic nerves. Rarely, involvement of other single nerves results in paresis and paraesthesiae in the thorax and trunk (truncal radiculopathies).

Nerve compression palsies commonly affect the median nerve, giving the clinical picture of carpal tunnel syndrome, and less commonly the ulnar nerve. Lateral popliteal nerve compression occasionally causes foot drop.

Autonomic neuropathy

This is not necessarily associated with peripheral somatic neuropathy. Either parasympathetic or sympathetic

21.48 Clinical features of autonomic neuropathy

Cardiovascular

- Postural hypotension
- Resting tachycardia
- Fixed heart rate

Gastrointestinal

- Dysphagia, due to oesophageal atony
- Abdominal fullness, nausea and vomiting, unstable glycaemia, due to delayed gastric emptying ('gastroparesis')
- Nocturnal diarrhoea ± faecal incontinence
- Constipation, due to colonic atony

Genitourinary

- Difficulty in micturition, urinary incontinence, recurrent infection, due to atonic bladder
- Erectile dysfunction and retrograde ejaculation

Sudomotor

- Gustatory sweating
- Nocturnal sweats without hypoglycaemia
- Anhidrosis; fissures in the feet

Vasomotor

- Feet feel cold, due to loss of skin vasomotor responses
- Dependent oedema, due to loss of vasomotor tone and increased vascular permeability
- Bullous formation

Pupillary

- Decreased pupil size
- Resistance to mydriatics
- Delayed or absent reflexes to light

21.49 How to test cardiovascular autonomic function

	Normal	Borderline	Abnormal
Simple reflex tests			
Heart rate responses			
• to Valsalva manœuvre (15 secs)[1]: ratio of longest to shortest R–R interval	≥1.21		≤1.20
• to deep breathing (6 breaths over 1 min): maximum–minimum heart rate	≥15	11–14	≤10
• to standing after lying: ratio of R–R interval of 30th to 15th beats	≥1.04	1.01–1.03	≤1.00
Blood pressure response[2]			
• to standing: systolic BP fall (mmHg)	≤10	11–29	≥30
Specialised tests			

Specialised tests

- Heart rate and blood pressure responses to sustained handgrip
- Heart rate variability using power spectral analysis of ECG monitoring
- Heart rate and blood pressure variability using time-domain analysis of ambulatory monitoring
- MIBG (met-iodobenzylguanidine) scan of the heart

[1]Omit in patients with previous laser therapy for proliferative retinopathy.
[2]Avoid arm with A-V fistula in dialysed patients.

nerves may be predominantly affected in one or more visceral systems. The resulting symptoms and signs are listed in Box 21.48. Tests of autonomic function are listed in Box 21.49. The development of autonomic neuropathy is less clearly related to poor metabolic control than somatic neuropathy, and improved control rarely results in amelioration of symptoms. Within 10 years of developing overt symptoms of autonomic neuropathy, 30–50% of patients are dead—many from sudden cardiorespiratory arrest, the cause of which is unknown. Patients with postural hypotension (a drop in systolic pressure of ≥30 mmHg on standing from the supine position) have the highest subsequent mortality.

21.50 Management options for peripheral sensorimotor and autonomic neuropathies

Pain and paraesthesiae from peripheral somatic neuropathies

- Intensive insulin therapy (strict glycaemic control)
- Anticonvulsants (gabapentin, pregabalin, carbamazepine, phenytoin)
- Tricyclic antidepressants (amitriptyline, imipramine)
- Other antidepressants (duloxetine)
- Substance P depleter (capsaicin—topical)
- Opiates (tramadol, oxycodone)
- Membrane stabilisers (mexiletine, intravenous lidocaine)
- Antioxidant (α-lipoic acid)

Postural hypotension

- Support stockings
- Fludrocortisone
- α-adrenoceptor agonist (midodrine)
- Non-steroidal anti-inflammatory drugs (NSAIDs)

Gastroparesis

- Dopamine antagonists (metoclopramide, domperidone)
- Erythromycin
- Gastric pacemaker; percutaneous enteral (jejunal) feeding (Fig. 5.16, p. 124)

Diarrhoea (p. 856)

- Loperamide
- Broad-spectrum antibiotics
- Clonidine
- Octreotide

Constipation

- Stimulant laxatives (senna)

Atonic bladder

- Intermittent self-catheterisation (p. 1168)

Excessive sweating

- Anticholinergic drugs (propantheline, poldine)
- Clonidine
- Topical antimuscarinic agent (glycopyrrolate cream)

Erectile dysfunction (impotence) (p. 477)

- Phosphodiesterase type 5 inhibitors (sildenafil, vardenafil, tadalafil)—oral
- Dopamine agonist (apomorphine) —sublingual
- Prostaglandin E1 (alprostadil) —injected into corpus cavernosum, or intra-urethral administration of pellets
- Vacuum tumescence devices
- Implanted penile prosthesis
- Psychological counselling; psychosexual therapy

Erectile dysfunction

Erectile failure (impotence) affects 30% of diabetic males and is often multifactorial. Although neuropathy and vascular causes are common, psychological factors, including depression, anxiety and reduced libido, may be partly responsible. Alcohol and antihypertensive drugs such as thiazide diuretics and β-adrenoceptor antagonists (β-blockers) may cause sexual dysfunction and, rarely, patients have an endocrine cause such as testosterone deficiency or hyperprolactinaemia. For further information, see page 477.

Management

Management of neuropathies is outlined in Box 21.50.

The diabetic foot

The foot is a frequent site for complications in patients with diabetes and for this reason foot care is particularly important. Tissue necrosis in the feet is a common reason for hospital admission in diabetic patients. Such admissions tend to be prolonged and may end with amputation.

Aetiology

Foot ulceration occurs as a result of trauma (often trivial) in the presence of neuropathy and/or peripheral vascular disease (p. 599), with infection occurring as a secondary phenomenon following disruption of the protective epidermis. The interplay between these factors is shown in Figure 21.19. Most ulcers develop at the site of a plaque of callus skin beneath which tissue necrosis occurs and eventually breaks through to the surface. In most cases multiple components are involved, but sometimes neuropathy or ischaemia predominate, as illustrated in Box 21.51. Ischaemia alone accounts for a minority of foot ulcers in diabetic patients, with most being either neuropathic or neuro-ischaemic in type.

21.51 Clinical features of the diabetic foot

	Neuropathy	Ischaemia
Symptoms	None	None
	Paraesthesiae	Claudication
	Pain	Rest pain
	Numbness	
Structural damage	Ulcer	Ulcer
	Sepsis	Sepsis
	Abscess	Gangrene
	Osteomyelitis	
	Digital gangrene	
	Charcot joint	

Management

The main components of medical management are listed in Box 21.52. Removal of callus skin with a scalpel is usually best done by a podiatrist who has specialist training and experience in diabetic foot problems. Effective treatment of local infection with appropriate antibiotics is essential, and may have to be continued for protracted periods; osteomyelitis may be extremely difficult to eradicate. Charcot neuroarthropathy with disorganisation of joints may cause serious deformity. Angiography may be necessary if the foot is ischaemic or ulcers are very slow to heal. Measures to improve glycaemic control may also promote healing. Amputation may be unavoidable if there is extensive tissue and/or bony destruction or intractable ischaemic pain at rest in a limb in which vascular reconstruction has failed or is impossible due to extensive large blood vessel disease. Further information is given on the management of peripheral arterial disease on page 601. Preventative measures are shown in Box 21.52.

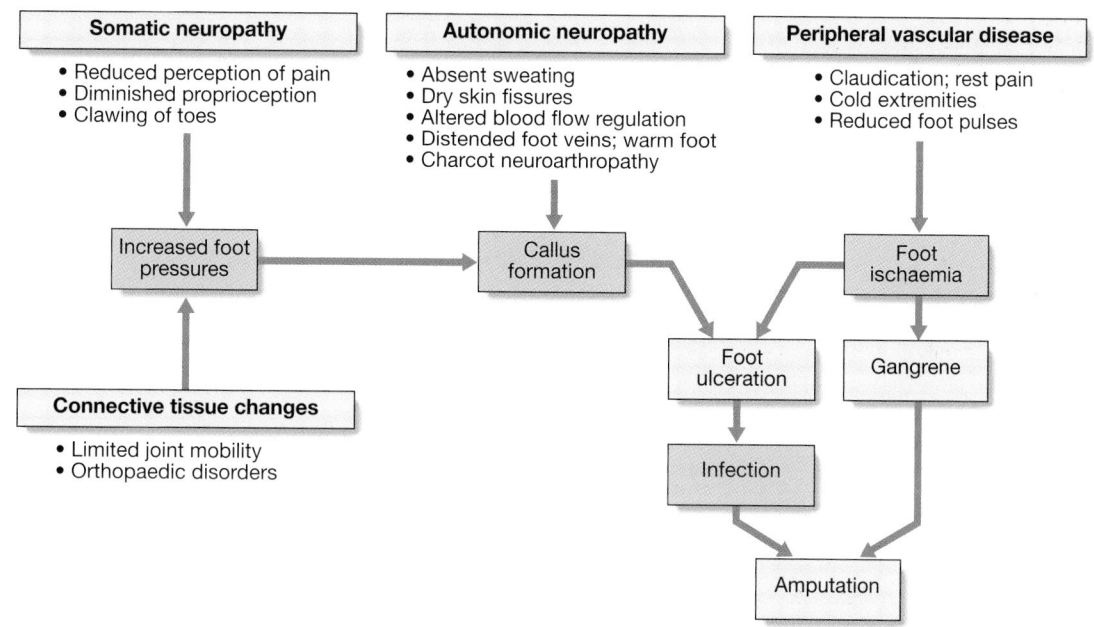

Fig. 21.19 Pathways leading to foot ulceration and amputation in diabetic foot disease.

Box 21.52 Management of diabetic foot ulcers

Prevention

- Prevention is the most effective way of dealing with the problem of tissue necrosis in the diabetic foot. Advice to all diabetic patients includes:
    Inspect feet every day
    Wash feet every day
    Moisturise skin if dry
    Cut or file toenails regularly
    Change socks or stockings every day
    Avoid walking barefoot
    Check footwear for foreign bodies
    Wear suitable good-fitting shoes
    Cover minor cuts with sterile dressings
    Do not burst blisters
    Avoid over-the-counter corn/callus remedies
- Advice to high-risk patients is as above plus:
    Do not attempt corn removal
    Avoid high and low temperatures
- A podiatrist is an integral part of the diabetes team to ensure regular and effective podiatry and to educate patients in care of the feet
- Specially manufactured and fitted orthotic footwear is required to prevent recurrence of ulceration and protect the feet of patients with Charcot neuroarthropathy

Treatment

- Remove callus
- Treat infection
- Avoid weight-bearing
- Ensure good glycaemic control
- Control oedema
- Undertake angiogram to assess feasibility of vascular reconstruction where indicated

Further information

www.cdc.gov/diabetes *Diabetes Public Health Resource. Useful American site with resources for patients and health-care professionals.*

www.diabetes.org *American Diabetes Association. Includes information on research and advocacy issues.*

www.diabetes.org.uk *Diabetes UK. Includes information for patients and leaflets.*

www.diabetologists-abcd.org.uk *Association of British Clinical Diabetologists. Up-to-date information on new treatments.*

www.idf.org *International Diabetes Federation. Useful information on international aspects of care and education.*

www.jdrf.org *Juvenile Diabetes Research Foundation. Excellent resource for patients with type 1 diabetes.*

www.joslin.org *Joslin Diabetes Center. Well-written resource for patients and health-care professionals, and information on diabetes research.*

www.ndei.org *National Diabetes Education Initiative. Web-based education for health-care professionals, including case studies and slides.*

www.ndep.nih.gov *National Diabetes Education Program. Education aimed mainly at people with diabetes.*

www.nlm.nih.gov/medlineplus/diabetes.html *Medline Plus Diabetes. Detailed information for patients and health-care professionals.*

www.sign.ac.uk *Scottish Intercollegiate Guidelines Network. Internationally renowned evidence-based guidelines, including updated guidelines in diabetes.*

K.R. Palmer
I.D. Penman

Alimentary tract and pancreatic disease

22

CLINICAL EXAMINATION OF THE GASTROINTESTINAL TRACT

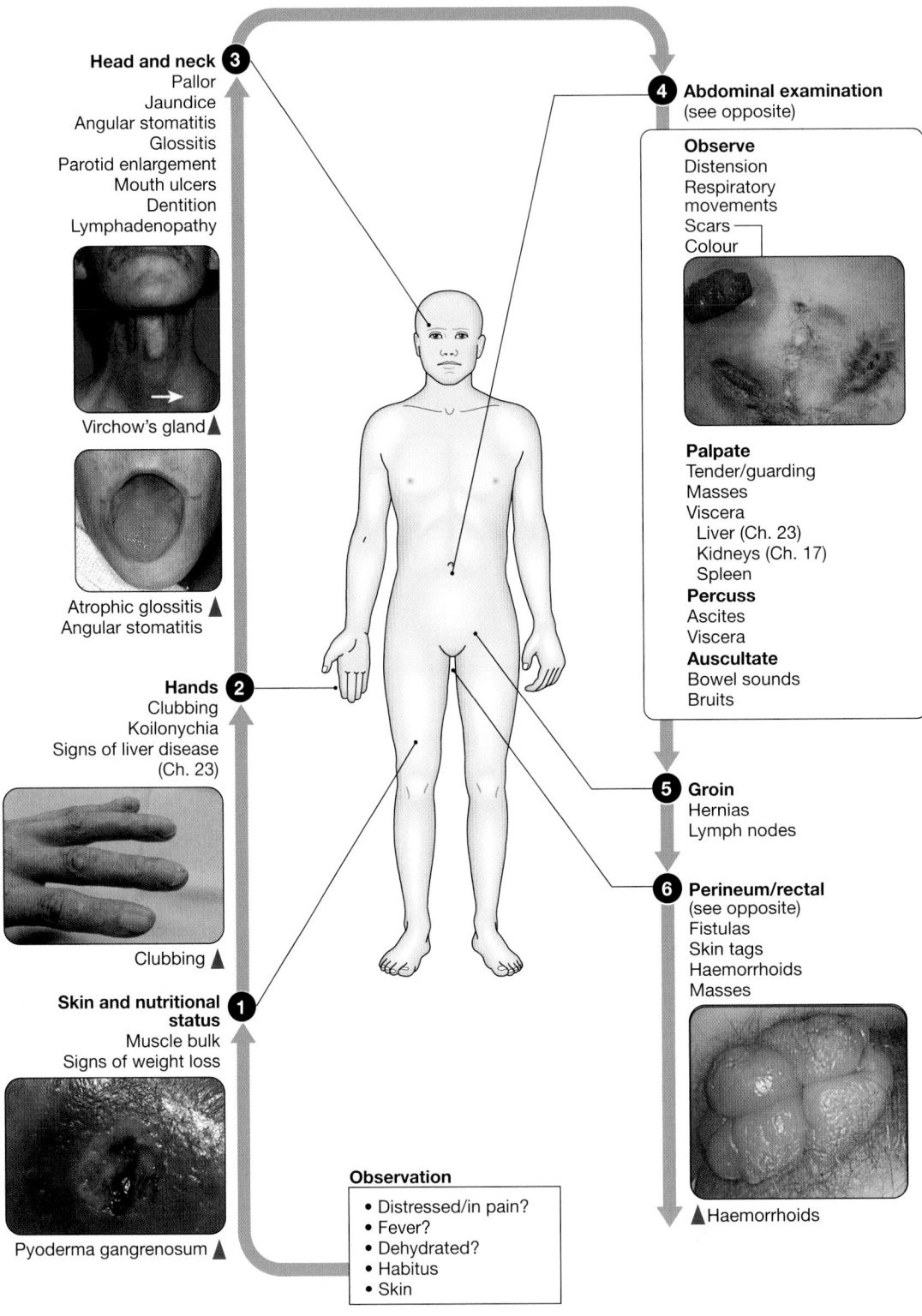

Head and neck ③
Pallor
Jaundice
Angular stomatitis
Glossitis
Parotid enlargement
Mouth ulcers
Dentition
Lymphadenopathy

Virchow's gland ▲

Atrophic glossitis ▲
Angular stomatitis

Hands ②
Clubbing
Koilonychia
Signs of liver disease
(Ch. 23)

Clubbing ▲

**Skin and nutritional
status** ①
Muscle bulk
Signs of weight loss

Pyoderma gangrenosum ▲

Observation

• Distressed/in pain?
• Fever?
• Dehydrated?
• Habitus
• Skin

Abdominal examination ④
(see opposite)

Observe
Distension
Respiratory
movements
Scars
Colour

Palpate
Tender/guarding
Masses
Viscera
  Liver (Ch. 23)
  Kidneys (Ch. 17)
  Spleen
Percuss
Ascites
Viscera
Auscultate
Bowel sounds
Bruits

Groin ⑤
Hernias
Lymph nodes

Perineum/rectal ⑥
(see opposite)
Fistulas
Skin tags
Haemorrhoids
Masses

▲ Haemorrhoids

4 **Abdominal examination: possible findings**

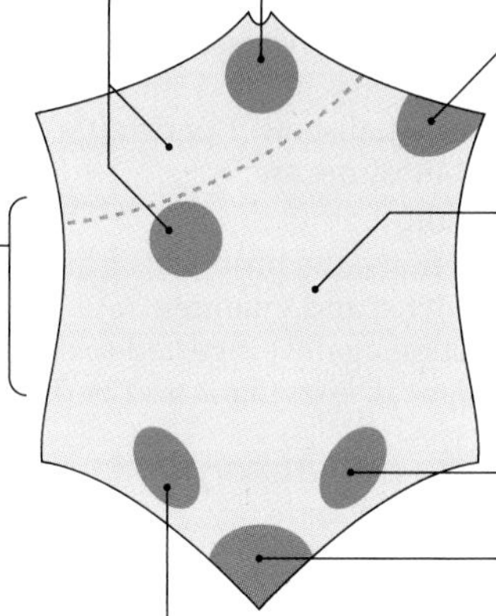

Hepatomegaly
Palpable gallbladder

(Ch. 23)

Epigastric mass

Gastric cancer
Pancreatic cancer
Aortic aneurysm

Left upper quadrant mass

?Spleen
  Edge
  Can't get above it
  Moves towards right
  iliac fossa
  Dull percussion note
  Notch

?Kidney
  Rounded
  Can get above it
  Moves down

  Resonant to percussion
  Ballotable

Tender to palpation

?Peritonitis
  Guarding and rebound
  Absent bowel sounds
  Rigidity

?Obstruction
  Distended
  Tinkling bowel sounds
  Visible peristalsis

Left iliac fossa mass

Sigmoid colon cancer
Constipation
Diverticular mass

Generalised distension

Fat (obesity)
Fluid (ascites)
Flatus (obstruction/ileus)
Faeces (constipation)
Fetus (pregnancy)

Right iliac fossa mass

Caecal carcinoma
Crohn's disease
Appendix abscess

Suprapubic mass

Bladder
Pregnancy
Fibroids/carcinoma

6 **Rectal examination: common findings**

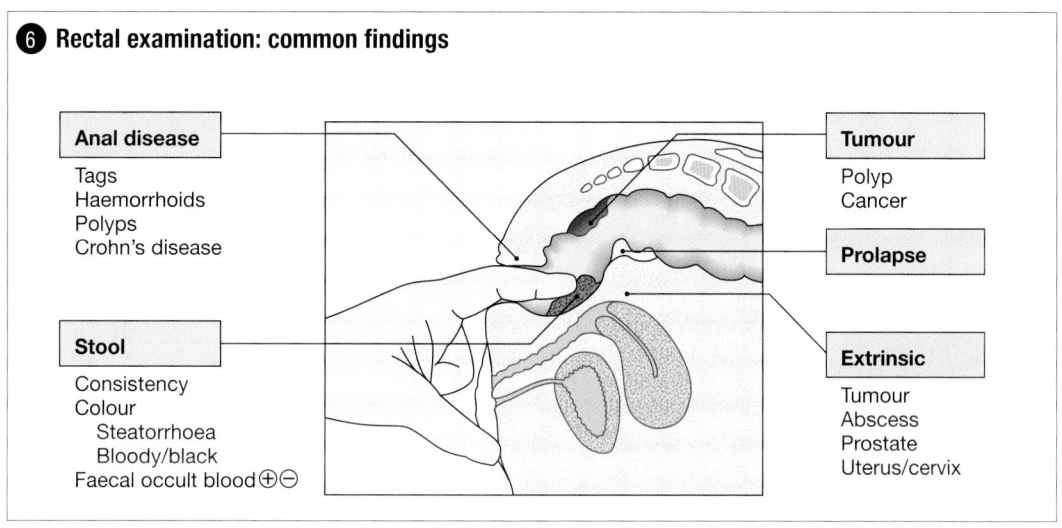

Anal disease

Tags
Haemorrhoids
Polyps
Crohn's disease

Tumour

Polyp
Cancer

Prolapse

Stool

Consistency
Colour
  Steatorrhoea
  Bloody/black
Faecal occult blood $\oplus\ominus$

Extrinsic

Tumour
Abscess
Prostate
Uterus/cervix

22

Diseases of the gastrointestinal tract are a major cause of morbidity and mortality. Approximately 10% of all general practitioner consultations in the United Kingdom are for indigestion, and 1 in 14 is for diarrhoea. Infective diarrhoea and malabsorption are responsible for much ill health and many deaths in the developing world. The gastrointestinal tract is the most common site for cancer development.

FUNCTIONAL ANATOMY AND PHYSIOLOGY

Functional anatomy

Oesophagus

This muscular tube extends 25 cm from the cricoid cartilage to the cardiac orifice of the stomach. It has an upper and a lower sphincter. A peristaltic swallowing wave propels the food bolus into the stomach (Fig. 22.1).

Stomach and duodenum (Fig. 22.2)

The stomach acts as a 'hopper', retaining and grinding food, then actively propelling it into the upper small bowel.

Gastric secretion

Hydrogen and chloride ions are secreted from the apical membrane of gastric parietal cells into the lumen of the stomach by a hydrogen-potassium ATPase ('proton pump') (Fig. 22.3). The hydrochloric acid sterilises the upper gastrointestinal tract and converts pepsinogen—which is secreted by chief cells—to pepsin. The glycoprotein intrinsic factor, secreted in parallel with acid, is necessary for vitamin B_{12} absorption.

Gastrin and somatostatin

The hormone gastrin is produced by G cells in the antrum whereas somatostatin is secreted from D cells through-out the stomach. Gastrin stimulates whilst somatostatin suppresses acid secretion.

Protective factors

Bicarbonate ions and mucus together protect the gastroduodenal mucosa from the ulcerative properties of acid and pepsin.

Small intestine

The small bowel extends from the ligament of Treitz to the ileocaecal valve (Fig. 22.4). During fasting, a wave of peristaltic activity passes down the small bowel every 1–2 hours. Entry of food into the gastrointestinal tract stimulates small bowel peristaltic activity. Functions of the small intestine are:

- digestion
- absorption—the products of digestion, water, electrolytes and vitamins
- protection against ingested toxins—immunological, mechanical, enzymatic and peristaltic.

Digestion and absorption

Fat

Dietary lipids comprise long chain triglycerides, cholesterol esters and lecithin. Lipids are insoluble in water and undergo lipolysis and incorporation into mixed micelles before they can be absorbed into enterocytes along with the fat-soluble vitamins A, D, K and E. The lipids are processed within enterocytes and pass via lymphatics into the systemic circulation. Fat absorption and digestion can be considered as a stepwise process:

- *Luminal phase* (Fig. 22.5, step 1). Fatty acids stimulate cholecystokinin (CCK) release from the duodenum and upper jejunum. The CCK stimulates release of amylase, lipase, colipase and proteases from the pancreas, causes gallbladder contraction and relaxes the sphincter of Oddi, causing bile to flow into the intestine. Pancreatic lipase, in the presence of its co-factor colipase, cleaves long chain triglycerides,

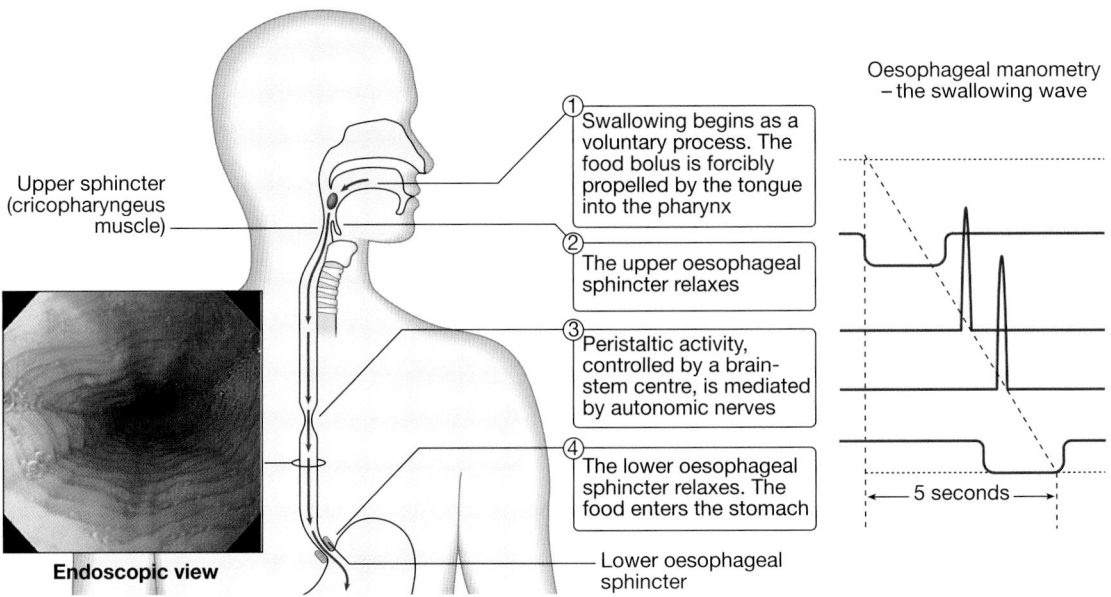

Upper sphincter (cricopharyngeus muscle)

Oesophageal manometry – the swallowing wave

① Swallowing begins as a voluntary process. The food bolus is forcibly propelled by the tongue into the pharynx

② The upper oesophageal sphincter relaxes

③ Peristaltic activity, controlled by a brain-stem centre, is mediated by autonomic nerves

④ The lower oesophageal sphincter relaxes. The food enters the stomach

← 5 seconds →

Lower oesophageal sphincter

Endoscopic view

Fig. 22.1 The oesophagus: anatomy and function. The swallowing wave.

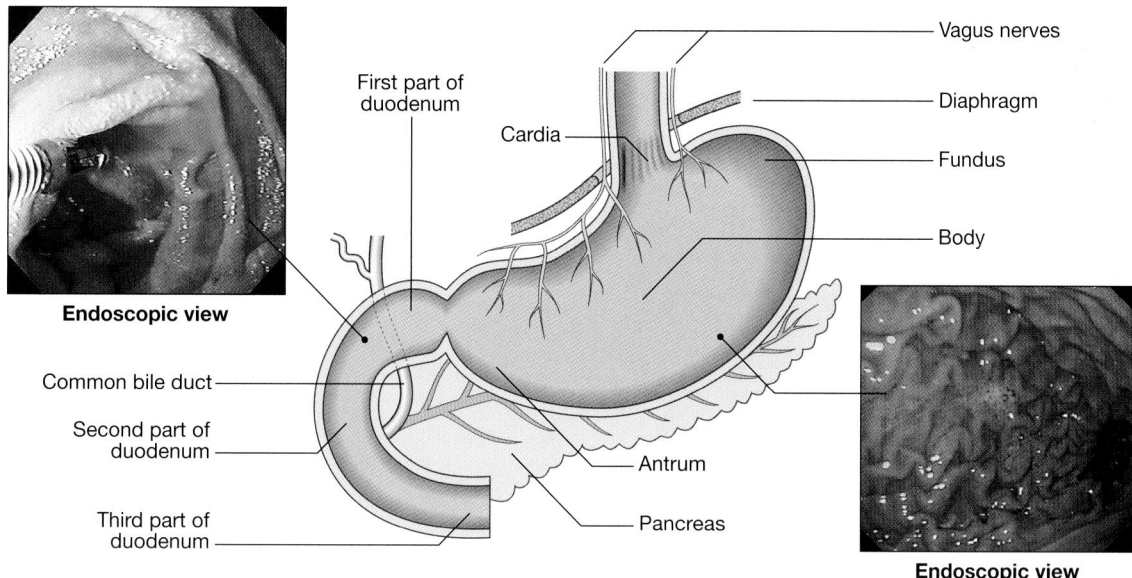

First part of duodenum

Cardia

Vagus nerves

Diaphragm

Fundus

Body

Endoscopic view

Common bile duct

Second part of duodenum

Third part of duodenum

Antrum

Pancreas

Endoscopic view

Fig. 22.2 Normal gastric and duodenal anatomy.

22

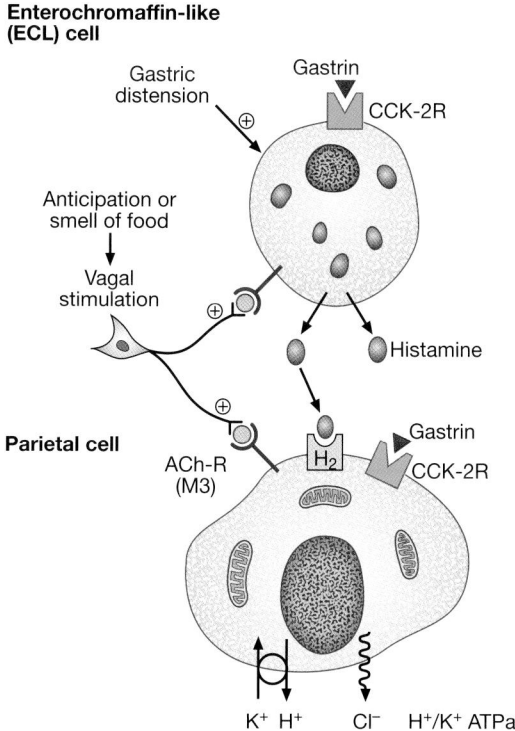

Enterochromaffin-like (ECL) cell

Gastric distension

Gastrin

CCK-2R

Anticipation or smell of food

Vagal stimulation

Histamine

Parietal cell

ACh-R (M3)

H₂

Gastrin

CCK-2R

K⁺ H⁺   Cl⁻   H⁺/K⁺ ATPase

Fig. 22.3 Control of acid secretion. Gastrin released from antral G cells in response to food binds to cholecystokinin receptors (CCK-2R) on the surface of enterochromaffin-like (ECL) cells, which in turn release histamine. The histamine binds to H_2 receptors on parietal cells and this leads to secretion of hydrogen ions, in exchange for potassium ions at the apical membrane. Parietal cells also express CCK-2R and it is thought that activation of these receptors by gastrin is involved in regulatory proliferation of parietal cells. Cholinergic (vagal) activity and gastric distension also stimulate acid secretion; somatostatin, vasoactive intestinal polypeptide (VIP) and gastric inhibitory polypeptide (GIP) inhibit it.

yielding fatty acids and monoglycerides (Fig. 22.5, step 2). These are solubilised by interacting with bile salts and phospholipids to form mixed micelles. Mixed micelles also contain cholesterol and fat-soluble vitamins.

- *Absorption.* Mixed micelles diffuse to the brush border of the enterocytes (Fig. 22.5, step 3). Long chain fatty acids there bind to fatty acid-binding proteins and are transported into the cell. Cholesterol, short chain fatty acids, phospholipids and fat-soluble vitamins enter the enterocytes by obscure mechanisms. Bile salts remain in the small intestinal lumen and are actively transported from the terminal ileum into the portal circulation and returned to the liver (the enterohepatic circulation, step 4).
- *Re-esterification* (Fig. 22.5, step 5). Within the enterocyte, fatty acids are re-esterified to form triglycerides. Triglycerides combine with cholesterol ester, fat-soluble vitamins, phospholipids and apoproteins to form chylomicrons.
- *Transport* (Fig. 22.5, step 6). Chylomicrons leave the enterocytes by exocytosis, enter mesenteric lymphatics, pass into the thoracic duct, and eventually reach the systemic circulation.

Carbohydrates

Starch is hydrolysed by salivary and pancreatic amylases to alpha-limit dextrins containing 4–8 glucose molecules; to the disaccharide maltose; and to the trisaccharide maltotriose.

Disaccharides are digested by enzymes fixed to the microvillous membrane to form the monosaccharides glucose, galactose and fructose. Glucose and galactose enter the cell by an energy-requiring process involving a carrier protein, and fructose enters by simple diffusion.

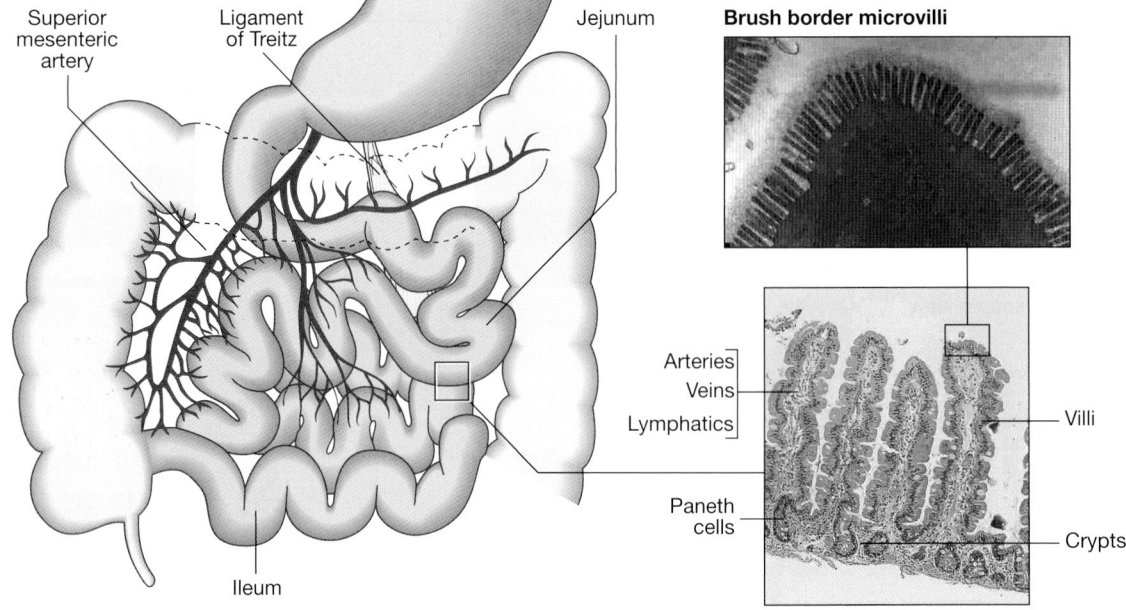

Fig. 22.4 **Small intestine: anatomy.** Epithelial cells are formed in crypts and differentiate as they migrate to the tip of the villi to form enterocytes (absorptive cells) and goblet cells.

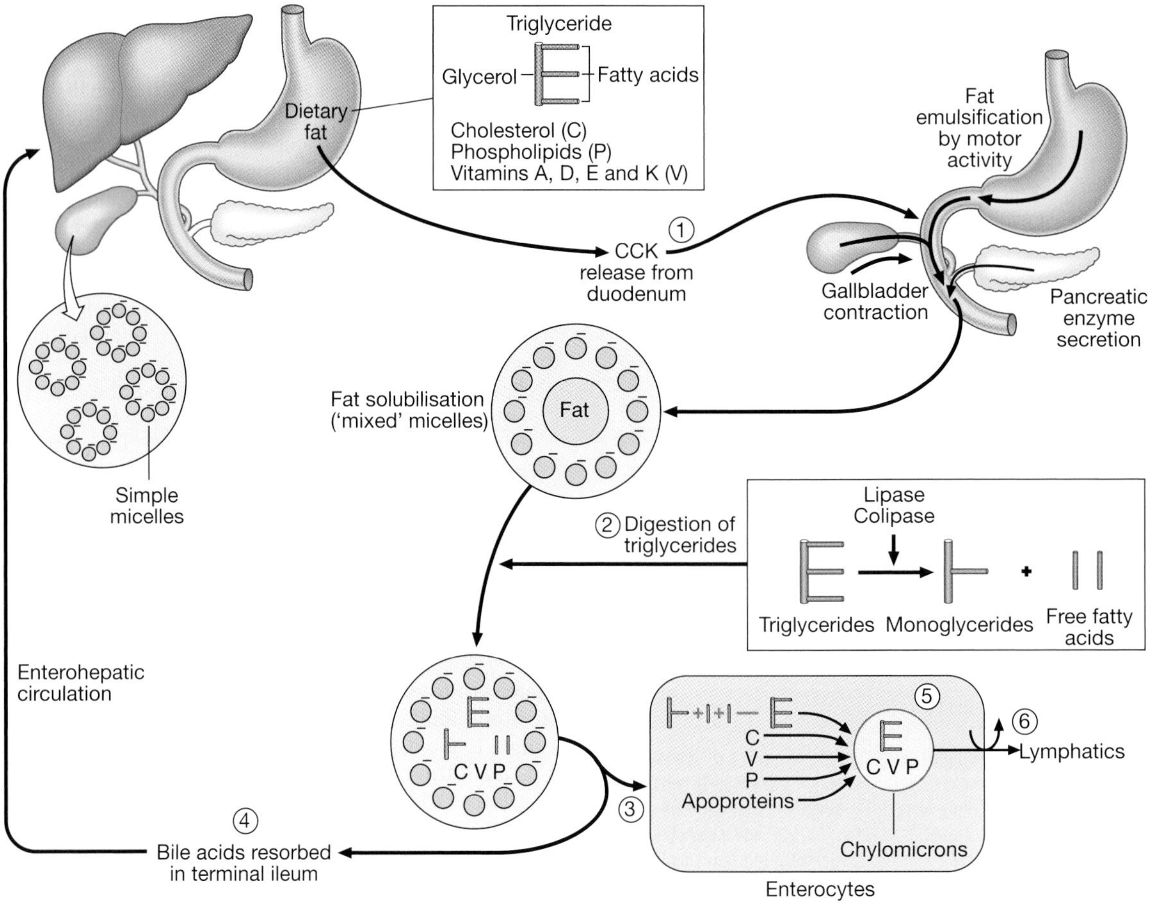

Fig. 22.5 Fat digestion.

Protein

The steps in protein digestion are shown in Figure 22.6. Intragastric digestion by pepsin is quantitatively modest but important because the resulting polypeptides and amino acids stimulate CCK release from the mucosa of the proximal jejunum, which in turn stimulates release of pancreatic proteases including trypsinogen, chymotrypsinogen, pro-elastases and procarboxypeptidases from the pancreas. On exposure to brush border enterokinase, inert trypsinogen is converted to the active proteolytic enzyme trypsin which activates the other pancreatic proenzymes. Trypsin digests proteins to produce oligopeptides, peptides and amino acids. Oligopeptides are further hydrolysed by brush border enzymes to yield dipeptides, tripeptides and amino acids. These small peptides and the amino acids are actively transported into the enterocytes where intracellular peptidases further digest peptides to amino acids. Amino acids are then actively transported across the basal cell membrane of the enterocyte into the portal circulation and the liver.

Water and electrolytes

Absorption and secretion of electrolytes and water occur throughout the intestine. Electrolytes and water are transported by two pathways:

- *the paracellular route*, in which passive flow through tight junctions between cells is a consequence of osmotic, electrical or hydrostatic gradients
- *the transcellular route* across apical and basolateral membranes by energy-requiring specific active transport carriers (pumps).

In healthy individuals, fluid balance is tightly controlled such that only 100 mL of the 8 litres of fluid entering the gastrointestinal tract daily is excreted in stools (Fig. 22.7).

Vitamins and trace elements

Water-soluble vitamins are absorbed throughout the intestine. The absorption of folic acid, vitamin B$_{12}$, calcium and iron is described on pages 1020–1022.

Protective function of the small intestine

Physical defence mechanisms

There are several levels of defence in the small bowel (Fig. 22.8). Firstly, the gut lumen contains host bacteria, mucins and secreted antibacterial products including defensins and immunoglobulins which help combat pathogenic infections. Secondly, epithelial cells have relatively impermeable brush border membranes and passage between cells is prevented by tight and adherens junctions. These cells can react to foreign peptides ('innate immunity') using pattern recognition receptors

22

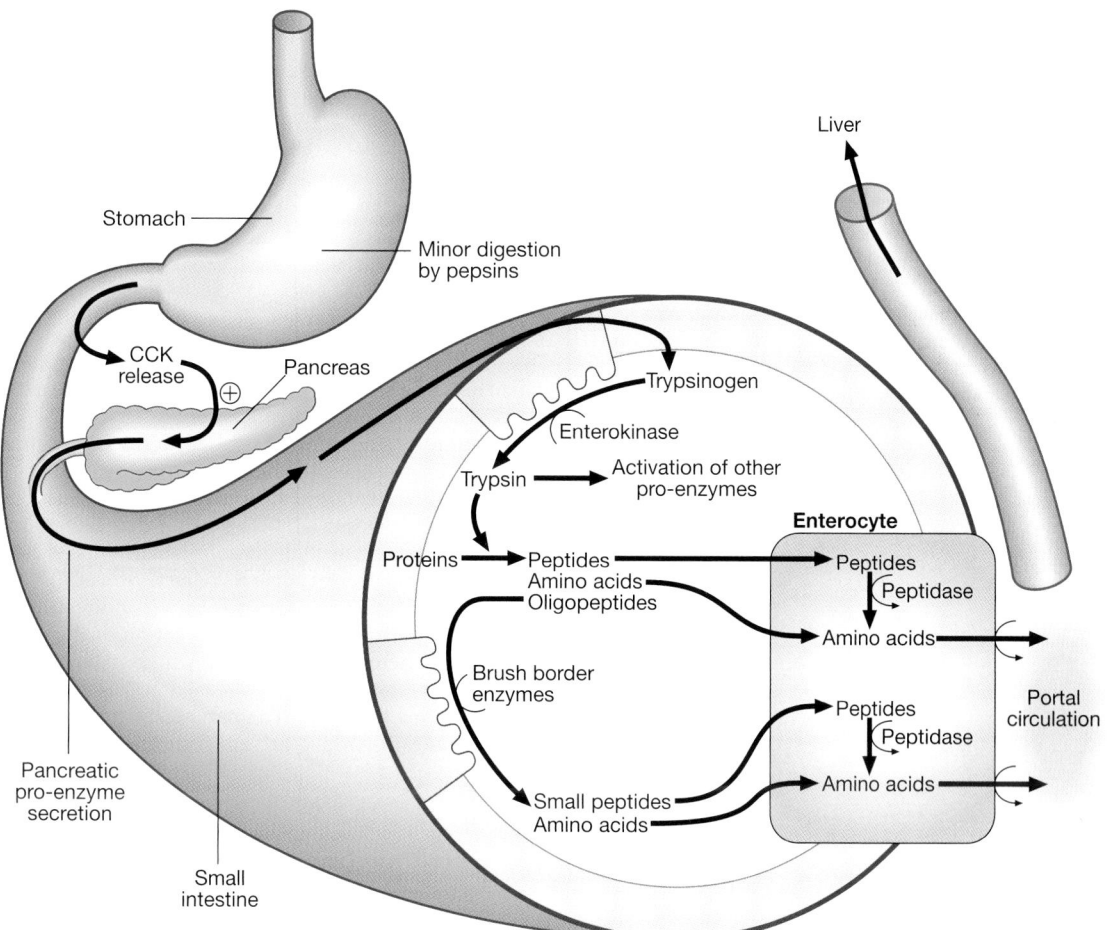

Fig. 22.6 Protein digestion.

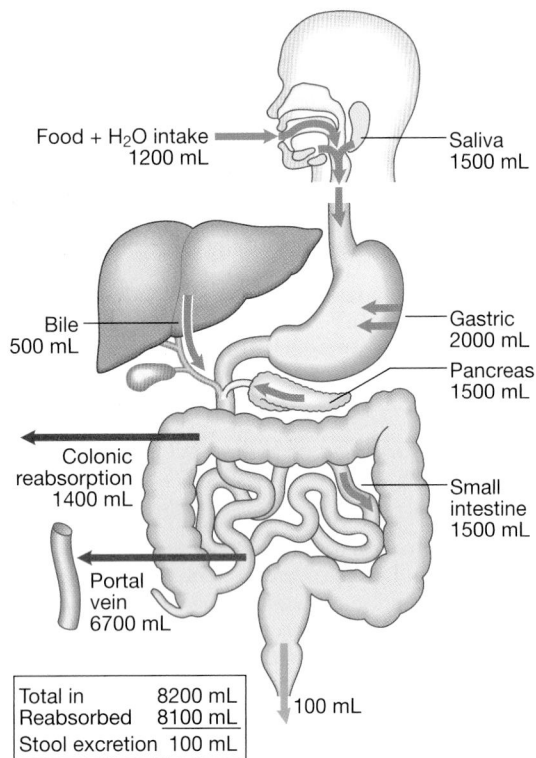

Food + H₂O intake
1200 mL

Saliva
1500 mL

Bile
500 mL

Gastric
2000 mL

Pancreas
1500 mL

Colonic
reabsorption
1400 mL

Small
intestine
1500 mL

Portal
vein
6700 mL

100 mL

Total in	8200 mL
Reabsorbed	8100 mL
Stool excretion	100 mL

Fig. 22.7 Fluid homeostasis in the gastrointestinal tract.

found on cell surfaces (Toll receptors) or intracellularly. Lastly, in the subepithelial layer immune responses occur under control of the adaptive immune system in response to pathogenic compounds.

Immunological defence mechanisms

Gastrointestinal mucosa-associated lymphoid tissue (MALT) constitutes 25% of the total lymphatic tissue of the body and is at the heart of adaptive immunity. B lymphocytes within Peyer's patches differentiate to plasma cells following exposure to antigens, and these cells migrate to mesenteric lymph nodes, and thence to the blood stream via the thoracic duct, then returning

to the lamina propria of the gut, bronchial tree and other lymph nodes. They release IgA which is transported into the lumen of the intestine. Intestinal T lymphocytes probably help localise plasma cells to the site of antigen exposure, as well as producing inflammatory mediators. Macrophages phagocytose foreign materials and secrete a range of cytokines which mediate inflammation. Similarly, activation of mast cell surface IgE receptors leads to degranulation and release of other molecules involved in inflammation.

Pancreas

The exocrine pancreas (Box 22.1) is necessary for the digestion of fat, protein and carbohydrate. Inactive pro-enzymes are secreted from acinar cells in response to circulating gastrointestinal hormones (Fig. 22.9) and are then activated by trypsin. Bicarbonate-rich fluid is secreted from ductular cells to produce an optimum alkaline pH for enzyme activity.

ℹ 22.1 Pancreatic enzymes

Enzyme	Substrate	Product
Amylase	Starch and glycogen	Limit dextrans Maltose Maltriose
Lipase Colipase	Triglycerides	Monoglycerides and free fatty acids
Proteolytic enzymes	Proteins and polypeptides	Short polypeptides
Trypsinogen Chymotrypsinogen Proelastase Procarboxypeptidases		

Colon

The colon (Fig. 22.10) absorbs water and electrolytes. It also acts as a storage organ and has contractile activity. Two types of contraction occur. The first of these is segmentation (ring contraction), which leads to mixing but not propulsion; this promotes absorption of water and electrolytes. Propulsive (peristaltic contraction) waves occur several times a day and propel faeces to the rectum. All activity is stimulated after meals, probably in response to release of motilin and CCK. Faecal continence depends upon maintenance of the anorectal angle and tonic contraction of the external anal sphincters. On defecation there is relaxation of the anorectal muscles, increased intra-abdominal pressure from the Valsalva manœuvre and contraction of abdominal muscles, and relaxation of the anal sphincters.

Control of gastrointestinal function

Secretion, absorption, motor activity, growth and differentiation of the gut are all modulated by a combination of neuronal and hormonal factors.

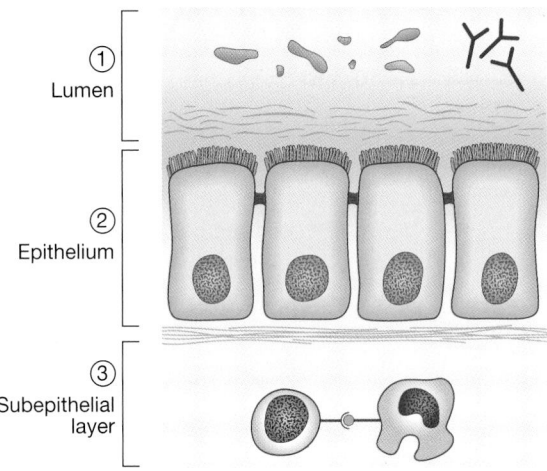

① Lumen

② Epithelium

③ Subepithelial layer

Fig. 22.8 Intestinal defence mechanisms. See text for details.

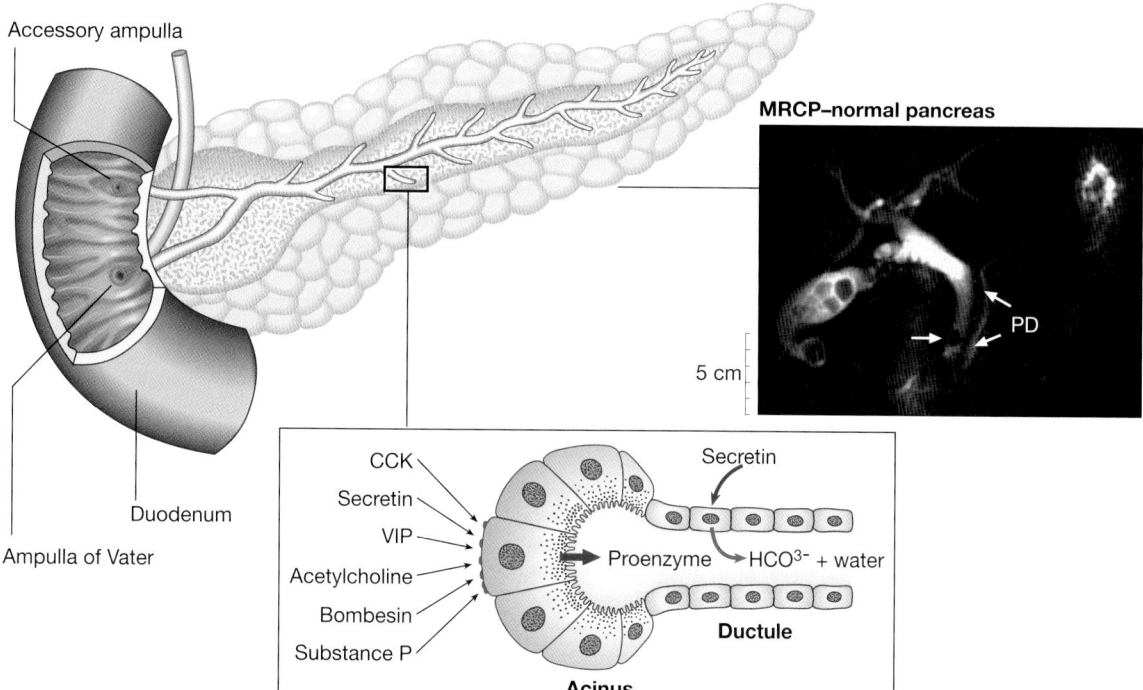

Fig. 22.9 Pancreatic structure and function. Ductular cells secrete alkaline fluid in response to secretin. Acinar cells secrete digestive enzymes from zymogen granules in response to a range of secretagogues. The photograph shows a normal pancreatic duct (PD) and side branches as defined at magnetic resonance cholangiopancreatography (MRCP). Note the incidental calculi in the gallbladder and common bile duct (arrow).

22

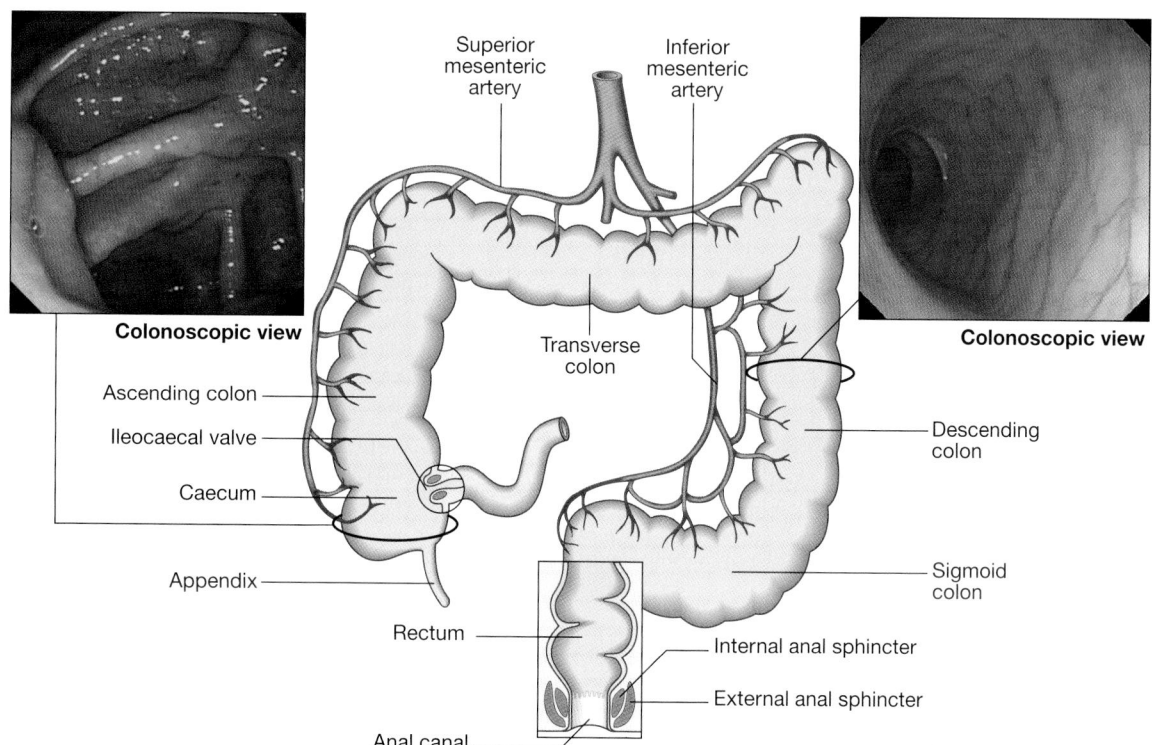

Fig. 22.10 The normal colon, rectum and anal canal.

22

The nervous system and gastrointestinal function

The central nervous system (CNS), the autonomic system (ANS) and the enteric nervous system (ENS) interact to regulate gut function. The ANS comprises:

- *parasympathetic pathways* (vagal and sacral efferent), which are cholinergic and generally increase smooth muscle tone and promote sphincter relaxation
- *sympathetic pathways*, which release noradrenaline (norepinephrine), reduce smooth muscle tone and stimulate sphincter contraction.

The enteric nervous system

This comprises two major networks intrinsic to the gut wall. The myenteric (Auerbach's) plexus in the smooth muscle layer regulates motor control; and the submucosal (Meissner's) plexus exerts secretory control over the epithelium, enteroendocrine cells and submucosal vessels. Together these plexuses form a two-layered neuronal mesh along the length of the gut. Although connected centrally via the ANS, the ENS can function autonomously, using a variety of transmitters including acetylcholine, noradrenaline (norepinephrine), 5-hydroxytryptamine (5-HT, serotonin), nitric oxide, substance P and calcitonin gene-related peptide (CGRP). There are local reflex loops within the ENS but also loops involving the coeliac and mesenteric ganglia and the paravertebral ganglia too.

The parasympathetic system generally stimulates motility and secretion while the sympathetic system generally acts in an inhibitory manner.

Peristalsis

Peristalsis is a reflex triggered by gut wall distension, which consists of a wave of circular muscle contraction to propel contents from the oesophagus to the rectum. It can be influenced by innervation but functions independently. It results from a basic electrical rhythm originating from the interstitial cells of Cajal in the circular layer of intestinal smooth muscle. These are stellate cells of mesenchymal origin with smooth muscle features, which act as the 'pacemaker' of the gut.

Migrating motor complexes

Migrating motor complexes (MMC) are powerful waves of contraction spreading from the stomach to the ileum and occurring at a frequency of about 5 per minute every 90 minutes or so, between meals and during fasting. They may serve to sweep intestinal contents distally in preparation for the next meal and are inhibited by eating.

Gut hormones

The origin, action and control of the major gut hormones, peptides and non-peptide signalling transmitters are summarised in Box 22.2.

22.2 Gut hormones and peptides

Hormone	Origin	Stimulus	Action
Gastrin	Stomach (G cell)	Products of protein digestion Suppressed by acid and somatostatin	Stimulates gastric acid secretion Stimulates growth of gastrointestinal mucosa
Somatostatin	Throughout GI tract (D cell)	Fat ingestion	Inhibits gastrin and insulin secretion Decreases acid secretion Decreases absorption Inhibits pancreatic secretion
Cholecystokinin (CCK)	Duodenum and jejunum (I cells); also ileal and colonic nerve endings	Products of protein digestion Fat and fatty acids Suppressed by trypsin	Stimulates pancreatic enzyme secretion Gallbladder contraction Sphincter of Oddi relaxation Satiety Decreases gastric acid secretion Reduces gastric emptying Regulates pancreatic growth
Secretin	Duodenum and jejunum (S cells)	Duodenal acid Fatty acids	Stimulates pancreatic fluid and bicarbonate secretion Decreases acid secretion Reduces gastric emptying
Motilin	Duodenum, small intestine and colon (Mo cells)	Fasting Dietary fat	Regulates peristaltic activity including migrating motor complexes (MMC)
Gastric inhibitory polypeptide (GIP)	Duodenum (K cells) and jejunum	Glucose and fat	Stimulates insulin release (also known as glucose-dependent insulinotrophic polypeptide) Inhibits acid secretion
Vasoactive intestinal peptide (VIP)	Nerve fibres throughout GI tract	Unknown	Vasodilator Smooth muscle relaxation Water and electrolyte secretion
Ghrelin	Stomach	Fasting Inhibited by eating	May regulate food intake
Guanylin	Small intestine	Unknown	Chloride secretion

INVESTIGATION OF GASTROINTESTINAL DISEASE

A wide range of tests are available for the investigation of patients with gastrointestinal symptoms. These can be classified broadly into tests of structure, tests for infection and tests of function.

Imaging

Plain X-rays

Plain X-rays of the abdomen are useful in the diagnosis of intestinal obstruction or paralytic ileus where dilated loops of bowel and (in the erect position) fluid levels may be seen. Calcified lymph nodes, gallstones and renal stones can also be detected. Chest X-ray is useful in the diagnosis of suspected perforation as it shows sub-diaphragmatic free air.

Contrast studies

X-rays with contrast medium are usually performed under fluoroscopic control to assess motility and to ensure that the patient is positioned correctly. Barium sulphate provides good mucosal coating and excellent opacification but can precipitate impaction proximal to an obstructive lesion. Water-soluble contrast is used to opacify bowel prior to abdominal computed tomography and in cases of suspected perforation. The double contrast technique improves mucosal visualisation by using gas to distend the barium-coated intestinal surface. Contrast studies are useful for detecting filling defects such as tumours, strictures, ulcers and motility disorders but they are being replaced by endoscopic procedures and by more sophisticated cross-sectional imaging techniques such as computed tomography and magnetic resonance imaging. The major uses and limitations of various contrast studies are shown in Box 22.3 and Figure 22.11.

Ultrasound, computed tomography (CT) and magnetic resonance imaging (MRI)

These are increasingly used in the evaluation of intra-abdominal disease. They are non-invasive and offer detailed images of the abdominal contents. Their main applications are summarised in Box 22.4 and Figure 22.12.

Endoscopy

Videoendoscopes have controls to allow steering of the tip and also possess channels for suction and insufflation of air and water. Accessories can be passed down the endoscope to allow both diagnostic and therapeutic

22

22.3 Contrast radiology in the investigation of gastrointestinal disease

	Barium swallow/meal	Barium follow-through	Barium enema
Indications and major uses	Possible motility disorder, e.g. achalasia or gastroparesis Suspected perforation or fistula (non-ionic contrast)	Diarrhoea and abdominal pain of small bowel origin Possible obstruction by strictures Suspected malabsorption Crohn's disease assessment	Altered bowel habit Evaluation of strictures or diverticular disease Megacolon Chronic constipation Suspected colon cancer (but superseded by colonoscopy in practice)
Limitations	Risk of aspiration Poor mucosal detail Low sensitivity for early cancer Inability to biopsy	Time-consuming Radiation exposure Relative insensitivity	Difficulty in frail elderly or incontinent patients Sigmoidoscopy necessary to evaluate rectum Low sensitivity for lesions < 1 cm

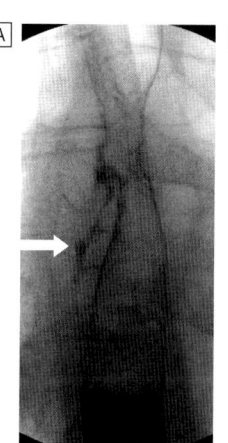
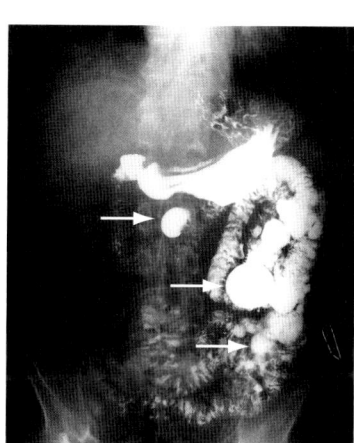
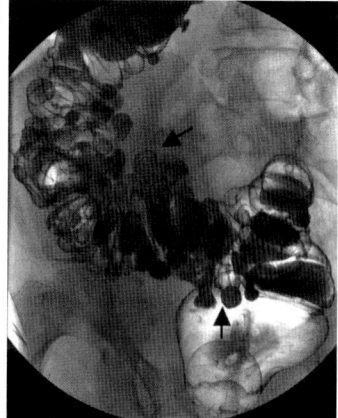

Fig. 22.11 Examples of contrast radiology. [A] Non-ionic contrast swallow shows leakage of contrast (arrow) into the mediastinum following stricture dilatation. [B] Barium follow-through. There are multiple diverticula (arrows) in this patient with jejunal diverticulosis. [C] Barium enema showing severe diverticular disease. There is tortuosity and narrowing of the sigmoid colon with multiple diverticula (arrows).

22.4 Ultrasound, computed tomography (CT), magnetic resonance imaging (MRI) and positron emission tomography (PET) in gastroenterology

	Ultrasound	CT	MRI	(CT)-PET
Indications and major uses	Abdominal masses, e.g. cysts, tumours, abscesses Organomegaly Ascites Biliary tract dilatation Gallstones Guided biopsy of lesions	Assessment of pancreatic disease Hepatic tumour deposits CT colonography ('virtual colonoscopy') Tumour staging Assessment of vascularity of lesions Abscesses and collections	Hepatic tumour staging Magnetic resonance cholangiopancreatography (MRCP) Pelvic/perianal disease Crohn's fistulas Small bowel visualisation	Detection of metastases not seen on ultrasound or CT Images can be fused with CT to form composite image (Fig. 22.12D)
Limitations	Low sensitivity for small lesions Little functional information Operator-dependent Gas and obesity may obscure view	Cost Radiation dose Availability	Availability Time-consuming 'Claustrophobic' for some Contraindicated in presence of metallic prostheses, cardiac pacemaker, cochlear implants	Relatively poor localisation of lesions unless combined with CT Signal detection depends on metabolic activity within tumour—not all are metabolically active

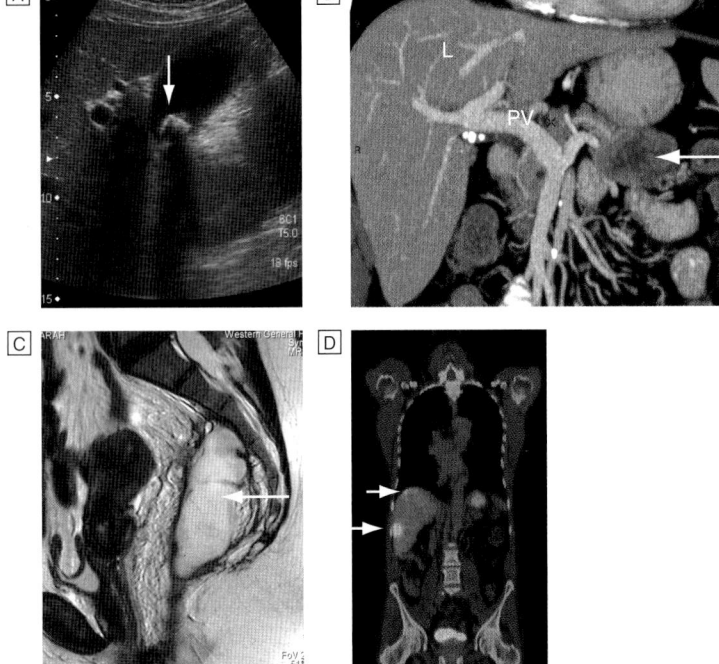

Fig. 22.12 Examples of ultrasound, CT and MRI. **A** Ultrasound showing large gallstone (arrow) with acoustic shadowing. **B** Multidetector coronal CT showing large solid and cystic malignant tumour in the pancreatic tail (P). (PV = portal vein; L = liver) **C** Pelvic MRI showing large pelvic abscess (arrow) posterior to the rectum in a patient with Crohn's disease. **D** Fused CT-PET image showing two liver metastases (arrows).

procedures, some of which are illustrated in Figure 22.13. New high-definition endoscopes with magnifying lenses allow almost microscopic detail to be observed, and newer imaging modalities such as autofluorescence and 'narrow band imaging' are increasingly used to detect subtle abnormalities not visible by standard 'white light' endoscopy.

Upper gastrointestinal endoscopy

This is performed under light intravenous benzodiazepine sedation, or using only local anaesthetic throat spray after the patient has fasted for at least 4 hours. With the patient in the left lateral position the entire oesophagus (excluding pharynx), stomach and first two parts of duodenum can be seen. Indications, contraindications and complications are given in Box 22.5.

Capsule endoscopy

Capsule endoscopy (Fig. 22.14) employs a 26 mm capsule containing an imaging device, battery, transmitter and antenna, which transmits images as it traverses the small intestine to a battery-powered recorder worn on a belt round the patient's waist. After approximately 8 hours the capsule is excreted. Images from the capsule are analysed as a video sequence and it is usually possible to

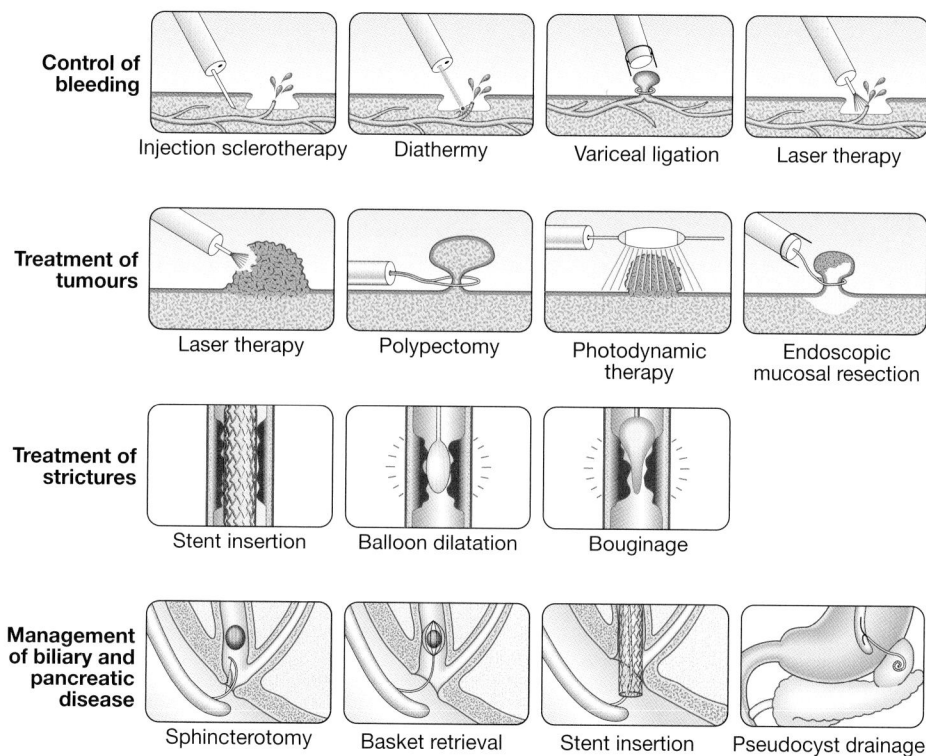

Fig. 22.13 **Examples of therapeutic techniques in endoscopy.**

22.5 Upper gastrointestinal endoscopy

Indications

- Dyspepsia over 55 years of age or with alarm symptoms
- Atypical chest pain
- Dysphagia
- Vomiting
- Weight loss
- Acute or chronic gastrointestinal bleeding
- Suspicious barium meal
- Duodenal biopsies in the investigation of malabsorption

Contraindications

- Severe shock
- Recent myocardial infarction, unstable angina, cardiac arrhythmia*
- Severe respiratory disease*
- Atlantoaxial subluxation*
- Possible visceral perforation

Complications

- Cardiorespiratory depression due to sedation
- Aspiration pneumonia
- Perforation

*These are 'relative' contraindications; in experienced hands, endoscopy can be safely performed.

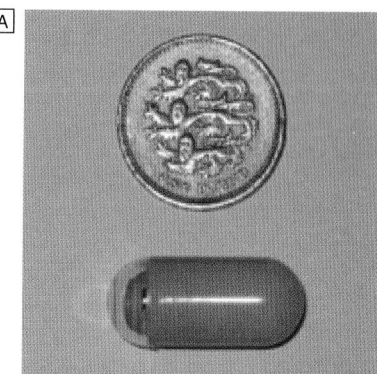

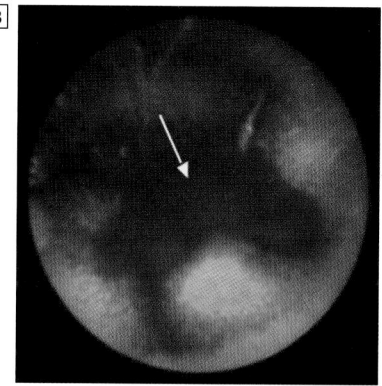

Fig. 22.14 **Wireless capsule endoscopy.** [A] Wireless capsule. [B] Capsule endoscopy image of bleeding jejunal vascular malformation (arrow).

localise the segment of small bowel in which lesions are seen. Abnormalities detected usually require enteroscopy for confirmation and therapy. Indications, contraindications and complications are listed in Box 22.6.

22.6 Capsule endoscopy

Indications

- Obscure gastrointestinal bleeding
- Small bowel Crohn's disease
- Assessment of coeliac disease and its complications
- Screening and surveillance in familial polyposis syndromes

Contraindications

- Known or suspected small bowel stricture (risk of capsule retention)
- Caution in people with pacemakers or implantable defibrillators

Complications

- Capsule retention (< 1%)

22.7 Double balloon enteroscopy

Indications

Diagnostic
- Obscure gastrointestinal bleeding
- Malabsorption or unexplained diarrhoea
- Suspicious radiological findings
- Suspected small bowel tumour
- Surveillance of polyposis syndromes

Therapeutic
- Coagulation/diathermy of bleeding lesions
- Jejunostomy placement

Contraindications

- As for upper gastrointestinal endoscopy

Complications

- As for upper gastrointestinal endoscopy
- Post-procedure abdominal pain (up to 20%)
- Pancreatitis (1–3%)
- Perforation (especially after resection of large polyps)

Double balloon endoscopy

While standard endoscopy can reach the proximal small intestine in most patients, a newer technique called double balloon enteroscopy (DBE, Fig. 22.15) is also available, which uses a long endoscope with a flexible overtube. Sequential and repeated inflation and deflation of balloons on the tip of the overtube and enteroscope allow the operator to push and pull along the entire length of the small intestine to the terminal ileum to diagnose or treat small bowel lesions detected by capsule endoscopy or other imaging modalities. Indications, contraindications and complications are listed in Box 22.7.

Sigmoidoscopy and colonoscopy

Sigmoidoscopy can be carried out either in the out-patient clinic using a 20 cm rigid plastic sigmoidoscope or in the endoscopy suite using a 60 cm flexible colonoscope following bowel preparation. When sigmoidoscopy is combined with proctoscopy, accurate detection of haemorrhoids, ulcerative colitis and distal colorectal neoplasia is possible. After full bowel cleansing it is possible to examine the entire colon and often the terminal ileum using a longer colonoscope. Indications, contraindications and complications of colonoscopy are listed in Box 22.8.

Endoscopic retrograde cholangiopancreatography (ERCP)

Using a side-viewing duodenoscope, it is possible to cannulate the main pancreatic duct and common bile duct. ERCP visualises the ampulla of Vater and produces

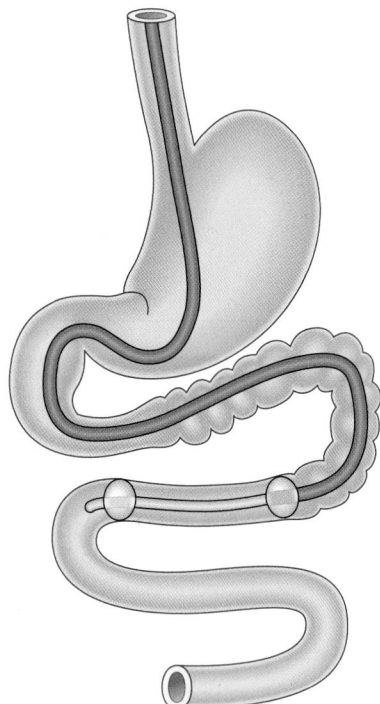

Fig. 22.15 Double balloon enteroscopy. The enteroscope and an overtube both have balloons at their tips. Sequential inflation and deflation of the balloons, combined with push and pull movements, allows deep intubation of the small intestine.

22.8 Colonoscopy

Indications*

- Suspected inflammatory bowel disease
- Chronic diarrhoea
- Altered bowel habit
- Rectal bleeding or anaemia
- Assessment of abnormal barium enema
- Colorectal cancer screening
- Colorectal adenoma follow-up
- Therapeutic procedures

Contraindications

- Severe, active ulcerative colitis
- As for upper gastrointestinal endoscopy

Complications

- Cardiorespiratory depression due to sedation
- Perforation
- Bleeding following polypectomy

*Colonoscopy is not useful in the investigation of constipation.

22.9 Endoscopic retrograde cholangiopancreatography (ERCP)

Indications

Diagnostic ERCP
- Rarely indicated—MRCP/EUS/CT provide excellent images of biliary tree and pancreas
- Occasionally performed when images are equivocal or MRCP is contraindicated

Therapeutic ERCP
- Biliary disease
  Removal of CBD calculi (N.B. In fit individuals who also require cholecystectomy laparoscopic surgery may be preferred)
  Palliation of biliary obstruction due to advanced malignant disease
  Management of biliary leaks/damage complicating biliary surgery
  Dilatation of benign strictures (e.g. primary sclerosing cholangitis)
- Pancreatic disease
  Drainage of pancreatic disruption (e.g. pseudocysts, pancreatic fistulas)
  Removal of pancreatic calculi (selected cases)

Contraindications
- Severe cardiopulmonary comorbidity
- Coagulopathy

Complications
- Occur in 5–10% with a 30-day mortality of 0.5–1%

General
- As for upper endoscopy

Specific
- Biliary disease
  Bleeding following sphincterotomy
  Cholangitis (only when biliary obstruction is not achieved at ERCP)
  Gallstone impaction
- Pancreatic disease
  Acute pancreatitis
  Infection of pseudocyst

22.10 Endoscopy in old age

- **Tolerance:** endoscopic procedures are generally well tolerated, even in very old people.
- **Side-effects from sedation:** older people are more sensitive, and respiratory depression, hypotension and prolonged recovery times are more common.
- **Bowel preparation for colonoscopy:** can be difficult in frail, immobile people. Sodium phosphate-based preparations can cause dehydration or hypotension and should be avoided in those with underlying cardiac or renal failure.
- **Antiperistaltic agents:** hyoscine should be avoided in those with glaucoma and can also cause tachyarrhythmias. Glucagon is preferred if an antiperistaltic agent is needed.

22.11 Reasons for biopsy or cytological examination

- Suspected malignant lesions
- Assessment of mucosal abnormalities
- Diagnosis of infection (e.g. *Candida, Helicobacter pylori, Giardia lamblia*)
- Measurement of enzyme contents (e.g. disaccharidases)
- Analysis of genetic mutations (e.g. oncogenes, tumour suppressor genes)

22

radiological images of the biliary tree and pancreas. Diagnostic ERCP has largely been replaced by magnetic resonance cholangiopancreatography (MRCP), which provides comparable images of the biliary tree and pancreas. MRCP complements CT and endoscopic ultrasound (EUS) in the evaluation of obstructive jaundice, biliary pain and suspected pancreatic disease, and therapeutic ERCP is then used to treat a range of biliary and pancreatic diseases identified by these non-invasive imaging techniques. Indications for and risks of ERCP are listed in Box 22.9.

Histology

Biopsy material obtained during endoscopy or percutaneously can provide useful information (Box 22.11).

Tests of infection
Bacterial cultures

Stool cultures are essential in the investigation of diarrhoea, especially when it is acute or bloody, to identify pathogenic organisms (Ch. 13).

Serology

Detection of antibodies plays a limited role in the diagnosis of gastrointestinal infection caused by organisms such as *Helicobacter pylori, Salmonella* species and *Entamoeba histolytica*.

Breath tests

Non-invasive breath tests for *H. pylori* infection are discussed on page 850. Breath tests for suspected small intestinal bacterial overgrowth are discussed on page 881.

Tests of function

A number of dynamic tests can be used to investigate aspects of gut function, including digestion, absorption, inflammation and epithelial permeability. Some of the more commonly used ones are listed in Box 22.12. In the assessment of suspected malabsorption, blood tests (full blood count, erythrocyte sedimentation rate (ESR), folate, B$_{12}$, iron status, albumin, calcium and phosphate) are essential, and endoscopy is undertaken to obtain mucosal biopsies.

Oesophageal motility

A barium swallow can give useful information about oesophageal motility. Videofluoroscopy, with joint assessment by a speech and language therapist and a radiologist, may be necessary in difficult cases. Oesophageal manometry (see Fig. 22.1, p. 838), often in conjunction with 24-hour pH measurements, is of value in diagnosing cases of refractory gastro-oesophageal reflux, achalasia and non-cardiac chest pain. Oesophageal impedance testing is useful for detecting non-acid or gas reflux events, especially in patients with atypical symptoms or those who respond poorly to acid suppression.

22.12 Dynamic tests of gastrointestinal function

Process	Test	Principle	Comments
Absorption			
Fat	^{14}C-triolein breath test	Measurement of $^{14}CO_2$ in breath after oral ingestion of radio-labelled fat	Non-invasive but not quantitative
Lactose	Lactose H$_2$ breath test	Measurement of breath H$_2$ content after 50 g oral lactose. Undigested sugar is metabolised by colonic bacteria in hypolactasia, and expired hydrogen is measured	Non-invasive and accurate. May provoke pain and diarrhoea in sufferers
Bile acids	^{75}SeHCAT test	Isotopic quantification of 7-day whole-body retention of oral dose ^{75}Se-labelled homocholyltaurine ($> 15\%$ = normal, $< 5\%$ = abnormal)	Accurate and specific but requires two visits and involves radiation. Can be equivocal. Serum 7α-hydroxycholestenone is as sensitive and specific
Pancreatic exocrine function	Pancreolauryl test	Pancreatic esterases cleave fluoroscein dilaurate after oral ingestion. Fluoroscein is absorbed and quantified in urine	Accurate and avoids duodenal intubation Takes 2 days. Accurate urine collection essential. Rarely performed
	Faecal elastase	Immunoassay of pancreatic enzymes on stool sample	Simple, quick and avoids urine collection Does not detect mild disease
Mucosal inflammation/ permeability	Calprotectin	A protein secreted non-specifically by neutrophils into the colon in response to inflammation or neoplasia	Useful screening test for colonic disease

Gastric emptying

This involves administering a test meal containing solids and liquids labelled with different radioisotopes and measuring the amount retained in the stomach afterwards (Box 22.13). It is useful in the investigation of suspected delayed gastric emptying (gastroparesis) when other studies are normal.

Colonic and anorectal motility

A plain abdominal X-ray taken on day 5 after ingestion of different-shaped inert plastic pellets on days 1–3 gives an estimate of whole gut transit time. The test is useful in the evaluation of chronic constipation when the position of

22.13 Commonly used radioisotope tests in gastroenterology

Test	Isotope	Major uses and principle of test
Gastric emptying study	^{99m}Tc-sulphur ^{111}In-DTPA	Used in assessment of gastric emptying, particularly for possible gastroparesis
Urea breath test	^{13}C-urea	Used in non-invasive diagnosis of *H. pylori*. Bacterial urease enzyme splits urea to ammonia and CO_2 which is detected in expired air
Meckel's scan	^{99m}Tc-pertechnate	Diagnosis of Meckel's diverticulum in cases of obscure gastrointestinal bleeding. Isotope is injected i.v. and localises in ectopic parietal mucosa within diverticulum
Somatostatin receptor scan (SRS)	^{111}In-DTPA-DPhe-octreotide	Labelled somatostatin analogue binds to cell surface somatostatin receptors on pancreatic neuroendocrine tumours

any retained pellets can be observed, and helps to differentiate cases of slow transit from those due to obstructed defecation. The mechanism of defecation and anorectal function can be assessed by anorectal manometry, electrophysiological tests and defecating proctography.

Radioisotope tests

Many different radioisotope tests are used (see Box 22.13). In some, structural information is obtained, e.g. localisation of a Meckel's diverticulum. Others use radioisotopes for functional information, e.g. rates of gastric emptying or ability to reabsorb bile acids. Yet others are tests of infection and rely on the presence of bacteria to hydrolyse a radio-labelled test substance followed by detection of the radioisotope in expired air (e.g. urea breath test for *H. pylori*).

PRESENTING PROBLEMS IN GASTROINTESTINAL DISEASE

Dysphagia

Dysphagia is defined as difficulty in swallowing. It may coexist with heartburn or vomiting but should be distinguished from both globus sensation (in which anxious people feel a lump in the throat without organic cause) and odynophagia (pain during swallowing, usually from gastro-oesophageal reflux or candidiasis).

Dysphagia can occur due to problems in the oropharynx or oesophagus (Fig. 22.16). Oropharyngeal disorders affect the initiation of swallowing at the pharynx and upper oesophageal sphincter. The patient has difficulty initiating swallowing and complains of choking, nasal regurgitation or tracheal aspiration. Drooling, dysarthria, hoarseness and cranial nerve or other neurological signs may be present. Oesophageal disorders cause dysphagia by obstructing the lumen or by

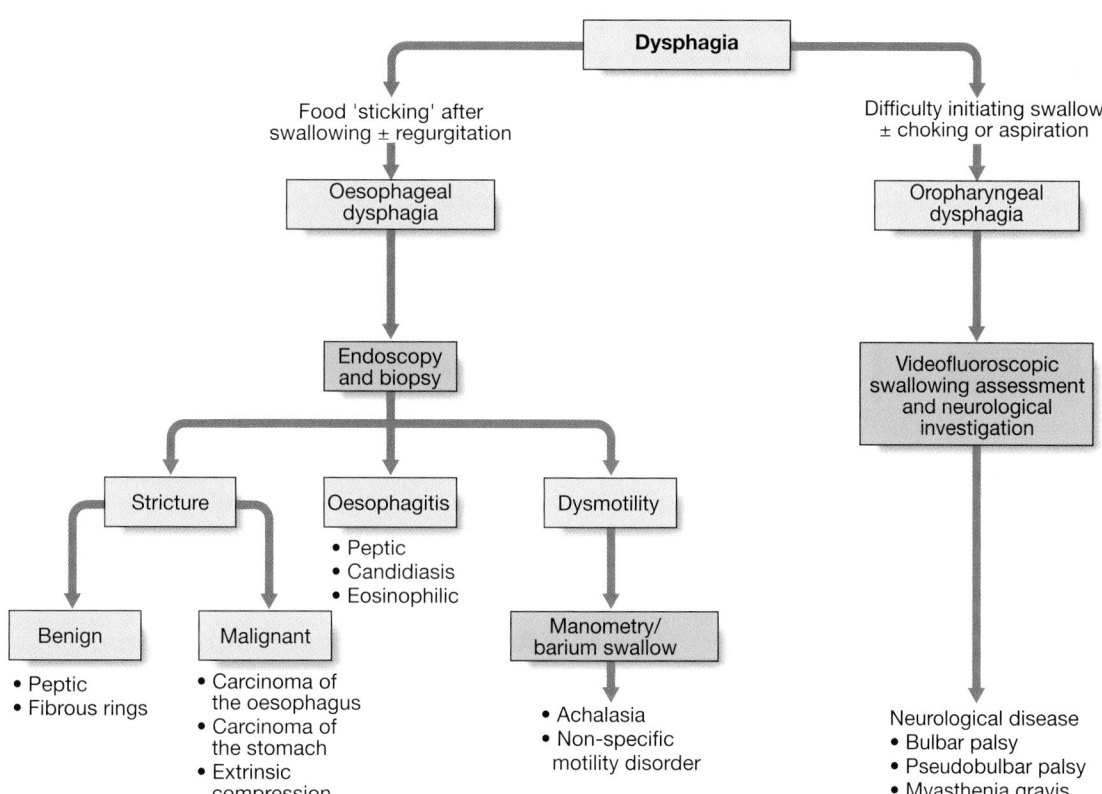

Fig. 22.16 Investigation of dysphagia.

affecting motility. Patients with oesophageal disease complain of food 'sticking' after swallowing, although the level at which this is felt correlates poorly with the true site of obstruction. Swallowing of liquids is normal until strictures become extreme.

Investigations

Dysphagia should always be investigated. Endoscopy is the investigation of choice because it allows biopsy and dilatation of suspicious strictures. If no abnormality is found, then barium swallow with videofluoroscopic swallowing assessment is indicated to detect motility disorders. In a few cases oesophageal manometry is required. Figure 22.16 summarises a diagnostic approach to dysphagia and lists the major causes.

Dyspepsia

Dyspepsia is the term used to describe symptoms such as bloating and nausea which are thought to originate from the upper gastrointestinal tract. There are many causes (Box 22.14), including some arising outside the digestive system. Heartburn and other 'reflux' symptoms are separate entities and are considered elsewhere. Although symptoms often correlate poorly with the underlying diagnosis, a careful history is important to detect 'alarm' features requiring urgent investigation (Box 22.15) and to detect atypical symptoms which might be due to problems outside the gastrointestinal tract.

Dyspepsia affects up to 80% of the population at some time in life and many patients have no serious underlying disease. Patients who present with new dyspepsia at an age of more than 55 years and younger

22.14 Causes of dyspepsia

Upper gastrointestinal disorders

- Peptic ulcer disease
- Acute gastritis
- Gallstones
- Motility disorders, e.g. oesophageal spasm
- 'Functional' (non-ulcer dyspepsia and irritable bowel syndrome)

Other gastrointestinal disorders

- Pancreatic disease (cancer, chronic pancreatitis)
- Hepatic disease (hepatitis, metastases)
- Colonic carcinoma

Systemic disease

- Renal failure
- Hypercalcaemia

Drugs

- Non-steroidal anti-inflammatory drugs (NSAIDs)
- Iron and potassium supplements
- Corticosteroids
- Digoxin

Others

- Alcohol
- Psychological, e.g. anxiety, depression

22.15 'Alarm' features in dyspepsia

- Weight loss
- Anaemia
- Vomiting
- Haematemesis and/or melaena
- Dysphagia
- Palpable abdominal mass

22

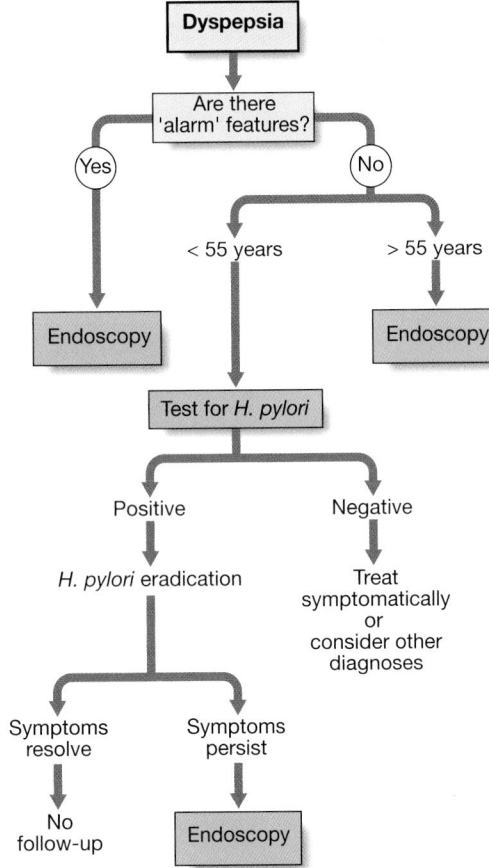

Fig. 22.17 Investigation of dyspepsia.

patients unresponsive to empirical treatment require investigation to exclude serious disease. An algorithm for the investigation of dyspepsia is outlined in Figure 22.17.

Vomiting

Vomiting is a complex reflex involving both autonomic and somatic neural pathways. Synchronous contraction of the diaphragm, intercostal muscles and abdominal muscles raises intra-abdominal pressure and, combined with relaxation of the lower oesophageal sphincter, results in forcible ejection of gastric contents. It is important to distinguish true vomiting from regurgitation and to elicit whether the vomiting is acute or chronic (recurrent), as the underlying causes may differ. The major causes are shown in Figure 22.18.

Gastrointestinal bleeding

Acute upper gastrointestinal haemorrhage

This is the most common gastrointestinal emergency, accounting for 50–170 admissions to hospital per 100 000 of the population each year in the UK. The mortality of patients admitted to hospital is about 10% but there is some evidence that outcome is better when patients are treated in specialised units. Risk factors for death are shown in Box 22.16 and the common causes of upper gastrointestinal bleeding are shown in Figure 22.19.

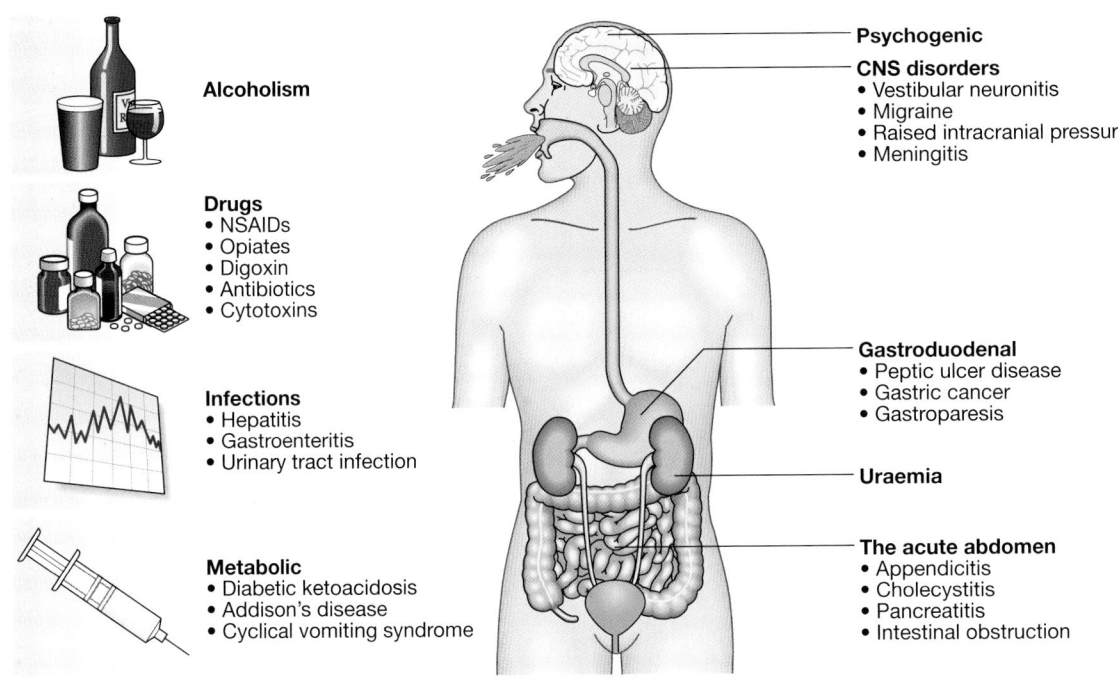

Fig. 22.18 Causes of vomiting.

✚ 22.16 Rockall score for risk stratification in acute upper gastrointestinal haemorrhage

Variable	Score 0	Score 1	Score 2	Score 3	Score
Calculate on admission					
Age	< 60	60–79	> 80		
Shock	No shock	Pulse > 100	SBP < 100		
Comorbidity	Nil major	CCF, IHD, major comorbidity	Renal/liver failure	Metastatic cancer	
Calculate after endoscopy					
Diagnosis	Mallory-Weiss tear or normal	All other diagnoses	GI malignancy[1]		
Evidence of bleeding	None	Blood in stomach	Adherent clot Visible or spurting vessel[2]		
					Final score (range 0–11)

[1] Malignancy and varices have the worst prognosis.
[2] These features are associated with a high risk of rebleeding. Rebleeding (fresh haematemesis or melaena associated with shock or a fall of haemoglobin > 20 g/L over 24 hours) is associated with a 10-fold increased risk of death.

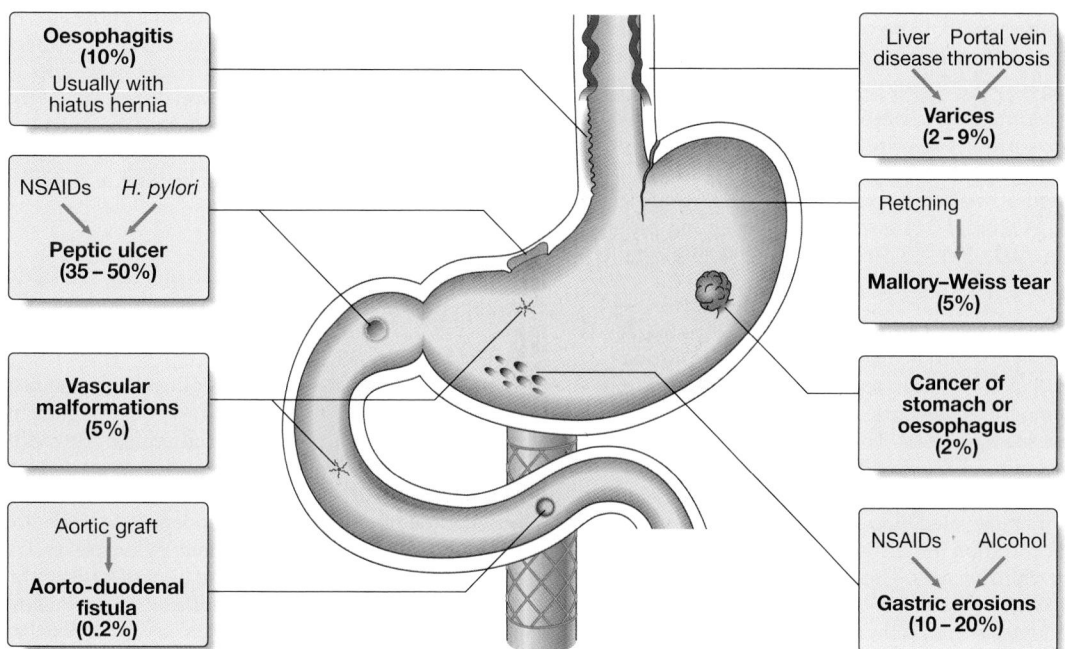

Fig. 22.19 Causes of acute upper gastrointestinal haemorrhage. (Frequency in parentheses.)

Clinical assessment

Haematemesis is red with clots when bleeding is profuse, or black ('coffee grounds') when less severe. Syncope may occur and is due to hypotension from intravascular volume depletion. Symptoms of anaemia suggest chronic bleeding. Melaena is the passage of black, tarry stools containing altered blood; it is usually caused by bleeding from the upper gastrointestinal tract, although haemorrhage from the right side of the colon is occasionally responsible. The characteristic colour and smell are the result of the action of digestive enzymes and of bacteria upon haemoglobin. Severe acute upper gastrointestinal bleeding can sometimes cause maroon or bright red stool.

Management

The principles of emergency management of non-variceal bleeding are summarised in Box 22.17 and are discussed in detail below. Management of variceal bleeding is discussed on page 939.

1. Intravenous access

The first step is to gain intravenous access using at least one large-bore cannula.

2. Initial clinical assessment

- *Define circulatory status.* Severe bleeding causes tachycardia, hypotension and oliguria. The patient is cold and sweating, and may be agitated.

22

✚ 22.17 Emergency management of acute non-variceal upper gastrointestinal haemorrhage

- Gain intravenous access with large-bore cannula
- Check full blood count and routine biochemistry; cross-match blood
- Perform hourly measurements of blood pressure, pulse and urine output; consider central venous pressure (CVP) monitoring in severe bleeding
- Give intravenous colloids or crystalloids in patients with hypotension and tachycardia
- Transfuse with blood if blood pressure remains low and patient is actively bleeding
- Organise endoscopy for diagnosis and treatment
- Give i.v. PPI therapy for bleeding peptic ulcer
- Consider surgery or arterial embolisation if bleeding recurs

- *Seek evidence of liver disease.* Jaundice, cutaneous stigmata, hepatosplenomegaly and ascites may be present in decompensated cirrhosis.
- *Identify comorbidity.* The presence of cardiorespiratory, cerebrovascular or renal disease is important, both because these may be worsened by acute bleeding and because they increase the hazards of endoscopy and surgical operations.

These factors can be combined using the Rockall scoring system to predict severity (see Box 22.16). An initial score can be calculated, endoscopic findings can be added later and a final score may be obtained, ranging from 0 to 11. A score < 3 is associated with a good prognosis while a total score > 8 carries a high risk of mortality.

3. Basic investigations

- *Full blood count.* Chronic or subacute bleeding leads to anaemia, but the haemoglobin concentration may be normal after sudden, major bleeding until haemodilution occurs.
- *Urea and electrolytes.* This test may show evidence of renal failure. The blood urea rises as the absorbed products of luminal blood are metabolised by the liver; an elevated blood urea with normal creatinine concentration implies severe bleeding.
- *Liver function tests.* These may show evidence of chronic liver disease.
- *Prothrombin time*, if there is clinical suggestion of liver disease or in anticoagulated patients.
- *Cross-matching* of at least 2 units of blood.

4. Resuscitation

Intravenous crystalloid fluids or colloid should be given to raise the blood pressure, and blood should be transfused when the patient is actively bleeding with low blood pressure and tachycardia. Comorbidities should be managed as appropriate. Patients with suspected chronic liver disease should receive broad-spectrum antibiotics. Central venous pressure (CVP) monitoring is useful in severe bleeding, particularly in patients who have cardiac disease, to assist in defining the volume of fluid replacement and in identification of rebleeding.

5. Oxygen

This should be given by facemask to all patients in shock.

6. Endoscopy

This should be carried out after adequate resuscitation, ideally within 24 hours, and will yield a diagnosis in 80% of cases. Patients who are found to have major endoscopic stigmata of recent haemorrhage (Fig. 22.20) can be treated endoscopically using a thermal modality such as a 'heater probe', by injection of dilute adrenaline (epinephrine) into the bleeding point, or by application of metallic clips. Endoscopic therapy may stop active bleeding and, combined with intravenous PPI (PPI) therapy, prevent rebleeding, thus avoiding the need for surgery (Boxes 22.18 and 22.19). Patients found to have bled from varices are treated by band ligation as described in Chapter 23.

7. Monitoring

Patients should be closely observed, with hourly pulse, blood pressure and urine output measurements.

8. Surgery

Surgery is indicated when endoscopic haemostasis fails to stop active bleeding and if rebleeding occurs on one occasion in an elderly or frail patient, or twice in a younger, fitter patients.

The choice of operation depends on the site and diagnosis of the bleeding lesion. Duodenal ulcers are treated by under-running with or without pyloroplasty. Under-running for gastric ulcers can also be carried out (a biopsy must be taken to exclude carcinoma). Local excision may also be performed, but when neither is possible, partial gastrectomy will be required. Following successful surgery for ulcer bleeding, all patients should be treated with

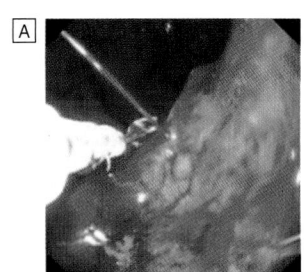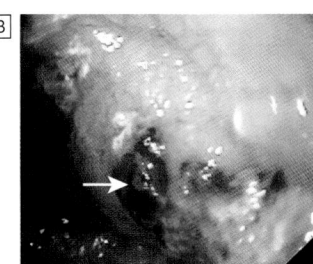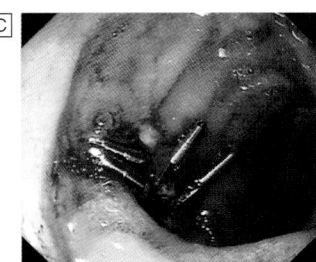

Fig. 22.20 Major stigmata of recent haemorrhage and endoscopic treatment. **A** Active arterial spurting from a gastric ulcer. An endoscopic clip is about to be placed on the bleeding vessel. When associated with shock, 80% of cases will continue to bleed or rebleed. **B** 'Visible vessel' (arrow). In reality, this is a pseudoaneurysm of the feeding artery seen here in a pre-pyloric peptic ulcer. It carries a 50% chance of rebleeding. **C** Haemostasis is achieved after endoscopic clipping of the bleeding vessel in the duodenum.

EBM **22.18 Endoscopic therapy in acute upper gastrointestinal haemorrhage**

'Peptic ulcers that are actively bleeding or have a protruberant vessel or adherent blood clot are treated endoscopically using a combination of injection (adrenaline (epinephrine)), application of thermal energy or clips.'

• Scottish Intercollegiate Guideline Network. Guideline 105. Management of acute upper and lower gastrointestinal bleeding, 2008.

For further information: www.sign.ac.uk

EBM **22.19 Adjunctive drug therapy for bleeding ulcers**

'Intravenous proton pump inhibitor infusions reduce rebleeding ($NNT_B = 12$) and need for surgery ($NNT_B = 20$) but not mortality in patients who have been subjected to endoscopic therapy for major peptic ulcer haemorrhage. When given prior to endoscopy they reduce the need for endoscopic therapy and hospital stay but not need for surgery or mortality.'

• Leontiadis GI, et al. BMJ 2005; 330:568–575.
• Lau JY, et al. New Engl J Med 2007; 356:1631–1640.

For further information: www.sign.ac.uk

H. pylori eradication therapy if positive and should avoid NSAIDs. Ulcer patients need confirmation of successful eradication by urea breath testing.

Lower gastrointestinal bleeding

This may be due to haemorrhage from the colon, anal canal or small bowel. It is useful to distinguish those patients who present with profuse, acute bleeding from those who present with chronic or subacute bleeding of lesser severity (Box 22.20).

Severe acute lower gastrointestinal bleeding

Patients present with profuse red or maroon diarrhoea and with shock. Diverticular disease is the most common cause and is often due to erosion of an artery within the mouth of a diverticulum. Bleeding almost always stops spontaneously, but if it does not, the diseased segment of colon should be resected after confirmation of the site by angiography or colonoscopy. Angiodysplasia is a disease of the elderly in which vascular malformations develop in the proximal colon. Bleeding can be acute and profuse; it usually stops spontaneously but commonly recurs. Diagnosis is often difficult. Colonoscopy may reveal characteristic vascular spots, and in the acute

 22.20 Causes of lower gastrointestinal bleeding

Severe acute

• Diverticular disease
• Angiodysplasia
• Ischaemia
• Meckel's diverticulum
• Inflammatory bowel disease (rarely)

Moderate, chronic/subacute

• Anal disease, e.g. fissure, haemorrhoids
• Inflammatory bowel disease
• Carcinoma
• Large polyps
• Angiodysplasia
• Radiation enteritis
• Solitary rectal ulcer

phase visceral angiography can show bleeding into the intestinal lumen and an abnormal large, draining vein. In some patients, diagnosis is only achieved by laparotomy with on-table colonoscopy. The treatment of choice is endoscopic thermal ablation, but resection of the affected bowel may be required if bleeding continues. Bowel ischaemia due to occlusion of the inferior mesenteric artery can present with abdominal colic and rectal bleeding. It should be considered in patients (particularly the elderly) who have evidence of generalised atherosclerosis. The diagnosis is made at colonoscopy. Resection is required only in the presence of peritonitis. Meckel's diverticulum with ectopic gastric epithelium may ulcerate and erode into a major artery. The diagnosis should be considered in children or adolescents who present with profuse or recurrent lower gastrointestinal bleeding. A Meckel's [99mTc]-pertechnate scan is sometimes positive but the diagnosis is commonly made only by laparotomy, at which time the diverticulum is excised.

Subacute or chronic lower gastrointestinal bleeding

This is common at all ages and is usually due to haemorrhoids or anal fissure. Haemorrhoidal bleeding is bright red and occurs during or after defecation. Proctoscopy is used to make the diagnosis but in subjects who also have altered bowel habit and in all patients presenting at over 40 years of age, colonoscopy is necessary to exclude coexisting colorectal cancer. Anal fissure should be suspected when fresh rectal bleeding and anal pain occur during defecation.

Obscure major gastrointestinal bleeding

In some patients who present with major gastrointestinal bleeding, upper endoscopy and colonoscopy fail to reveal a diagnosis. When severe life-threatening bleeding continues, urgent mesenteric angiography is indicated. This will usually identify the site if the bleeding rate exceeds 1 mL/min and embolisation can often stop the bleeding. If angiography is negative or bleeding is less severe, push or double balloon enteroscopy can visualise the small intestine (Fig. 22.21,

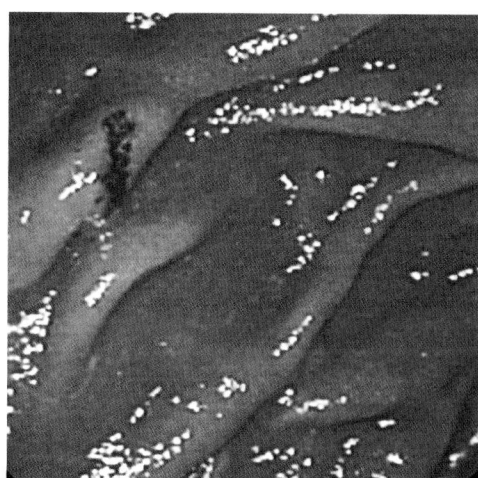

Fig. 22.21 Jejunal angiodysplastic lesion seen at enteroscopy in a patient with recurrent obscure bleeding.

and see Figs 22.14 and 22.15) and treat the bleeding source. Wireless capsule endoscopy is often used to define a source of bleeding prior to enteroscopy. When all else fails, laparotomy with on-table endoscopy is indicated.

Occult gastrointestinal bleeding

In this context occult means that blood or its breakdown products are present in the stool but cannot be seen by the naked eye. Occult bleeding may reach 200 mL per day, cause iron deficiency anaemia and signify serious gastrointestinal disease. Any cause of gastrointestinal bleeding may be responsible but the most important is colorectal cancer, particularly carcinoma of the caecum which may have no gastrointestinal symptoms. In clinical practice, investigation of the gastrointestinal tract should be considered whenever a patient presents with unexplained iron deficiency anaemia. Testing the stool for the presence of blood is unnecessary and should not influence whether or not the gastrointestinal tract is imaged because bleeding from tumours is often intermittent and a negative faecal occult blood (FOB) test does not exclude important gastrointestinal disease. Many colorectal cancer patients are FOB-negative at presentation, and the only value of FOB testing is as a means of screening for colonic disease in asymptomatic populations (p. 912).

Diarrhoea

Gastroenterologists define diarrhoea as the passage of more than 200 g of stool daily, and measurement of stool volume is helpful in confirming this. The most severe symptom in many patients is urgency of defecation, and faecal incontinence is a common event in acute and chronic diarrhoeal illnesses.

Acute diarrhoea

This is extremely common and usually due to faecal–oral transmission of bacteria, their toxins, viruses or parasites (Ch. 13). Infective diarrhoea is usually short-lived and patients who present with a history of diarrhoea lasting more than 10 days rarely have an infective cause. A variety of drugs, including antibiotics, cytotoxic drugs, PPIs and NSAIDs, may be responsible for acute diarrhoea.

Chronic or relapsing diarrhoea

The most common cause is irritable bowel syndrome (p. 904), which can present with increased frequency of defecation and loose, watery or pellety stools. Diarrhoea rarely occurs at night and is most severe before and after breakfast. At other times the patient is constipated and there are other characteristic symptoms of irritable bowel syndrome. The stool often contains mucus but never blood, and 24-hour stool volume is less than 200 g. Chronic diarrhoea can be categorised as disease of the colon or small bowel, or malabsorption (Box 22.21). Clinical presentation, examination of the stool, routine blood tests and imaging reveal a diagnosis in many cases. A series of negative investigations usually implies irritable bowel syndrome but some patients clearly have organic disease and need more extensive investigations.

Malabsorption

Diarrhoea and weight loss in patients with a normal diet should always lead to the suspicion of malabsorption. The symptoms are diverse in nature and variable in severity. A few patients have apparently normal bowel habit but diarrhoea is usual and may be watery and voluminous. Bulky, pale and offensive stools which float in the toilet (steatorrhoea) signify fat malabsorption. Abdominal distension, borborygmi, cramps, weight loss and undigested food in the stool may be present. Some patients complain only of malaise and lethargy. In others, symptoms related to deficiencies of specific vitamins, trace elements and minerals (e.g. calcium, iron, folic acid) may occur (Fig. 22.22).

22.21 Chronic or relapsing diarrhoea			
	Colonic	**Malabsorption**	**Small bowel**
Clinical features	Blood and mucus in stool Cramping lower abdominal pain	Steatorrhoea Undigested food in the stool Weight loss and nutritional disturbances	Large-volume, watery stool Abdominal bloating Cramping mid-abdominal pain

Some causes	Inflammatory bowel disease
	Neoplasia
	Ischaemia
	Irritable bowel syndrome
		Pancreatic
		    Chronic pancreatitis
		    Cancer of pancreas
		    Cystic fibrosis
		Enteropathy
		    Coeliac disease
		    Tropical sprue
		    Lymphoma
		    Lymphangiectasia
			VIPoma
			Drug-induced
			    NSAIDs
			    Aminosalicylates
			    Selective serotonin re-uptake inhibitors (SSRIs)

Investigations	Colonoscopy with biopsies	Ultrasound, CT and MRCP Small bowel biopsy Barium follow-through	Stool volume Gut hormone profile Barium follow-through

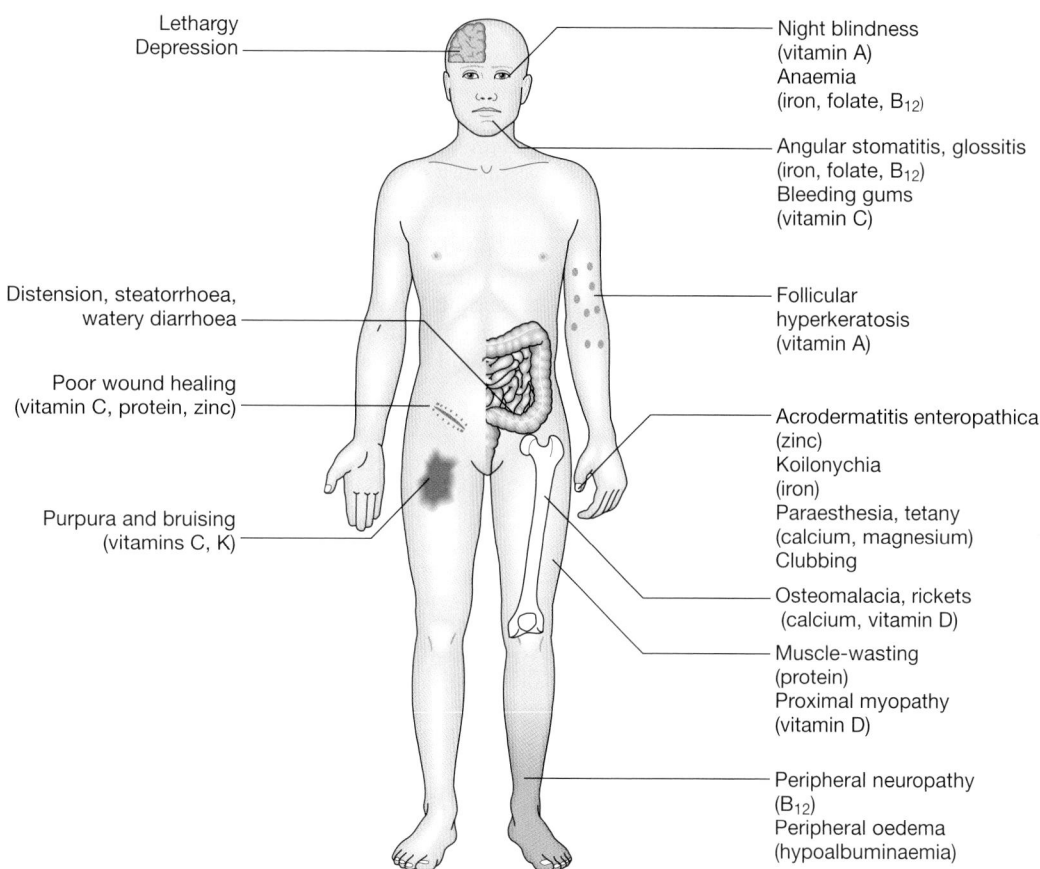

Lethargy
Depression

Night blindness
(vitamin A)
Anaemia
(iron, folate, B$_{12}$)

Angular stomatitis, glossitis
(iron, folate, B$_{12}$)
Bleeding gums
(vitamin C)

Distension, steatorrhoea,
watery diarrhoea

Follicular
hyperkeratosis
(vitamin A)

Poor wound healing
(vitamin C, protein, zinc)

Acrodermatitis enteropathica
(zinc)
Koilonychia
(iron)
Paraesthesia, tetany
(calcium, magnesium)
Clubbing

Purpura and bruising
(vitamins C, K)

Osteomalacia, rickets
(calcium, vitamin D)

Muscle-wasting
(protein)
Proximal myopathy
(vitamin D)

Peripheral neuropathy
(B$_{12}$)
Peripheral oedema
(hypoalbuminaemia)

Fig. 22.22 Possible physical consequences of malabsorption.

Pathophysiology

Malabsorption results from abnormalities of the three processes which are essential to normal digestion:

1. *Intraluminal maldigestion* occurs when deficiency of bile or pancreatic enzymes results in inadequate solubilisation and hydrolysis of nutrients. Fat and protein malabsorption results. This may also occur in the presence of small bowel bacterial overgrowth.
2. *Mucosal malabsorption* results from small bowel resection or conditions which damage the small intestinal epithelium, thereby diminishing the surface area for absorption and depleting brush border enzyme activity.
3. *'Postmucosal' lymphatic obstruction* prevents the uptake and transport of absorbed lipids into lymphatic vessels. Increased pressure in these vessels results in leakage into the intestinal lumen, leading to protein-losing enteropathy.

Investigations

Investigations are performed to confirm that malabsorption is present and then to determine the cause. Routine blood tests may show one or more of the abnormalities listed in Box 22.22. Tests to confirm fat and protein malabsorption are performed as described on page 850. An approach to the investigation of malabsorption is shown in Figure 22.23.

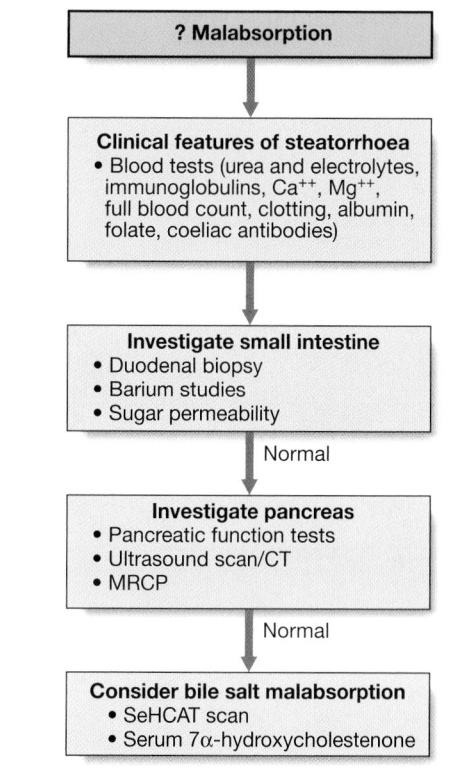

? Malabsorption

Clinical features of steatorrhoea
• Blood tests (urea and electrolytes, immunoglobulins, Ca^{++}, Mg^{++}, full blood count, clotting, albumin, folate, coeliac antibodies)

Investigate small intestine
• Duodenal biopsy
• Barium studies
• Sugar permeability

Normal

Investigate pancreas
• Pancreatic function tests
• Ultrasound scan/CT
• MRCP

Normal

Consider bile salt malabsorption
• SeHCAT scan
• Serum 7α-hydroxycholestenone

Fig. 22.23 Investigation for suspected malabsorption.

22

22.22 Routine blood test abnormalities in malabsorption
Haematology
• Microcytic anaemia (iron deficiency)
• Macrocytic anaemia (folate or B_{12} deficiency)
• Increased prothrombin time (vitamin K deficiency)
Biochemistry
• Hypoalbuminaemia
• Hypocalcaemia (p. 765)
• Hypomagnesaemia
• Deficiencies of phosphate, zinc

Weight loss

Weight loss may be 'physiological' due to dieting, exercise, starvation, or the decreased nutritional intake which accompanies old age. Alternatively, weight loss may signify disease and in this case a loss of more than 3 kg over 6 months is significant. Hospital and general practice weight records may be valuable in confirming that weight loss has occurred, as may reweighing patients at intervals; sometimes weight is regained or stabilises in those with no obvious cause. Pathological weight loss can be due to psychiatric illness, systemic disease, gastrointestinal causes or advanced disease of many organ systems (Fig. 22.24).

Physiological

Weight loss can occur in the absence of serious disease in healthy individuals who have changes in physical activity or social circumstances. It may be difficult to be sure of this diagnosis in older patients when the dietary history may be unreliable and professional help from a dietitian is often valuable under these circumstances.

Psychiatric illness

Features of anorexia nervosa (p. 249), bulimia (p. 250) and affective disorders (p. 250) may only be apparent after formal psychiatric input. Alcoholic patients lose weight as a consequence of self-neglect and poor dietary intake. Depression may cause weight loss.

Systemic diseases

Chronic infections, including tuberculosis (p. 688), recurrent urinary or chest infections, and a range of parasitic and protozoan infections (Ch. 13), should be considered. A history of foreign travel, high-risk activities and specific features such as fever, night sweats, rigors, productive cough and dysuria must be sought. Promiscuous sexual activity and drug misuse suggest HIV-related illness (Ch. 14). Weight loss is a late feature of disseminated malignancy but by the time the patient presents other features of cancer are often present.

Gastrointestinal disease

Almost any disease of the gastrointestinal tract can cause weight loss. Dysphagia and gastric outflow

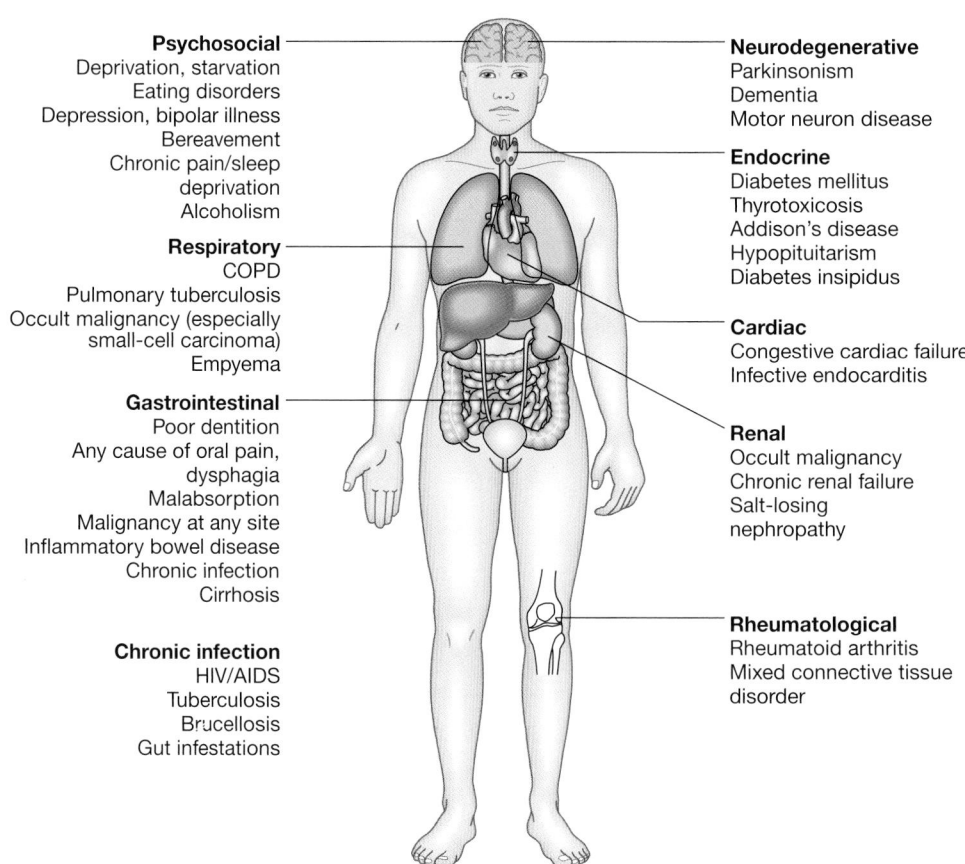

Fig. 22.24 Some important causes of weight loss.

22.23 Some easily overlooked causes of unexplained weight loss

- Depression/anxiety
- Chronic pain or sleep deprivation
- Psychosocial deprivation/malnutrition in the elderly
- Existing conditions (severe chronic obstructive pulmonary disease, cardiac failure)
- Diabetes mellitus/hyperthyroidism
- Occult malignancy (e.g. proximal colon, renal, lymphoma)
- Anorexia nervosa in atypical groups, e.g. young men
- Rare endocrine disorders, e.g. Addison's disease, panhypopituitarism

22.24 Causes of constipation

Gastrointestinal disorders

Dietary
- Lack of fibre and/or fluid intake

Motility
- Slow-transit constipation (p. 913)
- Irritable bowel syndrome
- Drugs (see below)
- Chronic intestinal pseudo-obstruction

Structural
- Colonic carcinoma
- Diverticular disease
- Hirschsprung's disease

Defecation
- Obstructed defecation (p. 913)
- Anorectal disease (Crohn's, fissures, haemorrhoids)

Non-gastrointestinal disorders

Drugs
- Opiates
- Anticholinergics
- Calcium antagonists
- Iron supplements
- Aluminium-containing antacids

Neurological
- Multiple sclerosis
- Spinal cord lesions
- Cerebrovascular accidents
- Parkinsonism

Metabolic/endocrine
- Diabetes mellitus
- Hypercalcaemia
- Hypothyroidism
- Pregnancy

Others
- Any serious illness with immobility, especially in the elderly
- Depression

obstruction (pp. 851 and 874) cause defective dietary intake. Malignancy at any site may cause weight loss by mechanical obstruction, anorexia or cytokine-mediated systemic effects. Malabsorption from pancreatic diseases (p. 888) or small bowel causes may lead to profound weight loss with specific nutritional deficiencies (Ch. 5). Inflammatory diseases such as Crohn's disease or ulcerative colitis (p. 895) cause anorexia, fear of eating and loss of protein, blood and nutrients from the gut.

Metabolic disorders and miscellaneous causes

Weight loss may occur in association with metabolic disorders as well as end-stage respiratory and cardiac disease. Some easily overlooked causes of weight loss are listed in Box 22.23.

Investigations

In cases where the cause of weight loss is not obvious after thorough history-taking and physical examination, or where it is considered that an existing condition is unlikely, the following investigations are indicated: urinalysis for sugar, protein and blood; blood tests including liver function tests, random blood glucose, and thyroid function tests; and ESR (may be raised in unsuspected infections such as tuberculosis, connective tissue disorders and malignancy). Sometimes invasive tests such as bone marrow aspiration or liver biopsy may be necessary to identify conditions like cryptic miliary tuberculosis (p. 689). Rarely, abdominal and pelvic imaging by CT may be necessary, but before embarking on invasive or very costly investigations it is always worth revisiting the patient's history and reweighing at intervals.

Constipation

Constipation is defined as infrequent passage of hard stools. Patients may also complain of straining, a sensation of incomplete evacuation and either perianal or abdominal discomfort. Constipation may be the end result of many gastrointestinal and other medical disorders (Box 22.24).

Clinical assessment and management

The onset, duration and characteristics are important; for example, a neonatal onset suggests Hirschsprung's disease, while a recent change in bowel activity in middle age should raise the suspicion of organic disorders such as colonic carcinoma. The presence of symptoms such as rectal bleeding, pain and weight loss is important, as are excessive straining, symptoms suggestive of irritable bowel syndrome, a history of childhood constipation and emotional distress.

Careful examination contributes more to the diagnosis than extensive investigation. A search should be made for general medical disorders as well as signs of intestinal obstruction. Neurological disorders, especially spinal cord lesions, should be sought. Perineal inspection and rectal examination are essential and may reveal abnormalities of the pelvic floor (e.g. abnormal descent, impaired sensation), anal canal or rectum (masses, faecal impaction, prolapse).

It is neither possible nor appropriate to investigate every person with this very common complaint. Most will respond to dietary fibre supplementation and the judicious use of laxatives. Middle-aged or elderly patients with a short history or worrying symptoms (rectal bleeding, pain or weight loss) must be investigated promptly, by either barium enema or colonoscopy. For those with simple constipation, investigation will usually proceed along the following lines.

Initial visit

Digital rectal examination, proctoscopy and sigmoidoscopy (to detect anorectal disease), routine biochemistry, including serum calcium and thyroid function tests, and

22

a full blood count should be carried out. If these are normal, a 1-month trial of dietary fibre and/or laxatives is justified.

Next visit

If symptoms persist, then examination of the colon by barium enema or colonoscopy is indicated to look for structural disease.

Further investigation

If no cause is found and disabling symptoms are present, then specialist referral for investigation of possible dysmotility may be necessary. The problem may be one of infrequent desire to defecate ('slow transit') or else may result from excessive straining ('obstructed defecation', p. 913). Intestinal marker studies, anorectal manometry, electrophysiological studies and defecating proctography can all be used to define the problem.

Abdominal pain

There are four types of abdominal pain:
- *Visceral.* Gut organs are insensitive to stimuli such as burning and cutting but are sensitive to distension, contraction, twisting and stretching. Pain from unpaired structures is usually but not always felt in the midline.
- *Parietal.* The parietal peritoneum is innervated by somatic nerves, and its involvement by inflammation, infection or neoplasia causes sharp, well-localised and lateralised pain.
- *Referred pain.* (For example, gallbladder pain is referred to the back or shoulder tip.)
- *Psychogenic.* Cultural, emotional and psychosocial factors influence everyone's experience of pain. In some patients, no organic cause can be found despite investigation, and psychogenic causes (depression or somatisation disorder) may be responsible (pp. 242 and 250).

The acute abdomen

This accounts for approximately 50% of all urgent admissions to general surgical units. The acute abdomen is a consequence of one or more pathological processes (Box 22.25):

22.25 Causes of acute abdominal pain

Inflammation

• Appendicitis	• Pancreatitis
• Diverticulitis	• Pyelonephritis
• Cholecystitis	• Intra-abdominal abscess
• Pelvic inflammatory disease	

Perforation/rupture

• Peptic ulcer	• Ovarian cyst
• Diverticular disease	• Aortic aneurysm

Obstruction

• Intestinal obstruction	• Ureteric colic
• Biliary colic	

Other (rare)

• See 'extraintestinal' causes (see Box 22.28)

- *Inflammation.* Pain develops gradually, usually over several hours. It is initially rather diffuse until the parietal peritoneum is involved, when it becomes localised. Movement exacerbates the pain; abdominal rigidity and guarding occur.
- *Perforation.* When a viscus perforates, pain starts abruptly; it is severe and leads to generalised peritonitis.
- *Obstruction.* Pain is colicky, with spasms which cause the patient to writhe around and double up. Colicky pain which does not disappear between spasms suggests complicating inflammation.

Initial clinical assessment

If there are signs of peritonitis (guarding and rebound tenderness with rigidity), adequate resuscitation should be arranged. In other circumstances further investigations are required (Fig. 22.25).

Investigations

Patients should have a full blood count, urea and electrolytes, and amylase taken to look for evidence of dehydration, leucocytosis and pancreatitis. An erect chest X-ray may show air under the diaphragm suggestive of perforation and a plain abdominal film may show evidence of obstruction. An abdominal ultrasound may help if gallstones or renal stones are suspected. Ultrasonography is also useful in the detection of free fluid and any possible intra-abdominal abscess. Contrast studies, by either mouth or anus, are useful in the further evaluation of intestinal obstruction, and essential in the differentiation of pseudo-obstruction from mechanical large bowel obstruction. Other investigations commonly used include CT (seeking evidence of pancreatitis, retroperitoneal collections or masses, including an aortic aneurysm) and angiography (mesenteric ischaemia).

Diagnostic laparotomy should be considered when the diagnosis has not been revealed by other investigations. All patients must be carefully and regularly reassessed (every 2–4 hours) so that any change in condition which might alter both the suspected diagnosis and clinical decision can be observed and acted upon early.

Management

In general, and depending on the organ affected, perforations are closed, inflammatory conditions are treated with antibiotics or resection, and obstructions are relieved. The speed of intervention and the necessity for surgery depend on a number of factors, of which the presence or absence of peritonitis is the most important. A treatment summary of some of the more common surgical conditions follows.

Acute appendicitis

Although non-operative treatment can be successful in some patients, the risk of perforation and subsequent recurrent attacks dictates that early surgery is undertaken. The appendix can be removed through a conventional right iliac fossa skin crease incision or by laparoscopic techniques.

Acute cholecystitis

This can be successfully treated non-operatively but the high risk of recurrent attacks and the low morbidity of surgery have made early laparoscopic cholecystectomy the treatment of choice.

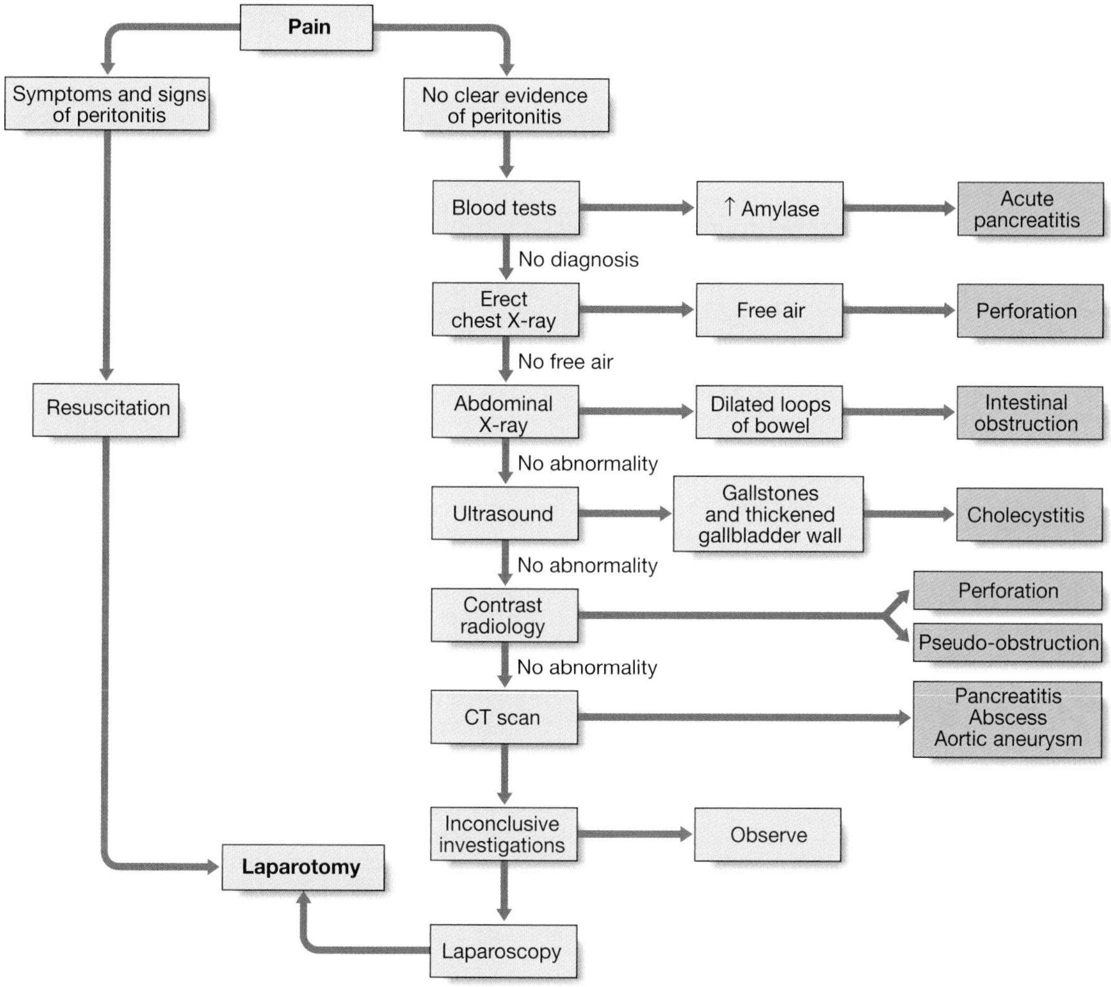

```
                           ┌──────────────┐
                    ┌──────│     Pain     │──────┐
                    │      └──────────────┘      │
                    ▼                            ▼
        ┌──────────────────┐         ┌──────────────────┐
        │ Symptoms and signs│         │ No clear evidence │
        │   of peritonitis  │         │   of peritonitis  │
        └──────────────────┘         └──────────────────┘
                    │                            │
                    │                            ▼
                    │                 ┌──────────────┐      ┌──────────────┐      ┌──────────────┐
                    │                 │  Blood tests │─────▶│  ↑ Amylase   │─────▶│     Acute    │
                    │                 └──────────────┘      └──────────────┘      │  pancreatitis │
                    │                        │ No diagnosis                       └──────────────┘
                    ▼                        ▼
        ┌──────────────────┐       ┌──────────────┐      ┌──────────────┐      ┌──────────────┐
        │   Resuscitation  │       │    Erect     │─────▶│   Free air   │─────▶│  Perforation │
        └──────────────────┘       │ chest X-ray  │      └──────────────┘      └──────────────┘
                    │              └──────────────┘
                    │                    │ No free air
                    │                    ▼
                    │              ┌──────────────┐      ┌──────────────┐      ┌──────────────┐
                    │              │  Abdominal   │─────▶│ Dilated loops│─────▶│   Intestinal │
                    │              │    X-ray     │      │   of bowel   │      │  obstruction │
                    │              └──────────────┘      └──────────────┘      └──────────────┘
                    │                    │ No abnormality
                    │                    ▼              ┌──────────────┐
                    │              ┌──────────────┐     │  Gallstones  │      ┌──────────────┐
                    │              │  Ultrasound  │────▶│ and thickened│─────▶│ Cholecystitis│
                    │              └──────────────┘     │gallbladder wall│    └──────────────┘
                    │                    │ No abnormality└──────────────┘
                    │                    ▼                           ┌──────────────┐
                    │              ┌──────────────┐                  │  Perforation │
                    │              │   Contrast   │──────────────────┤──────────────┤
                    │              │   radiology  │                  │Pseudo-obstruction│
                    │              └──────────────┘                  └──────────────┘
                    │                    │ No abnormality
                    │                    ▼                           ┌──────────────┐
                    │              ┌──────────────┐                  │  Pancreatitis│
                    │              │   CT scan    │─────────────────▶│   Abscess    │
                    │              └──────────────┘                  │Aortic aneurysm│
                    │                    │                           └──────────────┘
                    │                    ▼
                    │              ┌──────────────┐      ┌──────────────┐
                    │              │ Inconclusive │─────▶│   Observe    │
                    │              │investigations│      └──────────────┘
                    │              └──────────────┘
                    │                    │
              ┌──────────────┐           ▼
              │  Laparotomy  │◀──── ┌──────────────┐
              └──────────────┘      │  Laparoscopy │
                                    └──────────────┘
```

Fig. 22.25 Management of abdominal pain: an algorithm.

Acute diverticulitis

Conservative therapy is usually recommended, but if perforation has occurred, resection is advisable. Depending on peritoneal contamination and the state of the patient, primary anastomosis is preferable to a Hartmann's procedure (oversew of rectal stump and end colostomy).

22.26 Acute abdominal pain in old age

- **Presentation:** severity and localisation may blunt with age. Presentation may be atypical, even with perforation of a viscus.
- **Cancer:** a more common cause of acute pain in those over 70 years than in those under 50 years. Older people with vague abdominal symptoms should therefore be carefully assessed.
- **Non-specific symptoms:** intra-abdominal inflammatory conditions such as diverticulitis may present with non-specific symptoms such as acute confusion or anorexia and relatively little abdominal tenderness. The reasons for this are not clear but may result from altered sensory perception.
- **Outcome of abdominal surgery:** determined by the degree of comorbid disease and whether surgery is elective or emergency, rather than by chronological age.

Small bowel obstruction

If the cause is obvious and surgery inevitable (e.g. for an external hernia) an early operation is appropriate. If the suspected cause is adhesions from previous surgery, only those patients who do not resolve within the first 48 hours or who develop signs of strangulation (colicky pain becomes constant, peritonitis, tachycardia, fever, leucocytosis) will require surgery.

Large bowel obstruction

Pseudo-obstruction is treated non-operatively. Some patients benefit from colonoscopic decompression, but mechanical obstruction merits surgical resection, usually with primary anastomosis. Differentiation between the two is made by a water-soluble contrast enema.

Perforated peptic ulcer

Although surgical closure of the perforation is standard practice, some patients without generalised peritonitis in whom a water-soluble contrast meal has confirmed spontaneous sealing of the perforation can be treated non-operatively. Adequate and aggressive resuscitation is mandatory before surgery.

For a more detailed discussion of acute abdominal pain the reader is referred to the sister volume of this text, *Principles and Practice of Surgery.*

Chronic or recurrent abdominal pain

A detailed history, with particular attention to the features of the pain and any associated symptoms (Boxes 22.27 and 22.28), is essential.

Note should be made of the patient's general demeanour, mood and emotional state, signs of weight loss, fever, jaundice or anaemia. If a thorough abdominal and rectal examination is normal, a careful search should be made for evidence of disease affecting other structures, particularly the vertebral column, spinal cord, lungs and cardiovascular system.

Investigations will depend to a large extent on the clinical features elicited during the history and examination:

- Endoscopy and ultrasound are indicated for epigastric pain, and for dyspepsia and symptoms suggestive of gallbladder disease

- Colonoscopy is indicated for patients with altered bowel habit, rectal bleeding or features of obstruction suggesting colonic disease.
- Angiography should be considered when pain is provoked by food in a patient with widespread atherosclerosis since this may indicate mesenteric ischaemia.
- Persistent symptoms require exclusion of colonic or small bowel disease. However, young patients with pain relieved by defecation, bloating and alternating bowel habit are likely to have irritable bowel syndrome (p. 904). Simple investigations (blood tests, faecal calprotectin and sigmoidoscopy) are sufficient in the absence of rectal bleeding, weight loss and abnormal physical findings.
- Ultrasound, CT and faecal elastase are required for patients with upper abdominal pain radiating to the back. A history of alcohol misuse, weight loss and diarrhoea suggest chronic pancreatitis or pancreatic cancer.
- Recurrent attacks of pain in the loins radiating to the flanks with urinary symptoms should prompt investigation for renal or ureteric stones by abdominal X-ray, ultrasound and intravenous urography.
- A past history of psychiatric disturbance, repeated negative investigations or vague symptoms which do not fit any particular disease or organ pattern suggest a psychological origin for the patient's pain (p. 238). Careful review of case notes and previous investigations, along with open and honest discussion with the patient, reduces the need for further cycles of unnecessary and invasive tests. Care must always be taken, however, not to miss rare pathology or atypical presentations of common diseases.

Constant abdominal pain

Patients with chronic pain which is constant or nearly always present will usually have features to suggest the underlying diagnosis. In a minority no cause will be found despite thorough investigation, leading to the diagnosis of 'chronic functional abdominal pain'. In these patients a psychological cause is highly likely (p. 238) and the most important tasks are to provide symptom control, if not relief, and to minimise the effects of the pain on social, personal and occupational life. Patients are best managed in specialised pain clinics where, in addition to psychological support, appropriate use of drugs including amitriptyline, gabapentin, ketamine and opioids may be necessary.

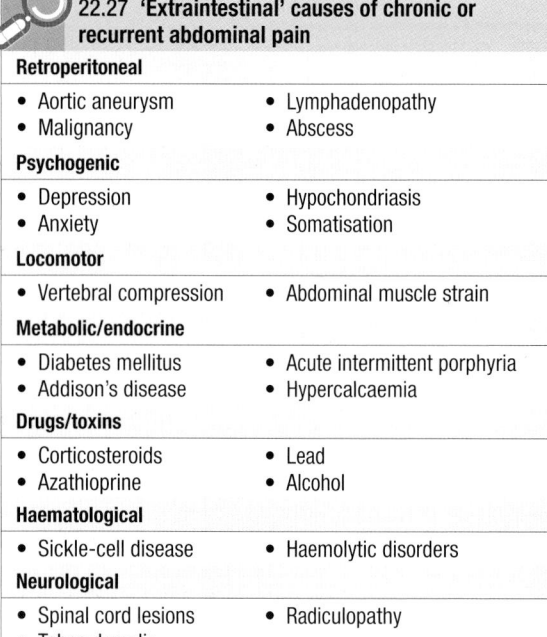

22.27 'Extraintestinal' causes of chronic or recurrent abdominal pain

Retroperitoneal

- Aortic aneurysm	- Lymphadenopathy
- Malignancy	- Abscess

Psychogenic

- Depression	- Hypochondriasis
- Anxiety	- Somatisation

Locomotor

- Vertebral compression	- Abdominal muscle strain

Metabolic/endocrine

- Diabetes mellitus	- Acute intermittent porphyria
- Addison's disease	- Hypercalcaemia

Drugs/toxins

- Corticosteroids	- Lead
- Azathioprine	- Alcohol

Haematological

- Sickle-cell disease	- Haemolytic disorders

Neurological

- Spinal cord lesions	- Radiculopathy
- Tabes dorsalis	

22.28 How to assess abdominal pain

- Duration
- Site and radiation
- Severity
- Precipitating and relieving factors (food, drugs, alcohol, posture, movement, defecation)
- Nature (colicky, constant, sharp or dull, wakes patient at night)
- Pattern (intermittent or continuous)
- Associated features (vomiting, dyspepsia, altered bowel habit)

DISEASES OF THE MOUTH AND SALIVARY GLANDS

Aphthous ulceration

Aphthous ulcers are superficial and painful; they occur in any part of the mouth. Recurrent ulcers afflict up to 30% of the population and are particularly common in women prior to menstruation. The cause is unknown, but in severe cases other causes of oral ulceration must be considered (Box 22.29). Occasionally, biopsy is necessary for diagnosis.

22.29 Causes of oral ulceration

Aphthous

- Idiopathic
- Premenstrual

Infection

- Fungal, e.g. candidiasis
- Viral, e.g. herpes simplex
- Bacterial, including syphilis

Gastrointestinal diseases

- Crohn's disease
- Coeliac disease

Dermatological conditions

- Lichen planus
- Pemphigoid
- Pemphigus

Drugs

- Hypersensitivity, e.g. Stevens–Johnson syndrome (p. 1285)
- Cytotoxic drugs

Systemic diseases

- Systemic lupus erythematosus (SLE, p. 1107)
- Behçet's syndrome (p. 1114)

Neoplasia

- Carcinoma
- Leukaemia
- Kaposi's sarcoma

Management is with topical corticosteroids (such as 0.1% triamcinolone in Orabase) or choline salicylate (8.7%) gel. Symptomatic relief is achieved using local anaesthetic mouthwashes. Rarely, patients with very severe, recurrent aphthous ulcers may need oral corticosteroids.

Oral cancer

Squamous carcinoma of the oral cavity is common world-wide and the incidence has increased by 19% since the mid-1990s in the UK. The mortality rate is around 50%, largely as a result of late diagnosis. Poor diet, alcohol excess and smoking or tobacco chewing are the main risk factors. In parts of Asia the disease is common among people who chew areca nuts wrapped in leaves of the betel plant ('betel nuts'). Oral cancer may present in many ways (Box 22.30) and a high index of suspicion is required. Patients with suspicious lesions should have all possible sources of local trauma or infection treated and be reviewed after 2 weeks. If the lesion persists, biopsy is advisable. Small cancers can be resected but extensive surgery with neck dissection to remove involved lymph nodes may be necessary. Some patients can be treated with radical radiotherapy alone, and radiotherapy is sometimes also given after surgery to treat microscopic residual disease. Some tumours may be amenable to photodynamic therapy (PDT), avoiding the need for surgery.

22.30 Symptoms and signs of oral cancer

- Solitary ulcer without precipitant, e.g. local trauma
- Solitary white patch ('leukoplakia') which fails to wipe off
- Solitary red patch
- Fixed lump
- Lip numbness in absence of trauma or infection
- Trismus (painful/difficult mouth opening)
- Cervical lymphadenopathy

Candidiasis

The yeast *Candida albicans* is a normal mouth commensal but it may proliferate to cause thrush. This occurs in babies, debilitated patients, patients receiving corticosteroid or antibiotic therapy, patients with diabetes and immunosuppressed patients, especially those receiving cytotoxic therapy and those with AIDS. White patches are seen on the tongue and buccal mucosa. Odynophagia or dysphagia suggests pharyngeal and oesophageal candidiasis. A clinical diagnosis is sufficient to instigate therapy, although brushings or biopsies can be obtained for mycological examination. Oral thrush is treated using nystatin or amphotericin suspensions or lozenges. Resistant cases or immunosuppressed patients may require oral fluconazole.

Parotitis

Parotitis is due to viral or bacterial infection. Mumps causes a self-limiting acute parotitis (p. 315). Bacterial parotitis usually occurs as a complication of major surgery. It is a consequence of dehydration and poor oral hygiene, and can be avoided by good post-operative care. Patients present with painful parotid swelling and this can be complicated by abscess formation. Broad-spectrum antibiotics are required, whilst surgical drainage is necessary for abscesses. Other causes of salivary gland enlargement are listed in Box 22.31.

22

22.31 Causes of salivary gland swelling

- Infection
  Mumps
  Bacterial (post-operative)
- Calculi
- Sjögren's syndrome (p. 1111)
- Sarcoidosis
- Tumours
  Benign: pleomorphic adenoma (95% of cases)
  Intermediate: mucoepidermoid tumour
  Malignant: carcinoma

22.32 Oral health in old age

- **Dry mouth:** affects around 40% of healthy older people.
- **Gustatory and olfactory sensation:** declines and chewing power is diminished.
- **Salivation:** baseline salivary flow falls but stimulated salivation is unchanged.
- **Root caries and periodontal disease:** common partly because oral hygiene deteriorates with increasing frailty.
- **Bacteraemia and septicaemia:** may complicate Gram-negative anaerobic infection in the periodontal pockets of the very frail.

DISEASES OF THE OESOPHAGUS

Gastro-oesophageal reflux disease

Gastro-oesophageal reflux resulting in heartburn affects approximately 30% of the general population.

Pathophysiology

Occasional episodes of gastro-oesophageal reflux are common in health. Reflux is normally followed by oesophageal peristaltic waves which efficiently clear

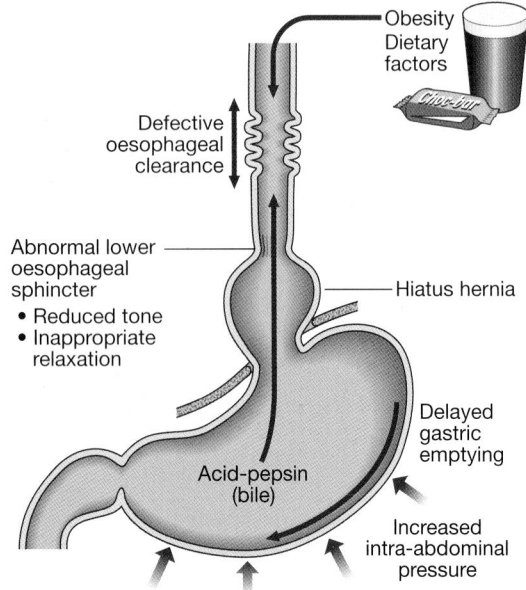

Fig. 22.26 Factors associated with the development of gastro-oesophageal reflux disease.

┌───┐
i │ **22.33 Important features of hiatus hernia**

- Herniation of the stomach through the diaphragm into the chest
- Occurs in 30% of the population over the age of 50 years
- Often asymptomatic
- Heartburn and regurgitation can occur
- Gastric volvulus may complicate large para-oesophageal hernias
└───┘

the gullet, alkaline saliva neutralises residual acid, and symptoms do not occur. Gastro-oesophageal reflux disease develops when the oesophageal mucosa is exposed to gastroduodenal contents for prolonged periods of time, resulting in symptoms and, in a proportion of cases, oesophagitis. Several factors are known to be involved (Fig. 22.26).

Abnormalities of the lower oesophageal sphincter

In health, the lower oesophageal sphincter is tonically contracted, relaxing only during swallowing (p. 838).

Some patients with gastro-oesophageal reflux disease have reduced lower oesophageal sphincter tone, permitting reflux when intra-abdominal pressure rises. In others, basal sphincter tone is normal but reflux occurs in response to frequent episodes of inappropriate sphincter relaxation.

Hiatus hernia

Hiatus hernia (Box 22.33 and Fig. 22.27) causes reflux because the pressure gradient between the abdominal and thoracic cavities, which normally pinches the hiatus,

is lost. In addition, the oblique angle between the cardia and oesophagus disappears. Many patients who have large hiatus hernias develop reflux symptoms, but the relationship between the presence of a hernia and symptoms is poor. Hiatus hernia is very common in individuals who have no symptoms, and some symptomatic patients have only a very small or no hernia. Nevertheless, almost all patients who develop oesophagitis, Barrett's oesophagus or peptic strictures have a hiatus hernia.

Delayed oesophageal clearance

Defective oesophageal peristaltic activity is commonly found in patients who have oesophagitis. It is a primary abnormality, since it persists after oesophagitis has been healed by acid-suppressing drug therapy. Poor oesophageal clearance leads to increased acid exposure time.

Gastric contents

Gastric acid is the most important oesophageal irritant and there is a close relationship between acid exposure time and symptoms.

Defective gastric emptying

Gastric emptying is delayed in patients with gastro-oesophageal reflux disease. The reason for this is unknown.

Increased intra-abdominal pressure

Pregnancy and obesity are established predisposing causes. Weight loss may improve symptoms.

Dietary and environmental factors

Dietary fat, chocolate, alcohol and coffee relax the lower oesophageal sphincter and may provoke symptoms.

Patient factors

Visceral sensitivity and patient vigilance play a role in determining symptom severity and consulting behaviour in individual patients.

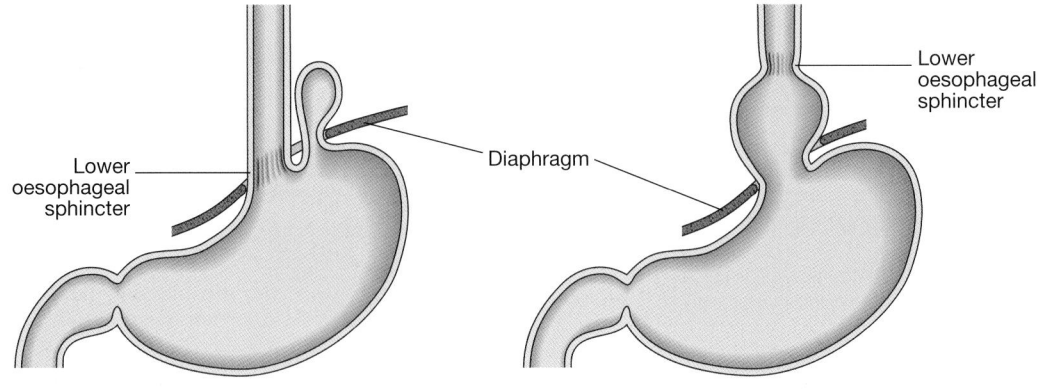

Fig. 22.27 Types of hiatus hernia.

Clinical features

The major symptoms are heartburn and regurgitation, often provoked by bending, straining or lying down. 'Waterbrash', which is salivation due to reflex salivary gland stimulation as acid enters the gullet, is often present. The patient is often overweight. Some patients are woken at night by choking as refluxed fluid irritates the larynx. Others develop odynophagia or dysphagia. A variety of 'extra-oesophageal' features have been described such as atypical chest pain which may be severe, can mimic angina and may be due to reflux-induced oesophageal spasm. Others include so-called 'acid laryngitis', recurrent chest infections, chronic cough and asthma (Box 22.34). The true relationship of these to gastro-oesophageal reflux disease remains unclear.

Complications

Oesophagitis

A range of endoscopic findings, from mild redness to severe, bleeding ulceration with stricture formation, are recognised, although appearances may be completely normal (Fig. 22.28). There is a poor correlation between symptoms and histological and endoscopic findings.

Barrett's oesophagus

Barrett's oesophagus is a pre-malignant condition in which the normal squamous lining of the lower oesophagus is replaced by columnar mucosa (columnar lined oesophagus; CLO) containing areas of intestinal metaplasia (Fig. 22.29). It occurs as an adaptive

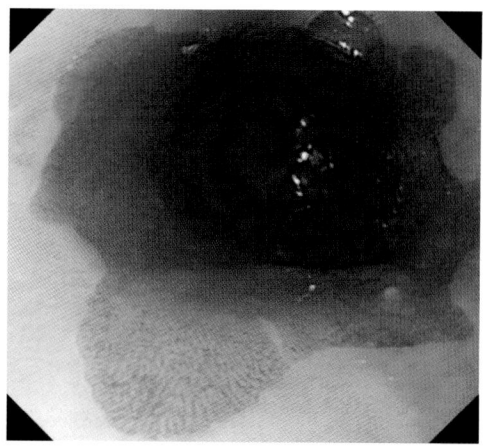

Fig. 22.29 Barrett's oesophagus. Pink columnar mucosa is seen extending upwards above the oesophago-gastric junction.

response to chronic gastro-oesophageal reflux and is found in 10% of patients undergoing gastroscopy for reflux symptoms. Community-based epidemiological and autopsy studies suggest the true prevalence may be up to 20 times greater, as the condition is often asymptomatic until first discovered when the patient presents with oesophageal cancer. CLO is a major risk factor for oesophageal adenocarcinoma, with a lifetime cancer risk of around 10%. The absolute risk is low, however, and more than 95% of patients with CLO die from causes other than oesophageal cancer. The epidemiology and aetiology of CLO are poorly understood. The prevalence is increasing, and it is more common in men (especially white) and those over 50 years of age. It is weakly associated with smoking but not alcohol. Cancer risk is more closely related to the severity and duration of reflux rather than the presence of CLO per se. Recent attention has focused on the importance of duodenogastro-oesophageal reflux, containing bile, pancreatic enzymes and pepsin in addition to acid. The molecular events underlying the progression of CLO from metaplasia to dysplasia to cancer are not well understood but E-cadherin polymorphisms, p53 mutations, transforming growth factor-β (TGF-β), epidermal growth factor (EGF) receptors, COX-2 and tumour necrosis factor-α (TNF-α) may play roles in neoplastic progression.

Diagnosis This requires multiple systematic biopsies to maximise the chance of detecting intestinal metaplasia and/or dysplasia.

Management Neither potent acid suppression nor anti-reflux surgery will stop progression or induce regression of CLO, and treatment is only indicated for symptoms of reflux or complications such as stricture. Endoscopic therapies such as argon plasma coagulation, radiofrequency ablation or photodynamic therapy can induce regression but remain experimental. Regular endoscopic surveillance can detect dysplasia and malignancy at an early stage and may improve survival but, because most CLO is undetected until cancer develops, surveillance strategies are unlikely to influence the overall mortality rate of oesophageal cancer. Surveillance is expensive and cost-effectiveness studies have been conflicting, but currently it is recommended that patients with CLO without

---

EBM 22.34 **The association between gastro-oesophageal reflux disease and asthma**

'Reflux is significantly more common in asthma patients (odds ratio 5.5) and asthma is more common in GORD patients (odds ratio 2.3), compared to controls. Evidence for the direction of causality, however, is lacking.'

• Havemann BD, et al. Gut 2007; 56:1654–1664.

For further information: 💻 www.evidbasedgastro.com

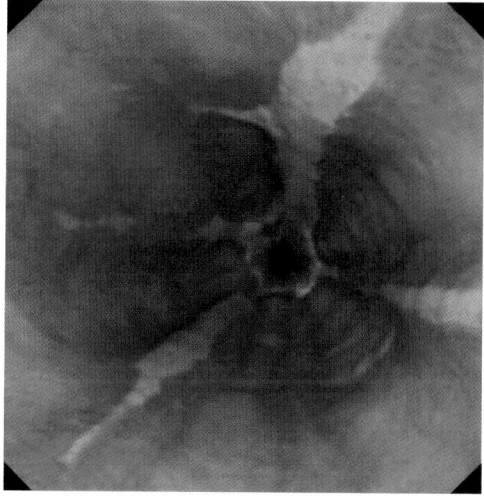

Fig. 22.28 Reflux oesophagitis. There are numerous linear streaks of superficial ulceration extending up the gullet.

dysplasia should undergo endoscopy every 2–3 years and those with low-grade dysplasia at 6–12-monthly intervals.

Oesophagectomy is widely recommended for those with high-grade dysplasia (HGD), as the resected specimen harbours cancer in up to 40%. This may be an over-estimate and recent data suggest that HGD often remains stable and may not progress to cancer, at least in the medium term. A combination of endoscopic mucosal resection (EMR) of any visibly abnormal areas and ablation of the remaining Barrett's mucosa shows promise as an 'organ-preserving' alternative to surgery.

Anaemia

Iron deficiency anaemia occurs as a consequence of chronic, insidious blood loss from long-standing oesophagitis. Most patients have a large hiatus hernia and bleeding can occur from subtle erosions in the neck of the sac ('Cameron lesions'). Nevertheless, hiatus hernia is very common and other causes of blood loss, particularly colorectal cancer, must be considered in anaemic patients, even when endoscopy reveals oesophagitis and a hiatus hernia.

Benign oesophageal stricture

Fibrous strictures develop as a consequence of long-standing oesophagitis. Most patients are elderly and have poor oesophageal peristaltic activity. They present with dysphagia which is worse for solids than for liquids. Bolus obstruction following ingestion of meat causes absolute dysphagia. A history of heartburn is common but not invariable; many elderly patients presenting with strictures have no preceding heartburn.

Diagnosis is by endoscopy, when biopsies of the stricture can be taken to exclude malignancy. Endoscopic balloon dilatation or bouginage is helpful. Subsequently, long-term therapy with a PPI drug at full dose should be started to reduce the risk of recurrent oesophagitis and stricture formation. The patient should be advised to chew food thoroughly, and it is important to ensure adequate dentition.

Gastric volvulus

Occasionally a massive intrathoracic hiatus hernia may twist upon itself, in either the organo-axial or the lateral axis, leading to a gastric volvulus. This leads to complete oesophageal or gastric obstruction and the patient presents with severe chest pain, vomiting and dysphagia. The diagnosis is made by chest X-ray (air bubble in the chest) and barium swallow. Most cases spontaneously resolve but tend to recur and surgery is usually advised after nasogastric decompression.

Investigations

Young patients who present with typical symptoms of gastro-oesophageal reflux, without worrying features such as dysphagia, weight loss or anaemia, can be treated empirically without investigation. Investigation is advisable if patients present in middle or late age, if symptoms are atypical or if a complication is suspected. Endoscopy is the investigation of choice. This is performed to exclude other upper gastrointestinal diseases which can mimic gastro-oesophageal reflux, and to identify complications. A normal endoscopy in a patient with compatible symptoms should not preclude treatment for gastro-oesophageal reflux disease.

Twenty-four-hour pH monitoring is indicated if the diagnosis is unclear or surgical intervention is under consideration. This involves tethering a slim catheter with a terminal radiotelemetry pH-sensitive probe above the gastro-oesophageal junction. The intraluminal pH is recorded whilst the patient undergoes normal activities, and episodes of pain are noted and related to pH. A pH of less than 4 for more than 6–7% of the study time is diagnostic of reflux disease. In a few patients with difficult reflux, impedance testing can detect weakly acidic or alkaline reflux that is not revealed by standard pH testing.

Management

Lifestyle advice, including weight loss, avoidance of dietary items which the patient finds worsen symptoms, elevation of the bed head in those who experience nocturnal symptoms, avoidance of late meals and giving up smoking, are recommended but rarely heeded. PPIs are the treatment of choice. Symptoms usually resolve and oesophagitis heals in the majority of patients. Recurrence of symptoms is common when therapy is stopped and some patients require life-long treatment at the lowest acceptable dose. There is no evidence that *H. pylori* eradication has any therapeutic value. Proprietary antacids and alginates also provide symptomatic benefit. H_2-receptor antagonist drugs also help symptoms without healing oesophagitis.

Patients who fail to respond to medical therapy, those who are unwilling to take long-term PPIs and those whose major symptom is severe regurgitation should be considered for laparoscopic anti-reflux surgery. Although heartburn and regurgitation are alleviated in most patients, a small minority develop complications such as inability to vomit and abdominal bloating ('gas-bloat' syndrome'). A treatment algorithm is outlined in Figure 22.30.

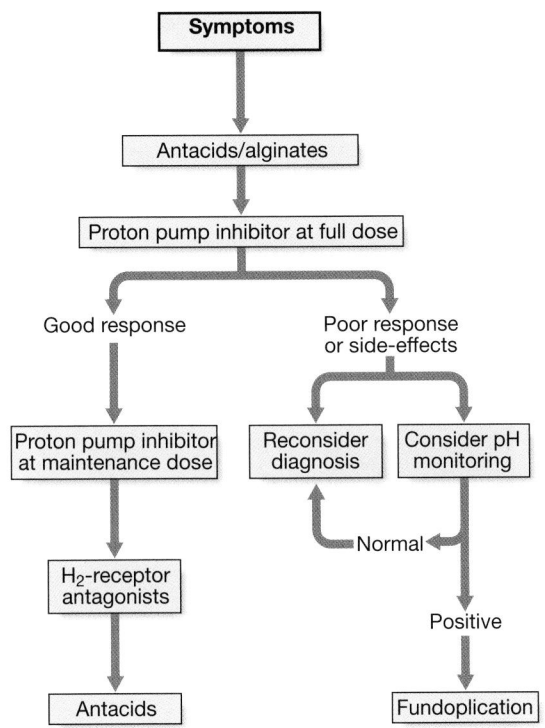

Fig. 22.30 Treatment of gastro-oesophageal reflux disease: a 'step-down' approach.

22.35 Gastro-oesophageal reflux disease in old age

- **Prevalence:** higher.
- **Severity of symptoms:** does not correlate with the degree of mucosal inflammation.
- **Complications:** late complications such as peptic strictures or bleeding from oesophagitis are more common.
- **Recurrent pneumonia:** consider aspiration from occult gastro-oesophageal reflux disease.

Other causes of oesophagitis

Infection

Oesophageal candidiasis occurs in debilitated patients and those taking broad-spectrum antibiotics or cytotoxic drugs. It is a particular problem in AIDS patients, who are also susceptible to a spectrum of other oesophageal infections (p. 393).

Corrosives

Suicide attempt by strong household bleach or battery acid is followed by painful burns of the mouth and pharynx and by extensive erosive oesophagitis. This is complicated by oesophageal perforation with mediastinitis and by stricture formation. At the time of presentation treatment is conservative, based upon analgesia and nutritional support; vomiting and endoscopy should be avoided because of the high risk of oesophageal perforation. Following the acute phase, a barium swallow should be performed to demonstrate the extent of stricture formation. Endoscopic dilatation is usually necessary, although it is difficult and hazardous because strictures are often long, tortuous and easily perforated.

Drugs

Potassium supplements and NSAIDs may cause oesophageal ulcers when the tablets are trapped above an oesophageal stricture. Liquid preparations of these drugs should be used in such patients. Bisphosphonates, especially alendronate, cause oesophageal ulceration and should be used with caution in patients with known oesophageal disorders.

Eosinophilic oesophagitis

This is more common in children but increasingly recognised in young adults. It occurs more often in atopic individuals and is characterised by eosinophilic infiltration of the oesophageal mucosa. Patients present with dysphagia more often than heartburn, and other symptoms such as chest pain and vomiting may be present. Endoscopy is usually normal although mucosal rings (that sometimes need endoscopic dilatation), strictures or a narrow-calibre oesophagus sometimes occur. Children may respond to elimination diets, but these are less successful in adults who should first be treated with PPIs. Good responses are reported with 8–12 weeks of therapy with topical corticosteroids (fluticasone or betamethasone); a metered dose inhaler is used but sprayed into the mouth and swallowed, rather than inhaled. Refractory symptoms sometimes respond to monteleukast, a leukotriene inhibitor.

Motility disorders

Pharyngeal pouch

Incoordination of swallowing within the pharynx leads to herniation through the cricopharyngeus muscle and formation of a pouch. Most patients are elderly and have no symptoms, although regurgitation, halitosis and dysphagia can occur. Some notice gurgling in the throat after swallowing. A barium swallow demonstrates the pouch and reveals incoordination of swallowing, often with pulmonary aspiration. Endoscopy may be hazardous since the instrument may enter and perforate the pouch. Surgical myotomy and resection of the pouch are indicated in symptomatic patients.

Achalasia of the oesophagus

Achalasia is a rare disease affecting 1:100000 people. It usually develops in middle life but can occur at any age.

Pathophysiology

Achalasia is characterised by:
- a hypertonic lower oesophageal sphincter which fails to relax in response to the swallowing wave
- failure of propagated oesophageal contraction, leading to progressive dilatation of the gullet.

The cause is unknown. Defective release of nitric oxide by inhibitory neurons in the lower oesophageal sphincter has been reported, and there is degeneration of ganglion cells within the sphincter and the body of the oesophagus. Loss of the dorsal vagal nuclei within the brain stem can be demonstrated in later stages. Infection with *Trypanosoma cruzi* in Chagas disease (p. 354) causes a syndrome that is clinically indistinguishable from achalasia.

Clinical features

The presentation is with dysphagia. This develops slowly, is initially intermittent, and is worse for solids and eased by drinking liquids, and by standing and moving around after eating. Heartburn does not occur because the closed oesophageal sphincter prevents gastro-oesophageal reflux. Some patients experience episodes of chest pain due to oesophageal spasm. As the disease progresses, dysphagia worsens, the oesophagus empties poorly and nocturnal pulmonary aspiration develops. Achalasia predisposes to squamous carcinoma of the oesophagus.

Investigations

Endoscopy should always be carried out because carcinoma of the cardia can mimic the presentation and radiological and manometric features of achalasia ('pseudo-achalasia'). A barium swallow shows tapered narrowing of the lower oesophagus and in late disease the oesophageal body is dilated, aperistaltic and food-filled (Fig. 22.31A). Manometry confirms the high-pressure, non-relaxing lower oesophageal sphincter with poor contractility of the oesophageal body (Fig. 22.31C).

Management

Endoscopic

Forceful pneumatic dilatation using a 30–35 mm diameter fluoroscopically positioned balloon disrupts the

22

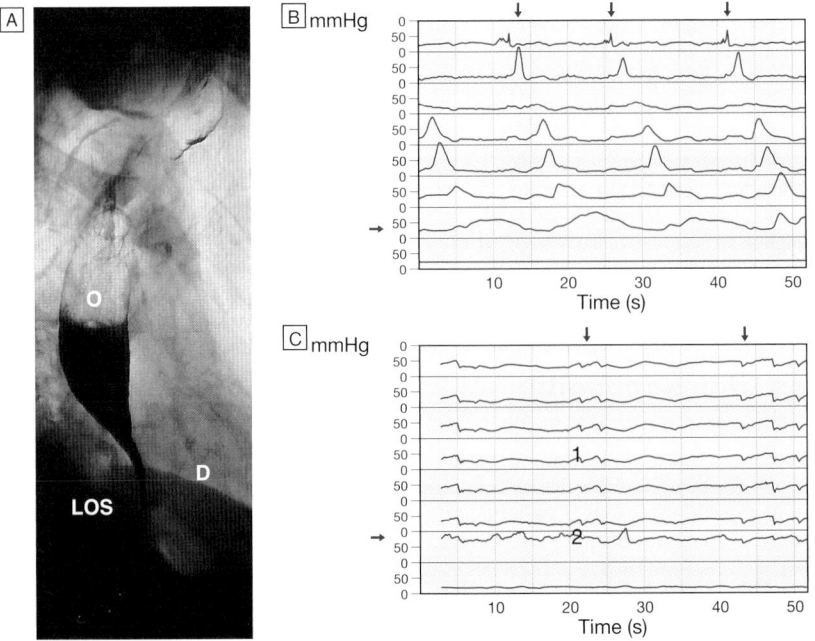

Fig. 22.31 Achalasia. [A] X-ray showing a dilated, barium-filled oesophagus (O) with fluid level and distal tapering, and a closed lower oesophageal sphincter (LOS). (D = diaphragm) [B] Normal oesophageal manometry showing propagated swallows and normal LOS pressure with relaxation on swallowing. [C] Manometry in achalasia showing non-propagated, ineffective contractions (1) and raised LOS pressure with failure of relaxation on swallowing (2). Compare with Figure 22.1, page 838.

oesophageal sphincter and improves symptoms in 80% of patients. Some patients require more than one dilatation but those requiring frequent dilatation are best treated surgically. Endoscopically directed injection of botulinum toxin into the lower oesophageal sphincter induces clinical remission, but relapse is common.

Surgical

Surgical myotomy ('Heller's operation'), performed either laparoscopically or as an open operation, is an extremely effective, although more invasive option. Both pneumatic dilatation and myotomy may be complicated by gastro-oesophageal reflux, and this can lead to severe oesophagitis because oesophageal clearance is so poor. For this reason Heller's myotomy is accompanied by a partial fundoplication anti-reflux procedure. PPI therapy is often necessary after surgery.

Other oesophageal motility disorders

Diffuse oesophageal spasm presents in late middle age with episodic chest pain which may mimic angina, but is sometimes accompanied by transient dysphagia. Some cases occur in response to gastro-oesophageal reflux. Treatment is based upon the use of PPI drugs when gastro-oesophageal reflux is present. Oral or sublingual nitrates or nifedipine may relieve attacks of pain. Drug therapy is often disappointing, as are the alternatives, pneumatic dilatation and surgical myotomy. 'Nutcracker' oesophagus is a condition in which extremely forceful peristaltic activity leads to episodic chest pain and dysphagia. Treatment is with nitrates or nifedipine. Some patients present with oesophageal motility disorders which do not fit into a specific disease entity. The patients are usually elderly and present

with dysphagia and chest pain. Manometric abnormalities ranging from poor peristalsis to spasm occur. Treatment is with dilatation and/or vasodilators for chest pain.

Secondary causes of oesophageal dysmotility

In systemic sclerosis the muscle of the oesophagus is replaced by fibrous tissue which causes failure of peristalsis leading to heartburn and dysphagia. Oesophagitis is often severe, and benign fibrous strictures occur. These patients require long-term therapy with PPIs. Dermatomyositis, rheumatoid arthritis and myasthenia gravis may also cause dysphagia.

Benign oesophageal stricture

Benign oesophageal stricture is usually a consequence of gastro-oesophageal reflux disease (Box 22.36) and occurs most often in elderly patients who have poor oesophageal clearance. Rings, due to submucosal fibrosis, occur at the

---

22.36 Causes of oesophageal stricture

- Gastro-oesophageal reflux disease
- Webs and rings
- Carcinoma of the oesophagus or cardia
- Eosinophilic oesophagitis
- Extrinsic compression from bronchial carcinoma
- Corrosive ingestion
- Post-operative scarring following oesophageal resection
- Post-radiotherapy
- Following long-term nasogastric intubation

oesophago-gastric junction ('Schatzki ring') and cause intermittent dysphagia, often starting in middle age. A post-cricoid web is a rare complication of iron deficiency anaemia (Paterson–Kelly or Plummer–Vinson syndrome), and may be complicated by the development of squamous carcinoma. Benign strictures are treated by endoscopic dilatation, in which wire-guided bougies or balloons are used to disrupt the fibrous tissue of the stricture.

Tumours of the oesophagus

Benign tumours

The most common is a gastrointestinal stromal tumour (GIST). This is usually asymptomatic but may cause bleeding or dysphagia.

Carcinoma of the oesophagus

Squamous oesophageal cancer (Box 22.37) is relatively rare in Caucasians (4/100 000), whilst in Iran, parts of Africa and China it is much more common (200 per 100 000). Squamous cancer can arise in any part of the oesophagus, and almost all tumours in the upper oesophagus are squamous cancers. Adenocarcinomas typically arise in the lower third of the oesophagus from Barrett's oesophagus or from the cardia of the stomach. The incidence is increasing and is now approximately 5:100 000 in the UK; this is possibly because of the high prevalence of gastro-oesophageal reflux and Barrett's oesophagus in Western populations. Despite modern treatment, the overall 5-year survival of patients presenting with oesophageal cancer is only 9–13%.

Clinical features

Most patients have a history of progressive, painless dysphagia for solid foods. Others present acutely because of food bolus obstruction. In late stages weight loss is often extreme; chest pain or hoarseness suggests mediastinal invasion. Fistulation between the oesophagus and the trachea or bronchial tree leads to coughing after swallowing, pneumonia and pleural effusion. Physical signs may be absent, but even at initial presentation cachexia, cervical lymphadenopathy or other evidence of metastatic spread is common.

Investigations

The investigation of choice is upper gastrointestinal endoscopy (Fig. 22.32) with cytology and biopsy. A barium swallow demonstrates the site and length of the stricture but adds little useful information. Once a diagnosis has been achieved, investigations are performed

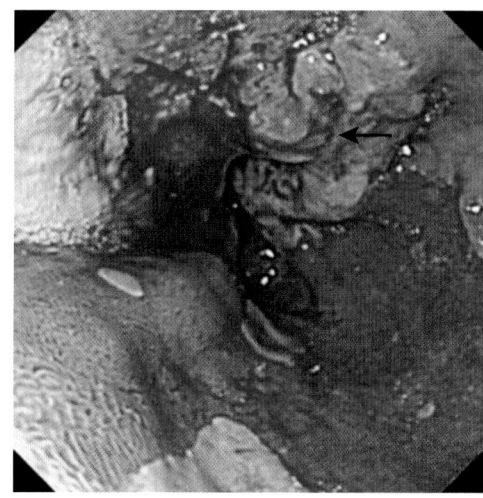

Fig. 22.32 Adenocarcinoma of the lower oesophagus. Adenocarcinoma in association with Barrett's oesophagus (arrow).

to stage the tumour and define operability. Thoracic and abdominal CT are carried out to identify metastatic spread and local invasion. Invasion of the aorta and other local structures may preclude surgery. EUS is the most sensitive method for determining depth of penetration of the tumour into the oesophageal wall and for detecting involved locoregional lymph nodes (Fig. 22.33). These investigations will define the TNM stage of the disease (Ch. 11).

Management

The treatment of choice is surgery if the patient presents at a point at which resection is possible. Tumours which have extended beyond the wall of the oesophagus and have lymph node involvement (T3,N1) are associated with a 5-year survival of around 10%. However, this figure improves significantly if the tumour is confined to the oesophageal wall and there is no spread to lymph nodes. Overall survival following 'potentially curative'

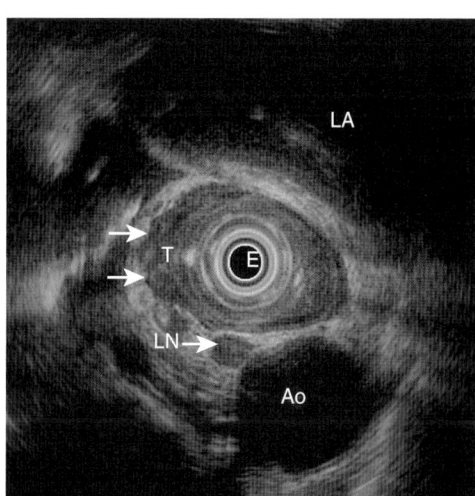

Fig. 22.33 Endoscopic ultrasound staging of oesophageal carcinoma. The tumour (T) has extended through the oesophageal wall (stage T3, arrows). A small peritumoral lymph node (LN) is also seen. (Ao = aorta; LA = left atrium; E = echoendoscope)

22.37 Squamous carcinoma: aetiological factors

- Smoking
- Alcohol excess
- Chewing betel nuts or tobacco
- Coeliac disease
- Achalasia of the oesophagus
- Post-cricoid web
- Post-caustic stricture
- Tylosis (familial hyperkeratosis of palms and soles)

surgery (all macroscopic tumour removed) is about 30% at 5 years, but recent studies have suggested that this can be improved by neoadjuvant (pre-operative) chemotherapy with agents such as cisplatin and 5-fluorouracil. Although squamous carcinomas are radiosensitive, radiotherapy alone is associated with a 5-year survival of only 5%, but combined chemoradiotherapy for these tumours can achieve 5-year survival rates of 25–30%.

Approximately 70% of patients have extensive disease at presentation; in these, treatment is palliative and based upon relief of dysphagia and pain. Endoscopic laser therapy or self-expanding metallic stents are used to improve swallowing. Palliative radiotherapy may induce shrinkage of both squamous cancers and adeno-carcinomas but symptomatic response may be slow. Quality of life can be improved by nutritional support and appropriate analgesia.

Perforation of the oesophagus

The most common cause is endoscopic perforation complicating dilatation or intubation. Malignant, corrosive or post-radiotherapy strictures are more likely to be perforated than peptic strictures. A perforated peptic stricture is usually managed conservatively using broad-spectrum antibiotics and parenteral nutrition; most heal within days. Malignant, caustic and radiotherapy stricture perforations require surgical resection or intubation.

Spontaneous oesophageal perforation ('Boerhaave's syndrome') results from forceful vomiting and retching. Severe chest pain and shock occur as oesophago-gastric contents enter the mediastinum and thoracic cavity. Subcutaneous emphysema, pleural effusions and pneumothorax develop. The diagnosis is made using a water-soluble contrast swallow, but in difficult cases both CT and careful endoscopy (usually in an intubated patient) may be required. Treatment is surgical. Delay in diagnosis is a key factor in the high mortality associated with this condition.

DISEASES OF THE STOMACH AND DUODENUM

Gastritis

Gastritis is a histological diagnosis, although it can sometimes be recognised at endoscopy.

Acute gastritis

Acute gastritis is often erosive and haemorrhagic. Neutrophils are the predominant inflammatory cell in the superficial epithelium. Many cases result from aspirin or NSAID ingestion (Box 22.38). Acute gastritis often produces no symptoms but may cause dyspepsia, anorexia, nausea or vomiting, and haematemesis or melaena. Many cases resolve quickly and do not merit investigation; in others, endoscopy and biopsy may be necessary to exclude peptic ulcer or cancer. Treatment should be directed to the underlying cause. Short-term symptomatic therapy with antacids, and acid suppression using PPIs or antiemetics (e.g. metoclopramide) may be necessary.

22.38 Common causes of gastritis
Acute gastritis (often erosive and haemorrhagic)
• Aspirin, NSAIDs
• *H. pylori* (initial infection)
• Alcohol
• Other drugs, e.g. iron preparations
• Severe physiological stress, e.g. burns, multi-organ failure, CNS trauma
• Bile reflux, e.g. following gastric surgery
• Viral infections, e.g. cytomegalovirus (CMV), herpes simplex virus in AIDS (pp. 393–394)
Chronic non-specific gastritis
• *H. pylori* infection
• Autoimmune (pernicious anaemia)
• Post-gastrectomy
Chronic 'specific' forms (rare)
• Infections, e.g. CMV, tuberculosis
• Gastrointestinal diseases, e.g. Crohn's disease
• Systemic diseases, e.g. sarcoidosis, graft-versus-host disease
• Idiopathic, e.g. granulomatous gastritis

Chronic gastritis due to *Helicobacter pylori* infection

This is the most common cause of chronic gastritis (see Box 22.38). The predominant inflammatory cells are lymphocytes and plasma cells. Correlation between symptoms and endoscopic or pathological findings is poor. Most patients are asymptomatic and do not require any treatment, but patients with dyspepsia may benefit from *H. pylori* eradication.

Autoimmune chronic gastritis

This involves the body of the stomach but spares the antrum; it results from autoimmune activity against parietal cells. The histological features are diffuse chronic inflammation, atrophy and loss of fundic glands, intestinal metaplasia and sometimes hyperplasia of enterochromaffin-like (ECL) cells. Circulating antibodies to parietal cell and intrinsic factor may be present. In some patients the degree of gastric atrophy is severe, and loss of intrinsic factor secretion leads to pernicious anaemia (p. 1021). The gastritis itself is usually asymptomatic. Some patients have evidence of other organ-specific autoimmunity, particularly thyroid disease. There is a fourfold increase in the risk of gastric cancer (see also p. 876).

Ménétrier's disease

In this rare condition the gastric pits are elongated and tortuous, with replacement of the parietal and chief cells by mucus-secreting cells. As a result, the mucosal folds of the body and fundus are greatly enlarged. Most patients are hypochlorhydric. Whilst some patients have upper gastrointestinal symptoms, the majority present in middle or old age with protein-losing enteropathy (p. 885) due to exudation from the gastric mucosa. Barium meal shows enlarged, nodular and coarse folds which are also seen at endoscopy, although biopsies may not be deep enough to show all the histological features. Treatment with antisecretory drugs may reduce protein loss but unresponsive patients require partial gastrectomy.

Peptic ulcer disease

The term 'peptic ulcer' refers to an ulcer in the lower oesophagus, stomach or duodenum, in the jejunum after surgical anastomosis to the stomach or, rarely, in the ileum adjacent to a Meckel's diverticulum. Ulcers in the stomach or duodenum may be acute or chronic; both penetrate the muscularis mucosae but the acute ulcer shows no evidence of fibrosis. Erosions do not penetrate the muscularis mucosae.

Gastric and duodenal ulcer

The prevalence of peptic ulcer is decreasing in many Western communities as a result of widespread use of *H. pylori* eradication therapy but it remains high in developing countries. The male to female ratio for duodenal ulcer varies from 5:1 to 2:1, whilst that for gastric ulcer is 2:1 or less. Chronic gastric ulcer is usually single; 90% are situated on the lesser curve within the antrum or at the junction between body and antral mucosa. Chronic duodenal ulcer usually occurs in the first part of the duodenum just distal to the junction of pyloric and duodenal mucosa; 50% are on the anterior wall. Gastric and duodenal ulcers coexist in 10% of patients and more than one peptic ulcer is found in 10–15% of patients.

Pathophysiology

H pylori

Peptic ulceration is strongly associated with *H. pylori* infection. The prevalence of *H. pylori* infection in developed nations rises steadily with age, and in the UK approximately 50% of people over the age of 50 years are infected. In many parts of the developing world infection is more common, affecting up to 90% of the adult population. These infections are probably acquired in childhood. The vast majority of colonised people remain healthy and asymptomatic and only a minority develop clinical disease. Around 90% of duodenal ulcer patients and 70% of gastric ulcer patients are infected with *H. pylori*; the remaining 30% of gastric ulcers are due to NSAIDs. *H. pylori* is Gram-negative and spiral, and has multiple flagella at one end which make it motile, allowing it to burrow and live deep beneath the mucus layer closely adherent to the epithelial surface. It uses an adhesin molecule (BabA) to bind to the Lewis b antigen on epithelial cells. Here the surface pH is close to neutral and any acidity is buffered by the organism's production of the enzyme urease. This produces ammonia from urea and raises the pH around the bacterium and between its two cell membrane layers. The bacteria spread by person-to-person contact via gastric refluxate or vomit. *H. pylori* exclusively colonises gastric-type epithelium and is only found in the duodenum in association with patches of gastric metaplasia. The bacterium stimulates chronic gastritis by provoking a local inflammatory response in the underlying epithelium (Fig. 22.34). This depends on numerous factors, notably expression of bacterial *cagA* and *vacA* genes. The cagA gene product is injected into epithelial cells, ultimately interacting with numerous cell-signalling pathways involved in cell replication and apoptosis. *H. pylori* strains expressing cagA (cagA⁺) are more often associated with disease than cagA⁻ strains. Most strains also secrete a large pore-forming protein called vacA which causes large vacuoles to form

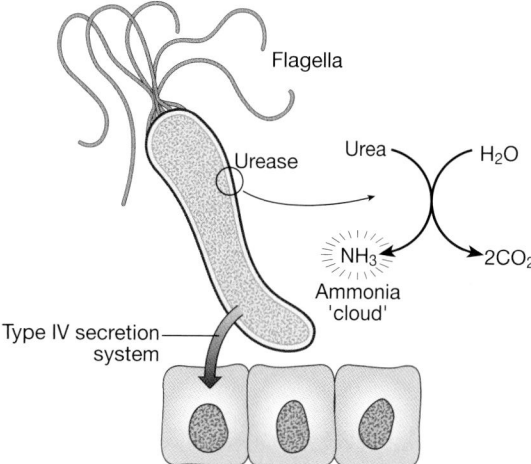

Other factors
- Vacuolating cytotoxin (vacA)
- Cytotoxin-associated gene (cagA)
- Adhesins (BabA)
- Outer inflammatory protein A (oipA)

Fig. 22.34 Factors which influence the virulence of *H. pylori*.

in cells in vitro. In vivo, vacA has many effects, including increased cell permeability, efflux of micronutrients from the epithelium, induction of apoptosis and suppression of local immune cell activity. Several forms of vacA exist and pathology is most strongly associated with the s1/ml form of the toxin. Host genetic polymorphisms are also important—for example, those that lead to greater levels of expression of the proinflammatory cytokine interleukin-1β (IL-1β) are associated with greater risk of gastric atrophy and subsequent carcinoma. In most people *H. pylori* causes antral gastritis associated with depletion of somatostatin (from D cells) and increased gastrin release from G cells. The subsequent hypergastrinaemia stimulates acid production by parietal cells, but in the majority of cases this has no clinical consequences. In a minority of patients (perhaps smokers) this effect is exaggerated, leading to duodenal ulceration (Fig. 22.35). The role of *H. pylori* in the pathogenesis of gastric ulcer is less clear

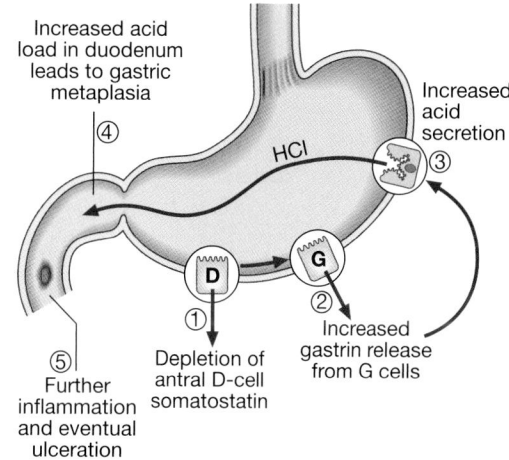

Fig. 22.35 Sequence of events in the pathophysiology of duodenal ulceration.

but it probably acts by reducing gastric mucosal resistance to attack from acid and pepsin. In approximately 1% of infected people, *H. pylori* causes a pangastritis leading to gastric atrophy and hypochlorhydria. This allows bacteria to proliferate within the stomach; these may produce mutagenic nitrites from dietary nitrates, predisposing to the development of gastric cancer (Fig. 22.36). Most duodenal ulcer patients have exaggerated acid secretion in response to stimulation by gastrin, and *H. pylori* exacerbates this by stimulating gastrin production. The effects of *H. pylori* are more complex in gastric ulcer patients; here the ulcer probably occurs because of impaired mucosal defence resulting from a combination of *H. pylori* infection, NSAIDs and smoking.

NSAIDs

NSAIDs are associated with peptic ulcers due to impairment of mucosal defences, as discussed on page 1076.

Smoking

Smoking confers an increased risk of gastric ulcer and, to a lesser extent, duodenal ulcer. Once the ulcer has formed, it is more likely to cause complications and less likely to heal if the patient continues to smoke.

Clinical features

Peptic ulcer disease is a chronic condition with a natural history of spontaneous relapse and remission lasting for decades, if not for life. Although they are different diseases, duodenal and gastric ulcers share common symptoms which will be considered together. The most common presentation is that of recurrent abdominal pain which has three notable characteristics: localisation to the epigastrium, relationship to food and episodic occurrence. Occasional vomiting occurs in about 40% of ulcer subjects; persistent daily vomiting suggests gastric outlet obstruction. In one-third of patients the history is less characteristic. This is especially true in elderly subjects under treatment with NSAIDs. In these patients pain may be absent or so slight that it is experienced only as a vague sense of epigastric unease. Occasionally, the only symptoms are anorexia and nausea, or a sense of undue repletion after meals. In some patients the ulcer is completely 'silent', presenting for the first time with anaemia from chronic undetected blood loss, as an abrupt haematemesis or as acute perforation; in others there is recurrent acute bleeding without ulcer pain between the attacks. The diagnostic value of individual symptoms for peptic ulcer disease is poor; the history is therefore a poor predictor of the presence of an ulcer.

Investigations

Endoscopy is the preferred investigation. Gastric ulcers may occasionally be malignant and therefore must always be biopsied and followed up to ensure healing. Patients should also be screened for *H. pylori* infection. The current options available are listed in Box 22.39. Some are invasive and require endoscopy; others are non-invasive. They vary in sensitivity and specificity. Overall, breath tests are best because of their accuracy, simplicity and non-invasiveness.

Management

The aims of management are to relieve symptoms, induce healing and prevent recurrence. *H. pylori* eradication is the cornerstone of therapy for peptic ulcers, as this will successfully prevent relapse and eliminate the need for long-term therapy in the majority of patients.

H pylori eradication

All patients with proven acute or chronic duodenal ulcer disease and those with gastric ulcers who are *H. pylori*-positive should be offered eradication as primary therapy. Treatment is based upon a PPI taken simultaneously with two antibiotics (from amoxicillin, clarithromycin and metronidazole) for 7 days (Box 22.40). Success is achieved in over 90% of patients, although compliance, side-effects (Box 22.41) and metronidazole resistance influence the success of therapy.

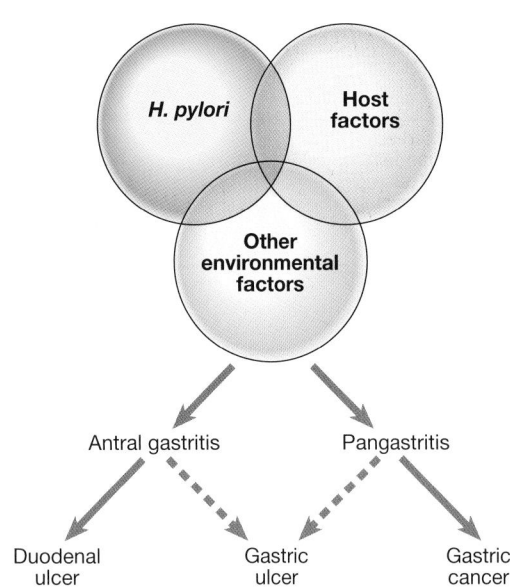

Fig. 22.36 Consequences of *H. pylori* infection.

22.39 Methods for the diagnosis of *Helicobacter pylori* infection

Test	Advantages	Disadvantages
Non-invasive		
Serology	Rapid office kits available Good for population studies	Lacks sensitivity and specificity Cannot differentiate current from past infection
^{13}C-urea breath tests	High sensitivity and specificity	Requires expensive mass spectrometer
Faecal antigen test	Cheap, specific (> 95%)	Acceptability
Invasive (antral biopsy)		
Histology	Sensitivity and specificity	False negatives occur Takes several days to process
Rapid urease tests	Cheap, quick, specific (> 95%)	Sensitivity 85%
Microbiological culture	'Gold standard' Defines antibiotic sensitivity	Slow and laborious Lacks sensitivity

EBM 22.40 **Antibiotic regimens for *H. pylori* eradication**

'First-line therapy is a proton pump inhibitor (12-hourly), clarithromycin 500 mg 12-hourly, and amoxicillin 1 g 12-hourly or metronidazole 400 mg 12-hourly, for 7 days. This is superior to ulcer-healing drugs for duodenal ulcer healing (relative risk of ulcer persistence 0.66, 95% confidence interval 0.58–0.78).'

● Ford, AC, et al. (Cochrane Review). Cochrane Library, issue 2, 2006. Oxford: Update Software.

For further information: www.cochrane.org/reviews

 22.41 Common side-effects of *H. pylori* eradication therapy

- Diarrhoea
- 30–50% of patients; usually mild but *Clostridium difficile*-associated colitis can occur
- Flushing and vomiting when taken with alcohol (metronizadole)
- Nausea, vomiting
- Abdominal cramp
- Headache
- Rash

Second-line therapy should be offered to those patients who remain infected after initial therapy once the reasons for failure of first-line therapy have been established. For those who are still colonised after two treatments, the choice lies between a third attempt with quadruple therapy (bismuth, PPI and two antibiotics) or long-term maintenance therapy with acid suppression.

H. pylori and NSAIDs are independent risk factors for ulcer disease but it is not clear whether patients requiring long-term NSAID therapy should first undergo eradication therapy to reduce ulcer risk. Current evidence suggests that this is not necessary in young, fit patients with no history of ulcer disease or dyspepsia, but a 'test and treat' strategy for older patients with major comorbidity or a previous ulcer history is recommended. Subsequent co-prescription of a PPI along with the NSAID is advised but is not always necessary for patients being given low-dose aspirin in whom the risk of ulcer complications is lower.

Other indications for *H. pylori* eradication are shown in Box 22.42.

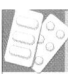 **22.42 Indications for *H. pylori* eradication**

Definite

● Peptic ulcer	● *H. pylori*-positive dyspepsia
● MALToma	

Not indicated

● Gastro-oesophageal reflux disease	● Asymptomatic

Uncertain

● Family history of gastric cancer	● Non-ulcer dyspepsia
	● Long-term NSAID users

General measures

Cigarette smoking, aspirin and NSAIDs should be avoided. Alcohol in moderation is not harmful and no special dietary advice is required.

Maintenance treatment

Continuous maintenance treatment should not be necessary after successful *H. pylori* eradication. For the minority who do require it, the lowest effective dose of PPI should be used.

Surgical treatment

The cure of most peptic ulcers by *H. pylori* eradication therapy and the availability of safe, potent acid-suppressing drugs have made elective surgery for peptic ulcer disease a rare event. Indications for surgery are listed in Box 22.43.

The operation of choice for a chronic non-healing gastric ulcer is partial gastrectomy, preferably with a Billroth I anastomosis, in which the ulcer itself and the ulcer-bearing area of the stomach are resected. The reason for this is to exclude an underlying cancer. In an emergency situation 'under-running' the ulcer for bleeding or 'oversewing' (patch repair) for perforation is all that is required, in addition to taking a biopsy. In the presence of giant duodenal ulcers partial gastrectomy using a 'Polya' or Billroth II reconstruction may be required.

Complications of gastric resection or vagotomy

Although gastric surgery is now rarely undertaken for benign disease, many patients underwent ulcer operations in the pre-*H. pylori* era and some degree of disability is seen in up to 50% of these. In most, the effects are minor, but in 10% of cases they significantly impair quality of life.

- *Dumping.* Rapid gastric emptying leads to distension of the proximal small intestine as the hypertonic contents draw fluid into the lumen. This leads to abdominal discomfort and diarrhoea after eating. Autonomic reflexes release a range of gastrointestinal hormones which lead to vasomotor features such as flushing, palpitations, sweating, tachycardia and hypotension. Patients should therefore avoid large meals with high carbohydrate content.
- *Bile reflux gastritis.* Duodenogastric bile reflux leads to chronic gastritis. This is usually asymptomatic but dyspepsia can occur. Symptomatic treatment with aluminium-containing antacids or sucralfate may be effective. A few patients require revisional surgery with creation of a Roux en Y loop to prevent bile reflux into the stomach.

22

 22.43 Indications for surgery in peptic ulcer

Emergency

- Perforation
- Haemorrhage

Elective

- Complications, e.g. gastric outflow obstruction
- Recurrent ulcer following gastric surgery

• *Diarrhoea and maldigestion.* Diarrhoea may develop after any peptic ulcer operation and usually occurs 1–2 hours after eating. Poor mixing of food in the stomach, with rapid emptying, inadequate mixing with pancreatic biliary secretions, reduced small intestinal transit times and bacterial overgrowth, may lead to malabsorption. Diarrhoea often responds to dietary advice to eat small, dry meals with a reduced intake of refined carbohydrates. Antidiarrhoeal drugs such as codeine phosphate (15–30 mg 4–6 times a day) or loperamide (2 mg after each loose stool) are helpful.

• *Weight loss.* Most patients lose weight shortly after surgery and 30–40% are unable to regain all the weight which is lost. The usual cause is reduced intake because of a small gastric remnant, but diarrhoea and mild steatorrhoea also contribute.

• *Anaemia.* Anaemia is common many years after subtotal gastrectomy. Iron deficiency is the most common cause; folic acid and B_{12} deficiency are much less frequent. Inadequate dietary intake of iron and folate, lack of acid and intrinsic factor secretion, mild chronic low-grade blood loss from the gastric remnant and recurrent ulceration are responsible.

• *Metabolic bone disease.* Both osteoporosis and osteomalacia can occur as a consequence of calcium and vitamin D malabsorption.

• *Gastric cancer.* An increased risk of gastric cancer has been reported from several epidemiological studies. The risk is highest in those with hypochlorhydria, duodenogastric reflux of bile, smoking and *H. pylori* infection. Although the relative risk is increased, the absolute risk of cancer remains low and endoscopic surveillance is not indicated following gastric surgery.

Complications of peptic ulcer disease

Perforation

When perforation occurs, the contents of the stomach escape into the peritoneal cavity, leading to peritonitis. This is more common in duodenal than in gastric ulcers, and is usually found with ulcers on the anterior wall. About one-quarter of all perforations occur in acute ulcers and NSAIDs are often incriminated. Perforation can be the first sign of ulcer, and a history of recurrent epigastric pain is uncommon. The most striking symptom is sudden, severe pain; its distribution follows the spread of the gastric contents over the peritoneum. The pain initially develops in the upper abdomen and rapidly becomes generalised; shoulder tip pain is due to irritation of the diaphragm. The pain is accompanied by shallow respiration due to limitation of diaphragmatic movements, and by shock. The abdomen is held immobile and there is generalised 'board-like' rigidity. Bowel sounds are absent and liver dullness to percussion decreases due to the presence of gas under the diaphragm. After some hours symptoms may improve, although abdominal rigidity remains. Later the patient's condition deteriorates as general peritonitis develops. In at least 50% of cases an erect chest X-ray shows free air beneath the diaphragm. If not, a water-soluble contrast swallow will confirm leakage of gastroduodenal contents. After resuscitation, the acute perforation is treated surgically, either by simple closure, or by converting the perforation into a pyloroplasty if it is large. On rare occa-

22.44 Peptic ulcer disease in old age

• **Gastroduodenal ulcers**: have a greater incidence, admission rate and mortality.
• **Causes**: high prevalence of *H. pylori*, NSAID use and impaired defence mechanisms.
• **Atypical presentations**: pain and dyspepsia are frequently absent or atypical. Older people often develop complications such as bleeding or perforation without a dyspeptic history.
• **Bleeding**: older patients require more intensive management (including CVP measurement) than younger patients because they tolerate hypovolaemic shock poorly.

sions a 'Polya' partial gastrectomy is required. Following surgery, *H. pylori* should be treated (if present) and NSAIDs avoided. Perforation carries a mortality of 25%. This high figure reflects the advanced age and significant comorbidity of this population.

Gastric outlet obstruction

The causes are shown in Box 22.45. The most common is an ulcer in the region of the pylorus. The presentation is with nausea, vomiting and abdominal distension. Large quantities of gastric content are often vomited, and food eaten 24 hours or more previously may be recognised. Physical examination may show evidence of wasting and dehydration. A succussion splash may be elicited 4 hours or more after the last meal or drink. Visible gastric peristalsis is diagnostic of gastric outlet obstruction. Loss of gastric contents leads to dehydration with low serum chloride and potassium, and raised serum bicarbonate and urea concentrations. This results in enhanced renal absorption of Na^+ in exchange for H^+ and paradoxical aciduria. Nasogastric aspiration of at least 200 mL of fluid from the stomach after an overnight fast suggests the diagnosis. Endoscopy should be performed after the stomach has been emptied by a wide-bore nasogastric tube. Nasogastric suction and intravenous correction of dehydration are undertaken. In severe cases at least 4 L of isotonic saline and 80 mmol of potassium may be necessary during the first 24 hours. In some patients PPI drugs heal ulcers, relieve pyloric oedema and overcome the need for surgery. Endoscopic balloon dilatation of benign stenoses may be possible in some patients, but in others partial gastrectomy is necessary, although this is best done after a 7-day period of nasogastric aspiration which enables the stomach to return to normal size. A gastroenterostomy is an alternative operation

22.45 Differential diagnosis and management of gastric outlet obstruction

Cause	Management
Fibrotic stricture from duodenal ulcer, i.e. 'pyloric stenosis'	Balloon dilatation or surgery
Oedema from pyloric channel or duodenal ulcer	PPI therapy
Carcinoma of antrum	Surgery
Adult hypertrophic pyloric stenosis	Surgery

but, unless this is accompanied by vagotomy, patients will require long-term PPI therapy to prevent stomal ulceration.

Bleeding

See pages 852–856.

Zollinger–Ellison syndrome

This is a rare disorder characterised by the triad of severe peptic ulceration, gastric acid hypersecretion and a non-beta cell islet tumour of the pancreas ('gastrinoma'). It probably accounts for about 0.1% of all cases of duodenal ulceration. The syndrome occurs in either sex at any age, although it is most common between 30 and 50 years of age.

Pathophysiology

The tumour secretes large amounts of gastrin, which stimulates the parietal cells of the stomach to secrete acid to their maximal capacity and increases the parietal cell mass three- to sixfold. The acid output may be so great that it reaches the upper small intestine, reducing the luminal pH to 2 or less. Pancreatic lipase is inactivated and bile acids are precipitated. Diarrhoea and steatorrhoea result. Around 90% of tumours occur in the pancreatic head or proximal duodenal wall. At least half are multiple, and tumour size can vary from 1 mm to 20 cm. Approximately one-half to two-thirds are malignant but are often slow-growing. Adenomas of the parathyroid and pituitary glands (multiple endocrine neoplasia, MEN type 1; p. 793) are present in 20–60% of patients.

Clinical features

The presentation is with severe and often multiple peptic ulcers in unusual sites such as the post-bulbar duodenum, jejunum or oesophagus. There is a poor response to standard ulcer therapy. The history is usually short; bleeding and perforations are common. The syndrome may present as severe recurrent ulceration following a standard operation for peptic ulcer. Diarrhoea is seen in one-third or more of patients and can be the presenting feature.

Investigations

Hypersecretion of acid under basal conditions with little increase following pentagastrin may be confirmed by gastric aspiration. Serum gastrin levels are grossly elevated (10- to 1000-fold). Injection of the hormone secretin normally causes no change or a slight decrease in circulating gastrin concentrations, but in Zollinger–Ellison syndrome produces a paradoxical and dramatic increase in gastrin. Tumour localisation is best achieved by EUS and radio-labelled somatostatin receptor scintigraphy.

Management

Approximately 30% of small and single tumours can be localised and resected but many tumours are multifocal. Some patients present with metastatic disease and surgery is inappropriate. PPIs have made total gastrectomy unnecessary, and in the majority of patients continuous therapy with omeprazole heals ulcers and alleviates diarrhoea. Larger doses (60–80 mg daily) than those used to treat duodenal ulcer are required. The synthetic somatostatin analogue, octreotide, given by subcutaneous injection, reduces gastrin secretion and is sometimes of value. Overall 5-year survival is 60–75% and all

patients should be monitored for the later development of other manifestations of MEN 1.

Functional disorders

Non-ulcer dyspepsia

This is defined as chronic dyspepsia in the absence of organic disease. Other commonly reported symptoms include early satiety, fullness, bloating and nausea. 'Ulcer-like' and 'dysmotility-type' subgroups are reported, but there is great overlap between these and also with irritable bowel syndrome.

Pathophysiology

The cause is poorly understood but probably covers a spectrum of mucosal, motility and psychiatric disorders.

Clinical features

Patients are usually young (< 40 years) and women are affected twice as commonly as men. Abdominal pain is associated with a variable combination of other 'dyspeptic' symptoms, the most common being nausea and bloating after meals. Morning symptoms are characteristic and pain or nausea may occur on waking. Direct enquiry may elicit symptoms suggestive of irritable bowel syndrome. Peptic ulcer disease must be considered, whilst in older subjects intra-abdominal malignancy is a prime concern. There are no diagnostic signs, apart perhaps from inappropriate tenderness on abdominal palpation. Symptoms may appear disproportionate to clinical well-being and there is no weight loss. Patients often appear anxious. A drug history should be taken and the possibility of a depressive illness should be considered. Pregnancy should be ruled out in young women before radiological studies are undertaken. Alcohol misuse should be suspected when early morning nausea and retching are prominent.

Investigations

The history will often suggest the diagnosis but in older subjects an endoscopy is necessary to exclude mucosal disease. While an ultrasound scan may detect gallstones, these are rarely responsible for dyspeptic symptoms.

Management

The most important elements are explanation and reassurance. Possible psychological factors should be explored and the concept of psychological influences on gut function should be explained. Idiosyncratic and restrictive diets are of little benefit, but fat restriction may help.

Drug treatment is not especially successful but merits trial. Antacids are sometimes helpful. Prokinetic drugs such as metoclopramide (10 mg 8-hourly) or domperidone (10–20 mg 8-hourly) may be given before meals if nausea, vomiting or bloating is prominent. Metoclopramide may induce extrapyramidal side-effects, including tardive dyskinesia in young subjects. H_2-receptor antagonist drugs may be tried if night pain or heartburn is troublesome. Low-dose amitriptyline is sometimes of value. The role of *H. pylori* eradication remains controversial, although up to 10% may benefit and a minority (5–15%) avoid ulcer development in the next 3 years. Eradication

22

also removes a major risk factor for gastric cancer but at the cost of a small risk of side-effects and worsening symptoms of underlying gastro-oesophageal reflux disease.

Symptoms which can be associated with an identifiable cause of stress resolve with appropriate counselling. Some patients have major chronic psychological disorders resulting in persistent or recurrent symptoms and need behavioural or other formal psychotherapy (p. 239).

Functional causes of vomiting

Psychogenic retching or vomiting may occur in anxiety. It typically occurs on wakening or immediately after breakfast and only rarely later in the day. The disorder is probably a reaction to facing up to the worries of everyday life; in the young it can be due to school phobia. Early morning vomiting also occurs in pregnancy, alcohol misuse and depression. Although functional vomiting may occur regularly over long periods, there is little or no weight loss. Children, and less often adults, sometimes suffer from acute and recurrent disabling bouts of vomiting for days at a time. The cause of this 'cyclical vomiting syndrome' is unknown.

In all patients it is essential to exclude other common causes (p. 852). Tranquillisers and antiemetic drugs (e.g. metoclopramide 10 mg 8-hourly, domperidone 10 mg 8-hourly, prochlorperazine 5–10 mg 8-hourly) have only a secondary place in management. Antidepressants in full dose may be effective (p. 852).

Gastroparesis

Defective gastric emptying without mechanical obstruction of the stomach or duodenum can occur as a primary event, due to inherited or acquired disorders of the gastric pacemaker, or can be secondary to disorders of autonomic nerves (particularly diabetic neuropathy) or the gastroduodenal musculature (e.g. systemic sclerosis, myotonic dystrophies and amyloidosis). Drugs such as opiates, calcium channel antagonists and those with anticholinergic activity (tricyclics, phenothiazines) can also cause gastroparesis. Early satiety and recurrent vomiting are the major symptoms; abdominal fullness and a succussion splash may be present on examination. Treatment is based upon small, frequent, low-fat meals and the use of metoclopramide and domperidone. In severe cases nutritional failure can occur and long-term jejunostomy feeding or total parenteral nutrition is required. Surgical insertion of a gastric pacing device has been successful in some cases but remains experimental.

Tumours of the stomach

Gastric carcinoma

This remains the leading cause of cancer death worldwide, but there is marked geographical variation in incidence. It is extremely common in China, Japan and parts of South America (mortality rate 30–40 per 100 000), less common in the UK (12–13 deaths per 100 000) and uncommon in the USA. Studies of Japanese migrants to the USA have revealed a much lower incidence in second-generation migrants, confirming the importance of environmental factors. Gastric cancer is more common

in men and the incidence rises sharply after 50 years of age. The overall prognosis is poor, with less than 30% surviving 5 years, and the best hope for improved survival lies in greater detection of tumours at an earlier stage.

Pathophysiology

H. pylori is associated with chronic atrophic gastritis and gastric cancer (Fig. 22.37). *H. pylori* infection may be responsible for 60–70% of cases and acquisition of infection at an early age may be important. Although *H. pylori* infection is common in Africa, gastric cancer is uncommon and this 'enigma' may be explained by lower life expectancy in this part of the world. Although the majority of *H. pylori*-infected individuals have normal or increased acid secretion, a few become hypo- or achlorhydric and these people are thought to be at greatest risk. Chronic inflammation with generation of reactive oxygen species and depletion of the normally abundant antioxidant ascorbic acid are also important.

Diets rich in salted, smoked or pickled foods and the consumption of nitrites and nitrates may increase cancer risk. Carcinogenic N-nitroso-compounds are formed from nitrates by the action of nitrite-reducing bacteria which colonise the achlorhydric stomach. Diets lacking fresh fruit and vegetables as well as vitamins C and A may also contribute. Other risk factors are listed in Box 22.46. No predominant genetic abnormality has been identified, although cancer risk is increased two- to threefold in first-degree relatives of patients, and links with blood group A have been reported. Rare 'gastric cancer families' have also been described, in which diffuse gastric cancers occur in association with mutations of the *E-cadherin* (CDH1) gene. This is inherited as an autosomal dominant trait. Virtually all tumours are adenocarcinomas arising from mucus-secreting cells in the base of the gastric crypts. Most develop upon a background of

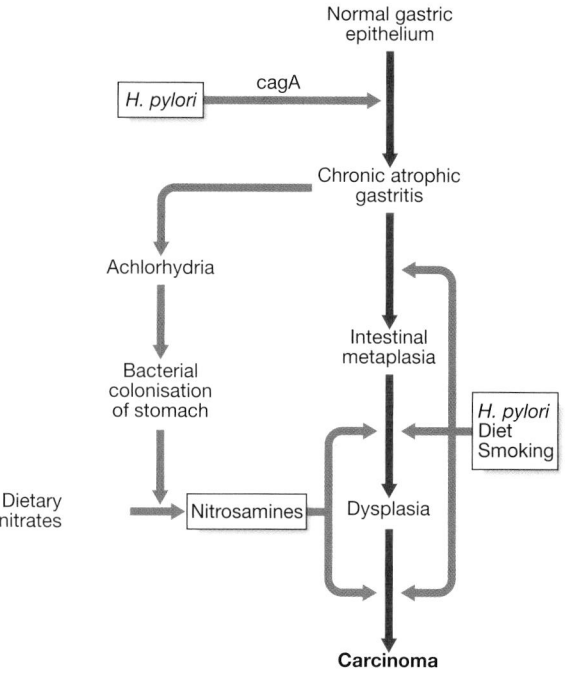

Fig. 22.37 Gastric carcinogenesis: a possible mechanism.

22.46 Risk factors for gastric cancer

- *H. pylori*
- Smoking
- Alcohol
- Dietary associations (see text)
- Autoimmune gastritis (pernicious anaemia)
- Adenomatous gastric polyps
- Previous partial gastrectomy (> 20 years)
- Ménétrier's disease
- Hereditary diffuse gastric cancer families (HDC-1 mutations)
- Familial adenomatous polyposis (FAP, p. 908)

chronic atrophic gastritis with intestinal metaplasia and dysplasia. Cancers are either 'intestinal', arising from areas of intestinal metaplasia with histological features reminiscent of intestinal epithelium, or 'diffuse', arising from normal gastric mucosa. Intestinal carcinomas are more common, and arise against a background of chronic mucosal injury. Diffuse cancers tend to be poorly differentiated and occur in younger patients. In the developing world 50% of gastric cancers develop in the antrum, 20–30% occur in the gastric body, often on the greater curve, and 20% are found in the cardia. In Western populations, however, proximal gastric tumours are becoming more common than those arising in the body and distal stomach. This change in disease pattern may be a reflection of changes in lifestyle or the decreasing prevalence of *H. pylori* in the West. Diffuse submucosal infiltration by a scirrhous cancer (linitis plastica) is uncommon. Macroscopically, tumours may be classified as polypoid, ulcerating, fungating or diffuse. Early gastric cancer is defined as cancer confined to the mucosa or submucosa (Fig. 22.38A). It is more often recognised in Japan, where widespread screening is practised, but is increasingly seen in Western countries. Some cases can be cured by endoscopic mucosal resection (Fig. 22.38B) or endoscopic submucosal dissection (ESD). The majority of patients (> 80%) in the West, however, present with advanced gastric cancer.

Clinical features

Early gastric cancer is usually asymptomatic but may occasionally be discovered during endoscopy for investigation of dyspepsia. Two-thirds of patients with advanced cancers have weight loss and 50% have ulcer-like pain. Anorexia and nausea occur in one-third, while early satiety, haematemesis, melaena and dyspepsia alone are less common features. Dysphagia occurs in tumours of the gastric cardia which obstruct the gastro-oesophageal junction. Anaemia from occult bleeding is also common. Examination may reveal no abnormalities, but signs of weight loss, anaemia or a palpable epigastric mass are not infrequent. Jaundice or ascites may signify metastatic spread. Occasionally, tumour spread occurs to the supraclavicular lymph nodes (Troisier's sign), umbilicus ('Sister Joseph's nodule') or ovaries (Krukenberg tumour). Paraneoplastic phenomena, such as acanthosis nigricans, thrombophlebitis (Trousseau's sign) and dermatomyositis, occur rarely. Metastases occur most commonly in the liver, lungs, peritoneum and bone marrow.

Investigations

There are no laboratory markers of sufficient accuracy for the diagnosis of gastric cancer. Upper gastrointestinal endoscopy is the investigation of choice and should be performed promptly in any dyspeptic patient with 'alarm features' (see Box 22.15, p. 851). Multiple biopsies from the edge and base of a gastric ulcer are required. Barium meal is a poor alternative approach and any abnormalities must be followed by endoscopy to obtain biopsy. Once the diagnosis is made, further imaging is necessary for accurate staging and assessment of resectability. CT may not demonstrate small involved lymph nodes, but will show evidence of intra-abdominal spread or liver metastases. Even with these techniques, laparoscopy is required to determine whether the tumour is resectable, as it is the only modality that will reliably detect peritoneal spread.

Management

Surgery

Resection offers the only hope of cure, which can be achieved in 90% of patients with early gastric cancer. For the majority who have locally advanced disease

22

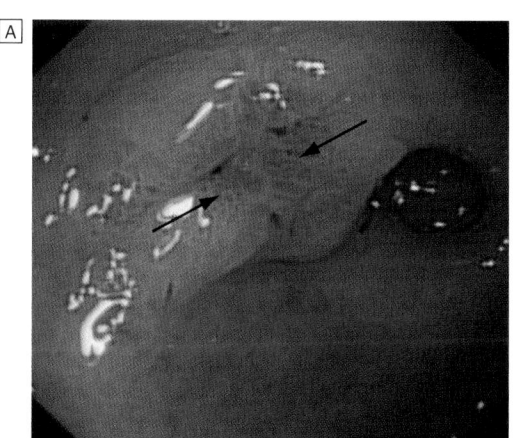 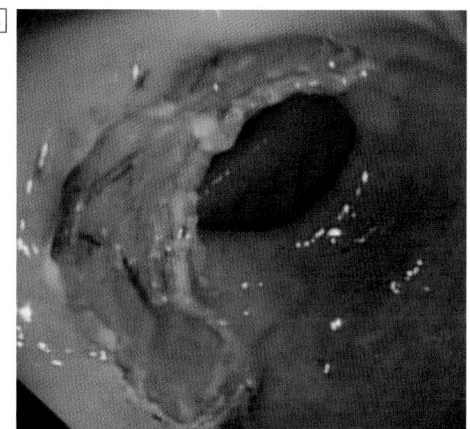

Fig. 22.38 Gastric carcinoma. [A] Endoscopic image of a small superficial prepyloric cancer (arrows). [B] Appearance after endoscopic mucosal resection (EMR). The tumour has been completely removed.

radical and total gastrectomy with lymphadenectomy is the operation of choice, preserving the spleen if possible. Proximal tumours involving the oesophago-gastric junction require an associated distal oesophagectomy. Small, distally sited tumours can be managed by a partial gastrectomy with lymphadenectomy and either a Billroth I or a Roux en Y reconstruction. More extensive lymph node resection may increase survival rates but carries greater morbidity. Even for those who cannot be cured, palliative resection may be necessary when patients present with bleeding or gastric outflow obstruction. Following surgery, recurrence is much more likely if serosal penetration has occurred, although complete removal of all macroscopic tumour combined with lymphadenectomy will achieve a 50–60% 5-year survival. Recent evidence suggests that perioperative chemotherapy with epirubicin, cisplatin and fluorouracil (ECF) improves survival rates.

Palliative treatment

In patients with inoperable tumours, palliation of symptoms can sometimes be achieved with chemotherapy using FAM (5-fluorouracil, doxorubicin and mitomycin C) or ECF. Endoscopic laser ablation for control of dysphagia or recurrent bleeding benefits some patients. Carcinomas at the cardia or pylorus may require endoscopic dilatation, laser therapy or insertion of expandable metallic stents for relief of dysphagia or vomiting. A nasogastric tube may offer temporary relief of vomiting from gastric outlet obstruction (Box 22.47).

Gastric lymphoma

Primary gastric lymphoma accounts for less than 5% of all gastric malignancies. The stomach is, however, the most common site for extranodal non-Hodgkin's lymphoma and 60% of all primary gastrointestinal lymphomas occur at this site. Lymphoid tissue is not found in the normal stomach but lymphoid aggregates develop in the presence of *H. pylori* infection. Indeed, *H. pylori* infection is closely associated with the development of a low-grade lymphoma ('MALToma'). EUS plays an important role in accurately staging these lesions.

The clinical presentation is similar to that of gastric cancer, and endoscopically the tumour appears as a polypoid or ulcerating mass. While initial treatment of low-grade MALTomas consists of *H. pylori* eradication and close observation, 25% contain t(11:18) chromosomal translocations and will rarely respond. In these cases, radiotherapy or chemotherapy is necessary. High-grade B-cell lymphomas are treated by a combination of chemotherapy, surgery and radiotherapy. The choice depends on the site and extent of tumour, the presence of comorbid illnesses, and other factors such as symptoms of bleeding and gastric outflow obstruction. The prognosis depends on the stage at diagnosis. Features predicting a favourable prognosis are stage I or II disease, small resectable tumours, tumours with low-grade histology, and age below 60 years.

Other tumours of the stomach

Gastrointestinal stromal cell tumours (GIST) arising from the interstitial cells of Cajal are occasionally found at upper gastrointestinal endoscopy. They are

22.47 How to insert a nasogastric (NG) tube

Equipment

- 8–9F 'fine-bore' tube for feeding or 16–18F 'wide-bore' tube for drainage
- Lubricant jelly
- Cup of water and straw for sipping
- Adhesive tape
- pH (not litmus) paper
- Sickness bowl and tissues
- Catheter drainage bag and clamp (for drainage)

Technique

- A clear explanation and a calm patient are essential
- Establish a 'stop signal' for the patient to use, if needed
- Ask the patient to sit semi-upright
- Examine the nose for deformity or blockage to determine which side to use
- Measure the distance from ear to xiphoid process via the nose and mark the position on the tube
- Advance the lubricated tube tip slowly along the floor of the nasal passage to the oropharynx
- Ask the patient to sip water and advance the tube 2–3 cm with each swallow
- Stop, withdraw and retry if the patient is distressed or coughing, as the tube may have entered the larynx
- Advance until the mark on the tube reaches the tip of the nose and secure with tape
- Aspirate the contents and check pH (gastric acid confirmed if pH < 5). If in doubt, perform a chest X-ray to confirm tube position (usually necessary with feeding tubes)
- Attach the catheter drainage bag, if necessary, and clamp

Aftercare

- Flush the tube daily after feeding or drug dosing
- Check position regularly and look for signs of displacement
- Check with the pharmacist what drugs, if any, can be safely given via the tube

differentiated from other mesenchymal tumours by expression of the *c-kit* proto-oncogene, which encodes a tyrosine kinase receptor. GISTs are usually benign and asymptomatic, but may occasionally be responsible for dyspepsia; they can also ulcerate and cause gastrointestinal bleeding.

A variety of polyps occur. Hyperplastic polyps and fundic cystic gland polyps are common and of no consequence. Adenomatous polyps are rare; they have malignant potential and should be removed endoscopically.

Occasionally, gastric carcinoid tumours are seen in the fundus and body in patients with long-standing pernicious anaemia. These benign tumours arise from ECL or other endocrine cells, and are often multiple but rarely invasive. Unlike carcinoid tumours arising elsewhere in the gastrointestinal tract, they usually run a benign and favourable course. However, large (> 2 cm) carcinoids may metastasise and should be removed. Rarely, small nodules of ectopic pancreatic exocrine tissue are found. These 'pancreatic rests' may be mistaken for gastric neoplasms and usually cause no symptoms. EUS is the most useful investigation.

DISEASES OF THE SMALL INTESTINE

Disorders causing malabsorption

Coeliac disease

Coeliac disease is an immunologically mediated inflammatory disorder of the small bowel occurring in genetically susceptible individuals and resulting from intolerance to wheat gluten and similar proteins found in rye, barley and, to a lesser extent, oats. It can result in malabsorption and responds to a gluten-free diet. The condition occurs world-wide but is more common in northern Europe. The prevalence in the UK is approximately 1%, although 50% of these people are asymptomatic. These include both undiagnosed 'silent' cases of the disease and cases of 'latent' coeliac disease—genetically susceptible people who may later develop clinical coeliac disease.

Pathophysiology

The precise mechanism of mucosal damage is unclear but immunological responses to gluten play a key role (Fig. 22.39). Tissue transglutaminase (tTG) is now recognised as the autoantigen for anti-endomysial antibodies, often used in serological diagnosis.

Clinical features

Coeliac disease can present at any age. In infancy it occurs after weaning on to cereals and typically presents with diarrhoea, malabsorption and failure to thrive. In older children it may present with non-specific features such as delayed growth. Features of malnutrition are often found on examination and mild abdominal distension may be present. Affected children have both growth and pubertal delay, leading to short stature in adulthood.

In adults peak onset is in the third or fourth decade and females are affected twice as often as males. The presentation is highly variable, depending on the severity and extent of small bowel involvement. Some patients have florid malabsorption while others develop non-specific symptoms such as tiredness, weight loss, folate deficiency or iron deficiency anaemia. Other recognised presentations include oral ulceration, dyspepsia and bloating. Unrecognised coeliac disease is associated with mild undernutrition and increased risk of osteoporosis.

Coeliac disease is associated with other human leucocyte antigen (HLA)-linked autoimmune disorders and with certain other diseases (Box 22.48).

Investigations

These are performed to confirm the diagnosis and to look for consequences of malabsorption.

> **22.48 Disease associations of coeliac disease**
>
> - Insulin-dependent diabetes mellitus (2–8%)
> - Thyroid disease (5%)
> - Primary biliary cirrhosis (3%)
> - Sjögren's syndrome (3%)
> - IgA deficiency (2%)
> - Pernicious anaemia
> - Inflammatory bowel disease
> - Sarcoidosis
> - Myasthenia gravis
> - Neurological complications: encephalopathy, cerebellar atrophy, peripheral neuropathy, epilepsy
> - Dermatitis herpetiformis
> - Down's syndrome
> - Enteropathy-associated T-cell lymphoma
> - Small bowel carcinoma
> - Squamous carcinoma of oesophagus
> - Ulcerative jejunitis
> - Pancreatic insufficiency
> - Microscopic colitis
> - Splenic atrophy

22

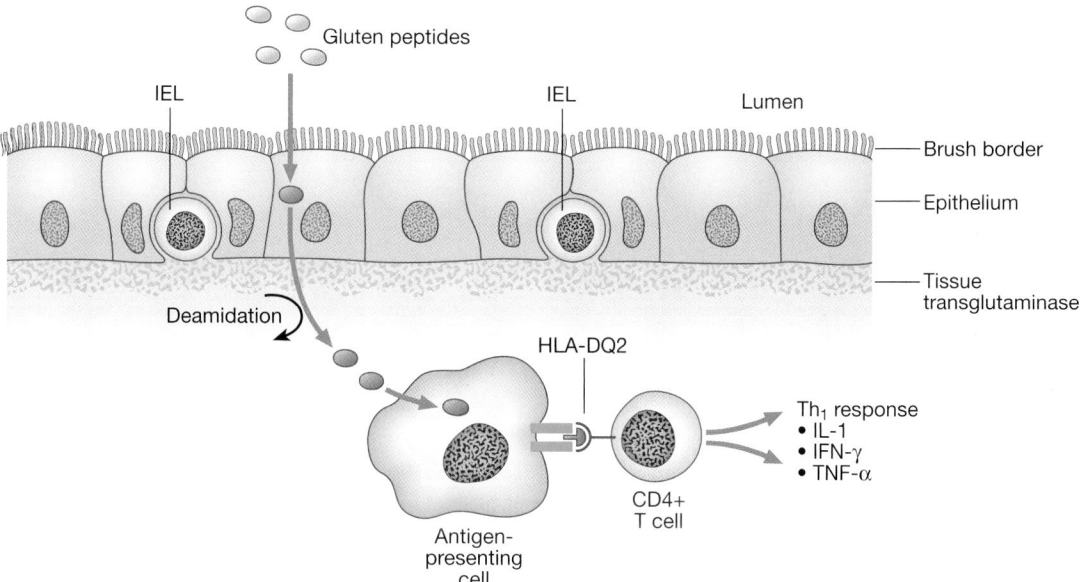

Fig. 22.39 Pathophysiology of coeliac disease. After being taken up by epithelial cells, gluten peptides are deamidated by the enzyme tissue transglutaminase in the subepithelial layer. They are then able to fit the antigen-binding motif on HLA-DQ2-positive antigen-presenting cells. Recognition by CD4+ T cells triggers a Th$_1$ immune response with generation of pro-inflammatory cytokines (IL-1, IFN-γ and TNF-α). Lymphocytes infiltrate the lamina propria, and increased intraepithelial lymphocytes (IEL), crypt hyperplasia and villous atrophy ensue.

22.49 Important causes of subtotal villous atrophy

- Coeliac disease
- Tropical sprue
- Dermatitis herpetiformis
- Lymphoma
- AIDS enteropathy
- Giardiasis
- Hypogammaglobulinaemia
- Radiation
- Whipple's disease
- Zollinger–Ellison syndrome

Duodenal biopsy

Endoscopic small bowel biopsy is the gold standard. The histological features are usually characteristic but other causes of villous atrophy should also be considered (Box 22.49 and Fig. 22.40). Sometimes the villi appear normal but there are excess numbers of intra-epithelial lymphocytes present.

Antibodies

IgA anti-endomysial antibodies are detectable by immunofluorescence in most untreated cases. They are not quantitative, but are sensitive (85–95%) and specific (approximately 99%) for the diagnosis, except in very young infants. IgG antibodies, however, must be analysed in patients with coexisting IgA deficiency. The tTG assay has replaced other blood tests in many countries as it is easier to perform, semi-quantitative and more accurate in patients with IgA deficiency. These antibody tests constitute a valuable screening tool in patients with diarrhoea but are not a substitute for small bowel biopsy; they usually become negative with successful treatment.

Haematology and biochemistry

A full blood count may show microcytic or macrocytic anaemia from iron or folate deficiency and features of hyposplenism (target cells, spherocytes and Howell–Jolly bodies). Biochemical tests may reveal reduced concentrations of calcium, magnesium, total protein, albumin or vitamin D.

Other investigations

Measurement of bone density should be considered to look for evidence of osteoporosis, especially in older patients and post-menopausal women.

Management

The aims are to correct existing deficiencies of iron, folate, calcium and/or vitamin D, and to commence a life-long gluten-free diet. This requires the exclusion of wheat, rye, barley and initially oats, although oats may be reintroduced safely in most patients after 6–12 months. Initially, frequent dietary counselling is required to make sure the diet is being observed, as the most common reason for failure to improve with dietary treatment is accidental or unrecognised gluten ingestion. Mineral and vitamin supplements are also given when indicated but are seldom necessary when a strict gluten-free diet is adhered to. Booklets produced by coeliac societies in many countries, containing diet sheets and recipes for the use of gluten-free flour, are of great value. Regular monitoring of symptoms, weight and nutrition is essential. Patients who have an excellent clinical response, with disappearance of circulating anti-endomysial antibodies, probably do not need to undergo repeat jejunal biopsies. These should be reserved for patients who do not symptomatically improve or whose antibodies remain persistently positive.

Rarely, patients are 'refractory' and require treatment with corticosteroids or immunosuppressive drugs to induce remission. Dietary compliance should be carefully assessed in patients who fail to respond, but if their diet is satisfactory, other conditions such as pancreatic insufficiency or microscopic colitis should be sought, as should complications of coeliac disease such as ulcerative jejunitis or enteropathy-associated T-cell lymphoma.

Complications

A twofold increased risk of malignancy, particularly of enteropathy-associated T-cell lymphoma, small bowel carcinoma and squamous carcinoma of the oesophagus, has been reported, but recent studies have found only modest increases compared to the general population. A few patients develop ulcerative jejuno-ileitis; fever, pain, obstruction or perforation may then supervene. The diagnosis of small bowel complications is rarely made by barium studies or enteroscopy, and laparotomy and full-thickness biopsy are usually necessary.

Treatment is difficult. Corticosteroids are used with mixed success and some patients require surgical resection and parenteral nutrition. The course is often progressive and relentless.

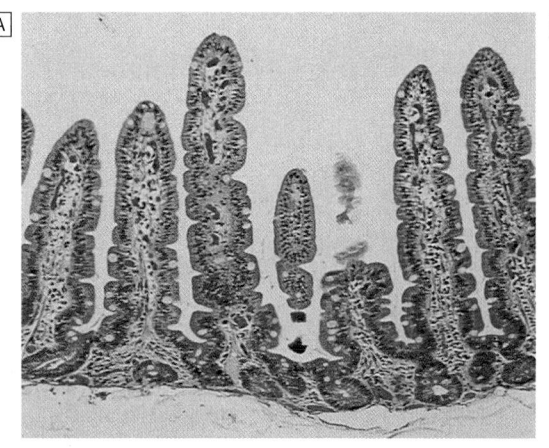
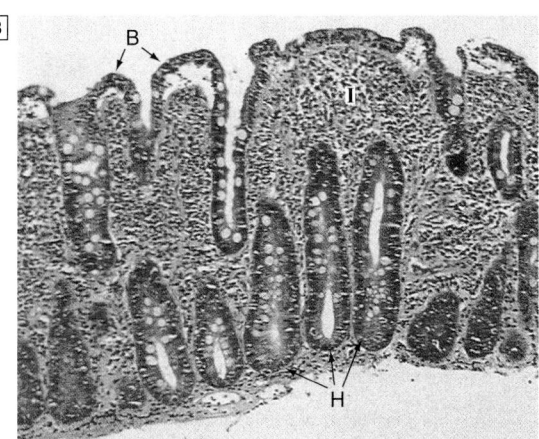

Fig. 22.40 Jejunal mucosa. [A] Normal. [B] Subtotal villous atrophy in coeliac disease. There is blunting of villi (B), crypt hyperplasia (H) and inflammatory infiltration of the lamina propria (I).

Osteoporosis and osteomalacia may occur in patients with long-standing, poorly controlled coeliac disease. These complications are less common in patients who adhere strictly to a gluten-free diet.

Dermatitis herpetiformis

This is characterised by crops of intensely itchy blisters over the elbows, knees, back and buttocks (p. 1276). Immunofluorescence shows granular or linear IgA deposition at the dermo-epidermal junction. Almost all patients have partial villous atrophy on jejunal biopsy, even though they usually have no gastrointestinal symptoms. In contrast, fewer than 10% of coeliac patients have evidence of dermatitis herpetiformis, although both disorders are associated with the same histocompatibility antigen groups. The rash usually responds to a gluten-free diet but some patients require additional treatment with dapsone (100–150 mg daily).

Tropical sprue

Tropical sprue is defined as chronic, progressive malabsorption in a patient in or from the tropics, associated with abnormalities of small intestinal structure and function. The disease occurs mainly in the West Indies and in Asia, including southern India, Malaysia and Indonesia.

Pathophysiology

The epidemiological pattern and occasional epidemics suggest that an infective agent may be involved. Although no single bacterium has been isolated, the condition often begins after an acute diarrhoeal illness. Small bowel bacterial overgrowth with *Escherichia coli, Enterobacter* and *Klebsiella* is frequently seen. The changes closely resemble those of coeliac disease.

Clinical features

There is diarrhoea, abdominal distension, anorexia, fatigue and weight loss. In visitors to the tropics the onset of severe diarrhoea may be sudden and accompanied by fever. When the disorder becomes chronic, the features of megaloblastic anaemia (folic acid malabsorption) and other deficiencies, including ankle oedema, glossitis and stomatitis, are common. Remissions and relapses may occur. The differential diagnosis in the indigenous tropical population is an infective cause of diarrhoea. The important differential diagnosis in visitors to the tropics is giardiasis (p. 363).

Management

Tetracycline 250 mg 6-hourly for 28 days is the treatment of choice and brings about long-term remission or cure. In most patients pharmacological doses of folic acid (5 mg daily) improve symptoms and jejunal morphology. In some cases treatment must be prolonged before improvement occurs, and occasionally patients must leave the tropics.

Small bowel bacterial overgrowth ('blind loop syndrome')

The normal duodenum and jejunum contain less than 10^4/mL organisms which are usually derived from saliva. The count of coliform organisms never exceeds 10^3/mL. In bacterial overgrowth there may be 10^8–10^{10}/mL organisms, most of which are normally found only in the colon. Disorders which impair the normal physiological mechanisms controlling bacterial proliferation

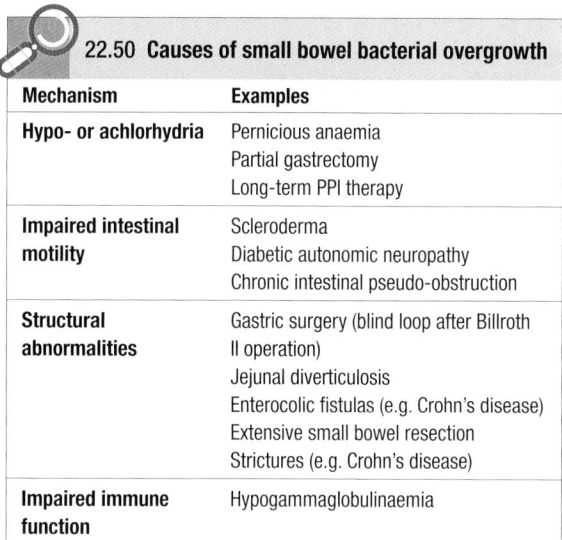

22.50 Causes of small bowel bacterial overgrowth

Mechanism	Examples
Hypo- or achlorhydria	Pernicious anaemia Partial gastrectomy Long-term PPI therapy
Impaired intestinal motility	Scleroderma Diabetic autonomic neuropathy Chronic intestinal pseudo-obstruction
Structural abnormalities	Gastric surgery (blind loop after Billroth II operation) Jejunal diverticulosis Enterocolic fistulas (e.g. Crohn's disease) Extensive small bowel resection Strictures (e.g. Crohn's disease)
Impaired immune function	Hypogammaglobulinaemia

in the intestine predispose to bacterial overgrowth (Box 22.50). The most important are loss of gastric acidity, impaired intestinal motility and structural abnormalities which allow colonic bacteria to gain access to the small intestine or provide a secluded haven from the peristaltic stream.

Pathophysiology

Bacterial overgrowth can occur in patients with small bowel diverticuli. Another cause is diabetic autonomic neuropathy (p. 831), which reduces small bowel motility and affects enterocyte secretion. In scleroderma, bacterial overgrowth occurs because the circular and longitudinal layers of the intestinal muscle are fibrosed, and motility is abnormal. In idiopathic hypogammaglobulinaemia the IgA and IgM levels in serum and jejunal secretions are reduced. Chronic diarrhoea and malabsorption occur because of bacterial overgrowth and recurrent gastrointestinal infections (particularly giardiasis, p. 363).

Clinical features

The patient presents with watery diarrhoea and/or steatorrhoea with anaemia due to B_{12} deficiency. These arise because of deconjugation of bile acids, which impairs micelle formation, and because of bacterial utilisation of vitamin B_{12}. There may also be symptoms from the underlying intestinal cause.

Investigations

Serum vitamin B_{12} concentration is low, whilst folate levels are normal or elevated because the bacteria produce folic acid. Barium follow-through or small bowel enema may reveal blind loops or fistulas. Endoscopic duodenal biopsies exclude mucosal disease such as coeliac disease. Jejunal contents for bacteriological examination can be aspirated at endoscopy; the laboratory analysis requires anaerobic and aerobic culture techniques. The diagnosis can often be made non-invasively using the glucose hydrogen or ^{14}C-glycocholic acid breath tests. In these tests breath samples are serially measured after oral ingestion of the test material. Bacteria within the small bowel cause an early rise in breath hydrogen from glucose or ^{14}C from ^{14}C-glycocholate. Hypogammaglobulinaemia can be diagnosed by measurement of serum immunoglobulins and by intestinal biopsy which shows reduced or absent plasma cells and nodules of lymphoid tissue (nodular lymphoid hyperplasia).

Management

The underlying cause of small bowel bacterial overgrowth should be addressed. Tetracycline 250 mg 6-hourly for 7 days is then the treatment of choice, although up to 50% of patients do not respond adequately. Metronidazole 400 mg 8-hourly or ciprofloxacin 250 mg 12-hourly is an alternative. Some patients require up to 4 weeks of treatment and, in a few, continuous rotating courses of antibiotics are necessary. Intramuscular vitamin B_{12} supplementation is needed in chronic cases. Patients with motility disorders such as diabetes and scleroderma may benefit from antidiarrhoeal drugs (diphenoxylate 5 mg 8-hourly orally or loperamide 2 mg 4–6-hourly orally). In hypogammaglobulinaemia treatment should focus on control of giardiasis and, if necessary, immunoglobulin infusions.

Whipple's disease

This rare condition is characterised by infiltration of small intestinal mucosa by 'foamy' macrophages which stain positive with periodic acid–Schiff (PAS) reagent. The disease is a multisystem one and almost any organ can be affected, sometimes long before gastrointestinal involvement becomes apparent (Box 22.52).

Pathophysiology

The disease is caused by infection with the Gram-positive bacillus *Tropheryma whipplei* which is resident within macrophages in the bowel mucosa. Villi are widened and flattened; densely packed macrophages occur in the lamina propria. These may obstruct lymphatic drainage, causing fat malabsorption. Molecular characterisation of the bacillus has led to development of polymerase chain reaction (PCR)-based diagnosis.

Clinical features

Middle-aged men are most commonly affected and the presentation depends on the pattern of organ involvement. Low-grade fever is common and most patients have joint symptoms to some degree, often as the first manifestation. Occasionally, neurological manifestations may predominate.

Management

Whipple's disease is often fatal if untreated but responds well, at least initially, to intravenous ceftriaxone 2 g daily

22.52 Clinical features of Whipple's disease
Gastrointestinal (> 70%)
• Diarrhoea (75%), steatorrhoea, weight loss (90%), bloating, protein-losing enteropathy, ascites, hepatosplenomegaly (< 5%)
Musculoskeletal (65%)
• Seronegative large joint arthropathy, sacroiliitis
Cardiac (10%)
• Pericarditis, myocarditis, endocarditis, coronary arteritis
Neurological (10–40%)
• Apathy, fits, dementia, myoclonus, meningitis, cranial nerve lesions
Pulmonary (10–20%)
• Chronic cough, pleurisy, pulmonary infiltrates
Haematological (60%)
• Anaemia, lymphadenopathy
Other (40%)
• Fever, pigmentation

for 2 weeks, followed by oral co-trimoxazole for at least 1 year. Symptoms usually resolve quickly and biopsy changes revert to normal in a few weeks. Long-term follow-up is essential, as relapse occurs in up to one-third of patients. This often occurs within the central nervous system, in which case the same therapy is repeated or else treatment with doxycycline and hydroxychloroquine is necessary.

Ileal resection

Malabsorption may occur as a complication of small bowel resection. Ileal resection is usually found after surgery for Crohn's disease. Vitamin B_{12} and bile salt malabsorption develops (Fig. 22.41). Unabsorbed bile salts pass into the colon, stimulating water and electrolyte secretion and resulting in diarrhoea. If hepatic synthesis of new bile salts cannot keep pace with faecal losses, fat malabsorption occurs. Another consequence is the formation of lithogenic bile, leading to gallstones. Renal calculi, rich in oxalate, develop. Normally, oxalate in the colon is bound to and precipitated by calcium. Unabsorbed bile salts preferentially bind calcium, leaving free oxalate to be absorbed with subsequent development of urinary oxalate calculi.

Patients have urgent watery diarrhoea or mild steatorrhoea. Contrast studies of the small bowel and tests of B_{12} and bile acid absorption (p. 850) are useful investigations. Parenteral vitamin B_{12} supplementation is necessary. Diarrhoea usually responds well to colestyramine, a resin which binds bile salts in the intestinal lumen. Aluminium hydroxide is an alternative therapy.

Short bowel syndrome

Short bowel syndrome is defined as malabsorption resulting from extensive small intestinal resection or disease. The syndrome has many causes (Box 22.53) but in adults it usually results from extensive surgery undertaken for Crohn's disease or mesenteric infarction. Irrespective of the cause, three main types of patient are seen:

22.51 Malabsorption in old age
• **Coeliac disease:** symptoms such as dyspepsia tend to be vague; only 25% present classically with diarrhoea and weight loss. Metabolic bone disease, folate or iron deficiency, coagulopathy and small bowel lymphoma are more common.
• **Small bowel bacterial overgrowth:** more prevalent: Atrophic gastritis resulting in hypo- or achlorhydria becomes more common Jejunal diverticulosis is prevalent The long-term effects of gastric surgery for ulcer disease are now being seen in older people.

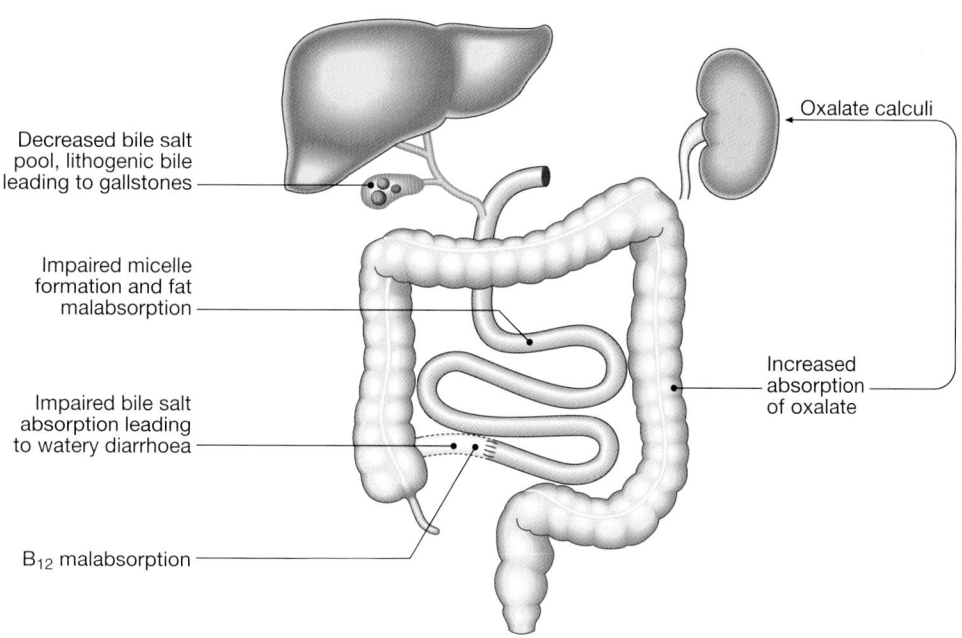

Decreased bile salt
pool, lithogenic bile
leading to gallstones

Impaired micelle
formation and fat
malabsorption

Impaired bile salt
absorption leading
to watery diarrhoea

B_{12} malabsorption

Oxalate calculi

Increased
absorption
of oxalate

Fig. 22.41 Consequences of ileal resection.

22

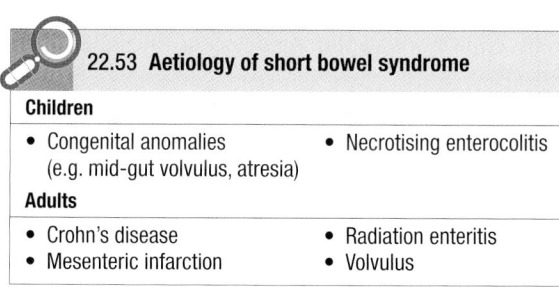

22.53 Aetiology of short bowel syndrome

Children

- Congenital anomalies
  (e.g. mid-gut volvulus, atresia)
- Necrotising enterocolitis

Adults

- Crohn's disease
- Mesenteric infarction
- Radiation enteritis
- Volvulus

- *Jejunal resection with intact ileum and colon.* This is uncommon and nutritional support is rarely needed.
- *Jejunum–colon patients* (jejuno-ileal resection with jejunocolic anastomosis).
- *Jejunostomy patients* (jejuno-ileal resection and colectomy).

Pathophysiology

Important differences occur between jejunum–colon and jejunostomy patients (Box 22.54) but in both groups loss of surface area for digestion and absorption is the key problem. These processes are normally completed within the first 100 cm of jejunum, and enteral feeding is usually possible if this amount of small intestine remains. The proximal small bowel normally reabsorbs most of the 8 L of fluid it receives daily, and patients with a high jejunostomy are at great risk of hypovolaemia, dehydration and electrolyte losses. The presence of some or all of the colon may markedly improve these losses by increased water reabsorption. The presence of an intact ileocaecal valve ameliorates the clinical picture by slowing small intestinal transit and reducing bacterial overgrowth.

Clinical features

Severely affected patients have large volumes of jejunostomy fluid losses or, if the colon is preserved, diarrhoea and steatorrhoea. Dehydration and signs of hypovolaemia are common, as are weight loss, loss of muscle bulk and malnutrition. Some patients remain in satisfactory but precarious fluid balance until a minor intercurrent illness or intestinal upset occurs, when they can rapidly become dehydrated.

Management

In the immediate post-operative period, total parenteral nutrition (TPN) should be started. PPI therapy is given to reduce gastric secretions. Enteral feeding can be cautiously introduced after 1–2 weeks under careful supervision and slowly increased as tolerated. For patients with a jejunostomy, parenteral saline is likely to be necessary if less than 100 cm of jejunum remains. If less than 75 cm of small bowel remains, TPN is also needed.

22.54 Effects of a short bowel

	Jejunum–colon	Jejunostomy
Clinical	Gradual diarrhoea, weight loss	Rapid fluid losses
Water/electrolyte depletion	+/–	++
Malabsorption nutrients	++	+++
D-lactic acidosis	+/–	–
Oxalate renal calculi	++	–
Pigment gallstones	++	++
Gut adaptation	+	–
Impact on quality of life	Diarrhoea	High output, dehydration, parenteral nutrition

The principles of long-term management are:
- Detailed nutritional assessments at regular intervals.
- Monitoring of fluid and electrolyte balance. Patients can usually be taught how to do this for themselves. A readily available supply of oral rehydration solution is useful for intercurrent illness.
- Adequate calorie and protein intake. Fats are a good energy source and should be taken as tolerated. Medium-chain triglyceride supplements are often given first because they are more easily absorbed.
- Use of oral/enteral rather than parenteral nutrition whenever possible.
- Replacement of vitamin B_{12}, calcium, vitamin D, magnesium, zinc and folic acid.
- Antidiarrhoeal agents, e.g. loperamide (2–4 mg 6-hourly) or codeine phosphate (30 mg 4–6-hourly).

Some patients are unable to maintain positive fluid balance. Octreotide (50–200 µg 8–12-hourly by subcutaneous injection) reduces gastrointestinal secretions and is useful in such individuals. Despite these measures, some patients require long-term home TPN for survival and this is best managed in specialist centres. Small bowel transplantation is an option but rejection and 'graft-versus-host' disease (p. 1014) remain significant hurdles.

Radiation enteritis and proctocolitis

Intestinal damage occurs in 10–15% of patients undergoing radiotherapy for abdominal or pelvic malignancy. The risk varies with total dose, dosing schedule and the use of concomitant chemotherapy.

Pathophysiology

The rectum, sigmoid colon and terminal ileum are most frequently involved. Radiation causes acute inflammation, shortening of villi, oedema and crypt abscess formation. These usually resolve completely but in some patients an obliterative endarteritis affecting the endothelium of submucosal arterioles develops over 2–12 months. Fibroblastic proliferation produces progressive ischaemic fibrosis over years and may lead to adhesions, ulceration, strictures, obstruction or fistula to adjacent organs.

Clinical features

In the acute phase there is nausea, vomiting, cramping abdominal pain and diarrhoea. When the rectum and colon are involved, rectal mucus, bleeding and tenesmus occur. The chronic phase develops after 5–10 years in some patients and produces one or more of the problems listed in Box 22.55.

Investigations

In the acute phase the rectal changes at sigmoidoscopy resemble those of ulcerative proctitis (see Fig. 22.57, p. 900). The extent of the lesion is determined by colonoscopy. Barium follow-through examination shows small bowel strictures, ulcers and fistulas.

Management

Diarrhoea in the acute phase is treated with codeine phosphate, diphenoxylate or loperamide in standard dosage. Local corticosteroid enemas help proctitis, and antibiotics may be required for bacterial overgrowth. Nutritional supplements are necessary when malab-

22.55 Chronic complications of intestinal irradiation

- Proctocolitis
- Bleeding from telangiectasia
- Small bowel strictures
- Fistulas: rectovaginal, colovesical, enterocolic
- Adhesions
- Malabsorption: bacterial overgrowth, bile salt malabsorption (ileal damage)

sorption is present. Colestyramine (4 g as a single sachet) is useful for bile salt malabsorption. Endoscopic laser or argon plasma coagulation therapy may reduce bleeding from proctitis. Surgery should be avoided, if possible, because the injured intestine is difficult to resect and anastomose, but it may be necessary for obstruction, perforation or fistula.

Abetalipoproteinaemia

This rare autosomal recessive disorder is caused by deficiency of apolipoprotein B which results in failure of chylomicron formation. It leads to fat malabsorption and deficiency of fat-soluble vitamins. Jejunal biopsy reveals enterocytes distended with resynthesised triglyceride and normal villous morphology. Serum cholesterol and triglyceride levels are low. A number of other abnormalities occur in this syndrome, including acanthocytosis, retinitis pigmentosa and a progressive neurological disorder with cerebellar and dorsal column signs. Symptoms may be improved by a low-fat diet supplemented with medium-chain triglycerides and vitamins A, D, E and K.

Motility disorders

Chronic intestinal pseudo-obstruction

Small intestinal motility is disordered in conditions which affect the smooth muscle or nerves of the intestine. Many cases are 'primary' (idiopathic), while others are 'secondary' to a variety of disorders or drugs (Box 22.56).

Clinical features

There are recurrent episodes of nausea, vomiting, abdominal discomfort and distension, often worse after

22.56 Causes of chronic intestinal pseudo-obstruction

Primary or idiopathic

- Rare familial visceral myopathies or neuropathies
- Congenital aganglionosis

Secondary

- Drugs, e.g. opiates, tricyclic antidepressants, phenothiazines
- Smooth muscle disorders, e.g. scleroderma, amyloidosis, mitochondrial myopathies
- Myenteric plexus disorders, e.g. paraneoplastic syndrome in small-cell lung cancer
- CNS disorders, e.g. Parkinsonism, autonomic neuropathy
- Endocrine and metabolic disorders, e.g. hypothyroidism, phaeochromocytoma, acute intermittent porphyria

food. Alternating constipation and diarrhoea occur and weight loss results from malabsorption (due to bacterial overgrowth) and fear of eating. There may also be symptoms of dysmotility affecting other parts of the gastrointestinal tract, such as dysphagia, and, in primary cases, features of bladder dysfunction. Some patients have obscure but severe abdominal pain which is extremely difficult to manage.

Investigations

The diagnosis is often delayed and a high index of suspicion is needed. Plain X-rays show distended loops of bowel and air–fluid levels, but barium studies demonstrate no mechanical obstruction. Laparotomy is sometimes performed to exclude obstruction and to obtain full-thickness biopsies of the intestine. Electron microscopy, histochemistry and special stains define rare, specific syndromes.

Management

This is often difficult. Underlying causes should be addressed and further surgery avoided if at all possible. Metoclopramide or domperidone may enhance motility, and antibiotics are given for bacterial overgrowth. Nutritional and psychological support is also necessary.

Miscellaneous disorders of the small intestine

Protein-losing enteropathy

This term is used when there is excessive loss of protein into the gut lumen, sufficient to cause hypoproteinaemia. Protein-losing enteropathy occurs in many gut disorders but is most common in those where ulceration occurs (Box 22.57). In other disorders protein loss results from increased mucosal permeability or obstruction of intestinal lymphatic vessels. Patients present with peripheral oedema and hypoproteinaemia in the presence of normal liver function and without proteinuria. The diagnosis is confirmed by measurement of faecal clearance of α_1-antitrypsin or ^{51}Cr-labelled albumin after intravenous injection. Other investigations are performed to determine the underlying cause. Treatment is that of the underlying disorder, with nutritional support and measures to control peripheral oedema.

22.57 Causes of protein-losing enteropathy	
With mucosal erosions or ulceration	
• Crohn's disease	• Oesophageal, gastric or
• Ulcerative colitis	colonic cancer
• Radiation damage	• Lymphoma
Without mucosal erosions or ulceration	
• Ménétrier's disease	• Tropical sprue
• Bacterial overgrowth	• Eosinophilic gastroenteritis
• Coeliac disease	• SLE
With lymphatic obstruction	
• Intestinal lymphangiectasia	• Lymphoma
• Constrictive pericarditis	• Whipple's disease

Intestinal lymphangiectasia

This may be primary, resulting from congenital malunion of lymphatics, or secondary to lymphatic obstruction due to lymphoma, filariasis or constrictive pericarditis. Impaired drainage of intestinal lymphatic vessels leads to discharge of protein and fat-rich lymph into the gastrointestinal lumen. The condition presents with peripheral lymphoedema, pleural effusions or chylous ascites, and steatorrhoea. Investigations reveal hypoalbuminaemia, lymphocytopenia and reduced serum immunoglobulin concentrations. Jejunal biopsies show greatly dilated lacteals, and lymphangiography shows lymphatic obstruction. Treatment consists of a low-fat diet with medium-chain triglyceride supplements.

Ulceration of the small intestine

Small bowel ulcers are uncommon and are either idiopathic or secondary to underlying intestinal disorders (Box 22.58). Ulcers are more common in the ileum, and cause bleeding, perforation, stricture formation or obstruction. Barium studies and enteroscopy confirm the diagnosis.

22

22.58 Causes of small intestinal ulcers
• Idiopathic
• Inflammatory bowel disease, e.g. Crohn's
• Drugs, e.g. NSAIDs, enteric-coated potassium tablets
• Ulcerative jejuno-ileitis
• Lymphoma and carcinoma
• Infections, e.g. tuberculosis, typhoid, *Yersinia enterocolitica*
• Others, e.g. radiation, vasculitis

NSAID-associated small intestinal toxicity

These drugs cause a spectrum of small intestinal lesions ranging from erosions and ulcers to mucosal webs, strictures and, rarely, a condition known as 'diaphragm disease' in which intense submucosal fibrosis results in circumferential stricturing. The condition can present with pain, obstruction, bleeding or anaemia, and may mimic Crohn's disease, carcinoma or lymphoma. Enteroscopy or capsule endoscopy can reveal the diagnosis but sometimes this is only discovered at laparotomy.

Eosinophilic gastroenteritis

This disorder of unknown aetiology can affect any part of the gastrointestinal tract; it is characterised by eosinophil infiltration affecting the gut wall in the absence of parasitic infection or eosinophilia of other tissues. Peripheral blood eosinophilia is present in 80% of cases.

Clinical features

There are features of obstruction and inflammation, such as colicky pain, nausea and vomiting, diarrhoea and weight loss. Protein-losing enteropathy occurs and up to 50% of patients have a history of other allergic disorders. Serosal involvement may produce eosinophilic ascites.

Diagnosis and management

The diagnosis is made by histological assessment of multiple endoscopic biopsies, although full-thickness biopsies are occasionally required. Other investigations are performed to exclude parasitic infection and other causes of eosinophilia. A raised serum IgE concentration is often seen. Dietary manipulations are rarely effective, although elimination diets, especially of milk, may benefit a few patients. Severe symptoms are treated with prednisolone 20–40 mg daily and/or sodium cromoglicate, which stabilises mast cell membranes. The prognosis is good in the majority of patients.

Meckel's diverticulum

This is the most common congenital anomaly of the gastrointestinal tract and occurs in 0.3–3% of people. Most patients are asymptomatic. The diverticulum results from failure of closure of the vitelline duct, with persistence of a blind-ending sac arising from the antimesenteric border of the ileum; it usually occurs within 100 cm of the ileocaecal valve, and is up to 5 cm long. Approximately 50% contain ectopic gastric mucosa; rarely, colonic, pancreatic or endometrial tissue is present. Complications most commonly occur in the first 2 years of life but are occasionally seen in young adults. Bleeding results from ulceration of ileal mucosa adjacent to the ectopic parietal cells and presents as recurrent melaena or altered blood per rectum. Diagnosis can be made by scanning the abdomen using a gamma counter following an intravenous injection of ^{99m}Tc-pertechnate, which is concentrated by ectopic parietal cells. Other complications include intestinal obstruction, diverticulitis, intussusception and perforation. Intervention is unnecessary unless complications occur. The vast majority of patients remain asymptomatic throughout life.

Adverse food reactions

Adverse food reactions are common and are subdivided into food intolerance and food allergy, the former being much more common. In food intolerance there is an adverse reaction to food which is not immune-mediated and results from pharmacological (e.g. histamine, tyramine or monosodium glutamate), metabolic (e.g. lactase deficiency) or other mechanisms (e.g. toxins or chemical contaminants in food).

Lactose intolerance

Human milk contains around 200 mmol/L (68 g/L) of lactose which is normally digested to glucose and galactose by the brush border enzyme lactase prior to absorption. In most populations enterocyte lactase activity declines throughout childhood. The enzyme is deficient in up to 90% of adult Africans, Asians and South Americans, but only 5% of northern Europeans.

In cases of genetically determined (primary) lactase deficiency, jejunal morphology is normal. 'Secondary' lactase deficiency occurs as a consequence of disorders which damage the jejunal mucosa, such as coeliac disease and viral gastroenteritis. Unhydrolysed lactose enters the colon, where bacterial fermentation produces volatile short-chain fatty acids, hydrogen and carbon dioxide.

Clinical features

In most people lactase deficiency is completely asymptomatic. However, some complain of colicky pain, abdominal distension, increased flatus, borborygmi and diarrhoea after ingesting milk or milk products. Irritable bowel syndrome is often suspected but the diagnosis is suggested by clinical improvement on lactose withdrawal. The lactose hydrogen breath test is a useful non-invasive confirmatory investigation.

Dietary exclusion of lactose is recommended, although most sufferers are able to tolerate small amounts of milk without symptoms. Addition of commercial lactase preparations to milk has been effective in some studies but is costly.

Intolerance of other sugars

'Osmotic' diarrhoea can be caused by sorbitol, an unabsorbable carbohydrate which is used as an artificial sweetener. Fructose may also cause diarrhoea if consumed in greater quantities than can be absorbed (e.g. in fruit juices).

Food allergy

Food allergies are immune-mediated disorders, most commonly due to IgE antibodies and type I hypersensitivity reactions, although type IV delayed reactions are also seen. Up to 20% of the population perceive themselves as suffering from food allergy but only 1–2% of adults and 5–7% of children have genuine food allergies. The most common culprits are peanuts, milk, eggs, soya and shellfish.

Clinical manifestations occur immediately on exposure and range from trivial to life-threatening or even fatal anaphylaxis. The common 'oral allergy syndrome' results from contact with benzoic acid in certain fresh fruit juices leading to urticaria and angioedema of the lips and oropharynx. This is not, however, an immune-mediated reaction. 'Allergic gastroenteropathy' has features similar to eosinophilic gastroenteritis, while 'gastrointestinal anaphylaxis' consists of nausea, vomiting, diarrhoea and sometimes cardiovascular and respiratory collapse. Fatal reactions to trace amounts of peanuts are well documented.

The diagnosis of food allergy is difficult to prove or refute. Skin prick tests and measurements of antigen-specific IgE antibodies in serum have limited predictive value. Double-blind placebo-controlled food challenges are the gold standard, but are laborious and are not readily available. In many cases clinical suspicion and trials of elimination diets are used.

Treatment of proven food allergy consists of detailed patient education and awareness, strict elimination of the offending antigen, and in some cases antihistamines or sodium cromoglicate. Anaphylaxis should be treated as a medical emergency with resuscitation, airway support and intravenous adrenaline (epinephrine). Teachers and other carers of affected children should be trained to deal with this. Patients should wear an information bracelet and be taught to carry and use a preloaded adrenaline (epinephrine) syringe.

Infections of the small intestine

Travellers' diarrhoea, giardiasis and amoebiasis

See pages 306, 363 and 362.

Abdominal tuberculosis

Mycobacterium tuberculosis is a rare cause of abdominal disease in Caucasians but must be considered in people in and from the developing world and in AIDS patients. Gut infection usually results from human *M. tuberculosis* which is swallowed after coughing. Many patients have no pulmonary symptoms and a normal chest X-ray.

The area most commonly affected is the ileocaecal region; presentation and radiological findings may be very similar to those of Crohn's disease. Abdominal pain can be acute or of several months' duration, but diarrhoea is less common in tuberculosis than in Crohn's disease. Low-grade fever is common but not invariable. Like Crohn's disease, tuberculosis can affect any part of the gastrointestinal tract, and perianal disease with fistula is recognised. Peritoneal tuberculosis may result in peritonitis with exudative ascites, associated with abdominal pain and fever. Granulomatous hepatitis occurs.

Diagnosis

Abdominal tuberculosis causes an elevated ESR; a raised serum alkaline phosphatase concentration suggests hepatic involvement. Histological confirmation should be sought by endoscopy, laparoscopy or liver biopsy. Caseation of granulomas is not always seen and acid- and alcohol-fast bacteria are often scanty. Culture may be helpful but identification of the organism may take 6 weeks and diagnosis is now possible on biopsy specimens by PCR-based techniques.

Management

When the presentation is very suggestive of abdominal tuberculosis, chemotherapy with four drugs—isoniazid, rifampicin, pyrazinamide and ethambutol (p. 694)—should be commenced, even if bacteriological or histological proof is lacking.

Cryptosporidiosis

Cryptosporidiosis and other protozoal infections, including isosporiasis *(Isospora belli)* and microsporidiosis, are dealt with on pages 393–394.

Tumours of the small intestine

The small intestine is rarely affected by neoplasia, and fewer than 5% of all gastrointestinal tumours occur here.

Benign tumours

The most common are adenomas, GIST, lipomas and hamartomas. Adenomas are most often found in the periampullary region and are usually asymptomatic, although occult bleeding or obstruction due to intussusception may occur. Transformation to adenocarcinoma is rare. Multiple adenomas are common in the duodenum of patients with familial adenomatous polyposis (FAP), who merit regular endoscopic surveillance. Hamartomatous polyps with almost no malignant potential occur in Peutz–Jeghers syndrome (p. 909).

Malignant tumours

These are rare and include, in decreasing order of frequency, adenocarcinoma, carcinoid tumour, malignant GIST and lymphoma. The majority occur in middle age or later. Kaposi's sarcoma is seen in patients with AIDS.

Adenocarcinomas occur with increased frequency in patients with FAP, coeliac disease and Peutz–Jeghers syndrome. The non-specific presentation and rarity of these lesions often lead to delay in diagnosis. Barium follow-through examination or small bowel enema studies will demonstrate most lesions of this type. Enteroscopy, capsule endoscopy, mesenteric angiography and CT also play a role in investigation. Treatment is by surgical resection.

Carcinoid tumours

These are derived from enterochromaffin cells and are most common in the appendix. Localised spread and the potential for metastasis to the liver increase with primary lesions over 2 cm in diameter. Carcinoid tumours also occur in the rectum and in the appendix; those in the latter are usually benign. Overall, these tumours are less aggressive than carcinomas and their growth is usually slow.

The term 'carcinoid syndrome' refers to the systemic symptoms produced when secretory products of the neoplastic enterochromaffin cells reach the systemic circulation (Box 22.59). When produced by the primary tumour they are usually metabolised in the liver and do not reach the systemic circulation. The syndrome is therefore only seen when 5-HT, bradykinin and other peptide hormones are released by hepatic metastases.

Management

The treatment of a carcinoid tumour is surgical resection. The treatment of carcinoid syndrome is palliative because hepatic metastases have occurred, although prolonged survival is common. Surgical removal of the primary tumour is usually attempted and the hepatic metastases can be excised as reduction of tumour mass improves symptoms. Hepatic artery embolisation retards growth of hepatic deposits. Octreotide 200 μg 8-hourly by subcutaneous injection is used to reduce tumour release of secretagogues. Cytotoxic chemotherapy has only a minor role.

22.59 Clinical features of carcinoid tumours*

- Small-bowel obstruction due to the tumour mass
- Intestinal ischaemia (due to mesenteric infiltration or vasospasm)
- Hepatic metastases causing pain, hepatomegaly and jaundice
- Flushing and wheezing
- Diarrhoea
- Cardiac involvement (tricuspid regurgitation, pulmonary stenosis, right ventricular endocardial plaques) leading to heart failure
- Facial telangiectasia

*The diagnosis is made by detecting excess levels of the 5-HT metabolite, 5-HIAA, in a 24-hour urine collection.

22

Lymphoma

Non-Hodgkin lymphoma (p. 1039) may involve the gastrointestinal tract as part of more generalised disease or may rarely arise in the gut, with the small intestine being most commonly affected. Lymphomas occur with increased frequency in patients with coeliac disease, AIDS and other immunodeficiency states. Most are of B-cell origin, although lymphoma associated with coeliac disease is derived from T cells (enteropathy-associated T-cell lymphoma).

Colicky abdominal pain, obstruction and weight loss are the usual presenting features, and perforation is also occasionally seen. Malabsorption is only a feature of diffuse bowel involvement and hepatosplenomegaly is rare.

The diagnosis is made by small bowel biopsy, radiological contrast studies and CT. Staging investigations are performed. Surgical resection where possible is the treatment of choice, with radiotherapy and combination chemotherapy reserved for those with advanced disease. The prognosis depends largely on the stage at diagnosis, cell type, patient age and the presence of 'B' symptoms (fever, weight loss, night sweats).

Immunoproliferative small intestinal disease (IPSID)

Also known as 'alpha heavy chain disease', this rare condition occurs mainly in the Mediterranean, Middle East, India and Pakistan, and North America. The aetiology is unknown but it may be a response to chronic stimulation by bacterial antigens. The condition varies in severity from relatively benign to frankly malignant.

The small intestinal mucosa is diffusely affected, especially proximally, by a dense lymphoplasmacytic infiltrate. Enlarged mesenteric lymph nodes are also common. Most patients are young adults who present with malabsorption, anorexia and fever. Serum electrophoresis confirms the presence of alpha heavy chains (from the F_c portion of IgA). Prolonged remissions can be obtained with long-term antibiotic therapy, but chemotherapy is required for those who fail to respond or who have aggressive disease.

DISEASES OF THE PANCREAS

Acute pancreatitis

Acute pancreatitis accounts for 3% of all cases of abdominal pain admitted to hospital. It affects 2–28 per 100 000 of the population and may be increasing in incidence. Despite recent advances in management, mortality has remained unchanged at 10%. About 80% of all cases are mild with a mortality of less than 5%; 98% of deaths occur in the 20% of severe cases. One-third occur within the first week, usually from multi-organ failure. After this time the majority of deaths result from sepsis, especially that complicating infected necrosis. At admission it is possible to predict patients at risk of these complications (Box 22.60). Patients with predicted or actual severe pancreatitis (Box 22.61), those with necrosis or other complications should be managed in a specialist centre with an intensive therapy unit and multidisciplinary hepatobiliary specialists.

22.60 Adverse prognostic factors in acute pancreatitis (Glasgow criteria)*

- Age > 55 years
- PO_2 < 8 kPa (60 mmHg)
- White blood cell count (WBC) > 15 × 10⁹/L
- Albumin < 32 g/L
- Serum calcium < 2 mmol/L (8 mg/dL) (corrected)
- Glucose > 10 mmol/L (180 mg/dL)
- Urea > 16 mmol/L (45 mg/dL) (after rehydration)
- Alanine aminotransferase (ALT) > 200 U/L
- Lactate dehydrogenase (LDH) > 600 U/L

*Severity and prognosis worsen as the number of these factors increases. More than three implies severe disease.

22.61 Factors that may predict severe pancreatitis within 48 hours of admission

Initial assessment

- Clinical impression of severity
- Body mass index > 30
- Pleural effusion on chest X-ray
- APACHE II score > 8

24 hrs after admission

- Clinical impression of severity
- APACHE II score > 8
- Glasgow score ≥ 3
- Persisting organ failure, especially if multiple
- CRP > 150 mg/L

48 hrs after admission

- Clinical impression of severity
- Glasgow score ≥ 3
- CRP > 150 mg/L
- Persisting organ failure for 48 hrs
- Multiple or progressive organ failure

Pathophysiology

Acute pancreatitis occurs as a consequence of premature activation of zymogen granules, releasing proteases which digest the pancreas and surrounding tissue (Fig. 22.42). The normal pancreas has only a poorly developed capsule, and adjacent structures, including the common bile duct, duodenum, splenic vein and transverse colon, are commonly involved in the inflammatory process. The severity of acute pancreatitis is dependent upon the balance between activity of released proteolytic enzymes and antiproteolytic factors. The latter comprise an intracellular pancreatic trypsin inhibitor protein and circulating β_2-macroglobulin, α_1-antitrypsin and Cl-esterase inhibitors. Causes of acute pancreatitis are given in Box 22.62. Acute pancreatitis is often self-limiting. In some patients, however, it is severe, with local complications such as necrosis, pseudocyst or abscess, and systemic complications leading to multi-organ failure.

Clinical features

Severe, constant upper abdominal pain which radiates to the back in 65% of cases builds up over 15–60 minutes. Nausea and vomiting are common. There is marked epigastric tenderness, but in the early stages (and in contrast to a perforated peptic ulcer) guarding and rebound tenderness are absent because the inflammation is principally retroperitoneal. Bowel sounds become quiet

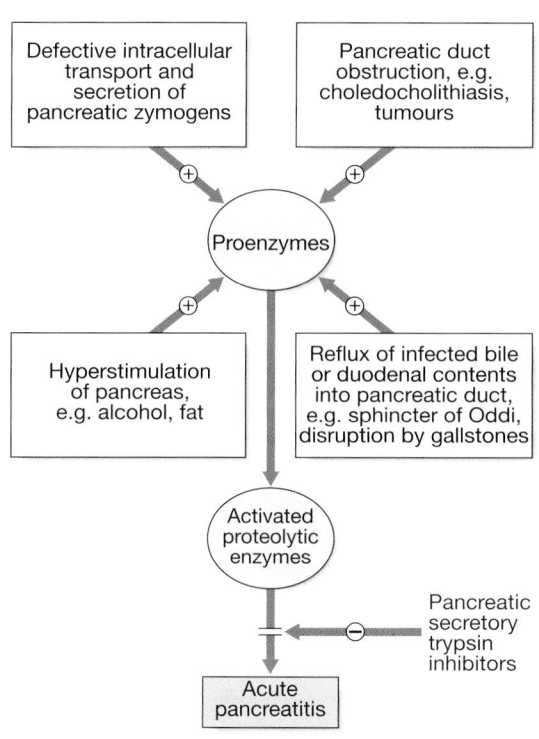

Fig. 22.42 **Pathophysiology of acute pancreatitis.**

22.62 Causes of acute pancreatitis

Common (90% of cases)

- Gallstones
- Alcohol
- Idiopathic
- Post-ERCP

Rare

- Post-surgical (abdominal, cardiopulmonary bypass)
- Trauma
- Drugs (azathioprine, thiazide diuretics, sodium valproate)
- Metabolic (hypercalcaemia, hypertriglyceridaemia)
- Pancreas divisum (p. 893)
- Sphincter of Oddi dysfunction
- Infection (mumps, Coxsackie virus)
- Hereditary
- Renal failure
- Organ transplantation (kidney, liver)
- Severe hypothermia
- Petrochemical exposure

22.63 Complications of acute pancreatitis

Complication	Cause
Systemic	
Systemic inflammatory response syndrome (SIRS)	Increased vascular permeability from cytokine, platelet aggregating factor and kinin release
Hypoxia	Acute respiratory distress syndrome (ARDS) due to microthrombi in pulmonary vessels
Hyperglycaemia	Disruption of islets of Langerhans with altered insulin/glucagon release
Hypocalcaemia	Sequestration of calcium in fat necrosis, fall in ionised calcium
Reduced serum albumin concentration	Increased capillary permeability
Pancreatic	
Necrosis	Non-viable pancreatic tissue and peripancreatic tissue death; frequently infected
Abscess	Circumscribed collection of pus close to the pancreas and containing little or no pancreatic necrotic tissue
Pseudocyst	Disruption of pancreatic ducts
Pancreatic ascites or pleural effusion	Disruption of pancreatic ducts
Gastrointestinal	
Upper gastrointestinal bleeding	Gastric or duodenal erosions
Variceal haemorrhage	Splenic or portal vein thrombosis
Erosion into colon	
Duodenal obstruction	Compression by pancreatic mass
Obstructive jaundice	Compression of common bile duct

22

or absent as paralytic ileus develops. In severe cases the patient becomes hypoxic and develops hypovolaemic shock with oliguria. Discoloration of the flanks (Grey Turner's sign) or the periumbilical region (Cullen's sign) is a feature of severe pancreatitis with haemorrhage. The differential diagnosis includes a perforated viscus, acute cholecystitis and myocardial infarction. Various complications may occur and these are listed in Box 22.63. An acute pancreatic pseudocyst is a localised peripancreatic collection of pancreatic juice and debris which usually develops in the lesser sac following inflammatory rupture of the pancreatic duct. The pseudocyst is initially contained within a poorly defined, fragile wall of granulation tissue which matures over a 6-week period to form a fibrous capsule (Fig. 22.43). Small intrapancreatic cysts

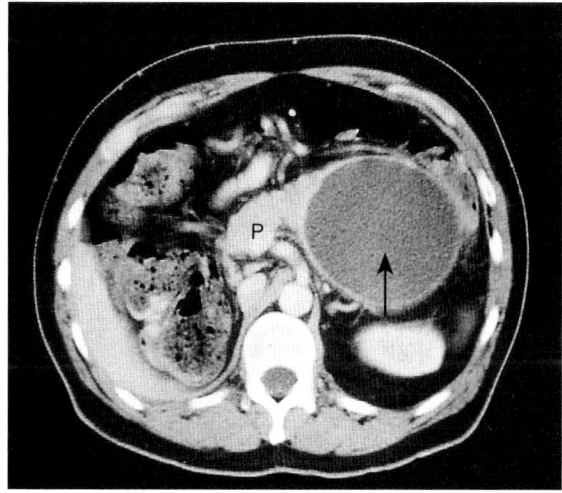

Fig. 22.43 **CT showing large pancreatic pseudocyst (arrow) developing from the body of the pancreas (P).**

and pseudocysts are common and resolve as the pancreatitis recovers, but those greater than 6 cm seldom disappear spontaneously and can cause abdominal pain and may compress or erode surrounding structures including blood vessels to form pseudoaneurysms. Pancreatic ascites occurs when fluid leaks from a disrupted pancreatic duct into the peritoneal cavity. Leakage into the thoracic cavity can result in a pleural effusion or a pleuro-pancreatic fistula.

Investigations

The diagnosis of acute pancreatitis is based upon finding raised serum amylase or lipase concentrations and ultrasound or CT evidence of pancreatic swelling. Plain X-rays are taken to exclude other diagnoses such as perforation or obstruction and to identify pulmonary complications. Amylase is efficiently excreted by the kidneys, and concentrations may have returned to normal if measured 24–48 hours after the onset of pancreatitis. In this situation the diagnosis can be made by demonstrating an elevated urinary amylase:creatinine ratio. A persistently elevated serum amylase concentration suggests pseudocyst formation. Peritoneal amylase concentrations are massively elevated in pancreatic ascites. Serum amylase concentrations are also elevated (but less so) in intestinal ischaemia, perforated peptic ulcer and ruptured ovarian cyst, whilst the salivary isoenzyme of amylase is elevated in parotitis. If available, serum lipase measurements are preferable to amylase as they have greater diagnostic accuracy for acute pancreatitis.

Ultrasound scanning confirms the diagnosis, although in the earlier stages the gland may not be grossly swollen. The ultrasound scan is also useful because it may show gallstones, biliary obstruction or pseudocyst formation.

Contrast-enhanced pancreatic CT 6–10 days after admission is used to define the viability of the pancreas if persisting organ failure, sepsis or clinical deterioration is present, as these may indicate pancreatic necrosis. Necrotising pancreatitis is associated with decreased pancreatic enhancement following intravenous injection of contrast material. The presence of gas within necrotic material (Fig. 22.44) suggests infection and impending abscess formation, in which case percutaneous aspira-

tion of material for bacterial culture should be carried out and appropriate antibiotics prescribed. Involvement of the colon, blood vessels and other adjacent structures by the inflammatory process is best seen by CT.

Certain investigations stratify the severity of acute pancreatitis and have important prognostic value at the time of presentation (Box 22.64). In addition, serial assessment of C-reactive protein (CRP) is a useful indicator of progress. A peak CRP > 210 mg/L in the first 4 days predicts severe acute pancreatitis with 80% accuracy. It is worth noting that the serum amylase concentration has no prognostic value.

Management

Management of acute pancreatitis comprises several related steps:
- establishing the diagnosis and stratifying disease severity
- early treatment (resuscitation) according to whether the disease is mild or severe
- detection and treatment of complications
- treating the underlying cause—specifically gallstones.

The initial management is based upon analgesia using pethidine and correction of hypovolaemia using normal saline and/or colloids. All severe cases should be managed in a high-dependency or intensive care unit. A central venous line or Swan–Ganz catheter and urinary catheter are used to monitor patients with shock. Hypoxic patients need oxygen and patients who develop acute respiratory distress syndrome (ARDS) may require ventilatory support. Hyperglycaemia is corrected using insulin, but it is not necessary to correct hypocalcaemia by intravenous calcium injection unless tetany occurs.

Nasogastric aspiration is only necessary if paralytic ileus is present. Enteral feeding, if tolerated, should be started at an early stage in patients with severe pancreatitis because they are in a severely catabolic state and need nutritional support (Box 22.65). In addition enteral feeding decreases endotoxaemia and thereby may

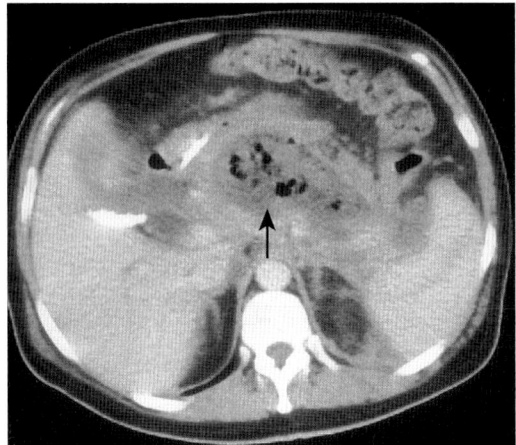

Fig. 22.44 Pancreatic necrosis. Lack of vascular enhancement of the pancreas during contrast-enhanced CT indicates necrosis (arrow). The presence of gas suggests infection has occurred.

EBM 22.64 **ERCP in acute pancreatitis**

'In patients with actual or predicted severe pancreatitis of suspected biliary origin, emergency ERCP with biliary sphincterotomy improves outcome and is best undertaken within 72 hours of onset. Greatest benefit occurs in those patients who have ascending cholangitis.'

- UK Working Party on Acute Pancreatitis. Gut 2005; 54(Suppl III):iii1–iii9.

For further information: www.bsg.org.uk

EBM 22.65 **Nutritional support in acute pancreatitis**

'Nutritional support is not necessary in all patients with severe pancreatitis. If it is required, the enteral route (if tolerated) is superior to parenteral feeding, and the nasogastric route can be used as it appears to be effective in 80% of cases.'

- UK Working Party on Acute Pancreatitis. Gut 2005;54(Suppl III):iii1–iii9

For further information: www.bsg.org.uk

reduce systemic complications. Nasogastric feeding is just as effective as the nasojejunal route. Prophylaxis of thromboembolism with low-dose subcutaneous heparin is also advisable. The use of prophylactic, broad-spectrum intravenous antibiotics such as imipenem or cefuroxime to prevent infection of pancreatic necrosis is controversial but they are often given.

Patients who present with cholangitis or jaundice in association with severe acute pancreatitis should undergo urgent ERCP to diagnose and treat choledocholithiasis. In less severe cases of gallstone pancreatitis, biliary imaging (using MRCP or EUS) can be carried out after the acute phase has resolved. If the liver function tests return to normal and ultrasound has not demonstrated a dilated biliary tree, laparoscopic cholecystectomy with an on-table cholangiogram is appropriate because any common bile duct stones have probably passed. When the operative cholangiogram detects residual common bile duct stones, these are removed by laparoscopic exploration of the duct or by post-operative ERCP. Cholecystectomy should be undertaken within 2 weeks following resolution of pancreatitis—and preferably during the same admission—to prevent further potentially fatal attacks of pancreatitis. Patients who have developed necrotising pancreatitis or pancreatic abscess require urgent endoscopic or surgical necrosectomy to débride all cavities of necrotic material. Pancreatic pseudocysts are treated by drainage into the stomach, duodenum or jejunum (Roux en Y). This is usually performed after an interval of at least 6 weeks, once a pseudocapsule has matured, using open surgery or endoscopic methods.

Chronic pancreatitis

Chronic pancreatitis is a chronic inflammatory disease characterised by fibrosis and destruction of exocrine pancreatic tissue. Diabetes mellitus occurs in advanced cases because the islets of Langerhans are involved.

22.66 Causes of chronic pancreatitis ('TIGAR-O')

Toxic-metabolic

- Alcohol
- Tobacco
- Hypercalcaemia
- Chronic renal failure

Idiopathic

- Tropical
- Early/late onset types

Genetic

- Hereditary pancreatitis (cationic trypsinogen mutation)
- *SPINK-1* mutation
- Cystic fbrosis

Autoimmune

- Isolated or as part of multi-organ problem

Recurrent and severe acute pancreatitis

- Post-necrotic
- Recurrent acute pancreatitis

Obstructive

- Ductal adenocarcinoma
- Intraductal papillary mucinous neoplasia
- Pancreas divisum
- Sphincter of Oddi stenosis

N.B. Many patients have gallstones but these do not cause chronic pancreatitis.

Pathophysiology

Around 80% of cases in Western countries result from alcohol misuse. In southern India severe chronic calcific pancreatitis occurs in non-alcoholics, possibly as a result of malnutrition and cassava consumption. Other causes are listed in Box 22.66. The pathophysiology of chronic pancreatitis is shown in Figure 22.45.

Clinical features

Chronic pancreatitis predominantly affects middle-aged alcoholic men. Almost all present with abdominal pain. In

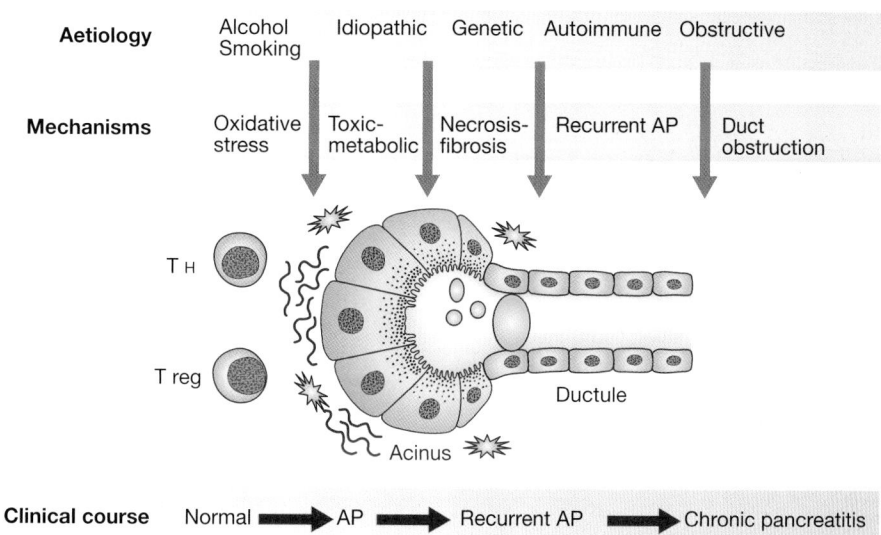

Fig. 22.45 Pathophysiology of chronic pancreatitis. Alcohol and other risk factors may trigger acute pancreatitis (AP) through multiple mechanisms. The first (or 'sentinel') episode of acute pancreatitis initiates an inflammatory response involving T-helper cells. Ongoing exposure to alcohol drives further inflammation but this is modified by regulatory T cells with subsequent fibrosis, via activation of pancreatic stellate cells. A cycle of inflammation and fibrosis ensues, with development of chronic pancreatitis. Alcohol is the most relevant risk factor as it is involved at multiple steps.

22

50% this occurs as episodes of 'acute pancreatitis', although each attack results in a degree of permanent pancreatic damage. Relentless, slowly progressive chronic pain without acute exacerbations affects 35% of patients, whilst the remainder have no pain but present with diarrhoea. Pain is due to a combination of increased pressure within the pancreatic ducts and direct involvement of pancreatic and peripancreatic nerves by the inflammatory process. Pain may be relieved by leaning forwards or by drinking alcohol. Approximately one-fifth of patients chronically consume opiate analgesics. Weight loss is common and results from a combination of anorexia, avoidance of food because of post-prandial pain, malabsorption and/or diabetes. Steatorrhoea occurs when more than 90% of the exocrine tissue has been destroyed; protein malabsorption only develops in the most advanced cases. Overall, 30% of patients are diabetic, but this figure rises to 70% in those with chronic calcific pancreatitis. Physical examination reveals a thin, malnourished patient with epigastric tenderness. Skin pigmentation over the abdomen and back is common and results from chronic use of a hot water bottle (erythema ab igne). Many patients have features of other alcohol- and smoking-related diseases. Complications are listed in Box 22.67.

Investigations

Investigations (Box 22.68 and Fig. 22.46) are carried out to:

- make a diagnosis of chronic pancreatitis
- define pancreatic function
- demonstrate anatomical abnormalities prior to surgical intervention.

22.67 Complications of chronic pancreatitis

- Pseudocysts and pancreatic ascites, which occur in both acute and chronic pancreatitis
- Extrahepatic obstructive jaundice due to a benign stricture of the common bile duct as it passes through the diseased pancreas
- Duodenal stenosis
- Portal or splenic vein thrombosis leading to segmental portal hypertension and gastric varices
- Peptic ulcer

22.68 Investigations in chronic pancreatitis

Tests to establish the diagnosis

- Ultrasound
- CT (may show atrophy, calcification or ductal dilatation)
- Abdominal X-ray (may show calcification)
- MRCP
- Endoscopic ultrasound

Tests of pancreatic function

- Collection of pure pancreatic juice after secretin injection (gold standard but invasive and seldom used)
- Pancreolauryl or PABA test (Box 22.12, p. 850)
- Faecal pancreatic elastase

Tests of anatomy prior to surgery

- MRCP

Management

Alcohol misuse

Alcohol avoidance is crucial in halting the progression of the disease and reducing pain.

Pain relief

A range of analgesic drugs, particularly NSAIDs, are valuable, but the severe and unremitting nature of the pain often leads to opiate use with the risk of addiction. Oral pancreatic enzyme supplements suppress pancreatic secretion and their regular use reduces analgesic consumption in some patients. Patients who are abstinent from alcohol and who have severe chronic pain which is resistant to conservative measures are considered for surgical or endoscopic pancreatic therapy (Box 22.69). Coeliac plexus neurolysis or minimally invasive thoracoscopic splanchnicectomy sometimes produces long-lasting pain relief, although relapse eventually occurs in the majority of cases. In some patients MRCP does not show a surgically or endoscopically correctable abnormality and in these patients the only surgical approach is total pancreatectomy. Unfortunately, even after this operation, some patients will continue to experience pain. Moreover, the procedure causes diabetes which may be difficult to control, with a high risk of

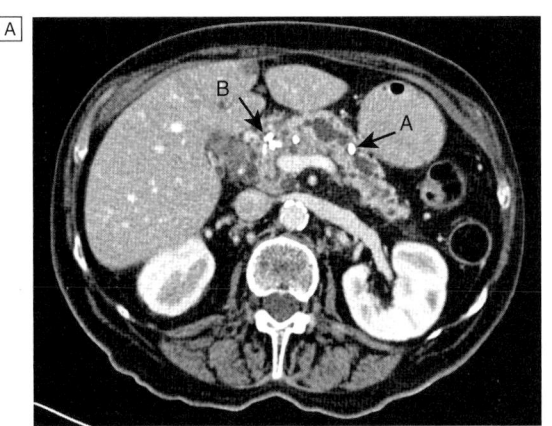
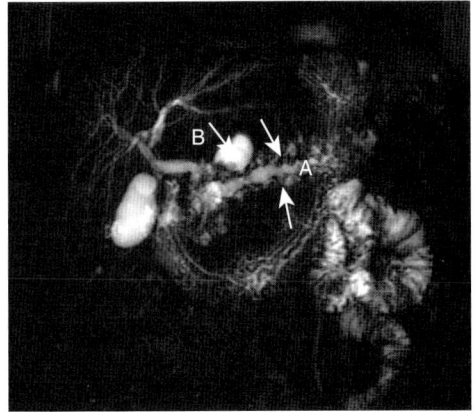

Fig. 22.46 Imaging in chronic pancreatitis. **A** CT scan showing a grossly dilated and irregular duct with a calcified stone (arrow A). Note the calcification in the head of the gland (arrow B). **B** MRCP of the same patient showing marked ductal dilatation with abnormal dilated side branches (arrows A). A small cyst is also present (arrow B).

22.69 Intervention in chronic pancreatitis

Endoscopic therapy

- Dilatation or stenting of pancreatic duct strictures
- Removal of calculi (mechanical or shock-wave lithotripsy)
- Drainage of pseudocysts

Surgical methods

- Partial pancreatic resection, preserving the duodenum
- Pancreatico-jejunostomy

hypoglycaemia (since both insulin and glucagon release are absent), and significant morbidity and mortality.

Malabsorption

This is treated by dietary fat restriction (with supplementary medium-chain triglyceride therapy in malnourished patients) and oral pancreatic enzyme supplements. A PPI is added to optimise duodenal pH for pancreatic enzyme activity.

Management of complications

Surgical or endoscopic therapy may be necessary for the management of pseudocysts, pancreatic ascites, common bile duct or duodenal stricture and the consequences of portal hypertension. Many patients with chronic pancreatitis also require treatment for other alcohol- and smoking-related diseases and for the consequences of self-neglect and malnutrition.

Autoimmune pancreatitis (AIP)

This is a form of chronic pancreatitis that can mimic cancer but which responds to corticosteroids. AIP is characterised by abdominal pain, weight loss or obstructive jaundice, without acute attacks of pancreatitis. Blood tests reveal increased serum immunoglobulin G (IgG) or IgG4, and the presence of other autoantibodies. Imaging shows a diffusely enlarged pancreas, narrowing of the pancreatic duct and stricturing of the lower bile duct on ERCP. AIP may occur alone or in association with other autoimmune disorders such as Sjögren's syndrome, primary sclerosing cholangitis (PSC) or inflammatory bowel disease. The response to steroids is usually excellent but some patients require azathioprine.

Congenital abnormalities of the pancreas

Pancreas divisum

This is due to failure of the primitive dorsal and ventral ducts to fuse during embryonic development of the pancreas. As a consequence, most of the pancreatic drainage occurs through the smaller accessory ampulla rather than through the major ampulla. The condition occurs in 7–10% of the normal population and is usually asymptomatic, but some patients develop acute pancreatitis, chronic pancreatitis or atypical abdominal pain.

Annular pancreas

In this congenital anomaly, the pancreas encircles the second/third part of the duodenum, leading to gastric outlet obstruction. Annular pancreas is associated with malrotation of the intestine, atresias and cardiac anomalies.

Cystic fibrosis

This disease is considered in detail on page 678. The major gastrointestinal manifestations of cystic fibrosis are pancreatic insufficiency and meconium ileus. Peptic ulcer, and hepatic and biliary disease also occur. In cystic fibrosis pancreatic secretions are protein- and mucus-rich. The resultant viscous juice forms plugs which obstruct the pancreatic ductules, leading to progressive destruction of acinar cells. Steatorrhoea is universal and the large-volume bulky stools predispose to rectal prolapse. Malnutrition is compounded by the metabolic demands of respiratory failure and by diabetes which develops in 40% of patients by adolescence.

The majority of patients now survive well into adulthood and heart/lung transplantation can further prolong life. Optimal treatment of the cystic fibrosis patient depends upon an assiduous team approach to respiratory, nutritional and hepatobiliary complications. Nutritional counselling and supervision are important to ensure intake of high-energy foods, providing 120–150% of the recommended intake for normal subjects. Fats are an important calorie source and, despite the presence of steatorrhoea, fat intake should not be restricted. Supplementary fat-soluble vitamins are also necessary. High-dose oral pancreatic enzymes are required, in doses sufficient to control steatorrhoea and stool frequency. A PPI aids fat digestion by producing an optimal duodenal pH. Diabetic patients usually require insulin injections rather than oral hypoglycaemic agents.

Meconium ileus

Mucus-rich plugs within intestinal contents can obstruct the small or large intestine. Meconium ileus is treated by the mucolytic agent N-acetylcysteine given orally, by gastrografin enema or by gut lavage using polyethylene glycol. In resistant cases of meconium ileus surgical resection may be necessary.

Tumours of the pancreas

Pancreatic carcinoma affects 10–15 per 100 000 in Western populations, rising to 100 per 100 000 in those over the age of 70. Men are affected twice as often as women. The disease is associated with increasing age, smoking and chronic pancreatitis. Between 5 and 10% of patients have a genetic predisposition (hereditary pancreatitis, MEN, hereditary non-polyposis colon cancer (HNPCC) and familial atypical mole multiple melanoma syndrome (FAMMM)). Overall survival is only 3–5% with median survival of 6–10 months for those with locally advanced disease and 3–5 months if metastases are present.

Pathophysiology

Approximately 90% of pancreatic neoplasms are adenocarcinomas which arise from the pancreatic ducts. These tumours involve local structures and metastasise to regional lymph nodes at an early stage. The majority of patients have advanced disease at the time of presentation.

22

Clinical features

The clinical features of pancreatic cancer are pain, weight loss and obstructive jaundice (Fig. 22.47). The pain results from invasion of the coeliac plexus and is characteristically incessant and boring. It often radiates from the upper abdomen through to the back and may be eased a little by bending forwards. Almost all patients lose weight and many are cachectic. Around 60% of tumours arise from the head of the pancreas, and involvement of the common bile duct results in the development of obstructive jaundice, often with severe pruritus. A few patients present with diarrhoea, vomiting from duodenal obstruction, diabetes mellitus, recurrent venous thrombosis, acute pancreatitis or depression. Physical examination reveals clear evidence of weight loss. An abdominal mass due to the tumour itself, a palpable gallbladder or hepatic metastasis is commonly found. A palpable gallbladder in a jaundiced patient is usually the consequence of distal biliary obstruction by a pancreatic cancer (Courvoisier's sign).

Investigations

When a patient presents with biochemically confirmed obstructive jaundice, the diagnosis is usually made by ultrasound and contrast-enhanced CT (Fig. 22.48). Diagnosis in non-jaundiced patients is often delayed because presenting symptoms are relatively non-specific. Fit patients with small localised tumours should undergo staging to define operability. EUS or laparoscopy with laparoscopic ultrasound will define tumour size, involvement of blood vessels and metastatic spread. In patients unsuitable for surgery because of advanced disease, frailty or comorbidity, endoscopic ultrasound (EUS) or CT-guided cytology or biopsy may be used to confirm the diagnosis. MRCP and ERCP are sensitive methods of diagnosing pancreatic cancer and are valuable when the diagnosis is in doubt, although differentiation between cancer and localised chronic pancreatitis can be difficult. The main role of ERCP is to insert a stent into the common bile duct to relieve obstructive jaundice in inoperable patients.

Management

Surgical resection is the only method of effecting cure, and 5-year survival in patients undergoing a complete resection is around 12%. Recent trials have demonstrated improved survival (21–29%) with adjuvant chemotherapy using 5-fluorouracil and folinic acid or gemcitabine.

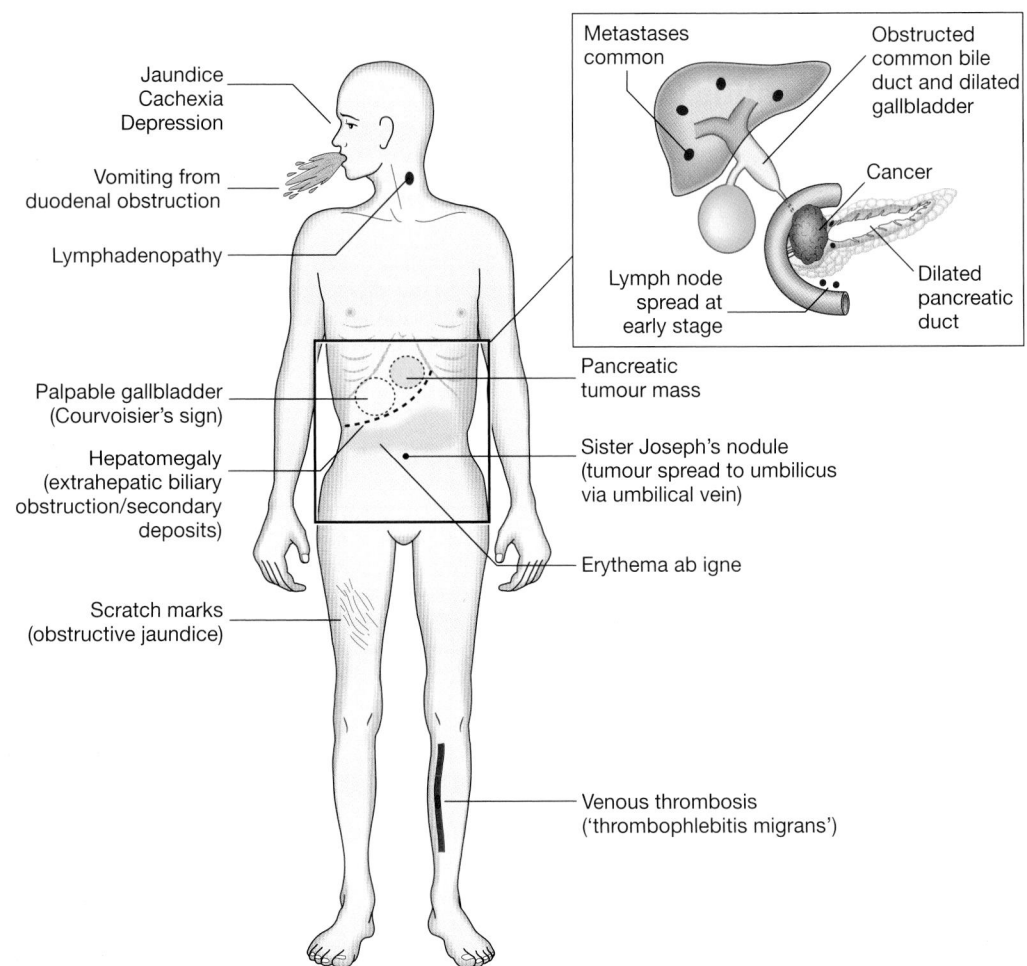

Jaundice
Cachexia
Depression

Vomiting from
duodenal obstruction

Lymphadenopathy

Palpable gallbladder
(Courvoisier's sign)

Hepatomegaly
(extrahepatic biliary
obstruction/secondary
deposits)

Scratch marks
(obstructive jaundice)

Metastases
common

Obstructed
common bile
duct and dilated
gallbladder

Cancer

Lymph node
spread at
early stage

Dilated
pancreatic
duct

Pancreatic
tumour mass

Sister Joseph's nodule
(tumour spread to umbilicus
via umbilical vein)

Erythema ab igne

Venous thrombosis
('thrombophlebitis migrans')

Fig. 22.47 Features of pancreatic cancer.

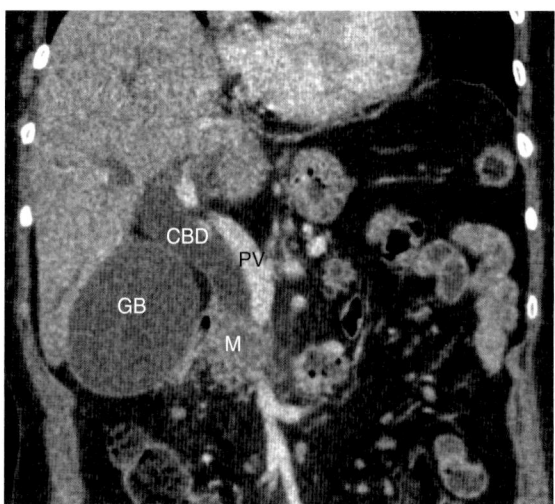

Fig. 22.48 Carcinoma of the pancreatic head. A large mass (M) in the head of pancreas involves the portal vein (PV) and obstructs the common bile duct (CBD). (GB = gallbladder)

Unfortunately, a mere 10–15% of tumours are amenable to curative resection since most neoplasms are locally advanced at the time of diagnosis. For the great majority of patients treatment is palliative. Pain relief is achieved using analgesic drugs and, in some patients, coeliac plexus neurolysis by a percutaneous or EUS-guided alcohol injection. Jaundice is relieved by choledochojejunostomy in fit patients; percutaneous or endoscopic stenting is used in the elderly or in patients who have very advanced disease. Ampullary or periampullary adenocarcinomas are rare neoplasms which arise from the ampulla of Vater or adjacent duodenum. They are often polypoid and may ulcerate; they frequently infiltrate the duodenum but behave less aggressively than pancreatic adenocarcinoma. Around 25% of patients undergoing resection of ampullary or periampullary tumours survive for 5 years in contrast to patients with pancreatic ductal cancer.

Cystic neoplasms of the pancreas are increasingly being seen with widespread use of CT. These are a heterogeneous group; serous cystadenomas rarely, if ever, become malignant and do not require surgery. Mucinous cysts occur more often in women, are usually in the pancreatic head and display a spectrum of behaviour from benign to borderline to frankly malignant. EUS with aspiration of cyst contents for cytology and measurement of carcinoembryonic antigen (CEA) and amylase concentrations can help determine whether a lesion is mucinous or not. In fit patients, all mucinous lesions should be resected. A variant, called intraductal papillary mucinous neoplasia (IPMN) is often discovered coincidentally on CT, often in elderly men. IPMN may affect the main pancreatic duct with marked dilatation and plugs of mucus, or may affect a side-branch. The histology varies from villous adenomatous change to dysplasia to carcinoma. IPMN is premalignant but indolent, and the decision to resect or to monitor depends on many factors, including age and fitness of the patient and location, size and evolution of lesions.

Endocrine tumours

These arise from neuroendocrine tissue within the pancreas and can occur in association with parathyroid and pituitary adenomas (MEN 1, p. 793). The majority of endocrine tumours are non-secretory and, although malignant, grow slowly and metastasise late. Other tumours secrete hormones and present because of their endocrine effects (see Box 20.52, p. 782). Neuroendocrine pancreatic tumours may be single, but are frequently multifocal and arise from other clusters of neuroendocrine cells derived from neural crest tissues. They are localised by CT and endoscopic ultrasound. ^{111}In-labelled DTPA is very sensitive in the diagnosis of glucagonoma.

INFLAMMATORY BOWEL DISEASE

Ulcerative colitis and Crohn's disease are chronic inflammatory bowel diseases which pursue a protracted relapsing and remitting course, usually extending over years. The diseases have many similarities and it is sometimes impossible to differentiate between them. A crucial distinction is that ulcerative colitis only involves the colon, while Crohn's disease can involve any part of the gastrointestinal tract from mouth to anus. A summary of the main features of ulcerative colitis and Crohn's disease is provided in Box 22.70.

22.70 Comparison of ulcerative colitis and Crohn's disease

	Ulcerative colitis	Crohn's disease
Age group	Any	Any
Gender	M = F	M = F
Ethnic group	Any	Any; more common in Ashkenazi Jews
Genetic factors	HLA-DR103 associated with severe disease	CARD 15/NOD-2 mutations predispose
Risk factors	More common in non-/ex-smokers Appendicectomy protects	More common in smokers
Anatomical distribution	Colon only; begins at anorectal margin with variable proximal extension	Any part of gastrointestinal tract; perianal disease common; patchy distribution—'skip lesions'
Extraintestinal manifestations	Common	Common
Presentation	Bloody diarrhoea	Variable; pain, diarrhoea, weight loss all common
Histology	Inflammation limited to mucosa; crypt distortion, cryptitis, crypt abscesses, loss of goblet cells	Submucosal or transmural inflammation common; deep fissuring ulcers, fistulas; patchy changes; granulomas
Management	5-ASA; corticosteroids; azathioprine; colectomy is curative	Corticosteroids; azathioprine; methotrexate; biologic therapy (anti-TNF); nutritional therapy; surgery for complications is not curative

22

The incidence of inflammatory bowel disease (IBD) varies widely between populations. Crohn's disease appears to be very rare in the developing world yet ulcerative colitis, although still unusual, is becoming more common. In the West, the incidence of ulcerative colitis is stable at 10–20 per 100 000, with a prevalence of 100–200 per 100 000, while the incidence of Crohn's disease is increasing and is now 5–10 per 100 000, with a prevalence of 50–100 per 100 000. Both diseases most commonly start in young adults, with a second smaller incidence peak in the seventh decade. Approximately 240 000 people are affected by IBD in the UK. Life expectancy in patients with IBD is similar to that of the general population. Although many patients require surgery and admission to hospital for other reasons, the majority have an excellent work record and pursue a normal life. Around 90% of ulcerative colitis patients have intermittent disease activity, whilst 10% have continuous symptoms.

Pathophysiology

It is thought that IBD develops because of an abnormal host response to an environmental trigger in genetically susceptible individuals (Box 22.71). This causes inflammation of the intestine and release of inflammatory mediators, such as TNF, IL-12 and IL-23, which cause tissue damage. These mediators are targets for therapeutic intervention (Fig. 22.49). In both diseases the intestinal wall is infiltrated with acute and chronic inflammatory cells. There are important differences in the distribution of disease and in histological features (Fig. 22.50).

Ulcerative colitis

Inflammation invariably involves the rectum (proctitis) but can spread to involve the sigmoid colon (proctosigmoiditis) or the whole colon (pancolitis). Inflammation is confluent and is more severe distally. In long-standing pancolitis the bowel can become shortened and 'pseudopolyps' develop which are normal or hypertrophied residual mucosa within areas of atrophy. The inflammatory process

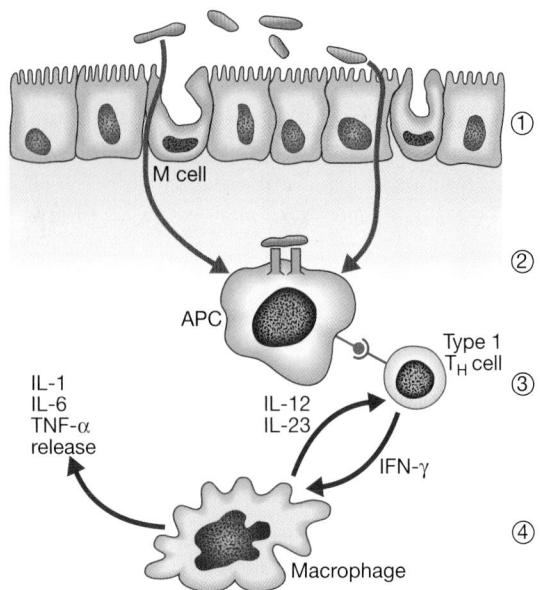

Fig. 22.49 Pathogenesis of inflammatory bowel disease.
(1) Bacterial antigens are taken up by specialised M cells, pass between leaky epithelial cells or enter the lamina propria through ulcerated mucosa. (2) After processing they are presented to type 1 T-helper cells by antigen-presenting cells (APC) in the lamina propria. (3) T-cell activation and differentiation results in a Th_1 T cell-mediated cytokine response (4) with secretion of cytokines including gamma interferon (IFN-γ). Further amplification of T cells perpetuates the inflammatory process with activation of non-immune cells and release of other important cytokines, e.g. interleukin (IL)-12, IL-23, IL-1, IL-6 and tumour necrosis factor (TNF). These pathways occur in all normal individuals exposed to an inflammatory insult and this is self-limiting in healthy subjects. In genetically predisposed persons, dysregulation of innate immunity may trigger inflammatory bowel disease.

is limited to the mucosa and spares the deeper layers of the bowel wall (Fig. 22.51). Both acute and chronic inflammatory cells infiltrate the lamina propria and the crypts ('cryptitis'). Crypt abscesses are typical. Goblet cells lose their mucus and in long-standing cases glands become distorted. Dysplasia, characterised by heaping of cells within the crypts, nuclear atypia and increased mitotic rate may herald the development of colon cancer.

Crohn's disease

The sites most commonly involved, in order of frequency, are terminal ileum and right side of colon, colon alone, terminal ileum alone, ileum and jejunum. The entire wall of the bowel is oedematous and thickened, and there are deep ulcers which often appear as linear fissures; thus the mucosa between them is described as 'cobblestone'. These may penetrate through the bowel wall to initiate abscesses or fistulas involving the bowel, bladder, uterus, vagina and skin of the perineum. The mesenteric lymph nodes are enlarged and the mesentery is thickened. Crohn's disease has a patchy distribution and the inflammatory process is interrupted by islands of normal mucosa. On histological examination, the bowel wall is thickened with a chronic inflammatory infiltrate throughout all layers (Fig. 22.52).

Clinical features

Ulcerative colitis

The major symptom is bloody diarrhoea. The first attack is usually the most severe and thereafter the disease is followed by relapses and remissions. Emotional stress,

---

22.71 Factors associated with the development of inflammatory bowel disease

Genetic

- More common in Ashkenazi Jews
- 10% have a first-degree relative or at least one close relative with IBD
- High concordance between identical twins
- Both ulcerative colitis and Crohn's disease are associated with the HLA locus and the genes encoding MST-1 and IL-23
- Crohn's disease is associated with the *NOD2*, *ATG16L1* and *IRGM* genes
- Ulcerative colitis is associated with the *ECM-1* gene
- Associated with autoimmune thyroiditis and SLE
- HLA-DR103 associated with severe ulcerative colitis
- Ulcerative colitis and Crohn's patients with HLA-B27 commonly develop ankylosing spondylitis

Environmental

- Ulcerative colitis is more common in non-smokers and ex-smokers
- Most Crohn's patients are smokers (relative risk = 3)
- Associated with low-residue, high refined sugar diet
- Appendicectomy protects against ulcerative colitis

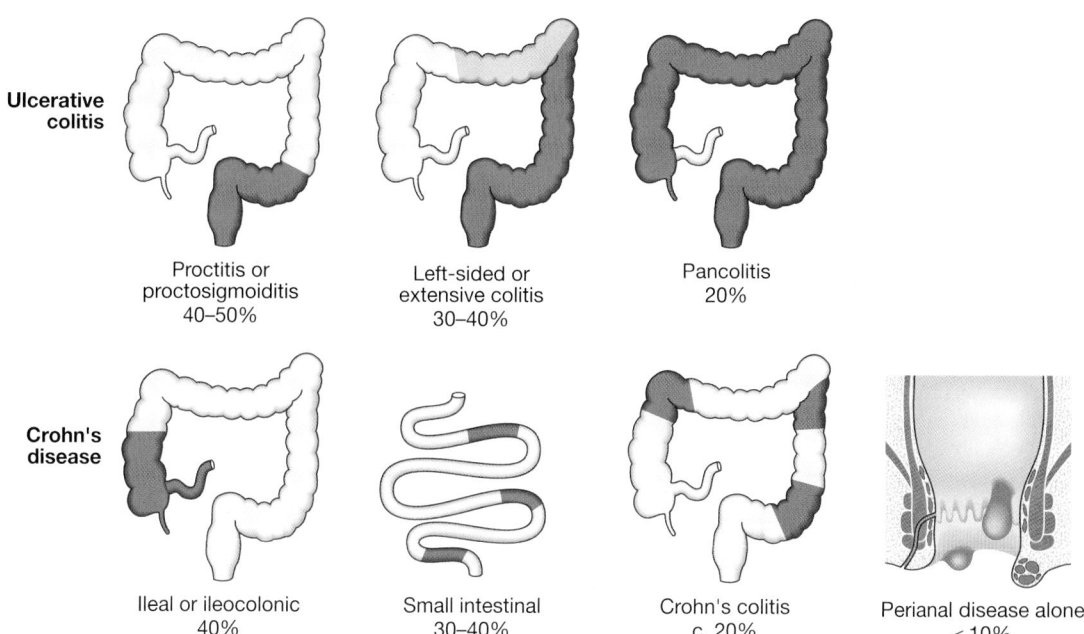

Ulcerative colitis

Proctitis or proctosigmoiditis
40–50%

Left-sided or extensive colitis
30–40%

Pancolitis
20%

Crohn's disease

Ileal or ileocolonic
40%

Small intestinal
30–40%

Crohn's colitis
c. 20%

Perianal disease alone
< 10%

Fig. 22.50 Common patterns of disease distribution in inflammatory bowel disease.

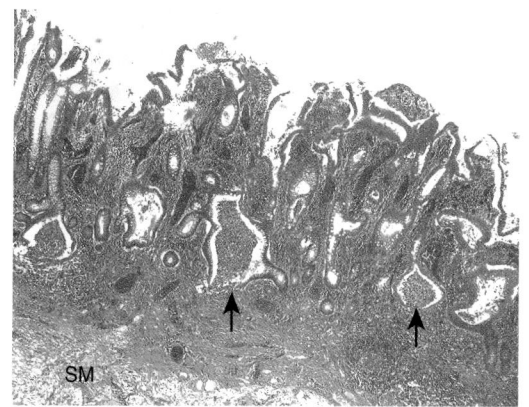

Fig. 22.51 Histology of ulcerative colitis. There is surface ulceration and inflammation is confined to the mucosa with excess inflammatory cells in the lamina propria, loss of goblet cells, and crypt abscesses (arrows). (SM = submucosa)

intercurrent infection, gastroenteritis, antibiotics or NSAID therapy may all provoke a relapse. Proctitis causes rectal bleeding and mucus discharge, sometimes accompanied by tenesmus. Some patients pass frequent, small-volume fluid stools, while others are constipated and pass pellety stools. Constitutional symptoms do not occur. Proctosigmoiditis causes bloody diarrhoea with mucus. Almost all patients are constitutionally well, but a small minority who have very active, limited disease develop fever, lethargy and abdominal discomfort.

Extensive colitis causes bloody diarrhoea with passage of mucus. In severe cases anorexia, malaise, weight loss and abdominal pain occur, and the patient is toxic with fever, tachycardia and signs of peritoneal inflammation (Box 22.72).

Crohn's disease

The major symptoms are abdominal pain, diarrhoea and weight loss. Ileal Crohn's disease (Figs 22.53 and 22.54)

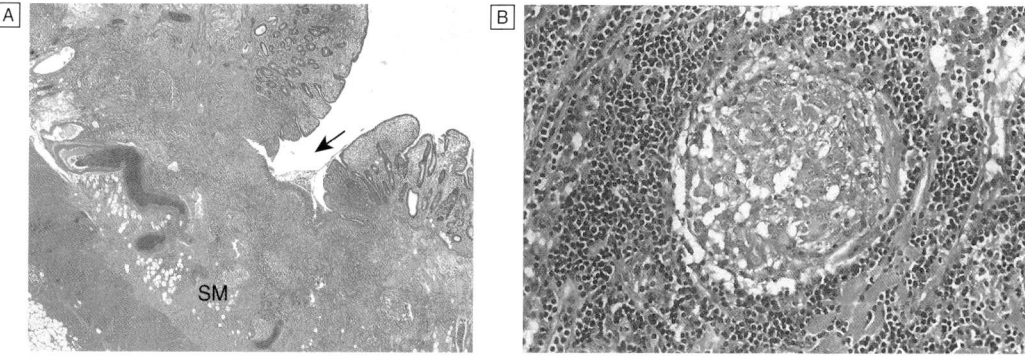

Fig. 22.52 Histology of Crohn's disease. A Inflammation is 'transmural'; there is fissuring ulceration (arrow) with inflammation extending into the submucosa (SM). B At higher power a characteristic non-caseating granuloma is seen.

	Mild	Severe
Daily bowel frequency	< 4	> 6
Blood in stools	+/–	+++
Stool volume	< 200 g/24 hrs	> 400 g/24 hrs
Pulse	< 90 bpm	> 90 bpm
Temperature	Normal	> 37.8°C, 2 days out of 4
Sigmoidoscopy	Normal or granular mucosa	Blood in lumen
Abdominal X-ray	Normal	Dilated bowel and/or mucosal islands
Haemoglobin	Normal	< 100 g/L (< 10 g/dL)
ESR	Normal	> 30 mm/hr
Serum albumin	> 35 g/L (> 3.5 g/dL)	< 30 g/L (< 3 g/dL)

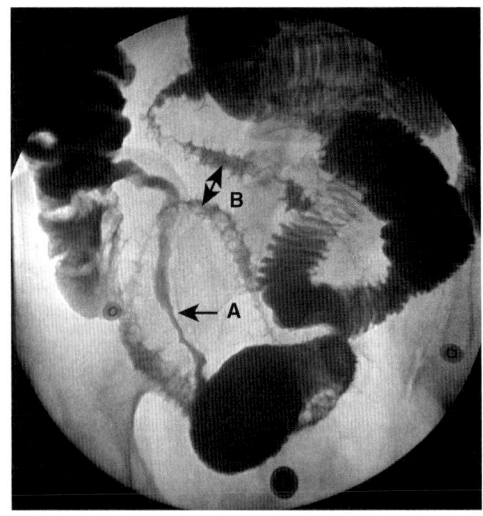

Fig. 22.54 Barium follow-through showing terminal ileal Crohn's disease. A long stricture is present (arrow A), and more proximally there is ulceration with characteristic 'rose thorn' ulcers (arrow B).

may cause subacute or even acute intestinal obstruction. The pain is often associated with diarrhoea which is usually watery and does not contain blood or mucus. Almost all patients lose weight because they avoid food since eating provokes pain. Weight loss may also be due to malabsorption, and some patients present with features of fat, protein or vitamin deficiencies. Crohn's colitis presents in an identical manner to ulcerative colitis, but rectal sparing and the presence of perianal disease are features which favour a diagnosis of Crohn's disease. Many patients present with symptoms of both small bowel and colonic disease. A few have isolated perianal disease, vomiting from jejunal strictures or severe oral ulceration.

Physical examination often reveals evidence of weight loss, anaemia with glossitis and angular stomatitis. There is abdominal tenderness, most marked over the inflamed area. An abdominal mass due to matted loops of thickened bowel or an intra-abdominal abscess may occur. Perianal skin tags, fissures or fistulas are found in at least 50% of patients.

Differential diagnosis

The differential diagnosis is summarised in Box 22.73. The most important issue is to distinguish the first attack of an acute colitis from infection. In general, diarrhoea lasting longer than 10 days in Western countries is

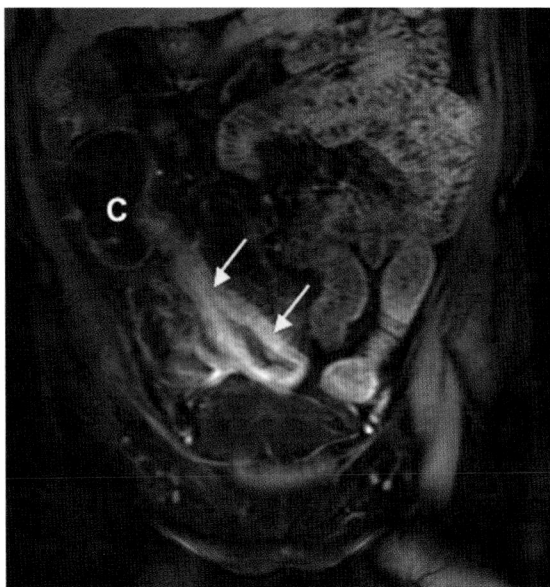

Fig. 22.53 Ileal Crohn's disease. MRI scan showing a thickened, narrowed loop of ileum with enhancement after MR contrast (arrows), consistent with active Crohn's disease. Normal small bowel can be seen at the top right of the image. (C = caecum)

ℹ 22.73 Conditions which can mimic ulcerative or Crohn's colitis

Infective

Bacterial
- *Salmonella*
- *Shigella*
- *Campylobacter jejuni*
- *E. coli* O157
- Gonococcal proctitis
- Pseudomembranous colitis
- *Chlamydia* proctitis

Viral
- Herpes simplex proctitis
- Cytomegalovirus

Protozoal
- Amoebiasis

Non-infective

Vascular
- Ischaemic colitis
- Radiation proctitis

Idiopathic
- Collagenous colitis
- Behçet's disease

Drugs
- NSAIDs

Neoplastic
- Colonic carcinoma

Other
- Diverticulitis

> **22.74 Differential diagnosis of small bowel Crohn's disease**
>
> - Other causes of right iliac fossa mass
>   Caecal carcinoma*
>   Appendix abscess*
> - Infection (tuberculosis, *Yersinia*, actinomycosis)
> - Mesenteric adenitis
> - Pelvic inflammatory disease
> - Lymphoma
>
> *Common; other causes are rare.

unlikely to be the result of infection, whereas a history of foreign travel, antibiotic exposure (pseudomembranous colitis) or homosexual contact increases the possibility of infection, which should be excluded by the appropriate investigations (see below). The diagnosis of Crohn's disease is usually more straightforward on the basis of imaging and clinical presentation, but in atypical cases biopsy or surgical resection is necessary to exclude other diseases (Box 22.74).

Complications

Life-threatening colonic inflammation

This can occur in both ulcerative colitis and Crohn's disease. In the most extreme cases the colon dilates (toxic megacolon) and bacterial toxins pass freely across the diseased mucosa into the portal then systemic circulation. This complication occurs most commonly during the first attack of colitis and is recognised by the features described in Box 22.72. An abdominal X-ray should be taken daily because when the transverse colon is dilated to more than 6 cm (Fig. 22.55) there is a high risk of colonic

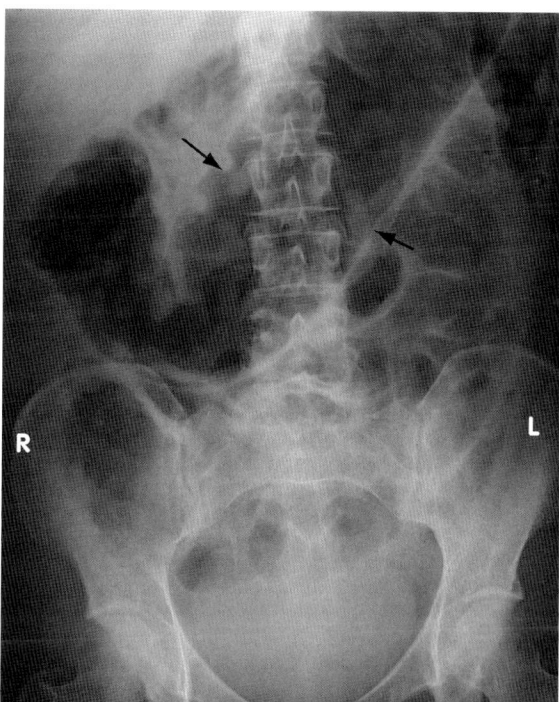

Fig. 22.55 Plain abdominal X-ray showing a grossly dilated colon due to severe ulcerative colitis. There is also marked mucosal oedema and 'thumb-printing' (arrows).

perforation, although this complication can also occur in the absence of toxic megacolon.

Haemorrhage

Haemorrhage due to erosion of a major artery is rare but can occur in both conditions.

Fistulas

These are specific to Crohn's disease. Enteroenteric fistulas can cause diarrhoea and malabsorption due to blind loop syndrome. Enterovesical fistulation causes recurrent urinary infections and pneumaturia. An enterovaginal fistula causes a feculent vaginal discharge. Fistulation from the bowel may also cause perianal or ischiorectal abscesses, fissures and fistulas.

Cancer

The risk of colon cancer is increased in patients with active colitis of more than 8 years' duration. The cumulative risk for ulcerative colitis may be as high as 20% after 30 years but is probably lower for Crohn's colitis. Tumours develop in areas of dysplasia and may be multiple. Patients with long-standing, extensive colitis are therefore entered into surveillance programmes beginning 8–10 years after diagnosis during which biopsies are taken throughout the colon at colonoscopy. If mild to moderate dysplastic changes are identified, the frequency of screening is increased to 1–2-yearly, but if high-grade dysplasia is found, panproctocolectomy should be considered because of the high risk of colon cancer.

Extraintestinal

Extraintestinal complications are common in IBD and may dominate the clinical picture. Some of these occur during relapse of intestinal disease; others appear unrelated to intestinal disease activity (Fig. 22.56).

Investigations

These are necessary to confirm the diagnosis, define disease distribution and activity, and identify complications. Full blood count may show anaemia resulting from bleeding or malabsorption of iron, folic acid or vitamin B_{12}. Serum albumin concentration falls as a consequence of protein-losing enteropathy, inflammatory disease or poor nutrition. The ESR and CRP are elevated in exacerbations and in response to abscess formation.

Bacteriology

At the time of initial presentation, stool microscopy, culture and examination for *Clostridium difficile* toxin or for ova and cysts, blood cultures and serological tests should be performed to exclude infection. These investigations may need to be repeated in established disease to exclude superimposed enteric infection in patients who present with exacerbations of IBD.

Endoscopy

Sigmoidoscopy (Fig. 22.57) with biopsy is an essential investigation in all patients who present with diarrhoea. In ulcerative colitis sigmoidoscopy is almost always abnormal with loss of vascular pattern, granularity, friability and ulceration. In Crohn's disease patchy inflammation with discrete, deep ulcers, perianal disease (fissures, fistulas and skin tags) or rectal sparing occurs. Colonoscopy may show active inflammation with pseudopolyps or a complicating carcinoma. Biopsies are

22

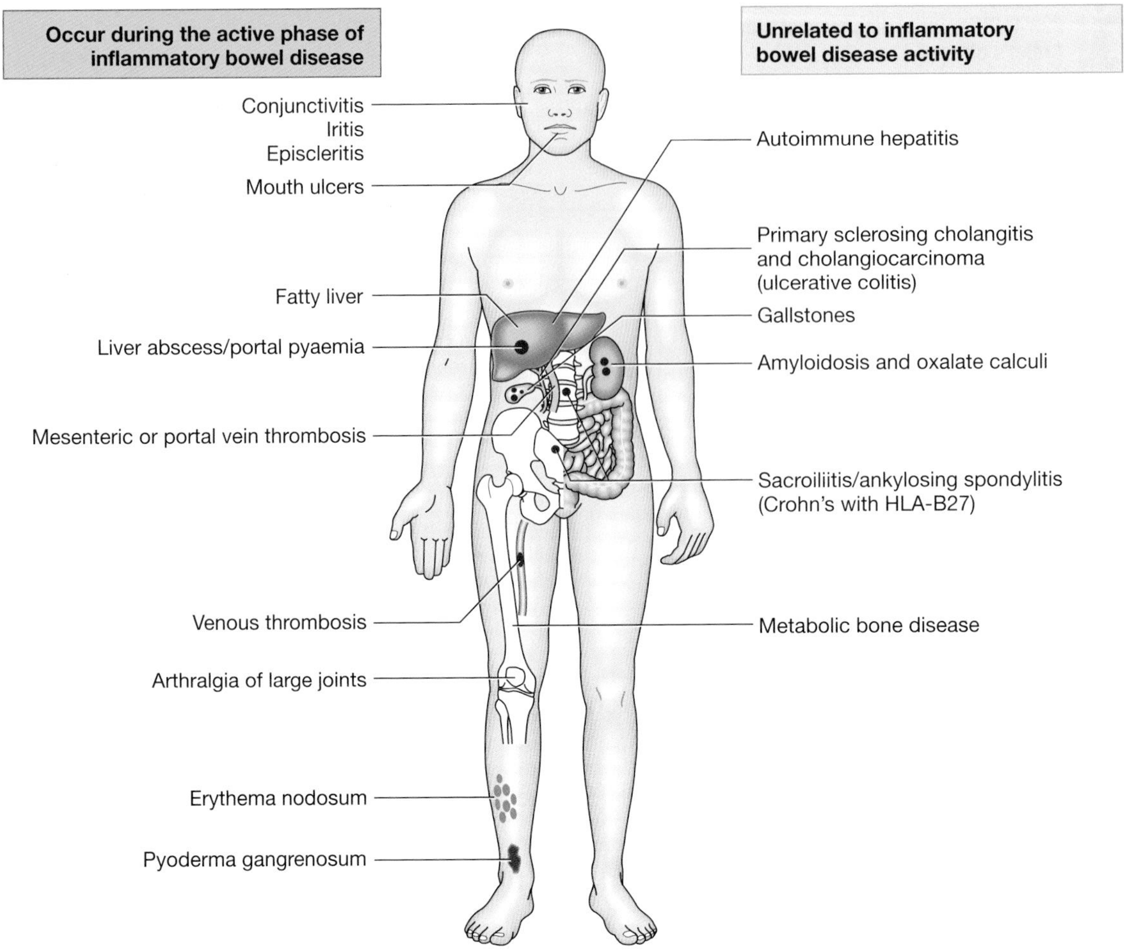

Occur during the active phase of inflammatory bowel disease	Unrelated to inflammatory bowel disease activity

Conjunctivitis
Iritis
Episcleritis
Mouth ulcers

Fatty liver

Liver abscess/portal pyaemia

Mesenteric or portal vein thrombosis

Venous thrombosis

Arthralgia of large joints

Erythema nodosum

Pyoderma gangrenosum

Autoimmune hepatitis

Primary sclerosing cholangitis and cholangiocarcinoma (ulcerative colitis)

Gallstones

Amyloidosis and oxalate calculi

Sacroiliitis/ankylosing spondylitis (Crohn's with HLA-B27)

Metabolic bone disease

Fig. 22.56 Systemic complications of inflammatory bowel disease. (See also Chs 19 and 20.)

taken to define disease extent, as this is underestimated by endoscopic appearances alone, and to seek dysplasia in patients with long-standing colitis. In ulcerative colitis the macroscopic and histological abnormalities are confluent and most severe in the distal colon and rectum. Stricture formation does not occur in the absence of a carcinoma. In Crohn's colitis the endoscopic abnormalities are patchy, with normal mucosa between the areas of abnormality. Aphthoid or deeper ulcers and strictures are common. Capsule endoscopy is useful in the identification of small bowel inflammation, but should be avoided in the presence of strictures.

Radiology

Barium enema is a less sensitive investigation than colonoscopy in patients with colitis and is now little used. Contrast studies of the small bowel can be helpful in the investigation of Crohn's disease; affected areas are narrowed and ulcerated, and multiple strictures are common (see Fig. 22.54). MRI scans provide comparable information without radiation exposure or risking small bowel obstruction and are useful in delineating pelvic or perineal involvement. A plain abdominal X-ray is essential in the management of patients who present with severe active disease. Dilatation of the colon (see Fig. 22.55), mucosal oedema ('thumb-printing') or evidence of perforation may be found. In small bowel Crohn's disease there may be evidence of intestinal obstruction or displacement of bowel loops by a mass. Ultrasound may identify thickened small bowel loops and abscess development in Crohn's disease.

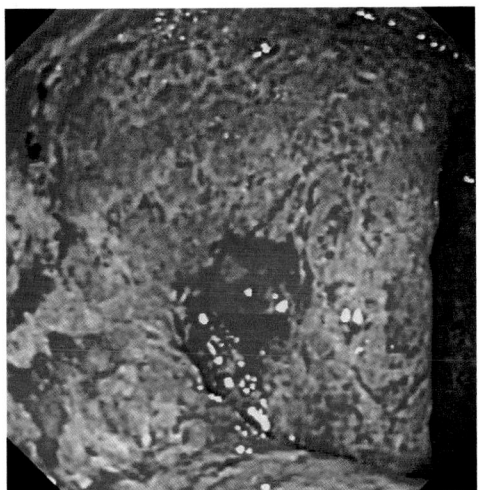

Fig. 22.57 Sigmoidoscopic view of moderately active ulcerative colitis. Mucosa is erythematous and friable with contact bleeding. Submucosal blood vessels are no longer visible.

Management

For optimal treatment, a team-based approach should be employed involving physicians, surgeons, radiologists, nurse specialists and dietitians. Both ulcerative colitis and Crohn's disease are life-long conditions and have psychosocial implications; counsellors and patient support groups have important roles in education, reassurance and coping. The key aims are to:

- treat acute attacks
- prevent relapses
- detect carcinoma at an early stage
- select patients for surgery.

Drugs used in the treatment of IBD are listed in Box 22.75.

Ulcerative colitis

Active proctitis In mild to moderate disease mesalazine enemas or suppositories combined with oral mesalazine are effective first-line therapy. Topical corticosteroids are less effective and are reserved for patients who are intolerant of topical mesalazine. Patients who fail to respond are treated with oral prednisolone 40 mg daily.

Active left-sided or extensive ulcerative colitis In mildly active cases, high-dose aminosalicylates combined with topical aminosalicylate and corticosteroids are effective. Oral prednisolone 40 mg daily is indicated for more active disease or when initial aminosalicylate therapy is ineffective.

22.75 Drugs used in the treatment of inflammatory bowel disease

Class	Mechanism of action	Notes
Aminosalicylates (mesalazine (Asacol, Salofalk, Pentasa), olsalazine, sulfasalazine, balsalazide)	Modulate cytokine release from mucosa Delivered to colon by one of three mechanisms: (1) pH-dependent (Asacol, Salofalk) (2) time-dependent (Pentasa) (3) bacterial breakdown by colonic bacteria from a carrier molecule (sulfasalazine, balsalazide)	No proven value in Crohn's Available as oral or topical (enema/suppository) preparation Sulfasalazine causes side-effects in 10–45%: headache, nausea, diarrhoea, blood dyscrasias Other aminosalicylates much better tolerated; diarrhoea, headache in 2–5% Rarely, renal impairment All safe during pregnancy
Corticosteroids (prednisolone, hydrocortisone, budesonide)	Anti-inflammatory Budesonide is a potent corticosteroid efficiently cleared from circulation by liver, thereby minimising adrenocortical suppression and steroid side-effects	Topical, oral or i.v., according to disease severity Bisphosphonates are co-prescribed to prevent osteopenia Budesonide considered for active ileitis and ileocolitis
Thiopurines (azathioprine, 6-mercaptopurine)	Immunomodulation by inducing T-cell apoptosis Azathioprine is metabolised in the liver to 6-mercaptopurine, then by thiopurine methyltransferase (TPMT) to thioguanine nucleotides	Effective after 12 weeks of starting therapy Complications in 20%. Flu-like syndrome with myalgia Leucopenia in 3%, particularly in inherited TPMT deficiency No increased risk of cancer but probable increase in lymphoma Safe during pregnancy
Methotrexate	Anti-inflammatory	Intolerance in 10–18%. Nausea, stomatitis, diarrhoea, hepatotoxicity and pneumonitis
Ciclosporin	Suppresses T-cell expansion	'Rescue' therapy to prevent surgery in ulcerative colitis responding poorly to corticosteroids. No value in Crohn's disease Major side-effects in 0–17%: nephrotoxicity, infections, neurotoxicity (including fits) Minor complications in up to 50%: tremor, paraesthesiae, abnormal liver function tests, hirsutism
Anti-TNF antibodies (infliximab and adalimumab)	Suppress inflammation and induce apoptosis of inflammatory cells	Moderately to severely active Crohn's disease, especially fistulating Severe active ulcerative colitis Anaphylactic reactions after multiple infusions Contraindicated in the presence of infections; reactivation of tuberculosis Increased risk of infections and malignancy
Antibiotics	Antibacterial	Useful in perianal Crohn's disease Major concern is peripheral neuropathy with long-term metronidazole
Antidiarrhoeal agents (codeine phosphate, loperamide, lomotil)	Reduce gut motility and small bowel secretion Loperamide improves anal function	Avoided in acute flare-ups of disease May precipitate colonic dilatation

22

Severe ulcerative colitis Patients who fail to respond to maximal oral therapy and those who present with severe colitis are best managed in hospital and should be monitored jointly by a physician and surgeon:

- clinically: for the presence of abdominal pain, temperature, pulse rate, stool blood and frequency
- in the laboratory; haemoglobin, white cell count, albumin, electrolytes, ESR and CRP
- radiologically: for colonic dilatation on plain abdominal X-rays.

Supportive treatment includes intravenous fluids to correct dehydration along with nutritional support, usually as enteral rather than intravenous feeding, for malnourished patients (Box 22.76).

Intravenous corticosteroids (methylprednisolone 60 mg or hydrocortisone 400 mg/day) are given as a constant infusion. Topical and oral aminosalicylates are also used, although their value in severe disease is unclear. Patients who do not promptly respond to corticosteroids are considered for intravenous ciclosporin or infliximab, which, in approximately 30% of cases, overcomes the need for urgent colectomy.

Patients who develop colonic dilatation (> 6 cm), those whose clinical and laboratory measurements deteriorate and those who do not respond after 7–10 days' maximal medical treatment usually require urgent colectomy.

Maintenance of remission Life-long maintenance therapy is recommended for all patients with extensive disease and patients with distal disease who relapse more than once a year. Oral aminosalicylates—either mesalazine or balsalazide—are first-line agents (Box 22.77). Sulfasalazine has a higher incidence of side-effects, but should be considered in patients with co-existent arthropathy. Patients who frequently relapse despite aminosalicylate drugs are treated with thiopurines.

Crohn's disease

Active disease Patients with active colitis or ileocolitis are initially treated in a similar manner to those with active ulcerative colitis. Aminosalicylates and corticosteroids are both effective and usually induce remission in active ileocolitis and colitis. In severe disease intravenous steroids are indicated, but abscess or fistulating disease should be excluded before instituting therapy. In contrast to ulcerative colitis, nutritional therapy using polymeric or elemental diets induces remission in Crohn's disease. Possible mechanisms include avoidance of dietary antigens, other ill-defined immunological effects and the non-specific effects of nutritional support. Prolonged nutritional therapy, which involves exclusion of a normal diet, is onerous for the patient; remission rates are comparable to those achieved by corticosteroids but relapse rates are higher and, except in paediatric practice, primary nutritional therapy is now seldom used.

Patients with isolated ileal disease should be treated with corticosteroids. Budesonide is appropriate for treating moderately active disease, although it is marginally less effective than prednisolone. Aminosalicylates have little added value but there is some evidence to support the use of oral metronidazole. Poorly responding patients should, at an early stage, be considered for surgical resection since this is associated with prolonged remission in most cases.

Therapy with the anti-TNF antibodies infliximab (given as an intravenous infusion 4–8-weekly on three occasions) or adalimumab (a subcutaneous injection given two weekly) can induce remission in patients with active Crohn's disease at any site within the gastrointestinal tract (Box 22.78). Interestingly, however, etanercept (a decoy receptor for TNF) is ineffective in Crohn's disease. These drugs also effectively treat some extraintestinal complications, including pyoderma gangrenosum and inflammatory arthritis. Infliximab and adalimumab are contraindicated in the presence of infection, including tuberculosis, and may be complicated by allergic reactions (Box 22.79). Relapse commonly occurs approximately 12 weeks after treatment and for this reason biological agents are usually combined with immunosuppressive drugs such as the thiopurines (azathioprine and 6-mercaptopurine) or methotrexate, to maintain remission. These drugs can induce remarkable mucosal healing but scarring can occur, and they should therefore be used with caution in patients with stenosing disease. Biological agents, particularly when combined with thiopurines, predispose to malignancy. Although this risk is relatively small and has to be balanced against the considerable value in transforming the quality of life for

---

✚ 22.76 Medical management of fulminant ulcerative colitis

- Intravenous fluids
- Transfusion if Hb < 100 g/L
- I.v. methylprednisolone (60 mg daily) or hydrocortisone (400 mg daily)
- Antibiotics for proven infection
- Nutritional support
- Subcutaneous heparin for prophylaxis of venous thromboembolism
- Avoidance of opiates and antidiarrhoeal agents
- Consider infliximab (5 mg/kg) in stable patients not responding to 3–5 days of corticosteroids

---

EBM 22.77 Aminosalicylates and remission in ulcerative colitis

'Higher doses of 5-ASA (4 g/day) are superior to placebo at inducing remission in mild ulcerative colitis and Crohn's disease. Maintenance with 5-ASA reduces the risk of colorectal cancer by 75% in ulcerative colitis.'

- Carter MJ, et al. Gut 2004; 53 (suppl. V):1–16.

For further information: www.bsg.org.uk

EBM 22.78 Infliximab in Crohn's disease

'Anti-TNF antibody treatment (infliximab) improves remission rates in Crohn's disease refractory to conventional therapies including corticosteroids (NNT 4), heals enterocutaneous Crohn's fistulas and maintains longer remissions.'

- Akobeng AK, et al. (Cochrane Review). Cochrane Library, issue 1, 2005. Oxford: Update Software.

For further information: www.cochrane.org

22.79 Biological drugs and inflammatory bowel disease

- Inhibit activity of TNF-α, resulting in suppression of T-cell-mediated immunity
- Two commercially available agents are infliximab and adalimumab
- Induce remission in 70% of cases of active Crohn's disease, with mucosal healing
- Fistulas heal in most patients
- Clinical relapse is frequent after about 12 weeks
- Efficacy is improved by corticosteroid co-treatment
- Maintenance therapy is necessary for aggressive disease
- Side-effects may be serious and related to suppression of cell-mediated immunity
    Infection: tuberculosis and active sepsis of any sort are absolute contraindications
    Malignancy: avoid in patients with a history of cancer or lymphoma. Increased incidence of malignant disease in patients on maintenance therapy, particularly if combined with thiopurines

many sufferers, the risk–benefit analysis should be discussed with all patients before therapy is started.

Patients with diffuse and extensive ileocolonic involvement present considerable therapeutic challenges. A combination of drug therapies, nutritional support (which in the most severe cases involves prolonged parenteral nutrition), surgical intervention and endoscopic balloon dilatation of strictures may all be needed at different times.

Fistulas and perianal disease Fistulas usually develop in association with active Crohn's disease and are often associated with sepsis. The first step in management is to define the site of fistulation by imaging. Surgical intervention is then required, although treatment of underlying active disease with corticosteroids and nutritional support, usually by TPN, are required in many cases. For simple perianal disease metronidazole and/or ciprofloxacin are first-line therapies. Thiopurines are used in chronic disease. In many patients examination under anaesthetic is needed to determine the site of complicating abscess, fissure and fistula. Infliximab and adalimumab heal enterocutaneous fistulas and perianal disease in many patients.

Maintenance of remission The most effective step, and one greater than any pharmacological intervention, is smoking cessation. Aminosalicylates have minimal efficacy. Patients who relapse more than once a year should be treated with thiopurines (Box 22.80). Patients who are intolerant of or resistant to thiopurines should be treated with once-weekly methotrexate combined with folic acid. Patients with aggressive disease are managed using a combination of immunosuppressives and anti-TNF therapy. Chronic use of corticosteroids should be

avoided since this leads to osteoporosis and other side-effects, without preventing relapse.

Surgical treatment

Ulcerative colitis

Up to 60% of patients with extensive ulcerative colitis eventually require surgery. The indications are listed in Box 22.81. Impaired quality of life, with impact upon occupation and on social and family life, is the most important of these. Surgery involves removal of the entire colon and rectum, and cures the patient. One-third of those with pancolitis undergo colectomy within 5 years of diagnosis. Before surgery, patients must be counselled by doctors, stoma nurses and patients who have undergone similar surgery. The choice of procedure is either panproctocolectomy with ileostomy, or proctocolectomy with ileal–anal pouch anastomosis. The sister surgical text to this book, *Principles and Practice of Surgery*, should be consulted for further details.

Crohn's disease

The indications for surgery are similar to those for ulcerative colitis. Operations are often necessary to deal with fistulas, abscesses and perianal disease, and may also be required to relieve small or large bowel obstruction. In contrast to ulcerative colitis, surgery is not curative and disease recurrence is the rule. Surgical intervention should therefore be as conservative as possible in order to minimise loss of viable intestine and to avoid creation of a short bowel syndrome. Obstructing or fistulating small bowel disease may require resection of affected tissue. Patients who have localised segments of Crohn's colitis may be managed by segmental resection and/or multiple stricturoplasties in which the stricture is not resected but instead incised in its longitudinal axis and sutured transversely. Others who have extensive colitis require total colectomy but ileal–anal pouch formation should be avoided because of the high risk of disease recurrence within the pouch and subsequent fistulas, abscess formation and pouch failure.

Patients who have perianal Crohn's disease should be managed as conservatively as possible. Seton drainage, fistulectomy and use of advancement flaps are appropriate for complex fistulas in combination with medical therapies. Around 80% of Crohn's patients undergo surgery at some stage, and 70% of these require more than one operation during their lifetime. Clinical recurrence following resectional surgery is present in 50% of all cases at 10 years.

22.81 Indications for surgery in ulcerative colitis

Impaired quality of life
- Loss of occupation or education
- Disruption of family life

Failure of medical therapy
- Dependence upon oral corticosteroids
- Complications of drug therapy

Fulminant colitis

Disease complications unresponsive to medical therapy
- Arthritis
- Pyoderma gangrenosum

Colon cancer or severe dysplasia

EBM 22.80 Azathioprine (thiopurine) in Crohn's disease

'Azathioprine is effective in preventing exacerbation of Crohn's disease.'

- Feagan BG, et al. In: McDonald J, et al., eds. Evidence-based gastroenterology and hepatology, 2nd edn. London: BMJ Books; 2003.

For further information: www.bsg.org.uk

22

IBD in special circumstances

Childhood

Ulcerative colitis and Crohn's disease can develop before adolescence. Chronic ill health results in growth failure, metabolic bone disease and delayed puberty. Loss of schooling and social contact, as well as frequent hospitalisation, can have important psychosocial consequences. Treatment is similar to that described for adults and may require the use of corticosteroids, immunosuppressive drugs, biological agents and surgery. Monitoring of height, weight and sexual development is crucial.

Pregnancy

The activity of IBD is not usually affected by pregnancy, although relapse may be more common after parturition. Drug therapy, including aminosalicylates, corticosteroids and azathioprine, can be safely continued throughout the pregnancy (Box 22.82).

Metabolic bone disease

Patients with IBD are prone to developing osteoporosis due to effects of chronic inflammation, corticosteroids, weight loss, malnutrition and malabsorption. Osteomalacia can also occur in Crohn's disease which is complicated by malabsorption, but is less common than osteoporosis. The risk of osteoporosis increases with age and with the dose and duration of corticosteroid therapy.

22.82 Pregnancy and inflammatory bowel disease

Pre-conception

- Outcomes are best when pregnancy is carefully planned and disease is in remission
- IBD drugs should be continued until discussed with a specialist
- Aminosalicylates, antidiarrhoeals and azathioprine are safe in pregnancy
- Corticosteroids are probably safe
- Safety of biological therapy in pregnancy is unclear; use only when absolutely necessary
- Daily folic acid supplements are recommended

Pregnancy

- Two-thirds of patients in remission will remain so during pregnancy
- Active disease is likely to remain active
- Severe active disease carries an increased risk of premature delivery and low birth weight
- Gentle flexible sigmoidoscopy is safe after the first trimester
- Colonoscopy and X-rays should be avoided

Labour

- Needs careful discussion between patient, gastroenterologist and obstetrician
- Normal labour and vaginal delivery are possible for most women
- Caesarean section may be preferred for patients with perianal Crohn's or an ileo-anal pouch to reduce risks of pelvic floor damage, fistulation and late incontinence

Breastfeeding

- Safe and does not exacerbate IBD
- Data on the risk to babies from drugs excreted in breast milk are limited; most are probably safe
- Patients should discuss breastfeeding and drug therapy carefully with their doctor

Diagnosis and management of osteomalacia and osteoporosis are discussed in Chapter 25.

Microscopic colitis

Some patients experience watery diarrhoea as a consequence of microscopic ('lymphocytic') colitis. The colonoscopic appearances are normal but histological examination of biopsies shows a range of abnormalities.

Collagenous colitis is characterised by the presence of a thick submucosal band of collagen; a chronic inflammatory infiltrate is usually seen. The disease is more common in women and is associated with rheumatoid arthritis, diabetes and coeliac disease. Patients have a history of intermittent watery diarrhoea and treatment is based on antidiarrhoeal drugs and budesonide.

IRRITABLE BOWEL SYNDROME

Irritable bowel syndrome (IBS) is a functional bowel disorder in which abdominal pain is associated with defecation or a change in bowel habit. Approximately 20% of the general population fulfil diagnostic criteria for IBS but only 10% of these consult their doctors because of gastrointestinal symptoms. Nevertheless, IBS is the most common cause of gastrointestinal referral and accounts for frequent absenteeism from work and impaired quality of life. Young women are affected 2–3 times more often than men. Co-existing conditions such as non-ulcer dyspepsia, chronic fatigue syndrome, dysmenorrhoea and fibromyalgia are common. A significant proportion of patients have a history of physical or sexual abuse.

Pathophysiology

IBS encompasses a wide range of symptoms and a single cause is unlikely. It is generally believed that most patients develop symptoms in response to psychosocial factors, altered gastrointestinal motility, altered visceral sensation or luminal factors.

Psychosocial factors

Most patients seen in general practice do not have psychological problems but about 50% of patients referred to hospital meet the criteria for a psychiatric diagnosis. A range of disturbances are identified, including anxiety, depression, somatisation and neurosis. Panic attacks are also common. Acute psychological stress and overt psychiatric disease are known to alter visceral perception and gastrointestinal motility in both irritable bowel patients and healthy people. There is an increased prevalence of abnormal illness behaviour with frequent consultations for minor symptoms and reduced coping ability (p. 238). These factors contribute to but do not cause IBS.

Altered gastrointestinal motility

A range of motility disorders are found but none is diagnostic. Patients with diarrhoea as a predominant symptom exhibit clusters of rapid jejunal contraction waves, rapid intestinal transit and an increased number of fast and propagated colonic contractions. Those who are predominantly constipated have decreased orocaecal transit and a reduced number of high-amplitude, propagated colonic contraction waves but there is no consistent evidence of abnormal motility.

Abnormal visceral perception

IBS is associated with increased sensitivity to intestinal distension induced by inflation of balloons in the ileum, colon and rectum, a consequence of altered central nervous system processing of visceral sensation. This is more common in women and in diarrhoea-predominant IBS.

Infection and allergy

Between 7 and 32% of patients develop IBS following an episode of gastroenteritis, more commonly young women and those with existing background psychological problems. Others may be intolerant of specific dietary components, particularly lactose and wheat. Abnormalities of gut microflora leading to increased fermentation and gas production and minimal inflammation have also been postulated. Some patients have subtle, histologically undetectable mucosal inflammation, possibly leading to activation of inflammatory cells and release of cytokines, nitric oxide and histamine. These may trigger abnormal secretomotor function and sensitise enteric sensory nerve endings.

Clinical features

The most common presentation is that of recurrent abdominal pain (Box 22.83). This is usually colicky or 'cramping', felt in the lower abdomen and relieved by defecation. Abdominal bloating worsens throughout the day; the cause is unknown but it is not due to excessive intestinal gas. The bowel habit is variable. Most patients alternate between episodes of diarrhoea and constipation, but it is useful to classify patients as having predominantly constipation or predominantly diarrhoea. Those with constipation tend to pass infrequent pellety stools, usually in association with abdominal pain or proctalgia. Those with diarrhoea have frequent defecation but produce low-volume stools and rarely have nocturnal symptoms. Passage of mucus is common but rectal bleeding does not occur. Despite apparently severe symptoms, patients do not lose weight and are constitutionally well. Physical examination is generally unremarkable, with the exception of variable tenderness to palpation.

Diagnosis

The diagnosis is clinical in nature and can be made confidently in most patients under the age of 40 years without resorting to complicated tests (Box 22.84). Full blood count, faecal calprotectin and sigmoidoscopy are usually done routinely and are normal in IBS. Colonoscopy should be undertaken in older patients to exclude colorectal cancer. Those who present atypically require investigations to exclude organic gastrointestinal disease. Diarrhoea-predominant patients justify investigations to exclude microscopic colitis (p. 904), lactose intolerance (p. 886), bile acid malabsorption (p. 850),

22.84 Supporting diagnostic features and alarm features in IBS

Features supporting a diagnosis of IBS

- Symptoms > 6 months
- Frequent consultations for non-GI problems
- Previous medically unexplained symptoms
- Stress worsens symptoms

Alarm features

- Age > 50 years; male gender
- Weight loss
- Nocturnal symptoms
- Family history of colon cancer
- Anaemia
- Rectal bleeding

coeliac disease (p. 879), thyrotoxicosis and, in developing countries, parasitic infection. All patients who give a history of rectal bleeding should undergo colonoscopy to exclude colonic cancer or IBD.

Management

The most important steps are to make a positive diagnosis and reassure the patient. Many patients are concerned that they have developed cancer, and a cycle of anxiety leading to colonic symptoms, which further heighten anxiety, can be broken by explanation that symptoms are not due to organic disease but are the result of altered bowel motility and sensation. In patients who fail to respond to reassurance, treatment is tailored to the predominant symptoms (Fig. 22.58). Elimination diets are generally unhelpful but up to 20% may benefit from a wheat-free diet, some may respond to lactose exclusion, and excess intake of caffeine or artificial sweeteners such as sorbitol should be addressed. The role of probiotics has yet to be clearly established.

Patients with intractable symptoms sometimes benefit from several months of therapy with amitriptyline (10–25 mg orally at night) (Box 22.85). Side-effects include dry mouth and drowsiness but these are usually mild and the drug is generally well tolerated, although patients with features of somatisation tolerate the drug poorly and lower doses should be used. It may act by reducing visceral sensation and by altering gastrointestinal motility. Other drugs may overcome abnormalities of 5-HT signalling which have been identified in some IBS patients. These include 5-HT4 agonists. Active anxiety or affective disorders should be separately treated. Psychological interventions such as cognitive behavioural therapy, relaxation and gut-directed hypnotherapy are reserved for the most difficult cases. A range of complementary and alternative therapies exist; most lack a good evidence base but are popular and help some patients (Box 22.86).

22

22.83 Features of irritable bowel syndrome

- Colicky abdominal pain
- Altered bowel habit
- Abdominal distension
- Rectal mucus
- Feeling of incomplete defecation

EBM 22.85 Drug therapy for IBS

'Evidence for efficacy of drug therapy for IBS is weak. There is evidence of benefit for antispasmodic drugs for abdominal pain and overall response but there is no clear evidence of benefit for antidepressants or bulking agents. For each individual, treatment should be aimed at the most debilitating symptom.'

- (Cochrane Review). Cochrane Library, issue 2, 2005. Oxford: Update Software.

For further information: 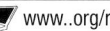 www..org/reviews

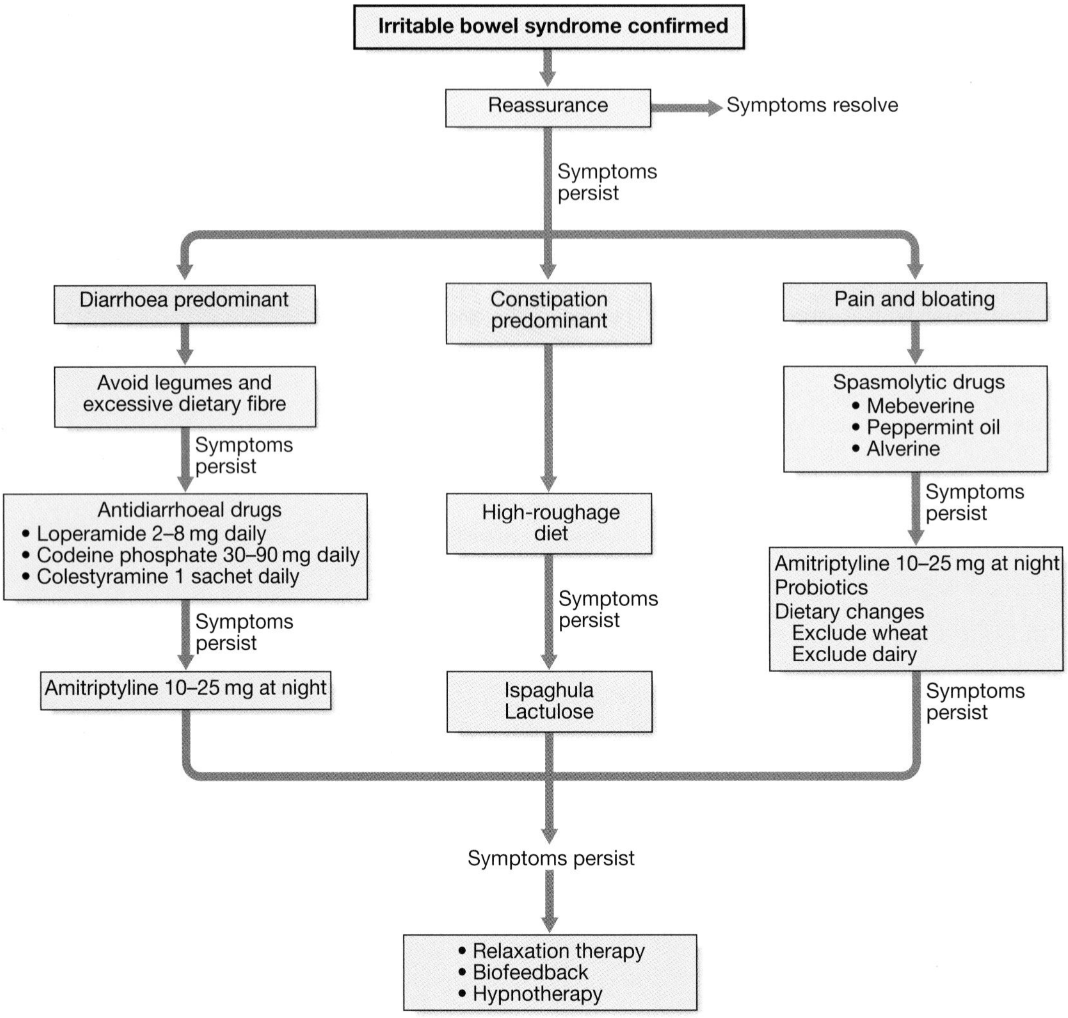

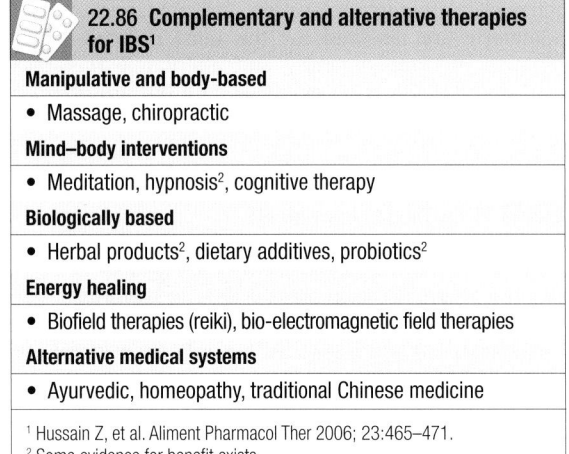

Fig. 22.58 Management of irritable bowel syndrome.

Most patients have a relapsing and remitting course. Exacerbations often follow stressful life events, occupational dissatisfaction and difficulties with interpersonal relationships.

22.86 Complementary and alternative therapies for IBS[1]
Manipulative and body-based
• Massage, chiropractic
Mind–body interventions
• Meditation, hypnosis[2], cognitive therapy
Biologically based
• Herbal products[2], dietary additives, probiotics[2]
Energy healing
• Biofield therapies (reiki), bio-electromagnetic field therapies
Alternative medical systems
• Ayurvedic, homeopathy, traditional Chinese medicine
[1] Hussain Z, et al. Aliment Pharmacol Ther 2006; 23:465–471.
[2] Some evidence for benefit exists.

AIDS AND THE GASTROINTESTINAL TRACT

See page 393.

ISCHAEMIC GUT INJURY

Ischaemic gut injury is usually the result of arterial occlusion. Severe hypotension and venous insufficiency are less frequent causes (p. 199). The presentation is variable depending on the different vessels involved and the acuteness of the event. Diagnosis is often difficult.

Acute small bowel ischaemia

An embolus from the heart or aorta to the superior mesenteric artery is responsible for 40–50% of cases, thrombosis of underlying atheromatous disease for approximately 25% and non-occlusive ischaemia due to hypotension complicating myocardial infarction, heart failure, arrhythmias or sudden blood loss for approximately 25%. Vasculitis or venous occlusion is a rare cause. The pathological spectrum ranges from transient alteration of bowel function to transmural haemorrhagic necrosis and gangrene. Patients usually have evidence of cardiac disease and arrhythmia. Almost all develop abdominal pain that is more impressive than the physical findings. In the early stages the only physical signs may be a silent, distended abdomen or diminished bowel sounds, peritonitis only developing later.

Leucocytosis, metabolic acidosis, hyperphosphataemia and hyperamylasaemia are typical. Plain abdominal X-rays show 'thumb-printing' due to mucosal oedema. Mesenteric or CT angiography reveals an occluded or narrowed major artery with spasm of arterial arcades, although most patients undergo laparotomy on the basis of a clinical diagnosis without angiography. Resuscitation, management of cardiac disease and intravenous antibiotic therapy, followed by laparotomy, are key steps. If treatment is instituted early, embolectomy and vascular reconstruction may salvage some small bowel. In these rare cases a 'second look' laparotomy is undertaken 24 hours later and further necrotic bowel resected. In patients at high surgical risk thrombolysis may sometimes be effective. The results of therapy depend on early intervention; patients treated late have a 75% mortality rate. Survivors often have nutritional failure from short bowel syndrome (p. 882) and require intensive nutritional support, sometimes including home parenteral nutrition, as well as anticoagulation. Small bowel transplantation is promising in selected patients. Patients with mesenteric venous thrombosis also require surgery if there are signs of peritonitis but are otherwise treated with anticoagulation. Investigations for underlying prothrombotic disorders should be performed (p. 1049).

Acute colonic ischaemia

The splenic flexure and descending colon have little collateral circulation and lie in 'watershed' areas of arterial supply. The spectrum of injury ranges from reversible colopathy to transient colitis, colonic stricture, gangrene and fulminant pancolitis. Arterial thromboembolism is usually responsible but colonic ischaemia can also follow severe hypotension, colonic volvulus, strangulated hernia, systemic vasculitis or hypercoagulable states. Ischaemia of the descending and sigmoid colon is also a complication of abdominal aortic aneurysm surgery (where the inferior mesenteric artery is ligated). The patient is usually elderly and presents with sudden onset of cramping left-sided lower abdominal pain and rectal bleeding. Symptoms usually resolve spontaneously over 24–48 hours and healing occurs within 2 weeks. Some have a residual fibrous stricture or segment of colitis. A minority develop gangrene and peritonitis. The diagnosis is established by colonoscopy within 48 hours of presentation; otherwise, mucosal ulceration and oedema may have resolved. Resection is required for peritonitis.

Chronic mesenteric ischaemia

This results from atherosclerotic stenosis affecting at least two of the coeliac axis, superior mesenteric and inferior mesenteric arteries. Dull but severe mid- or upper abdominal pain develops about 30 minutes after eating. Patients lose weight because of reluctance to eat, and some experience diarrhoea. Physical examination invariably shows evidence of generalised arterial disease. An abdominal bruit is sometimes audible but is non-specific. Mesenteric angiography confirms at least two affected mesenteric arteries. Vascular reconstruction

or percutaneous angioplasty is sometimes possible. Left untreated, many patients eventually develop intestinal infarction.

DISORDERS OF THE COLON AND RECTUM

Tumours of the colon and rectum

Polyps and polyposis syndromes

Polyps may be neoplastic or non-neoplastic. The latter include hamartomas, metaplastic ('hyperplastic') polyps and inflammatory polyps. These have no malignant potential. Polyps may be single or multiple and vary from a few millimetres to several centimetres in size.

Colorectal adenomas are extremely common in the Western world and the prevalence rises with age; 50% of people over 60 years of age have adenomas, and in half of these the polyps are multiple. They are more common in the rectum and distal colon and are either pedunculated or sessile. Histologically, they are classified as either tubular, villous or tubulovillous, according to the glandular architecture. Nearly all forms of colorectal carcinoma develop from adenomatous polyps over 5–10 years, although not all polyps carry the same degree of risk. Features associated with a higher risk of subsequent malignancy in colonic polyps are listed in Box 22.87.

Adenomas are usually asymptomatic and discovered incidentally. Occasionally, they cause bleeding and anaemia. Villous adenomas sometimes secrete large amounts of mucus, causing diarrhoea and hypokalaemia.

Discovery of a polyp at sigmoidoscopy is an indication for colonoscopy because proximal polyps are present in 40–50% of such patients. Colonoscopic polypectomy should be carried out wherever possible, as this considerably reduces subsequent colorectal cancer risk (Fig. 22.59). Very large or sessile polyps can sometimes be removed safely by endoscopic mucosal resection (EMR) but will otherwise require surgery. Once all polyps have been removed, patients should undergo surveillance colonoscopy at 3–5-year intervals, as new polyps develop in 50% of patients. Patients over 75 years of age do not require repeated colonoscopies, as their subsequent lifetime cancer risk is low.

Between 10 and 20% of polyps show histological evidence of malignancy. When cancer cells are found within 2 mm of the resection margin of the polyp, when the polyp cancer is poorly differentiated or when lymphatic invasion is present, segmental colonic resection is recommended because residual tumour or lymphatic spread (in up to 10%) may be present. Malignant polyps without these features can be followed up by surveillance colonoscopy.

Polyposis syndromes are classified by histopathology (Box 22.88). It should be noted that, while the hamarto-

22.87 Risk factors for malignant change in colonic polyps

- Large size (> 2 cm)
- Villous architecture
- Multiple polyps
- Dysplasia

22

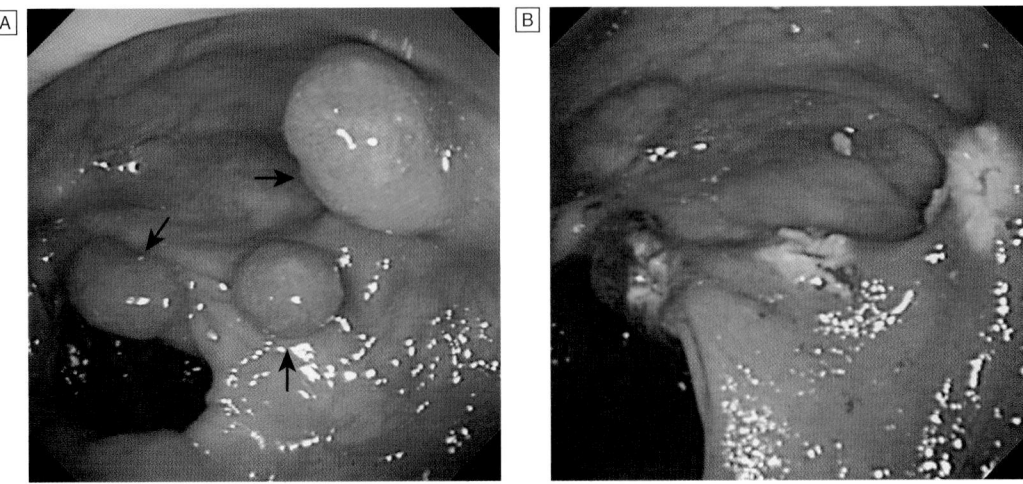

Fig. 22.59 Adenomatous colonic polyps. A Before colonoscopic polypectomy (arrows show polyps). B After polypectomy.

matous polyps in Peutz–Jeghers syndrome and juvenile polyposis are not themselves neoplastic, these disorders are associated with an increased risk of certain malignancies, e.g. breast, colon, ovary and thyroid.

Familial adenomatous polyposis

Familial adenomatous polyposis (FAP) is an uncommon autosomal dominant disorder affecting 1 in 13 000 of the population and accounting for 1% of all colorectal cancer. It results from germline mutation of the tumour suppressor *APC* gene followed by acquired mutation of the remaining allele (Ch. 3). *APC* is a large gene and over 1400 different mutations have been reported, but most result in a truncated APC protein. This protein has many functions in the regulation of colonic epithelial turnover. It normally binds to and sequesters β-catenin and is unable to do so when mutated, allowing β-catenin to translocate to the nucleus where it upregulates the expression of many genes.

Around 20% of cases arise as new mutations and have no family history. Hundreds to thousands of adeno-matous colonic polyps will develop in 80% of patients by age 15 (Fig. 22.60), with symptoms such as rectal bleeding beginning a few years later. In those affected, cancer will develop within 10–15 years of the appearance of adenomas and 90% of patients will develop colorectal cancer by the age of 50 years. Despite surveillance, approximately 1 in 4 patients with FAP has cancer by the time they undergo colectomy.

Recently, a second gene involved in base excision repair (MutY homolog, *MYH*) has been identified which may give rise to colonic polyposis. *MYH* displays autosomal recessive inheritance and leads to tens to hundreds of polyps and a tendency to proximal colon cancer. This variant is referred to as *MYH*-associated polyposis (MAP).

Non-neoplastic cystic fundic gland polyps occur in the stomach but adenomatous polyps also occur uncommonly. Duodenal adenomas occur in over 90% and are most common around the ampulla of Vater. Malignant transformation to adenocarcinoma occurs in 10% and is the leading cause of death in those who have had

22.88 Gastrointestinal polyposis syndromes

	Neoplastic	Non-neoplastic			
	Familial adenomatous polyposis	**Peutz–Jeghers syndrome**	**Juvenile polyposis**	**Cronkhite–Canada syndrome**	**Cowden's disease**
Inheritance	Autosomal dominant	Autosomal dominant	Autosomal dominant in 1/3	None	Autosomal dominant
Oesophageal polyps	–	–	–	+	+
Gastric polyps	+	+	+	+++	+++
Small bowel polyps	++	+++	++	++	++
Colonic polyps	+++	++	++	+++	+
Other features	See text	See text	See text	Hair loss, pigmentation, nail dystrophy, malabsorption	Many congenital anomalies, oral and cutaneous hamartomas, thyroid and breast tumours

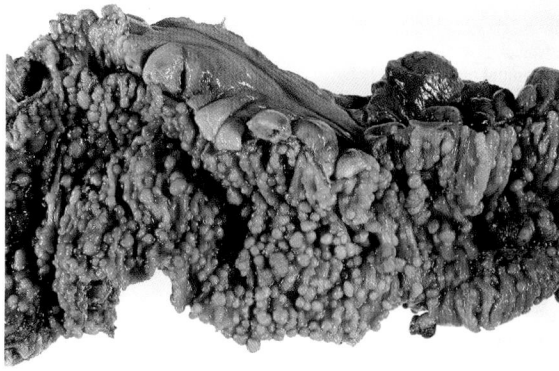

Fig. 22.60 Familial adenomatous polyposis. There are hundreds of adenomatous polyps throughout the colon.

prophylactic colectomy. Many extraintestinal features are also seen in FAP and these are summarised in Box 22.89.

Desmoid tumours occur in up to one-third of patients and usually arise in the mesentery or abdominal wall. Although benign, they may become very large, causing compression of adjacent organs, intestinal obstruction or vascular compromise, and are difficult to remove. They sometimes respond to hormonal therapy with tamoxifen, and the NSAID sulindac may lead to regression in some, by unknown mechanisms. Congenital hypertrophy of the retinal pigment epithelium (CHRPE) occurs in some and is seen as dark, round, pigmented retinal lesions. When present in an at-risk individual, they are 100% predictive of the presence of FAP. A variant, Turcot's syndrome, is characterised by FAP with primary central nervous system tumours (astrocytoma or medulloblastoma).

Early identification of affected individuals before symptoms develop is essential. The diagnosis can be excluded if sigmoidoscopy is normal. In newly diagnosed cases with new mutations, genetic testing confirms the diagnosis, and all first-degree relatives should also undergo testing (p. 57). In families with known FAP, at-risk family members should undergo direct mutation testing at 13–14 years of age. This is less invasive than regular sigmoidoscopy, which is reserved for those known to have the mutation. Affected individuals should undergo colectomy after school or college education has been completed. The operation of choice is total proctocolectomy with ileal pouch–anal anastomosis. Periodic upper gastrointestinal endoscopy is recommended to detect duodenal adenomas.

22.89 Extraintestinal features of familial adenomatous polyposis
• Congenital hypertrophy of the retinal pigment epithelium (CHRPE, 70–80%) • Epidermoid cysts (extremities, face, scalp)* (50%) • Benign osteomas, especially skull and angle of mandible* (50–90%) • Dental abnormalities (15–25%)* • Desmoid tumours (10–15%) • Other malignancies (brain, thyroid, liver, 1–3%)
*Gardner's syndrome.

Peutz–Jeghers syndrome

This is characterised by multiple hamartomatous polyps in the small intestine and colon, as well as melanin pigmentation of the lips, mouth and digits (Fig. 22.61). Most cases are asymptomatic, although chronic bleeding, anaemia or intussusception can be seen. There is a significant risk of small bowel or colonic adenocarcinoma and of cancer of the pancreas, lung, ovary, breast and endometrium. It is an autosomal dominantly inherited disorder most commonly resulting from truncating mutations in a serine-threonine kinase gene on chromosome 19p (*STRK11-LKB1*).

Diagnosis requires two of the following:
- small bowel polyposis
- mucocutaneous pigmentation
- a family history suggesting autosomal dominant inheritance.

Genetic testing is also available but may be inconclusive since mutants in genes other than *STRK11-LKB1* can cause the disorder. Affected people should undergo regular upper endoscopy, colonoscopy, and small bowel and pancreatic imaging. Polyps > 1 cm in size should be removed. Testicular examination is essential for men while women should undergo pelvic examination, cervical smears and regular mammography. Asymptomatic relatives of affected patients should also undergo screening.

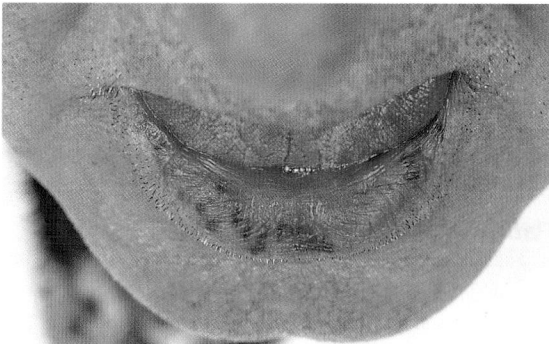

Fig. 22.61 Peutz–Jeghers syndrome. Typical lip pigmentation.

Juvenile polyposis (JPS)

In this condition, tens to hundreds of mucus-filled hamartomatous polyps are found in the colorectum. One-third of cases are inherited in an autosomal dominant manner and up to 20% of patients develop colorectal cancer before the age of 40. The criteria for diagnosis are:
- 10 or more colonic juvenile polyps
- juvenile polyps elsewhere in the gut, *or*
- any number of polyps in those with a family history.

Germline mutations in the tumour suppressor gene *SMAD4* are often found, as are *PTEN* mutations. Colonoscopy with polypectomy should be performed every 1–3 years and colectomy considered for extensive involvement.

Colorectal cancer

Although relatively rare in the developing world, colorectal cancer is the second most common internal malignancy and the second leading cause of cancer deaths in Western countries. In the UK the incidence is 50–60 per 100 000, equating to 30 000 cases per year. The condition becomes increasingly common over the age of 50.

22

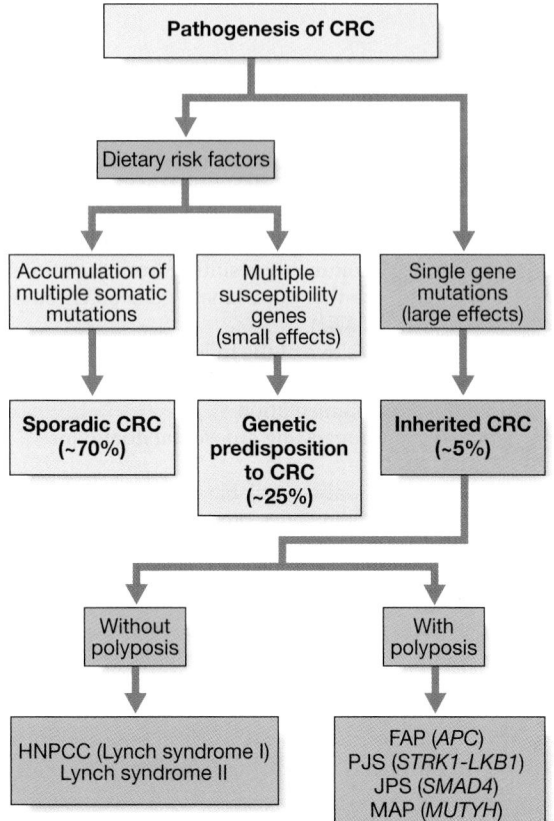

Fig. 22.62 Pathogenesis of colorectal cancer (CRC). (FAP = familial adenomatous polyposis; HNPCC = hereditary non-polyposis colon cancer); JPS = juvenile polyposis syndrome; MAP = *MUTYH*-associated polyposis; PJS = Peutz–Jeghers syndrome

Pathophysiology

Both environmental and genetic factors are important in colorectal carcinogenesis (Fig. 22.62).

Environmental factors probably account for 70% of all 'sporadic' colorectal cancers. This figure is based on the

22.90 Dietary risk factors for colorectal cancer development

Risk factor	Comments
Increased risk	
Red meat*	High saturated fat and protein content. Carcinogenic amines formed during cooking
Saturated animal fat*	High faecal bile acid and fatty acid levels. May affect colonic prostaglandin turnover
Decreased risk	
Dietary fibre*	Effects vary with fibre type; shortened transit time, binding of bile acids and effects on bacterial flora proposed
Fruit and vegetables	Green vegetables contain anticarcinogens, such as glucosinolates and flavonoids. Little evidence for protection from vitamins A, C, E
Calcium	Binds and precipitates faecal bile acids
Folic acid	Reverses DNA hypomethylation
Omega-3 fatty acids	May be of modest benefit; trials awaited

*Evidence is inconsistent and a clear relationship is unproven.

22.91 Non-dietary risk factors in colorectal cancer

Medical conditions

- Colorectal adenomas (p. 907)
- Long-standing extensive ulcerative colitis or Crohn's colitis (p. 895), especially if associated with primary sclerosing cholangitis (PSC)
- Ureterosigmoidostomy
- Acromegaly
- Pelvic radiotherapy

Others

- Obesity and sedentary lifestyle—may be related to dietary factors
- Smoking (relative risk 1.5–3.0)
- Alcohol (weak association)
- Cholecystectomy (effect of bile acids in right colon)
- Type 2 diabetes (hyperinsulinaemia)
- Use of aspirin or NSAIDs (COX-2 inhibition) and perhaps statins associated with *reduced* risk

wide geographic variation in incidence and the decrease in risk seen in migrants who move from high- to low-risk countries. Dietary factors are believed to be most important and these are summarised in Box 22.90; other recognised risk factors are listed in Box 22.91.

Colorectal cancer development results from the accumulation of multiple genetic mutations arising from two major pathways: chromosomal instability and microsatellite instability (Fig. 22.63).

- *Chromosomal instability.* This involves mutations or deletions of portions of chromosomes with loss of heterozygosity (LOH) and inactivation of specific tumour suppressor genes. In LOH, one allele of a gene is deleted but gene inactivation only occurs when a subsequent unrelated mutation affects the other allele.
- *Microsatellite instability.* This involves germline mutations in one of six genes encoding enzymes involved in repairing errors that occur normally during DNA replication (DNA mismatch repair); these genes are designated *hMSH2*, *hMSH6*, *hMLH1*, *hMLH3*, *hPMS1* and *hPMS2*. Replication errors accumulate and can be detected in 'microsatellites' of repetitive DNA sequences. Replication errors also occur in important regulatory genes, resulting in a genetically unstable phenotype and accumulation of multiple somatic mutations throughout the genome that eventually lead to cancer formation. A minority of sporadic cancers develop this way, as do almost all cases of HNPCC.

HNPCC accounts for 5–10% of cancers; it occurs in those with a family history and often at a young age. Pedigrees of HNPCC families indicate an autosomal dominant pattern of inheritance. The criteria necessary for diagnosing this condition are given in Box 22.92. The lifetime risk of colorectal cancer in affected individuals is 80%. The mean age of cancer development is 45 years, and in contrast to sporadic colon cancer two-thirds of tumours occur proximally. In a subset of patients, there is also an increased incidence of cancers of the endometrium, ovary, urinary tract, stomach, pancreas, small intestine and central nervous system, related to inheritance of different mismatch repair gene mutations.

Those who fulfil the criteria for diagnosis should be referred for pedigree assessment, genetic testing and

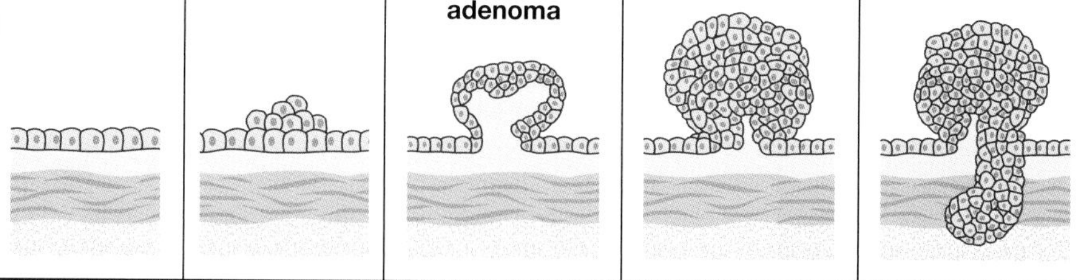

	Normal	Early adenoma	Intermediate adenoma	Late adenoma	Carcinoma
Key gene		APC (adenomatous polyposis coli)	K-ras	DCC (SMAD4) (deleted in colon cancer)	p53
Chromosome		5q	12p	18q	17p
Normal function		'Gatekeeper'	Transmembrane GTP-binding protein mediating mitogenic signals (p21)	Multiple: role in apoptosis, tumour suppressor gene; TGF signalling	Upregulated during cell damage to arrest cell cycle and allow DNA repair or apoptosis to occur
Alteration		Truncating mutations	Gain in function mutations	Allelic deletion	Allelic deletion; gain in function mutations
Effect		Progression to early adenoma development	Cell proliferation	? Role in invasion and metastasis	Cell proliferation; impaired apoptosis

Further mutations
- Anchorage independence
- Protease synthesis
- Telomerase synthesis
- Multidrug resistance
- Evasion of immune system

Fig. 22.63 The multistep origin of cancer: molecular events implicated in colorectal carcinogenesis. (GTP = guanine triphosphate)

22.92 Criteria for the diagnosis of hereditary non-polyposis colon cancer ('modified Amsterdam II criteria')*

- Three or more relatives with colon cancer (at least one first-degree)
- Colorectal cancer in two or more generations
- At least one member affected under 50 years of age
- FAP excluded

*These criteria are strict and may miss some families with mutations. HNPCC should also be considered in individuals with colorectal or endometrial cancer under 45 years of age.

colonoscopy. These should begin around 25 years of age or 5–10 years earlier than the youngest case of cancer in the family. Colonoscopy needs to be repeated every 1–2 years, but even then, interval cancers can still occur.

A further 20% of patients who do not have HNPCC still have a family history of colorectal cancer. The lifetime risk of developing cancer with one or two affected first-degree relatives is 1 in 12 and 1 in 6, respectively. The risk is even higher if relatives were affected at an early age. The genes mediating this increased risk are unknown. Most tumours arise from malignant transformation of a benign adenomatous polyp. Over 65% occur in the rectosigmoid and a further 15% recur in the caecum or ascending colon. Synchronous tumours are present in 2–5% of patients. Macroscopically, the majority of cancers are either polyp-oid and 'fungating', or annular and constricting. Spread occurs through the bowel wall. Rectal cancers may invade the pelvic viscera and side walls. Lymphatic invasion is common at presentation, as is spread through both portal and systemic circulations to reach the liver and, less commonly, the lungs. Tumour stage at diagnosis is the most important determinant of prognosis (see Fig. 22.65, p. 912).

Clinical features

Symptoms vary depending on the site of the carcinoma. In tumours of the left colon, fresh rectal bleeding is common and obstruction occurs early. Tumours of the right colon present with anaemia from occult bleeding or with altered bowel habit, but obstruction is a late feature. Colicky lower abdominal pain is present in two-thirds of patients and rectal bleeding occurs in 50%. A minority present with features of either obstruction or perforation, leading to peritonitis, localised abscess or fistula formation. Carcinoma of the rectum usually causes early bleeding, mucus discharge or a feeling of incomplete emptying. Between 10 and 20% of patients present with iron deficiency anaemia or weight loss. On examination there may be a palpable mass, signs of anaemia or hepatomegaly from metastases. Low rectal tumours may be palpable on digital examination.

Investigations

Colonoscopy (Fig. 22.64) is the investigation of choice because it is more sensitive and specific than barium enema. Furthermore, lesions can be biopsied and polyps removed. Rigid sigmoidoscopy will detect less than one-third of tumours. Endoanal ultrasound or pelvic MRI stages rectal cancers accurately. CT colonography ('virtual colonoscopy') is a sensitive non-invasive technique for diagnosing tumours and polyps greater than 1 cm that can be used if colonoscopy is incomplete or high-risk. CT is valuable for detecting hepatic metastases, although intraoperative ultrasound is increasingly being used for this purpose. A proportion of patients have raised serum carcinoembryonic antigen (CEA) concentrations but this is variable and so of little use in diagnosis. Measurements of CEA are valuable, however, during follow-up and can help to detect early recurrence.

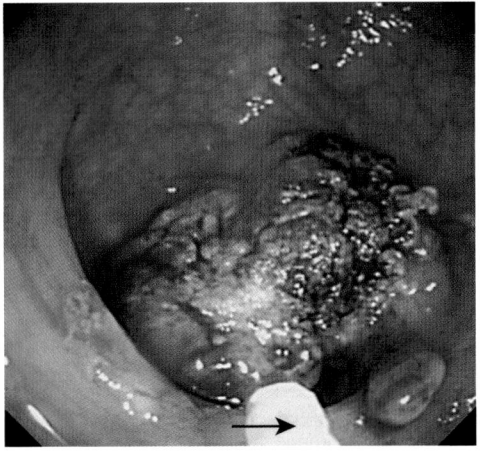

Fig. 22.64 Colonoscopic view of a polypoid rectal carcinoma undergoing laser therapy (arrow) in a patient unfit for surgery.

Management

Surgery

The tumour is removed, along with adequate resection margins and pericolic lymph nodes. Continuity is restored by direct anastomosis wherever possible. Carcinomas within 2 cm of the anal verge may require abdominoperineal resection and formation of a colostomy. All patients should be counselled pre-operatively about the possible need for a stoma. Total mesorectal excision (TME) reduces recurrence rates and increases survival in rectal cancer. Solitary hepatic or lung metastases are sometimes resected at a later stage. Post-operatively, patients should undergo colonoscopy after 6–12 months and periodically thereafter to search for local recurrence or development of new 'metachronous' lesions, which occur in 6% of cases.

Adjuvant therapy

Two-thirds of patients have lymph node or distant spread (Dukes stage C, Fig. 22.65) at presentation and are, therefore, beyond cure with surgery alone. Most recurrences are within 3 years of diagnosis. Colonic cancers recur locally at the site of resection, in lymph nodes, liver and peritoneum. Adjuvant chemotherapy with 5-fluorouracil and folinic acid (to reduce toxicity) for 6 months improves both disease-free and overall survival in patients with Dukes C colon cancer by around 4–13%. Pre-operative radiotherapy can be given to patients with large, fixed rectal cancers to 'downstage' the tumour, making it resectable and reducing local recurrence. Dukes C and some Dukes B rectal cancers are given post-operative radiotherapy to reduce the risk of local recurrence if operative resection margins are involved. In some countries, patients with metastatic disease are treated with monoclonal antibodies using bevacizumab or cetuximab either alone or with chemotherapeutic agents such as irinotecan.

Chemotherapy

Surgical resection of the primary tumour is appropriate for some patients with metastases to treat obstruction, bleeding or pain. Palliative chemotherapy with 5-fluorouracil and folinic acid improves survival, and second-line therapy with irinotecan is used when this fails. Pelvic radiotherapy is sometimes useful for distressing rectal symptoms such as pain, bleeding or severe tenesmus. Endoscopic laser therapy or insertion of an expandable metal stent can be used to relieve obstruction.

Prevention and screening

Secondary prevention aims to detect and remove lesions at an early or pre-malignant stage. Several potential methods exist:

- Widespread screening by regular *faecal occult blood (FOB) testing* reduces colorectal cancer mortality (Box 22.93) and increases the proportion of early cancers detected. These tests currently lack sensitivity and specificity and need to be improved. FOB screening is recommended after the age of 50 years.
- *Colonoscopy* remains the gold standard but is expensive and carries risks; many countries lack the resources to offer this form of screening.
- *Flexible sigmoidoscopy* is an alternative option and has been shown to reduce overall colorectal cancer mortality by approximately 35% (70% for cases arising in the rectosigmoid). It is recommended in the USA every 5 years in all persons over the age of 50.

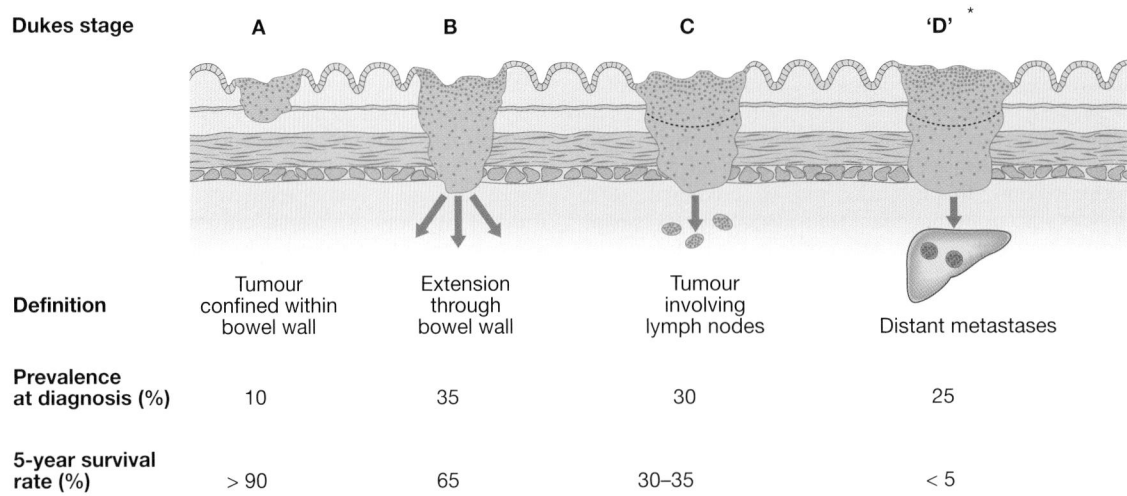

Dukes stage	A	B	C	'D' *
Definition	Tumour confined within bowel wall	Extension through bowel wall	Tumour involving lymph nodes	Distant metastases
Prevalence at diagnosis (%)	10	35	30	25
5-year survival rate (%)	> 90	65	30–35	< 5

Fig. 22.65 **Staging and survival in colorectal cancer.** (Modified Dukes classification. *Dukes' original staging only had stages A–C.)

EBM 22.93 Faecal occult blood (FOB) testing and colon cancer mortality

'Combined results from four randomised controlled trials show that participants allocated to screening by FOB testing had a 16% reduction in the relative risk of colorectal cancer mortality (RR 0.84, CI: 0.78–0.90). When adjusted for screening attendance, there was a 25% relative risk reduction (RR 0.75, CI: 0.66–0.84) for those attending at least one round of FOB screening.'

● (Cochrane Review). Cochrane Library, issue 4, 2006. Oxford: Update Software.

For further information: www.cochrane.org/reviews

● Screening for high-risk patients by *molecular genetic analysis* is an exciting prospect but is not yet available.

Diverticulosis

Diverticula are acquired and are most common in the sigmoid and descending colon of middle-aged people. Asymptomatic diverticula (diverticulosis) are present in over 50% of people above the age of 70. Symptomatic diverticular disease supervenes in 10–25% of cases while complicated diverticulosis (acute diverticulitis, pericolic abscess, bleeding, perforation or stricture) is uncommon.

Pathophysiology

A life-long refined diet with a relative deficiency of fibre is widely thought to be responsible and the condition is rare in populations with a high dietary fibre intake, such as in Asia, where it more often affects the right side of the colon. It is postulated that small-volume stools require high intracolonic pressures for propulsion and this leads to herniation of mucosa between the taeniae coli (Fig. 22.66). Diverticula consist of protrusions of mucosa covered by peritoneum. There is commonly hypertrophy of the circular muscle coat. Inflammation is thought to result from impaction of diverticula with faecoliths. This may resolve spontaneously or progress to cause haemorrhage, perforation, local abscess formation, fistula and peritonitis. Repeated attacks of inflammation lead to thickening of the bowel wall, narrowing of the lumen and eventual obstruction.

Clinical features

Symptoms are usually the result of associated constipation or spasm. Colicky pain is usually suprapubic or felt in the left iliac fossa. The sigmoid colon may be palpable and, in attacks of diverticulitis, there is local tenderness, guarding, rigidity ('left-sided appendicitis') and sometimes a palpable mass. During these episodes there may also be diarrhoea, rectal bleeding or fever. The differential diagnosis includes colorectal cancer, ischaemic colitis, inflammatory bowel disease and infection. Diverticular disease is complicated by perforation, pericolic abscess, fistula formation (usually colovesical) and acute rectal bleeding. These complications are more common in patients who take NSAIDs or aspirin. After one attack of diverticulitis, the recurrence rate is around 3% per year. Over 10–30 years, perforation, obstruction or bleeding will each affect around 5% of patients.

Investigations

These are usually performed to exclude colorectal neoplasia. Barium enema confirms the presence of diverticula (see Fig. 22.11C, p. 845). Strictures and fistulas may also be seen. Flexible sigmoidoscopy is performed to exclude a coexisting neoplasm which is easily missed radiologically. Colonoscopy requires expertise and carries a risk of perforation. CT is used to assess complications.

Management

Diverticulosis which is asymptomatic and discovered coincidentally requires no treatment. Constipation can be relieved by a high-fibre diet with or without a bulking laxative (ispaghula husk, 1–2 sachets daily) taken with plenty of fluids. Stimulants should be avoided. Antispasmodics may sometimes help. An acute attack of diverticulitis requires 7 days of metronidazole (400 mg 8-hourly orally), along with either a cephalosporin or ampicillin (500 mg 6-hourly orally). Severe cases require intravenous fluids, intravenous antibiotics, analgesia and nasogastric suction, but randomised trials show no benefit from acute resection compared to conservative management, and emergency surgery is reserved for severe haemorrhage or perforation. Percutaneous drainage of acute paracolic abscesses can be effective and avoids the need for emergency surgery. Elective surgery is performed in patients after recovery from repeated acute attacks of obstruction, and resection of the affected segment with primary anastomosis is the procedure of choice.

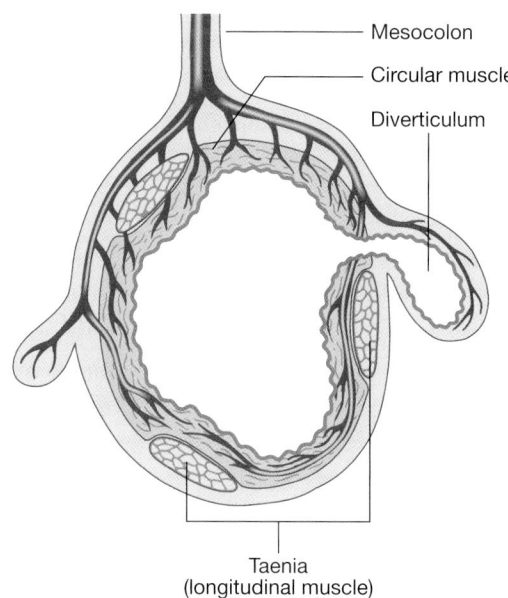

Mesocolon

Circular muscle

Diverticulum

Taenia
(longitudinal muscle)

Fig. 22.66 The human colon in diverticulosis. The colonic wall is weak between the taeniae. The blood vessels that supply the colon pierce the circular muscle and weaken it further by forming tunnels. Diverticula usually emerge through these points of least resistance.

Constipation and disorders of defecation

The clinical approach to patients with constipation and its aetiology have been described on page 859.

22

Simple constipation

This is extremely common and does not imply underlying organic disease. It usually responds to increased dietary fibre or the use of bulking agents; an adequate fluid intake is also essential. Many types of laxative are available, and these are listed in Box 22.94.

Severe idiopathic constipation

This occurs almost exclusively in young women and often begins in childhood or adolescence. The cause is unknown but some have 'slow transit' with reduced motor activity in the colon. Others have 'obstructed defecation' resulting from inappropriate contraction of the external anal sphincter and puborectalis muscle (anismus). The condition is often resistant to treatment. Bulking agents may exacerbate symptoms but prokinetic agents or balanced solutions of polyethylene glycol '3350' benefit some patients with slow transit. Glycerol suppositories and biofeedback techniques are used for those with obstructed defecation. Rarely, subtotal colectomy is necessary as a last resort.

Faecal impaction

In faecal impaction a large, hard mass of stool fills the rectum. This tends to occur in disabled, immobile or institutionalised patients, especially the frail elderly or those with dementia. Constipating drugs, autonomic neuropathy and painful anal conditions also contribute. Megacolon, intestinal obstruction and urinary tract infections may supervene. Perforation and bleeding from pressure-induced ulceration are occasionally seen. Treatment involves adequate hydration and careful digital disimpaction after softening the impacted stool with arachis oil enemas. Stimulants should be avoided.

Melanosis coli and laxative misuse syndromes

Long-term consumption of stimulant laxatives leads to accumulation of lipofuscin pigment in macrophages in the lamina propria. This imparts a brown discoloration to the colonic mucosa, often described as resembling 'tiger

22.95 Constipation in old age

- **Evaluation:** particular attention should be paid to immobility, dietary fluid and fibre intake, drugs and depression.
- **Immobility:** predisposes to constipation by increasing the colonic transit time; the longer this is, the greater the fluid absorption and the harder the stool.
- **Bulking agents:** can make matters worse in patients with slow transit times and should be avoided.
- **Overflow diarrhoea:** if faecal impaction develops, paradoxical overflow diarrhoea may occur. If antidiarrhoeal agents are given, the underlying impaction may worsen and result in serious complications such as stercoral ulceration and bleeding.

skin'. The condition is benign and resolves when the laxatives are stopped. Prolonged laxative use may rarely result in megacolon or 'cathartic colon', in which barium enema demonstrates a featureless mucosa, loss of haustra and shortening of the bowel. Surreptitious laxative misuse is a psychiatric condition seen in young women, some of whom have a history of bulimia or anorexia nervosa (pp. 249–250). They complain of refractory watery diarrhoea. Laxative use is usually denied and may continue even when patients are undergoing investigation. Screening of urine for laxatives may reveal the diagnosis.

Hirschsprung's disease

This disease is characterised by constipation and colonic dilatation (megacolon) due to congenital absence of ganglion cells in the large intestine. The incidence is 1:5000 and a family history is present in one-third of cases. The main gene contributing to susceptibility is the *RET* gene, but often other genetic mutations need to be present for the disease to occur. These genes are implicated in the regulation of enteric neurogenesis, and the mutations cause failure of migration of neuroblasts into the gut wall during embryogenesis. Ganglion cells are absent from nerve plexuses, most commonly in a short segment of the rectum and/or sigmoid colon. As a result, the internal anal sphincter fails to relax. Constipation, abdominal distension and vomiting usually develop immediately after birth but a few cases do not present until childhood or adolescence. The rectum is empty on digital examination.

Barium enema shows a small rectum and colonic dilatation above the narrowed segment. Full-thickness biopsies are required to demonstrate nerve plexuses and confirm the absence of ganglion cells. Histochemical stains for acetylcholinesterase are also used. Anorectal manometry demonstrates failure of the rectum to relax with balloon distension. Treatment involves resection of the affected segment.

Acquired megacolon

This may develop in childhood as a result of voluntary withholding of stool during toilet training. In such cases it presents after the first year of life and is distinguished from Hirschsprung's disease by the urge to defecate and the presence of stool in the rectum. It usually responds to osmotic laxatives.

In adults, acquired megacolon has several causes. It is seen in depressed or demented patients, either as part of

22.94 Laxatives

Class	Examples
Bulk-forming	Ispaghula husk Methylcellulose
Stimulants	Bisacodyl Dantron (only for terminally ill patients) Docusate Senna
Faecal softeners	Docusate Arachis oil enema
Osmotic laxatives	Lactulose Lactitol Magnesium salts
Others	Polyethylene glycol (PEG)* Phosphate enema*

*Used mainly for bowel preparation prior to investigation or surgery.

the condition or as a side-effect of antidepressant drugs. Prolonged misuse of stimulant laxatives may cause degeneration of the myenteric plexus, while interruption of sensory or motor innervation may be responsible in a number of neurological disorders. Scleroderma and hypothyroidism are other recognised causes.

Most patients can be managed conservatively by treatment of the underlying cause, high-residue diets, laxatives and the judicious use of enemas. Prokinetics are helpful in a minority of patients. Subtotal colectomy is a last resort for the most severely affected patients.

Acute colonic pseudo-obstruction (Ogilvie's syndrome)

This condition has many causes (Box 22.96) and is characterised by relatively sudden onset of painless, massive enlargement of the proximal colon accompanied by distension; there are no features of mechanical obstruction. Bowel sounds are normal or high-pitched rather than absent. Left untreated, it may progress to perforation, peritonitis and death.

Plain abdominal X-rays show colonic dilatation with air extending to the rectum. A caecal diameter greater than 10–12 cm is associated with a high risk of perforation. Single-contrast or water-soluble barium enemas demonstrate the absence of mechanical obstruction.

Management consists of treating the underlying disorder and correcting any biochemical abnormalities. The anticholinesterase, neostigmine, is often effective in enhancing parasympathetic activity and gut motility. Decompression either with a rectal tube or by careful colonoscopy may be effective but needs to be repeated until the condition resolves. In severe cases, surgical or fluoroscopic defunctioning caecostomy is necessary.

22.96	Causes of acute colonic pseudo-obstruction

- Trauma, burns
- Recent surgery
- Drugs, e.g. opiates, phenothiazines
- Respiratory failure
- Electrolyte and acid–base disorders
- Diabetes mellitus
- Uraemia

Colonic infections

These are discussed on pages 302–305.

Anorectal disorders

Faecal incontinence

The normal control of anal continence is described on page 842. Common causes of incontinence are listed in Box 22.97.

Patients are often embarrassed to admit incontinence and may complain only of 'diarrhoea'. A careful history and examination, especially of the anorectum and perineum, may help to establish the underlying cause. Endoanal ultrasound is valuable for defining the integrity of the anal sphincters, while anorectal manometry and electrophysiology are also useful investigations if available.

22.97	Causes of faecal incontinence

- Obstetric trauma: childbirth, hysterectomy
- Severe diarrhoea
- Faecal impaction
- Congenital anorectal anomalies
- Anorectal disease: haemorrhoids, rectal prolapse, Crohn's disease
- Neurological disorders: spinal cord or cauda equina lesions, dementia

Management

This is often very difficult. Underlying disorders should be treated and diarrhoea managed with loperamide, diphenoxylate or codeine phosphate. Pelvic floor exercises and biofeedback techniques help some patients, and those with confirmed anal sphincter defects may benefit from sphincter repair operations.

Haemorrhoids ('piles')

Haemorrhoids arise from congestion of the internal and/or external venous plexuses around the anal canal (Fig. 22.67). They are extremely common in adults. The aetiology is unknown, although they are associated with constipation and straining and may develop for the first time during pregnancy. First-degree piles bleed, while second-degree piles prolapse but retract spontaneously. Third-degree piles are those which require manual replacement after prolapsing. Bright red rectal bleeding occurs after defecation. Other symptoms include pain, pruritus ani and mucus discharge. Treatment involves measures to prevent constipation and straining. Injection sclerotherapy or band ligation is effective for most, but a minority of patients require haemorrhoidectomy, which is usually curative.

Pruritus ani

This is common and can stem from many causes (Box 22.98), most of which result in contamination of the perianal skin with faecal contents.

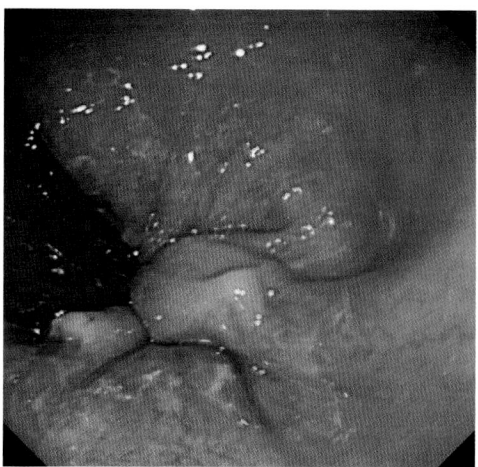

Fig. 22.67 Internal haemorrhoids seen as bluish cushions of prominent veins at sigmoidoscopy.

22.98 Causes of pruritus ani

Local anorectal conditions

- Haemorrhoids
- Fistula, fissures
- Poor hygiene

Infections

- Threadworms
- Candidiasis

Skin disorders

- Contact dermatitis
- Psoriasis
- Lichen planus

Other

- Diarrhoea or incontinence of any cause
- Irritable bowel syndrome
- Anxiety

Itching may be trivial or severe, and results in an itch-scratch-itch cycle which exacerbates the problem. When no underlying cause is found, all local barrier ointments and creams must be stopped. Good personal hygiene is essential, with careful washing after defecation. The perineal area must be kept dry and clean. Bulk-forming laxatives may reduce faecal soiling.

Solitary rectal ulcer syndrome

This is most common in young adults and occurs on the anterior rectal wall. It is thought to result from localised chronic trauma and/or ischaemia associated with disordered puborectalis function and mucosal prolapse. The ulcer is seen at sigmoidoscopy and biopsies show a characteristic accumulation of collagen.

Symptoms include minor bleeding and mucus per rectum, tenesmus and perineal pain. Treatment is often difficult but avoidance of straining at defecation is important and treatment of constipation may help. Marked mucosal prolapse is treated surgically.

Anal fissure

In this common problem traumatic or ischaemic damage to the anal mucosa results in a superficial mucosal tear, most commonly in the midline posteriorly. Spasm of the internal anal sphincter exacerbates the condition. Severe pain occurs on defecation and there may be minor bleeding, mucus discharge and pruritus. The skin may be indurated and an oedematous skin tag, or 'sentinel pile', adjacent to the fissure is common.

Avoidance of constipation with bulk-forming laxatives and increased fluid intake is important. Relaxation of the internal sphincter is normally mediated by nitric oxide, and 0.2% glyceryl trinitrate or diltiazem ointment, which donates nitric oxide and improves mucosal blood flow, is effective in 60–80% of patients. Resistant cases may respond to injection of botulinum toxin into the internal anal sphincter to induce sphincter relaxation. Manual dilatation under anaesthesia leads to long-term incontinence and should not be considered. The majority of cases can now be treated without surgery, but where these measures fail, healing can usually be achieved surgically by lateral internal anal sphincterotomy or advancement anoplasty.

Anorectal abscesses and fistulas

Perianal abscesses develop between the internal and external anal sphincters and may point at the perianal skin. Ischiorectal abscesses occur lateral to the sphincters in the ischiorectal fossa. They usually result from infection of anal glands by normal intestinal bacteria. Crohn's disease (p. 895) is sometimes responsible.

Patients complain of extreme perianal pain, fever and/or discharge of pus. Spontaneous rupture may also lead to the development of fistulas. These may be superficial or may track through the anal sphincters to reach the rectum. Abscesses are drained surgically and superficial fistulas are laid open with care to avoid sphincter damage.

Diseases of the peritoneal cavity

Peritonitis

Surgical peritonitis occurs as the result of a ruptured viscus (see surgical textbooks). Peritonitis may also complicate ascites (spontaneous bacterial peritonitis) or may occur in children in the absence of ascites, due to infection with pneumococci or β-haemolytic streptococci.

Chlamydial peritonitis is a complication of pelvic inflammatory disease. The affected woman presents with right upper quadrant abdominal pain, pyrexia and a hepatic rub (the Fitz-Hugh–Curtis syndrome). Tuberculosis may cause peritonitis and ascites.

Tumours

The most common is secondary adenocarcinoma from the ovary or gastrointestinal tract. Mesothelioma is a rare tumour complicating asbestos exposure. It presents as a diffuse abdominal mass, due to omental infiltration, and with ascites. The prognosis is extremely poor.

Other disorders

Endometriosis

Ectopic endometrial tissue can become embedded on the serosal aspect of the intestine, most frequently in the sigmoid and rectum. The overlying mucosa is usually intact. Cyclical engorgement and inflammation result in pain, bleeding, diarrhoea, constipation, and adhesions or obstruction. Low backache is frequent. The onset is usually between 20 and 45 years and is more common in nulliparous women. Bimanual examination may reveal tender nodules in the pouch of Douglas. Endoscopic studies only reveal the diagnosis if carried out during menstruation, when a bluish mass with intact overlying mucosa is apparent. In some patients laparoscopy is required. Treatment options include laparoscopic diathermy and hormonal therapy with progestogens (e.g. norethisterone), gonadotrophin-releasing hormone analogues or danazol.

Pneumatosis cystoides intestinalis

In this rare condition multiple gas-filled submucosal cysts line the colonic and small bowel walls. The cause is unknown, but the condition may be seen in patients with chronic cardiac or pulmonary disease, pyloric obstruction, scleroderma or dermatomyositis. Most patients are asymptomatic, although there may be abdominal cramp, diarrhoea, tenesmus, rectal bleeding and mucus discharge. The cysts are recognised on sigmoidoscopy, plain abdominal X-rays or barium enema. Fasting breath hydrogen levels are elevated and fall with treatment. Therapies reported to be effective include prolonged high-flow oxygen, elemental diets and antibiotics.

Further information

Books and journal articles

Cotton PB, Williams CB. Practical gastrointestinal endoscopy: the fundamentals. 6th edn. Oxford: Wiley–Blackwell; 2008.

Feldman M, Friedman LS, Brandt LJ. Sleisenger and Fordtran's gastrointestinal and liver disease. 8th edn. Philadelphia: Saunders Elsevier; 2006.

Websites

www.bsg.org.uk *British Society of Gastroenterology.*
www.coeliac.org.uk *UK Coeliac Society.*
www.gastro.org *American Gastroenterological Association and American Digestive Health Foundation.*
www.gastrohep.com
www.isg.org.in *Indian Society of Gastroenterology.*
www.nacc.org.uk *National Association for Colitis and Crohn's disease (NACC).*

22

J.D. Collier
G. Webster

Liver and biliary tract disease

23

CLINICAL EXAMINATION OF THE ABDOMEN FOR LIVER AND BILIARY DISEASE

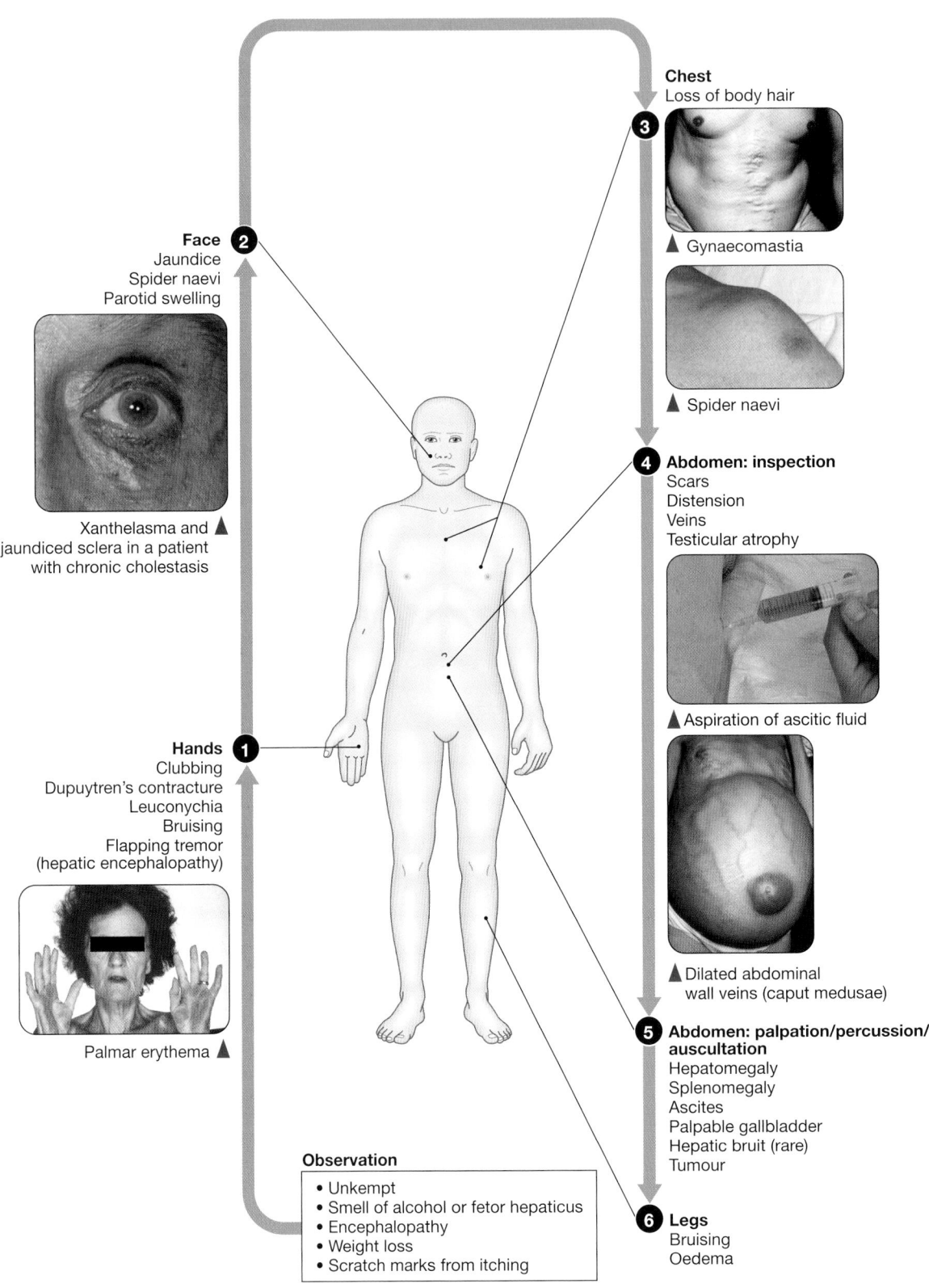

Chest
Loss of body hair

3

▲ Gynaecomastia

▲ Spider naevi

Face **2**
Jaundice
Spider naevi
Parotid swelling

Xanthelasma and ▲
jaundiced sclera in a patient
with chronic cholestasis

4 Abdomen: inspection
Scars
Distension
Veins
Testicular atrophy

▲ Aspiration of ascitic fluid

▲ Dilated abdominal
wall veins (caput medusae)

Hands **1**
Clubbing
Dupuytren's contracture
Leuconychia
Bruising
Flapping tremor
(hepatic encephalopathy)

Palmar erythema ▲

**5 Abdomen: palpation/percussion/
auscultation**
Hepatomegaly
Splenomegaly
Ascites
Palpable gallbladder
Hepatic bruit (rare)
Tumour

Observation

- Unkempt
- Smell of alcohol or fetor hepaticus
- Encephalopathy
- Weight loss
- Scratch marks from itching

6 Legs
Bruising
Oedema

History and significance of abdominal signs

❶ Flapping tremor

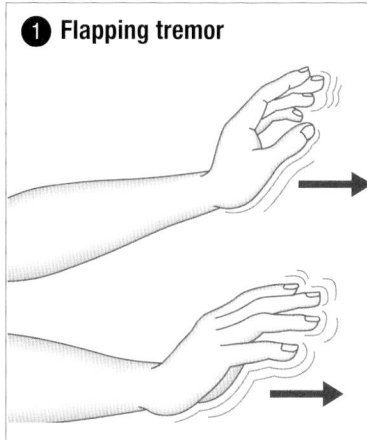

Jerky forward movements every 2–3 minutes when arms are outstretched and hands are dorsiflexed suggest hepatic encephalopathy.

❺ Assessment of liver size

- Start in the right iliac fossa.
- Progress up the abdomen 2 cm with each breath (through open mouth).
- Confirm the lower border of the liver by percussion.
- Detect if smooth or irregular, tender or non-tender; ascertain shape.
- Identify the upper border by percussion.
- Clinical assessment of hepatomegaly important in diagnosing liver disease

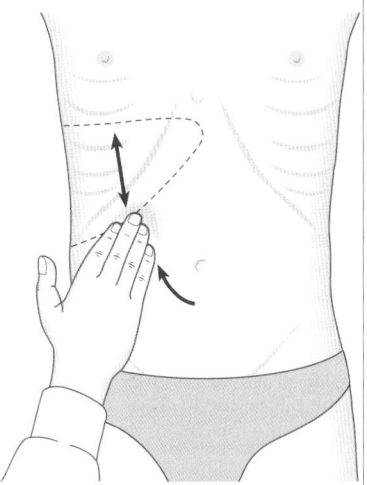

Liver size

Large liver (hepatomegaly)

- Liver metastases
- Multiple or large hepatic cysts
- Cirrhosis
   - Alcohol
   - Haemochromatosis
- Hepatic vein outflow obstruction
- Infiltration
   - Amyloid

Small liver

- Cirrhosis

Ascites

Causes	Associated clinical findings
Exudative (high protein)*	
Carcinoma	Weight loss ± hepatomegaly
Tuberculosis	Weight loss + fever
Transudative (low protein)	
Cirrhosis	Hepatomegaly
	Splenomegaly
	Spider naevi
Renal failure (including nephrotic syndrome)	Generalised oedema
Congestive heart failure	Peripheral oedema
	Elevated jugular venous pulse (JVP)

*See ascites (p. 936)

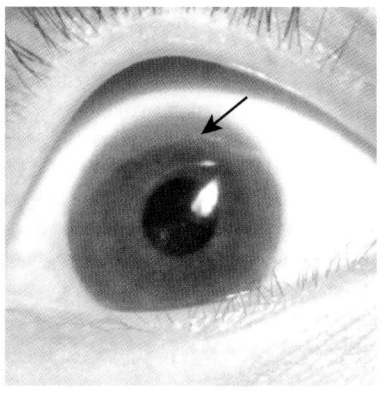

Kayser–Fleischer rings in Wilson's disease.

Key history points

Symptoms*

- Itching preceding jaundice
- Abdominal pain (suggests stones)
- Weight loss (chronic liver disease and malignancy)
- Dark urine and pale stools
- Fever ± rigors
- Dry eyes/dry mouth
- Fatigue

Recent drug history

Other

- Exposure to intravenous drug or blood transfusions
- Travel history and country of birth
- Family history of liver disease
- Autoimmune disease history
- Alcohol history
- Inflammatory bowel disease
- Metabolic syndrome (increased body mass index ± type 2 diabetes/hypertension)

*Symptoms may be absent and abnormal liver function tests detected incidentally.

The liver is the largest organ in the body. It plays a central role in digestion and in the regulation of protein, carbohydrate and lipid metabolism, and is responsible for the metabolism of drugs and environmental toxins. In view of this, it is not surprising that diseases of the liver are a major cause of morbidity and mortality; worldwide, 1 in 40 deaths are due to liver disease or primary liver cell cancer. In developed countries, the most common cause of liver disease is alcohol abuse, although in keeping with the rise in obesity rates, the incidence of non-alcoholic fatty liver disease (NAFLD) is rapidly increasing. In the developing world, infections caused by hepatitis viruses, often complicated by hepatobiliary cancer, and those caused by parasites, are responsible for most chronic liver disease. In the UK, liver disease is responsible for about 5000 deaths per year and is the fifth most common cause of death. This figure has doubled over the last decade. About a quarter of liver disease in the UK is due to chronic viral hepatitis, and alcohol is responsible for 70% of deaths from cirrhosis.

FUNCTIONAL ANATOMY AND PHYSIOLOGY

Applied anatomy

Normal liver structure and blood supply

The liver is one of the heaviest organs in the body, weighing 1.2–1.5 kg. It is classically divided into left and right lobes by the falciform ligament, but a more useful functional division is into the right and left hemilivers, based on the hepatic blood supply (Fig. 23.1). The right and left hemilivers are further divided into a total of eight segments in accordance with subdivisions of the hepatic and portal veins. Each segment has its own branch of the hepatic artery and biliary tree, and this segmental classification is used clinically to describe the position of

liver tumours on radiological imaging. A liver segment is made up of multiple smaller units known as lobules, comprised of a central vein, radiating sinusoids separated from each other by single liver cell (hepatocyte) plates, and peripheral portal tracts. The functional unit of the liver is the hepatic acinus (Fig. 23.2).

Blood flows into the hepatic acinus via a single branch of the portal vein and hepatic artery situated centrally in the portal tracts. The blood flows outwards along the hepatic sinusoids into one of several tributaries of the hepatic vein at the periphery of the acinus. Bile flows in the opposite direction from the periphery of the acinus through channels termed cholangioles, which converge in interlobular bile ducts in the portal tracts. The hepatocytes in each acinus lie in three zones, depending on their position relative to the portal tract. The hepatocytes in zone 1 are closest to the terminal branches of the portal vein and hepatic artery, and are richly supplied with oxygenated blood, and blood containing the highest concentration of nutrients and toxins. Conversely, hepatocytes in zone 3 are furthest from the portal tracts and closest to the hepatic veins, and are therefore relatively hypoxic and exposed to lower concentrations of nutrients and toxins compared with the zone 1 hepatocytes.

Liver cells

Hepatocytes comprise 80% of liver cells and the remainder is made up of sinusoidal endothelial cells (10%), bile duct endothelial cells (1%) and cells of the immune system (9%). Endothelial cells line the hepatic sinusoids (Fig. 23.3), which constitute a network of capillary vessels that differ from other capillary beds in the body in that there is no basement membrane. The endothelial cells have gaps between them (fenestrae) of about 0.1 micron in diameter, allowing free flow of fluid and particulate matter to the hepatocytes.

Individual hepatocytes are separated from the leaky endothelial lining of the sinusoids by the space of Disse, which contains non-parenchymal cells called stellate (Ito) cells (see Fig. 23.3) Stellate cells store vitamin A and play an important part in regulating liver blood flow. They also have a role in causing hepatic fibrosis, since they differentiate into myofibroblasts in response to cytokines produced by Kupffer cells and hepatocytes following liver injury (Fig. 23.4).

Blood supply

The liver receives 80% of its blood supply via the portal vein and 20% via the hepatic artery, which drains blood from the gut via the splanchnic circulation. The normal portal venous pressure is 2–5 mmHg and is determined by the portal blood flow and portal vascular resistance. When portal venous pressure rises above 12 mm, portal hypertension is said to be present.

Biliary system and gallbladder

Hepatocytes provide the driving force for bile flow by creating osmotic gradients of bile acids, which form micelles in bile (bile acid-dependent bile flow), and of sodium (bile acid-independent bile flow). Bile is secreted by hepatocytes and flows from cholangioles to the biliary canaliculi in the portal tracts. The canaliculi join together to form larger intrahepatic bile ducts, which in turn merge to form the right and left hepatic ducts. These ducts join as they emerge from the liver to form

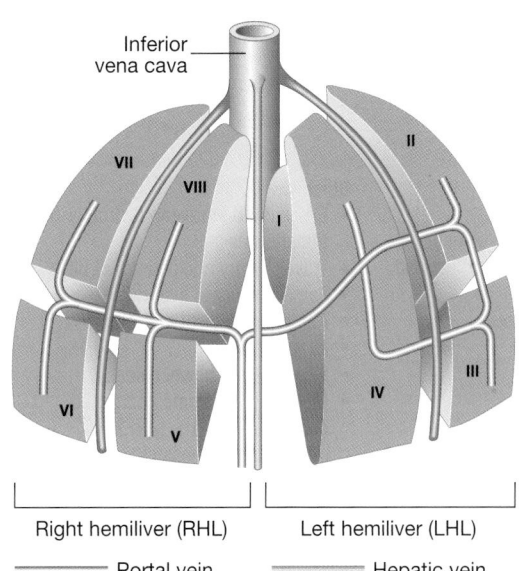

Inferior vena cava

VII · VIII · I · II · III · IV · V · VI

Right hemiliver (RHL) · Left hemiliver (LHL)

═══ Portal vein ═══ Hepatic vein

Fig. 23.1 Liver blood supply.

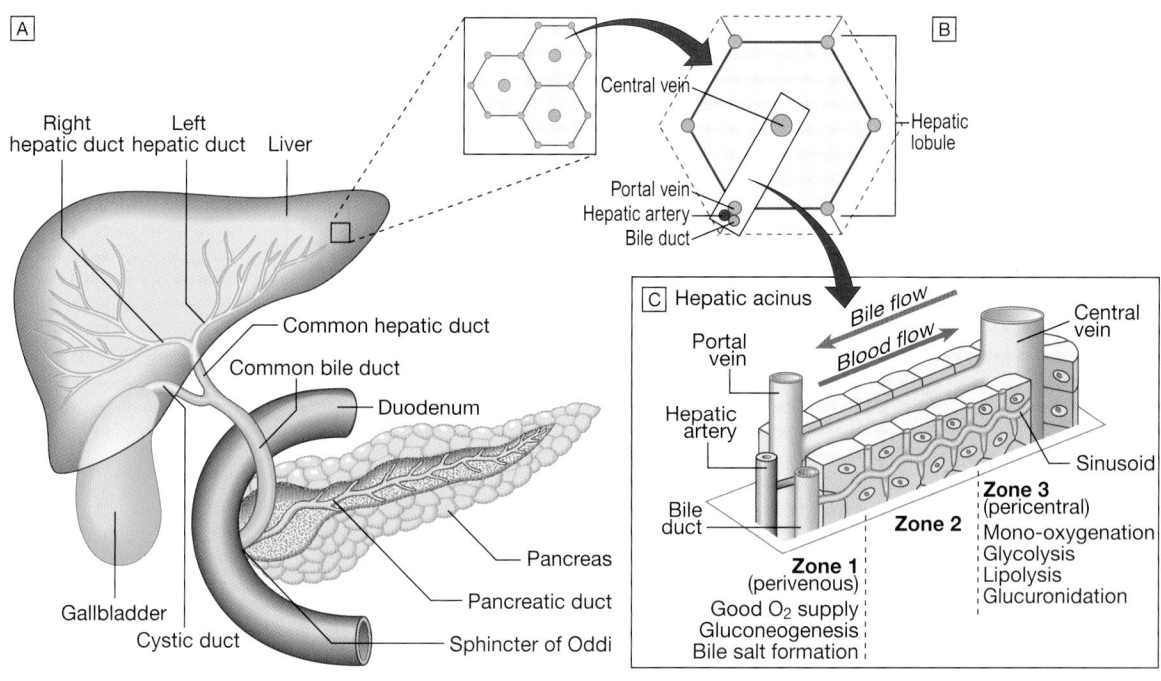

Fig. 23.2 Liver structure and microstructure. [A] Liver anatomy showing relationship with pancreas, bile duct and duodenum. [B] Hepatic lobule. [C] Hepatic acinus.

23

the common hepatic duct, which becomes the common bile duct after joining the cystic duct (see Fig. 23.2). The common bile duct is approximately 5 cm long and 4–6 mm wide. The distal portion of the duct passes through the head of the pancreas and usually joins the pancreatic duct before entering the duodenum through the sphincter of Oddi. Common bile duct pressure is maintained by rhythmic contraction and relaxation of the ampullary sphincter (sphincter of Oddi); this pressure exceeds gallbladder pressure in the fasting state, so that bile normally flows into the gallbladder, where it is concentrated tenfold by resorption of water and electrolytes.

The gallbladder is a pear-shaped sac lying under the right hemiliver, with its fundus located anteriorly behind the tip of the 9th costal cartilage. Its function is to concentrate and provide a reservoir for bile. Gallbladder tone is maintained by vagal activity, and cholecystokinin released from the duodenal mucosa during feeding causes gallbladder contraction and reduces sphincter pressure, so that bile flows into the duodenum. The body and neck of the gallbladder pass posteromedially towards the porta hepatis, and the cystic duct then joins it to the common hepatic duct. The cystic duct mucosa has prominent crescentic folds (valves of Heister), giving it a beaded appearance on cholangiography.

Hepatic function

Carbohydrate, amino acid and lipid metabolism

The liver plays a central role in carbohydrate, lipid and amino acid metabolism, and is involved in metabolising drugs and environmental toxins (Fig. 23.5).

- Amino acids from dietary proteins are used by hepatocytes for endogenous protein synthesis and for production of plasma proteins including albumin. The liver produces 8–14 g of albumin per day. Albumin plays a critical role in maintaining oncotic pressure in the vascular space and in the transport of small molecules like bilirubin, hormones and drugs throughout the body. Amino acids which are not required for the production of new proteins are broken down to urea. Production of urea and endogenous liver proteins is suppressed during fasting and hepatic amino acid release is reduced.

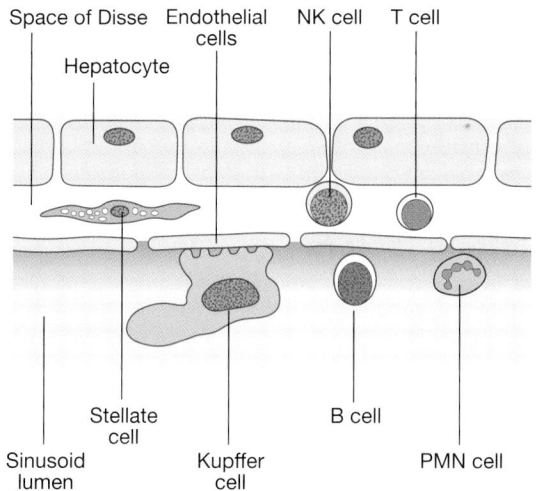

Fig. 23.3 Non-parenchymal liver cells. (NK= natural killer cells; PMN= polymorphonuclear leucocytes; B = B lymphocytes; T = T lymphocytes)

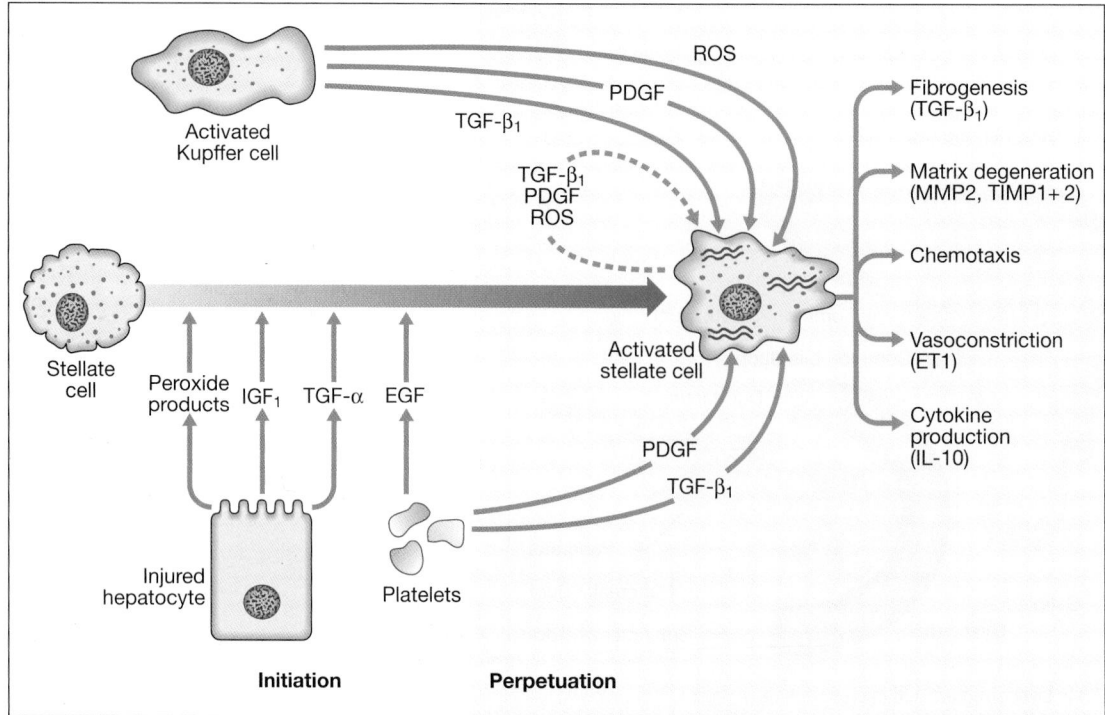

Fig. 23.4 Pathogenic mechanisms in hepatic fibrosis. Stellate cell activation occurs under the influence of cytokines released by other cell types in the liver, including hepatocytes, Kupffer cells (tissue macrophages), platelets and lymphocytes. Once stellate cells become activated, they can perpetuate their own activation by synthesis of transforming growth factor-beta (TGF-β_1) and platelet-derived growth factor (PDGF) through autocrine loops. Activated stellate cells produce TGF-β_1, stimulating the production of collagen matrix as well as inhibitors of collagen breakdown. The inhibitors of collagen breakdown, matrix metalloproteinase 2 and 9 (MMP2 and MMP9), are inactivated in turn by tissue inhibitors TIMP1 and TIMP2, which are increased in fibrosis. Inflammation also contributes to fibrosis with the cytokine profile produced by Th2 lymphocytes, such as interleukin-6 and 13 (IL-6 and IL-13). Activated stellate cells also produce endothelin 1 (ET1), which may contribute to portal hypertension. (ROS = reactive oxygen species; IGF$_1$ = insulin-like growth factor 1; EGF = epidermal growth factor)

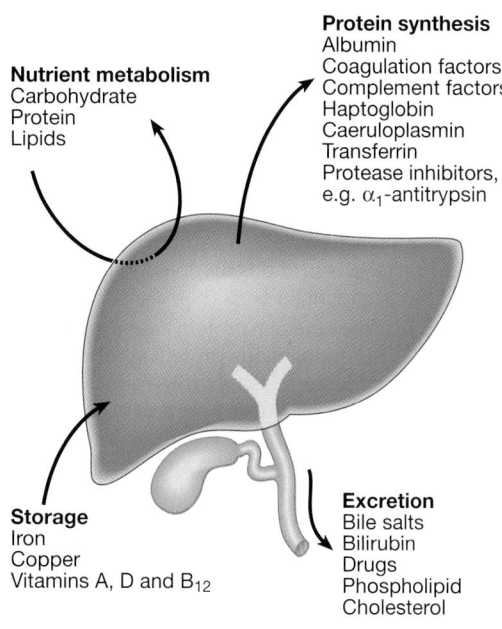

Nutrient metabolism
Carbohydrate
Protein
Lipids

Protein synthesis
Albumin
Coagulation factors
Complement factors
Haptoglobin
Caeruloplasmin
Transferrin
Protease inhibitors,
e.g. α_1-antitrypsin

Storage
Iron
Copper
Vitamins A, D and B$_{12}$

Excretion
Bile salts
Bilirubin
Drugs
Phospholipid
Cholesterol

Fig. 23.5 Important liver functions.

- Following a meal, more than half of the glucose absorbed is taken up by the liver and stored as glycogen or converted to glycerol and fatty acids, thus preventing hyperglycaemia. During fasting, glycogen in the liver and that in other tissues, such as skeletal muscle, is broken down to release glucose (gluconeogenesis), thereby preventing hypoglycaemia (p. 798).
- The liver plays a central role in lipid metabolism, producing very low-density lipoproteins and further metabolising low- and high-density lipoproteins (p. 449).

Clotting factors

The liver plays a key role in the regulation of blood clotting by producing proteins that are involved in the coagulation cascade. Many of these coagulation factors (II, VII, IX and X) are post-translationally modified by vitamin K-dependent enzymes, and their synthesis is impaired in the presence of vitamin K deficiency (p. 993).

Bilirubin metabolism and bile

The liver plays a central role in the metabolism of bilirubin and is responsible for the production of bile (Fig. 23.6). Between 425 and 510 mmol (250–300 mg) of

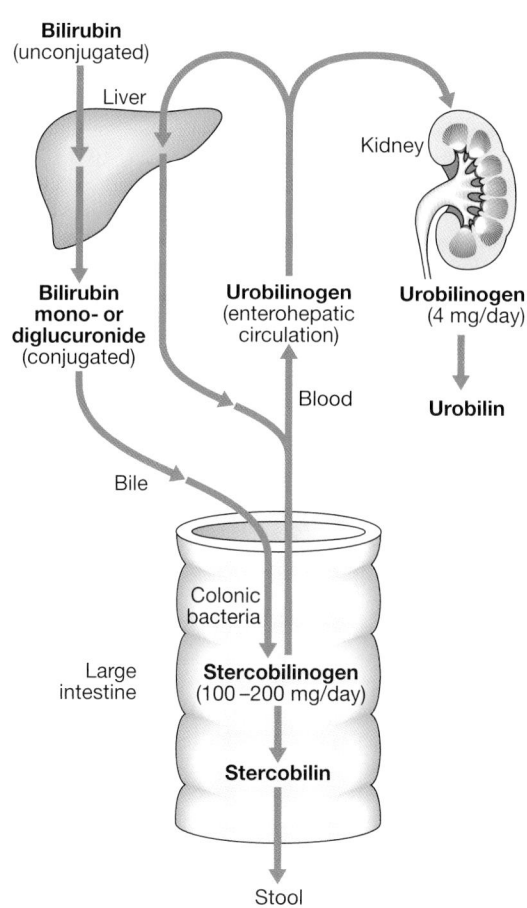

Fig. 23.6 Pathway of bilirubin excretion.

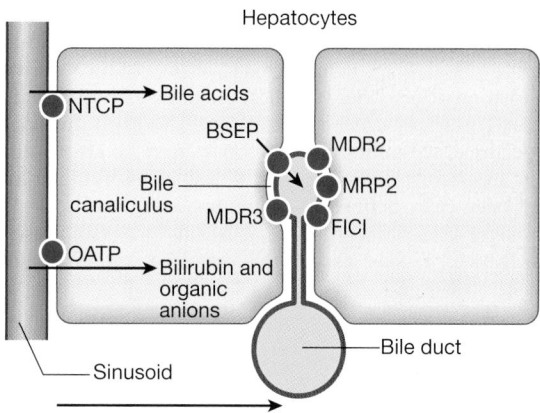

Fig. 23.7 Biliary transporter proteins. On the hepatocyte basolateral membrane, NTCP (sodium taurocholate cotransporting polypeptide) mediates uptake of conjugated bile acids from portal blood. At the canalicular membrane, these bile acids are secreted via BSEP (bile salt export pump) into bile. MDR3 (multidrug resistance protein 3), also situated on the canalicular membrane, transports phospholipid to the outer side of the membrane. This solubilises bile acids, forming micelles and protecting bile duct membranes from bile salt damage. FIC1 (familial intrahepatic cholestasis 1) moves phosphatidylserine from the inside to the outside of the canalicular membrane; mutations result in familial cholestasis syndrome in childhood. MDR2 (multidrug resistance 2) regulates transport of glutathione. MRP2 (multidrug resistance protein 2) transports bilirubin and is induced by rifampicin. OATP (organic anion transporter protein) transports bilirubin and organic anions.

23

unconjugated bilirubin is produced from the catabolism of haem every day. Bilirubin in the blood is normally almost all unconjugated and, because it is not water-soluble, is bound to albumin and does not pass into the urine. Unconjugated bilirubin is taken up by hepatocytes at the sinusoidal membrane, where it is conjugated in the endoplasmic reticulum by UDP-glucuronyl transferase, producing bilirubin mono- and diglucuronide. Impaired conjugation by this enzyme is a cause of inherited hyperbilirubinaemias (see Box 23.10, p. 932). These bilirubin conjugates are water-soluble and are exported into the bile canaliculus by specific carriers on the hepatocyte membrane. The conjugated bilirubin is excreted in the bile and passes into the bowel lumen.

Once in the bowel, conjugated bilirubin is metabolised by colonic bacteria to form stercobilinogen, which may be further oxidised to stercobilin. Both stercobilinogen and stercobilin are then excreted in the stool, contributing to its brown colour. Blockage to the biliary system results in reduced stercobilinogen in the stool, and the stools become pale. A small amount of stercobilinogen (4 mg/day) is absorbed from the bowel, passes through the liver and is excreted in the urine, where it is known as urobilinogen or, following further oxidisation, urobilin. The liver secretes 1–2 L of bile daily. Bile contains bile acids (formed from cholesterol), phospholipids, bilirubin and cholesterol. Several biliary transporter proteins have now been identified that are involved in transporting bilirubin and bile acids from the hepato-cyte and into the biliary system (Fig. 23.7). Mutations in the genes encoding these proteins have been identified in inherited intrahepatic biliary diseases presenting in childhood, as well as in adult-onset disease such as intrahepatic cholestasis of pregnancy and gallstone formation.

Storage of vitamins and minerals

Vitamins A, D and B$_{12}$ are stored by the liver in large amounts, while others, such as vitamin K and folate, are stored in smaller amounts and disappear rapidly if dietary intake is reduced. The liver is also able to metabolise vitamins to more active compounds, e.g. 7-dehydrocholesterol to 25(OH) vitamin D. Vitamin K is a fat-soluble vitamin and so the inability to absorb fat-soluble vitamins, as occurs in biliary obstruction, results in a coagulopathy. The liver also stores minerals such as iron, in ferritin and haemosiderin, and copper, which is excreted in bile.

Immune regulation

Approximately 9% of the normal liver is composed of immune cells (see Fig. 23.3). Cells of the innate immune system include Kupffer cells derived from blood monocytes (4%), the liver macrophages and natural killer (NK) cells (2.5%), as well as B and T cells of the adaptive immune response (p. 74). Kupffer cells constitute the largest single mass of tissue-resident macrophages in the body and account for 80% of the phagocytic capacity of this system. They remove aged and damaged red blood cells, bacteria, viruses, antigen–antibody complexes and endotoxin. In addition, they are able to produce a wide variety of inflammatory mediators that can act locally or may be released into the systemic circulation.

The immunological environment of the liver is unique in that antigens presented within it tend to induce immunological tolerance. This is of importance in liver transplantation, where classical major histocompatibility (MHC) barriers may be crossed, and also in chronic viral infections, when immune responses may be attenuated. The mechanisms which underlie this phenomenon have not been fully defined but include a significant role for the liver sinusoidal endothelial cells, which may present antigen to T cells, as well as specialist innate subsets within the organ.

INVESTIGATION OF HEPATOBILIARY DISEASE

The aims of investigation in patients with suspected liver disease are shown in Box 23.1.

Liver function tests

Liver function tests (LFTs) include the measurement of serum bilirubin, aminotransferases, alkaline phosphatase, gamma-glutamyl transferase and albumin. Most analytes measured by LFTs are not truly 'function' tests, but rather provide biochemical markers of liver cell damage. Liver function is best assessed by the serum albumin, prothrombin time and bilirubin. Although abnormalities on LFTs are often non-specific, the patterns are frequently helpful in directing further investigations. Also levels of bilirubin, albumin and the prothrombin are related to clinical outcome in patients with severe liver disease, reflected by their use in several prognostic scores: the Child–Pugh and MELD score in cirrhosis (see Boxes 23.29 and 23.31, p. 945), the Maddrey score in alcoholic hepatitis (see Box 23.49, p. 956) and the King's College Hospital criteria for liver transplantation in acute liver failure (see Box 23.16, p. 935).

Bilirubin and albumin

The degree of elevation of bilirubin reflects the degree of liver damage. A raised bilirubin often occurs earlier in the natural history of biliary disease (e.g. primary biliary cirrhosis) than in disease of the liver parenchyma (e.g. cirrhosis) where the hepatocytes are primarily involved.

Serum albumin levels are often reduced in patients with liver disease. This is due to a change in the volume of distribution of albumin, as well as a reduction in synthesis. Since the plasma half-life of albumin is about 2 weeks, serum albumin levels may be normal in acute liver failure but are almost always reduced in chronic liver failure.

Alanine aminotransferase and aspartate aminotransferase

Alanine aminotransferase (ALT) and aspartate aminotransferase (AST) normally transfer the amino group from an amino acid—alanine in the case of ALT and aspartate in the case of AST—to a ketoacid, producing pyruvate and oxalo-acetate respectively. Both ALT and AST are located in the cytoplasm of the hepatocyte; AST is also located in the hepatocyte mitochondria. Although both transaminase enzymes are widely distributed, expression of ALT outside the liver is relatively low and therefore this enzyme is considered more specific for hepatocellular damage. Large increases of aminotransferase activity favour hepatocellular damage, and this pattern of LFT abnormality is known as 'hepatitic'.

Alkaline phosphatase and gamma-glutamyl transferase

Alkaline phosphatase (ALP) is the collective name given to several different enzymes that are capable of hydrolysing phosphate esters at alkaline pH. These enzymes are widely distributed in the body, but the main sites of production are the liver, gastrointestinal tract, bone, placenta and kidney. ALPs are post-translationally modified, resulting in the production of several different isoenzymes which differ in abundance in different tissues. ALP enzymes in the liver are located in cell membranes of the hepatic sinusoids and the biliary canaliculi. Accordingly, levels rise with intrahepatic and extrahepatic biliary obstruction and with sinusoidal obstruction, as occurs in infiltrative liver disease.

Gamma-glutamyl transferase (GGT) is a microsomal enzyme found in many cells and tissues of the body. The highest concentrations are found in the liver, where it is produced by hepatocytes and by the epithelium lining small bile ducts. The function of GGT is to transfer glutamyl groups from gamma-glutamyl peptides to other peptides and amino acids.

The pattern of a modest increase in aminotransferase activity and large increases in ALP and GGT activity favours biliary obstruction and is commonly described as 'cholestatic' or 'obstructive' (Box 23.2). Isolated elevation of the serum GGT is relatively common, and may occur during ingestion of microsomal enzyme-inducing drugs (Box 23.3), including alcohol.

Other biochemical tests

Other widely available biochemical tests may become altered in patients with liver disease:

- Hyponatraemia occurs in severe liver disease due to increased production of antidiuretic hormone (ADH) (p. 944).

23.1 Aims of investigations in patients with suspected liver disease

- Detect hepatic abnormality
- Measure the severity of liver damage
- Detect the pattern of liver function test abnormality: hepatitic or obstructive/cholestatic
- Identify the specific cause
- Investigate possible complications

23.2 'Hepatitic' and 'cholestatic'/'obstructive' LFTs

Pattern	AST/ALT	GGT	ALP
Biliary obstruction	↑	↑↑	↑↑↑
Hepatitis	↑↑↑	↑	↑
Alcohol/enzyme-inducing drugs	N/↑	↑↑	N

N = normal; ↑ mild elevation (< twice normal); ↑↑ moderate elevation (2–5 times normal); ↑↑↑ marked elevation (> 5 times normal).

23.3 Drugs that increase levels of GGT

- Barbiturates
- Carbamazepine
- Ethanol
- Griseofulvin
- Isoniazid
- Rifampicin
- Phenytoin

23.4 Chronic liver disease screen

- Hepatitis B surface antigen
- Hepatitis C antibody
- Liver autoantibodies (antinuclear factor, smooth muscle antibody, antimitochondrial antibody)
- Immunoglobulins
- Ferritin
- α_1-antitrypsin
- Caeruloplasmin

- Serum urea may be reduced in hepatic failure, whereas levels of urea may be increased following gastrointestinal haemorrhage.
- When high levels of urea are accompanied by raised bilirubin, high serum creatinine and low urinary sodium, this suggests hepatorenal failure, which carries a grave prognosis.

Haematological tests

Routine haematology

Routine haematological investigations are often abnormal in patients with liver disease and can give a clue to the underlying diagnosis:

- *A normochromic normocytic anaemia* may reflect recent gastrointestinal haemorrhage, whereas chronic blood loss is characterised by a hypochromic microcytic anaemia secondary to iron deficiency. A high erythrocyte mean cell volume (macrocytosis) is associated with alcohol misuse, but target cells in any jaundiced patient also result in a macrocytosis.
- *Leucopenia* may complicate portal hypertension and hypersplenism, whereas leucocytosis may occur with cholangitis, alcoholic hepatitis and hepatic abscesses. Atypical lymphocytes are seen in infectious mononucleosis, which may be complicated by an acute hepatitis.
- *Thrombocytopenia* is common in cirrhosis and is due to reduced platelet production, and increased breakdown because of hypersplenism. Thrombopoietin, required for platelet production, is produced in the liver and levels fall with worsening liver function. Thus platelet levels are usually more depressed than white cells and haemoglobin in the presence of hypersplenism in patients with cirrhosis. A low platelet count is often an indicator of chronic liver disease, particularly in the context of hepatomegaly. Thrombocytosis is unusual in patients with liver disease but may occur in those with active gastrointestinal haemorrhage and, rarely, in association with hepatocellular carcinoma.

Coagulation tests

Tests of the coagulation system are often abnormal in patients with liver disease. The normal half-lives of the vitamin K-dependent coagulation factors in the blood are short (5–72 hours) and so changes in the prothrombin time occur relatively quickly following liver damage; these changes provide valuable prognostic information in patients with both acute and chronic liver failure. An increased prothrombin time is evidence of severe liver damage in chronic liver disease. Vitamin K does not reverse this deficiency if it is due to liver disease, but will reverse the prothrombin time if due to vitamin K deficiency, as may occur with biliary obstruction due to non-absorption of fat-soluble vitamins.

Immunological tests

A variety of immunological tests, often known as a 'chronic liver disease screen' (Box 23.4), are available to evaluate the aetiology of hepatic disease (Box 23.5). These are discussed in more detail under specific diseases later in this chapter. In certain clinical situations, positive blood tests may require further assessment by performing a liver biopsy to confirm the diagnosis and assess the degree of liver scarring.

Radiological imaging

Several imaging techniques can be used to determine the site and general nature of structural lesions in the liver and biliary tree.

Ultrasound

Ultrasound is a non-invasive technique most commonly used to identify gallstones (Fig. 23.8) and biliary obstruction. It is also very useful in the initial assessment of patients with liver disease to determine whether further, more invasive investigations are required. Ultrasound is good for the identification of splenomegaly and abnormalities in liver texture, but is less effective at identifying diffuse parenchymal disease. Focal lesions, such as

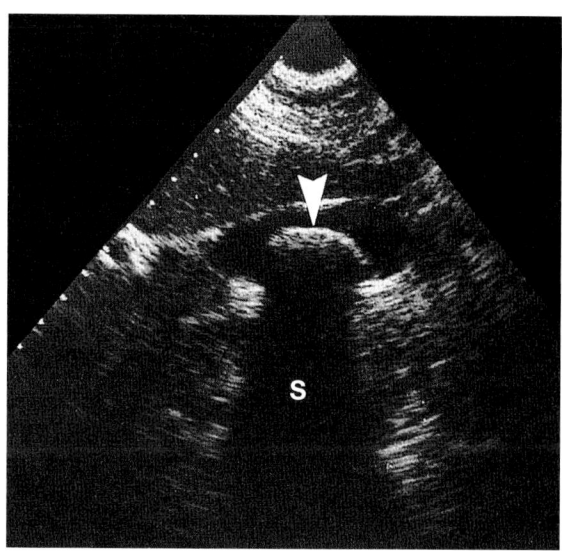

Fig. 23.8 Ultrasound showing a stone in the gallbladder. Stone (arrow) with acoustic shadow (S).

Diagnosis	Clinical clue	Initial test	Additional tests
Alcoholic liver disease	History	LFTs AST > ALT; high MCV	Random blood alcohol
Non-alcoholic fatty liver disease (NAFLD)	Metabolic syndrome (central obesity, diabetes, hypertension)	LFTs	Liver biopsy
Chronic hepatitis B	Injection drug use; blood transfusion	HBsAg	HBeAg, HBeAb HBV-DNA
Chronic hepatitis C		HCV antibody	HCV-RNA
Primary biliary cirrhosis	Itching; raised ALP	AMA	Liver biopsy
Primary sclerosing cholangitis	Inflammatory bowel disease	MRCP	ANCA
Autoimmune hepatitis	Other autoimmune diseases	ASMA, ANA, LKM, immunoglobulin	Liver biopsy
Haemochromatosis	Diabetes/joint pain	Transferrin saturation, ferritin	HFE gene test
Wilson's disease	Neurological signs; haemolysis	Caeruloplasmin	24-hr urinary copper
α_1-antitrypsin	Lung disease	α_1-antitrypsin level	α_1-antitrypsin genotype
Drug-induced liver disease	Drug/herbal remedy history	LFTs	Liver biopsy
Coeliac disease	Malabsorption	Endomysial antibody	Small bowel biopsy

(ALP = alkaline phosphatase; ALT = alanine aminotransferase; AMA = antimitochondrial antibody; ANA = antinuclear antibody; ANCA = antineutrophil cytoplasmic antibodies; ASMA = anti-smooth muscle antibody; AST = aspartate aminotransferase; HBeAb = antibody to hepatitis B e antigen; HBeAg = hepatitis B e antigen; HBsAg = hepatitis B surface antigen; HBV = hepatitis B virus; HCV = hepatitis C virus; LKM = liver-kidney microsomal antibody; MCV = mean cell volume; MRCP = magnetic resonance cholangiopancreatography)

tumours, may not be detected unless they are more than 2 cm in diameter and have echogenic characteristics sufficiently different from normal liver tissue. Colour Doppler ultrasound allows blood flow in the hepatic artery, portal vein and hepatic veins to be investigated. Endoscopic and laparoscopic ultrasound provides high-resolution images of the pancreas, biliary tree and liver.

Computed tomography and magnetic resonance imaging

Computed tomography (CT) can be used for the same purpose as ultrasound but detects smaller focal lesions in the liver, especially when combined with contrast injection (Fig. 23.9). Magnetic resonance imaging (MRI) can also be

used to localise and confirm the aetiology of focal liver lesions, particularly primary and secondary tumours.

Hepatic angiography is seldom used nowadays as a diagnostic tool, since CT and MRI are both able to provide images of hepatic vasculature, but it still has a therapeutic role in the embolisation of vascular tumours such as hepatoma. Hepatic venography is also rarely performed, but may be necessary to image the hepatic veins further in patients with suspected hepatic venous outflow obstruction (Budd–Chiari syndrome, p. 973).

Cholangiography

Cholangiography can be undertaken by magnetic resonance cholangiopancreatography (MRCP, Fig 23.10)

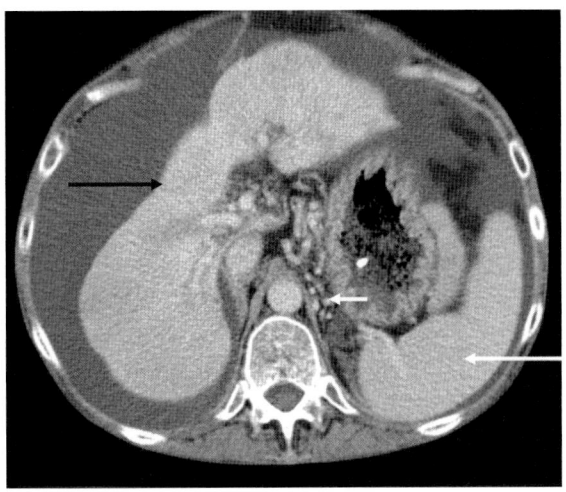

Fig. 23.9 CT scan in a patient with cirrhosis. The liver is small and has an irregular outline (black arrow), the spleen is enlarged (long white arrow), fluid (ascites) is seen around the liver, and collateral vessels are present around the proximal stomach (short white arrow).

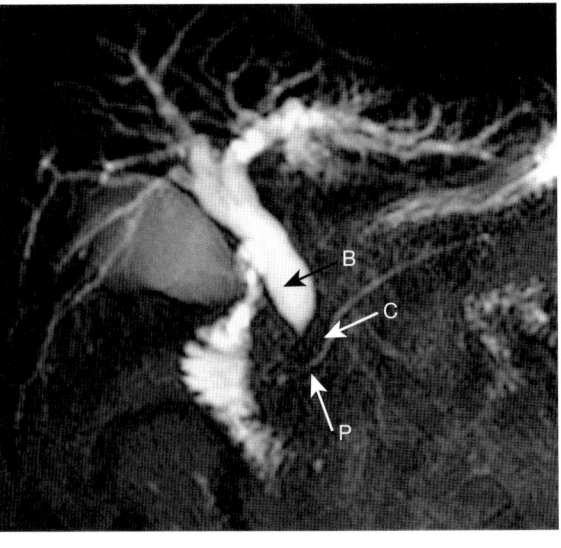

Fig. 23.10 MRCP showing a cholangiocarcinoma in the distal common bile duct (C). The proximal common bile duct (B) is dilated but the pancreatic duct (P) is normal.

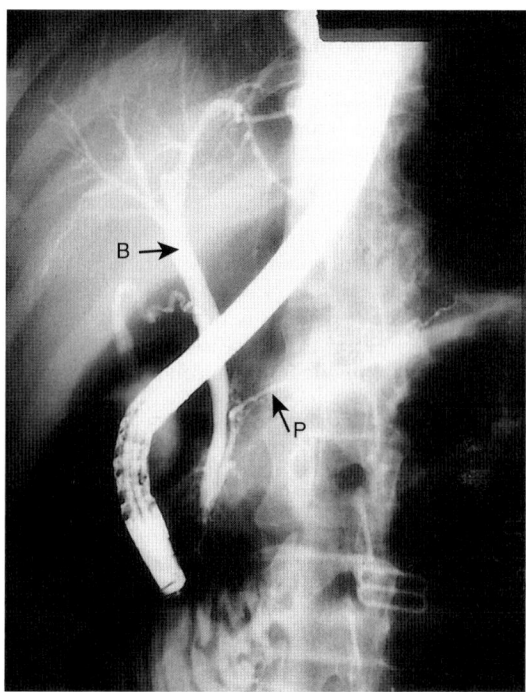

Fig. 23.11 ERCP showing the normal biliary (B) and pancreatic (P) duct system.

endoscopy (endoscopic retrograde cholangiopancreatography, ERCP, Fig 23.11) or the percutaneous approach (percutaneous transhepatic cholangiography, PTC). The latter does not allow the ampulla of Vater or pancreatic duct to be visualised. MRCP is as good as ERCP at providing images of the biliary tree but has fewer complications and is the diagnostic test of choice. Both endoscopic and percutaneous approaches allow therapeutic interventions such as the insertion of biliary stents across malignant bile duct strictures. The percutaneous approach is only used if it is not possible to access the bile duct endoscopically.

Liver biopsy

An ultrasound-guided liver biopsy can confirm the severity of liver damage and provide aetiological information; it is performed percutaneously with a Trucut or Menghini needle, usually through an intercostal space, under local anaesthesia.

Percutaneous liver biopsy is a relatively safe procedure if the conditions detailed in Box 23.6 are met, but carries a mortality of about 0.01% and should never be undertaken lightly. The main complications are abdominal and/or shoulder pain, bleeding and biliary peritonitis. Biliary peritonitis is rare and usually occurs when a biopsy is performed in a patient with obstruction of a large bile duct. Liver biopsies can be carried out in patients with defective haemostasis if:

- the defect is corrected with fresh frozen plasma and platelet transfusion

23.6 Conditions required for safe percutaneous liver biopsy

- Cooperative patient
- Prothrombin time < 4 seconds prolonged
- Platelet count $> 80 \times 10^9$/L
- Exclusion of bile duct obstruction, localised skin infection, advanced chronic obstructive pulmonary disease, marked ascites and severe anaemia

- the biopsy is obtained by the transjugular route, *or*
- the procedure is conducted percutaneously under ultrasound control and the needle track is then plugged with procoagulant material.

In patients with potentially resectable malignancy, biopsy should be avoided due to the potential risk of tumour dissemination. Operative or laparoscopic liver biopsy may sometimes be valuable.

Histological assessment of liver biopsy tissue is enhanced by discussion between clinicians and pathologists. Although the pathological features of liver disease are complex with several features occurring together, liver disorders can be broadly classified histologically into fatty liver (steatosis), hepatitis and cirrhosis. The use of special histological stains can help in determining the aetiology of liver disorders. The clinical features and prognosis of these changes are dependent on the underlying aetiology, and are discussed in the relevant sections below.

Non-invasive markers of hepatic fibrosis

Non-invasive markers of liver fibrosis have been developed and can obviate the need for liver biopsy when it is being used to evaluate progression of liver fibrosis or where the underlying diagnosis, such as hepatitis C or non-alcoholic fatty liver disease, is clear.

Serological markers of hepatic fibrosis, such as procollagen-type peptide and metalloproteinases (see Fig. 23.4, p. 924), are used in the 'Fibrotest'. The ELF (European Liver Fibrosis) serological assay uses a combination of hyaluronic acid, procollagen peptide III (PIIINP) and tissue inhibitor of metalloproteinase 1 (TIMP1). All these tests are good at differentiating severe fibrosis from mild scarring, but are limited in their ability to detect subtle changes.

An alternative to serological markers is the 'Fibroscan' test, in which ultrasound-based shock waves are sent through the liver, allowing hepatic fibrosis to be detected and quantitated.

PRESENTING PROBLEMS IN LIVER DISEASE

Liver injury may be either acute or chronic. The main causes are listed in Figure 23.12 and discussed in detail later in the chapter.

23

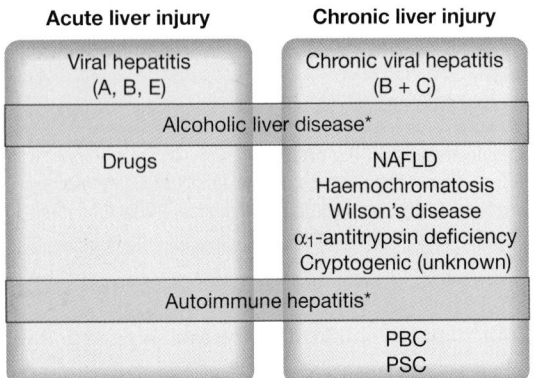

Acute liver injury	Chronic liver injury
Viral hepatitis (A, B, E)	Chronic viral hepatitis (B + C)
Alcoholic liver disease*	
Drugs	NAFLD Haemochromatosis Wilson's disease α₁-antitrypsin deficiency Cryptogenic (unknown)
Autoimmune hepatitis*	
	PBC PSC

Fig. 23.12 Causes of acute and chronic liver injury. *Although there is often evidence of chronic liver disease at presentation, may present acutely with jaundice. In alcoholic liver disease this is due to superimposed alcoholic hepatitis (NAFLD = non-alcoholic fatty liver disease; PBC = primary biliary cirrhosis; PSC = primary sclorosing cholangitis).

- *Acute liver injury* may present with non-specific symptoms of fatigue and abnormal LFTs, or with jaundice and acute liver failure.
- *Chronic liver injury* is defined as hepatic injury, inflammation and/or fibrosis occurring in the liver for more than 6 months. In the early stages patients can be asymptomatic with abnormal LFTs. With more severe liver damage, however, the presentation can be with jaundice, portal hypertension or other signs of cirrhosis (Box 23.7).

Abnormal liver function tests

Frequently, LFTs are requested in patients who have no symptoms or signs of liver disease, as part of routine health checks, insurance medicals and drug monitoring. When abnormal results are found, it is important for the clinician to be able to interpret them and to investigate patients appropriately. Many patients with chronic liver disease are asymptomatic or have vague non-specific symptoms. Since effective medical treatments are now available for many types of chronic liver disease, further evaluation is often warranted to make sure the patient does not have a treatable condition. Indeed, when thorough investigations are performed, the majority of

patients with abnormal LFTs will be found to have significant liver disease that merits treatment or follow-up, whereas those who do not have significant disease can be reassured and safely discharged.

Asymptomatic abnormal LFTs are quite common. When LFTs are measured routinely prior to elective surgery, 3.5% of patients have elevated transaminase concentrations and 0.3% have values greater than twice normal. The prevalence of abnormal LFTs has been reported to be as high as 10% in some studies. Although transient mild abnormalities in LFTs are seldom clinically significant, the majority of patients with persistently abnormal LFTs have significant liver disease. The most common abnormality is alcoholic or non-alcoholic fatty liver disease (pp. 954–958).

When abnormal LFTs are detected, a thorough history should be taken to determine the patient's alcohol consumption, drug use (prescribed or otherwise), risk factors for viral hepatitis (e.g. blood transfusion, injection drug use), the presence of autoimmune diseases, family history, neurological symptoms, and the presence of diabetes and/or obesity (see Box 23.5). Surprisingly, the presence or absence of stigmata of chronic liver disease (pp. 920 and 943) does not reliably identify patients with significant chronic liver disease, and further investigations may be indicated, even in absence of these signs.

Most hepatologists investigate patients with LFTs that are greater than twice the normal range. Both the pattern of LFT abnormality, hepatitic or obstructive, and the degree of elevation are helpful in determining the cause of underlying liver disease (Boxes 23.8 and 23.9). The investigations that make up a standard liver screen and additional or confirmatory tests are shown in Boxes 23.4 and 23.5. An algorithm for investigating abnormal LFTs is provided in Figure 23.13.

Jaundice

Jaundice is usually detectable clinically when the plasma bilirubin exceeds 50 µmol/L (~3 mg/dL). The causes of jaundice overlap with the causes of abnormal LFTs, discussed above. In a patient with jaundice it is useful to consider whether the cause might be pre-hepatic, hepatic or post-hepatic.

23.7 Presentation of liver disease

Severity	Acute liver injury	Chronic liver injury
Mild/moderate	Abnormal LFTs	Abnormal LFTs
Severe	Jaundice	Signs of cirrhosis ± portal hypertension
Very severe	Acute liver failure	Chronic liver failure* Jaundice Ascites Hepatic encephalopathy Portal hypertension with variceal bleeding

*May not occur until several years after cirrhosis has presented.

23.8 Common causes of elevated serum transaminases

Minor elevation (< 100 U/L)

- Chronic hepatitis C
- Chronic hepatitis B
- Haemochromatosis
- Fatty liver disease

Moderate elevation (100–300 U/L)

As above plus:
- Alcoholic hepatitis
- Non-alcoholic steatohepatitis
- Autoimmune hepatitis
- Wilson's disease

Major elevation (> 300 U/L)

- Drugs (e.g. paracetamol)
- Acute viral hepatitis
- Autoimmune liver disease
- Ischaemic liver
- Toxins (e.g. *Amanita phalloides* poisoning)
- Flare of chronic hepatitis B

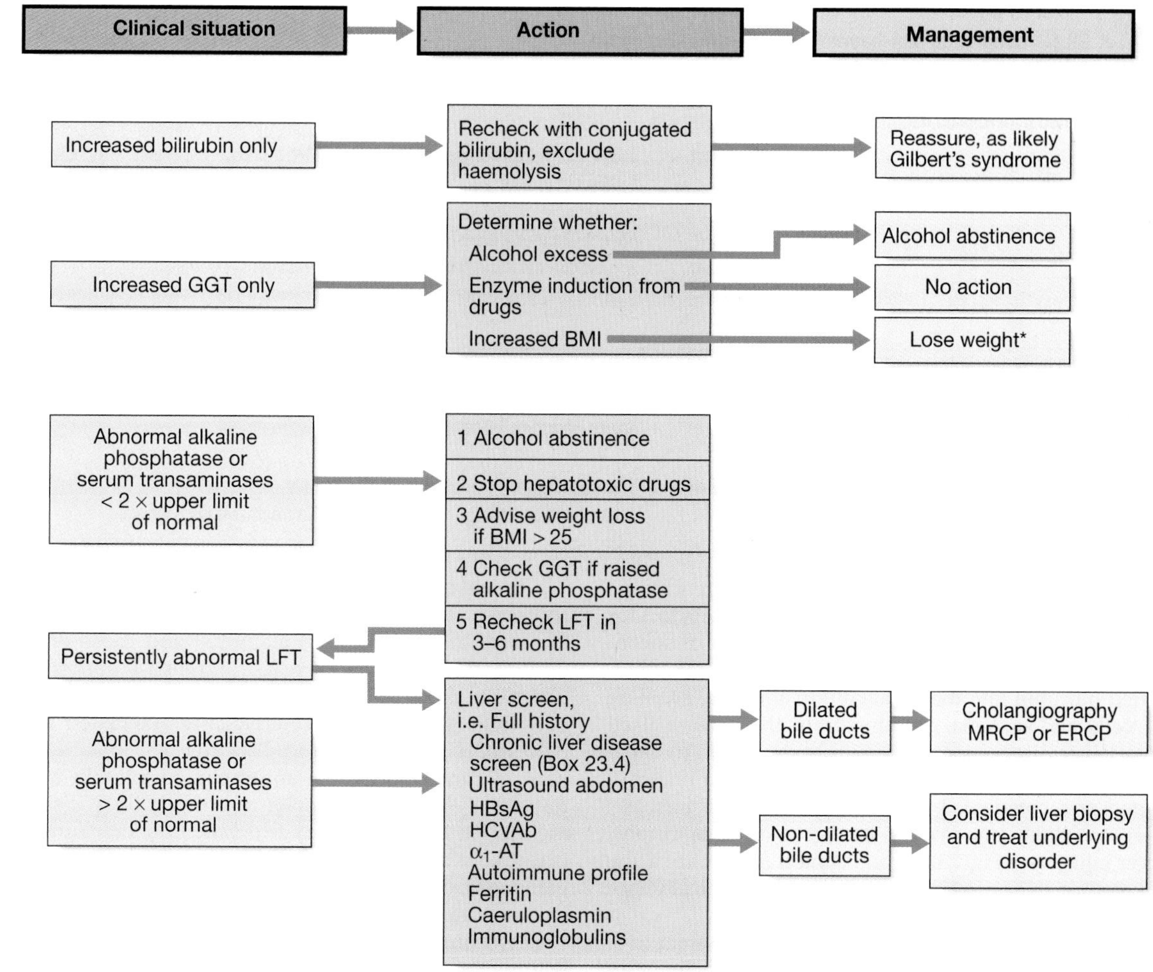

Clinical situation	→	Action	→	Management

Increased bilirubin only → Recheck with conjugated bilirubin, exclude haemolysis → Reassure, as likely Gilbert's syndrome

Increased GGT only → Determine whether:
- Alcohol excess → Alcohol abstinence
- Enzyme induction from drugs → No action
- Increased BMI → Lose weight*

Abnormal alkaline phosphatase or serum transaminases < 2 × upper limit of normal →
1 Alcohol abstinence
2 Stop hepatotoxic drugs
3 Advise weight loss if BMI > 25
4 Check GGT if raised alkaline phosphatase
5 Recheck LFT in 3–6 months

Persistently abnormal LFT

Abnormal alkaline phosphatase or serum transaminases > 2 × upper limit of normal →
Liver screen, i.e. Full history
Chronic liver disease screen (Box 23.4)
Ultrasound abdomen
HBsAg
HCVAb
α_1-AT
Autoimmune profile
Ferritin
Caeruloplasmin
Immunoglobulins

→ **Dilated bile ducts** → Cholangiography MRCP or ERCP

→ **Non-dilated bile ducts** → Consider liver biopsy and treat underlying disorder

Fig. 23.13 Suggested management of abnormal LFTs in asymptomatic patients. *No further investigation needed.

23

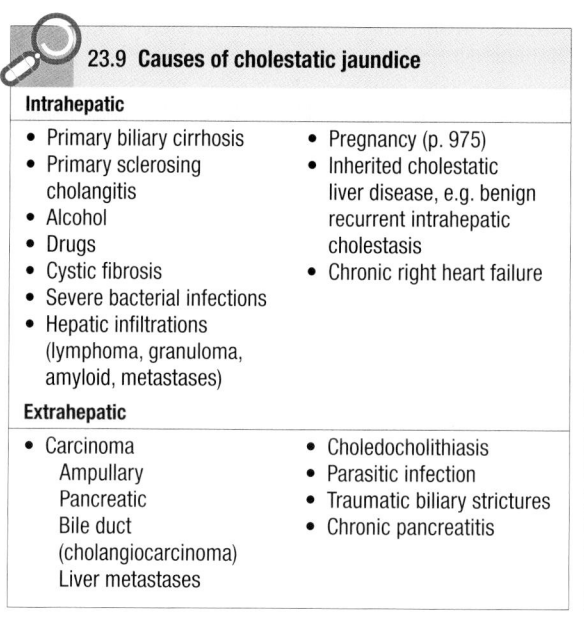

23.9 Causes of cholestatic jaundice

Intrahepatic

- Primary biliary cirrhosis
- Primary sclerosing cholangitis
- Alcohol
- Drugs
- Cystic fibrosis
- Severe bacterial infections
- Hepatic infiltrations (lymphoma, granuloma, amyloid, metastases)

- Pregnancy (p. 975)
- Inherited cholestatic liver disease, e.g. benign recurrent intrahepatic cholestasis
- Chronic right heart failure

Extrahepatic

- Carcinoma
  Ampullary
  Pancreatic
  Bile duct (cholangiocarcinoma)
  Liver metastases

- Choledocholithiasis
- Parasitic infection
- Traumatic biliary strictures
- Chronic pancreatitis

Pre-hepatic jaundice

This is caused either by haemolysis or by congenital hyperbilirubinaemia, and is characterised by an isolated raised bilirubin level.

- In haemolysis, destruction of red blood cells or their precursors in the marrow causes increased bilirubin production. Jaundice due to haemolysis is usually mild because a healthy liver can excrete a bilirubin load six times greater than normal before unconjugated bilirubin accumulates in the plasma. This does not apply to the newborn, who have a reduced capacity to metabolise bilirubin.
- The most common form of non-haemolytic hyperbilirubinaemia is Gilbert's syndrome, an inherited disorder of bilirubin metabolism (Box 23.10). Other inherited disorders of bilirubin metabolism also exist but they are very rare.

Hepatocellular jaundice

Hepatocellular jaundice results from an inability of the liver to transport bilirubin across the hepatocyte into

23.10 Congenital non-haemolytic hyperbilirubinaemia

Syndrome	Inheritance	Abnormality	Clinical features/treatment
Unconjugated hyperbilirubinaemia			
Gilbert's	Autosomal dominant	↓ Glucuronyl transferase ↓ Bilirubin uptake	Mild jaundice, especially with fasting No treatment necessary
Crigler–Najjar			
Type I	Autosomal recessive	Absent glucuronyl transferase	Rapid death in neonate (kernicterus)
Type II	Autosomal dominant	↓↓ Glucuronyl transferase	Presents in neonate Phenobarbital, ultraviolet light or liver transplant as treatment
Conjugated hyperbilirubinaemia			
Dubin–Johnson	Autosomal recessive	↓ Canalicular excretion of organic anions, including bilirubin	Mild No treatment necessary
Rotor's	Autosomal recessive	↓ Bilirubin uptake ↓ Intrahepatic binding	Mild No treatment necessary

the bile, occurring as a consequence of parenchymal liver disease. Bilirubin transport across the hepatocytes may be impaired at any point between uptake of unconjugated bilirubin into the cells and transport of conjugated bilirubin into the canaliculi. In addition, swelling of cells and oedema resulting from the disease itself may cause obstruction of the biliary canaliculi. In hepatocellular jaundice the concentrations of both unconjugated and conjugated bilirubin in the blood increase. Hepatocellular jaundice can be due to acute or chronic liver injury (see Fig. 23.12), and clinical features of acute or chronic liver disease may be detected clinically (see Box 23.7, p. 930).

Characteristically, jaundice due to parenchymal liver disease is associated with increases in transaminases (AST, ALT), but increases in other LFTs, including cholestatic enzymes (GGT, ALP) may occur, and suggest specific aetiologies (see below). Acute jaundice in the presence of AST > 1000 U/L is highly suggestive of an infectious cause (e.g. hepatitis A, B), drugs (e.g. paracetamol) or hepatic ischaemia. Imaging is essential, in particular to identify features suggestive of cirrhosis (e.g. irregular liver outline, splenomegaly), to define the patency of hepatic arteries and veins, and of the portal vein, and to obtain evidence of portal hypertension. Liver biopsy has an important role in defining the aetiology of hepatocellular jaundice and the extent of established liver injury.

Obstructive (cholestatic) jaundice

Cholestatic jaundice may be caused by:
- failure of hepatocytes to initiate bile flow
- obstruction of bile flow in the bile ducts or portal tracts
- obstruction of bile flow in the extrahepatic bile ducts between the porta hepatis and the papilla of Vater.

In the absence of treatment, cholestatic jaundice tends to become progressively more severe because conjugated bilirubin is unable to enter the bile canaliculi and passes back into the blood, and also because there is a failure of clearance of unconjugated bilirubin arriving at the liver cells. The causes of cholestatic jaundice are listed in Box 23.9. Cholestasis may result from defects at more than one of these levels. Those confined to the extrahepatic bile ducts may be amenable to surgical correction.

Clinical features in cholestatic jaundice (Box 23.11) comprise those due to cholestasis itself, those due to secondary infection (cholangitis) and those of the underlying condition (Box 23.12). Obstruction of the bile duct drainage due to blockage of the extrahepatic biliary tree is characteristically associated with pale stools and dark urine. Pruritus may be a dominant feature, and can be accompanied by skin excoriations. Peripheral stigmata of chronic liver disease are absent. If the gallbladder is palpable, the jaundice is unlikely to be caused by biliary obstruction due to gallstones, probably because a chronically inflamed stone-containing gallbladder cannot readily dilate. This is Courvoisier's Law, and suggests that jaundice is due to a malignant biliary obstruction (e.g. pancreatic cancer). Cholangitis is characterised by 'Charcot's triad' of jaundice, right upper quadrant pain and fever. Cholestatic jaundice is characterised by a relatively greater elevation of ALP and GGT than the aminotransferases.

Ultrasound evaluation is indicated in all cases to determine whether there is evidence of mechanical obstruction and dilatation of the biliary tree (Fig. 23.14). Management of cholestatic jaundice depends on the

23.11 Clinical features and complications of cholestatic jaundice

Cholestasis

Early features
- Jaundice
- Dark urine
- Pale stools
- Pruritus

Late features
- Malabsorption (vitamins A, D, E and K)
  Weight loss
  Steatorrhoea
  Osteomalacia
  Bleeding tendency
- Xanthelasma and xanthomas

Cholangitis
- Fever
- Rigors
- Pain (if gallstones are present)

23.12 Clinical features suggesting an underlying cause of cholestatic jaundice*

Clinical feature	Causes
Jaundice	
Static or increasing	Carcinoma
	Primary biliary cirrhosis
	Primary sclerosing cholangitis
Fluctuating	Choledocholithiasis
	Stricture
	Pancreatitis
	Choledochal cyst
	Primary sclerosing cholangitis
Abdominal pain	Choledocholithiasis
	Pancreatitis
	Choledochal cyst
Cholangitis	Stone
	Stricture
	Choledochal cyst
Abdominal scar	Stone
	Stricture
Irregular hepatomegaly	Hepatic carcinoma
Palpable gallbladder	Carcinoma below cystic duct (usually pancreas)
Abdominal mass	Carcinoma
	Pancreatitis (cyst)
	Choledochal cyst
Occult blood in stools	Ampullary tumour

*Each of the diseases listed here can give rise to almost any of the clinical features shown, but the box indicates the most likely cause of the clinical features listed.

underlying cause of the cholestasis and is discussed in detail in the relevant sections below.

Acute liver failure

Acute liver failure is an uncommon but serious syndrome. The presentation is with mental changes progressing from confusion to stupor and coma, and a progressive deterioration in liver function. The syndrome was originally defined further as occurring within 8 weeks of onset of the precipitating illness, in the absence of evidence of pre-existing liver disease. This distinguishes it from instances in which hepatic encephalopathy represents a deterioration in chronic liver disease. More recently, newer classifications have been developed to reflect differences in presentation and outcome of acute liver failure. One such classification divides acute liver failure into hyperacute, acute and subacute according to the interval between onset of jaundice and encephalopathy (Box 23.13).

Pathophysiology

Any cause of liver damage can produce acute liver failure, provided it is sufficiently severe (Fig. 23.15). Acute viral hepatitis is the most common cause world-wide, whereas paracetamol toxicity (p. 209) is the most frequent cause in the UK. Acute liver failure occurs occasionally with other drugs, or from *Amanita phalloides* (mushroom) poisoning,

in pregnancy, in Wilson's disease, following shock (p. 186) and, rarely, in extensive malignant disease of the liver. In 10% of cases the cause of acute liver failure remains unknown and these patients are often labelled as having non-A–E viral hepatitis or cryptogenic acute liver failure.

Clinical assessment

Cerebral disturbance (hepatic encephalopathy) is the cardinal manifestation of acute liver failure, but in the early stages this can be mild and episodic. The initial clinical features are often subtle and include reduced alertness and poor concentration, progressing through behavioural abnormalities such as restlessness and aggressive outbursts, to drowsiness and coma (Box 23.14). Cerebral oedema may occur due to increased intracranial pressure causing unequal or abnormally reacting pupils, fixed pupils, hypertensive episodes, bradycardia, hyperventilation, profuse sweating, local or general myoclonus, focal fits or decerebrate posturing. Papilloedema occurs rarely and is a late sign. More general symptoms include weakness, nausea and vomiting. Right hypochondrial discomfort is an occasional feature.

The patient is usually jaundiced, except in Reye's syndrome when jaundice is rare. Occasionally, death may occur in fulminant cases of acute liver failure before jaundice develops. Fetor hepaticus can be present. The liver is usually of normal size but later becomes smaller. Hepatomegaly is unusual and, in the presence of a sudden onset of ascites, suggests venous outflow obstruction as the cause (Budd–Chiari syndrome). Splenomegaly is uncommon and never prominent. Ascites and oedema are late developments and may be a consequence of fluid therapy. Other features are related to the development of complications, which are considered below.

23.13 Classification of acute liver failure

Type	Time: jaundice to encephalopathy	Cerebral oedema	Common causes
Hyperacute	< 7 days	Common	Viral, paracetamol
Acute	8–28 days	Common	Cryptogenic, drugs
Subacute	29 days–12 weeks	Uncommon	Cryptogenic, drugs

23.14 How to grade hepatic encephalopathy clinically

Clinical grade	Clinical signs
Grade 1	Poor concentration, slurred speech, slow mentation, disordered sleep rhythm
Grade 2	Drowsy but easily rousable, occasional aggressive behaviour, lethargic
Grade 3	Marked confusion, drowsy, sleepy but responds to pain and voice, gross disorientation
Grade 4	Unresponsive to voice, may or may not respond to painful stimuli, unconscious

23

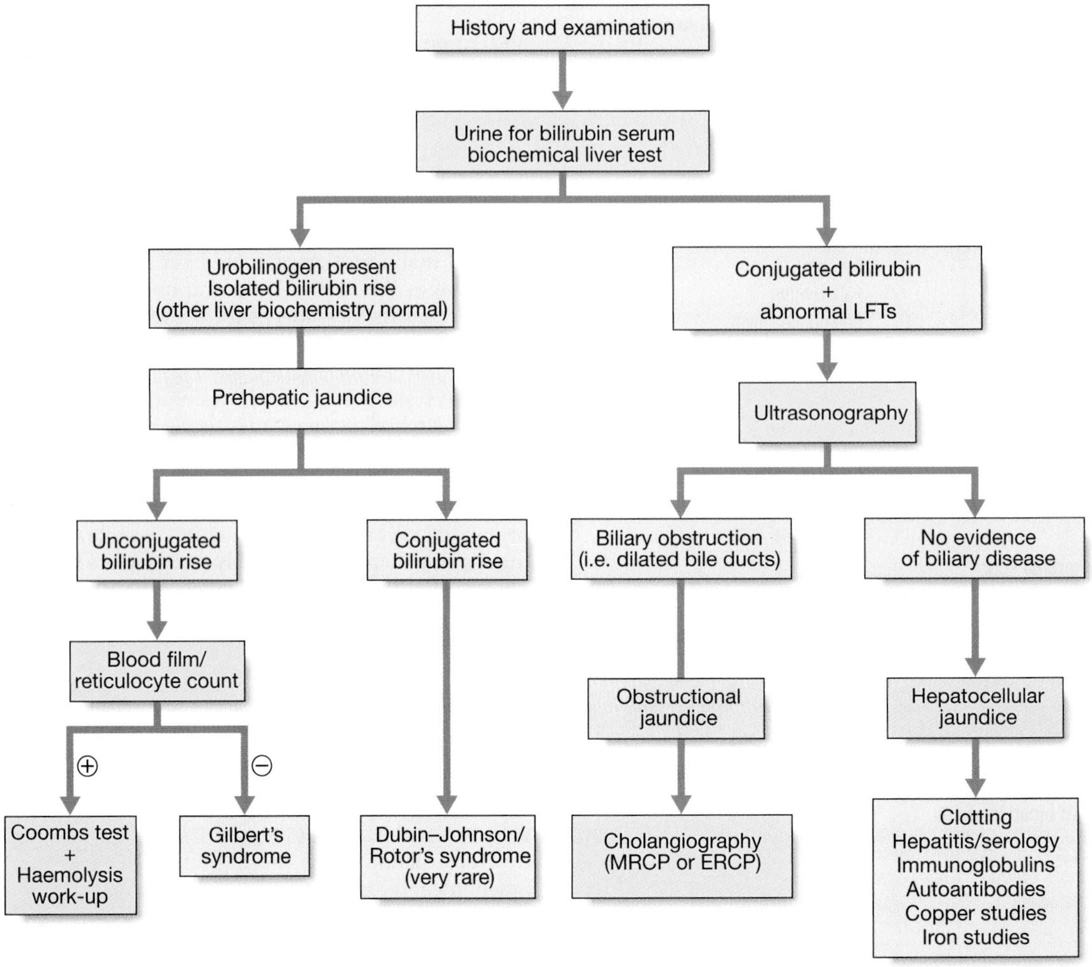

History and examination

↓

Urine for bilirubin serum
biochemical liver test

Urobilinogen present
Isolated bilirubin rise
(other liver biochemistry normal)

Conjugated bilirubin
+
abnormal LFTs

↓

Prehepatic jaundice

↓

Ultrasonography

Unconjugated
bilirubin rise

Conjugated
bilirubin rise

Biliary obstruction
(i.e. dilated bile ducts)

No evidence
of biliary disease

↓

Blood film/
reticulocyte count

Obstructional
jaundice

Hepatocellular
jaundice

⊕   ⊖

Coombs test
+
Haemolysis
work-up

Gilbert's
syndrome

Dubin–Johnson/
Rotor's syndrome
(very rare)

Cholangiography
(MRCP or ERCP)

Clotting
Hepatitis/serology
Immunoglobulins
Autoantibodies
Copper studies
Iron studies

Fig. 23.14 Investigation of jaundice.

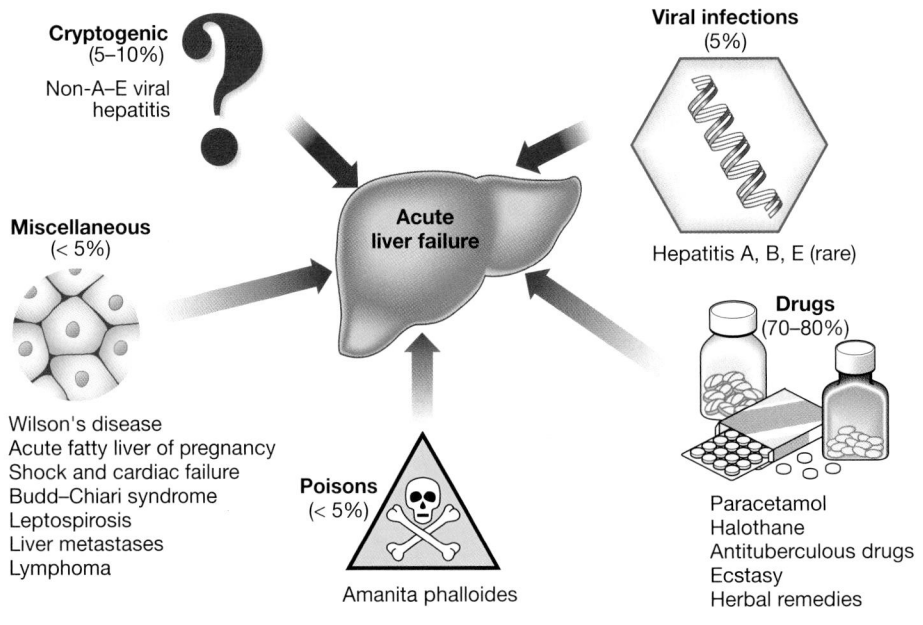

Cryptogenic
(5–10%)

Non-A–E viral
hepatitis

Viral infections
(5%)

Hepatitis A, B, E (rare)

Miscellaneous
(< 5%)

**Acute
liver failure**

Wilson's disease
Acute fatty liver of pregnancy
Shock and cardiac failure
Budd–Chiari syndrome
Leptospirosis
Liver metastases
Lymphoma

Poisons
(< 5%)

Amanita phalloides

Drugs
(70–80%)

Paracetamol
Halothane
Antituberculous drugs
Ecstasy
Herbal remedies

Fig. 23.15 Causes of acute liver failure in the UK. The relative frequency of the different causes varies according to geographical area.

Investigations

The patient should be investigated to determine the cause of the liver failure and the prognosis (Boxes 23.15 and 23.16). Hepatitis B core IgM antibody is the best screening test for acute hepatitis B infection, as liver damage is due to the immunological response to the virus which has often been eliminated and the test for HBsAg may be negative. The prothrombin time rapidly becomes prolonged as coagulation factor synthesis fails; this is the laboratory test of greatest prognostic value and should be carried out at least twice daily. Its prognostic importance emphasises the necessity of avoiding the use of fresh frozen plasma to correct raised prothrombin time in acute liver failure, except in the setting of frank bleeding. Factor V levels can be used instead of the prothrombin time to assess the degree of liver impairment. The plasma bilirubin reflects the degree of jaundice. Plasma aminotransferase activity is particularly high after paracetamol overdose, reaching 100–500 times normal, but falls as liver damage progresses and is not helpful in determining prognosis. Plasma albumin remains normal unless the course is prolonged. Percutaneous liver biopsy is contraindicated because of the severe coagulopathy, but biopsy can be undertaken using the transjugular route.

Management

Patients with acute liver failure should be treated in a high-dependency or intensive care unit as soon as progressive prolongation of the prothrombin time occurs or hepatic encephalopathy is identified (Box 23.17), so that prompt treatment of complications can be initiated (Box 23.18). Conservative treatment aims to maintain life in the hope that hepatic regeneration will occur, but early transfer to a specialised transplant unit should always be considered. N-acetylcysteine therapy may improve outcome, particularly in patients with acute liver failure due to paracetamol poisoning. Liver transplantation is an increasingly important treatment option for acute liver failure, and criteria have been developed to identify patients unlikely to survive without a transplant (see Box 23.16). Patients should, wherever possible, be transferred to a transplant centre before these criteria are met to allow time for assessment and to maximise the time for a donor liver to become available. Survival following liver transplantation for acute liver failure is improving, and 1-year survival rates of about 60% can be expected.

23

23.15 Investigations to determine the cause of acute liver failure

- Toxicology screen of blood and urine
- HBsAg, IgM anti-HBc
- IgM anti-HAV
- Anti-HEV, HCV, cytomegalovirus, herpes simplex, Epstein–Barr virus
- Ceruloplasmin, serum copper, urinary copper, slit-lamp eye examination
- Autoantibodies: ANF, ASMA, LKM
- Immunoglobulins
- Ultrasound of liver and Doppler of hepatic veins

(ANF = antinuclear factor; ASMA = anti-smooth muscle antibody; LKM = liver-kidney microsomal antibody)

23.17 Monitoring in acute liver failure

Neurological

- Intracranial pressure monitoring (specialist units, p. 199)
- Conscious level

Cardiorespiratory

- Pulse
- Blood pressure
- Central venous pressure
- Respiratory rate

Fluid balance

- Hourly output (urine, vomiting, diarrhoea)
- Input: oral, intravenous

Blood analyses

- Arterial blood gases
- Peripheral blood count (including platelets)
- Sodium, potassium, HCO_3^-, calcium, magnesium
- Creatinine, urea
- Glucose (2-hourly in acute phase)
- Prothrombin time

Infection surveillance

- Cultures: blood, urine, throat, sputum, cannula sites
- Chest X-ray
- Temperature

23.16 Adverse prognostic criteria in acute liver failure*

- $H^+ > 50$ nmol/L (pH < 7.3) at or beyond 24 hours following the overdose
  or
- Serum creatinine > 300 μmol/L ($\cong$ 3.38 mg/dL) *plus* prothrombin time > 100 seconds *plus* encephalopathy grade 3 or 4

Non-paracetamol cases

- Prothrombin time > 100 seconds
  or
- Any three of the following:
  Jaundice to encephalopathy time > 7 days
  Age < 10 or > 40 years
  Indeterminate or drug-induced causes
  Bilirubin > 300 μmol/L ($\cong$ 17.6 mg/dL)
  Prothrombin time > 50 seconds
  or
- Factor V level < 15% and encephalopathy grade 3 or 4

*Predict a mortality rate of ≥ 90% and are an indication for referral for possible liver transplantation.

23.18 Complications of acute liver failure

- Encephalopathy and cerebral oedema
- Hypoglycaemia
- Metabolic acidosis
- Infection (bacterial, fungal)
- Renal failure
- Multi-organ failure (hypotension and respiratory failure)

Hepatomegaly

Hepatomegaly may occur as the result of a general enlargement of the liver or because of primary or secondary liver tumour. The most common liver tumour in the West is liver metastasis, whereas primary liver cancer complicating chronic viral hepatitis is more common in the Far East. Unlike metastases, neuro-endocrine tumours typically cause massive hepatomegaly but without significant weight loss. Cirrhosis often presents with hepatomegaly, although in end-stage disease the liver may be reduced in size. Although all causes of cirrhosis can involve hepatomegaly, it is much more common in alcoholic liver disease and haemochromatosis. Hepatomegaly may resolve in patients with alcoholic cirrhosis when they stop drinking.

Ascites

Ascites is present when there is accumulation of free fluid in the peritoneal cavity. Small amounts of ascites are asymptomatic, but with larger accumulations of fluid (> 1 L) there is abdominal distension, fullness in the flanks, shifting dullness on percussion and, when the ascites is marked, a fluid thrill. In obese patients, much larger volumes of ascites may accumulate before they are detectable clinically. Other features include distortion or eversion of the umbilicus, herniae, abdominal striae, divarication of the recti and scrotal oedema. Dilated superficial abdominal veins may be seen if the ascites is due to portal hypertension.

Pathophysiology

Ascites may result from several different causes, the most common of which are malignant disease, cirrhosis or heart failure. Many primary disorders of the peritoneum and visceral organs can also cause ascites, and these need to be considered even in a patient with chronic liver disease (Box 23.19). Splanchnic vasodilata-

tion is thought to be the main factor leading to ascites in cirrhosis. This is mediated by vasodilators (mainly nitric oxide) that are released when portal hypertension causes shunting of blood into the systemic circulation. Systemic arterial pressure falls due to pronounced splanchnic vasodilatation as cirrhosis advances. This leads to activation of the renin–angiotensin system with secondary aldosteronism, increased sympathetic nervous activity, increased atrial natriuretic hormone secretion and altered activity of the kallikrein–kinin system (Fig. 23.16). These systems tend to normalise arterial pressure but produce salt and water retention. In this setting, the combination of splanchnic arterial vasodilatation and portal hypertension alters intestinal capillary permeability, promoting accumulation of fluid within the peritoneum.

Investigations

Ultrasonography is the best means of detecting ascites, particularly in the obese and those with small volumes of fluid. Paracentesis (if necessary under ultrasonic guidance) can also be used to confirm the presence of ascites but is most useful for obtaining ascitic fluid for analysis. The appearance of ascitic fluid may point to the underlying cause (Box 23.20). Pleural effusions are found in about 10% of patients, usually on the right side (hepatic hydrothorax); most are small and only identified on chest X-ray, but occasionally a massive hydrothorax occurs. Pleural effusions, particularly those on the left side, should not be assumed to be due to the ascites.

Measurement of the protein concentration and the serum–ascites albumin gradient (SAAG) are used to

23.19 **Causes of ascites**	
Common causes	

• Malignant disease
    Hepatic
    Peritoneal
	• Cardiac failure
	• Hepatic cirrhosis

Other causes	

• Hypoproteinaemia
    Nephrotic syndrome
    Protein-losing enteropathy
    Malnutrition
• Hepatic venous occlusion
    (p. 973)
    Budd–Chiari syndrome
    Veno-occlusive disease
	• Pancreatitis
	• Lymphatic obstruction
	• Infection
	    Tuberculosis

Rare causes	
• Meigs' syndrome*	• Hypothyroidism

*Meigs' syndrome is the association of a right pleural effusion with or without ascites and a benign ovarian tumour. The ascites resolves on removal of the tumour.

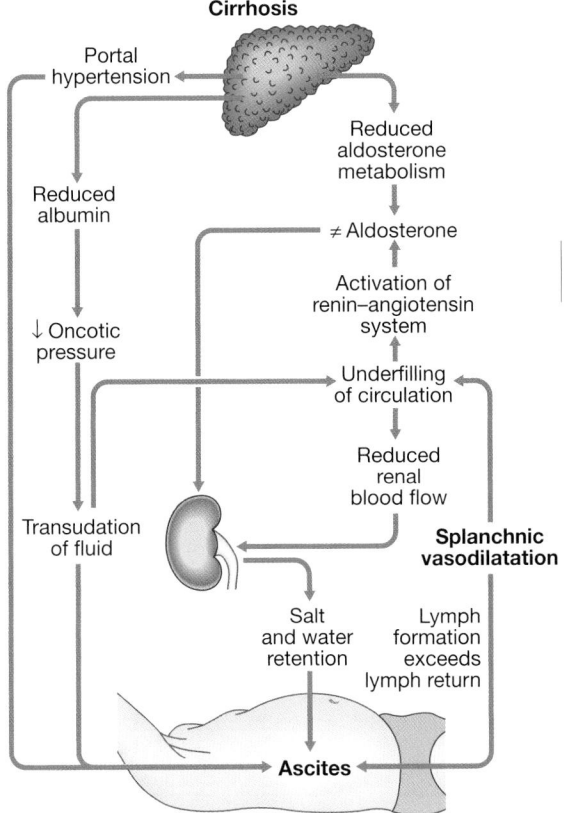

Fig. 23.16 Pathogenesis of ascites.

23.20 Ascitic fluid: appearance and analysis

Cause/appearance

- Cirrhosis: clear, straw-coloured or light green
- Malignant disease: bloody
- Infection: cloudy
- Biliary communication: heavy bile staining
- Lymphatic obstruction: milky-white (chylous)

Useful investigations

- Total albumin (plus serum albumin) and protein*
- Amylase
- Neutrophil count
- Cytology
- Microscopy and culture

*To calculate the serum–ascites albumin gradient (SAAG).

23.21 Some drugs containing relatively large amounts of sodium or causing sodium retention

High sodium content

- Antacids
- Alginates
- Antibiotics
- Phenytoin
- Sodium valproate
- Effervescent preparations (e.g. aspirin, calcium, paracetamol)

Sodium retention

- Carbenoxolone
- Corticosteroids
- Metoclopramide
- NSAIDs
- Oestrogens

distinguish a transudate from an exudate. Cirrhotic patients typically develop a transudate with a total protein concentration below 25 g/L and relatively few cells. However, in up to 30% of patients, the total protein concentration is more than 30 g/L. In these cases it is useful to calculate the SAAG by subtracting the concentration of the ascites fluid albumin from the serum albumin. A gradient of more than 11 g/L is 96% predictive that ascites is due to portal hypertension. Venous outflow obstruction due to cardiac failure or hepatic venous outflow obstruction can also cause a transudative ascites, as indicated by an albumin gradient above 11 g/L, but unlike in cirrhosis the total protein content is usually above 25 g/L.

Exudative ascites (ascites protein concentration above 25 g/L or a SAAG of less than 11 g/L) raises the possibility of infection (especially tuberculosis), malignancy, hepatic venous obstruction, pancreatic ascites or, rarely, hypothyroidism. Ascites amylase activity above 1000 U/L identifies pancreatic ascites, and low ascites glucose concentrations suggest malignant disease or tuberculosis. Cytological examination may reveal malignant cells (one-third of cirrhotic patients with a bloody tap have a hepatoma). Polymorphonuclear leucocyte counts above 250×10^6/L strongly suggest infection (spontaneous bacterial peritonitis, see below). Laparoscopy can be valuable in detecting peritoneal disease.

Management

Successful treatment of ascites relieves discomfort but does not prolong life, and if over-vigorous, can produce serious disorders of fluid and electrolyte balance and precipitate hepatic encephalopathy (p. 938). Treatment of transudative ascites is based on restricting sodium and water intake, promoting urine output with diuretics and, if necessary, removing ascites directly by paracentesis. Exudative ascites due to malignancy should be treated with paracentesis but fluid replacement is generally not required. In ovarian cancer, however, paracentesis usually needs to be guided by ultrasound, as the need for frequent paracentesis often results in the fluid becoming loculated. During management of ascites, the patient should be weighed regularly. It is important to avoid removing more than 1 L of fluid daily, so body weight should not fall by more than 1 kg daily if fluid depletion in the rest of the body is to be avoided.

Sodium and water restriction

Restriction of dietary sodium intake is essential to achieve negative sodium balance in ascites, and a few patients can be managed satisfactorily on this treatment alone. Restriction of sodium intake to 100 mmol/day ('no added salt diet') is usually adequate. Drugs containing relatively large amounts of sodium and those promoting sodium retention, such as non-steroidal anti-inflammatory drugs, must be avoided (Box 23.21). Restriction of water intake to 1.0–1.5 L/day is necessary only if the plasma sodium falls below 125 mmol/L.

Diuretics

Most patients require diuretics in addition to sodium restriction. Spironolactone (100–400 mg/day) is the drug of choice for long-term therapy because it is a powerful aldosterone antagonist; unfortunately, it can cause painful gynaecomastia and hyperkalaemia. Some patients also require loop diuretics, such as furosemide, but these can cause fluid and electrolyte imbalance and renal dysfunction. Diuresis is improved if patients are rested in bed, perhaps because renal blood flow increases in the horizontal position. Patients who do not respond to doses of 400 mg spironolactone and 160 mg furosemide are considered to have refractory or diuretic-resistant ascites and should be treated by other therapeutic measures.

Paracentesis

The first-line treatment of refractory ascites is large-volume paracentesis with intravenous albumin replacement. Paracentesis to dryness or the removal of 3–5 L daily is safe, provided the circulation is supported with an intravenous colloid such as human albumin (6–8 g per litre of ascites removed, usually as 100 mL of 20% human albumin solution (HAS) for every 3 L of ascites drained) or another plasma expander. Paracentesis can therefore be used as an initial therapy or when other treatments fail.

Peritoneo-venous shunt

The peritoneo-venous shunt is a long tube with a non-return valve running subcutaneously from the peritoneum to the internal jugular vein in the neck; it allows ascitic fluid to pass directly into the systemic circulation. It is effective in ascites resistant to conventional treatment but complications, including infection, superior vena caval thrombosis, pulmonary oedema, bleeding from oesophageal varices and disseminated intravascular

23

coagulopathy, limit its use and insertion of these shunts is now rare.

Transjugular intrahepatic portosystemic stent shunt (TIPSS)

TIPSS (pp. 941–942) can relieve resistant ascites but does not prolong life; it may be an option where the only alternative is frequent, large-volume paracentesis. It can be used when liver function is reasonable or in patients awaiting liver transplantation.

Renal failure

Renal failure can occur in patients with ascites. It can be pre-renal due to vasodilatation from sepsis and/or diuretic therapy, or due to hepatorenal failure, which is discussed on page 944.

Spontaneous bacterial peritonitis

Patients with cirrhosis are highly susceptible to spontaneous bacterial peritonitis (SBP). This usually presents suddenly with abdominal pain, rebound tenderness, absent bowel sounds and fever in a patient with obvious features of cirrhosis and ascites. Abdominal signs are mild or absent in about one-third of patients, and in these patients hepatic encephalopathy and fever are the main features. Diagnostic paracentesis may show cloudy fluid, and an ascites neutrophil count above $250 \times 10^6/$L almost invariably indicates infection. The source of infection cannot usually be determined, but most organisms isolated from ascitic fluid or blood cultures are of enteric origin and *Escherichia coli* is the organism most frequently found. Ascitic culture in blood culture bottles gives the highest yield of organisms. SBP needs to be differentiated from other intra-abdominal emergencies, and the finding of multiple organisms on culture should arouse suspicion of a perforated viscus.

Treatment should be started immediately with broad-spectrum antibiotics, such as cefotaxime. Recurrence of SBP is common but may be reduced with prophylactic quinolones such as norfloxacin (400 mg daily) or ciprofloxacin (250 mg 12-hourly) (Box 23.22).

Prognosis

Only 10–20% of patients survive 5 years from the first appearance of ascites due to cirrhosis. The outlook is not universally poor, however, and is best in those with well-maintained liver function and a good response to therapy. The prognosis is also better when a treatable cause for the underlying cirrhosis is present or when a precipitating cause for ascites, such as excess salt intake, is found. The mortality at 1 year is 50% following the first episode of bacterial peritonitis.

EBM | **23.22 Antibiotics and spontaneous bacterial peritonitis (SBP)**

'In patients with a previous episode of SBP and continued ascites, norfloxacin 400 mg/day prevents recurrence (NNT$_B$ 4.5).'

'In patients with cirrhosis who have had a gastrointestinal haemorrhage, prophylactic antibiotics reduce the risk of bacterial peritonitis (NNT$_B$ 12.5) and improve survival (NNT$_B$ 11).'

- Gines P, et al. Hepatology 1990; 12:716.
- Bernard B, et al. Hepatology 1999; 29:1655–1661.

Hepatic encephalopathy

Hepatic encephalopathy is a neuropsychiatric syndrome caused by chronic liver disease. As encephalopathy progresses, confusion is followed by coma. Confusion needs to be differentiated from delirium tremens and Wernicke's encephalopathy, and coma from subdural haematoma which can occur in alcoholics after a fall (Box 23.23). Features include changes of intellect, personality, emotions and consciousness, with or without neurological signs. The degree of encephalopathy can be graded from 1 to 4, depending on these features, and this is useful in assessing response to therapy (see Box 23.14, p. 933). When an episode develops acutely, a precipitating factor may be found (Fig. 23.17). The earliest features are very mild and easily overlooked but, as the condition becomes more severe, apathy, inability to concentrate, confusion, disorientation, drowsiness, slurring of speech and eventually coma develop. Convulsions sometimes occur. Examination usually shows a flapping tremor (asterixis, p. 921), inability to perform simple mental arithmetic tasks (Fig. 23.18) or to draw objects such as a star (constructional apraxia, Fig. 23.19), and, as the condition progresses, hyper-reflexia and bilateral extensor plantar responses. Hepatic encephalopathy rarely causes focal neurological signs, and if these are present, other causes must be sought. Fetor hepaticus, a sweet musty odour to the breath, is usually present but is more a sign of liver failure and portosystemic shunting than of hepatic encephalopathy. Rarely, chronic hepatic encephalopathy (hepatocerebral degeneration) gives rise to variable combinations of cerebellar

---

i | **23.23 Differential diagnosis of hepatic encephalopathy**

- Intracranial bleed (subdural, extradural haematoma, p. 1191)
- Drug or alcohol intoxication (pp. 246–247)
- Delirium tremens/alcohol withdrawal (p. 246)
- Wernicke's encephalopathy (p. 246)
- Primary psychiatric disorders (p. 240)
- Hypoglycaemia (p. 812)
- Neurological Wilson's disease (p. 1203)
- Post-ictal state

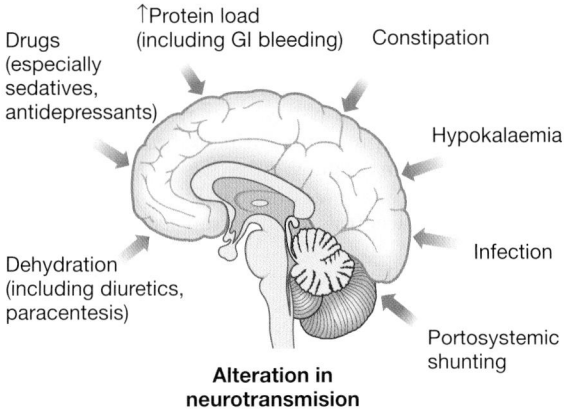

Fig. 23.17 Factors precipitating hepatic encephalopathy.

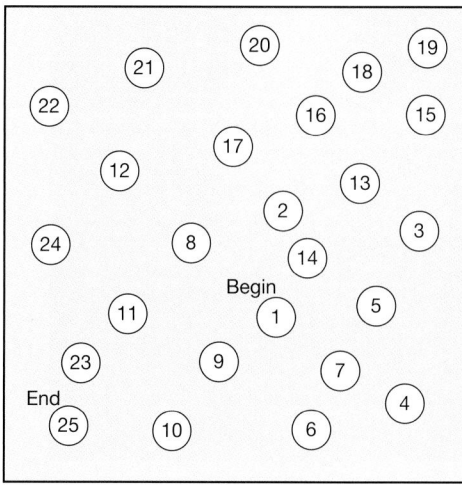

Fig. 23.18 Number connection test used in assessing encephalopathy. These 25 numbered circles can normally be joined together within 30 seconds. Serial observations may provide useful information as long as the position of the numbers is varied to avoid the patient learning their pattern.

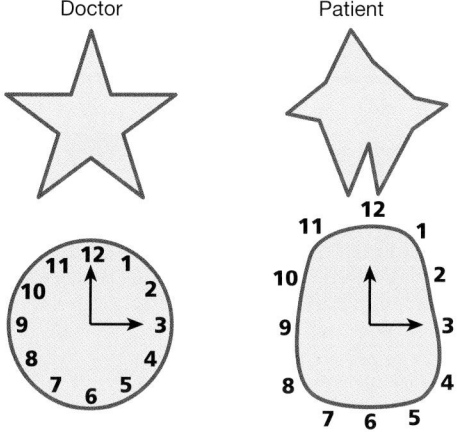

Fig. 23.19 Constructional apraxia in encephalopathy. Drawing stars and clocks may reveal marked abnormality.

dysfunction, Parkinsonian syndromes, spastic paraplegia and dementia.

Pathophysiology

Hepatic encephalopathy is thought to be due to a disturbance of brain function provoked by circulating neurotoxins that are normally metabolised by the liver. Accordingly, most affected patients have evidence of liver failure and portosystemic shunting of blood, but the balance between these varies from individual to individual. Some degree of liver failure is a key factor, as portosystemic shunting of blood alone hardly ever causes encephalopathy. Little is known of the biochemical 'neurotoxins' causing the encephalopathy, but they are thought to be mainly nitrogenous substances produced in the gut, at least in part by bacterial action. These substances are normally metabolised by the healthy liver and therefore excluded from the systemic circulation. Ammonia has traditionally been considered an important factor and ammonia-induced alteration in astrocyte glutamine and glutamate concentrations may be important. Recent interest has focused on γ-aminobutyric acid as a mediator, along with other factors such as octopamine, amino acids, mercaptans and fatty acids which can act as neurotransmitters. Some factors appear to precipitate hepatic encephalopathy by increasing the availability of these substances; in addition, the brain in cirrhosis may be sensitised to other factors such as drugs that are able to precipitate hepatic encephalopathy (see Fig. 23.17). Disruption of the function of the blood–brain barrier is a feature of acute hepatic failure and may lead to cerebral oedema.

Investigations

The diagnosis can usually be made clinically, but when doubt exists, an electroencephalogram (EEG) shows diffuse slowing of the normal alpha waves with eventual development of delta waves. The arterial ammonia is usually increased in patients with hepatic encephalopathy. However, increased concentrations can occur in the absence of clinical encephalopathy, so this investigation is of little or no diagnostic value.

Management

The principles of management are to treat or remove precipitating causes (see Fig. 23.17) and to suppress the production of neurotoxins by bacteria in the bowel. Dietary protein restriction is rarely needed and is no longer recommended as first-line treatment because it is unpalatable and can lead to a worsening nutritional state in already malnourished patients. Lactulose (15–30 mL 8-hourly) is a disaccharide which is taken orally and reaches the colon intact, to be metabolised by colonic bacteria. The dose is increased gradually until the bowels are moving twice daily. It produces an osmotic laxative effect, reduces the pH of the colonic content, thereby limiting colonic ammonia absorption, and promotes the incorporation of nitrogen into bacteria. Lactitol is a rather more palatable alternative to lactulose, with a less explosive action on bowel function. Neomycin (1–4 g 4–6-hourly) is an antibiotic which acts by reducing the bacterial content of the bowel. It can be used in addition or as an alternative to lactulose if diarrhoea becomes troublesome. Neomycin is poorly absorbed from the bowel but sufficient gains access to the body to contraindicate its use when uraemia is present. It is less desirable than lactulose for long-term use; ototoxicity is the main deleterious effect and so neomycin is now rarely used. Chronic or refractory hepatic encephalopathy is one of the main indications for liver transplantation.

Variceal bleeding

Acute upper gastrointestinal haemorrhage from oesophagogastric varices (Fig. 23.20) is a common manifestation of chronic liver disease. However, gastrointestinal bleeding can also occur as the result of peptic ulceration, which is more common in patients with liver disease than in the general population. The investigation and management of gastrointestinal bleeding are dealt with in more detail on pages 852–856, but the specific management of variceal bleeding is discussed here.

23

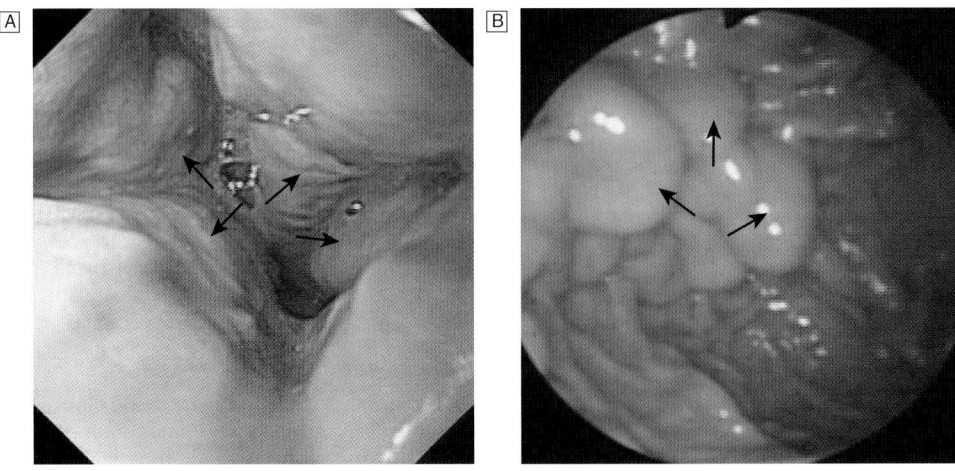

Fig. 23.20 **Varices: endoscopic views.** A Oesophageal varices (arrows) at the lower end of the oesophagus. B Gastric varices (arrows).

Management

Principles

The priority in acute bleeding from oesophageal varices is to restore the circulation with blood and plasma, not least because shock reduces liver blood flow and causes further deterioration of liver function. Even in patients with known varices, the source of bleeding should always be confirmed by endoscopy because about 20% of patients are bleeding from some other lesion, especially acute gastric erosions. Management of acute variceal bleeding is described in Box 23.24 and illustrated in Figure 23.21. All patients with cirrhosis and gastrointestinal bleeding should receive prophylactic broad-spectrum antibiotics, such as oral ciprofloxacin or intravenous cephalosporin, because sepsis is common and treatment with antibiotics has been shown to improve outcome. The measures used to control acute variceal bleeding include endoscopic therapy (banding or sclerotherapy), balloon tamponade and oesophageal transection.

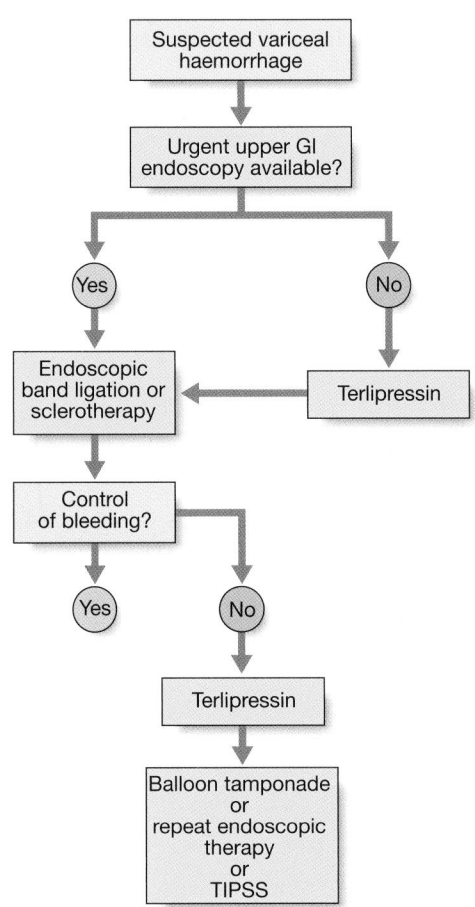

Fig. 23.21 **Management of acute bleeding from oesophageal varices.** (TIPSS = transjugular intrahepatic portosystemic stent shunt)

Banding ligation and sclerotherapy

This is the most widely used initial treatment and is undertaken if possible at the time of diagnostic endoscopy (Fig. 23.22). It stops variceal bleeding in 80% of patients and can be repeated if bleeding recurs. Band ligation involves the varices being sucked into a cap placed on the end of the endoscope, allowing them to

23.24 Emergency management of bleeding	
Management	**Reason**
0.9% saline (1–2 L)	Extracellular volume replacement
Vasopressor (terlipressin)	Reduces portal pressure, acute bleeding and risk of early rebleeding
Prophylactic antibiotics (cephalosporin i.v.)	Reduces incidence of SBP
Emergency endoscopy	Confirm variceal rather than ulcer bleed
Variceal band ligation	To stop bleeding
Proton pump inhibitor	To prevent peptic ulcers
Phosphate enema and/or lactulose	To prevent hepatic encephalopathy

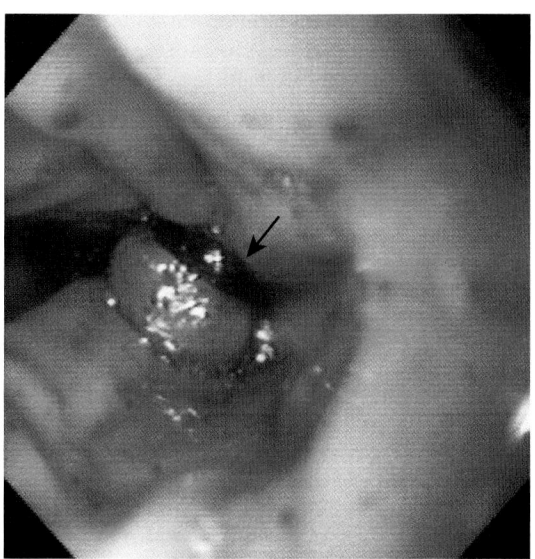

Fig. 23.22 Appearance of oesophageal varices following application of strangulating bands (band ligation, arrow).

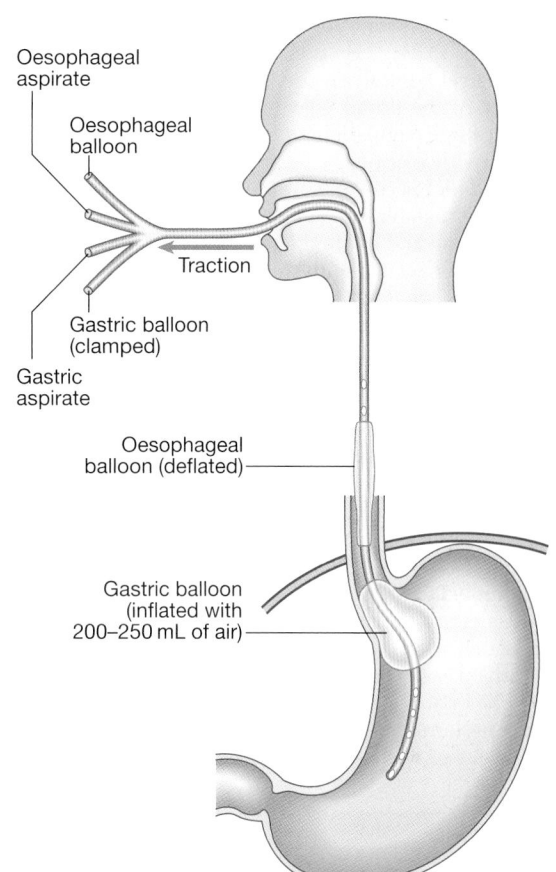

Fig. 23.23 Sengstaken–Blakemore tube.

23

be occluded with a tight rubber band. The occluded varix subsequently sloughs with variceal obliteration. Banding is repeated every 1–2 weeks until the varices are obliterated. Regular follow-up endoscopy is required to identify and treat any recurrence of varices. Band ligation has fewer side-effects than sclerotherapy, a technique in which varices are injected with a sclerosing agent, which has now been largely abandoned in preference to banding ligation. Banding is associated with less risk of oesophageal perforation and oesophageal strictures. Prophylactic acid suppression with proton pump inhibitors reduces the risk of secondary bleeding from banding-induced ulceration.

Active bleeding at endoscopy may make endoscopic therapy difficult; in such cases, bleeding should be controlled by balloon tamponade prior to endoscopic therapy. Protection of the patient's airway with endotracheal intubation may allow an improved endoscopic view, facilitating endoscopic therapy, and significantly reduce the risk of pulmonary aspiration.

Pharmacological reduction of portal venous pressure

Pharmacological reduction of portal pressure is less important than banding in preventing rebleeding, but is useful in reducing active bleeding while endoscopy is being arranged. Terlipressin is the current drug of choice and releases the vasoconstrictor, vasopressin, over several hours in amounts sufficient to reduce the portal pressure without producing systemic effects. It is given in a dose of 2 mg i.v. 6-hourly until bleeding stops, and then 1 mg 6-hourly for a further 24 hours.

Balloon tamponade

This technique employs a Sengstaken–Blakemore tube possessing two balloons which exert pressure in the fundus of the stomach and in the lower oesophagus respectively (Fig. 23.23). Current modifications incorporate additional lumens to allow material to be aspirated from the stomach and from the oesophagus above the oesophageal balloon.

The tube should be passed through the mouth and its presence in the stomach should be checked by auscultating the upper abdomen while injecting air into the stomach and by radiology. Gentle traction is essential to maintain pressure on the varices. Initially, only the gastric balloon should be inflated with 200–250 mL of air, as this will usually control bleeding. Inflation of the gastric balloon must be stopped if the patient experiences pain because inadvertent inflation in the oesophagus can cause oesophageal rupture. If the oesophageal balloon needs to be used because of continued bleeding, it should be deflated for about 10 minutes every 3 hours to avoid oesophageal mucosal damage. Pressure in the oesophageal balloon should be monitored with a sphygmomanometer and should not exceed 40 mmHg. Balloon tamponade will almost always stop oesophageal and gastric fundal variceal bleeding, but only creates time for the use of more definitive therapy. Particular care should be taken to avoid pulmonary aspiration whilst inserting the tube; as mentioned above, patients unable to protect their airway should be intubated.

Self-expanding removable oesophageal stents are a new alternative to the Sengstaken tube in patients with bleeding oesophageal, in contrast to gastric, varices.

Transjugular intrahepatic portosystemic stent shunting (TIPSS)

This technique uses a stent placed between the portal vein and the hepatic vein within the liver to provide a portosystemic shunt and therefore reduce portal pressure (Fig. 23.24). The procedure is carried out under radiological control via the internal jugular vein; prior patency of the portal vein must be determined angiographically, coagulation deficiencies may require correction with fresh frozen plasma, and antibiotic cover is provided. Successful shunt placement stops and prevents variceal bleeding. Further bleeding necessitates investigation and treatment (e.g. angioplasty) because it is usually associated with shunt narrowing or occlusion. Hepatic encephalopathy may occur following TIPSS and is managed by reducing the shunt diameter. Although TIPSS is associated with less rebleeding than endoscopic therapy, survival is not improved (Box 23.25).

Portosystemic shunt surgery

Surgery prevents recurrent bleeding, but carries a high mortality and often leads to encephalopathy. Non-selective portacaval shunts can divert the majority of the portal blood away from the liver, rendering patients liable to post-operative liver failure and hepatic encephalopathy. This led to the development of more selective shunts (such as the distal splenorenal shunt); such devices are associated with less post-operative encephalopathy, but with the passage of time liver portal blood flow falls and encephalopathy may supervene. Furthermore, survival is not prolonged, as death from liver failure may occur.

In practice, portosystemic shunts are now reserved for patients in whom other treatments have not been successful and are offered only to those with good liver function.

Oesophageal transection

Transection of the varices can be performed with a stapling gun, although this carries some risk of subsequent oesophageal stenosis and is normally combined with splenectomy. The operation is used when TIPSS is not available and when bleeding cannot be controlled by the other therapies described. The operative morbidity and mortality are considerable and the procedure is now rarely used.

Prognosis

In the presence of portal hypertension, the risk of a variceal bleed occurring within 2 years varies from 7% for small varices up to 30% for large varices. The mortality following a variceal bleed has improved to around 15% overall but still is about 45% in those with poor liver function, i.e. Child–Pugh C patients.

CIRRHOSIS

Hepatic cirrhosis is a common disease characterised by diffuse hepatic fibrosis and nodule formation. It can occur at any age, has significant morbidity and is an important cause of premature death. World-wide, the most common causes of cirrhosis are chronic viral hepatitis and prolonged excessive alcohol consumption. Cirrhosis is the most common cause of portal hypertension and its associated complications.

The causes of cirrhosis are listed in Box 23.26; any condition leading to persistent or recurrent hepatocyte death, such as chronic hepatitis C infection, may lead to cirrhosis. It may also occur in prolonged biliary damage or obstruction, as is found in primary biliary cirrhosis, primary sclerosing cholangitis and post-surgical biliary strictures. Persistent blockage of venous return from the liver, such as occurs in veno-occlusive disease and Budd–Chiari syndrome, can also result in liver cirrhosis.

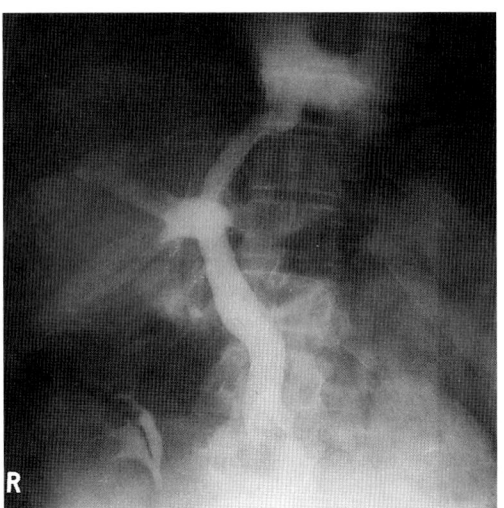

Fig. 23.24 Transjugular intrahepatic portosystemic stent shunt (TIPSS). X-ray showing placement of TIPSS within the portal vein (PV), allowing blood to flow from the portal vein into the hepatic vein (HV) and then the inferior vena cava (IVC). (H = heart)

EBM **23.25 Secondary prevention of variceal bleeding in patients with cirrhosis**

'While TIPSS is more effective than endoscopic treatment in reducing variceal rebleeding, it does not improve survival and is associated with more encephalopathy.'

• Jalan R, et al. Gut 2000; 6:1–15.
• Laine L. Hepatology 1995; 22:663–665.

For further information: www.bsg.org.uk

23.26 Causes of cirrhosis

• Alcohol
• Chronic viral hepatitis (B or C)
• Non-alcoholic fatty liver disease
• Immune
  Primary sclerosing cholangitis
  Autoimmune liver disease
• Biliary
  Primary biliary cirrhosis
  Secondary biliary cirrhosis
  Cystic fibrosis

• Genetic
  Haemochromatosis
  Wilson's disease
  α_1-antitrypsin deficiency
• Cryptogenic (unknown—15%)
• Chronic venous outflow obstruction

Pathophysiology

The cardinal feature of cirrhosis is an increase in fibrous tissue, progressive and widespread death of liver cells, and inflammation leading to loss of the normal liver architecture. Following liver injury, stellate cells in the space of Disse (see Fig. 23.3, p. 923) are activated by cytokines produced by Kupffer cells and hepatocytes. This transforms the stellate cell into a myofibroblast-like cell, capable of producing collagen, pro-inflammatory cytokines and other mediators which promote hepatocyte damage and cause tissue fibrosis (see Fig. 23.4, p. 924).

Destruction of the liver architecture causes distortion and loss of the normal hepatic vasculature with the development of portosystemic vascular shunts and the formation of nodules. Cirrhosis evolves slowly over years to decades, and normally continues to progress even after removal of the aetiological agent (e.g. abstinence from alcohol, venesection in haemochromatosis). Cirrhosis is a histological diagnosis characterised by diffuse hepatic fibrosis and nodule formation (Fig. 23.25). These changes usually affect the whole liver, but in biliary cirrhosis (e.g. primary biliary cirrhosis) they can be patchy.

Cirrhosis can be classified histologically into two types:

- *Micronodular cirrhosis*, characterised by small nodules about 1 mm in diameter and seen in alcoholic cirrhosis.
- *Macronodular cirrhosis*, characterised by larger nodules of various sizes. Areas of previous collapse of the liver architecture are evidenced by large fibrous scars.

Clinical features

The clinical presentation of cirrhosis is highly variable. Some patients are completely asymptomatic and the diagnosis is made incidentally at ultrasound or at surgery. Others present with isolated hepatomegaly, splenomegaly or signs of portal hypertension (p. 945). When symptoms are present, they are often non-specific and include weakness, fatigue, muscle cramps, weight loss, anorexia, nausea, vomiting and upper abdominal discomfort (Box 23.27). Occasionally, cirrhosis presents with features of hepatic insufficiency. Cirrhosis will occasionally present to a chest physician because of shortness of breath and a large right pleural effusion, without accompanying ascites or with hepatopulmonary syndrome (p. 973).

Hepatomegaly is common when the cirrhosis is due to alcoholic liver disease and haemochromatosis. Progressive hepatocyte destruction and fibrosis gradually reduce liver size as the disease progresses in other causes of cirrhosis. A reduction in liver size is especially common if the cause of cirrhosis is viral hepatitis or autoimmune liver disease. The liver is often hard, irregular and non-tender. Jaundice is usually mild when it first appears and is due primarily to a failure to excrete bilirubin. Mild haemolysis may occur due to hypersplenism but is not a major contributor to the jaundice. Palmar erythema can be seen early in the disease but is of limited diagnostic value, as it occurs in many other conditions associated with a hyperdynamic circulation including normal pregnancy, as well as being found in some normal people. Spider telangiectasias occur and comprise a central arteriole (which occasionally raises the skin surface), from which small vessels radiate. They vary in

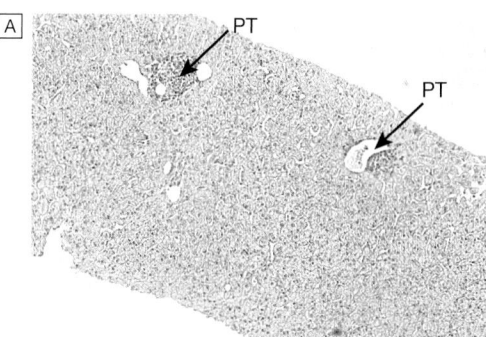

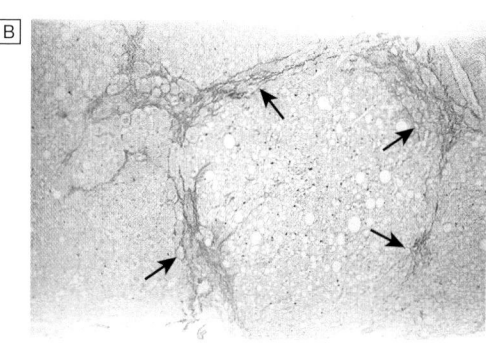

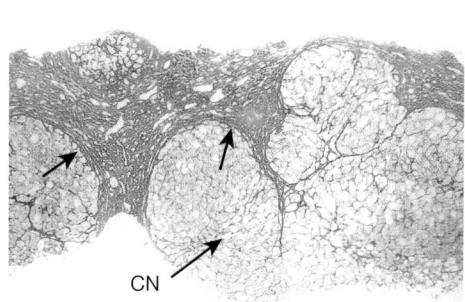

Fig. 23.25 Histological features in normal liver, hepatic fibrosis and cirrhosis. A Normal liver. Columns of hepatocytes 1–2 cells thick radiate from the portal tracts (PT) to the central veins. The portal tract contains a normal intralobular bile duct branch of the hepatic artery and portal venous radical. B Bridging fibrosis (stained pink, arrows) spreading out around the hepatic vein and single liver cells (pericellular), and linking adjacent portal tracts and hepatic veins. C A cirrhotic liver. The liver architecture is disrupted. The normal arrangement of portal tracts and hepatic veins is now lost and nodules of proliferating hepatocytes are broken up by strands of pink/orange-staining fibrous tissue (arrows) forming cirrhotic nodules (CN).

size from 1 to 2 mm in diameter, are usually found only above the nipples, and can occur early in the disease. One or two small spider telangiectasias can be found in about 2% of healthy people and can occur transiently in greater numbers in the third trimester of pregnancy, but otherwise they are a strong indicator of liver disease. Florid spider telangiectasia, gynaecomastia and parotid enlargement are most common in alcoholic cirrhosis. Pigmentation is most striking in haemochromatosis and in any cirrhosis associated with prolonged cholestasis. Pulmonary arteriovenous shunts also develop, leading to hypoxaemia and eventually to central cyanosis, but this is a late feature.

23

23.27 Clinical features of hepatic cirrhosis

- Hepatomegaly (although liver may also be small)
- Jaundice
- Ascites
- Circulatory changes
  Spider telangiectasia, palmar erythema, cyanosis
- Endocrine changes
  Loss of libido, hair loss
  Men: gynaecomastia, testicular atrophy, impotence
  Women: breast atrophy, irregular menses, amenorrhoea
- Haemorrhagic tendency
  Bruises, purpura, epistaxis
- Portal hypertension
  Splenomegaly, collateral vessels, variceal bleeding
- Hepatic (portosystemic) encephalopathy
- Other features
  Pigmentation, digital clubbing, Dupuytren's contracture

Endocrine changes are noticed more readily in men, who show loss of male hair distribution and testicular atrophy. Gynaecomastia is common and can be due to drugs such as spironolactone. Easy bruising becomes more frequent as cirrhosis advances. Epistaxis is common and sometimes severe; it can mimic upper gastrointestinal bleeding if the blood is swallowed.

Splenomegaly and collateral vessel formation are features of portal hypertension, which occurs in more advanced disease (see below). Ascites is due to a combination of liver failure and portal hypertension (p. 945), and signifies advanced disease. Evidence of hepatic encephalopathy also becomes increasingly common with advancing disease. Non-specific features of chronic liver disease include clubbing of the fingers and toes. Dupuytren's contracture is traditionally regarded as a complication of cirrhosis, but the evidence for this is weak. Chronic liver failure develops when the metabolic capacity of the liver is exceeded. It is characterised by the presence of encephalopathy and/or ascites. The term 'hepatic decompensation' or 'decompensated liver disease' is often used when chronic liver failure occurs.

A variety of clinical and laboratory features may be present (Box 23.28), in addition to encephalopathy and ascites; these include peripheral oedema, renal failure, jaundice, and hypoalbuminaemia and coagulation abnormalities due to defective protein synthesis.

Management

This includes treatment of the underlying cause, maintenance of nutrition and treatment of complications,

23.28 Features of chronic liver failure

- Worsening synthetic liver function
  Prolonged prothrombin time
  Low albumin
- Jaundice
- Portal hypertension
- Variceal bleeding
- Hepatic encephalopathy
- Ascites
  Spontaneous bacterial peritonitis
  Hepatorenal failure

which are discussed in detail below. Chronic liver failure due to cirrhosis can also be treated by orthotopic liver transplantation, which currently accounts for about three-quarters of all liver transplant operations (p. 976).

Ascites

Management of ascites is discussed on page 937. In patients with cirrhosis, ascites may be complicated by renal failure and also by spontaneous infections which are often precipitated by a variceal bleed. Blood in the gastrointestinal tract appears to affect permeability of the gastrointestinal tract to bacteria. Both of these complications have adverse prognostic significance and may prompt referral for transplantation.

Hepatorenal syndrome

This occurs in 10% of patients with advanced cirrhosis complicated by ascites. There are two clinical types; both are mediated by renal vasoconstriction due to underfilling of the arterial circulation.

- *Type 1 hepatorenal syndrome* is characterised by progressive oliguria, a rapid rise of the serum creatinine and a very poor prognosis (without treatment, median survival is less than 1 month). There is usually no proteinuria, a urine sodium excretion below 10 mmol/day and a urine/plasma osmolarity ratio of > 1.5. Other non-functional causes of renal failure must be excluded before the diagnosis is made. Treatment consists of albumin infusions in combination with terlipressin and is effective in about two-thirds of patients. Haemodialysis should not be used routinely because it does not improve the outcome. Patients who survive should be considered for liver transplantation.
- *Type 2 hepatorenal syndrome* usually occurs in patients with refractory ascites, is characterised by a moderate and stable increase in serum creatinine, and has a better prognosis.

Varices and hepatocellular carcinoma surveillance

Once the diagnosis of cirrhosis is made, endoscopy should be performed to screen for oesophageal varices (p. 947) and ultrasound performed to check for hepatocellular carcinoma (p. 968).

Prognosis

The overall prognosis in cirrhosis is poor. Many patients present with advanced disease and/or serious complications that carry a high mortality. Overall, only 25% of patients survive 5 years from diagnosis but, where liver function is good, 50% survive for 5 years and 25% for up to 10 years. The prognosis is more favourable when the underlying cause of the cirrhosis can be corrected, as in alcohol misuse, haemochromatosis and Wilson's disease.

Laboratory tests give only a rough guide to prognosis in individual patients. Deteriorating liver function, as evidenced by jaundice, ascites or encephalopathy, indicates a poor prognosis unless a treatable cause such as infection is found. Increasing bilirubin, falling albumin (or an albumin concentration < 30 g/L), marked hyponatraemia (< 120 mmol/L) not due to diuretic therapy, and a prolonged prothrombin time are all bad prognostic features (Boxes 23.29 and 23.30). The

23.29 Child–Pugh classification of prognosis in cirrhosis

Score	1	2	3
Encephalopathy	None	Mild	Marked
Bilirubin (μmol/L)*			
PBC/sclerosing cholangitis	< 68	68–170	> 170
Other causes of cirrhosis	< 34	34–50	> 50
Albumin (g/L)	> 35	28–35	< 28
Prothrombin time (seconds prolonged)	< 4	4–6	> 6
Ascites	None	Mild	Marked

Add the individual scores: < 7 = Child's A, 7–9 = Child's B, > 9 = Child's C

*To convert bilirubin in μmol/L to mg/dL, divide by 17.

23.30 Survival in cirrhosis

Child–Pugh grade	Survival (%) 1 year	5 years	10 years	Hepatic deaths (%)
A	82	45	25	43
B	62	20	7	72
C	42	20	0	85

Child–Pugh score and, more recently, the MELD (Model for End-stage Liver Disease) score can be used to assess prognosis. The MELD is more difficult to calculate at the bedside but, unlike the Child–Pugh score, includes renal function; if this is impaired, it is known to be a poor prognostic feature in end-stage liver disease (Box 23.31). Although these scores give a guide to prognosis, the course of cirrhosis can be unpredictable, as unforeseen complications such as variceal bleeding may unexpectedly lead to death.

23.31 1-year survival rate depending on MELD score

MELD score	1-year survival (%) No complications	Complications*
< 9	97	90
10–19	90	85
20–29	70	65
30–39	70	50

MELD from SI units

$10 \times (0.378[\ln \text{serum bilirubin } (\mu mol/L) + 1.12[\ln \text{INR}] + 0.957[\ln \text{serum creatinine } (\mu mol/L)] + 0.643)$

MELD from non-SI units

$3.8 [\ln \text{serum bilirubin } (mg/dL)] + 11.2 [\ln \text{INR}] + 9.3 [\ln \text{serum creatinine } (mg/dL)] + 6.4$

ln = natural log. To calculate online, go to www.unos.org/resources/meldPeldCalculator.asp.

*Complications are the presence of ascites, encephalopathy or variceal bleeding.

PORTAL HYPERTENSION

Portal hypertension is an invariable complication of cirrhosis but also can occur as the result of other causes. It is defined as a portal venous pressure above 7 mmHg; however, clinical features or complications do not usually develop until the portal venous pressure exceeds 12 mmHg. Increased vascular resistance is the cause in most cases, but the underlying causes are classified in accordance with the main sites of obstruction to blood flow in the portal venous system (Fig. 23.26). Extrahepatic portal vein obstruction is the usual source of portal hypertension in childhood and adolescence, while cirrhosis causes at least 90% of cases of portal hypertension in adults in developed countries. Schistosomiasis is the most common cause of portal hypertension world-wide but is infrequent outside endemic areas (e.g. Egypt; p. 370).

Clinical features

The clinical features of portal hypertension result principally from portal venous congestion and collateral vessel formation (Box 23.32). Splenomegaly is a cardinal finding, and a diagnosis of portal hypertension is unusual when splenomegaly cannot be detected clinically or by ultrasonography. The spleen is rarely enlarged more than 5 cm below the left costal margin in adults, but more marked splenomegaly can occur in childhood and adolescence. Collateral vessels may be visible on the anterior abdominal wall and occasionally several radiate from the umbilicus to form a caput medusae. Rarely, a large umbilical collateral vessel has a blood flow sufficient to give a venous hum on auscultation (Cruveilhier–Baumgarten syndrome). The most important collateral vessel formation occurs in the oesophagus and stomach, and this can be a source of severe bleeding. Rectal varices also cause bleeding and are often mistaken for haemorrhoids, which are no more common in portal hypertension than in the general population. Fetor hepaticus results from portosystemic shunting of blood, which allows mercaptans to pass directly to the lungs.

Ascites can occur as a result of portal hypertension when intrahepatic sinusoidal distension is present, as occurs with post-hepatic portal hypertension (hepatic outflow obstruction, p. 973) or cirrhosis. Pre-sinusoidal portal hypertension does not cause ascites, as there is no distension of the sinusoids.

The most important clinical feature of portal hypertension is variceal bleeding, which commonly arises from oesophageal varices located within 3–5 cm of the oesophagogastric junction, or from gastric varices. The size of the varices, endoscopic variceal features such as red spots and red stripes, high portal pressure and liver failure are all general factors that predispose to bleeding. Drugs capable of causing mucosal erosion, such as salicylates and other non-steroidal anti-inflammatory drugs (NSAIDs), can also precipitate bleeding. Variceal bleeding is often severe, and recurrent bleeding occurs if preventative treatment is not given. Bleeding from varices at other sites is comparatively uncommon but most often occurs from varices in the rectum or intestinal stomas.

Pathophysiology

Increased portal vascular resistance leads to a gradual reduction in the flow of portal blood to the liver and simultaneously to the development of collateral vessels,

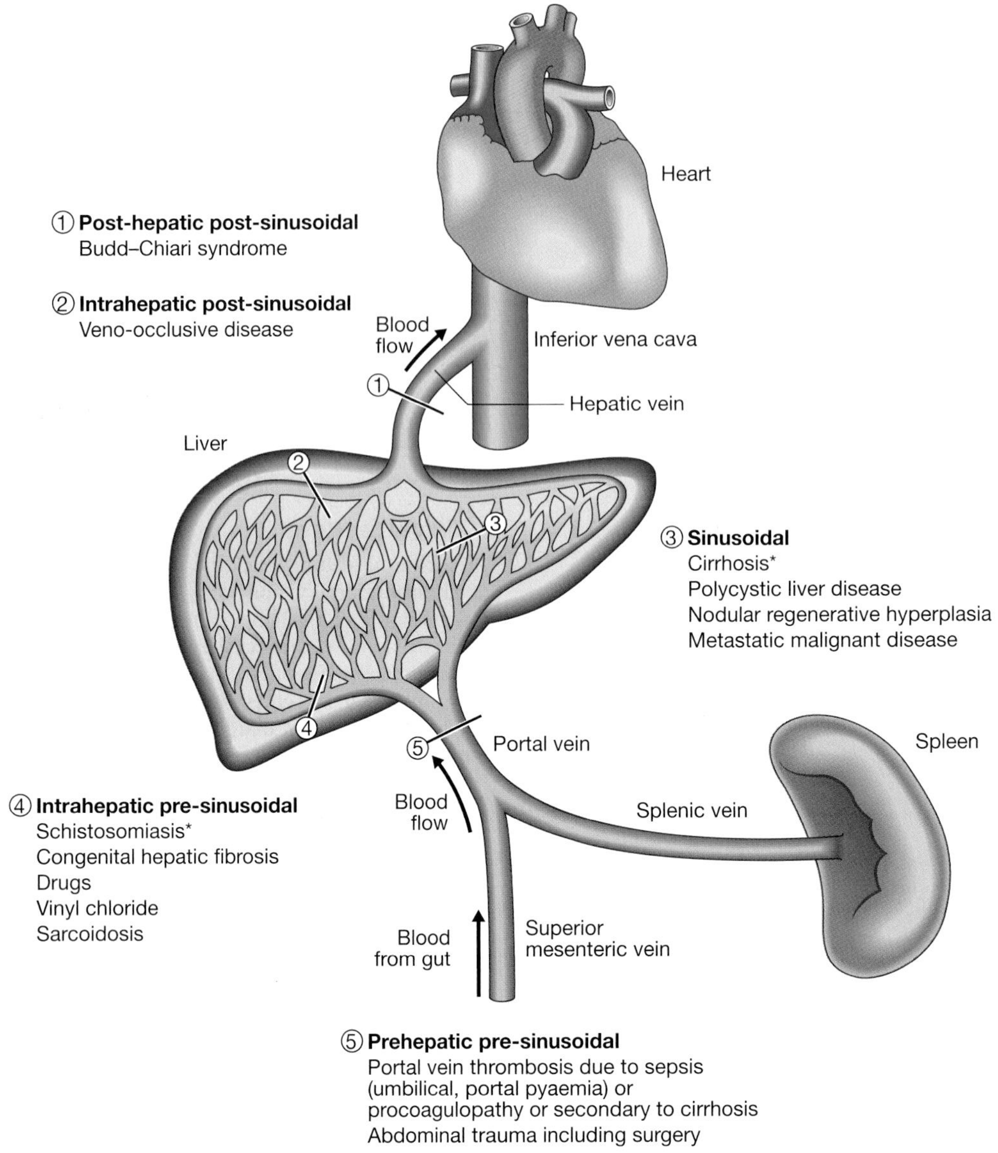

① **Post-hepatic post-sinusoidal**
Budd–Chiari syndrome

② **Intrahepatic post-sinusoidal**
Veno-occlusive disease

Blood flow

Heart

Inferior vena cava

Hepatic vein

Liver

③ **Sinusoidal**
Cirrhosis*
Polycystic liver disease
Nodular regenerative hyperplasia
Metastatic malignant disease

④ **Intrahepatic pre-sinusoidal**
Schistosomiasis*
Congenital hepatic fibrosis
Drugs
Vinyl chloride
Sarcoidosis

Blood flow

Portal vein

Spleen

Splenic vein

Blood from gut

Superior mesenteric vein

⑤ **Prehepatic pre-sinusoidal**
Portal vein thrombosis due to sepsis
(umbilical, portal pyaemia) or
procoagulopathy or secondary to cirrhosis
Abdominal trauma including surgery

Fig. 23.26 Classification of portal hypertension according to site of vascular obstruction. *Most common cause. Note that splenic vein occlusion can also follow pancreatitis leading to gastric varices.

23.32 Complications of portal hypertension

- Variceal bleeding: oesophageal, gastric, other (rare)
- Congestive gastropathy
- Hypersplenism
- Ascites*
- Iron deficiency anaemia
- Renal failure
- Hepatic encephalopathy

*Except in post-hepatic.

---

allowing portal blood to bypass the liver and enter the systemic circulation directly. Portosystemic shunting occurs, particularly in the gastrointestinal tract and especially the distal oesophagus, stomach and rectum, in the anterior abdominal wall, and in the renal, lumbar, ovarian and testicular vasculature. Stomal varices can also occur at the site of an ileostomy. Normally, virtually all the portal blood flows through the liver but, as collateral vessel formation progresses, more than half of the portal blood flow may be shunted directly to the systemic circulation. Increased portal flow contributes to portal hypertension but is not the dominant factor.

Investigations

The diagnosis is often made on clinical grounds. Portal venous pressure measurements are rarely needed for clinical assessment or routine management, but can be used to confirm portal hypertension and to differentiate sinusoidal and pre-sinusoidal forms. Pressure measurements are usually made by using a balloon catheter inserted using the transjugular route (via the inferior vena cava into a hepatic vein and then hepatic venule) to measure the wedged hepatic venous pressure (WHVP). This is used as an indirect measurement of portal vein pressure. Thrombocytopenia is common due to hypersplenism, and platelet counts are usually in the region of $100 \times 10^9/\text{L}$; values below $50 \times 10^9/\text{L}$ are uncommon. Leucopenia occurs occasionally but anaemia is seldom attributed directly to hypersplenism; if anaemia is found, a source of bleeding should be sought.

The most useful investigation is endoscopic examination of the upper gastrointestinal tract to determine whether gastro-oesophageal varices are present (see Fig. 23.20, p. 940). This establishes the presence of portal hypertension but not its cause. Ultrasonography often shows features of portal hypertension, such as splenomegaly and collateral vessels, and can sometimes indicate the cause, such as liver disease or portal vein thrombosis. CT and MRI angiography can identify the extent of portal vein clot and are used to identify hepatic vein patency.

Management

Management of variceal bleeding

This is discussed on page 940.

Primary prevention of variceal bleeding

Propranolol (80–160 mg/day) or nadolol is effective in reducing portal venous pressure. Administration of these drugs at doses which reduce the heart rate by 25% has been shown to be effective in the primary prevention of variceal bleeding, which is the most important complication of portal hypertension (Box 23.33). The efficacy of β-adrenoceptor antagonists (β-blockers) in primary prevention is similar to that of prophylactic banding.

Secondary prevention of variceal bleeding

Beta-blockers have also been used as a secondary measure to prevent recurrent variceal bleeding following banding.

EBM **23.33 Primary prevention of variceal bleeding**

'In patients with cirrhosis, treatment with propranolol reduces variceal bleeding by 47% (NNT_B 10), death from bleeding by 45% (NNT_B 25) and overall mortality by 22% (NNT_B 16).'

- Hayes PC, et al. Lancet 1990; 336:153–156.

For further information: www.bsg.org.uk

Congestive gastropathy

Long-standing portal hypertension causes chronic gastric congestion recognisable at endoscopy as multiple areas of punctate erythema ('snake skin gastropathy'). Rarely, similar lesions occur more distally in the gastrointestinal tract. These areas may become eroded, causing bleeding from multiple sites. Acute bleeding can occur, but repeated minor bleeding causing iron-deficiency anaemia is more common. Anaemia may be prevented by oral iron supplements but repeated blood transfusions can become necessary. Reduction of the portal pressure using propranolol 80–160 mg/day is the best initial treatment. If this is ineffective, a TIPSS procedure can be undertaken.

INFECTIONS AND THE LIVER

Viral hepatitis

Viral hepatitis is a common cause of jaundice and must be considered in anyone presenting with hepatitic liver blood tests (high transaminases). The causes are listed in Box 23.34.

All these viruses cause illnesses with similar clinical and pathological features and which are frequently anicteric or even asymptomatic. They differ in their tendency to cause acute and chronic infections. The features of the major hepatitis viruses are shown in Box 23.35.

23.34 Causes of viral hepatitis

Common

- Hepatitis A
- Hepatitis B ± hepatitis D
- Hepatitis C
- Hepatitis E

Less common

- Cytomegalovirus
- Epstein–Barr virus

Rare

- Herpes simplex
- Yellow fever

23.35 Features of the main hepatitis viruses

	Hepatitis A	Hepatitis B	Hepatitis C	Hepatitis D	Hepatitis E
Virus					
Group	Enterovirus	Hepadna virus	Flavivirus	Incomplete virus	Calicivirus
Nucleic acid	RNA	DNA	RNA	RNA	RNA
Size (diameter)	27 nm	42 nm	30–38 nm	35 nm	27 nm
Incubation					
(weeks)	2–4	4–20	2–26	6–9	3–8
Spread					
Faeces	Yes	No	No	No	Yes
Blood	Uncommon	Yes	Yes	Yes	No
Saliva	Yes	Yes	Yes	Unknown	Unknown
Sexual	Uncommon	Yes	Uncommon	Yes	Unknown
Vertical	No	Yes	Uncommon	Yes	No
Chronic infection	No	Yes	Yes	Yes	No
Prevention					
Active	Vaccine	Vaccine	No	Prevented by	No
Passive	Immune serum globulin	Hyperimmune serum globulin	No	hepatitis B vaccination	No

Note All body fluids are potentially infectious, although some (e.g. urine) are less infectious than others.

23

23

Clinical features of acute infection

A non-specific prodromal illness characterised by headache, myalgia, arthralgia, nausea and anorexia usually precedes the development of jaundice by a few days to 2 weeks. Vomiting and diarrhoea may follow, and abdominal discomfort is common. Dark urine and pale stools may precede jaundice. There are usually few physical signs. The liver is often tender but only minimally enlarged. Occasionally, mild splenomegaly and cervical lymphadenopathy are seen. These are more frequent in children or those with Epstein–Barr virus infection.

Jaundice may be mild and the diagnosis may be suspected only after finding abnormal liver blood tests in the setting of non-specific symptoms. Symptoms rarely last longer than 3–6 weeks. Complications may occur, as listed in Box 23.36, but these are rare.

23.36 Complications of acute viral hepatitis

- Acute liver failure
- Cholestatic hepatitis (hepatitis A)
- Aplastic anaemia
- Chronic liver disease and cirrhosis (hepatitis B and C)
- Relapsing hepatitis

Investigations

A hepatitic pattern of LFTs develops, with serum transaminases typically between 200 and 2000 U/L. The plasma bilirubin reflects the degree of liver damage. The ALP rarely exceeds twice the upper limit of normal. Prolongation of the prothrombin time indicates the severity of the hepatitis but, except in rare cases of acute liver failure, rarely exceeds 25 seconds. The white cell count is usually normal with a relative lymphocytosis. Serological tests confirm the aetiology of the infection.

Management

Most individuals do not need hospital care. Drugs such as sedatives and narcotics, which are metabolised in the liver, should be avoided. No specific dietary modifications are needed. Alcohol should be avoided during the acute illness. Elective surgery should be avoided in cases of acute viral hepatitis, as there is a risk of post-operative liver failure.

Liver transplantation is very rarely indicated for acute viral hepatitis complicated by liver failure, but is commonly performed for complications of cirrhosis resulting from chronic hepatitis B and C infection.

Hepatitis A

The hepatitis A virus (HAV) belongs to the picornavirus group of enteroviruses. HAV is highly infectious and is spread by the faecal–oral route. Infected individuals, who may be asymptomatic, excrete the virus in faeces for about 2–3 weeks before the onset of symptoms and then for a further 2 weeks or so. Infection is common in children but often asymptomatic, and so up to 30% of adults will have serological evidence of past infection but give no history of jaundice. Infection is also more common in areas of overcrowding and poor sanitation. In occasional outbreaks water and shellfish have been the vehicles of transmission. In contrast to hepatitis B, a chronic carrier state does not occur.

Investigations

Only one HAV antigen has been found; individuals infected with HAV make an antibody to this antigen (anti-HAV). Anti-HAV is important in diagnosis, as HAV is only present in the blood transiently during the incubation period. Excretion in the stools occurs for only 7–14 days after the onset of the clinical illness and the virus cannot be grown readily. Anti-HAV of the IgM type, indicating a primary immune response, is already present in the blood at the onset of the clinical illness and is diagnostic of an acute HAV infection. Titres of this antibody fall to low levels within about 3 months of recovery. Anti-HAV of the IgG type is of no diagnostic value as HAV infection is common and this antibody persists for years after infection, but it can be used as a marker of previous HAV infection. Its presence indicates immunity to HAV.

Management

Infection in the community is best prevented by improving social conditions, especially overcrowding and poor sanitation. Individuals can be given substantial protection from infection by active immunisation with an inactivated virus vaccine.

Immunisation should be considered for individuals with chronic hepatitis B or C infections. Immediate protection can be provided by immune serum globulin if this is given soon after exposure to the virus. The protective effect of immune serum globulin is attributed to its anti-HAV content. Immunisation should be considered for those at particular risk, such as close contacts, the elderly, those with other major disease and perhaps pregnant women.

Immune serum globulin can be effective in an outbreak of hepatitis, in a school or nursery, as injection of those at risk prevents secondary spread to families. People travelling to endemic areas are best protected by vaccination.

Acute liver failure is rare in hepatitis A (0.1%) and chronic infection does not occur. However, HAV infection in patients with chronic liver disease may cause serious or life-threatening disease. In adults a cholestatic phase with elevated ALP levels may complicate infection.

Hepatitis B

The hepatitis B virus consists of a core containing DNA and a DNA polymerase enzyme needed for virus replication. The core of the virus is surrounded by surface protein (Fig. 23.27). The virus, also called a Dane particle, and an excess of its surface protein (known as hepatitis B surface antigen) circulate in the blood. Humans are the only source of infection.

Hepatitis B infection affects 300 million people and is one of the most common causes of chronic liver disease and hepatocellular carcinoma world-wide.

Hepatitis B may cause an acute viral hepatitis; however, the acute infection is often asymptomatic, particularly when acquired at birth. Many individuals with chronic hepatitis B are also asymptomatic. Chronic hepatitis, associated with elevated serum transaminases, may occur and can lead to cirrhosis, usually after decades of infection (Fig. 23.28).

The risk of progression to chronic liver disease depends on the source of infection (Box 23.37). Vertical transmission from mother to child in the perinatal period

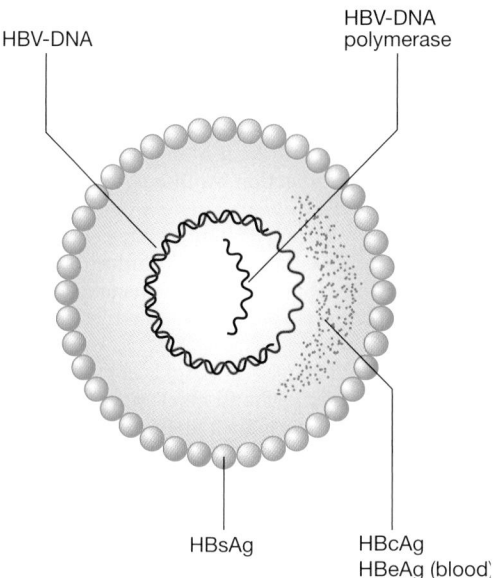

HBV-DNA

HBV-DNA polymerase

HBsAg

HBcAg
HBeAg (blood)

Fig. 23.27 Schematic diagram of hepatitis B virus. Hepatitis B surface antigen (HBsAg) is a protein which makes up part of the viral envelope. Hepatitis B core antigen (HBcAg) is a protein which makes up the capsid or core part of the virus (found in the liver but not in blood). Hepatitis B e antigen (HBeAg) is part of the HBcAg which can be found in the blood and indicates infectivity.

23.37 Source of hepatitis B infection and risk of chronic infection
Horizontal transmission (10%)
• Injection drug use
• Infected unscreened blood products
• Tattoos/acupuncture needles
• Sexual (homosexual and heterosexual)
• Close living quarters/playground play as a toddler (may contribute to high rate of horizontal transmission in Africa)
Vertical transmission (90%)
• HBsAg-positive mother

is the most common cause of infection world-wide and carries the highest risk.

In this setting, adaptive immune responses to HBV may be absent initially, with apparent immunological tolerance. Several mechanisms contribute towards this.
- Firstly, the introduction of antigen in the neonatal period is tolerogenic.
- Secondly, the presentation of such antigen within the liver, as described above, promotes tolerance; this is particularly evident in the absence of a significant innate or inflammatory response.
- Finally, very high loads of antigen may lead to so-called 'exhaustion' of cellular immune responses.

23

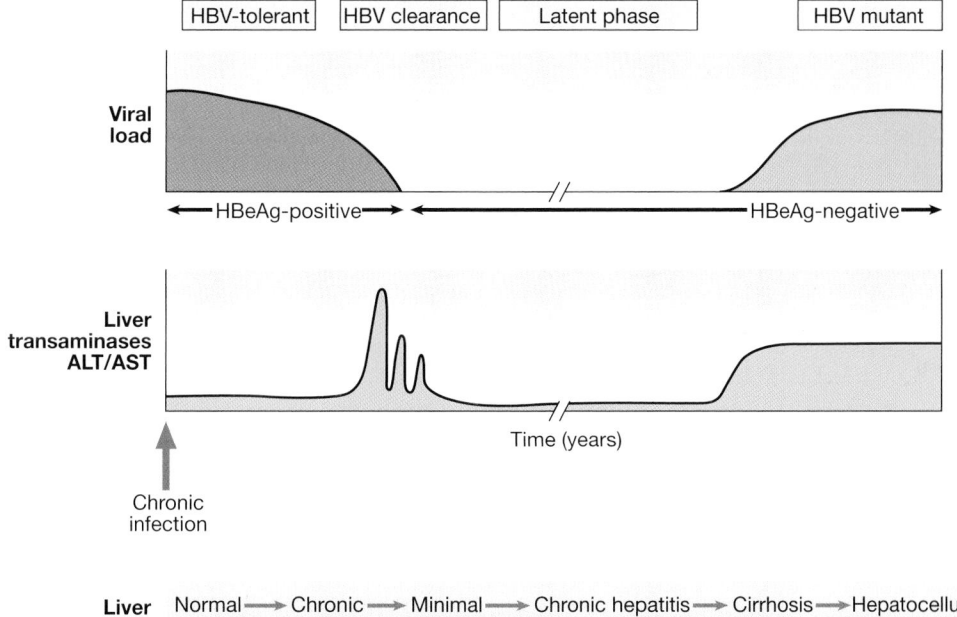

Fig. 23.28 Natural history of chronic hepatitis B infection. There is an initial immunotolerant phase with high levels of virus and normal liver biochemistry. An immunological response to the virus then occurs, with elevation in serum transaminases which causes liver damage: chronic hepatitis. If this response is sustained over many years and viral clearance does not occur promptly, chronic hepatitis may result in cirrhosis. In individuals where the immunological response is successful, viral load falls, HBe antibody develops and there is no further liver damage. Some individuals may subsequently develop HBV-DNA mutants, which escape from immune regulation, and viral load again rises with further chronic hepatitis. Mutations in the core protein result in the virus's inability to secrete HBe antigen despite high levels of viral replication; such individuals have HBeAg-negative chronic hepatitis. (ALT = alanine aminotransferase; AST = aspartate aminotransferase)

However, the state of tolerance is not permanent and may be reversed as a result of therapy, or through spontaneous changes in innate responses such as interferon-alpha and NK cells, accompanied by host-mediated immunopathology.

Investigations

Serology

HBV contains several antigens to which infected persons can make immune responses (Fig. 23.29); these antigens and their antibodies are important in identifying HBV infection (Box 23.38).

- *The hepatitis B surface antigen* (HBsAg) is an indicator of active infection, and a negative test for HBsAg makes HBV infection very unlikely. In acute liver failure from hepatitis B the liver damage is mediated by viral clearance and so HBsAg is negative, with evidence of recent infection shown by the presence of hepatitis B core IgM. HBsAg appears in the

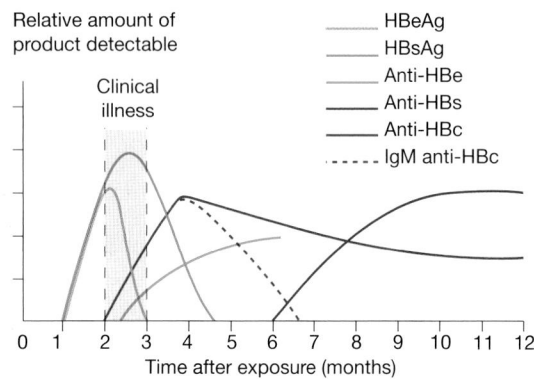

Fig. 23.29 Serological responses to hepatitis B virus infection. (HBsAg = hepatitis B surface antigen; anti-HBs = antibody to HBsAg; HBeAg = hepatitis B e antigen; anti-HBe = antibody to HBeAg; anti-HBc = antibody to hepatitis B core antigen)

blood late in the incubation period but before the prodromal phase of acute type B hepatitis; it may be present for a few days only, disappearing even before jaundice has developed, but usually lasts for 3–4 weeks and can persist for up to 5 months. The persistence of HBsAg for longer than 6 months indicates chronic infection. Antibody to HBsAg (anti-HBs) usually appears after about 3–6 months and persists for many years or perhaps permanently. Anti-HBs implies either a previous infection, in which case anti-HBc (see below) is usually also present, or previous vaccination, in which case anti-HBc is not present.

- *The hepatitis B core antigen* (HBcAg) is not found in the blood, but antibody to it (anti-HBc) appears early in the illness and rapidly reaches a high titre, which subsides gradually but then persists. Anti-HBc is initially of IgM type with IgG antibody appearing later. Anti-HBc (IgM) can sometimes reveal an acute HBV infection when the HBsAg has disappeared and before anti-HBs has developed (see Fig. 23.29 and Box 23.38).

- *The hepatitis B e antigen* (HBeAg) is an indicator of viral replication. In acute hepatitis B it may appear only transiently at the outset of the illness; its appearance is followed by the production of antibody (anti-HBe). The HBeAg reflects active replication of the virus in the liver.

Chronic HBV infection (see below) is marked by the presence of HBsAg and anti-HBc (IgG) in the blood. Usually, HBeAg or anti-HBe is also present; HBeAg indicates continued active replication of the virus in the liver. Although the presence of anti-HBe usually implies low viral replication, the exception is HBeAb-positive replicating chronic hepatitis B (also called 'pre-core mutant' infection and discussed below), in which high levels of serum HBV-DNA are seen, despite negative HBeAg.

Viral load

HBV-DNA can be measured by polymerase chain reaction (PCR) in the blood. Viral loads are usually in excess of 10^5 copies/mL in the presence of active viral replication, as indicated by the presence of e antigen. In contrast, in those with low viral replication, HBsAg- and anti-HBe-positive, viral loads are less than 10^5 copies/mL. The exception is in patients who have a mutation in the pre-core protein, which means they cannot secrete e antigen into serum (Fig. 23.30). Such individuals will be anti-HBe-positive but have a high viral load and often evidence of chronic hepatitis. These mutations are common in the Far East and those patients affected are classified as having e antigen-negative chronic hepatitis. They respond differently to antiviral drugs from those with classical e antigen-positive chronic hepatitis.

Measurement of viral load is important in monitoring antiviral therapy and identifying patients with pre-core mutants. Specific HBV genotypes can also be identified using PCR. Genotypes B and C appear to have more aggressive disease that responds less well to interferon.

Management

Acute hepatitis B

Treatment is supportive with monitoring for acute liver failure, which occurs in less than 1% of cases. There is no definitive evidence that antiviral therapy (e.g. lamivudine) reduces the severity or duration of acute hepatitis B.

23.38 How to interpret the main investigations used in the serological diagnosis of hepatitis B virus infection				
		Anti-HBc		
Interpretation	**HBsAg**	**IgM**	**IgG**	**Anti-HBs**
Incubation period	+	+	−	−
Acute hepatitis				
Early	+	+	−	−
Established	+	+	+	−
Established (occasional)	−	+	+	−
Convalescence				
(3–6 months)	−	±	+	±
(6–9 months)	−	−	+	+
Post-infection				
> 1 year	−	−	+	+
Uncertain	−	−	+	−
Chronic infection				
Usual	+	−	+	−
Occasional	−	−	+	−
Immunisation without infection	−	−	−	+

+ Positive; − negative; ± present at low titre or absent.

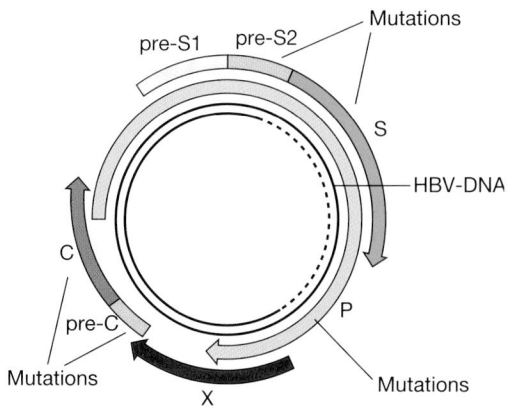

Fig. 23.30 The site of HBV-DNA mutations. HBV-DNA encodes four proteins: a DNA polymerase needed for viral replication (P), a surface protein (S), a core protein (C) and an X protein. The pre-C and C regions encode a core protein and an e antigen. Although mutations in the hepatitis B virus are frequent, certain mutations have important clinical consequences. Pre-C encodes a signal sequence needed for the C protein to be secreted from the liver cell into serum as e antigen. A mutation in the pre-core region leads to a failure of secretion of e antigen into serum, and so individuals have high levels of viral production but no detectable e antigen in the serum. Mutations can also occur in the surface protein and may lead to the failure of vaccination to prevent infection since surface antibodies are produced against the native S protein. Mutations also occur in the DNA polymerase during antiviral treatment with lamivudine.

Full recovery occurs in 90–95% of adults following acute HBV infection. The remaining 5–10% develop a chronic infection which usually continues for life, although later recovery occasionally occurs. Infection passing from mother to child at birth leads to chronic infection in the child in 90% of cases and recovery is rare. Chronic infection is also common in immunodeficient individuals, such as those with Down's syndrome or HIV infection. Fulminant liver failure due to acute hepatitis B occurs in less than 1% of cases.

Recovery from acute HBV infection occurs within 6 months and is characterised by the appearance of antibody to viral antigens. Persistence of HBeAg beyond this time indicates chronic infection. Combined HBV and HDV infection causes more aggressive disease.

Chronic hepatitis B

Treatments are still limited, as no drug is able to eradicate hepatitis B infection completely (i.e. render the patient HBsAg-negative). The goals of treatment are HBeAg seroconversion, reduction in HBV-DNA and normalisation of the LFTs. The indication for treatment is a high viral load in the presence of active hepatitis, as demonstrated by elevated serum transaminases and/or histological evidence of inflammation and fibrosis. The oral antiviral agents are more effective in reducing viral loads in patients with e antigen-negative chronic hepatitis B than in those with e antigen-positive chronic hepatitis B, as the pre-treatment viral loads are lower.

Most patients with chronic hepatitis B are asymptomatic and develop complications such as cirrhosis and hepatocellular carcinoma only after many years (see Fig. 23.28). Cirrhosis develops in 15–20% of patients with chronic HBV over 5–20 years. This proportion is higher in those who are e antigen-positive.

Interferon-alfa. This is most effective in selected patients with a low viral load and serum transaminases greater than twice the upper limit of normal, in whom it acts by augmenting a native immune response. In HBeAg-positive chronic hepatitis, 33% lose e antigen after 4–6 months of treatment, compared to 12% of controls. Response rates are lower in HBeAg-negative chronic hepatitis, even when patients are given longer courses of treatment. Interferon is contraindicated in the presence of cirrhosis, as it may cause a rise in serum transaminases and precipitate liver failure. Longer-acting pegylated interferons which can be given once weekly have been evaluated in both HBeAg-positive and HBeAg-negative chronic hepatitis (Box 23.39). Other antiviral therapies are required because many patients with chronic hepatitis B have high levels of viraemia and/or low transaminase levels, and are therefore not candidates for interferon. Side-effects are common and include fatigue, depression, irritability, bone marrow suppression and thyroid disease. The drug appears to be better tolerated in patients with hepatitis B compared to those with hepatitis C.

Lamivudine. This is a nucleoside analogue which inhibits DNA polymerase and suppresses HBV-DNA levels. It is effective in improving liver function in patients with decompensated cirrhosis and may prevent the need for transplantation. Long-term therapy is complicated by the development of HBV-DNA polymerase mutants (known as 'YMDD variants'), which may occur after 9 months of treatment and is characterised by a rise in viral load during treatment. These viral mutants are less hepatotoxic than native virus. Elevations in transaminases occur when lamivudine is stopped if mutant virus is present, as native virus replaces mutant virus. In the event of mutations occurring, other antiviral agents can be added (add-on therapy) but are less effective than when used in lamivudine-naïve patients.

Adefovir. This is a nucleotide analogue that is phosphorylated to yield active drug which inhibits HBV-DNA polymerase. It reduces HBV-DNA levels by 3–4 logs, enhances the frequency of HBeAg seroconversion and leads to histological improvement, but is contraindicated in renal failure. The HBV-DNA mutants develop at a lower rate than with lamivudine; 2% are identified after 2 years of treatment but this figure increases to 18% after 3 years. Relapse occurs on stopping treatment, and the optimum length of treatment remains unknown. Adefovir is effective in suppressing most of the lamivudine-induced DNA polymerase mutant viruses.

23

> **EBM** **23.39 Pegylated interferons in chronic hepatitis B infection**
>
> 'In HBeAg-positive chronic hepatitis, treatment with pegylated interferon for 6 months eliminates HBeAg in 35%, and normalises liver biochemistry in 25% of patients. In HBeAg-negative chronic hepatitis, treatment with pegylated interferon for 12 months leads to normal liver biochemistry in 60%, and sustained suppression of hepatitis B virus load below 400 copies/mL in 20% of patients.'
>
> • Cooksley WG, et al. J Viral Hep 2003; 10:298–302.
> • Marcellin P. N Engl J Med 2004; 351:1206–1217.
>
> For further information: www.aasld.org
>
> www.nice.org.uk

EBM **23.40 Entecavir and telbivudine in chronic hepatitis B infection**

'In HBeAg-positive patients, 48 weeks of treatment with entecavir suppresses HBV-DNA levels in 67%, compared to 36% with lamivudine and 60% with telbivudine. Anti-HBe seroconversion occurs in 21% following a year of entecavir, lamivudine or telbivudine. In HBeAg-negative chronic hepatitis, HBV-DNA negativity is achieved in 90% with entecavir, compared to 72% with lamivudine and 88% with telbivudine at 1 year. Treatment also improves histology and liver biochemistry.'

• Chang T-T. N Engl J Med 2006; 354:1001–1010.
• Lai C-L. N Engl J Med 2007; 357:2576–2588.
• Lai C-L. N Engl J Med 2006; 354:1011–1020.

For further information: www.aasld.org

Entecavir and telbivudine. These drugs are more effective than lamivudine and adefovir in reducing viral load in HBeAg-positive and HBeAg-negative chronic hepatitis (Box 23.40). Antiviral resistance mutations occur in only 1% after 3 years of entecavir drug exposure. Entecavir, unlike telbivudine, may have anti-HIV action and is contraindicated in HIV patients who are not on antiretroviral therapy.

Tenofovir and other drugs. Other drugs which also have action against chronic hepatitis B include tenofovir and emcitabine; these also have anti-HIV efficacy. Tenofovir has recently been shown to be superior to adefovir in the treatment of chronic hepatitis B (Box 23.41). The role of combination antiviral therapy, as used in HIV infection, is still unclear.

Liver transplantation. Historically, liver transplantation was contraindicated in the presence of hepatitis B because infection often recurred in the graft. However, the use of post-liver transplant prophylaxis with lamivudine and hepatitis B immunoglobulins has reduced the reinfection rate to 10% and increased 5-year survival to 80%, making transplantation an acceptable treatment option in selected cases.

Prevention

Individuals are most infectious when markers of continuing viral replication, such as HBeAg, and high levels of HBV-DNA are present in the blood; they are least infectious when only anti-HBe is present with low levels of virus. HBV-DNA can be found in saliva, urine, semen and vaginal secretions. The virus is about ten times more infectious than hepatitis C, which in turn is about ten times more infectious than HIV.

A recombinant hepatitis B vaccine containing HBsAg is available (Engerix) and is capable of producing active

EBM **23.41 Tenofovir for chronic hepatitis B**

'Among patients with chronic HBV infection, tenofovir at a daily dose of 300 mg had superior antiviral efficacy with a similar safety profile as compared with adefovir 10 mg daily. In HBeAg-positive patients, tenofovir suppressed HBV DNA to < 400 copies/mL in 76% of patients, compared with 13% of those given adefovir (p < 0.001).

• Marcellin P, et al. NEJM 2008; 359:2442–2445.

immunisation in 95% of normal individuals. The vaccine gives a high degree of protection and should be offered to those at special risk of infection who are not already immune, as evidenced by anti-HBs in the blood (Box 23.42). The vaccine is ineffective in those already infected by HBV. Infection can also be prevented or minimised by the intramuscular injection of hyperimmune serum globulin prepared from blood containing anti-HBs. This should be given within 24 hours, or at most a week, of exposure to infected blood in circumstances likely to cause infection (e.g. needlestick injury, contamination of cuts or mucous membranes). Vaccine can be given together with hyperimmune globulin (active-passive immunisation).

Neonates born to hepatitis B-infected mothers should be immunised at birth and given immunoglobulin. Hepatitis B serology should then be checked at 12 months of age.

23.42 At-risk groups meriting hepatitis B vaccination in low endemic areas

• Parenteral drug users
• Men who have sex with men
• Close contacts of infected individuals
    Newborn of infected mothers
    Regular sexual partners
• Patients on chronic haemodialysis
• Patients with chronic liver disease
• Medical, nursing and laboratory personnel

Hepatitis D (Delta virus)

The hepatitis D virus (HDV) is an RNA-defective virus which has no independent existence; it requires HBV for replication and has the same sources and modes of spread. It can infect individuals simultaneously with HBV, or can superinfect those who are already chronic carriers of HBV. Simultaneous infections give rise to acute hepatitis, which is often severe but is limited by recovery from the HBV infection. Infections in individuals who are chronic carriers of HBV can cause acute hepatitis with spontaneous recovery, and occasionally simultaneous cessation of the chronic HBV infection occurs. Chronic infection with HBV and HDV can also occur, and this frequently causes rapidly progressive chronic hepatitis and eventually cirrhosis.

HDV has a world-wide distribution. It is endemic in parts of the Mediterranean basin, Africa and South America, where transmission is mainly by close personal contact and occasionally by vertical transmission from mothers who also carry HBV. In non-endemic areas, transmission is mainly a consequence of parenteral drug misuse.

Investigations

HDV contains a single antigen to which infected individuals make an antibody (anti-HDV). Delta antigen appears in the blood only transiently, and in practice diagnosis depends on detecting anti-HDV. Simultaneous infection with HBV and HDV followed by full recovery is associated with the appearance of low titres of anti-HDV of IgM type within a few days of the onset of the illness. This antibody generally disappears within 2 months but persists in a few patients. Superinfection of patients with chronic HBV infection leads to the production of high titres of anti-HDV, initially IgM and later IgG. Such patients may then develop chronic infection with both viruses, in which case anti-HDV titres plateau at high levels.

Management

Effective managemnt of hepatitis B effectively prevents hepatitis D.

Hepatitis C

This is caused by an RNA flavivirus. Acute symptomatic infection with hepatitis C is rare. Most individuals are unaware of when they became infected and are only identified when they develop chronic liver disease.

Eighty per cent of individuals exposed to the virus become chronically infected and late spontaneous viral clearance is rare.

Hepatitis C is the cause of what used to be known as 'non-A, non-B hepatitis', a syndrome of acute hepatitis often with jaundice seen after a transfusion of blood or blood products. Following the identification of the virus in 1990, blood donors are now screened for infection in many parts of the world. New cases of post-transfusion hepatitis C no longer occur in the UK.

Hepatitis C infection is usually now identified in asymptomatic individuals screened because they have risk factors for infection such as previous injection drug use (Box 23.43) or they have incidentally been found to have abnormal liver blood tests. Although most individuals remain asymptomatic until progression to cirrhosis occurs, fatigue can complicate chronic infection and appears to be unrelated to the degree of liver damage.

Investigations

Serology and virology

The HCV protein contains several antigens that give rise to antibodies in an infected person, and these are used in diagnosis. It may take 6–12 weeks for antibodies to appear in the blood following acute infection such as a needlestick injury. In these cases hepatitis C RNA can be identified in the blood as early as 2–4 weeks after infection. Active infection is confirmed by the presence of serum hepatitis C RNA in anyone who is antibody-positive. Anti-HCV antibodies persist in serum even after viral clearance, whether spontaneous or post-treatment.

Molecular analysis

There are six common viral genotypes whose distribution varies world-wide. Genotype has no effect on progression of liver disease but does affect response to treatment. Genotype 1 is most common in north-ern Europe and is less easy to eradicate with current treatments.

Liver function tests

LFTs may be normal or show fluctuating serum transaminases between 50 and 200 U/L. Jaundice is rare and only usually appears in end-stage cirrhosis.

Liver histology

Serum transaminase levels in hepatitis C are a poor predictor of the degree of liver fibrosis, and so a liver biopsy is often required to stage the degree of liver damage. Non-invasive methods of assessing liver fibrosis in hepatitis C infection remain an area of active research. The degree of inflammation and fibrosis can be scored histologically. The most common scoring system used in hepatitis C is the Metavir system, which scores fibrosis from 1 to 4, the latter equating to cirrhosis.

Management

The aim of treatment is to eradicate infection. The treatment of choice is pegylated α-interferon given weekly subcutaneously, together with oral ribavirin, a synthetic nucleotide analogue (Box 23.44). The main side-effect of ribavirin is haemolytic anaemia. Side-effects of interferon are significant and include flu-like symptoms, irritability, and depression which can affect quality of life. Virological relapse can occur in the first 3 months after stopping treatment, and cure is defined as loss of virus from serum 6 months after completing therapy (sustained virological response, or SVR). The length of treatment and efficacy depend on viral genotype (12 months' treatment for genotype 1 results in a 40% SVR, whereas 6 months' treatment for genotype 2/3 leads to an SVR in > 70%). Response to treatment is better in patients who have an early virological response, as defined by negativity of HCV-RNA in serum 1 month after starting therapy, and it may be possible to shorten the duration of therapy in this patient group. Protease inhibitors are currently in clinical trials; when given in combination with interferon and ribavirin, they appear to increase efficacy.

Liver transplantation should be considered when complications of cirrhosis occur, such as diuretic-resistant ascites. Unfortunately, hepatitis C almost always recurs in the transplanted liver and up to 15% of patients will develop cirrhosis in the liver graft within 5 years of transplantation.

There is no active or passive protection against HCV. Progression from chronic hepatitis to cirrhosis occurs over 20–40 years. Risk factors for progression include male gender, immunosuppression (such as co-infection with HIV) and heavy alcohol misuse. Not everyone with hepatitis C infection will necessarily develop cirrhosis, but approximately 20% do so within 20 years. Once cirrhosis

23.43 Risk factors for the acquisition of chronic hepatitis C infection

- Intravenous drug misuse (95% of new cases in the UK)
- Unscreened blood products
- Vertical transmission (3% risk)
- Needlestick injury (3% risk)
- Iatrogenic parenteral transmission, (i.e. contaminated vaccination needles)
- Sharing toothbrushes/razors

EBM 23.44 Treatment of hepatitis C

'The addition of ribavirin to pegylated α-interferon therapy improves the overall sustained virological response from 33% to 55%.'

- Manns MP, et al. Lancet 2001; 358:958–965.
- Hadziyannis SJ, et al. Ann Intern Med 2004; 140:346–553.

For further information: www.nice.org.uk

has developed, the 5- and 10-year survival rates are 95% and 81% respectively. One-quarter of people with cirrhosis will develop complications within 10 years and, once complications like ascites have arisen, the 5-year survival is around 50%. Once cirrhosis is present, 2–5% per year will develop primary hepatocellular carcinoma.

Hepatitis E

Hepatitis E is caused by an RNA virus which is endemic in India and the Middle East. An increase in prevalence has recently been noted in northern Europe and infection is no longer seen only in travellers from an endemic area.

The clinical presentation and management of hepatitis E are similar to that of hepatitis A. Disease is spread via the faecal–oral route; in most cases, it presents as a self-limiting acute hepatitis and does not cause chronic liver disease.

Hepatitis E differs from hepatitis A in that infection during pregnancy is associated with the development of acute liver failure, which has a high mortality. In acute infection, IgM antibodies to HEV are positive.

Other forms of viral hepatitis

Non-A, non-B, non-C (NANBNC) or non-A–E hepatitis is the term used to describe hepatitis thought to be due to a virus that is not HAV, HBV, HCV or HEV. Other viruses which affect the liver probably do exist, but the hepatitis viruses described above now account for the majority of hepatitis virus infections. Cytomegalovirus and Epstein–Barr virus infection causes abnormal LFTs in most patients, and occasionally icteric hepatitis occurs. Herpes simplex is a rare cause of hepatitis in adults, and most of these patients are immunocompromised. Abnormal LFTs are also common in chickenpox, measles, rubella and acute HIV infection.

HIV infection and the liver

Several causes of abnormal LFTs occur in HIV infection, as shown in Box 23.45. This topic is discussed in more detail on page 394.

> **23.45 Causes of abnormal liver blood tests in HIV infection**
>
> **Hepatitic blood tests**
> - Chronic hepatitis C
> - Chronic hepatitis B
> - Antiretroviral drugs
> - Cytomegalovirus
>
> **Cholestatic blood tests**
> - Tuberculosis
> - Atypical mycobacterium
> - Sclerosing cholangitis due to *Cryptosporidia*

ALCOHOLIC LIVER DISEASE

Alcohol is one of the most common causes of chronic liver disease. In the UK mortality from alcoholic liver disease is rising, with over 3000 deaths/year; the mean age at presentation is falling.

The risk of alcoholic liver disease is variable and not everyone who drinks heavily will develop liver disease. Only 10% of alcoholics have evidence of cirrhosis at postmortem. Alcoholic liver disease does not occur below a threshold of 21 units/week in women and 28 units/week

Alcohol type	% alcohol by volume	Amount	Units*
23.46 Amount of alcohol in an average drink			
Beer	3.5	440 mL (1 pint)	2
	9	440 mL (1 pint)	4
Wine	10	125 mL	1
	12	750 mL	9
'Alcopops'	6	330 mL	2
Sherry	17.5	750 mL	13
Vodka/rum/gin	37.5	25 mL	1
Whisky/brandy	40	700 mL	28

*1 unit = 8 g.

in men (Box 23.46). Most individuals with liver disease will have drunk heavily for more than 5 years.

Although the average alcohol consumption of an individual with cirrhosis is 160 g/day for an average of 8 years, there is no clear linear relationship between dose and liver damage.

Some of the risk factors for alcoholic liver disease are:

- *Drinking patterns.* The type of beverage does not affect risk, but liver damage is more likely to occur in continuous rather than binge drinkers.
- *Gender.* The incidence of alcoholic liver disease is increasing in women, who often conceal alcohol misuse and have higher blood ethanol levels than men after drinking because their body mass is lower.
- *Genetics.* Alcoholism is more common in monozygotic than dizygotic twins. However, polymorphisms in the genes involved in alcohol metabolism, such as aldehyde dehydrogenase (ALD), have yet to be linked to alcoholic liver disease.
- *Nutrition.* Animals given a choline-deficient diet are more likely to develop alcoholic liver disease.

Pathophysiology

Alcohol is metabolised almost exclusively by the liver via one of two main pathways (Fig. 23.31).

- Eighty per cent of alcohol is metabolised to acetaldehyde by the mitochondrial enzyme, alcohol dehydrogenase (ADH). Acetaldehyde forms adducts with cellular proteins in hepatocytes which activate the immune system, leading to cell injury. Acetaldehyde is then metabolised to acetyl-CoA and acetate by ALD. This generates NADH from NAD (nicotinamide adenine dinucleotide), which changes the redox potential of the cell.
- The remaining 20% is metabolised by the mixed function oxidase enzymes of the smooth endoplasmic reticulum. Cytochrome CYP2E1 is an enzyme which oxidises ethanol to acetate. It is induced by alcohol, and during metabolism of ethanol it releases oxygen free radicals, leading to lipid peroxidation which can induce mitochondrial damage. The CYP2E1 enzyme also metabolises acetaminophen and hence chronic alcoholics are more susceptible to hepatotoxicity from low doses of paracetamol.

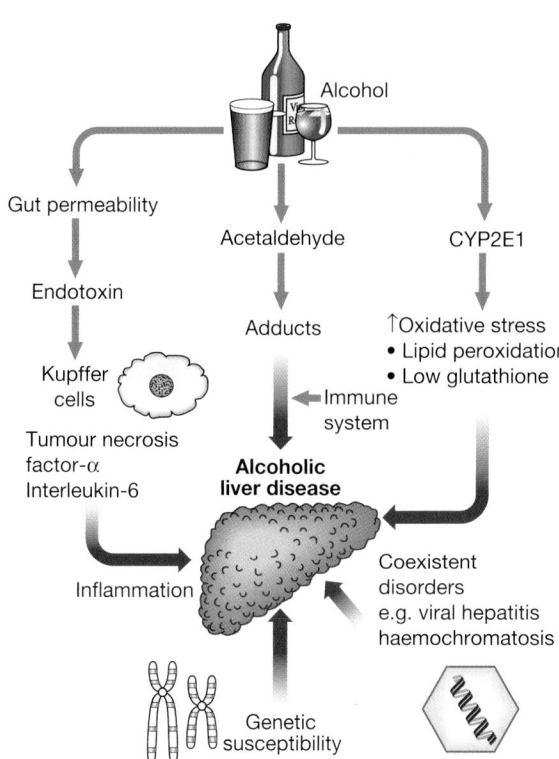

Fig. 23.31 Factors involved in the pathogenesis of alcoholic liver disease.

It is thought that pro-inflammatory cytokines may also be involved in inducing hepatic damage in alcoholic hepatitis, since endotoxin is released into the blood because of increased gut permeability, leading to release of TNF-α, IL-1, IL-2 and IL-8 from immune cells. All of these cytokines have been implicated in the pathogenesis of liver fibrosis (see Fig. 23.4, p. 924).

The pathological features of alcoholic liver disease are shown in Box 23.47. In about 80% of patients with severe alcoholic hepatitis, cirrhosis will coexist at presentation. Iron deposition is common and does not necessarily indicate haemochromatosis. Figure 23.33 (p. 958) shows the histological features of alcoholic liver disease, which are identical to those of non-alcoholic steatohepatitis.

Clinical features

Alcoholic liver disease has a wide clinical spectrum ranging from mild abnormalities of LFTs on biochemical testing to advanced cirrhosis. The liver is often enlarged in alcoholic liver disease, even in the presence of cirrhosis. Peripheral stigmata of chronic liver

---

 23.47 Pathological features of alcoholic liver disease

- Alcoholic hepatitis
  Lipogranuloma
  Neutrophil infiltration
  Mallory's hyaline
  Pericellular fibrosis
- Macrovesicular steatosis
- Fibrosis and cirrhosis
- Central hyaline sclerosis

23.48 Clinical syndromes of alcoholic liver disease

Fatty liver

• Asymptomatic abnormal liver biochemistry	• Normal/large liver

Alcoholic hepatitis

• Jaundice • Malnutrition • Hepatomegaly	• Features of portal hypertension (e.g. ascites, encephalopathy)

Cirrhosis

• Stigmata of chronic liver disease • Ascites/varices/ encephalopathy	• Large, normal or small liver • Hepatocellular carcinoma

---

disease, such as palmar erythema, are more common in alcoholic cirrhosis than in cirrhosis of other aetiologies. Alcohol misuse may also cause damage of other organs and this should be specifically looked for (see Box 10.31, p. 247). Three types of alcoholic liver disease are recognised (Box 23.48), but in reality these overlap considerably, as do the pathological changes seen in the liver.

Alcoholic fatty liver disease (AFLD)

This usually presents with elevated transaminases in the absence of hepatomegaly. It has a good prognosis and steatosis usually disappears after 3 months of abstinence.

Alcoholic hepatitis

This presents with jaundice and hepatomegaly; complications of portal hypertension may also be present. It has a significantly worse prognosis than AFLD. About one-third of patients die in the acute episode, particularly those with hepatic encephalopathy or a prolonged prothrombin time. Cirrhosis often coexists; if not present, it is the likely outcome if drinking continues. Patients with acute alcoholic hepatitis often deteriorate during the first 1–3 weeks in hospital. Even if they abstain, it may take up to 6 months for jaundice to resolve. In patients presenting with jaundice who subsequently abstain, the 3- and 5-year survival is 70%. In contrast, those who continue to drink have 3- and 5-year survival rates of 60% and 34% respectively.

Alcoholic cirrhosis

Alcohol-induced cirrhosis often presents with a serious complication such as variceal haemorrhage or ascites, and only half of such patients will survive 5 years from presentation. However, most who survive the initial illness and who become abstinent will survive beyond 5 years.

Investigations

Investigations aim to establish alcohol misuse, exclude alternative or coexistent causes of liver disease, such as hepatitis C or haemochromatosis, and assess the severity of liver disease. The clinical history from patient, relatives and friends is most important in establishing alcohol misuse, duration and severity. Biological markers, particularly macrocytosis in the absence of anaemia, may suggest and support a history of alcohol misuse. A raised GGT is not specific for alcohol misuse and will be elevated in the presence of hepatic steatosis and fibrosis. The level may not therefore return to normal with abstinence if chronic liver disease is present. Unexplained rib fractures, particularly bilateral, on a chest X-ray are also suggestive of alcohol misuse. The presence of jaundice suggests alcoholic hepatitis. Determining the extent of liver damage often requires a liver biopsy.

Prothrombin time and bilirubin are used to give a 'discriminant function' (DF), also known as the Maddrey score, which enables the clinician to assess prognosis in alcoholic hepatitis (PT = prothrombin time; serum bilirubin in µmol/L is divided by 17 to convert to mg/dL):

$$DF = [4.6 \times \text{Increase in PT (sec)}] + \text{Bilirubin (mg/dL)}$$

A value over 32 implies severe liver disease with a poor prognosis.

A second scoring system, the Glasgow score, uses the age, white cell count and renal function in addition to PT and bilirubin to assess prognosis with a cutoff of 9 (Box 23.49).

Management

Cessation of alcohol consumption is the single most important treatment; without this, all other therapies are of limited value. Abstinence is even effective at preventing progression of liver disease and death when cirrhosis is present. Life-long abstinence is the best advice and is essential for those with more severe liver disease. Treatment of alcohol dependency is discussed on pages 246–247. In the acute presentation of alcoholic liver disease it is also important to identify and anticipate alcohol withdrawal and Wernicke's encephalopathy, which need treating in parallel with the liver disease (pp. 246 and 1199).

Treatment for complications of cirrhosis, such as variceal bleeding, encephalopathy and ascites, may also be needed.

The most important prognostic factor is the patient's ability to stop drinking alcohol. General health and life expectancy are improved when this occurs, irrespective of the form of alcoholic liver disease.

Nutrition

Good nutrition is very important, and enteral feeding via a fine-bore nasogastric tube may be needed in severely ill patients.

Corticosteroids

These are of value in patients with severe alcoholic hepatitis (Maddrey's discriminative score > 32) and increase

23.49 How to assess prognosis using the Glasgow alcoholic hepatitis score

Score	1	2	3
Age	< 50	> 50	
WCC (× 10⁹/L)	< 15	> 15	> 2.0
Urea (mmol/L)	< 5	> 5	> 250
PT ratio	< 1.5	1.5–2.0	
Bilirubin (µmol/L)	< 125	125–250	

A score > 9 is associated with a 40% 28-day survival, compared to 80% for patients with a score < 9.

(PT = prothrombin time; WCC = white cell count)

EBM 23.50 Corticosteroids in alcoholic hepatitis

'In severe alcoholic hepatitis, corticosteroids improve survival at 28 days from 65% to 85% (NNT$_B$ 5).'

• Mathurin P, et al. J Hepatol 2002; 36:480–487.

For further information: www.aasld.org

survival (Box 23.50). A similar improvement in 28-day survival from 52% to 78% is seen when steroids are given to those with a Glasgow score of > 9. Sepsis is the main side-effect of steroids, and existing sepsis and variceal haemorrhage are the main contraindications to their use. If the bilirubin has not fallen 7 days after starting steroids, the drugs are unlikely to reduce mortality and should be stopped.

Pentoxifylline

Pentoxifylline, which has a weak anti-TNF action, may be beneficial in severe alcoholic hepatitis. It appears to reduce the incidence of hepatorenal failure and its use is not complicated by sepsis (Box 23.51).

EBM 23.51 Pentoxifylline in alcoholic hepatitis

'In severe alcoholic hepatitis, oral pentoxifylline reduces inpatient mortality, particularly from hepatorenal failure, from 46% to 25% (NNT$_B$ 5).'

• Akriviadis E, et al. Gastroenterology 2000; 119:1637–1648.

For further information: www.aasld.org

Liver transplantation

The role of liver transplantation in the management of alcoholic liver disease remains controversial. In many centres, however, alcoholic liver disease is a common indication for liver transplantation. The challenge is to identify patients with an unacceptable risk of returning to harmful alcohol consumption. Many programmes require a 6-month period of abstinence from alcohol before a patient is considered for transplantation. Although this relates poorly to the incidence of alcohol relapse after transplantation, liver function may improve to the extent that transplantation is no longer necessary. The outcome of transplantation for alcoholic liver disease is good (if the patient remains abstinent) because minimal immunosuppression is often required and there is no risk of disease recurrence. Transplantation for alcoholic hepatitis has a poorer outcome than for complications of alcoholic cirrhosis.

NON-ALCOHOLIC FATTY LIVER DISEASE

Non-alcoholic fatty liver disease (NAFLD) is a disease of affluent societies which increases in prevalence in proportion to the rise in obesity. It has become the most common cause of chronic liver disease after hepatitis B, hepatitis

C and alcohol. It can be classified into simple fatty liver disease (or non-alcoholic fatty liver, NAFL) and non-alcoholic steatohepatitis (NASH). The former has a benign prognosis, but the latter is associated with fibrosis and progression to cirrhosis. Many consider NAFLD to be a liver complication of the metabolic syndrome (hypertriglyceridaemia, hypertension, diabetes mellitus, an elevated body mass index (BMI) > 25 and especially truncal obesity; see Box 21.4, p. 802).

NAFLD affects about 3% of the population in the USA. The prevalence is higher in those with diabetes and those with the metabolic syndrome. Rare causes of NAFLD include tamoxifen, amiodarone and exposure to certain petrochemicals. NAFLD has also been reported following weight-reducing jejunal bypass surgery. Many cases of cirrhosis that were previously labelled cryptogenic (i.e. cause unknown) are now thought to be due to NAFLD.

Pathophysiology

Most individuals with NAFLD have insulin resistance (see Box 21.4, p. 802) but not necessarily overt glucose intolerance. The current two-hit hypothesis (Fig. 23.32) explains why not everyone with fatty liver disease develops hepatic fibrosis. The 'first hit' results in steatosis (fatty liver), which is only complicated by inflammation if a 'second hit' occurs. Leptin (p. 108), which, as well as reducing appetite, is fibrogenic in vitro, is probably then needed to cause hepatic fibrosis. The components of the first hit include release of free fatty acids from central adipose tissue, which, along with adipokines, drain into the portal vein as well as causing insulin resistance. Together, these processes result in reduced hepatic fatty acid oxidation and increased fatty acid synthesis (p. 802 and Figure 21.2, p. 799).

Clinical features

Most patients present with asymptomatic abnormal LFTs, particularly elevation of the transaminases or isolated elevation of the GGT. Occasionally, the condition presents with a complication of cirrhosis such as variceal haemorrhage or hepatocellular carcinoma. In contrast to alcoholic liver disease, jaundice only occurs when cirrhosis is established. NAFLD is the most likely diagnosis in a patient with mild to moderately elevated serum transaminases, no history of alcohol abuse and a negative chronic liver disease screen.

Investigations

Liver function tests

Unfortunately, there is no single diagnostic blood test but, in contrast to alcoholic liver disease, the ALT is normally higher than the AST. Elevated ALP levels are seen in about 30% of cases. It is important to differentiate NAFL, which does not require follow-up, from NASH. Elevated serum transaminases greater than twice the upper limit of normal and the presence of the metabolic syndrome are useful predictors of NASH.

Ultrasound

Ultrasound cannot differentiate NAFL from NASH; in both cases the liver will appear bright on ultrasound.

Liver biopsy

Individuals with serum transaminases greater than twice the upper limit of normal and features of the metabolic

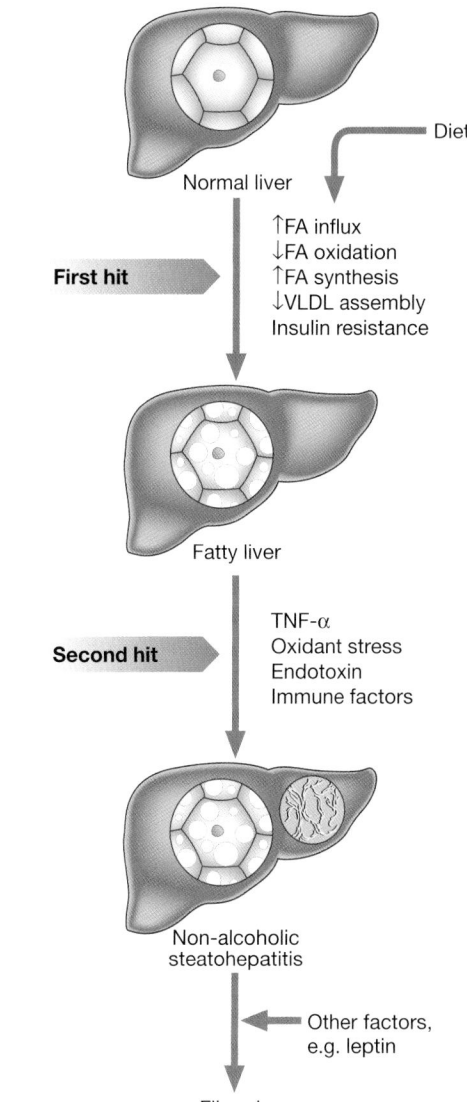

Fig. 23.32 Pathogenesis of non-alcoholic fatty liver disease: the 'two-hit' hypothesis. Fatty liver occurs as a result of increased fat import into hepatocytes and reduced fat export. Insulin resistance causes hepatic steatosis, which also perpetuates insulin resistance. Subsequent activation of TNF-α, oxidant stress through the production of reactive oxygen species, and production of endotoxin then result in inflammation and eventually fibrosis. Factors including leptin are probably needed for fibrosis. (FA = fatty acids; VLDL = very low-density lipoproteins)

syndrome should be offered a liver biopsy to determine whether inflammation and fibrosis are present. Histologically, fat deposition is usually macrovesicular (Fig. 23.33), in contrast to the microvesicular fat seen in acute fatty liver disease of pregnancy. NASH is characterised by fat, Mallory bodies, neutrophil infiltration and pericellular fibrosis. These features are indistinguishable histologically from alcoholic hepatitis, so a diagnosis of NASH relies on excluding alcohol misuse, the absence of jaundice, and the presence of risk factors such as obesity and diabetes. Fat often disappears by the time cirrhosis develops.

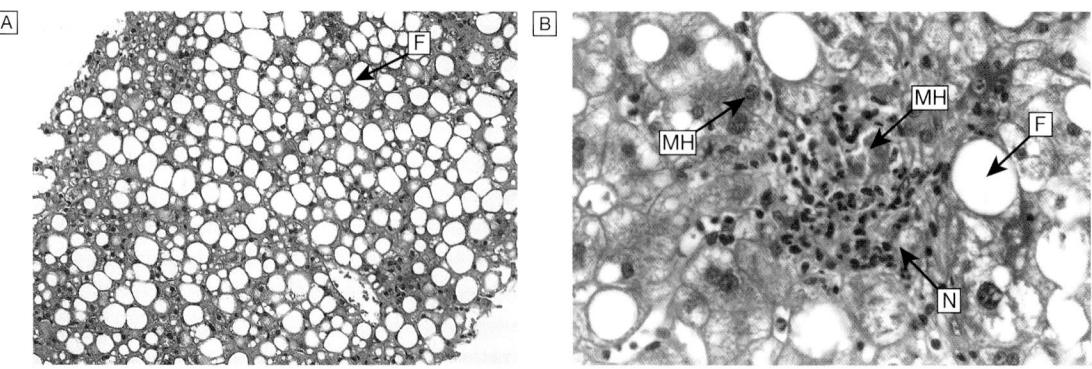

Fig. 23.33 Histology of non-alcoholic fatty liver disease. [A] Macroscopic steatosis (NAFL). Large fat droplets (F) fill hepatocytes but there is no inflammation. [B] Non-alcoholic steatohepatitis at higher power. Fat is associated with an inflammatory infiltrate of neutrophils (N) and dense pink Mallory's hyaline (MH).

Management

Current treatments are aimed at reducing BMI and insulin resistance. Metformin (p. 820) has been shown to improve LFTs and should be the first-line treatment in type 2 diabetes with NAFLD. Metformin can be used safely in patients with cirrhosis who have good liver function (Child–Pugh A). Thiazolidinediones such as pioglitazone (p. 821) also improve LFTs in NAFLD and early data suggest they may improve inflammation and fibrosis. Weight loss (pp. 118–121) will also reduce serum transaminase levels, improve liver fibrosis and reduce insulin resistance. Antioxidants such as vitamin E are not effective. There is no evidence that HMG-CoA reductase inhibitors (statins) are of value in the treatment of NAFLD but they are not contraindicated for treatment of coexistent hyperlipidaemia. The role of anti-obesity (bariatric) surgery in patients with morbid obesity and NAFLD has yet to be defined, but can result in improvement in liver fibrosis.

Once cirrhosis has occurred, survival is similar to that in hepatitis C cirrhosis with 5- and 10-year survival rates of 90% and 84% respectively. Hepatocellular carcinoma can complicate NAFLD cirrhosis. Although fewer than 5% of liver transplants are currently performed for NAFLD, this is likely to increase. Unfortunately, the condition may recur in the graft.

DRUGS, TOXINS AND THE LIVER

The liver is the primary site of drug metabolism. Liver disease may affect the capacity of the liver to metabolise drugs, and unexpected toxicity may occur when patients with liver disease are given drugs in normal doses (p. 28). Box 23.52 also shows drugs that should be avoided in patients with cirrhosis, as they can exacerbate known complications of cirrhosis.

Hepatotoxic drug reactions

Drug toxicity should be high in the differential diagnosis of acute liver failure, jaundice and abnormal liver biochemistry. Some typical patterns of drug toxicity are listed in Box 23.53; the most common picture is of a mixed cholestatic hepatitis. The presence of jaundice indicates more severe liver damage. Although acute liver failure

23.52 Drugs to be avoided in cirrhosis

Drug	Problem	Toxicity
NSAIDs	Reduced renal blood flow Ulceration	Hepatorenal failure Bleeding varices
ACE inhibitors	Reduced renal blood flow	Hepatorenal failure
Codeine	Constipation	Hepatic encephalopathy
Narcotics	Constipation, drug accumulation	Hepatic encephalopathy
Anxiolytics	Drug accumulation	Hepatic encephalopathy

23.53 Examples of common causes of drug-induced hepatotoxicity

Pattern	Drug
Cholestasis	Chlorpromazine High-dose oestrogens
Cholestatic hepatitis	NSAIDs Co-amoxiclav Statins
Acute hepatitis	Rifampicin Isoniazid
Non-alcoholic steatohepatitis	Amiodarone
Venous outflow obstruction	Busulfan Azathioprine
Fibrosis	Methotrexate

can occur, most drug reactions are self-limiting and chronic liver damage is rare. Abnormal LFTs often take weeks to normalise following a drug-induced hepatitis, and it may take months for them to normalise following a cholestatic hepatitis. Occasionally permanent bile duct loss (ductopenia) follows a cholestatic drug reaction, such as that due to co-amoxiclav, resulting in chronic cholestasis with persistent symptoms such as itching.

The key to diagnosing acute drug-induced liver disease is to take a detailed drug history (Box 23.54). A liver biopsy should be considered if there is suspicion of

23.54 The diagnosis of acute drug-induced liver disease

- Tabulate drugs taken
  Prescribed
  Self-administered
- Establish if reported hepatotoxicity in the literature
- Relate time drugs taken to onset of illness
  4 days–8 weeks (usual)
- Effect of stopping drugs on normalisation of liver biochemistry
  Hepatitic LFTs (2 months)
  Cholestatic/mixed LFTs (6 months)
- Exclude other causes
  Viral hepatitis
  Biliary disease
- Consider liver biopsy

N.B. Challenge tests with drugs should be avoided.

pre-existing liver disease or if blood tests fail to improve when the suspect drug is withdrawn.

Types of liver injury

Different histological patterns of liver injury may occur.

Cholestasis

Pure cholestasis (selective interference with bile flow in the absence of liver injury) can occur with oestrogens; this was seen quite frequently when high concentrations of oestrogens (50 μg/day) were used as contraceptives. Both the current oral contraceptive pill and hormone replacement therapy can be safely used in chronic liver disease.

Chlorpromazine and antibiotics such as flucloxacillin are examples of drugs that cause cholestatic hepatitis, which is characterised by inflammation and canalicular injury. Co-amoxiclav is the most common antibiotic to cause abnormal LFTs but, unlike other antibiotics, it may not produce symptoms until 10–42 days after it is stopped. Anabolic steroids used by body-builders may also cause a cholestatic hepatitis. In some cases (e.g. NSAIDs and COX-2 inhibitors) there is overlap with acute hepatocellular injury.

Hepatocyte necrosis

Many drugs cause an acute hepatocellular necrosis with high serum transaminase concentrations; paracetamol (p. 209) is the best known. Inflammation is not always present but does accompany necrosis in liver injury due to diclofenac (an NSAID) and isoniazid (an anti-tuberculous drug). Granuloma may be seen in liver injury following the use of allopurinol. Acute hepatocellular necrosis has also been described following the use of several herbal remedies including germander, comfrey and jin bu huan. Recreational drugs, including cocaine and ecstasy, can also cause severe acute hepatitis.

Steatosis

Microvesicular hepatocyte fat deposition, due to direct effects on mitochondrial beta-oxidation, can follow exposure to tetracyclines and sodium valproate (see Box 23.66, p. 975). Macrovesicular hepatocyte fat deposition has been described with tamoxifen, and amiodarone toxicity can produce a similar histological picture to NASH (p. 958).

Vascular/sinusoidal lesions

Drugs such as alkylating agents used in oncology can damage the vascular endothelium and lead to hepatic venous outflow obstruction. Chronic overdose of vitamin A can damage the sinusoids and trigger local fibrosis that can result in portal hypertension.

Hepatic fibrosis

Most drugs cause reversible liver injury and hepatic fibrosis is very uncommon. Methotrexate, however, as well as causing acute liver injury when it is started, can lead to cirrhosis when used in high doses over a long period of time. Risk factors for drug-induced hepatic fibrosis include pre-existing liver disease and a high alcohol intake.

INHERITED LIVER DISEASES

Haemochromatosis

Haemochromatosis is a condition in which the amount of total body iron is increased; the excess iron is deposited in, and causes damage to, several organs, including the liver. It may be primary or secondary to other diseases (Box 23.55).

23

Hereditary haemochromatosis

In hereditary haemochromatosis (HHC) iron is deposited throughout the body and total body iron may reach 20–60 g (normally 4 g). The important organs involved are the liver, pancreatic islets, endocrine glands and heart. In the liver, iron deposition occurs first in the periportal hepatocytes, extending later to all hepatocytes. The gradual development of fibrous septa leads to the formation of irregular nodules, and finally regeneration results in macronodular cirrhosis. An excess of liver iron can occur in alcoholic cirrhosis but this is mild by comparison with haemochromatosis.

Pathophysiology

The disease is caused by increased absorption of dietary iron and is inherited as an autosomal recessive trait.

23.55 Causes of haemochromatosis

Primary haemochromatosis

- Hereditary haemochromatosis
- Congenital acaeruloplasminaemia
- Congenital atransferrinaemia

Secondary iron overload

- Parenteral iron-loading (e.g. repeated blood transfusion)
- Iron-loading anaemia (thalassaemia, sideroblastic anaemia, pyruvate kinase deficiency)
- Liver disease

Complex iron overload

- Juvenile haemochromatosis
- Neonatal haemochromatosis
- Alcoholic liver disease
- Porphyria cutanea tarda
- African iron overload (Bantu siderosis)

Approximately 90% of patients are homozygous for a single-point mutation resulting in a cysteine to tyrosine substitution at position 282 (C282Y) in the HFE protein which has structural and functional similarity to the human leucocyte antigen (HLA) proteins. The mechanisms by which HFE regulates iron absorption are unclear. However, it is believed that HFE normally interacts with the transferrin receptor in the basolateral membrane of intestinal epithelial cells. In HHC, it is thought that the lack of functional HFE causes a defect in uptake of transferrin-associated iron, leading to up-regulation of enterocyte iron-specific divalent metal transporters and excessive iron absorption. A histidine to aspartic acid mutation at position 63 (H63D) in HFE causes a less severe form of haemochromatosis that is most commonly found in patients who are compound heterozygotes also carrying a C282Y mutated allele. Fewer than 50% of C282Y homozygotes will develop clinical features of haemochromatosis; therefore other factors must also be important. HHC may promote accelerated liver disease in patients with alcohol excess or hepatitis C infection. Iron loss in menstruation and pregnancy protects females from developing clinical manifestations of HHC, as 90% of patients are male.

Clinical features

Symptomatic disease usually presents in men over 40 years with features of liver disease (often with hepatomegaly), diabetes mellitus or heart failure. Fatigue and arthropathy are early symptoms. Leaden-grey skin pigmentation due to excess melanin occurs, especially in exposed parts, axillae, groins and genitalia; hence the term 'bronzed diabetes'. Impotence, loss of libido, testicular atrophy and arthritis with chondrocalcinosis secondary to calcium pyrophosphate deposition are also common. Cardiac failure or cardiac dysrhythmia may occur due to iron deposition in the heart.

Investigations

Serum iron studies show a greatly increased ferritin, a raised plasma iron and saturated plasma iron-binding capacity. Transferrin saturation > 45% is suggestive of iron overload. Significant liver disease is unusual in patients with ferritin < 1000 µg/L. MRI has high specificity for iron overload, but poor sensitivity. Liver biopsy allows assessment of fibrosis and distribution of iron (hepatocyte iron characteristic of haemochromatosis). The Hepatic Iron Index (HII) provides quantification of liver iron (µmol of iron per g dry weight of liver/age in years). HII > 1.9 suggests genetic haemochromatosis (Fig. 23.34). Both the C282Y and H63D mutations can be identified by genetic testing.

Management

Treatment consists of weekly venesection of 500 mL blood (250 mg iron) until the serum iron is normal; this may take 2 years or more. The aim is to reduce ferritin to < 50 µg/L. Thereafter, venesection is continued as required to keep the serum ferritin normal. Liver and cardiac problems improve after iron removal, but joint pain is less predictable and can improve or worsen after iron removal. Diabetes mellitus does not resolve after venesection. Other therapy includes that for cirrhosis and diabetes mellitus. First-degree family members should be investigated, preferably by

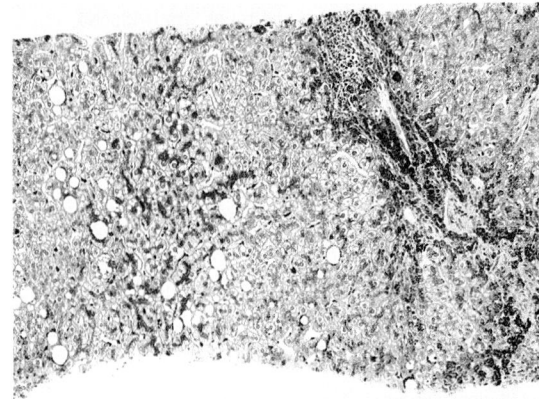

Fig. 23.34 Liver histology: haemochromatosis. This Perls stain shows accumulating iron within hepatocytes, which is stained blue. There is also accumulation of large fat globules in some hepatocytes (macrovesicular steatosis). Iron also accumulates in Kupffer cells and biliary epithelial cells.

genetic screening and also by checking the plasma ferritin and iron-binding saturation. Liver biopsy is only indicated in asymptomatic relatives if the LFTs are abnormal and/or the serum ferritin is greater than 1000 µg/L because these features are associated with significant fibrosis or cirrhosis. Asymptomatic disease should also be treated by venesection until the serum ferritin is normal.

Pre-cirrhotic patients with HHC have a normal life expectancy, and even cirrhotic patients have a good prognosis, compared with other forms of cirrhosis (three-quarters of patients are alive 5 years after diagnosis). This is probably because liver function is usually well preserved at diagnosis and improves with therapy. Screening for hepatocellular carcinoma (p. 968) is mandatory because this is the main cause of death, affecting about one-third of patients with cirrhosis irrespective of therapy. Venesection reduces but does not abolish the risk of hepatocellular carcinoma in the presence of cirrhosis.

Secondary haemochromatosis

Many conditions, including chronic haemolytic disorders, sideroblastic anaemia, other conditions requiring multiple blood transfusion (generally over 50 L), porphyria cutanea tarda, dietary iron overload and occasionally alcoholic cirrhosis, are associated with widespread secondary siderosis. The features are similar to primary haemochromatosis, but the history and clinical findings point to the true diagnosis. Some patients are heterozygotes for the *HFE* gene and this may contribute to the development of iron overload.

Wilson's disease

Wilson's disease (hepatolenticular degeneration) is a rare but important autosomal recessive disorder of copper metabolism that is caused by a variety of mutations in the *ATP7B* gene on chromosome 13. Total body copper is increased, with excess copper deposited in, and causing damage to, several organs.

Pathophysiology

Normally, dietary copper is absorbed from the stomach and proximal small intestine and is rapidly taken into the liver, where it is stored and incorporated into caeruloplasmin, which is secreted into the blood. The accumulation of excessive copper in the body is ultimately prevented by its excretion, the most important route being via the bile. In Wilson's disease, there is almost always a failure of synthesis of caeruloplasmin; however, some 5% of patients have a normal circulating caeruloplasmin concentration and this is not the primary pathogenic defect. The amount of copper in the body at birth is normal, but thereafter it increases steadily; the organs most affected are the liver, basal ganglia of the brain, eyes, kidneys and skeleton.

The *ATP7B* gene encodes a member of the copper-transporting P-type adenosine triphosphatase family, which functions to export copper from various cell types. At least 200 different mutations have been described. Although most of these are rare, their relative frequency varies in different populations. The histidine to glycine single-base mutation at position 1069 is most common in Polish and Austrian patients, but rare in India, other Asian countries and Sardinia. In contrast, approximately 60% of Sardinian patients have a 15 nucleotide deletion in the 5′ untranslated region of the Wilson's gene. Most cases are compound heterozygotes with two different mutations in *ATP7B*. Attempts to correlate the genotype with the mode of presentation and clinical course have not shown any consistent patterns.

Clinical features

Symptoms usually arise between the ages of 5 and 45 years. Hepatic disease occurs predominantly in childhood and early adolescence, although it can present in adults in their fifties. Neurological damage causes basal ganglion syndromes and dementia which tends to present in later adolescence. These features can occur alone or simultaneously. Other manifestations include renal tubular damage and osteoporosis, but these are rarely presenting features.

Liver disease

Episodes of acute hepatitis, sometimes recurrent, can occur, especially in children, and may progress to acute fulminant liver failure. The latter is characterised by the liberation of free copper into the blood stream, causing massive haemolysis and renal tubulopathy. Chronic hepatitis can also develop insidiously and eventually present with established cirrhosis; liver failure and portal hypertension may supervene. Recurrent acute hepatitis of unknown cause, especially when accompanied by haemolysis, or chronic liver disease of unknown cause in a patient under 40 years old suggests Wilson's disease.

Neurological disease

Clinical features include a variety of extrapyramidal features, particularly tremor, choreoathetosis, dystonia, parkinsonism and dementia (p. 1203). Unusual clumsiness for age may be an early symptom.

Kayser–Fleischer rings

These are the most important single clinical clue to the diagnosis and can be seen in 60% of adults with Wilson's disease (less often in children but almost always in neurological Wilson's disease), albeit sometimes only by slit-lamp examination. Kayser–Fleischer rings are characterised by greenish-brown discoloration of the corneal margin appearing first at the upper periphery (Fig. 23.35). They eventually disappear with treatment.

Investigations

A low serum caeruloplasmin is the best single laboratory clue to the diagnosis. However, advanced liver failure from any cause can reduce the serum caeruloplasmin, and occasionally it is normal in Wilson's disease. Other features of disordered copper metabolism should therefore be sought; these include a high free serum copper concentration, a high urine copper excretion of greater than 0.6 µmol/24 hrs (38 µg/24 hrs) and a very high hepatic copper content. Measuring 24-hour urinary copper excretion whilst giving D-penicillamine is a useful confirmatory test; more than 25 µmol/24 hrs is considered diagnostic of Wilson's disease.

Genetic testing may be useful in screening families once the abnormality has been identified in an affected individual.

Management

The copper-binding agent, penicillamine, is the drug of choice. The dose given must be sufficient to produce cupriuresis and most patients require 1.5 g/day (range 1–4 g). The dose can be reduced once the disease is in remission but treatment must continue for life, even through pregnancy. Care must be taken to ensure that reaccumulation of copper does not occur. Abrupt discontinuation of treatment must be avoided because this may precipitate acute liver failure. Toxic effects occur in one-third of patients and include rashes, protein-losing nephropathy, lupus-like syndrome and bone marrow depression. If these do occur, trientine dihydrochloride (1.2–2.4 g/day) and zinc (50 mg 8-hourly) are alternative effective therapies.

Liver transplantation is indicated for fulminant liver failure or for advanced cirrhosis with liver failure. The value of liver transplantation in severe neurological Wilson's disease is highly controversial.

The prognosis is excellent, provided treatment is started before there is irreversible damage. Siblings and children of patients with Wilson's disease must

23

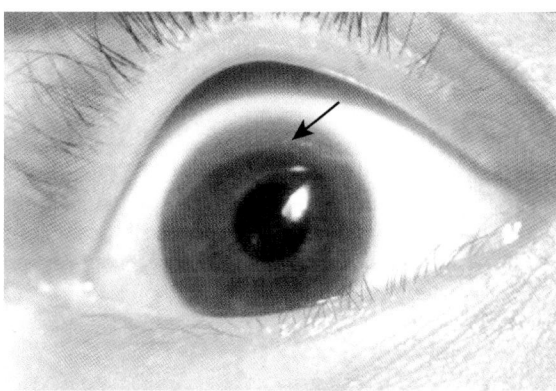

Fig. 23.35 Kayser–Fleischer rings at the junction of the cornea and sclera (arrow) in a patient with Wilson's disease.

be investigated and treatment should be given to all affected individuals, even if they are asymptomatic.

Alpha₁-antitrypsin deficiency

Alpha₁-antitrypsin (α_1-AT) is a serine protease inhibitor (Pi) produced by the liver. The mutated form of α_1-AT (PiZ) cannot be secreted into the blood by liver cells because it is retained within the endoplasmic reticulum of the hepatocyte. Homozygous individuals (PiZZ) have low plasma α_1-AT concentrations, although globules containing α_1-AT are found in the liver, and they may develop hepatic and pulmonary disease. Liver manifestations include cholestatic jaundice in the neonatal period (neonatal hepatitis), which can resolve spontaneously, chronic hepatitis and cirrhosis in adults, and in the long term hepatocellular carcinoma.

There are no clinical features distinguishing liver disease due to α_1-AT deficiency from liver disease due to other causes, and the diagnosis is made from the low plasma α_1-AT concentration and genotyping for the presence of the mutation. Alpha₁-AT-containing globules can be demonstrated in the liver (Fig. 23.36) but this is not necessary to make the diagnosis. Occasionally, patients with liver disease and minor reductions of plasma α_1-AT concentrations have α_1-AT variants other than PiZZ, but the relationship of these to liver disease is uncertain.

No specific treatment is available; the concurrent risk of severe and early-onset emphysema means that all patients should be advised to abandon cigarette smoking.

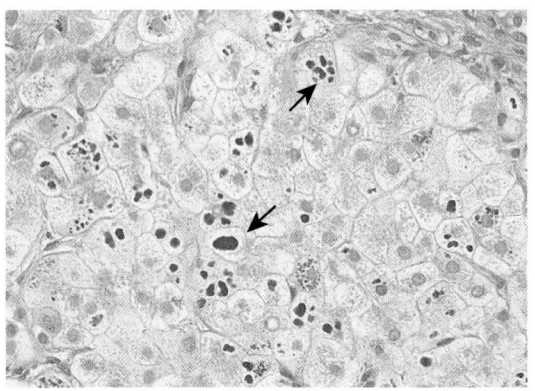

Fig. 23.36 Liver histology in α_1-antitrypsin deficiency. Accumulation of periodic acid-Schiff-positive granules (arrows) within individual hepatocytes is shown in this section from a patient with α_1-AT deficiency.

Gilbert's syndrome

Gilbert's syndrome is by far the most common inherited disorder of bilirubin metabolism (see Box 23.10, p. 932). It is inherited as an autosomal dominant trait and is caused by a mutation in the promoter region of the UDP-glucuronyl transferase enzyme, which leads to reduced enzyme expression. This results in decreased conjugation of bilirubin, which accumulates as unconjugated bilirubin in the blood. The levels of unconjugated bilirubin increase during fasting, as fasting reduces levels of UDP-glucuronyl transferase.

Clinical features

There are no stigmata of chronic liver disease other than jaundice. Increased excretion of bilirubin and hence stercobilinogen leads to normal-coloured or dark stools, and increased urobilinogen excretion causes the urine to turn dark on standing as urobilin is formed. In the presence of haemolysis, pallor due to anaemia and splenomegaly due to excessive reticulo-endothelial activity are usually present.

Investigations

In Gilbert's syndrome the plasma bilirubin is usually less than 100 µmol/L (~6 mg/dL) and the LFTs are otherwise normal. There is no bilirubinuria because the hyperbilirubinaemia is predominantly unconjugated. Other LFTs and hepatic histology are normal. The condition has an excellent prognosis, needs no treatment, and is clinically important only because it may be mistaken for more serious liver disease.

AUTOIMMUNE HEPATITIS

Autoimmune hepatitis is a liver disease of unknown aetiology characterised by a strong association with other autoimmune diseases (Box 23.56), high levels of serum immunoglobulins (hypergammaglobulinaemia) and autoantibodies in the serum. It occurs most often in women, particularly in the second and third decades of life, but may develop in either sex at any age.

Pathophysiology

Several subtypes of this disorder have been proposed which have differing immunological markers:

- *Classical (type I) autoimmune hepatitis* is characterised by a high frequency of other autoimmune disorders, such as Graves' disease. Type I autoimmune hepatitis is associated with HLA-DR3 and DR4, particularly HLA-DRB3*0101 and HLA-DRB1*0401. These patients have high titres of antinuclear and anti-smooth muscle antibodies, but none of these antibodies is cytotoxic. A suggested hypothesis for the development of type I autoimmune hepatitis is the aberrant expression on the hepatocyte of HLA antigen, influenced by viral, genetic and environmental factors.
- *Type II autoimmune hepatitis* is characterised by the presence of anti-LKM (liver-kidney microsomal) antibodies and lack of antinuclear and anti-smooth muscle antibodies. Anti-LKM antibodies recognise cytochrome P450-IID6, which is expressed on the hepatocyte membrane.
- *Type III autoimmune hepatitis* is characterised by elevated serum immunoglobulin levels; the

23.56 Conditions associated with autoimmune hepatitis

• Migrating polyarthritis	• Coombs-positive haemolytic
• Urticarial rashes	anaemia
• Lymphadenopathy	• Transient pulmonary
• Hashimoto's thyroiditis	infiltrates
• Thyrotoxicosis	• Ulcerative colitis
• Myxoedema	• Glomerulonephritis
• Pleurisy	• Nephrotic syndrome

antibodies described above are absent, whilst antibodies against soluble liver antigen are present. The histopathological features of all forms of autoimmune hepatitis are similar.

Clinical features

The onset is usually insidious, with fatigue, anorexia and jaundice. In about one-quarter of patients the onset is acute, resembling viral hepatitis, but resolution does not occur. This acute presentation can lead to extensive liver necrosis and liver failure. Other features include fever, arthralgia, vitiligo and epistaxis. Amenorrhoea is the rule but general health may be good. Jaundice is mild to moderate or occasionally absent, but signs of chronic liver disease, especially spider naevi and hepatosplenomegaly, are usually present. Some patients have a 'Cushingoid' face with acne, hirsutism and pink cutaneous striae, especially on the thighs and abdomen.

Approximately two-thirds of patients have associated autoimmune disease such as Hashimoto's thyroiditis, renal tubular acidosis and rheumatoid arthritis.

Investigations

Serological tests for autoantibodies are often positive (Box 23.57), but low titres of these antibodies occur in some healthy people. Antinuclear antibodies also occur in connective tissue diseases and other autoimmune diseases, while anti-smooth muscle antibody has been reported in infectious mononucleosis and a variety of malignant diseases. Antimicrosomal antibodies (anti-LKM) occur particularly in children and adolescents. Elevated levels of serum IgG immunoglobulins are invariable and are an important diagnostic feature. If the diagnosis of autoimmune hepatitis is suspected, liver biopsy should be performed. It typically shows interface hepatitis, with or without cirrhosis.

Management

Treatment with corticosteroids is life-saving in autoimmune hepatitis, particularly during exacerbations of active and symptomatic disease. Initially, prednisolone 40 mg/day is given orally; the dose is then gradually reduced as the patient and LFTs improve. Maintenance therapy is required for at least 2 years after LFTs have returned to normal, and withdrawal of treatment should

---

EBM 23.58 Immunosuppression in autoimmune hepatitis

'In autoimmune hepatitis, treatment with prednisolone ± azathioprine improves serum biochemistry and hepatic histology. It also improves survival at 10 years from 27% to 63% (NNT$_B$ 2.7).'

'In patients who have been in remission for more than 1 year, increasing the dose of azathioprine (from 1 to 2 mg/kg) and withdrawing prednisolone reduces steroid side-effects and does not increase the risk of relapse.'

- Kirk AP, et al. Gut 1980; 21:78–83.
- Johnson PJ, et al. N Engl J Med 1995; 333:958–963.

---

not be considered unless a liver biopsy is also normal. Most individuals require long-term immunosuppression. Azathioprine 1.0–1.5 mg/kg/day orally may allow the dose of prednisolone to be reduced (Box 23.58). Azathioprine can also be used as the sole maintenance immunosuppressive agent. Corticosteroids treat acute exacerbations but do not prevent cirrhosis; they are therefore less important in mild asymptomatic autoimmune hepatitis.

The disease is characterised by exacerbations and remissions, but most patients eventually develop cirrhosis and its complications. Hepatocellular carcinoma is uncommon. Approximately 50% of symptomatic patients will die of liver failure within 5 years if no treatment is given, but this falls to about 10% with therapy.

INTRAHEPATIC BILIARY DISEASES

Primary biliary cirrhosis

Primary biliary cirrhosis (PBC) is a chronic, progressive cholestatic liver disease of unknown cause which predominantly affects middle-aged women. The condition is strongly associated with the presence of antimitochondrial antibodies (AMA), which are diagnostic. It is characterised by a granulomatous inflammation of the portal tracts, leading to progressive damage and eventually loss of the small and middle-sized bile ducts. This in turn leads to fibrosis and cirrhosis of the liver. The condition typically presents with an insidious onset of itching and/or tiredness; it may also be found incidentally as the result of routine blood tests.

Epidemiology

The prevalence of PBC varies across the world. It is relatively common in northern Europe and North America (the prevalence in north-east England is 245/million), but is rare in Africa and Asia. There is a strong female to male predominance of 9:1; it is also more common amongst cigarette smokers. Clustering of cases has been reported, suggesting an infectious agent.

Pathophysiology

The cause of PBC is unknown but immune mechanisms are clearly involved. The condition is closely associated with other autoimmune non-hepatic diseases, such as thyroid disease, and there is a weak association with HLA-DR8. Antimitochondrial and antinuclear (nuclear pore antigens gp210) antibodies are found in the serum with elevations in serum immunoglobulin levels, particularly IgM; cellular immunity is impaired

---

23.57 Frequency of autoantibodies in chronic non-viral liver diseases and in healthy people

Disease	Antinuclear antibody (%)	Anti-smooth muscle antibody (%)	Antimitochondrial antibody*
Healthy controls	5	1.5	0.01
Autoimmune hepatitis	80	70	15
Primary biliary cirrhosis	25	35	95
Cryptogenic cirrhosis	40	30	15

*Patients with antimitochondrial antibody frequently have cholestatic LFTs and may have primary biliary cirrhosis (see text).

and abnormal cellular immune reactions have been described. Infectious agents, such as retroviruses and bacteria, including *E. coli* and mycobacteria, have been suggested as the trigger for the disease process, but this hypothesis remains unproven.

The primary pathological lesion is a chronic granulomatous inflammation which damages and destroys the interlobular bile ducts; progressive lymphocyte-mediated inflammatory damage causes fibrosis, which spreads from the portal tracts to the liver parenchyma and eventually leads to cirrhosis. A model of the natural history of the disease process is shown in Figure 23.37.

Clinical features

Non-specific symptoms, such as lethargy and arthralgia, are common and may precede diagnosis for years. Pruritus is the most common initial complaint, pointing to hepatobiliary disease, and may precede jaundice by months or years; jaundice is rarely a presenting feature. The itching is usually worse on the limbs. Although there may be right upper abdominal discomfort, fever and rigors do not occur. Bone pain or fractures can rarely result from osteomalacia (fat-soluble vitamin malabsorption) or, more commonly, from osteoporosis (hepatic osteodystrophy).

Initially, patients are well nourished but considerable weight loss can occur as the disease progresses. Scratch marks may be found. Jaundice is only prominent late in the disease and can become intense. Xanthomatous deposits occur in a minority, especially around the eyes, in the hand creases and over the elbows, knees and buttocks. Hepatomegaly is virtually constant, and splenomegaly becomes increasingly common as portal hypertension develops. Liver failure may supervene.

Associated diseases

Autoimmune and connective tissue diseases occur with increased frequency in PBC, particularly the sicca syndrome (p. 1090), systemic sclerosis, coeliac disease (p. 879) and thyroid diseases. Hypothyroidism should always be considered in patients with fatigue.

Diagnosis and investigations

The LFTs show a pattern of cholestasis (p. 930). Hypercholesterolaemia is common and worsens as disease progresses; however, it is of no diagnostic value. The antimitochondrial antibody is present in over 95% of patients, and when it is absent the diagnosis should not be made without obtaining histological evidence and considering cholangiography (MRCP or ERCP) to exclude other biliary disease. Antinuclear and anti-smooth muscle antibodies are present in around 15% of patients (see Box 23.57); autoantibodies found in associated diseases may also be present. Ultrasound examination shows no sign of biliary obstruction. Liver biopsy is only necessary if there is diagnostic uncertainty. The histological features of PBC correlate poorly with the clinical features; portal hypertension can develop before the histological onset of cirrhosis.

Management

Asymptomatic patients require monitoring on a yearly basis to assess the onset of symptoms and associated disease. Immunosuppressants such as corticosteroids, azathioprine, penicillamine and ciclosporin have all been tried in PBC, but none is effective and all may have serious adverse effects. The hydrophilic bile acid, ursodeoxycholic acid (UDCA), improves bile flow, replaces toxic hydrophobic bile acids in the bile acid pool, and reduces apoptosis of the biliary epithelium. Clinically, UDCA improves LFTs, may slow down histological progression and has few side-effects (Box 23.59); it is therefore widely used in the treatment of PBC at a dose of 13–15 mg/kg/day.

Liver transplantation should be considered once liver failure has developed and may be indicated in patients with intractable pruritus. Prognostic models are available but serum bilirubin remains the most reliable marker of

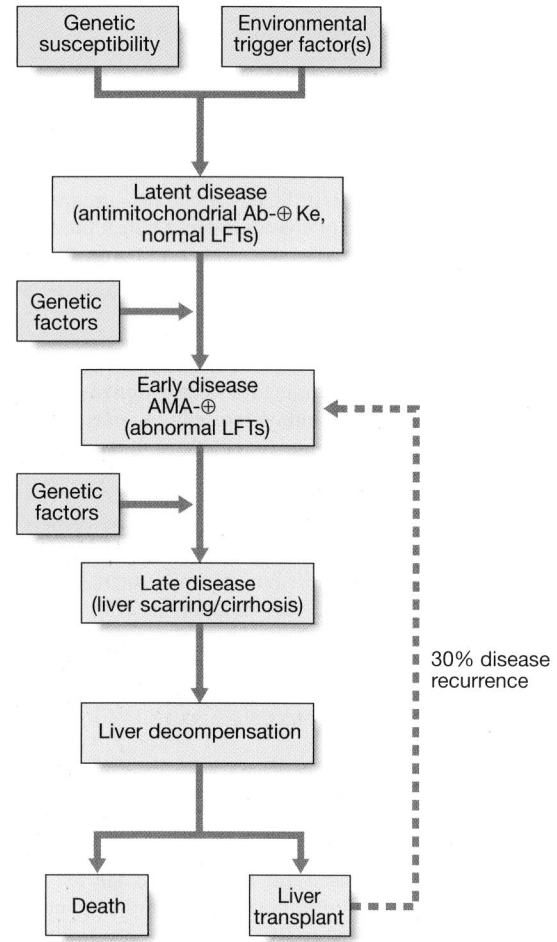

Fig. 23.37 Natural history of primary biliary cirrhosis.

| EBM | **23.59 Ursodeoxycholic acid (UDCA) in primary biliary cirrhosis (PBC)** |

'In PBC UDCA therapy (13–15 mg/kg/day) improves biochemical markers of cholestasis and jaundice. Some randomised trials have shown that UDCA treatment significantly slows disease progression, but whether it affects mortality or transplantation rates remains controversial.'

• Poupon RE, et al. Gastroenterology 1997; 113:884–890.
• Corpechot C, et al. Hepatology 2000; 32:1196–1199.
• Goulis J, et al. Lancet 1999; 354:1053–1060.

declining liver function. Transplantation is associated with an excellent 5-year survival of over 80%, although the disease will recur in over one-third of patients at 10 years.

Pruritus

This is the main symptom requiring treatment. The cause of itching is unknown but current research suggests that it is due to up-regulation of opioid receptors and increased levels of endogenous opioids. It is best treated with the anion-binding resin colestyramine, which probably acts by binding potential pruritogens in the intestine and increasing their excretion in the stool. A dose of 4–16 g/day orally is used. The powder is mixed in orange juice and the main dose (8 g) taken before and after breakfast when maximal duodenal bile acid concentrations occur. Colestyramine may bind other drugs in the gut (e.g. anticoagulants), which should therefore be taken 1 hour before the binding agent. Colestyramine is sometimes ineffective, especially in complete biliary obstruction. Alternative treatments include rifampicin 300 mg/day, naltrexone (an opioid antagonist) 25 mg/day initially increasing up to 300 mg/day, plasmapheresis and a liver support device (e.g. a molecular adsorbent recirculating system (MARS) machine).

Fatigue

Fatigue affects about one-third of patients with PBC. The cause is unknown but it may reflect intracerebral changes due to cholestasis. Unfortunately, once depression and hypothyroidism have been excluded, there is no treatment.

Malabsorption

Prolonged cholestasis is associated with steatorrhoea and malabsorption of fat-soluble vitamins, which should be replaced as necessary. Coeliac disease should be excluded since its incidence is increased in PBC.

Bone disease

Osteopenia and osteoporosis are common, and normal post-menopausal bone loss is accelerated. Baseline bone density should be measured (p. 1118) and treatment started with replacement calcium and vitamin D_3. Bisphosphonates should be used if there is evidence of osteoporosis. Osteomalacia is rare.

Overlap syndromes

AMA-negative PBC ('autoimmune cholangitis')

A few patients demonstrate the clinical, biochemical and histological features of PBC but do not have detectable antimitochondrial antibodies in the serum. Serum transaminases, serum Ig levels and titres of antinuclear antibodies tend to be higher than in AMA-positive PBC. However, the clinical course mirrors classical PBC and these patients should be considered to have a variant of PBC.

PBC/autoimmune hepatitis overlap

A small minority of patients with AMA and cholestatic LFTs have elevated transaminases, high serum immunoglobulins and interface hepatitis on liver histology; in such patients a trial of corticosteroids may be beneficial.

Secondary biliary cirrhosis

This develops after prolonged large duct biliary obstruction due to gallstones, benign bile duct strictures or sclerosing cholangitis (see below). Carcinomas rarely cause secondary biliary cirrhosis because few patients survive long enough. The clinical features are of chronic cholestasis with episodes of ascending cholangitis or even liver abscess (p. 972). Cirrhosis, ascites and portal hypertension are late features. Relief of biliary obstruction may require endoscopic or surgical intervention. Cholangitis requires treatment with antibiotics, which can be given continuously if attacks recur frequently.

Primary sclerosing cholangitis

Primary sclerosing cholangitis is a cholestatic liver disease caused by diffuse inflammation and fibrosis; it can involve the entire biliary tree and leads to the gradual obliteration of intrahepatic and extrahepatic bile ducts, and ultimately biliary cirrhosis, portal hypertension and hepatic failure. The incidence is about 6.3/100 000 in Caucasians. Cholangiocarcinoma develops in about 10–30% of patients during the course of the disease.

Primary sclerosing cholangitis occurs mainly in young men (male:female ratio 2:1). Most patients present at age 25–40 years, although the condition may be diagnosed at any age and is an important cause of chronic liver disease in children. The generally accepted diagnostic criteria are:
- generalised beading and stenosis of the biliary system on cholangiography (Fig. 23.38)
- absence of choledocholithiasis (or history of bile duct surgery)

23

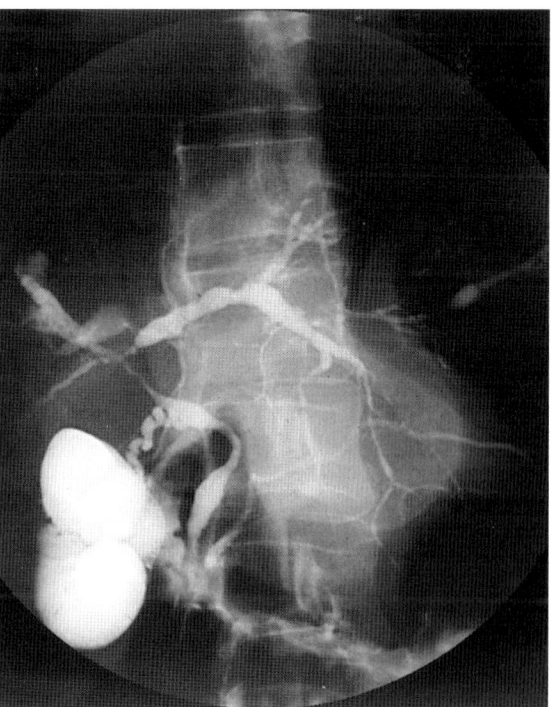

Fig. 23.38 A percutaneous cholangiogram in sclerosing cholangitis showing characteristic irregularity of the biliary tree.

• exclusion of bile duct cancer, usually by prolonged follow-up.

The term 'secondary sclerosing cholangitis' is used to describe the typical bile duct changes described above when a clear predisposing factor for duct fibrosis can be identified. The causes of secondary sclerosing cholangitis are shown in Box 23.60.

Pathophysiology

The cause of primary sclerosing cholangitis is unknown but there is a close association with inflammatory bowel disease, particularly ulcerative colitis (Box 23.61). About two-thirds of patients with primary sclerosing cholangitis have coexisting ulcerative colitis, and primary sclerosing cholangitis is the most common form of chronic liver disease in ulcerative colitis. Between 3% and 10% of patients with ulcerative colitis develop primary sclerosing cholangitis, particularly those with substantial or total colitis. The prevalence of primary sclerosing cholangitis is lower in patients with Crohn's colitis (about 1%). Patients with primary sclerosing cholangitis and ulcerative colitis are at greater risk of colorectal neoplasia than those with ulcerative colitis alone, and those who develop colorectal neoplasia are at greater risk of cholangiocarcinoma.

It is currently believed that primary sclerosing cholangitis is an immunologically mediated disease, triggered in genetically susceptible individuals by toxic or infectious agents, which may gain access to the biliary tract through a leaky diseased colon.

Immunogenic factors

A close link with HLA haplotype A1 B8 DR3 DRW52A has been identified. This haplotype is commonly found in association with other organ-specific autoimmune diseases (e.g. autoimmune hepatitis). The prevalence of HLA-DR2 and HLA-DR6 is greater in patients who are DR3-negative.

23.60 Causes of secondary sclerosing cholangitis

• Previous bile duct surgery with stricturing and cholangitis
• Bile duct stones causing cholangitis
• Intrahepatic infusion of 5-fluorodeoxyuridine
• Insertion of formalin into hepatic hydatid cysts
• Insertion of alcohol into hepatic tumours
• Parasitic infections (e.g. *Clonorchis*)
• Autoimmune pancreatitis/IgG4-associated cholangitis
• AIDS (probably infective as a result of cytomegalovirus or *Cryptosporidium*)

23.61 Diseases associated with primary sclerosing cholangitis

• Ulcerative colitis
• Crohn's colitis
• Chronic pancreatitis
• Retroperitoneal fibrosis
• Riedel's thyroiditis
• Retro-orbital tumours
• Immune deficiency states
• Sjögren's syndrome
• Angio-immunoplastic lymphadenopathy
• Histiocytosis X
• Autoimmune haemolytic anaemia
• Autoimmune pancreatitis/ IgG4-associated cholangitis

The importance of immunological factors has been emphasised by reports showing humoral and cellular abnormalities in primary sclerosing cholangitis. Perinuclear antineutrophil cytoplasmic antibodies (ANCA) have been detected in the sera of about 60–80% of patients with primary sclerosing cholangitis with or without ulcerative colitis, and in about 30–40% of patients with ulcerative colitis alone. The antibody is not specific for primary sclerosing cholangitis and is found in other chronic liver diseases (e.g. 50% of patients with autoimmune hepatitis).

Clinical features

The diagnosis is often made incidentally when persistently raised serum ALP is discovered in an individual with ulcerative colitis. Common symptoms include fatigue, intermittent jaundice, weight loss, right upper quadrant abdominal pain and pruritus. Attacks of acute cholangitis are uncommon and usually follow biliary instrumentation. Physical examination is abnormal in about 50% of symptomatic patients; the most common findings are jaundice and hepatomegaly/splenomegaly. The condition may be associated with many other diseases (see Box 23.61).

Investigations

Biochemical screening usually reveals a cholestatic pattern of LFTs but ALP and bilirubin levels may vary widely in individual patients during the course of the disease. For example, ALP and bilirubin values increase during acute cholangitis, decrease after therapy, and sometimes fluctuate for no apparent reason. Modest elevations in serum transaminases are usually seen, whereas hypoalbuminaemia and clotting abnormalities are found only at a late stage. In addition to ANCA, low titres of serum antinuclear and anti-smooth muscle antibodies may be found in primary sclerosing cholangitis but have no diagnostic significance; serum antimitochondrial antibody is absent. IgM concentrations are increased in about 50% of symptomatic patients and elevations of IgG are found in about 30% of adults.

The key investigation is ERCP, which is usually diagnostic, revealing multiple irregular stricturing and dilatation (see Fig. 23.38). MRCP is a non-invasive method of imaging the biliary tree; it is being assessed and will probably become the standard method of diagnosis.

On liver biopsy the characteristic early features of primary sclerosing cholangitis are periductal 'onion-skin' fibrosis and inflammation, with portal oedema and bile ductular proliferation resulting in expansion of the portal tracts (Fig. 23.39). Later fibrosis spreads, leading inevitably to biliary cirrhosis; obliterative cholangitis leads to the so-called 'vanishing bile duct syndrome'.

Management

There is no cure for primary sclerosing cholangitis, but management of cholestasis and its complications and specific treatment of the disease process are indicated.

The course of primary sclerosing cholangitis is variable. In symptomatic patients, median survival from presentation to death or liver transplantation is about 12 years. About 75% of asymptomatic patients survive 15 years or more. Most patients die from liver failure, about 30% die from bile duct carcinoma, and the

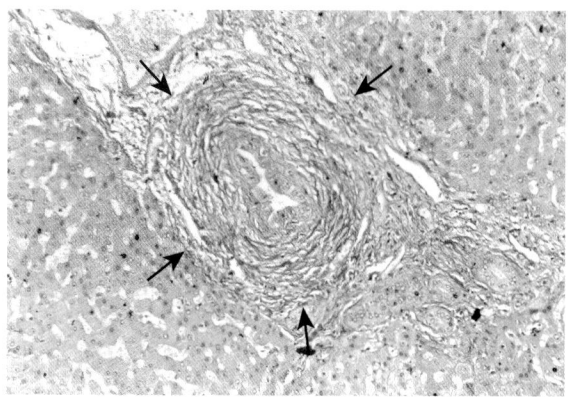

Fig. 23.39 Primary sclerosing cholangitis. Note onion-skin scarring (arrows) surrounding a bile duct.

remainder die from colonic cancer or complications of colitis.

Management of cholestasis

Symptomatic patients often have pruritus, which is best managed initially with colestyramine; the dose should be increased until relief is obtained.

Management of complications

Broad-spectrum antibiotics (e.g. ciprofloxacin) should be given for acute attacks of cholangitis but have no proven value in preventing attacks. If cholangiography shows a well-defined obstruction to the extrahepatic bile ducts ('dominant stricture'), mechanical relief can be obtained by placement of a plastic stent or by balloon dilatation performed at ERCP. Fat-soluble vitamin replacement is necessary in jaundiced patients. Metabolic bone disease (usually osteoporosis) is a common complication that requires treatment (p. 1116).

Specific treatment

Ursodeoxycholic acid (UDCA) is a non-hepatotoxic hydrophilic bile acid that has been used widely for treatment of cholestasis; it reduces levels of cholestatic liver enzymes, but controlled trials in conventional doses have shown no effect on symptoms, histology or survival. Larger doses (20–25 mg/kg daily) have beneficial effects on liver histology and cholangiographic appearance. Immunosuppressive agents, including prednisolone, azathioprine, methotrexate and ciclosporin, have been tried; generally, results have been disappointing but combination therapy with UDCA may be beneficial.

Surgical treatment

Orthotopic transplantation is the only option in young patients with primary sclerosing cholangitis and advanced liver disease; 5-year survival is 80–90% in most centres. Unfortunately, the condition may recur in the graft. Cholangiocarcinoma is a contraindication to transplantation.

Cystic and fibropolycystic disease

Fibropolycystic diseases of the liver and biliary system constitute a heterogeneous group of rare disorders, some of which are inherited. They are not distinct entities and combined lesions occur.

Solitary hepatic cysts

Isolated hepatic cysts may be discovered by chance; rarely, they give rise to complications, including pain or jaundice from cyst enlargement, haemorrhage or infection. Portal hypertension and bleeding from varices are exceptional.

Diagnosis is best made by ultrasonography. Resection of a large cyst or groups of cysts is only required if symptoms are troublesome. The prognosis is excellent.

Adult hepatorenal polycystic disease

The kidneys are predominantly affected in this condition (Fig. 23.40), which is inherited as an autosomal dominant trait (p. 506). Hepatic cysts which do not communicate with the biliary system are present in over half of patients with renal cysts, and cysts can also be found in other organs. Cerebrovascular aneurysms may develop. Cysts restricted to the liver constitute a separate rare genetic disorder.

Caroli's syndrome

This is very rare and is characterised by segmental saccular dilatations of the intrahepatic biliary tree. The whole liver is usually affected, and extrahepatic biliary dilatation occurs in about one-quarter of patients. Recurrent attacks of cholangitis (see Box 23.11, p. 932) occur and may cause hepatic abscesses. Complications include biliary stones and cholangiocarcinoma. Antibiotics are required for episodes of cholangitis. Occasionally, localised disease can be treated by segmental liver resection and liver transplantation may sometimes be required.

Congenital hepatic fibrosis

This is characterised by broad bands of fibrous tissue linking the portal tracts in the liver, abnormalities of the interlobular bile ducts, and sometimes a lack of portal venules. The renal tubules may show cystic dilatation (medullary sponge kidney, p. 507), and eventually renal cysts may develop. The condition can be inherited as an

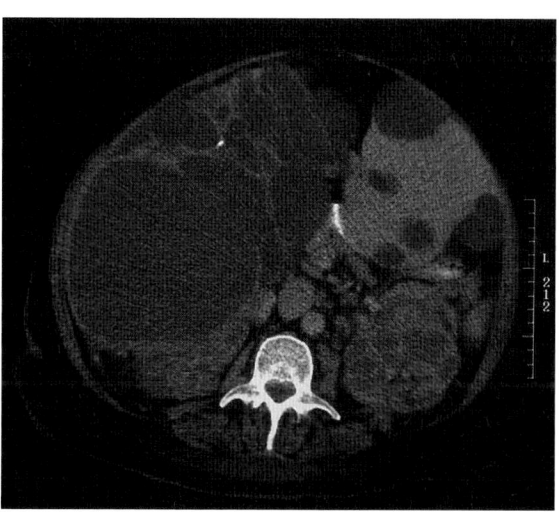

Fig. 23.40 CT showing multiple cysts in the liver and kidneys in polycystic disease.

23

autosomal recessive trait. Liver involvement causes portal hypertension with splenomegaly and bleeding from oesophageal varices that usually presents in adolescence or in early adult life. The prognosis is good because liver function is preserved. Treatment may be required for variceal bleeding and occasionally cholangitis. Patients can present during childhood with renal failure if the kidneys are severely affected.

Choledochal cysts

This term applies to cysts anywhere in the biliary tree (Fig. 23.41). The great majority cause diffuse dilatation of the common bile duct (type I), but others take the form of biliary diverticula (type II), dilatation of the intraduodenal bile duct (type III) and multiple biliary cysts (type IV). The last type merges with Caroli's syndrome (see above). In the neonate they may present with jaundice or biliary peritonitis. Recurrent jaundice, abdominal pain and cholangitis may arise in the adult. Liver abscess and biliary cirrhosis may develop, and there is an increased incidence of cholangiocarcinoma. Excision of the cyst with hepatico-jejunostomy is the treatment of choice.

Cystic fibrosis

Cystic fibrosis (p. 678) is associated with a biliary cirrhosis in about 5% of individuals. Splenomegaly and an elevated ALP are characteristic. Complications do not normally arise until late adolescence or early adulthood, when bleeding due to variceal haemorrhage may occur. UDCA improves liver blood tests but it is not known whether the drug can prevent progression of liver disease. Deficiency of fat-soluble vitamins (A, D, E and K) may need to be treated in view of both biliary and pancreatic disease (pancreatic exocrine insufficiency occurs in 90% of individuals with cystic fibrosis).

Intrahepatic cholestasis

Mutations in the biliary transporter proteins on the hepatocyte canalicular membrane (FIC1—familial intrahepatic cholestasis 1), illustrated in Figure 23.7 (p. 925), have been shown to cause an inherited intrahepatic biliary disease in childhood characterised by raised ALP levels and progression to a biliary cirrhosis. It is also becoming increasingly clear that these proteins contribute to intrahepatic biliary disease in adulthood.

Benign recurrent intrahepatic cholestasis

This rare condition usually presents in adolescence and is characterised by recurrent episodes of cholestasis, lasting 1–6 months. It is now known to be mediated by mutations in the *ATP8B1* gene, which lies on chromosome 18 and encodes FIC1. The same gene is thought to be responsible for a cholestatic condition that causes cirrhosis in childhood.

Episodes start with pruritus, while painless jaundice develops later. LFTs show a cholestatic pattern. Liver biopsy shows cholestasis (bilirubin in hepatocytes) during an episode but is normal between episodes. Treatment is required to relieve pruritus and the long-term prognosis is good.

LIVER TUMOURS AND FOCAL LIVER LESIONS

Hepatocellular carcinoma

Hepatocellular carcinoma (HCC) is the most common primary liver tumour, and the sixth most common cause of cancer world-wide. The age-adjusted incidence rates vary from 28 per 100 000 in South-east Asia (reflecting the prevalence of hepatitis B) to 10 per 100 000 in southern Europe and 5 per 100 000 in northern Europe. The incidence in Europe and North America has risen recently; this is probably related to an increase in hepatitis C cirrhosis.

Hepatitis B vaccination has led to a fall in HCC in countries with a high prevalence of hepatitis B, such as Taiwan.

Chronic hepatitis B infection increases the risk of HCC 100-fold and is the major risk factor for HCC world-wide. The risk of HCC is 0.4% per year in the absence of cirrhosis and 2–6% in cirrhosis. The risk is four times higher in HBeAg-positive than in HBeAg-negative individuals.

Cirrhosis is present in 75–90% of individuals with HCC and is an important risk factor for the disease. The risk is between 1 and 5% in cirrhosis caused by hepatitis B and C. There is also an increased risk in cirrhosis due to haemochromatosis, alcohol, NASH and α_1-antitrypsin deficiency. In northern Europe 90% of those with HCC have underlying cirrhosis, compared to 30% in Taiwan where hepatitis B is the main risk factor.

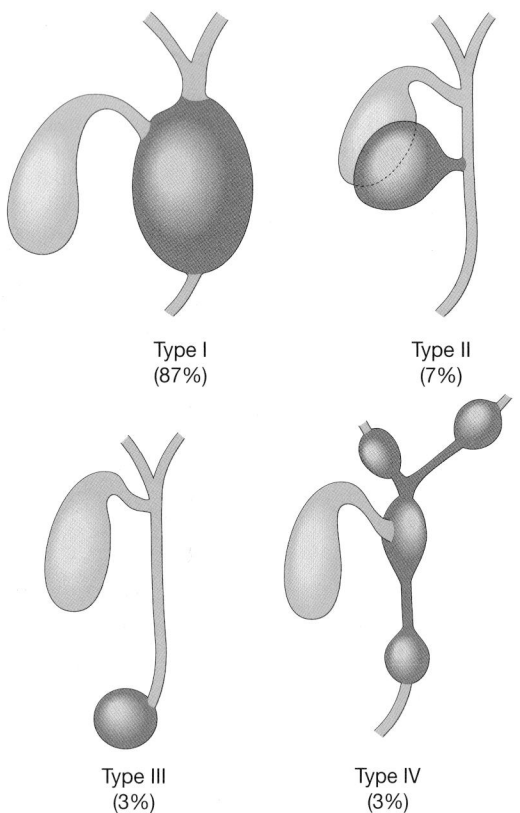

Type I
(87%)

Type II
(7%)

Type III
(3%)

Type IV
(3%)

Fig. 23.41 Classification and frequency of choledochal cysts.

The risk is higher in men and rises with age. Women with PBC do not seem to be at an increased risk of HCC.

Macroscopically, the tumour usually appears as a single mass in the absence of cirrhosis, or as a single or multiple nodules in the presence of cirrhosis. It takes its blood supply from the hepatic artery and tends to spread by invasion into the portal vein and its radicals. Lymph node metastases are common, but lung and bone metastases are rare.

Well-differentiated tumours can resemble normal hepatocytes and can be difficult to distinguish from normal liver.

Clinical features

In patients with underlying cirrhosis there may be ascites, jaundice and variceal haemorrhage. Other symptoms include weight loss, anorexia and abdominal pain. Many tumours detected through screening programmes are asymptomatic. In patients without cirrhosis, tumours are often much larger at presentation (usually > 5 cm), in which case abdominal pain and weight loss are more common.

Examination may reveal hepatomegaly or a right hypochondrial mass. Tumour vascularity can lead to an abdominal bruit, and hepatic rupture with intra-abdominal bleeding may occur.

Investigations

Serum markers

Alpha-fetoprotein (AFP) is produced by 60% of HCCs. Levels increase with the size of the tumour and are often normal in small tumours detected by ultrasound screening. Serum AFP also rises in the presence of active hepatitis B and C viral replication; very high levels are seen in acute hepatic necrosis, such as that following paracetamol toxicity. AFP is used in conjunction with ultrasound in screening but, in view of low sensitivity and specificity, levels need to be interpreted with caution. Nevertheless, in the absence of a marked hepatic flare of disease, a progressively rising AFP, or AFP > 400 ng/mL (normal < 10 ng/mL) necessitates an aggressive search for HCC.

Imaging

Ultrasound scanning will detect focal liver lesions as small as 2–3 cm. The use of ultrasound contrast agents has increased sensitivity and specificity, but the technique is highly user-dependent. Ultrasound may also show evidence of portal vein involvement and features of coexistent cirrhosis. Helical CT, following intravenous contrast, identifies HCC by its classical hypervascular appearance (Fig. 23.42). Small lesions of less than 2 cm can be difficult to differentiate from hyperplastic nodules in cirrhosis. MRI can be used instead of helical CT. Hepatocellular cancers are characteristically hypo-intense on T1-weighted imaging and hyperintense on T2-weighted imaging. Imaging techniques tend to underestimate the multifocal nature of the tumour and combinations of ultrasound scanning and CT or MRI are often helpful. Angiography is now seldom performed and has been superseded by the above techniques.

Liver biopsy

Histological confirmation is advisable in patients with large tumours who do not have cirrhosis or hepatitis B, in order to confirm the diagnosis and exclude metastatic tumour. Biopsy should be avoided in patients who

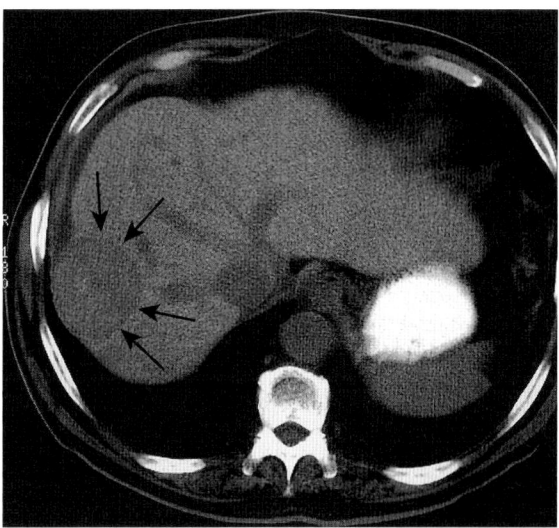

Fig. 23.42 CT showing a large hepatocellular carcinoma (arrows).

may be eligible for transplantation or surgical resection because there is a small (< 2%) risk of tumour seeding along the needle tract.

Role of screening

Screening for HCC, by ultrasound scanning and AFP measurements at 3–6-month intervals, is indicated in high-risk patients, such as those with cirrhosis due to hepatitis B and C, haemochromatosis, alcohol and α_1-AT deficiency. It may also be indicated in individuals with chronic hepatitis B (who carry an increased risk of HCC, even in the absence of cirrhosis). Although no randomised controlled studies of outcome have been undertaken, screening has been shown to identify smaller tumours, often less than 3 cm in size, which are more likely to be cured by surgical resection, local ablative therapy or transplantation (Box 23.62).

Management

This is different for patients with cirrhosis and those without (see Box 23.62). An algorithm for managing those with cirrhosis is shown in Figure 23.43; it is integral to the European and American Study of the Liver

---

EBM | **23.62 Guidelines for screening and management of hepatocellular carcinoma**

'Cirrhotic patients who would be suitable for curative therapy if diagnosed with hepatocellular carcinoma should be offered screening with 6-monthly ultrasound and AFP testing.'

'Curative therapies for hepatocellular carcinoma include liver transplantation, hepatic resection and ablative therapy. Treatment depends on the presence/absence of cirrhosis, underlying liver function, tumour size and tumour multicentricity.'

- Bruix J, et al. (European Association for the Study of the Liver consensus conference). J Hepatol 2001; 35:421–430.
- Bruix J, et al. (American Association for the Study of the Liver practice guidelines). Hepatology 2005; 42:1208–1236.

For further information: 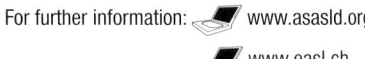 www.asasld.org

www.easl.ch

23

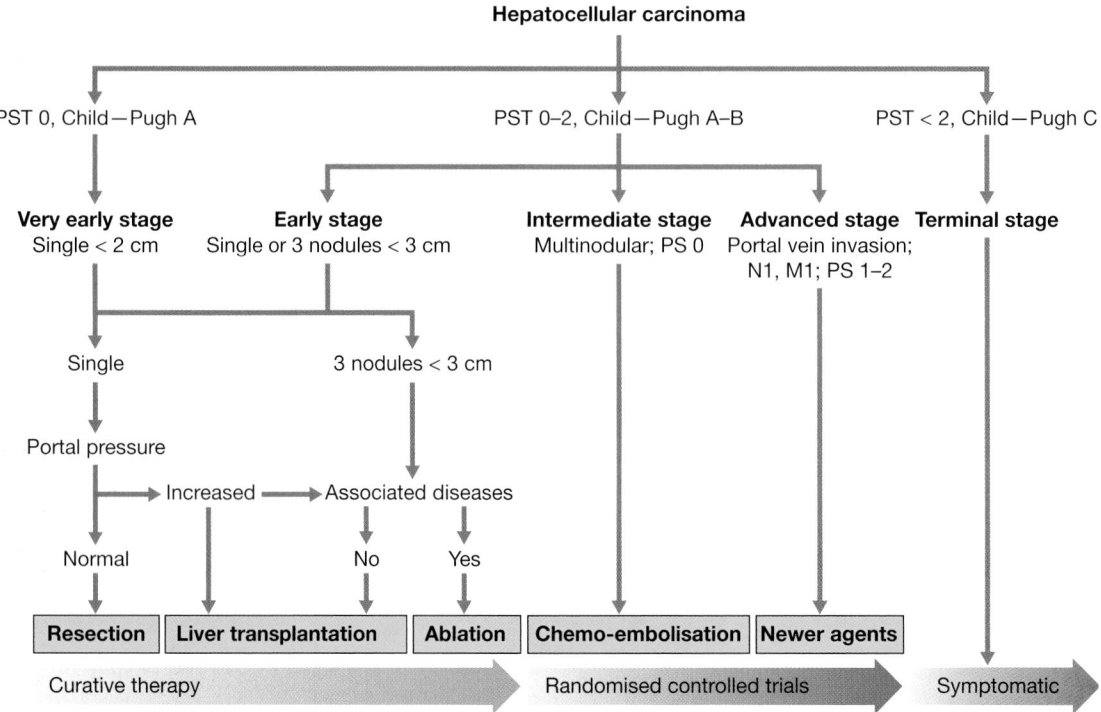

Fig. 23.43 Management of hepatocellular carcinoma (HCC) complicating cirrhosis. Performance status (PST; see Box 11.4, p. 263): 0 = fully active, no symptoms; > 2 = limited self-care, confined to bed or chair for 50% of waking hours. Child-Pugh score: see Box 23.29, p. 945. N1, M1: lymph node involvement and metastases (for TNM classification, see Box 11.1, p. 261).

guidelines. In the presence of cirrhosis, tumour size, multicentricity, extent of liver disease (Child–Pugh score) and performance status dictate appropriate therapy.

Prognosis depends on tumour size, the presence of vascular invasion, and liver function in those with cirrhosis. Screening has improved the outlook through early detection.

Hepatic resection

This is the treatment of choice for non-cirrhotic patients. The 5-year survival in this group is about 50%. However, there is a 50% recurrence rate at 5 years; this may be due to a second de novo tumour or recurrence of the original tumour. Few patients with cirrhosis are amenable to hepatic resection because of the high risk of hepatic failure; nevertheless, surgery is offered, particularly in the Far East, to some cirrhotic patients with small tumours and good liver function (Child–Pugh A with no portal hypertension).

Liver transplantation

Transplantation has the benefit of curing the cirrhosis and removing the risk of a second de novo tumour. The 5-year survival following liver transplantation is 75% for single tumours less than 5 cm in size or three tumours smaller than 3 cm. Unfortunately, the underlying liver disease, such as hepatitis B and C, may recur in the transplanted liver.

Percutaneous ablation

Percutaneous ethanol injection into the tumour under ultrasound guidance is efficacious (80% cure rate) for tumours of 3 cm or smaller. Recurrence rates (50% at 3 years) are similar to those following surgical resection. Radiofrequency ablation, using a single electrode inserted into the tumour under radiological guidance, is an alternative means of ablation that takes longer to perform but appears to cause more complete tumour necrosis.

Transarterial chemo-embolisation (TACE)

Hepatocellular cancers are not radiosensitive and the response rate to chemotherapy with drugs such as doxorubicin is only around 30%. In contrast, hepatic artery embolisation with Gelfoam and doxorubicin is more effective, with survival rates of 60% in cirrhotic patients with unresectable HCC and good liver function (compared with 20% in untreated patients) at 2 years. Unfortunately, any survival benefit is lost at 4 years. TACE is contraindicated in decompensated cirrhosis and multifocal HCC.

Chemotherapy

A phase III trial has indicated an improvement in survival from 7.9 to 10.7 months in cirrhotic patients given intravenous sorafenib. The drug is a multikinase inhibitor with activity against Raf, VEGF and PDGF signalling, and is the first systemic therapy to prolong survival in this tumour.

Fibrolamellar hepatocellular carcinoma

This rare variant differs from the more common HCC in that it occurs in young adults, equally in males and females, in the absence of hepatitis B infection and cirrhosis. The tumours are often large at presentation and the AFP is usually normal. Histology of the tumour reveals malignant hepatocytes that are surrounded by a dense fibrous stroma. The treatment of choice is surgical resection. This variant of HCC has a better prognosis following surgery than an equivalent-sized HCC, two-thirds of patients surviving beyond 5 years.

Other primary malignant tumours

These are rare but include haemangio-endothelial sarcomas.

Secondary malignant tumours

These are common and usually originate from carcinomas in the lung, breast, abdomen or pelvis. They may be single or multiple. Peritoneal dissemination frequently results in ascites.

Clinical features

The primary neoplasm is asymptomatic in about 50% of patients. There is usually liver enlargement and weight loss; jaundice may be present.

Investigations

A raised ALP activity is the most common biochemical abnormality, but LFTs may be normal. Ascitic fluid, if present, has a high protein content and may be blood-stained; cytology sometimes reveals malignant cells. Imaging (p. 928) usually shows up filling defects (Fig. 23.44); laparoscopy may reveal the tumour and facilitates liver biopsy.

Management

Hepatic resection can improve survival for slow-growing tumours such as colonic carcinomas. Patients with neuro-endocrine tumours, such as gastrinomas, insulinomas and glucagonomas, and those with lymphomas may benefit from surgery, hormonal treatment or chemotherapy. Unfortunately, palliative treatment to relieve pain is all that is available for most patients; this may include arterial embolisation of the tumour masses.

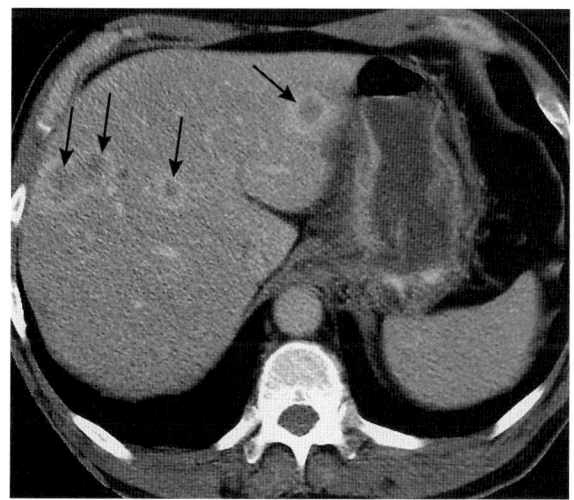

Fig. 23.44 CT showing multiple liver metastases (arrows).

Benign tumours

The increasing use of ultrasound scanning has led to more frequent identification of incidental benign focal liver lesions.

Haemangiomas

These are the most common benign liver tumours and are present in 1–20% of the population. Most are smaller than 5 cm and rarely cause symptoms (Fig. 23.45). The diagnosis is usually made by ultrasound, but CT may show a low-density lesion with delayed arterial filling. Surgery is only needed for very large symptomatic lesions, or where the diagnosis is in doubt.

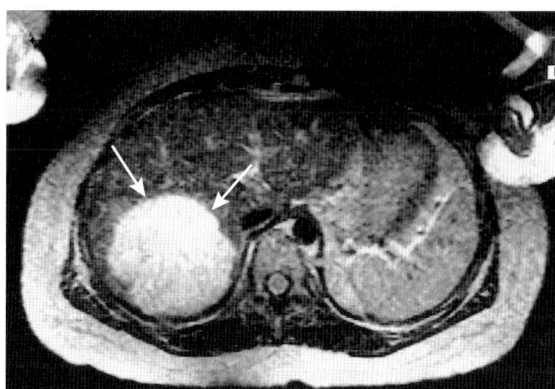

Fig. 23.45 MRI showing a haemangioma (arrows) in the liver.

Hepatic adenomas

These are rare vascular tumours which may present as an abdominal mass, or with abdominal pain or intraperitoneal bleeding. They are more common in women and may be caused by oral contraceptives, androgens and anabolic steroids. Resection is indicated for the relief of symptoms. Hepatic adenomas can increase in size during pregnancy.

Focal nodular hyperplasia

Focal nodular hyperplasia (FNH) is common in women less than 40 years old. The lesions are usually asymptomatic but can be up to 10 cm in diameter; they can be differentiated from adenoma because of a focal central scar seen on CT or MRI. Histologically, they consist of nodular regeneration of hepatocytes but without fibrosis. They may be multiple but rarely need resection.

Liver abscess

Liver abscesses can be classified as pyogenic, hydatid or amoebic.

Pyogenic liver abscess

Pyogenic liver abscesses are uncommon but important because they are potentially curable, inevitably fatal if untreated, and readily overlooked.

The mortality of liver abscesses is 20–40%; failure to make the diagnosis is the most common cause of death. Older patients and those with multiple abscesses also have a higher mortality.

23

Pathophysiology

Infection can reach the liver in several ways (Box 23.63). Pyogenic abscesses are most common in older patients and usually result from ascending infection due to biliary obstruction (cholangitis) or contiguous spread from an empyema of the gallbladder. Abscesses complicating suppurative appendicitis used to be common in young adults but are now rare. Immunocompromised patients are particularly likely to develop liver abscesses. Single lesions are more common in the right liver; multiple abscesses are usually due to infection secondary to biliary obstruction. Abscesses vary greatly in size. *E. coli* and various streptococci, particularly *Strep. milleri*, are the most common organisms; anaerobes, including streptococci and *Bacteroides*, can often be found when infection has been transmitted from large bowel pathology via the portal vein, and multiple organisms are present in one-third of patients.

Clinical features

Patients are generally ill with fever, and sometimes rigors and weight loss. Abdominal pain is the most common symptom and is usually in the right upper quadrant, sometimes with radiation to the right shoulder. The pain may be pleuritic in nature. Hepatomegaly is found in more than 50% of patients, and tenderness can usually be elicited by gentle percussion over the organ. Mild jaundice may be present but is severe only when large abscesses cause biliary obstruction. Abnormalities are present at the base of the right lung in about one-quarter of patients. Atypical presentations are common and explain the frequency with which the diagnosis is made only at postmortem. This is a particular problem in patients with gradually developing illnesses or pyrexia of unknown origin without localising features. Necrotic colorectal metastases can be misdiagnosed as hepatic abscess.

Investigations

Liver imaging is the most revealing investigation and shows 90% or more of symptomatic abscesses. Needle aspiration under ultrasound guidance confirms the diagnosis and provides pus for culture. A leucocytosis is frequently found, plasma ALP activity is usually increased, and the serum albumin is often low. The chest X-ray may show a raised right diaphragm and lung collapse, or an effusion at the base of the right lung. Blood cultures are positive in 50–80%. Abscesses due to gut-derived organisms require active exclusion of significant colonic pathology, such as a colonoscopy to exclude colorectal carcinoma.

Management

This includes prolonged antibiotic therapy and drainage of the abscess. Associated biliary obstruction and cholangitis require biliary drainage (preferably endoscopically). Pending the results of culture of blood and pus from the abscess, treatment should be commenced with a combination of antibiotics such as ampicillin, gentamicin and metronidazole. Aspiration or drainage with a catheter placed in the abscess under ultrasound guidance is required if the abscess is large or if it does not respond to antibiotics. Surgical drainage is rarely undertaken, although hepatic resection may be indicated for a chronic persistent abscess or 'pseudotumour'.

Hydatid cysts

Hydatid cysts are caused by *Echinococcus granulosus* infection (p. 375). They have an outer layer derived from the host, an intermediate laminated layer and an inner germinal layer. They can be single (Fig. 23.46) or multiple. Chronic cysts become calcified. The cysts may be asymptomatic but may present with abdominal pain or a mass. Peripheral blood eosinophilia is present in 20% of cases, whilst X-rays may show calcification of the rim of the abscess. CT reliably shows the cyst(s), and *Echinococcus* ELISA has 90% sensitivity for hepatic hydatid cysts. Rupture or secondary infection of cysts can occur, and a communication with the intrahepatic biliary tree can then result, with associated biliary obstruction.

All patients should be treated medically with albendazole or mebendazole prior to definitive therapy. In the absence of communications with the biliary tree, treatment consists of percutaneous aspiration of the cyst followed by the injection of 100% ethanol into the cysts and then re-aspiration of the cyst contents (PAIR). Where there is communication between the cyst and biliary system, surgical removal of the intact cyst is the preferred treatment.

Amoebic liver abscesses

Amoebic liver abscesses are caused by *Entamoeba histolytica* infection (p. 362). Up to 50% of cases do not have a previous history of intestinal disease. Although

---

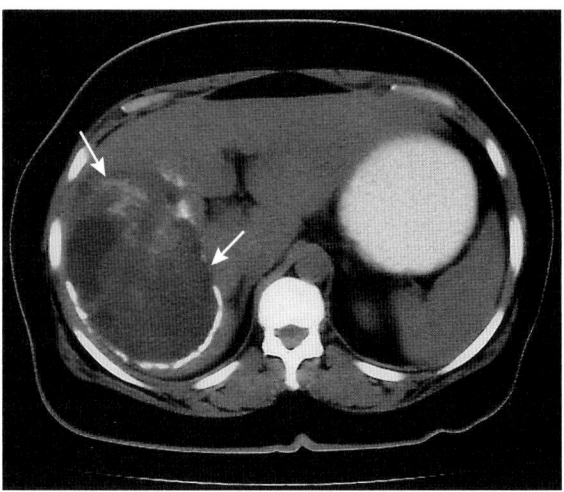

Fig. 23.46 Hydatid cyst of the liver on CT (arrows).

🔍 **23.63 Causes of pyogenic liver abscesses**

- Biliary obstruction (cholangitis)
- Haematogenous
    Portal vein (mesenteric infections)
    Hepatic artery (bacteraemia)
- Direct extension
- Trauma
    Penetrating or non-penetrating
- Infection of liver tumour or cyst

amoebic liver abscesses are most often found in endemic areas, patients can present with no history of travel to these places. Abscesses are usually large, single and located in the right lobe; multiple abscesses may occur in advanced disease. Fever and abdominal pain or swelling are the most common symptoms. Diagnosis may depend on cyst aspiration revealing the classic anchovy sauce appearance of the cyst fluid. Analysis of serum for *Entamoeba* antibodies by immunoassay carries 99% sensitivity and > 90% specificity, and is more accurate than stool analysis in amoebic liver disease. Treatment is described on page 363.

VASCULAR LIVER DISEASES

Hepatic arterial disease

Hepatic arterial disease is rare and difficult to diagnose, but can cause serious liver damage. Hepatic artery occlusion may result from inadvertent injury during biliary surgery or may be caused by emboli, neoplasms, polyarteritis nodosa, blunt trauma or radiation. It usually causes severe upper abdominal pain with or without signs of circulatory shock. LFTs show raised transaminases (AST or ALT usually > 1000 U/L), as in other causes of acute liver damage. Patients usually survive if the liver and portal blood supply are otherwise normal.

Hepatic artery aneurysms are extrahepatic in three-quarters of cases and intrahepatic in one-quarter. Atheroma, vasculitis, bacterial endocarditis, and surgical or biopsy trauma are the main causes. These aneurysms usually cause bleeding into the biliary tree, peritoneum or intestine, and are best diagnosed by arteriography. Treatment is radiological or surgical. Any of the vasculitides can affect the hepatic artery, but this rarely causes symptoms.

Portal venous thrombosis

Portal venous thrombosis is rare but can occur in any condition predisposing to thrombosis. It may also complicate intra-abdominal inflammatory or neoplastic disease, and is a recognised cause of portal hypertension. Acute portal venous thrombosis causes abdominal pain and diarrhoea, and may lead to bowel infarction. This rare complication of infarction requires surgical management. Treatment is otherwise based on anticoagulation, although there are no randomised data on efficacy. An underlying thrombophilia needs to be excluded. Subacute thrombosis can be asymptomatic but may subsequently lead to extrahepatic portal hypertension (p. 945). Ascites is unusual in non-cirrhotic portal hypertension, unless the albumin is particularly low.

Hepatopulmonary syndrome

This is characterised by resistant hypoxaemia (PaO_2 < 9.3 kPa or 70 mmHg), intrapulmonary vascular dilatation and chronic liver disease with portal hypertension. Clinical features include digital clubbing, cyanosis, spider naevi and a characteristic reduction in arterial oxygen saturation on standing. The hypoxia is due to intrapulmonary shunting through direct arteriovenous communications. It is believed that nitric oxide overproduction may be important in pathogenesis, as exhaled NO correlates with the severity of hypoxia. The hepatopulmonary syndrome can be treated by liver transplantation but, if severe (PaO_2 < 6.7 kPa or 50 mmHg), is associated with an increased operative risk.

Portopulmonary hypertension

This unusual complication of portal hypertension is similar to 'primary pulmonary hypertension' (p. 720); it is defined as pulmonary hypertension with increased pulmonary vascular resistance and a normal pulmonary artery wedge pressure in a patient with portal hypertension. It is caused by vasoconstriction and obliteration of the pulmonary arterial system, and leads to breathlessness and fatigue.

Hepatic venous outflow obstruction

Obstruction to hepatic venous blood flow can occur in the small central hepatic veins, the large hepatic veins, the inferior vena cava or the heart. The clinical features depend on the cause and on the speed with which obstruction develops, but congestive hepatomegaly and ascites are consistent features.

Budd–Chiari syndrome
Pathophysiology

This uncommon condition is caused by thrombosis of the larger hepatic veins and sometimes the inferior vena cava. Some patients have haematological disorders such as primary proliferative polycythaemia, paroxysmal nocturnal haemoglobinuria and antithrombin III, protein C or protein S deficiencies (Ch. 24). Pregnancy and oral contraceptive use, obstruction due to tumours (particularly carcinomas of the liver, kidneys or adrenals), congenital venous webs and occasionally inferior vena caval stenosis are the other main causes. The underlying cause cannot be found in about 50% of patients. Hepatic congestion affecting the centrilobular areas is the initial consequence; centrilobular fibrosis develops later and eventually cirrhosis supervenes in those who survive long enough.

Clinical features

Acute venous occlusion causes rapid development of upper abdominal pain, marked ascites and occasionally acute liver failure. More gradual occlusion causes gross ascites and often upper abdominal discomfort. Hepatomegaly, frequently with tenderness over the liver, is almost always present. Peripheral oedema occurs only when there is inferior vena cava obstruction. Features of cirrhosis and portal hypertension develop in those who survive the acute event.

Investigations

The LFTs vary considerably, depending on the presentation, and can show the features of acute hepatitis (p. 926). Ascitic fluid analysis typically shows a protein concentration above 25 g/L (exudate) in the early stages;

23

973

however, this often falls later in the disease. Doppler ultra-sound examination may reveal obliteration of the hepatic veins and reversed flow or associated thrombosis in the portal vein. CT may show enlargement of the caudate lobe, as it often has a separate venous drainage system that is not involved in the disease. CT and MRI may also demonstrate occlusion of the hepatic veins and inferior vena cava. Liver biopsy demonstrates centrilobular congestion with fibrosis, depending on the duration of the illness. Venography is only needed if CT and MRI are unable to demonstrate the hepatic venous anatomy clearly.

Management

Predisposing causes should be treated as far as possible; where recent thrombosis is suspected, treatment with streptokinase followed by heparin and oral anticoagulation should be considered. Ascites is initially treated medically but often with limited success. Short hepatic venous strictures can be treated with angioplasty. In the case of more extensive hepatic vein occlusion, many patients can be managed successfully by insertion of a covered TIPSS followed by anticoagulation. Surgical shunts, such as portacaval shunts, are less commonly performed now that TIPSS is available. Occasionally, a web can be resected or an inferior vena caval stenosis dilated. Progressive liver failure is an indication for liver transplantation and life-long anticoagulation.

The prognosis without transplantation or shunting is poor, particularly following an acute presentation with liver failure. A 3-year survival of 50% is reported in those who survive the initial acute event. The 1- and 10-year survival following liver transplantation is 85% and 69% respectively, and this compares with a 5- and 10-year survival of 87% and 37% following surgical shunting.

Veno-occlusive disease

Veno-occlusive disease (VOD) is a rare condition character-ised by widespread occlusion of the small central hepatic veins. Pyrrolizidine alkaloids in *Senecio* and *Heliotropium* plants used to make teas, cytotoxic drugs and hepatic irra-diation are all recognised causes. VOD may develop in 10–20% of patients following bone marrow transplanta-tion (usually within the first 20 days), and carries a 90% mortality in severe cases. Pathogenesis involves oblitera-tion and fibrosis of terminal hepatic venules, due to depo-sition of red cells, haemosiderin-laden macrophages and coagulation factors. In this setting VOD is thought to relate to pre-conditioning therapy with irradiation and cytotoxic chemotherapy. The clinical features are similar to those of the Budd–Chiari syndrome (see above). Investigations show evidence of venous outflow obstruction histologi-cally but, in contrast to Budd–Chiari, the large hepatic veins appear patent radiologically. Transjugular liver biopsy (with portal pressure measurements) may make the diagnosis. Traditionally, treatment has been support-ive, but defibrotide shows promise (the drug binds to vascular endothelial cells, promoting fibrinolysis and sup-pressing coagulation).

Cardiac disease

Hepatic damage due primarily to congestion may develop in all forms of right heart failure (p. 543); the clinical features are usually dominated by the cardiac disease. Very rarely, long-standing cardiac failure and hepatic congestion cause cardiac cirrhosis.

Ischaemic hepatitis ('shock liver')

Acute heart failure sometimes causes a syndrome sim-ilar to acute hepatitis. This is usually mediated by a reduction in hepatic perfusion, and is termed 'shock liver'. Pre-existing right heart dysfunction is often pres-ent. Common causes include heart surgery, myocardial infarction, decompensation of any chronic myocardial disease, respiratory conditions associated with cor pul-monale and tamponade. The patient is generally very ill with an enlarged, tender liver, jaundice and LFTs show-ing very high serum transaminases (often over 2000 U/L). The correct diagnosis is made by recognising that the cardiac output is low, the jugular venous pressure is high and other signs of cardiac disease are present.

Ascites

Chronic congestive cardiac failure sometimes causes hep-atomegaly and ascites disproportionate to the degree of peripheral oedema, and in the circumstances can mimic ascites due to liver disease. Constrictive pericarditis (p. 639) is easy to overlook as the heart size is normal, but the diagnosis can be confirmed by echocardiography.

Management

Treatment is that of the underlying heart disease.

Nodular regenerative hyperplasia of the liver

This is the most common cause of non-cirrhotic portal hypertension in developed countries; it is characterised by small hepatocyte nodules throughout the liver with-out fibrosis, which can result in sinusoidal compres-sion. The condition is believed to be due to damage to small hepatic arterioles and portal venules. It occurs in older people and has been associated with many con-ditions, including connective tissue disease, haemato-logical diseases and immunosuppressive drugs such as azathioprine used in transplant recipients. The condi-tion is usually asymptomatic, but occasionally presents with portal hypertension or with an abdominal mass. The diagnosis is made by liver biopsy, which, in contrast to cirrhosis, shows nodule formation in the absence of fibrous septa. Liver function is good and the prognosis

23.64 Liver disease in old age

- **Alcoholic liver disease:** 10% of cases present over the age of 70 years, when disease is more likely to be severe and has a worse prognosis.
- **Hepatitis A:** causes more severe illness and runs a more protracted course.
- **Primary biliary cirrhosis:** one-third of cases are over 65 years and age is an adverse prognostic factor.
- **Liver abscess:** more than 50% of all cases in the UK are over 60 years.
- **Hepatocellular carcinoma:** approximately 50% of cases present over the age of 65 years in the UK.
- **Surgery:** older people are less likely to survive liver surgery (including transplantation) because comorbidity is more prevalent.

is very favourable. Management is based on treatment of the portal hypertension.

PREGNANCY AND THE LIVER

Intercurrent and pre-existing liver disease

When elevated serum transaminases are present, acute viral hepatitis and drug causes need to be excluded. Acute hepatitis A can occur during pregnancy but has no effect on the fetus. Chronic hepatitis B requires identification in pregnancy, because of long-term health implications for the mother and the effectiveness of perinatal vaccination (with or without pre-delivery maternal antiviral therapy) in reducing neonatal acquisition of chronic hepatitis B. Maternal transmission of hepatitis C occurs in 1% of cases, and there is no convincing evidence that the mode of delivery affects this. Hepatitis E is reported to progress to acute liver failure much more commonly in pregnancy, with a 20% maternal mortality. Pregnancy may be associated with both worsening and improvement of autoimmune liver disease (e.g. autoimmune hepatitis). Cirrhosis often leads to infertility, but full-term delivery can occur. Complications of portal hypertension may be a particular issue in the second and third trimesters.

Gallstones (p. 977) are more common during pregnancy, and may present with cholecystitis or biliary obstruction. The diagnosis can usually be made with ultrasound. In biliary obstruction due to gallstones, therapeutic ERCP can be safely performed, but lead protection for the fetus is essential and X-ray screening must be kept to an absolute minimum.

Pregnancy-associated liver disease

These conditions only occur during pregnancy, may recur in subsequent pregnancies and resolve after delivery of the baby. The causes of abnormal LFTs in pregnancy, which include pregnancy-associated liver disease, are shown in Box 23.65.

Intrahepatic cholestasis of pregnancy

This accounts for 20% of cases of jaundice in pregnancy; it usually occurs in the third trimester of pregnancy but can occur earlier. It is associated with intrauterine growth retardation and premature birth. There is a high prevalence in Chile. The condition characteristically presents with itching and cholestatic LFTs; however, the bilirubin may be normal and the liver biochemistry hepatitic. Bile salts are elevated in the serum. Delivery leads to resolution, and pregnancy should not continue beyond term. UDCA effectively controls itching and probably prevents premature birth; it should be given at a daily dose of 15 mg/kg. Recurrence of cholestasis occurs in 60% of future pregnancies.

Acute fatty liver of pregnancy

This is more common in twin and first pregnancies; it occurs in 1 in 14 000 pregnancies in the USA. It typi-

23.65 Abnormal liver function tests in pregnancy

- **Liver function tests:** ALT levels and albumin normally fall in pregnancy. ALP levels can rise due to the contribution of placental ALP.
- **Pre-existing liver disease:** pregnancy is uncommon in cirrhosis due to infertility. Variceal bleeding can occur if varices present prior to conception, and ascites or polyhydramnios should be treated with amiloride rather than spironolactone. Penicillamine for Wilson's disease and azathioprine for autoimmune liver disease should be continued during pregnancy. Autoimmune liver disease can flare up post-partum.
- **Unrelated liver disease:** viral- and drug-induced hepatitis must be excluded in the presence of an elevated ALT. Immunoglobulin/vaccination given to the fetus at birth prevents transmission of hepatitis B to the mother if the mother is infected. Gallstones are more common in pregnancy and post-partum, and are a cause of a raised ALP level. Biliary imaging with ultrasound and MRCP is safe. ERCP can be performed safely to remove stones with shielding of the fetus from radiation.
- **Pregnancy-related liver diseases:** occur predominantly in the third trimester and resolve post-partum. Maternal and fetal mortality and morbidity are prevented by early delivery.

cally presents between 31 and 38 weeks of pregnancy with vomiting and abdominal pain followed by jaundice. In severe cases this may be followed by lactic acidosis, a coagulopathy, encephalopathy and renal failure. Hypoglycaemia can also occur. The features are characteristic of a defect in beta-oxidation of fatty acids in the mitochondria that leads to the formation of small fat droplets in liver cells (known as microvesicular fatty liver). Some women are heterozygous for loss-of-function mutations in the long-chain 3-hydroxyacyl-CoA dehydrogenase (*LCHAD*) gene. Other causes of microvesicular steatosis due to defects in mitochondrial beta-oxidation of fatty acids that have a similar clinical presentation outside pregnancy are shown in Box 23.66. Differentiation from toxaemia of pregnancy (which is more common) can be achieved by the finding of high serum uric acid levels and the absence of haemolysis. Overlap between acute fatty liver of pregnancy, HELLP (see below) and toxaemia of pregnancy can occur. Early diagnosis, specialist care and delivery of the fetus have led to a fall in maternal and perinatal mortality to 1% and 7% respectively.

Toxaemia of pregnancy and HELLP

The HELLP syndrome (haemolysis, elevated liver enzymes and low platelets) is a variant of pre-eclampsia that tends to affect multiparous women. It usually presents at 27–36 weeks of pregnancy with hypertension, proteinuria and

23.66 Hepatic mitochondrial cytopathies

- Acute fatty liver of pregnancy
- Drugs
  Sodium valproate
  Tetracyclines
- Reye's syndrome (aspirin toxicity in childhood)
- Toxins
  Bacillus cereus

23

fluid retention. Jaundice only occurs in 5% of cases. Blood tests may show low haemoglobin, with fragmented red cells, markedly elevated serum transaminases and raised D-dimers. The condition can be complicated by hepatic infarction and rupture. Maternal complications also include disseminated intravascular coagulation and placental abruption. Maternal mortality is 1% and perinatal mortality can be up to 30%. Delivery usually leads to prompt resolution, and disease recurs in < 5% of subsequent pregnancies.

LIVER TRANSPLANTATION

The outcome following liver transplantation has improved significantly over the last decade and this is now an effective treatment for end-stage liver disease. The number of procedures is limited by cadaveric donor availability, and in many parts of the world this has led to living donor transplant programmes. Despite this, 10% of those listed for liver transplantation will die while awaiting a donor liver. The main complications of liver transplantation relate to disease recurrence in the liver graft.

Indications and contraindications

Currently, around 9500 liver transplants are undertaken in Europe and the USA per year. About 10% are performed for acute liver failure, 6% for metabolic diseases, 71% for cirrhosis and 11% for hepatocellular carcinoma. Most patients are under 60 years of age, and only 10% are aged between 60 and 70 years. In North America the most common indication is hepatitis C cirrhosis, about 10–20% of transplants being for alcoholic cirrhosis (Fig. 23.47). Patients with alcoholic liver disease need to show a capacity for abstinence.

Liver transplantation in cirrhosis is considered when the anticipated mortality without transplantation exceeds 50% at 1 year (Box 23.67).

The main contraindications to transplantation are sepsis, extrahepatic malignancy, active alcohol or other substance misuse, and marked cardiorespiratory dysfunction.

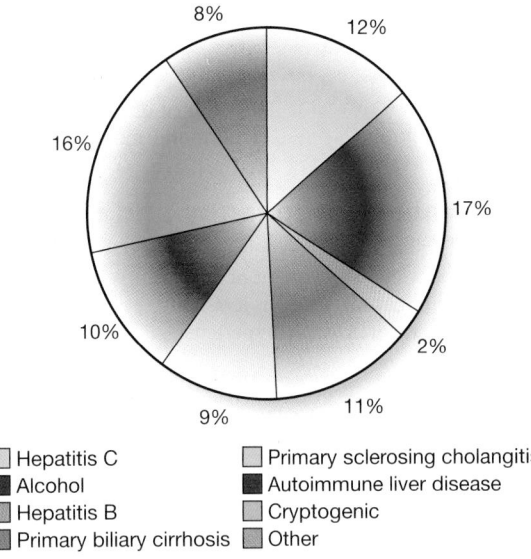

Fig. 23.47 Indications for liver transplantation in the UK between 2001 and 2005.

Legend:
- Hepatitis C
- Alcohol
- Hepatitis B
- Primary biliary cirrhosis
- Primary sclerosing cholangitis
- Autoimmune liver disease
- Cryptogenic
- Other

23.67 Indications for liver transplant assessment for cirrhosis

Complications

- First episode of bacterial peritonitis
- Diuretic-resistant ascites
- Recurrent variceal haemorrhage
- Hepatocellular carcinoma < 5 cm
- Persistent hepatic encephalopathy

Poor liver function

- Bilirubin > 100 µmol/L (5.8 mg/dL) in primary biliary cirrhosis
- MELD score > 12
- Child–Pugh C

In many parts of the world the MELD score (see Box 23.31, p. 945) is used to identify and prioritise patients for transplantation. Patients are ABO- and size-matched, but not HLA-matched with donors.

Two types of transplant are increasingly used because of insufficient cadaveric donors:

- **Split liver transplantation.** A cadaveric donor liver can be split into two, with the larger right lobe used in an adult and the smaller left lobe used in a child. This practice has led to an increase in donor organs.
- **Living donor transplantation.** This is normally performed using the left lateral segment or the right lobe. The donor mortality is significant at 0.5%–1%. Pre-operative assessment includes looking at donor liver size and psychological status.

Complications

Early complications

Less immunosuppression is needed following liver transplantation than with kidney and heart/lung grafting. Initial immunosuppression is usually with tacrolimus or ciclosporin, prednisolone and azathioprine or mycophenolate. Some patients can eventually be maintained on a single agent.

- **Acute rejection.** This occurs in up to 60% of patients, usually within the first 6 weeks after transplantation, and normally responds to 3 days of high-dose methylprednisolone.
- **Surgical complications.** These include hepatic artery thrombosis, which may necessitate retransplantation. Anastomotic biliary strictures can also occur, and may respond to balloon dilatation or require surgical reconstruction. Portal vein thrombosis is rare.
- **Infections.** Bacterial infections such as pneumonia and wound infections can occur in the first few weeks after transplantation. Cytomegalovirus (primary infection or reactivation) is a common infection in the 3 months after transplantation and can cause hepatitis. Patients who have never had cytomegalovirus infection but who receive a liver from a donor who has been exposed are at greatest risk of infection, and are usually given prophylactic antiviral therapy such as valciclovir. Tuberculous prophylaxis is given to recipients who have had previous exposure to tuberculosis for the first 6 months after transplantation to prevent reactivation.

Late complications

These include recurrence of the initial disease in the graft and complications due to the immunosuppressive therapy, such as renal impairment from ciclosporin. Chronic vascular rejection is rare, occurring in only 5% of cases.

Prognosis

The outcome following transplantation for acute liver failure is worse than for chronic liver disease because most patients have multi-organ failure at the time of transplantation. The 1-year survival is 65% and falls only a little to 59% at 5 years. The 1-year survival for patients with cirrhosis is 80–90%, falling to 70–75% at 5 years.

GALLBLADDER AND EXTRAHEPATIC BILIARY DISEASE

Gallstones

Gallstone formation is the most common disorder of the biliary tree and it is unusual for the gallbladder to be diseased in the absence of gallstones. In developed countries gallstones are common and occur in 7% of males and 15% of females aged 18–65 years, with an overall prevalence of 11%. In those under 40 years there is a 3:1 female preponderance, whereas in the elderly the sex ratio is about equal. In developed countries the incidence of symptomatic gallstones appears to be increasing and they occur at an earlier age. Gallstones are less frequent in India, the Far East and Africa.

There has been much debate over the role of diet in cholesterol gallstone disease; an increase in dietary cholesterol, fat, total calories and refined carbohydrate or lack of dietary fibre has been implicated. At present, the best data support an association between simple refined sugar in the diet and gallstones. There is a negative association between a moderate alcohol intake (2–3 units daily) and gallstones.

Pathophysiology

Gallstones are conveniently classified into cholesterol or pigment stones, although the majority are of mixed composition. Cholesterol stones are most common in developed countries, whereas pigment stones are more frequent in developing countries. Gallstones contain varying quantities of calcium salts, including calcium bilirubinate, carbonate, phosphate and palmitate, which are radio-opaque.

Gallstone formation is multifactorial, and the factors involved are related to the type of gallstone (Boxes 23.68 and 23.69).

Cholesterol gallstones

Cholesterol is held in solution in bile by its association with bile acids and phospholipids in the form of micelles and vesicles. Biliary lipoproteins may also have a role in solubilising cholesterol. In gallstone disease the liver produces bile which contains an excess of cholesterol, because there is either a relative deficiency of bile salts or a relative excess of cholesterol. Bile, which is supersaturated with cholesterol, is termed 'lithogenic'. Disorders with the potential to induce the production of lithogenic bile are shown in Box 23.70. Factors initiating crystallisation of cholesterol in lithogenic bile

23.68 Risk factors and mechanisms for cholesterol gallstones

↑ **Cholesterol secretion**

- Old age
- Female gender
- Pregnancy
- Obesity
- Rapid weight loss

Impaired gallbladder emptying

- Pregnancy
- Gallbladder stasis
- Fasting
- Total parenteral nutrition
- Spinal cord injury

↓ **Bile salt secretion**

- Pregnancy

23.69 Composition of and risk factors for pigment stones

	Black	Brown
Composition	Polymerised calcium bilirubinates* Mucin glycoprotein Calcium phosphate Calcium carbonate Cholesterol	Calcium bilirubinate crystals* Mucin glycoprotein Cholesterol Calcium palmitate/stearate
Risk factors	Haemolysis Age Hepatic cirrhosis Ileal resection/disease	Infected bile Stasis

*Major component.

23

(nucleation factors) are also important; patients with cholesterol gallstones have gallbladder bile which forms cholesterol crystals more rapidly than equally saturated bile from patients who do not form gallstones. Factors favouring nucleation (mucus, calcium, fatty acids, other proteins) and antinucleating factors (apolipoproteins) have been described.

Pigment stones

Brown crumbly pigment stones are almost always the consequence of bacterial or parasitic infection in the biliary tree. They are common in the Far East, where infection of the biliary tree allows bacterial β-glucuronidase to hydrolyse conjugated bilirubin to its free form, which then precipitates as calcium bilirubinate. The mechanism of black pigment gallstone formation in developed countries is not satisfactorily explained. Haemolysis is important, as these stones occur in chronic haemolytic disease.

23.70 Pathogenic factors leading to the production of lithogenic bile

- Defective bile salt synthesis
- Excessive intestinal loss of bile salts
- Over-sensitive bile salt feedback
- Excessive cholesterol secretion
- Abnormal gallbladder function

Biliary sludge

The term 'biliary sludge' describes gelatinous bile that contains numerous microspheroliths of calcium bilirubinate granules and cholesterol crystals, as well as glycoproteins; it is an important precursor to the formation of gallstones in the majority of patients. Biliary sludge is frequently formed under normal conditions, but then either dissolves or is cleared by the gallbladder; only in about 15% of patients does it persist to form cholesterol stones. Fasting, parenteral nutrition and pregnancy are also associated with sludge formation.

Clinical features

The majority of gallstones are asymptomatic and only about 10% of those with gallstones develop clinical evidence of gallstone disease.

Symptomatic stones within the gallbladder (Box 23.71) manifest as either biliary pain ('biliary colic') or cholecystitis (see below). If a gallstone becomes acutely impacted in the cystic duct, the patient will experience pain. The term 'biliary colic' is a misnomer because the pain does not rhythmically increase and decrease in intensity like other forms of colic. Typically, the pain occurs suddenly and persists for about 2 hours; if it continues for more than 6 hours, a complication such as cholecystitis or pancreatitis may be present. Pain is usually felt in the epigastrium (70% of patients) or right upper quadrant (20% of patients), and radiates to the interscapular region or the tip of the right scapula, but other sites include the left upper quadrant and the lower chest. The pain can mimic intrathoracic disease, oesophagitis, myocardial infarction or dissecting aneurysm.

Combinations of fatty food intolerance, dyspepsia and flatulence not attributable to other causes have been referred to as 'gallstone dyspepsia'. These symptoms are not now recognised as being caused by gallstones and are best regarded as non-ulcer dyspepsia (p. 851).

Acute and chronic cholecystitis is described below.

A mucocele may develop if there is slow distension of the gallbladder from continuous secretion of mucus; if this material becomes infected, an empyema supervenes. Calcium may be secreted into the lumen of the hydropic gallbladder, causing 'limey' bile, and if calcium salts are precipitated in the gallbladder wall, the radiological appearance of 'porcelain' gallbladder results.

Gallstones in the gallbladder (cholecystolithiasis) migrate to the common bile duct (choledocholithiasis, p. 980) in approximately 15% of patients and cause biliary colic. Rarely, fistulae develop between the gallbladder and the duodenum, colon or stomach. If this occurs, air will be seen in the biliary tree on plain abdominal X-rays. If a stone larger than 2.5 cm in diameter has migrated into the gut, it may impact either at the terminal ileum or occasionally in the duodenum or sigmoid colon. The resultant intestinal obstruction may be followed by 'gallstone ileus'. Gallstones impacted in the cystic duct may cause stricturing of the common hepatic duct and obstructive jaundice (Mirizzi's syndrome), which may be confused with a malignant bile duct stricture. The more common cause of jaundice due to gallstones is a stone passing from the cystic duct into the common bile duct (choledocholithiasis), which may also result in cholangitis or acute pancreatitis. It is usually very small stones that precipitate acute pancreatitis, due (it is thought) to oedema at the ampulla as the stone passes into the duodenum (no stone is seen within the bile duct in 80% of cases of presumed gallstone pancreatitis, suggesting stone passage). Previous stone passage is also the likely cause of most cases of benign papillary fibrosis, which is most commonly seen in patients with previous or present gallstone disease (it may present with jaundice, obstructive LFTs with biliary dilatation, post-cholecystectomy pain or acute pancreatitis).

Cancer of the gallbladder is uncommon (p. 981) but in over 95% of cases is associated with gallstones. The diagnosis is usually made as an incidental histological finding following cholecystectomy for gallstone disease.

Investigations

Ultrasound is the investigation of choice for diagnosing gallstones. Most stones are diagnosed by transabdominal ultrasound, which has a > 92% sensitivity and 99% specificity for gallbladder stones (see Fig. 23.8, p. 927). CT (Fig. 23.48) and MRCP are excellent modalities for detecting complications of gallstones (distal bile duct stone or gallbladder empyema), but are inferior to ultrasound in defining their presence in the gallbladder.

23.71 Clinical features and complications of gallstones	
Clinical features	
• Asymptomatic (80%)	• Acute cholecystitis
• Biliary colic	• Chronic cholecystitis
Complications	
• Empyema of the gallbladder	• Pressure on/inflammation of the common bile duct by a gallstone in the cystic duct (Mirizzi's syndrome)
• Porcelain gallbladder	
• Choledocholithiasis	
• Acute pancreatitis	
• Fistulae between the gallbladder and duodenum or colon	• Cancer of the gallbladder
• Gallstone ileus	

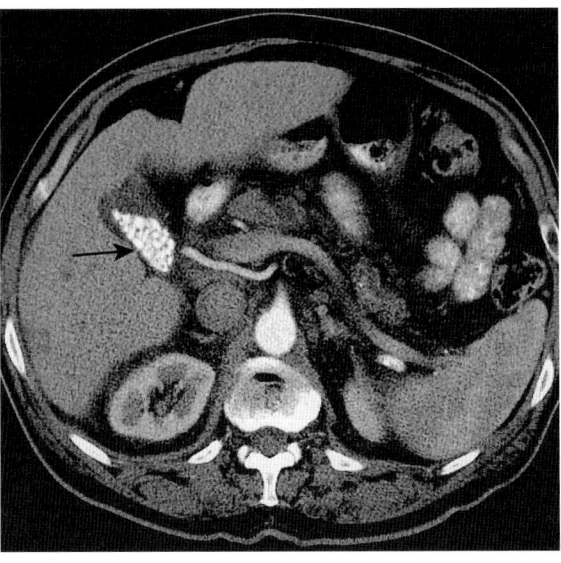

Fig. 23.48 CT showing a gallstone within the gallbladder (arrow).

Management

Asymptomatic gallstones found incidentally should not be treated because the majority will never cause symptoms. Symptomatic gallstones are best treated surgically by laparoscopic cholecystectomy. Non-surgical methods to dissolve gallstones or fragment gallbladder stones may be tried if surgery is not an option. Various techniques can be used to treat common bile duct stones (Box 23.72).

23.72 Treatment of gallstones

Gallbladder stones

- Cholecystectomy: open or laparoscopic
- Oral bile acids: chenodeoxycholic or ursodeoxycholic (low rate of stone dissolution)

Bile duct stones

- Lithotripsy (endoscopic or extracorporeal shock wave, ESWL)
- Endoscopic sphincterotomy and balloon trawl
- Surgical bile duct exploration

Medical dissolution of gallstones can be attempted by long-term oral administration of the bile acid UDCA. Medical treatment should be considered in those with radiolucent gallstones, a gallbladder that opacifies on oral cholecystography, stones smaller than 15 mm in diameter, moderate obesity and no or at most mild symptoms. Success can be expected in approximately 75% of patients who fulfil these criteria. An alternative is extracorporeal shock-wave lithotripsy (ESWL) but this is expensive and not widely available. Bile salt therapy is necessary following lithotripsy to dissolve the gallstone fragments within the gallbladder. Only 30% of patients with gallbladder disease are suitable for lithotripsy. All therapeutic regimens which retain the gallbladder have a 50% recurrence of stones after 5 years.

Cholecystitis

Acute cholecystitis

Pathophysiology

Acute cholecystitis is almost always associated with obstruction of the gallbladder neck or cystic duct by a gallstone. Occasionally, obstruction may be by mucus, parasitic worms or a bile tumour, or may follow endoscopic stent insertion. The pathogenesis is unclear, but the initial inflammation is possibly chemically induced. This leads to gallbladder mucosal damage which releases phospholipase, converting biliary lecithin to lysolecithin, a recognised mucosal toxin. At the time of surgery, approximately 50% of cultures of the gallbladder contents are sterile. Infection occurs eventually and in elderly patients or those with diabetes mellitus a severe infection with gas-forming organisms can cause emphysematous cholecystitis. Acalculous cholecystitis can occur in the intensive care setting and in association with parenteral nutrition, sickle cell disease and diabetes mellitus.

Clinical features

The cardinal feature is pain in the right upper quadrant but also in the epigastrium, the right shoulder tip or the interscapular region. Differentiation between biliary colic (p. 978) and acute cholecystitis may be difficult; features suggesting cholecystitis include severe and prolonged pain, fever and leucocytosis.

Examination shows right hypochondrial tenderness, rigidity worse on inspiration (Murphy's sign) and occasionally a gallbladder mass (30% of cases). Fever is present but rigors are unusual. Jaundice occurs in less than 10% of patients and is usually due to passage of stones into the common bile duct or to Mirizzi's syndrome. Gallbladder perforation occurs in 10–15% of cases, and gallbladder empyema may occur.

Investigations

Peripheral blood leucocytosis is common, except in the elderly patient in whom the signs of inflammation may be minimal. Minor increases of transaminases and amylase may be encountered. Amylase should be measured to detect acute pancreatitis (p. 888), which may be a potentially serious complication of gallstones. Only when the amylase is > 1000 U/L can pain be confidently attributed to acute pancreatitis, since moderately elevated levels of amylase can occur in many other causes of abdominal pain. Plain X-rays of the abdomen and chest may show radio-opaque gallstones, and rarely intrabiliary gas due to fistulation of a gallstone into the intestine; they are important in excluding lower lobe pneumonia and a perforated viscus. Ultrasonography detects gallstones and gallbladder thickening due to cholecystitis, but gallbladder empyema or perforation is best excluded with CT.

Management
Medical

This consists of bed rest, pain relief, antibiotics and maintenance of fluid balance. Moderate pain can be treated with NSAID but more severe pain should be treated with pethidine. A cephalosporin (such as cefuroxime) is the antibiotic of choice, but metronidazole is usually added in severely ill patients. Fluid balance is maintained by intravenous therapy, and nasogastric aspiration is only needed for persistent vomiting. Cholecystitis usually resolves with medical treatment, but the inflammation may progress to an empyema or perforation and peritonitis.

Surgical

Urgent surgery is the optimal treatment when cholecystitis progresses in spite of medical therapy and when complications such as empyema or perforation develop. Operation should be carried out within 5 days of the onset of symptoms. Delayed surgery after 2–3 months is no longer favoured. In patients in whom cholecystectomy may be difficult due to extensive inflammatory change, percutaneous gallbladder drainage can be performed, with subsequent cholecystectomy 4–6 weeks later. Recurrent biliary colic or cholecystitis is frequent if the gallbladder is not removed.

Chronic cholecystitis

Chronic inflammation of the gallbladder is almost invariably associated with gallstones. The usual symptoms are those of recurrent attacks of upper abdominal pain, often at night and following a heavy meal. The clinical features are similar to those of acute calculous cholecystitis but milder. The patient may recover spontaneously or following analgesia and antibiotics. Patients are usually advised to undergo elective laparoscopic cholecystectomy.

Acute cholangitis

Acute cholangitis is caused by bacterial infection of bile ducts and occurs in patients with other biliary problems such as choledocholithiasis (see below), biliary strictures or tumours, or after ERCP. Jaundice, rigors and abdominal pain are the main presenting features. Treatment is with antibiotics, relief of biliary obstruction and removal (if possible) of the underlying cause.

Choledocholithiasis

Stones in the common bile duct (choledocholithiasis) occur in 10–15% of patients with gallstones (Fig. 23.49) which have usually migrated from the gallbladder. Primary bile duct stones are rare but can develop within the common bile duct many years after a cholecystectomy, and are sometimes related to biliary sludge arising from dysfunction of the sphincter of Oddi. In Far Eastern countries, where bile duct infection is common, primary common bile duct stones are thought to follow bacterial infection secondary to parasitic infections with *Clonorchis sinensis*, *Ascaris lumbricoides* or *Fasciola hepatica* (pp. 365 and 373). Common bile duct stones can cause partial or complete bile duct obstruction and may be complicated by cholangitis due to secondary bacterial infection, septicaemia, liver abscess and biliary stricture.

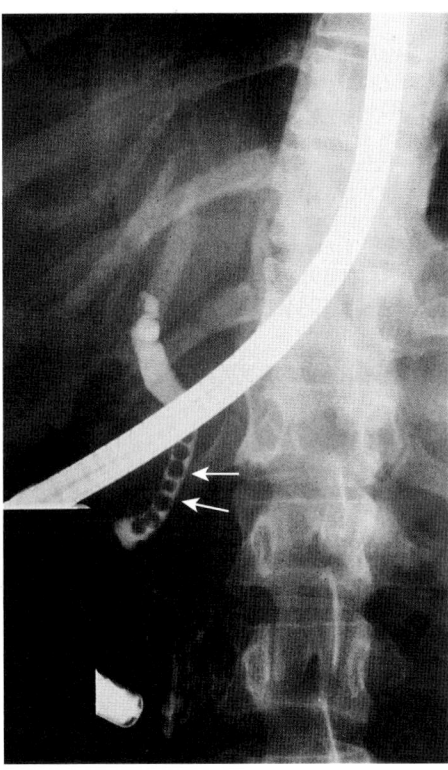

Fig. 23.49 ERCP showing common duct stones (arrows).

Clinical features

Choledocholithiasis may be asymptomatic, may be found incidentally by operative cholangiography at cholecystectomy, or may manifest as recurrent abdominal pain with or without jaundice. The pain is usually in the right upper quadrant, and fever, pruritus and dark urine may be present. Rigors may be a feature; jaundice is common and usually associated with pain. Physical examination may show the scar of a previous cholecystectomy; if the gallbladder is present, it is usually small, fibrotic and impalpable.

Investigations

The LFTs show a cholestatic pattern and there is bilirubinuria. If cholangitis is present, the patient usually has a leucocytosis. The most convenient method of demonstrating obstruction to the common bile duct is by transabdominal ultrasound; this shows dilated extrahepatic and intrahepatic bile ducts, together with gallbladder stones (Fig. 23.50), but does not always reveal the cause of the obstruction in the common bile duct as 50% of bile duct stones are missed on ultrasound, particularly those in the distal common bile duct. Endoscopic ultrasound is extremely accurate at identifying bile duct stones. MRCP is non-invasive, and is indicated when intervention is not necessarily mandatory (e.g. the patient with possible bile duct stones, but no jaundice or sepsis). ERCP can be used to diagnose obstruction and its cause, and to remove bile duct stones (see Fig. 23.49). If ERCP fails, PTC may be undertaken.

Management

Cholangitis should be treated with analgesia, intravenous fluids and broad-spectrum antibiotics such as cefuroxime and metronidazole. Blood cultures should be taken before the antibiotics are administered. Patients also require urgent decompression of the biliary tree and stone removal. ERCP with biliary sphincterotomy and

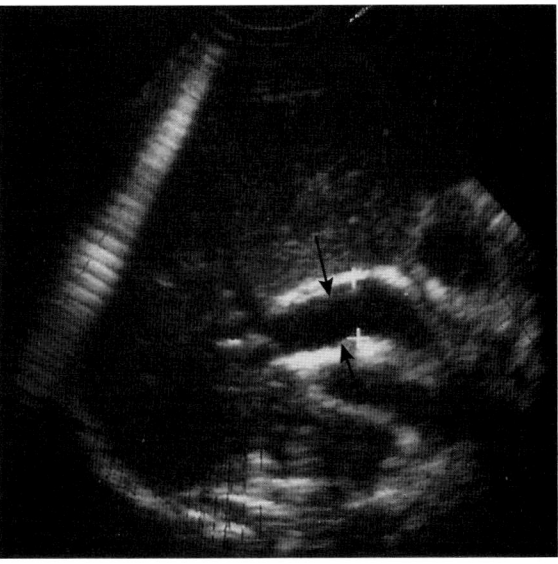

Fig. 23.50 Ultrasound showing dilated bile ducts (between arrows) in obstructive jaundice secondary to obstruction of the common bile duct.

stone extraction is the treatment of choice and is successful in about 90% of patients. Failure of stone extraction may relate to stone size or number, or difficult biliary access. Depending upon the clinical scenario, other approaches include percutaneous transhepatic drainage and combined ('rendez-vous') endoscopic procedures, ESWL and surgery.

Surgical treatment of choledocholithiasis is performed less frequently than ERCP because it carries higher morbidity and mortality. Before the common bile duct is explored, the diagnosis of choledocholithiasis should be confirmed by intraoperative cholangiography. If gallstones are found, the bile duct is explored, all stones are removed, stone clearance is checked by cholangiography or choledochoscopy, and a T-tube is inserted into the common bile duct. It is now possible to achieve these goals in specialist centres by laparoscopic means.

Recurrent pyogenic cholangitis

This disease occurs predominantly in South-east Asia. Biliary sludge, calcium bilirubinate concretions and stones accumulate in the intrahepatic bile ducts, with secondary bacterial infection. Patients present with recurrent attacks of upper abdominal pain, fever and cholestatic jaundice. Investigation of the biliary tree demonstrates that both the intrahepatic and the extrahepatic portions are filled with soft biliary mud. Eventually, the liver becomes scarred and liver abscesses and secondary biliary cirrhosis develop. The condition is difficult to manage, and requires drainage of the biliary tract with extraction of stones, antibiotics and, in certain patients, partial resection of damaged areas of the liver.

Tumours of the gallbladder and bile duct

Carcinoma of the gallbladder

This is an uncommon tumour, occurring more often in females and usually encountered above the age of 70 years. More than 90% are adenocarcinomas; the remainder are anaplastic or, rarely, squamous tumours. Gallstones are present in 70–80% of cases and are thought to be important in the aetiology of the tumour. Individuals with a calcified gallbladder ('porcelain gallbladder', p. 978) are at high risk of malignant change, and gallbladder polyps > 1 cm are associated with increased risk of malignancy.

The condition may be diagnosed incidentally and is found in 1–3% of gallbladders removed at cholecystectomy for gallstone disease. It may manifest as repeated attacks of biliary pain and later persistent jaundice and weight loss. A gallbladder mass may be palpable in the right hypochondrium. LFTs show cholestasis, and gallbladder calcification (porcelain gallbladder) may be found on X-ray. The tumour can be diagnosed by ultrasonography and staged by CT. The treatment is surgical excision, but local extension of the tumour beyond the wall of the gallbladder into the liver, lymph nodes and surrounding tissues is invariable and palliative management is usually all that can be offered. Survival is generally short, death typically occurring within 1 year.

Cholangiocarcinoma (CCA)

This uncommon tumour can arise anywhere in the biliary tree from the intrahepatic bile ducts (20–25% of cases) and the confluence of the right and left hepatic ducts at the liver hilum (50–60%) to the distal common bile duct (20%). It accounts for only 1.5% of all cancers but the rate is increasing. The cause is unknown but the tumour is associated with gallstones, primary and secondary sclerosing cholangitis, Caroli's disease and choledochal cysts (see Fig. 23.41, p. 968). In the Far East, particularly northern Thailand, chronic liver fluke infection (*Clonorchis sinensis*) is a major risk factor for the development of CCA in men. Primary sclerosing cholangitis carries a lifetime risk of CCA of approximately 20%, although only 5% of CCAs relate to primary sclerosing cholangitis. Chronic biliary inflammation appears to be a common factor in the development of biliary dysplasia and cancer that is shared by all the predisposing causes.

Tumours typically invade the lymphatics and adjacent vessels, with a predilection for spread within perineural sheaths.

The presentation is with obstructive jaundice. About 50% of patients also have upper abdominal pain and weight loss. The diagnosis is made by a combination of CT and MRI but can be difficult to confirm in patients with sclerosing cholangitis. Serum levels of the tumour marker CA19-9 are elevated in up to 80% of cases, although this may occur in biliary obstruction of any cause. In the setting of biliary obstruction, ERCP may result in positive biliary cytology. CCAs can be treated surgically in about 20% of patients, which improves 5-year survival from less than 5% to 20–40%. Surgery involves excision of the extrahepatic biliary tree with or without a liver resection and a Roux loop reconstruction. However, most patients are treated by stents inserted across the biliary stricture caused by the tumour, using endoscopic or transhepatic techniques (Fig. 23.51). Combination chemotherapy is increasingly used and palliation with photodynamic therapy has provided encouraging results.

Carcinoma at the ampulla of Vater

Nearly 40% of all adenocarcinomas of the small intestine arise in relationship to the ampulla of Vater, and present with pain, anaemia, vomiting and weight loss. Jaundice may be intermittent or persistent. The diagnosis is made by duodenal endoscopy and biopsy of the tumour, but staging by CT/MRI is essential. Ampullary carcinoma must be differentiated from carcinoma of the head of the pancreas and a cholangiocarcinoma because these latter conditions both have a worse prognosis. Imaging may show a 'double duct sign' with stricturing of both the common bile duct and pancreatic duct at the ampulla indicated by a dilated common bile duct and pancreatic duct down to the level of the ampulla.

Curative surgical treatment can be undertaken by pancreaticoduodenectomy, and the 5-year survival may be as high as 50%. When resection is impossible, a palliative surgical bypass or stent insertion may be necessary.

Benign gallbladder tumours

These are uncommon, often asymptomatic and usually found incidentally at operation or postmortem. Cholesterol polyps, sometimes associated with cholesterolosis, papillomas and adenomas, are the main types.

23

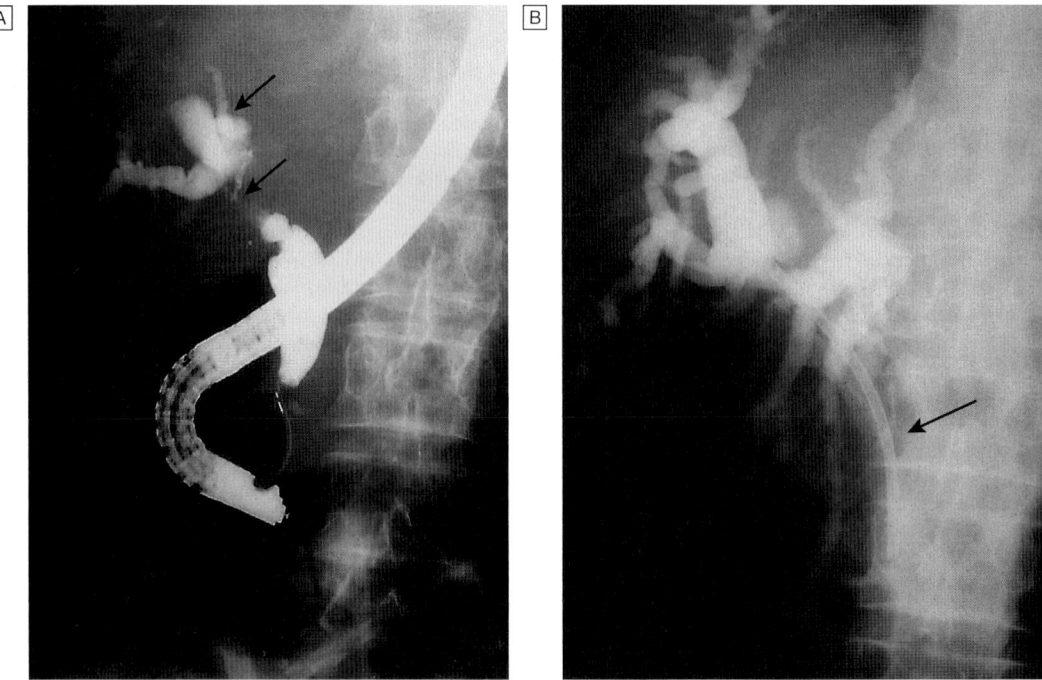

Fig. 23.51 Cholangiocarcinoma. [A] ERCP showing malignant biliary stricture (bottom arrow) and dilated intrahepatic bile ducts above (top arrow). [B] Post-ERCP stenting showing plastic endobiliary stent (arrow) which will draw bile from the dilated ducts above the stricture into the duodenum.

Miscellaneous biliary disorders

Post-cholecystectomy syndrome

Dyspeptic symptoms following cholecystectomy (post-cholecystectomy syndrome) occur in about 30% of patients, depending on how the condition is defined, how actively symptoms are sought and the original indication for cholecystectomy. The syndrome occurs most frequently in women, in patients who have had symptoms for more than 5 years before cholecystectomy, and in patients in whom the operation was undertaken for non-calculous gallbladder disease. An increase in bowel habit occurs in about 5–10% of patients after cholecystectomy, which often responds to colestyramine 4–8 g daily. Severe post-cholecystectomy syndrome occurs in only 2–5% of patients. The main causes are listed in Box 23.73.

The usual symptoms include right upper quadrant abdominal pain, flatulence, fatty food intolerance, and occasionally jaundice and cholangitis. The LFTs may be abnormal and sometimes show cholestasis. Ultrasonography is used to detect biliary obstruction, and ERCP or MRCP is used to seek common bile duct stones. If retained bile duct stones are excluded, sphincter of Oddi dysfunction should be considered (see below). Other investigations that may be required include upper gastrointestinal endoscopy, barium examination of the small intestine, pancreatic function tests, cholescintigraphy and a liver biopsy. The possibility of a functional illness should also be considered (p. 238).

23.73 Causes of post-cholecystectomy symptoms

Immediate post-surgical

- Bleeding
- Biliary peritonitis
- Abscess
- Bile duct trauma/transection
- Fistula

Biliary

- Common bile duct stones
- Benign stricture
- Tumour
- Cystic duct stump syndrome
- Disorders of the ampulla of Vater (e.g. benign papillary fibrosis; sphincter of Oddi dysfunction)

Extrabiliary

- Non-ulcer dyspepsia
- Peptic ulcer
- Pancreatic disease
- Gastro-oesophageal reflux
- Irritable bowel syndrome
- Functional abdominal pain

Sphincter of Oddi dysfunction

The sphincter of Oddi (SO) is a small smooth muscle sphincter situated at the junction of the bile duct and pancreatic duct in the duodenum. Sphincter of Oddi dysfunction (SOD) is characterised by an increase in contractility that produces a benign non-calculous obstruction to the flow of bile or pancreatic juice. This may cause pancreatico-biliary pain, deranged LFTs or recurrent pancreatitis. A clinical classification system, based on clinical history, laboratory results and ERCP findings, is widely used (Boxes 23.74 and 23.75).

23.74 Classification of biliary sphincter of Oddi dysfunction

Biliary type I

- Biliary-type pain
- Abnormal liver enzymes (ALT/AST > twice normal on two or more occasions)
- Dilated common bile duct (> 12 mm diameter)
- Delayed drainage of ERCP contrast beyond 45 minutes

Biliary type II

- Biliary-type pain with one or two of the above criteria

Biliary type III

- Biliary-type pain with no other abnormalities

23.75 Classification of pancreatic sphincter of Oddi dysfunction

Pancreatic type I

- Pancreatic-type pain
- Twice normal amylase or lipase
- Pancreatic duct > 6 mm in the head or 5 mm in the body

Pancreatic type II

- Pancreatic-type pain with only one of the above criteria

Pancreatic type III

- Pancreatic-type pain with no other abnormalities

Clinical features

Patients with SOD, who are predominantly female, present with symptoms and signs suggestive of either biliary or pancreatic disease.

- *Patients with biliary-type SOD* experience recurrent episodic biliary-type pain. They have often had a cholecystectomy but the gallbladder may be intact.
- *Patients with pancreatic SOD* usually present with unexplained recurrent attacks of pancreatitis.

Investigations

The diagnosis is established by excluding gallstones and demonstrating a dilated or slowly draining bile duct. The gold standard for diagnosis is SO manometry. However, this is not widely available and is associated with a high rate of procedure-related pancreatitis.

Management

All biliary SOD patients with type I disease are treated with endoscopic sphincterotomy. The results are good but patients should be warned that there is a high risk of complications, particularly acute pancreatitis. Manometry should ideally be performed in all suspected SOD type II and III patients, and 'speculative' sphincterotomy should be avoided. In type III patients without documented evidence of sphincter hypertension (who should undergo sphincterotomy), medical therapy with nifedipine and/or low-dose amitriptyline may be tried. The role of botulinum toxin ('botox') injection into the sphincter to improve sphincter function remains unclear.

Pancreatic SOD can be treated with pancreatic stenting followed by pancreatic sphincterotomy, carried out in specialised units. Emerging evidence suggests that all patients undergoing ERCP for suspected SOD should undergo prophylactic pancreatic stenting, because this significantly reduces the rate of procedure-related acute pancreatitis.

Cholesterolosis of the gallbladder

In this condition lipid deposits in the submucosa and epithelium appear as multiple yellow spots on the pink mucosa, giving rise to the description 'strawberry gallbladder'. The condition is usually asymptomatic but may occasionally present with right upper quadrant pain. Small, fixed filling defects may be visible on cholecystography or ultrasonography; the radiologist can usually differentiate between gallstones and cholesterolosis. The condition is usually diagnosed at cholecystectomy; if the diagnosis is made radiologically, cholecystectomy may be indicated, depending on symptoms.

Adenomyomatosis of the gallbladder

In this condition there is hyperplasia of the muscle and mucosa of the gallbladder. The projection of pouches of mucous membrane through weak points in the muscle coat produces Rokitansky–Aschoff sinuses. There is much disagreement over whether adenomyomatosis is a cause of right upper quadrant pain or other gastrointestinal symptoms. It may be diagnosed by oral cholecystography, when a halo or ring of opacified diverticula can be seen around the gallbladder. Other appearances include deformity of the body of the gallbladder or marked irregularity of the outline. Localised adenomyomatosis in the region of the gallbladder fundus causes the appearance of a 'Phrygian cap'. Most patients are treated by cholecystectomy but only after excluding other diseases in the upper gastrointestinal tract.

IgG4-associated cholangitis

This recently reported disease (as well as its nomenclature) is closely related to autoimmune pancreatitis (which is present in > 90% of the patients). IgG4-associated cholangitis (IAC) often presents with obstructive jaundice (due to either hilar stricturing/intrahepatic sclerosing cholangitis or a low bile duct stricture), and cholangiographic appearances suggest

23.76 Gallbladder disease in old age

- **Gallstones:** by the age of 70 years, prevalence is around 30% in women and 19% in men.
- **Acute cholecystitis:** tends to be severe, may have few localising signs, and is associated with a high frequency of empyema and perforation. If such complications supervene, mortality may reach 20%.
- **Cholecystectomy:** mortality after urgent cholecystectomy for acute uncomplicated cholecystitis is not significantly higher than in younger patients.
- **Endoscopic sphincterotomy and removal of common duct stones:** well tolerated by older patients and has a substantially lower mortality than surgical common bile duct exploration.
- **Cancer of the gallbladder:** a disease of old age, with a 1-year survival of 10%.

23

primary sclerosing cholangitis with or without hilar cholangiocarcinoma. The serum IgG4 is often raised, and liver biopsy shows a lymphoplasmacytic infiltrate, with IgG4-positive plasma cells. An important observation is that, compared to primary sclerosing cholangitis, IAC appears to respond well to steroid therapy.

Further information

Books and journal articles

Day CP. Non-alcoholic fatty liver disease: current concepts and management strategies. Clinical Medicine 2008; 6:19–25.

Friedman SL. Liver fibrosis—from bench to bedside. Journal of Hepatology 2003; 38:S38–53.

Guruprasad P, et al. Clinical diagnostic scale: a useful tool in the evaluation of suspected hepatotoxic adverse drug reactions. Journal of Hepatology 2000; 33:949–952.

Hoofnagle JH, Doo ED, Liang TJ, et al. Management of hepatitis B: summary of a clinical workshop. Hepatology 2007; 45:1056–1075.

Neuberger J, Gimson A, Davies M, et al. Selection of patients for liver transplantation and allocation of donated livers in the UK. Gut 2008; 57:252–257.

Pietrangelo A. Hereditary haemochromatosis. A new look at an old disease. New England Journal of Medicine 2004; 350:2383–2397.

Websites

www.aasld.org *American Association for the Study of Liver Diseases (guidelines available).*

www.bsg.org.uk *British Society of Gastroenterology (guidelines available).*

www.easl.ch *European Association for the Study of the Liver (guidelines available).*

www.eltr.org *European Liver Transplant Registry.*

www.unos.org *United Network for Organ Sharing: US transplant register.*

J.I.O. Craig
D.B.L. McClelland
H.G. Watson

Blood disease

CLINICAL EXAMINATION IN BLOOD DISEASE

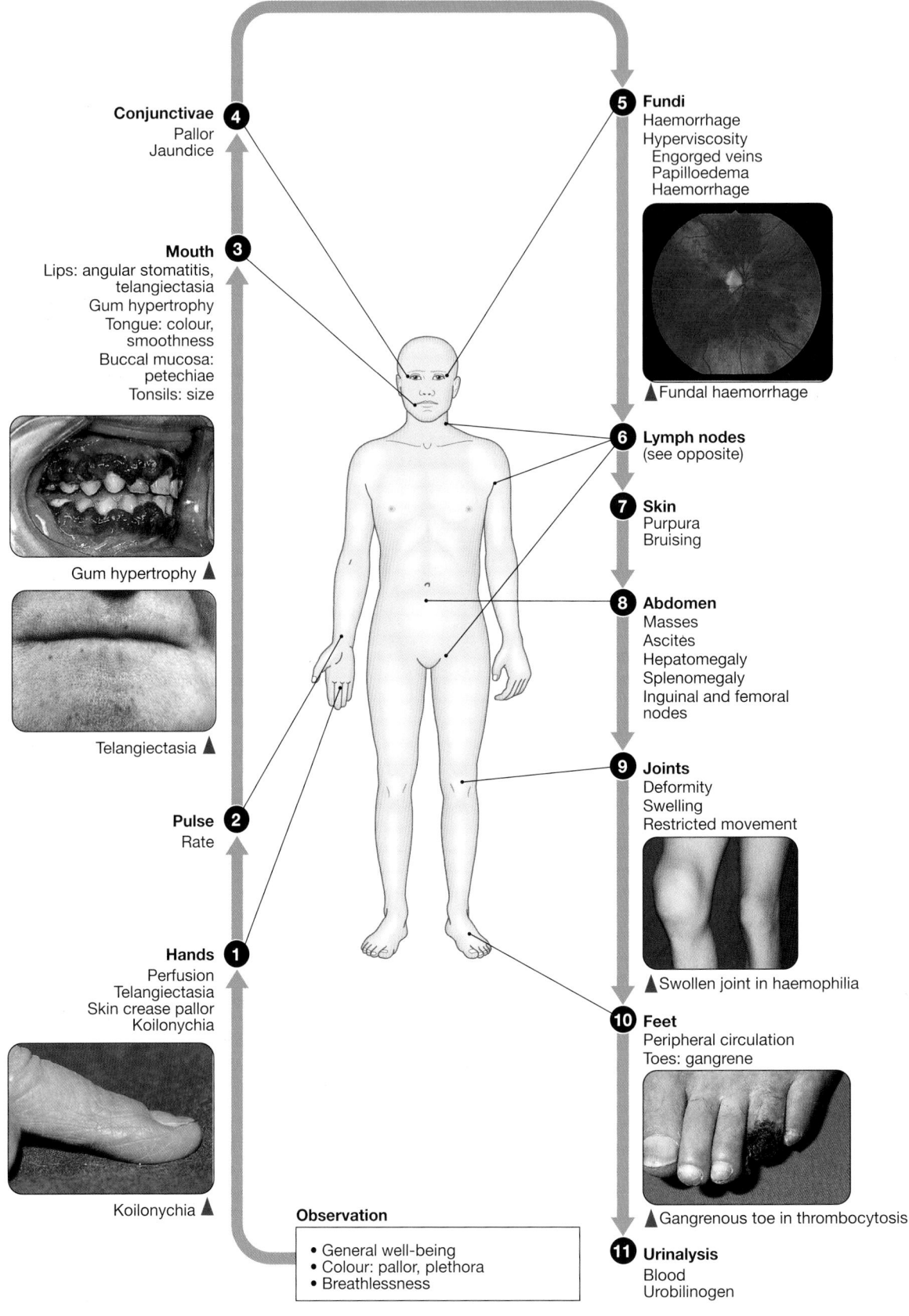

4 Conjunctivae
Pallor
Jaundice

3 Mouth
Lips: angular stomatitis,
  telangiectasia
Gum hypertrophy
Tongue: colour,
  smoothness
Buccal mucosa:
  petechiae
Tonsils: size

Gum hypertrophy ▲

Telangiectasia ▲

2 Pulse
Rate

1 Hands
Perfusion
Telangiectasia
Skin crease pallor
Koilonychia

Koilonychia ▲

Observation
• General well-being
• Colour: pallor, plethora
• Breathlessness

5 Fundi
Haemorrhage
Hyperviscosity
  Engorged veins
  Papilloedema
  Haemorrhage

▲ Fundal haemorrhage

6 Lymph nodes
(see opposite)

7 Skin
Purpura
Bruising

8 Abdomen
Masses
Ascites
Hepatomegaly
Splenomegaly
Inguinal and femoral
nodes

9 Joints
Deformity
Swelling
Restricted movement

▲ Swollen joint in haemophilia

10 Feet
Peripheral circulation
Toes: gangrene

▲ Gangrenous toe in thrombocytosis

11 Urinalysis
Blood
Urobilinogen

Abnormalities detected in the blood are caused not only by primary diseases of the blood and lymphoreticular systems, but also by diseases affecting other systems of the body. The clinical assessment of patients with haematological abnormalities must include a general history and examination, as well as a search for symptoms and signs of abnormalities of red cells, white cells, platelets, bleeding and clotting systems, lymph nodes and lymphoreticular tissues.

Anaemia

The box shows the symptoms and signs that will help to indicate the clinical severity of anaemia. A full history and examination is needed to identify clues to the underlying cause.

---

6 Lymphadenopathy

Lymphadenopathy can be caused by benign or malignant disease. The clinical points to clarify are shown in the box.

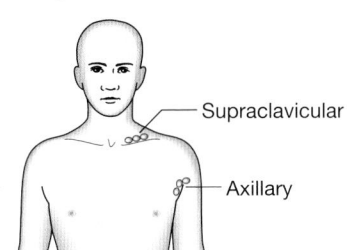
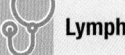

Supraclavicular

Axillary

Epitrochlear

Inguinal

Femoral

Popliteal fossa

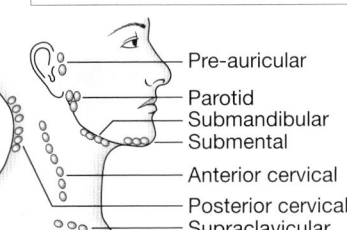

Pre-auricular
Parotid
Submandibular
Submental
Anterior cervical
Posterior cervical
Supraclavicular

Lymphadenopathy

History

- Speed of onset, rate of enlargement
- Painful or painless
- Associated symptoms: weight loss, night sweats, itch

Examination

- Sites: localised, generalised
- Size (cm)
- Character: hard, soft, rubbery
- Fixed, mobile
- Search area that node drains for abnormalities (e.g. tooth abscess)
- Other general examination (e.g. joints, rashes, finger clubbing)

Anaemia

Non-specific symptoms

- Tiredness
- Lightheadedness
- Breathlessness
- Ankle-swelling
- Development/worsening of ischaemic symptoms e.g. angina or claudication

Non-specific signs

- Mucous membrane pallor
- Tachypnoea
- Raised jugular venous pressure
- Flow murmurs
- Ankle oedema
- Postural hypotension
- Tachycardia

Bleeding

Bleeding can be due to congenital or acquired abnormalities in components of the clotting system. The history and examination will help to clarify the severity and underlying cause of the bleeding problem.

---

8 Examination of the spleen

- Move hand up from right iliac fossa, towards left upper quadrant on expiration.

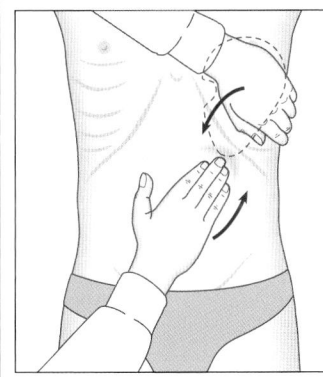

- Keep hand still and ask patient to take a deep breath through the mouth to feel spleen edge being displaced downwards.
- Place your left hand around patient's lower ribs and approach costal margin to pull spleen forward.
- To help palpate small spleens, roll patient on to the right side and examine as before.

Characteristics of the spleen

- Notch
- Superficial
- Dull to percussion
- Cannot get between ribs and spleen
- Moves well with respiration

Bleeding

History

- Site of bleed
- Duration of bleed
- Precipitating causes, including previous surgery or trauma
- Family history
- Drug history
- Other medical conditions, e.g. liver disease

Examination

There are two major patterns of bleeding:

1. **Mucosal bleeding**
   Reduced number or function of platelets (e.g. bone marrow failure or aspirin) or von Willebrand factor (e.g. von Willebrand disease)
   - Skin: petechiae, bruises, post-surgical bleeding
   - Gum and mucous membrane bleeding
   - Fundal haemorrhage
2. **Coagulation factor deficiency**
   (e.g. haemophilia or warfarin)
   - Bleeding into joints (haemarthrosis) or muscles
   - Bleeding into soft tissues
   - Intracranial haemorrhage
   - Post-surgical bleeding

Disorders of the blood cover a wide spectrum of illnesses, ranging from some of the most common disorders affecting mankind (anaemias), to relatively rare conditions such as leukaemias and congenital coagulation disorders. Although the latter are uncommon, advances in cellular and molecular biology have had major impacts on their diagnosis, treatment and prognosis. Haematological changes occur as a consequence of diseases affecting any system and give important information in the diagnosis and monitoring of many conditions.

FUNCTIONAL ANATOMY AND PHYSIOLOGY

Blood flows throughout the body in the vascular system, and consists of plasma and three cellular components:

- red cells, which transport oxygen from the lungs to the tissues
- white cells, which protect against infection
- platelets, which interact with blood vessels and clotting factors to maintain vascular integrity and prevent bleeding.

Haematopoiesis

Haematopoiesis describes the formation of blood cells, an active process that must maintain normal numbers of circulating cells and be able to respond rapidly to increased demands such as bleeding or infection. During development, haematopoiesis occurs in the liver and spleen and subsequently in red bone marrow in the medullary cavity of all bones. In childhood, red marrow is progressively replaced by fat (yellow marrow), so that in adults normal haematopoiesis is restricted to the vertebrae, pelvis, sternum, ribs, clavicles, skull, upper humeri and proximal femora. However, red marrow can expand in response to increased demands for blood cells.

Bone marrow contains a range of immature haematopoietic precursor cells and a storage pool of mature cells for release at times of increased demand. Haematopoietic cells interact closely with surrounding connective tissue stroma, made of reticular cells, macrophages, fat cells, blood vessels and nerve fibres (Fig. 24.1). In normal marrow, nests of red cell precursors cluster around a central macrophage, which provides iron and phagocytoses extruded nuclei. Megakaryocytes are large cells which produce and release platelets into vascular sinuses. White cell precursors are clustered next to the bone trabeculae; maturing cells migrate into the marrow spaces towards the vascular sinuses. Plasma cells are antibody-secreting mature B cells which normally represent < 5% of the marrow population and are scattered throughout the intertrabecular spaces.

Stem cells

All blood cells are derived from pluripotent stem cells. These comprise only 0.01% of the total marrow cells, but they can self-renew (i.e. make more stem cells) or differentiate to produce a hierarchy of lineage-committed stem cells. The resulting primitive progenitor cells cannot be identified morphologically, so they are named according to the types of cell (or colony) they form during cell culture experiments. CFU–GM (colony-forming unit–granulocyte, monocyte) is a stem cell that produces granulocytic and monocytic lines, CFU–E produces erythroid cells, and CFU–Meg produces megakaryocytes and ultimately platelets (Fig. 24.2).

A range of growth factors, produced in bone marrow stromal cells and elsewhere, controls the survival, proliferation, differentiation and function of stem cells and their progeny. Some, such as granulocyte macrophage–colony stimulating factor (GM–CSF), interleukin-3 (IL-3) and stem cell factor (SCF), act on a wide number of

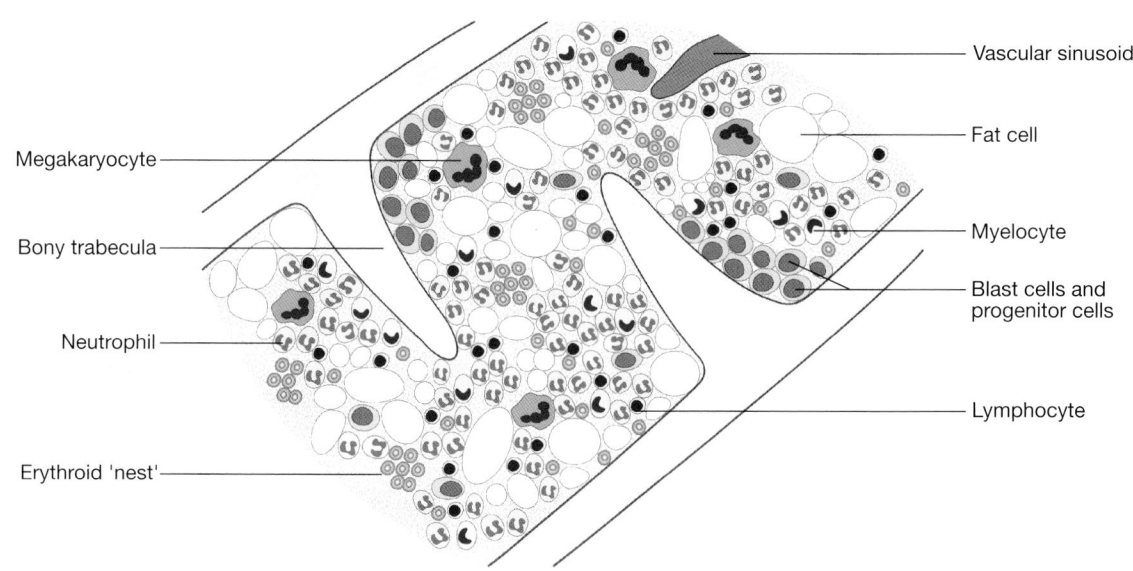

Fig. 24.1 Structural organisation of normal bone marrow.

Megakaryocyte

Bony trabecula

Neutrophil

Erythroid 'nest'

Vascular sinusoid

Fat cell

Myelocyte

Blast cells and progenitor cells

Lymphocyte

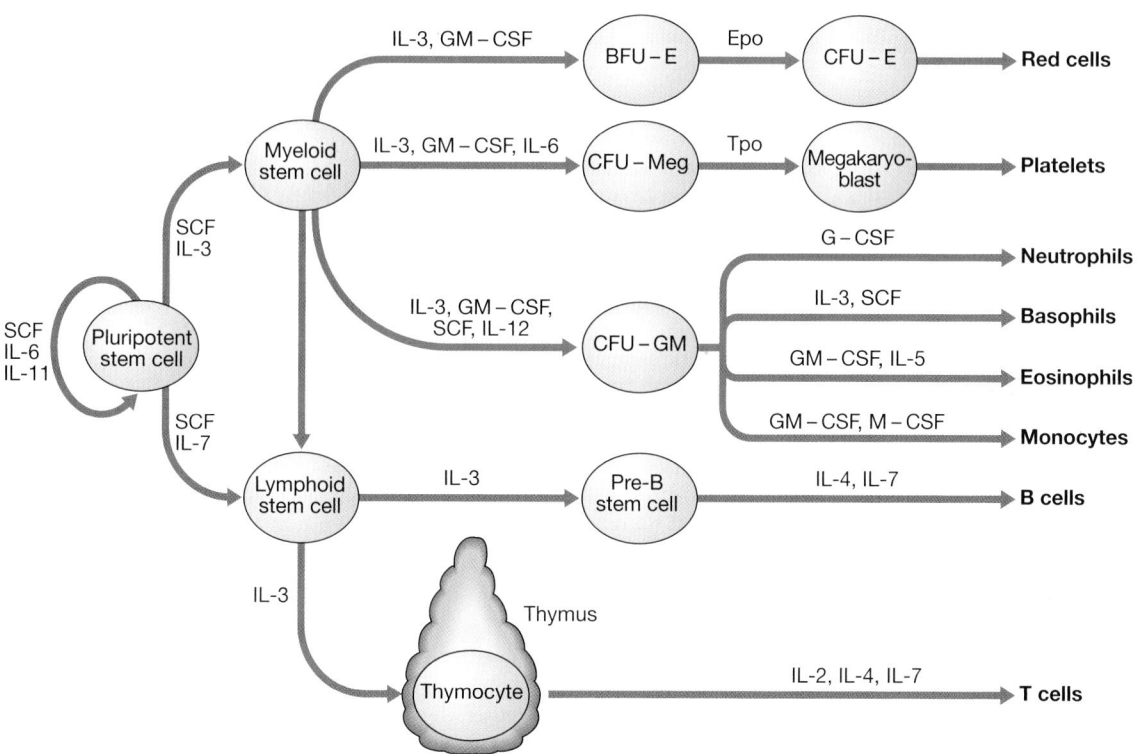

Fig. 24.2 Stem cells and growth factors in haematopoietic cell development. (BFU–E = burst-forming unit–erythroid; CFU–E = colony-forming unit–erythroid; CFU–GM = colony-forming unit–granulocyte, monocyte; CFU–Meg = colony-forming unit–megakaryocyte; Epo = erythropoietin; G–CSF = granulocyte–colony-stimulating factor; GM–CSF = granulocyte macrophage–colony-stimulating factor; IL = interleukin; M–CSF = macrophage–colony-stimulating factor; SCF = stem cell factor; Tpo = thrombopoietin)

cell types at various stages of differentiation. Others, such as erythropoietin (Epo), granulocyte–colony stimulating factor (G–CSF) and thrombopoietin (Tpo), are lineage-specific. Many of these growth factors are now synthesised by recombinant DNA technology and used as treatments.

Recent evidence suggests that the bone marrow contains stem cells which can differentiate into non-haematological cells, such as nerve, skeletal muscle, cardiac muscle, liver and blood vessel endothelium. This is termed stem-cell plasticity and may have exciting clinical applications in the future (Ch. 3).

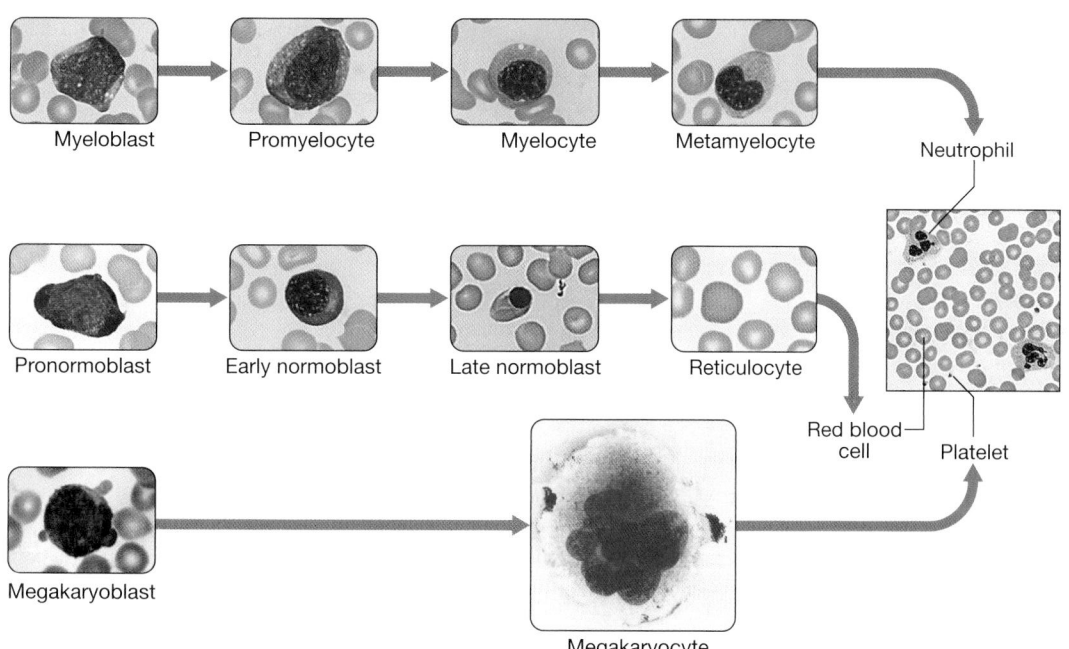

Fig. 24.3 Maturation pathway of red cells, granulocytes and platelets.

24

Blood cells and their functions

Red cells

Red cell precursors formed in the bone marrow from the erythroid (CFU–E) progenitor cells are called erythroblasts or normoblasts (Fig. 24.3). These divide and acquire haemoglobin which turns the cytoplasm pink; the nucleus condenses and is extruded from the cell. The first non-nucleated red cell is a reticulocyte which still contains ribosomal material in the cytoplasm, giving these large cells a faint blue tinge ('polychromasia'). Reticulocytes lose their ribosomal material and mature over 3 days, during which time they are released into the circulation. Increased numbers of circulating reticulocytes (reticulocytosis) reflect increased erythropoiesis. Proliferation and differentiation of red cell precursors is stimulated by erythropoietin, a polypeptide hormone produced by renal tubular cells in response to hypoxia. Failure of erythropoietin production in patients with renal failure (p. 482) causes anaemia, which can be treated with exogenous recombinant erythropoietin.

Mature red cells circulate for about 120 days. They are 8 μm biconcave discs lacking a nucleus but filled with haemoglobin, which delivers oxygen to the tissues from the lungs. In order to pass through the smallest capillaries the red cell membrane is adapted to be deformable, with a lipid bilayer to which a 'skeleton' of filamentous proteins is attached via special linkage proteins (Fig. 24.4). Inherited abnormalities of any of these proteins result in loss of membrane as cells pass through the spleen, and the formation of abnormally shaped red cells called spherocytes or elliptocytes (see Fig. 24.8D, p. 995).

Red cells are exposed to osmotic stress in the pulmonary and renal circulation; to maintain homeostasis, the membrane contains ion pumps which control intracellular levels of sodium, potassium, chloride and bicarbonate. In the absence of mitochondria, the energy for these functions is provided by anaerobic glycolysis and the pentose phosphate pathway in the cytosol. Membrane glycoproteins inserted into the lipid bilayer also form the antigens recognised by blood grouping (see Fig. 24.4). The ABO and Rhesus systems are the most commonly recognised (pp. 1008–1010), but over 400 blood group antigens have been described.

Haemoglobin

Haemoglobin is a protein specially adapted for oxygen transport. It is composed of four globin chains, each surrounding an iron-containing porphyrin pigment molecule termed haem. Globin chains are a combination of two alpha and two non-alpha chains; haemoglobin A ($\alpha\alpha/\beta\beta$) represents over 90% of adult haemoglobin, whereas haemoglobin F ($\alpha\alpha/\gamma\gamma$) is the predominant type in the fetus. Each haem molecule contains a ferrous ion (Fe^{2+}) to which oxygen reversibly binds; the affinity for oxygen increases as successive oxygen molecules bind. When oxygen is bound, the beta chains 'swing' closer together; they move apart as oxygen is lost. In the 'open' deoxygenated state, 2,3 diphosphoglycerate (DPG), a product of red cell metabolism, binds to the haemoglobin molecule and lowers its oxygen affinity. These complex interactions produce the sigmoid shape of the oxygen dissociation curve (Fig. 24.5). The position of this curve depends upon the concentrations of 2,3 DPG, H^+ ions and CO_2; increased levels shift the curve to the right and cause oxygen to be released more readily, e.g.

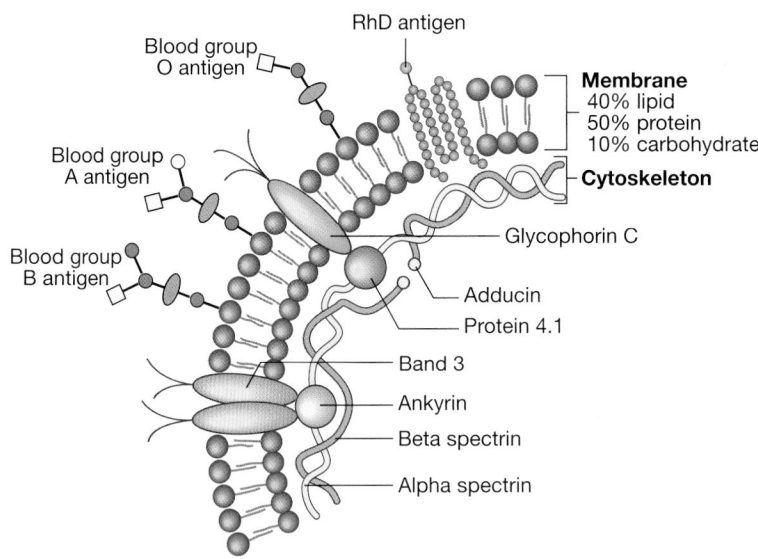

Fig. 24.4 Normal structure of red cell membrane. Red cell membrane flexibility is conferred by attachment of cytoskeletal proteins. Important transmembrane proteins include band 3 (an ion transport channel) and glycophorin (involved in cytoskeletal attachment and gas exchange, and a receptor for *Plasmodium falciparum* in malaria). Antigens on the red blood cell determine an individual's blood group. There are about 22 blood group systems (groups of carbohydrate or protein antigens controlled by a single gene or by multiple closely linked loci); the most important clinically are the ABO and Rhesus (Rh) systems (p. 1007). The ABO genetic locus has three main allelic forms: A, B and O. The A and B alleles encode glycosyltransferases that introduce N-acetylgalactosamine (open circle) and D-galactose (blue circle), respectively, on to antigenic carbohydrate molecules on the membrane surface. People with the O allele produce an O antigen which lacks either of these added sugar groups. Rh antigens are transmembrane proteins.

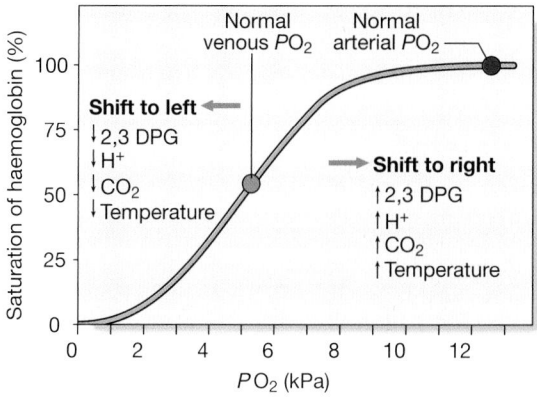

Fig. 24.5 The haemoglobin oxygen dissociation curve. Factors are listed which shift the curve to the right (more oxygen released from blood) and to the left (less oxygen released) at given PO_2. (To convert kPa to mmHg, multiply by 7.5.)

when red cells reach hypoxic tissues. Haemoglobin F is unable to bind 2,3 DPG and has a left-shifted oxygen dissociation curve which, together with the low pH of fetal blood, ensures fetal oxygenation.

Genetic mutations affecting the haem-binding pockets of globin chains or the 'hinge' interactions between globin chains result in haemoglobinopathies or unstable haemoglobins. Alpha globin chains are produced by two genes on chromosome 16 and beta globin chains by a single gene on chromosome 11; imbalance in the production of globin chains produces the thalassaemias (p. 1029). Defects in haem synthesis cause the porphyrias (p. 456).

Destruction

Red cells at the end of their lifespan of approximately 120 days are phagocytosed by the reticulo-endothelial system. Amino acids from globin chains are recycled and iron is removed from haem for reuse in haemoglobin synthesis. The remnant haem structure is degraded to bilirubin and conjugated with glucuronic acid before being excreted in bile. In the small bowel, bilirubin is converted to stercobilin; most of this is excreted, but a small amount is reabsorbed and excreted by the kidney as urobilinogen. Increased red cell destruction due to haemolysis or ineffective haematopoiesis results in jaundice and increased urinary urobilinogen. Free intravascular haemoglobin is toxic and is normally bound by haptoglobins, which are plasma proteins produced by the liver.

White cells

White cells or leucocytes in the blood consist of granulocytes (neutrophils, eosinophils and basophils), monocytes and lymphocytes (see Fig. 24.12, p. 1000). Granulocytes and monocytes are formed from bone marrow CFU–GM progenitor cells. The first recognisable granulocyte in the marrow is the myeloblast, a large cell with a small amount of basophilic cytoplasm and a primitive nucleus with open chromatin and nucleoli. As the cells divide and mature, the nucleus segments and the cytoplasm acquires specific neutrophilic, eosinophilic or basophilic granules (see Fig. 24.3). This takes about 14 days. The cytokines G–CSF, GM–CSF and M–CSF are involved in the production of myeloid cells and G–CSF can be used clinically to hasten recovery of blood neutrophil counts after chemotherapy.

Myelocytes or metamyelocytes are normally only found in the marrow but may appear in the circulation in infection or toxic states. The appearance of more primitive myeloid precursors in the blood is often associated with the presence of nucleated red cells and is termed a 'leucoerythroblastic' picture; this indicates a serious disturbance of marrow function.

Neutrophils

Neutrophils, the most common white blood cells in the blood of adults, are 10–14 µm in diameter with a multilobular nucleus containing 2–5 segments and granules in their cytoplasm. Their main function is to recognise, ingest and destroy foreign particles and microorganisms (p. 70). A large storage pool of mature neutrophils exists in the bone marrow. Every day some 10^{11} neutrophils enter the circulation, where cells may be freely circulating or attached to endothelium in the marginating pool. These two pools are equal in size; factors such as exercise or catecholamines increase the number of cells flowing in the blood. Neutrophils spend 6–10 hours in the circulation before being removed, principally by the spleen. Alternatively, they pass into the tissues and either are consumed in the inflammatory process or undergo apoptotic cell death and phagocytosis by macrophages.

Eosinophils

Eosinophils represent 1–6% of the circulating white cells. They are a similar size to neutrophils but have a bilobed nucleus and prominent orange granules on Romanowsky staining. Eosinophils are phagocytic and their granules contain a peroxidase capable of generating reactive oxygen species and proteins involved in the intracellular killing of protozoa and helminths (p. 307). They are also involved in allergic reactions (e.g. atopic asthma, p. 662; see also p. 86).

Basophils

These cells are less common than eosinophils, representing less than 1% of circulating white cells. They contain dense black granules which obscure the nucleus. Mast cells resemble basophils but are only found in the tissues. These cells are involved in hypersensitivity reactions (p. 73).

Monocytes

Monocytes are the largest of the white cells, with a diameter of 12–20 µm and an irregular nucleus in abundant pale blue cytoplasm containing occasional cytoplasmic vacuoles. These cells circulate for a few hours and then migrate into the tissue where they become macrophages, Kupffer cells or antigen-presenting dendritic cells. The former phagocytose debris, apoptotic cells and microorganisms (see Box 4.1, p. 72).

Lymphocytes

Lymphocytes are derived from pluripotent haematopoietic stem cells in the bone marrow. There are two main types: T cells (which mediate cellular immunity) and B cells (which mediate humoral immunity) (pp. 75–76). Lymphoid cells which migrate to the thymus develop into T cells, whereas B cells develop in the bone marrow.

The majority of lymphocytes (approximately 80%) in the circulation are T cells. Lymphocytes are heterogeneous, the smallest cells being the size of red cells and

24

the largest being the size of neutrophils. Small lymphocytes are circular with scanty cytoplasm but the larger cells are more irregular with abundant blue cytoplasm. Lymphocyte subpopulations can be defined with specific functions and their lifespan can vary from a few days to many years.

Haemostasis

Blood must be maintained in a fluid state in order to function as a transport system, but must be able to solidify to form a clot following vascular injury to prevent excessive bleeding, a process known as haemostasis. Successful haemostasis is localised to the area of tissue damage and is followed by removal of the clot and tissue repair. This is achieved by complex interactions between the vascular endothelium, platelets,

coagulation factors, natural anticoagulants and fibrinolytic enzymes, as detailed in Figure 24.6. Dysfunction of any of these components may result in haemorrhage or thrombosis.

Platelets

Platelets are formed in the bone marrow from megakaryocytes. Megakaryocytic stem cells (CFU–Meg) divide to form megakaryoblasts, which undergo a process called 'endomitotic reduplication', in which there is division of the nucleus but not the cell. This creates mature megakaryocytes, large cells with several nuclei and cytoplasm containing platelet granules. Up to 3000 platelets then fragment off from each megakaryocyte into the circulation in the marrow sinusoids. The formation and maturation of megakaryocytes are stimulated by thrombopoietin produced in the liver. Platelets circulate for 8–10 days before they are destroyed in the reticulo-

Fig. 24.6 The stages of normal haemostasis. **A** *Stage 1 Pre-injury conditions encourage flow* The vascular endothelium produces substances (including nitric oxide, prostacyclin and heparans) to prevent adhesion of platelets and white cells to the vessel wall. Platelets and coagulation factors circulate in a non-activated state.

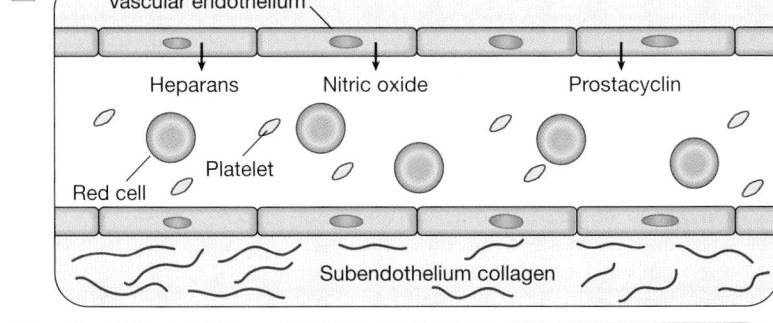

B *Stage 2 Early haemostatic response: platelets adhere; coagulation is activated.* At the site of injury the endothelium is breached, exposing subendothelial collagen. Small amounts of tissue factor (TF) are released. Platelets bind to collagen via a specific receptor, glycoprotein Ia (GPIa), causing a change in platelet shape and its adhesion to the area of damage by the binding of other receptors (GPIb and GPIIb/IIIa) to von Willebrand factor and fibrinogen respectively. Coagulation is activated by the tissue factor (extrinsic) pathway, generating small amounts of thrombin.

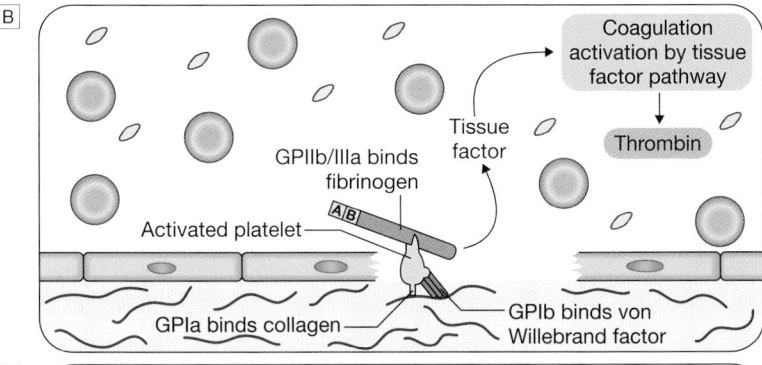

C *Stage 3 Fibrin clot formation: platelets become activated and aggregate; fibrin formation is supported by the platelet membrane; stable fibrin clot forms.* The adherent platelets are activated by many pathways, including binding of ADP, collagen, thrombin and adrenaline (epinephrine) to surface receptors. The cyclo-oxygenase pathway converts arachidonic acid from the platelet membrane into thromboxane A_2, which causes aggregation of platelets. Activation of the platelets results in release of the platelet granule contents, enhancing coagulation further (see Fig. 24.7). Thrombin plays a key role in the control of coagulation: the small amount generated via the TF pathway massively amplifies its own production; the 'intrinsic' pathway becomes activated and large amounts of thrombin are generated. Thrombin enhances clot formation by cleaving fibrinogen to produce fibrin. Fibrin monomers are cross-linked by factor XIII, which is also activated by thrombin. Having had a key role in clot formation and stabilisation, thrombin then starts to regulate clot formation in

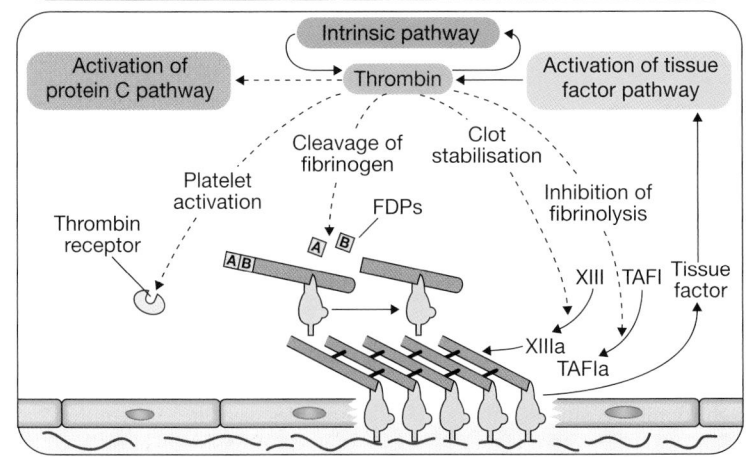

endothelial system. Some 30% of peripheral platelets are normally pooled in the spleen and do not circulate.

Under normal conditions platelets are discoid, with a diameter of 2–4 μm (Fig. 24.7). The surface membrane invaginates to form a tubular network, the canalicular system, which provides a conduit for the discharge of the granule content following platelet activation. Drugs which inhibit platelet function and thrombosis include aspirin (cyclo-oxygenase inhibitor), clopidogrel (inhibits adenosine diphosphate (ADP)-mediated activation), dipyridamole (inhibits phosphodiesterase), and the IIb/IIIa inhibitors abciximab, tirofiban and eptifibatide (prevent fibrinogen binding) (p. 592).

Clotting factors

The coagulation system consists of a cascade of soluble inactive zymogen proteins designated by Roman numerals. When proteolytically cleaved and activated, each is capable of activating one or more components of the cascade. Activated factors are designated by the suffix 'a'. Some of these reactions require phospholipid and calcium. Coagulation occurs by two pathways; it is initiated by the extrinsic (or tissue factor) pathway and amplified by the intrinsic pathway (see Fig. 24.6).

Clotting factors are synthesised by the liver, although factor V is also produced by platelets and endothelial cells. Factors II, VII, IX and X require post-translational carboxylation to allow them to participate in coagulation. The carboxylase enzyme responsible for this in the liver is vitamin K-dependent. Vitamin K is converted to an epoxide in this reaction and must be reduced to its active form by a reductase enzyme. This reductase is inhibited by warfarin, and this is the basis of the anticoagulant effect of coumarins (p. 1015). Congenital

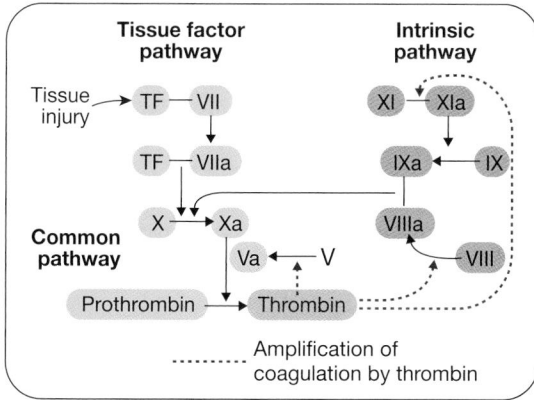

two main ways: (a) activation of the protein C (PC) pathway (a natural anticoagulant), which reduces further coagulation; (b) activation of thrombin-activatable fibrinolysis inhibitor (TAFI), which inhibits fibrinolysis (see D and E).

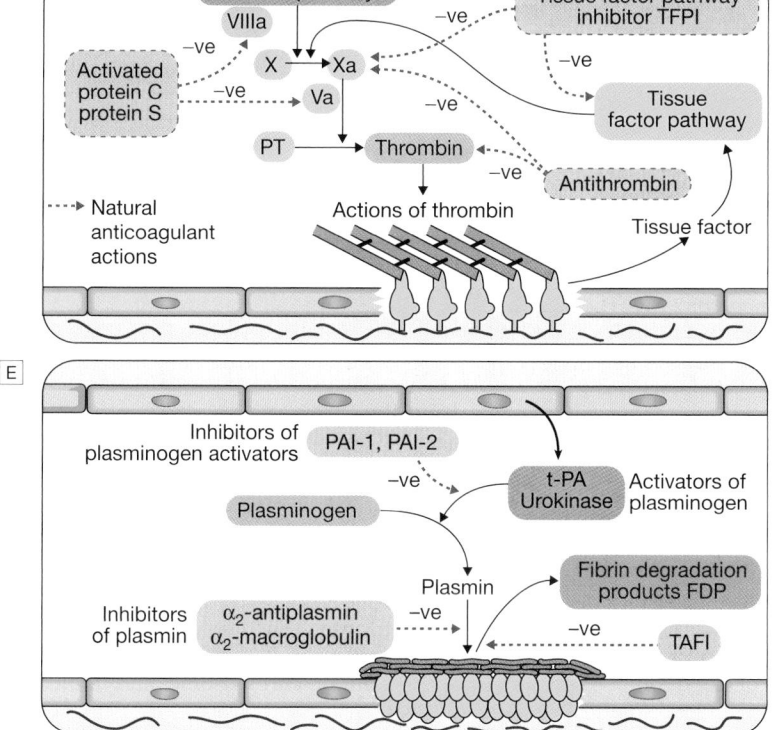

D *Stage 4 Limiting clot formation: natural anticoagulants reverse activation of coagulation factors.* Once haemostasis has been secured, the propagation of clot is curtailed by anticoagulants. Antithrombin is a serine protease inhibitor synthesised by the liver, which destroys activated factors such as XIa, Xa and thrombin (IIa). Its major activity against thrombin and Xa is enhanced by heparin and fondaparinux, explaining their anticoagulant effect. Tissue factor pathway inhibitor (TFPI) binds to and inactivates VIIa and Xa. Activation of PC occurs following binding of thrombin to membrane-bound thrombomodulin; activated protein C (aPC) binds to its co-factor protein S (PS), and cleaves Va and VIIIa. PC and PS are vitamin K-dependent and are depleted by coumarin anticoagulants such as warfarin.

E *Stage 5 Fibrinolysis: plasmin degrades fibrin to allow vessel recanalisation and tissue repair.* The insoluble clot needs to be broken down for vessel recanalisation. Plasmin, the main fibrinolytic enzyme, is produced when plasminogen is activated, e.g. by tissue plasminogen activator (t-PA) or urokinase in the clot. Plasmin hydrolyses the fibrin clot, producing fibrin degradation products including the D-dimer. This process is highly regulated; the plasminogen activators are controlled by an inhibitor called plasminogen activator inhibitor (PAI), the activity of plasmin is inhibited by α_2-antiplasmin and α_2-macroglobulin, and fibrinolysis is further inhibited by the thrombin-activated TAFI.

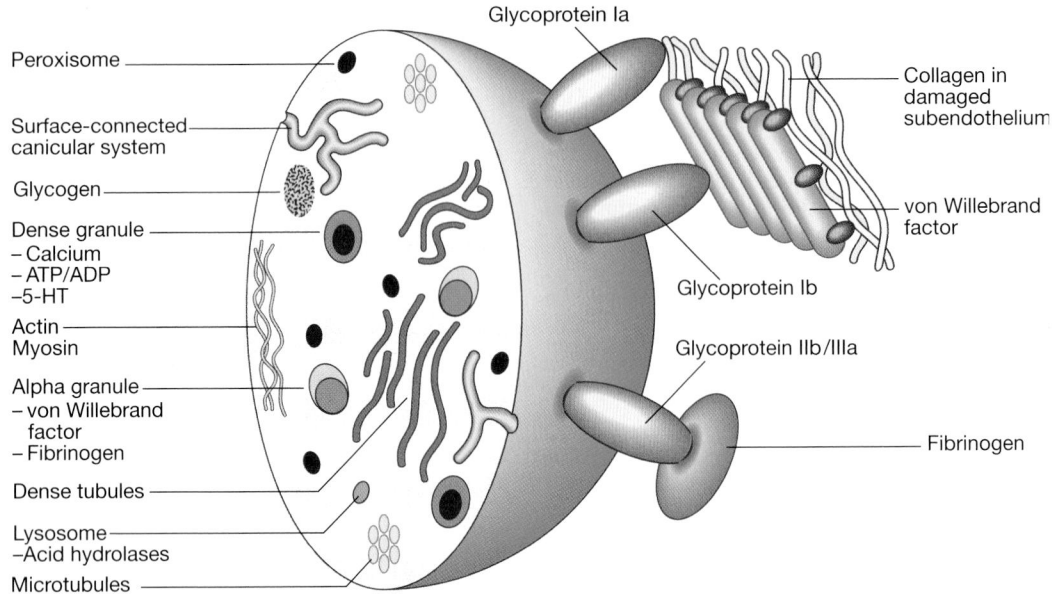

Fig. 24.7 Normal platelet structure. (5-HT = 5-hydroxytryptamine, serotonin; ADP = adenosine diphosphate; ATP = adenosine triphosphate)

(e.g. haemophilia) and acquired (e.g. liver failure) causes of coagulation factor deficiency are associated with bleeding.

INVESTIGATION OF DISEASES OF THE BLOOD

The full blood count (FBC)

To obtain an FBC, anticoagulated blood is processed through automatic blood analysers which use a variety of technologies (particle-sizing, radiofrequency and laser instrumentation) to measure the haematological parameters. These include numbers of circulating cells and platelets, the proportion of whole blood volume occupied by red cells (the haematocrit, Hct), and the red cell indices which give information about the size of red cells (mean cell volume, MCV) and the amount of haemoglobin present in the red cells (mean cell haemoglobin, MCH). Modern blood analysers can differentiate types of white blood cell and give automated counts of neutrophils, lymphocytes, monocytes, eosinophils and basophils. It is important to appreciate, however, that a number of conditions can lead to spurious results (Box 24.1). The reference values for a number of common haematological parameters in adults are given in Chapter 28.

Blood film examination

Although the technical advances of modern full blood count analysers have resulted in fewer blood samples requiring manual examination, scrutiny of blood components prepared on a microscope slide (the 'blood film') can often yield invaluable information (Box 24.2 and Fig. 24.8). Analysers cannot identify abnormalities of red cell

24.1 Spurious FBC results from autoanalysers

Result	Explanation
Increased haemoglobin	Lipaemia, jaundice, very high white cell count
Reduced haemoglobin	Improper sample mixing, blood taken from vein into which an infusion is flowing
Increased red cell volume (MCV)	Cold agglutinins, non-ketotic hyperosmolarity
Increased white cell count	Nucleated red cells present
Reduced platelet count	Clot in sample, platelet clumping

shape and content (e.g. Howell–Jolly bodies, basophilic stippling, malaria parasites) or fully define abnormal white cells such as blasts.

Bone marrow examination

In adults bone marrow for examination is usually obtained from the posterior iliac crest. After a local anaesthetic, marrow may be sucked out from the medullary space, stained and examined under the microscope (bone marrow aspirate). In addition, a core of bone may be removed (trephine biopsy), fixed and decalcified before sections are cut for staining (Fig. 24.9). A bone marrow aspirate is used to assess the composition and morphology of haematopoietic cells or abnormal infiltrates. Further investigations may be performed, such as cell surface marker analysis (immunophenotyping), chromosome and molecular studies to assess malignant disease, or marrow culture for suspected tuberculosis. A trephine biopsy is superior for assessing marrow cellularity, marrow

24.2 How to interpret red cell appearances

Microcytosis (reduced average cell size, MCV < 76 fL) A
- Iron deficiency
- Thalassaemia
- Sideroblastic anaemia

Macrocytosis (increased average cell size, MCV > 100 fL) B
- Vitamin B$_{12}$ or folate deficiency
- Liver disease, alcohol
- Hypothyroidism
- Drugs (e.g. zidovudine)

Target cells (central area of haemoglobinisation) C
- Liver disease
- Thalassaemia
- Post-splenectomy
- Haemoglobin C disease

Spherocytes (dense cells, no area of central pallor) D
- Autoimmune haemolysis
- Post-splenectomy
- Hereditary spherocytosis

Red cell fragments (intravascular haemolysis) E
- Disseminated intravascular coagulation (DIC)
- Haemolytic uraemic syndrome (HUS)/thrombotic thrombocytopenic purpura (TTP)

Nucleated red blood cells (normoblasts) F
- Marrow infiltration
- Severe haemolysis
- Myelofibrosis
- Acute haemorrhage

Howell–Jolly bodies (small round nuclear remnants) G
- Hyposplenism
- Post-splenectomy
- Dyshaematopoiesis

Polychromasia (young red cells—reticulocytes present) H
- Haemolysis, acute haemorrhage
- Increased red cell turnover

Basophilic stippling (abnormal ribosomes appear as blue dots) I
- Dyshaematopoiesis
- Lead poisoning

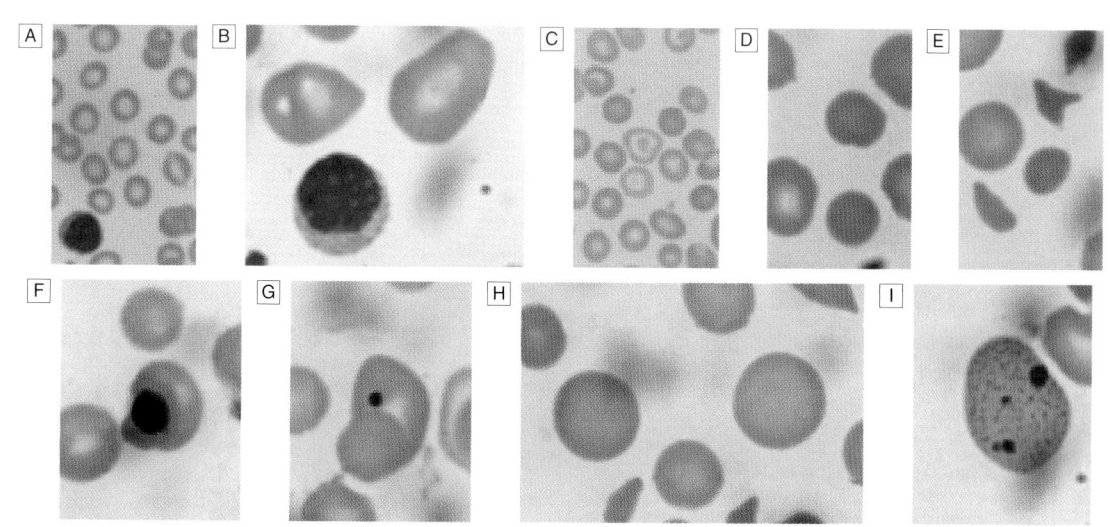

Fig. 24.8 A Microcytosis. B Macrocytosis. C Target cells. D Spherocytes. E Red cell fragments. F Nucleated red blood cells. G Howell–Jolly bodies. H Polychromasia. I Basophilic stippling.

fibrosis, and infiltration by abnormal cells such as metastatic carcinoma. Bone marrow aspiration can usually be performed safely in a thrombocytopenic patient.

Investigation of coagulation

Bleeding disorders

In patients with clinical evidence of a bleeding disorder (p. 987), there are recommended screening tests (Box 24.3).

Coagulation tests measure the time to clot formation in vitro in a plasma sample after the clotting process is initiated by activators and calcium. The result of the test sample is compared with normal controls. The extrinsic pathway is assessed by the prothrombin time (PT) and the intrinsic pathway by the activated partial thromboplastin time (APTT), sometimes known as the partial thromboplastin time with kaolin, (PTTK). Clotting is delayed by deficiencies of coagulation factors and the presence of inhibitors of coagulation, e.g. heparin. The approximate normal ranges and causes of abnormalities are shown in Box 24.3. If both the PT and APTT are prolonged, there is deficiency or inhibition of the final common pathway which includes factors X, V, prothrombin and fibrinogen, or global coagulation factor deficiency involving more than one factor. Further specific tests may be performed based on interpretation of the clinical scenario and results of these screening tests. A mixing test with normal plasma allows differentiation between a coagulation factor deficiency (the prolonged time corrects) and the presence of an inhibitor of coagulation (the prolonged time does not correct); the latter may be chemical (heparins) or an antibody (most often a lupus anticoagulant but occasionally a specific inhibitor of one of the coagulation factors, typically factor VIII). Von Willebrand disease may present with a normal APTT; further investigation of suspected cases is detailed on page 64.

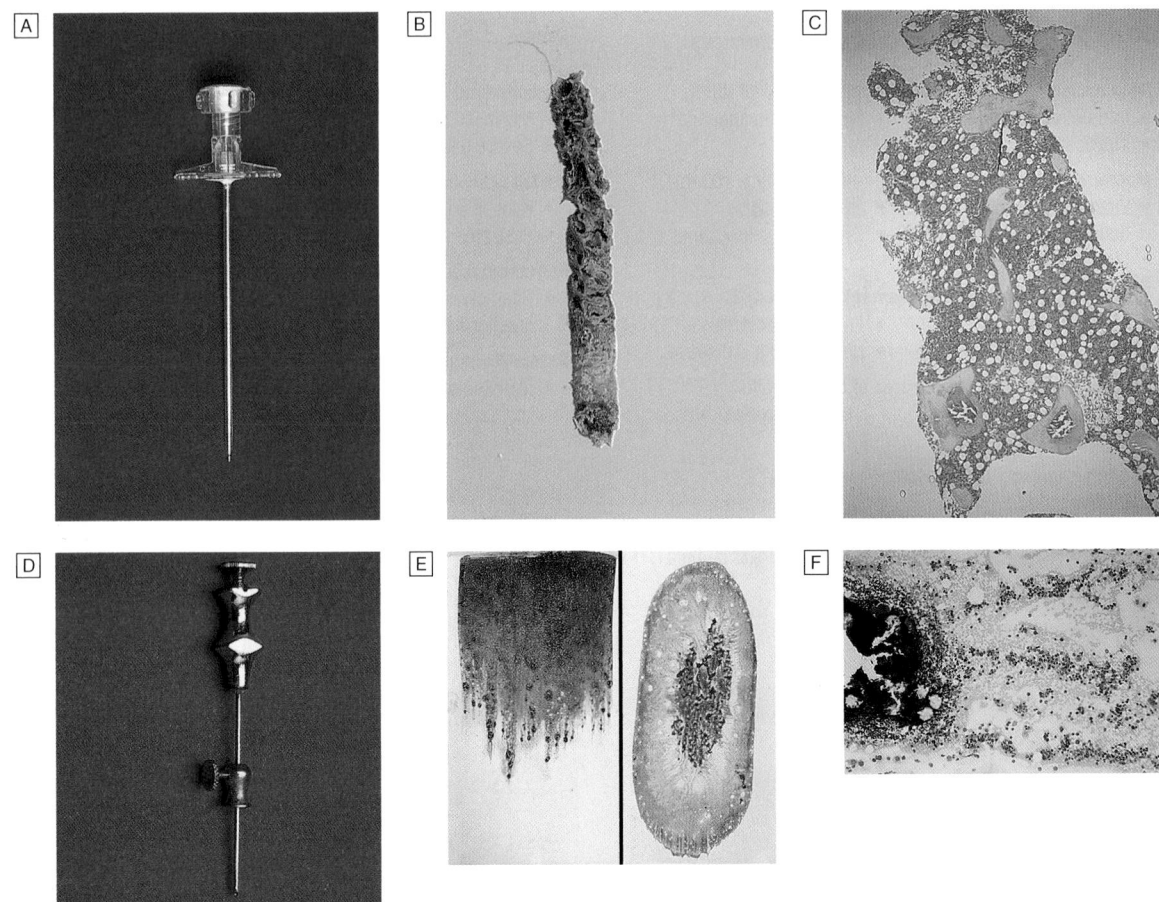

Fig. 24.9 Bone marrow aspirate and trephine. [A] Trephine biopsy needle. [B] Macroscopic appearance of a trephine biopsy. [C] Microscopic appearance of stained section of trephine. [D] Bone marrow aspirate needle. [E] Stained macroscopic appearance of marrow aspirate: smear (left) and squash (right). [F] Microscopic appearance of stained marrow particles and trails of haematopoietic cells.

24.3 Coagulation screening tests

Investigation	Normal range	Situations in which tests may be abnormal
Platelet count	150–400 × 10⁹/L	Thrombocytopenia
Bleeding time	< 8 mins	Thrombocytopenia Abnormal platelet function von Willebrand disease Vascular and connective tissue abnormalities
Prothrombin time (PT)	9–12 secs	Deficiencies of factors II, V, VII or X Severe fibrinogen deficiency
Activated partial thromboplastin time (APTT)	26–36 secs	Deficiencies of factors II, V, VIII, IX, X, XI, XII Severe fibrinogen deficiency Unfractionated heparin therapy Antibodies against clotting factors Lupus anticoagulant
Fibrinogen concentration	1.5–4.0 g/L	Hypofibrinogenaemia, e.g. liver failure, disseminated intravascular coagulation

N.B. International normalised ratio (INR) is used only to monitor coumarin therapy and is not a coagulation screening test.

Platelet function has historically been assessed by the bleeding time, using a standardised incision. However, many centres have abandoned this test as it is non-specific, being affected by the coagulation factor disorders shown in Box 24.3. Platelet function can be assessed in vitro by measuring aggregation in response to various agonists such as adrenaline (epinephrine), collagen, thrombin or ADP, or by measuring the constituents of the intracellular granules, e.g. ATP/ADP.

Coagulation screening tests are also performed in patients with suspected disseminated intravascular coagulation (DIC, p. 190) when clotting factors and platelets are consumed, resulting in thrombocytopenia and prolonged PT and APTT. In addition, there is evidence of active coagulation with consumption of fibrinogen and generation of fibrin degradation products (D-dimers). Note, however, that fibrinogen is an acute phase protein which may also be elevated in inflammatory disease (p. 81).

Monitoring anticoagulant therapy

The international normalised ratio (INR) is validated only to assess the therapeutic effect of coumarin anticoagulants, including warfarin. INR is the ratio of the patient's prothrombin time to that of a normal control, raised to the power of the international sensitivity index of the thromboplastin used in the test (ISI, derived by comparison with an international reference standard material).

Monitoring of heparin therapy is on the whole only required with unfractionated heparins. Therapeutic anticoagulation prolongs the APTT relative to a control sample by a ratio of ~1.5–2.5. Low molecular weight heparins have such a predictable dose response that monitoring of the anticoagulant effect is not required, except in patients with renal impairment (GFR < 30 mL/min).

Thrombotic disorders

Measurement of plasma levels of D-dimers derived from fibrin degradation is useful in excluding the diagnosis of active thrombosis in some patients (see Fig. 24.15, p. 1006).

A variety of tests exist which may help to explain an underlying propensity to thrombosis, especially venous thromboembolism (Box 24.4). Examples of indications for testing are given in Box 24.5. In most patients, the results do not affect clinical management (p. 1049) but they may influence the duration and intensity of anticoagulation (e.g. antiphospholipid antibodies, p. 1050), justify family screening in inherited thrombophilias (p. 1049), or suggest additional management strategies to reduce thrombosis risk (e.g. in myeloproliferative disease and paroxysmal nocturnal haemoglobinuria; p. 1027). Anticoagulants can interfere with some of these assays; for example, warfarin reduces protein C and S levels and affects measurement of lupus anticoagulant, while heparin interferes with antithrombin and lupus anticoagulant assays.

24.4 Investigation of possible thrombophilia

Full blood count

Plasma levels
- Antithrombin
- Protein C
- Protein S (free)

- Antiphospholipid antibodies/ lupus anticoagulant and anticardiolipin antibody

Thrombin/reptilase time (for dysfibrinogenaemia)

Genetic testing
- Factor V Leiden
- Prothrombin G20210A

- *JAK-2* mutation

Flow cytometry
- Screen for GPI-linked cell surface proteins (CD 14, 16, 55, 59), deficient in paroxysmal nocturnal haemoglobinuria

---

24.5 Indications for thrombophilia testing*

- Venous thrombosis < 45 years
- Recurrent venous thrombosis
- Family history of unprovoked or recurrent thrombosis
- Combined arterial and venous thrombosis

- Venous thrombosis at an unusual site
  Cerebral venous thrombosis
  Hepatic vein (Budd–Chiari syndrome)
  Portal vein, mesenteric vein

*Antiphospholipid antibodies should be sought where clinical criteria for antiphospholipid syndrome (APS) are fulfilled (p. 1050).

24.6 Haematological investigations in old age

- **Blood cell counts and film components**: not altered by ageing alone.
- **Ratio of bone marrow cells to marrow fat**: falls.
- **Neutrophils**: maintained throughout life, although leucocytes may be less readily mobilised by bacterial invasion in old age.
- **Lymphocytes**: functionally compromised by age due to a T cell-related defect in cell-mediated immunity.
- **Clotting factors**: no major changes, although mild congenital deficiencies may be first noticed in old age.
- **Erythrocyte sedimentation rate (ESR)**: raised above the normal range, but usually in association with chronic or subacute disease. In truly healthy older people the ESR range is very similar to that in younger people.

PRESENTING PROBLEMS IN BLOOD DISEASE

Anaemia

Anaemia refers to a state in which the level of haemoglobin in the blood is below the normal range appropriate for age and sex. Other factors, including pregnancy and altitude, also affect haemoglobin levels and must be taken into account when considering whether an individual is anaemic. The clinical features of anaemia reflect diminished oxygen supply to the tissues (p. 987). A rapid onset of anaemia (e.g. due to blood loss) causes more profound symptoms than a gradually developing anaemia. Individuals with cardiorespiratory disease are more susceptible to symptoms of anaemia.

The clinical assessment and investigation of anaemia must not only assess its severity but also define the underlying cause (Box 24.7).

Clinical assessment

- *Iron deficiency anaemia* (p. 1017) is the most common type of anaemia world-wide. A thorough gastrointestinal history is important, looking in particular for symptoms of blood loss. Menorrhagia is a common cause of anaemia in pre-menopausal females, so women should always be asked about their periods.
- *A dietary history* should assess the intake of iron and folate which may become deficient in comparison to needs (e.g. in pregnancy or during periods of rapid growth; pp. 1020 and 114).

24.7 Causes of anaemia

Decreased or ineffective marrow production

- Lack of iron, vitamin B$_{12}$ or folate
- Hypoplasia

- Invasion by malignant cells
- Renal failure
- Anaemia of chronic disease

Peripheral causes

- Blood loss
- Haemolysis

- Hypersplenism

24

- *Past medical history* may reveal a disease which is known to be associated with anaemia, such as rheumatoid arthritis (the anaemia of chronic disease), or previous surgery (e.g. resection of the stomach or small bowel which may lead to malabsorption of iron and/or vitamin B$_{12}$).
- *Family history and ethnic background* may raise suspicion of haemolytic anaemias such as the haemoglobinopathies and hereditary spherocytosis. Pernicious anaemia may also be familial.
- *A drug history* may reveal the ingestion of drugs which cause blood loss (e.g. aspirin and anti-inflammatory drugs), haemolysis or aplasia.

On examination, as well as the general physical findings of anaemia shown on page 987, there may be specific findings related to the aetiology of the anaemia; for example, a patient may be found to have a right iliac fossa mass due to an underlying caecal carcinoma. Haemolytic anaemias can cause jaundice. Vitamin B$_{12}$ deficiency may be associated with neurological signs including peripheral neuropathy, dementia and signs of subacute combined degeneration of the cord (p. 1021). Sickle-cell anaemia (p. 1028) may result in leg ulcers, stroke or features of pulmonary hypertension. Anaemia may be multifactorial and the lack of specific symptoms and signs does not rule out silent pathology.

Investigations

Schemes for the investigation of anaemias are often based on the size of the red cells, which is most accurately indicated by the MCV in the FBC. Commonly, in the presence of anaemia:

- A normal MCV (normocytic anaemia) suggests either acute blood loss or the anaemia of chronic disease (ACD) (Fig. 24.10).
- A low MCV (microcytic anaemia) suggests iron deficiency or thalassaemia (see Fig. 24.10).
- A high MCV (macrocytic anaemia) suggests vitamin B$_{12}$ or folate deficiency or myelodysplasia (Fig. 24.11).

Specific types of anaemia and their management are described later in this chapter (pp. 1017–1027).

High haemoglobin

A haemoglobin level greater than the upper limit of normal (adult females 165 g/L or haematocrit > 0.48; adult males 180 g/L or haematocrit > 0.52) may be due

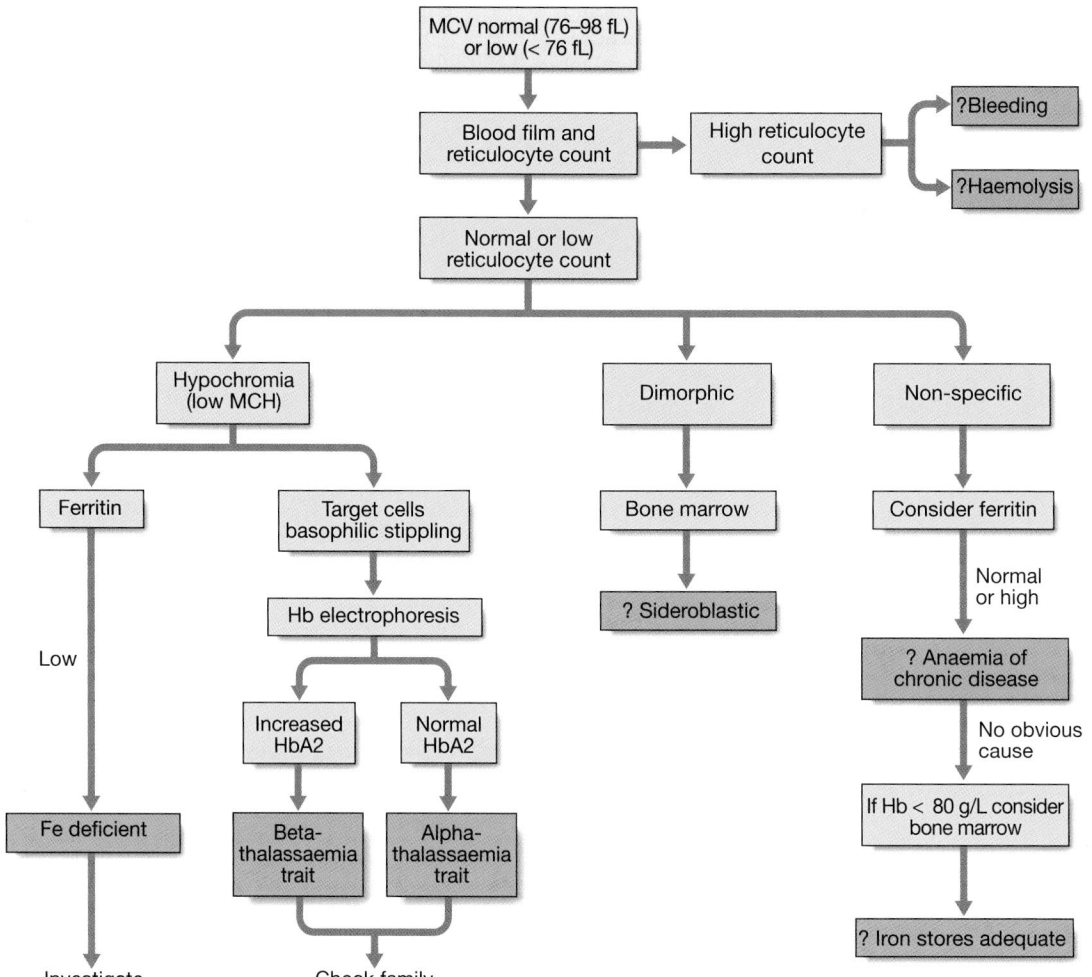

Fig. 24.10 Investigation of anaemia with normal or low MCV.

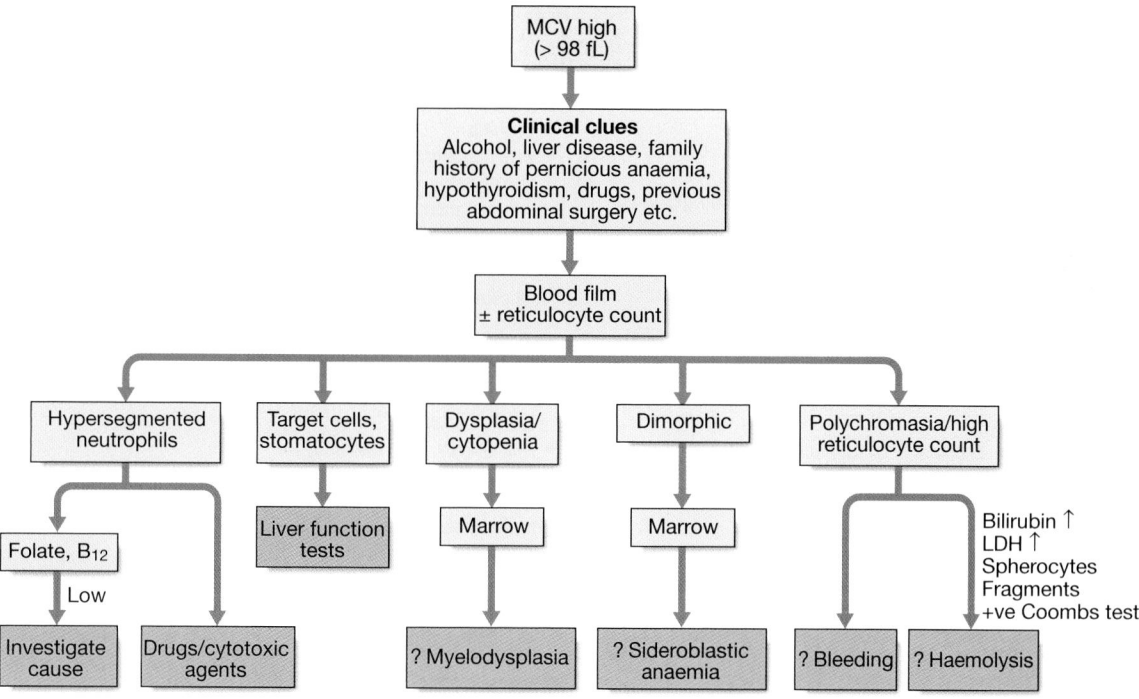

Fig. 24.11 Investigation of anaemia with high MCV. (LDH = lactate dehydrogenase)

to an increase in the number of red blood cells (true polycythaemia) or a reduction in the plasma volume (relative or apparent polycythaemia; Box 24.8). Circulating red cell mass is measured by radio-labelling an aliquot of the patient's red cells with ^{51}Cr, re-injecting the cells and measuring the dilution of the isotope. The plasma volume is measured by a similar dilution technique using albumin labelled with ^{125}I.

Causes of true polycythaemia are shown in Box 24.9. These involve increased erythropoiesis in the bone marrow, either due to a primary increase in marrow activity, in response to increased erythropoietin (Epo) levels in chronic hypoxaemia, or due to inappropriate secretion of Epo. Athletes who seek to benefit from increased oxygen-carrying capacity may be found guilty of doping offences as a result of their use of Epo.

Relative polycythaemia with a reduction in plasma volume is usually a consequence of dehydration, diuretic use or alcohol consumption.

Clinical assessment and investigations

A clinical history and examination will provide clues as to the aetiology of true polycythaemia. Those with PRV may have arterial thromboses, pruritus worse after a hot bath, hepatosplenomegaly and gout (due to high red cell turnover). The cardiovascular and respiratory systems should be assessed for evidence and causes of hypox-

24.9 Causes of true polycythaemia

	Aetiology	Examples
Primary	Myeloproliferative disorder	Polycythaemia rubra vera (PRV; primary proliferative polycythaemia)
Secondary	Increased Epo due to tissue hypoxia	High altitude Lung disease Cyanotic heart disease High-affinity haemoglobins

	Inappropriately increased Epo	Renal disease
		  Hydronephrosis
		  Cysts
		  Carcinoma
		Other tumours
		  Hepatoma
		  Bronchogenic carcinoma
		  Uterine fibroids
		  Phaeochromocytoma
		  Cerebellar haemangioblastoma
		Exogenous administration (e.g. endurance athletes)

aemia. In PRV a mutation in *JAK-2* is found in over 97% of cases (p. 1044). If no other cause is identified, further investigations to exclude inappropriate erythropoietin secretion should be performed.

Leucopenia (low white cell count)

A reduction in the total numbers of circulating white cells is called leucopenia. This may be due to a reduction in all types of white cell or in individual cell types

24.8 Classification of polycythaemia

	Red cell mass	Plasma volume
True polycythaemia	Increased	Normal
Relative polycythaemia	Normal	Decreased

24.10 How to interpret white blood cell results

Neutrophils A

Neutrophilia
- Infection: bacterial, fungal
- Trauma: surgery, burns
- Infarction: myocardial infarct, pulmonary embolus, sickle-cell crisis
- Inflammation: gout, rheumatoid arthritis, ulcerative colitis, Crohn's disease
- Malignancy: solid tumours, Hodgkin lymphoma
- Myeloproliferative disease: polycythaemia, chronic myeloid leukaemia
- Physiological: exercise, pregnancy

Neutropenia
- Infection: viral, bacterial (e.g. *Salmonella*), protozoal (e.g. malaria)
- Drugs: see Box 24.11
- Autoimmune: connective tissue disease
- Alcohol
- Bone marrow infiltration: leukaemia, myelodysplasia
- Congenital: Kostmann's syndrome

Eosinophils B

Eosinophilia
- Allergy: hay fever, asthma, eczema
- Infection: parasitic
- Drug hypersensitivity: e.g. gold, sulphonamides
- Skin disease
- Connective tissue disease: polyarteritis nodosa
- Malignancy: solid tumours, lymphomas
- Primary bone marrow disorders: myeloproliferative disorders, hypereosinophilia syndrome (HES), acute myeloid leukaemia

Basophils C

Basophilia
- Myeloproliferative disease: polycythaemia, chronic myeloid leukaemia
- Inflammation: acute hypersensitivity, ulcerative colitis, Crohn's disease
- Iron deficiency

Monocytes D

Monocytosis
- Infection: bacterial (e.g. tuberculosis)
- Inflammation: connective tissue disease, ulcerative colitis, Crohn's disease
- Malignancy: solid tumours

Lymphocytes E

Lymphocytosis
- Infection: viral, bacterial (e.g. *Bordetella pertussis*)
- Lymphoproliferative disease: chronic lymphocytic leukaemia, lymphoma
- Post-splenectomy

Lymphopenia
- Inflammation: connective tissue disease
- Lymphoma
- Renal failure
- Sarcoidosis
- Drugs: corticosteroids, cytotoxics
- Congenital: severe combined immunodeficiency

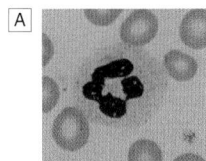 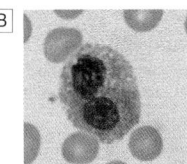 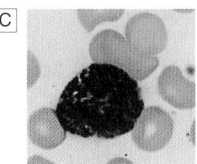 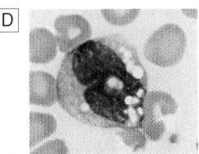 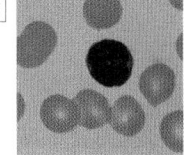

Fig. 24.12 A Neutrophil. B Eosinophil. C Basophil. D Monocyte. E Lymphocyte.

(usually neutrophils or lymphocytes). Leucopenia may occur in isolation or as part of a reduction in all three haematological lineages (pancytopenia; p. 1004).

Neutropenia

A reduction in neutrophil count (usually less than 1.5×10^9/L, but dependent on age and race) is called neutropenia. The main causes are listed in Box 24.10. Drug-induced neutropenia is not uncommon (Box 24.11). Clinical manifestations range from no symptoms to overwhelming sepsis. The risk of bacterial infection is related to the degree of neutropenia, with counts lower than 0.5×10^9/L considered to be critically low. Fever is the first and often only manifestation of infection. A sore throat, perianal pain or skin inflammation may be present. The lack of neutrophils allows the patient to become septicaemic and shocked within hours if immediate antibiotic therapy is not commenced. The management of such patients is discussed on page 1033.

Lymphopenia

This occurs when the absolute lymphocyte count is less than 1×10^9/L. The causes are shown in Box 24.10. Although minor deficiencies may be asymptomatic, deficiencies in cell-mediated immunity may cause infections (with organisms such as fungi, viruses and mycobacteria) and a propensity to lymphoid and other malignancies (particularly those associated with viral infections such as Epstein–Barr virus (EBV), human papillomavirus (HPV) and human herpes virus 8 (HHV-8)).

Leucocytosis (high white cell count)

An increase in the total numbers of circulating white cells is called leucocytosis. This is usually due to an increase in a specific type of cell (see Box 24.10). It is important to realise that an increase in a single type of white cell (e.g. eosinophils or monocytes) may not

24.11 Drugs which can induce neutropenia

Group	Examples
Analgesics/anti-inflammatory agents	Gold, penicillamine, naproxen
Antithyroid drugs	Carbimazole, propylthiouracil
Anti-arrhythmics	Quinidine, procainamide
Antihypertensives	Captopril, enalapril, nifedipine
Antidepressants/psychotropics	Amitriptyline, dosulepin, mianserin
Antimalarials	Pyrimethamine, dapsone, sulfadoxine, chloroquine
Anticonvulsants	Phenytoin, sodium valproate, carbamazepine
Antibiotics	Sulphonamides, penicillins, cephalosporins
Miscellaneous	Cimetidine, ranitidine, chlorpropamide, zidovudine

increase the total white cell count (WCC) above the upper limit of normal and will only be apparent if the 'differential' of the white count is examined.

Neutrophilia

An increase in the number of circulating neutrophils is called a neutrophilia or a neutrophil leucocytosis. It can result from an increased production of cells from the bone marrow or redistribution from the marginated pool. The normal neutrophil count depends upon age, race and certain physiological parameters. During pregnancy, not only is there an increase in neutrophils but also earlier forms such as metamyelocytes can be found in the blood. The causes of a neutrophilia are shown in Box 24.10.

Eosinophilia

A high eosinophil count $> 0.5 \times 10^9/L$ is usually secondary to infection (especially parasites; p. 307), allergy (e.g. eczema, asthma, reactions to drugs; p. 86), immunological disorders (e.g. polyarteritis, sarcoidosis) or malignancy (e.g. lymphomas)(see Box 24.10). Usually, such eosinophilia is short-lived.

In the rarer primary disorders, there is a persistently raised, often clonal, eosinophilia: for example, in myeloproliferative disorders, subtypes of acute myeloid leukaemia and idiopathic hypereosinophilic syndrome (HES). Recently, specific mutations in receptor tyrosine kinase genes have been found in some primary eosinophilias (e.g. causing rearrangements of platelet-derived growth factor receptors α and β or c-kit), which allow diagnosis and, in some cases, specific therapy with tyrosine kinase inhibitors such as imatinib.

Eosinophil infiltration can damage many organs (e.g. heart, lungs, gastrointestinal tract, skin, musculoskeletal system); therefore evaluation of eosinophilia includes not only the identification of any underlying cause and its appropriate treatment, but also assessment of any related organ damage.

Lymphocytosis

A lymphocytosis is an increase in circulating lymphocytes above that expected for the patient's age. In adults this is $> 3.5 \times 10^9/L$. Infants and children have higher counts; age-related normal ranges should be consulted. Causes are shown in Box 24.10; the most common is viral infection.

Lymphadenopathy

Enlarged lymph glands may be an important indicator of haematological disease but they are not uncommon in reaction to infection or inflammation (Box 24.12). The sites of lymph node groups, and symptoms and signs that may help elucidate the underlying cause are shown on page 987. Nodes which enlarge in response to local infection or inflammation ('reactive nodes') usually expand rapidly and are painful, whereas those due to haematological disease are more frequently painless. Localised lymphadenopathy should elicit a search for a source of inflammation in the appropriate drainage area:

- the scalp, ear, mouth, face or teeth for neck nodes
- the breast for axillary nodes
- the perineum or external genitalia for inguinal nodes.

Generalised lymphadenopathy may be secondary to infection, connective tissue disease or extensive skin disease, but is more likely to signify underlying haematological malignancy. Weight loss and drenching night sweats which may require a change of night clothes are associated with haematological malignancies, particularly lymphoma.

Initial investigations in lymphadenopathy include an FBC (to detect neutrophilia in infection or evidence of haematological disease), an ESR and a chest X-ray (to detect mediastinal lymphadenopathy). If the findings suggest malignancy, a formal cutting needle or excision biopsy of a representative node is indicated to obtain a histological diagnosis.

24.12 Causes of lymphadenopathy

Infective
- Bacterial: streptococcal, tuberculosis, brucellosis
- Viral: Epstein-Barr virus (EBV), human immunode ficiency virus (HIV)
- Protozoal: toxoplasmosis
- Fungal: histoplasmosis, coccidioidomycosis

Neoplastic
- Primary: lymphomas, leukaemias
- Secondary: lung, breast, thyroid, stomach

Connective tissue disorders
- Rheumatoid arthritis
- Systemic lupus erythematosus (SLE)

Sarcoidosis

Amyloidosis

Drugs
- Phenytoin

24

Splenomegaly

The spleen may be enlarged due to involvement by lymphoproliferative disease, the resumption of extra-medullary haematopoiesis in myeloproliferative disease, enhanced reticulo-endothelial activity in autoimmune haemolysis, expansion of the lymphoid tissue in response to infections or vascular congestion as a result of portal hypertension (Box 24.13). Hepatosplenomegaly is suggestive of lympho- or myeloproliferative disease, liver disease or infiltration (e.g. with amyloid). Associated lymphadenopathy is suggestive of lymphoproliferative disease. An enlarged spleen may cause abdominal discomfort, accompanied by back pain and abdominal bloating due to stomach compression. Splenic infarction may occur and produces severe abdominal pain radiating to the left shoulder tip, associated with a splenic rub on auscultation. Rarely, spontaneous or traumatic rupture and bleeding may occur.

Investigation will focus on the suspected cause. Imaging of the spleen by ultrasound or computed tomography (CT) will detect variations in density in the spleen which may be a feature of lymphoproliferative disease; it also allows imaging of the liver and abdominal lymph nodes. Biopsy of enlarged abdominal or superficial lymph nodes may provide the diagnosis. A chest X-ray or CT of the thorax will detect mediastinal lymphadenopathy. An FBC may show pancytopenia secondary to hypersplenism, when the enlarged spleen has become overactive, destroying blood cells prematurely. If other abnormalities are present, such as abnormal lymphocytes or a leuco-erythroblastic blood film, a bone marrow examination is indicated. Screening for infectious or liver disease (pp. 307 and 926) may be appropriate. If all investigations are unhelpful, splenectomy may be diagnostic.

Bleeding

Normal bleeding is seen following surgery and trauma. Pathological bleeding occurs when structurally abnormal vessels rupture or when a vessel is breached in the presence of a defect in haemostasis. This may be due to a deficiency or dysfunction of platelets, the coagulation factors, or occasionally to excessive fibrinolysis, which is most commonly observed following therapeutic thrombolysis (p. 594).

Clinical assessment

'Screening' blood tests (see Box 24.3, p. 996) do not reliably detect all causes of pathological bleeding (e.g. von Willebrand disease, scurvy and the causes of purpura in Box 24.14) and should not be used indiscriminately. A careful clinical evaluation is the key to diagnosis of bleeding disorders (see pp. 1044–1049).

It is important to consider the following points:

- *Site of bleeding.* Bleeding into muscle and joints, along with retroperitoneal and intracranial haemorrhage, indicates a likely defect in coagulation factors. Purpura, prolonged bleeding from superficial cuts, epistaxis, gastrointestinal haemorrhage or menorrhagia is more likely to be due to thrombocytopenia, a platelet function disorder or von Willebrand disease. Recurrent

24.13 Causes of splenomegaly

Congestive

Intrahepatic portal hypertension
- Cirrhosis
- Hepatic vein occlusion

Extrahepatic portal hypertension
- Thrombosis
- Stenosis or malformation of the portal or splenic vein

Cardiac
- Chronic congestive cardiac failure
- Constrictive pericarditis

Infective

Bacterial
- Endocarditis
- Septicaemia
- Tuberculosis
- Brucellosis
- Salmonella

Viral
- Hepatitis
- Epstein–Barr
- Cytomegalovirus

Protozoal
- Malaria*
- Leishmaniasis (kala-azar)*
- Trypanosomiasis

Fungal
- Histoplasmosis

Inflammatory/granulomatous disorders
- Felty's syndrome in rheumatoid arthritis
- Systemic lupus erythematosus
- Sarcoidosis

Haematological

Red cell disorders
- Megaloblastic anaemia
- Haemoglobinopathies

Autoimmune haemolytic anaemias

Myeloproliferative disorders
- Chronic myeloid leukaemia*
- Myelofibrosis*
- Polycythaemia rubra vera
- Essential thrombocythaemia

Neoplastic
- Leukaemias, including chronic myeloid leukaemia*
- Lymphomas

Other malignancies
- Metastatic cancer—rare

Lysosomal storage diseases
- Gaucher's disease
- Niemann–Pick disease

Miscellaneous
- Cysts, amyloid, thyrotoxicosis

Causes of massive splenomegaly.

bleeds at a single site suggest a local structural abnormality.
- *Duration of history.* It may be possible to assess whether the disorder is congenital or acquired.
- *Precipitating causes.* Bleeding arising spontaneously indicates a more severe defect than bleeding that occurs only after trauma.

24.14 Causes of non-thrombocytopenic purpura

- Senile purpura
- Factitious purpura
- Henoch–Schönlein purpura (pp. 501 and 1114)
- Vasculitis (p. 1112)
- Paraproteinaemias
- Purpura fulminans

- *Surgery.* Ask about all operations. Dental extractions, tonsillectomy and circumcision are particularly stressful tests of the haemostatic system. Immediate post-surgical bleeding suggests defective platelet plug formation and primary haemostasis, while delayed haemorrhage is more suggestive of a coagulation defect. However, in post-surgical patients, persistent bleeding from a single site is more likely to indicate surgical bleeding than a bleeding disorder.
- *Family history.* While a positive family history may be present in patients with inherited disorders, the absence of affected relatives does not exclude a hereditary bleeding diathesis; about one-third of cases of haemophilia arise in individuals without a family history and deficiencies of factor VII, X and XIII are recessively inherited. Recessive disorders are more common in cultures where there is consanguineous marriage.
- *Drugs.* Use of antithrombotic, anticoagulant and fibrinolytic drugs must be elicited. Drug interactions with warfarin and drug-induced thrombocytopenia should be considered. Some 'herbal' remedies may result in a bleeding diathesis.

Superficial clinical examination may reveal different patterns of skin bleeding. Petechial purpura is minor bleeding into the dermis that is flat and non-blanching (Fig. 24.13). Petechiae are typically found in patients with thrombocytopenia or platelet dysfunction. Palpable purpura occurs in vasculitis. Ecchymosis, or bruising, is more extensive bleeding into deeper layers of the skin. The lesions are initially dark red or purple but become yellow as haemoglobin is degraded. Retroperitoneal bleeding presents with a flank haematoma. Telangiectasia of lips and tongue points to hereditary haemorrhagic telangiectasia (p. 1045). Joints should be examined for evidence of haemarthroses. A full exam-

ination is important, as it may give clues to an underlying associated systemic illness such as a haematological or other malignancy, liver disease, renal failure, connective tissue disease and possible causes of splenomegaly.

Investigations

Screening investigations and their interpretation are described on pages 995–997. If the patient has a history strongly suggestive of a bleeding disorder and all the preliminary screening tests give normal results, further investigations, such as measurement of von Willebrand factor and assessment of platelet function, should be performed (p. 1048).

Thrombocytopenia (low platelet count)

A reduced platelet count may arise by one of two mechanisms:

Box 24.15 Causes of thrombocytopenia

Decreased production

Marrow hypoplasia
- Childhood bone marrow failure syndromes, e.g. Fanconi's anaemia, dyskeratosis congenita, amegakaryocytic thrombocytopenia
- Idiopathic aplastic anaemia
- Drug-induced: cytotoxics, antimetabolites
- Transfusion-associated graft-versus-host disease

Marrow infiltration
- Leukaemia
- Myeloma
- Carcinoma (rare)
- Myelofibrosis
- Osteopetrosis
- Lysosomal storage disorders, e.g. Gaucher's disease

Haematinic deficiency
- Vitamin B_{12} and/or folate deficiency

Familial (macro-)thrombocytopathies
- Myosin heavy chain abnormalities, e.g. Alport's syndrome, Fechner's syndrome
- Bernard Soulier disease
- Montreal platelet syndrome
- Wiskott–Aldrich syndrome (small platelets)

Increased consumption of platelets

Immune mechanisms
- Idiopathic thrombocytopenic purpura (ITP)*
- Post-transfusion purpura
- Neonatal alloimmune thrombocytopenia
- Drug-associated, especially quinine

Coagulation activation
- Disseminated intravascular coagulation (DIC) (see Box 24.70, p. 1050)

Mechanical pooling
- Hypersplenism

Thrombotic microangiopathies
- Haemolytic uraemic syndrome
- Liver disease
- Thrombotic thrombocytopenic purpura

Others
- Gestational thrombocytopenia
- Type 2B von Willebrand disease

*Associated conditions include collagen vascular diseases (particularly SLE), B cell malignancy, HIV infection, antiphospholipid syndrome

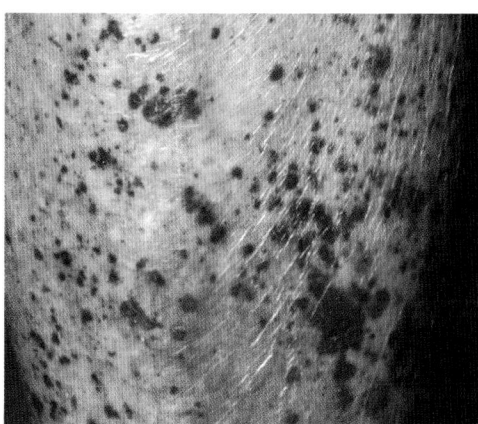

Fig. 24.13 Petechial purpura.

24

- decreased or abnormal production (bone marrow failure and hereditary thrombocytopathies)
- increased consumption following release into the circulation (immune-mediated, disseminated intravascular coagulation (DIC) or sequestration).

Spontaneous bleeding does not usually occur until the platelet count falls below $20 \times 10^9/L$, unless their function is also compromised. Purpura and spontaneous bruising are characteristic but there may also be oral, nasal, gastrointestinal or genitourinary bleeding. Severe thrombocytopenia ($< 10 \times 10^9/L$) may result in retinal haemorrhage and potentially fatal intracranial bleeding.

Investigations are directed at the possible causes listed in Box 24.15. A blood film is the single most useful initial investigation. Examination of the bone marrow may reveal increased megakaryocytes in consumptive causes of thrombocytopenia, or the underlying cause of bone marrow failure in leukaemia, hypoplastic anaemia or myelodysplasia.

Treatment (if required) depends on the underlying cause. Platelet transfusion is rarely required and is usually confined to patients with bone marrow failure and platelet counts $< 10 \times 10^9/L$, or to clinical situations with actual or predicted serious haemorrhage.

Thrombocytosis (high platelet count)

The most common reason for a raised platelet count is that it is reactive to another process such as infection, connective tissue disease, malignancy, iron deficiency, acute haemolysis or gastrointestinal bleeding (Box 24.16). The presenting clinical features are usually those of the underlying disorder and haemostasis is rarely affected. Reactive thrombocytosis is distinguished from the myeloproliferative disorders by the presence of uniform small platelets and lack of splenomegaly. The key to diagnosis is the clinical history and examination, combined with observation of the platelet count over time.

The platelets are a product of an abnormally expanding clone of cells in the myeloproliferative disorders, chronic myeloid leukaemia and some forms of myelodysplasia. Patients with PRV, essential thrombocythaemia and occasionally myelofibrosis may present with thrombosis or rarely bleeding. Stroke and transient ischaemic attacks, amaurosis fugax, or digital ischaemia or gangrene are also features. In addition, patients with myeloproliferative disorders present with features such

as itching after exposure to water (aquagenic pruritus), splenomegaly and systemic upset.

Pancytopenia

Pancytopenia refers to the combination of anaemia, leucopenia and thrombocytopenia. It may be due to reduced production of blood cells as a consequence of bone marrow suppression or infiltration, or there may be peripheral destruction or splenic pooling of mature cells. Causes are shown in Box 24.17. A bone marrow aspirate and trephine are usually required to establish the diagnosis.

24.17 Causes of pancytopenia
Bone marrow failure
• Hypoplastic/aplastic anaemia (p. 1043): inherited, idiopathic, viral, drugs
Bone marrow infiltration
• Acute leukaemia
• Myeloma
• Lymphoma
• Carcinoma
• Haemophagocytic syndrome
• Myelodysplastic syndromes
Ineffective haematopoiesis
• Megaloblastic anaemia
• Acquired immunodeficiency syndrome (AIDS)
Peripheral pooling/destruction
• Hypersplenism: portal hypertension, Felty's syndrome, malaria, myelofibrosis
• Systemic lupus erythematosus (SLE)

Infection

Infection is a major complication of haematological disorders. The type of infection relates to the immunological deficit caused by the disease itself, or its treatment with chemotherapy and/or immunotherapy (pp. 1000 and 298).

Venous thrombosis

While the most common presentation of venous thromboembolic disease (VTE) is with deep vein thrombosis (DVT) of the leg and/or pulmonary embolism (PE; see also p. 717), similar principles apply to rarer manifestations such as jugular vein thrombosis, upper limb DVT, cerebral sinus thrombosis (p. 1191) and intra-abdominal venous thrombosis (e.g. Budd–Chiari syndrome; p. 973).

DVT has an annual incidence of approximately 1:1000 in Western populations and the case mortality is 1–3%. It is increasingly common with ageing, and many of the deaths are related to coexisting medical conditions. Risk factors for DVT and PE are often present (Box 24.18). Figure 24.14 illustrates some of the causes and consequences of VTE disease.

24.16 Causes of a raised platelet count	
Reactive thrombocytosis	
• Chronic inflammatory disorders	• Haemolytic anaemias
• Malignant disease	• Post-splenectomy
• Tissue damage	• Post-haemorrhage
Clonal thrombocytosis	
• Primary thrombocythaemia	• Myelodysplastic syndromes (refractory anaemia with sideroblasts (RARS) with thrombocytosis, 5q⁻ syndrome)
• Polycythaemia rubra vera (PRV)	
• Myelofibrosis	
• Chronic myeloid leukaemia	

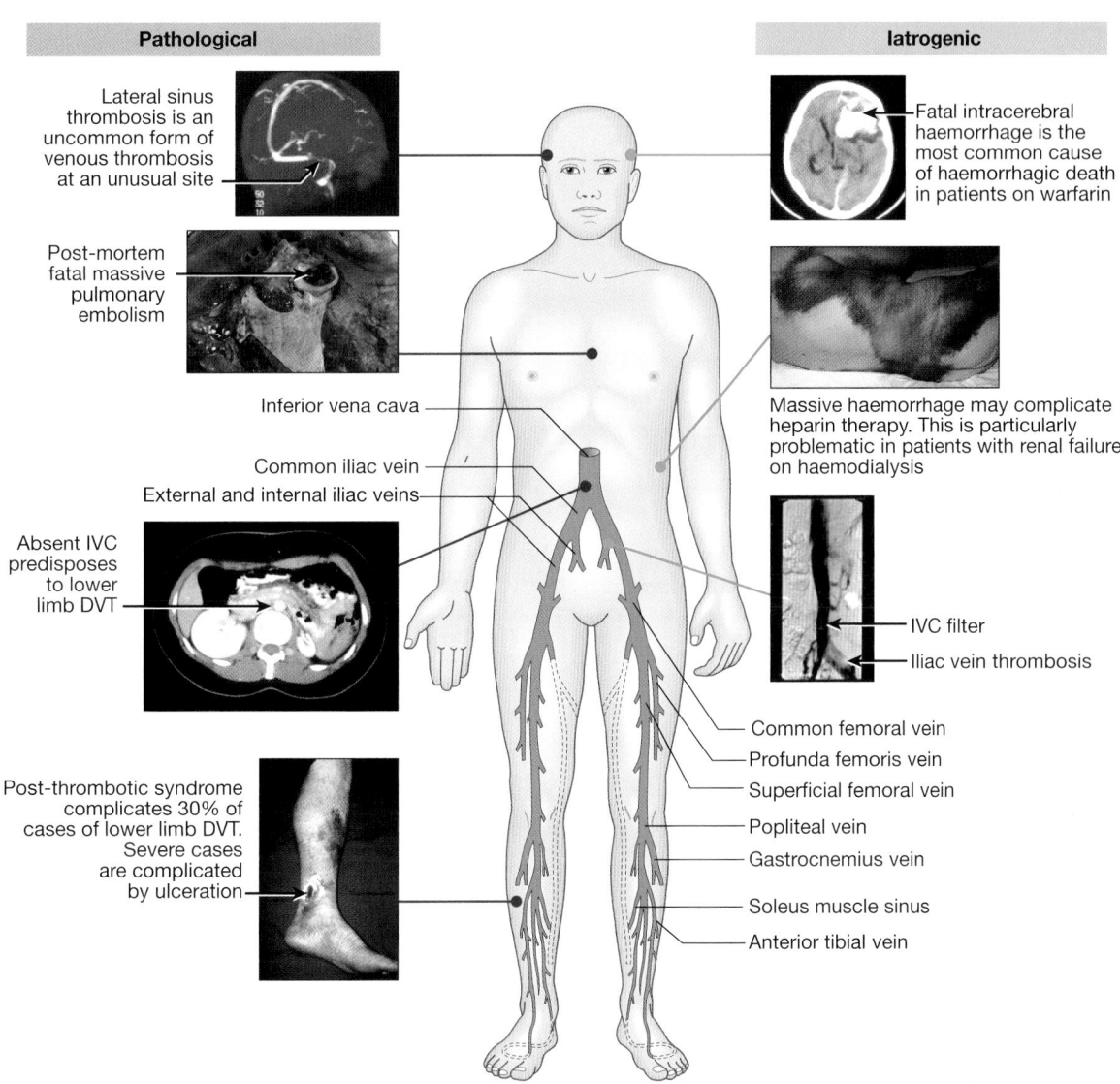

Pathological

Lateral sinus thrombosis is an uncommon form of venous thrombosis at an unusual site

Post-mortem fatal massive pulmonary embolism

Inferior vena cava

Common iliac vein

External and internal iliac veins

Absent IVC predisposes to lower limb DVT

Post-thrombotic syndrome complicates 30% of cases of lower limb DVT. Severe cases are complicated by ulceration

Iatrogenic

Fatal intracerebral haemorrhage is the most common cause of haemorrhagic death in patients on warfarin

Massive haemorrhage may complicate heparin therapy. This is particularly problematic in patients with renal failure on haemodialysis

IVC filter

Iliac vein thrombosis

Common femoral vein

Profunda femoris vein

Superficial femoral vein

Popliteal vein

Gastrocnemius vein

Soleus muscle sinus

Anterior tibial vein

Fig. 24.14 Causes and consequences of venous thromboembolic disease.

Clinical assessment

Lower limb DVT characteristically starts in the distal veins, causing pain, swelling, an increase in temperature and dilatation of the superficial veins. Often, however, there are only minimal symptoms and signs. It is typically unilateral but may be bilateral when clot extends proximally into the inferior vena cava. Bilateral DVT is more commonly seen in patients with underlying malignancy or anomalies of the inferior vena cava. The differential diagnosis of unilateral leg swelling includes a spontaneous or traumatic calf muscle tear or a ruptured Baker's cyst, both characterised by sudden onset and by localised tenderness. Baker's cysts usually occur in patients with rheumatoid arthritis. Infective cellulitis is usually distinguished by marked skin erythema and heat which is localised within a well-demarcated area of the leg and may be associated with an obvious source of entry of infection (e.g. an insect bite or leg ulcer).

Risk factors for DVT should be considered (see Box 24.18), and examination should include assessment for malignancy. Symptoms and signs of PE should be sought (p. 717), particularly in those with proximal thrombosis; asymptomatic PE is thought to be present in approximately 30% of patients with lower limb DVT.

Clinical criteria can be used to rank patients according to their likelihood of DVT using the Wells scoring system (Box 24.19).

Investigations

Figure 24.15 gives an algorithm for investigation of suspected DVT based on initial Wells score (see Box 24.19). In patients with a low pre-test probability of DVT, D-dimer levels can be measured; if these are normal, further investigation for DVT is unnecessary. In those with moderate or high probability of DVT or with elevated D-dimer levels, objective diagnosis of DVT should be obtained using appropriate imaging.

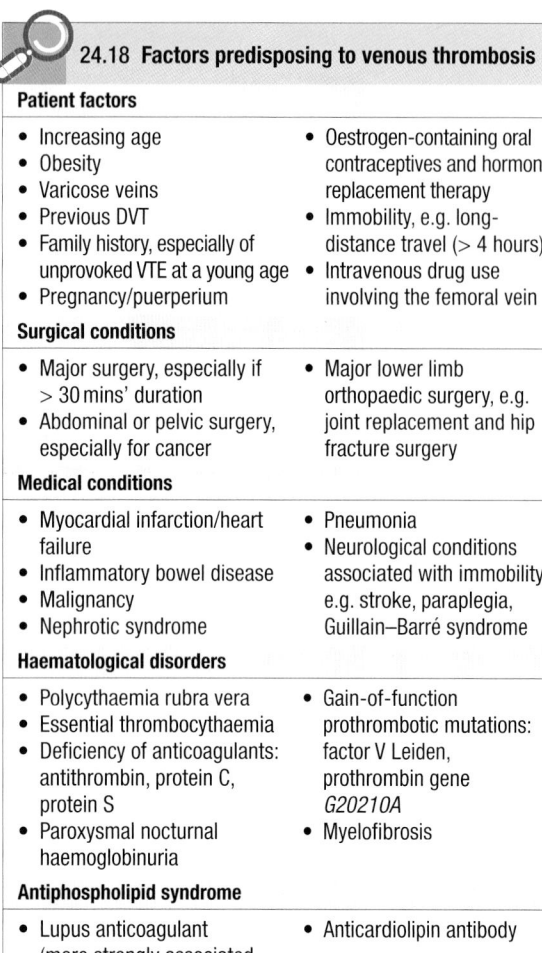

24.18 Factors predisposing to venous thrombosis

Patient factors

- Increasing age
- Obesity
- Varicose veins
- Previous DVT
- Family history, especially of unprovoked VTE at a young age
- Pregnancy/puerperium
- Oestrogen-containing oral contraceptives and hormone replacement therapy
- Immobility, e.g. long-distance travel (> 4 hours)
- Intravenous drug use involving the femoral vein

Surgical conditions

- Major surgery, especially if > 30 mins' duration
- Abdominal or pelvic surgery, especially for cancer
- Major lower limb orthopaedic surgery, e.g. joint replacement and hip fracture surgery

Medical conditions

- Myocardial infarction/heart failure
- Inflammatory bowel disease
- Malignancy
- Nephrotic syndrome
- Pneumonia
- Neurological conditions associated with immobility, e.g. stroke, paraplegia, Guillain–Barré syndrome

Haematological disorders

- Polycythaemia rubra vera
- Essential thrombocythaemia
- Deficiency of anticoagulants: antithrombin, protein C, protein S
- Paroxysmal nocturnal haemoglobinuria
- Gain-of-function prothrombotic mutations: factor V Leiden, prothrombin gene *G20210A*
- Myelofibrosis

Antiphospholipid syndrome

- Lupus anticoagulant (more strongly associated with thrombosis than anticardiolipin antibodies)
- Anticardiolipin antibody

24.19 Predicting the pre-test probability of deep vein thrombosis

Clinical characteristic	Score
Active cancer (patient receiving treatment for cancer within the previous 6 months or currently receiving palliative treatment)	1
Paralysis, paresis or recent plaster immobilisation of the lower extremities	1
Recently bedridden for 3 days or more, or major surgery within the previous 4 weeks	1
Localised tenderness along the distribution of the deep venous system	1
Entire leg swollen	1
Calf swelling at least 3 cm larger than that on the asymptomatic side (measured 10 cm below the tibial tuberosity)	1
Pitting oedema confined to the symptomatic leg	1
Collateral superficial veins (non-varicose)	1
Alternative diagnosis at least as likely as DVT	–2
Clinical probability	**Total score**
DVT low probability	< 1
DVT moderate probability	1–2
DVT high probability	> 2

an alternative that is now rarely used. In patients with suspected PE, further investigation is described on pages 717–719.

Predisposing factors, particularly pelvic malignancy and those listed in Box 24.18, should be considered and investigation pursued as appropriate. In occasional patients, further investigation for an underlying thrombophilic condition may be considered (see Boxes 24.4 and 24.5, p. 997).

Management

The management of leg DVT includes elevation and analgesia. Thrombolysis may be considered for limb-threatening DVT, but the mainstay of treatment is anticoagulation with low molecular weight heparin (LMWH) followed by a coumarin anticoagulant, such as warfarin, to achieve a target INR of 2.5 (range 2–3; pp. 996 and 1014).

Compression ultrasound is the imaging modality of choice in most centres. It has a sensitivity for proximal DVT (clot involving the popliteal vein or above) of 99.5%. Sensitivity and specificity are lower for diagnosing calf vein thrombosis. Contrast venography is

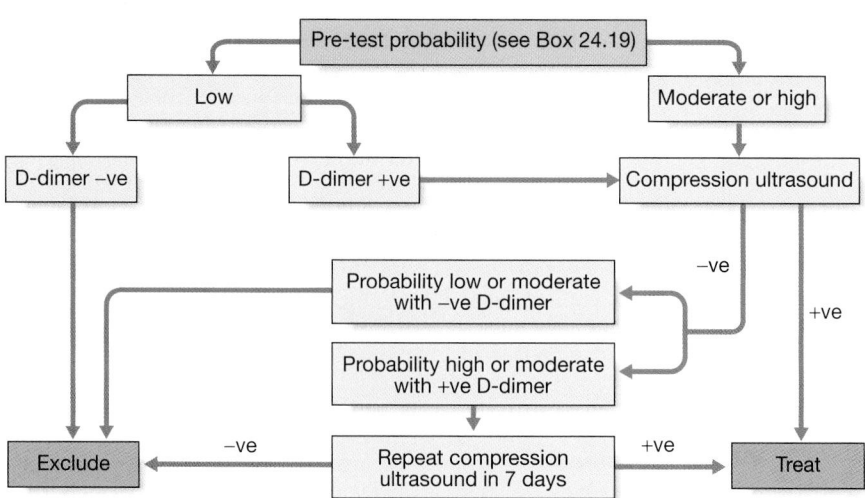

Fig. 24.15 Investigation of suspected DVT. Pre-test probability is calculated in Box 24.19.

EBM 24.20 Treatment of venous thromboembolism

'In patients with active cancer, treatment of DVT with LMWH for 6 months is superior in preventing recurrence of thrombosis to short-period LMWH followed by warfarin.'

• Lee AY, et al. N Engl J Med 2003; 349(2):146–153.

EBM 24.21 Red cell transfusion in critically ill patients

'In patients in intensive care, mortality and morbidity are similar or better in patients in whom Hb is maintained at 70–90 g/L than in those who received approximately twice as many red cell units to maintain Hb at 100–200 g/L.'

• Scottish Intercollegiate Guidelines Network (SIGN) guideline 54: Perioperative blood transfusion for elective surgery; revised 2004.

For further information: www.transfusionguidelines.org.uk
www.sign.ac.uk

Treatment of acute VTE with heparin should continue for a minimum of 5 days. If a coumarin is being introduced, the heparin should continue until the INR has been in the target range for 2 days. Patients who have had a DVT and have a strong contraindication to anticoagulation, and those who, despite therapeutic anticoagulation, continue to have new pulmonary emboli, should have an inferior vena cava filter inserted to prevent life-threatening PE.

The optimal duration of anticoagulation is between 6 weeks and 6 months. Patients who have thrombosis in the presence of a temporary risk factor which is then removed can usually be treated for shorter periods (e.g. 3 months) than those who sustain unprovoked thrombosis. In patients with active cancer and VTE, there is evidence that LMWH should be continued for 6 months rather than being replaced by a coumarin (Box 24.20). Evidence indicates that periods of anticoagulation of more than 6 months do not alter the rate of recurrence following discontinuation of therapy.

Recurrence of DVT is about 2–3% per annum in patients who have a medical temporary risk factor at presentation and about 10% per annum in those with apparently unprovoked DVT. This plateaus at around 30–40% recurrence at 5 years. Post-thrombotic syndrome is due to damage of venous valves by the thrombus. It results in persistent leg swelling, heaviness and discoloration. The most severe complication of this syndrome is ulceration around the medial malleolus.

BLOOD PRODUCTS AND TRANSFUSION

Blood is a tissue; transfusion from an unrelated donor to a recipient is a form of allogeneic transplant and inevitably carries some risk, including adverse immunological interactions between the host and graft (p. 93) and transmission of infectious agents. Although there are many compelling clinical indications for blood component transfusion, there are also many clinical circumstances in which transfusion is conventional but the evidence for its effectiveness is very limited. In these settings, allogeneic transfusion may be avoided by following protocols that recommend use of low haemoglobin thresholds for red cell transfusion (Box 24.21), perioperative blood salvage, antifibrinolytic drugs or recombinant coagulation proteins.

Blood products

Blood components are prepared from blood collected from individual human donors and include whole blood, red cells, platelets, plasma or cryoprecipitate (see Box 24.23 overleaf).

Plasma derivatives are licensed pharmaceutical products produced on a factory scale from large volumes of human plasma obtained from many individuals and treated to remove virus contamination. Examples include the following:

• *Coagulation factors.* Concentrates of factors VIII and IX were used for the treatment of conditions such as haemophilia A, haemophilia B and von Willebrand disease. Coagulation factors made by recombinant DNA technology are now preferred due to perceived lack of infection risk.

• *Immunoglobulins.* Intravenous immunoglobulin (IVIgG) is administered as regular replacement therapy to reduce infective complications in patients with antibody deficiencies. A short high-dose course of IVIgG may also be effective in some immunological disorders, including immune thrombocytopenia (p. 1045) and Guillain–Barré syndrome (p. 1229). However, IVIgG can cause acute renal failure, especially in the elderly, and acute reactions. It must be infused strictly according to the manufacturer's product information. Anti-zoster immunoglobulin has a role in the prophylaxis of varicella zoster (p. 313). Anti-Rhesus D immunoglobulin is used in pregnancy to prevent haemolytic disease of the newborn (see Box 24.25).

• *Human albumin.* This is available in two strengths. The 5% solution can be used as a colloid resuscitation fluid, but it is no more effective and is more expensive than crystalloid solutions (Box 24.22). Human albumin 20% solution is used in the management of hypoproteinaemic oedema with nephrotic syndrome (p. 479), and ascites in chronic liver disease (p. 936). It is hyperoncotic and expands plasma volume by more than the amount infused.

• Blood components and their use are summarised in Box 24.23.

Blood donation

A safe supply of blood products depends on a well-organised system with regular donation by healthy individuals who have no excess risk of infections transmissible

EBM 24.22 Fluid resuscitation in critically ill patients

'In patients with trauma, burns or following surgery there is no evidence that resuscitation with albumin or other colloid solutions reduces the risk of death compared to resuscitation with crystalloid solutions.'

• Perel P, Roberts I. (Cochrane Review). Cochrane Library, issue 4, 2007. Oxford: Update Software.

24

24.23 Blood components and their use

	Major haemorrhage	Other indications
Red cell concentrate[1] Most of the plasma is removed and replaced with a solution of glucose and adenine in saline to maintain viability of red cells ABO compatibility with recipient essential	Replace acute blood loss: increase circulating red cell mass to relieve clinical features caused by insufficient oxygen delivery	**Severe anaemia** If no cardiovascular disease, transfuse to maintain Hb at 70–90 g/L If known or likely to have cardiovascular disease, maintain Hb 90–100 g/L
Platelet concentrate One adult dose is made from 4–5 donations of whole blood, or from a single platelet apheresis ABO compatibility with recipient preferable	Maintain platelet count $> 50 \times 10^9$/L, or in multiple or CNS trauma $> 100 \times 10^9$/L Each adult dose has ~ 2.5–3×10^{11} platelets, which raises platelet count by $\sim 50 \times 10^9$/L unless there is consumptive coagulopathy, e.g. disseminated intravascular coagulation (DIC)	**Thrombocytopenia**, e.g. in acute leukaemia Maintain platelet count $>10 \times 10^9$/L if not bleeding Maintain platelet count $> 20 \times 10^9$/L if bleeding or at risk (sepsis, concurrent use of antibiotics, abnormal clotting) Increase platelet count $> 50 \times 10^9$/L for minor invasive procedure (e.g. lumbar puncture, gastroscopy and biopsy, insertion of indwelling lines, liver biopsy, laparotomy) Increase platelet count $> 100 \times 10^9$/L for operations in critical sites such as brain or eyes
Fresh frozen plasma (FFP)[2] 150–300 mL plasma from one donation of whole blood ABO compatibility with recipient recommended	Dilutional coagulopathy with a prothrombin time prolonged $> 50\%$ is likely after replacement of 1–1.5 blood volumes with red cell concentrate Initial dose of FFP 15 mL/kg Further doses only if bleeding continues and guided by PT and APTT	**Replacement of coagulation factor deficiency** If no virally inactivated or recombinant product is available **Thrombotic thrombocytopenic purpura (TTP)** Plasma exchange (or plasma infusion in HIV-related TTP) is frequently effective
Cryoprecipitate[2] Fibrinogen and coagulation factor concentrated from plasma by controlled thawing 10–20 mL pack contains fibrinogen 150–300 mg, factor VIII 80–120 U, von Willebrand factor 80–120 U In UK supplied as pools of 5 units	May be indicated if fibrinogen < 1 g/L due to dilution and DIC Pooled units containing 3–6 g fibrinogen in 200–500 mL raise fibrinogen by ~ 1 g/L	**von Willebrand disease and haemophilia** If virus-inactivated or recombinant products are not available

[1]**Whole blood** is an alternative to red cell concentrate. ABO compatibility with recipient essential.
[2]Use only if an alternative virus-inactivated plasma is unavailable: Pooled plasma can be treated with solvent and detergent or single units treated with methylene blue.

in blood (Fig. 24.16). Blood donations are obtained by either venesection of a unit of whole blood or collection of a specific component, such as platelets, by apheresis. During apheresis the donor's blood is drawn via a closed system into a machine which separates the components by centrifugation and collects the desired fraction into a bag, returning the rest of the blood to the donor. Each donation must be tested for hepatitis B (HBV), hepatitis C (HCV), HIV and human T lymphotropic (HTLV) virus nucleic acid and/or antibodies. Platelet concentrates may be tested for bacterial contamination. The need for other microbiological tests depends on local epidemiology. For example, testing for *Trypanosoma cruzi* (Chagas disease; p. 354) is required in areas of South America and the USA where infection is prevalent; tests for West Nile virus have been required in the USA since this agent became prevalent; plasma donated in the UK is not used at present for producing pooled plasma derivatives in view of concerns about transmission of variant Creutzfeldt–Jakob disease (vCJD; p. 1214).

Adverse effects of transfusion

Death directly attributable to transfusion is rare, at < 0.5 per 100 000 transfusions. However, relatively minor symptoms of transfusion reactions (fever, itch or urticaria) occur during about 1% of transfusions, usually in patients who have had repeated transfusions. Any symptoms or signs that arise during a transfusion must be taken seriously, as they may be the first warnings of a serious reaction. Figure 24.18 (p. 1012) outlines the symptoms and signs, management and investigation of acute reactions to blood products.

Red cell incompatibility

Red blood cell membranes contain numerous cell surface molecules which are potentially antigenic (see Fig. 24.4, p. 990). The ABO and Rh(D) antigens are the most important in routine transfusion and antenatal practice.

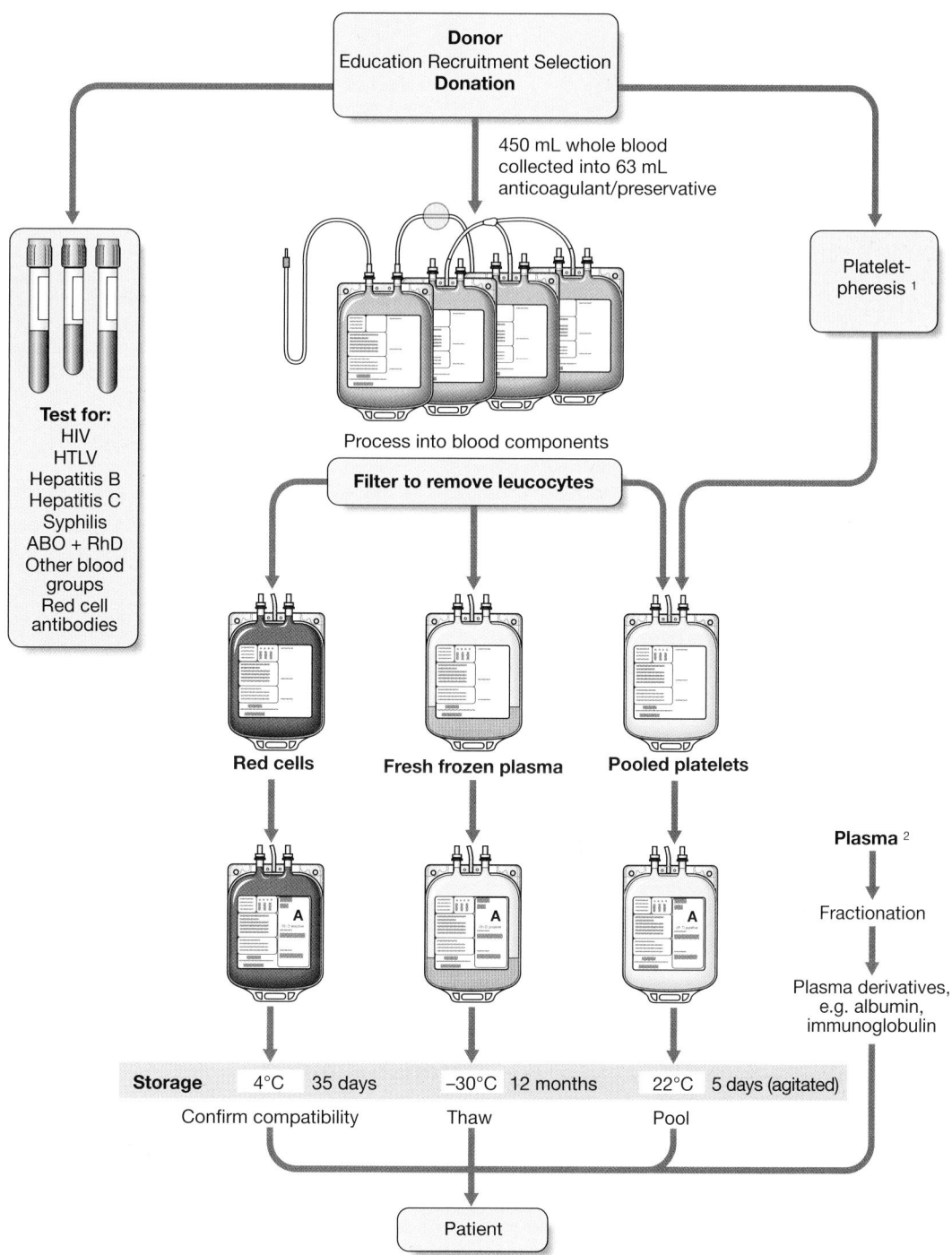

Fig. 24.16 Blood donation, processing and storage. [1]Platelet-pheresis involves circulating the donor's blood through a cell separator to remove platelets before returning other blood components to the donor. [2]In the UK, plasma for fractionation is imported as a precautionary measure against vCJD.

ABO blood groups

The frequency of the ABO antigens varies among different populations. The ABO blood group antigens are oligosaccharide chains that project from the red cell surface. These chains are attached to proteins and lipids that lie in the red cell membrane. The ABO gene encodes a glycosyltransferase that catalyses the final step in the synthesis of the chain which has three common alleles: A, B and O. The O allele encodes an inactive enzyme, leaving the ABO antigen precursor (called the H antigen) unmodified. The A and B alleles encode enzymes that differ by four amino acids and hence attach different sugars to the end of the chain. Individuals are tolerant to their own ABO antigens, but do not suppress B cell clones producing antibodies against ABO antigens that they do not carry themselves (Box 24.24). They are therefore capable of mounting a humoral immune response to these 'foreign' antigens.

24

i **24.24 ABO blood group antigens and antibodies**

ABO blood group	Red cell A or B antigens	Antibodies in plasma	UK frequency (%)
O	None	Anti-A and anti-B	46
A	A	Anti-B	42
B	B	Anti-A	9
AB	A and B	None	3

24.25 Rhesus D blood groups in pregnancy

- **Haemolytic disease of the newborn (HDN):** occurs when the mother has anti-red cell IgG antibodies that cross the placenta and haemolyse fetal red cells.
- **Screening for HDN in pregnancy:** at the time of booking (12–16 weeks) every pregnant woman should have a blood sample sent for determination of ABO and RhD group and testing for red cell allo-antibodies that may be directed against paternal blood group antigens.
- **Anti-D immunoglobulin prophylaxis in a mother who is RhD-negative:** following delivery of an RhD-positive baby, the mother is given anti-D within 72 hours; a maternal sample is checked for remaining fetal red cells and extra anti-D given if indicated. Anti-D is also given after other antenatal events (e.g. early bleeding). Doses vary according to national recommendations.

ABO-incompatible red cell transfusion

If red cells of an incompatible ABO group are transfused (especially if a group O recipient is transfused with group A, B or AB red cells), the *recipient's* IgM anti-A, anti-B or anti-AB binds to the *transfused* red cells. This activates the full complement pathway (p. 73), creating pores in the red cell membrane and destroying the transfused red cells in the circulation (intravascular haemolysis). The anaphylatoxins C3a and C5a, released by complement activation, liberate cytokines such as tumour necrosis factor (TNF), interleukin 1 (IL-1) and IL-8, and stimulate degranulation of mast cells with release of vasoactive mediators. All these substances may lead to inflammation, increased vascular permeability and hypotension, which may in turn cause shock and renal failure. Inflammatory mediators can also cause platelet aggregation, lung peribronchial oedema and smooth muscle contraction. About 20–30% of ABO-incompatible transfusions cause some degree of morbidity, and 5–10% cause or contribute to a patient's death. The main reason for this relatively low morbidity is the lack of potency of ABO antibodies in group A or B subjects; even if the recipient is group O, those who are very young or very old usually have weaker antibodies that do not lead to the activation of large amounts of complement.

The Rhesus D blood group and haemolytic disease of the newborn

About 15% of Caucasians are Rhesus-negative: that is, they lack the Rhesus D (RhD) red cell surface antigen (see Fig. 24.4, p. 990). In other populations (e.g. in Chinese and Bengalis), only 1–5% may be Rhesus-negative. RhD-negative individuals do not normally produce substantial amounts of anti-RhD antibodies. However, if RhD-positive red cells enter the circulation of an RhD-negative individual, then IgG antibodies are produced. This can occur during pregnancy if the mother is exposed to fetal cells via fetomaternal haemorrhage, or following transfusion. If a woman is so sensitised, during a subsequent pregnancy anti-RhD antibodies can cross the placenta; if the fetus is RhD-positive, haemolysis with severe fetal anaemia and hyperbilirubinaemia can result. This can cause severe neurological damage or death due to haemolytic disease of the newborn (HDN). Therefore, an RhD-negative female who may subsequently become pregnant should never be transfused with RhD-positive blood.

In RhD-negative women, administration of anti-RhD immunoglobulin (anti-D) perinatally can block the immune response to RhD antigen on fetal cells and is the only effective product for preventing the development of Rhesus antibodies (Box 24.25).

HDN can also be caused by other alloantibodies against red cell antigens, usually after previous pregnancies or transfusions. These antigens include RhC, Rhc, RhE, Rhe, and the Kidd, Kell and Duffy antigen systems.

Other immunological complications of transfusion

Rare but serious complications include transfusion-associated lung injury (TRALI) and transfusion-associated graft-versus-host disease (TA GVHD). The latter occurs when there is sharing of a human leucocyte antigen (HLA) haplotype between donor and recipient which allows transfused lymphocytes to engraft, proliferate and recognise the recipient as foreign, resulting in acute GVHD (p. 1014). Prevention is by gamma irradiation of blood components to prevent lymphocyte proliferation. Patients at risk of TA GVHD who must receive irradiated blood components include those with congenital T cell immunodeficiencies or Hodgkin lymphoma, recipients of stem-cell transplants or of blood from a family member, neonates and patients taking T lymphocyte-suppressing drugs such as fludarabine.

Infections transmitted by transfusion

Over the past 30 years, the viruses that cause HBV, AIDS and HCV have been identified and effective tests introduced to detect and exclude infected blood units. Where blood is from 'safe' donors and correctly tested, the current risk of a donation being infectious is very small. By 2002–3 in the UK, the estimated chances that a unit of blood might transmit one of the viruses for which blood is tested, was 0.25 per million units for HIV, 0.02 for HCV and 1.62 for HBV. However, some patients who received transfusions before these tests were available have suffered very serious consequences from these infections; this is a reminder to avoid non-essential transfusions since it is impossible to exclude the possibility that some new or currently unrecognised transfusion-transmissible infection may emerge. Licensed plasma derivatives that have been virus-inactivated do not transmit HIV, HTLV, HBV, HCV, cytomegalovirus or other lipid-enveloped viruses.

vCJD is a human prion disease linked to bovine spongiform encephalitis (BSE; p. 1214). The risk of a recipient acquiring the agent of vCJD from a transfusion is uncertain, but of 16 surviving recipients of blood from donors who later developed the disease, 3 have died with clinical vCJD and 1 of unrelated causes who had postmortem immunohistological signs of infection.

Bacterial contamination of a blood component—usually platelets—is extremely rare (2 reports in the UK in 2005 and in 2006) but can cause very severe and often lethal transfusion reactions.

Safe transfusion procedures

The proposed transfusion and any alternatives should be discussed with the patient or, if that is not possible, with a relative, and this should be documented. Some patients, e.g. Jehovah's Witnesses, may refuse transfusion and require specialised management to survive profound anaemia following blood loss.

Pre-transfusion testing

To ensure that red cells supplied for transfusion are compatible with the intended recipient, the transfusion laboratory will perform either a 'group and screen' procedure or a 'cross-match'.

In the group and screen procedure, the red cells from the patient's blood sample are tested to determine the ABO and RhD type, and the patient's serum is also tested against an array of red cells expressing the most important antigens to detect any red cell antibodies. Any antibody detected can be identified by further testing, so that red cell units that lack the corresponding antigen

can be selected. The patient's sample can be held in the laboratory for up to a week, so that the hospital blood bank can quickly prepare compatible blood without the need for a further patient sample. In the so-called 'electronic cross-match' blood can be issued for suitable patients on the basis of blood group information held in the laboratory's computer.

Conventional cross-matching consists of the group and antibody screen, followed by direct confirmation of the compatibility of individual units of red cell with the patient's serum. Full cross-matching takes about 45 minutes if no red cell antibodies are present, but may require hours if a patient has multiple antibodies.

Bedside procedures for safe transfusion

Errors leading to patients receiving the wrong blood are an important avoidable cause of mortality and morbidity. Most incompatible transfusions result from failure to adhere to standard procedures for taking correctly labelled blood samples from the patient and ensuring that the correct pack of blood component is transfused into the intended patient. In the UK in 2003/4, there were 787 reports of transfusion of an incorrect blood component (12 per 100 000 units transfused). Every hospital where blood is transfused should have a written transfusion policy that is used by all staff who order, check or administer blood products (Fig. 24.17).

Management of suspected transfusion reactions is described in Figure 24.18.

Taking blood for pre-transfusion testing

Positively identify the patient at the bedside
Label the sample tube and complete
the request form clearly and accurately
after identifying the patient
Do not write forms and labels in advance

Administering blood

Positively identify the patient at the bedside
Ensure that the identification of each blood pack matches the patient's identification
Check that the ABO and RhD groups of each pack are compatible with the patient's
Check each pack for evidence of damage
If in doubt, do not use and return to the blood bank
Complete the forms that document the transfusion of each pack

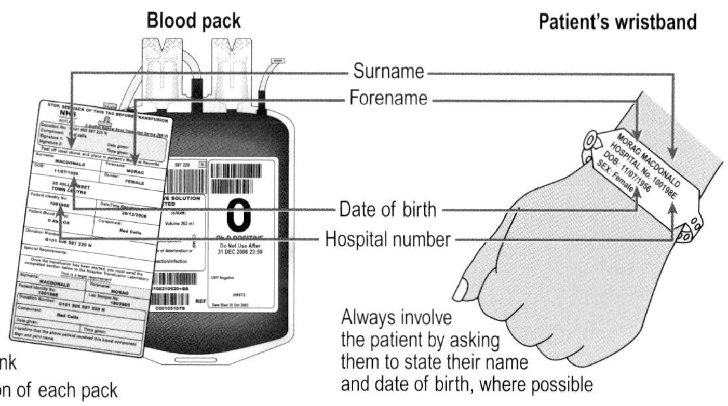

Record-keeping

Record in the patient's notes the reason for transfusion, the product given, dose, any adverse effects and the clinical response

Observations

Transfusions should only be given when the patient can be observed
Blood pressure, pulse and temperature should be monitored before and 15 minutes after starting each pack
In conscious patients, further observations are only needed if the patient has symptoms or signs of a reaction
In unconscious patients, check pulse and temperature at intervals during transfusion
Signs of abnormal bleeding during the transfusion could be due to disseminated intravascular coagulation resulting from an acute haemolytic reaction

Check the compatibility label on the pack against the patient's wristband

Blood pack   **Patient's wristband**

Surname
Forename
Date of birth
Hospital number

Always involve
the patient by asking
them to state their name
and date of birth, where possible

Fig. 24.17 Bedside procedures for safe blood transfusion. The patient's safety depends on adherence to standard procedures for taking samples for compatibility testing, administering blood, record-keeping and observations.

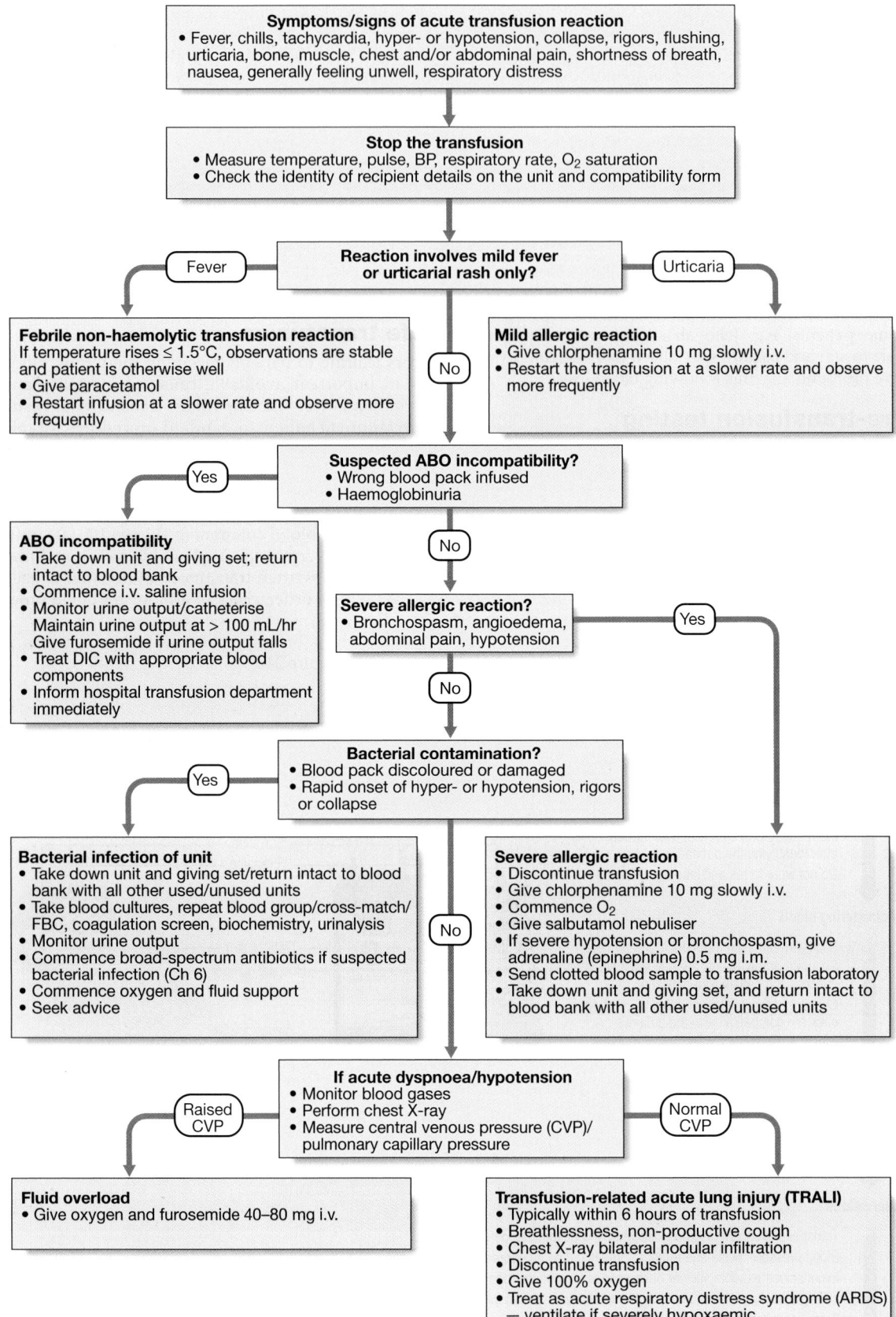

Symptoms/signs of acute transfusion reaction
- Fever, chills, tachycardia, hyper- or hypotension, collapse, rigors, flushing, urticaria, bone, muscle, chest and/or abdominal pain, shortness of breath, nausea, generally feeling unwell, respiratory distress

Stop the transfusion
- Measure temperature, pulse, BP, respiratory rate, O_2 saturation
- Check the identity of recipient details on the unit and compatibility form

Fever

Reaction involves mild fever or urticarial rash only?

Urticaria

Febrile non-haemolytic transfusion reaction
If temperature rises ≤ 1.5°C, observations are stable and patient is otherwise well
- Give paracetamol
- Restart infusion at a slower rate and observe more frequently

No

Mild allergic reaction
- Give chlorphenamine 10 mg slowly i.v.
- Restart the transfusion at a slower rate and observe more frequently

Yes

Suspected ABO incompatibility?
- Wrong blood pack infused
- Haemoglobinuria

No

ABO incompatibility
- Take down unit and giving set; return intact to blood bank
- Commence i.v. saline infusion
- Monitor urine output/catheterise Maintain urine output at > 100 mL/hr Give furosemide if urine output falls
- Treat DIC with appropriate blood components
- Inform hospital transfusion department immediately

Severe allergic reaction?
- Bronchospasm, angioedema, abdominal pain, hypotension

Yes

No

Yes

Bacterial contamination?
- Blood pack discoloured or damaged
- Rapid onset of hyper- or hypotension, rigors or collapse

Bacterial infection of unit
- Take down unit and giving set/return intact to blood bank with all other used/unused units
- Take blood cultures, repeat blood group/cross-match/FBC, coagulation screen, biochemistry, urinalysis
- Monitor urine output
- Commence broad-spectrum antibiotics if suspected bacterial infection (Ch 6)
- Commence oxygen and fluid support
- Seek advice

No

Severe allergic reaction
- Discontinue transfusion
- Give chlorphenamine 10 mg slowly i.v.
- Commence O_2
- Give salbutamol nebuliser
- If severe hypotension or bronchospasm, give adrenaline (epinephrine) 0.5 mg i.m.
- Send clotted blood sample to transfusion laboratory
- Take down unit and giving set, and return intact to blood bank with all other used/unused units

Raised CVP

If acute dyspnoea/hypotension
- Monitor blood gases
- Perform chest X-ray
- Measure central venous pressure (CVP)/pulmonary capillary pressure

Normal CVP

Fluid overload
- Give oxygen and furosemide 40–80 mg i.v.

Transfusion-related acute lung injury (TRALI)
- Typically within 6 hours of transfusion
- Breathlessness, non-productive cough
- Chest X-ray bilateral nodular infiltration
- Discontinue transfusion
- Give 100% oxygen
- Treat as acute respiratory distress syndrome (ARDS) — ventilate if severely hypoxaemic

Fig. 24.18 Investigation and management of reactions to blood products.

BONE MARROW AND PERIPHERAL BLOOD STEM CELL TRANSPLANTATION

Blood and marrow transplantation (BMT) refers to the transplantation of haematopoietic stem cells and has offered the only hope of 'cure' in a variety of haematological and non-haematological disorders (Box 24.26). As standard treatment improves, the indications for BMT are being refined and extended, although its use remains most common in haematological malignancies. The type of BMT is defined according to the donor and source of stem cells:

- In *allogeneic* BMT the stem cells come from a *donor*— either related (usually an HLA-identical sibling) or from a closely HLA-matched volunteer unrelated donor (VUD).
- In an *autologous* transplant the stem cells are harvested from the *patient* and stored in the vapour phase of liquid nitrogen until required. Stem cells can be harvested from the bone marrow or from the blood.

Allogeneic BMT

Healthy marrow or blood stem cells from a donor are infused intravenously into the recipient, who has been suitably 'conditioned'. The conditioning treatment (chemotherapy with or without radiotherapy) destroys malignant cells and immunosuppresses the recipient, as well as ablating the recipient's haematopoietic tissues. The injected donor cells 'home' to the marrow, engraft and produce enough erythrocytes, granulocytes and platelets for the patient's needs after about 3–4 weeks. During this period of aplasia patients are at risk of infection and bleeding, and require intensive supportive care as described on page 1033. It may take several years to regain normal immunological function and patients remain at risk from opportunistic infections, in particular in the first year.

An advantage of receiving allogeneic donor stem cells is that the donor's immunological system can recognise residual malignant recipient cells and destroy them. This immunological 'graft versus disease' effect is a powerful tool against many haematological tumours and can be boosted post-transplantation by the infusion of T cells taken from the donor, so-called donor lymphocyte infusion (DLI).

Haematological indications for allogeneic transplantation are shown in Box 24.27. There is considerable morbidity and mortality associated with BMT. The best results are obtained in patients with minimal residual

disease, and in those under 20 years of age who have an HLA-identical sibling donor. Older patients can be transplanted, but results become progressively worse with age and an upper age limit of 55 years is usually applied.

Complications

These are outlined in Boxes 24.28 and 24.29. The risks and outcomes of transplantation depend upon several patient- and disease-related factors. In general, 25% die from procedure-related complications such as graft-versus-host disease (see below), and there remains a significant risk of relapse in haematological malignancy. The

24.27 Haematological indications for bone marrow transplantation

Allogeneic transplant

- Acute myeloid leukaemia (AML) high-risk CR1, CR2
- Adult acute lymphoblastic leukaemia (ALL) CR1, CR2
- Chronic myeloid leukaemia (CML) resistant to imitanib
- Myelodysplastic syndrome
- Severe aplastic anaemia
- Myelofibrosis
- Severe immune deficiency syndromes

Autologous transplant

- AML CR2
- Myeloma
- Poor-risk Hodgkin lymphoma
- High-grade non-Hodgkin lymphoma second response
- Mantle cell lymphoma

24.28 Complications of allogeneic bone marrow transplantation

- Mucositis
- Infection
- Bleeding
- Cataract formation
- Pneumonitis
- Infertility
- Chronic graft-versus-host disease
- Acute graft-versus-host disease
- Secondary malignant disease

24.29 Infection during recovery from bone marrow transplantation

Infection	Time after BMT	Management
Herpes simplex (p. 321)	0–4 weeks	Aciclovir
Bacterial, fungal	0–4 weeks	As for acute leukaemia (p. 1031)
Cytomegalovirus (CMV; p. 317)	7–21 weeks	Hyperimmune immunoglobulin and ganciclovir for documented infections
Varicella zoster (p. 313)	After 13 weeks	Aciclovir i.v.
Pneumocystis jirovecii (p. 395)	8–26 weeks	Co-trimoxazole
Interstitial pneumonitis (non-infective)	6–18 weeks	No specific therapy Prednisolone may be tried

24.26 General indications for allogeneic BMT

- Neoplastic disorders affecting stem cell compartments (e.g. leukaemias)
- Failure of haematopoiesis (e.g. aplastic anaemia)
- Major inherited defects in blood cell production (e.g. thalassaemia, immunodeficiency diseases)
- Inborn errors of metabolism with missing enzymes or cell lines

24

long-term survival for patients undergoing allogeneic BMT in acute leukaemia is around 50%.

Graft-versus-host disease (GVHD)

GVHD is due to the cytotoxic activity of donor T lymphocytes which become sensitised to their new host, regarding it as foreign. This may cause either an acute or a chronic form of GVHD.

Acute GVHD occurs in the first 100 days after transplant in about one-third of patients. It can affect the skin, causing rashes, the liver, causing jaundice, and the gut, causing diarrhoea, and may vary from mild to lethal. Prevention includes HLA-matching of the donor, immunosuppressant drugs, including methotrexate and ciclosporin, and antithymocyte globulin. The more severe forms are very difficult to control and, despite high-dose corticosteroids, may result in death.

Chronic GVHD may follow acute GVHD or arise independently; it occurs later than acute GVHD. It often resembles a connective tissue disorder, although in mild cases a rash may be the only manifestation. Chronic GVHD is usually treated with corticosteroids and prolonged immunosuppression with, for example, ciclosporin. Associated with chronic GVHD is the graft-versus-leukaemia effect, which results in a lower relapse rate.

Reduced-intensity BMT

This concept has been developed in an attempt to reduce the mortality of allografting. Rather than use very intensive conditioning which causes morbidity from organ damage, relatively low doses of drugs such as fludarabine and cyclophosphamide are used simply to immunosuppress the recipient and allow donor stem cells to engraft. The emerging donor immune system then eliminates malignant cells via the 'graft versus disease' effect, which may be boosted by the elective use of donor T cell infusions post-transplant. This approach is less toxic and allows BMT to be offered to an older group of patients. However, relapse and infections post-transplant remain a concern and the role of this type of transplant is still under investigation.

Autologous BMT

This procedure can also be used in haematological malignancies. The patient's own stem cells from blood or marrow are first harvested and frozen. After conditioning therapy, the autologous stem cells are reinfused in order to rescue the patient from the marrow damage and aplasia caused by chemotherapy. Autologous BMT may be used for disorders which do not primarily involve the haematopoietic tissues, or in patients in whom very good remissions have been achieved. The preferred source of stem cells for autologous transplants is peripheral blood. These stem cells engraft more quickly, marrow recovery occurring within 2–3 weeks. There is no risk of GVHD and no immunosuppression is required. Thus autologous stem cell transplantation carries a lower procedure-related mortality rate than allogeneic BMT at around 5%, but there is a higher rate of recurrence of malignancy. The issue of whether the stem cells should be treated (purged) in an attempt to remove any residual leukaemia cells is controversial.

ANTICOAGULANT AND ANTITHROMBOTIC THERAPY

There are numerous indications for anticoagulant and antithrombotic medications (Box 24.30). The guiding principles are outlined here, but management in specific indications is discussed elsewhere in the book. Broadly speaking, antiplatelet medications are of greater efficacy in the prevention of arterial thrombosis and of less value in the prevention of venous thromboembolism. Thus, anti-platelet agents such as aspirin and clopidogrel are the drugs of choice in acute coronary events, and in ischaemic cerebrovascular disease, while warfarin and other anticoagulants are favoured in venous thromboembolism. In some extremely prothrombotic situations, such as coronary artery stenting, a combination of anticoagulant and anti-platelet drugs is used.

A wide range of anticoagulant and antithrombotic drugs are used in clinical practice. These drugs and their modes of action are given in Box 24.31. The ultimate aim is to produce antithrombotics for oral anticoagulation which can be given at fixed doses with predictable effects and no need for monitoring. A variety of drugs are presently undergoing clinical trials in the prevention and treatment of thrombosis. Initial studies show that dabigatran and rivaroxaban are effective in preventing venous thromboembolism following high-risk orthopaedic surgery.

24.30 Indications for anticoagulation

Heparin

- Prevention and treatment of VTE
- Percutaneous coronary intervention
- Post thrombolysis for myocardial infarction
- Unstable angina pectoris
- Non-Q wave myocardial infarction
- Acute peripheral arterial occlusion
- Cardiopulmonary bypass
- Haemodialysis and haemofiltration

Coumarins (warfarin etc.)

- Prevention and treatment of VTE ⎤
- Arterial embolism
- Atrial fibrillation with specific stroke risk factors (p. 562)
- Mobile mural thrombus post-myocardial infarction
- Extensive anterior myocardial infarction — Therapeutic INR 2.5
- Dilated cardiomyopathy
- Cardioversion
- Ischaemic stroke in antiphospholipid syndrome
- Mitral stenosis and mitral regurgitation with atrial fibrillation ⎦
- Recurrent venous thrombosis whilst on warfarin ⎤ INR 3.5
- Mechanical prosthetic cardiac valves ⎦

(INR= International normalised ratio)

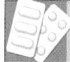

24.31 Modes of action of anticoagulant and antithrombotic drugs

Drug	Mode of action
Antiplatelet drugs	
Aspirin	Cyclo-oxygenase (COX) inhibition
Clopidogrel	Adenosine diphosphate (ADP) receptor inhibition
Abciximab	Glycoprotein IIb/IIIa inhibition
Tirofiban	Glycoprotein IIb/IIIa inhibition
Eptifibatide	Glycoprotein IIb/IIIa inhibition
Dipyridamole	Phosphodiesterase inhibition
Oral anticoagulants	
Warfarin/coumarins	Vitamin K antagonism
Dabigatran	Direct thrombin inhibition
Rivaroxaban	Direct Xa inhibition
Apixaban	Direct Xa inhibition
Intravenous anticoagulants	
Heparin	Antithrombin-dependent inhibition of thrombin and Xa
Fondaparinux/idraparinux	Antithrombin-dependent inhibition of Xa
Lepirudin	Direct thrombin inhibition
Argatroban	Direct thrombin inhibition
Bivalirudin	Direct thrombin inhibition

Heparins

Unfractionated heparin (UFH) and low molecular weight heparins (LMWH) both act by binding to a specific pentasaccharide on antithrombin which potentiates its natural anticoagulant activity (see Fig. 24.6, pp. 992–993). Increased cleavage of activated proteases, particularly factor Xa and thrombin (IIa), accounts for the anticoagulant effect. LMWHs preferentially augment antithrombin activity against factor Xa. For the licensed indications, LMWHs are at least as efficacious as UFH but have several advantages.

- LMWHs are nearly 100% bioavailable and therefore produce reliable dose-dependent anticoagulation.
- LMWHs do not require monitoring of their anticoagulant effect (except possibly in patients with very low body weight and with GFR < 30 mL/min).
- LMWHs have a half-life of around 4 hours when given subcutaneously, compared with 1 hour for UFH. This permits once-daily dosing by the subcutaneous route, rather than the therapeutic continuous intravenous infusion or prophylactic twice-daily subcutaneous administration required for UFH.
- While rates of bleeding are similar between products, the risk of osteoporosis and heparin-induced thrombocytopenia is much lower for LMWH.
- However, UFH is more completely reversed by protamine sulphate in the event of bleeding and at the end of cardiopulmonary bypass, for which UFH remains the drug of choice.

LMWHs are widely used for the prevention and treatment of VTE, the management of acute coronary syndromes and for most other scenarios listed in Box 24.30. In some situations, UFH is still favoured by some clinicians, though there is little evidence that it is advantageous except when rapid reversibility is required. UFH is useful in patients with a high risk of bleeding, e.g. who have peptic ulceration or may require surgery. It is also favoured in treatment of life-threatening thromboembolism, e.g. major PE with significant hypoxaemia, hypotension and right-sided heart strain. In this situation UFH is started with a loading dose of 5000 U i.v., followed by a continuous infusion of 20 U/kg/hr initially. The level of anticoagulation should be assessed by the APTT after 6 hours and, if satisfactory, twice daily thereafter. It is usual to aim for a patient time which is 1.5–2.5 times the control time of the test.

Heparin-induced thrombocytopenia (HIT)

HIT is a rare complication of heparin therapy, caused by induction of anti-heparin/PF4 antibodies which bind to and activate platelets via an Fc receptor. This results in platelet activation and a prothrombotic state, with a paradoxical thrombocytopenia. HIT is more common in surgical than medical patients (especially cardiac and orthopaedic patients), with use of UFH rather than LMWH, and with higher doses of heparin.

Clinical features

Patients present, typically 5–14 days after starting heparin treatment, with a fall in platelet count of > 30% from baseline. The count may still be in the normal range. They may be asymptomatic, or develop venous or arterial thrombosis and skin lesions, including overt skin necrosis. Affected patients may complain of pain or itch at injection sites and of systemic symptoms such as shivering following heparin injections. Patients who have received heparin in the preceding 100 days and who have preformed antibodies may develop acute systemic symptoms and an abrupt fall in platelet count in the first 24 hours after re-exposure.

Investigations

The pre-test probability of the diagnosis is assessed using the 4Ts scoring system. This assigns a score based on:
- the **t**hrombocytopenia
- the **t**iming of the fall in platelet count
- the presence of new **t**hrombosis
- the likelihood of ano**t**her cause for the thrombocytopenia.

Individuals at low risk need no further test; those with intermediate and high likelihood scores should have the diagnosis confirmed or refuted using an anti-PF4 enzyme-linked immunosorbent assay (ELISA).

Management

Heparin should be discontinued as soon as HIT is diagnosed and an alternative anticoagulant which does not cross-react with the antibody substituted. Lepirudin (a hirudin analogue) and danaparoid (a heparin analogue) are licensed for use in the UK. In asymptomatic patients with HIT who do not receive an alternative anticoagulant, around 50% will sustain a thrombosis in the subsequent 30 days. Patients with established thrombosis have a poor prognosis.

Coumarins (e.g. warfarin)

Although several coumarin anticoagulants are used around the world, warfarin is the most common.

24

Coumarins inhibit the vitamin K-dependent post-translational carboxylation of factors II, VII, IX and X in the liver. This results in anticoagulation due to an effective deficiency of these factors. This is monitored by the INR, a standardised test based on measurement of the prothrombin time (p. 996). Recommended target INR values for specific indications are given in Box 24.30.

Warfarin anticoagulation typically takes more than 3 days to become established, even using initial loading doses. Patients who require rapid initiation of therapy may receive higher initiation doses of warfarin. A typical regime is to give 10 mg warfarin on the first and second days, with 5 mg on the third day; subsequent doses are titrated against the INR. Patients with risk factors requiring prophylactic anticoagulation (e.g. atrial fibrillation) can have warfarin introduced slowly using lower doses. Low-dose regimens are associated with a lower risk of the patient developing a supratherapeutic INR, and hence a lower bleeding risk. The duration of warfarin therapy depends on the clinical indication, and while treatment of DVT or preparation for cardioversion requires a limited duration, anticoagulation to prevent cardioembolic stroke in atrial fibrillation or from heart valve disease is long-term.

The major problems with warfarin are:
- it has a narrow therapeutic window
- its metabolism is affected by many factors.

Drug interactions are common through protein binding and metabolism by the cytochrome P-450 system. Naturally occurring polymorphisms in the *CYP2C9* and the *VKORC1* genes account for many of the observed differences in dose requirements between races. Dietary intake of vitamin K also affects dose requirements.

Major bleeding is the most common serious side-effect of warfarin and occurs in about 1.0% of patients each year. Fatal haemorrhage, which is most commonly intracranial, occurs in about 0.25% per annum. There are scoring systems which predict the annual bleeding risk and these can be used to help compare the risks and benefits of warfarin for an individual patient (Box .32). There are also some specific contraindications to anticoagulation (see Box 24.32). Management of warfarin includes strategies for over-anticoagulation and for bleeding.

- If the INR is above the therapeutic level, warfarin should be withheld or the dose reduced. If the patient is not bleeding, it may be appropriate to give a small dose of vitamin K either orally or intravenously (1–2.5 mg), especially if the INR is > 8.
- In the event of bleeding, withhold further warfarin. Minor bleeding can be treated with 1–2.5 mg of vitamin K intravenously. Major haemorrhage should be treated as an emergency with vitamin K 5–10 mg slowly i.v., combined with coagulation factor replacement. This should optimally be a prothrombin complex concentrate (30–50 U/kg) which contains factors II, VII, IX and X; if that is not available, fresh frozen plasma (15–30 mL/kg) should be given.

Prophylaxis of venous thrombosis

All patients admitted to hospital should be assessed for their risk of developing VTE. Both medical and surgical patients are at increased risk. A summary of the risk categories is given in Box 24.33. Early mobilisation of all patients is important to prevent DVT. Patients at medium or high risk require additional antithrombotic measures;

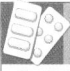

24.32 Assessing risks of anticoagulation

Contraindications

• Recent surgery, especially to eye or central nervous system	• Pre-existing structural lesions, e.g. peptic ulcer
• Pre-existing haemorrhagic state, e.g. liver disease, haemophilia, thrombocytopenia	• Recent cerebral haemorrhage • Uncontrolled hypertension • Cognitive impairment • Frequent falls in old age

Bleeding risk score

- Age > 65 years (1 point)
- Previous gastrointestinal bleed (1 point)
- Previous stroke (1 point)
- Medical illness (1 point)
    Recent myocardial infarction
    Renal failure
    Anaemia
    Diabetes mellitus

Score: annual rate of major haemorrhage

0 = 3%

1–2 = 12%

3–4 = 30–48%

24.33 Antithrombotic prophylaxis

Patients in the following categories should be considered for specific antithrombotic prophylaxis:

Moderate risk of DVT

Major surgery
- In patients > 40 years or with other risk factor for VTE

Major medical illness, e.g.

• Heart failure	• Inflammatory bowel disease
• Myocardial infarction with complications	• Nephrotic syndrome
• Sepsis	• Stroke and other conditions leading to lower limb paralysis
• Active malignancy	

High risk of DVT

• Major abdominal or pelvic surgery for malignancy or with history of DVT or known thrombophilia (Box 24.4, p. 997)	• Major hip or knee surgery • Neurosurgery

Methods of VTE prophylaxis

Mechanical

• Intermittent pneumatic compression	• Graduated compression stockings
• Mechanical foot pumps	

Pharmacological

• Low molecular weight heparins	• Dabigatran
• Unfractionated heparin	• Rivaroxaban
• Fondaparinux	• Warfarin
	• Aspirin

these may be pharmacological or mechanical. There is increasing evidence in high-risk groups, such as patients who have had major lower limb orthopaedic surgery, for protracted thromboprophylaxis extending out to 30 days after the procedure. Particular care should be taken with the use of pharmacological prophylaxis in patients with a high risk of bleeding or with specific risks of haemorrhage related to the site of surgery or the use of spinal or epidural anaesthesia.

ANAEMIAS

Around 30% of the total world population is anaemic and half of these, some 600 million people, have iron deficiency. The classification of anaemia by the size of the red cells (MCV) indicates the likely cause (see Figs 24.10 and 24.11, pp. 998–999).

Red cells in the bone marrow must acquire a minimum level of haemoglobin before being released into the blood stream (Fig. 24.19). Whilst in the marrow compartment, red cell precursors undergo cell division driven by erythropoietin. If red cells cannot acquire haemoglobin at a normal rate, they will undergo more divisions than normal and will have a low MCV when finally released into the blood. The MCV is low because component parts of the haemoglobin molecule are not fully available: that is, iron in iron deficiency, globin chains in thalassaemia, haem ring in congenital sideroblastic anaemia and, occasionally, poor iron utilisation in the anaemia of chronic disease.

In megaloblastic anaemia the biochemical consequence of vitamin B_{12} or folate deficiency is an inability to synthesise new bases to make DNA. A similar defect of cell division is seen in the presence of cytotoxic drugs or haematological disease in the marrow such as myelodysplasia. In these states, cells haemoglobinise normally but undergo fewer cell divisions, resulting in circulating red cells with a raised MCV. The red cell membrane is composed of a lipid bilayer which will freely exchange with the plasma pool of lipid. Conditions such as liver disease, hypothyroidism, hyperlipidaemia and pregnancy are associated with raised lipids and may also cause a raised MCV. Reticulocytes are larger than mature red cells, so when the reticulocyte count is raised—for example, in haemolysis—this may also increase the MCV.

Iron deficiency anaemia

This occurs when iron losses or physiological requirements exceed absorption.

Blood loss

The most common explanation in men and postmenopausal women is gastrointestinal blood loss (p. 852). This may result from occult gastric or colorectal malignancy, gastritis, peptic ulceration, inflammatory bowel disease, diverticulitis, polyps and angiodysplastic lesions. World-wide, hookworm and schistosomiasis are the most common causes of gut blood loss (pp. 364

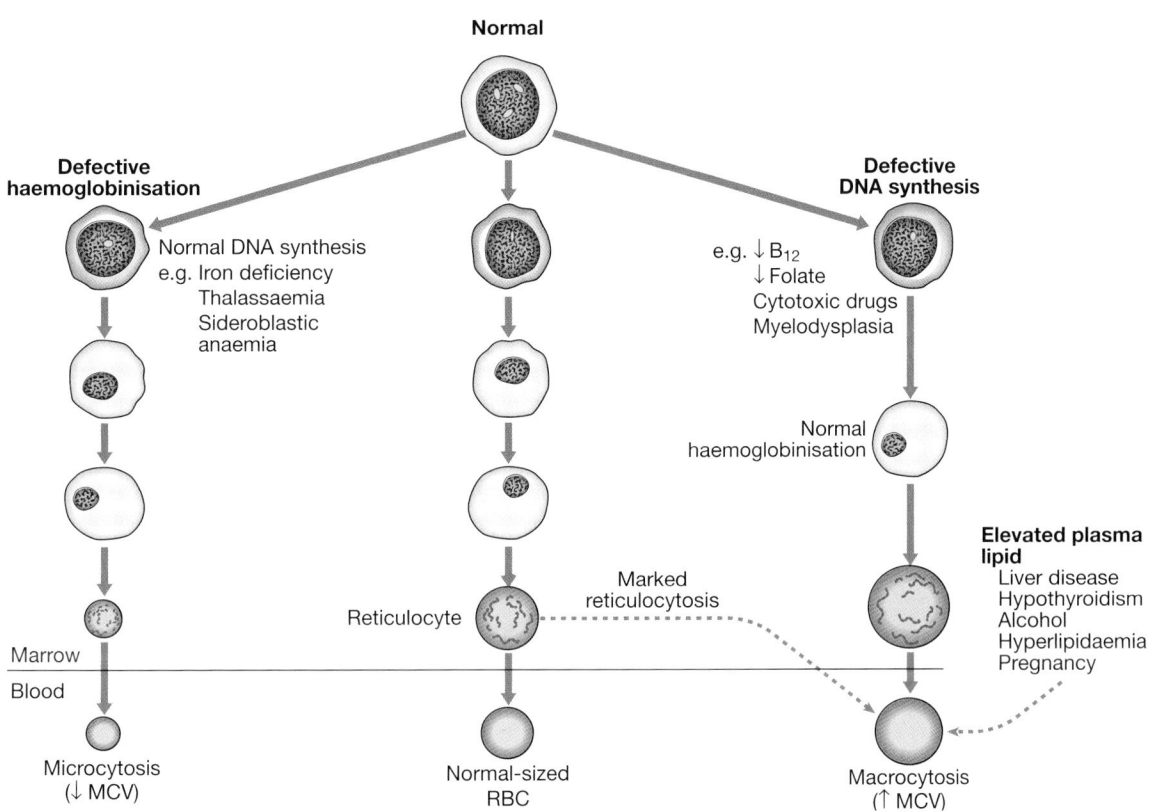

Fig. 24.19 Factors which influence the size of red cells in anaemia. ↓ MCV is < 76 fL; ↑ MCV is > 100 fL.

and 370). Gastrointestinal blood loss may be exacerbated by the chronic use of aspirin or non-steroidal anti-inflammatory drugs (NSAIDs), which cause intestinal erosions and impair platelet function. In women of child-bearing age, menstrual blood loss, pregnancy and breastfeeding contribute to iron deficiency by depleting iron stores; in developed countries one-third of pre-menopausal women have low iron stores but only 3% display iron-deficient haematopoiesis. Very rarely, chronic haemoptysis or haematuria may cause iron deficiency.

Malabsorption

A dietary assessment should be made in all patients to ascertain their iron intake (p. 114). Gastric acid is required to release iron from food and helps to keep iron in the soluble ferrous state (Fig. 24.20). Hypochlorhydria in the elderly or that due to drugs such as proton pump inhibitors may contribute to the lack of iron availability from the diet, as may previous gastric surgery. Iron is absorbed actively in the upper small intestine and hence can be affected by coeliac disease (p. 879).

Physiological demands

At times of rapid growth, such as infancy and puberty, iron demands increase and may outstrip absorption. In pregnancy, iron is diverted to the fetus, the placenta and the increased maternal red cell mass, and is lost with bleeding at parturition (Box 24.34).

Investigations
Confirmation of iron deficiency

Plasma ferritin is a measure of iron stores in tissues and is the best single test to confirm iron deficiency (Box 24.35). It is a very specific test; a subnormal level is due to iron deficiency, hypothyroidism or vitamin C deficiency. Levels can be raised by liver disease and in an acute phase response; in these conditions a ferritin level of up to 100 μg/L may still be compatible with low bone marrow iron stores.

Plasma iron and total iron binding capacity (TIBC) are measures of iron availability; hence they are affected by many factors besides iron stores. Plasma iron has a marked diurnal and day-to-day variation and becomes very low during an acute phase response but is raised in liver disease and haemolysis. Levels of transferrin, the binding protein for iron, are lowered by malnutrition, liver disease, an acute phase response and nephrotic syndrome, but raised by pregnancy or the oral contraceptive pill. A transferrin saturation (i.e. iron/TIBC × 100) of less than 16% is consistent with iron deficiency but is less specific than a ferritin measurement.

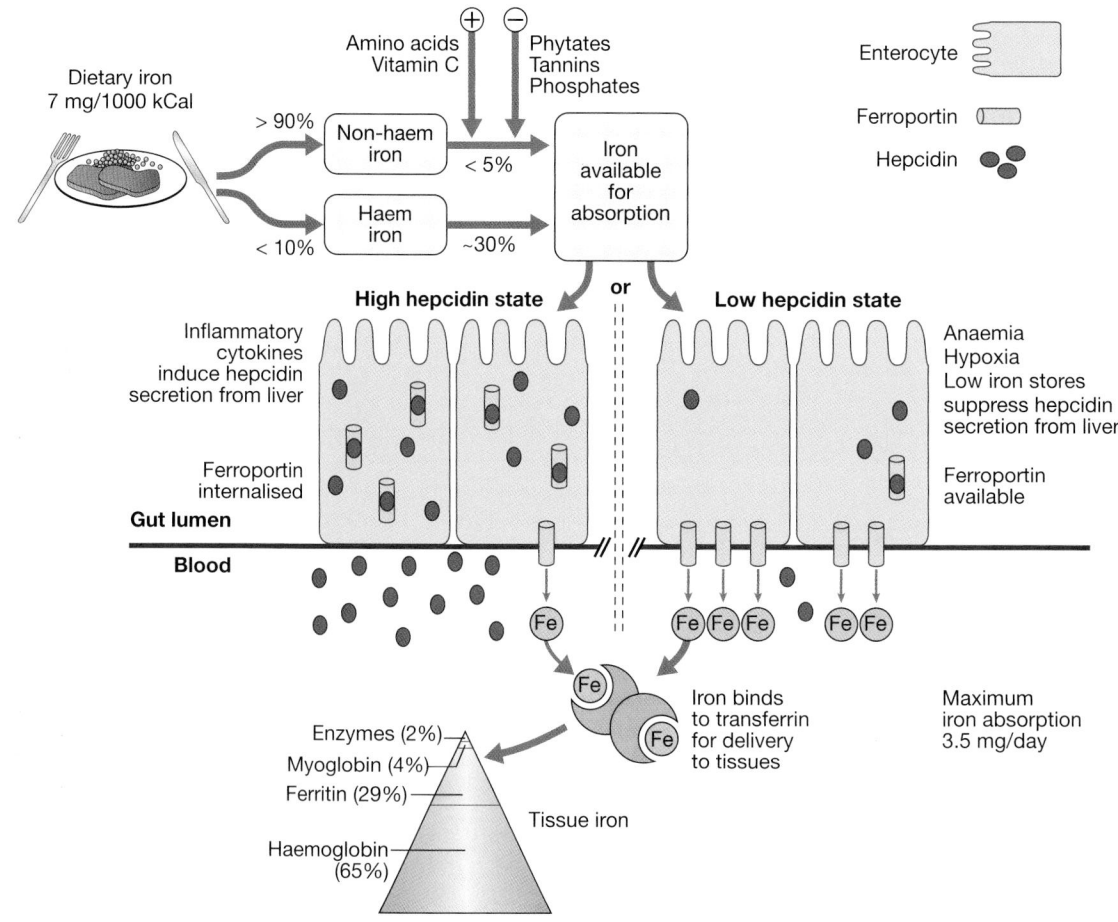

Fig. 24.20 The regulation of iron absorption, uptake and distribution in the body. The transport of iron is regulated in a similar fashion to enterocytes in other iron-transporting cells such as macrophages.

24.34 Haematological physiology in pregnancy

- **Full blood count:** increased plasma volume (40%) lowers normal Hb (reference range reduced to > 105 g/L at 28 weeks). The MCV may increase by 5 fL. A progressive neutrophilia occurs. Gestational thrombocytopenia (rarely < 60 × 10⁹/L) is a benign phenomenon.
- **Depletion of iron stores:** iron deficiency is a common cause of anaemia in pregnancy and, if present, should be treated with oral iron supplement.
- **Vitamin B₁₂:** serum levels are physiologically low in pregnancy but deficiency is uncommon.
- **Folate:** tissue stores may become depleted, and folate supplementation is recommended in all pregnancies (see Box 5.20, p. 113).
- **Coagulation factors:** from the second trimester, procoagulant factors increase approximately three-fold, particularly fibrinogen, von Willebrand factor and factor VIII. This causes activated protein C resistance and a shortened APTT, and contributes to a prothrombotic state.
- **Anticoagulants:** levels of protein C increase from the second trimester while levels of free protein S fall as C4b binding protein increases.

24.35 Investigations to differentiate anaemia of chronic disease from iron deficiency anaemia

	Ferritin	Iron	TIBC	Transferrin saturation	Soluble transferrin receptor
Iron deficiency anaemia	↓	↓	↑	↓	↑
Anaemia of chronic disease	↑/Normal	↓	↓	↓	↓/Normal

(TIBC = total iron binding capacity)

All proliferating cells express membrane transferrin receptors to acquire iron; a small amount of this receptor is shed into blood, where it can be detected in a free soluble form. At times of poor iron stores, cells up-regulate transferrin receptor expression and the levels of soluble plasma transferrin receptor increase. This can now be measured by immunoassay and used to distinguish storage iron depletion in the presence of an acute phase response or liver disease when a raised level indicates iron deficiency. In difficult cases it may still be necessary to examine a bone marrow aspirate for iron stores.

Investigation of the cause

This will depend upon the age and sex of the patient, as well as the history and clinical findings. In men and in post-menopausal women with a normal diet, the upper and lower gastrointestinal tract should be investigated by endoscopy or barium studies. Serum anti-endomysial antibodies and possibly a duodenal biopsy are indicated (p. 894) to detect coeliac disease in iron-deficient patients who have features of malabsorption or recurrent deficiency in the absence of other expla-nations, or who are young men with normal diet or young women with normal menstruation and diet. In the tropics, stool and urine should be examined for parasites (p. 307).

Management

Unless the patient has angina, heart failure or evidence of cerebral hypoxia, transfusion is not necessary and oral iron supplementation is appropriate. Ferrous sulphate 200 mg 8-hourly (195 mg of elemental iron per day) is more than adequate and should be continued for 3–6 months to replete iron stores. The occasional patient is intolerant of ferrous sulphate, with dyspepsia and altered bowel habit. In this case a reduction in dose to 200 mg 12-hourly or a switch to ferrous gluconate 300 mg 12-hourly (70 mg of elemental iron per day) should be made. Delayed-release preparations are not useful, since they release iron beyond the upper small intestine where it cannot be absorbed.

The haemoglobin should rise by 10 g/L every 7–10 days and a reticulocyte response will be evident within a week. A failure to respond adequately may be due to non-compliance, continued blood loss, malabsorption or an incorrect diagnosis. The occasional patient with malabsorption or chronic gut disease may need parenteral iron therapy with single or multiple doses of intravenous iron dextran or iron sucrose. Doses required can be calculated based on the patient's starting Hb and body weight. Observation for anaphylaxis following an initial test dose is recommended.

Anaemia of chronic disease (ACD)

This is a common type of anaemia, particularly in hospital populations. It occurs in the setting of chronic infection, chronic inflammation or neoplasia. The anaemia is not related to bleeding, haemolysis or marrow infiltration, is mild, with Hb in the range of 85–115 g/L, and is usually associated with a normal MCV (normocytic, normochromic), though this may be reduced in long-standing inflammation. The serum iron is low but iron stores are normal or increased, as indicated by the ferritin or stainable marrow iron.

Pathogenesis

It has recently become clear that the key regulatory protein that accounts for the findings characteristic of ACD is hepcidin, which is produced by the liver (see Fig. 24.20). High levels of production are encouraged by pro-inflammatory cytokines, especially IL-6. Hepcidin binds to ferroportin on the membrane of iron exporting cells, such as small intestinal enterocytes and macrophages, internalising the ferroportin and thereby inhibiting the export of iron from these cells into the blood (and hence to the main target cells and proteins of iron). The iron remains trapped inside the cells in the form of ferritin, levels of which are therefore normal or high in the face of significant anaemia. Inhibition or blockade of hepcidin is a likely target for potential treatment of this form of anaemia.

Diagnosis and management

It is often difficult to distinguish ACD associated with a low MCV from iron deficiency. Box 24.35 summarises the investigations and results. Examination of the marrow may ultimately be required to assess iron stores directly. A trial of oral iron can be given in difficult situations. A positive response occurs in true iron deficiency but not in ACD. Measures which reduce the severity of the underlying disorder generally help to improve the ACD.

Megaloblastic anaemia

This results from a deficiency of vitamin B_{12} or folic acid, or from disturbances in folic acid metabolism. Folate is an important substrate of, and vitamin B_{12} a co-factor for, the generation of the essential amino acid methionine from homocysteine. This reaction produces tetrahydrofolate, which is converted to thymidine monophosphate for incorporation into DNA. Deficiency of either vitamin B_{12} or folate will therefore produce high plasma levels of homocysteine and impaired DNA synthesis.

The end result is cells with arrested nuclear maturation but normal cytoplasmic development: so-called nucleocytoplasmic asynchrony. All proliferating cells will exhibit megaloblastosis; hence changes are evident in the buccal mucosa, tongue, small intestine, cervix, vagina and uterus. The high proliferation rate of bone marrow results in striking changes in the haematopoietic system in megaloblastic anaemia. Cells become arrested in development and die within the marrow; this ineffective erythropoiesis results in an expanded hypercellular marrow. The megaloblastic changes are most evident in the early nucleated red cell precursors, and haemolysis within the marrow results in a raised bilirubin and lactate dehydrogenase (LDH), but without the reticulocytosis characteristic of other forms of haemolysis (p. 1022). Iron stores are usually raised. The mature red cells are large and oval, and sometimes contain nuclear remnants. Nuclear changes are seen in the immature granulocyte precursors and a characteristic appearance is that of 'giant' metamyelocytes with a large 'sausage-shaped' nucleus. The mature neutrophils show hypersegmentation of their nuclei, with cells having six or more nuclear lobes. If severe, a pancytopenia may be present in the peripheral blood.

Vitamin B_{12} deficiency, but not folate deficiency, is associated with neurological disease in up to 40% of cases. The main pathological finding is focal demyelination affecting the spinal cord, peripheral nerves, optic nerves and cerebrum. The most common manifestations are sensory, with peripheral paraesthesiae and ataxia of gait. The clinical and diagnostic features of megaloblastic anaemia are summarised in Boxes 24.36 and 24.37, and the neurological findings of B_{12} deficiency in Box 24.38.

Vitamin B_{12}

Vitamin B_{12} absorption

The average daily diet contains 5–30 µg of vitamin B_{12}, mainly in meat, fish, eggs and milk—well in excess of the 1 µg daily requirement. In the stomach, gastric enzymes release vitamin B_{12} from food and at gastric pH it binds to a carrier protein termed R protein. The gastric parietal cells produce intrinsic factor, a vitamin B_{12}-binding protein which optimally binds vitamin B_{12}

24.36 Clinical features of megaloblastic anaemia

Symptoms

- Malaise (90%)
- Breathlessness (50%)
- Paraesthesiae (80%)
- Sore mouth (20%)
- Weight loss
- Altered skin pigmentation
- Grey hair

- Impotence
- Poor memory
- Depression
- Personality change
- Hallucinations
- Visual disturbance

Signs

- Smooth tongue
- Angular cheilosis
- Vitiligo

- Skin pigmentation
- Heart failure
- Pyrexia

24.37 Investigations in megaloblastic anaemia

Investigation	Result
Haemoglobin	Often reduced, may be very low
MCV	Usually raised, commonly > 120 fL
Erythrocyte count	Low for degree of anaemia
Blood film	Oval macrocytosis, poikilocytosis, red cell fragmentation, neutrophil hypersegmentation
Reticulocyte count	Low for degree of anaemia
Leucocyte count	Low or normal
Platelet count	Low or normal
Bone marrow	Increased cellularity, megaloblastic changes in erythroid series, giant metamyelocytes, dysplastic megakaryocytes, increased iron in stores, pathological non-ring sideroblasts
Serum ferritin	Elevated
Plasma lactate dehydrogenase (LDH)	Elevated, often markedly

24.38 Neurological findings in B_{12} deficiency

Peripheral nerves
- Glove and stocking paraesthesiae
- Loss of ankle reflexes

Spinal cord
- Subacute combined degeneration of the cord
    Posterior columns—diminished vibration sensation and proprioception
    Corticospinal tracts—upper motor neuron signs

Cerebrum
- Dementia
- Optic atrophy

Autonomic neuropathy

at pH 8. As gastric emptying occurs, pancreatic secretion raises the pH and vitamin B_{12} released from the diet switches from the R protein to intrinsic factor. Bile also contains vitamin B_{12} which is available for reabsorption in the intestine. The vitamin B_{12} intrinsic factor complex binds to specific receptors in the terminal ileum and vitamin B_{12} is actively transported by the enterocytes to plasma, where it binds to transcobalamin II, a transport protein produced by the liver, which carries it to the tissues for utilisation. The liver stores enough vitamin B_{12} for 3 years and this, together with the enterohepatic circulation, means that vitamin B_{12} deficiency takes years to become manifest, even if all dietary intake is stopped.

Blood levels of vitamin B_{12} provide a reasonable indication of tissue stores and are usually diagnostic of deficiency. Levels of cobalamins fall in normal pregnancy. Each laboratory must validate its own normal range but levels below 150 ng/L are common and in the last trimester 5–10% of women have levels below 100 ng/L. Paraproteins can interfere with vitamin B_{12} assays and so myeloma may be associated with a spuriously low vitamin B_{12}.

Causes of vitamin B_{12} deficiency

Dietary deficiency

This only occurs in strict vegans but the onset of clinical features can occur at any age between 10 and 80 years. Less strict vegetarians often have slightly low vitamin B_{12} levels but are not tissue vitamin B_{12}-deficient.

Gastric factors

Release of vitamin B_{12} from the food requires normal gastric acid and enzyme secretion, and this is impaired by hypochlorhydria in elderly patients or following gastric surgery. Total gastrectomy invariably results in vitamin B_{12} deficiency within 5 years, often combined with iron deficiency; these patients need life-long 3-monthly vitamin B_{12} injections. After partial gastrectomy vitamin B_{12} deficiency only develops in 10–20% of patients by 5 years; an annual injection of vitamin B_{12} should prevent deficiency in this group.

Pernicious anaemia

This is an autoimmune disorder in which the gastric mucosa is atrophic, with loss of parietal cells causing intrinsic factor deficiency. In the absence of intrinsic factor, less than 1% of dietary vitamin B_{12} is absorbed. Pernicious anaemia has an incidence of 25/100000 population over the age of 40 years in developed countries, but an average age of onset of 60 years. It is more common in individuals with other autoimmune disease (Hashimoto's thyroiditis, Graves' disease, vitiligo, hypoparathyroidism or Addison's disease; Ch. 20) or a family history of these or pernicious anaemia. The finding of anti-intrinsic factor antibodies in the context of B_{12} deficiency is diagnostic of pernicious anaemia without further investigation. Antiparietal cell antibodies are present in over 90% of cases but are also present in 20% of normal females over the age of 60 years; a negative result makes pernicious anaemia less likely but a positive result is not diagnostic. Patients with low B_{12} levels and negative anti-intrinsic factor antibodies should have a Schilling test performed to determine whether there is B_{12} malabsorption, and if so, where it is occurring (Fig. 24.21).

Part One

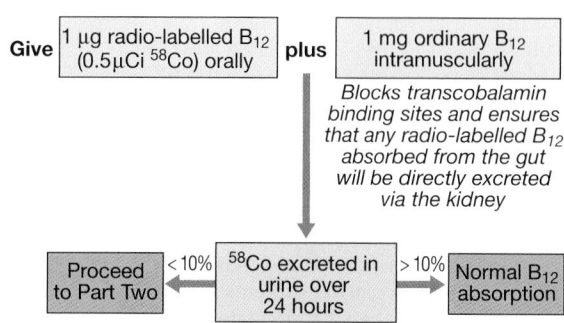

Part Two (if excretion ↓ in Part One)

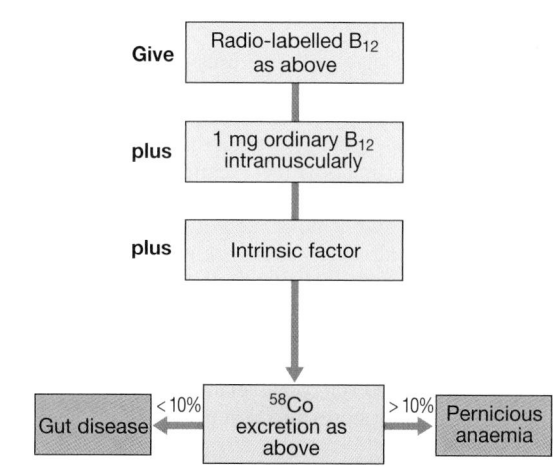

Fig. 24.21 The two-part Schilling test in the diagnosis of the cause of vitamin B_{12} deficiency.

Small bowel factors

One-third of patients with pancreatic exocrine insufficiency fail to transfer dietary vitamin B_{12} from R protein to intrinsic factor. This usually results in slightly low vitamin B_{12} values but no tissue evidence of vitamin B_{12} deficiency.

Motility disorders or hypogammaglobulinaemia can result in bacterial overgrowth and the ensuing competition for free vitamin B_{12} can lead to deficiency. This is corrected to some extent by appropriate antibiotics.

A small number of people heavily infected with the fish tapeworm (p. 373) develop vitamin B_{12} deficiency.

Inflammatory disease of the terminal ileum, such as Crohn's disease, may impair the interaction of the vitamin B_{12}–intrinsic factor complex with its receptor, as will surgery on part of the bowel. Both may result in vitamin B_{12} malabsorption.

It is possible to distinguish pernicious anaemia from intestinal problems with a two-part Schilling test (see Fig. 24.21). The patient must be vitamin B_{12}-replete, have normal renal function and be able to comply with a 24-hour urine collection. This latter criterion is important, as up to 25% of tests are invalidated by an incomplete urine collection. It is important to note that this is not a test of gut function, but simply distinguishes pernicious anaemia from the other causes of vitamin B_{12} deficiency.

24

Folate

Folate absorption

Folates are produced by plants and bacteria; hence dietary leafy vegetables (spinach, broccoli, lettuce), fruits (bananas, melons) and animal protein (liver, kidney) are a rich source. An average Western diet contains more than the minimum daily intake of 50 µg but excess cooking for longer than 15 minutes destroys folates. Most dietary folate is present as polyglutamates; these are converted to monoglutamate in the upper small bowel and actively transported into plasma. Plasma folate is loosely bound to plasma proteins such as albumin and there is an enterohepatic circulation. Total body stores of folate are small and deficiency can occur in a matter of weeks.

Folate deficiency

The causes and diagnostic features of folate deficiency are shown in Boxes 24.39 and 24.40. The edentulous elderly or psychiatric patient is particularly susceptible to dietary deficiency and this is exacerbated in the presence of gut disease or malignancy. Pregnancy-induced folate deficiency is the most common cause of megaloblastosis world-wide and is more likely in the context of twin pregnancies, multiparity and hyperemesis gravidarum. Serum folate is very sensitive to dietary intake; a single meal can normalise it in a patient with true folate deficiency, whereas anorexia, alcohol and anticonvulsant therapy can reduce it in the absence of megaloblastosis. For this reason red cell folate levels are a more accurate indicator of folate stores and tissue folate deficiency.

24.39 Causes of folate deficiency

Diet

- Poor intake of vegetables

Malabsorption

- e.g. Coeliac disease

Increased demand

- Cell proliferation, e.g. haemolysis
- Pregnancy

Drugs*

- Certain anticonvulsants (e.g. phenytoin)
- Certain cytotoxic drugs (e.g. methotrexate)
- Contraceptive pill

*Usually only a problem in patients deficient in folate from another cause.

24.40 Investigation of folic acid deficiency

Diagnostic findings

- Low serum folate levels (fasting blood sample)
- Red cell folate levels low (but may be normal if folate deficiency is of very recent onset)

Corroborative findings

- Macrocytic dysplastic blood picture
- Megaloblastic marrow

Management of megaloblastic anaemia

If a patient with a severe megaloblastic anaemia is very ill and treatment must be started before vitamin B_{12} and red cell folate results are available, treatment should always include both folic acid and vitamin B_{12}. The use of folic acid alone in the presence of vitamin B_{12} deficiency may result in worsening of neurological deficits.

Rarely, if severe angina or heart failure is present, transfusion can be used in megaloblastic anaemia. The cardiovascular system is adapted to the chronic anaemia present in megaloblastosis, and the volume load imposed by transfusion may result in decompensation and severe cardiac failure. In such circumstances, exchange transfusion or slow administration of 1 unit each day with diuretic cover may be given cautiously.

Vitamin B_{12} deficiency

Vitamin B_{12} deficiency is treated with hydroxycobalamin 1000 µg i.m. in five doses 2 or 3 days apart, followed by maintenance therapy of 1000 µg every 3 months for life. The reticulocyte count will peak by the 5th–10th day after therapy and may be as high as 50%. The haemoglobin will rise by 10 g/L every week. The response of the marrow is associated with a fall in plasma potassium levels and rapid depletion of iron stores. If an initial response is not maintained and the blood film is dimorphic (i.e. shows a mixture of microcytic and macrocytic cells), the patient may need additional iron therapy. A sensory neuropathy may take 6–12 months to correct; long-standing neurological damage may not improve.

Folate deficiency

Oral folic acid 5 mg daily for 3 weeks will treat acute deficiency and 5 mg once weekly is adequate maintenance therapy. Prophylactic folic acid in pregnancy prevents megaloblastosis in women at risk, and reduces the risk of fetal neural tube defects (p. 113). Prophylactic supplementation is also given in chronic haematological disease associated with reduced red cell lifespan (e.g. autoimmune haemolytic anaemia or haemoglobinopathies). There is some evidence that supraphysiological supplementation (400 µg/day) can reduce the risk of coronary and cerebrovascular disease by reducing plasma homocysteine levels. This has led the US Food and Drug Administration to introduce fortification of bread, flour and rice with folic acid.

Haemolytic anaemia

The normal red cell lifespan of 120 days may be shortened by a variety of abnormalities. The bone marrow may increase its output of red cells six- to eight-fold by increasing the proportion of red cells produced, expanding the volume of active marrow and releasing reticulocytes prematurely. If the rate of destruction exceeds this increased production rate, then anaemia will develop.

Investigation and differential diagnosis of haemolysis are outlined in Figure 24.22. Red cell destruction overloads pathways for haemoglobin breakdown, causing a modest rise in unconjugated bilirubin in the blood and mild jaundice. Increased reabsorption of urobilinogen

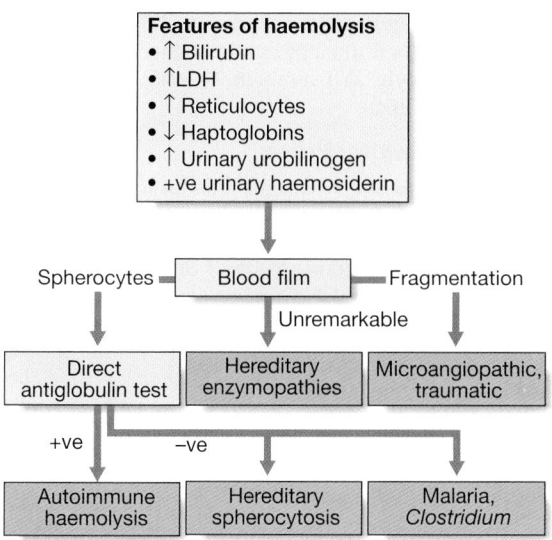

Features of haemolysis
- ↑ Bilirubin
- ↑LDH
- ↑ Reticulocytes
- ↓ Haptoglobins
- ↑ Urinary urobilinogen
- +ve urinary haemosiderin

Spherocytes ◄ Blood film ► Fragmentation

Unremarkable

| Direct antiglobulin test | Hereditary enzymopathies | Microangiopathic, traumatic |

+ve / −ve

| Autoimmune haemolysis | Hereditary spherocytosis | Malaria, *Clostridium* |

Fig. 24.22 Laboratory features and classification of the causes of haemolysis. (LDH = lactate dehydrogenase; DAT = direct antiglobulin test)

from the gut results in an increase in urinary urobilinogen (pp. 930 and 990). Red cell destruction releases LDH into the serum. The bone marrow compensation results in a reticulocytosis, and nucleated red cell precursors may also appear in the blood. Activation of the bone marrow can result in a neutrophilia and immature granulocytes appearing in the blood to cause a leuco-erythroblastic blood film. The appearances of the red cells may give an indication of the likely cause of the haemolysis (see Box 24.2, p. 995).

- Spherocytes are small, dark red cells which suggest autoimmune haemolysis or hereditary spherocytosis.
- Sickle cells suggest haemoglobinopathy.
- Red cell fragments indicate microangiopathic haemolysis.

The compensatory erythroid hyperplasia may give rise to folate deficiency, when the blood findings will be complicated by the presence of megaloblastosis. Measurement of red cell folate is unreliable in the presence of haemolysis and serum folate will be elevated.

Intravascular haemolysis

When rapid red cell destruction occurs, free haemoglobin is released into the plasma. Free haemoglobin is toxic to cells and binding proteins have evolved to minimise this risk. Haptoglobin is an α_2-globulin produced by the liver which binds free haemoglobin, resulting in a fall in levels of haptoglobin. Once haptoglobins are saturated, free haemoglobin is oxidised to form methaemoglobin which binds to albumin, in turn forming methaemalbumin which can be detected spectrophotometrically in the Schumm's test. Methaemoglobin is degraded and any free haem is bound to a second binding protein termed haemopexin. If all the protective mechanisms are overloaded, free haemoglobin may appear in the urine. When fulminant, this gives rise to black urine, as in severe *falciparum* malaria infection (p. 348). In smaller amounts, renal tubular cells absorb the haemoglobin, degrade it and store the iron as haemosiderin. When the tubular cells are subsequently sloughed into the urine, they give rise to haemosiderinuria, which is always indicative of intravascular haemolysis.

Extravascular haemolysis

Physiological red cell destruction occurs in the fixed reticulo-endothelial cells in the liver or spleen, so avoiding free haemoglobin in the plasma. In most haemolytic states, haemolysis is predominantly extravascular.

To confirm the haemolysis, patients' red cells can be labelled with [51]Chromium. When re-injected, they can be used to determine red cell survival; when combined with body surface radioactivity counting this test may indicate whether the liver or the spleen is the main source of red cell destruction. However, this is seldom performed in clinical practice.

Causes of haemolytic anaemia

These can be classified as congenital or acquired.

- *Inherited* red cell abnormalities resulting in chronic haemolytic anaemia may arise from pathologies of the red cell membrane (hereditary spherocytosis or elliptocytosis), of the haemoglobin (haemoglobinopathies) or of protective enzymes which prevent cellular oxidative damage, such as glucose-6-phosphate dehydrogenase (G6PD).
- *Acquired* causes include auto- and allo-antibody-mediated destruction of red blood cells and other mechanical, toxic and infective causes, as detailed below.

Red cell membrane defects

The structure of the red cell membrane is shown in Figure 24.4 (p. 990). The basic structure is a cytoskeleton 'stapled' on to the lipid bilayer by special protein complexes. This structure ensures great deformability and elasticity; the red cell diameter is 8 μm but the narrowest capillaries in the circulation are in the spleen, measuring just 2 μm in diameter. When the normal red cell structure is disturbed, usually by a quantitative or functional deficiency of one or more proteins in the cytoskeleton, cells lose their elasticity. Each time such cells pass through the spleen, they lose membrane relative to their cell volume. This results in an increase in mean cell haemoglobin concentration (MCHC), abnormal cell shape (see Box 24.2, p. 995) and reduced red cell survival due to extravascular haemolysis.

Hereditary spherocytosis

This is usually inherited as an autosomal dominant condition, although 25% of cases have no family history and represent new mutations. The incidence is approximately 1:5000 in developed countries but this may be an underestimate, since the disease may present de novo in patients aged over 65 years and is often discovered as a chance finding on a blood count. The most common abnormalities are deficiencies of beta spectrin or ankyrin (see Fig. 24.4, p. 990). The severity of spontaneous haemolysis varies. Most cases are associated with an asymptomatic compensated chronic haemolytic state with spherocytes present on the blood film, a reticulocytosis and mild hyperbilirubinaemia. Pigment gallstones are present in up to 50% of patients and may cause symptomatic cholecystitis. Occasional cases are associated with more severe haemolysis; these may be due to coincidental polymorphisms in alpha spectrin or

24

co-inheritance of a second defect involving a different protein.

The clinical course may be complicated by crises:

- A *haemolytic crisis* occurs when the severity of haemolysis increases; this is rare, and usually associated with infection.
- A *megaloblastic crisis* follows the development of folate deficiency; this may occur as a first presentation of the disease in pregnancy.
- An *aplastic crisis* occurs in association with erythrovirus infection (p. 311). Erythrovirus causes a common exanthem in children, but if individuals with chronic haemolysis become infected, the virus directly invades red cell precursors and temporarily switches off red cell production. Patients present with severe anaemia and a low reticulocyte count.

Investigations

The patient and other family members should be screened for features of compensated haemolysis (see Fig. 24.22). This may be all that is required to confirm the diagnosis. Haemoglobin levels are variable, depending on the degree of compensation. The blood film will show spherocytes but the direct Coombs test (see Fig. 24.23 below) is negative, excluding immune haemolysis. An osmotic fragility test may show increased sensitivity to lysis in hypotonic saline solutions but is limited by lack of sensitivity and specificity. More specific flow cytometric tests, detecting binding of eosin-5-maleimide to red cells, are recommended in borderline cases.

Management

Folic acid prophylaxis, 5 mg once weekly, should be given for life. Consideration may be given to splenectomy, which improves but does not normalise red cell survival. Potential indications include moderate to severe haemolysis with complications (anaemia and gallstones), although splenectomy should be delayed until after 6 years of age in view of the risk of sepsis. Guidelines for the management of patients after splenectomy are presented in Box 24.41.

24.41 Management of the splenectomised patient

- Vaccinate with pneumococcal, *Haemophilus influenzae* type B, meningococcal group C and influenza vaccines at least 2–3 weeks before elective splenectomy. Vaccination should be given after emergency surgery, but may be less effective
- Pneumococcal re-immunisation should be given at least 5-yearly and influenza annually. Vaccination status must be documented
- Life-long prophylactic penicillin V 500 mg 12-hourly is recommended. In penicillin-allergic patients, consider erythromycin
- A card or bracelet should be carried by splenectomised patients to alert health professionals to the risk of overwhelming sepsis
- In septicaemia, splenectomised patients should be resuscitated and given intravenous antibiotics to cover pneumococcus, *Haemophilus* and meningococcus
- The risk of malaria is increased
- Animal bites should be promptly treated with local disinfection and antibiotics, to prevent serious soft tissue infection and septicaemia

Acute, severe haemolytic crises require transfusion support, but blood must be cross-matched carefully and transfused slowly as haemolytic transfusion reactions may occur (p. 1012).

Hereditary elliptocytosis

This term refers to a heterogeneous group of disorders that produce an increase in elliptocytic red cells on the blood film and a variable degree of haemolysis. This is due to a functional abnormality of one or more anchor proteins in the red cell membrane, e.g. alpha spectrin or protein 4.1. Inheritance may be autosomal dominant or recessive. It is less common than hereditary spherocytosis in Western countries, with an incidence of 1/10 000, but is more common in equatorial Africa and parts of South-east Asia. The clinical course is variable and depends upon the degree of membrane dysfunction caused by the inherited molecular defect(s); most cases present as an asymptomatic blood film abnormality, but occasional cases result in neonatal haemolysis or a chronic compensated haemolytic state. Management of the latter is the same as for hereditary spherocytosis.

A characteristic variant of hereditary elliptocytosis occurs in South-east Asia, particularly Malaysia and Papua New Guinea, with stomatocytes and ovalocytes in the blood. This has a prevalence of up to 30% in some communities because it offers relative protection from malaria and thus has sustained a high gene frequency. The differential diagnosis includes iron deficiency, thalassaemia, myelofibrosis, myelodysplasia and pyruvate kinase deficiency.

Red cell enzymopathies

The mature red cell must produce energy via ATP to maintain a normal internal environment and cell volume whilst protecting itself from the oxidative stress presented by oxygen carriage. Anaerobic glycolysis via the Embden–Meyerhof pathway generates ATP, and the hexose monophosphate shunt produces NADPH and glutathione to protect against oxidative stress. The impact of functional or quantitative defects in the enzymes in these pathways depends upon the importance of the steps affected and the presence of alternative pathways. In general, defects in the hexose monophosphate shunt pathway result in periodic haemolysis induced by oxidative stress, whilst those in the Embden–Meyerhof pathway result in shortened red cell survival and chronic haemolysis.

Glucose-6-phosphate dehydrogenase (G6PD) deficiency

This enzyme is pivotal in the hexose monophosphate shunt pathway. Deficiencies result in the most common human enzymopathy, affecting 10% of the world's population, with a geographical distribution which parallels the malaria belt because heterozygotes are protected from malarial parasitisation. The enzyme is a heteromeric structure made of catalytic subunits which are encoded by a gene on the X chromosome. The deficiency therefore affects males and rare homozygotic females (p. 50), but it is carried by females. Carrier heterozygous females are usually only affected in the neonatal period or in the presence of extreme lyonisation, producing selective inactivation of one of the X chromosomes.

There are over 400 subtypes of G6PD described. The most common types associated with normal activity

24.42 Glucose-6-phosphate dehydrogenase deficiency

Clinical features

- Acute drug-induced haemolysis to (e.g.)
  Analgesics: aspirin, phenacetin
  Antimalarials: primaquine, quinine, chloroquine, pyrimethamine
  Antibiotics: sulphonamides, nitrofurantoin, ciprofloxacin
  Miscellaneous: quinidine, probenecid, vitamin K, dapsone
- Chronic compensated haemolysis
- Infection or acute illness
- Neonatal jaundice: may be a feature of the B⁻ enzyme
- Favism, i.e. acute haemolysis after ingestion of the broad bean *Vicia faba*

Laboratory features

Non-spherocytic intravascular haemolysis during an attack
The blood film will show:

- Bite cells (red cells with a 'bite' of membrane missing)
- Blister cells (red cells with surface blistering of the membrane)
- Irregularly shaped small cells
- Polychromasia reflecting the reticulocytosis
- Denatured haemoglobin visible as Heinz bodies within the red cell cytoplasm, if stained with a supravital stain such as methyl violet

G6PD level

- Can be indirectly assessed by screening methods which usually depend upon the decreased ability to reduce dyes
- Direct assessment of G6PD is made in those with low screening values
- Care must be taken close to an acute haemolytic episode because reticulocytes may have higher enzyme levels and give rise to a false normal result

are the B⁺ enzyme present in most Caucasians and 70% of Afro-Caribbeans, and the A⁺ variant present in 20% of Afro-Caribbeans. The two common variants associated with reduced activity are the A⁻ variety in approximately 10% of Afro-Caribbeans, and the Mediterranean or B⁻ variety in Caucasians. In East and West Africa, up to 20% of males and 4% of females (homozygotes) are affected and have enzyme levels of approximately 15% of normal. The deficiency in Caucasian and Oriental populations is more severe, with enzyme levels as low as 1%.

Clinical features and investigation findings are shown in Box 24.42.

Management aims to stop any precipitant drugs and treat any underlying infection. Acute transfusion support may be life-saving.

Pyruvate kinase deficiency

This is the second most common red cell enzyme defect. It results in deficiency of ATP production and a chronic haemolytic anaemia. It is inherited as an autosomal recessive trait. The extent of anaemia is variable; the blood film shows characteristic 'prickle cells' which resemble holly leaves. Enzyme activity is only 5–20% of normal. Transfusion support may be necessary.

Pyrimidine 5′ nucleotidase deficiency

This enzyme catalyses the dephosphorylation of nucleoside monophosphates and is important during the degradation of RNA in reticulocytes. It is inherited as an autosomal recessive trait and is as common as pyruvate kinase deficiency in Mediterranean, African and Jewish populations. The accumulation of excess ribonucleoprotein results in coarse basophilic stippling (see Box 24.2, p. 998) associated with a chronic haemolytic state. The enzyme is very sensitive to inhibition by lead and this is the reason why basophilic stippling is a feature of lead poisoning.

Autoimmune haemolytic anaemia

This results from increased red cell destruction due to red cell autoantibodies. The antibodies may be IgG or M, or more rarely IgE or A. If an antibody avidly fixes complement, it will cause intravascular haemolysis, but if complement activation is weak, the haemolysis will be extravascular. Antibody-coated red cells lose membrane to macrophages in the spleen and hence spherocytes are present in the blood. The optimum temperature at which the antibody is active (thermal specificity) is used to classify immune haemolysis:

- *Warm antibodies* bind best at 37°C and account for 80% of cases. The majority are IgG and often react against Rhesus antigens.
- *Cold antibodies* bind best at 4°C but can bind up to 37°C in some cases. They are usually IgM and bind complement. They account for the other 20% of cases.

Warm autoimmune haemolysis

The incidence of warm autoimmune haemolysis is approximately 1/100000 population per annum; it occurs at all ages but is more common in middle age and in females. No underlying cause is identified in up to 50% of cases. The remainder are secondary to a wide variety of other conditions:

- lymphoid neoplasms: lymphoma, chronic lymphocytic leukaemia, myeloma
- solid tumours: lung, colon, kidney, ovary, thymoma
- connective tissue disease: SLE, rheumatoid arthritis
- drugs: methyldopa, mefenamic acid, penicillin, quinidine
- miscellaneous: ulcerative colitis, HIV.

Investigations

There is evidence of haemolysis and spherocytes on the blood film. The diagnosis is confirmed by the direct Coombs or antiglobulin test (Fig. 24.23). The patient's red cells are mixed with Coombs reagent, which contains antibodies against human IgG/M/complement. If the red cells have been coated by antibody in vivo, the Coombs reagent will induce their agglutination and this can be detected visually. The relevant antibody can be eluted from the red cell surface and tested against a panel of typed red cells to determine against which red cell antigen it is directed. The most common specificity is Rhesus and most often anti-e; this is helpful when choosing blood to cross-match. The direct Coombs test can be negative in the presence of brisk haemolysis. A positive test requires about 200 antibody molecules to attach to each red cell; with a very avid complement-fixing antibody, haemolysis may occur at lower levels of antibody-binding. The standard Coombs reagent will miss IgA or IgE antibodies.

24

A Direct antiglobulin test (DAT) (Coombs test)

Detects the presence of antibody bound to
the red cell surface, e.g.
1. Autoimmune haemolytic anaemia
2. Haemolytic disease of newborn (HDN)
3. Transfusion reactions

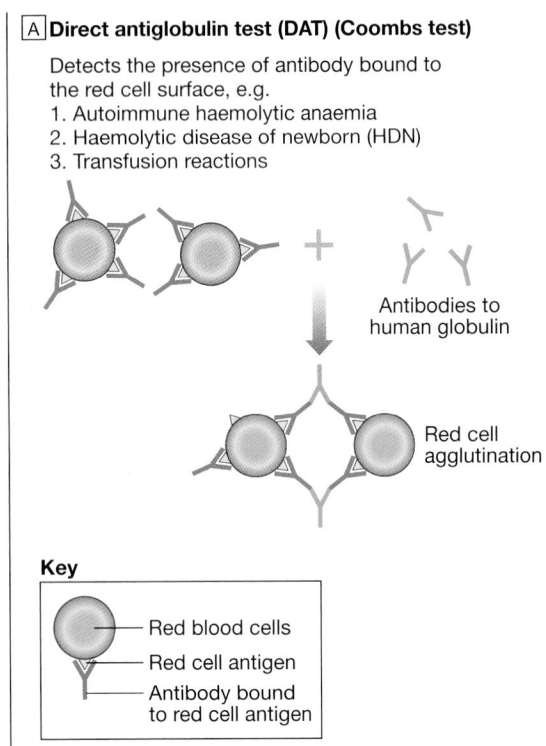

Key
- Red blood cells
- Red cell antigen
- Antibody bound
  to red cell antigen

B Indirect antiglobulin test (IAT) (indirect Coombs test)

Detects antibodies in the plasma, e.g.
1. Antibody screen in pre-transfusion testing
2. Screening in pregnancy for antibodies that may cause
   haemolytic disease of the newborn

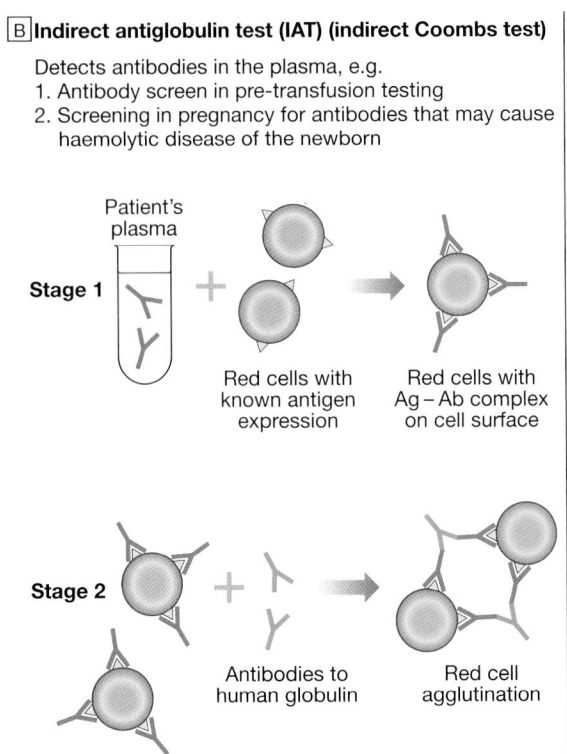

Fig. 24.23 Direct and indirect antiglobulin tests.

Management

If the haemolysis is secondary to an underlying cause, this must be treated and any offending drugs stopped.

It is usual to treat patients initially with prednisolone 1 mg/kg orally. A response is seen in 70–80% of cases but may take up to 3 weeks; a rise in haemoglobin will be matched by a fall in bilirubin, LDH and reticulocyte levels. Once the haemoglobin has normalised and the reticulocytosis resolved, the corticosteroid dose can be reduced slowly over about 10 weeks. Corticosteroids work by decreasing macrophage destruction of antibody-coated red cells and reducing antibody production.

Transfusion support may be required for life-threatening problems, such as the development of heart failure or rapid unabated falls in Hb. The least incompatible blood should be used but this may still give rise to transfusion reactions or the development of alloantibodies.

If the haemolysis fails to respond to corticosteroids or can only be stabilised by large doses, then splenectomy should be considered. This removes a main site of red cell destruction and antibody production, with a good response in 50–60% of cases. The operation can be performed laparoscopically with reduced morbidity. If splenectomy is not appropriate, alternative immunosuppressive therapy with azathioprine or cyclophosphamide may be considered. This is least suitable for young patients, in whom long-term immunosuppression carries a risk of secondary neoplasms. The anti-CD20 (B cell) monoclonal antibody, rituximab, has shown some success in difficult cases.

Cold agglutinin disease

This is due to antibodies, usually IgM, which bind to the red cells at 4 °C and cause them to agglutinate. It may cause intravascular haemolysis if complement fixation occurs. This can be chronic when the antibody is monoclonal, or acute or transient when the antibody is polyclonal.

Chronic cold agglutinin disease

This affects elderly patients and may be associated with an underlying low-grade B cell lymphoma. It causes a low-grade intravascular haemolysis with cold, painful and often blue fingers, toes, ears or nose (so-called acrocyanosis). The latter is due to red cell agglutination in the small vessels in these colder exposed areas. The blood film shows red cell agglutination and the MCV may be spuriously raised because the automated analysers count aggregates as single cells. The monoclonal IgM usually has specificity against the I or, more rarely, i red cell antigen and is present in a very high titre. Treatment is directed at any underlying lymphoma but if the disease is idiopathic, then patients must keep extremities warm, especially in winter. Some patients respond to corticosteroid therapy and blood transfusion may be considered, but the cross-match sample must be placed in a transport flask at a temperature of 37 °C and blood administered via a blood-warmer.

Other causes of cold agglutination

Cold agglutination can occur in association with *Mycoplasma pneumoniae* or with infectious mononucleosis. Paroxysmal cold haemoglobinuria is a very rare cause seen in children in association with congenital syphilis. An IgG antibody binds to red cells in the peripheral circulation but lysis occurs in the central circulation when complement fixation takes place. This antibody is termed the Donath–Landsteiner antibody and has specificity against the P antigen on the red cells.

Alloimmune haemolytic anaemia

Alloimmune haemolytic anaemia is due to an antibody against non-self red cells. It has two main causes:

- an unmatched transfusion of red cells (a haemolytic transfusion reaction, p. 1012)
- maternal sensitisation to paternal antigens on fetal cells (haemolytic disease of the newborn, p. 1010).

Non-immune haemolytic anaemia

Physical trauma

Physical disruption of red cells may occur in a number of conditions and is characterised by the presence of red cell fragments on the blood film and markers of intravascular haemolysis:

- *Mechanical heart valves.* High flow through incompetent valves or periprosthetic leaks through the suture ring holding a valve in place result in shear stress damage.
- *March haemoglobinuria.* Vigorous exercise, such as prolonged marching or marathon running, can cause red cell damage in the capillaries in the feet.
- *Thermal injury.* Severe burns cause thermal damage to red cells characterised by fragmentation and the presence of microspherocytes in the blood.
- *Microangiopathic haemolytic anaemia.* Fibrin deposition in capillaries can cause severe red cell disruption. It may occur in a wide variety of conditions: disseminated carcinomatosis, malignant or pregnancy-induced hypertension, haemolytic uraemic syndrome (p. 498), thrombotic thrombocytopenic purpura (p. 1051) and disseminated intravascular coagulation (p. 1050).

Infection

Plasmodium falciparum malaria (p. 348) may be associated with intravascular haemolysis; when severe, this is termed blackwater fever due to the associated haemoglobinuria. *Clostridium perfringens* septicaemia (p. 301), usually in the context of ascending cholangitis, may cause severe intravascular haemolysis with marked spherocytosis due to bacterial production of a lecithinase which destroys the red cell membrane.

Chemicals or drugs

Dapsone and sulfasalazine cause haemolysis by oxidative denaturation of haemoglobin. Denatured haemoglobin forms Heinz bodies in the red cells, visible on supravital staining with brilliant cresyl blue. Arsenic gas, copper, chlorates, nitrites and nitrobenzene derivatives may all cause haemolysis.

Paroxysmal nocturnal haemoglobinuria (PNH)

This rare acquired non-malignant clonal expansion of haematopoietic stem cells deficient in GPI-anchor protein results in intravascular haemolysis and anaemia because of increased sensitivity of red cells to lysis by complement. Episodes of intravascular haemolysis result in haemoglobinuria, most noticeable in early morning urine which has a characteristic red-brown colour. The disease is associated with an increased risk of venous thrombosis in unusual sites such as the liver or abdomen. PNH is also associated with hypoplastic bone marrow failure, aplastic anaemia and myelodysplastic syndrome (pp. 1043 and 1036). Management is supportive with transfusion and treatment of thrombosis. Recently the anti-complement C5 monoclonal antibody ecluzimab was shown to be effective in reducing haemolysis.

HAEMOGLOBINOPATHIES

These diseases are caused by dysfunction of the genes encoding the globin chains of the haemoglobin molecule. Normal haemoglobin is comprised of two alpha and two non-alpha globin chains. Alpha globin chains are produced throughout life, so severe mutations may cause intrauterine death. Production of non-alpha chains varies with age; fetal haemoglobin (HbF-$\alpha\alpha/\gamma\gamma$) has two gamma chains, while the predominant adult haemoglobin (HbA-$\alpha\alpha/\beta\beta$) has two beta chains. Thus, disorders affecting the beta chains do not present until after 6 months of age. A constant small amount of haemoglobin A$_2$ (HbA$_2$-$\alpha\alpha/\delta\delta$, usually < 2%) is made from birth.

The geographical distribution of the common haemoglobinopathies is shown in Figure 24.24. The

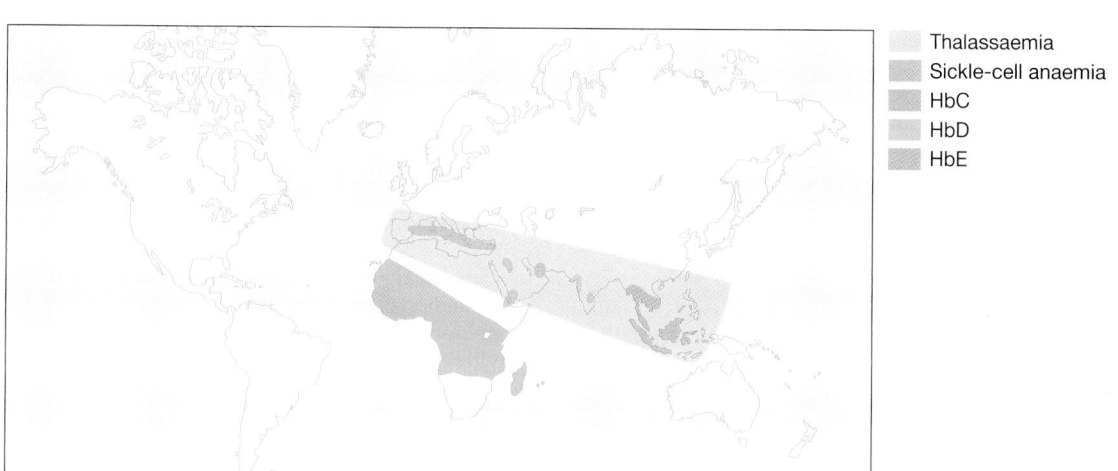

Thalassaemia
Sickle-cell anaemia
HbC
HbD
HbE

Fig. 24.24 The geographical distribution of the haemoglobinopathies.

haemoglobinopathies can be classified into qualitative or quantitative abnormalities.

Qualitative abnormalities—abnormal haemoglobins

In qualitative abnormalities (called the abnormal haemoglobins), there is a functionally important alteration in the amino acid structure of the polypeptide chains of the globin chains. Several hundred such variants are known; they were originally designated by letters of the alphabet, e.g. S, C, D or E, but are now described by names usually taken from the town or district in which they were first described. The best-known example is haemoglobin S, found in sickle-cell anaemia. Mutations around the haem-binding pocket cause the haem ring to fall out of the structure and produce an unstable haemoglobin. These substitutions often change the charge of the globin chains, producing different electrophoretic mobility, and this forms the basis for the diagnostic use of haemoglobin electrophoresis to identify haemoglobinopathies.

Quantitative abnormalities—thalassaemias

In quantitative abnormalities (the thalassaemias) there are mutations causing a reduced rate of production of one or other of the globin chains, altering the ratio of alpha to non-alpha chains. In alpha-thalassaemia excess beta chains are present, whilst in beta-thalassaemia excess alpha chains are present. The excess chains precipitate, causing red cell membrane damage and reduced red cell survival.

Sickle-cell anaemia

Sickle-cell disease results from a single glutamic acid to valine substitution at position 6 of the beta globin polypeptide chain. It is inherited as an autosomal recessive trait (p. 50). Homozygotes only produce abnormal beta chains that make haemoglobin S (HbS, termed SS), and this results in the clinical syndrome of sickle-cell disease. Heterozygotes produce a mixture of normal and abnormal beta chains that make normal HbA and HbS (termed AS), and this results in the clinically asymptomatic sickle-cell trait.

Epidemiology

The heterozygote frequency is over 20% in tropical Africa (see Fig. 24.24). In black American populations, sickle-cell trait has a frequency of 8%. Individuals with sickle-cell trait are relatively resistant to the lethal effects of *falciparum* malaria in early childhood; the high prevalence in equatorial Africa can be explained by the selective survival advantage it confers in areas where *falciparum* malaria is endemic. However, homozygous patients with sickle-cell anaemia do not have correspondingly greater resistance to *falciparum* malaria.

Pathogenesis

When haemoglobin S is deoxygenated, the molecules of haemoglobin polymerise to form pseudocrystalline structures known as 'tactoids'. These distort the red cell membrane and produce characteristic sickle-shaped cells (Fig. 24.25). The polymerisation is reversible when reoxygenation occurs. The distortion of the red cell membrane, however, may become permanent and the red cell 'irreversibly sickled'. The greater the concentration of sickle-cell haemoglobin in the individual cell, the more easily tactoids are formed, but this process may be enhanced or retarded by the presence of other haemoglobins. Thus, the abnormal haemoglobin C variant participates in the polymerisation more readily than haemoglobin A, whereas haemoglobin F strongly inhibits polymerisation.

Clinical features

Sickling is precipitated by hypoxia, acidosis, dehydration and infection. Irreversibly sickled cells have a shortened survival and plug vessels in the microcirculation. This results in a number of acute syndromes, termed 'crises', and chronic organ damage, as shown in Figure 24.25:

- *Vaso-occlusive crisis.* Plugging of small vessels in the bone produces acute severe bone pain. This affects areas of active marrow: the hands and feet in children (so-called dactylitis) or the femora, humeri, ribs, pelvis and vertebrae in adults. Patients usually have a systemic response with tachycardia, sweating and a fever. This is the most common crisis.
- *Sickle chest syndrome.* This may follow on from a vaso-occlusive crisis and is the most common cause of death in adult sickle disease. Bone marrow infarction results in fat emboli to the lungs which cause further sickling and infarction, leading to ventilatory failure if not treated.
- *Sequestration crisis.* Thrombosis of the venous outflow from an organ causes loss of function and acute painful enlargement. In children the spleen is the most common site. Massive splenic enlargement may result in severe anaemia, circulatory collapse and death. Recurrent sickling in the spleen in childhood results in infarction and adults may have no functional spleen. In adults the liver may undergo sequestration with severe pain due to capsular stretching.
- *Aplastic crisis.* Infection of adult sicklers with human erythrovirus 19 results in a severe but self-limiting red cell aplasia. This produces a very low haemoglobin which may cause heart failure. Unlike in all other sickle crises, the reticulocyte count is low.

Investigations

Patients with sickle-cell disease have a compensated anaemia, usually around 60–80 g/L. The blood film shows sickle cells, target cells and features of hyposplenism. A reticulocytosis is present. The presence of HbS can be demonstrated by exposing red cells to a reducing agent such as sodium dithionite; HbA gives a clear solution, whereas HbS polymerises to produce a turbid solution. This forms the basis of emergency screening tests before surgery in appropriate ethnic groups but cannot distinguish between sickle-cell trait and disease. The definitive diagnosis requires haemoglobin electrophoresis to demonstrate the absence of HbA, 2–20% HbF and the predominance of HbS. Both parents of the affected individual will have sickle-cell trait.

Management

All patients with sickle-cell disease should receive prophylaxis with daily folic acid, and penicillin V to protect against pneumococcal infection which may be lethal in the presence of hyposplenism. These patients should be

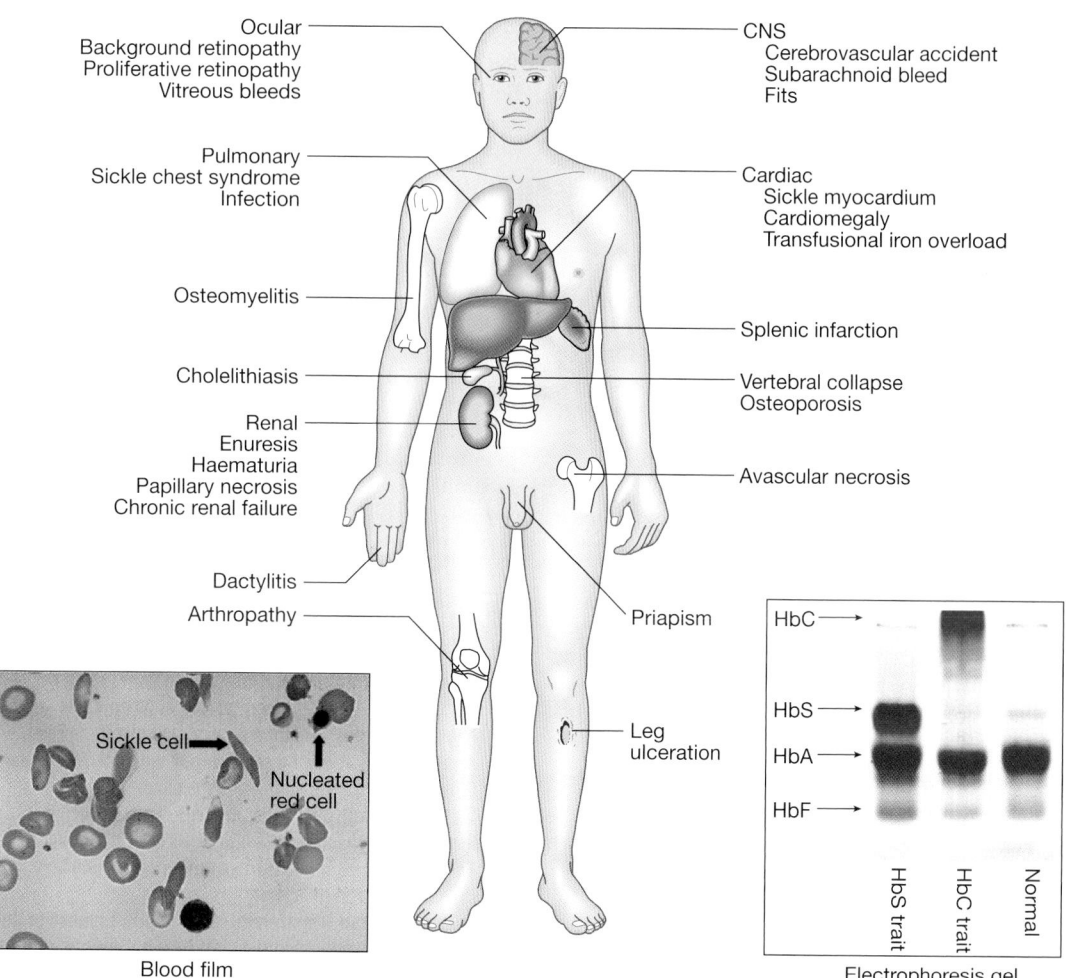

Fig. 24.25 Clinical manifestations of sickle-cell disease.

vaccinated against pneumococcus and, where vaccine is available, *Haemophilus influenzae* B and hepatitis B.

Vaso-occlusive crises are managed by aggressive rehydration, oxygen therapy, adequate analgesia (which often requires opiates) and antibiotics. Transfusion should be with fully genotyped blood wherever possible. Simple top-up transfusion may be used in a sequestration or aplastic crisis. A regular transfusion programme to suppress HbS production and maintain the HbS level below 30% may be indicated in patients with recurrent severe complications such as cerebrovascular accidents in children or chest syndromes in adults. Exchange transfusion, in which a patient is simultaneously venesected and transfused to replace HbS with HbA, may be used in life-threatening crises or to prepare patients for surgery.

A high HbF level inhibits polymerisation of HbS and reduces sickling. Patients with sickle-cell disease and high HbF levels have a mild clinical course with few crises. Some agents are able to increase synthesis of HbF and this has been used to reduce the frequency of severe crises. The oral cytotoxic agent hydroxycarbamide has been shown to have clinical benefit with acceptable side-effects in children and adults who have recurrent severe crises.

Relatively few allogeneic stem-cell transplants from HLA-matched siblings have been performed but this procedure appears to be potentially curative (p. 1013).

Prognosis

In Africa few children with sickle-cell anaemia survive to adult life without medical attention. Even with standard medical care, approximately 15% die by the age of 20 years and 50% by the age of 40 years.

Other abnormal haemoglobins

Another beta chain haemoglobinopathy, haemoglobin C (HbC) disease, is clinically silent but associated with microcytosis and target cells on the blood film. Compound heterozygotes inheriting one HbS gene and one HbC gene from their parents have haemoglobin SC disease, which behaves like a mild form of sickle-cell disease. It is associated with a reduced frequency of crises but is not uncommonly associated with complications in pregnancy and retinal vein thrombosis.

The thalassaemias

Thalassaemia is an inherited impairment of haemoglobin production, in which there is partial or complete failure to synthesise a specific type of globin chain. In alpha-thalassaemia, disruption of one or both alleles on chromosome 16 may occur, with production of some or no alpha globin chains. In beta-thalassaemia, defective production usually results from disabling point mutations causing no (β^0) or reduced (β^-) beta chain production.

Beta-thalassaemia

Failure to synthesise beta chains (beta-thalassaemia) is the most common type of thalassaemia, most prevalent in the Mediterranean area. Heterozygotes have thalassaemia minor, a condition in which there is usually mild anaemia and little or no clinical disability, which may be detected only when iron therapy for a mild microcytic anaemia fails. Homozygotes (thalassaemia major) either are unable to synthesise haemoglobin A or at best produce very little; after the first 4–6 months of life they develop profound hypochromic anaemia. The diagnostic features are summarised in Box 24.43. Intermediate grades of severity occur.

Management and prevention

See Box 24.44. Cure is now a possibility for selected children, with allogeneic bone marrow transplantation (p. 1013).

It is possible to identify a fetus with homozygous beta-thalassaemia by obtaining chorionic villous material for DNA analysis sufficiently early in pregnancy to allow termination. This examination is only appropriate if both parents are known to be carriers (beta-thalassaemia minor) and will accept a termination.

24.43 Diagnostic features of beta-thalassaemia

Beta-thalassaemia major (homozygotes)

- Profound hypochromic anaemia
- Evidence of severe red cell dysplasia
- Erythroblastosis
- Absence or gross reduction of the amount of haemoglobin A
- Raised levels of haemoglobin F
- Evidence that both parents have thalassaemia minor

Beta-thalassaemia minor (heterozygotes)

- Mild anaemia
- Microcytic hypochromic erythrocytes (not iron-deficient)
- Some target cells
- Punctate basophilia
- Raised haemoglobin A_2 fraction
- Evidence that one parent has thalassaemia minor

24.44 Treatment of beta-thalassaemia major

Problem	Management
Erythropoietic failure	Allogeneic bone marrow transplantation from human leucocyte antigen (HLA)-compatible sibling Transfusion to maintain Hb > 100 g/L Folic acid 5 mg daily
Iron overload	Iron therapy forbidden Iron chelation therapy
Splenomegaly causing mechanical problems, excessive transfusion needs	Splenectomy

Alpha-thalassaemia

Reduced or absent alpha chain synthesis is common in Southeast Asia. There are two alpha gene loci on chromosome 16 and therefore each individual carries four alpha gene alleles.

- If one is deleted, there is no clinical effect.
- If two are deleted, there may be a mild hypochromic anaemia.
- If three are deleted, the patient has haemoglobin H disease.
- If all four are deleted, the baby is stillborn (hydrops fetalis).

Haemoglobin H is a beta-chain tetramer, formed from the excess of beta chains, which is functionally useless, so that patients rely on their low levels of HbA for oxygen transport. Treatment of haemoglobin H disease is similar to that of beta-thalassaemia of intermediate severity, involving folic acid supplementation, transfusion if required and avoidance of iron therapy.

24.45 Anaemia in old age

- **Mean haemoglobin**: falls with age in both sexes, but remains well within the normal range. When a low haemoglobin does occur, it is generally due to disease.
- **Anaemia can never be considered 'normal' in old age.**
- **Symptoms**: may be subtle and insidious. Cardiovascular features such as dyspnoea and oedema, and cerebral features such as dizziness and apathy, tend to predominate.
- **Ferritin**: if less than 45 μg/L in older people, is highly predictive of iron deficiency.
- **Serum iron and transferrin**: fall with age because of the prevalence of other disorders, and are not reliable indicators of deficiency.
- **Most common cause of iron deficiency**: gastrointestinal blood loss.
- **Most common cause of vitamin B_{12} deficiency:** pernicious anaemia, as the prevalence of chronic atrophic gastritis rises in old age.
- **Neuropsychiatric symptoms associated with vitamin B_{12} deficiency**: well established association but a causal relationship has not been clearly shown. Dementia associated with vitamin B_{12} deficiency in the absence of haematological abnormalities is rare.
- **Anaemia of chronic disease**: frequent in old age because of the rising prevalence of diseases that inhibit iron transport.

HAEMATOLOGICAL MALIGNANCIES

Haematological malignancies arise when the processes controlling proliferation or apoptosis are corrupted in blood cells. If mature differentiated cells are involved, the cells will have a low growth fraction and produce indolent neoplasms, such as the low-grade lymphomas or chronic leukaemias, when patients have an expected survival of many years. In contrast, if more primitive stem cells are involved, the cells can have the highest growth fractions of all human neoplasms, producing rapidly progressive life-threatening illnesses such as the acute leukaemias or high-grade lymphomas. Involvement of pluripotent stem cells produces the most aggressive acute leukaemias. In general, haematological neoplasms are diseases of elderly patients, the exceptions being acute lymphoblastic leukaemia which predominantly affects children, and Hodgkin lymphoma which affects people aged 20–40 years.

Leukaemias

Leukaemias are malignant disorders of the haematopoietic stem cell compartment, characteristically associated with increased numbers of white cells in the bone marrow and/or peripheral blood. The course of leukaemia may vary from a few days or weeks to many years, depending on the type.

Epidemiology and aetiology

The incidence of leukaemia of all types in the population is approximately 10/100 000 per annum, of which just under half are cases of acute leukaemia. Males are affected more frequently than females, the ratio being about 3:2 in acute leukaemia, 2:1 in chronic lymphocytic leukaemia and 1.3:1 in chronic myeloid leukaemia. Geographical variation in incidence does occur, the most striking being the rarity of chronic lymphocytic leukaemia in the Chinese and related races. Acute leukaemia occurs at all ages. Acute lymphoblastic leukaemia shows a peak of incidence in children aged 1–5 years. All forms of acute myeloid leukaemia have their lowest incidence in young adult life and there is a striking rise over the age of 50. Chronic leukaemias occur mainly in middle and old age.

The cause of the leukaemia is unknown in the majority of patients. Several risk factors, however, are known (Box 24.46).

Terminology and classification

Leukaemias are traditionally classified into four main groups:

- acute lymphoblastic leukaemia (ALL)
- acute myeloid leukaemia (AML)
- chronic lymphocytic leukaemia (CLL)
- chronic myeloid leukaemia (CML).

In acute leukaemia there is proliferation of primitive stem cells leading to an accumulation of blasts, predominantly in the bone marrow, which causes bone marrow failure. In chronic leukaemia the malignant clone is able to differentiate, resulting in an accumulation of more mature cells. Lymphocytic and lymphoblastic cells are those derived from the lymphoid stem cell (B cells and T cells). Myeloid refers to the other lineages, i.e. precursors of red cells, granulocytes, monocytes and platelets (see Fig. 24.2, p. 989).

The diagnosis of leukaemia is usually suspected from an abnormal blood count, often a raised white count, and is confirmed by examination of the bone marrow. This includes the morphology of the abnormal cells, analysis of cell surface markers (immunophenotyping), clone-specific chromosome abnormalities and molecular changes. These results are incorporated in the World Health Organization (WHO) classification of tumours of haematopoietic and lymphoid tissues; the subclassification of acute leukaemias is shown in Box 24.47. The features in the bone marrow not only provide an accurate diagnosis but also give valuable prognostic information, allowing therapy to be tailored to the patient's disease.

Acute leukaemia

There is a failure of cell maturation in acute leukaemia. Proliferation of cells which do not mature leads to an accumulation of useless cells which take up more and more marrow space at the expense of the normal haematopoietic elements. Eventually, this proliferation spills into the blood. Acute myeloid leukaemia (AML) is about four times more common than acute lymphoblastic leukaemia (ALL) in adults. In children the proportions are reversed, the lymphoblastic variety being more common. The clinical features are usually those of bone marrow failure (anaemia, bleeding or infection— pp. 997, 1002 and 1004).

24.46 Risk factors for leukaemia

Ionising radiation

- After atomic bombing of Japanese cities (myeloid leukaemia)
- Radiotherapy for ankylosing spondylitis
- Diagnostic X-rays of the fetus in pregnancy

Cytotoxic drugs

- Especially alkylating agents (myeloid leukaemia, usually after a latent period of several years)
- Industrial exposure to benzene

Retroviruses

- One rare form of T-cell leukaemia/lymphoma appears to be associated with a retrovirus similar to the viruses causing leukaemia in cats and cattle

Genetic

- Identical twin of patients with leukaemia
- Down's syndrome and certain other genetic disorders

Immunological

- Immune deficiency states (e.g. hypogammaglobulinaemia)

24.47 WHO classification of acute leukaemia

Acute myeloid leukaemia (AML) with recurrent genetic abnormalities

- AML with t(8;21) gene product AML/ETO
- AML with eosinophilia inv(16) or t(16;16), gene product CBFβ/MYH11
- Acute promyelocytic leukaemia t(15;17), gene product PML/RARA
- AML with 11q23 abnormalities (MLL)

Acute myeloid leukaemia with multilineage dysplasia

- e.g. Following a myelodysplastic syndrome

Acute myeloid leukaemia and myelodysplastic syndromes, therapy-related

- e.g. Alkylating agent or topoisomerase II inhibitor

Acute myeloid leukaemia not otherwise specified

- e.g. AML with or without differentiation, acute myelomonocytic leukaemia, erythroleukaemia, megakaryoblastic leukaemia, myeloid sarcoma

Acute lymphoblastic leukaemia (ALL)

- Precursor B ALL
- Precursor T ALL

24

Investigations

Blood examination usually shows anaemia with a normal or raised MCV. The leucocyte count may vary from as low as 1×10^9/L to as high as 500×10^9/L or more. In the majority of patients the count is below 100×10^9/L. Severe thrombocytopenia is usual but not invariable. The appearance of blast cells in the blood film is usually diagnostic. Sometimes the blast cell count may be very low in the peripheral blood and a bone marrow examination is necessary to confirm the diagnosis.

The bone marrow is usually hypercellular, with replacement of normal elements by leukaemic blast cells in varying degrees (but more than 20% of the cells)(Fig. 24.26). The presence of Auer rods in the cytoplasm of blast cells indicates a myeloblastic type of leukaemia. Illustrations of immunophenotyping and chromosome analysis are shown in Figure 24.27.

Management

The general strategy for acute leukaemia is shown in Figure 24.28. The first decision must be whether or not to give specific treatment. This is generally aggressive, has a number of side-effects, and may not be appropriate for the very elderly or patients with other serious disorders

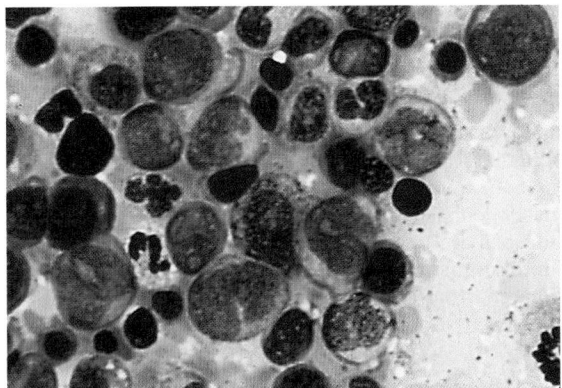

Fig. 24.26 Acute myeloid leukaemia. Bone marrow aspirate showing infiltration with large blast cells which display nuclear folding and prominent nucleoli.

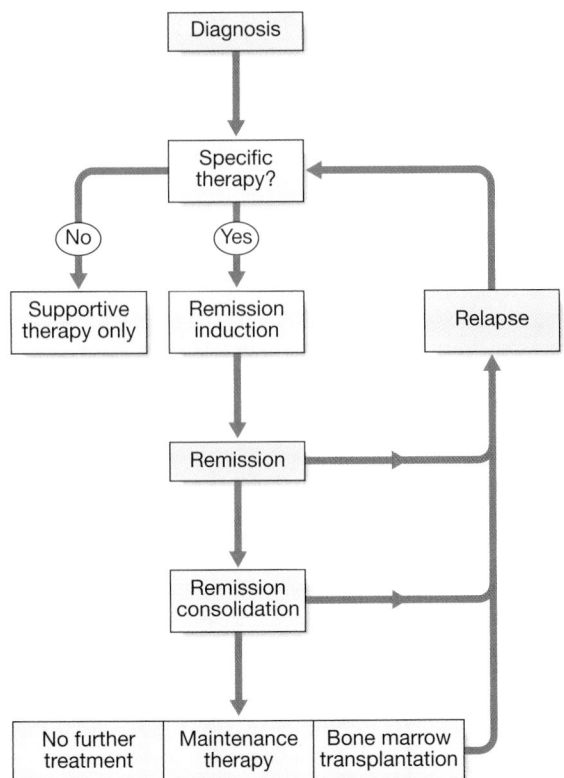

Fig. 24.28 Treatment strategy in acute leukaemia.

(Chs 7 and 11). In these patients supportive treatment can effect considerable improvement in well-being.

Specific therapy

If a decision to embark on specific therapy has been taken, the patient should be prepared as recommended in Box 24.48. It is unwise to attempt aggressive management of acute leukaemia unless adequate services are available for the provision of supportive therapy.

The aim of treatment is to destroy the leukaemic clone of cells without destroying the residual normal stem cell compartment from which repopulation of

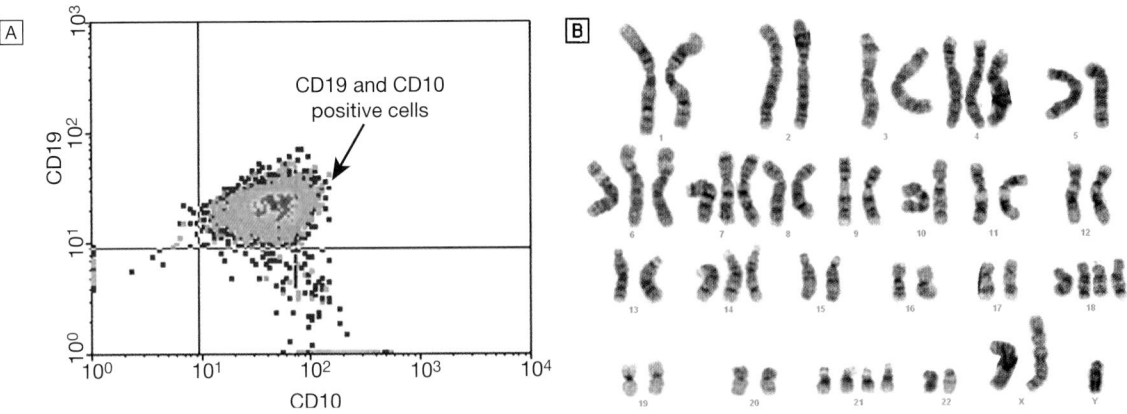

Fig. 24.27 Investigation of acute lymphoblastic leukaemia (ALL). **A** Flow cytometric analysis of blasts labelled with the fluorescent antibodies anti-CD19 (y axis) and anti-CD10 (x axis). ALL blasts are positive for both CD19 and CD10 (arrow). **B** Chromosome analysis (karyotype) of blasts showing additional chromosomes X, 4, 6, 7, 14, 18 and 21.

24.48 Preparation for specific therapy in acute leukaemia

- Existing infections identified and treated (e.g. urinary tract infection, oral candidiasis, dental, gingival and skin infections)
- Anaemia corrected with red cell concentrate tranfusion
- Thrombocytopenic bleeding controlled with platelet transfusions
- If possible, central venous catheter (e.g. Hickman line) inserted to facilitate access to the circulation for delivery of chemotherapy
- Therapeutic regimen carefully explained to the patient and informed consent obtained

the haematopoietic tissues will occur. There are three phases:

- *Remission induction.* In this phase, the bulk of the tumour is destroyed by combination chemotherapy. The patient goes through a period of severe bone marrow hypoplasia, requiring intensive support and inpatient care from a specially trained multidisciplinary team.
- *Remission consolidation.* If remission has been achieved, residual disease is attacked by therapy during the consolidation phase. This consists of a number of courses of chemotherapy, again resulting in periods of marrow hypoplasia. In poor-prognosis leukaemia this may include bone marrow transplantation.
- *Remission maintenance.* If the patient is still in remission after the consolidation phase for ALL, a period of maintenance therapy is given, consisting of a repeating cycle of drug administration. This may extend for up to 3 years if relapse does not occur and is usually given on an outpatient basis.

In patients with ALL it is necessary to give prophylactic treatment to the central nervous system, as this is a sanctuary site where standard therapy does not penetrate. This usually consists of a combination of cranial irradiation, intrathecal chemotherapy and high-dose methotrexate, which crosses the blood–brain barrier.

Thereafter, specific therapy is discontinued and the patient observed.

The detail of the schedules for these treatments can be found in specialist texts. The drugs most commonly employed are listed in Box 24.49. Generally, if a patient

24.49 Drugs commonly used in the treatment of acute leukaemia

Phase	ALL	AML
Induction	Vincristine (i.v.) Prednisolone (oral) L-asparaginase (i.m.) Daunorubicin (i.v.) Methotrexate (intrathecal)	Daunorubicin (i.v.) Cytarabine (i.v.) Etoposide (i.v. and oral)
Consolidation	Daunorubicin (i.v.) Cytarabine (i.v.) Etoposide (i.v.) Methotrexate (i.v.)	Cytarabine (i.v.) Amsacrine (i.v.) Mitoxantrone (i.v.)
Maintenance	Prednisolone (oral) Vincristine (i.v.) Mercaptopurine (oral) Methotrexate (oral)	

fails to go into remission with induction treatment, alternative drug combinations may be tried but the outlook is poor unless remission can be achieved. Disease which relapses during treatment or soon after the end of treatment carries a poor prognosis and is difficult to treat. The longer after the end of treatment that relapse occurs, the more likely it is that further treatment will be effective.

In some patients, alternative chemotherapy, not designed to achieve remission, may be used to curb excessive leucocyte proliferation. Drugs used for this purpose include hydroxycarbamide and mercaptopurine. The aim is to reduce the leucocyte count without inducing bone marrow failure.

Supportive therapy

Aggressive and potentially curative therapy which involves periods of severe bone marrow failure would not be possible without adequate and skilled supportive care. The following problems commonly arise.

Anaemia. Anaemia is treated with red cell concentrate transfusions.

Bleeding. Thrombocytopenic bleeding requires platelet transfusions, unless the bleeding is trivial. Prophylactic platelet transfusion should be given to maintain the platelet count above $10 \times 10^9/L$. Coagulation abnormalities occur and need accurate diagnosis and treatment as appropriate (p. 1049).

Infection. Fever ($> 38°C$) lasting over 1 hour in a neutropenic patient indicates possible septicaemia. Parenteral broad-spectrum antibiotic therapy is essential. Empirical therapy is given with a combination of an aminoglycoside (e.g. gentamicin) and a broad-spectrum penicillin (e.g. piperacillin/tazobactam). This combination is synergistic and bactericidal and should be continued for at least 3 days after the fever has resolved. The organisms most commonly associated with severe neutropenia are Gram-positive bacteria, such as *Staphylococcus aureus* and *Staph. epidermidis*, which are present on the skin and gain entry via cannulae and central lines. Gram-negative infections often originate from the gastrointestinal tract, which is affected by chemotherapy-induced mucositis; organisms such as *Escherichia coli*, *Pseudomonas* and *Klebsiella* spp. are more likely to cause rapid clinical deterioration and must be covered with the initial empirical therapy. Gram-positive infection may require vancomycin therapy.

Patients with ALL are susceptible to infection with *Pneumocystis jirovecii* (p. 395), which causes a severe pneumonia. Prophylaxis with co-trimoxazole is given during chemotherapy. Diagnosis can be difficult and may require either bronchoalveolar lavage or open lung biopsy. Treatment is with high-dose co-trimoxazole, initially intravenously, changing to oral treatment as soon as possible.

Oral and pharyngeal monilial infection is common. Fluconazole is effective for the treatment of established local infection. Prophylaxis against systemic fungal infections with either fluconazole or itraconazole is usual practice during intensive chemotherapy.

For systemic fungal infection with *Candida* or aspergillosis, intravenous amphotericin is required for at least 3 weeks, but is nephrotoxic and hepatotoxic. Lipid formulations of amphotericin have a lower incidence of renal toxicity and allow high-dose therapy for aspergillosis. New antifungal agents such as caspofungin and voriconazole are also available (p. 157).

24

Herpes simplex infection (p. 321) occurs frequently around the lips and nose during ablative therapy for acute leukaemia, and is treated with aciclovir. This may also be prescribed prophylactically to patients with a history of cold sores or elevated antibody titres to herpes simplex. Herpes zoster manifesting as chicken pox or, after reactivation, as shingles (p. 314) should be treated in the early stage with high-dose aciclovir, as it can be fatal in immunocompromised patients.

The value of isolation facilities, such as laminar flow rooms, is debatable but may contribute to staff awareness of careful reverse barrier nursing practice. The isolation is often psychologically stressful for the patient.

Metabolic problems. Frequent monitoring of fluid balance and renal, hepatic and haemostatic function is necessary. Patients are often severely anorexic as a consequence of the side-effects of therapy; they may find drinking difficult and hence require intravenous fluids and electrolytes. Renal toxicity occurs with some antibiotics (e.g. aminoglycosides) and antifungal agents (amphotericin). Cellular breakdown during induction therapy (tumour lysis syndrome) releases intracellular ions and nucleic acid breakdown products, causing hyperkalaemia, hyperuricaemia, hyperphosphataemia and hypocalcaemia. This may cause renal failure. Allopurinol and intravenous hydration are given to try to prevent this. In patients at high risk of tumour lysis syndrome prophylactic rasburicase (a recombinant urate oxidase enzyme) can be used. Occasionally, dialysis may be required.

Psychological problems. Psychological support is a key aspect of care. Patients should be kept informed, and their questions answered and fears allayed as far as possible. An optimistic attitude from the staff is vital. Delusions, hallucinations and paranoia are not uncommon during periods of severe bone marrow failure and septicaemic episodes, and should be met with patience and understanding.

Bone marrow transplantation

This is described on pages 1013–1014. Indications for BMT are shown in Box 24.27 (p. 1013). In patients with high-risk acute leukaemia, allogeneic BMT can improve 5-year survival from 20% to around 50%.

i | **24.50 Outcome in adult acute leukaemia**

Disease/risk	Risk factors	5-year overall survival
AML		
Good risk	Promyelocytic leukaemia t(15;17) t(8;21) inv 16 or t(16;16)	76%
Poor risk	Cytogenetic abnormalities −5,−7,del 5q, abn(3q), complex (≥ 5)	21%
Intermediate risk	AML with none of the above	48%
ALL		
Poor risk	Philadelphia chromosome High white count > 100 × 10⁹/L Abnormal short arm of chromosome 11 t(1;19)	20%
Standard	ALL with none of the above	37%

Prognosis

Without treatment, the median survival of patients with acute leukaemia is about 5 weeks. This may be extended to a number of months with supportive treatment. Patients who achieve remission with specific therapy have a better outlook. Around 80% of adult patients under 60 years of age with ALL or AML achieve remission, although remission rates are lower for older patients. However, the relapse rate continues to be high. Box 24.50 shows the survival in ALL and AML and the influence of prognostic features.

Advances in treatment have led to steady improvement in survival from leukaemia. Advances include the introduction of drugs such as ATRA (all transretinoic acid) in acute promyelocytic leukaemia, which has greatly reduced induction deaths from bleeding in this good-risk leukaemia. Current trials aim to improve survival, especially in standard and poor-risk disease, with strategies that include allogeneic BMT.

Chronic myeloid leukaemia (CML)

Chronic myeloid leukaemia is a myeloproliferative stem-cell disorder resulting in proliferation of all haematopoietic lineages but manifesting predominantly in the granulocytic series. Maturation of cells proceeds fairly normally. The disease occurs chiefly between the ages of 30 and 80 years, with a peak incidence at 55 years. It is rare, with an annual incidence in the UK of 1.8/100 000, and accounts for 20% of all leukaemias. The disease is found in all races.

Approximately 95% of patients with CML have a chromosome abnormality known as the Philadelphia (Ph) chromosome. This is a shortened chromosome 22 resulting from a reciprocal translocation of material with chromosome 9. The break on chromosome 22 occurs in the breakpoint cluster region (BCR). The fragment from chromosome 9 that joins the BCR carries the *abl* oncogene, which forms a chimeric gene with the remains of the BCR. This *BCR ABL* chimeric gene codes for a 210 kDa protein with tyrosine kinase activity, which plays a causative role in the disease as an oncogene (p. 56), influencing cellular proliferation, differentiation and survival. In some patients in whom conventional chromosomal analysis does not detect a Ph chromosome, the BCR ABL gene product is detectable by molecular techniques.

Natural history

The disease has three phases:

- *A chronic phase*, in which the disease is responsive to treatment and is easily controlled, typically lasting 3–5 years. With the introduction of imatinib therapy this phase has been prolonged to longer than 5 years in many patients.
- *An accelerated phase* (not always seen), in which disease control becomes more difficult.
- *Blast crisis*, in which the disease transforms into an acute leukaemia, either myeloid (70%) or lymphoblastic (30%), which is relatively refractory to treatment. This is the cause of death in the majority of patients; therefore survival is dictated by the timing of blast crisis, which cannot be predicted. Prior to imatinib therapy (see below) approximately 10% of patients per year would transform. In those treated with imatinib for up to 5 years, only between 0.5-2.5% have transformed each year.

24.51 Symptoms at presentation of chronic myeloid leukaemia	
Symptom	**Present (%)**
Tiredness	37
Weight loss	26
Breathlessness	21
Abdominal pain and discomfort	21
Lethargy	13
Anorexia	12
Sweating	11
Abdominal fullness	10
Bruising	7
Vague ill health	7

EBM 24.52 Imatinib and chronic myeloid leukaemia

'As first-line therapy in CML, imatinib is better tolerated and induces a cytogenetic response in ~87% of cases at 18 months, compared with ~35% response to interferon + cytarabine.'

• O'Brien SG for the IRIS Investigators. N Engl J Med 2003; 348:994–1004.

Patients who are Ph chromosome-negative and *BCR ABL*-negative tend to be older, mostly male, with lower platelet counts and higher absolute monocyte counts, and respond poorly to treatment, with a median survival of less than 1 year.

Clinical features

The common symptoms at presentation are shown in Box 24.51; about 25% of patients are asymptomatic at diagnosis. Splenomegaly is present in 90%; in about 10% the enlargement is massive, extending to over 15 cm below the costal margin. A friction rub may be heard in cases of splenic infarction. Hepatomegaly occurs in about 50%. Lymphadenopathy is unusual.

Investigations

FBC results are variable between patients. There is usually a normocytic, normochromic anaemia. The leucocyte count can vary from 10 to $600 \times 10^9/L$. In about one-third of patients there is a very high platelet count, sometimes as high as $2000 \times 10^9/L$. In the blood film the full range of granulocyte precursors from myeloblasts to mature neutrophils is seen but the predominant cells are neutrophils and myelocytes (see Fig. 24.3, p. 989). Myeloblasts usually constitute less than 10% of all white cells. There is often an absolute increase in eosinophils and basophils, and nucleated red cells are common. If the disease progresses through an accelerated phase, the percentage of more primitive cells increases. Blast transformation is characterised by a dramatic increase in the number of circulating blasts. In patients with thrombocytosis, very high platelet counts may persist during treatment, in both chronic and accelerated phases, but usually drop dramatically at blast transformation. Basophilia tends to increase as the disease progresses.

Bone marrow should be obtained to confirm the diagnosis and phase of disease by morphology, chromosome analysis to demonstrate the presence of the Ph chromosome, and RNA analysis to demonstrate the presence of the BCR ABL gene product. Blood LDH levels are elevated and the uric acid level may be high due to increased cell breakdown.

Management

Chronic phase

Imatinib specifically inhibits BCR ABL tyrosine kinase activity and reduces the uncontrolled proliferation of white cells. It is recommended as first-line therapy in chronic phase CML, producing complete cytogenetic response (disappearance of the Ph chromosome) in 76% at 18 months of therapy (Box 24.52). Patients are monitored by repeated bone marrow examination until in a complete cytogenetic response, and then by 3-monthly real-time quantitative polymerase chain reaction (PCR) for BCR ABL mRNA transcripts in blood. For those failing to respond or progress on imatinib, options include second-generation tyrosine kinase inhibitors such as dasatinib or nilotinib, allogeneic bone marrow transplantation (p. 1013) or classical cytotoxic drugs such as hydroxycarbamide (hydroxyurea) or interferon. Hydroxycarbamide was previously used widely for initial control of disease, and is still useful in this context or in palliative situations. It does not diminish the frequency of the Ph chromosome or affect the onset of blast cell transformation. Interferon-alfa was considered first-line treatment before imatinib was developed. It was given alone or with the chemotherapy agent Ara-C, and controlled CML chronic phase in about 70% of patients.

Accelerated phase and blast crisis

Management is more difficult. For patients presenting in accelerated phase, imatinib is indicated if the patient has not already received it. Hydroxycarbamide can be an effective single agent and low-dose cytarabine can also be tried. When blast transformation occurs, the type of blast cell should be determined. Response to appropriate acute leukaemia treatment (see Box 24.49) is better if disease is lymphoblastic than if myeloblastic. Given the very poor response in myeloblastic transformation, there is a strong case for supportive therapy only, particularly in older patients.

Patients progressing to advanced-phase disease on imatinib may respond to a second-generation tyrosine kinase inhibitor and may be considered for allogeneic BMT (p. 1013).

Chronic lymphocytic leukaemia (CLL)

This is the most common variety of leukaemia, accounting for 30% of cases. The male:female ratio is 2:1 and the median age at presentation is 65–70 years. In this disease B lymphocytes, which would normally respond to antigens by transformation and antibody formation, fail to do so. An ever-increasing mass of immuno-incompetent cells accumulates, to the detriment of immune function and normal bone marrow haematopoiesis.

Clinical features

The onset is very insidious. Indeed, in around 70% of patients the diagnosis is made incidentally on a routine FBC. Presenting problems may be anaemia, infections, painless lymphadenopathy, and systemic symptoms such as night sweats or weight loss. However, these more often occur later in the progress of the disease.

24

Investigations

The diagnosis is based on the peripheral blood findings of a mature lymphocytosis ($>5 \times 10^9/L$) with characteristic morphology and cell surface markers. Immunophenotyping reveals the lymphocytes to be monoclonal B cells expressing the B cell antigens CD19 and CD23, with either kappa or lambda immunoglobulin light chains and, characteristically, an aberrant T cell antigen, CD5.

Other useful investigations in CLL include a reticulocyte count and a direct Coombs test as autoimmune haemolytic anaemia may occur (p. 1025). Serum immunoglobulin levels should be estimated to establish the degree of immunosuppression, which is common and progressive. Bone marrow examination by aspirate and trephine is not essential for the diagnosis of CLL, but may be helpful in difficult cases, for prognosis (patients with diffuse marrow involvement have a poorer prognosis) and to monitor response to therapy. The main prognostic factor is stage of disease (Box 24.53); however, newer markers such as CD38 expression, mutations of IgV_H genes, and cytogenetic abnormalities of chromosome 11 or 17 may also suggest a poorer prognosis.

> ### 24.53 Staging of chronic lymphocytic leukaemia
>
> **Clinical stage A (60% patients)**
> - No anaemia or thrombocytopenia and fewer than three areas of lymphoid enlargement
>
> **Clinical stage B (30% patients)**
> - No anaemia or thrombocytopenia, with three or more involved areas of lymphoid enlargement
>
> **Clinical stage C (10% patients)**
> - Anaemia and/or thrombocytopenia, regardless of the number of areas of lymphoid enlargement

Management

No specific treatment is required for most clinical stage A patients unless progression occurs. Life expectancy is usually normal in older patients. The patient should be offered clear information about CLL, and be reassured about the 'benign' nature of the disease, as the diagnosis of leukaemia inevitably causes anxiety.

Treatment is only required if there is evidence of bone marrow failure, massive or progressive lymphadenopathy or splenomegaly, systemic symptoms such as weight loss or night sweats, a rapidly increasing lymphocyte count or autoimmune haemolytic anaemia or thrombocytopenia. Initial therapy for those requiring treatment (stages B and C) may consist of oral chemotherapy with the alkylating agent chlorambucil. This will reduce the abnormal lymphocyte mass and produce symptomatic improvement in most patients. More recently, the purine analogue fludarabine, in combination with the alkylating agent cyclophosphamide, has increased remission rates and disease-free survival, although there is an increased risk of infection. Bone marrow failure or autoimmune cytopenias may respond to corticosteroid treatment.

Supportive care is increasingly required in progressive disease, e.g. transfusions for symptomatic anaemia or thrombocytopenia, prompt treatment of infections and, for some patients with hypogammaglobulinaemia, immunoglobulin replacement. Radiotherapy may be used for lymph nodes causing discomfort or local obstruction, and for symptomatic splenomegaly. Splenectomy may be required to improve low blood counts due to autoimmune destruction or to hypersplenism, and can relieve massive splenomegaly.

Prognosis

The overall median survival for patients with CLL is about 6 years. The majority of clinical stage A patients have a normal life expectancy but stage C patients have a median survival of between 2 and 3 years. Approximately 50% of patients die from infection and 30% of causes unrelated to CLL. Rarely, CLL transforms to an aggressive high-grade lymphoma, called Richter's transformation.

Prolymphocytic leukaemia

This is a variant of chronic lymphatic leukaemia found mainly in males over the age of 60 years; 25% of cases are of the T cell variety. There is massive splenomegaly with little lymphadenopathy and a very high leucocyte count, often in excess of $400 \times 10^9/L$; the characteristic cell is a large lymphocyte with a prominent nucleolus. Treatment is generally unsuccessful and the prognosis very poor. Leukapheresis, splenectomy and chemotherapy may be tried.

Hairy cell leukaemia

This is a rare chronic lymphoproliferative B cell disorder. The male:female ratio is 6:1 and the median age at diagnosis is 50 years. Presenting symptoms are those of general ill health and recurrent infections. Splenomegaly occurs in 90% but lymph node enlargement is unusual.

Severe neutropenia, monocytopenia and the characteristic hairy cells in the blood and bone marrow are typical. These cells usually have a B lymphocyte immunotype but they also characteristically express CD25 and CD103. A useful test is the demonstration that the acid phosphatase staining reaction in the cells is resistant to the action of tartrate.

Over recent years a number of treatments, including cladribine and deoxycoformycin, have been shown to produce long-lasting remissions.

Myelodysplastic syndrome (MDS)

This syndrome consists of a group of clonal haematopoietic disorders which represent steps in the progression to the development of leukaemia. It presents with consequences of bone marrow failure (anaemia, recurrent infections or bleeding), usually in older people (median age at diagnosis is 69 years). The overall incidence is 4/100 000 in the population, rising to more than 30/100 000 in the over-seventies. The blood film is characterised by cytopenias and abnormal-looking (dysplastic) blood cells, including macrocytic red cells and hypogranular neutrophils with nuclear hyper- or hyposegmentation. The bone marrow is hypercellular with dysplastic changes in all three cell lines. Blast cells may be increased but do not reach the 20% level which indicates acute leukaemia. Chromosome analysis frequently reveals abnormalities, particularly of chromosome 5 or 7. The WHO classification of MDS is shown in Box 24.54.

24.54 WHO classification of myelodysplastic syndromes

Disease	Bone marrow findings
Refractory anaemia (RA)	Blasts < 5% Erythroid dysplasia only
Refractory anaemia with sideroblasts (RARS)	Blasts < 5% Ringed sideroblasts > 15%
Refractory cytopenias with multilineage dysplasia (RCMD)	Blasts < 5% 2–3 lineage dysplasia
Refractory anaemia with excess blasts (RAEB)	Blasts 5–20% 2–3 lineage dysplasia
Myelodysplastic syndrome with 5q–	Myelodysplastic syndrome associated with a del (5q) cytogenetic abnormality Blasts < 5% Often normal or increased blood platelet count
Myelodysplastic syndrome unclassified	None of the above or inadequate material

Management

For the majority of patients the disease is incurable, and supportive care with red cell and platelet transfusions is the mainstay of treatment. A trial of erythropoietin and granulocyte–colony-stimulating factor (G–CSF) is recommended in some patients with early disease to improve haemoglobin and white cell counts. Allogeneic bone marrow transplantation may afford a cure in younger patients. Transplantation should be preceded by intensive chemotherapy in those with more advanced disease.

Prognosis

Inevitably, MDS progresses to acute myeloid leukaemia, although the time to progression varies (from months to years) with the subtype of MDS, being slowest in refractory anaemia and most rapid in refractory anaemia with excess of blasts. Poor prognostic factors include blasts > 10% in the marrow, certain cytogenetic abnormalities and more than one cytopenia in the blood.

Lymphomas

These neoplasms arise from lymphoid tissues, and are diagnosed from the pathological findings on biopsy as Hodgkin or non-Hodgkin lymphoma. The majority are of B cell origin. Non-Hodgkin lymphomas are classified as low- or high-grade tumours on the basis of their proliferation rate.

- *High-grade tumours* divide rapidly, are typically present for a matter of weeks before diagnosis and may be life-threatening.
- *Low-grade tumours* divide slowly, may be present for many months before diagnosis and typically behave in an indolent fashion.

Hodgkin lymphoma (HL)

The histological hallmark of HL is the presence of Reed–Sternberg cells, large malignant lymphoid cells of B cell origin (Fig. 24.29). They are often only present in small

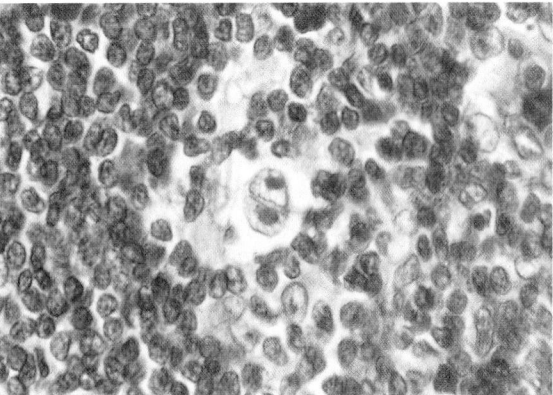

Fig. 24.29 Hodgkin lymphoma. In the centre of this lymph node biopsy is a large typical Reed–Sternberg cell with two nuclei containing a prominent eosinophilic nucleolus.

numbers but are surrounded by large numbers of reactive non-malignant T cells, plasma cells and eosinophils.

The epidemiology of HL is shown in Box 24.55 and its histological WHO classification in Box 24.56.

Nodular lymphocyte-predominant HL is slow-growing, localised and rarely fatal. Classical HL is divided into four histological subtypes from the appearance of the Reed–Sternberg cells and surrounding reactive cells. The nodular sclerosing type is more common in young patients and in women. Mixed cellularity is more common in the

24.55 Epidemiology and aetiology of Hodgkin lymphoma

Incidence
- Approximately 4 new cases/100 000 population/year

Sex ratio
- Slight male excess (1.5:1)

Age
- Median age 31 years; first peak at 20–35 years and second at 50–70 years

Aetiology
- Unknown
- More common in patients from well-educated backgrounds and small families
- Three times more likely with a past history of infectious mononucleosis but no causal link to Epstein–Barr virus infection proven

24.56 WHO pathological classification of Hodgkin lymphoma (HL)

Type	Histology classification	Proportion of HL
Nodular lymphocyte-predominant HL		5%
Classical HL	Nodular sclerosing	70%
	Mixed cellularity	20%
	Lymphocyte-rich	5%
	Lymphocyte-depleted	Rare

elderly. Lymphocyte-rich HL usually presents in men. Lymphocyte-depleted HL is rare and probably represents large-cell or anaplastic non-Hodgkin lymphoma.

Clinical features

There is painless rubbery lymphadenopathy, usually in the neck or supraclavicular fossae; the lymph nodes may fluctuate in size. Young patients with nodular sclerosing disease may have large mediastinal masses which are surprisingly asymptomatic but may cause dry cough and some breathlessness. Isolated subdiaphragmatic nodes occur in fewer than 10% at diagnosis. Hepatosplenomegaly may be present but does not always indicate disease in those organs. Spread is contiguous from one node to the next and extranodal disease, such as bone, brain or skin involvement, is rare.

24.57 Clinical stages of Hodgkin lymphoma (Ann Arbor classification)	
Stage	**Definition**
I	Involvement of a single lymph node region (I) or extralymphatic* site (I_E)
II	Involvement of two or more lymph node regions (II) or an extralymphatic site and lymph node regions on the same side of (above or below) the diaphragm (II_E)
III	Involvement of lymph node regions on both sides of the diaphragm with (III_E) or without (III) localised extralymphatic involvement or involvement of the spleen (III_S) or both (III_{SE})
IV	Diffuse involvement of one or more extralymphatic tissues, e.g. liver or bone marrow
Each stage is subclassified:	
A	No systemic symptoms
B	Weight loss >10%, drenching sweats, fever

*The lymphatic structures are defined as the lymph nodes, spleen, thymus, Waldeyer's ring, appendix and Peyer's patches.

Investigations

Treatment of HL depends upon the stage at presentation; therefore investigations aim not only to diagnose lymphoma but also to determine the extent of disease (Box 24.57).
- *FBC* may be normal. If a normochromic, normocytic anaemia or lymphopenia is present, this is a poor prognostic factor. An eosinophilia or a neutrophilia may be present.
- *ESR* may be raised.
- *Renal function tests* are required to ensure function is normal prior to treatment.
- *Liver function* may be abnormal in the absence of disease or may reflect hepatic infiltration. An obstructive pattern may be caused by nodes at the porta hepatis.
- *LDH measurements* showing raised levels are an adverse prognostic factor.
- *Chest X-ray* may show a mediastinal mass.
- *CT scan* of chest, abdomen and pelvis permits staging. Bulky disease (> 10cm in a single node mass) is an adverse prognostic feature.
- *Lymph node biopsy* may be undertaken surgically or by percutaneous needle biopsy under radiological guidance (Fig. 24.30).

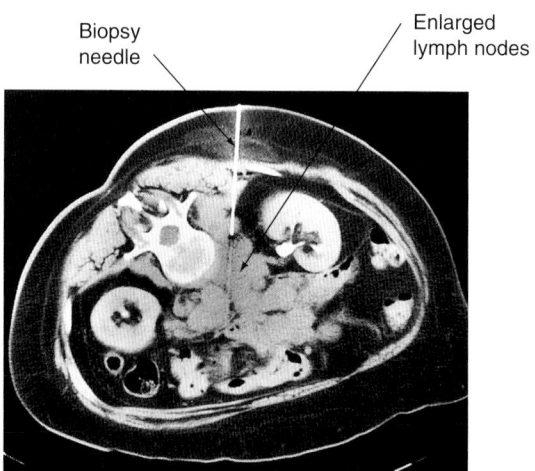

Biopsy needle — Enlarged lymph nodes

Fig. 24.30 CT-guided percutaneous needle biopsy of retroperitoneal nodes involved by lymphoma.

Management

Historically, radiotherapy to lymph nodes alone has been used to treat localised stage IA or stage IIA disease effectively with no adverse prognostic features. Careful planning of radiotherapy is required to limit the doses delivered to normal tissues. Fertility is usually preserved after radiotherapy. Young women receiving breast irradiation during the treatment of chest disease have an increased risk of breast cancer and should participate in a screening programme. Patients continuing to smoke after lung irradiation are at particular risk of lung cancer.

Recent data have, however, shown that patients with early-stage disease have better outcomes if chemotherapy is included in their treatment. The majority of HL patients are now treated with chemotherapy and adjunctive radiotherapy. The ABVD regimen (doxorubicin, vinblastine, bleomycin and dacarbazine) is widely used in the UK. Standard therapy of early-stage patients usually includes additional treatment with radiotherapy to the involved lymph nodes after four courses of ABVD. Treatment response is assessed clinically and by repeat CT and newer scanning modalities such as positron emission tomography (PET). ABVD chemotherapy can cause cardiac and pulmonary toxicity, due to doxorubicin and bleomycin, respectively. The incidence of infertility and secondary myelodysplasia/AML is low with this regime.

Patients with advanced-stage disease are most commonly managed with chemotherapy alone. Standard treatment in the UK is 6–8 cycles of ABVD, followed by an assessment of response. As with early disease, achieving PET-negative remission predicts a better long-term remission rate. Overall, the long-term disease control/cure rates are lower with advanced disease.

Patients with disease which is resistant to therapy may be considered for autologous bone marrow transplantation (BMT) (p. 1014).

Prognosis

Over 90% of patients with early-stage HL achieve complete remission when treated with chemotherapy followed by involved field radiotherapy, and the great majority are cured. The major challenge is how to reduce treatment intensity, and hence long-term toxicity, without reducing the excellent cure rates in this group.

24.58 The Hasenclever prognostic index for advanced Hodgkin lymphoma

Score 1 for each of the following risk factors present at diagnosis:

- Age > 45 years
- Male gender
- Serum albumin < 40 g/L
- Hb < 105 g/L
- Stage IV disease
- WBC > 15×10^9/L
- Lymphopenia < 0.6×10^9/L

Score	5-year rate of freedom from progression (%)	5-year rate of overall survival (%)
0–1	79	90
≥ 2	60	74
≥ 3	55	70
≥ 4	47	59

24.59 Epidemiology and aetiology of non-Hodgkin lymphoma

Incidence

- 12 new cases/100 000 people/year

Sex ratio

- Slight male excess

Age

- Median age 65–70 years

Aetiology

- No single causative abnormality described
- Lymphoma is a late manifestation of HIV infection (p. 401)
- Specific lymphoma types are associated with EBV, human herpes virus 8 (HHV8) and human T-cell lymphotropic virus (HTLV) infection
- Gastric lymphoma can be associated with *Helicobacter pylori* infection
- Some lymphomas are associated with specific chromosome lesions; the t(14:18) translocation in follicular lymphoma results in the dysregulated expression of the BCL-2 gene product, which inhibits apoptotic cell death
- Lymphoma occurs in congenital immunodeficiency states and in immunosuppressed patients after organ transplantation

Between 50 and 70% of those with advanced-stage HL can be cured. The Hasenclever index (Box 24.58) can be helpful in assigning approximate chances of cure when discussing treatment plans with patients. Patients who fail to respond to initial chemotherapy have a poor prognosis but some may achieve long-term survival after autologous BMT. Patients relapsing within a year of initial chemotherapy have a good salvage rate with autologous BMT. Patients relapsing after 1 year may obtain long-term survival with further chemotherapy alone.

Non-Hodgkin lymphoma (NHL)

NHL represents a monoclonal proliferation of lymphoid cells of B cell (70%) or T cell (30%) origin. The incidence of these tumours increases with age, to 62.8/million population per annum at age 75 years, and the overall rate is increasing at about 3% per year.

The epidemiology of NHL is shown in Box 24.59. It has been difficult to establish a reproducible and clinically useful histological classification. The current WHO classification stratifies according to cell lineage. Clinically, the most important factor is grade, which is a reflection of proliferation rate. High-grade NHL has high proliferation rates, rapidly produces symptoms, is fatal if untreated, but is potentially curable. Low-grade NHL has low proliferation rates, may be asymptomatic for many months before presentation, runs an indolent course, but is not curable by conventional therapy. Of all cases of NHL, 85% are either high-grade diffuse large B-cell NHL or low-grade follicular NHL (Fig. 24.31). Other forms of NHL, including mantle cell lymphoma and MALT lymphomas, are less common.

Clinical features

Unlike Hodgkin lymphoma, NHL is often widely disseminated at presentation, including in extranodal sites. Patients present with lymph node enlargement which may be associated with systemic upset: weight loss, sweats, fever and itching. Hepatosplenomegaly may be present. Extranodal involvement is more common in T cell disease and involves the bone marrow, gut, thyroid, lung, skin, testis, brain and, more rarely, bone. Bone marrow involvement is more common in low-grade (50–60%) than high-grade (10%) disease. Compression syndromes may occur, including gut obstruction, ascites, superior vena caval obstruction and spinal cord compression.

The same staging system (see Box 24.57) is used for both HL and NHL, but NHL is more likely to be stage III or IV at presentation.

24

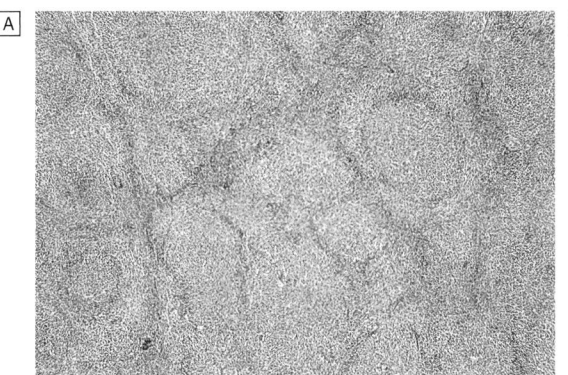

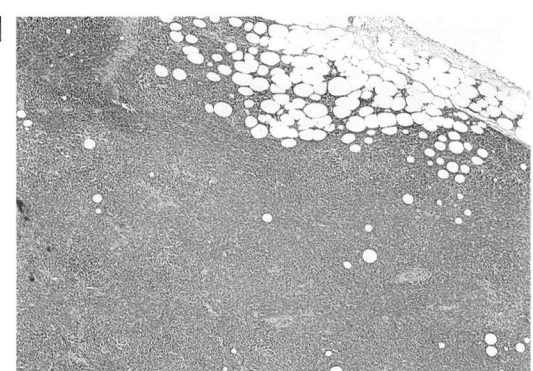

Fig. 24.31 **Histology of non-Hodgkin lymphoma.** [A] (Low-grade) follicular or nodular pattern. [B] (High-grade) diffuse pattern.

Investigations

These are as for HL, but in addition the following should be performed:

- *Routine bone marrow aspiration and trephine.*
- *Immunophenotyping of surface antigens to distinguish T and B cell tumours.* This may be done on blood, marrow or nodal material.
- *Immunoglobulin determination.* Some lymphomas are associated with IgG or IgM paraproteins, which serve as markers for treatment response.
- *Measurement of uric acid levels.* Some very aggressive high-grade NHLs are associated with very high urate levels, which can precipitate renal failure when treatment is started.
- *HIV testing.* This may be appropriate if risk factors are present (p. 385).

Management

Low-grade NHL

Asymptomatic patients may not require therapy. Indications for treatment include marked systemic symptoms, lymphadenopathy causing discomfort or disfigurement, bone marrow failure or compression syndromes. The options are:

- *Radiotherapy.* This can be used for localised stage I disease, which is rare.
- *Chemotherapy.* Most patients will respond to oral therapy with chlorambucil, which is well tolerated but not curative. More intensive intravenous chemotherapy in younger patients produces better quality of life but no survival benefit.
- *Monoclonal antibody therapy.* Humanised monoclonal antibodies can be used to target surface antigens on tumour cells, and induce tumour cell apoptosis directly. The anti-CD20 antibody rituximab has been shown to induce durable clinical responses in up to 60% of patients when given alone, and acts synergistically when given with chemotherapy. Rituximab in combination with cyclophosphamide, vincristine and prednisolone (R-CVP) is recommended as first-line therapy.
- *Transplantation.* Particular interest centres on the role of high-dose chemotherapy and bone marrow transplantation in patients with relapsed disease. Such high-dose therapy improves disease-free survival but longer follow-up is awaited before conclusions can be drawn about cure.

High-grade NHL

Patients with high-grade NHL need treatment at initial presentation:

- *Chemotherapy.* The majority (> 90%) are treated with intravenous combination chemotherapy, typically with the CHOP regimen (cyclophosphamide, doxorubicin, vincristine and prednisolone).
- *Radiotherapy.* A few stage I patients without bulky disease may be suitable for radiotherapy. Radiotherapy is also indicated for a residual localised site of bulk disease after chemotherapy, and for spinal cord and other compression syndromes.
- *Monoclonal antibody therapy.* When combined with CHOP chemotherapy, rituximab (R) increases the complete response rates and improves overall survival. R-CHOP is currently recommended as first-

EBM 24.60 **Autologous bone marrow transplantation in non-Hodgkin lymphoma**

'The addition of autologous bone marrow transplantation to conventional salvage chemotherapy improves survival from 32% to 54% in relapsed high-grade NHL.'

- Philip T, et al. N Engl J Med 1995; 333:1540–1545.

For further information: www.lymphoma.org.uk

line therapy for those with stage II or greater diffuse large-cell lymphoma.

- *Bone marrow transplantation.* Autologous BMT benefits patients with relapsed chemosensitive disease (Box 24.60).

Prognosis

Low-grade NHL runs an indolent remitting and relapsing course, with an overall median survival of 10 years. Transformation to a high-grade NHL is associated with poor survival.

In high-grade NHL, some 80% of patients overall respond initially to therapy but only 35% will have disease-free survival at 5 years. The prognosis for patients with NHL is further refined according to the international prognostic index (IPI). For high-grade NHL, 5-year survival ranges from 75% in those with low-risk scores (age < 60 years, stage I or II, one or fewer extranodal sites, normal LDH and good performance status) to 25% in those with high-risk scores (increasing age, advanced stage, concomitant disease and a raised LDH).

Relapse is associated with a poor response to further chemotherapy (< 10% 5-year survival), but in patients under 65 years, bone marrow transplantation improves survival.

Paraproteinaemias

A gammopathy refers to over-production of one or more classes of immunoglobulin. It may be polyclonal in association with acute or chronic inflammation, such as infection, sarcoidosis, autoimmune disorders or some malignancies. Alternatively, a monoclonal increase in a single immunoglobulin class may occur in association with normal or reduced levels of the other immunoglobulins. Such monoclonal proteins (also called M-proteins, paraproteins or monoclonal gammopathies) occur as a feature of myeloma, lymphoma and amyloidosis, in connective tissue disease such as rheumatoid arthritis or polymyalgia rheumatica, in infection such as HIV, and in solid tumours. In addition, they may be present with no underlying disease. Gammopathies are detected by plasma immunoelectrophoresis.

Monoclonal gammopathy of uncertain significance (MGUS)

In this condition (also known as benign monoclonal gammopathy or monoclonal gammopathy unclassified (MGu)), a paraprotein is present in the blood but with no other features of myeloma, Waldenström macroglobulinaemia (see below), lymphoma or related disease. It is a common condition associated with increasing age; a paraprotein can be found in 1% of the population aged over 50 years, increasing to 5% over 80 years.

Clinical features and investigations

Patients are usually asymptomatic, and the paraprotein is found on blood testing for other reasons. The routine blood count and biochemistry are normal, the paraprotein is usually present in small amounts with no associated immune paresis, and there are no lytic bone lesions. The bone marrow may have increased plasma cells but these usually constitute less than 10% of nucleated cells.

Prognosis

After follow-up of 20 years, only one-quarter will progress to myeloma or a related disorder. There is no way of predicting progression in an individual patient, and if investigations remain stable, annual monitoring is all that is required.

Waldenström macroglobulinaemia

This is a low-grade lymphoplasmacytoid lymphoma associated with an IgM paraprotein, causing clinical features of hyperviscosity syndrome. It is a rare tumour occurring in the elderly and affects a slight excess of males.

Patients classically present with features of hyperviscosity, such as nosebleeds, bruising, confusion and visual disturbance. However, presentation may be with anaemia, systemic symptoms, splenomegaly or lymphadenopathy. Patients are found on investigation to have an IgM paraprotein associated with a raised plasma viscosity. The bone marrow has a characteristic appearance, with infiltration of lymphoid cells and prominent mast cells.

Management

Severe hyperviscosity and anaemia may necessitate plasmapheresis to remove IgM and make blood transfusion possible. Treatment with alkylating agents, such as chlorambucil, is effective but rather slow; fludarabine may be more effective in this disease. The monoclonal anti-CD20 antibody rituximab can also be effective. The median survival is 5 years.

Multiple myeloma

This is a malignant proliferation of plasma cells. Normal plasma cells are derived from B cells and produce immunoglobulins which contain heavy and light chains. Normal immunoglobulins are polyclonal, which means that a variety of heavy chains are produced and each may be of kappa or lambda light chain type (p. 75). In myeloma, plasma cells produce immunoglobulin of a single heavy and light chain, a monoclonal protein commonly referred to as a paraprotein. In some cases only light chain is produced and this appears in the urine as Bence Jones proteinuria. The frequency of different paraprotein types in myeloma is shown in Box 24.61.

Although a small number of malignant plasma cells are present in the circulation, the majority are present in the bone marrow. The malignant plasma cells produce cytokines which stimulate osteoclasts and result in net bone reabsorption. The resulting lytic lesions cause bone pain, fractures and hypercalcaemia. Marrow involvement can result in anaemia or pancytopenia.

Clinical features and investigations

The incidence of myeloma is 4/100 000 new cases per annum, with a male:female ratio of 2:1. The median age of diagnosis is 60–70 years and the disease is more common in Afro-Caribbeans. The clinical features are demonstrated in Figure 24.32.

Diagnosis of myeloma requires two of the following criteria:
- increased malignant plasma cells in the bone marrow
- serum and/or urinary paraprotein
- skeletal lytic lesions.

Bone marrow aspiration, plasma and urinary electrophoresis, and a skeletal survey are thus required. Other investigations are listed in Box 24.62. Normal immunoglobulin levels, i.e. the absence of immunoparesis, should cast doubt on the diagnosis. Paraproteinaemia can cause an elevated ESR (p. 82), but this is a non-specific test; only approximately 5% of patients with a persistently elevated ESR above 100 mm/hr have underlying myeloma.

Management

If patients are asymptomatic, treatment may not be required.

24.61 Classification of multiple myeloma

Type of paraprotein	Relative frequency (%)
IgG	55
IgA	21
Light chain only	22
Others (D, E, non-secretory)	2

24.62 Rationale for investigations in multiple myeloma

Question	Investigations
Presence of lytic lesions, bone fractures?	X-rays (skeletal survey)[1] Alkaline phosphatase[1]
Spinal cord compression?	MRI spine[2]
Presence of urine or plasma paraprotein?	Blood and urine protein electrophoresis
Type of paraprotein?	Blood and urine immunoelectrophoresis
Amount of paraprotein?	Quantification of paraprotein
Degree of immune paresis?	Plasma immunoglobulins
Presence of plasma cells in bone marrow?	Bone marrow aspiration and trephine
Degree of bone marrow failure?	Full blood count
Renal function?	Urea and electrolytes, creatinine, urate
Presence of hypercalcaemia?	Blood calcium and albumin
Degree of haemostasis?	Coagulation screen
Poor prognostic factors at diagnosis?	β_2 microglobulin > 5.5 mg/L, albumin < 35 g/L

[1]In the absence of fractures, the plasma alkaline phosphatase and isotope bone scan will be normal despite the lytic lesions.
[2]All investigations shown above are routine in myeloma, except the MRI spine, which is reserved for those with clinical indications.

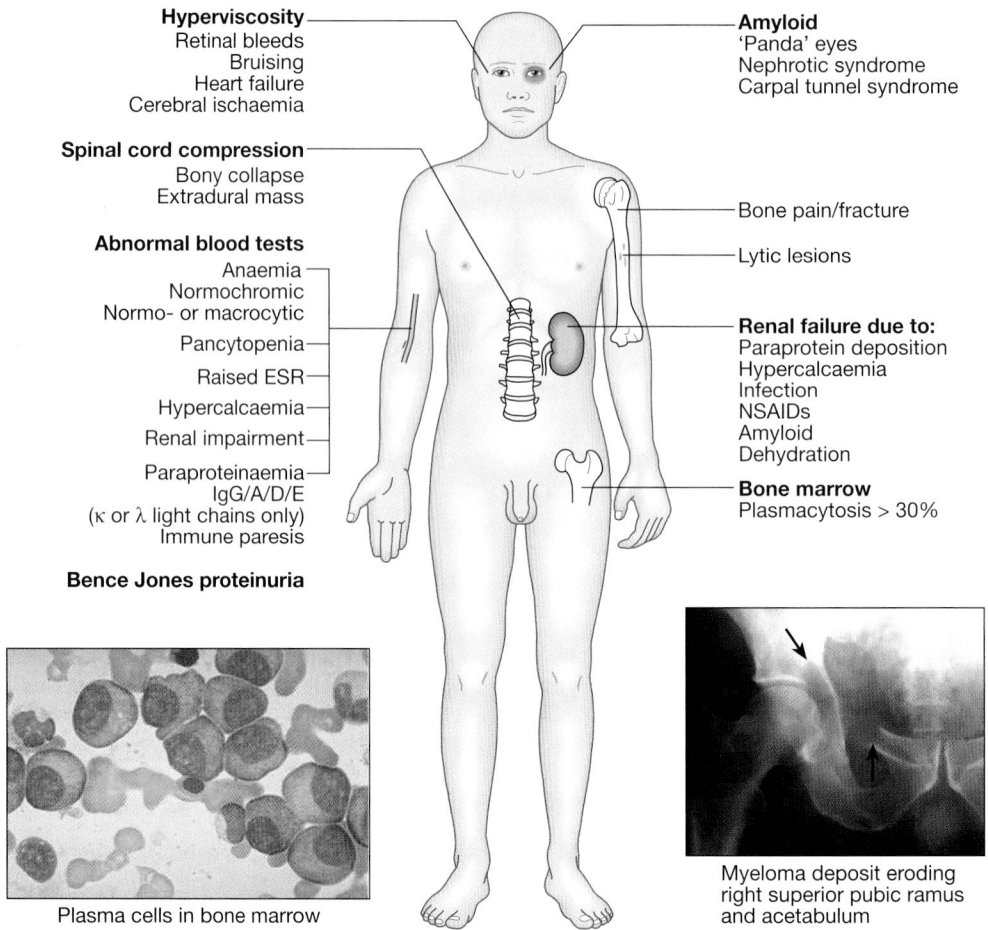

Hyperviscosity
Retinal bleeds
Bruising
Heart failure
Cerebral ischaemia

Spinal cord compression
Bony collapse
Extradural mass

Abnormal blood tests
Anaemia
Normochromic
Normo- or macrocytic

Pancytopenia

Raised ESR

Hypercalcaemia

Renal impairment

Paraproteinaemia
IgG/A/D/E
(κ or λ light chains only)
Immune paresis

Bence Jones proteinuria

Amyloid
'Panda' eyes
Nephrotic syndrome
Carpal tunnel syndrome

Bone pain/fracture

Lytic lesions

Renal failure due to:
Paraprotein deposition
Hypercalcaemia
Infection
NSAIDs
Amyloid
Dehydration

Bone marrow
Plasmacytosis > 30%

Plasma cells in bone marrow

Myeloma deposit eroding
right superior pubic ramus
and acetabulum

Fig. 24.32 Manifestations of multiple myeloma.

Immediate support

- High fluid intake to treat renal impairment and hypercalcaemia (p. 764).
- Analgesia for bone pain.
- Bisphosphonates for hypercalcaemia and to delay other skeletal related events (p. 1119).
- Allopurinol to prevent urate nephropathy.
- Plasmapheresis, as necessary, for hyperviscosity.

Chemotherapy ± bone marrow transplantation

Myeloma therapy has improved with the addition of thalidomide to first-line treatments. In older patients, thalidomide combined with the alkylating agent melphalan and prednisolone has increased the median overall survival to 51 months. Thalidomide has both anti-angiogenic effects against tumour blood vessels and immunomodulatory effects. It can cause somnolence, constipation and a peripheral neuropathy. It is vital that females of child-bearing age use adequate contraception, as thalidomide is teratogenic. Treatment is administered until paraprotein levels have stopped falling. This is termed 'plateau phase' and can last for weeks or years.

In younger, fitter patients standard treatment includes first-line chemotherapy to maximum response and then an autologous stem-cell transplantation, which improves quality of life and prolongs survival (Box 24.63) but does not cure myeloma. The role of allogeneic transplantation (p. 1013) remains under evaluation. Studies are in progress on the role of reduced-intensity allografting after autologous transplantation in younger patients.

When myeloma progresses, treatment is given to induce a further plateau phase. In the UK at present, the proteosome inhibitor bortezomib is recommended. Successive relapses respond less well to treatment and the interval between them tends to be shorter.

Radiotherapy

This is effective for localised bone pain not responding to simple analgesia and for pathological fractures. It is also useful for the emergency treatment of spinal cord compression complicating extradural plasmacytomas.

EBM 24.63 **Autologous bone marrow transplantation in multiple myeloma**

'The addition of autologous bone marrow transplantation to conventional intravenous chemotherapy improves survival from 42 to 54 months.'

- Child JA, et al. N Engl J Med 2003; 348:1875–1883.

For further information: www.ukmf.org.uk

Bisphosphonates

Long-term bisphosphonate therapy reduces bone pain and skeletal events. These drugs protect bone (p. 1119) and may cause apoptosis of malignant plasma cells. Osteonecrosis of the jaw may be associated with long-term use; therefore regular dental review is advisable.

Prognosis

Poor prognostic features include high β_2-microglobulin, low albumin, low haemoglobin or high calcium at presentation. Although new treatments have increased overall survival, fewer than 5% of patients survive longer than 10 years with standard treatment. The recent advances in therapy with thalidomide and bortezomib and the development of other new drugs, such as the thalidomide derivative lenalidomide, may improve this in future.

24.64 Haematological malignancy in old age

- **Median age:** approximately 70 years for most haematological malignancies.
- **Poor-risk biological features:** adverse cytogenetics or the presence of a multidrug resistance phenotype are more frequent.
- **Prognosis:** increasing age is an independent adverse variable in acute leukaemia and aggressive lymphoma.
- **Chemotherapy:** may be less well tolerated. Older people are more likely to have antecedent cardiac, pulmonary or metabolic problems, tolerate systemic infection less well and metabolise cytotoxic drugs differently.
- **Cure rates:** similar to those in younger patients, in those who do tolerate treatment.
- **Decision to treat:** should be based on the individual's biological status, the level of social support available, and the patient's wishes and those of the immediate family, but not on chronological age.

APLASTIC ANAEMIA

Primary idiopathic acquired aplastic anaemia

This is a rare disorder in Europe and North America, with 2–4 new cases per million population per annum; the disease is much more common in certain other parts of the world: for example, east Asia. The basic problem is failure of the pluripotent stem cells, producing hypoplasia of the bone marrow with a pancytopenia in the blood. The diagnosis rests on exclusion of other causes of secondary aplastic anaemia (see below) and rare congenital causes such as Fanconi's anaemia.

Clinical features and investigations

Patients present with symptoms of bone marrow failure, usually anaemia or bleeding, and less commonly infections. An FBC demonstrates pancytopenia, low reticulocytes and often macrocytosis. Bone marrow aspiration and trephine reveal hypocellularity.

Management

All patients will require blood product support and aggressive management of infection. The prognosis of severe aplastic anaemia managed with supportive therapy only is poor and more than 50% of patients die, usually in the first year. The curative treatment for patients under 30 years of age with severe idiopathic aplastic anaemia is allogeneic bone marrow transplantation if there is an available donor (p. 1013). Those with a compatible sibling donor should proceed to transplantation as soon as possible; they have a 75–90% chance of long-term cure. In older patients, immunosuppressive therapy with ciclosporin and antithymocyte globulin gives 5-year survival rates of 75%. Such patients may relapse or other clonal disorders of haematopoiesis may evolve, such as paroxysmal nocturnal haemoglobinuria (p. 1027), myelodysplastic syndrome (p. 1036) and even acute myeloid leukaemia (p. 1031). They must be followed up long-term.

Secondary aplastic anaemia

Causes of this condition are listed in Box 24.65. It is not practical to list all the drugs which have been suspected of causing aplasia. It is important to check the reported side-effects of all drugs taken over the preceding months. In some instances the cytopenia is more selective and affects only one cell line, most often the neutrophils. Frequently, this is an incidental finding with no ill health. It probably has an immune basis but this is difficult to prove.

The clinical features and methods of diagnosis are the same as for primary idiopathic aplastic anaemia. An underlying cause should be treated or removed but otherwise management is as for the idiopathic form.

24.65 Causes of acquired aplastic anaemia

- Drugs
    Cytotoxic drugs
    Antibiotics—chloramphenicol, sulphonamides
    Antirheumatic agents—penicillamine, gold, phenylbutazone, indometacin
    Antithyroid drugs
    Anticonvulsants
    Immunosuppressives—azathioprine
- Chemicals
    Benzene toluene solvent misuse—glue-sniffing
    Insecticides—chlorinated hydrocarbons (DDT), organophosphates and carbamates (p. 218)
- Radiation
- Viral hepatitis
- Pregnancy
- Paroxysmal nocturnal haemoglobinuria

MYELOPROLIFERATIVE DISORDERS

These make up a group of chronic conditions characterised by clonal proliferation of marrow erythroid precursors (polycythaemia rubra vera, PRV), megakaryocytes (essential thrombocythaemia and myelofibrosis) or myeloid cells (chronic myeloid leukaemia; p. 1034). Although the majority of patients are classifiable as having one of these disorders, some have overlapping features and there is often progression from one to another, e.g. PRV to myelofibrosis. The recent discovery of the molecular basis of these disorders will lead to changes in classification and treatment; a mutation in the gene on chromosome 9 encoding the signal transduction molecule *JAK-2* has been found in 97% of PRV cases and 50% of those with essential thrombocythaemia and myelofibrosis.

Myelofibrosis

In myelofibrosis the marrow is initially hypercellular, with an excess of abnormal megakaryocytes which release growth factors, e.g. platelet-derived growth factor, to the marrow microenvironment, resulting in a reactive proliferation of fibroblasts. As the disease progresses, the marrow becomes fibrosed.

Most patients present over the age of 50 years with lassitude, weight loss and night sweats. The spleen can be massively enlarged due to extramedullary haematopoiesis (blood cell formation outside the bone marrow), and painful splenic infarcts may occur.

The characteristic blood picture is a leucoerythroblastic anaemia, with circulating immature red blood cells (increased reticulocytes and nucleated red blood cells) and granulocyte precursors (myelocytes). The red cells are shaped like teardrops (teardrop poikilocytes), and giant platelets may be seen in the blood. The white count varies from low to moderately high, and the platelet count may be high, normal or low. Urate levels may be high due to increased cell breakdown, and folate deficiency is common. The marrow is often difficult to aspirate and a trephine biopsy shows an excess of megakaryocytes, increased reticulin and fibrous tissue replacement. The presence of a *JAK-2* mutation supports the diagnosis.

Management and prognosis

Median survival is 4 years from diagnosis, but ranges from 1 year to over 20 years. Treatment is directed at control of symptoms, e.g. red cell transfusions for anaemia. Folic acid should be given to prevent deficiency. Cytotoxic therapy with hydroxycarbamide may help control spleen size, the white cell count or systemic symptoms. Splenectomy may be required for a grossly enlarged spleen or symptomatic pancytopenia secondary to splenic pooling of cells and hypersplenism. Bone marrow transplantation may be considered for younger patients.

Essential thrombocythaemia

Malignant proliferation of megakaryocytes results in a raised level of circulating platelets that are often dysfunctional. Prior to making a diagnosis of essential thrombocythaemia, reactive causes of increased platelets must be excluded (p. 1004). The presence of a *JAK-2* mutation supports the diagnosis. Patients present at a median age of 60 years with vascular occlusion or bleeding events, or with an asymptomatic isolated raised platelet count. In most individuals the condition is chronic, with the platelet count gradually increasing. A very small percentage may transform to acute leukaemia and others to myelofibrosis.

Low-risk patients (age < 40 years, platelet count < 1000×10^9/L and no bleeding or thrombosis) may not require treatment to reduce the platelet count. For those with a platelet count > 1000×10^9/L, with symptoms, or with other risk factors for thrombosis such as diabetes or hypertension, treatment to control platelets should

be given. Agents include oral hydroxycarbamide or anagrelide, an inhibitor of megakaryocyte maturation. Intravenous radioactive phosphorus (^{32}P) may be useful in old age. Aspirin therapy is recommended for all patients to reduce the risk of thrombosis and is particularly useful for those with digital ischaemia.

Polycythaemia rubra vera (PRV)

PRV occurs mainly in patients over the age of 40 years and presents either as an incidental finding of a high haemoglobin, or with symptoms of hyperviscosity, such as lassitude, loss of concentration, headaches, dizziness, blackouts, pruritus and epistaxis. Some patients present with manifestations of peripheral arterial disease or a cerebrovascular accident. Venous thromboembolism may also occur. Peptic ulceration is common, sometimes complicated by bleeding. Patients are often plethoric and the majority have a palpable spleen at diagnosis.

Investigation of polycythaemia is discussed on page 998. The diagnosis of PRV now rests upon the demonstration of a high haematocrit and the presence of the *JAK-2* mutation. In the occasional *JAK-2*-negative cases, a raised red cell mass and absence of causes of a secondary erythrocytosis must be established. The spleen is enlarged, neutrophil and platelet counts are frequently raised, an abnormal karyotype may be found in the marrow, and in vitro culture of the marrow can be used to demonstrate autonomous growth in the absence of added growth factors.

Management and prognosis

Aspirin reduces the risk of thrombosis. Venesection gives prompt relief of hyperviscosity symptoms. Between 400 and 500 mL of blood (less if the patient is elderly) are removed and the venesection is repeated every 5–7 days until the haematocrit is reduced to below 45%. Less frequent but regular venesection will maintain this level until the haemoglobin remains reduced because of iron deficiency.

Suppression of marrow proliferation with hydroxycarbamide or α-interferon may reduce the risk of vascular occlusion, control spleen size and reduce transformation to myelofibrosis. Radioactive phosphorus (5 mCi of ^{32}P i.v.) is reserved for older patients, as it increases the risk of transformation to acute leukaemia by 6- to 10-fold.

Median survival after diagnosis in treated patients exceeds 10 years. Some patients survive more than 20 years; however, cerebrovascular or coronary events occur in up to 60% of patients. The disease may convert to another myeloproliferative disorder, with about 15% developing myelofibrosis. Acute leukaemia develops principally in those patients who have been treated with radioactive phosphorus.

BLEEDING DISORDERS

Disorders of primary haemostasis

The initial formation of the platelet plug (see Fig. 24.6A, p. 993; also known as 'primary haemostasis') may fail in thrombocytopenia (p. 1003), von Willebrand disease (p. 1048), and also in platelet function disorders and diseases affecting the vessel wall.

Vessel wall abnormalities

Vessel wall abnormalities may be:

- congenital, such as hereditary haemorrhagic telangiectasia
- acquired, as in a vasculitis (p. 1112) or scurvy.

Hereditary haemorrhagic telangiectasia (HHT)

HHT is a dominantly inherited condition caused by mutations in the genes encoding endoglin and activin receptor-like kinase, which are endothelial cell receptors for transforming growth factor-beta (TGF-β), a potent angiogenic cytokine. Telangiectasia and small aneurysms are found on the fingertips, face and tongue, and in the nasal passages, lung and gastrointestinal tract. A significant proportion of these patients develop larger pulmonary arteriovenous malformations (PAVMs) that cause arterial hypoxaemia due to a right-to-left shunt. These predispose to paradoxical embolism, resulting in stroke or cerebral abscess. All patients with HHT should be screened for PAVMs; if these are found, ablation by percutaneous embolisation should be considered.

Patients present either with recurrent bleeds, particularly epistaxis, or with iron deficiency due to occult gastrointestinal bleeding. Treatment can be difficult because of the multiple bleeding points but regular iron therapy often allows the marrow to compensate for blood loss. Local cautery or laser therapy may prevent single lesions from bleeding. A variety of medical therapies have been tried but none has been found to be universally effective.

Ehlers–Danlos disease

Vascular Ehlers–Danlos syndrome (type 4) is a rare autosomal dominant disorder (1 in 100 000) caused by a defect in type 3 collagen which results in fragile blood vessels and organ membranes, leading to bleeding and organ rupture. Classical joint hypermobility (p. 1128) is often limited in this form of the disease but skin changes and facial appearance are typical. The diagnosis should be considered when there is a history of bleeding but normal laboratory tests.

Scurvy

Vitamin C deficiency affects the normal synthesis of collagen and results in a bleeding disorder characterised by perifollicular and petechial haemorrhage, bruising and subperiosteal bleeding. The key to diagnosis is the dietary history (p. 128).

Platelet functional disorders

Bleeding may result from thrombocytopenia (see Box 24.15, p. 1003) or from congenital or acquired abnormalities of platelet function. The most common acquired disorders are iatrogenic, resulting from the use of aspirin, clopidogrel, dipyridamole and the IIb/IIIa inhibitors to prevent arterial thrombosis (see Box 24.31, p. 1015). Inherited platelet function abnormalities are relatively rare. Congenital abnormalities may be due to deficiency of the membrane glycoproteins, e.g. Glanzmann's thrombasthenia (IIb/IIIa) or Bernard–Soulier disease (Ib), or due to the presence of defective platelet granules, e.g. a deficiency of dense (delta) granules (see Fig. 24.6A, p. 992) giving rise to storage pool disorders. The congenital macrothrombocytopathies, which are due to mutations in the myosin heavy chain gene MYH-9, are characterised by large platelets, inclusion bodies in the neutrophils (Döhle bodies) and a variety of other features, including sensorineural deafness and renal abnormalities.

Apart from Glanzmann's thrombasthenia, these conditions are mild disorders with bleeding typically occurring after trauma or surgery but rarely spontaneously. Glanzmann's is an autosomal recessive condition associated with a variable but often severe bleeding disorder. These conditions are usually managed by local mechanical measures, but antifibrinolytics such as tranexamic acid may be useful and in severe bleeding platelet transfusion may be required. Recombinant VIIa is licensed for the treatment of resistant bleeding in Glanzmann's thrombasthenia.

Thrombocytopenia

Thrombocytopenia occurs in many disease processes, listed in Box 24.15 (p. 1003), many of which are discussed elsewhere in this chapter.

Idiopathic thrombocytopenic purpura (ITP)

ITP is mediated by autoantibodies, most often directed against the platelet membrane glycoprotein IIb/IIIa, which sensitise the platelet, resulting in premature removal from the circulation by cells of the reticuloendothelial system. It is not a single disorder; some cases occur in isolation while others are associated with underlying immune dysregulation in conditions such as connective tissue diseases, HIV infection, B cell malignancies, pregnancy and certain drug therapies. However, the clinical presentation and pathogenesis are similar, whatever the cause of ITP.

Clinical features and investigations

The presentation depends on the degree of thrombocytopenia. Spontaneous bleeding typically occurs only when the platelet count is $< 20 \times 10^9/L$. At higher counts the patient may complain of easy bruising or sometimes epistaxis or menorrhagia. Many cases with counts of $> 50 \times 10^9/L$ are discovered by chance.

In adults ITP more commonly affects females and has an insidious onset. Unlike ITP in children, it is unusual for there to be a history of a preceding viral infection. Symptoms or signs of a connective tissue disease may be apparent at presentation or emerge several years later. Patients aged over 65 years should have a bone marrow examination to look for an accompanying B cell malignancy and appropriate autoantibody testing performed if a diagnosis of connective tissue disease is likely. HIV testing should be considered. The peripheral blood film is normal, apart from a greatly reduced platelet number, whilst the bone marrow reveals an obvious increase in megakaryocytes.

Management

Many patients with stable compensated ITP and a platelet count $> 30 \times 10^9/L$ do not require treatment to raise the platelet count, except at times of increased bleeding risk such as surgery and biopsy. First-line therapy for patients with spontaneous bleeding is with prednisolone 1 mg/kg daily to suppress antibody production and inhibit phagocytosis of platelets by reticuloendothelial cells. Administration of intravenous immunoglobulin (IVIg) can raise the platelet count by blocking antibody receptors on reticuloendothelial cells, and is combined

24

with corticosteroid therapy if there is severe haemostatic failure or a slow response to steroids alone. A similar effect can be obtained by administering intravenous anti-D which will bind red cells and saturate antibody receptors in RhD-positive individuals who have a spleen. Persistent or potentially life-threatening bleeding should be treated with platelet transfusion in addition to the other therapies.

The condition may become chronic, with remissions and relapses. Relapses should be treated by re-introducing corticosteroids. If a patient has two relapses, or primary refractory disease, splenectomy is considered with the precautions shown in Box 24.41 (p. 1024). Splenectomy produces complete remission in about 70% of patients and improvement in a further 20–25%, so that following splenectomy only 5–10% of patients require further medical therapy. If significant bleeding persists despite splenectomy, low-dose corticosteroid therapy, immunosuppressive therapy such as rituximab, ciclosporin and tacrolimus should be considered.

Coagulation disorders

Normal coagulation is explained in Figure 24.6 (p. 992). Coagulation factor deficiency may be congenital or acquired and may affect one or several of the coagulation factors (Box 24.66). Inherited disorders are almost uniformly related to decreased synthesis, as a result of mutation in the gene encoding a key protein in coagulation. Von Willebrand disease is the most common inherited bleeding disorder. Haemophilia A and B are the most common single coagulation factor deficiencies, but deficiencies of all the other coagulation factors are seen. Acquired disorders may be due to under-production (e.g. in liver failure), increased consumption (e.g. in disseminated intravascular coagulation) or inhibition of function (such as heparin therapy or immune inhibitors of coagulation, e.g. acquired haemophilia A).

Haemophilia A

Factor VIII deficiency resulting in haemophilia A affects 1/10 000 individuals. It is the most common congenital coagulation factor deficiency. Factor VIII is primarily synthesised by the liver and endothelial cells, and has a half-life of about 12 hours. It is protected from proteolysis in the circulation by binding to von Willebrand factor (vWF).

Genetics

The factor VIII gene is located on the X chromosome. Severe haemophilia is associated with large deletions in the gene, while single-base changes more often result in moderate or mild disease (Box 24.67). As the factor VIII gene is on the X chromosome, haemophilia A is a sex-linked disorder (p. 50). Thus all daughters of haemophiliacs are obligate carriers and they, in turn, have a 1 in 4 chance of each pregnancy resulting in the birth of an affected male baby, a normal male baby, a carrier female or a normal female. Antenatal diagnosis by chorionic villous sampling is possible in families with a known mutation.

Haemophilia 'breeds true' within a family; all members have the same factor VIII gene mutation and a similarly severe or mild phenotype. Female carriers of haemophilia may have reduced factor VIII levels because of random inactivation of their normal X chromosome in the developing fetus (lyonisation). This can result in a mild bleeding disorder; thus all known or suspected carriers of haemophilia should have their factor VIII level measured.

Clinical features

The extent and patterns of bleeding are closely related to residual factor VIII levels. Patients with severe haemophilia (< 1% of normal factor VIII levels) present with spontaneous bleeding into skin, muscle and joints. Retroperitoneal and intracranial bleeding is also a feature. Babies with severe haemophilia have an increased

24.66 Causes of coagulopathy

Congenital

X-linked
- Haemophilia A and B

Autosomal
- Von Willebrand disease
- Factor II, V, VII, X, XI and XIII deficiencies
- Combined II, VII, IX and X deficiency
- Combined V and VIII deficiency
- Hypofibrinogenaemia
- Dysfibrinogenaemia

Acquired

Underproduction
- Liver failure

Increased consumption
- Coagulation activation
  Disseminated intravascular coagulation (DIC)
- Immune-mediated
  Acquired haemophilia and von Willebrand syndrome
- Others
  Acquired factor X deficiency (in amyloid)
  Acquired von Willebrand syndrome in Wilms tumour

Drug-induced
- Inhibition of function
  Heparins
  Lepirudin
  Fondaparinux
  Rivaroxaban
  Dabigatran
- Inhibition of synthesis
  Warfarin

24.67 Severity of haemophilia (ISTH criteria)

Degree of severity	Factor VIII or IX level	Clinical presentation
Severe	< 0.01 U/mL	Spontaneous haemarthroses and muscle haematomas
Moderate	0.01–0.05 U/mL	Mild trauma or surgery causes bleeding
Mild	> 0.05 < 0.4 U/mL	Major injury or surgery results in excess bleeding

(ISTH = International Society on Thrombosis and Haemostasis)

risk of intracranial haemorrhage and, although there is insufficient evidence to recommend routine caesarean section for these births, it is appropriate to avoid head trauma and to perform imaging of the newborn within the first 24 hours of life. Individuals with moderate and mild haemophilia (factor VIII levels 1–40%) present with the same pattern of bleeding, but usually after trauma or surgery when bleeding is greater than would be expected from the severity of the insult.

The major morbidity of recurrent bleeding in severe haemophilia is musculoskeletal. Bleeding is typically into large joints, especially knees, elbows, ankles and hips. Muscle haematomas are also characteristic, most commonly in the calf and psoas muscles. If early treatment is not given to arrest bleeding, a hot, swollen and very painful joint or muscle haematoma develops. Recurrent bleeding into joints leads to synovial hypertrophy, destruction of the cartilage and secondary osteoarthrosis (Fig. 24.33). Complications of muscle haematomas depend on their location. A large psoas bleed may extend to compress the femoral nerve; calf haematomas may increase pressure within the inflexible fascial sheath causing a compartment syndrome with

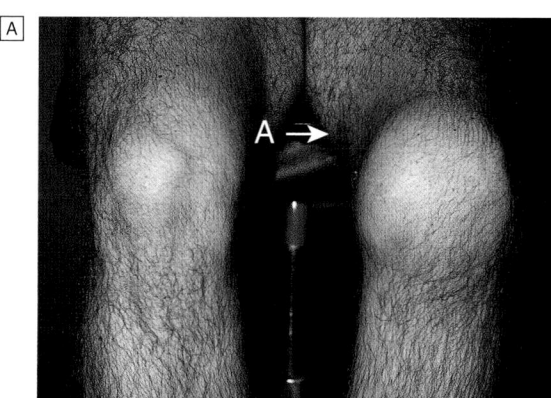

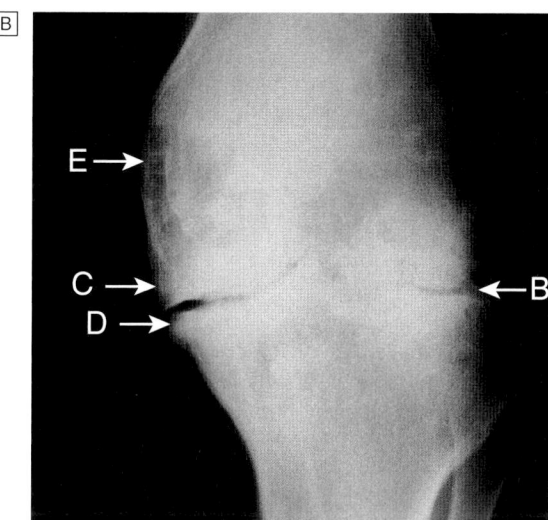

Fig. 24.33 Chronic haemophilic arthropathy of the left knee.
A Repeated bleeds have led to broadening of the femoral epicondyles. Unilateral atrophy of the quadriceps (A) is easily seen. **B** X-ray confirms broadening of femoral epicondyles. There is no cartilage present, as evidenced by the close proximity of the femur and tibia (B); sclerosis (C), osteophyte (D) and bony cysts (E) are present.

ischaemia, necrosis, fibrosis, and subsequent contraction and shortening of the Achilles tendon.

Management

In severe haemophilia A, bleeding episodes should be treated by raising the factor VIII level, usually by intravenous infusion of factor VIII concentrate. Factor VIII concentrates are freeze-dried and stable at 4°C and can therefore be stored in domestic refrigerators, allowing patients to treat themselves at home at the earliest indication of bleeding. Factor VIII concentrate prepared from blood donor plasma is now screened for HBV, HCV and HIV, and undergoes two separate viral inactivation processes during manufacture; these preparations have a good safety record. However, factor VIII concentrates prepared by recombinant technology are now widely available and, although more expensive, are perceived as being safer than those derived from human plasma. In addition to raising factor VIII concentrations, resting of the bleeding site by either bed rest or a splint reduces continuing haemorrhage. Once bleeding has settled, the patient should be mobilised and physiotherapy used to restore strength to the surrounding muscles. All non-immune potential recipients of pooled blood products should be offered hepatitis A and B immunisation.

The vasopressin receptor agonist DDAVP (p. 793) raises the vWF and factor VIII levels by 3–4-fold, which is useful in arresting bleeding in patients with mild or moderate haemophilia A. The dose required for this purpose is high, typically 0.3 µg/kg given intravenously or subcutaneously. Alternatively, the same effect can be achieved by intranasal administration of 300 µg. Following repeated administration of DDAVP, patients need to be monitored for evidence of water retention which can result in significant hyponatraemia (p. 793).

In addition to treatment 'on demand' for bleeding, factor VIII can be administered 2 or 3 times per week as 'prophylaxis' to prevent bleeding in severe haemophilia. This is most appropriate in children, but its widespread use is limited by the high cost of factor VIII preparations.

Complications of coagulation factor therapy

Before 1986, coagulation factor concentrates from human plasma were not virally inactivated with heat or chemicals, and many patients became infected with HIV and the hepatitis viruses HBV and HCV. In exposed patients with severe haemophilia, infection with HCV is almost universal, 80–90% have evidence of HBV exposure, and 60% became HIV-positive. Management of these is described in Chapters 23 and 14. Since 1986, viral inactivation of these blood products has eradicated the risk of viral infection.

Concern that the infectious agent which causes vCJD (p. 1214) might be transmissible by blood and blood products has been confirmed in recipients of red cell transfusion, and in at least one recipient of factor VIII. Pooled plasma products, including factor VIII concentrate, are now manufactured from plasma collected in countries with a low incidence of bovine spongiform encephalopathy.

Another serious complication of factor VIII infusion is the development of anti-factor VIII antibodies, which arise in about 20% of severe haemophiliacs. Such antibodies rapidly neutralise therapeutic infusions, making

24

treatment relatively ineffective. Infusions of activated clotting factors, e.g. VIIa or FEIBA, may stop bleeding.

Haemophilia B (Christmas disease)

Aberrations of the factor IX gene, which is also present on the X chromosome, result in a reduction of the plasma factor IX level, giving rise to haemophilia B. This disorder is clinically indistinguishable from haemophilia A but is less common. The frequency of bleeding episodes is related to the severity of the deficiency of the plasma factor IX level. Treatment is with a factor IX concentrate, used in much the same way as factor VIII for haemophilia A. Although factor IX concentrates shared the problems of virus transmission seen with factor VIII, they do not commonly induce inhibitor antibodies (< 1% patients); when this does occur, however, it may be heralded by the development of a severe allergic-type reaction.

von Willebrand disease

Von Willebrand disease is a common but usually mild bleeding disorder caused by impaired function of von Willebrand factor (vWF). vWF is a protein synthesised by endothelial cells and megakaryocytes, which is involved in both platelet function and coagulation. vWF normally forms a multimeric structure which is essential for its interaction with subendothelial collagen and platelets (see Fig. 24.7, p. 994). vWF acts as a carrier protein for factor VIII, to which it is non-covalently bound; deficiency of vWF lowers the plasma factor VIII level. vWF also forms bridges between platelets and subendothelial components (e.g. collagen; see Fig. 24.6, p. 992), allowing platelets to adhere to damaged vessel walls; deficiency of vWF therefore leads to impaired platelet plug formation. Blood group antigens (A and B) are expressed on vWF. This reduces its susceptibility to proteolysis; as a result, people with blood group O have lower circulating vWF levels than individuals with non-O groups. This needs to be borne in mind when making a diagnosis of von Willebrand disease.

Most patients with von Willebrand disease have type 1 vWD which is characterised by a quantitative decrease in a normal functional protein. Patients with type 2 disorders inherit vWF molecules which are functionally abnormal. The type of abnormality depends on the site of the mutation in the vWD gene; patients with mutations in platelet binding have type 2A disease, those with mutations in the platelet glycoprotein 1b binding site have type 2B, those with mutations in the factor VIII binding site have type 2N disease, and those with other abnormalities in platelet binding have type 2M. The patterns of laboratory abnormality accompanying these types is described in Box 24.68. The gene for vWF is located on chromosome 12 and the disease is usually inherited as an autosomal dominant, except in cases of type 2N when it is recessive. Rare patients carrying two defective copies of the vWF gene ('compound heterozygosity') develop a clinically severe form with almost undetectable levels of vWF.

Clinical features

Patients present with haemorrhagic manifestations similar to those in individuals with reduced platelet function. Superficial bruising, epistaxis, menorrhagia and gastrointestinal haemorrhage are common. Bleeding episodes are usually much less common than in severe

	24.68 Classification of von Willebrand disease			
Type	**Defect**	**Inheritance**	**Investigations**	
1	Partial quantitative	AD	Parallel decrease in vWF: Ag and VIII:c	
2A	Qualitative	AD	Absent HWM of vWF Ratio of vWF activity to antigen < 0.7	
2B	Qualitative	AD	Reduced HWM of vWF Enhanced platelet agglutination (RIPA)	
2M	Qualitative	AD	Normal multimers of vWF Abnormal platelets interactions	
2N	Qualitative	AR	Defective binding of vWF to VIII	
3	Severe quantitative	AD or CH	Very low vWF activity and VIII:c Absent multimers	

(AD = autosomal dominant; AR = autosomal recessive; CH = compound heterozygote; HWM = high-weight multimers of vWF; RIPA = ristocetin-induced platelet agglutination; VIII: c = coagulation factor VIII activity in functional assay vWF = von Willebrand factor; vWF: Ag = vWF antigen measured by ELISA)

haemophilia and excessive haemorrhage may only be observed after trauma or surgery. Within a single family the disease has variable penetrance, so that some members may have quite severe and frequent bleeds, whereas others are relatively asymptomatic.

Investigations

The disorder is characterised by reduced activity of vWF and factor VIII, and a prolongation of the bleeding time. The disease can be classified using a combination of assays which include functional and antigenic measures of vWF, multimeric analysis of the protein, and specific tests of function to determine binding to platelet glycoprotein 1b (RIPA) and factor VIII (see Box 24.68).

Management

Many episodes of mild haemorrhage can be successfully treated by local means or with DDAVP, which raises the vWF level, resulting in a secondary increase in factor VIII. Tranexamic acid may be useful in mucosal bleeding. For more serious or persistent bleeds, haemostasis can be achieved with selected factor VIII concentrates which contain considerable quantities of vWF in addition to factor VIII. Young children and patients with severe arterial disease should not receive DDAVP, and patients with type 2B disease develop thrombocytopenia which may be troublesome following DDAVP. Bleeding in type 3 patients responds to nothing apart from concentrates.

Rare inherited bleeding disorders

Deficiencies of factor VII, X and XIII occur as autosomal recessive disorders. They are rare but are associated with severe bleeding. Typical features include haemorrhage from the umbilical stump and intracranial haemorrhage.

Factor XIII deficiency is typically associated with female infertility.

Factor XI deficiency may occur in heterozygous or homozygous individuals. Bleeding is very variable and is not accurately predicted by coagulation factor levels. In general, severe bleeding is confined to patients with levels below 15% of normal.

Acquired bleeding disorders

Disseminated intravascular coagulation (DIC) is an important cause of bleeding which begins with exaggerated coagulation. It is discussed under thrombotic disease on page 1050.

Liver disease

In severe parenchymal liver disease (Ch. 23), bleeding may arise from many different causes. Pathological sources of potential major bleeding, such as oesophageal varices or peptic ulcer, are more likely. There is reduced hepatic synthesis, e.g. of factors V, VII, VIII, IX, X, XI, prothrombin and fibrinogen. Clearance of plasminogen activator is reduced. Thrombocytopenia may occur secondary to hypersplenism in portal hypertension. In cholestatic jaundice there is reduced vitamin K absorption, leading to deficiency of factors II, VII, IX and X. Treatment with plasma products or platelet transfusion should be reserved for acute bleeds or to cover interventional procedures such as liver biopsy. Vitamin K deficiency can be readily corrected with parenteral administration of vitamin K.

Renal failure

The severity of the haemorrhagic state in renal failure is proportional to the plasma urea concentration (p. 482). Bleeding manifestations are those of platelet dysfunction, with gastrointestinal haemorrhage being particularly common. The causes are multifactorial, including anaemia, mild thrombocytopenia and the accumulation of low molecular weight waste products, normally excreted by the kidney, which inhibit platelet function. Treatment is by dialysis to reduce the urea concentration. Rarely, in severe or persistent bleeding, platelet concentrate infusions and red cell transfusions are indicated. Increasing the concentration of vWF, either by cryoprecipitate or by DDAVP, may promote haemostasis.

THROMBOTIC DISORDERS

Venous thromboembolic disease (VTE) and its treatment have many clinical manifestations. The approach to patients with the most common presentation, deep venous thrombosis of the leg, is described on pages 1004–1006. Pulmonary embolism is discussed on page 717. Anticoagulant therapy is discussed on pages 1014–1016.

Predisposing factors for VTE are listed in Box 24.18 (p. 1006). In a small proportion of cases, there is an underlying haematological disorder predisposing to venous thrombosis, detected using the screening tests described in Boxes 24.4 and 24.5 (p. 997). These disorders include myeloproliferative disorders and paroxysmal nocturnal haemoglobinuria, which are discussed above (pp. 1027 and 1043–1044). They also include inherited acquired conditions, described below.

Inherited abnormalities of coagulation

Several inherited conditions predispose to VTE, with several points in common which are worth noting:

- None of them is strongly associated with arterial thrombosis.
- All are associated with a slightly increased incidence of adverse outcome of pregnancy, including recurrent early fetal loss, but there are no data to indicate that any specific intervention changes that outcome.
- Apart from in antithrombin deficiency and homozygous factor V Leiden, most carriers of these genes will never have an episode of VTE; if they do, it will be associated with the presence of an additional temporary risk factor.
- There is little evidence that detection of these abnormalities predicts recurrence of VTE.
- None of these conditions per se requires treatment with anticoagulants. Patients with thrombosis should receive LMWH followed by a coumarin, as discussed on page 1006. Patients who are deemed to be at high risk of thrombosis, e.g. those with antithrombin deficiency in pregnancy, should receive treatment or prophylactic doses of heparin (p. 1006) to cover the period of risk only.

Antithrombin deficiency

Antithrombin (AT) is a serine protease inhibitor (SERPIN) which inactivates factors IIa, IXa, Xa and XIa. Heparins, fondaparinux and idraparinux achieve their therapeutic effect by potentiating the activity of AT. Familial deficiency of AT is inherited as an autosomal dominant; homozygosity for mutant alleles is not compatible with life. Around 70% of affected individuals will have an episode of VTE before the age of 60 years and the relative risk for thrombosis compared with the background population is 10–20. Pregnancy is a high-risk period for VTE and this requires fairly aggressive management with doses of LMWH which are greater than the usual prophylactic doses ($\geq 100\,U/kg/day$). AT concentrate (either plasma-derived or recombinant) is available; this is required for cardiopulmonary bypass and may be used as an adjunct to heparin in surgical prophylaxis.

Protein C and S deficiencies

Protein C and S are vitamin K-dependent natural anticoagulants involved in switching off coagulation factor activation and thrombin generation (see Fig. 24.6E, p. 993). Inherited deficiency of either protein C or S results in a prothrombotic state with a five-fold relative risk of VTE compared with the background population.

Factor V Leiden

Factor V Leiden results from a gain of function single-base pair mutation which prevents the cleavage and hence inactivation of activated factor Va. This results in a relative risk of venous thrombosis of 5 in heterozygotes and ≥ 50 in rare homozygotes. The mutation is found in about 5% of Northern Europeans, 2% of Hispanics, 1.2% of African-Americans, 0.5% of Asian-Americans and 1.25% of Native Americans, and is rare in Chinese and Malay people.

24

Prothrombin G20210A

This gain-of-function mutation in the non-coding 3′ end of the prothrombin gene is associated with an increased plasma level of prothrombin. It is present in about 2% of Northern Europeans but is rare in native populations of Korea, China, India and Africa. In the heterozygous state it is associated with a 2–3-fold increase in risk of VTE compared with background population.

Antiphospholipid syndrome (APS)

APS is a clinicopathological entity in which a constellation of clinical conditions, alone or in combination, is found in association with a persistently positive test for an antiphospholipid antibody. The antiphospholipid antibodies are heterogeneous and typically are directed against proteins which bind to phospholipids (Box 24.69). Although causal roles for these antibodies have been proposed, the mechanisms underlying the clinical features of APS are not clear. In clinical practice, two types of test are used, which detect:

- antibodies which bind to negatively charged phospholipid on an ELISA plate (called an anticardiolipin antibody test)
- those which interfere with phospholipid-dependent coagulation tests like the APPT or the dilute Russell viper venom time (DRVVT; called a lupus anticoagulant test).

The term antiphospholipid antibody encompasses both a lupus anticoagulant and an anticardiolipin antibody; individuals may be positive for one or both of these activities.

Clinical features and management

APS may present in isolation (primary APS) or in association with one of the conditions shown in Box 24.69, most typically SLE (secondary APS). Most patients present with a single manifestation and APS is now most frequently diagnosed in women with adverse outcomes of pregnancy. It is extremely important to make the diagnosis in patients with APS, whatever the manifesta-tion, because it affects the prognosis and management of arterial thrombosis, VTE and pregnancy.

Arterial thrombosis, typically stroke, associated with APS should be treated with warfarin as opposed to aspirin. APS-associated VTE is one of the situations where the predicted recurrence rate is high enough to indicate long-term anticoagulation after a first event. In women with APS it is likely that intervention with heparin and possibly aspirin increases the chance of a successful pregnancy outcome.

Disseminated intravascular coagulation (DIC)

DIC may complicate a range of illnesses (Box 24.70). It is characterised by systemic activation of the pathways involved in coagulation and its regulation. This may result in the generation of intravascular fibrin clots causing organ failure, with simultaneous coagulation factor and platelet consumption causing bleeding. The systemic coagulation activation is induced either through cytokine pathways which are activated as part of a systemic inflammatory response, or by the release of procoagulant substances such as tissue factor. In addition, suboptimal function of the natural anticoagulant pathways and dysregulated fibrinolysis contribute to DIC. There is consumption of platelets, coagulation factors (notably factors V and VIII) and fibrinogen. The

---

24.70 Disseminated intravascular coagulation

Underlying conditions

- Infection/sepsis
- Trauma
- Obstetric, e.g. amniotic fluid embolism, placental abruption, pre-eclampsia
- Severe liver failure
- Malignancy, e.g. solid tumours and leukaemias
- Tissue destruction, e.g. pancreatitis, burns
- Vascular abnormalities, e.g. vascular aneurysms, liver haemangiomas
- Toxic/immunological, e.g. ABO incompatibility, snake bites, recreational drugs

ISTH scoring system for diagnosis of DIC

Presence of an associated disorder	Essential
Platelets	> 100 = 0
	< 100 = 1
	< 50 = 2
Elevated fibrin degradation products	No increase = 0
	Moderate = 2
	Strong = 3
Prolonged prothrombin time	< 3 s = 0
	> 3 s but < 6 s = 1
	> 6 s = 2
Fibrinogen	> 1 g/L = 0
	< 1 g/L = 1

Total score:
≥ 5 = Compatible with overt DIC
< 5 = Repeat monitoring over 1–2 days

(ISTH = International Society for Thrombosis and Haemostasis)

24.69 Antiphospholipid syndrome (APS)

Clinical manifestations

- Adverse pregnancy outcome Recurrent first trimester abortion (≥ 3) Unexplained death of morphologically normal fetus after 10 weeks' gestation Severe early pre-eclampsia
- Venous thromboembolism
- Arterial thromboembolism
- Livedo reticularis, catastrophic APS, transverse myelitis, skin necrosis, chorea

Conditions associated with secondary APS

- SLE
- Rheumatoid arthritis
- Systemic sclerosis
- Behçet's syndrome
- Temporal arteritis
- Sjögren's syndrome

Targets for antiphospholipid antibodies

- β₂-glycoprotein 1
- Protein C
- Annexin V
- Prothrombin (may result in haemorrhagic presentation)

lysis of fibrin clot results in production of fibrin degradation products (FDP), including D-dimers.

Investigations

DIC should be suspected when any of the conditions listed in Box 24.70 are met. Measurement of coagulation times (APTT and PT; p. 997), along with fibrinogen, platelet count and FDPs, helps in the assessment and aids clinical decision-making with regard to both bleeding and thrombotic complications.

Management

Therapy is primarily aimed at the underlying cause. These patients will often require intensive care to deal with concomitant issues, such as acidosis, dehydration, renal failure and hypoxia. Blood component therapy, such as fresh frozen plasma, cryoprecipitate and platelets, should be given if the patient is bleeding or to cover interventions with high bleeding risk, but should not be given routinely based on coagulation tests and platelet counts alone. Prophylactic doses of heparin should be given, unless there is a clear contraindication. Established thrombosis should be treated cautiously with therapeutic doses of unfractionated heparin, unless clearly contraindicated. Some patients with sepsis-associated DIC benefit from treatment with activated protein C concentrate. Patients with DIC should not in general be treated with antifibrinolytic therapy, e.g. tranexamic acid.

Thrombotic thrombocytopenic purpura

Like DIC and also heparin-induced thrombocytopenia (p. 1015), this is a disorder in which thrombosis is accompanied by paradoxical thrombocytopenia. Thrombotic thrombocytopenic purpura is characterised by a pentad of findings, although few patients have all five components:

- thrombocytopenia
- microangiopathic haemolytic anaemia
- neurological sequelae
- fever
- renal impairment.

It is an acute autoimmune disorder mediated by antibodies against ADAMTS-13 (A disintegrin and metalloproteinase with a thrombospondin type-1 motif).

This enzyme normally cleaves vWF multimers to produce normal functional units and its deficiency results in large vWF multimers which cross-link platelets. The features are of microvascular occlusion by platelet thrombi affecting key organs, principally brain and kidneys. It is a rare disorder (1 in 750 000 per annum) which may occur alone or in association with drugs (ticlopidine, ciclosporin), HIV, shiga toxins and malignancy. It should be treated by emergency plasma exchange. Corticosteroids, aspirin and rituximab also have a role in management. Untreated mortality rates are 90% in the first 10 days, and even with appropriate therapy the mortality rate is 20–30% at 6 months.

24.71 Haemostasis and thrombosis in old age

- **Thrombocytopenia**: not uncommon because of the rising prevalence of disorders in which it may be a secondary feature, and also because of the greater use of drugs which can cause it.
- **'Senile' purpura**: presumed to be due to an age-associated loss of subcutaneous fat and the collagenous support of small blood vessels, making them more prone to damage from minor trauma.
- **Thrombosis**: more frequent in old age. This may be due to stasis, to which older people are prone; some studies show increased platelet aggregation with age, and others age-associated hyperactivity of the haemostatic system which could create a prothrombotic state.

FURTHER INFORMATION

www.bcshguidelines.com *British Committee for Standards in Haematology guidelines.*

www.cibmtr.org *International Bone Marrow Transplant Registry.*

www.transfusionguidelines.org.uk *Contains the UK Transfusion Services' Handbook of Transfusion Medicine and links to other relevant sites.*

www.ukhcdo.org *UK Haemophilia Centre Doctors' organisation.*

24

M. Doherty
S.H. Ralston

Musculoskeletal disease

25

CLINICAL EXAMINATION OF THE MUSCULOSKELETAL SYSTEM

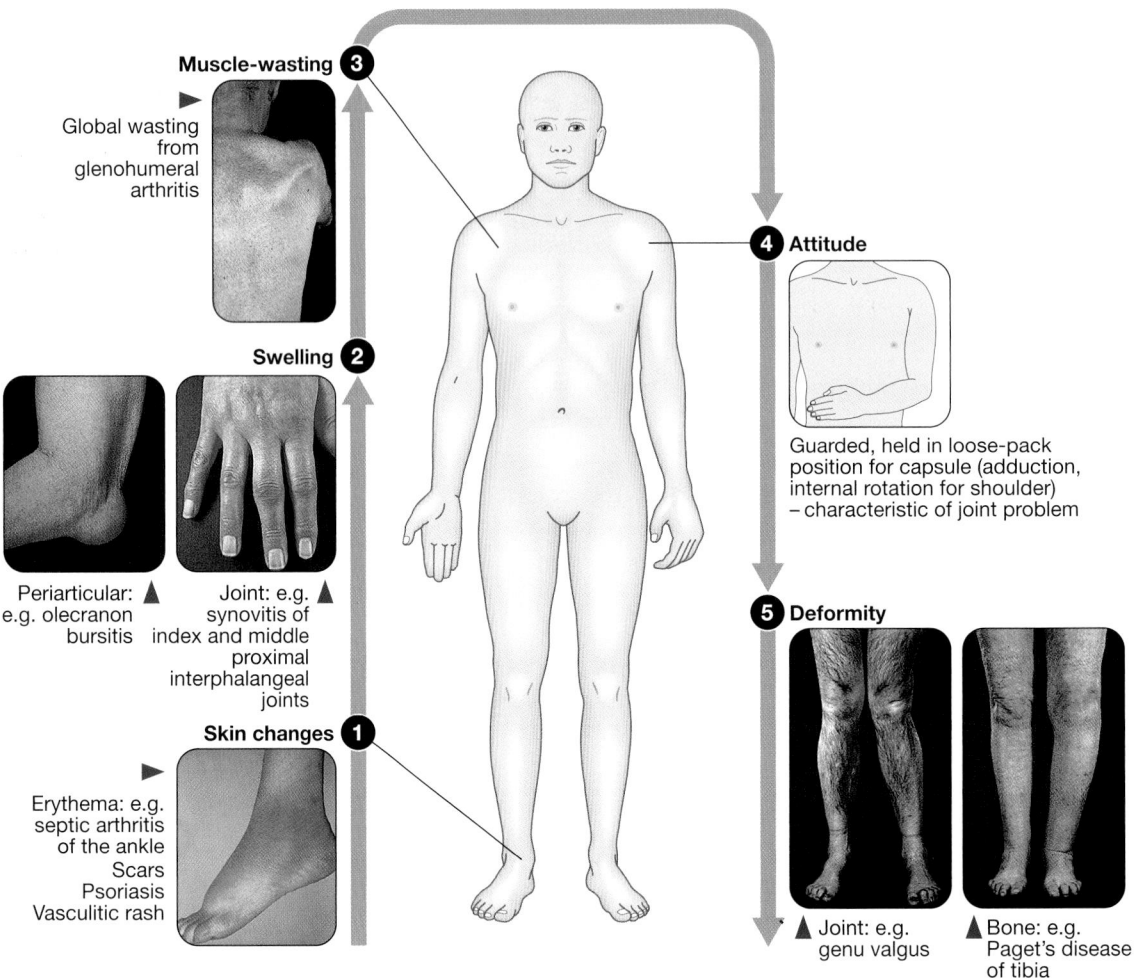

Muscle-wasting **3**

Global wasting from glenohumeral arthritis

Swelling **2**

Periarticular: e.g. olecranon bursitis

Joint: e.g. synovitis of index and middle proximal interphalangeal joints

Skin changes **1**

Erythema: e.g. septic arthritis of the ankle
Scars
Psoriasis
Vasculitic rash

4 Attitude

Guarded, held in loose-pack position for capsule (adduction, internal rotation for shoulder) – characteristic of joint problem

5 Deformity

Joint: e.g. genu valgus

Bone: e.g. Paget's disease of tibia

Detailed regional examination involves 'look' (at rest and during movement), 'feel' and 'move'

A. Inspection at rest
(See figure above for examples)
- Skin changes
- Swelling
- Wasting of muscle
- Attitude
- Deformity

B. Inspection during movement
- Restriction
  Limited to one plane–periarticular lesion
  Affecting most or all movements–joint problem
- Increased range
  Hypermobility, instability
- Pain on usage
  Stress pain = increasing pain towards extremes of movement
  Universal stress pain (in most/all directions) –synovitis
  Selective stress pain (one plane only) –periarticular lesion

C. Palpation with movement
- Tenderness
  Joint line–intra-articular/joint problem
  Periarticular–periarticular lesion
- Increased warmth
  Inflammation (e.g. synovitis, bursitis)
- Swelling
  Fluid (fluctuant)
  Soft tissue (soft, non-fluctuant)
  Bone (hard)
- Crepitus
  Coarse, easily felt, may be readily audible–joint damage
  Fine, localised, heard with stethoscope–tendon sheath, bursa
- Stability
- Resisted active movements
  Reproduce pain from muscle, tendon, enthesis
- Stress tests
  Reproduce pain from ligament or tendon sheath

Important MSK symptoms

Pain

- Usage pain: worse on use, relieved by rest (mechanical strain, damage)
- Rest pain: worse after rest, improved by movement (inflammation)
- Night or 'bone' pain: mostly at night, poorly related to movement (bone origin)

Stiffness

- Subjective feeling of inability to move freely
- Duration and severity of early morning and inactivity stiffness that can be 'worn off' suggest degree of inflammation

Weakness

- Consider primary or secondary muscle abnormality

Swelling

- Fluid
- Soft tissue
- Bone

Deformity

- Joint
- Bone

Non-specific symptoms of systemic illness

- Weight loss ± reduction in appetite
- Fatigability, poor concentration
- Sweats and chills, particularly at night
- Feeling ill, low, irritable

Regional examination differences between joint and periarticular lesions

Sign	Joint	Periarticular
Tenderness	Over joint line	Away from joint line
Restricted movement	Active and passive movement affected equally	Active more restricted than passive
Resisted active	Not painful	May reproduce muscle, tendon, ligament or enthesis pain
Stress pain	Present in all tight-pack positions (several directions)	Present in direction of use of ligament, tendon or enthesis (mainly one direction)
Swelling	Capsular pattern	Localised, periarticular
Crepitus	Coarse or fine	Fine

Features that differentiate joint inflammation ('synovitis') from joint damage

Feature	Synovitis	Joint damage
Stiffness (early morning, inactivity)	+++	±
Increased warmth	+	−
Stress pain	+	−
Soft tissue swelling	+	−
Effusion	+++	±
Crepitus	−	+++
Deformity	−	+
Instability	−	+

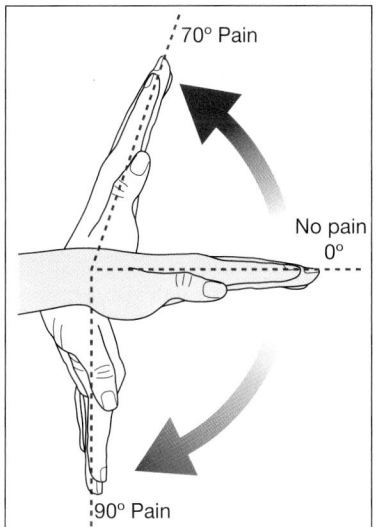

70° Pain

No pain 0°

90° Pain

Example of 'stress pain' at the wrist.
Pain worsens as the wrist moves towards the 'tight-pack' positions (flexion and extension) because of increased intracapsular pressure from inflammatory swelling and effusion. In the mid 'loose-pack' position, when the capsule is at its slackest, there is no pain. Stress pain is the earliest and most sensitive sign of synovitis, occurring before visible swelling or reduction of movement. With joint damage, pain is more evenly spread throughout the range.

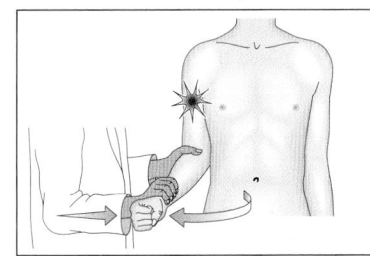

Example of resisted active movement.
Attempted external rotation reproduces upper arm pain resulting from an infraspinatus/teres minor rotator cuff lesion.

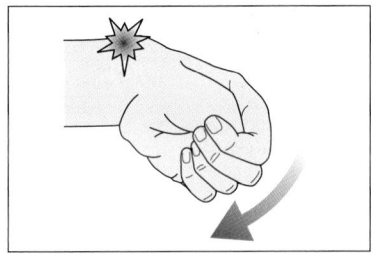

Example of a stress test. Passive ulnar flexion reproduces pain from de Quervain's tenosynovitis.

Disorders of the musculoskeletal (MSK) system are prevalent throughout the world, affecting all ages and ethnic groups. In the UK, up to 1 in 4 new consultations in general practice are for MSK symptoms. The principal manifestations are pain and impairment of locomotor function.

Most MSK conditions predominate in women and show a strong association with age; 40% of those over 65 have a significant MSK disorder. They are the single most common cause of physical disability in older people and account for one-third of physical disability at all ages.

Non-inflammatory conditions are far more prevalent than inflammatory disease (Box 25.1). Most regional MSK pain arises from muscles, tendons and periarticular structures. Osteoarthritis (OA) is the most common joint disorder, with knee involvement a major cause of disability. Osteoporosis is the most prevalent bone disorder and in developed countries about 30% of women and 12% of men sustain a fracture related to osteoporosis during their lifetime.

FUNCTIONAL ANATOMY AND PHYSIOLOGY

The MSK system is responsible for body movements, provides a structural framework to protect internal organs and acts as a reservoir for storage of calcium and phosphate in the regulation of mineral homeostasis. Individual components are depicted in Figure 25.1.

Bone

Bones are of two main types based on their embryonic development. Flat bones, such as the skull, develop by intramembranous ossification, in which embryonic fibroblasts differentiate directly into bone within condensations of mesenchymal tissue during early fetal life. Long bones, such as the femur and radius, develop by endochondral ossification from a cartilage template. During development, the cartilage is invaded by vascular tissue containing osteoprogenitor cells and is gradually replaced by bone from centres of ossification situated in the middle and at the ends of the bone. A thin remnant of cartilage called the growth plate or epiphysis remains at each end of long bones, and chondrocyte proliferation here is responsible for skeletal growth during childhood and adolescence. During puberty, the rise in levels of sex hormones halts cell division in the growth plate. The cartilage remnant then disappears as the epiphysis fuses and longitudinal bone growth ceases.

The normal skeleton has two types of bone (see Fig. 25.1). Cortical bone is formed from Haversian systems, comprising concentric lamellae of bone tissue surrounding a central canal that contains blood vessels. Cortical bone is dense and forms a hard envelope around the long bones. Trabecular or cancellous bone fills the centre of the bone and consists of an interconnecting meshwork of trabeculae, separated by spaces filled with bone marrow.

There are three main cell types in bone:

- *Osteoclasts*: multinucleated cells of haemopoietic origin, responsible for bone resorption
- *Osteoblasts*: mononuclear cells of mesenchymal origin, responsible for bone formation
- *Osteocytes*: these differentiate from osteoblasts during bone formation and become embedded in bone matrix. Osteocytes play a critical role in regulating phosphate metabolism by producing the hormone FGF23 (Fig. 25.2) and are thought to be responsible for sensing and responding to mechanical loading of the skeleton.

Bone matrix and mineral

The most abundant protein of bone is type I collagen, which is formed from two α1 peptide chains and one α2 chain wound together in a triple helix. Type I collagen is proteolytically processed inside the cell before being laid down in the extracellular space, releasing propeptide fragments that can be used as biochemical markers of bone formation (p. 1064). Subsequently, the collagen fibrils become 'cross-linked' to one another by pyridinium molecules, a process which enhances bone strength. When bone is broken down by osteoclasts, the cross-links are released, providing biochemical markers of bone resorption (p. 1064). Bone is normally laid down in an orderly fashion, but when bone turnover is high, as in Paget's disease or severe hyperparathyroidism, it is laid down in a chaotic pattern, giving rise to 'woven bone' which is mechanically weak. Bone matrix also contains growth factors, other structural proteins and proteoglycans, thought to be involved in helping bone cells attach to bone matrix and in regulating bone cell activity. The other major component of bone is mineral, comprised of calcium and phosphate crystals deposited between the collagen fibrils in the form of hydroxyapatite $[Ca_{10}(PO_4)_6(OH)_2]$. Mineralisation is essential for bone's rigidity and strength, but over-mineralisation can increase brittleness which contributes to bone fragility in diseases like osteogenesis imperfecta (p. 1126).

Bone remodelling

Bone remodelling is responsible for renewal and repair of the skeleton during adult life (see Fig. 25.2). It starts with attraction of osteoclast precursors in peripheral blood to the target site, probably by local release of chemotactic

---

ℹ 25.1 Relative prevalence of musculoskeletal disorders

	Prevalence	Female: male	Age association
'Non-inflammatory' conditions			
Neck and back pain	20%	=	–
Osteoarthritis			
Knee	10%	F > M	++
Hip	4%	=	+
Osteoporosis	15%	F > M	++
Regional 'soft tissue' pain	10%	F > M	++
Fibromyalgia	3%	F > M	++
'Inflammatory' conditions			
Rheumatoid arthritis	1.5%	F > M	+
Gout	1.5%	M > F	–
Seronegative spondyloarthritis	0.8%	=	–
Polymyalgia rheumatica	0.04%	F > M	++
Connective tissue diseases (mainly lupus)	0.02%	F > M	–

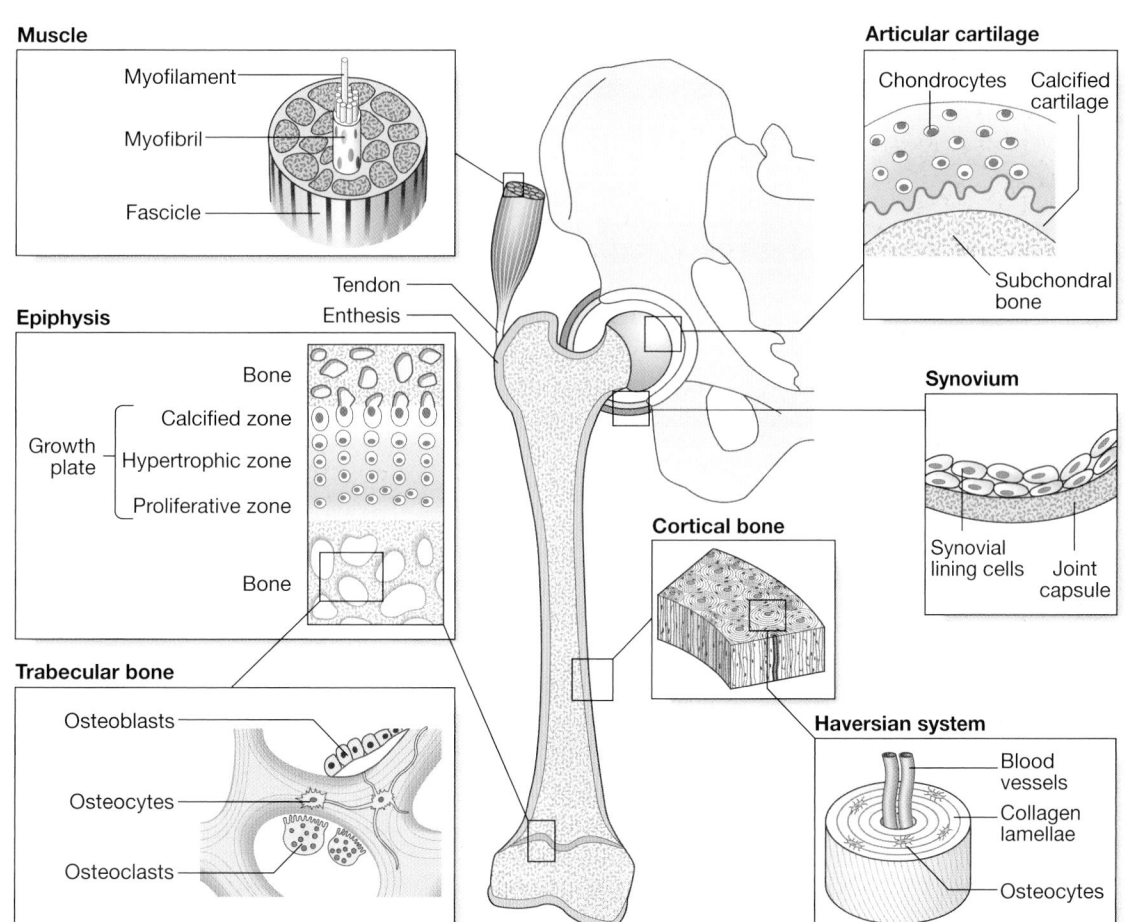

Muscle
- Myofilament
- Myofibril
- Fascicle

Articular cartilage
- Chondrocytes
- Calcified cartilage
- Subchondral bone

Tendon
Enthesis

Epiphysis
- Bone
- Growth plate
  - Calcified zone
  - Hypertrophic zone
  - Proliferative zone
- Bone

Synovium
- Synovial lining cells
- Joint capsule

Cortical bone

Trabecular bone
- Osteoblasts
- Osteocytes
- Osteoclasts

Haversian system
- Blood vessels
- Collagen lamellae
- Osteocytes

Fig. 25.1 Structure of major musculoskeletal tissues.

25

factors from areas of microdamage. The osteoclast precursors differentiate into mature osteoclasts in response to RANK ligand (RANKL), which is expressed by bone marrow stromal cells. RANKL activates the RANK receptor, which is expressed on osteoclasts and precursors. This is blocked by osteoprotegerin (OPG), a decoy receptor for RANKL that inhibits osteoclast formation. Mature osteoclasts attach to the bone surface by a tight sealing zone, and secrete hydrochloric acid and proteolytic enzymes such as cathepsin K into the space underneath. The acid dissolves the mineral and cathepsin K degrades collagen. When resorption is complete, osteoclasts undergo programmed cell death, and bone formation begins with the attraction of osteoblast precursors to the resorption site. These differentiate into mature osteoblasts, which deposit new bone matrix in the resorption lacuna, until the hole is filled. Some osteoblasts become trapped in bone matrix and differentiate into osteocytes. These act as biomechanical sensors and produce several molecules that influence bone remodelling and phosphate metabolism. Bone formation is stimulated by Wnt proteins which bind to and activate lipoprotein-related receptor protein 5 (LRP5), expressed on osteoblasts. This process is inhibited by other molecules such as sclerostin (SOST) (see Fig. 25.2). Initially, the newly formed bone matrix (osteoid) is uncalcified but subsequently becomes mineralised to form mature bone. Alkaline phosphatase (ALP), produced by osteoblasts, plays an important role

in bone mineralisation by degrading pyrophosphate, an inhibitor of mineralisation. Bone remodelling is regulated by circulating hormones, such as parathyroid hormone (PTH) and oestrogen, and locally produced factors such as cytokines (Box 25.2). Many systemic hormones exert

i | **25.2 Regulators of bone remodelling**

Factor	Bone resorption	Bone formation
Parathyroid hormone (PTH)	↑	↑
RANKL	↑	↔
Osteoprotegerin (OPG)	↑	↔
Wnt/LRP5	↓	↑
Sclerostin (SOST)	↔	↓
Interleukin-1 (IL-1)	↑	↓
Tumour necrosis factor-α (TNF-α)	↑	↓
Thyroid hormone	↑	↔
Glucocorticoids	↑	↓↓
Oestrogen/testosterone	↓	↑
Mechanical loading	↓	↑

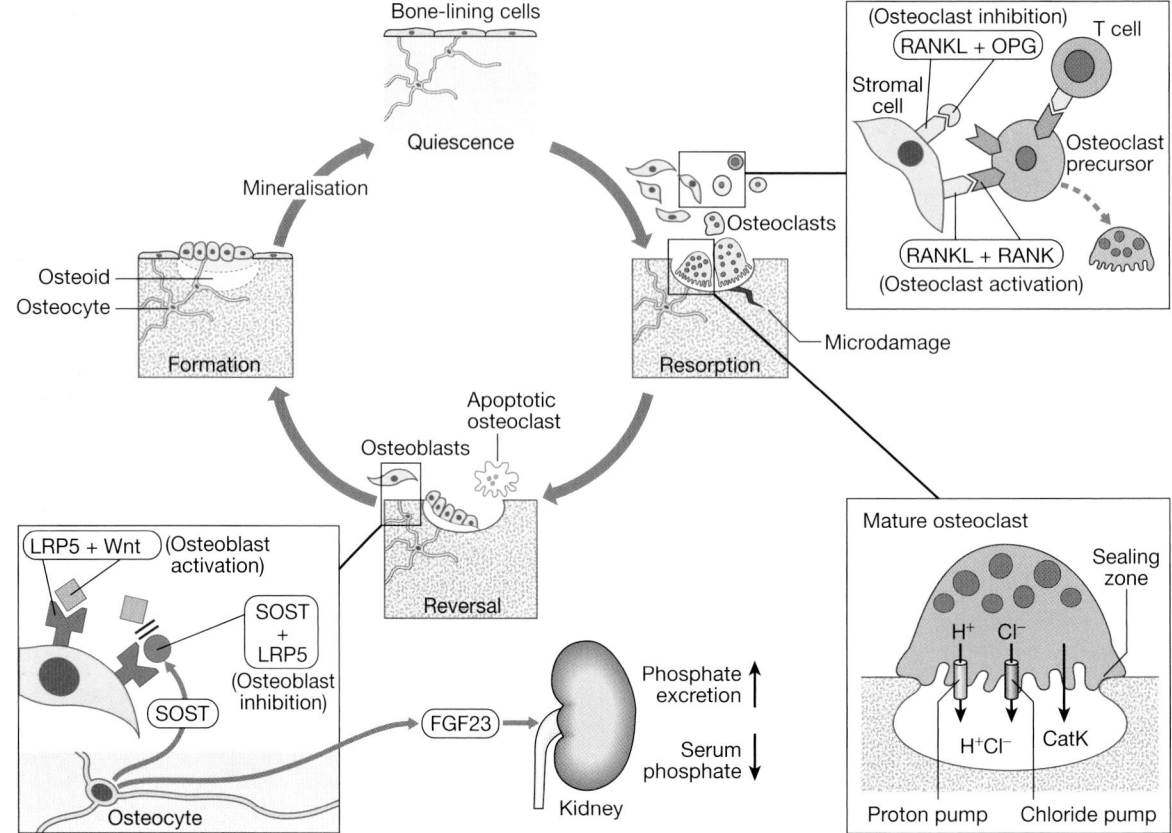

Fig. 25.2 The bone remodelling cycle. (CatK = cathepsin K; LRP5 = lipoprotein receptor protein 5; OPG = osteoprotegerin; RANK = receptor activator of nuclear factor κB; RANKL = RANK ligand; SOST = sclerostin)

effects on bone turnover by affecting local expression of RANK, RANKL, OPG, sclerostin (SOST) and molecules in the Wnt/LRP5 pathway (see Fig. 25.2).

Joints

Bones are linked by joints. There are three main subtypes: fibrous, fibrocartilaginous and synovial (Box 25.3).

Fibrous and fibrocartilaginous joints

These comprise a simple bridge of fibrous or fibrocartilaginous tissue joining two bones together where there is little requirement for movement. The intervertebral disc is a special type of fibrocartilaginous joint in which an amorphous area, the nucleus pulposus, lies in the centre of the fibrocartilaginous bridge. The nucleus has a high water content and acts as a cushion to improve the disc's shock-absorbing properties.

Synovial joints

These are complex structures containing several cell types and are found where a wide range of movement is required.

Articular cartilage

This avascular tissue covers the bone ends in synovial joints. Cartilage cells (chondrocytes) are responsible for synthesis and turnover of cartilage, which consists of a mesh of type II collagen fibrils that extend through a hydrated 'gel' of proteoglycan molecules. The most important proteoglycan is aggrecan, which consists of a core protein to which several glycosaminoglycan (GAG) side-chains are attached (Fig. 25.3). The GAGs are polysaccharides that consist of long chains of disaccharide repeats comprising one normal sugar and an amino sugar. The most abundant GAGs in aggrecan are chondroitin sulphate and keratan sulphate. Hyaluronan is another important GAG which binds to aggrecan molecules to form very large complexes with a total molecular weight more than 100 million. Aggrecan has a strong negative charge and avidly binds water molecules to assume a shape that occupies the maximum possible volume available. The expansive force of the hydrated aggrecan, combined with the restrictive strength of the collagen mesh, gives articular cartilage excellent shock-absorbing properties.

25.3 Types of joint		
Type	**Range of movement**	**Examples**
Fibrous	Minimal	Skull sutures
Fibrocartilaginous	Limited	Symphysis pubis Costochondral junctions Intervertebral discs Sacroiliac joints
Synovial	Large	Most limb joints Temporomandibular Costovertebral

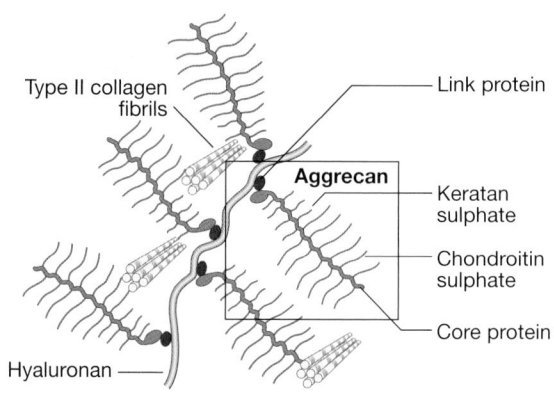

Fig. 25.3 Ultrastructure of articular cartilage.

With ageing, the concentration of chondroitin sulphate decreases, whereas that of keratan sulphate increases, resulting in reduced water content and shock-absorbing properties. These changes differ from those found in OA (p. 1083), where there is abnormal chondrocyte division, loss of proteoglycan from matrix and an increase in water content. Cartilage matrix is constantly turning over and in health there is a perfect balance between synthesis and degradation. Degradation is mediated by enzymes such as aggrecanase and matrix metalloproteinases that degrade the proteins, and glycosidases that degrade GAGs. Pro-inflammatory cytokines such as interleukin-1 (IL-1) and tumour necrosis factor (TNF), which are released during joint inflammation, stimulate production of aggrecanase and metalloproteinases that promote cartilage degradation.

Synovial fluid

The surfaces of articular cartilage are separated by a space filled with synovial fluid, a viscous liquid that lubricates the joint. Synovial fluid is an ultrafiltrate of plasma into which synovial cells secrete hyaluronan and proteoglycans.

Intra-articular discs

Some joints contain fibrocartilaginous discs within the joint space (e.g. the menisci of the knee) that act as shock absorbers. These are avascular and remain viable by diffusion of oxygen and nutrients from the synovial fluid.

The synovial membrane, joint capsule and bursae

The bones of synovial joints are connected by the joint capsule, a fibrous structure richly supplied with blood vessels, nerves and lymphatics which encases the joint. Ligaments are discrete, regional thickenings of the capsule that act to stabilise joints. The inner surface of the joint capsule is the synovial membrane, comprising an outer layer of blood vessels and loose connective tissue, and an inner layer 1–4 cells thick consisting of two main cell types. Type A synoviocytes are phagocytic cells derived from the monocyte/macrophage lineage and are responsible for removing particulate matter from the joint cavity; type B synoviocytes are fibroblast-like cells that secrete synovial fluid. Most inflammatory and degenerative joint diseases associate with thickening of the synovial membrane and infiltration by lymphocytes, polymorphs and macrophages.

Bursae are hollow sacs lined with synovium and contain a small amount of synovial fluid. They help tendons and muscles move smoothly in relation to bones and other articular structures.

Skeletal muscle

Skeletal muscles are responsible for body movements and respiration. Muscle consists of bundles of cells (myocytes) embedded in fine connective tissue containing nerves and blood vessels. Myocytes are large, elongated, multinucleated cells formed by fusion of mononuclear precursors (myoblasts) in early embryonic life. The nuclei lie peripherally and the centre of the cell contains actin and myosin molecules which interdigitate with one another to form the myofibrils that are responsible for muscle contraction. The molecular mechanisms of skeletal muscle contraction are the same as for cardiac muscle (p. 526). Myocytes contain many mitochondria which provide the large amounts of adenosine triphosphate (ATP) necessary for muscle contraction, and are rich in the protein myoglobin which acts as a reservoir for oxygen during contraction.

Individual myofibrils are organised into bundles (fasciculi) that are bound together by a thin layer of connective tissue (the perimysium). The surface of the muscle is surrounded by a thicker layer of connective tissue, the epimysium, which merges with the perimysium to form the muscle tendon. Tendons are tough, fibrous structures that attach muscles to the point of insertion on the bone surface that is called the enthesis.

INVESTIGATION OF MUSCULOSKELETAL DISEASE

For most MSK conditions, clinical enquiry and examination alone give sufficient information for diagnosis and management. Investigations may be helpful in confirming the diagnosis, assessing disease activity or indicating prognosis.

Synovial fluid analysis

This is the pivotal investigation when septic arthritis, crystal-associated arthritis or intra-articular bleeding is suspected, and should be performed in all patients with acute monoarthritis, especially with overlying erythema.

Synovial fluid (SF) can be obtained by aspiration from most peripheral joints and only a small volume is required for diagnostic purposes. Normal SF is present in small volume, contains few cells, is clear and either colourless or pale yellow, and has high viscosity. With joint inflammation, the volume increases, the cell count and the proportion of neutrophils rise (causing turbidity), and the viscosity reduces (due to enzymatic degradation of hyaluronan and aggrecan). However, there is considerable overlap between arthropathies, and these features alone have little diagnostic value. High concentrations of crystals, mainly urate or cholesterol, can make SF appear white.

Non-uniform blood-staining of SF is common, usually reflecting needle trauma to the synovium. Uniform blood-staining (haemarthrosis) often accompanies florid synovitis but may also result from a bleeding diathesis,

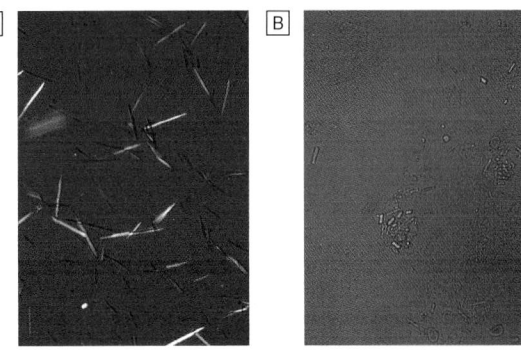

Fig. 25.4 Compensated polarised light microscopy of synovial fluids (× 400). A Monosodium urate crystals showing bright birefringence (negative sign) and needle-shaped morphology. B Calcium pyrophosphate crystals showing weak birefringence (positive sign), scant numbers and a predominantly rhomboid morphology. These are clearly more difficult to detect than urate crystals.

25.4 Abnormalities seen on plain X-ray

Soft tissue swelling

- e.g. Altered skin contours, displaced fat planes and intracapsular fat pads (fat appears dark on X-ray)

Bone density

- Decreased (osteopenia) or increased (osteosclerosis)
- Localised or generalised change

Bone enlargement and deformity

- e.g. Paget's disease, fracture, tumour

Joint erosion

- Non-proliferative or proliferative
- Marginal or central

Joint-space narrowing

- Focal: osteoarthritis
- Generalised: inflammatory arthritis

New bone formation

- e.g. Osteophyte, enthesophyte, syndesmophyte and periosteal reaction

Calcification

- Cartilage (chondrocalcinosis), synovium, capsule, ligament, tendon, muscle, fat, blood vessels, skin
- Intra-articular osteochondral bodies

trauma or pigmented villonodular synovitis. A lipid layer floating above blood-stained fluid is diagnostic of intra-articular fracture and is caused by release of bone marrow fat into the joint.

If sepsis is suspected, SF should be sent for urgent Gram stain and culture in a sterile container. If gonococcus or uncommon organisms are suspected, especially in immunocompromised patients, the microbiologist should be asked to ensure optimal cultures and that molecular techniques of antigen detection are used, if appropriate.

Crystals are identified by compensated polarised light microscopy of fresh unrefrigerated SF (to avoid crystal dissolution and post-aspiration crystallisation). Urate crystals are long and needle-shaped and show a strong light intensity and negative birefringence (Fig. 25.4A). Calcium pyrophosphate crystals are smaller, rhomboid in shape and usually less numerous than urate, and have weak intensity and positive birefringence (Fig. 25.4B).

Imaging

Plain radiography

X-rays can show anatomical changes that reflect important pathological processes (Box 25.4). Although most changes have low specificity, combinations of features and targeting of certain bones or joints (Fig. 25.5) result in characteristic patterns that have high diagnostic specificity.

Joints to be X-rayed are usually selected on the basis of involvement identified at clinical assessment. An exception is seronegative spondyloarthritis where sacroiliac involvement is often asymptomatic. In this case, an anteroposterior (AP) view of the pelvis and a lateral view of the thoracolumbar spine are usually sufficient to show sacroiliitis or syndesmophytes (bony spurs that bridge adjacent vertebral bodies), if present. The selection of X-rays often differs depending on whether they are taken for diagnostic or disease assessment purposes. For example, to determine whether a patient with inflammatory polyarthritis has erosions typical of rheumatoid arthritis (RA), postero-anterior (PA) views of hands and feet are appropriate, since erosions appear first in wrists and

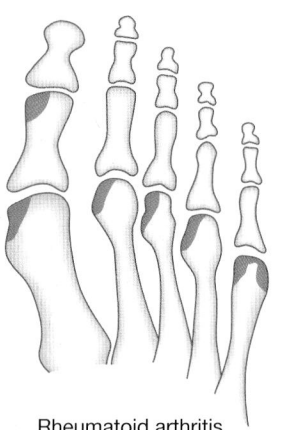

Rheumatoid arthritis

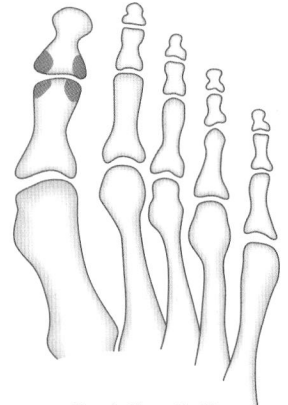

Psoriatic arthritis

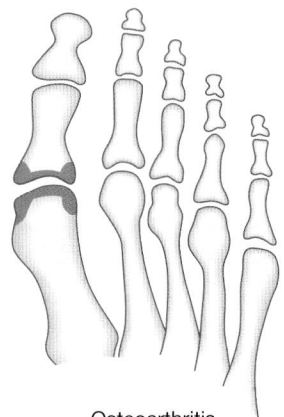

Osteoarthritis

Fig. 25.5 Examples of different target sites of involvement in the forefoot for arthritis.

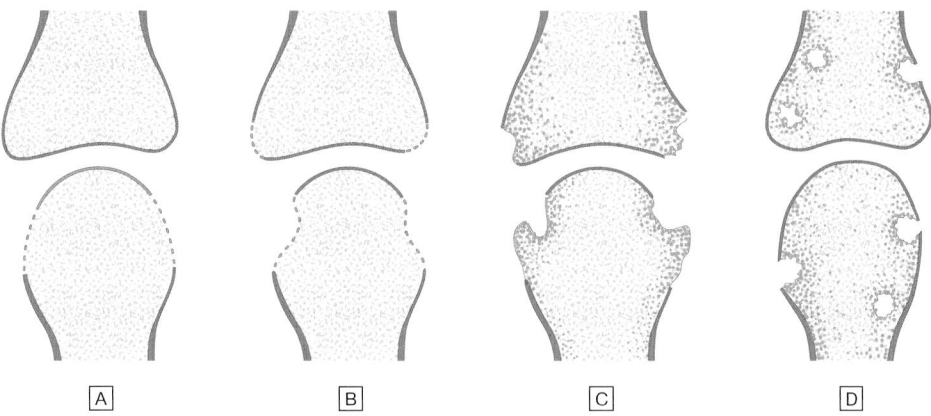

Fig. 25.6 Metacarpophalangeal joint. [A] Early dot-dash erosion of rheumatoid arthritis. [B] Later definite non-proliferative erosion of rheumatoid arthritis. [C] The proliferative erosion of psoriatic arthritis. [D] The intra- and extracapsular 'pressure erosions' of gout.

small joints of hands and feet. However, if the degree of structural damage in one large joint is a cause for concern, an X-ray of that joint is required.

Arthrography is mainly used to demonstrate a ruptured popliteal ('Baker's') cyst as the cause of calf pain and swelling. It may be combined with computed tomography (CT) or magnetic resonance imaging (MRI) to facilitate anatomical assessment.

Erosions

Cartilage and bone erosion is a hallmark of major inflammatory arthropathies. Intracapsular bone erosion first occurs at the joint margin ('marginal erosion') where bone is exposed directly to inflammatory synovium without the protection of overlying cartilage. Loss of the sharp cortical line is the first radiographic sign and precedes more definite scalloping of the bony contour (Fig. 25.6). Cartilage erosion also starts at the margin and slowly works centrally, resulting in loss of 'joint space'. Both RA and seronegative spondyloarthritis (especially psoriatic arthritis) can cause marginal erosions. In RA there is no bone or periosteal reaction, resulting in atrophic 'non-proliferative' erosions (Fig. 25.6B), often with juxta-articular osteopenia and soft tissue swelling. By contrast, in seronegative spondyloarthritis new bone formation and periosteal reaction with retained bone density are more common, resulting in 'proliferative' erosions (Fig. 25.6C). Accompanying ossifying enthesopathy (enthesophytes) and the targeting of different joints further assist differentiation.

In the first 1–2 weeks of acute septic arthritis the X-ray is often normal, apart from osteopenia and soft tissue swelling. However, erosion proceeds rapidly and results in generalised loss of joint space with loss of cortical integrity centrally (central erosion) as well as marginally. In chronic gout, bony defects develop slowly as massive crystal deposits ('tophi') cause pressure necrosis to surrounding bone. Such 'pressure erosions' (Fig. 25.6D) occur at extracapsular as well as intracapsular sites and are not accompanied by osteopenia.

Osteoarthritis

The two cardinal features of OA are joint space narrowing and osteophytes. Joint space narrowing in OA is focal rather than widespread as in inflammatory arthritis

(Fig. 25.7). Osteophytes are most noticeable at the joint margins. Subchondral sclerosis (focal increased density of bone), 'cysts' and osteochondral 'loose' bodies within the synovium are additional features, and there is an association with chondrocalcinosis. Bone density is normal or increased and there are no marginal erosions.

Calcification

Calcification of fibrocartilage and hyaline cartilage (chondrocalcinosis) is most commonly due to calcium pyrophosphate crystals. Calcification at extracapsular sites is mainly apatite. Spotty, multiple calcifications of soft tissues (calcinosis) mainly target peripheral and intermediate sites such as finger pulps, wrists and forearms, and are a feature of connective tissue disease.

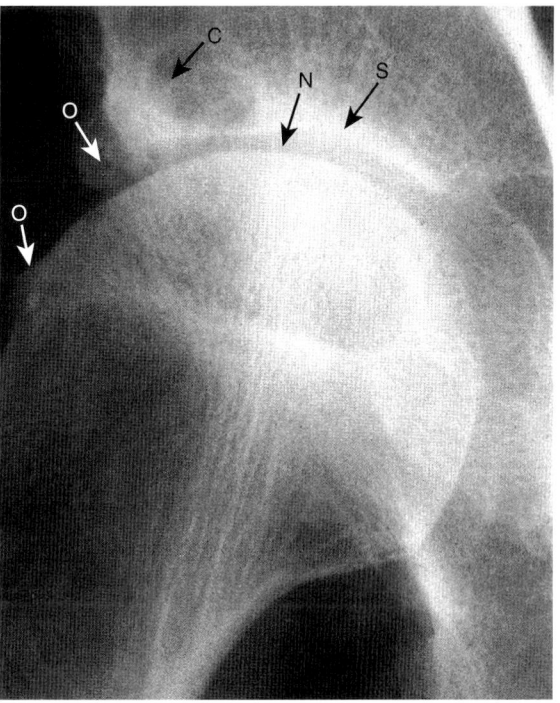

Fig. 25.7 X-ray of hip showing changes of osteoarthritis. Note the superior joint space narrowing (N), subchondral sclerosis (S), marginal osteophytes (white arrows) and cysts (C).

25

Radionuclide bone scan

This is a useful investigation in patients who have bone pain. It involves gamma-camera imaging following an intravenous injection of ^{99m}Tc-bisphosphonate. Early post-injection images reflect vascularity and can show increased perfusion of inflamed synovium, Pagetic bone, or primary or secondary bone tumours (Fig. 25.8). Delayed images taken a few hours later reflect bone remodelling as the bisphosphonate localises to sites of active bone turnover. Scintigraphy has a high sensitivity for detecting important bone and joint pathology that is not apparent on plain X-rays (Box 25.5).

Computerised tomography (CT) and magnetic resonance imaging (MRI)

These techniques give detailed information on anatomy, allowing three-dimensional visualisation of anatomically complex structures such as the spinal canal and facet joints which may be inadequately assessed by plain X-rays. Drawbacks of CT are limited soft tissue resolution and a high radiation dose, and MRI is frequently preferred. It provides detailed information on both structure and physiology of cartilage, bone and other locomotor tissues, allows multiplanar imaging and avoids radiation exposure. T1-weighted short sequences are useful for defining anatomy and T2-weighted long sequences for assessing pathology. MRI, with or without enhancement with gadolinium, is particularly useful to detect and assess:

- early osteonecrosis
- intervertebral disc disease, root entrapment and spinal cord compression
- osteoarticular and soft tissue sepsis

25.5 Pathology detected by isotope bone scanning

- Presence and extent of Paget's disease of bone
- Bone metastases
- Bone or joint sepsis
- Early osteonecrosis
- Bone fractures (including stress fractures)
- Reflex sympathetic dystrophy (algodystrophy, p. 1125)
- Hypertrophic osteoarthropathy (p. 1127)

- osteoarticular and soft tissue malignancy
- bone marrow oedema in patients with recent fractures and reflex sympathetic dystrophy
- internal derangement of joints such as the knee
- soft tissue and periarticular pathology (e.g. early synovitis, rotator cuff tears, bursitis, tenosynovitis).

Ultrasonography

Ultrasonography is inferior to CT or MRI for definition of deep structures and abnormalities within bone, but is a useful outpatient investigation for confirmation of small joint synovitis/erosion, for anatomical confirmation of periarticular lesions, and for assistance in guiding accurate aspiration and injection of joints and bursae.

Bone mineral density

Measurement of bone mineral density (BMD) plays a pivotal role in the investigation and management of osteoporosis. The investigation of choice is dual energy X-ray absorptiometry (DEXA) of the spine and hip. Further details are discussed on page 1118.

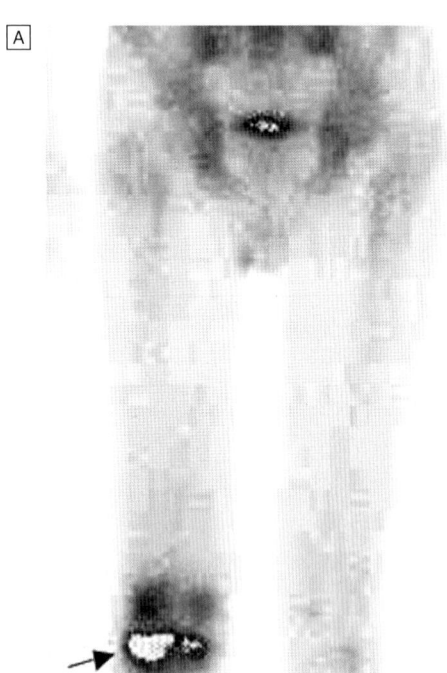

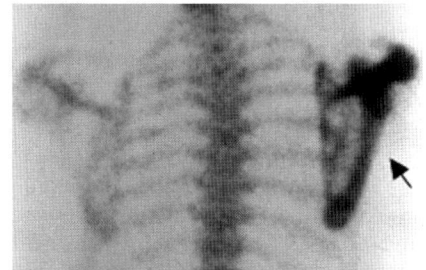

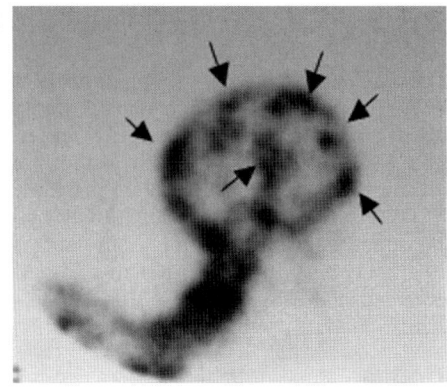

Fig. 25.8 Isotope bone scan appearances in different bone diseases. **A** Patchy tracer uptake in the distal femur in a patient with reflex sympathetic dystrophy. **B** Homogeneous tracer uptake in the scapula in a patient with Paget's disease. **C** Multiple focal areas of tracer uptake in the skull and cervical spine of a patient with metastatic breast cancer.

Blood tests

C-reactive protein and erythrocyte sedimentation rate

Infections, inflammation and malignancy can trigger an acute phase response (APR) with alterations in C-reactive protein (CRP), full blood count (FBC) and erythrocyte sedimentation rate (ESR). CRP is the single most useful marker of the APR. A notable exception is in connective tissue diseases such as lupus and systemic sclerosis, where CRP may be normal in patients with active disease. However, patients with these diseases can mount an APR in response to sepsis, and elevations of CRP in a patient with lupus or scleroderma suggest an incidental cause such as sepsis rather than active disease. A discussion of the interpretation of CRP and ESR changes is given on page 82.

Full blood count

Changes in the FBC can occur in inflammatory rheumatic diseases but are non-specific (e.g. neutrophilia in vasculitis, acute gout and sepsis; neutropenia in lupus). Many disease-modifying antirheumatic drugs (DMARDs) have marrow toxicity and require regular monitoring of the FBC.

Autoantibodies

Autoantibody tests are a useful adjunct to clinical evaluation in the diagnosis of rheumatic diseases but false positive results are common. Those most commonly used in rheumatology are described below; antiphospholipid antibodies, which occur in systemic lupus erythematosus (SLE), are discussed on page 1050. High antibody titres or concentrations are generally of greater clinical significance but the results must be interpreted in light of the clinical picture and the different detection and assay systems used in different hospitals.

Rheumatoid factor

Rheumatoid factor (RF) is an antibody directed against the Fc fragment of human IgG and was so named because it was first identified in patients with RA. RFs may be of any immunoglobulin class but IgM is most commonly tested. RF also occurs in a wide variety of other conditions and in some normal adults (Box 25.6); it

therefore has low diagnostic specificity for RA and also lacks sensitivity, since about 30% of patients with typical signs of RA are negative for RF (so-called seronegative RA). The principal use of RF testing is for prognosis, since a high RF titre at presentation associates with more severe disease.

Antibodies to cyclic citrullinated peptides (anti-CCP antibodies)

Anti-CCP antibodies bind to peptides in which the amino acid arginine has been converted to citrulline by peptidylarginine deiminase, an enzyme abundant in inflamed synovium. They have similar sensitivity to RF for RA (70%) but much higher specificity (> 95%). Anti-CCP antibodies are increasingly being used in preference to RF to support a diagnosis of RA in patients with early polyarthritis. Anti-CCP antibodies are associated with more severe disease and can be detected in asymptomatic patients several years before the development of RA.

Antinuclear antibodies (ANA)

These are directed against one or more components of the nucleus. Box 25.7 gives the many causes of a positive ANA. Low titre ANA is common in normal individuals. The higher the ANA titre, the greater its diagnostic significance, but high titres do not imply more severe disease. The most common indication for ANA testing is in the diagnosis of SLE. ANA has high sensitivity for SLE (virtually 100%) but low specificity (10–40%); a negative ANA virtually excludes SLE but a positive result does not confirm it.

If an ANA result is positive, it is usual to test for the specific antigen. Anti-DNA antibodies bind to double-stranded DNA and are highly specific (95%) but only moderately sensitive (30%) for SLE. They can be useful in disease monitoring since very high titres are associated with more severe disease, including renal or central nervous system (CNS) involvement, and an increase in antibody titre may precede relapse.

Antibodies to specific 'extractable' nuclear antigens can have higher specificity for certain diagnoses or certain patterns of system involvement, although their sensitivity is low (Box 25.8). They are useful in the

25.6 Conditions associated with a positive rheumatoid factor

Disease	Frequency (%)
Rheumatoid arthritis with nodules and extra-articular manifestations	100
Rheumatoid arthritis (overall)	70
Sjögren's syndrome	90
Mixed essential cryoglobulinaemia	90
Primary biliary cirrhosis	50
Subacute bacterial endocarditis	40
Systemic lupus erythematosus	30
Tuberculosis	15
Old age (> 65 yrs)	20

N.B. Normal healthy people can be seropositive.

25.7 Conditions associated with a positive antinuclear antibody

Disease	Approximate frequency
Diseases for which an ANA is useful in diagnosis	
SLE	~100%
Systemic sclerosis	60–80%
Sjögren's syndrome	40–70%
Dermatomyositis or polymyositis	30–80%
Mixed connective tissue disease	100%
Autoimmune hepatitis	Part of diagnostic criteria
Diseases for which an ANA is not useful in diagnosis	
Rheumatoid arthritis	30–50%
Autoimmune thyroid disease	30–50%
Malignancy	Varies widely
Infectious diseases	Varies widely

N.B. 5% of healthy individuals have an ANA titre > 1:80.

25

25.8 Conditions associated with antibodies to extractable nuclear antigens

Antibody	Disease association
Anti-centromere antibody	CREST variant of systemic sclerosis (sensitivity 60%, specificity 98%) Also occasionally found in primary Raynaud's syndrome
Anti-histone antibody	Drug-induced lupus
Anti-Jo-1 (anti-histidyl-tRNA synthetase)	Polymyositis, dermatomyositis or polymyositis-systemic sclerosis overlap (20–30%). Particularly associated with interstitial lung disease
Anti-La antibody (anti-SS-B)	Sjögren's syndrome SLE (20–60%)
Anti-ribonucleoprotein antibody (anti-RNP)	Mixed connective tissue disease SLE, usually in conjunction with anti-Sm antibodies
Anti-Ro antibody (anti-SS-A)	SLE (35–60%): associated with photosensitivity, thrombocytopenia and subacute cutaneous lupus Maternal anti-Ro antibodies associated with neonatal lupus and congenital heart block Sjögren's syndrome (40–80%)
Anti-RNA polymerase I	Rapidly progressive diffuse systemic sclerosis
Anti-Smith antibody (Anti-Sm)	Very specific for SLE (15–30%); associated with renal disease
Anti-topoisomerase I antibody (Anti-Scl-70)	Diffuse systemic sclerosis: associated with more severe organ involvement, including pulmonary fibrosis

evaluation of SLE and other connective tissue diseases and can give clues to the underlying diagnosis, especially when combined with clinical findings. For example, antibodies to Sm occur in 10% of Caucasian and 30% of black and Chinese patients with SLE. They have high diagnostic specificity and are associated with renal disease. Antibodies to Ro occur in SLE and in Sjögren's syndrome (in association with anti-La antibodies), and are associated with a high frequency of photosensitive rashes and risk of congenital heart block. Antibodies to ribonuclear protein (RNP) occur in SLE and also in mixed connective tissue disease, where features of lupus, myositis and systemic sclerosis coexist. Anti-topoisomerase 1 (also termed Scl-70) antibodies are specific for diffuse systemic sclerosis, whereas anti-centromere antibodies are more specific for limited systemic sclerosis.

Antineutrophil cytoplasmic antibodies (ANCA)

ANCA are IgG antibodies to the cytoplasmic constituents of granulocytes and are useful in the diagnosis of suspected systemic vasculitis. Two common patterns are described by immunofluorescence: cytoplasmic fluorescence (c-ANCA) and perinuclear fluorescence

(p-ANCA). c-ANCA are associated with antibodies to proteinase-3 (PR3), and occur in > 90% of patients with Wegener's granulomatosis with renal involvement. p-ANCA are associated with antibodies to other cytoplasmic enzymes, particularly myeloperoxidase (MPO), lactoferrin and elastase. A positive p-ANCA alone is a non-specific finding but, if due to MPO antibodies, is associated with microscopic polyarteritis and Churg–Strauss vasculitis. Atypical p-ANCA, which is not due to anti-myeloperoxidase antibodies, are commonly found in patients with ulcerative colitis and autoimmune liver disease but are not of diagnostic or prognostic significance. Serial measurement of anti-PR3 or anti-MPO antibodies may be useful for disease monitoring. Although ANCA are useful, they are not specific for vasculitis and may be found in malignancy, infection (bacterial and HIV), inflammatory bowel disease, rheumatoid arthritis, lupus and pulmonary fibrosis.

Biochemistry

Routine biochemistry is useful in the assessment of metabolic bone disease, muscle diseases and gout. Serum levels of uric acid are usually raised in gout but a normal level does not exclude the diagnosis, especially during an acute attack when urate levels temporarily fall. Equally, an elevated serum uric acid does not confirm the diagnosis, since most hyperuricaemic people never develop gout.

Serum creatine kinase (CK) levels are useful in the diagnosis of myopathy or myositis, but the specificity and sensitivity are poor and raised levels may occur in a variety of conditions (Box 25.9).

Several bone diseases, including Paget's disease, renal bone disease and osteomalacia give a characteristic pattern on biochemical testing which can be useful diagnostically (Box 25.10). Other, more specific biochemical markers can reflect levels of bone resorption and bone formation. The best markers of bone resorption are N-telopeptide (NTX) and C-telopeptide (CTX) collagen cross-links, which can be measured in blood or urine samples, or deoxypyridinoline (DPD), which is measured in urine. Bone formation can be assessed by serum alkaline phosphatase (ALP), but this is non-specific and levels can also be raised in liver and kidney disease. Bone-specific alkaline phosphatase (BSAP) and the amino terminal fragment of procollagen (PINP) are more specific markers of bone formation. Measurement of these markers can be useful in patients with unusual presentations and to monitor the response to treatment, especially in osteoporosis.

25.9 Causes of an elevated serum creatine kinase

- Inflammatory myositis ± vasculitis
- Muscular dystrophy
- Motor neuron disease
- Alcohol, drugs
- Trauma, strenuous exercise
- Myocardial infarction*
- Hypothyroidism, metabolic myopathy

*The CK-MB cardiac-specific isoform is disproportionately elevated compared with total CK.

25.10 Biochemical abnormalities in various bone diseases

	Serum calcium	Serum phosphate	Serum alkaline phosphatase	Serum PTH	Serum 25(OH)D
Osteoporosis	N	N	N	N	N or ↓
Paget's disease	N	N	↑↑	N or ↑	N
Renal osteodystrophy	↓	↑↑	↑	↑↑↑	N
Vitamin D-deficient osteomalacia	N or ↓	N or ↓	↑↑	↑↑	↓
Hypo-phosphataemic rickets	N	↓↓↓	↑↑	N	N

N = normal.

Tissue sampling

Bone biopsy is helpful in the differential diagnosis of bone diseases when less invasive tests have proved inconclusive. If a systemic disease is suspected, the biopsy should be taken from the iliac crest using a large diameter (8 mm) trephine needle under local anaesthetic. For focal lesions, the biopsy should be taken under X-ray guidance or at open surgery, from an affected site. If osteomalacia is suspected, the sample should be processed without decalcification.

Synovial biopsy may be required in patients with chronic inflammatory monoarthritis or tenosynovitis to identify specific causes such as chronic mycobacterial infection or pigmented villonodular synovitis (p. 1129). It may be obtained arthroscopically or using ultrasound guidance under local anaesthetic.

Muscle biopsy is useful in the investigation of myopathy, myositis and systemic vasculitis. It is usually taken from the quadriceps or deltoid under local anaesthetic through a small skin incision. Immunohistochemical staining, together with plain histology, gives information on primary and secondary muscle and neuromuscular disease, as well as some forms of systemic vasculitis. Repeat biopsy can be useful for monitoring treatment response.

Electromyography

Electromyography (EMG, p. 1142) is used in the investigation of suspected myopathy or myositis. In inflammatory polymyositis, it may show a diagnostic triad of:

- spontaneous fibrillation
- short-duration action potentials in a polyphasic disorganised outline
- repetitive bouts of high-voltage oscillations produced by needle contact with diseased muscle.

PRESENTING PROBLEMS IN MUSCULOSKELETAL DISEASE

Pain in a single joint

Acute inflammatory monoarthritis

This is most commonly due to crystals or sepsis. Other causes are listed in Box 25.11. Acute monoarthritis can be the presentation of what subsequently evolves into oligo- or polyarthritis. Consideration of the following suggests the most likely diagnosis:

- *Age and gender of the patient.* Reactive arthritis is the most common cause in young men; gout typically presents in middle-aged men; pseudogout mainly targets older women.
- *Joint involved.* Classic target sites include the first metatarsophalangeal (MTP) joint (gout); the big toe interphalangeal joint (reactive/psoriatic arthritis); the elbow and ankle (haemarthrosis, seronegative spondyloarthritis); the wrist and shoulder (pseudogout); and finger joints (psoriasis, plant thorn synovitis). The knee can be affected in almost any disease.
- *Speed of onset.* Crystal synovitis develops very rapidly, often reaching maximum severity with extreme pain within just 6–12 hours, whereas sepsis is more subacute and continues to progress until treated.
- *Periarticular inflammation.* Synovitis with soft tissue swelling and erythema is a classic feature of sepsis and crystals, but may also occur with seronegative spondyloarthritis and erythema nodosum. Haemarthrosis can cause a very tense effusion, often splinting the joint in its loose-pack position, but there is no surrounding swelling or skin change. The combination of small joint synovitis and adjacent periarticular swelling in a digit ('dactylitis') is characteristic of psoriasis (fingers, toes) or reactive arthritis (toes).
- *Features preceding the onset of pain.* These include dysentery or new sexual contact preceding reactive arthritis; intercurrent illness or surgery triggering crystal synovitis; clinical features or a family history of psoriasis; and streptococcal sore throat triggering erythema nodosum.

25.11 Principal causes of acute monoarthritis in a previously normal joint

- Septic arthritis*
- Crystal synovitis: gout, pseudogout
- Monoarticular presentation of oligo- or polyarthritis
    Reactive, psoriatic or other seronegative spondarthritis
    Erythema nodosum
    Rheumatoid arthritis
    Juvenile idiopathic arthritis*
- Trauma: especially if associated with haemarthrosis
- Haemarthrosis associated with clotting abnormality
- Foreign body reaction (e.g. plant thorn)

*In children, sepsis and juvenile idiopathic arthritis are the most common causes, but osteomyelitis and leukaemia also present with monoarthritis.

25.12 Common causes of acute arthritis in a previously abnormal joint

Damaged joint

- Pseudogout in association with osteoarthritis
- Bone pathology
    Secondary avascular necrosis
    Subchondral collapse or fracture
- Cartilage damage
    Fibrocartilage tear, cartilage debris
- Haemarthrosis
- Septic arthritis

Existing inflammatory disease (with or without damage)

- Septic arthritis
- Exacerbation of underlying disease

25.13 Causes of chronic single site synovitis

- Foreign body (e.g. plant thorn)
- Infection, including tuberculosis, fungi
- Chronic sarcoidosis (p. 708)
- Enteropathic arthritis (mainly Crohn's)
- Amyloidosis
- Pigmented villonodular synovitis
- Synovial chondromatosis
- Synovial sarcoma
- Monoarticular presentation of oligo-/polyarticular disease
    Rheumatoid arthritis
    Seronegative spondarthritis
    Juvenile idiopathic arthritis

The differential diagnosis changes when acute monoarthritis occurs in a joint that is already abnormal (Box 25.12). For example, an acute flare of inflammation in a single joint in a patient with known RA suggests sepsis, as RA has a strong negative association with crystal deposition. Investigation of acute monoarthritis varies depending on the presentation, but joint aspiration is required if there is a possibility of sepsis or crystals.

Chronic inflammatory monoarthritis

There are various causes of chronic inflammatory monoarthritis that persists for more than 6 weeks (Box 25.13). The knee is the most common site but almost any joint may be involved. If no cause is apparent by 6 months, or if there are radiographic signs of osteopenia, erosion or periostitis, synovial biopsy is usually undertaken to exclude chronic infection or rare causes that have specific treatments. Retrospective studies suggest that about 25% of cases evolve to OA and about 25% to RA but 30% remain undiagnosed.

Oligoarthritis

Oligoarthritis affects 2–4 joints or joint groups (the wrist has many joints but counts as a single site). By far the most common cause is OA, which causes non-inflammatory symptoms that usually affect just one or a few sites at any one time, even though asymptomatic multiple joint OA may be apparent on examination.

Acute or subacute inflammatory oligoarthritis that targets the lower limbs in an asymmetric pattern is usually

25.14 Causes of inflammatory oligoarthritis

- Seronegative spondyloarthritis
    Reactive arthritis
    Psoriatic arthritis
    Ankylosing spondylitis
    Enteropathic arthritis
- Erythema nodosum
- Juvenile idiopathic arthritis
- Oligoarticular presentation of polyarthritis
- Infection, including
    Infective endocarditis
    Neisseria
    Mycobacteria

due to seronegative spondyloarthritis (Box 25.14). Sequential joint involvement that ascends a limb—for example, a midfoot, followed by the ankle and then the knee—is almost always due to sepsis.

Polyarthritis

Polyarthritis is defined as the involvement of five or more joints or joint groups. Features helpful in determining the cause (Box 25.15) are:
- symmetry
- involvement of the upper and/or lower limbs
- involvement of large and/or small joints
- periarticular involvement
- extra-articular features (Box 25.16).

25.15 Causes of polyarthritis

Cause	Characteristics
Non-inflammatory	
Generalised osteoarthritis	Very common; symmetrical, small and large joints with only a few symptomatic at any one time, Heberden's nodes
Haemochromatosis (p. 959)	Rare; small and large joints
Acromegaly (p. 790)	Rare; mainly large joints, spine
Inflammatory	
Viral arthritis	Very acute, self-limiting
Rheumatoid arthritis	Symmetrical, small and large joints, upper and lower limbs
Seronegative spondyloarthritis (psoriasis, reactive, ankylosing spondylitis, enteropathic arthropathy)	Asymmetrical, large > small joints, lower > upper limbs, spondylitis
Systemic lupus erythematosus (SLE)	Symmetrical, small > large joints, joint damage uncommon
Chronic gout	Distal > proximal joints, preceded by acute attacks
Juvenile idiopathic arthritis	Symmetrical, small and large joints, upper and lower limbs
Chronic sarcoidosis	Symmetrical, small and large joints
Systemic sclerosis and polymyositis	Rare; small and large joints
Hypertrophic osteoarthropathy	Rare; large > small joints, clubbing

25.16 Extra-articular features of inflammatory arthritis

Clinical feature	Disease association
Skin, nails and mucous membranes	
Psoriasis, nail pitting and dystrophy	Psoriatic arthritis
Raynaud's phenomenon	SLE, systemic sclerosis
Photosensitivity	SLE
Livedo reticularis	SLE
Splinter haemorrhages, nail-fold infarcts	Vasculitis
Oral ulcers	SLE, reactive arthritis, Behçet's syndrome
Large nodules (mainly extensor surfaces)	RA, gout
Clubbing	Enteropathic arthritis, metastatic lung cancer, endocarditis
Eyes	
Uveitis	Seronegative spondyloarthritis
Conjunctivitis	Reactive arthritis
Episcleritis, scleritis	RA, vasculitis
Heart, lungs	
Pleuro-pericarditis	SLE, RA
Fibrosing alveolitis	RA, SLE, other connective tissue disease
Abdominal organs	
Hepatosplenomegaly	RA, SLE
Haematuria, proteinuria	SLE, vasculitis, systemic sclerosis
Urethritis	Reactive arthritis
Fever, lymphadenopathy	Infection, systemic juvenile idiopathic arthritis

Many viral infections can cause arthralgia (joint pain without abnormal examination findings), and an acute symmetrical inflammatory polyarthritis affecting small and large joints of upper and lower limbs that is usually self-limiting within 6 weeks. They include parvovirus, hepatitis B and C, mumps, rubella, chickenpox and infectious mononucleosis. The rapidity of onset, the presence of fever and the characteristic rash usually suggest the diagnosis. Arthritis usually precedes jaundice from hepatitis B. Rubella arthritis mainly affects girls and women, occurring 1–7 days after the rash or 2–6 weeks after vaccination. Rubella is exceptional in that although the symmetrical polyarthritis settles, oligoarthritis may persist for some months.

Polyarthritis that persists for more than 6 weeks is unlikely to be viral (see Box 25.15). A definitive diagnosis may initially be difficult but often becomes clearer as characteristic features develop. However, certain patterns are characteristic and may be present at or soon after presentation (Fig. 25.9). RA is by far the most common cause of chronic inflammatory, symmetrical polyarthritis affecting small and large joints of upper and lower limbs. Tenosynovitis and bursitis are the main periarticular manifestations. Marked asymmetry, lower limb predominance and greater involvement of large joints are all more characteristic of seronegative spondyloarthritis (p. 1092). Systemic lupus erythematosus (SLE) usually causes arthralgia and tenosynovitis rather than synovitis (p. 1107). Chronic polyarthritis due to gout is invariably preceded by a long history of acute attacks. Other causes of polyarthritis are rare.

A detailed history and examination often reveal the likely diagnosis and direct investigation. For inflammatory polyarthritis present for less than 6 weeks, an FBC, liver

25

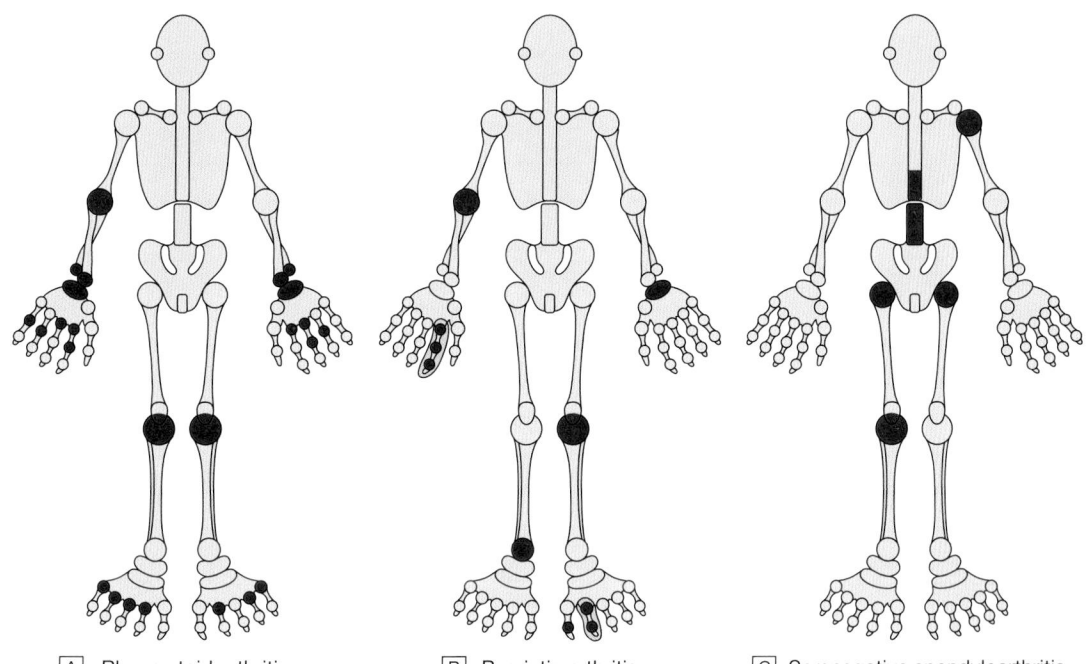

| A | Rheumatoid arthritis | B | Psoriatic arthritis | C | Seronegative spondyloarthritis |

Fig. 25.9 Contrasting patterns of involvement in polyarthritis. A Rheumatoid arthritis (symmetrical, small and large joints, upper and lower limbs). B Seronegative psoriatic arthritis (asymmetrical, large > small joints, associated periarticular inflammation giving dactylitis). C Seronegative spondyloarthritis (axial involvement, large > small joints, asymmetrical).

function tests and viral serology are useful. For early persistent polyarthritis of indeterminate cause, initial investigation should also include an ESR, CRP, anti-CCP, RF and anti-nuclear antibodies, and X-rays of hands and feet.

Fracture

The presentation is with localised bone pain usually occurring after trauma, which is worsened by movement of the affected limb or region. Fractures are divisible into three subtypes:

- *Fragility fractures* result from relatively minor trauma and are typical of osteoporosis. With vertebral fractures, the precipitating factor is often bending or lifting but with long bone fractures the trigger is usually a fall.
- *Pathological fractures* occur in bone that is structurally abnormal, such as in Paget's disease, osteomalacia, bone metastases and parathyroid bone disease. Like fragility fractures, they can occur spontaneously or follow minor trauma.
- *High-energy fractures* result from major trauma and can affect normal bones. The same is true of *stress (fatigue) fractures* in healthy individuals such as athletes and military recruits who are exposed to repetitive trauma.

The main differential diagnosis is soft tissue injury, but fracture should be suspected when there is marked pain and swelling, abnormal movement of the affected limb, crepitus or deformity. Femoral neck fractures typically produce a shortened, externally rotated leg that is painful to move. Presentation of vertebral fractures is highly variable. Some cause acute severe back pain with radiation to the anterior chest or abdominal wall. Others cause few symptoms and present insidiously with intermittent back pain and height loss. Osteoporotic rib fractures are characterised by aggravation of the pain by movement, local tenderness and pain on springing the rib cage.

Investigations include X-rays of the affected bone which should be taken in at least two planes and examined for discontinuity of the cortical outline (Box 25.17). If these are normal but clinical suspicion remains high, other imaging techniques may be used such as radioisotope bone scans for fatigue fractures or scaphoid fractures, and CT or MRI scans for fractures of the pelvis or spine. CT or MRI can also help differentiate pathological fractures of the spine due to tumour from fractures due to osteoporosis.

Treatment includes adequate pain relief with opiates, if necessary, reduction of the fracture to restore normal anatomy, and immobilisation to promote healing, either by plaster cast or by internal fixation. Femoral neck fractures present a special management problem since non-union and avascular necrosis are common complications. This is especially true with intracapsular hip fractures, and these require surgical replacement of the femoral head with a prosthesis.

Rehabilitation is as important as reduction and fixation in determining outcome. A supervised exercise programme is required to avoid muscle-wasting and joint stiffness which impair long-term mobility, especially in old age. Older patients with hip fracture also benefit from nutritional supplementation. Patients with high-energy and fatigue fractures generally require no further investigation or treatment once the fracture has healed. Patients with fragility fractures, vertebral fractures and pathological fractures should be investigated for secondary causes (p. 1117).

Bone pain without fracture

Causes of this are shown in Box 25.18. It is often difficult to differentiate bone pain from joint or periarticular pain, but in the absence of fracture, bone pain is characteristically:

- localised to the affected bone, rather than the joint
- present at rest and worse at night
- not reproduced by joint movement

Relentlessly progressive pain suggests a destructive disease like malignancy or chronic infection. Malignancy may be associated with weight loss, fatigue and symptoms relating to the primary site. Pain experienced over a wider area associated with deformity suggests Paget's disease (p. 1124). Osteomalacia (p. 1121) is associated with bone tenderness and limb girdle weakness. Pain from osteonecrosis is initially bony and progressive but may change its characteristics as the adjacent joint cartilage collapses, with pain worse on usage or weight-bearing, with or without radiation, (mainly hips, shoulders or elbows). Investigation of bone pain includes plain X-rays of the symptomatic site, MRI, or radioisotope bone scan and other tests directed by the presumptive diagnosis.

25.18 Causes of bone pain without fracture

- Metastatic bone disease or primary bone tumour
- Paget's disease
- Osteomalacia
- Chronic infection (osteomyelitis)
- Osteonecrosis

Regional periarticular pain

Single regional pain

This usually results from an over-usage strain or injury affecting a periarticular structure. The patient can often identify an obvious provoking event or injury. The pain is non-progressive and reproduced by just one or a few movements; the patient is otherwise well. Examination reveals localised periarticular tenderness without signs of florid inflammation, and the pain may be reproduced by resisted active movement or by stress testing the

25.17 How to investigate a suspected fracture

- Order X-rays in two projections at right angles to one another
- Include the whole bone and the joints at either end (this may reveal an additional unsuspected fracture)
- Check for evidence of displacement
- Check for a break in the cortex
- In suspected vertebral fracture, check for depression of the end-plate
- If clinical suspicion is high but no fracture is seen, consider further imaging (e.g. bone scan, CT, MRI)

involved structure. Predisposing factors include increasing age, obesity, generalised hypermobility, and occupational and recreational usage.

Muscle injuries usually settle within days, whereas fibrous structures such as tendons and ligaments can take weeks or months to return to normal. The diagnosis is usually made clinically, although imaging, especially ultrasound and MRI, may confirm the anatomical structure involved and the extent of injury. Management is aimed towards:

- identifying and avoiding predisposing or adverse mechanical factors if possible
- pain relief (topical and/or oral analgesics, local injection for severe pain)
- appropriate exercise and rehabilitation to restore movement and function.

Surgery is only occasionally required for very resistant or disabling lesions.

Shoulder pain

Shoulder pain is a common complaint in both genders over the age of 40, principally due to rotator cuff lesions (Box 25.19). Varying pain patterns of common lesions are shown in Figure 25.10.

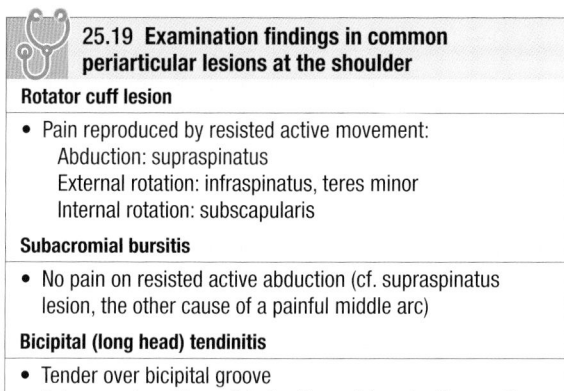

25.19 Examination findings in common periarticular lesions at the shoulder

Rotator cuff lesion

- Pain reproduced by resisted active movement:
  Abduction: supraspinatus
  External rotation: infraspinatus, teres minor
  Internal rotation: subscapularis

Subacromial bursitis

- No pain on resisted active abduction (cf. supraspinatus lesion, the other cause of a painful middle arc)

Bicipital (long head) tendinitis

- Tender over bicipital groove
- Pain reproduced by resisted active wrist supination or elbow flexion

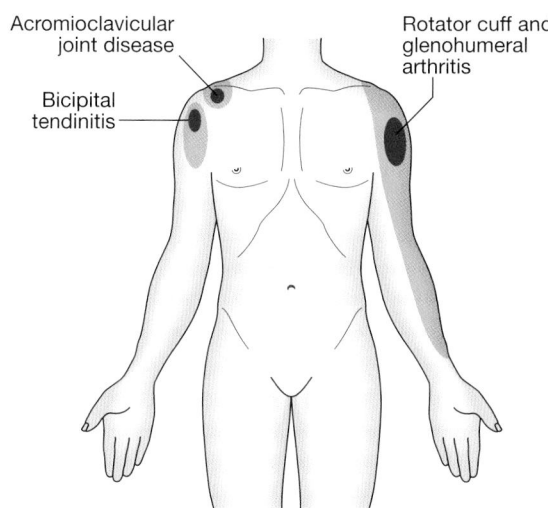

Fig. 25.10 Pain patterns around the shoulder. The dark shading indicates sites of maximum pain.

Labels on figure:
Acromioclavicular joint disease
Bicipital tendinitis
Rotator cuff and glenohumeral arthritis

Adhesive capsulitis ('frozen shoulder') presents with upper arm pain that progresses over 4–10 weeks before subsiding over a similar time course. Glenohumeral restriction is present from the outset but progresses to its maximum as the pain settles. In the early phase, there is marked anterior joint/capsular tenderness and stress pain in a capsular pattern; later there is painless restriction, often of all movements. Frozen shoulder is more common in diabetes mellitus, and may be triggered by a rotator cuff tear, local trauma, myocardial infarction or hemiplegia. Treatment in the early stage is with analgesia, intra- and extracapsular steroid injection, and regular 'pendulum' exercises of the arm to prevent the capsule from over-tightening. Mobilising and strengthening exercises are the sole treatment in the painless 'frozen' stage. The natural history is for slow but complete recovery, sometimes taking up to 2 years.

Elbow pain

Pain from the three joint compartments is felt maximally at the elbow, close to its origin, with occasional radiation down the forearm. Lateral epicondylitis is the most common periarticular lesion (Box 25.20). Olecranon bursitis can follow local repetitive trauma but infection, gout and RA may also be responsible.

25.20 Periarticular lesions presenting as elbow pain

Lesion	Pain	Examination findings
Tennis elbow	Lateral epicondyle Radiation to extensor forearm	Tender over epicondyle Pain reproduced by resisted active wrist extension
Golfer's elbow	Medial epicondyle Radiation to flexor forearm	Tender over epicondyle Pain reproduced by resisted active wrist flexion
Olecranon bursitis	Olecranon	Fluctuant tender swelling over olecranon

Hand and wrist pain

Pain from hand or wrist joints is well localised to the affected joint, except for pain from the first carpometacarpal joint, commonly targeted by OA which, although maximal at the thumb base, often radiates down the thumb and back over the radial wrist. Non-articular causes of hand pain include:

- tenosynovitis: flexor or extensor (pain and swelling, with or without fine crepitus on volar or extensor aspect)
- median nerve compression (carpal tunnel syndrome, p. 1228)
- Raynaud's phenomenon (p. 601)
- C8/T1 radiculopathy
- algodystrophy (reflex sympathetic dystrophy, p. 1125).

Trigger finger results from stenosing tenosynovitis in the flexor tendon sheath, with intermittent locking of the finger in flexion. A local steroid injection often relieves the problem and surgical decompression is only occasionally required.

De Quervain's tenosynovitis involves the tendon sheaths of abductor pollicis longus and extensor pollicis brevis, and produces pain maximal over the radial aspect of the distal forearm and wrist. There is tenderness (with or without warmth, linear swelling and fine crepitus) over the distal radius and marked pain on forced ulnar deviation of the wrist with the thumb held across the patient's palm (Finkelstein's sign). It is usually caused by over-usage.

Dupuytren's contracture results from fibrosis and contracture of the superficial palmar fascia. The patient is unable to extend the fingers fully and there is puckering of the skin with palpable nodules. The ring and little fingers are usually the first and worst affected. It is usually painless and the main symptoms relate to the curled fingers becoming snagged in pockets. It is age-related and usually bilateral, strongly predominates in men, and is often familial with dominant inheritance. It can be associated with plantar fibromatosis, Peyronie's disease, alcohol misuse and chronic vibration injury. It is very slowly progressive. Often no treatment is required, but fasciotomy may be necessary if symptoms are troublesome.

Hip pain

Pain from the hip joint is usually maximal deep in the anterior groin, with variable radiation to the buttock, anterolateral thigh, knee or shin (Fig. 25.11). Trochanteric bursitis is the most common periarticular lesion (Box 25.21), typically affecting obese women, and occurring in isolation or secondary to an abnormal gait, such as in hip or knee OA.

Hip pain may be referred from other structures. Back pain commonly radiates to the buttock and posterior thigh but the site of maximal pain is close to the spine or pelvic brim. Root entrapment can cause pain in the lateral thigh (T12–L1) or the inguinal region and lateral thigh (L2–4) but is worsened by coughing and straining

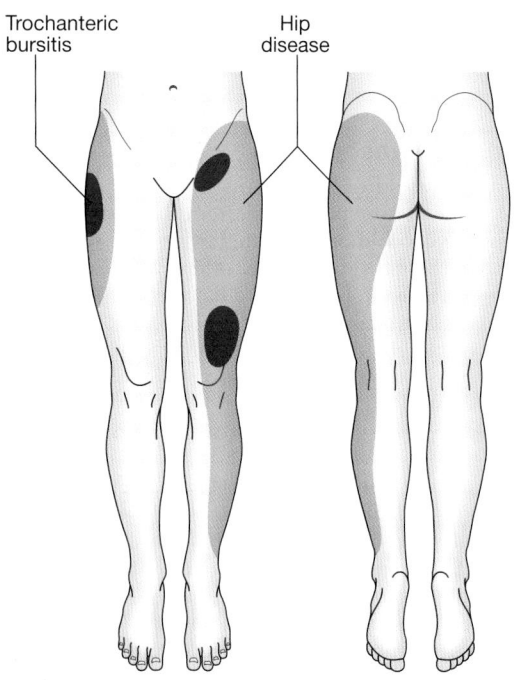

Trochanteric bursitis | Hip disease

Fig. 25.11 Pain patterns of hip disease and trochanteric bursitis. The dark shading indicates sites of maximum pain.

25.21 Periarticular lesions at the hip

Lesion	Pain	Examination findings
Trochanteric bursitis	Upper lateral thigh, worse on lying on that side at night	Tender over greater trochanter
Gluteal enthesopathy	Upper lateral thigh, worse on lying on that side at night	Tender over greater trochanter Pain reproduced by resisted active hip abduction
Adductor tendinitis	Upper inner thigh Usually clearly sports-related	Tender over adductor origin/tendon/muscle Pain reproduced by resisted active hip adduction
Ischiogluteal bursitis	Buttock, worse on sitting	Tender over ischial prominence
Iliopectineal bursitis	Anterior groin	Tender (± fluctuant swelling) lateral to femoral pulse, not worsened by internal rotation of hip (cf. hip pain)

more than by movement and is often accompanied by sensory disturbance. A psoas abscess, retroperitoneal haemorrhage or pelvic inflammation can cause inguinal and lateral thigh pain that is aggravated by resisted hip flexion. Sacroiliac pain is maximal in the buttock, with radiation down the posterior thigh, worse on standing on that leg.

Knee pain

Pain arising from the patello-femoral or medial and lateral tibio-femoral compartments is anterior and well localised to the involved compartment. Patello-femoral pain is worse going up and down stairs or inclines. Locking—sudden painful inability to extend fully that often spontaneously unlocks, followed by aching—is usually due to mechanical derangement such as a meniscal tear or osteochondritis dissecans. Referred pain from the hip may present at the knee but is more diffuse and often relieved by rubbing; on examination, it is reproduced by hip not knee movement.

Pain from periarticular lesions is well localised to the involved structure (Box 25.22). Inflammation of any of the three bursae around the patella usually results from repetitive occupational kneeling, but also infection and gout.

Anterior knee pain syndrome is common, especially in adolescent girls. The pain has patello-femoral characteristics and is often aggravated by sports. In a small proportion, there is evidence of non-progressive fibrillation of the retropatellar cartilage ('chondromalacia patellae'). It is usually self-limiting and treatment is conservative.

Anterior tibial compartment syndrome is characterised by severe pain in the front of the lower leg, aggravated by exercise and relieved by rest. Symptoms result from fascial compression of the muscles in the anterior tibial compartment and may be associated with foot drop. Treatment is urgent surgical decompression.

25.22 Periarticular lesions at the knee

Lesion	Pain	Examination findings
Pre-patellar bursitis	Anterior patella	Tender fluctuant swelling in front of patella
Superficial and deep infrapatellar bursitis	Anterior knee, inferior to patella	Tender fluctuant swelling in front of (superficial) or behind (deep) patella tendon
Anserine bursitis	Upper medial tibia	Tenderness (± warmth, swelling) over upper medial tibia
Inferior medial collateral ligament enthesopathy	Upper medial tibia	Localised tenderness of upper medial tibia. Pain reproduced by valgus stress on mildly flexed knee
Popliteal ('Baker's') cyst	Popliteal fossa	Tender swelling of popliteal fossa, usually reducible by massage with knee in mid-flexion
Patella tendon enthesopathy (Osgood–Schlatter disease)	Anterior upper tibia. Mainly energetic adolescents	Tenderness and firm swelling of tibial tubercle. Pain on resisted active knee extension

Foot and ankle pain

Pain from the ankle joint is felt anteriorly between the two malleoli and is worse on standing or walking. Subtalar pain is mainly posterior between the malleoli and is particularly aggravated by walking on uneven surfaces, requiring eversion/inversion. Periarticular lesions that cause hindfoot pain are listed in Box 25.23.

25.23 Periarticular lesions causing hindfoot pain

Lesion	Pain	Examination findings
Plantar fasciitis	Under heel, worse on standing and walking	Tender under distal calcaneus/plantar fascia insertion site
Subcalcaneal bursitis	Under heel, worse on standing and walking	Tender under middle of calcaneus
Achilles tendinitis	Localised to tendon	Tender on squeezing tendon, ± swelling of tendon. Pain reproduced by standing on toes or resisted plantar flexion
Achilles enthesopathy	Localised to tendon insertion	Tender over insertion site, ± firm swelling. Pain reproduced by standing on toes or resisted plantar flexion
Retro-Achilles bursitis	Posterior heel	Tenderness and soft swelling posterior to tendon
Pre-Achilles bursitis	Posterior heel	Tenderness and fluctuant swelling anterior to tendon

Midtarsal disease causes pain in the 'bootlace' area, mainly during the late stance and toe-off phase of walking. Loss of the normal arches—pes planus ('flat foot')—may cause pain in the mid-sole. This is often congenital, but acquired causes include trauma, constitutional hyper-mobility, RA and neuropathic arthropathy. Medial arch supports in well-fitting shoes and/or intrinsic muscle-strengthening exercises usually relieve symptoms, but rigid splints may be required for hyperpronated feet, provided the foot is not rigid from fusion of the tarsal bones (tarsal coalition).

MTP joint pain is felt below the metatarsal heads (metatarsalgia) and is often described as 'like walking on marbles'. Hallux valgus deformity with secondary bursitis (bunions) and OA of the first MTP joint is often associated with flattening of the transverse metatarsal arch and is a common cause of forefoot pain. It predominates in women as a consequence of wearing narrow high-heeled shoes. Severe restriction of first MTP joint extension (hallux rigidus), usually due to OA, may cause marked pain during attempted toe-off. For both hallux problems, conservative treatment and appropriate footwear usually suffice, although surgery is required in a minority.

Pes cavus ('claw foot') is characterised by a high medial arch, secondary clawing of toes and metatarsal callosities. It can be caused by neurological disorders such as Friedreich's ataxia, spina bifida or poliomyelitis. Associated pain is often helped by medial arch supports and metatarsal insoles, and fasciotomy or osteotomy is rarely indicated.

Morton's neuroma is an entrapment neuropathy of the interdigital nerves, mostly between the third and fourth metatarsal heads in middle-aged women with ill-fitting shoes. The neuralgic, lancinating pain occurs mainly when the patient is wearing shoes and may associate with local sensory loss and a palpable tender swelling between the metatarsal heads. Footwear adjustment, with or without a local corticosteroid injection, is often sufficient but excision is occasionally required.

Multiple regional pain

Widespread pain localised to the soft tissues is most commonly due to fibromyalgia (p. 1105). Another important cause is joint hypermobility. This tends to be more common in women and in Afro-Caribbeans, and declines with age. The 10% of adults at the lax end of the spectrum of joint mobility are predisposed to ligament strain, traumatic enthesopathy, mechanical back pain, arthralgia and dislocation (mainly glenohumeral). For epidemiological purposes, generalised hypermobility is recognised in adults by a modified Beighton score (Box 25.24). Within this 10%

25.24 Modified Beighton score

- Extend little finger > 90° — (1 point each side)
- Bring thumb back parallel to/touching forearm — (1 point each side)
- Extend elbow > 10° — (1 point each side)
- Extend knee > 10° — (1 point each side)
- Touch floor with flat of hands, legs straight — (1 point)

Hypermobile = 6 or more out of a possible 9 points for epidemiological studies, or 4 or more (with arthralgia in four or more joints) for clinical diagnosis of the benign joint hypermobility syndrome.

25

25

25.25 Causes of chronic multiple regional pain without arthritis

- Fibromyalgia (p. 1105)
- Joint hypermobility
- Seronegative spondyloarthritis (p. 1092)
- Osteomalacia (p. 1121)
- Polymyalgia rheumatica (p. 1115)
- Polymyositis (p. 1111)
- Diffuse idiopathic skeletal hyperostosis (DISH, p. 1129)
- Endocrine disease
  Primary hyperparathyroidism (p. 766)
  Hypothyroidism (p. 741)
  Addison's disease (p. 775)
- Parkinson's disease (p. 1199)
- Drugs, e.g. retinoids (p. 1264), statins (p. 455)

25.26 Specific causes of low back pain

- Spondylolysis (p. 1128)
- Spondylolisthesis (p. 1128)
- Spinal stenosis
- Prolapsed intervertebral disc
- Arachnoiditis
- Scheuermann's disease (p. 1129)
- Vertebral fracture (p. 1068)

are individuals with disease-associated hypermobility, such as in Marfan's syndrome (p. 602), Ehlers–Danlos syndrome (p. 1128) and acromegaly. For clinical purposes, the benign joint hypermobility syndrome (BJHS) has been defined and validated as a Beighton score of 4/9 or more (currently or historically) plus arthralgia for longer than 3 months in four or more joints. Other causes of multiple regional pain without arthropathy are shown in Box 25.25.

Back and neck pain

Low back pain

Back pain affects 60–80% of people at some time in their lives. Although the prevalence has not increased, reported disability from back pain has increased significantly in the last 30 years. In Western countries, back pain is the most common cause of sickness-related work absence, and in the UK 7% of adults consult their GP each year with back pain.

Only a small number of patients with back pain have a clear diagnosis. All structures in the spinal column, other than cartilage, are pain-sensitive. Although the exact mechanism of pain is often unclear, some specific causes are recognised (Box 25.26). The main purpose of clinical assessment is to identify the small number who have a serious spinal disorder. This should address the questions in Figure 25.12.

Mechanical pain

Mechanical pain accounts for more than 90% of episodes, usually affecting patients aged 20–55 years. The onset is often acute and associated with lifting or bending. It is related to activity and is generally relieved by rest (Box 25.27). It is usually confined to the lumbosacral region, buttock or thigh, is asymmetrical, and does not radiate beyond the knee (this implies nerve root irritation). On examination, there may be asymmetric local paraspinal muscle spasm and tenderness, and painful restriction of some but not all movements. Back pain precipitated by extension may relate to facet joint hypertrophy or spinal stenosis. Low back pain is more common in heavy

25.27 Features of simple mechanical low back pain

- Pain varies with physical activity (improved with rest)
- Sudden onset, precipitated by lifting or bending
- Recurrent episodes
- Pain limited to back or upper leg
- No clear-cut nerve root distribution
- No systemic features
- Prognosis good (90% recovery at 6 wks)

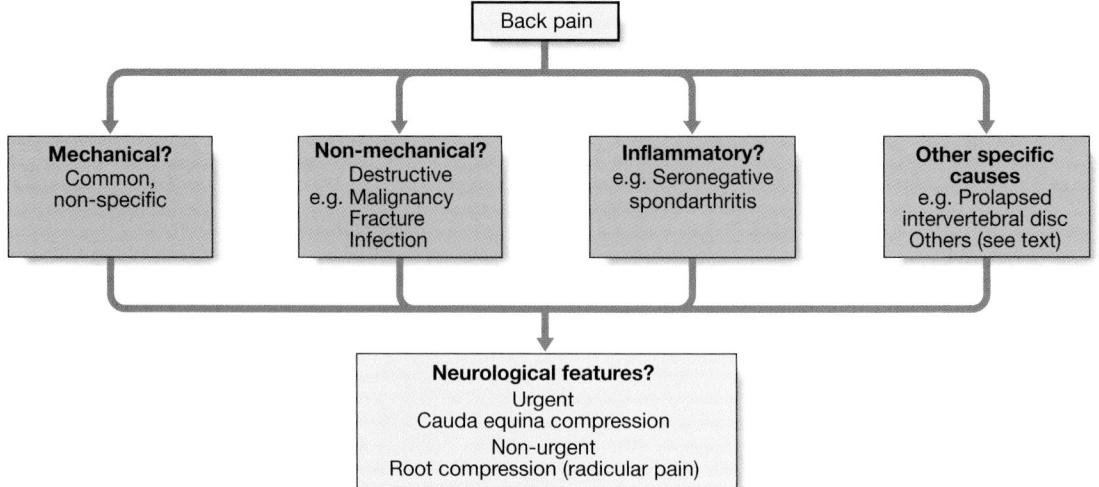

Fig. 25.12 Initial triage assessment of back pain.

manual workers, particularly those in occupations that involve heavy lifting and twisting. Psychological factors (e.g. job dissatisfaction, depression, anxiety) are important risk factors for both acute back pain and the transition to chronic pain and disability.

Non-mechanical pain

This is constant and often progressive, and has little variation in intensity or with activity. Anorexia, dyspepsia, change in bowel habit, prostatism or abnormal vaginal bleeding may indicate specific malignancies. Other 'red flags' for possible serious spinal pathology are indicated in Box 25.28. If there is evidence of a spinal cord or cauda equina lesion (Box 25.29), urgent neurosurgical assessment is required.

Inflammatory pain

Inflammatory pain due to spondylitis ('inflamed vertebrae/spine') has a more gradual onset and often occurs before the age of 30. It is usually axial, symmetrical and spread over many segments which may include the thoracic region. Pain from sacroiliitis is maximal in the buttock, with radiation down the posterior thigh. Inflammatory pain associates with marked morning and inactivity stiffness, and improves rather than worsens with activity.

25.28 Red flags for possible spinal pathology

History

- *Age:* presentation < 20 yrs or > 55 yrs
- *Character:* constant, progressive pain unrelieved by rest
- *Location:* thoracic pain
- *Past medical history:* carcinoma, tuberculosis, HIV, systemic corticosteroid use
- *Constitutional:* systemic upset, sweats, weight loss
- *Major trauma*

Examination

- Painful spinal deformity
- Severe/symmetrical spinal deformity
- Saddle anaesthesia
- Progressive neurological signs/muscle-wasting
- Multiple levels of root signs

25.29 Features of radicular pain

Nerve root pain

- Unilateral leg pain worse than low back pain
- Pain radiates beyond knee
- Paraesthesia in same distribution
- Nerve irritation signs (reduced straight leg raising which reproduces leg pain)
- Motor, sensory or reflex signs (limited to one nerve root)
- Prognosis reasonable (50% recovery at 6 wks)

Cauda equina syndrome

- Difficulty with micturition
- Loss of anal sphincter tone or faecal incontinence
- Saddle anaesthesia
- Gait disturbance
- Pain, numbness or weakness affecting one or both legs

Spinal stenosis

Spinal stenosis occurs when there is narrowing of the vertebral canal. The most common presentation is 'pseudoclaudication' with discomfort in the legs on walking that is relieved by rest, bending forwards or walking uphill. Common causes include Paget's disease where enlargement of the vertebrae may encroach on the spinal canal, and spondylosis of the spine where osteophytes can have the same effect. Patients may adopt a characteristic simian posture, with a forward stoop and slight flexion at the hips and knees. Decompression is indicated if mobility or quality of life is significantly impaired.

Prolapsed intervertebral disc

Age-related reductions in proteoglycans within the nucleus pulposus diminish its viscoelasticity, leading to focal damage and disc herniation. These changes occur most frequently at L4 and L5 due to the increased mechanical forces across this area. Most patients have their first episode between the ages of 20 and 30 years. Presentation is with radicular pain (invariably felt below the knee) in combination with evidence of root involvement (sensory deficit, motor weakness, asymmetrical reflexes) and a positive sciatic or femoral stretch test. About 70% of patients improve by 4 weeks. Persistent neurological deficit at 6 weeks is an indication for surgery.

Radicular pain

Radicular (nerve root) pain has a severe, sharp, lancinating quality, radiates down the back of the leg beyond the knee, and is aggravated by coughing, sneezing and straining at stool more than by back movement. On examination, there are signs of lumbar nerve root irritation (see Box 25.29). In contrast, referred pain is usually a dull, deep ache, poorly localised with indistinct boundaries.

Symptoms and signs of compression of multiple nerve roots in the cauda equina are shown in Box 25.29. It is vital to exclude compression of the spinal cord (p. 1223).

Arachnoiditis

Chronic inflammation of nerve root sheaths in the spinal canal can cause severe low back pain, sometimes combined with nerve root symptoms. Arachnoiditis can complicate meningitis or spinal surgery, but most frequently occurs as a late complication of myelography with oil-based contrast agents. No satisfactory treatment is available.

Investigations

Plain X-rays are rarely helpful in acute mechanical back pain unless red flags are present (see Box 25.28). Although advanced lumbar 'spondylosis' frequently accompanies low back pain, there is a poor correlation between pain and X-ray changes. Indeed, by the age of 50, 60% of women and 80% of men have radiographic features of spondylosis. Plain X-rays may be helpful in persistent pain in a young patient to confirm a diagnosis of ankylosing spondylitis, and in an older patient to detect vertebral osteoporotic fracture.

If red flags are present, MRI should be undertaken, even if plain X-rays are normal. CT is inferior to MRI for assessing soft tissue structures and nerves, but is useful for detecting minor abnormalities of bone architecture and in cases where MRI is contraindicated (e.g. pacemaker or metallic clips).

25

A low haemoglobin and raised CRP or ESR suggest inflammation or malignancy. A raised prostate-specific antigen (PSA) may indicate prostatic carcinoma, and raised alkaline phosphatase can occur in patients with bone metastases, osteomalacia and Paget's disease. Myeloma (p. 1041) is associated with a monoclonal band on serum immunoelectrophoresis and the presence of urinary light chains (Bence Jones proteinuria). EMG and nerve conduction studies are occasionally required to confirm and localise nerve root lesions.

Management

Most episodes of mechanical low back pain settle spontaneously with explanation, reassurance and simple analgesics. After 2 days, 30% are better and at 6 weeks 90% have recovered. Recurrences of pain are common, however, and the 10–15% of patients with acute back pain who develop chronic pain consume 85% of back pain resources.

Patient education is paramount and should emphasise that pain does not imply harm to the underlying structures and that exercise is helpful rather than damaging. Regular analgesia and/or non-steroidal anti-inflammatory drugs (NSAIDs) may be required to improve mobility and facilitate exercise. Return to work and normal activity should take place as soon as possible. Bed rest is not helpful and may increase the risk of chronic disability. Referral for physiotherapy or manipulation should be considered if a return to normal activities has not been achieved by 6 weeks. Low-dose tricyclic antidepressant drugs may help pain, sleep and mood.

Other treatment modalities occasionally used include epidural and facet joint injection, traction and lumbar supports. There is currently no evidence to support these (Box 25.30). Surgery is required in less than 1% of patients with low back pain.

EBM 25.30 **Management of low back pain**

'There is a reasonable evidence to support the following:
- Reassure patients (favourable prognosis)
- Advise patients to stay active
- Prescribe medication if necessary (preferably at fixed time intervals)
    Paracetamol
    NSAID
    Consider opioids, muscle relaxants
- Discourage bed rest
- Consider spinal manipulation for pain relief
- Do not advise lumbar supports, back-specific exercises, traction, acupuncture, epidural or facet injections.'

• Koes BW. BMJ 2006; 332:1430–1434.

Neck pain

Neck pain is usually due to mechanical or degenerative problems, although serious spinal disease needs to be excluded using the same principles as for back pain. Most episodes of transient mechanical neck pain are not associated with demonstrable spinal pathology. Other causes of neck pain are listed in Box 25.31.

Pain arising from neck structures is often poorly localised. Pain from upper segments may radiate to the occiput, temple or face, and pain from lower segments to

---

25.31 **Causes of neck pain**

Mechanical

• Postural	• Disc prolapse
• Whiplash injury	• Cervical spondylosis

Inflammatory

• Infections	• RA
• Spondylitis	• Polymyalgia rheumatica
• Juvenile idiopathic arthritis	

Metabolic

• Osteoporosis	• Paget's disease
• Osteomalacia	

Neoplasia

• Metastases	• Lymphoma
• Myeloma	• Intrathecal tumours

Other

• Fibromyalgia	• Torticollis

Referred pain

• Pharynx	• Aortic aneurysm
• Cervical lymph nodes	• Pancoast tumour
• Teeth	• Diaphragm
• Angina pectoris	

---

the scapula, shoulder, arm and occasionally chest wall. Mechanical neck pain is often acute in onset and associated with asymmetrical restriction of neck movements and a history of awkward posture or trauma. Radicular pain may arise from compression from osteophyte or disc prolapse. Most (70%) affect the C6 disc, compressing the C7 root, but 20% affect C5 and compress the C6 root. Massive cervical osteophytes or DISH (p. 1129) occasionally cause dysphagia due to oesophageal indentation.

The principles of investigation and management are identical to those for low back pain. Surgery is only required when there are neurological signs of radiculopathy or progressive cervical myelopathy (p. 1222).

Muscle pain and weakness

Acute muscle weakness can arise from a variety of causes. It is important to distinguish between a subjective feeling of generalised weakness or fatigue, and an objective weakness with loss of muscle power and function. The former is a non-specific manifestation of many diseases, whereas the latter is often a sign of primary muscle disease.

Proximal muscle weakness suggests a proximal myopathy, which typically causes difficulty with standing from a seated position, squatting and lifting overhead. Distal power, such as grip, is usually preserved. The causes of proximal myopathy (Box 25.32) are either inflammatory (myositis) or non-inflammatory (endocrine or metabolic abnormalities or toxins).

Serum CK may be elevated with myopathy due to hypothyroidism, but is usually normal with Cushing's disease and steroid myopathy. Exercise intolerance, with post-exertional cramps (with or without a family history), suggests a metabolic myopathy, most commonly glycogen storage disorder (p. 448). A strong family history and

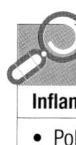

25.32 Causes of proximal muscle pain and weakness

Inflammatory

- Polymyositis
- Dermatomyositis
- Inclusion body myositis

Endocrine (Ch. 20)

- Hypothyroidism
- Hyperthyroidism
- Osteomalacia
- Cushing's syndrome (usually iatrogenic)
- Addison's disease

Metabolic (Ch. 16)

- Myophosphorylase deficiency
- Phosphofructokinase deficiency
- Hypokalaemia
- Carnitine deficiency
- Myoadenylate deaminase deficiency

Drugs/toxins

- Alcohol
- Cocaine
- Fibrates
- Statins
- Penicillamine
- Zidovudine

Infections (Ch. 13)

- Viral (HIV, cytomegalovirus, rubella, Epstein–Barr, echo)
- Bacterial (*Clostridia*, staphylococci, tuberculosis, *Mycoplasma*)
- Parasitic (schistosomiasis, cysticercosis, toxoplasmosis)

25.33 Clinical features of multisystem rheumatic disease

Systemic

- Malaise
- Fever
- Night sweats
- Weight loss with arthralgia and myalgia

Rashes

- Palpable purpura
- Pulp infarcts
- Ulceration
- Livedo reticularis

Ear, nose and throat

- Epistaxis
- Recurrent sinusitis
- Deafness

Respiratory

- Haemoptysis
- Cough
- Wheeze (uncontrolled asthma)

Gastrointestinal

- Abdominal pain (due to mucosal inflammation or enteric ischaemia)
- Mouth ulcers
- Diarrhoea

Neurological

- Sensory or motor neuropathy

onset in childhood or early adulthood suggest muscular dystrophy (p. 1233). A drug history is important, notably alcohol, which can cause both inflammatory myopathy and muscle atrophy of type 2 fibres. Myopathy can associate with viral infections, including HIV, due to the virus itself or treatment with zidovudine.

Distal or generalised weakness usually indicates a neurological cause, which is even more likely if there are sensory abnormalities or if weakness is unilateral or focal. The weakness of myasthenia gravis (p. 1231) is characteristically worsened by repeated exertion (fatigability) and improved by rest, and usually involves the ocular muscles.

Physical examination should establish the presence, pattern and severity of muscle weakness, graded according to the Medical Research Council (MRC) 1–5 scale, and the presence of fasciculation, evidence of endocrine disease, malignancy, arthropathy or connective tissue disease.

Investigations and management

The most sensitive biochemical test is CK (p. 1064). A raised level suggests muscle pathology but does not establish the cause. Muscle biopsy and EMG are usually required to make the diagnosis, but MRI can be used to identify focal areas of muscle abnormality and increase the diagnostic yield from muscle biopsies. Management is determined by the cause. In all patients with muscle disease, physical therapy to maximise muscle function and conditioning may be helpful.

Rheumatic disease presenting as systemic illness

Systemic illness may be a dominant feature of rheumatic disease, with symptoms such as arthralgia and myalgia in combination with weight loss, night sweats, fever, skin rashes, raised inflammatory markers and abnormal urinalysis. The differential diagnosis is potentially wide but important conditions to consider include sepsis, systemic vasculitis (p. 1112), adult-onset Still's disease (p. 1129), disseminated malignancy, atrial myxoma, cholesterol emboli and antiphospholipid syndrome (p. 1050).

If the patient is febrile, unwell or hypotensive, empirical broad-spectrum antibiotics should be initiated after appropriate samples have been taken for culture. Symptoms suggesting vasculitis are shown in Box 25.33. If these are present and there is evidence of critical organ involvement, immediate treatment with high-dose steroids may be required prior to diagnostic confirmation.

PRINCIPLES OF MANAGEMENT OF MUSCULOSKELETAL DISORDERS

The aims of management of MSK disorders are to:

- educate the patient
- control pain
- optimise function
- modify the disease process where possible.

These aims are interrelated and success in one often benefits the others. Successful management requires careful assessment of the whole person as well as his or her MSK system. The management plan needs to be individualised and patient-centred, to be agreed and understood by both patient and practitioner, and take into account:

- the person's daily activity requirements, and work and recreational aspirations
- risk factors and associations of the MSK condition (e.g. obesity, muscle weakness, non-restorative sleep)
- the person's perceptions and knowledge of their condition
- medications and coping strategies already tried by the patient

25

- comorbid disease and its therapy
- the availability, costs and logistics of appropriate evidence-based interventions.

Simple and safe interventions should be tried first. Symptoms and signs will change with time, so the plan requires review and possible readjustment. Effective management may require the expertise of a variety of health professionals, with a coordinated multidisciplinary team approach.

The core interventions that should be considered for everyone with a painful MSK condition are listed in Box 25.34. There are also other non-pharmacological and drug options, the choice depending largely on the nature and severity of the diagnosis.

Core interventions

Education

All doctors should inform patients about the nature of their condition and its investigation, treatment and prognosis, as education can improve outcome. Information and therapist contact can reduce pain and disability, improve self-efficacy and reduce the health-care costs of many MSK conditions, including osteoarthritis and RA. The mechanisms are unclear but in part may result from improved adherence. Benefits are modest but potentially long-lasting, safe and cost-effective (Box 25.35). Education can be provided though one-to-one discussion, written literature, patient-led group education classes and interactive computer programs. Inclusion of the patient's partner or carer is often appropriate; this is essential for childhood conditions but also helps in many chronic adult conditions such as RA or fibromyalgia.

Exercise

Two types of exercise should be prescribed (see Box 25.35):

- Aerobic fitness training can produce long-term reduction in pain and disability. It improves well-being, encourages restorative sleep and benefits common comorbidity such as obesity, diabetes, chronic heart failure and hypertension.
- Local strengthening exercise for muscles that act over compromised joints also reduces pain and disability, with improvements in the reduced muscle

> **25.34 Interventions for patients with musculoskeletal pain**
>
> **Core**
>
> | | |
> |---|---|
> | • Education | • Reduction of adverse |
> | • Exercise | mechanical factors |
> | Aerobic conditioning | Pacing of activities |
> | Strengthening | Appropriate footwear |
> | • Simple analgesia | • Weight reduction if obese |
>
> **Other options**
>
> | | |
> |---|---|
> | • Other analgesic drugs | • Corticosteroids |
> | Oral NSAIDs | • Local injections |
> | Topical agents | • Physical treatments |
> | Opioid analgesics | Heat, cold, aids, appliances |
> | Amitriptyline | • Surgery |
> | • Slow-acting | • Coping strategies |
> | antirheumatic drugs | |

EBM   **25.35 Education and exercise in the management of arthritis**

'Both patient education and exercise regimens have a modest, yet clinically important influence on patients' well-being.'

'Both aerobic walking and home-based quadriceps-strengthening exercises reduce pain and disability from knee osteoarthritis.'

- Devos-Combey L, et al. J Rheumatol 2006; 33:744–756.
- Roddy E, et al. Ann Rheum Dis 2005; 64:544–548.

strength, proprioception, coordination and balance that associate with chronic arthritis. 'Small amounts often' of strengthening exercise are better than protracted sessions performed infrequently.

Joint protection

Excessive impact-loading and adverse repetitive use of a compromised joint or periarticular tissue can often be reduced: for example, cessation of contact sports, or altered use of machinery or tools at the workplace. Simple 'pacing' of activities—dividing physically onerous tasks into shorter segments with brief breaks in between—is helpful. Use of shock-absorbing footwear with thick soft soles can reduce impact-loading through feet, knees, hips and back, and improve symptoms at these sites. A walking stick held on the contralateral side takes weight off a painful hip, knee or foot.

Weight loss

Obesity aggravates pain at most sites of the body through increased mechanical strain and is a risk factor for more rapid progression of joint damage in patients with arthritis. Obese patients should receive an explanation of this and be offered strategies on how to lose and then maintain an appropriate weight (p. 118).

Pharmacological options for direct symptom control

Analgesia

Paracetamol (1 g 6–8-hourly) is the oral analgesic of choice and, if successful, the preferred long-term oral analgesic. It inhibits prostaglandin synthesis in the brain but has less effect on peripheral prostaglandin production. It is generally well tolerated and has few adverse effects and drug interactions. There is a possible increased risk of both gastrointestinal events and cardiovascular disease with chronic usage, but it is uncertain whether this is due to the underlying disease or the drug itself.

Non-steroidal anti-inflammatory drugs (NSAIDs)

These are among the most commonly prescribed drugs, although their use has declined recently because of growing concern over their gastrointestinal and cardiorenal risk. Oral NSAIDs are particularly useful in the management of inflammatory arthritis, and a long-acting NSAID taken in the evening may help reduce early morning stiffness. There is marked variability in individual tolerance and response; patients who do not respond to one may still gain relief from another.

The mechanism of NSAID action is through inhibition of prostaglandin H synthase and cyclo-oxygenase (COX) enzymes. Arachidonic acid, derived from membrane phospholipids, is metabolised to produce prostaglandins and leukotrienes by the COX and 5-lipoxygenase pathways respectively (Fig. 25.13). There are two isoforms of COX, encoded by different genes. COX-1 is constitutively expressed and fulfills a 'housekeeping' function in the gastric mucosa, platelets and kidneys. The COX-2 enzyme is largely induced at sites of inflammation, producing prostaglandins that cause local pain and inflammation, but COX-2 is also upregulated in the CNS, where it plays a role in the central mediation of pain and fever. Traditional NSAIDs such as ibuprofen, diclofenac and naproxen inhibit both COX enzymes, whereas newer NSAIDs such as celecoxib and etoricoxib selectively inhibit COX-2. Whilst NSAIDs have anti-inflammatory activity, they do not reduce peripheral cytokine production, acute phase reactants or ESR, and are not thought to have a disease-modifying effect in OA or RA.

Adverse effects

Traditional NSAIDs can damage the gastric mucosal barrier and are an important aetiological factor in up to 30% of gastric ulcers. They also reduce the integrity of the duodenal mucosa but are probably responsible for only a small proportion of duodenal ulcers. They greatly increase the risk of bleeding or perforation from pre-existing gastric and duodenal ulcers. The risks of gastrointestinal events with NSAIDs are appreciable:

- Approximately 1% of patients with RA or OA are hospitalised each year because of NSAID-associated gastroduodenal bleeding.
- Endoscopic evidence of peptic ulceration is found in 20% of NSAID users, even in the absence of symptoms.

- About 2000 people in the UK and 16 000 in the USA die each year from NSAID-associated bleeding or perforation (i.e. higher than deaths from some cancers).

The adjusted increased risk (odds ratio) of bleeding or perforation from all NSAIDs is 4–5, though differences exist between NSAIDs (Box 25.36). Dyspepsia is a poor guide to the presence of NSAID-associated ulceration and bleeding, and the principal risk factors are shown in Box 25.37. Co-prescription of omeprazole (20 mg daily)

25.36 Commonly used NSAIDs and their relative risk of gastroduodenal bleeding and perforation

Drug	Daily adult dose	Doses/day	Idiosyncratic side-effects, comments
Very low risk			
Celecoxib	100–200 mg	1–2	Selective COX-2 inhibitor
Etoricoxib	60–120 mg	1	Selective COX-2 inhibitor
Low risk			
Ibuprofen	600–1600 mg	3–4	Weak anti-inflammatory effect at this dose
Etodolac	600 mg	1	Partially selective COX-2 inhibitor
Meloxicam	7.5–15 mg	1	Partially selective COX-2 inhibitor
Nabumetone	1–2 g	1–2	Partially selective COX-2 inhibitor
Medium risk			
Ibuprofen	1600–2400 mg	3–4	
Naproxen	500–1000 mg	1–2	
Diclofenac	75–150 mg	2–3	Abnormal liver function tests
High risk			
Indometacin	50–200 mg	3–4	High incidence of dyspepsia and CNS side-effects (headache, dizziness, confusion)
Ketoprofen	100–200 mg	2–4	
Highest risk			
Piroxicam	20–30 mg	1–2	Restricted use, esp. in those > 60 yrs
Azapropazone	600–1200 mg	2–4	Marked uricosuric action. Restricted use, esp. in those > 60 yrs

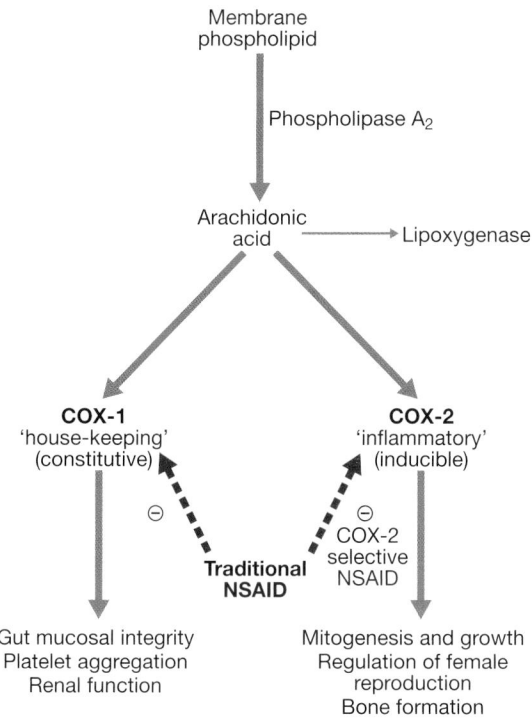

Membrane phospholipid

↓ Phospholipase A$_2$

Arachidonic acid → Lipoxygenase

COX-1
'house-keeping'
(constitutive)

COX-2
'inflammatory'
(inducible)

⊖ **Traditional NSAID**

⊖ COX-2 selective NSAID

Gut mucosal integrity
Platelet aggregation
Renal function

Mitogenesis and growth
Regulation of female reproduction
Bone formation
Renal function

Fig. 25.13 COX-1 and COX-2 pathways.

25.37 Risk factors for NSAID-induced ulcers

- Age > 60 yrs*
- Past history of peptic ulcer*
- Past history of adverse event with NSAIDs
- Concomitant corticosteroid use
- High-dose or multiple NSAIDs
- Individual NSAID: highest with azapropazone, piroxicam, ketoprofen; lower with ibuprofen

*The most important risk factors.

25

or misoprostol (200μg 8–12-hourly) reduces but does not eliminate NSAID-induced ulceration and bleeding, but H$_2$-antagonists are ineffective. The COX-2 selective NSAIDs celecoxib and etoricoxib are less likely to cause gastrointestinal toxicity but benefit is attenuated in patients on low-dose aspirin. In the UK, NICE guidelines advise that a proton pump inhibitor (PPI) should be co-prescribed with all NSAIDs, including COX-2 selective NSAID, even though the risk of gastrointestinal events with these is low. Since chronic PPI therapy is associated with an increased risk of hip fracture, the merits of giving PPI therapy with a COX-2 selective drug need to be weighed up carefully.

Chronic NSAID therapy has also been associated with an increased risk of cardiovascular disease. The mechanism is incompletely understood but may involve an increased risk of thrombosis due to inhibition of COX-2 in the endothelium. Other side-effects include fluid retention and renal impairment due to inhibition of renal prostaglandin production, non-ulcer-associated dyspepsia, abdominal pain and altered bowel habit, and rashes. Interstitial nephritis, asthma and anaphylaxis can also occur but are rare. Recommendations for NSAID prescribing are summarised in Box 25.38, and NSAIDs should generally be avoided altogether in the elderly (Box 25.39).

Nutriceuticals

A wide variety of nutritional supplements and health foods are marketed for relief of MSK symptoms. In most cases there is no rationale for their use, but some supplements including glucosamine sulphate (not the hydrochloride), chondroitin sulphate and avocado/soya bean unsaponifiable have been shown to provide modest pain relief in knee OA in some randomised clinical trials. There is also some evidence that regular glucosamine or chondroitin sulphate may slow further structural damage. Currently, these agents remain largely unlicensed and are not recommended by NICE.

Topical agents

NSAID creams and gels and capsaicin (chilli extract; 0.025%) cream are safe and effective for pain relief from OA and superficial periarticular lesions affecting hands, elbows and knees. They may be used as monotherapy or as an adjunct to oral analgesics. Topical NSAIDs can penetrate superficial tissues and even reach the joint capsule, though intrasynovial levels mainly reflect blood-borne drug delivery. Capsaicin selectively binds to the protein transient receptor potential vanilloid type 1 (TRPV1), which is a heat-activated calcium channel on the surface of peripheral type C nociceptor fibres. Initial application causes a burning sensation but continued use depletes presynaptic substance P, with subsequent pain reduction that is optimal after 1–2 weeks.

Other analgesics

Opioid analgesics are sometimes required for moderate to severe pain which is unresponsive to other approaches. Codeine and dihydrocodeine are relatively weak analgesics, but when combined with paracetamol give better analgesia than paracetamol alone. Side-effects include constipation, headache and confusion, especially in old age. The centrally acting analgesics tramadol and meptazinol may be useful for temporary control of severe pain unresponsive to other measures. Both may cause nausea, bowel upset, dizziness and somnolence, and withdrawal symptoms after chronic use. Patients with severe or intractable pain may require stronger opioid analgesics such as oxycodon and morphine. The non-opioid analgesic nefopam (30–90 mg 8-hourly) can help moderate pain, though side-effects (nausea, anxiety, dry mouth) often limit its use. Adjuvant analgesics are described on page 283.

Disease-modifying antirheumatic drugs (DMARDs)

DMARDs are widely used in the treatment of inflammatory rheumatic diseases (Box 25.40). They reduce clinical signs of inflammation and improve or normalise objective parameters of the APR. They have a delayed onset of action and must be taken for weeks or months before benefit occurs. For some agents, there is evidence that a successful response may reduce target tissue damage. The main indications for DMARDs are:
- persistent inflammatory synovitis (> 6 weeks)
- systemic vasculitis
- SLE with cardiac, renal or CNS involvement
- as an adjunct to corticosteroid therapy in polymyalgia rheumatica and myositis.

Regular monitoring of DMARD therapy is essential (see Box 25.40) and most DMARDs are contraindicated in pregnancy, especially during the first trimester (Box 25.41). Traditionally, DMARDs were given as single agents, but drug combinations are increasingly used for resistant RA. DMARDs are given in addition to, rather

---

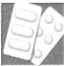

25.38 Recommendations for the use of NSAIDs

- Current use of anticoagulants is a contraindication to NSAID use
- Avoid NSAIDs in the elderly and in those with important comorbidity, including heart failure and hypertension
- Start with the lowest dose of one of the safer established NSAIDs (e.g. ibuprofen) and only increase the dose if required
- If an unsatisfactory result is obtained with one NSAID, a trial of another NSAID may be warranted
- Never prescribe more than one NSAID at a time
- Allow a 2–3-week trial to assess efficacy of any particular NSAID or dose
- For a patient with recognised risk factors for gastrointestinal ulceration (see Box 25.37), co-prescribe omeprazole or misoprostol; in the UK, this is recommended for all adults

---

25.39 Use of oral NSAIDs in old age

- **Gastrointestinal complications:** age is a strong risk factor for complications (bleeding, perforation) of NSAID-associated peptic ulceration.
- **Prognosis:** older people, especially those with cardiovascular comorbidity, are more likely to die if they suffer NSAID-associated bleeding or perforation.
- **Other side-effects:** older people are at greater risk of renal and cardiovascular side-effects of NSAIDs (peripheral oedema, cardiac failure).
- **Paracetamol:** for many, oral paracetamol is as effective as oral NSAID for pain relief. Because of its greater safety and low expense, paracetamol remains the oral analgesic of choice.

25.40 Commonly used disease-modifying antirheumatic drugs

Drug	Disease indications	Usual maintenance dose	Principal side-effects	Monitoring requirement	Monitoring frequency
Hydroxychloroquine	RA, SLE	200–400 mg/day	Rash, nausea, diarrhoea, headache, corneal deposits, retinopathy (rare)	Visual acuity, Amsler chart, fundoscopy	6–12-monthly
Sulfasalazine	RA, seroneg	2–4 g/day	Nausea, GI upset, rash, hepatitis, neutropenia, pancytopenia (rare)	FBC, LFTs	Monthly for 3 mths, then 3-monthly
D-penicillamine	RA	250–750 mg/day	Rash, stomatitis, metallic taste, proteinuria, thrombocytopenia	FBC, urine (protein)	Initially 1–2-weekly; 4–6-weekly for maintenance
Gold	RA	50 mg/mth by i.m. injection	Rash, stomatitis, alopecia, proteinuria, thrombocytopenia, myelosuppression	FBC, urine (protein)	Each injection
Methotrexate	RA, seroneg, SLE, CTD, vasculitis, PMR	5–30 mg/wk	GI upset, stomatitis, rash, alopecia, hepatotoxicity, acute pneumonitis	FBC, LFTs	Initially monthly, then every 3 months
Azathioprine	RA, seroneg, SLE, CTD, vasculitis, PMR	50–150 mg/day	GI upset, stomatitis, hepatitis, myelosuppression	FBC, LFTs	Initially weekly, then monthly
Leflunomide	RA	10–20 mg/day	Nausea, GI upset, rash, alopecia, hepatitis, hypertension	FBC, LFTs, blood pressure	2–4-weekly
Cyclophosphamide	Vasculitis, SLE, myositis	0.5–1 g by i.v. injection, 1–4-weekly	Nausea, GI upset, alopecia, cystitis, myelosuppression, azoospermia, anovulation	FBC, urine (blood)	Each i.v. injection
Ciclosporin	RA, psoriasis, SLE	150–300 mg/day	Nausea, GI upset, renal impairment, hypertension	FBC, LFTs, creatinine, blood pressure	2–4-weekly
Mycophenolate mofetil	SLE, vasculitis	1–3 g/day	Myelosuppression, GI upset (diarrhoea, vomiting, ulceration), hepatitis	FBC, LFTs	Initially weekly, then monthly in first year, then every 3 months

(CTD = connective tissue disease; FBC = full blood count; LFTs = liver function tests; PMR = polymyalgia rheumatica; RA = rheumatoid arthritis; seroneg = peripheral arthritis due to seronegative spondyloarthritis; SLE = systemic lupus erythematosus)

25

than instead of, the patient's pain-relieving drugs, but if treatment is successful, analgesic and NSAID requirements may fall. Box 25.40 gives the usual doses, principal toxicity and monitoring requirements of DMARDs.

Methotrexate

Methotrexate competitively inhibits dihydrofolate reductase, interfering with DNA synthesis and cell division. It is often the first-choice DMARD for RA and seronegative spondyloarthritis but is also used in SLE, vasculitis and other connective tissue disease. It works within 1–2 months. It is usually given as a weekly oral dose starting at 5–7.5 mg and increasing in 2.5 mg increments every 3–4 weeks until benefit occurs or toxicity develops. It is usually well tolerated but can cause nausea and malaise for 24–48 hours after ingestion. Marrow suppression is rare but hepatotoxicity and hepatic fibrosis may occur, especially at higher doses. Folic acid (5 mg/day) reduces the incidence of adverse effects without reducing efficacy. Patients should be warned of drug interaction with sulphonamides and to avoid excess alcohol, which enhances methotrexate hepatotox-

icity. Acute pulmonary toxicity (pneumonitis) is rare but can occur at any time during treatment. Patients should therefore be warned to seek early advice if they develop any new respiratory symptoms. Methotrexate should be stopped immediately if pneumonitis is suspected and high-dose steroids should be given.

Sulfasalazine

Sulfasalazine has a good benefit-to-risk profile and is used for RA and seronegative spondyloarthritis. Nausea and gastrointestinal intolerance are the main side-effects but can be reduced by use of enteric-coated tablets and taking them with food. The usual starting dose is 500 mg daily, building up to the maintenance dose over 2–4 weeks. The patient should be warned of possible orange staining of urine and contact lenses.

Hydroxychloroquine

This antimalarial is used for mild to moderate lupus, especially when skin or locomotor involvement predominates. It is also used for RA, usually in combination with other DMARDs, but has relatively weak activity and a

1079

25.41 Treatment of rheumatic disease in pregnancy

- **Immunological changes in pregnancy:** may influence disease activity.
  - Approximately 75% of patients with RA go into remission during pregnancy.
  - Most patients with SLE remain stable but some worsen, especially those with renal disease.
  - Most patients with psoriatic arthritis show improvement.
- **Conception:** patients with systemic rheumatic diseases should be in clinical remission, if possible, prior to conception (for at least 6 mths for those with associated renal disease).
- **Disease control:** paramount during pregnancy, as uncontrolled inflammatory disease is a significant risk to both mother and baby.
- **Use of medication:** minimise or discontinue as appropriate. Treat symptoms and signs, not the diagnosis (e.g. only use steroids in SLE patients if disease is active).
- **Paracetamol:** the oral analgesic of choice during pregnancy.
- **Oral NSAIDs and selective COX-2 inhibitors:** can be used after implantation up until the last trimester.
- **Corticosteroids:** may be used to control disease flares; the main maternal risks are hypertension, glucose intolerance and osteoporosis.
- **DMARDs that may be used:** sulfasalazine, hydroxychloroquine, azathioprine or ciclosporin if required to control inflammation.
- **DMARDs that must be avoided:** methotrexate, leflunomide, cyclophosphamide, gold and penicillamine. Women should not conceive while taking methotrexate or leflunomide.
- **Biologic agents:** safety during pregnancy is currently unclear.
- **Breastfeeding:** methotrexate, leflunomide, cyclophosphamide, ciclosporin, azathioprine, sulfasalazine and hydroxychloroquine are contraindicated.

slow onset of action (2–4 months). Despite a wide range of potential side-effects, it is usually well tolerated.

Azathioprine

Azathioprine is most commonly employed as a steroid-sparing agent and to prevent relapse in patients with SLE and vasculitis. It is metabolised to 6-mercaptopurine (6-MP), which is then converted intracellularly to active purine thioanalogues, which inhibit DNA and RNA biosynthesis. Nausea, diarrhoea and mouth ulcers are common, but hepatitis and marrow suppression less so. Since 6-MP requires oxidation by xanthine oxidase before renal excretion, co-administration of allopurinol increases toxicity; if both drugs are required, the azathioprine dose should be reduced by 75%. Genotyping for alleles of thiopurine methyltransferase (TPMT), which are associated with reduced activity of this enzyme, can help predict azathioprine toxicity.

Leflunomide

Leflunomide is used for RA. It inhibits uridine monophosphate production and tyrosine kinases, and is an inhibitor of activated lymphocytes. It is usually well tolerated and has low marrow toxicity, but may cause liver dysfunction.

Gold, penicillamine and ciclosporin A

These drugs are used in RA, but have a high incidence of side-effects and tend to be reserved for patients who have failed on other DMARDs.

Gold (sodium aurothiomalate) is given by deep intramuscular injection. After an initial 10 mg test dose, 50 mg is given weekly until benefit occurs, when the frequency is reduced to fortnightly and then monthly. If there is a flare, a temporary return to weekly frequency may recapture control. If there is no benefit after 6 months, treatment should be stopped. Side-effects are potentially serious and preclude further therapy.

Penicillamine is given in a starting dose of 125–250 mg daily on an empty stomach, and the dose increased in 125 mg increments every 6 weeks until benefit occurs. Rarely, drug-induced lupus, myasthenia gravis or pemphigus may occur.

Ciclosporin A (150–300 mg/day) is a fungal cyclic polypeptide that blocks resting lymphocytes in the G0 or G1 phase of the cell cycle, inhibiting lymphokine production and release.

Cyclophosphamide

Cyclophosphamide is mainly used as pulse therapy in the treatment of systemic vasculitis and in SLE where there is renal, cardiac or CNS involvement. It is an alkylating agent that binds DNA, RNA and proteins, and is both mutagenic and teratogenic. It is inactive until converted by the cytochrome P-450 oxidase system to phosphoramide mustard and acrolein. It is usually given as 'pulse' intravenous injections of $0.5–1.5\,g/m^2$ weekly or monthly. The risk of haemorrhagic cystitis can be minimised by good hydration and ingestion of mesna, which binds urotoxic metabolites of cyclophosphamide. Because of the high risk of azoospermia and anovulation, which may be permanent, pre-treatment sperm or ova collection and storage may need consideration.

Mycophenolate mofetil

Mycophenolate mofetil (MMF) is an alternative to cyclophosphamide in inducing remission in SLE and vasculitis, and is also used as maintenance therapy to prevent relapse. MMF works by inhibiting purine synthesis, but its effects are relatively specific for lymphocytes because the molecular target (inosine monophosphate dehydrogenase) plays a critical role in production of guanine nucleotides in lymphocytes. Other cells can use purine salvage pathways for nucleotide production. A dose of 3 g daily is used initially, usually with high-dose steroids, and then the dose is reduced to 1–2 g daily, depending on the clinical response. Adverse affects include diarrhoea and leucopenia.

Biologic disease-modifying antirheumatic drugs

These synthesised antibodies or natural cytokine inhibitors have specificity for single targets; because they are proteins they require subcutaneous or parenteral administration.

Anti-TNF therapy

Anti-TNF therapy is widely used in the treatment of patients with RA, psoriatic arthritis and ankylosing spondylitis who have had an inadequate response to standard treatments. Three anti-TNF agents are now in routine use. Infliximab is a chimeric human–murine anti-TNF-α monoclonal antibody which is administered by intravenous infusion (3 mg/kg), typically every 6–8 weeks. It requires co-prescription of methotrexate to reduce immunogenicity. Etanercept is a synthetic human TNF receptor–Fc fusion protein, administered subcutaneously, either 50 mg weekly or 25 mg twice weekly. Adalimumab is a fully human monoclonal antibody to TNF-α, administered subcutaneously, 40 mg every 2 weeks. Neither etanercept nor adalimumab requires the co-prescription of methotrexate, but combining either with methotrexate is more effective than either agent alone, without any increase in side-effects. All three drugs are more effective than standard DMARDs in RA but are much more expensive (approximately £7500 annually). Because of this, many countries have set guidelines restricting their use. Current UK recommendations are that anti-TNF therapy should be initiated only in active RA (DAS 28 > 5.1; see p. 1092) when an adequate trial of at least two other DMARDs (including methotrexate) has failed.

The main adverse effect of TNF blockade is the risk of serious infections, particularly reactivation of latent tuberculosis, which is more likely with infliximab than etanercept. There is also evidence of a possible increased risk of malignancy, but the contribution of TNF blockade as opposed to the underlying disease and other treatments is unclear.

Rituximab

Rituximab is an antibody directed against the CD20 receptor, expressed on B lymphocytes. It is given by two intravenous infusions (1 g each) 2 weeks apart, usually in combination with intravenous corticosteroid. It causes depletion of peripheral B cells which is sustained for several months after administration. The treatment is repeated usually when signs of improvement are wearing off (anything from 6 months to 3 years). It is mostly used in the treatment of patients with resistant RA who have failed to respond to TNF blockade.

Abatacept

Abatacept is a biologic agent in which the Fc domain of IgG is fused to the extracellular domain of CTLA4. Abatacept blocks the interaction between CD28 and CTLA-4 which is required for full activation of T cells following antigen presentation. It is generally used in patients who have failed to respond to other treatments.

Anakinra

Anakinra is an IL-1 receptor antagonist which is used in RA. It appears to be less effective than anti-TNF therapy and is generally reserved for those who have failed to respond to other treatments.

Tocilizumab

This agent is an antibody directed against the IL-6 receptor. It has recently been licensed for the treatment of RA and has effects similar to those of TNF blockade. Its role in therapy remains to be defined.

Corticosteroids

Corticosteroids have a very rapid and dramatic anti-inflammatory action and there is evidence that systemic steroids favourably modify the disease outcome in RA,

> **25.42 Principal indications for systemic corticosteroids**
>
> - Short-term control of inflammatory arthritis whilst awaiting efficacy from DMARD
> - Maintenance therapy in RA that cannot be adequately controlled by DMARD alone
> - Systemic vasculitis
> - SLE with involvement of CNS, renal or cardiovascular systems
> - Polymyalgia rheumatica and giant cell arteritis
> - Control of inflammatory disease during pregnancy

vasculitis and SLE. They are also used locally by injection in the treatment of soft tissue rheumatism and osteoarthritis. Since the adverse effects of corticosteroids are dose- and duration-dependent, the aim is always to use the smallest amount possible for the shortest time to achieve the desired therapeutic goal. Box 25.42 lists the main indications for oral or parenteral steroid. In RA, steroid therapy is initiated for rapid control of inflammatory disease at the same time as commencing a DMARD, and therapy is reduced and withdrawn as this takes effect.

Oral therapy

Prednisolone is the oral steroid of choice. It should be given as a single morning dose to coincide with peak levels of endogenous cortisol. Potential side-effects are numerous (p. 774) but osteoporosis, infection, diabetes, hypertension and cardiovascular disease are the major concerns. Patients receiving long-term oral corticosteroids (> 7.5 mg for more than 3 months) should be given prophylaxis against osteoporosis (p. 1119).

Parenteral therapy

Parenteral treatment with corticosteroids is used in the treatment of inflammatory arthritis, SLE and vasculitis. For inflammatory arthritis, a single intramuscular injection of methylprednisolone (80–120 mg) may quickly and effectively control inflammation for 2–6 weeks. Higher doses (500–1000 mg) are used intravenously along with cyclophosphamide in the treatment of SLE and vasculitis.

Local injections

Intra-articular steroid injections are useful adjunctive therapy for short-term pain relief in OA and inflammatory arthritis and for temporary control of synovitis. The duration of benefit varies according to joint size and the nature and severity of the arthritis, but is in the order of 2–8 weeks. Frequently repeated injections may result in joint tissue atrophy and Cushing's syndrome, and some advise no more than four injections per year into a large joint like the knee. As long as precautions are taken (Box 25.43), the incidence of iatrogenic infection is

> **25.43 Aseptic precautions with intra-articular corticosteroid injection**
>
> - Never inject if the diagnosis is in doubt
> - Never inject if there is local or systemic infection
> - Use an aseptic technique: single ampoules, sterile needle and syringe, clean hands (with gloves), clean skin (alcohol/antiseptic)
> - If aspirated fluid is very turbid, send it for culture

25

almost negligible. Other side-effects are facial flushing 24–72 hours post-injection, local skin atrophy, telangiectasia and permanent fat atrophy due to leakage along the needle track (especially with fluorinated triamcinolone preparations). Sometimes post-injection 'flare' in disease occurs, with temporary (1–3 days) exacerbation.

Injection of local steroid and/or anaesthetic can give rapid and effective control of pain from periarticular lesions such as bursitis, tenosynovitis and enthesopathy. It will not hasten, and may retard healing, but its analgesic effect may extend beyond the natural history of the lesion. Non-fluorinated steroids (e.g. hydrocortisone, methylprednisolone) should be used for superficial lesions (e.g. lateral epicondylitis, anserine bursitis) to avoid fat and skin atrophy. If anaesthetic is combined with the steroid, quick relief of pain confirms both the diagnosis and accurate placement of the injection. Injection of steroid into, or even adjacent to, certain tendons (e.g. long head of biceps tendon) can predispose to rupture and should be avoided. Steroid injection may also be used to confirm and temporarily relieve peripheral nerve entrapment syndromes (e.g. carpal tunnel injection for median nerve entrapment at the wrist).

Other treatments

Hyaluronan injections

In knee OA, intra-articular injection of one of several forms of hyaluronan (polymers of hyaluronate), mainly given as a course of weekly injections for 3–5 weeks, may give modest pain relief for several months. However, evidence for efficacy is heterogeneous and their expense and common requirement for serial injection mean that they are not recommended for OA in the UK.

Radiation-induced synovectomy

Intra-articular injection of radiocolloid (^{90}yttrium silicate for large to medium joints, ^{159}erbium for small joints) can give prolonged control of synovitis but should be avoided in patients under the age of 45. Joints should be immobilised for 24–72 hours post-injection to reduce spread to regional lymph nodes. The synovium often recovers with return of synovitis after 1–3 years. Indications include inflammatory synovitis where just one or a few joints are resistant to other measures, synovitis of chronic haemophilic arthropathy and pigmented villonodular synovitis.

Nerve blockade

Nerve blockade using steroids and/or long-acting anaesthetics may be helpful for control of severe chronic arthritis or periarticular pain resistant to other means (e.g. suprascapular nerve block for severe glenohumeral arthritis or chronic rotator cuff pain). Epidural injections of corticosteroid may also give temporary relief of troublesome root entrapment symptoms.

Non-pharmacological interventions

Physical therapy

Local heat, ice packs, wax baths and other local external applications can induce muscle relaxation and temporary relief of symptoms in a range of rheumatic diseases.

Hydrotherapy permits muscle relaxation and enhanced movement in a warm, pain-relieving environment without the restraints of gravity and normal load-bearing. Various manipulative techniques may also help improve restricted movement. The combination of these with education and therapist contact enhances their benefits.

Splints can give temporary rest and support for painful joints and periarticular tissues, and prevent disadvantageous involuntary postures during sleep. Prolonged rest, however, must be avoided.

Orthoses are more permanent appliances used to reduce instability and excessive abnormal movement. They include working wrist splints, knee orthoses, and iron and T-straps to control ankle instability. Orthoses are particularly suited to severely disabled patients in whom a surgical option is inappropriate, and often need to be custom-made for the individual.

Aids and appliances can provide dignity and independence to patients with respect to activities of daily living. Common examples are a raised toilet seat, raised chair height, extended handles on taps, a shower instead of a bath, thick-handled cutlery, and extended 'hands' to pull on tights and socks. Full assessment and advice from an occupational therapist can maximise the benefits.

Surgery

A variety of surgical interventions can relieve pain and conserve or restore function in patients with bone, joint and periarticular disease (Box 25.44). Soft tissue release and tenosynovectomy may reduce inflammatory symptoms, improve function and prevent or retard tendon damage for variable periods, sometimes indefinitely. Synovectomy of joints does not prevent disease progression but may be indicated for pain relief when drugs, physical therapy and intra-articular injections have provided insufficient relief. The main approaches for damaged joints are osteotomy (cutting bone to alter joint mechanics and load transmission), excision arthroplasty (removing part or all the joint), joint replacement (insertion of prosthesis in place of the excised joint) and arthrodesis (joint fusion). Surgical fixation of fractures is frequently required in patients with osteoporosis and other bone diseases.

The main aims of surgery are to provide pain relief and improve function and quality of life. If surgery is to be successful, the aims and consequences of each operation should be considered as part of an integrated programme of management and rehabilitation, by multidisciplinary teams of surgeons, allied health professionals and physicians, and carefully explained to the patient. Assessment of motivation, social support and environment is no less important than careful consideration of patients' general health, their risks for major surgery, the extent of disease in other joints and their ability to mobilise following surgery. For some severely compromised people, pain relief and functional independence are better served by provision of a suitable wheelchair, home adjustments and social services than by surgery that is technically successful but following which the patient cannot mobilise.

Self-help and coping strategies

These help patients to cope better with, and to adjust to chronic pain and disability. They may be useful at any stage but are particularly so for patients with incurable

25.44 Examples of surgical procedures for MSK disorders

Procedure	Indication
Soft tissue release	
Carpal tunnel	Median nerve compression
Tarsal tunnel	Posterior tibial nerve entrapment
Flexor tenosynovectomy	Relief of 'trigger' fingers
Ulnar nerve transposition	Ulnar nerve entrapment at elbow
Fasciotomy	Severe Dupuytren's contracture
Tendon repairs and transfers	
Hand extensor tendons	Extensor tendon rupture
Thumb and finger flexor tendons	Flexor tendon rupture
Synovectomy	
Wrist and extensor tendon sheath (+ excision of radial head)	Pain relief and prevention of extensor tendon rupture in RA, resistant inflammatory synovitis
Knee synovectomy	Resistant inflammatory synovitis
Osteotomy	
Femoral osteotomy	Early OA of hip
Tibial osteotomy	Unicompartmental knee OA
	Deformed tibia in OA
	Paget's disease
Excision arthroplasty	
First metatarsophalangeal joint (Keller's procedure)	Painful hallux valgus
Radial head	Painful distal radio-ulnar joint
Lateral end of clavicle	Painful acromioclavicular joint
Metatarsal head	Painful subluxed metatarsophalangeal joints
Joint replacement arthroplasty	
Knee, hip, shoulder, elbow	Painful damaged joints (mainly OA) Fractured neck of femur (hemiarthroplasty)
Arthrodesis	
Wrist	Damaged joint: pain relief, improvement of grip
Ankle/subtalar joints	Damaged joint: pain relief, stabilisation of hindfoot

problems, who have received all available treatment options. The aim is to increase self-management through self-assessment and problem-solving so that patients can recognise negative but potentially remediable aspects of their mood (stress, frustration, anger or low self-esteem) and their situation (physical, social, financial). These may then be addressed by changes in attitude and behaviour, as shown in Box 25.45.

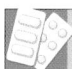

25.45 Self-help and coping strategies

- Yoga and relaxation techniques to reduce stress
- Avoiding negative situations or activities that produce stress, and increasing pleasant activities that give satisfaction
- Information and discussion to alter beliefs about and perspectives on disease
- Reducing or avoiding catastrophising and maladaptive pain behaviour
- Imagery and distraction techniques for pain
- Expanding social contact and better utilising social services

Involvement of the spouse or partner in mutual goal-setting can improve partnership adjustment. Such approaches are often an element of group education classes and pain clinics, but may require more formal clinical psychological input.

OSTEOARTHRITIS

Osteoarthritis (OA) is by far the most common form of arthritis. It is strongly associated with ageing and is a major cause of pain and disability in older people. Pathologically, it may be defined as a condition of synovial joints characterised by focal loss of articular hyaline cartilage with proliferation of new bone and remodelling of joint contour. Inflammation is not a prominent clinical feature. OA preferentially targets certain small and large joints (Fig. 25.14) but is not a disease or a single condition. It is best viewed as the dynamic repair process of synovial joints that may be triggered by a variety of insults, some but not all of which result in symptomatic 'joint failure'.

Epidemiology

The prevalence of OA rises progressively with age, such that by 65 years 80% of people have radiographic evidence of OA, though only 25–30% are symptomatic. The knee and hip are the principal large joints involved, affecting 10–25% of those aged over 65 years. Even for joints less frequently targeted by OA, such as the elbow or ankle, OA remains the most common cause of arthritis.

OA is a complex disorder with multiple risk factors (Fig. 25.15). Twin and family studies show that genetic factors play a major role, particularly for hand and generalised OA, but also for hip and knee OA. The genes responsible remain to be identified. Knee OA is

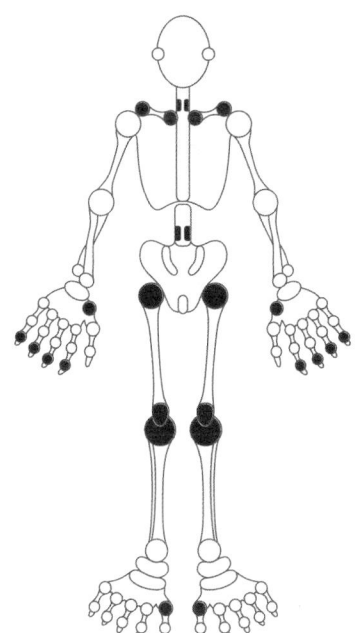

Fig. 25.14 The distribution of osteoarthritis. Although OA can affect any synovial joint, those shown in red are the most commonly targeted.

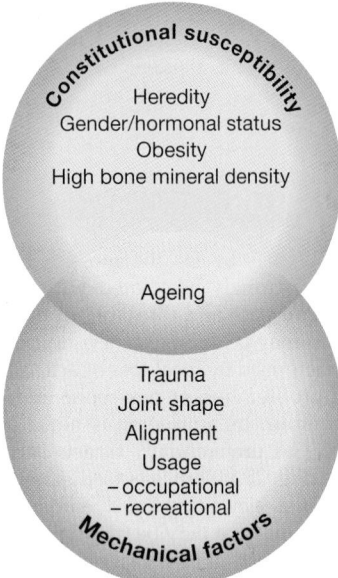

Fig. 25.15 Risk factors for the development of osteoarthritis.

prevalent in all racial groups but hip, hand and generalised OA are particularly prevalent in Caucasians. OA is more prevalent and more commonly symptomatic in women, except at the hip where men are equally affected. Trauma is a recognised predisposing factor and repetitive adverse loading of joints during occupation or competitive sports also appears important, such as in farmers (hip OA), miners (knee OA) and professional footballers (knee OA).

Aetiology and pathogenesis

A variety of mechanical, metabolic, genetic or constitutional insults may damage a synovial joint and trigger the need for repair. Most often this remains unclear ('primary' OA) but sometimes there is an obvious cause such as trauma ('secondary' OA). Since all the joint structures depend on each other for health and function, an insult to one will impact on the others, leading to effects on the whole joint. The OA process involves production of new tissue and remodelling of joint shape. Often this slow but efficient process compensates for the insults, resulting in an anatomically altered but pain-free functioning joint ('compensated' OA). Sometimes, however, because of an overwhelming insult or a defective repair response, the system fails, resulting in progressive tissue damage, more frequent association with symptoms, and presentation as 'joint failure'. This readily explains the clinical heterogeneity of OA.

Cartilage changes

There is enzymatic degradation of the major structural components aggrecan and collagen (see Fig. 25.3, p. 1059). Chondrocytes increase production of matrix components and divide to produce nests of metabolically active cells. Although the turnover of aggrecan components is increased, the concentration of aggrecan eventually falls. The decrease in size of the hydrophilic aggrecan molecules increases the water concentration and swelling pressure in cartilage, further disrupting the retaining scaffolding of type II collagen and making the cartilage vulnerable to load-bearing injury. Fissuring of the cartilage surface ('fibrillation') eventually occurs, leading to the development of deep vertical clefts, localised chondrocyte death and decreased cartilage thickness. Cartilage loss is focal rather than generalised and usually restricted to the maximum load-bearing part of the joint (Fig. 25.16). The changes in OA cartilage encourage deposition of calcium pyrophosphate and basic calcium phosphate crystals.

Bone changes

The subchondral bone shows a mixture of osteolysis and osteosclerosis. In some cases, this reflects healed trabecular microfractures. Subchondral 'cysts' often develop, possibly as the result of small areas of osteonecrosis caused by the increased pressure in bone as the cartilage fails in its load-transmitting function. There is production of new fibrocartilage at the joint margin which undergoes endochondral ossification to form osteophytes. With severe cartilage loss there may be attrition of bone as the two unprotected bone ends wear on each other. Such wear may ablate the trabeculae and lead to a smooth, shiny surface ('eburnation'), often with deep linear grooves.

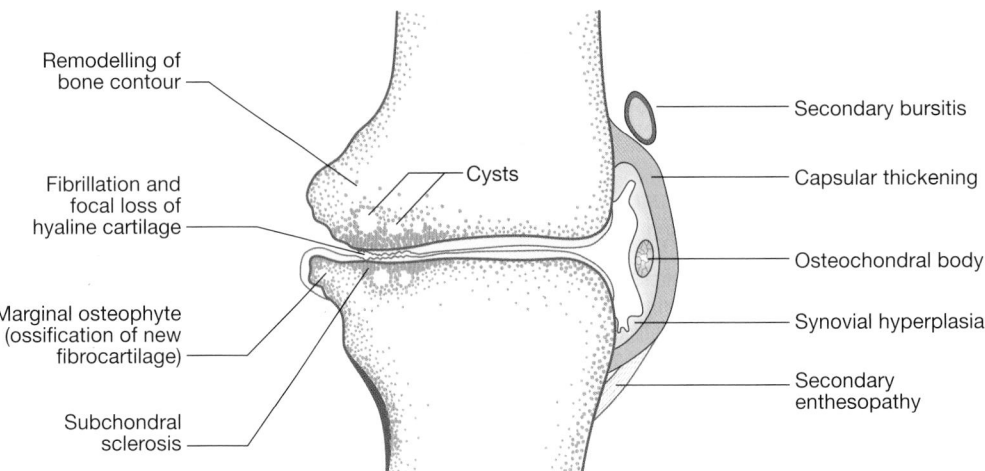

Fig. 25.16 Pathological changes in osteoarthritis.

Bone remodelling and cartilage thinning slowly alter the shape of the OA joint, increasing its surface area.

Other changes

The synovium undergoes variable degrees of hyperplasia. Sometimes histological changes are as florid, though less widespread, as those of RA. Osteochondral bodies commonly occur within the synovium, reflecting chondroid metaplasia or secondary uptake and growth of damaged cartilage fragments. The outer capsule also thickens and contracts, usually retaining the stability of the remodelling joint. The muscles that act over the joint commonly show non-specific type II fibre atrophy.

Clinical features

The main presenting symptoms are pain and functional restriction. Pain may directly relate to the OA process through increased pressure in subchondral bone (mainly causing night pain), trabecular microfractures, capsular distension and low-grade synovitis, or may result from bursitis and enthesopathy secondary to altered joint mechanics. Typical OA pain has the characteristics listed in Box 25.46. For many people, functional restriction of the hands, knees or hips is an equal, if not greater, problem than pain. The clinical findings vary according to severity but are principally those of joint damage.

The correlation between the presence of structural OA (clinical signs, radiographic changes) and pain and disability varies according to site. It is stronger at the hip than the knee, and poor at most small joints. Risk factors for pain and disability may differ from those for structural change. At the knee, for example, reduced quadriceps muscle strength and adverse psychosocial factors (anxiety, depression) correlate more strongly with pain and disability than the degree of radiographic change.

OA is prevalent and commonly asymptomatic in middle-aged and older people, so the presence of OA may not necessarily be the explanation of a patient's problem. Because of their high prevalence, generalised OA, knee OA and hip OA will be considered individu-

ally. Apophyseal joint OA is part of 'spondylosis', and its presentation and management are those of common mechanical back and neck pain (p. 1072).

Nodal generalised OA

Characteristics of this common form of OA are shown in Box 25.47. Presentation is typically in women between 40 and 50 who develop pain, stiffness and swelling of one or a few finger interphalangeal joints (IPJs). Gradually, over many months, more finger IPJs (distal > proximal) are affected. These joints develop posterolateral swellings on each side of the extensor tendon which slowly enlarge and harden to become Heberden's (distal IPJ) and Bouchard's (proximal IPJ) nodes (Fig. 25.17). Typically, each joint goes through a phase of episodic symptoms (1–5 years) while the node evolves and OA develops in the underlying IPJ. Once OA is fully established, symptoms may subside and hand function often remains good. Affected IPJs often show characteristic lateral deviation, reflecting the asymmetric focal cartilage loss of OA. Involvement of the first carpometacarpal joint is also common. At this site, marked osteophyte and subluxation may result in 'thumb-base squaring'. Unlike IPJ OA, thumb-base OA may associate with more persistent symptoms and more severe functional impairment.

People with nodal OA are at increased risk of OA at other sites ('generalised OA'), especially the knee. Nodal generalised OA has a very strong genetic predisposition, the daughter of an affected mother having approximately a 1 in 3 chance of developing nodal OA. Nodal OA with multiple nodes and symptom onset in middle age should not be confused with just one or two asymptomatic nodes related to past trauma, a common finding, particularly in old age.

25.46 Typical characteristics of pain and clinical signs of osteoarthritis

Pain

- Age > 45 yrs (often > 60)
- Insidious onset over months or years
- Variable or intermittent over time ('good days, bad days')
- Mainly related to movement and weight-bearing, relieved by rest
- Only brief (< 15 mins) morning stiffness and brief (< 1 min) 'gelling' after rest
- Usually only one or a few joints painful (not multiple regional pain)

Clinical signs

- Restricted movement due to capsular thickening, or blocking by osteophyte
- Palpable, sometimes audible, coarse crepitus due to rough articular surfaces
- Bony swelling (osteophyte) around joint margins
- Deformity, usually without instability
- Joint-line or periarticular tenderness
- Muscle weakness, wasting
- No or only mild synovitis (effusion, increased warmth)

25.47 Characteristics of nodal generalised osteoarthritis

- Polyarticular finger interphalangeal joint OA
- Heberden's (± Bouchard's) nodes
- Marked female preponderance
- Peak onset in middle age
- Good functional outcome for hands
- Predisposition to OA at other joints, especially knees
- Strong genetic predisposition

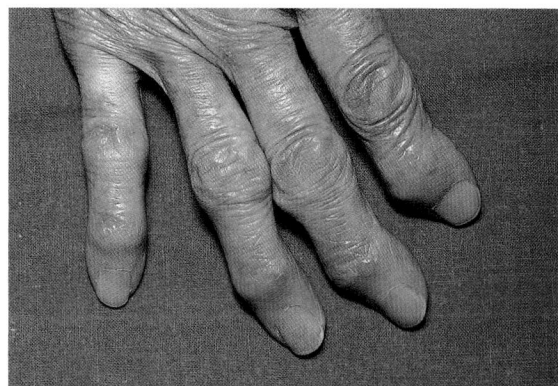

Fig. 25.17 Nodal osteoarthritis. Heberden's nodes and lateral (radial/ulnar) deviation of distal interphalangeal joints, with mild Bouchard's nodes at the proximal interphalangeal joints.

25

Knee OA

OA principally targets the patello-femoral and medial tibio-femoral compartments of the knee. It may be isolated or occur as part of nodal generalised OA. Most knee OA, particularly in women, is bilateral and symmetrical. Trauma is a more important risk factor in men and may result in unilateral OA.

OA knee pain is usually localised to the anterior or medial aspect of the knee and upper tibia. Patello-femoral pain is usually worse going up and down stairs or inclines. Posterior knee pain suggests a complicating popliteal 'cyst'. Prolonged walking, rising from a chair, getting in or out of a car, or bending to put on shoes and socks may be difficult. Local examination findings may include:

- a jerky, asymmetric (antalgic) gait: less time weightbearing on the painful side
- a varus (Fig. 25.18), less commonly valgus, and/or fixed flexion deformity
- joint-line and/or periarticular tenderness (secondary anserine bursitis and medial ligament enthesopathy (see Box 25.22, p. 1071) are common, giving tenderness of the upper medial tibia)
- weakness and wasting of the quadriceps muscle
- restricted flexion/extension with coarse crepitus
- bony swelling around the joint line.

Calcium pyrophosphate dihydrate (CPPD) crystal deposition in association with OA is most common at the knee. This may result in a more overt inflammatory component (stiffness, effusions) and super-added acute attacks of synovitis ('pseudogout', p. 1101), which may predict more rapid radiographic and clinical progression.

Hip OA

Hip OA most commonly targets the superior aspect of the joint (Fig. 25.19). Such 'superior pole' OA is often unilateral at presentation, often progresses with superolateral migration of the femoral head, and has a poor prognosis. The less common central (medial) OA shows more central cartilage loss and is largely confined to women. It is

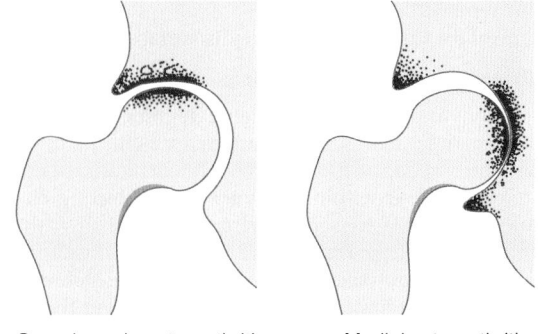

Superior pole osteoarthritis   Medial osteoarthritis

Fig. 25.19 Patterns of hip osteoarthritis.

often bilateral at presentation, may associate with nodal generalised OA, uncommonly progresses with axial femoral migration, and has a better prognosis.

The hip shows the best correlation between symptoms and radiographic change. Hip pain is usually maximal deep in the anterior groin, with variable radiation to the buttock, anterolateral thigh, knee or shin. Lateral hip pain, worse on lying on that side with tenderness over the greater trochanter, suggests secondary trochanteric bursitis. Common functional difficulties are the same as for knee OA; in addition, restricted hip abduction in women may cause pain on intercourse. Examination may reveal:

- an antalgic gait
- weakness and wasting of quadriceps and gluteal muscles
- pain and restriction of internal rotation with the hip flexed —the earliest and most sensitive sign of hip OA; other movements may subsequently be restricted and painful
- anterior groin tenderness just lateral to the femoral pulse
- fixed flexion, external rotation deformity of the hip
- ipsilateral leg shortening with severe joint attrition and superior femoral migration.

Although obesity is not a major risk factor for development of hip OA, it is associated with more rapid progression.

Early-onset OA

Unusually, typical symptoms and signs of OA may present before the age of 45. In most cases, a single joint is affected and there is a clear history of previous trauma. However, in people with early-onset OA affecting several joints, especially those not normally targeted by OA, rare causes need to be considered (Box 25.48). Patients with endemic OA, due to unknown environmental cartilage toxins, will have grown up in just a few specific areas of the world: for example, eastern Russia and northern China ('Kashin–Beck disease').

Erosive OA

This term is used in connection with rare patients with IPJ OA who have a more prolonged symptom phase, more overt IPJ inflammation, more disability and worse outcome than those with nodal OA. Distinguishing features from nodal OA include preferential targeting of proximal IPJs, common develop-

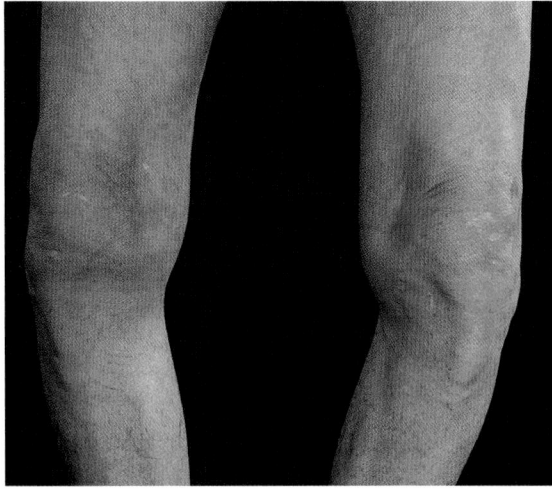

Fig. 25.18 Typical varus deformity resulting from marked medial tibio-femoral osteoarthritis.

25.48 Causes of early-onset osteoarthritis (< 45 years)

Monoarticular

- Previous trauma, localised instability

Pauciarticular or polyarticular

- Prior joint disease (e.g. juvenile idiopathic arthritis)
- Metabolic or endocrine disease
    Haemochromatosis (p. 959)
    Ochronosis
    Acromegaly (p. 790)
- (Spondylo-)epiphyseal dysplasia
- Late avascular necrosis
- Neuropathic joint
- Endemic OA

ment of IPJ lateral instability, subchondral erosions on X-rays, occasional eventual ankylosis of IPJs and lack of association with OA elsewhere. Some patients with nodal OA have one or a few joints with radiographic subchondral erosions, and whether erosive OA is part of the spectrum of hand OA or a discrete subset is uncertain.

Investigations

A plain X-ray may show one or more of the typical features of OA (see Fig. 25.7, p. 1061). Its main use is to assess severity of structural change, an issue if surgery is being considered. A non-weight-bearing PA view of the pelvis is adequate for assessing hip OA, but standing (stressed) AP radiographs are needed to assess tibio-femoral cartilage loss, and a flexed skyline view is best for assessing patello-femoral narrowing.

The FBC, ESR and CRP are normal in OA. Synovial fluid aspirated from OA knees shows variable characteristics but is predominantly viscous with low turbidity; accompanying CPPD and basic calcium phosphate may also be identified. Radioisotope bone scans performed for other reasons often show, as an incidental finding, discrete increased uptake in OA joints due to bone remodelling.

Unexplained early-onset OA requires additional investigation, guided by the suspected underlying condition. X-rays may show typical features of dysplasia or avascular necrosis, widening of joint spaces in acromegaly, multiple cysts and chondrocalcinosis in haemochromatosis (p. 959), or disorganised architecture in neuropathic joints.

Management

Treatment follows the principles on pages 1075–1082 and always requires:

- *Full explanation of the condition.* This should include relevant risk factors (obesity, heredity, trauma); the fact that established structural changes are permanent but that pain and function can improve; discussion of prognosis (good for nodal hand OA, more optimistic for knee than hip OA); and the fact that appropriate action can improve the prognosis of large joint OA.
- *Exercise.* This should cover both strengthening and aerobic exercise, preferably with reinforcement by a physiotherapist (see Box 25.35, p. 1076).
- *Reduction of adverse mechanical factors.* This includes weight loss if obese, shock-absorbing footwear,

pacing of activities, use of a walking stick for painful knee or hip OA, or provision of built-up shoes to equalise leg lengths.

- *Drug treatment.* Give an initial trial of paracetamol and consider the addition of a topical NSAID, and then capsaicin, for knee and hand OA. If required, consider escalating to combined analgesics or oral NSAIDs (p. 1076). Opiates may occasionally be required.

For temporary benefit of moderate to severe pain, consider intra-articular injection of corticosteroid (particularly for knee and thumb-base OA) and local physical therapies such as heat or cold. At present there are no licensed disease-modifying drugs for OA, but the measures above may reduce structural progression as well as improve symptoms. Box 25.49 describes the treatment aspects that are particularly pertinent in older people.

Surgery

Surgery should be considered for patients with OA whose pain, stiffness and reduced function impact significantly on their quality of life and are refractory to non-surgical core and adjunctive treatments. Osteotomy may prolong the life of malaligned joints and relieve pain by reducing intra-osseous pressure. Joint replacement, however, can transform the quality of life of people with severe knee or hip OA. Surgery for refractory OA should be considered before there is prolonged and established functional limitation and severe pain, since these may compromise the surgical outcome. Patient-specific factors such as age, gender, smoking and presence of obesity, should not be barriers to referral for joint replacement.

Total joint replacements are required for the minority of people with large joint OA. Over 95% of joint replacements continue to function well into the second decade after surgery and most provide life-long pain-free function. However, approximately 1 in 5 patients are not satisfied with the outcome, and a minority get little or no improvement in pain following surgery.

25.49 Osteoarthritis in old age

- **OA:** the major MSK cause of pain and disability in older people.
- **Functional impact:** the reduced muscle strength, proprioception and balance that accompany ageing all associate with and contribute to pain and disability from knee and hip OA.
- **Coexistent calcium pyrophosphate crystal deposition:** an age-associated phenomenon that may result in superimposed acute attacks of synovitis (pseudogout).
- **Regular strengthening exercise:** can safely reduce the pain and disability of knee OA with accompanying improvements in balance and reduced tendency to fall.
- **Oral paracetamol and topical NSAIDs:** safe in older people, with no important drug interactions or contraindications, and often effective for pain relief.
- **Intra-articular injection of corticosteroid:** a very safe and often effective treatment, particularly useful for tiding a patient over a special event.
- **Total joint replacement:** with appropriate rehabilitation, an excellent cost-effective treatment for severe disabling knee or hip OA in old age. Age per se is not a contraindication to considering joint replacement.

25

25

Rheumatoid arthritis

Rheumatoid arthritis (RA) is the most common persistent inflammatory arthritis, occurring throughout the world and in all ethnic groups. The prevalence is lowest in black Africans and Chinese, and highest in Pima Indians. In Caucasians, it is 1.0–1.5%, with a female to male ratio of 3:1. The clinical course is prolonged, with intermittent exacerbations and remissions. Patients with RA have an increased mortality when compared with age-matched controls, primarily due to cardiovascular disease. This is most marked in those with severe disease, with a reduction in expected lifespan by 8–15 years. Around 40% of RA patients are registered disabled within 3 years; around 80% are moderately to severely disabled within 20 years; and 25% will require a large joint replacement. Functional capacity decreases most rapidly at the beginning of disease and the functional status of patients within their first year of RA is often predictive of long-term outcome. Factors that associate with a poorer prognosis are disability at presentation, female gender, involvement of MTP joints, smoking and a positive RF and anti-CCP. It is hoped that the prognosis of RA will improve as more aggressive early treatment is used but this has yet to be demonstrated.

Pathophysiology

Both genetic and environmental factors appear to be involved in the pathogenesis of RA. The concordance rate of RA is higher in monozygotic (12–15%) than in dizygotic twins (3%), and there is an increased frequency of disease in first-degree relatives of patients. Up to 50% of the genetic susceptibility is due to genes in the HLA region. HLA-DR4 is the major susceptibility haplotype in most ethnic groups, occurring in 50–75% of Caucasian patients with RA compared to 20–25% of the normal population. However, DR1 is more important in Indians and Israelis, and DW15 in Japanese. Severity is also under genetic influence, with DR4 positivity being more common in those with severe erosive disease. Although it is thought that RA may be triggered by an infectious agent in a genetically susceptible host, a specific pathogen has not been indentified. Susceptibility is increased post-partum and by breastfeeding. Cigarette smoking is a strong risk factor for developing RA and also associates with greater severity.

Whatever the initiating stimulus, RA is characterised by infiltration of the synovial membrane with lymphocytes, plasma cells and macrophages. CD4+ T cells play a central role by interacting with other cells in the synovium. Activated T cells stimulate B cells to produce immunoglobulins including RF, and macrophages to produce proinflammatory cytokines. These act on endothelium, synovial fibroblasts, bone cells and chondrocytes to promote swelling and congestion of the synovial membrane and destruction of bone, cartilage and soft tissues (Fig. 25.20).

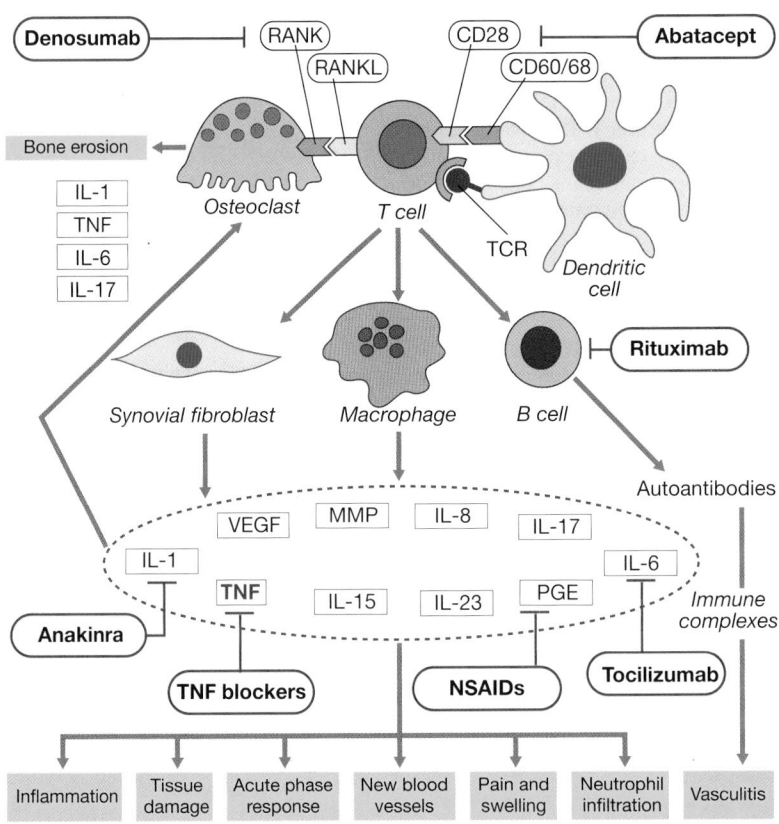

Fig. 25.20 Pathogenesis of rheumatoid arthritis. The figure summarises some of the cytokines and cellular interactions believed to be important in RA. The molecular targets for biologic agents currently used in the treatment of RA are shown. It is thought that TNF plays a particularly important role by orchestrating production of other cytokines. (IL = interleukins; MMP = matrix metalloproteinases; PGE = prostaglandin E; TCR = T-cell receptor; TNF = tumour necrosis factor; VEGF = vascular endothelial growth factor)

The pro-inflammatory cytokine TNF-α plays an important role in this process by regulating production of other cytokines, whose actions are shown in Figure 25.20. The B cells release immunoglobulins, including RF, which can form immune complexes within the joint and in extra-articular tissues, leading to vasculitis. Lymphoid follicles form within the synovial membrane. Inflammatory granulation tissue (pannus) spreads over and under the articular cartilage, which is progressively eroded and destroyed. Later, fibrous or bony ankylosis may occur. Muscles adjacent to inflamed joints atrophy and may be infiltrated with lymphocytes.

Rheumatoid nodules consist of a central area of fibrinoid material surrounded by a palisade of proliferating mononuclear cells. Similar granulomatous lesions may occur in the pleura, lung, pericardium and sclera. Lymph nodes in RA are often hyperplastic, showing many lymphoid follicles with large germinal centres and numerous plasma cells in the sinuses and medullary cords. Immunofluorescence confirms RF synthesis by plasma cells in synovium and lymph nodes.

Clinical features

The typical presentation is with pain, joint swelling and stiffness affecting the small joints of the hands, feet and wrists. Large joint involvement, systemic symptoms and extra-articular features may also occur. Clinical criteria for the diagnosis of RA are shown in Box 25.50, although it should be noted that these were designed for epidemiological studies rather than for the diagnosis of individual patients. By convention, symptoms need to have persisted for more than 6 weeks for the diagnosis of RA. Although somewhat arbitrary, this ensures that patients with viral or other types of self-limiting arthritis are not prematurely labelled as having RA.

Sometimes RA has a very acute onset, with florid morning stiffness, polyarthritis and pitting oedema. This occurs more commonly in old age. Other patients may present with proximal muscle stiffness mimicking polymyalgia rheumatica (p. 1115). Occasionally, the onset is palindromic, with relapsing and remitting episodes of pain, stiffness and swelling which last only for a few hours or days.

Examination of the hands often provides a good reflection of overall disease activity. The typical features are symmetrical swelling of the metacarpophalangeal (MCP) joints and proximal IPJs. These and other joints are actively inflamed if they are tender on pressure, and have stress pain on passive movement or effusion/soft tissue swelling. Erythema is not usually a feature and its presence implies coexistent sepsis. Characteristic deformities develop with long-standing disease, including 'swan neck' deformity, the boutonnière or 'button hole' deformity, and a Z deformity of the thumb (Fig. 25.21). Dorsal subluxation of the ulna at the distal radio-ulnar joint is common and may contribute to rupture of the fourth and fifth extensor tendons. Triggering of fingers may occur because of nodules in the flexor tendon sheaths.

In the foot, dorsal subluxation of the MTP joints may result in 'cock-up' toe deformities. This causes pain on weight-bearing on the exposed MTP heads and development of secondary adventitious bursae and callosities. In the hindfoot, calcaneovalgus (eversion) is the most common deformity, reflecting damage to the ankle and subtalar joint. This is often associated with loss of the longitudinal arch (flat foot) due to rupture of the tibialis posterior tendon.

Popliteal ('Baker's') cysts usually occur in combination with knee synovitis, where synovial fluid communicates with the cyst but is prevented from returning to the joint by a valve-like mechanism. Rupture, often induced by knee flexion in the presence of a large effusion, leads to calf pain and swelling.

Extra-articular features

Anorexia, weight loss and fatigue are common and may occur throughout the disease course. Generalised osteoporosis and muscle-wasting (sarcopenia) result from systemic inflammation. Extra-articular features are most

25.50 Criteria for diagnosis of rheumatoid arthritis*

Diagnosis of RA is made with four or more of the following:

- Morning stiffness (> 1 hr)
- Arthritis of three or more joint areas
- Arthritis of hand joints
- Symmetrical arthritis
- Rheumatoid nodules Rheumatoid factor
- Radiological changes

*American Rheumatism Association 1988 revision.
Note: symptoms must have been present for 6 weeks or more.

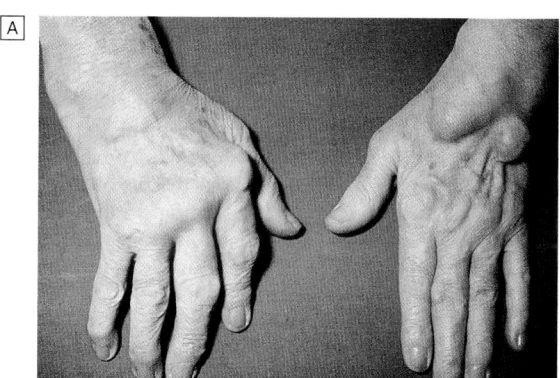 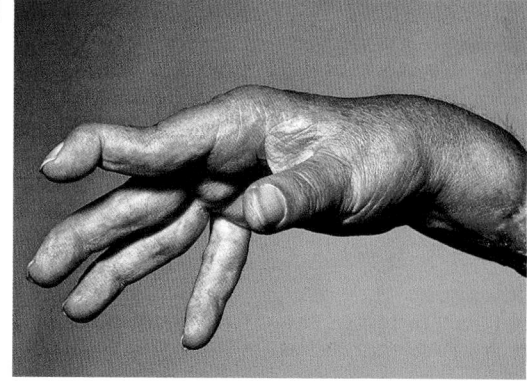

Fig. 25.21 The hand in rheumatoid arthritis. **A** Ulnar deviation of the fingers with wasting of the small muscles of the hands and synovial swelling at the wrists, the extensor tendon sheaths, the metacarpophalangeal and proximal interphalangeal joints. **B** 'Swan neck' deformity of the fingers.

common in patients with long-standing seropositive erosive disease but may occasionally occur at presentation, especially in men. Most are due to serositis, granuloma/nodule formation or vasculitis (Box 25.51).

Cutaneous and vascular features

Rheumatoid nodules occur almost exclusively in seropositive patients, usually at sites of pressure or friction such as the extensor surfaces of the forearm, sacrum, Achilles tendon and toes (Fig. 25.22). They may be complicated by ulceration and secondary infection.

Rheumatoid vasculitis usually occurs in older seropositive patients in the context of systemic symptoms and multiple extra-articular features. Vasculitis can vary from the relatively benign nail-fold infarcts to widespread cutaneous ulceration and skin necrosis. Involvement of medium-sized arteries can lead to mesenteric, renal or coronary artery occlusion.

Ocular involvement

The most common symptom is dry eyes (keratoconjunctivitis sicca) due to secondary Sjögren's syndrome. Painless

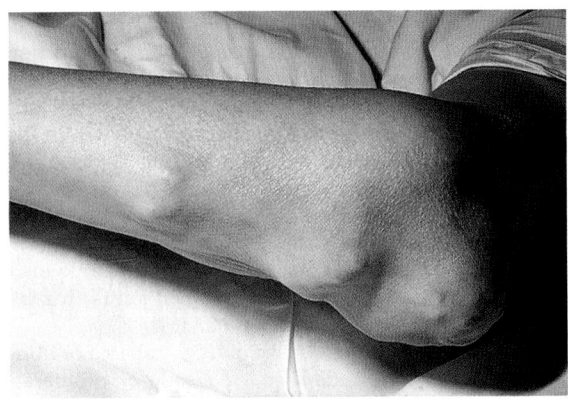

Fig. 25.22 Rheumatoid nodules and olecranon bursitis. Nodules were palpable within as well as outside the bursa.

episcleritis frequently accompanies nodular seropositive disease; it may cause intense redness of superficial vessels but sight is unimpaired. Scleritis is more serious and potentially sight-threatening; the eye is red and painful, vision is often impaired and the sclera shows a deep red blush beneath the individual red superficial vessels. Scleromalacia is painless bilateral thinning of the sclera, with the affected area appearing blue or grey (the colour of the underlying choroid). Corneal melting is a rare but devastating manifestation. It usually occurs in long-standing disease and is associated with systemic vasculitis. It causes pain, redness and blurred vision with corneal thinning. If it is untreated, progression to perforation is common, so urgent high-dose steroid and immunosuppressive therapy are indicated.

Cardiac and pulmonary involvement

Cardiac involvement occurs in about 30% of patients with seropositive RA but is usually asymptomatic. Symptomatic pericardial effusions and constrictive pericarditis are rare. Occasionally, granulomatous lesions can cause heart block, cardiomyopathy, coronary artery occlusion or aortic regurgitation. Serositis is commonly asymptomatic but may cause pleurisy or breathlessness. Pulmonary fibrosis can occur in advanced RA and may cause dyspnoea (p. 714).

Neurological complications

Peripheral entrapment neuropathies may result from compression by hypertrophied synovium or by joint subluxation. Median nerve compression in the carpal tunnel is most common and bilateral compression can occur as an early presenting feature of RA. Other syndromes include ulnar nerve compression at the elbow or wrist, compression of the lateral popliteal nerve at the head of the fibula, and tarsal tunnel syndrome (entrapment of the posterior tibial nerve in the flexor retinaculum) which causes burning, tingling and numbness in the distal sole and toes. Diffuse symmetrical peripheral neuropathy and mononeuritis multiplex may occur in patients with rheumatoid vasculitis.

Cervical cord compression can result from subluxation of the cervical spine at the atlanto-axial joint or at a subaxial level (Fig. 25.23). Atlanto-axial subluxation is a common finding in long-standing RA and is due to erosion of the transverse ligament that is posterior to

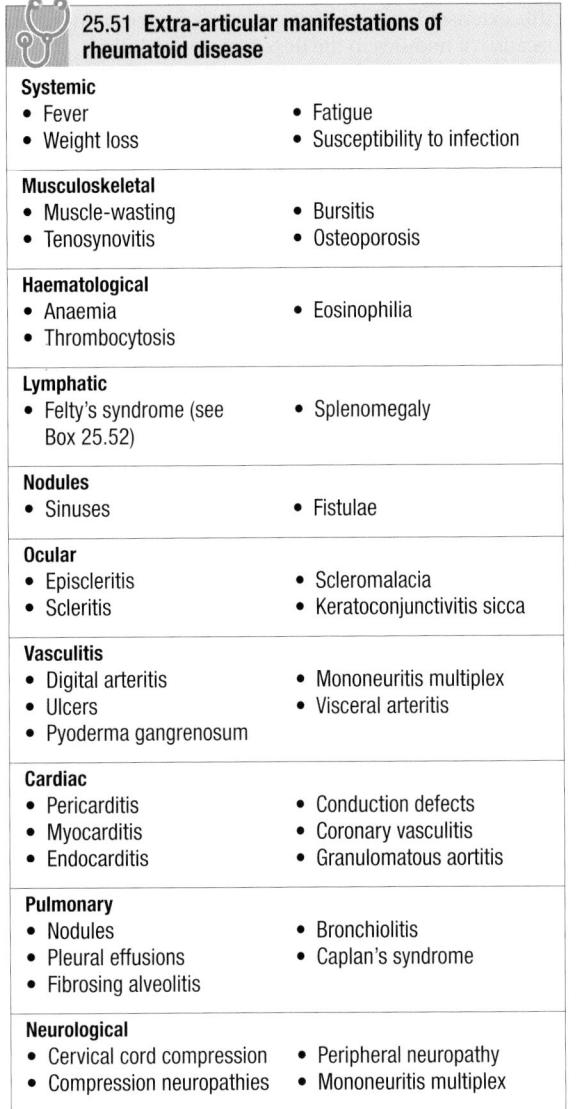

25.51 Extra-articular manifestations of rheumatoid disease	
Systemic	
• Fever	• Fatigue
• Weight loss	• Susceptibility to infection
Musculoskeletal	
• Muscle-wasting	• Bursitis
• Tenosynovitis	• Osteoporosis
Haematological	
• Anaemia	• Eosinophilia
• Thrombocytosis	
Lymphatic	
• Felty's syndrome (see Box 25.52)	• Splenomegaly
Nodules	
• Sinuses	• Fistulae
Ocular	
• Episcleritis	• Scleromalacia
• Scleritis	• Keratoconjunctivitis sicca
Vasculitis	
• Digital arteritis	• Mononeuritis multiplex
• Ulcers	• Visceral arteritis
• Pyoderma gangrenosum	
Cardiac	
• Pericarditis	• Conduction defects
• Myocarditis	• Coronary vasculitis
• Endocarditis	• Granulomatous aortitis
Pulmonary	
• Nodules	• Bronchiolitis
• Pleural effusions	• Caplan's syndrome
• Fibrosing alveolitis	
Neurological	
• Cervical cord compression	• Peripheral neuropathy
• Compression neuropathies	• Mononeuritis multiplex
Amyloidosis (p. 84)	

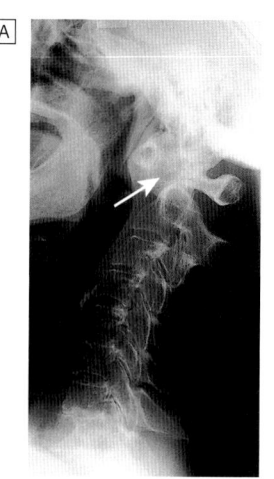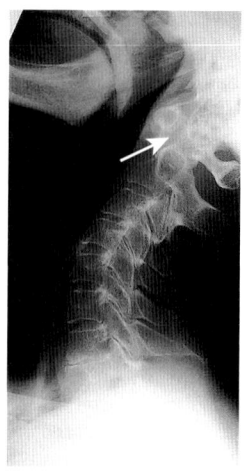

Fig. 25.23 Subluxation of cervical spine. [A] Flexion, showing widening of the space (arrow) between the odontoid peg of the axis (behind) and the anterior arch of the atlas (in front). [B] Extension, showing reduction in this space.

the odontoid peg. On neck flexion, this allows the peg to move posteriorly and indent the cord. If unrecognised, it can lead to cord compression or sudden death following minor trauma or manipulation. Atlanto-axial subluxation should be suspected in any RA patient who describes new onset of occipital headache, particularly if symptoms of paraesthesia or electric shock are present in the arms. In some patients, the onset may be insidious, with subtle loss of function that is initially attributed to active disease. Reflexes and power can be very difficult to assess in the presence of marked joint damage and therefore sensory or upper motor signs are the most important to elicit. Patients with spinal cord compression may require operative stabilisation and fixation, though the outcome is poor if the patient already has tetraparesis.

Other complications

Amyloidosis is a rare complication of prolonged active disease and usually presents with nephrotic syndrome. Microcytic anaemia can occur due to iron deficiency resulting from NSAID-induced gastrointestinal blood loss, and normochromic, normocytic anaemia with thrombocytosis occurs in active disease. Felty's syndrome is the association of splenomegaly and neutropenia with RA (Box 25.52). Generalised and local lymphadenopathy affecting nodes draining actively inflamed joints may both occur. Patients with persistent lymphadenopathy should be biopsied since there is an increased risk of lymphoma in patients with long-standing RA.

Investigations

The diagnosis of RA is based on clinical criteria and there is no single diagnostic test. However, investigations are useful in confirming the diagnosis and assessing disease activity (Box 25.53). The DAS 28 score is frequently used to assess the response to treatment and the need for biologic therapy. It involves counting the number of swollen and tender joints in the upper limbs and knees, and combining this with the ESR and the patient's assessment of his/her general health on a visual analogue scale, to generate a numerical score. The higher the value, the greater the disease activity.

25.52 Felty's syndrome

Risk factors

- Age of onset 50–70 yrs
- Female > male
- Caucasians > blacks
- Long-standing RA
- Deforming but inactive disease
- Seropositive for RF

Common clinical features

- Splenomegaly
- Lymphadenopathy
- Weight loss
- Skin pigmentation
- Keratoconjunctivitis sicca
- Vasculitis, leg ulcers
- Recurrent infections
- Nodules

Laboratory findings

- Anaemia (normochromic, normocytic)
- Neutropenia
- Abnormal liver function
- Thrombocytopenia
- Impaired T- and B-cell immunity

25.53 Investigations and monitoring of rheumatoid arthritis

To establish diagnosis

- Clinical criteria
- Acute phase response (APR)
- Serological tests
- X-rays

To monitor disease activity and drug efficacy

- Pain (visual analogue scale)
- Early morning stiffness (minutes)
- Joint tenderness
- Joint swelling
- DAS 28 score
- APR

To monitor disease damage

- X-rays
- Functional assessment

To monitor drug safety

- Urinalysis
- Biochemistry
- Haematology

ESR and CRP are usually raised (acute phase response), but may not be in patients with isolated small joint arthritis. RF and anti-CCP antibodies are detected in 60–80% of patients but their absence does not exclude the diagnosis. A positive anti-CCP antibody is highly specific for RA and can occur before clinical onset of the disease. RF is non-specific; low titres are found in about 10% of the normal population and in other diseases (p. 1063). Plain X-rays of the hands, wrist and feet are useful. Periarticular osteoporosis is common during the early stages of disease and may be present within 6 months of onset. Non-proliferative marginal joint erosions on X-ray are characteristic, but uncommon within the first year. Ultrasound and MRI are more sensitive than X-rays at detecting early erosions. Patients who are suspected of having atlanto-axial disease should have lateral X-rays taken in flexion and extension, and the degree of cord compression should be established with MRI. In patients with Baker's cyst, Doppler ultrasound and an arthrogram may be required to establish the diagnosis, since deep venous thrombosis (DVT) and Baker's cyst may coexist.

25

Management

This follows the principles outlined on pages 1075–1082. Physical rest, targeted anti-inflammatory therapy and passive exercises are the mainstays, with the aim of relieving symptoms, suppressing inflammation, and conserving and restoring function in affected joints. A multidisciplinary approach is required, including doctors, nurses, physiotherapists and occupational therapists, and patient education and counselling play a key role. During treatment, periodic assessment of disease activity, progression and disability is essential. In the vast majority, management is outpatient-based, but hospital admission can be helpful in patients with very active disease for a period of bed rest, multiple joint injections, splinting, regular hydrotherapy, physiotherapy and education.

Drug therapy

Prompt introduction of DMARD therapy plays a central role. The patient should be advised that this will not improve symptoms immediately, but in the longer term there is a good chance that symptoms will come under control and joint damage will be prevented. If the first-choice drug fails to control disease activity, other DMARDs can be added. If adverse effects occur, the patient should be switched to another DMARD. If disease activity persists despite an adequate trial of two DMARDs including methotrexate, anti-TNF therapy should be considered. Because of the delayed onset of action, corticosteroids (prednisolone 7.5–10 mg daily for 3 months, or methylprednisolone 80–120 mg i.m.) are often given when DMARDs are commenced to give symptomatic relief. Most patients also require NSAID and other analgesics. Early DMARD use reduces radiographic progression in RA, at least in the medium term (Box 25.54), but anti-TNF therapy seems more effective in preventing joint erosions. Box 25.55 lists the special considerations in old age.

EBM 25.54 DMARD therapy for rheumatoid arthritis

'There is a therapeutic window of opportunity early in the course of RA associated with sustained benefit in radiographic progression for up to 5 years. Prompt initiation of antirheumatic therapy in persons with RA may alter the long-term course of the disease.'

• Finckh A, et al. Arthritis Rheum 2006; 55:864–872.

25.55 Rheumatoid arthritis in old age

• **Presentation:** may be atypical—for example, with an initial polymyalgic picture or with synovitis and marked peripheral oedema.
• **Increasing age and comorbidity** (e.g. cardiac, renal, gastrointestinal tract disease): increase the risks of NSAID gastrotoxicity; comorbidity can also make overall management more difficult.
• **Corticosteroid-induced osteoporosis:** increased risk in those aged > 65 yrs. Bisphosphonates should be co-prescribed in those on corticosteroid therapy for > 3 mths.
• **DMARD and biologic therapy:** age alone is not a contraindication.

Surgery

Synovectomy of the wrist or finger tendon sheaths of the hands may be required for pain relief or to prevent tendon rupture when medical interventions have failed. In later stages when joint damage has occurred, osteotomy, arthrodesis or arthroplasty may be required (see Box 25.44, p. 1083).

Seronegative spondyloarthritis

This describes a group of related inflammatory joint diseases distinct from RA, which show considerable overlap in their clinical features and shared immunogenetic association with the HLA B27 antigen (Box 25.56). The diseases included are:
• ankylosing spondylitis
• reactive arthritis, including Reiter's syndrome
• psoriatic arthritis
• arthropathy associated with inflammatory bowel disease.

The synovitis is non-specific and, apart from absence of granulomas, is often indistinguishable from RA. However, the distinctive feature of this group of diseases is the marked degree of extrasynovial inflammation, especially of the enthesis but also affecting the joint capsule, periarticular periosteum, cartilage and subchondral bone. Large central cartilaginous joints (sacroiliac, intervertebral, symphysis pubis) are particularly involved, but even when synovial joints are affected (often spinal apophyseal joints, hips, knees, shoulders) extrasynovial inflammation is prominent. Apart from targeting entheses, the other characteristic features are resolution of inflammation by extensive fibrosis and a tendency for the resulting scar tissue to calcify. This chronic inflammation, which largely targets extrasynovial tissue, may characteristically lead to joint fusion in the relative absence of joint synovitis. Similarly, periarticular osteitis and periostitis may result in bony spurs that bridge adjacent vertebral bodies (syndesmophytes) or protrude at sites of ligament attachment (e.g. calcaneal or olecranon 'spurs').

There is a striking association with carriage of the HLA-B27 allele, particularly for ankylosing spondylitis (> 95%) and Reiter's disease (90%), and when there is sacroiliitis, uveitis or balanitis. The mechanism is

---

25.56 Clinical features common to seronegative spondyloarthritis

• Asymmetrical inflammatory oligoarthritis (lower > upper limb)
• Sacroiliitis and inflammatory spondylitis
• Inflammatory enthesitis
• Tendency for familial aggregation
• No association with seropositivity for RF
• Absence of nodules and other extra-articular features of RA
• Typical overlapping extra-articular features:
    Mucosal inflammation: conjunctivitis, buccal ulceration, urethritis, prostatitis, bowel ulceration
    Pustular skin lesions and nail dystrophy
    Anterior uveitis
    Aortic root fibrosis (aortic incompetence, conduction defects)
    Erythema nodosum

unclear. The suggested pathogenesis for the seronegative spondyloarthritides is an aberrant response to infection in genetically predisposed people: the 'reactive' concept. In some situations a triggering organism can be identified, as in Reiter's disease following bacterial dysentery or chlamydial urethritis, but in others the environmental trigger remains obscure. The seronegative spondyloarthritis 'group' concept is also supported by aggregation of the conditions within families, with each showing an increased familial incidence of the other conditions. Such families may thus share an inherited 'reactive' potential, but the phenotypic expression is modified according to the inciting trigger and other genetic and constitutional features of the individual.

Ankylosing spondylitis

Ankylosing spondylitis (AS) is characterised by a chronic inflammatory arthritis predominantly affecting the sacro-iliac joints and spine, which can progress to bony fusion of the spine. It has a peak onset in the second and third decades, with a male:female ratio of about 3:1. In Europe, more than 90% of those affected are HLA-B27-positive. The overall prevalence is less than 0.5% in most communities. Over 75% of patients are able to remain in employment and enjoy a good quality of life. Even if severe ankylosis develops, functional limitation may not be marked as long as the spine is fused in an erect posture.

AS is thought to result from exposure to a common environmental pathogen in genetically susceptible individuals, although no specific trigger has been identified. Chronic prostatitis is more common than expected but appears to be non-infective in origin. Increased faecal carriage of *Klebsiella aerogenes* occurs in patients with established AS and may relate to exacerbation of both joint and eye disease.

Clinical features

The onset is usually insidious, with recurring episodes of low back pain and marked stiffness. Radiation of pain to the buttocks or posterior thighs may be misdiagnosed as sciatica. Unlike mechanical back pain, symptoms extend over many segments and are axial and symmetrical in distribution. Symptoms are most marked in the early morning and after inactivity, and are relieved by movement. Although the lumbosacral area is usually the first and worst affected region, some patients present with mainly thoracic or neck symptoms. The disease tends to ascend the spine slowly and eventually, after several years, the whole spine may be affected. As the spine becomes progressively ankylosed, spinal rigidity and secondary osteoporosis predispose to spinal fracture. Spinal cord compression is rare.

Early physical signs include failure to obliterate the lumbar lordosis on forward flexion, restriction of movements of the lumbar spine in all directions, and possible pain on sacroiliac stressing. As the disease progresses, stiffness increases throughout the spine, and chest expansion frequently becomes restricted. Spinal fusion varies in its extent and in most cases does not cause a gross flexion deformity, but a few develop marked kyphosis of the dorsal and cervical spine that may interfere with forward vision. This may prove incapacitating, especially when associated with fixed flexion contractures of hips or knees. Pleuritic chest pain aggravated by breathing is common and results from costovertebral joint involve-

ment. Plantar fasciitis, Achilles tendinitis and tenderness over bony prominences such as the iliac crest and greater trochanter are common, reflecting inflammation at the sites of tendon insertions (enthesitis).

Peripheral arthritis

Up to 40% of patients have peripheral arthritis. This is usually asymmetrical at first, mainly affecting hips, knees, ankles or shoulders. Involvement of a peripheral joint, most commonly ankle, knee or elbow, may precede the development of spinal symptoms in around 10% of cases. In a further 10%, symptoms begin in childhood as one variety of pauciarticular juvenile idiopathic arthritis.

Extra-articular disease

Fatigue is often a major complaint and may result from both chronic interruption of sleep due to pain, as well as chronic systemic inflammation. Acute anterior uveitis is the most common extra-articular feature. Occasionally, this precedes joint disease. Other extra-articular features are rare (Box 25.57).

> **25.57 Extra-articular features of ankylosing spondylitis**
>
> - Anterior uveitis (25%) and conjunctivitis (20%)
> - Prostatitis (80% men): usually asymptomatic
> - Cardiovascular disease
>   Aortic incompetence
>   Mitral incompetence
>   Cardiac conduction defects
>   Pericarditis
> - Amyloidosis
> - Atypical upper lobe pulmonary fibrosis

Investigations

X-ray changes are characteristic but may take years to develop. Sacroiliitis is often the first abnormality, beginning in the lower synovial parts of the joints with irregularity and loss of cortical margins, widening of the joint space and subsequently sclerosis, narrowing and fusion. MRI is more sensitive for detection of early sacroiliitis, but is seldom required. Lateral thoracolumbar spine X-rays may show anterior 'squaring' of vertebrae due to erosion and sclerosis of the anterior corners and periostitis of the waist. Bridging syndesmophytes are fine and symmetrical, and follow the outermost fibres of the annulus (Fig. 25.24). Ossification of the anterior longitudinal ligament and facet joint fusion may also be visible. The combination of these features may result in the typical 'bamboo' spine (Fig. 25.25). Erosive changes may be seen in the symphysis pubis, the ischial tuberosities and peripheral joints. Osteoporosis and atlanto-axial dislocation can occur as late features.

The ESR and CRP are usually raised in active disease. RF and other autoantibodies are usually negative. Testing for HLA-B27 can be a helpful investigation for pauciarticular juvenile idiopathic arthritis but is unhelpful in adults with spinal symptoms.

Management

The aims are to relieve pain and stiffness, maintain a maximal range of skeletal mobility and avoid the

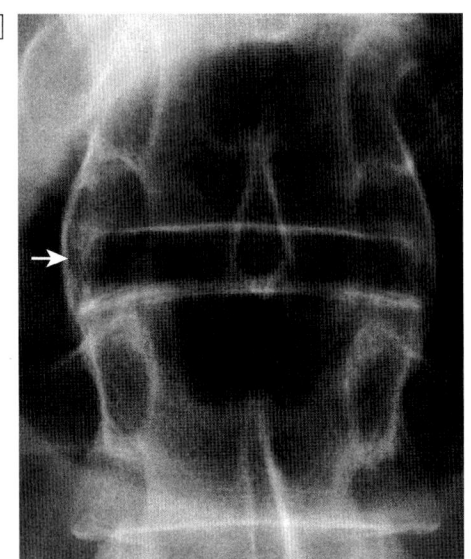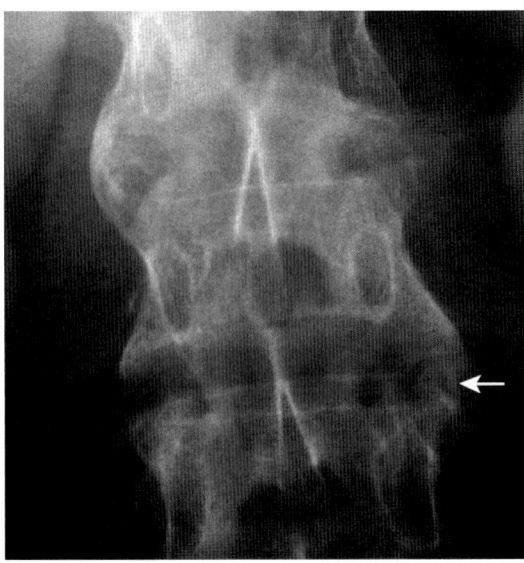

Fig. 25.24 Radiographic syndesmophyte (arrows). [A] Fine symmetrical marginal syndesmophytes typical of ankylosing spondylitis. [B] Coarse, asymmetrical non-marginal syndesmophytes typical of psoriatic/Reiter's spondylitis.

development of deformities. Education and appropriate physical activity are the cornerstones of management. Early in the disease, patients should be taught to perform daily back extension exercises, including a morning 'warm-up' routine, and to punctuate prolonged periods of inactivity with regular breaks. Swimming is ideal exercise. Poor posture must be avoided.

NSAIDs and analgesics are often effective in relieving symptoms but do not alter the course of the disease. A long-acting NSAID at night is helpful for marked morning stiffness. Peripheral arthritis can be treated with methotrexate or sulfasalazine, but these drugs have no effect on axial disease. Anti-TNF therapy should be considered for disease inadequately controlled by these measures since it often has a significant impact on axial symptoms.

Local corticosteroid injections can be useful for persistent plantar fasciitis, other enthesopathies and peripheral arthritis. Oral corticosteroids may be required for acute uveitis but do not help spinal disease. Severe hip, knee or shoulder restriction may require surgery. Total hip arthroplasty has largely removed the need for difficult spinal surgery in those with advanced deformity.

Reactive arthritis and Reiter's disease

Reactive arthritis is predominantly a disease of young men with a sex ratio of 15:1. It is the most common cause of inflammatory arthritis in men aged 16–35 but may

Fig. 25.25 'Bamboo' spine of severe late ankylosing spondylitis. Note the symmetrical marginal syndesmophytes (arrows), sacroiliac joint fusion and generalised osteopenia.

25.58 Reiter's disease
Classic triad*
• Non-specific urethritis • Conjunctivitis (~50%) • Reactive arthritis
Additional extra-articular features
• Circinate balanitis (20–50%) • Keratoderma blennorrhagica (15%) • Nail dystrophy • Buccal erosions (10%)
Precipitated by
• Bacterial dysentery, mainly *Salmonella*, *Shigella*, *Campylobacter* or *Yersinia* • Sexually acquired infection with *Chlamydia*
*Incomplete forms with just one or two of the classic triad are more frequent than the full syndrome.

occur at any age. Between 1 and 2% of patients with non-specific urethritis seen at genitourinary medicine clinics have reactive arthritis. Following an epidemic of *Shigella* dysentery, 20% of HLA-B27-positive men developed reactive arthritis. Reiter's disease is the triad described in Box 25.58 but many patients present with just arthritis.

Clinical features

The onset is typically acute or subacute, with an inflammatory oligoarthritis that is asymmetrical and targets lower limb joints, typically the ankles, midtarsal joints, metatarsophalangeal joints or knees. Achilles tendinitis or plantar fasciitis may also be present. There may be considerable systemic disturbance with fever and weight loss. It occasionally presents subacutely with single joint involvement and there may be no clear history of an infectious trigger. The first attack of arthritis is usually self-limiting, with spontaneous remission within 2–4 months. However, recurrent or chronic arthritis develops in more than 60% of patients. Low back pain and stiffness are common and 15–20% of patients develop spondylitis. Around 10% of patients have evidence of active disease 20 years after the onset. Spondylitis, chronic erosive arthritis, recurrent acute arthritis and uveitis are the major causes of long-term morbidity.

Extra-articular features (see Box 25.58)

Circinate balanitis starts as vesicles on the coronal margin of the prepuce and glans penis, later rupturing to form superficial erosions with minimal surrounding erythema, some coalescing to give the circular pattern. Lesions are often painless and may escape notice. Keratoderma blennorrhagica begins as discrete waxy yellow-brown vesico-papules with desquamating margins, occasionally coalescing to form large crusty plaques. The palms and soles are particularly affected but spread may occur to the scrotum, scalp and trunk. These lesions are indistinguishable from pustular psoriasis. Nail dystrophy with subungual hyperkeratosis is common and indistinguishable from psoriatic nail dystrophy. Mouth ulcers manifest as shallow red painless patches on tongue, palate, buccal mucosa and lips, lasting only a few days. Conjunctivitis may accompany the first acute episode. Uveitis is rare with the first attack but occurs in 30% of patients with recurring or chronic arthritis.

Other complications are rare but include aortic incompetence, conduction defects, pleuro-pericarditis, peripheral neuropathy, seizures and meningoencephalitis.

Investigations

The diagnosis is usually made clinically but joint aspiration may be required to exclude crystal arthritis and infection. Synovial fluid is inflammatory and often contains giant macrophages (Reiter's cells). ESR and CRP may be raised. Urethritis may be confirmed in the 'two-glass test' by demonstration of mucoid threads in the first-void specimen that clear in the second. High vaginal swabs may reveal *Chlamydia* on culture. Except for post-*Salmonella* arthritis, stool cultures are usually negative by the time the arthritis presents, but serum agglutinin tests may help confirm previous dysentery. RF, CCP and ANA are negative.

X-rays are seldom helpful during the acute attack, but in chronic or recurrent disease periarticular osteopenia, joint space narrowing and marginal prolifera-tive erosions may be observed. Another characteristic feature is periostitis, especially of metatarsals, phalanges and pelvis, and large 'fluffy' calcaneal spurs. In contrast to AS, radiographic sacroiliitis is often asymmetrical and sometimes unilateral, and syndesmophytes are predominantly coarse and asymmetrical, often extending beyond the contours of the annulus ('non-marginal') (see Fig. 25.24). X-ray changes in the peripheral joints and spine are identical to those in psoriasis.

Management

The acute attack should be treated with limited rest, oral NSAIDs and analgesics, and for marked synovitis, intra-articular injection of corticosteroids. Non-specific chlamydial urethritis is usually treated with a short course of tetracycline and this may reduce the frequency of arthritis in sexually acquired cases. Treatment with DMARDs should be considered for patients with persistent marked symptoms, recurrent arthritis or severe keratoderma blennorrhagica. Anterior uveitis is a medical emergency requiring topical, subconjunctival or systemic corticosteroids.

Psoriatic arthritis

Psoriatic arthritis (PsA) occurs in about 1 in 1000 of the general population and in 7% of patients with psoriasis. Approximately 20% of all patients with seronegative polyarthritis have PsA. The onset is usually between 25 and 40 years of age. Most patients (70%) have pre-existing psoriasis, but in 20% the arthritis predates its onset. Occasionally, the arthritis and psoriasis develop synchronously.

Clinical features

The presentation is with joint pain and swelling. Several different patterns of joint involvement are recognised but the course is generally one of intermittent exacerbation followed by varying periods of complete or near-complete remission. Destructive arthritis and disability are uncommon, except in the case of arthritis mutilans.

- *Asymmetrical inflammatory oligoarthritis* affects about 40% of patients and often presents abruptly with a combination of synovitis and adjacent periarticular inflammation; this occurs most characteristically in the hands and feet when synovitis of a finger or toe is coupled with tenosynovitis, enthesitis and inflammation of intervening tissue to give a 'sausage digit' or dactylitis (Fig. 25.26A). Large joints such as the knee and ankle may also be involved, sometimes with very large effusions.
- *Symmetrical polyarthritis* occurs in about 25% of cases. It predominates in women and may strongly resemble RA, with symmetrical involvement of small and large joints in both upper and lower limbs. Nodules and other extra-articular features of RA are absent and arthritis is generally less extensive and more benign. Much of the hand deformity often results from tenosynovitis and soft tissue contractures.
- *Distal IPJ arthritis* is an uncommon but characteristic pattern mainly affecting men. It targets finger distal IPJs and surrounding periarticular tissues, almost invariably with accompanying nail dystrophy (Fig. 25.26B).

25

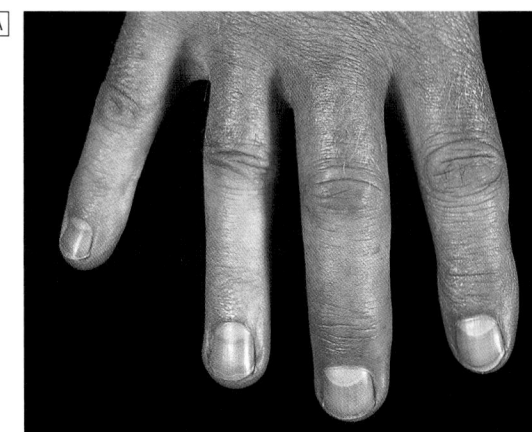

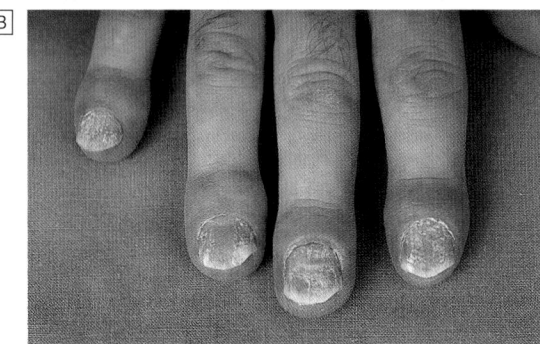

Fig. 25.26 Psoriatic arthropathy. [A] 'Sausage' middle finger of a patient with psoriatic arthritis. [B] Typical distal interphalangeal joint pattern with accompanying nail dystrophy (pitting and onycholysis).

- *Psoriatic spondylitis* presents a similar clinical picture to AS but with less severe involvement. It may occur alone or with any of the other clinical patterns.
- *Arthritis mutilans* is a deforming erosive arthritis targeting the fingers and toes which occurs in 5% of cases. Marked cartilage and bone destruction results in marked instability. The encasing skin appears invaginated and 'telescoped' ('main en lorgnette') and traction can pull the finger back to its original length.

Nail changes include pitting, onycholysis, subungual hyperkeratosis and horizontal ridging. They are found in 85% of those with PsA and only 30% of those with uncomplicated psoriasis, and can occur in the absence of skin disease. The characteristic rash of psoriasis (p. 1260) may be widespread, or confined to the scalp, natal cleft and umbilicus, where it is easily overlooked. Conjunctivitis can occur, whereas uveitis is mainly confined to HLA-B27-positive individuals with sacroiliitis and spondylitis.

Investigations

The diagnosis is clinical but ESR and CRP may be raised, especially in patients with extensive disease. RF, CCP and ANA are generally negative. X-rays may be normal or show erosive change with joint space narrowing. Features that favour PsA over RA include proliferative marginal erosions, absence of periarticular osteoporosis and osteosclerosis of the phalanges ('ivory phalanx'). Arthritis mutilans and peripheral joint ankylosis can occur. The changes in the axial skeleton resemble those of chronic reactive arthritis, with coarse, asymmetrical, non-marginal syndesmophytes and asymmetrical sacroiliitis.

Management

Therapy with NSAID and analgesics may be sufficient to control symptoms. Intra-articular injections of corticosteroid may help control synovitis in problem joints. In general, splints and prolonged rest should be avoided because of the tendency to fibrous and bony ankylosis. Patients with spondylitis should be prescribed the same exercise and posture regime as in AS.

Therapy with DMARDs should be considered for persistent synovitis unresponsive to conservative treatment. Methotrexate is the treatment of first choice since it may also help skin psoriasis, but other DMARDs may also be effective. Hydroxychloroquine is generally avoided, as it can cause exfoliative skin reactions. Anti-TNF treatment should be considered for patients with active synovitis who respond inadequately to standard DMARDs. This is effective for both PsA and psoriasis.

The retinoid acitretin (p. 1264) is effective for skin lesions and can also help the arthritis, but is teratogenic so must be avoided in young women. It also causes mucocutaneous side-effects, hyperlipidaemia, myalgias and extraspinal calcification. Photochemotherapy with methoxypsoralen and long-wave ultraviolet light (psoralen + UVA, PUVA) is primarily used for skin disease, but can also help those with synchronous exacerbations of inflammatory arthritis.

Arthritis associated with inflammatory bowel disease

An acute inflammatory oligoarthritis ('enteropathic arthritis') occurs in around 10% of patients with ulcerative colitis and 20% of those with Crohn's disease. It predominantly affects the large lower limb joints (knees, ankles, hips) but wrists and small joints of the hands and feet can also be involved. The arthritis usually coincides with exacerbations of the underlying bowel disease, and sometimes occurs with aphthous mouth ulcers, iritis and erythema nodosum. It improves with effective treatment of the bowel disease, and can be cured by total colectomy in patients with ulcerative colitis. Patients with inflammatory bowel disease may also develop sacroiliitis (16%) and AS (6%), which are clinically and radiologically identical to classic AS. These can predate or follow the onset of bowel disease and there is no correlation between activity of the spondylitis and bowel disease.

Crystal-associated disease

A variety of crystals can deposit in and around joints and associate with both acute inflammatory and chronic syndromes (Box 25.59). In some instances crystals are the primary pathogenic agents—true 'crystal deposition disease', e.g. gout. In others, MSK disease predisposes to secondary crystal formation: for example, predisposition to calcium pyrophosphate and apatite crystal formation in OA. Such crystals may subsequently amplify symptoms and damage, or be of no clinical consequence.

Several factors influence crystal formation (Fig. 25.27). There must be sufficient concentration of the chemical

25.59 Crystal-associated arthritis and deposition in connective tissue	
Crystal	**Associations**
Common	
Monosodium urate monohydrate	Acute gout
	Chronic tophaceous gout
Calcium pyrophosphate dihydrate	Acute 'pseudogout'
	Chronic (pyrophosphate) arthropathy
	Chondrocalcinosis
Basic calcium phosphates	Calcific periarthritis
	Calcinosis
Uncommon	
Cholesterol	Chronic effusions in RA
Calcium oxalate	Acute arthritis in dialysis patients
Extrinsic crystals/semi-crystalline particles	
Synthetic crystals	Acute synovitis
Plant thorns/sea urchin spines	Chronic monoarthritis, tenosynovitis

components (ionic product), but whether a crystal then forms depends on the balance of tissue factors that promote and inhibit crystal nucleation and growth. Many tissues are supersaturated for various products but depend on natural inhibitors to prevent crystallisation. Crystals can also dissolve and the yield of crystals at any one

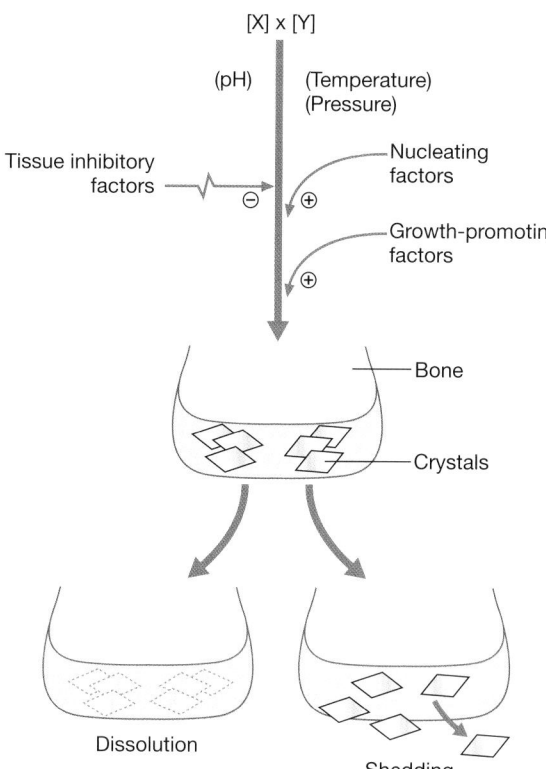

Fig. 25.27 Factors relating to crystal formation and tissue concentration at any one time.

time will depend on the relative rates of crystallisation, growth and dissolution.

The inflammatory potential of crystals resides in their physical irregularity and high negative surface charge, which can induce inflammation and damage cell membranes. Crystals may also cause mechanical damage to tissues and act as wear particles at the joint surface. Crystals forming deep within cartilage or tendon are prevented from interaction with proteins and cells, and can paradoxically reside in MSK tissues for years without causing inflammation or symptoms. It is only when they are released ('crystal shedding') from these protected sites that they are exposed to inflammatory mediators and trigger acute inflammation. Such attacks may occur spontaneously, result from mechanical loosening (local trauma), partial dissolution and reduced crystal size (e.g. initiation of hypouricaemic treatment), or occur in association with an acute phase response due to intercurrent illness or surgery.

Gout

Gout is a true crystal deposition disease, and is defined as the pathological reaction of the joint or periarticular tissues to the presence of monosodium urate monohydrate (MSU) crystals. MSU crystals preferentially deposit in peripheral connective tissues in and around synovial joints, initially favouring lower rather than upper limbs and especially targeting the first MTP joint and small joints of feet and hands. As the crystal deposits slowly increase and enlarge, there is progressive involvement of more proximal sites and the potential for cartilage and bone damage, with 'secondary' OA. MSU crystals take months or years to grow to a detectable size, implying a long asymptomatic phase.

Epidemiology

The prevalence of gout varies between populations but is approximately 1–2%, with a strong male predominance (> 5:1). It is the most common inflammatory arthritis in men and in older women. Prevalence increases with increasing serum uric acid (SUA) and with age. The incidence and prevalence of gout have increased in many countries in recent decades, in parallel with increased longevity and the higher prevalence of metabolic syndrome, of which hyperuricaemia is an integral component.

SUA levels are distributed in the community as a continuous variable (p. 4). Levels are higher in men than women; they rise from the age of 20 in men and after the menopause in women, positively correlate with obesity and vary according to ethnicity (highest in New Zealand Maoris). Hyperuricaemia is defined as an SUA level greater than 2 standard deviations above the mean for the population. Only a minority of hyperuricaemic people develop gout, emphasising the importance of tissue factors in crystal formation.

Aetiology

Primary gout

About one-third of the body uric acid pool is derived from dietary sources and two-thirds from endogenous purine metabolism (Fig. 25.28). The concentration of uric acid in body fluids depends on the balance between its synthesis and elimination by the kidneys (two-thirds) and gut (one-third). Purine nucleotide synthesis and

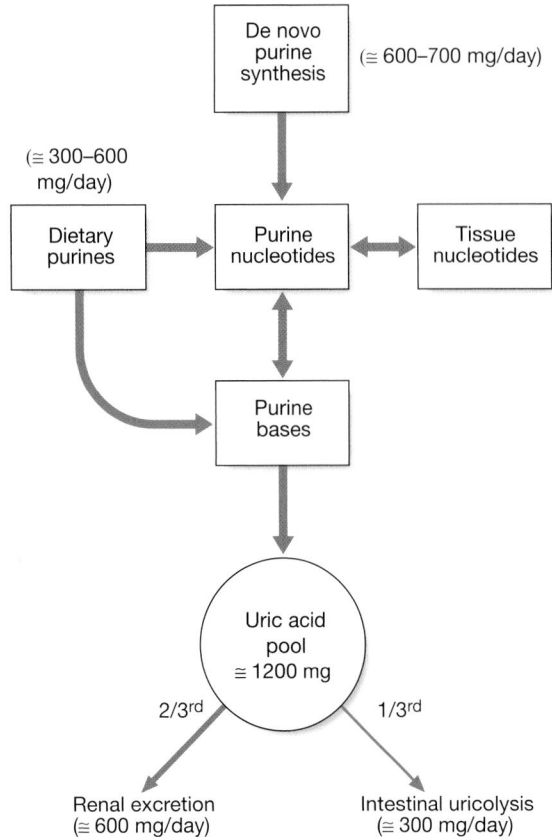

Fig. 25.28 The uric acid pool. Origins and disposal of uric acid in normal humans.

25.60 Factors that predispose to chronic hyperuricaemia and gout

Diminished renal excretion (common)

- Inherited isolated renal tubular defect ('under-excretors')
- Renal failure
- Chronic drug therapy
  Thiazide and loop diuretics
  Low-dose aspirin
  Ciclosporin
  Pyrazinamide
- Lead toxicity (e.g. in 'moonshine' drinkers)
- Lactic acidosis (alcohol)

Increased production of uric acid (uncommon)

- Increased purine turnover
  Chronic myeloproliferative or lymphoproliferative disorders (e.g. polycythaemia, chronic lymphatic leukaemia)
- Increased de novo synthesis ('over-producers')
  Unidentified abnormality (most common)
  Specific enzyme defect (rare)
    Hypoxanthine-guanine phosphoribosyl transferase deficiency
    Phosphoribosyl pyrophosphate synthetase over-activity
    Glucose-6-phosphatase deficiency

25.61 Gout in old age

- **Aetiology:** predominantly primary gout, but a higher proportion of secondary gout (chronic diuretic therapy or chronic kidney disease) than in middle-aged patients.
- **Nodal generalised OA:** an important additional risk factor for gout.
- **Presentation:** more often atypical (e.g. presentation with painful tophi and chronic symptoms, rather than as classic acute attacks; presentation in upper rather than lower limbs).
- **Treatment of acute attacks:** best treated by aspiration and intra-articular injection of long-acting corticosteroid followed by early mobilisation. Oral NSAID and colchicine are best avoided because of increased toxicity.
- **Allopurinol:** because of increased toxicity, should be started at the low dose of 50–100 mg/day.

degradation are regulated by a network of enzyme pathways; xanthine oxidase catalyses the end conversion of hypoxanthine to xanthine and then xanthine to uric acid.

Causes of hyperuricaemia are shown in Box 25.60. In over 90% of patients with primary gout, hyperuricaemia results from an inherited defect in fractional uric acid excretion which impairs their ability to increase urate excretion in response to a purine load ('under-excretors'). Recent studies have identified polymorphisms in several genes that encode urate transporters which are associated with gout, the most important of which is *SLC2A9*. Some primary gout patients are intrinsic 'over-producers' of uric acid through no identifiable cause. Very rarely (< 1%), there may be an inherited defect in purine metabolism, which should be suspected particularly if gout develops under age 25, in patients with uric acid renal calculi, or if there is a strong family history of early-onset gout.

Risk factors and associations for primary gout include metabolic syndrome (p. 802), high alcohol intake (predominantly beer which contains guanosine), and diets relatively high in red meat or fructose or relatively low in vitamin C or coffee.

Secondary gout

Secondary gout results from hyperuricaemia due to renal impairment or chronic diuretic use. In diuretic-induced gout, nodal generalised OA is a further risk factor, especially in elderly women (Box 25.61). This presumably relates to a non-specific predisposition to crystallisation in osteoarthritic cartilage, possibly due to reduced levels of proteoglycan and other inhibitors of crystal formation. Lead poisoning is a rare cause of hyperuricaemia and secondary ('saturnine') gout.

Clinical features

Acute gout

In almost all first attacks a single distal joint is affected. The first MTP joint is affected in over 50% of cases— 'podagra' ('seizing the foot', Fig. 25.29). Other common sites are, in order of decreasing frequency, the ankle, midfoot, knee, small joints of hands, wrist and elbow. The axial skeleton and large proximal joints are rarely involved and never as the first site. Typical attacks have the following characteristics:

- extremely rapid onset, reaching maximum severity in just 2–6 hours, often waking the patient in the early morning
- severe pain, often described as the 'worst pain ever'

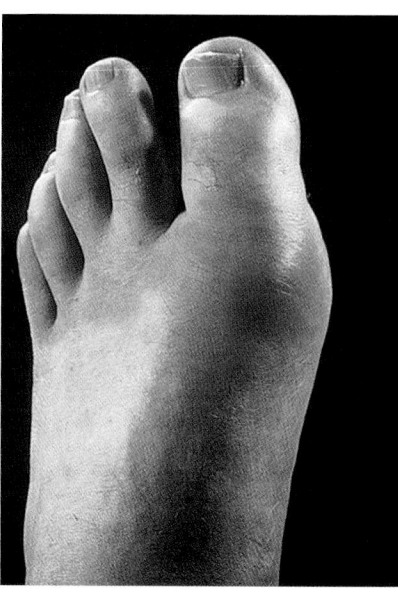

Fig. 25.29 Podagra. Acute gout causing swelling, erythema and extreme pain and tenderness of the first metatarsophalangeal joint.

- extreme tenderness: the patient is unable to wear a sock or to let bedding rest on the joint
- marked swelling with overlying red, shiny skin
- self-limiting over 5–14 days, with complete return to normality.

During the attack the joint shows signs of marked synovitis but also periarticular swelling and erythema. There may be accompanying fever, malaise and even confusion, especially if a large joint such as the knee is involved. As the attack subsides, pruritus and desquamation of overlying skin are common. The main differential diagnosis is septic arthritis, infective cellulitis or another crystal disease. Sepsis, however, is usually more subacute in onset and progresses in severity until treated.

Acute attacks may also manifest as bursitis, tenosynovitis or cellulitis, which have the same clinical characteristics. Many patients describe milder episodes lasting just a few days ('petite attacks'). Some have attacks in more than one joint; sometimes one attack, by triggering the APR, triggers attacks in other joints a few days later ('cluster attacks'). Polyarticular attacks are rare.

Recurrent and chronic gout

After an acute attack, some people never have a second episode; in others the next episode occurs after years. In most, however, a second attack occurs within 1 year and the frequency of attacks gradually increases with time. Later attacks are more likely to involve several joints and be more severe. Eventually, continued MSU deposition causes joint damage and chronic pain. The interval between the first attack and the development of chronic symptoms is variable but averages around 10 years. The main determinant is the SUA; the higher it is, the earlier and more extensive the development of joint damage and MSU deposits. The joints most commonly involved are the same as those affected by acute attacks. Occasionally there may be severe

deformity and marked functional impairment, especially of feet and hands. As with tophi, asymmetry is characteristic.

Chronic tophaceous gout

Large MSU crystal deposits produce irregular firm nodules ('tophi') around extensor surfaces of fingers, hands, forearm, elbows, Achilles tendons and sometimes the helix of the ear. The white colour of MSU crystals may be evident and permits distinction from rheumatoid nodules (Fig. 25.30). Large nodules may ulcerate, discharging white gritty material and associating with local inflammation (erythema, pus), even in the absence of secondary infection. Although clinically apparent tophi are usually a very late feature, they may appear surprisingly rapidly, in under 1 year, in patients with chronic renal failure.

Secondary gout may present with painful, sometimes discharging, tophi without preceding acute attacks. This is particularly seen in older, mainly female patients with nodal OA who develop tophi in and around their osteoarthritic finger joints as a consequence of chronic (> 1–2 years) diuretic therapy (see Fig. 25.30).

Renal and urinary tract manifestations

Uric acid (not MSU) stones cause renal colic (p. 473) in around 10% of gout patients in Europe. The incidence is higher in hot climates and is favoured by purine overproduction, uricosuric drugs, defects in tubular reabsorption of uric acid, dehydration and lowering of urine pH (e.g. chronic diarrhoea or ileostomy). Hyperuricaemia and gout also predispose to calcium oxalate, calcium phosphate or mixed stones.

Progressive renal disease is an important complication confined to untreated severe chronic tophaceous gout. This results from MSU crystal deposition in the interstitium of the medulla and pyramids with consequent chronic inflammation, giant-cell reaction, fibrosis, glomerulosclerosis and secondary pyelonephritis.

25

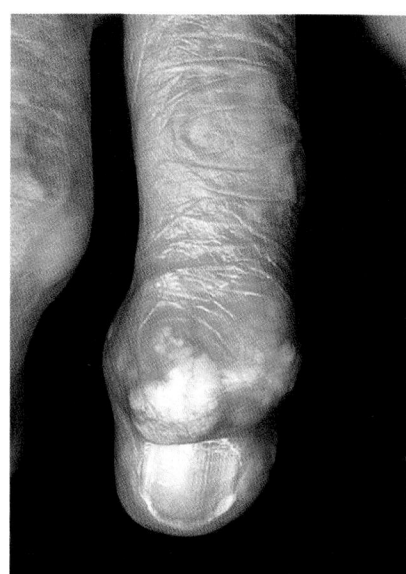

Fig. 25.30 Tophus with white MSUM crystals visible beneath the skin. Diuretic-induced gout in a patient with pre-existing nodal OA.

25

Investigations

Definitive diagnosis requires identification of MSU crystals in the aspirate from a joint, bursa or tophus (see Fig. 25.4A, p. 1060). In acute gout, synovial fluid shows increased turbidity due to the greatly elevated cell count (> 90% neutrophils); chronic gouty fluid is more variable but occasionally appears white due to the high crystal load. Between attacks, aspiration of an asymptomatic first MTP joint or knee may still permit crystal identification.

Although hyperuricaemia is usually present, it does not confirm gout. Equally, a normal SUA, especially during an attack, does not exclude gout since it falls as part of the APR. Measurement of 24-hour urinary uric acid excretion on a low purine diet will identify an over-producer. Assessment of renal function (serum creatinine, urinalysis), hypertension, blood glucose and serum lipid profile should be undertaken. An FBC and ESR should detect chronic myeloproliferative disorders during remission of acute gout. During an attack, an elevated CRP and neutrophilia are usual; the ESR is often modestly raised in tophaceous gout.

X-rays can assess the degree of joint damage. In early disease they are usually normal, but changes of OA may develop in affected joints with time, or be present as a predisposing factor in secondary gout. Gouty 'erosions' (bony tophi) are a less common but more specific feature occurring as para-articular 'punched-out' defects with well-delineated borders and retained bone density (see Fig. 25.6, p. 1061). Tophi may also be visible as eccentric soft tissue swellings. In late disease, changes are similar to other forms of inflammatory polyarthritis. Ultrasound can detect subclinical microtophi and MSU deposits within cartilage of the first MTP joint, even at first clinical presentation.

Management

The acute attack

A fast-acting oral NSAID (plus a PPI) (p. 1076) can give effective pain relief and is the standard treatment, together with local ice packs. Patients can keep a supply of an NSAID and take it as soon as the first symptoms occur, continuing until the attack resolves. Oral colchicine (a potent inhibitor of neutrophil microtubular assembly) is also very effective but often causes vomiting and severe diarrhoea at high doses; a low-dose regimen (0.5 mg 6-, 8- or 12-hourly) is therefore recommended. Joint aspiration can give instant relief and, when combined with an intra-articular steroid injection to prevent fluid reaccumulation, often effectively aborts the attack. For severe oligo- or polyarticular attacks, parenteral corticosteroid is sometimes used.

Long-term management

Once an acute attack has settled, predisposing factors should be corrected if possible. Weight loss and reduction of excess alcohol intake, especially beer, may significantly reduce hyperuricaemia. Diuretics should be stopped if possible. A very high purine diet (e.g. seafood, red meat, offal) should be tempered but there is no need for a highly restrictive diet. Associated comorbidity should be treated appropriately.

Indications for urate-lowering therapy (ULT) are shown in Box 25.62. Allopurinol is the drug of choice. It is a xanthine oxidase inhibitor, which reduces the

25.62 Indications for urate-lowering drugs

- Recurrent attacks of acute gout
- Tophi
- Evidence of bone or joint damage
- Associated renal disease and/or nephrolithiasis
- Gout with greatly elevated serum uric acid

conversion of hypoxanthine and xanthine to uric acid. The recommended starting dose is 100 mg daily, but 50 mg in older patients or if renal function is impaired. The reduction in tissue uric acid levels that follows initiation of ULT can partially dissolve MSU crystals and trigger acute attacks. The patient should be warned of this and told to continue ULT, even if an attack occurs. The risk can be minimised by using a low starting dose (50–100 mg rather than 300 mg), or by concurrent administration of oral colchicine (0.5 mg 12-hourly) or an NSAID for the first few months.

The aim of ULT is to bring the SUA below the therapeutic target of 360 μmol/L (i.e. the saturation point for MSU crystals) to ensure dissolution of existing crystals and to prevent new ones forming. The SUA should therefore be measured every 3–4 weeks and the dose of allopurinol increased in 100 mg increments (50 mg if the patient is elderly or there is renal impairment) until this is achieved (maximum 900 mg daily). The lower the SUA is brought below this target, the faster the velocity of MSU crystal dissolution, the reduction in tophus size and the eventual cessation of acute attacks. Annual monitoring is advised subsequently to ensure maintenance of effective treatment. In most cases ULT will need to be continued indefinitely.

Febuxostat is a recently introduced xanthine oxidase inhibitor that is useful in patients in whom allopurinol is not tolerated or contraindicated. It commonly provokes attacks at the recommended starting dose (80 mg daily) so prophylaxis with colchicine or NSAID is advised for the initial 6 months. It undergoes hepatic metabolism and so no dose adjustment is required for renal impairment.

Uricosuric drugs such as probenecid or sulfinpyrazone can be effective but require several doses each day and maintenance of a high urine flow to avoid uric acid crystallisation in renal tubules. Salicylates antagonise the uricosuric action of these drugs and should be avoided. Uricosurics are contraindicated in over-producers, in those with renal impairment and in urolithiasis (they increase stone formation). The uricosuric benzbromarone (50–200 mg daily) can be very effective and safe in mild to moderate renal impairment but can rarely cause hepatotoxicity; availability is limited in most countries.

Asymptomatic hyperuricaemia

Although hyperuricaemia is an independent risk factor for hypertension, vascular disease, renal disease and cardiovascular events, there is no evidence that ULT is effective in the treatment of these diseases.

Calcium pyrophosphate dihydrate (CPPD) crystal deposition

CPPD crystal deposition in hyaline and fibrocartilage of joints causes chondrocalcinosis. Sporadic, familial and metabolic disease-associated forms are recognised (Box 25.63). Radiographic chondrocalcinosis is rare under the

25.63 Associations of CPPD crystal deposition

	Chondro-calcinosis	Structural arthritis
Ageing (sporadic) (most common)	+	−
Osteoarthritis, joint damage (common)	+	+
Familial predisposition (rare)	+	Variable
Metabolic disease (rare)		
Haemochromatosis	+	+
Hyperparathyroidism	+	−
Hypophosphatasia	+	−
Hypomagnesaemia	+	−
Wilson's disease	+	−

age of 55, but rises from 10–15% in those aged 65–75 to 30–60% in those over 85. The knee (hyaline cartilage and menisci) is by far the most common site, followed by the wrist (triangular fibrocartilage) and pelvis (symphysis pubis). It is often clinically occult, but can cause acute self-limiting synovitis ('pseudogout') or occur as a chronic arthritis showing a strong association/overlap with OA, especially at the knee (Fig. 25.31).

Aetiology

In OA, CPPD crystal deposition is favoured by a reduction in concentration of proteoglycan and other natural inhibitors of crystal formation, and by increased extracellular pyrophosphate levels due to increased chondrocyte metabolism. Other metabolic diseases are associated with CPPD deposition, but of these only haemochromatosis also predisposes to OA-like structural change. All of these conditions are characterised by elevated levels of extracellular pyrophosphate in joint tissues, mainly

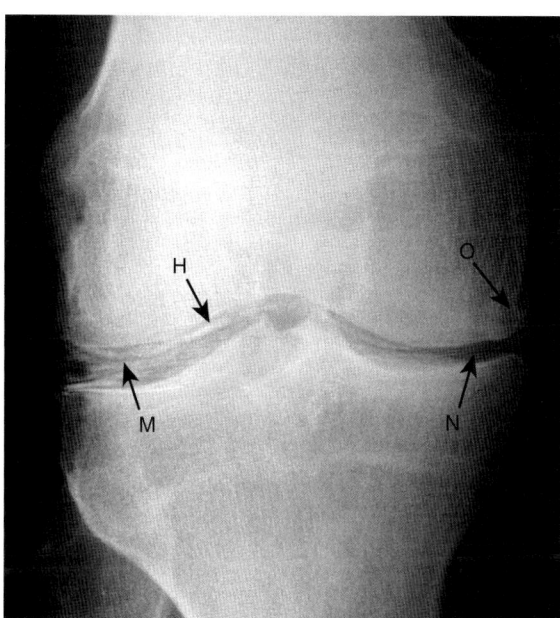

Fig. 25.31 Knee X-ray showing chondrocalcinosis of the fibrocartilaginous menisci (M) and articular hyaline cartilage (H). There is also narrowing (N) and osteophyte (O) of the medial tibio-femoral compartment.

through reduced concentrations or activity of alkaline phosphatase and other pyrophosphatases, resulting in ectopic mineralisation.

Clinical features

Acute synovitis: 'pseudogout'

This is a common cause of acute monoarthritis in the elderly. The knee is by far the most common site, followed by the wrist, shoulder, ankle and elbow. It may be the first presentation of disease in the joint, or occur on a background of chronic symptomatic arthritis. Triggering factors include direct trauma and intercurrent illness or surgery.

The typical attack resembles acute gout and develops rapidly, with severe pain, stiffness and swelling, maximal within 6–24 hours of onset. Overlying erythema is common and examination reveals a very tender joint held in the flexed 'loose-pack' position with signs of marked synovitis (large/tense effusion, warmth, restricted movement with stress pain). Fever is common and the patient may appear confused and ill. The attack is self-limiting but can take 1–3 weeks to resolve.

Sepsis and gout are the main differential diagnoses. Although sepsis is often more subacute in onset and progressive, it should be considered especially when pseudogout has been triggered by chest infection or surgery, or if the patient is unwell. Furthermore, sepsis and pseudogout can coexist, so Gram stain and culture should still be undertaken, even if CPPD crystals are identified in aspirated fluid. Gout is unlikely in patients over the age of 65 without a preceding history of primary gout or chronic diuretic therapy and seldom involves the knee in a first attack.

Chronic (pyrophosphate) arthritis

This largely affects elderly women. The distribution is similar to that of pseudogout, with knees being the worst affected, then wrists, shoulders, elbows, hips and midtarsals. In the hand, the second and third MCP joints are most affected. Symptoms are chronic pain, variable early morning and inactivity stiffness, and functional impairment. Acute attacks may be superimposed. Affected joints show features of OA (bony swelling, crepitus, restriction) with varying degrees of synovitis. Effusion and synovial thickening are usually most apparent at knees and wrists; wrist involvement may result in carpal tunnel syndrome. Examination often reveals more widespread but asymptomatic signs of OA.

Inflammatory features may be sufficiently pronounced to suggest RA, but tenosynovitis and extra-articular involvement are absent, and large and medium rather than small joints are targeted. Severe damage and instability of knees or shoulders may occasionally lead to consideration of a neuropathic joint, but neurological findings are normal.

Incidental findings

Due to its high prevalence, radiographic chondrocalcinosis often occurs as an incidental finding in older people. Thorough history and examination are always required to determine the relevance of such findings to symptom causation.

Investigations

In acute pseudogout, examination of synovial fluid using compensated polarised microscopy will demonstrate CPPD crystals (see Fig. 25.4B, p. 1060) and permit distinction from urate gout. The aspirated fluid is often turbid and may be uniformly blood-stained, reflecting the severity of inflammation. Gram stain and culture of the fluid will exclude sepsis. CPPD crystals may also be identified in fluid aspirated from chronic pyrophosphate arthritis.

X-rays may show chondrocalcinosis in hyaline cartilage and/or fibrocartilage (occasionally capsule or ligament) with or without associated structural changes of OA (see Fig. 25.31). Chondrocalcinosis is not always evident, especially in joints showing some degree of cartilage loss, and its absence does not exclude the diagnosis.

Screening for metabolic or familial predisposition (see Box 25.63) should be undertaken in patients with CPPD deposition aged under 55; florid polyarticular, as opposed to pauciarticular, chondrocalcinosis; recurrent acute attacks without chronic arthropathy; or additional clinical or radiographic features of predisposing disease.

Management

For acute pseudogout, aspiration quickly reduces pain and may be sufficient. Fluid reaccumulation, however, is common, particularly early in an attack, and intra-articular injection of corticosteroid is usually required. Oral NSAIDs (plus PPI) and colchicine are also effective, as in gout, but should be avoided if possible in older people. Early active mobilisation is also important. For chronic arthropathy, management is as for OA (p. 1087).

Basic calcium phosphate (BCP) deposition

Hydroxyapatite (apatite) is the principal mineral in bone and teeth. Apatite and other basic, as opposed to acidic, calcium phosphates (octacalcium phosphate, tricalcium phosphate) are also the usual minerals to deposit in extraskeletal tissues. In MSK tissues, abnormal deposition may occur in:

- periarticular tissues, particularly tendon
- hyaline cartilage in association with OA
- subcutaneous tissue and muscle, principally in connective tissue diseases.

Aetiology

Mineralisation of soft tissues is normally prevented by inhibitors such as pyrophosphate and proteoglycans. When these protective mechanisms break down, abnormal calcification due to BCP occurs. There are many causes (Box 25.64). In most situations, calcification is of no consequence, possibly because of encasement by protein and surrounding fibrous tissue. However, BCP crystals have inflammatory potential and their deposition in MSK tissues sometimes causes clinical problems. Individual apatite crystals are too small to be viewed by light microscopy but their aggregated spherulites can be seen using calcium stains. Sophisticated analytical techniques are required to identify individual BCPs, but for clinical purposes presumptive diagnosis based on radiographic calcification or non-specific calcium staining of synovial fluid or histological tissue is sufficient.

Calcific periarthritis

Deposition of BCP in the supraspinatus tendon (Fig. 25.32) is an incidental X-ray finding in around 7% of adults. It occasionally results in acute inflammation

25.64 Causes of ectopic calcification

High calcium [Ca²⁺] × phosphate [PO₄²⁻] ionic product (metastatic calcification)

- Hyperparathyroidism (especially tertiary, p. 766)
- Renal dialysis
- Vitamin D intoxication
- Basal ganglia in pseudohypoparathyroidism

Altered tissue balance of inhibitors and promoters of crystal formation (dystrophic calcification)

- Calcific periarthritis
- Atherosclerotic arteries
- Fibrotic lymph nodes
- Scarred lung parenchyma
- Scarred adrenal glands (tuberculosis)
- Polymyositis
- Systemic sclerosis (calcinosis)
- Tumours (e.g. craniopharyngioma)

of the subacromial/subdeltoid bursa and periarticular tissues through crystal shedding from the tendon into and around the bursa. Periarticular sites around the greater trochanter of the hip, foot or hand are less commonly affected.

The acute episode may occur spontaneously or follow local trauma. Within just a few hours, shoulder pain and tenderness are extreme and the area appears swollen, hot and sometimes red. Modest systemic upset and fever are common. X-rays show tendon calcification. If the subacromial bursa is aspirated, inflammatory fluid containing many calcium-staining (alizarin red S) aggregates may be obtained.

The condition usually resolves spontaneously over 1–3 weeks, often accompanied by radiographic dispersal and disappearance of small to modest-sized deposits (i.e. complete crystal shedding). Calcific periarthritis may

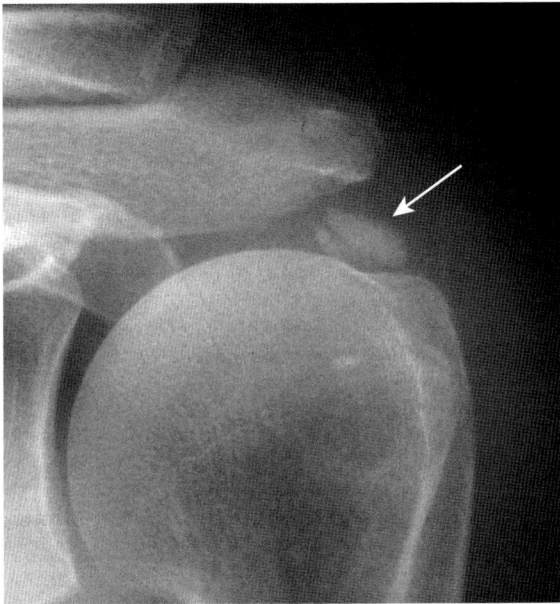

Fig. 25.32 Shoulder X-ray showing supraspinatus tendon calcification (arrow).

result from renal failure, hyperparathyroidism or hypo-phosphatasia, but measurements of serum creatinine, calcium and alkaline phosphatase are usually normal. The CRP is elevated during the episode.

Oral analgesics and NSAIDs ameliorate symptoms and the attack may be shortened by aspiration and injection of corticosteroid. Exceptionally large deposits may cause mechanical blocking and painful impingement on abduction rather than acute periarthritis, and require surgical removal.

Osteoarthritis and BCP crystal deposition

Modest amounts of BCP aggregates are commonly found in synovial fluid from osteoarthritic joints, either alone or with CPPD crystals ('mixed crystal deposition'). Whether they contribute to joint damage or cause minor inflammatory episodes remains unclear. Large amounts of BCP, however, have been associated with an uncommon but distinctive form of OA that is largely confined to elderly people, mainly women, and characterised by:

- involvement of knee, hip or shoulder (large joints) only
- rapid progression, leading to severe pain and disability in just a few months
- development of marked instability and large effusions of knees or shoulders
- atrophic X-ray appearances with marked loss of cartilage and bone.

Aspiration yields large volumes of relatively non-inflammatory fluid containing abundant BCP aggregates and often cartilage fragments. The differential diagnosis is end-stage avascular necrosis, chronic sepsis or neuro-pathic joint. Unlike in sepsis, the APR is not triggered and synovial fluid cultures are negative.

Treatment is with analgesics, intra-articular injection of corticosteroids, local physical treatments and physiotherapy. The clinical outcome, however, is poor and most patients require joint replacement. It is most likely that the BCP aggregates, rather than being causal pathogenic agents, are a marker of the speed of joint damage in such 'apatite-associated destructive arthritis', which represents the most severe end of the OA spectrum.

Bone and joint infection

Septic arthritis

Septic arthritis is a medical emergency. It is the most rapid and destructive joint disease, and has significant morbidity and a mortality of 10%. This has not improved over the last 20 years despite advances in antimicrobial therapy. The incidence is 2–10 per 100 000 in the general population and 30–70 per 100 000 in those with pre-existing joint disease or joint replacement.

Septic arthritis is usually due to haematogenous spread from either skin or upper respiratory tract; infection from direct puncture wounds or secondary to joint aspiration is uncommon. Risk factors include increasing age, pre-existing joint disease (principally RA), diabetes mellitus, immunosuppression (by drugs or disease) and intravenous drug misuse. In RA, the skin is a frequent portal of entry because of maceration of skin between the toes due to joint deformity and difficulties with foot hygiene due to hand deformity. Box 25.65 describes the particular considerations in old age.

25.65 Joint and bone infection in old age

- **Vertebral infection:** more common. Recognition may be delayed, as symptoms may be attributed to compression fractures caused by osteoporosis.
- **Peripheral vascular disease:** leads to more frequent involvement of the bones of the feet, and diabetic foot ulcers are also commonly complicated by osteomyelitis.
- **Prosthetic joint infections:** now more common because of the increased frequency of prosthetic joint insertion in older people.
- **Gram-negative bacilli:** more frequent pathogens than in youth.

Lyme disease (p. 329) may present with monoarthritis, often with headaches, neurological signs and fatigue. There is usually a history of rash (erythema migrans) occurring 7–10 days after a tick bite. Diagnosis is confirmed by *Borrelia* serology, although false positives may occur.

Clinical features

The usual presentation is with acute or subacute mono-arthritis and fever. The joint is usually swollen, hot and red and is held in the 'loose-pack' position, with an effusion, rest pain and stress pain on movement. Although any joint can be affected, lower limb joints, such as the knee and hip, are commonly targeted. In patients with pre-existing arthritis, involvement of one or more joints is not uncommon and all should be examined.

In adults, the most likely organism is *Staphylococcus aureus*, particularly in patients with RA and diabetes. In young, sexually active adults, disseminated gonococcal infection occurs in up to 3% of untreated gonorrhoea, usually presenting with migratory arthralgia, low-grade fever and tenosynovitis, which may precede the development of oligo- or monoarthritis. Painful pustular skin lesions may also be present. Amongst the elderly and intravenous drug misusers, Gram-negative bacilli or group B, C and G streptococci are important causes. Group A streptococci, pneumococci, meningococci and *Haemophilus influenzae* are occasionally isolated.

Investigations

The pivotal investigation is joint aspiration but blood cultures should also be taken. The synovial fluid is usually turbid or blood-stained but may appear normal. If the joint is not readily accessible, aspiration should be performed under imaging guidance or in theatre. Prosthetic joints should only be aspirated in theatre.

Synovial fluid should be sent for Gram stain and culture; cultures are positive in around 90% of cases, but the Gram stain is positive in only 50%. In contrast, synovial fluid culture is positive in only 30% of gonococcal infections, making it important to obtain concurrent cultures from the genital tract (positive in 70–90% of cases). There is a leucocytosis with raised ESR and CRP in most patients, but these features may be absent in elderly or immuno-compromised patients or early in the disease course.

Management (Box 25.66)

Hospitalisation is essential for:
- pain relief
- parenteral antibiotics

Box 25.66 Emergency management of suspected septic arthritis

Admit patient to hospital

Perform urgent investigations

- Aspirate joint
  Send synovial fluid for Gram stain and culture
  Use imaging guidance if required (e.g. for hip)
- Send blood for Gram stain and culture, FBC, CRP, LFTs, renal function
- Consider sending other samples (e.g. sputum, urine) for culture, depending on patient history, to determine primary source of infection

Commence intravenous antibiotic

- Flucloxacillin 2 g 6-hourly
- If penicillin allergic, give clindamycin 450–600 mg 6-hourly
- If at high risk of Gram-negative sepsis (e.g. elderly, frail, recurrent urinary tract infection), add a cephalosporin (e.g. cefuroxime 1.5 g 8-hourly)

Relieve pain

- Oral and/ or intravenous analgesics
- Consider local ice-packs

Keep joint decompressed

- Serial needle aspiration to dryness (1–3 times/day as required)
- If loculated fluid or technically difficult aspiration, consider lavage or arthroscopy

Physiotherapy from first day

- Early regular passive movement, progressing to active movements once pain controlled and effusion not re-accumulating

- adequate drainage
- early active rehabilitation.

Flucloxacillin (2 g i.v. 6-hourly) is the antibiotic of first choice since it will cover most staphylococcal and streptococcal infections until the organism is identified and its antibiotic sensitivity defined. Intravenous treatment is usually continued for 2–3 weeks, followed by oral treatment for 6 weeks in total. Initially, the joint should be aspirated once or twice daily to minimise the effusion. If this proves unsuccessful or the joint is inaccessible, surgical drainage may be required. Regular passive movement should be undertaken from the outset, and active movements encouraged once the condition has stabilised. Infected prosthetic joints require management by the orthopaedic team, but often prolonged antibiotic treatment on its own is ineffective and removal of the prosthesis is required for eradication of the infection.

Viral arthritis

Most forms of viral arthritis are self-limiting. The usual presentation is with acute polyarthritis, fever or viral prodrome and rash. Human parvovirus (mainly B19, p. 311) arthropathy is the most common in Europe; adults may not have the characteristic 'slapped cheek' facial rash, and joint symptoms with prominent stiffness may be recurrent or persistent for months or even years. Diagnosis is confirmed by a rise in specific IgM. Polyarthritis may also occur rarely with hepatitis B and C, rubella (including rubella vaccination) and HIV infection. A variety of mosquito-borne viruses may cause epidemics of acute polyarthritis, including Ross River

25.67 Arthritis associated with HIV

• Non-specific arthralgia	Most common; intermittent and polyarticular
• Reactive arthritis • Psoriatic arthritis • Idiopathic lower limb inflammatory oligoarthritis	Especially in men who have sex with men
• Osteonecrosis • Myositis • Vasculitis • Sjögren's-like disease	Unclear if related to HIV or its treatment, or intercurrent disease

virus (Australia, Pacific), Chikungunya and O'nyong-nyong viruses (Asia, Africa), and Mayaro virus (South America). A wide variety of articular symptoms have been associated with HIV, mainly in the later stages of infection (Box 25.67).

Osteomyelitis

Some degree of adjacent bone infection is usual with septic arthritis, but bone or bone marrow is the primary site of infection in osteomyelitis. Any part of a bone may be involved but there is preferential targeting of the juxta-epiphyseal regions of long bones adjacent to joints. The usual source is via haematogenous spread, although directly introduced infection may complicate trauma or orthopaedic surgery. Organisms most frequently implicated are staphylococci, *Pseudomonas* and *Mycobacterium tuberculosis*. Risk factors include childhood and adolescence, diabetes mellitus (especially involving the foot), compromised immunity (including AIDS) and sickle cell disease, which particularly increases the risk of *Salmonella* infection. Pathologically, the infection often results in a florid inflammatory response, greatly increased intra-osseous pressure and localised areas of osteonecrosis (bone death). A separated shard of dead bone in this context is called a 'sequestrum'. Eventual perforation of the cortex by pus stimulates local new bone formation ('involucrum') by the subperiosteum and periosteum, often with sinuses that discharge through the skin.

Clinical features and investigations

The presentation is with localised bone pain and tenderness, often with malaise, night sweats and pyrexia. The adjacent joint may be painful to move and may develop a sterile ('sympathetic') effusion or secondary septic arthritis. The earliest X-ray abnormality is localised osteopenia adjacent to an epiphysis, which may be followed by more obvious areas of bone lucency mixed with patchy sclerosis (osteonecrosis) and adjacent periosteal new bone formation. X-rays may be normal for the first few weeks, but bone technetium scans, labelled white cell scans and MRI are much more sensitive and show clear abnormalities at presentation. The diagnosis may be confirmed on blood cultures and/or culture of a bone aspirate or biopsy.

Management

Early recognition and management is critical; once osteomyelitis becomes established and chronic, it may prove very hard to eradicate the infection with antibiotics alone. The principles are those for septic arthritis, with parenteral antibiotics for at least 2 weeks, followed by oral antibiotics for at least 4 weeks. Resection of the infected bone and subsequent reconstruction are often required: e.g. with callus distraction and external fixators. Complications of chronic osteomyelitis include secondary amyloidosis (p. 84) and skin malignancy at the margin of a discharging sinus (Marjolin's ulcer).

Tuberculosis of bone and joints

This is discussed on page 691. X-ray changes are non-specific and mycobacteria are often not identified from synovial fluid, so definite diagnosis requires biopsy of synovium (peripheral joint) or bone (spinal involvement). Management is as for pulmonary tuberculosis (p. 693), although additional surgical débridement may be required for extensive joint or bone disease, and spinal involvement may require surgical stabilisation and decompression.

FIBROMYALGIA

This is a common cause of multiple regional pain and disability, which is commonly associated with medically unexplained symptoms in other systems (p. 238).

The prevalence in the UK and US is about 2–3%. Although fibromyalgia can occur at any age, including adolescence, it increases in prevalence with age, to reach a peak of 7% in women aged over 70. There is a strong female predominance of around 10:1. Risk factors include life events that cause psychosocial distress such as marital disharmony, alcoholism in the family, injury or assault, low income and self-reported childhood abuse (Box 25.68). The condition is reported in a wide variety of races and cultures.

Aetiology

Despite intensive investigation, no structural, inflammatory, metabolic or endocrine abnormality has been identified. However, two abnormalities which may interrelate (Fig. 25.33) have been reported consistently:

- *Sleep abnormality.* Delta waves are characteristic of deep stages of non-rapid eye movement (non-REM) sleep, usually occurring in the first few hours and thought to have an important restorative function. People with fibromyalgia have reduced delta sleep in a pattern distinct from that seen with depression. Furthermore, deprivation of delta but not REM sleep in normal volunteers produces the symptoms and signs of fibromyalgia, supporting fibromyalgia as a non-restorative sleep disorder.
- *Abnormal peripheral and central pain processing.* A reduced threshold to pain perception and tolerance at characteristic sites throughout the body is characteristic of fibromyalgia. Affected people have peripheral sensitisation and spinal cord 'wind-

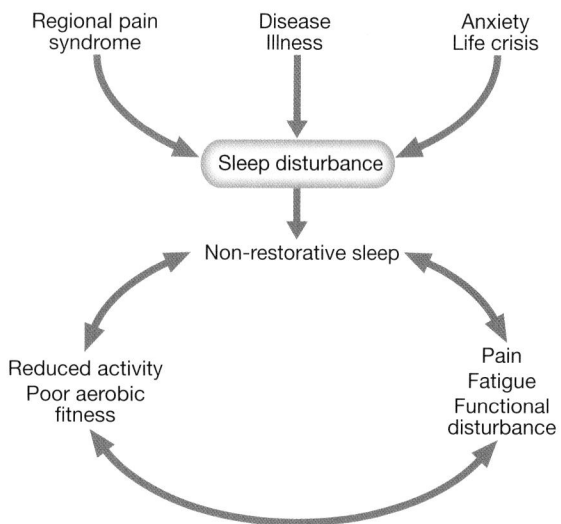

Fig. 25.33 Possible mechanisms involved in fibromyalgia.

up' (pain amplification), with an exaggerated skin flare response to topically applied capsaicin and frequent occurrence of dermatographism and allodynia (allodynia is when normally non-noxious stimuli become painful). Abnormal central pain processing is suggested by altered cerebrospinal fluid levels of substance P (increased) and 5-HT (5-hydroxytryptamine or serotonin—reduced); reduced basal levels of regional cerebral blood flow in the caudate and thalamus with an augmented processing response on functional MRI; low basal free cortisol and reduction in evening trough of cortisol; and altered descending inhibition via the hypothalamo-pituitary-adrenal and growth hormone somatomedin axes.

Clinical features

The main presenting feature is multiple regional pain, often focusing on the neck and back (Box 25.69). At presentation, just one or a few regions may dominate the

25.69 Symptoms of fibromyalgia

Usual symptoms

- Multiple regional pain
- Marked fatigability
- Marked disability
- Broken non-restorative sleep
- Low affect, irritability, weepiness
- Poor concentration, forgetfulness

Variable locomotor symptoms

- Early morning stiffness
- Swelling of hands, fingers
- Numbness, tingling of all fingers

Additional, variable, non-locomotor symptoms

- Non-throbbing bifrontal headache (tension headache)
- Colicky abdominal pain, bloating, variable bowel habit (irritable bowel syndrome)
- Bladder fullness, nocturnal frequency (irritable bladder)
- Hyperacusis, dyspareunia, discomfort when touched (allodynia)
- Frequent side-effects with drugs (chemical sensitivity)

EBM 25.68 **Associations of fibromyalgia**

'Epidemiological studies show that widespread body pain, fatigue, psychological distress and multiple hyperalgesic tender sites cluster together and associate with stressful life events.'

- Wolfe F, et al. Arthritis Rheum 1995; 38:19–28.
- Croft P, et al. BMJ 1994; 309:696–699.

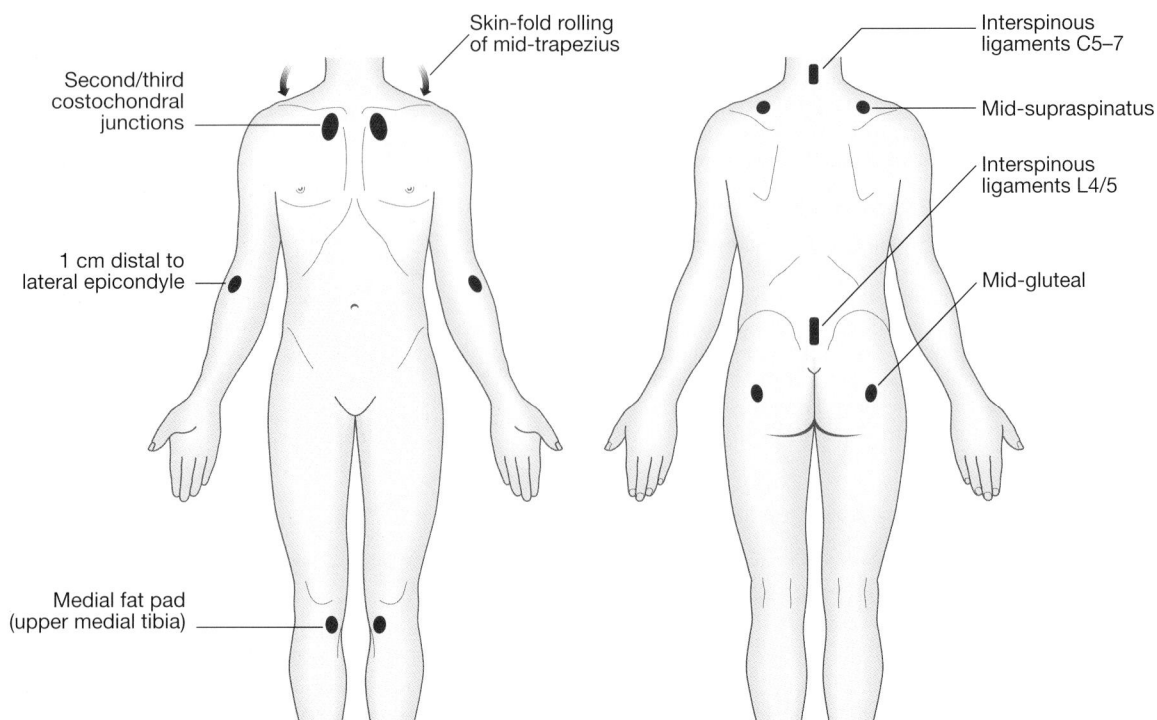

Fig. 25.34 Major tender sites that become hyperalgesic with fibromyalgia.

picture, but over the preceding months pain will have affected all body quadrants: both arms, both legs, neck and back. The pain is characteristically diffuse and unresponsive to analgesics and NSAIDs, and physiotherapy often makes it worse. Fatigability, most prominent in the morning, is another major problem and disability is often marked. Although people can usually dress, feed and groom themselves, they may be unable to perform tasks such as shopping or housework. They may have experienced major difficulties at work or even retired because of pain and fatigue.

Examination usually reveals no synovitis or damage, and no overt neurological defect or wasting. Depending on their age, people may have signs of OA or other prevalent MSK conditions, but of insufficient severity to explain such widespread symptoms and severe disability. The principal finding is hyperalgesia at tender sites (Fig. 25.34). Moderate digital pressure at each site may be uncomfortable in a normal subject but in fibromyalgia it produces a wince/withdrawal response. Metered dolorimeters are used for research purposes but moderate digital pressure, enough just to whiten the nail, is sufficient for clinical diagnosis.

People with other MSK diseases can develop fibromyalgia. Assessment may prove challenging since many of the symptoms could relate to activity of their multisystem disease. Marked discordance between the severity of reported and observed abnormality is an important feature that suggests fibromyalgia, and widespread hyperalgesic tender sites are not explained by polyarticular disease.

Investigations and management

There are no abnormalities on routine blood tests or imaging, but it is important to screen for other clinically occult conditions that could contribute to some of the symptoms (Box 25.70).

The aims of management are to educate the patient about the condition, to achieve pain control and to improve sleep. Principles of management of medically unexplained symptoms are outlined on pages 251–252.

Wherever possible, discussion should include the spouse, family or carer. It should be acknowledged that, although we recognise this condition, it is not fully understood but we do know that the chronic widespread pain does not reflect inflammation, damage or disease. The model of a self-perpetuating cycle of poor sleep and pain (see Fig. 25.33) is often readily accepted and is a useful framework for problem-based management. Ascribing the symptoms to a cause for which the patient cannot be blamed, and knowing that it is common often help. Repeat or drawn-out investigation may reinforce beliefs in occult serious pathology and should be avoided.

Low-dose amitriptyline (10–75 mg at night) with or without fluoxetine may help by encouraging delta sleep and reducing spinal cord wind-up. Many people with

25.70 Minimum investigation screen in fibromyalgia	
Test	**Condition screened**
FBC	Anaemia, lymphopenia of SLE
ESR, CRP	Inflammatory disease
Thyroid function	Hypothyroidism
Calcium, alkaline phosphatase	Hyperparathyroidism, osteomalacia
ANA	SLE

fibromyalgia, however, are intolerant of even small doses of amitriptyline. There is limited evidence for the use of tramadol, serotonin-noradrenaline (norepinephrine) reuptake inhibitors (SNRIs) such as duloxetine, and the anticonvulsants pregabalin and gabapentin. A graded increase in aerobic exercise can improve well-being and sleep quality. The use of self-help strategies and a cognitive behavioural approach with relaxation techniques should be encouraged. Sublimated anxiety relating to distressing life events should be specifically explored with appropriate counselling. There are patient organisations which provide additional information and support.

The prognosis for hospital-diagnosed fibromyalgia is poor. Although treatment may improve quality of life and ability to cope, most people do not lose their symptoms or diagnostic criteria over 5 years. Subjects diagnosed in primary care, or who have sublimated anxiety that can be successfully addressed, may fare better.

SYSTEMIC CONNECTIVE TISSUE DISEASE

The connective tissue diseases are a group of chronic inflammatory disorders that involve multiple body systems and exhibit a wide spectrum of clinical manifestations. Their aetiology is multifactorial, involving genetic and environmental factors. Although each disease displays different clinical and pathological features, the group shares enough characteristics to be considered a family of overlapping conditions.

Systemic lupus erythematosus (SLE)

SLE is the most common connective tissue disease. Its prevalence varies according to geographical and racial background from 3/10 000 in Caucasians to 20/10 000 in Afro-Caribbeans. Around 90% of affected individuals are women, and the peak age at onset is between 20 and 30 years. The overall 5-year survival of SLE is over 90%. Mortality within 5 years of diagnosis is usually due to organ failure or overwhelming sepsis, both of which are modifiable by early effective intervention. However, compared to the normal population, patients with lupus have a fivefold increased mortality. This mainly results from premature cardiovascular disease to which chronic steroid therapy makes a major contribution.

Pathophysiology

The cause of SLE is incompletely understood but genetic factors play an important role. There is a higher concordance in monozygotic twins and associations with multiple polymorphisms in the HLA locus on chromosome 6 have been identified. In a few instances, SLE is associated with inherited mutations in complement components C1q, C2, and C4; in the immunoglobulin receptor FcγRIIIb or in the DNA exonuclease *TREX1*. Recent studies have identified common polymorphisms that predispose to SLE, including the *ITGAM* gene which encodes an integrin; the *IRF5* and *STAT4* genes which are involved in interferon signalling; and the *BLK* gene which is involved in B-cell signalling. From an immunological standpoint, the characteristic feature of SLE is the production of autoantibodies. These have specificity for a wide range of targets but many are directed against antigens present within the cell or within the nucleus. This has led to the suggestion that patients with SLE have defects in apoptosis or in the clearance of apoptotic cells, which causes inappropriate exposure of intracellular antigens on the cell surface, leading to polyclonal B- and T-cell activation and autoantibody production. This is supported by the fact that environmental factors that cause flares of lupus, such as ultraviolet (UV) light, pregnancy and infections, increase oxidative stress and/or stimulate apoptosis; by the association with complement deficiency; and by the defect in the *TREX1* nuclease. Whatever the underlying cause, immune complex formation is thought to be an important mechanism of tissue damage in active SLE, leading to widespread vasculitis and organ damage.

Clinical features
General symptoms

Patients often have non-specific symptoms. Some, such as fever, weight loss and mild lymphadenopathy, reflect active inflammatory disease, whereas others, such as fatigue, malaise and fibromyalgia-like symptoms, are not necessarily associated with flares in disease activity, at least as assessed by standard laboratory tests.

Arthritis and arthralgia

A variety of joint problems occur, including migratory arthralgia and early morning stiffness, tenosynovitis and small joint synovitis that can mimic rheumatoid. However, joint deformities and erosions are rare and synovitis is seldom obvious clinically. When joint deformities do occur, they result more from tendon inflammation and damage than from bone destruction (Jaccoud's arthropathy).

Raynaud's phenomenon

Raynaud's (p. 601) is common and may antedate other symptoms by months or years. A common presentation is Raynaud's in combination with arthralgia or arthritis (Fig. 25.35). Raynaud's associated with SLE and other connective tissue disease needs to be differentiated from primary Raynaud's, which is common in healthy young women. Features in favour of secondary Raynaud's include age at onset of over 25 years, absence of a family history of

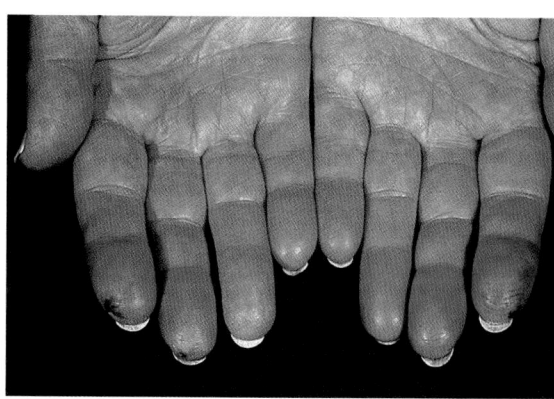

Fig. 25.35 Severe secondary Raynaud's phenomenon leading to digital ulceration.

Raynaud's, and occurrence in a male. Examination of capillary nail-fold loops using an ophthalmoscope (and oil placed on the skin) may help distinguish primary from secondary Raynaud's. Loss of the normal loop pattern, with capillary 'fallout' and dilatation and branching of loops, supports connective tissue disease.

Rash

This is common in SLE and is classically precipitated by exposure to UV light. Three distinct types of rash occur:

* The classic butterfly facial rash (up to 20% of patients). This is erythematous, raised and painful or itchy, and occurs over the cheeks with sparing of the nasolabial folds (Fig. 25.36).
* Subacute cutaneous lupus erythematosus (SCLE) rashes are migratory, non-scarring and either annular or psoriaform.
* Discoid lupus lesions are characterised by hyperkeratosis and follicular plugging, and may cause scarring alopecia if present on the scalp.

Diffuse, usually non-scarring alopecia may occur with active disease. Other skin manifestations include periungual erythema (reflecting dilated capillary loops), vasculitis and livedo reticularis, which is also a common feature of the antiphospholipid syndrome (Fig. 25.37).

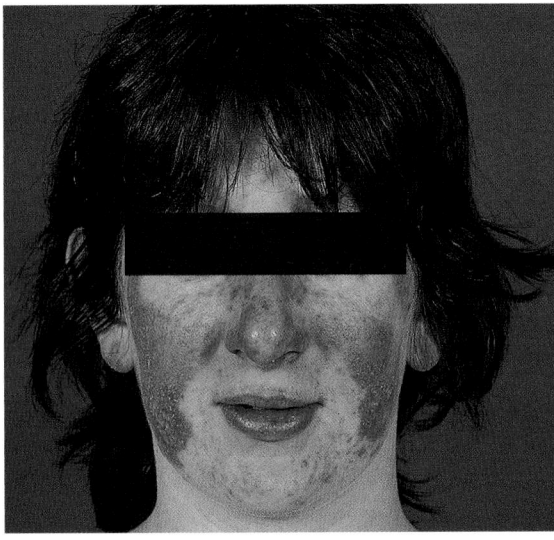

Fig. 25.36 Butterfly (malar) rash of systemic lupus erythematosus, sparing the nasolabial folds.

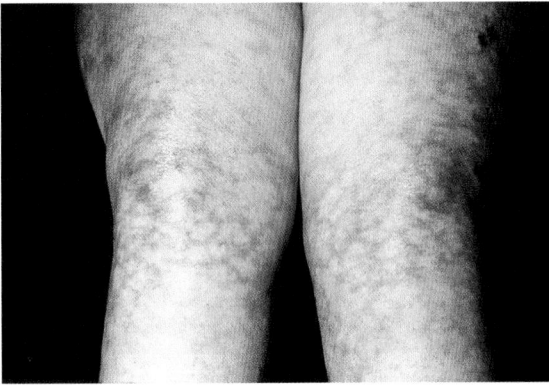

Fig. 25.37 Livedo reticularis in systemic lupus erythematosus.

Renal involvement

This is one of the main determinants of prognosis, and regular monitoring of urinalysis and blood pressure is essential. The typical renal lesion is a proliferative glomerulonephritis (p. 500), characterised by heavy haematuria, proteinuria and casts on urine microscopy.

Cardiovascular features

The most common manifestation is pericarditis. Myocarditis and Libman–Sacks endocarditis can also occur. The latter comprises non-infectious vegetations on the heart valves and is thought to be a manifestation of hypercoagulability associated with antiphospholipid antibodies. Cardiovascular disease is increased in patients with long-standing SLE.

Pulmonary features

These are common and most frequently manifest as pleurisy or pleural effusion. Other features include pneumonitis, atelectasis, reduced lung volume and pulmonary fibrosis leading to breathlessness. The risk of thromboembolism is increased, especially in patients with antiphospholipid antibodies.

Neurological features

Fatigue, headache and poor concentration are common, and often occur without laboratory evidence of active disease. More specific features of cerebral lupus include visual hallucinations, chorea, organic psychosis, transverse myelitis and lymphocytic meningitis.

Haematological features

A variety of abnormalities may occur, including neutropenia, lymphopenia, thrombocytopenia or haemolytic anaemia, due to antibody-mediated destruction of peripheral blood cells. The degree of lymphopenia is a good guide to disease activity.

Gastrointestinal features

Mouth ulcers may occur, which may or may not be painful. Mesenteric vasculitis is a serious complication which can present with abdominal pain, bowel infarction or perforation.

Investigations

The diagnosis is based on a combination of clinical features and laboratory abnormalities. To fulfil the classification criteria for SLE, at least 4 of the 11 factors shown in Box 25.71 must be present or have occurred in the past. Patients should be screened for ANA and antibodies to extractable nuclear antigens, and have complement levels checked along with routine haematology and biochemistry. Patients with active SLE almost always test positive for ANA, but ANA-negative SLE can very rarely occur in the presence of antibodies to the Ro antigen. Anti-dsDNA antibodies are characteristic of severe active SLE but occur in only around 30% of cases. Similarly, patients with active disease tend to have low levels of C3 and C4, but this may be the result of inherited complement deficiency which predisposes to SLE. Studies of other family members can help to differentiate inherited deficiency from complement consumption. A raised ESR, leucopenia and lymphopenia are typical of active SLE, along with anaemia, haemolytic anaemia and thrombocytopenia. CRP levels are often normal in

25.71 Revised American Rheumatism Association criteria for systemic lupus erythematosus[1]

Features	Characteristics
Malar rash	Fixed erythema, flat or raised, sparing the nasolabial folds
Discoid rash	Erythematous raised patches with adherent keratotic scarring and follicular plugging
Photosensitivity	Rash due to unusual reaction to sunlight
Oral ulcers	Oral or nasopharyngeal ulceration, which may be painless
Arthritis	Non-erosive, involving two or more peripheral joints
Serositis	Pleuritis (history of pleuritic pain or rub, or pleural effusion) *or* pericarditis (rub, ECG evidence or effusion)
Renal disorder	Persistent proteinuria > 0.5 g/day *or* cellular casts (red cell, granular or tubular)
Neurological disorder	Seizures or psychosis, in the absence of provoking drugs or metabolic derangement
Haematological disorder	Haemolytic anaemia *or* leucopenia[2] ($< 4 \times 10^9$/L), *or* lymphopenia[2] ($< 1 \times 10^9$/L), *or* thrombocytopenia[2] ($< 100 \times 10^9$/L) in the absence of offending drugs
Immunological disorder	Anti-DNA antibodies in abnormal titre *or* presence of antibody to Sm antigen *or* positive antiphospholipid antibodies
Antinuclear antibody (ANA) disorder	Abnormal titre of ANA by immunofluorescence

[1] A person has SLE if any 4 out of these 11 features are present serially or simultaneously.
[2] On two separate occasions.

active SLE, except in the presence of serositis, and an elevated CRP suggests co-existing infection.

Management

The therapeutic goals are to educate the patient about the nature of the illness, to control symptoms and to prevent organ damage. Patients should be advised to avoid sun and UV light exposure, and to employ sun blocks (factor 25–50). Cardiovascular risk factors, such as hypertension and hyperlipidaemia, should be controlled and patients advised to stop smoking. Patients with mild disease restricted to skin and joints can often be managed satisfactorily with analgesics and/or NSAIDs, and if necessary hydroxychloroquine (200–400 mg daily). Short courses of oral steroids may be required for rash, synovitis, pleurisy and pericarditis.

Life-threatening disease affecting the kidney, CNS or cardiovascular system requires high-dose steroids and immunosuppressives. A commonly used regimen is pulse methylprednisolone (500 mg–1 g i.v) coupled with cyclophosphamide (2 mg/kg i.v.), repeated at 2–3 weekly intervals on 6–8 occasions, depending on the clinical response. Mycophenolate mofetil (MMF) has been used successfully in combination with high-dose steroids for renal involvement in SLE, with results

equivalent to those of pulse cyclophosphamide but with fewer adverse effects. Following control of the acute episode, the patient should be switched to oral prednisolone (40–60 mg daily) and azathioprine, methotrexate or MMF. The long-term aim is to continue the lowest dose of corticosteroids and immunosuppressive required to maintain remission. Co-trimoxazole is sometimes given prophylactically (960 mg thrice weekly) with the aim of preventing *Pneumocystis* pneumonia, and mesna is given with bolus cyclophosphamide to reduce the risk of haemorrhagic cystitis. Lupus patients with the antiphospholipid antibody syndrome (p. 1050) who have had previous thrombosis require life-long warfarin. It has been suggested that if repeated thromboses occur despite warfarin, the INR target range should be 3.0–4.0.

Systemic sclerosis

Systemic sclerosis is a generalised disorder of connective tissue affecting the skin, internal organs and vasculature. It is characterised by sclerodactyly in combination with Raynaud's or digital ischaemia (Fig. 25.38). The peak age of onset is in the fourth and fifth decades, and overall prevalence is 10–20 per 100 000 with a 4:1 female preponderance. It is subdivided into diffuse cutaneous systemic sclerosis (DCSS; 30% of cases) and limited cutaneous systemic sclerosis (LCSS; 70% of cases). Many patients with LCSS have features which are phenotypically grouped into the 'CREST' syndrome (**C**alcinosis, **R**aynaud's, o**E**sophageal involvement, **S**clerodactyly and **T**elangiectasia). The prognosis in DCSS is poor, with a 5-year survival of approximately 70%. Features that associate with a poor prognosis include older age, diffuse skin disease, proteinuria, high ESR, a low TLCO (gas transfer factor for carbon monoxide) and pulmonary hypertension.

Pathophysiology

The cause of systemic sclerosis is poorly understood. There is evidence for a genetic component and associations with alleles at the HLA locus. The disease occurs in all ethnic groups, and race may influence severity since DCCS is significantly more common in black compared to white women. Isolated cases are reported of systemic sclerosis-like disease that has been triggered

25

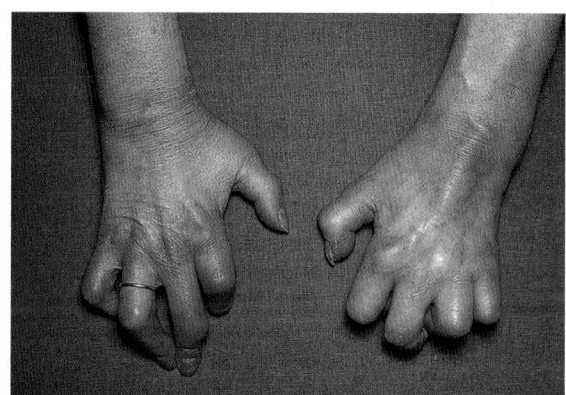

Fig. 25.38 Systemic sclerosis. Hands showing tight shiny skin, sclerodactyly, flexion contractures of the fingers and thickening of the left middle finger extensor tendon sheath.

by exposure to silica dust, vinyl chloride, hypoxyresins and trichloroethylene. There is clear evidence of immunological dysfunction; T lymphocytes infiltrate the skin and there is abnormal fibroblast activation leading to increased production of extracellular matrix in the dermis, primarily type I collagen. This results in symmetrical thickening, tightening and induration of the skin (sclerodactyly). Arterial and arteriolar narrowing occurs due to intimal proliferation and vessel wall inflammation. Endothelial injury causes release of vasoconstrictors and platelet activation, resulting in further ischaemia, which is thought to exacerbate the fibrotic process.

Clinical features

Skin

Initially there is non-pitting oedema of fingers and flexor tendon sheaths. Subsequently, the skin becomes shiny and taut, and distal skin creases disappear. This is accompanied by erythema and tortuous dilatation of capillary loops in the nail-fold bed, readily visible with an ophthalmoscope or dissecting microscope (and oil placed on the skin). The face and neck are usually involved next, with thinning of the lips and radial furrowing. In some patients, skin thickening stops at this stage. Skin involvement restricted to sites distal to the elbow or knee (apart from the face) is classified as 'limited disease' or CREST syndrome (Fig. 25.39). Involvement proximal to the knee and elbow and on the trunk is classified as 'diffuse disease'.

Raynaud's phenomenon

This is a universal feature and can precede other features by many years. Involvement of small blood vessels in the extremities may cause critical tissue ischaemia, leading to skin ulceration over pressure areas, localised areas of infarction and pulp atrophy at the fingertips.

Musculoskeletal features

Arthralgia, morning stiffness and flexor tenosynovitis are common. Restricted hand function is due to skin rather than joint disease and erosive arthropathy is uncommon. Muscle weakness and wasting can occur due to myositis.

Gastrointestinal involvement

Smooth muscle atrophy and fibrosis in the lower two-thirds of the oesophagus lead to reflux with erosive oesophagitis. Dysphagia and odynophagia may also occur. Involvement of the stomach causes early satiety and occasionally outlet obstruction. Recurrent occult upper gastrointestinal bleeding may indicate a 'watermelon' stomach (antral vascular ectasia), which occurs in up to 20% of patients. Small intestine involvement may lead to malabsorption due to bacterial overgrowth and intermittent bloating, pain or constipation. Dilatation of large or small bowel due to autonomic neuropathy may cause pseudo-obstruction with nausea, vomiting, abdominal discomfort and distension, often worse after food.

Pulmonary involvement

This is a major cause of morbidity and mortality. Pulmonary hypertension complicates long-standing disease and is six times more prevalent in LCSS than in DCSS. It presents with rapidly progressive dyspnoea (more rapid than interstitial lung disease), right heart failure and angina, often in association with severe digital ischaemia. Fibrosing alveolitis mainly affects patients with DCSS who have topoisomerase 1 antibodies.

Renal involvement

One of the main causes of death is hypertensive renal crisis characterised by rapidly developing malignant hypertension and renal failure. Hypertensive renal crisis is much more likely to occur in DCSS than in LCSS, and in patients with topoisomerase 1 antibodies.

Investigations

Scleroderma is a clinical diagnosis but various laboratory abnormalities are characteristic.

The ESR is usually elevated and raised levels of IgG are common, but CRP values tend to be normal unless there is severe organ involvement or coexisting infection. ANA is positive in about 70%, and approximately 30% of patients with DCSS have antibodies to topoisomerase 1 (Scl-70). About 60% of patients with CREST syndrome have anticentromere antibodies (p. 1064).

Management

The focus of management is to ameliorate the effects of the disease on target organs. No treatments are available that halt or reverse the fibrotic changes which underlie the disease.

- *Raynaud's syndrome and digital ulcers* should be treated by avoidance of cold exposure and use of mittens (heated mittens are available), supplemented if necessary with calcium antagonists or angiotensin II receptor blockers. Intermittent infusions of epoprostenol may benefit severe digital ischaemia. Infections occur commonly in ulcerated skin lesions and require treatment with antibiotics, but as these penetrate tissues poorly in scleroderma they need to be given at higher doses for longer courses than usual.
- *Oesophageal reflux* should be treated with PPIs and anti-reflux agents. Antibiotics may be required for bacterial overgrowth syndromes and metoclopramide or domperidone may help patients with symptoms of pseudo-obstruction.
- *Hypertension* should be treated aggressively with angiotensin-converting enzyme (ACE) inhibitors, even if renal impairment is present. The benefit of prophylactic ACE inhibitors in patients with DCSS to prevent deterioration of renal function is uncertain.

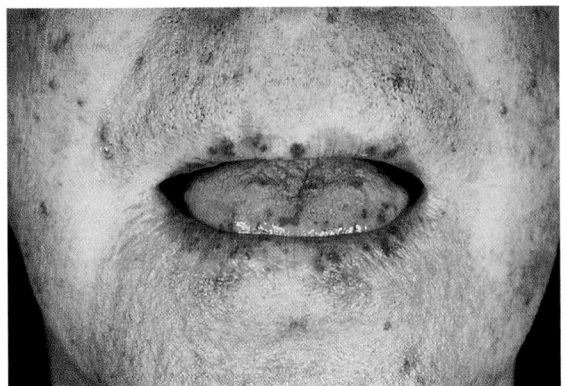

Fig. 25.39 Typical facial appearance in the CREST syndrome.

- *Joint involvement* may be treated with analgesics.
- *Pulmonary hypertension* may be treated with the endothelin 1 antagonist, bosentan, and in selected patients heart-lung transplantation may be considered. Corticosteroids and cytotoxic drugs are indicated in patients who have coexisting myositis or fibrosing alveolitis.

Mixed connective tissue disease

This is an overlap condition in which there are clinical features of SLE, systemic sclerosis and myositis. It commonly presents with synovitis and oedema of the hands in combination with Raynaud's phenomenon and muscle pain/weakness. Most patients have anti-ribonucleoprotein (RNP) antibodies, but these can occur in SLE without overlap features. Management focuses on treating the individual components of the syndrome.

Sjögren's syndrome

This is an autoimmune disorder of unknown cause characterised by lymphocytic infiltration of salivary and lachrymal glands, leading to glandular fibrosis and exocrine failure. The typical age of onset is between 40 and 50 with a 9:1 female preponderance. The disease may be primary or secondary to other autoimmune diseases.

Clinical features

The eye symptoms, termed keratoconjunctivitis sicca, are due to lack of lubricating tears. Conjunctivitis and blepharitis are frequent, and may lead to filamentary keratitis due to tenacious mucous filaments binding to the cornea and conjunctiva. Oral involvement manifests as a dry mouth and typically the patient needs water to swallow food. There is a high incidence of dental caries. Other sites of extraglandular involvement are listed in Box 25.72. The disease is associated with a 40-fold increased lifetime risk of lymphoma.

Investigations

The diagnosis can be established by the Schirmer tear test, which measures tear flow over 5 minutes using absorbent paper strips placed on the lower eyelid; a normal result is more than 6mm of wetting. Staining with rose Bengal may show punctate epithelial abnormalities over the area not covered by the open eyelid. If the diagnosis remains in doubt, it can be confirmed by lip biopsy which shows focal lymphocytic infiltrate of the minor salivary glands. Most patients have an elevated ESR and hypergammaglobulinaemia, and one or more autoantibodies, including ANF and RF. Anti-Ro and anti-La antibodies are commonly present (see Box 25.8, p. 1064).

Management

Treatment is symptomatic. Lachrymal substitutes such as hypromellose should be used during the day in combination with more viscous lubricating ointment at night. Soft contact lenses can be useful for corneal protection in patients with filamentary keratitis, and occlusion of the lachrymal ducts is occasionally needed. Artificial saliva and oral gels can be tried for xerostomia but are often not effective. Stimulation of saliva flow by sugar-

25.72 Features of Sjögren's syndrome

Risk factors

- Age of onset 40–60
- Female > Male
- HLA-B8/DR3

Common clinical features

- Keratoconjunctivitis sicca
- Xerostomia
- Salivary gland enlargement
- Non-erosive arthritis
- Raynaud's phenomenon
- Fatigue

Less common features

- Low-grade fever
- Interstitial lung disease
- Anaemia, leucopenia
- Thrombocytopenia
- Cryoglobulinaemia
- Vasculitis
- Peripheral neuropathy
- Lymphadenopathy
- Lymphoreticular lymphoma
- Glomerulonephritis
- Renal tubular acidosis

Autoantibodies frequently detected

- RF
- ANA
- SS-A (anti-Ro)
- SS-B (anti-La)
- Gastric parietal cell
- Thyroid

Associated autoimmune disorders

- SLE
- Progressive systemic sclerosis
- Primary biliary cirrhosis
- Chronic active hepatitis
- Myasthenia gravis

free chewing gum or lozenges may be helpful. Adequate post-prandial oral hygiene and prompt treatment of oral candidiasis are essential. Vaginal dryness is treated with lubricants such as K-Y jelly. Extraglandular and MSK manifestations may respond to steroids, and if so, immunosuppressive drugs can be added for their steroid-sparing effect. Fatigue is difficult to treat; this is usually due to non-restorative sleep (often because of xerostomia) and is unresponsive to steroids. Immunosuppression does not improve sicca symptoms. If lymphadenopathy or salivary gland enlargement develops, biopsy should be performed to exclude malignancy.

Polymyositis and dermatomyositis

Polymyositis is characterised by an inflammatory process affecting skeletal muscle. Dermatomyositis describes the same disease but with skin involvement. They are rare, with an incidence of 2–10 cases per million/year. Polymyositis can occur in isolation or in association with other autoimmune diseases such as SLE, systemic sclerosis and Sjögren's syndrome. The cause is unknown, although there is evidence for a genetic contribution.

Clinical features

The typical presentation of polymyositis is with symmetrical proximal muscle weakness, usually affecting the lower limbs more than the upper limbs. The onset is usually between 40 and 60 years of age and is typically gradual, over a few weeks. Myositis is usually widespread but focal disease can also occur (e.g. orbital myositis). Affected patients report difficulty rising from a chair, climbing stairs and lifting, sometimes in combination with muscle pain. Systemic features of fever, weight loss and fatigue are common. Respiratory

25

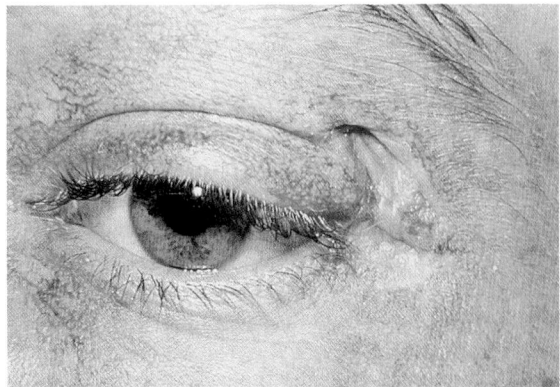

Fig. 25.40 Typical eyelid appearance in dermatomyositis. Note the oedema and telangiectasia.

or pharyngeal muscle involvement can lead to ventilatory failure or aspiration that requires urgent treatment. Interstitial lung disease occurs in up to 30% of patients and is strongly associated with the presence of antisynthetase (Jo-1) antibodies.

Dermatomyositis presents similarly but in combination with characteristic skin lesions. These include Gottron's papules, which are scaly erythematous or violaceous psoriaform plaques occurring over the extensor surfaces of proximal and distal IPJs, and a heliotrope rash which is a violaceous discoloration of the eyelid in combination with periorbital oedema (Fig. 25.40). Similar rashes occur on the upper back, chest and shoulders ('shawl' distribution). Periungual nail-fold capillaries are often enlarged and tortuous. There is about a three-fold increased risk of malignancy in patients with dermatomyositis and polymyositis. This may be apparent at the time of presentation, but the risk remains increased for at least 5 years following diagnosis.

Investigations

Muscle biopsy is a pivotal investigation and shows the typical features of fibre necrosis, regeneration and inflammatory cell infiltrate (Fig. 25.41). EMG can confirm the presence of myopathy and exclude neuropathy. Occasionally, however, a biopsy may be normal, particu-

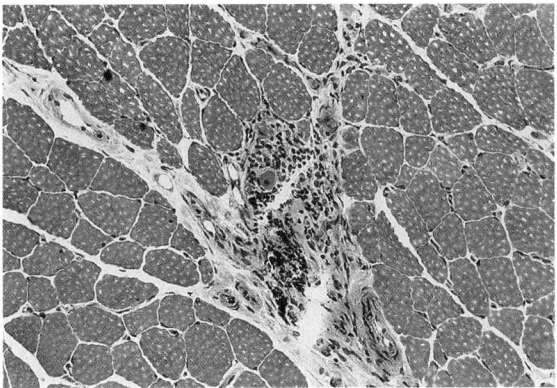

Fig. 25.41 Muscle biopsy from a patient with inflammatory myositis. The sample shows an intense inflammatory cell infiltrate in an area of degenerating and regenerating muscle fibres.

larly if myositis is patchy. In such cases, MRI will identify areas of abnormal muscle for biopsy. Serum levels of CK are usually raised and are a useful measure of disease activity, although a normal CK does not exclude the diagnosis, particularly in juvenile myositis. Screening for underlying malignancy should be undertaken routinely, and should include chest/abdomen/pelvis CT, gastrointestinal tract imaging and mammography (in women).

Management

Oral corticosteroids (e.g. prednisolone 40–60 mg daily) are the mainstay of initial treatment but high-dose intravenous methylprednisolone (1 g/day for 3 days) may be required in patients with respiratory or pharyngeal weakness. If there is a good response, steroids should be reduced by approximately 25% per month to a maintenance dose of 5–7.5 mg. Although most patients have an initial response to steroids, most need additional immunosuppressive therapy. Azathioprine and methotrexate are the agents of first choice, but ciclosporin, cyclophosphamide, tacrolimus or MMF can be used as alternatives. Intravenous immunoglobulin may be effective in refractory cases. Relapses may occur associated with a rising CK, and indicate the need for additional therapy. If the patient relapses or fails to respond to treatment, this may be due to steroid-induced myopathy. This is an indication for further biopsy which may show type 2 fibre atrophy in steroid-induced myopathy, as opposed to necrosis and regeneration in active myositis.

SYSTEMIC VASCULITIS

This is a heterogeneous group of diseases characterised by inflammation and necrosis of blood vessel walls, with associated damage to skin, kidney, lung, heart, brain and gastrointestinal tract. There is a wide spectrum of involvement and disease severity, ranging from mild and transient disease affecting the skin, to life-threatening fulminant disease with multiple organ failure. Vasculitis may occur secondary to a variety of inflammatory and infectious diseases, including SLE, Sjögren's syndrome, RA, endocarditis and hepatitis B or C, when it is thought to be due to deposition of immune complexes in small vessels. Primary vasculitis occurs in the absence of a known cause. It is uncommon, with an estimated incidence of 18–40 per million per year, and has a peak onset between the ages of 65 and 75. Vasculitis is usually classified on the basis of the size of vessel involved (Box 25.73).

i 25.73 Size of vessel involvement in vasculitis

Large vessel	
• Giant cell arteritis	• Takayasu's arteritis

Medium vessel	
• Classical polyarteritis nodosa	• Kawasaki disease (in childhood)

Small vessel	
• Microscopic polyangiitis	• Henoch-Schönlein purpura
• Wegener's granulomatosis	• Mixed essential cryoglobulinaemia
• Churg–Strauss syndrome	

The clinical features of vasculitis result from a combination of local tissue ischaemia (due to vessel inflammation and narrowing) and the systemic effects of widespread inflammation. Systemic vasculitis should be considered in any patient with fever, weight loss, fatigue, evidence of multisystem involvement, rashes, raised inflammatory markers and abnormal urinalysis. The symptoms of vasculitis are shown in Box 25.33 (p. 1075). Other conditions that may mimic vasculitis include sepsis (particularly infective endocarditis and meningococcaemia), malignancy, cholesterol emboli, atrial myxoma and the antiphospholipid syndrome. This may lead to diagnostic delay, but early diagnosis and management are essential to prevent irreversible organ damage.

Takayasu's arteritis

Takayasu's disease predominantly affects the aorta, its major branches and occasionally the pulmonary arteries. The typical age at onset is between 25 and 30 years, with an 8:1 female preponderance. It has a world-wide distribution but is most common in Asia. In contrast to other vasculitides, Takayasu's is characterised by granulomatous inflammation of the vessel wall leading to vessel occlusion or weakening of the vessel wall. It presents with claudication, fever, arthralgia and weight loss. The vessels most commonly affected are the aorta, carotid, ulnar, brachial, radial and axillary arteries. Clinical examination may reveal loss of pulses, bruits, hypertension and aortic incompetence. Investigation shows an APR and normocytic, normochromic anaemia, but the diagnosis is based on angiographic findings of coarctation, occlusion and aneurysmal dilatation. The distribution of involvement is classified into four types:
- type 1: localised to the aorta and its branches
- type 2: localised to the descending thoracic and abdominal aorta
- type 3: combines features of 1 and 2
- type 4: involves the pulmonary artery.

Treatment is with high-dose steroids and immunosuppressives. With appropriate treatment, the 5-year survival is 83%.

Polyarteritis nodosa (PAN)

PAN can affect any age group but the peak incidence is between 40 and 50, with a male preponderance of 2:1. The annual incidence is around 2/1 000 000. Hepatitis B is an important risk factor, and the incidence of PAN is 10 times higher in the Inuit of Alaska, in whom hepatitis B infection is endemic. Presentation is with fever, myalgia, arthralgia and weight loss, in combination with manifestations of multisystem disease. The most common skin lesions are palpable purpura (Fig. 25.42), ulceration, infarction and livedo reticularis (see Fig. 25.37, p. 1108). Pathological changes comprise necrotising inflammation and vessel occlusion, and in 70% of patients arteritis of the vasa nervorum leads to neuropathy which is typically symmetrical and affects both sensory and motor function. Severe hypertension and/or renal impairment may occur due to multiple renal infarctions but glomerulonephritis is rare (in contrast to microscopic polyangiitis). The diagnosis is confirmed by angiographic demonstration of multiple aneurysms and smooth narrowing of mesenteric, hepatic or renal systems, or by histology (muscle or sural nerve biopsy). Mortality is less

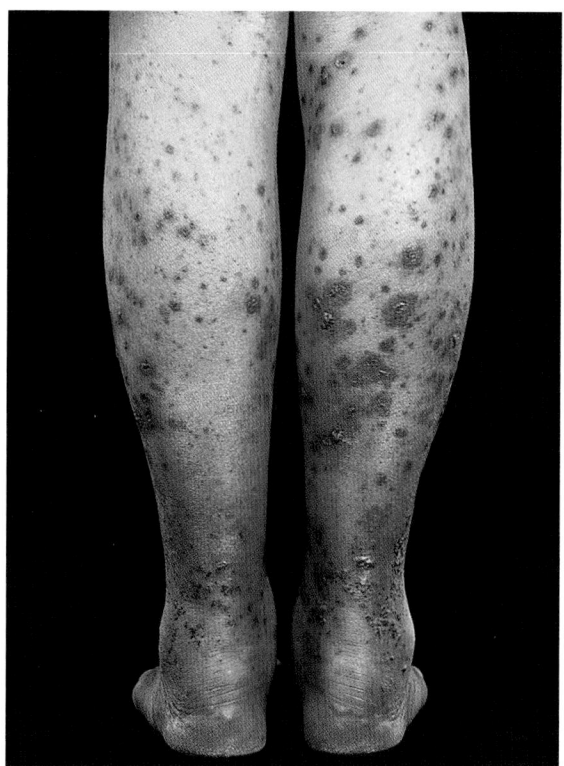

Fig. 25.42 Rash of systemic vasculitis (palpable purpura).

than 20% with treatment but relapse occurs in up to 50% of patients.

Kawasaki disease

Kawasaki disease is an acute systemic disorder of childhood that predominantly occurs in Japan. Presentation is with fever, generalised rash including the palms and soles, inflamed oral mucosa and conjunctival injection resembling a viral exanthem or Stevens–Johnson syndrome. Although the causative trigger is unknown, it has been associated with *Mycoplasma* and HIV infection. Cardiovascular complications include transient coronary dilatation, myocarditis, pericarditis, myocardial infarction, peripheral vascular insufficiency and gangrene. Treatment is with aspirin (5 mg/kg daily for 14 days) and intravenous gammaglobulin (400 mg/kg daily for 4 days).

Microscopic polyangiitis (MPA)

This has an annual incidence of about 8/1 000 000 and is characterised by necrotising vasculitis affecting small vessels. Typical presentation is with rapidly progressive glomerulonephritis, often associated with alveolar haemorrhage. Cutaneous and gastrointestinal involvement is common and other features include neuropathy (15%) and pleural effusions (15%). Patients are usually p-ANCA (myeloperoxidase)-positive (see below).

Wegener's granulomatosis (WG)

WG has an incidence of 5–10/1 000 000 and is characterised by granulomatous inflammation and necrotising vasculitis affecting the nasal passages, airways and kidney. The most common presentation is with upper airway involvement (typically epistaxis, nasal crusting and

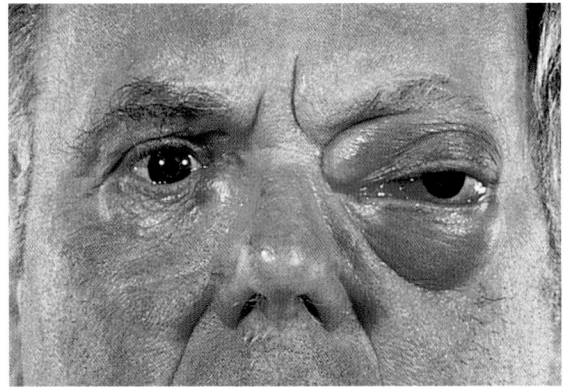

Fig. 25.43 Eye involvement in Wegener's granulomatosis.

sinusitis), haemoptysis, mucosal ulceration and deafness due to serous otitis media. Proptosis may occur due to inflammation of the retro-orbital tissue, causing diplopia due to entrapment of the extra-ocular muscles, or loss of vision due to optic nerve compression. Disturbance of colour vision is an early feature of optic nerve compression (Fig. 25.43). Untreated nasal disease ultimately leads to destruction of bone and cartilage. Migratory pulmonary infiltrates and nodules occur in 50% of patients. A minority of patients present with glomerulonephritis. Patients are usually c-ANCA-positive.

Churg–Strauss syndrome (CSS)

CSS has an incidence of 1–3/1 000 000. Pathologically, it is similar to WG but eosinophilic infiltration of the vessel wall also occurs. Most patients have a prodromal period for many years characterised by allergic rhinitis, nasal polyposis and late-onset asthma that is often difficult to control. The typical acute presentation is with a triad of skin lesions (purpura or nodules), asymmetric mononeuritis multiplex and eosinophilia on a background of resistant asthma. Pulmonary infiltrates and pleural or pericardial effusions due to serositis may be present. Up to 50% of patients have abdominal symptoms due to mesenteric vasculitis. Either c-ANCA or p-ANCA is present in around 40% of cases.

Henoch–Schönlein purpura (HSP)

HSP usually occurs in children and young adults and generally has a good prognosis. It is characterised by immune complex deposition in small vessels with associated vasculitis. The typical presentation is with purpura over the buttocks and lower legs, abdominal symptoms (pain and bleeding) and arthritis (knee or ankle) following an upper respiratory tract infection. Nephritis is found in 40% of patients and may occur up to 4 weeks after the onset of other symptoms. The diagnosis can be confirmed by tissue biopsy, which demonstrates IgA deposition within and around blood vessel walls. The prognosis is determined by the severity of renal involvement. Adverse prognostic features at presentation in adults include hypertension, abnormal renal function and proteinuria > 1.5 g/day, but only 1% of patients develop end-stage renal failure.

Cryoglobulinaemic vasculitis

Cryoglobulins are circulating immunoglobulins that precipitate out in the cold. They are classified into three types (Box 4.14, p. 87); types II and III are associated with cryoglobulinaemic vasculitis. Pathology is similar to HSP. The typical clinical features are palpable purpura over the lower extremities, arthralgia, Raynaud's phenomenon and neuropathy. Type II cryoglobulinaemia is secondary to hepatitis C virus (HCV) infection in most patients, the virus being present in the vasculitic lesions complexed with IgG and IgM. For HCV-positive patients, interferon-alpha (IFN-α) is currently the treatment of choice; for high HCV loads, combination with ribavirin may be more effective (p. 953).

Investigations in systemic vasculitis

Angiography and tissue biopsy are the pivotal investigations. Biopsies can be taken from the nasal septal tissue or from areas of ulceration in patients suspected of having WG, from muscle or nerve in PAN or CSS, from kidney in patients with renal involvement, or from skin in HSP and cryoglobulinaemic vasculitis. Angiography is useful in PAN and Takayasu's disease.

Complement levels are useful; C3 and C4 are typically reduced in active disease, reflecting complement consumption, and can be used as an index of disease activity. Screening for ANCA is important, although they are not specific for the diagnosis of vasculitis and can occur in other diseases (p. 1064). The presence of c-ANCA is particularly associated with WG and CSS, whereas p-ANCA is associated with MPA. Urinalysis for protein and blood should always be performed with subsequent microscopy, since the prognosis of vasculitis is often determined by the degree of renal involvement. Routine biochemistry should be performed to identify renal impairment. CRP and ESR are elevated in active disease and are useful in monitoring disease activity.

Management of systemic vasculitis

Treatment is with high-dose corticosteroids and immunosuppressives, as described for life-threatening involvement in SLE (p. 1109). If cyclophosphamide fails to induce a remission, the diagnosis should be reconsidered. ANCA-positive patients with acute renal failure have a better outcome when also treated with adjunctive plasma exchange. Patients with PAN who have evidence of hepatitis B infection should also be treated with antiviral therapy (p. 951). In Takayasu's arteritis, reconstructive vascular surgery may benefit selected patients, especially those with hypertension secondary to aortic or renal lesions.

Behçet's syndrome

This is a vasculitis of unknown aetiology that characteristically targets venules. It is rare in Western Europe but more common in 'Silk Route' countries around the Mediterranean and Japan, where there is a strong association with HLA-B51.

There is a wide range of clinical features, with unpredictable exacerbations. Oral ulcers are universal (Fig. 25.44). Unlike aphthous ulcers, they are usually deep and multiple, and last for 10–30 days. Genital ulcers are less common (60–80%). The usual skin lesions are erythema nodosum or acneiform lesions but migratory thrombophlebitis and vasculitis also occur. The pathergy reaction is hyper-reactivity at the site of minor trauma. A formal pathergy test involves intradermal skin pricking with a needle, and is positive if a pustule develops within 48 hours. Ocular involvement is usually bilateral

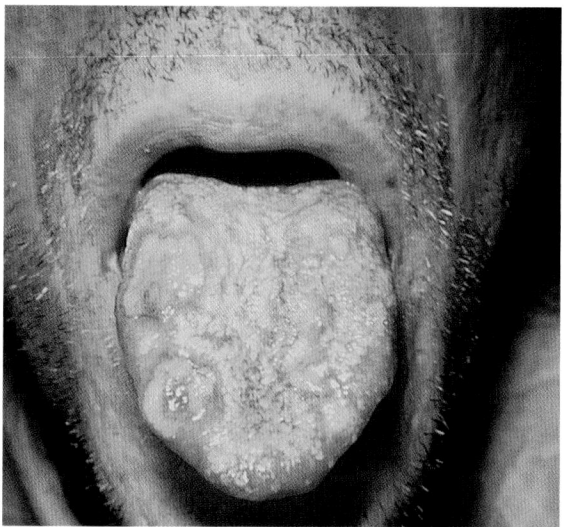

Fig. 25.44 Oral ulceration in Behçet's syndrome.

and may include anterior or posterior uveitis or retinal vasculitis. Neurological involvement occurs in 5% and mainly involves the brain stem, although the meninges, hemispheres and cord can also be involved, causing pyramidal signs, cranial nerve lesions, brain-stem symptoms or hemiparesis. Recurrent thromboses also occur. Renal involvement is extremely rare.

There are no defining investigations and the diagnosis is clinical (Box 25.74). Oral ulceration can be managed with topical steroid preparations (e.g. soluble prednisolone mouthwashes, steroid pastes). Colchicine can be effective for erythema nodosum and arthralgia. Thalidomide (100–300 mg per day for 28 days initially) is very effective for resistant oral and genital ulceration but is teratogenic and neurotoxic. Steroids and immunosuppressives are indicated for systemic disease.

25.74 Criteria for the diagnosis of Behçet's syndrome

- Recurrent oral ulceration: minor aphthous, major aphthous or herpetiform ulceration at least three times in a 12-month period

Plus two of the following:
- Recurrent genital ulceration
- Eye lesions: anterior uveitis, posterior uveitis, cells in vitreous on slit-lamp examination, retinal vasculitis
- Skin lesions: erythema nodosum, pseudofolliculitis, papulopustular lesions, acneiform nodules
- Positive pathergy test

Giant cell arteritis (GCA) and polymyalgia rheumatica (PMR)

GCA and PMR are related diseases associated with a granulomatous arteritis of medium-sized vessels of the head and neck. They are sometimes considered as separate diseases but many patients with PMR also have symptoms of GCA and vice versa. Since the management of both is similar, they are considered together here. Both are diseases of the elderly, with a prevalence of approximately 20 per 100 000 over the age of 50 years. The average age at onset is 70, and they are rare under the age of 60. There is a female preponderance of about 3:1. The clinical features result from occlusion of vessels and subsequent tissue ischaemia.

Clinical features

The cardinal features of PMR are symmetrical muscle pain and stiffness affecting the shoulder and pelvic girdles. Constitutional symptoms such as weight loss, fatigue, malaise and night sweats are common. The onset of symptoms is usually fairly sudden, over a few days, but may be more insidious. On examination, there may be stiffness and painful restriction of active shoulder movement but passive movements are preserved. Muscles may be tender to palpation but weakness and muscle-wasting are absent. The cardinal symptom of GCA is headache, which is often localised to the temporal or occipital region and may be accompanied by scalp tenderness. Jaw pain develops in some patients, brought on by chewing or talking, and due to ischaemia of the masseter muscles. Visual disturbance can occur and a catastrophic presentation is blindness in one eye due to occlusion of the posterior ciliary artery. On fundoscopy the optic disc may appear pale and swollen with haemorrhages, but these changes may take 24–36 hours to develop and the fundi may initially appear normal. Other visual symptoms include loss of visual acuity, reduced colour perception and papillary defects. Rarely, neurological involvement may occur, with transient ischaemic attacks, brain-stem infarcts and hemiparesis. Other conditions that mimic PMR are shown in Box 25.75.

Investigations

The typical laboratory abnormality is an elevated ESR, often with a normochromic, normocytic anaemia. CRP may also be elevated and in some cases this precedes elevation of the ESR. Occasionally, PMR and GCA occur with a normal ESR. The diagnosis is usually based on a combination of the typical clinical features, raised ESR and prompt response to steroid. However, if there is doubt concerning the diagnosis of GCA, a temporal artery biopsy may be undertaken. Characteristic biopsy findings are fragmentation of the internal elastic lamina with necrosis of the media in combination with a mixed inflammatory cell infiltrate. Whilst a positive biopsy is helpful, a negative biopsy does not exclude the diagnosis because the lesions are focal. Ultrasound or arteriography may be used to help guide the biopsy.

Management

Corticosteroids are the treatment of choice and should be commenced urgently in suspected GCA because of the risk of visual loss (Box 25.76). Response to treatment is dramatic, such that symptoms will have completely resolved within 48–72 hours of starting corticosteroid therapy in virtually all patients. It is customary to use higher doses in GCA (60 mg prednisolone) than in PMR (20–30 mg), although the

25.75 Conditions that may mimic polymyalgia rheumatica

- Fibromyalgia
- Hypothyroidism
- Cervical spondylosis
- RA
- Systemic vasculitis
- Inflammatory myopathy (particularly inclusion body myositis, p. 1128)
- Malignancy

25

Box 25.76 Emergency management of giant cell arteritis

- Take blood for ESR and CRP
- Commence prednisolone 40–60 mg daily
- Review patient in 3–4 days
- Continue steroids in patients whose symptoms have resolved, with gradual reduction in dose
- Organise temporal artery biopsy in patients with poor or equivocal response

evidence base for this is weak. In both conditions the steroid dose should be progressively reduced, guided by symptoms and ESR, with the aim of reaching a dose of 10–15 mg by about 8 weeks. Thereafter reduction is slower by 1 mg per month until an acceptable dose is achieved (5–7.5 mg daily). If symptoms recur, the dose should be increased to that which previously controlled the symptoms, and reduction attempted in another few months. Most patients need steroids for an average of 12–24 months. Some patients require steroid-sparing agents, such as methotrexate or azathioprine, if they require a maintenance dose of prednisolone of more than 7.5 mg daily. Osteoporosis prophylaxis should be given for the duration of treatment.

DISEASES OF BONE

Osteoporosis

The defining feature of osteoporosis is reduced bone density, which causes a micro-architectural deterioration of bone tissue and leads to an increased risk of fracture. The prevalence of osteoporosis increases with age, reflecting the fact that bone density declines with age, especially in women (Fig. 25.45). The age-related decline

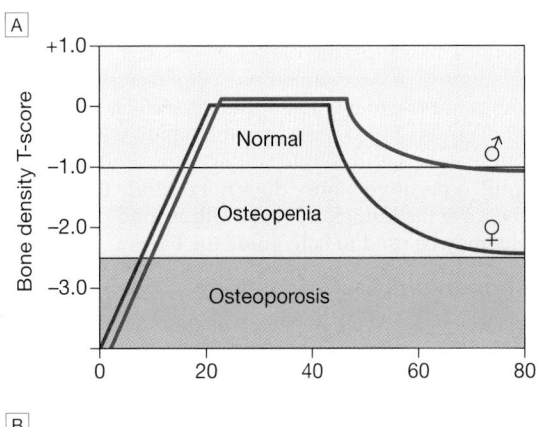

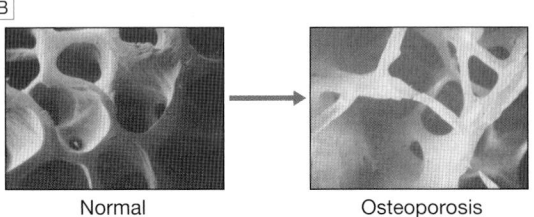

Fig. 25.45 Changes in bone mass and microstructure with age. **A** Changes in bone mass with age in men (blue line) and women (pink line). **B** Scanning electron micrographs of normal bone (left) and osteoporotic bone (right).

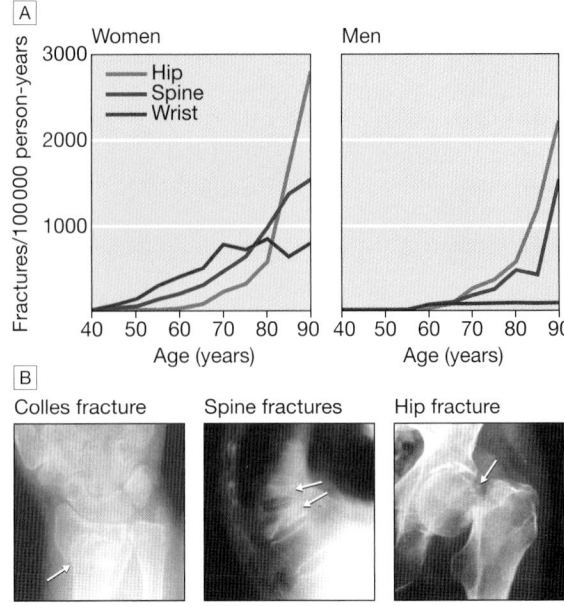

Fig. 25.46 Relation between age and the incidence of osteoporotic fractures. **A** Changes in the incidence of wrist fractures, vertebral fractures and hip fractures with age. **B** X-rays showing Colles fracture, vertebral fractures and hip fracture.

in bone mass is accompanied by an increased risk of fractures (Fig. 25.46A). This is due in part to the fall in bone density, but more importantly to the increased risk of falling which increases with age (p. 170). Fractures related to osteoporosis are estimated to affect around 30% of women and 12% of men at some point in developed countries and are a major public health problem. In the UK alone, fractures are sustained by over 250 000 individuals annually, with treatment costs of about £1.75 billion. Osteoporotic fractures can affect any bone, but the most common sites are the forearm (Colles fracture), spine (vertebral fracture) and hip (Fig. 25.46B); of these, hip fractures are the most serious. The immediate mortality is about 12% and there is a continued increase in mortality of about 20% when compared with age-matched controls. Treatment of hip fracture accounts for the majority of the health-care costs associated with osteoporosis.

Pathophysiology

Osteoporosis can occur because of a defect in attaining peak bone mass and/or because of accelerated bone loss. In normal individuals, bone mass increases during skeletal growth to reach a peak between the ages of 20 and 40 years but falls thereafter (see Fig. 25.45). In women there is an accelerated phase of bone loss after the menopause due to oestrogen deficiency which causes uncoupling of bone resorption and bone formation, such that the amount of bone removed by osteoclasts exceeds the rate of new bone formation by osteoblasts. Age-related bone loss is a distinct process that accounts for the gradual bone loss that occurs with advancing age in both genders. Bone resorption is not particularly increased but bone formation is reduced and fails to keep pace with bone resorption. Accumulation of fat in the bone marrow space also occurs because of an age-related decline in the ability of bone marrow stem cells to differentiate into osteoblasts and an increase in their ability to differentiate into adipocytes (see Fig. 25.45).

Peak bone mass and bone loss are regulated by both genetic and environmental factors. Genetic factors account for up to 80% of the population variance in peak bone mass and other determinants of fracture risk, such as bone turnover and bone size. Polymorphisms have been identified in several genes that contribute to the pathogenesis of osteoporosis, including the oestrogen receptor gene (*ESR1*); the lipoprotein receptor-related protein 5 gene (*LRP5*); and the genes that encode osteoprotegerin (*TNFRSF11B*), RANK (*TNFRSF11A*) and the alpha 1 chain of type I collagen (*COL1A1*). However, these account for only a small proportion of the genetic contribution to osteoporosis and many genetic variants remain to be discovered.

Environmental factors such as exercise and calcium intake during growth and adolescence are important in maximising peak bone mass and in regulating rates of post-menopausal bone loss. Smoking has a detrimental effect on BMD and is associated with an increased fracture risk, partly because female smokers have an earlier menopause than non-smokers. Heavy alcohol intake is a recognised cause of osteoporosis and fractures, but moderate intake does not substantially alter risk.

Postmenopausal osteoporosis

This is the most common cause of osteoporosis because of the effects of oestrogen deficiency, as described above. Early menopause (below the age of 45 years) is a particularly important risk factor.

Osteoporosis in men

Osteoporosis is less common in men and a secondary cause can be identified in about 50% of cases. The most common are hypogonadism, corticosteroid use (see below) and alcoholism. In hypogonadism, the pathogenesis is as described for postmenopausal osteoporosis, as testosterone deficiency results in an increase in bone turnover and uncoupling of bone resorption from bone formation. Genetic factors are probably important in the 50% of cases with no identifiable cause.

Corticosteroid-induced osteoporosis

This is an important cause of osteoporosis which relates to dose and duration of corticosteroid therapy. Although there is no 'safe' dose of corticosteroid, the risk increases when the dose of prednisolone exceeds 7.5 mg daily and is continued for more than 3 months. Corticosteroids have adverse effects on calcium metabolism and bone cell function. A key abnormality is reduced bone formation due to a direct inhibitory effect on osteoblast function and steroid-induced osteoblast and osteocyte apoptosis. Corticosteroids also inhibit intestinal calcium absorption and cause renal leak of calcium, and this tends to reduce serum calcium, leading to secondary hyperparathyroidism with increased osteoclastic bone resorption. Hypogonadism may also occur with high-dose steroids.

Pregnancy-associated osteoporosis

This is a rare condition that typically presents with back pain and multiple vertebral fractures during the second or third trimester. The cause is unknown but may relate to an exaggerated bone loss that normally occurs during pregnancy, in patients with pre-existing low bone mass.

Other causes

Osteoporosis can occur as a complication of many diseases and drug treatments (Box 25.77). Primary hyperparathyroidism causes bone loss because sustained elevation in PTH increases bone turnover, and bone formation cannot keep pace with resorption. A similar mechanism operates in thyrotoxicosis, driven by raised levels of thyroid hormones. Cushing's disease is a rare cause, identical in mechanism to corticosteroid-induced osteoporosis. Anorexia nervosa causes osteoporosis through calcium deficiency, weight loss and hypogonadism, whereas malabsorption predisposes to it through calcium and vitamin D deficiency and consequent secondary hyperparathyroidism. Chronic HIV infection predisposes to osteoporosis because of low body weight, chronic immune activation and anti-retroviral therapy. Inflammatory diseases increase bone resorption and suppress bone formation through release of pro-inflammatory cytokines such as IL-1 and TNF and increased expression of RANK by lymphocytes. Similar mechanisms operate in certain cancers which release a variety of bone-resorbing factors, including TNF, lymphotoxin and parathyroid hormone-related protein (PTHrP). Gaucher's disease (p. 449) and systemic mastocytosis also cause release of bone resorbing factors. Thiazolidinediones such as rosiglitazone inhibit osteoblast differentiation and promote adipocyte differentiation in the bone marrow, leading to reduced bone formation and bone loss. Aromatase inhibitors cause osteoporosis by reducing peripheral conversion of adrenal androgens to oestrogen, whereas gonadotrophin-releasing hormone agonists predispose to osteoporosis by causing hypogonadism.

Clinical features

Patients with osteoporosis are asymptomatic until a fracture occurs. Osteoporotic spinal fracture may

25

25.77 Causes of osteoporosis and osteoporotic fractures

Endocrine disease

• Hypogonadism	• Hyperparathyroidism
• Hyperthyroidism	• Cushing's syndrome

Inflammatory disease

• Inflammatory bowel disease	• RA
• Ankylosing spondylitis	

Drugs

• Corticosteroids	• Thiazolidinediones
• Gonadotrophin-releasing hormone (GnRH) agonists	• Sedatives
	• Anticonvulsants
• Aromatase inhibitors	• Alcohol excess
• Thyroxine over-replacement	• Heparin

Gastrointestinal disease

• Malabsorption	• Chronic liver disease

Miscellaneous

• Myeloma	• Gaucher's disease
• Homocystinuria	• Systemic mastocytosis
• Anorexia nervosa*	• Immobilisation
• Highly trained athletes*	• Poor diet/low body weight
• HIV infection	• Antibodies to OPG

*Hypogonadism plays an important role in osteoporosis associated with these conditions.

present with acute back pain or gradual onset of height loss and kyphosis with chronic pain. The pain of acute vertebral fracture can occasionally radiate to the anterior chest or abdominal wall and be mistaken for a myocardial infarction or intra-abdominal pathology, but worsening of pain by movement and local tenderness both suggest vertebral fracture. Peripheral osteoporotic fractures present with local pain, tenderness and deformity, often after an episode of minimal trauma. In patients with hip fracture, the affected leg is shortened and externally rotated. Many patients present with incidental osteopenia on an X-ray performed for other reasons.

Investigations

The pivotal investigation is dual energy X-ray absorptiometry (DEXA) at the lumbar spine and hip, which works on the principle that calcium in bone attenuates passage of X-ray beams in proportion to the amount of mineral present. The DEXA provides an image of the region studied, a BMD measurement (expressed as grams of hydroxyapatite/cm²) and T-score and Z-score values. The T-score is a measure of how many standard deviations the patient's BMD value differs from that of a young healthy control, whereas the BMD Z-score is a measure of how many standard deviations the BMD deviates from age-matched controls (Fig. 25.47). Osteoporosis is diagnosed when the T-score value falls to −2.5 or below (shaded red in the figure), whereas osteopenia is diagnosed when the T-score lies between −1.0 and −2.5 (pink in the figure). Many healthy people, especially above the age of 50, have BMD values in the osteopenic range and this is not considered an indication for drug treatment. Values of BMD above −1.0 are considered normal.

DEXA should be considered in patients with one or more clinical risk factors for osteoporosis (Box 25.78). Traditionally the presence of a single risk factor has been considered sufficient indication for DEXA, but recently a prediction tool has been developed (FRAX®; website listed at end of chapter) which synthesises information from several risk factors, allowing the calculation of a 10-year fracture probability in individuals. Figure 25.48 gives an algorithm for the investigation of patients with suspected osteoporosis using FRAX and DEXA.

A history should be taken to identify any predisposing causes, such as early menopause, excessive alcohol intake, smoking and corticosteroid therapy. Signs of endocrine disease, neoplasia and inflammatory disease should be sought on clinical examination. A falls history should be taken and a 'get up and go' test performed, especially in elderly patients (p. 165). Renal function, liver function, thyroid function, immunoglobulins and ESR, with screening for coeliac disease (TTG antibodies), should be performed. Serum 25(OH)D and PTH measurements are useful to exclude vitamin D deficiency and secondary hyperparathyroidism. Primary hyperparathyroidism should be suspected if hypercalcaemia is present (p. 766). Levels of sex hormones and gonadotrophins should be measured in men with osteoporosis and women under the age of 50. Transiliac bone biopsy is sometimes required in early-onset osteoporosis of unknown cause or when coexisting osteomalacia is suspected.

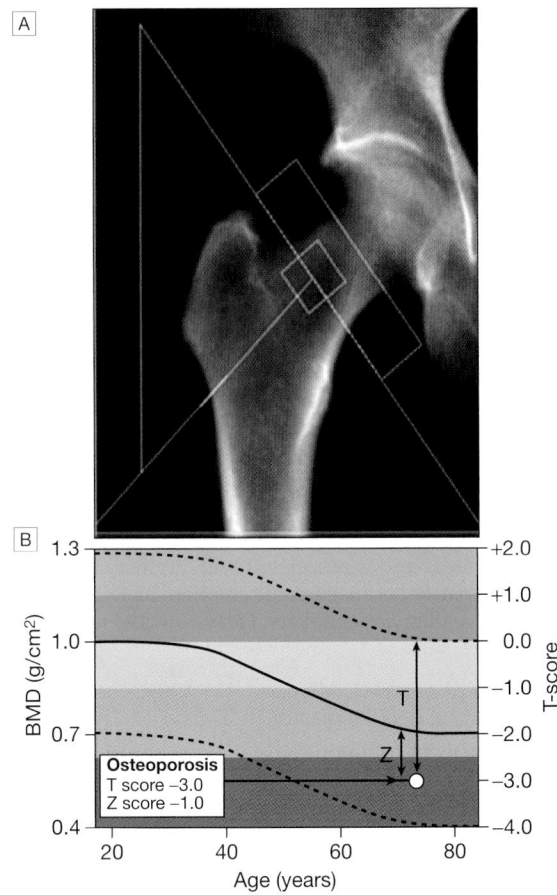

Fig. 25.47 Typical output from a DEXA scanner. **A** DEXA scan of the hip. **B** Bone mineral density (BMD) values plotted in g/cm² (left axis) and as the T-score values (right axis). The solid line represents the population average plotted against age, and the interrupted lines are ± 2 standard deviations from the average. The patient shown, aged 80, has an osteoporotic T-score of −3.0, but has a Z-score of −1.0, which is within the 'normal range' for that age, reflecting the fact that bone is lost with age.

25.78 Indications for bone densitometry

- Low trauma fracture (fall from standing height or less)
- Clinical features of osteoporosis (height loss, kyphosis)
- Osteopenia on plain X-ray
- Corticosteroid therapy (> 7.5 mg prednisolone daily for > 3 mths)
- Family history of osteoporotic fracture
- Low body weight (body mass index < 19)
- Early menopause (< 45 yrs)
- Diseases associated with osteoporosis
- Assessing response of osteoporosis to treatment
- High fracture risk on FRAX analysis

Management: lifestyle advice and falls prevention

The aim of treatment is to reduce the risk of fracture and this can be achieved by a combination of non-pharmacological and pharmacological approaches. Advice on lifestyle factors, such as smoking cessation, moderation of alcohol intake, dietary calcium intake and

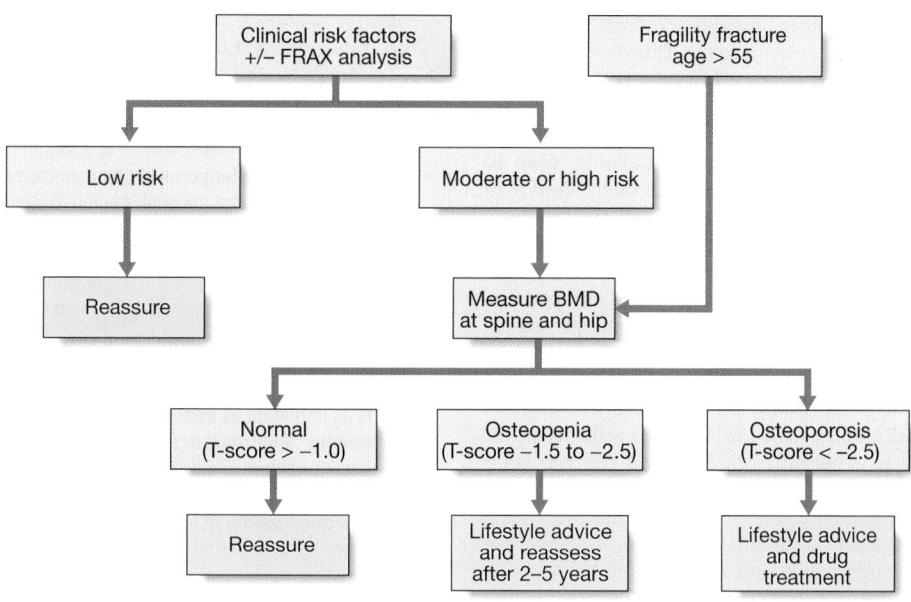

Fig. 25.48 Algorithm for the investigation of patients with suspected osteoporosis.

exercise, should be given. Those with recurrent falls or unsteadiness on a 'get up and go' test should be referred to a multidisciplinary falls prevention team (p. 170). Hip protectors can reduce the risk of hip fracture in selected patients but compliance is often poor.

Drug treatment

Several drugs have been shown to reduce the risk of osteoporotic fractures in randomised controlled trials (Box 25.79). Their effects on vertebral and non-vertebral fracture are summarised in Box 25.80.

Drug treatment should be considered in patients with BMD T-score values below −2.5 or below −1.5 in corticosteroid-induced osteoporosis because there is evidence that fractures occur at a higher BMD value in steroid users and that drugs prevent fracture in patients with T-scores at this level. Treatment should also be considered in patients with vertebral fractures, irrespective of BMD, unless they resulted from significant trauma.

Bisphosphonates

Bisphosphonates inhibit bone resorption by binding to hydroxyapatite crystals on the bone surface. When osteoclasts attempt to resorb bone that contains bisphosphonate, the drug is released within the cell, where it inhibits key signalling pathways that are essential for osteoclast function. Although bisphosphonates primarily target the osteoclast, bone formation is also suppressed because of coupling

between bone formation and bone resorption and an inhibitory effect on osteoblasts. However, the balance of effect on bone turnover is favourable, resulting in a gain in bone density due partly to increased mineralisation of bone. Bisphosphonate treatment typically leads to an increase in spine BMD of about 5–8% and hip BMD of 2–4% during the first 3 years of treatment and plateaus thereafter.

Alendronate is the bisphosphonate used most frequently. It reduces risk of vertebral fractures by 40%

EBM 25.79 Effective drug treatments for osteoporosis

'Alendronate, strontium ranelate, risedronate, parathyroid hormone zoledronate and denosumab have been shown to reduce the risk of both vertebral and non-vertebral fractures in randomised controlled trials.'

- Black DM, et al. Lancet 1996; 348:1535–1541.
- Reginster JY, et al. J Clin Endocrinol Metab 2005; 90:2816–2822.
- McClung MR, et al. N Engl J Med 2001; 344:333–340.
- Neer RM, et al. N Engl J Med 2001; 344:1434–1441.
- Black DM, et al. N Engl J Med 2007; 356:1809–1822.
- Cummings SR, et al. N Engl J Med 2009; 361:756–765.

25.80 Effects of drugs on the risk of osteoporotic fractures

Drug	Regimen	Vertebral fracture	Non-vertebral fracture
Alendronate	70 mg/week orally	+	+
Risedronate	35 mg/week orally	+	+
Ibandronate	150 mg/month orally 3 mg/3 mths i.v.	+	+/−
Zoledronate	5 mg/12 mths i.v.	+	+
Denosumab	60 mg/6 mths s.c.	+	+
Strontium ranelate	2 g daily orally	+	+
Calcitonin	200 U/day intranasally	+	+/−
HRT	Various preparations	+	+
PTH 1-34	20 µg/day s.c.	+	+
PTH 1-84	100 µg/day s.c.	+	−
Raloxifene	60 mg/day orally	+	−
Calcium/ vitamin D	500 mg calcium and 800 U vitamin D orally	−	+/−

+ effective; − not effective; +/− equivocal results, or efficacy based on post-hoc subgroup analysis of clinical trials.

and non-vertebral fractures by about 25% in postmeno-pausal women with osteoporosis. Risedronate is an alternative with similar efficacy, but may be better toler-ated in patients with a history of gastrointestinal upset. Both drugs are also effective in the treatment of cortico-steroid-induced osteoporosis. They can also be used to treat male osteoporosis but neither has been shown to prevent non-vertebral fractures in men. Ibandronate is sometimes used but the evidence for prevention of non-vertebral fractures is less robust. Zoledronate is effec-tive in the treatment of postmenopausal osteoporosis, corticosteroid-induced osteoporosis and osteoporosis in men. It is also useful for secondary prevention of frac-tures in elderly patients with hip fracture and reduces mortality in this group, being the only treatment that has been shown to modify this. Etidronate is still occasion-ally used and is generally well tolerated but has been largely superseded by the drugs mentioned above.

Oral bisphosphonates are poorly absorbed from the gastrointestinal tract and should be taken on an empty stomach with plain water and no food taken for 30–45 minutes after administration. Upper gastrointestinal upset occurs in about 5% and bisphosphonates should be used with caution in patients with existing gastro-oesoph-ageal reflux disease. They should be avoided in patients with oesophageal stricture or achalasia, since tablets may stick in the oesophagus, causing ulceration and perfo-ration. The most common side-effect with intravenous bisphosphonates is a transient influenza-like illness char-acterised by fever, malaise, anorexia and generalised aches which occurs 24–48 hours after administration. This is self-limiting but can be treated with paracetamol or NSAID if necessary. It predominantly occurs after the first exposure and tolerance develops thereafter. Rare side-effects of bisphosphonates include uveitis, atrial fibrillation (zoledronate), osteonecrosis of the jaw (ONJ) and subtrochanteric fractures. ONJ is characterised by the presence of necrotic bone in the mandible or maxilla, typically occurring after tooth extraction when the socket fails to heal. Most ONJ cases have occurred in cancer patients with coexisting morbidity such as infection and diabetes, who have received high doses of intravenous bisphosphonates; this complication is very rare in patients who are treated with the dose regimes used in osteoporo-sis. None the less, all patients receiving bisphosphonates for any reason should be advised to pay attention to good oral hygiene. Some advise that bisphosphonates should be temporarily stopped in patients undergoing tooth extraction but there is no evidence that this is necessary or alters the occurrence of ONJ. Atypical subtrochan-teric fractures have been described recently in patients who have received long-term bisphosphonates, and it is thought that this might result from over-suppression of normal bone remodelling. In the vast majority of patients with osteoporosis the benefits of bisphosphonate therapy far outweigh the risks, but it is important that treatment is targeted to patients with low BMD who are most likely to benefit.

Calcium and vitamin D

Calcium and vitamin D have limited efficacy in the pre-vention of osteoporotic fractures when given in isolation but are widely used as an adjunct to other treatments, most often as combination preparations containing 500 mg calcium and 800 U vitamin D (e.g. AdCalD3,

25.81 Osteoporosis in old age

- **Bone loss:** due to increased bone turnover, with an age-related defect switch in differentiation of bone marrow stromal cells to form adipocytes as opposed to osteoblasts.
- **Fractures due to osteoporosis:** common cause of morbidity and mortality, although fracture healing is not delayed by age.
- **Recurrent fractures:** those who suffer a fragility fracture are at increased risk of further fracture, so should be investigated for osteoporosis and treated if this is confirmed.
- **Falls:** risk factors for falls (such as visual and neuromuscular impairments) are independent risk factors for hip fracture in elderly women, so intervention to prevent falls is as important as treatment of osteoporosis (p. 170).
- **Intravenous zoledronic acid:** reduces mortality and subsequent fracture in elderly patients who have suffered hip fractures.
- **Calcium and vitamin D:** reduce the risk of fractures in those who are housebound or living in care homes.

Calcichew D3). They are of greatest value in preventing fragility fractures in elderly or institutionalised patients who are at high risk of calcium and vitamin D deficiency (Box 25.81).

Strontium ranelate

Strontium ranelate reduces vertebral fracture risk by about 40% after 3 years and non-vertebral fracture risk by 12%. The mechanism of action is poorly understood. It has a weak inhibitory effect on bone resorption, stimu-lates biochemical markers of bone formation and is incorporated within hydroxyapatite crystals in place of calcium. Large changes in BMD (12%) occur, although this is partly an artefact due to substitution of heavier strontium atoms for calcium atoms in bone mineral. The most common adverse effect is diarrhoea. There is also a slight increased risk of venous thromboembolism (VTE) for reasons that are unclear. Rarely, a severe rash occurs, and this is an indication to stop treatment.

Parathyroid hormone

PTH is an anabolic agent that works by stimulating new bone formation. The most widely used preparation is the 1-34 fragment of PTH given by single daily subcuta-neous injection of 20 μg. Teriparatide increases BMD by 10% or more in osteoporotic subjects and reduces risk of vertebral fractures by about 65% and non-vertebral fractures by 50%. It is also effective in corticosteroid-induced osteoporosis and appears superior to alen-dronate in terms of BMD gain and vertebral fracture reduction. It is also effective in male osteoporosis. PTH is expensive and is usually reserved for patients with severe osteoporosis (BMD T-score of −3.5 to −4.0 or below) and those who have failed to respond ade-quately to other treatments. The recommended duration of treatment is 24 months, after which patients should receive an anti-resorptive drug, such as a bisphospho-nate, to maintain the increase in BMD. Teriparatide should not be administered at the same time as bisphos-phonates, as this blunts the anabolic effect. In patients who are being treated with teriparatide because of fail-ure to respond, existing treatment is stopped. The 1-84 fragment of PTH acts in a similar way to teriparatide but the evidence for prevention of non-vertebral fracture is less robust than for 1-34 PTH.

Calcitonin

This osteoclast inhibitor is occasionally used for treatment of postmenopausal osteoporosis. Its efficacy in preventing fractures is less robust than that of the drugs described above. Calcitonin may have analgesic properties and it is therefore sometimes used in the short to medium term in patients with acute vertebral fracture. It can be given by subcutaneous or intramuscular injection (100–200 U daily) or by intranasal spray (200 U daily).

Hormone replacement therapy (HRT), raloxifene and tibolone

Cyclical HRT with oestrogen and progestogen prevents postmenopausal bone loss and reduces the risk of vertebral and non-vertebral fractures in postmenopausal women. It is primarily indicated for the prevention of osteoporosis in women with an early menopause (p. 757) and for treatment of women with osteoporosis in their early fifties who have troublesome menopausal symptoms. HRT should be avoided in older women with established osteoporosis because it significantly increases the risk of breast cancer and cardiovascular disease. Raloxifene acts as a partial agonist at oestrogen receptors in bone and liver but as an antagonist in breast and endometrium, and is classified as a selective oestrogen receptor modulator (SERM). It results in a modest increase in BMD (2%) and a 40% reduction in vertebral fractures, but does not influence the risk of non-vertebral fracture and can provoke muscle cramps and worsen hot flushes. It increases the risk of VTE to a similar extent as HRT but reduces the risk of breast cancer; it does not influence the risk of cardiovascular disease. Bazedoxifene is a related SERM which has similar effects to raloxifene. Tibolone is a steroid which has partial agonist activity at oestrogen, progestogen and androgen receptors. It has similar effects on BMD as raloxifene and has been found to prevent vertebral and non-vertebral fractures in postmenopausal osteoporosis. Treatment is associated with a slightly increased risk of stroke but a reduced risk of breast cancer.

Other drugs

Calcitriol ($1,25(OH)_2D_3$), the active metabolite of vitamin D, is licensed for treatment of osteoporosis, but it is seldom used since the data on fracture prevention are less robust than for other agents.

Denosumab is a monoclonal antibody which inhibits RANKL (see Fig. 25.2, p. 1058) and is a powerful inhibitor of bone resorption. It has recently been approved for the treatment of osteoporosis, with effects similar to those of zoledronate, and is given by subcutaneous injection every 6 months.

Surgery, kyphoplasty and vertebroplasty

Surgery is frequently required to reduce and immobilise osteoporotic fractures. Patients with intracapsular fracture of the femoral neck generally require partial or total hip replacement in view of the high risk of avascular necrosis. Kyphoplasty is used in the treatment of acute vertebral compression fractures where there is a significant degree of vertebral collapse and severe pain. It involves introducing a needle into the affected vertebral body and inflating a balloon filled with methyl methacrylate cement in an attempt to restore vertebral shape. The procedure often relieves pain, but potential adverse effects include spinal cord compression, fat embolus and triggering of vertebral fractures on either side of the injected vertebra. Vertebroplasty is similar but the injection is with cement alone and no attempt is made to restore vertebral shape. It is indicated for painful vertebral fractures which fail to settle with medical management.

Duration of treatment and monitoring response

For established osteoporosis, treatment is generally given long-term. Exceptions are teriparatide and 1-84 PTH, for which the course of treatment lasts for 24 months.

The response to drug treatment can be assessed by repeating BMD measurements after 2–3 years. However, changes in BMD do not predict anti-fracture efficacy well and there is little evidence that monitoring by BMD or markers improves adherence. It may, however, reassure the patient that the treatment is working. Since the precision of spine BMD (approximately 1%) is better than hip (approximately 2.5%), spine BMD is best for monitoring. To be sure that a change has occurred in a patient, about twice the precision (i.e. 2% for spine, 5% for hip) is required. Biochemical markers of bone turnover, such as NTX (p. 1064), respond more quickly than BMD and can be used to assess adherence, but the correlation with anti-fracture efficacy is modest. Treatment response can also be established by measuring change in height to assess progression of vertebral osteoporosis and documenting the occurrence of clinical fractures. However, a fracture during drug therapy does not necessarily indicate treatment failure, as even the most effective interventions only reduce fracture risk by 25–50%. A pragmatic approach is to restrict repeat BMD measurements to patients who have suffered a fracture on treatment, and to consider changing to another agent if there is evidence of bone loss, assuming that the patient has been complying with therapy.

Osteomalacia and rickets

These conditions are characterised by defective mineralisation of bone due to vitamin D deficiency, resistance to the effects of vitamin D or hypophosphataemia. Osteomalacia describes a syndrome in adults of defective bone mineralisation, bone pain, increased bone fragility and fractures. Rickets is the equivalent syndrome in children and is characterised by enlargement of the growth plate and bone deformity. The disease remains prevalent in frail older people who have a poor diet and limited sunlight exposure, and in some Muslim women who live in northern latitudes. There are four main causes of osteomalacia and rickets (Box 25.82).

Vitamin D deficiency

The most common cause is lack of sunlight exposure since maintenance of normal levels of vitamin D depends on UV sunlight exposure to catalyse synthesis of cholecalciferol from 7-dehydrocholesterol in the skin (p. 764). Dietary deficiency can also play a role, but vitamin D occurs in only small quantities in most foods,

25.82 Causes of osteomalacia and rickets

Cause	Predisposing factor	Mechanism
Vitamin D deficiency		
Classical	Lack of sunlight exposure and poor diet	Reduced cholecalciferol synthesis in the skin/low levels of vitamin D in diet
Gastrointestinal disease	Malabsorption	Malabsorption of dietary vitamin D and calcium
Failure of 1,25 vitamin D synthesis		
Chronic renal failure	Hyperphosphataemia and kidney damage	Impaired conversion of $25(OH)D_3$ to $1,25(OH)_2D_3$
Vitamin D-resistant rickets type I (autosomal recessive)	Mutation in renal 25(OH)D-1-alpha-hydroxylase enzyme	Impaired conversion of $25(OH)D_3$ to $1,25(OH)_2D_3$
Vitamin D receptor defects		
Vitamin D-resistant rickets type II (autosomal recessive)	Inactivating mutations in vitamin D receptor	Impaired response to $1,25(OH)_2D_3$
Defects in phosphate and pyrophosphate metabolism		
Hypophosphataemic rickets (X-linked dominant)	Mutations in *PHEX* gene	FGF23 not degraded normally
Autosomal dominant hypophosphataemic rickets	Mutation in *FGF23*	Mutant FGF23 is resistant to degradation
Autosomal recessive hypophosphataemic rickets	*DMP1* mutation	Increased expression of FGF23 by osteocytes and local effect of DMP1 deficiency on mineralisation
Tumour-induced hypophosphataemic osteomalacia	Ectopic production of FGF23 by tumour	Over-production of FGF23
Hypophosphatasia	Mutations in bone-specific alkaline phosphatase	Inhibition of bone mineralisation due to accumulation of pyrophosphate in bone
Iatrogenic and other		
Bisphosphonate therapy	High-dose etidronate/pamidronate	Drug-induced impairment of mineralisation
Aluminium	Use of aluminium-containing phosphate binders or aluminium in dialysis fluids	Aluminium-induced impairment of mineralisation
Fluoride	High fluoride in water	Fluoride inhibits mineralisation

except oily fish, so the amount present in average diets is insufficient to meet requirements. Lack of cholecalciferol results in reduced hepatic production of $25(OH)D_3$ and thus reduced renal production of the biologically active metabolite $1,25(OH)_2D_3$. The lack of $1,25(OH)_2D_3$ impairs intestinal calcium absorption and lowers serum calcium, which stimulates PTH secretion. This causes phosphate wasting and increased bone resorption in an attempt to maintain serum calcium levels within the normal range, causing progressive demineralisation of bone.

Clinical features

Vitamin D deficiency in children causes delayed development, muscle hypotonia, craniotabes (small unossified areas in membranous bones of the skull that yield to finger pressure with a cracking feeling), bossing of the frontal and parietal bones and delayed anterior fontanelle closure, enlargement of epiphyses at the lower end of the radius, and swelling of the rib costochondral junctions ('rickety rosary'). Osteomalacia in adults presents insidiously. Mild osteomalacia can be asymptomatic or present with fractures and mimic osteoporosis. More severe osteomalacia presents with muscle and bone pain, general malaise and fragility fractures. Proximal muscle weakness is prominent and the patient may walk with a waddling gait and struggle to climb stairs or get out of a chair. There may be bone and muscle tenderness on pressure and focal bone pain can occur due to fissure fractures of the ribs and pelvis.

Investigations

The diagnosis can usually be made on a routine biochemical screen with measurement of serum 25(OH)D and PTH. Typically, serum alkaline phosphatase levels are raised, 25(OH)D levels are low or undetectable, and PTH is elevated. Serum calcium and phosphate levels may also be low but normal values do not exclude the diagnosis. X-rays are normal until advanced disease, when focal radiolucent areas (pseudofractures or Looser's zones) may be seen in ribs, pelvis and long bones (Fig. 25.49A). Radiographic osteopenia is common and the presence of vertebral crush fractures may cause confusion with osteoporosis. In children, there is thickening and widening of the epiphyseal plate. Radionuclide bone scan can show multiple hot spots in the ribs and pelvis at the site of fractures and the appearance may be mistaken for metastases. Where there is doubt, the diagnosis can be confirmed by bone biopsy, which shows the pathognomonic features of increased thickness and extent of osteoid seams (Fig. 25.49B).

Management

Osteomalacia and rickets respond promptly to treatment with ergocalciferol (250–1000 µg daily), showing rapid clinical improvement, an elevation in 25(OH)D and a reduction in PTH. Serum alkaline phosphatase levels sometimes rise initially as mineralisation of bone increases, but eventually fall to within the normal range as the bone disease heals. After 3–4 months, treatment

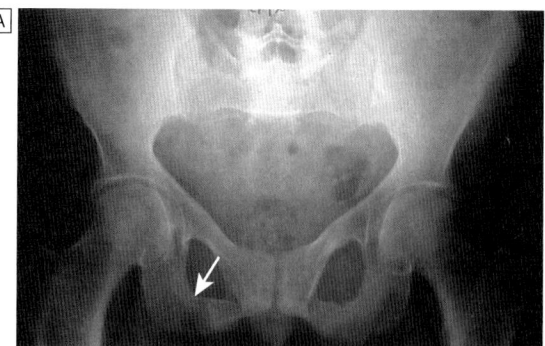

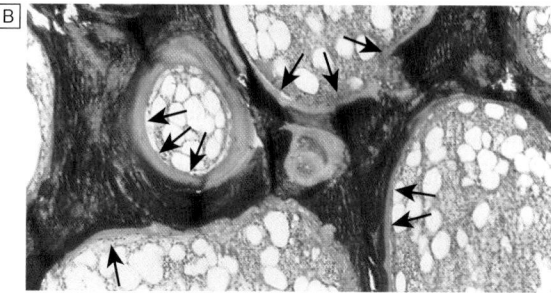

Fig. 25.49 Osteomalacia. [A] X-ray of the pelvis showing Looser's zones (arrow). [B] Photomicrograph of bone biopsy from osteomalacic patient showing thick osteoid seams (stained light blue) which cover almost all of the bone surface. Calcified bone is stained dark blue.

can generally be stopped or the dose of vitamin D reduced to a maintenance level of 10–20 µg cholecalciferol daily, except in patients with underlying disease such as malabsorption, in whom higher doses may be required.

Vitamin D-resistant rickets (VDRR)

This term describes osteomalacia and rickets caused by:

- inactivating mutations in the 25-hydroxyvitamin D-1-alpha-hydroxylase (*CYP27B1*) enzyme which converts 25(OH)D to the active metabolite $1,25(OH)_2D_3$ (type I VDRR)
- inactivating mutations in the vitamin D receptor which impair its ability to activate transcription (type II VDRR).

Clinical features are similar to those of infantile rickets and the diagnosis is usually first suspected when the patient fails to respond to vitamin D supplementation. Since both are recessive disorders, consanguinity is common but there may or may not be a positive family history. Biochemical features of type I disease are similar to vitamin D deficiency, except that levels of 25(OH)D are normal. In type II disease, 25(OH)D is normal but PTH and $1,25(OH)_2D_3$ values are raised. Type I can be treated with the active vitamin D metabolites, 1-alpha hydroxyvitamin D (1–2 µg daily orally) or 1,25 dihydroxyvitamin D (0.25–1.5 µg daily orally), with or without calcium supplements, depending upon the patient's diet. Type II VDRR is extremely difficult to treat but sometimes responds partially to very high doses of active vitamin D metabolites and calcium and phosphate supplements.

Renal rickets and osteomalacia

Osteomalacia and rickets occur in patients with chronic renal failure due to defects in synthesis of renal $1,25(OH)_2D_3$ or due to over-aggressive treatment with oral phosphate binders. Pathogenesis and management are discussed on page 490.

Hypophosphataemic rickets and osteomalacia

Rickets and osteomalacia can occur as the result of inherited or acquired defects in renal tubular phosphate reabsorption, and rarely in patients with tumours that secrete phosphaturic substances (see Box 25.82).

Pathophysiology

Circulating levels of FGF23 play a critical role in regulating serum phosphate by modulating expression of sodium-dependent phosphate transporters in the kidney which are responsible for renal tubular phosphate reabsorption. Osteocytes are the main source of FGF23 and levels of expression are regulated by the proteins DMP1 and PHEX, which are also produced by osteocytes (see Fig. 25.2, p. 1058). Inherited mutations affecting these proteins are summarised in Box 25.82 and account for most cases of hypophosphataemic rickets. Acquired hypophosphataemic rickets is mostly caused by over-production of FGF23 by tumours.

Clinical features and diagnosis

The hereditary disorders usually present in childhood with rickets. The diagnosis is made on the basis of the early age at onset and presence of hypophosphataemia with renal phosphate wasting in the absence of vitamin D deficiency. Molecular diagnosis can define the causal mutation. Tumour-induced hypophosphataemic osteomalacia presents with severe, rapidly progessive symptoms in patients with no obvious predisposing factor for osteomalacia. Strenuous efforts should be made to identify the underlying, usually occult tumour. This often requires whole-body MRI or CT.

Management

Treatment is with phosphate supplements (1–4 g daily) and active metabolites of vitamin D (1-alpha hydroxyvitamin D 1–2 µg daily or 1,25 dihydroxyvitamin D 0.25–1.5 µg daily) to promote intestinal calcium and phosphate absorption. The aim is to ameliorate symptoms, restore normal growth, maintain serum phosphate levels within the normal range and normalise alkaline phosphatase levels. Levels of calcium, phosphate and alkaline phosphatase, along with renal function, should be monitored. Tumour-induced osteomalacia can be managed in the same way but surgical excision of the tumour is curative.

Hypophosphatasia

Hypophosphatasia is an autosomal recessive disorder caused by inactivating mutations in the alkaline phosphatase gene that impair alkaline phosphatase function, resulting in accumulation of pyrophosphate and inhibition of bone mineralisation. Chondrocalcinosis may also occur. The diagnosis should be suspected in osteomalacic patients with low or undetectable levels of serum alkaline phosphatase but normal levels of calcium,

25

phosphate, PTH and vitamin D metabolites. There is no medical treatment but bone marrow transplantation has been used successfully in severe cases.

Other causes of osteomalacia

These are summarised in Box 25.82. Aluminium intoxication is now rare due to reduced use of aluminium-containing phosphate binders and removal of aluminium from water supplies used in dialysis. If aluminium intoxication is suspected, the diagnosis can be confirmed by demonstration of aluminium at the calcification front in a bone biopsy. Osteomalacia due to bisphosphonates has mostly been described in patients with Paget's disease receiving etidronate and high-dose pamidronate. It is usually asymptomatic and healing occurs when treatment is stopped. Excessive fluoride intake causes osteomalacia due to direct inhibition of mineralisation and is common in parts of the world where there is a high fluoride content in drinking water. The condition reverses when fluoride intake is reduced.

Paget's disease

Paget's disease of bone (PDB) is a common condition characterised by focal areas of increased and disorganised bone remodelling. It mostly affects the axial skeleton, and bones that are commonly affected include the pelvis, femur, tibia, lumbar spine, skull and scapula. It is seldom diagnosed before age 40, but gradually increases in incidence thereafter to affect up to 8% of the UK population by the age of 85. The disease is common in Caucasians from north-west and southern Europe but is rare in Scandinavians, Asians, Chinese and Japanese. These ethnic differences persist after migration, supporting the importance of genetic factors in the aetiology, but the incidence of PDB has fallen in some countries over the past 25 years, suggesting that environmental triggers also play a role.

Pathophysiology

The primary abnormality is increased osteoclastic bone resorption, accompanied by marrow fibrosis, increased vascularity of bone and increased osteoblast activity. Bone in PDB is architecturally abnormal and has reduced mechanical strength. Osteoclasts in PDB are increased in number, are unusually large, and contain characteristic nuclear inclusion bodies. Genetic factors are important and mutations in the *SQSTM1* gene are a common cause of classical PDB. The presence of nuclear inclusion bodies in osteoclasts has fuelled speculation that PDB might be cause by a slow virus infection with measles or distemper but the evidence is conflicting. Biomechanical factors may help determine the pattern of involvement, since PDB often starts at sites of muscle insertions into bone and, in some cases, localises to bones or limbs that have been subjected to repetitive trauma or overuse. Involvement of subchondral bone can compromise the joint and predispose to OA ('Pagetic arthropathy').

Clinical features

The classic presentation is with bone pain, deformity, deafness and pathological fractures, but many patients are asymptomatic and are diagnosed as a result of an abnormal X-ray or blood test performed for another reason. Clinical signs include bone deformity and expansion, increased warmth over affected bones, and pathological fracture. Bone deformity is most evident in weight-bearing bones such as the femur and tibia, but when the skull is affected the patient may complain that hats no longer fit properly due to cranial enlargement. Neurological problems, such as deafness, cranial nerve defects, nerve root pain, spinal cord compression and spinal stenosis, are recognised complications due to enlargement of affected bones and encroachment upon the spinal cord and nerve foraminae. Surprisingly, deafness seldom results from compression of the auditory nerve, but is conductive due to osteosclerosis of the temporal bone. The increased vascularity of Pagetic bone makes operative procedures difficult and, in extreme cases, can precipitate high-output cardiac failure in elderly patients with limited cardiac reserve. Osteosarcoma is a rare but serious complication which presents with subacute onset of increasing pain and swelling of an affected site.

Investigations

The characteristic features are an elevated serum alkaline phosphatase and, on X-ray, bone expansion with alternating areas of radiolucency and osteosclerosis (Fig. 25.50B). Alkaline phosphatase is normal in about 10% of cases, usually because of monostotic involvement. Radionuclide bone scanning is useful to define the presence and extent of disease (Fig. 25.50A). If the bone scan is positive, X-rays should be taken of an affected bone to confirm the diagnosis. Bone biopsy is not usually required but may help in cases of diagnostic uncertainty to exclude osteosclerotic metastases.

Management

The main indication for treatment is bone pain. Patients sometimes have pain due to the increase in bone turnover, but it is more commonly caused by complications such as deformity and coexisting OA. Pain secondary to OA should be managed as described on page 1087. Pain

			Inhibitory effect on bone turnover
Drug	**Route of administration**	**Dose**	
Etidronate	Oral	400 mg daily for 3–6 mths	+
Tiludronate	Oral	400 mg daily for 3–6 mths	++
Risedronate	Oral	30 mg daily for 2 months	+++
Pamidronate	Intravenous	1–3 × 60 mg	+++
Zoledronate	Intravenous	1 × 5 mg	++++
Calcitonin	Subcutaneous	100–200 U 3 times weekly for 2–3 mths	+

25.83 Medical management of Paget's disease

+ moderately effective; ++ effective; +++ highly effective; ++++ extremely effective

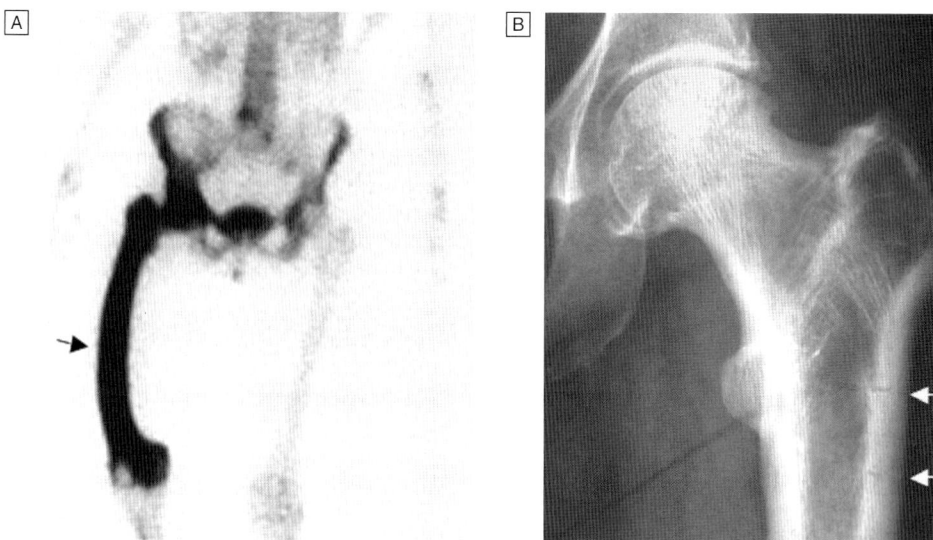

Fig. 25.50 Paget's disease. **A** Isotope bone scan from a patient with Paget's disease, illustrating the intense tracer uptake and deformity of the affected femur. **B** The typical radiographic features with expansion of the femur, alternating areas of osteosclerosis and radiolucency of the trochanter, and pseudofractures breaching the bone cortex (arrows).

due to increased bone turnover can be treated either by administration of analgesics and NSAIDs or by bisphosphonates (Box 25.83). The aminobisphosphonates pamidronate, zoledronate and risedronate are more effective than simple bisphosphonates such as etidronate and tiludronate at suppressing bone turnover in PDB, but their effects on pain are similar. Calcitonin can be used as an alternative but is less convenient to administer and more expensive. Repeated courses of bisphosphonates or calcitonin can be given if symptoms recur. The role of bisphosphonates in preventing complications is unclear, and no benefit has been demonstrated from 'intensive' bisphosphonate therapy aimed at suppressing bone turnover as compared with symptomatic treatment.

Primary tumours of the musculoskeletal system

Primary MSK tumours are rare, have a peak incidence in childhood and adolescence, and can be benign or malignant (Box 25.84). PDB accounts for most cases of osteosarcoma occurring above the age of 40. Presentation is with local pain, swelling and tenderness. Rapid growth and overlying erythema suggest malignancy. In the case of bone tumours, X-rays may show expansion of the bone with a surrounding soft tissue mass, often containing islands of calcification, but further evaluation by MRI or CT is necessary to determine the extent of tumour. The diagnosis can be confirmed by biopsy but this should be done after referral to a specialist team. Treatment depends on histological type but generally involves surgical removal of the tumour followed by chemotherapy and radiotherapy. The prognosis is excellent with benign tumours and also generally good in cases that present in childhood and adolescence. The prognosis is poor in elderly patients with osteosarcoma related to PDB.

Metastatic bone disease

This may present in a variety of ways with localised or generalised progressive bone pain, generalised regional pain, symptoms of spinal cord compression, or acute pain due to pathological fracture. Systemic features, such as weight loss and anorexia, and symptoms referable to the primary tumour are often present. Tumours which most commonly metastasise to bone are myeloma and tumours of the bronchus, breast, prostate, kidney and thyroid. Management is discussed in Chapter 11.

Other bone diseases

Reflex sympathetic dystrophy

Reflex sympathetic dystrophy (RSD) or algodystrophy presents with gradual onset of severe pain, swelling and local tenderness, usually affecting a limb extremity. It is characterised by localised osteoporosis of the affected limb and evidence of regional autonomic dysfunction, such as abnormal sweating, colour and temperature change. It is commonly triggered by fracture, occurring in up to 25% of patients with Colles' fracture. It can also associate with

25.84 Primary tumours of the musculoskeletal system		
Cell type	**Benign**	**Malignant**
Osteoblast	Osteoid osteoma	Osteosarcoma
Chondrocyte	Chondroma Osteochondroma	Chondrosarcoma
Fibroblast	Fibroma	Fibrosarcoma
Bone marrow cell	Eosinophilic granuloma	Ewing's sarcoma
Endothelial cell	Haemangioma	Angiosarcoma
Osteoclast precursor	Giant cell tumour	Malignant giant cell tumour

25

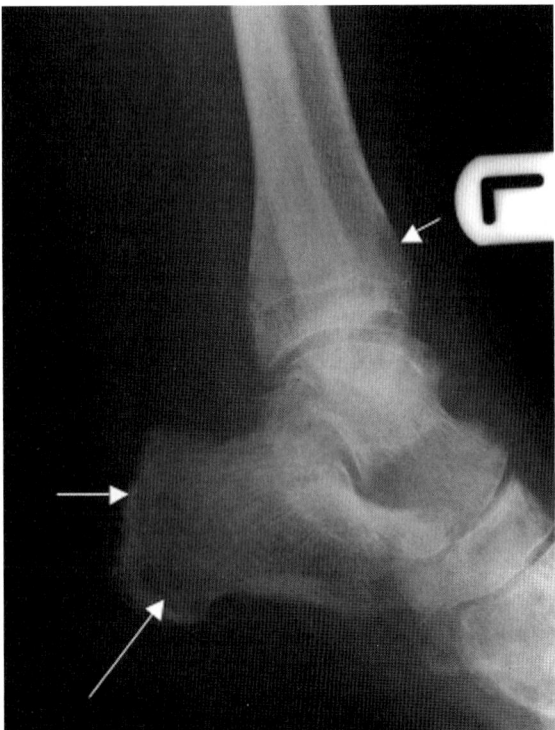

Fig. 25.51 Lateral X-ray of the foot in a patient with reflex sympathetic dystrophy. There is generalised osteopenia and also some more focal areas of patchy osteolysis (arrows).

soft tissue injury, pregnancy and intercurrent illness, or can develop spontaneously. The cause is unknown but overactivity of the sympathetic nervous system is thought to be responsible for many of its features.

The diagnosis is clinical but supported by patchy osteoporosis of the affected region on X-ray, by a local increase in isotope uptake on bone scanning (see Fig. 25.8A, p. 1062) and by bone marrow 'oedema' on MRI. The differential diagnosis includes infection, inflammation and malignancy. Usually, RSD is distinguished from infection and inflammation by the absence of an APR and lack of synovitis. The X-ray appearances in RSD are also distinct from those of focal osteolytic malignant lesions (Fig. 25.51), but in doubtful cases biopsy of the affected site can be undertaken. This usually shows non-specific changes and osteopenia.

Management is difficult but analgesics, NSAIDs, amitriptyline, gabapentin, calcitonin, corticosteroids, β-adrenoceptor antagonists (β-blockers), sympathectomy and bisphosphonates can all be tried. Typically, patients end up on a combination of these, as none is particularly effective. Although some cases resolve with time, many have persistent symptoms and fail to regain normal function.

Polyostotic fibrous dysplasia

This is an acquired disorder due to mutations in the GNAS1 gene, characterised by focal or multifocal bone pain, bone deformity and expansion, and pathological fractures. Associated features include endocrine dysfunction, especially precocious puberty, and café-au-lait skin pigmentation (McCune–Albright syndrome). The diagnosis is made by skeletal imaging, which shows

focal, predominantly osteolytic lesions and bone expansion on X-ray, and focal increased uptake on bone scan. The condition can resemble PDB but the earlier age of onset and pattern of involvement are usually distinctive. Management is symptomatic. Surgery is sometimes required for treatment of fracture and deformity. Very rarely, malignant change can occur and should be suspected by a sudden increase in pain and swelling. There is limited evidence that intravenous pamidronate may help bone pain and promote healing of lytic lesions.

Rare inherited disorders of bone

Osteogenesis imperfecta (OI)

This condition usually presents with severe osteoporosis and multiple fractures in infancy and childhood. Other common features include blue sclerae and abnormal dentition. Most cases are due to mutations in the COL1A1 and COL1A2 genes which encode the proteins that constitute type I collagen, resulting in reduced collagen production or formation of abnormal collagen chains that are rapidly degraded. Most cases of OI show dominant inheritance but recessive forms of OI have been described which are caused by mutations in the CRTAP and LEPRE genes which are involved in proline hydroxylation of collagen. Some have no family history and result from new mutations. Severity varies from neonatal lethal (type II), through very severe with multiple fractures in infancy and childhood (types III and IV), to mild (type I) which is classically accompanied by blue sclerae and less marked bone deformity. Severe OI is usually diagnosed clinically, but in milder cases osteoporosis enters the differential diagnosis. In these cases, mutation screening of COLIA1 and COLIA2 can be helpful but molecular testing is not widely available. Treatment is multidisciplinary, involving surgical reduction and fixation of fractures and correction of limb deformities, and physiotherapy and occupational therapy for rehabilitation of patients with bone deformity. Bisphosphonates are widely used but there is limited evidence that they prevent fractures or deformity.

Osteopetrosis

Osteopetrosis is the name given to a rare group of inherited diseases caused by failure of osteoclast function. Presentation is highly variable, ranging from a lethal disorder that presents with bone marrow failure in infancy to a milder and sometimes asymptomatic form that presents in adulthood. Severe osteopetrosis is inherited in an autosomal recessive manner and presents with failure to thrive, delayed dentition, cranial nerve palsies (due to absent cranial foramina), blindness, anaemia and recurrent infections due to bone marrow failure. The adult-onset type (Albers–Shonberg disease) shows autosomal dominant inheritance and presents with bone pain, cranial nerve palsies, osteomyelitis, OA or fracture, or is sometimes detected as an incidental radiographic finding. The responsible mutations either affect the genes that regulate osteoclast differentiation (RANK, RANKL), causing 'osteoclast-poor' osteopetrosis, or affect the genes involved in bone resorption, causing 'osteoclast-rich' osteopetrosis. These include mutations in the TCIRG1 gene which encodes a component of the osteoclast proton pump, and mutations in the CLCN7 gene which encodes the osteoclast chloride pump. Management is difficult. IFN-γ treatment can improve blood counts and reduce frequency of infections, but in severe cases bone marrow transplantation is required to provide a source of osteoclasts that resorb bone normally.

Sclerosing bone dysplasias

These constitute a rare heterogeneous group of diseases characterised by osteosclerosis due to increased bone formation.

Van Buchem's disease and sclerosteosis are recessive disorders caused by mutations of the *SOST* gene which normally suppresses bone formation. This is characterised by enlargement of the cranium and jaw, tall stature and cranial nerve palsies. Treatment is symptomatic.

Camurati–Engelmann disease is an autosomal dominant condition caused by activating mutations in the *TGFB1* gene, characterised by bone pain, muscle weakness and osteosclerosis mainly affecting the diaphysis of long bones. Corticosteroid treatment can help the bone pain but required doses are often unacceptably high.

High bone mass syndrome is characterised by unusually high bone density. Most patients are asymptomatic but bone overgrowth in the palate can occur. Treatment is not usually required.

MUSCULOSKELETAL PRESENTATIONS OF DISEASE IN OTHER SYSTEMS

Many systemic diseases can cause symptoms and signs in the MSK system and sometimes this may be the presentation of the disease. Furthermore, drugs used for other systemic disease may result in MSK complications

25.85 Drug-induced effects on the musculoskeletal system

Musculoskeletal problem	Principal drug
Secondary gout	Thiazides, furosemide, alcohol
Osteoporosis	Corticosteroids, heparin, glitazones, aromatase inhibitors, GnRH agonists
Osteomalacia	Anticonvulsants, etidronate and pamidronate (high-dose)
Osteonecrosis	Corticosteroids, alcohol
Drug-induced lupus syndrome	Procainamide, hydralazine, isoniazid, chlorpromazine
Arthralgias or arthritis	Corticosteroid withdrawal, glibenclamide, methyldopa, ciclosporin, isoniazid, barbiturates
Myalgias	Corticosteroid withdrawal, L-tryptophan, fibrates, statins
Myopathy	Corticosteroid, chloroquine
Myositis, myasthenia	Penicillamine, statins
Cramps	Corticosteroid, adrenocorticotrophic hormone (ACTH), diuretics, carbenoxolone
Vasculitis	Amphetamines, thiazides

25.86 Rheumatological manifestations of malignancy

- Polyarthritis
- Dermatomyositis/polymyositis
- Hypophosphataemic osteomalacia
- Hypertrophic osteoarthropathy
- Bone metastases, pathological fracture
- Polymyalgia rheumatica syndrome

(Box 25.85). The following examples illustrate the variety of conditions that may be encountered but the list is not exhaustive. Bone disease in sarcoidosis is described on page 709, in haemophilia on page 1047 and sickle cell anaemia on page 1028.

Malignant disease

MSK manifestations of malignancy are summarised in Box 25.86. An unusual but striking presentation is with hypertrophic osteoarthropathy, which is characterised by clubbing and painful swelling of the limbs, periosteal new bone formation and arthralgia/arthritis. The most common causes are bronchial carcinoma and mesothelioma (p. 729), but the condition can be inherited; in this case, it is caused by inactivating mutations in the *HPGD* gene, which is responsible for degradation of PGE$_2$, suggesting that over-production of prostaglandins may generally play a causal role in clubbing. Bone scans show increased periosteal uptake before new bone is apparent on X-ray. The course follows that of the underlying malignancy and resolves if this is cured.

Endocrine disease

Hypothyroidism (p. 741) may present with carpal tunnel syndrome, or rarely with severely painful, symmetrical proximal myopathy with muscle hypertrophy. Both resolve with thyroxine replacement. Hyperparathyroidism (p. 766) predisposes to chondrocalcinosis and pseudogout and to calcific periarthritis, especially in patients with renal disease.

Diabetes mellitus (Ch. 21) commonly causes diabetic 'stiff hands' (cheiroarthropathy) characterised by tightening of skin and periarticular structures, giving flexion deformities of the fingers which are sometimes painful. Diabetic osteopathy presents as forefoot pain and shows radiographic progression from osteopenia to complete osteolysis of the phalanges and metatarsals. Diabetes also predisposes to 'frozen shoulder', Dupuytren's contracture, septic arthritis and neuropathic joints.

Acromegaly (p. 790) can be associated with mechanical back pain, with normal or excessive (not restricted) movement; carpal tunnel syndrome; Raynaud's syndrome; and an arthropathy (50%). The arthropathy mainly affects the large joints and has clinical similarities to OA but with normal or increased movement. X-rays may show widening of joint spaces, squaring of bone ends, generalised osteopenia and tufting of terminal phalanges. It does not improve with treatment of the acromegaly.

Metabolic disease

Approximately 50% of people with haemochromatosis (p. 959) develop an arthropathy, usually between the age of 40 and 50, which may predate other features of the disease. It predominantly affects the small joints of the hands and wrists but hips, shoulders and knees are also commonly affected. X-ray changes resemble OA but cysts are often multiple and prominent, with little osteophyte formation, and atypical sites are targeted (radiocarpal joint, MCP joints). About 30% have pseudogout and radiographic chondrocalcinosis as additional diagnostic clues. Treatment of the haemochromatosis does not influence the arthropathy.

Neuropathic (Charcot) joints

Neurological disease may result in rapidly destructive arthritis of joints, first described by Charcot in association with syphilis. Although repetitive microtrauma following sensory loss was thought to be the cause, the more likely pathogenesis is altered blood flow secondary to impaired sympathetic nervous system control. The following are the principal predisposing diseases and sites of involvement:

- diabetic neuropathy (hindfoot)
- syringomyelia (shoulder, elbow, wrist)
- leprosy (hands, feet)
- tabes dorsalis (knees, spine).

The presentation is with subacute or insidious monoarthritis or dislocation. Pain can occur, especially at the onset, but once the joint is severely deranged, pain is often minimal and signs become disproportionately greater than symptoms. The joint is often grossly swollen, with effusion, crepitus, marked instability and deformity, though usually no increased warmth. It may eventually become flail and be complicated by peripheral nerve entrapment or spinal cord compression. X-rays show disorganisation of normal joint architecture and often multiple loose bodies (Fig. 25.52), and either no (atrophic) or gross (hypertrophic) new bone formation. Management principally involves orthoses and occasionally arthrodesis.

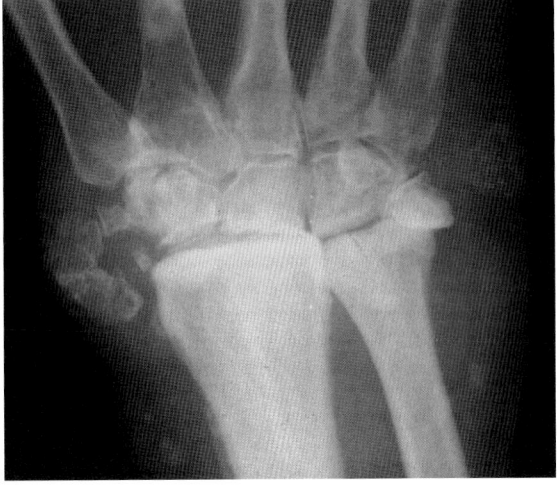

Fig. 25.52 Wrist X-ray showing a neuropathic (Charcot) joint in a patient with syringomyelia. Note the disorganised architecture with complete loss of the proximal carpal row, bony fragments and soft tissue swelling.

MISCELLANEOUS CONDITIONS

Inherited connective tissue diseases

Ehlers–Danlos syndrome is characterised by generalised hypermobility, skin laxity and easy bruising, with scoliosis, short stature, ocular fragility and visceral vascular catastrophes. It may result from mutations in several genes, including *COLIA2*, lysyl oxidase, fibronectin and elastin. Marfan's syndrome is described on page 602 and homocystinuria, which may cause osteoporosis, on page 447.

Relapsing polychondritis

Relapsing polychondritis is an idiopathic condition of cartilage that classically presents with acute pain and swelling of one or both ear pinnae, sparing the lower non-cartilaginous portion. Around 30% of patients have coexisting autoimmune or connective tissue disease. In a minority, involvement of tracheobronchial cartilage leads to hoarse voice, cough, stridor or expiratory wheeze. Manifestations at other cartilage sites include collapse of the bridge of the nose, scleritis, hearing loss and cardiac valve dysfunction. Diagnosis is made by ear cartilage biopsy. Pulmonary function tests, including flow volume loops, should be performed to assess the degree of laryngotracheal disease, since this is an important cause of mortality. Mild ear disease usually responds to low-dose steroid or NSAIDs. Major organ involvement requires high-dose steroids in combination with cytotoxic drugs. Rarely, tracheostomy or tracheal stents are required.

Inclusion body myositis

This is the most common muscle disease in patients aged over 50 and predominates in men. Although proximal weakness does occur, distal involvement is more usual and may be asymmetrical. Investigation is the same as for polymyositis (p. 1111). CK may be marginally elevated and both myopathic and neurogenic abnormalities may be present on EMG. The characteristic findings on muscle biopsy are abnormal fibres containing rimmed vacuoles and filamentous inclusions in the nucleus and cytoplasm. These inclusions contain paired helical filaments resembling those seen in the brain in Alzheimer's disease. Treatment is less successful than for polymyositis, but some patients respond to corticosteroids and immunosuppressives.

Mucopolysaccharidoses

This is a group of inborn errors of metabolism in which lysosomal enzyme defects lead to abnormal accumulation of glycosaminoglycans. All are associated with stiff joints and short stature, except for the Morquio syndrome, which is associated with hypermobility and atlanto-axial subluxation. The diagnoses are confirmed by identification of the urinary glycosaminoglycan metabolites and detection of the enzyme defects in fibroblast cultures.

Spondylolysis and spondylolisthesis

Spondylolysis describes a break in the integrity of the neural arch. The principal cause is an acquired defect in pars interarticularis due to a fracture, mainly seen in gymnasts, dancers and runners in whom it is an important cause of back pain. Spondylolisthesis is where a defect causes slippage of a vertebra on the one below. This may be congenital, post-traumatic or degenerative. Rarely, it can result from metastatic destruction of the posterior elements.

Uncomplicated spondylolysis does not cause symptoms but spondylolisthesis can cause low back pain aggravated by standing and walking. More severe cases can result in nerve root compression or a lumbar stenosis syndrome and the vertebral slip is occasionally palpable. Spondylolysis and spondylolisthesis can usually be diagnosed from lateral X-rays of the lumbar spine. MRI may be required if there is nerve root involvement. Advice on posture and muscle-strengthening exercises is required in mild cases. Surgical fusion is indicated for severe and recurrent low back pain, and surgical decompression is mandatory prior to fusion in patients with significant lumbar stenosis or symptoms of cauda equina compression.

Diffuse idiopathic skeletal hyperostosis (DISH)

DISH is a common disorder in old age, affecting 10% of men and 8% of women over the age of 65. It associates with obesity, hypertension and type 2 diabetes mellitus. It is characterised by florid new bone formation along the anterolateral aspect of at least four contiguous vertebral bodies (Fig. 25.53). It is distinguished from lumbar spondylosis by the absence of disc space narrowing and marginal vertebral body sclerosis, and from spondylitis by the absence of sacroiliitis or apophyseal joint fusion. It rarely causes pain and is usually an asymptomatic radiographic finding. Ossifying enthesopathy at peripheral sites may cause pain: for example, under the heel with calcaneal spur formation.

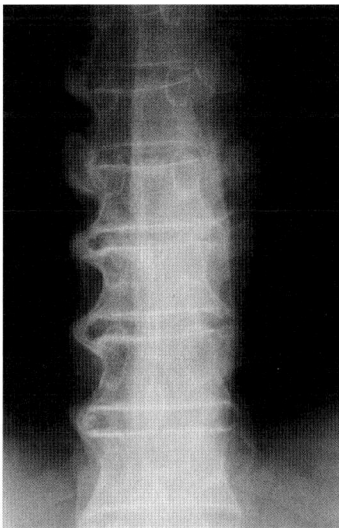

Fig. 25.53 Diffuse idiopathic skeletal hyperostosis (DISH).
Anteroposterior X-ray of thoracic spine showing right-sided flowing new bone joining more than four contiguous vertebrae. The disc spaces are preserved.

Scheuermann's osteochondritis

This disorder predominates in adolescent boys, who develop a painless dorsal kyphosis in association with irregular radiographic ossification of the vertebral end plates. Back pain, aggravated by exercise and relieved by rest, may occur if upper lumbar vertebrae are affected, and secondary spondylosis can follow in middle age. Excessive exercise and heavy manual labour before epiphyseal fusion has occurred may aggravate symptoms. Treatment is avoidance of excessive activity and protective postural exercises. Surgery may be required for severe deformity.

Pigmented villonodular synovitis

Pigmented villondular synovitis (PVNS) is an uncommon proliferative disorder of synovium which typically affects young adults. The presentation is with joint swelling, limitation of movement and pain. The diagnosis can be confirmed by synovial biopsy. Treatment is by surgical or radiation synovectomy.

Adult-onset Still's disease

This is a rare systemic inflammatory disorder of unknown cause typically affecting young adults, which presents with intermittent fever, rash and arthralgia.

Splenomegaly, hepatomegaly and lymphadenopathy may be present. Investigations typically show evidence of an acute phase response, with a markedly elevated serum ferritin. Tests for RF and ANA are negative. Most patients respond to corticosteroids but DMARDs may be required as steroid-sparing agents. Anecdotal reports indicate that anakinra (p. 1081) and anti-TNF therapy may be helpful in patients with resistant disease.

Further information

Journal articles

Brennan FM, McInnes IB. Evidence that cytokines play a role in rheumatoid arthritis. J Clin Invest 2008; 118:3537–3545.

Ralston SH, Langston AL, Reid IR. Pathogenesis and management of Paget's disease of bone. Lancet 2008; 378:155–163.

Zhang W, Doherty M, et al. EULAR recommendations for gout. Part 2: Management. Ann Rheum Dis 2006; 65:1312–1324.

Zhang W, Moskowitz RW, et al. OARSI recommendations for the management of hip and knee osteoarthritis. Part II: OARSI evidence-based, expert consensus guidelines. Osteoarthritis Cart 2008; 16:137–162.

Websites

www.eBandolier.com *Updates on management.*
www.kineret-eu.com/en/pro/pro/prodas.jsp *DAS 28 calculator.*
www.nice.org.uk/Guidance/Topic *Guidelines for management of osteoarthritis, rheumatoid arthritis and other musculoskeletal conditions.*
www.rheumatology.com *Updates on management.*
www.shef.ac.uk/FRAX/ *Fracture risk assessment tool.*
www.shef.ac.uk/NOGG/ *Guidelines for the management of osteoporosis.*

25

C.M.C. Allen
C.J. Lueck
M. Dennis

Neurological disease

26

CLINICAL EXAMINATION OF THE NERVOUS SYSTEM

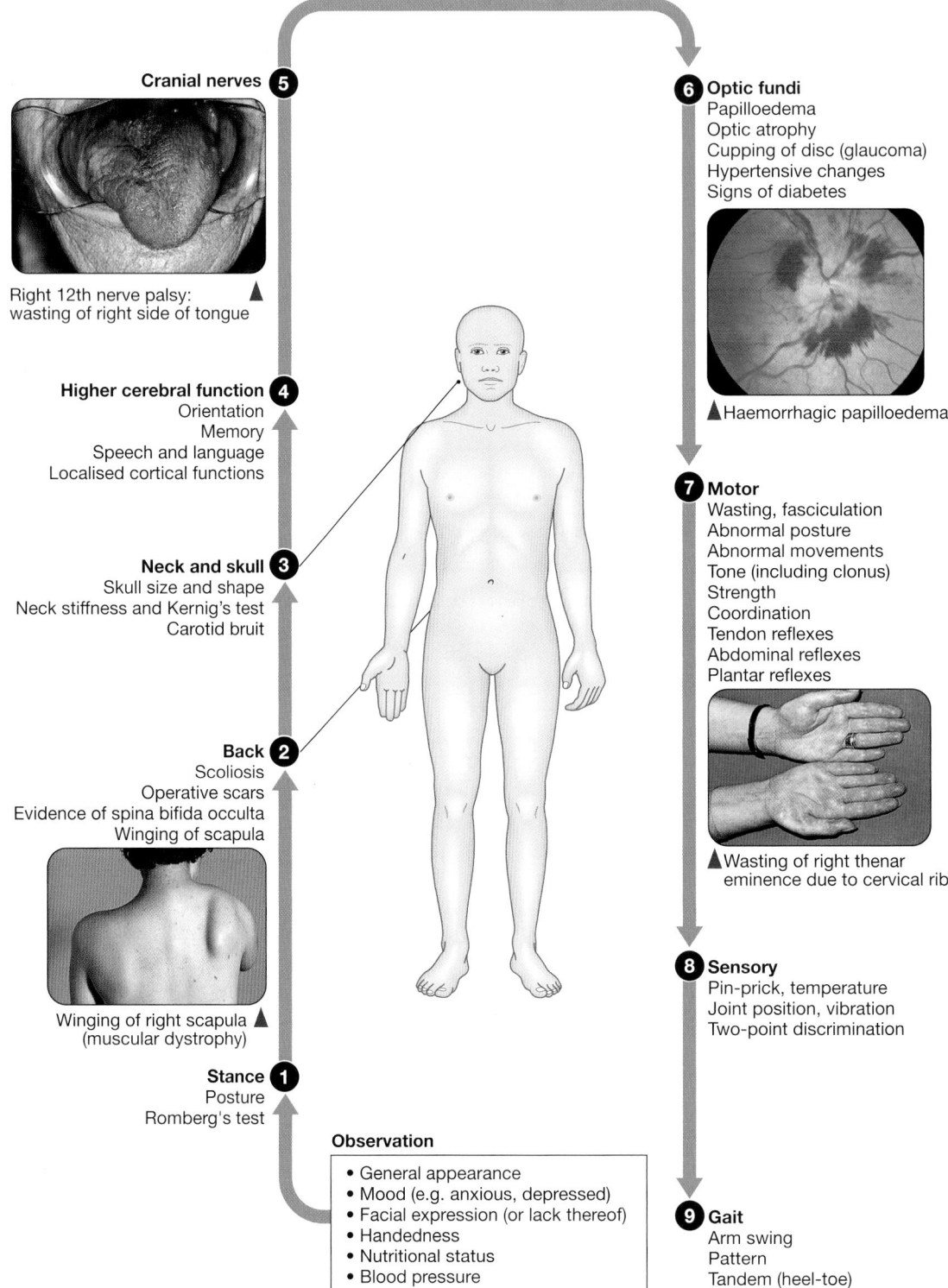

Cranial nerves 5

Right 12th nerve palsy:
wasting of right side of tongue ▲

Higher cerebral function 4
Orientation
Memory
Speech and language
Localised cortical functions

Neck and skull 3
Skull size and shape
Neck stiffness and Kernig's test
Carotid bruit

Back 2
Scoliosis
Operative scars
Evidence of spina bifida occulta
Winging of scapula

Winging of right scapula ▲
(muscular dystrophy)

Stance 1
Posture
Romberg's test

Observation
- General appearance
- Mood (e.g. anxious, depressed)
- Facial expression (or lack thereof)
- Handedness
- Nutritional status
- Blood pressure

6 **Optic fundi**
Papilloedema
Optic atrophy
Cupping of disc (glaucoma)
Hypertensive changes
Signs of diabetes

▲Haemorrhagic papilloedema

7 **Motor**
Wasting, fasciculation
Abnormal posture
Abnormal movements
Tone (including clonus)
Strength
Coordination
Tendon reflexes
Abdominal reflexes
Plantar reflexes

▲Wasting of right thenar
eminence due to cervical rib

8 **Sensory**
Pin-prick, temperature
Joint position, vibration
Two-point discrimination

9 **Gait**
Arm swing
Pattern
Tandem (heel-toe)

4.9 Examination of gait and posture

Step	Procedure	Abnormality	Disease
1	Examine posture	Stooped	Parkinsonism
	Axial tone	Axial tone increased	Parkinsonism (Parkinson's plus syndrome)
	Retropulsion/anteropulsion	Postural instability	Parkinsonism
2	Examine arms during walking	Reduced arm swing	Parkinsonism, upper motor neuron lesion
3	Examine routine walking	Circumduction (stiff leg moves outwards in 'circular' manner)	Upper motor neuron lesion
		'Slapping' due to foot drop	Lower motor neuron lesion
		Narrow-based, short strides	Parkinsonism
		Wide-based, short strides (marche à petits pas, magnetic gait)	Frontal lobe lesion
		Wide-based, irregular strides	Cerebellar lesion
		High-stepping gait	Dorsal column lesion/sensory neuropathy
4	Examine tandem gait	Inability to perform task	Cerebellar lesion, dorsal column lesion
5	Perform Romberg test	Patient falls with eyes shut	Loss of joint position sense at ankles

5 Examination of cranial nerves

Nerve	Name	Tests
I	Olfactory	Ask patient about sense of smell
II	Optic	Visual acuity
		Visual fields
		'Swinging' torch test for relative afferent pupillary defect
		Ophthalmoscopy
III	Oculomotor	Eye movements (nystagmus)
		Eyelid movement
		Pupil size, symmetry, reactions
IV	Trochlear	Eye movements (nystagmus)
V	Trigeminal	Sensation to face
		Corneal reflex
		Jaw movements (deviates on opening to side of lesion)
VI	Abducens	Eye movements (nystagmus)
VII	Facial	Facial symmetry and movements
		Ask patient about taste
VIII	Vestibulocochlear	Hearing (whisper to each ear)
		Tuning fork tests (Rinne and Weber)
		Look for nystagmus
IX	Glossopharyngeal	Gag reflex (sensory)
X	Vagus	Palatal elevation (uvula deviates to side opposite lesion)
		Gag reflex (motor)
		Cough (bovine cough)
XI	Accessory	Look for wasting
		Elevation of shoulders
		Turning head to right and left
XII	Hypoglossal	Look for wasting/fasciculation
		Tongue protrusion (deviates to side of lesion)

7 Root values of tendon reflexes

Reflex	Root value
Upper limb	
Biceps jerk	C5/C6
Supinator jerk	C5/C6
Triceps jerk	C7
Finger jerk	C8
Lower limb	
Knee jerk	L3/L4
Ankle jerk	S1/S2

Neurological examination in old age

- **Limb tone assessment:** often difficult because of increased difficulty in relaxing the limbs and concomitant joint disease.
- **Ankle reflexes:** may be bilaterally absent without diagnostic significance.
- **Gait assessment:** more difficult because of concurrent musculoskeletal disease and pre-existing neurological deficits.
- **Sensory testing:** especially difficult when there is cognitive impairment.
- **Vibration sense:** may be reduced in the lower extremities without diagnostic significance.

The brain, spinal cord and peripheral nerves constitute an organ responsible for perception of the environment, a person's behaviour within it, and the maintenance of the body's internal milieu in readiness for this behaviour. Some 10% of the population in the United Kingdom consult their general practitioner each year with a neurological symptom, and neurological disorders account for about one-fifth of acute medical admissions and a large proportion of chronic physical disability in the UK. However, neurological symptoms are often not associated with disease, and considerable clinical skill is needed to distinguish those with significant disease from those who need sympathetic reassurance.

A carefully taken history of the pattern of presenting neurological symptoms should suggest a short list of diagnoses that can then be tested on examination. During the neurological examination, knowledge of the relevant anatomy and physiology of the nervous system helps to determine the site of the lesion. The underlying pathology is often suggested by the time course of the symptoms and the epidemiological context. Increasingly sophisticated investigations, particularly imaging, are available to refine this clinical diagnosis.

Once the patient's neurological lesion (the deficit) is identified, the clinician needs to assess what impact this has had on the patient's functioning (the disability) and,

in turn, how this is affecting his or her life (the handicap). Even when a complete cure cannot be effected, much can be done to improve the disability by pharmacological correction of the pathophysiology and through rehabilitation (p. 174).

FUNCTIONAL ANATOMY AND PHYSIOLOGY

Cells of the nervous system

The nervous system comprises a complex network of specialised blood vessels, ependymal cells which line the cerebral ventricles, neurons and glial cells, of which there are three types. Astrocytes form the structural framework for neurons and control their biochemical environment. Astrocyte foot processes are intimately associated with blood vessels and form the blood–brain barrier (Fig. 26.1). Oligodendrocytes are responsible for the formation and maintenance of the myelin sheath, which surrounds axons and is essential for the rapid transmission of action potentials by saltatory conduction. Microglial cells are cells of the monocyte/macrophage lineage which play a role in fighting infection and removing damaged cells. Peripheral neurons have axons invested in myelin made by Schwann cells.

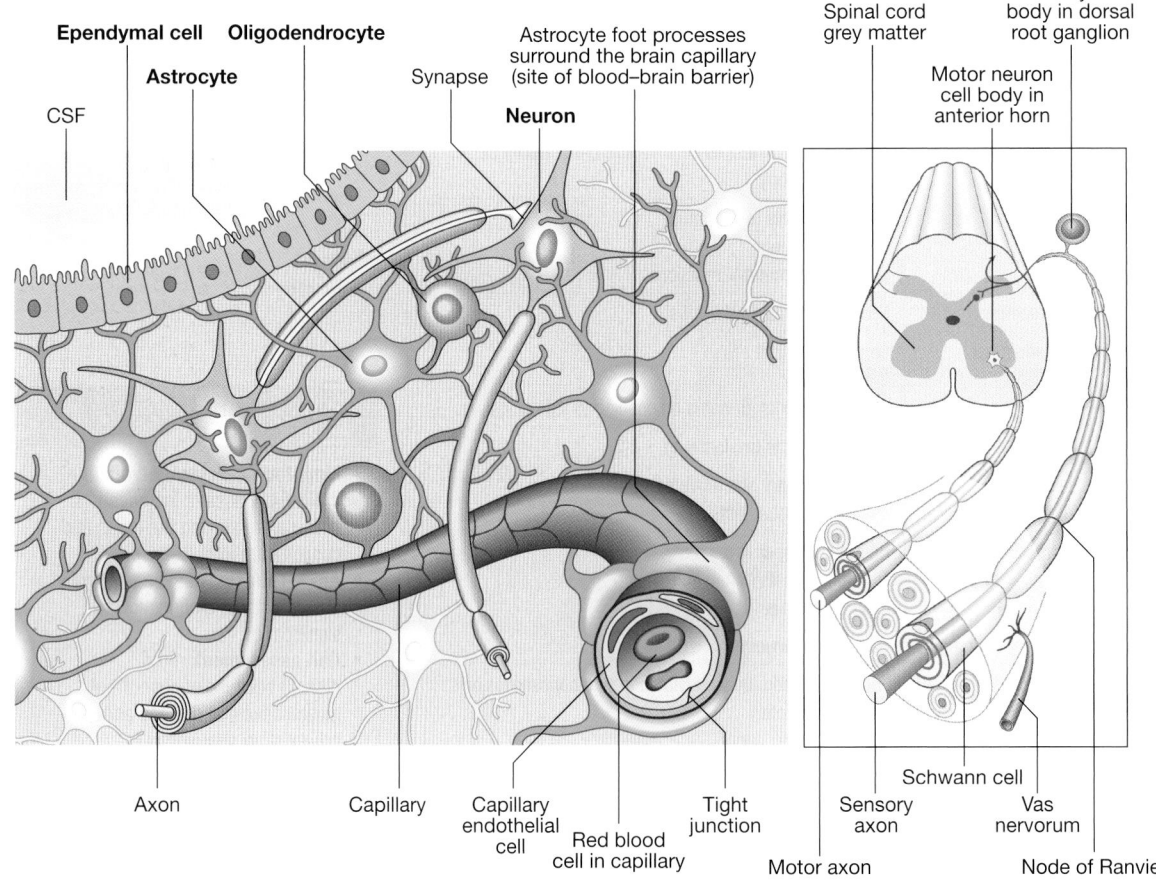

Fig. 26.1 Cells of the nervous system.

Generation and transmission of the nervous impulse

Function of the nervous system rests upon two physiological processes: the generation of an action potential and its conduction down axons, and the synaptic transmission of impulses between neurons and muscle cells. These processes depend upon the energy-demanding maintenance of an electrochemical gradient across neuron cell membranes, and alterations in this are effected by specialised ion channels in the membrane. Synaptic transmission involves the release of neurotransmitters. These modulate function of the target cell by interacting with various molecules on the cell surface, including ion channels and other cell surface receptors (Fig. 26.2). At least 20 different neurotransmitters have been identified which act at different sites in the nervous system, and all are potentially amenable to pharmacological manipulation.

The neuronal cell bodies are acted upon by synapses with large numbers of other neurons. Each neuron therefore acts as a microprocessor, reacting to the influences upon it by changes to its cell membrane potential, causing it to be more or less able to discharge an impulse down its axon(s). The synapsing neuron terminals are also subject to regulation by receptor sites on their pre-synaptic membrane, which modify the release of transmitter across the synaptic cleft. The effect of some neurotransmitters is to produce long-term modulation of metabolic function or gene expression rather than simply to change the membrane potential. This effect probably underlies more complex processes in cognition, such as long-term memory.

Functional anatomy of the nervous system

Major components of the nervous system and their inter-relationships are depicted in Figure 26.3.

Cerebral hemispheres

The cerebral hemispheres coordinate the highest level of nervous function, the anterior half dealing with executive ('doing') functions and the posterior half constructing a perception of the environment ('receiving and perceiving'). Each cerebral hemisphere has four functionally specialised lobes (Fig. 26.4 and Box 26.1). Many of the functions are lateralised and this depends on which of the two hemispheres is 'dominant', i.e. the one in which language function is represented. In right-handed

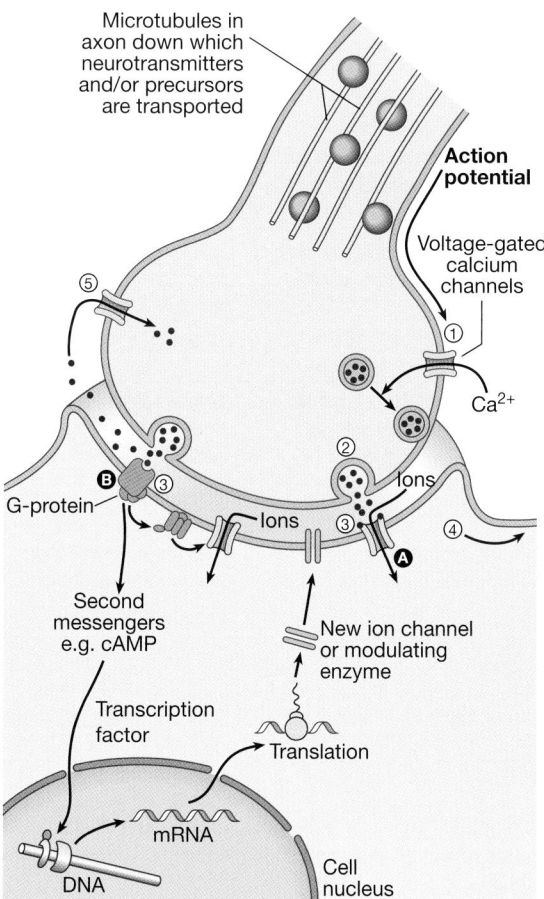

Fig. 26.2 Neurotransmission and neurotransmitters. (1) An action potential arriving at the nerve terminal depolarises the membrane and this opens voltage-gated calcium channels. (2) Entry of calcium causes the fusion of synaptic vesicles containing neurotransmitters with the pre-synaptic membrane and release of the neurotransmitter across the synaptic cleft. (3) The neurotransmitter binds to receptors on the postsynaptic membrane to either (A) open ligand-gated ion channels which, by allowing ion entry, depolarise the membrane and initiate an action potential (4), or (B) bind to metabotrophic receptors which activate an effector enzyme (e.g. adenylyl cyclase) and thus modulate gene transcription via the intracellular second messenger system leading to changes in synthesis of ion channels or modulating enzymes. (5) Neurotransmitters are taken up at the pre-synaptic membrane and/or metabolised.

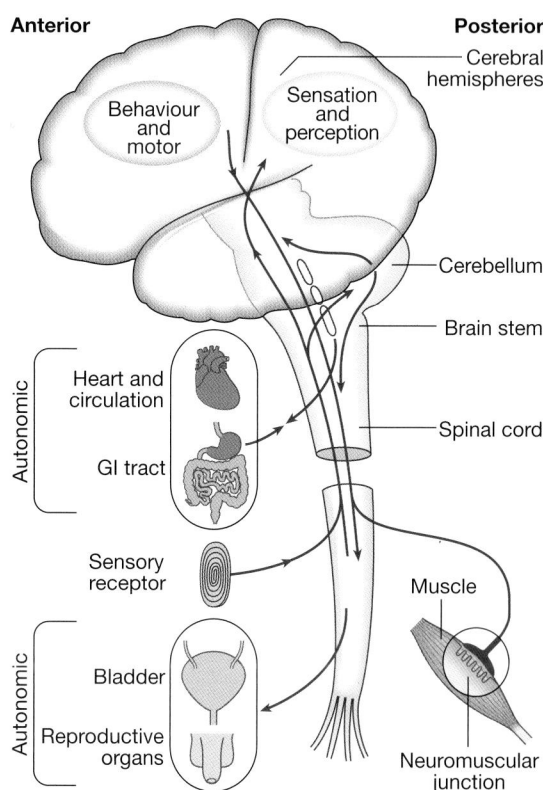

Fig. 26.3 The major anatomical components of the nervous system.

26

26.1 Cortical lobar functions

Lobe	Function	Effects of damage		
		Cognitive/behavioural	Associated physical signs	Positive phenomena
Frontal	Personality Emotional control Social behaviour Contralateral motor control Language Micturition	Disinhibition Lack of initiation Antisocial behaviour Impaired memory Expressive dysphasia Incontinence	Impaired smell Contralateral hemiparesis Frontal release signs[1]	Versive seizures Focal motor seizures (Jacksonian march) Continuous partial seizures (epilepsia partialis continua)
Parietal: dominant	Language Calculation	Dysphasia Dyscalculia Dyslexia Apraxia[4] Agnosia[5]	Contralateral hemisensory loss Astereognosis[2] Agraphaesthesia[3] Contralateral homonymous lower quadrantanopia Asymmetry of optokinetic nystagmus (OKN)	Focal sensory seizures
Parietal: non-dominant	Spatial orientation Constructional skills	Neglect of contralateral side Spatial disorientation Constructional apraxia Dressing apraxia	Contralateral hemisensory loss Astereognosis Agraphaesthesia Contralateral homonymous lower quadrantanopia Asymmetry of OKN	Focal sensory seizures
Temporal: dominant	Auditory perception Language Verbal memory Smell Balance	Receptive aphasia Dyslexia Impaired verbal memory	Contralateral homonymous lower quadrantanopia	Complex hallucinations (smell, sound, vision, memory)
Temporal: non-dominant	Auditory perception Melody/pitch perception Non-verbal memory Smell Balance	Impaired non-verbal memory Impaired musical skills (tonal perception)	Contralateral homonymous upper quadrantanopia	Complex hallucinations (smell, sound, vision, memory)
Occipital	Visual processing	Visual inattention Visual loss Visual agnosia	Homonymous hemianopia (macular sparing)	Simple visual hallucinations (e.g. phosphenes, zigzag lines)

[1] Grasp reflex, palmomental response, rooting reflex.
[2] Inability to determine 3-D shape by touch.
[3] Inability to 'read' numbers or letters drawn on hand, with eyes shut.
[4] Inability to perform complex movements in the presence of normal motor, sensory and cerebellar function.
[5] Inability to recognise or discriminate.

individuals the left hemisphere is almost always dominant, while in left-handers either hemisphere may be dominant with about equal frequency.

The frontal lobes are concerned with executive function, movement and behaviour. In addition to the primary and supplementary motor cortex, there are specialised areas for the control of eye movements, speech (Broca's area) and micturition.

The parietal lobes are concerned with the integration of sensory perception. The primary sensory cortex lies in the post-central gyrus of the parietal lobe. Much of the remainder is devoted to 'association' cortex, which integrates the input from the various sensory modalities. The supramarginal and angular gyri of the dominant parietal lobe form part of the language area (p. 1160). Close to these are regions dealing with numerical function. The non-dominant parietal lobe houses areas concerned with spatial awareness and orientation.

The temporal lobes contain the primary auditory cortex and primary vestibular cortex. On the medial side lie the olfactory cortex and the parahippocampal cortex which is involved in memory function. The temporal lobes also contain many structures associated with the limbic system, including the hippocampus and the amygdala, which are involved in the processing of memory and emotions. The dominant temporal lobe also participates in language functions, particularly verbal comprehension (Wernicke's area). Music processing occurs in both temporal lobes, rhythm being processed on the dominant side and melody/pitch more on the non-dominant side.

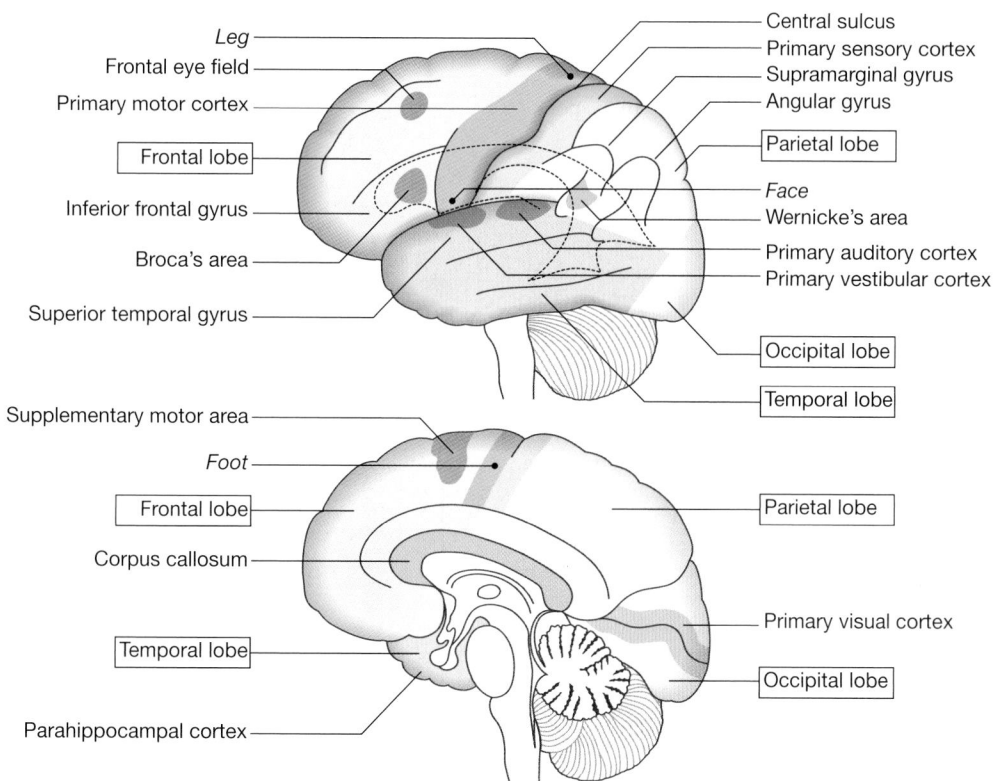

Fig. 26.4 The anatomy of the cerebral cortex.

The occipital lobes are principally concerned with visual processing. The contralateral visual hemifield is represented in the primary visual (striate) cortex, and areas immediately surrounding this are involved in the processing of specific visual submodalities such as colour, movement or depth, and the analysis of more complex visual patterns such as faces.

Collections of cells in the depths of the hemispheres deal with motor control (the basal ganglia), the appropriate attention to sensory perception (the thalamus), emotion and memory (the limbic system), and internal bodily functions such as temperature and appetite control (the hypothalamus). The cerebral ventricles contain the choroid plexus and this produces the cerebrospinal fluid (CSF), which cushions the brain within the cranium. The CSF flows through the third and fourth ventricles and exits the brain through foramina in the brain stem to circulate down and around the spinal cord and over the brain surface where it is reabsorbed into the cerebral venous system (see Fig. 26.51, p. 1220).

The brain stem

In addition to containing all the sensory and motor pathways entering and leaving the hemispheres, the brain stem houses the nuclei of the cranial nerves and nuclei projecting to the cerebrum and cerebellum, as well as other important collections of neurons in the reticular formation (Fig. 26.5). The cranial nerve nuclei provide motor control to muscles of the head (including the face and eyes) and some in the neck, along with coordinating sensory input from the special sense organs and the face, nose, mouth, larynx and pharynx. They also control autonomic functions including pupillary, salivary

and lacrimal functions. The reticular formation is predominantly involved in the control of conjugate eye movements, the maintenance of balance, cardiorespiratory control and the maintenance of arousal.

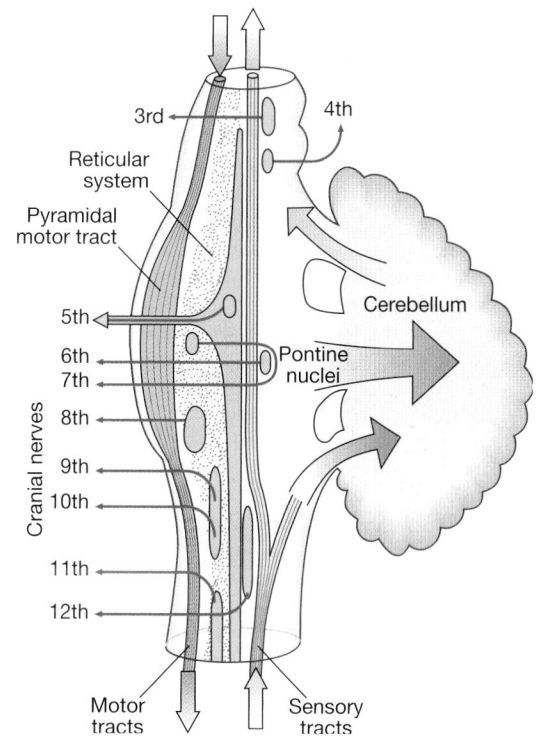

Fig. 26.5 Anatomy of the brain stem.

26

The spinal cord

The spinal cord contains not only the afferent and efferent fibres arranged in functionally discrete bundles but also, in the grey matter, collections of cells which are responsible for lower-order motor reflexes and the primary processing of sensory information, including pain.

The peripheral nervous system

The sensory cell bodies of peripheral nerves are situated in the dorsal root ganglia in the spinal exit foramina, whilst the distal ends of their neurons are invested with various specialised endings for the transduction of external stimuli into nervous impulses. The motor cell bodies are in the anterior horns of the spinal cord. Motor neurons initiate muscle contraction by the release of acetylcholine across the neuromuscular junction, which results in change in potential in the muscle end plate. To increase the speed of impulse conduction, peripheral nerve axons are variably invested in myelin sheaths consisting of the wrapped membranes of Schwann cells. Thus, any peripheral nerve is made up of a combination of large, fast, myelinated axons (which carry information about joint position sense and commands to muscles) and smaller, slower, unmyelinated axons (which carry information about pain and temperature, as well as autonomic function).

The autonomic system

The autonomic system plays a key role in regulating the cardiovascular and respiratory systems, the smooth muscle of the gastrointestinal tract, and many exocrine and endocrine glands throughout the body. The autonomic system is controlled centrally by diffuse modulatory systems in the brain stem, limbic system and frontal lobes, which are concerned with arousal and background behavioural responses to threat. The output of the autonomic system is divided functionally and pharmacologically into two divisions: the parasympathetic and sympathetic systems.

The motor system

A programme of movement formulated by the premotor cortex is converted into a series of signals in the motor cortex which are transmitted to the spinal cord in the pyramidal tract (Fig. 26.6). This passes through the internal capsule and the ventral brain stem before decussating in the medulla to enter the lateral columns of the spinal cord. The pyramidal tract 'upper motor neurons' end by synapsing with the anterior horn cells of the spinal cord grey matter, which form the 'lower motor neurons'.

Movement of a body part necessitates changes in posture and alteration in the tone of many muscles, some quite distant from the part being moved. The motor system consists of a hierarchy of control mechanisms that maintain body posture and baseline muscle tone upon which a specific movement is superimposed. The lowest order of this hierarchy resides in the grey matter of the spinal cord which controls the muscle tone response to stretch, and the reflex withdrawal response to noxious stimuli. The afferent side of the stretch reflex is detected by muscle spindles that sense lengthening of the muscle and initiate a monosynaptic reflex leading to muscle contraction. The predominantly inhibitory descending input from the brain stem and cerebral hemispheres

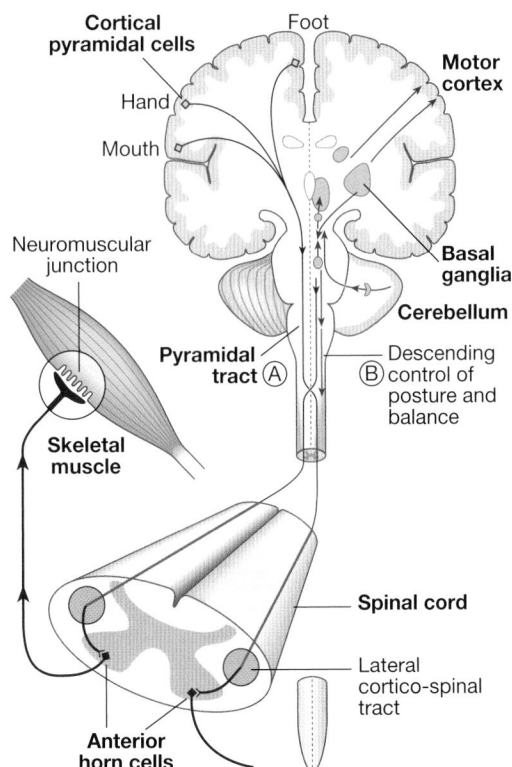

Fig. 26.6 The motor system. Neurons from the motor cortex descend as the pyramidal tract in the internal capsule and cerebral peduncle to the ventral brain stem, where most cross low in the medulla (A). In the spinal cord the upper motor neurons form the cortico-spinal tract in the lateral column before synapsing with the lower motor neurons in the anterior horns. The activity in the motor cortex is modulated by influences from the basal ganglia and cerebellum. Pathways descending from these structures control posture and balance (B).

modulates the sensitivity of the stretch reflex. It is the state of this stretch reflex that is tested clinically when a patient's tendon reflexes are elicited and muscle tone is assessed. Polysynaptic connections in the spinal cord grey matter control more complex reflex actions of flexion and extension of the limbs that form the basic building blocks of coordinated actions, but these require control from the extrapyramidal system and the cerebellum to function usefully.

Lower motor neurons

Lower motor neurons in the anterior horn of the spinal cord innervate a group of muscle fibres termed a 'motor unit'. Loss of function of lower motor neurons causes loss of contraction within this unit, resulting in weakness and reduced muscle tone. Subsequently, denervated muscle fibres atrophy, causing muscle wasting, and depolarise spontaneously, causing 'fibrillations'. Except in the tongue, these are usually only perceptible on an electromyelogram (EMG; p. 1143). With the passage of time, re-innervation from neighbouring intact motor neurons occurs but the neuromuscular junctions of the enlarged motor units are unstable and depolarise spontaneously, causing fasciculations (which are visible to the naked eye because the motor units are larger than normal). Fasciculations therefore imply chronic partial denervation with re-innervation.

Upper motor neurons

Upper motor neurons have an inhibitory influence on the function of anterior horn motor neurons. When upper motor neuron lesions occur, motor units have an exaggerated response to stretch. In the limbs, this results in reflex patterns of movement, such as flexion withdrawal to noxious stimuli and spasms of extension. An upper motor neuron lesion therefore manifests clinically with an increased muscle tone greater in the extensors of the lower limbs and the flexors of the upper limbs (spasticity), brisk tendon reflexes, and extensor plantar responses. On clinical examination, the increase in muscle tone varies with both the degree and the speed of stretch. The increased tone is more obvious with rapid stretch ('spastic catch'), but may suddenly give way with sustained tension (the 'clasp-knife' phenomenon). Spasticity takes time to develop and may not be present for weeks after the onset of an upper motor neuron lesion. Spasticity will be exacerbated by increased sensory input into the reflex arc, as may be caused by a pressure sore or urinary tract infection in a patient with a spinal cord lesion. The weakness found in upper motor neuron lesions is more pronounced in the extensors of the upper limbs and the flexors of the lower limbs.

The extrapyramidal system

Circuits between the basal ganglia and the motor cortex constitute the extrapyramidal system, which controls muscle tone, body posture and the initiation of movement (see Fig. 26.6). Lesions of the extrapyramidal system produce an increase in tone which is not an exaggerated response to stretch but is continuous throughout the range of movement at any speed of stretch ('lead pipe' rigidity). Involuntary movements are also a feature of extrapyramidal lesions (p. 1154), and tremor combined with rigidity produces typical 'cogwheel' rigidity. Rapid movements are slowed and clumsy (bradykinesia). Extrapyramidal lesions also cause postural instability which often precipitates falls.

The cerebellum

The cerebellum is responsible for fine-tuning and coordinating goal-directed movements initiated by the motor cortex. It also participates in the planning and learning of skilled movements through its reciprocal connections with the thalamus and cortex and in controlling speech. A lesion in a cerebellar hemisphere causes lack of coordination on the same side of the body. The initial part of movement is normal, but as the target is approached, the accuracy of the movement deteriorates, producing an 'intention tremor'. The distances of targets are misjudged (dysmetria), resulting in 'past-pointing'. The ability to produce rapid, accurate, regularly alternating movements is also impaired (dysdiadochokinesis). The central vermis of the cerebellum is concerned with the coordination of gait and posture. Disorders of this part therefore produce a characteristic ataxic gait (see below).

Speech

Speech is the process whereby vocal sounds are used to convey meaning between individuals. A large volume of the cerebral cortex is involved in this complex process, mostly in the dominant hemisphere (see Box 26.1,

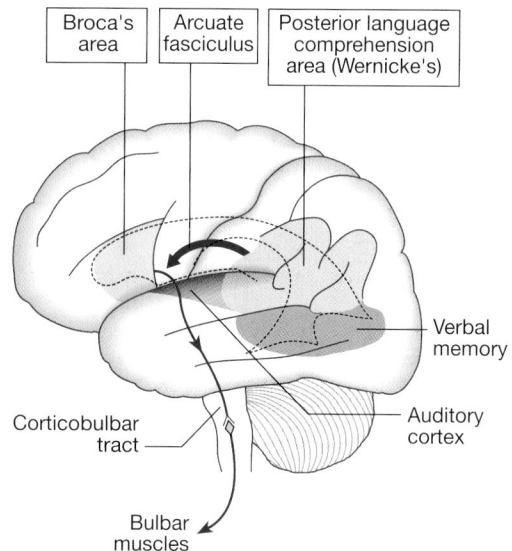

Fig. 26.7 Areas of the cerebral cortex involved in the generation of spoken language.

p. 1136). The decoding of speech sounds (phonemes) is a function of the upper part of the posterior temporal lobe. The perception of these sounds as meaningful language, as well as the formulation of the language required for the expression of ideas and concepts, occurs predominantly in the lower parts of the anterior parietal lobe (the angular and supramarginal gyri). The temporal speech comprehension region is referred to as Wernicke's area. Other parts of the temporal lobe contribute to language processing in areas specialising in verbal memory, where lexicons of meaningful words are 'stored'. Parts of the non-dominant parietal lobe appear to contribute to non-verbal aspects of language in the recognition of meaningful intonation patterns of spoken words (prosody).

The language information generated in the temporal and parietal lobes passes anteriorly via the arcuate fasciculus to Broca's area in the posterior end of the inferior frontal gyrus on the dominant side. The motor commands generated in Broca's area then pass to the cranial nerve nuclei in the pons and medulla, as well as to the anterior horn cells in the spinal cord. Nerve impulses then travel to the lips, tongue, palate, pharynx, larynx and respiratory muscles via the facial nerve and cranial nerves 9, 10 and 12, and result in the series of ordered sounds known as speech (Fig. 26.7). The cerebellum also plays an important role in coordinating speech, and lesions of the cerebellum lead to a speech disorder termed dysarthria.

The somatosensory system

Somatic sensory information from the limbs ascends the nervous system in two anatomically discrete systems (Fig. 26.8). Fibres from proprioceptive organs and those mediating well-localised touch (including vibration) enter the spinal cord at the posterior horn and pass without synapsing into the ipsilateral posterior columns. Neural fibres conveying pain and temperature sensory information (nociceptive neurons) synapse with second-order neurons which cross the midline in the spinal cord before ascending in the

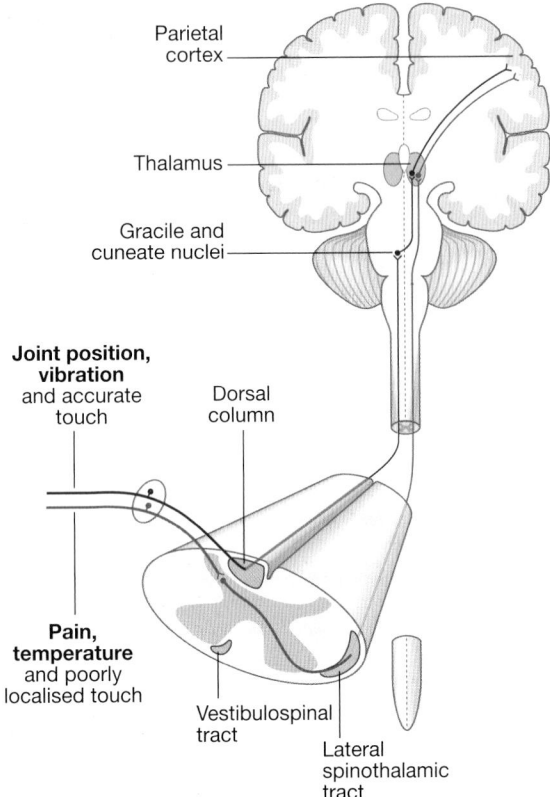

Parietal cortex

Thalamus

Gracile and cuneate nuclei

Joint position, vibration and accurate touch

Dorsal column

Pain, temperature and poorly localised touch

Vestibulospinal tract

Lateral spinothalamic tract

Fig. 26.8 The main somatic sensory pathways.

contralateral anterolateral spinothalamic tract to the brain stem.

The second-order neurons of the dorsal column sensory system cross the midline in the upper medulla to ascend through the brain stem. Here they lie just medial to the (already crossed) spinothalamic pathway. Brain-stem lesions can therefore cause sensory loss affecting all modalities of the contralateral side of the body. Sensory loss on the face due to brain-stem lesions is dependent upon the anatomy of the trigeminal fibres within the brain stem. Fibres from the back of the face (near the ears) descend within the brain stem to the upper part of the spinal cord before synapsing, the second-order neurons crossing the midline and then ascending with the spinothalamic fibres. Fibres conveying sensation from progressively more forward areas of the face descend a shorter distance in the brain stem. Thus, sensory loss in the face from low brain-stem lesions is in a 'balaclava helmet' distribution, as the longer descending trigeminal fibres are affected. Both the dorsal column and spinothalamic tracts end in the thalamus, relaying from there to the parietal cortex.

Pain

Pain is a complex percept that is only partly related to activity in nociceptor neurons (Fig. 26.9). In the posterior horn of the spinal cord, the second-order neuron of the spinothalamic tract is subject to modulation by a number of influences in addition to its synapse with the fibres from nociceptors. Branches from the larger mechanoceptor fibres destined for the posterior column also synapse with the second-order spinothalamic neurons and with interneurons of the grey matter of the posterior horn. The nociceptor neurons release neurotransmitters (such as substance P), in addition to excitatory transmitters, which influence the excitability of the spinothalamic neurons. Neurons in the posterior horn are also subject to modulation by fibres descending from the peri-aqueductal grey matter of the midbrain and raphe nuclei of the medulla. Neurons of this 'descending analgesia system' are activated by endogenous opiate (endorphin) peptides. The spinal cord's posterior horn is therefore much more than a way-station in the

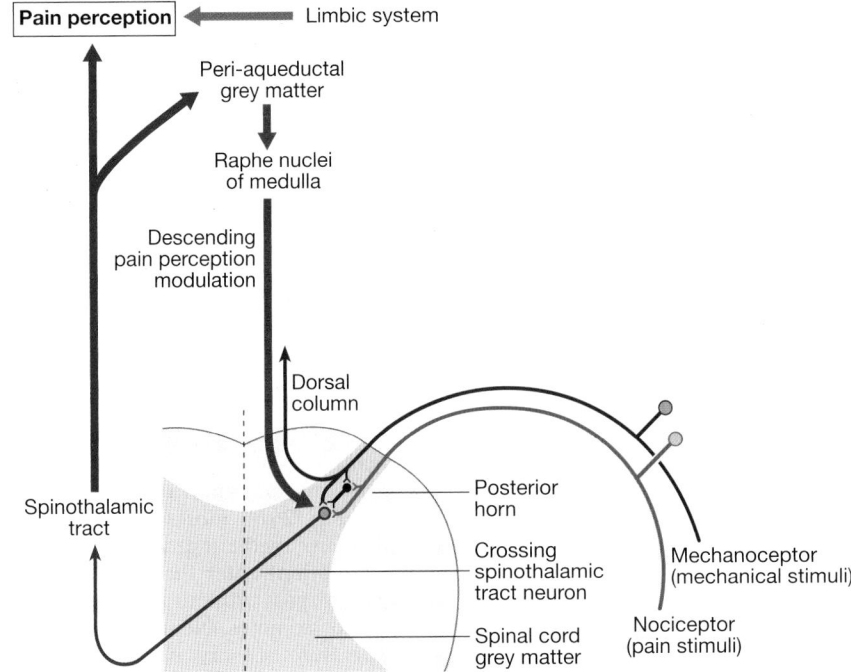

Pain perception ← Limbic system

Peri-aqueductal grey matter

Raphe nuclei of medulla

Descending pain perception modulation

Dorsal column

Posterior horn

Spinothalamic tract

Crossing spinothalamic tract neuron

Mechanoceptor (mechanical stimuli)

Spinal cord grey matter

Nociceptor (pain stimuli)

Fig. 26.9 The pain perception system.

transmission of nociceptive sensory information; it is a complex organ for gating and modulating information about painful stimuli before this ascends in the spinothalamic tract. In the diencephalon the perception of pain is further influenced by the rich interconnections of the thalamus with the limbic system.

Sleep

The function of sleep is unknown but it appears to be necessary for the normal functioning of the brain. Normal sleep is controlled by the reticular activating system in the upper brain stem and diencephalon. During overnight sleep, a series of repeated cycles of electroencephalogram (EEG) patterns can be recorded. As drowsiness occurs, alpha rhythm disappears and the EEG gradually becomes dominated by deepening slow-wave activity. After 60–80 minutes this slow-wave pattern is replaced by a short spell of low-amplitude EEG background on which are superimposed rapid eye movements (REM). After a few minutes of REM sleep, another slow-wave spell starts and the cycle repeats several times throughout the night. The REM periods tend to become longer as the sleep period progresses. Dreaming takes place mostly during REM sleep. This is accompanied by muscle relaxation, penile erection and loss of tendon reflexes. REM sleep seems to be the most important part of the sleep cycle for refreshing cognitive processes. Deprivation of REM sleep causes tiredness, irritability and impaired judgement.

INVESTIGATION OF NEUROLOGICAL DISEASE

In the investigation of neurological disease, tests of function have a somewhat more restricted application than tests of structure (imaging). Nevertheless, recording of electrical activity over the brain and assessment of nerve and muscle function are essential in certain conditions. The major tests are electroencephalography, evoked potentials, nerve conduction studies and electromyography.

Electroencephalography

The electroencephalogram (EEG) is used to detect electrical activity arising in the cerebral cortex. Although the EEG can only detect 0.1–1% of the brain's electrical activity at any one time, it is a clinically useful technique in the investigation of neurological disorders. The EEG involves placing an array of electrodes on the scalp to provide spatial information, and recording the resulting waveforms which are distinguished by their amplitude and frequency. When the eyes are shut, the most obvious frequency over the occipital cortex is 8–13 Hz; this is known as alpha rhythm, and disappears when the eyes are opened. Other frequency bands seen over different parts of the brain in different circumstances are beta (faster than 13/s), theta (4–8/s) and delta (slower than 4/s). Lower frequencies predominate in the very young and during sleep.

Various diseases cause abnormalities in the EEG. These may be continuous or episodic, focal or diffuse. Examples of continuous abnormalities include a global increase in fast frequencies (beta) seen with sedating drugs such as benzodiazepines, or marked focal slowing seen over a structural lesion such as a tumour or an infarct. The EEG is now seldom used to localise lesions, except in some patients with epilepsy (see p. 1176 and Fig. 26.10. It is useful in the investigation of patients who have disturbance of consciousness or disorders of sleep, in the diagnosis of cerebral diseases such as encephalitis, and in certain dementias such as sporadic Creutzfeldt–Jakob disease.

26

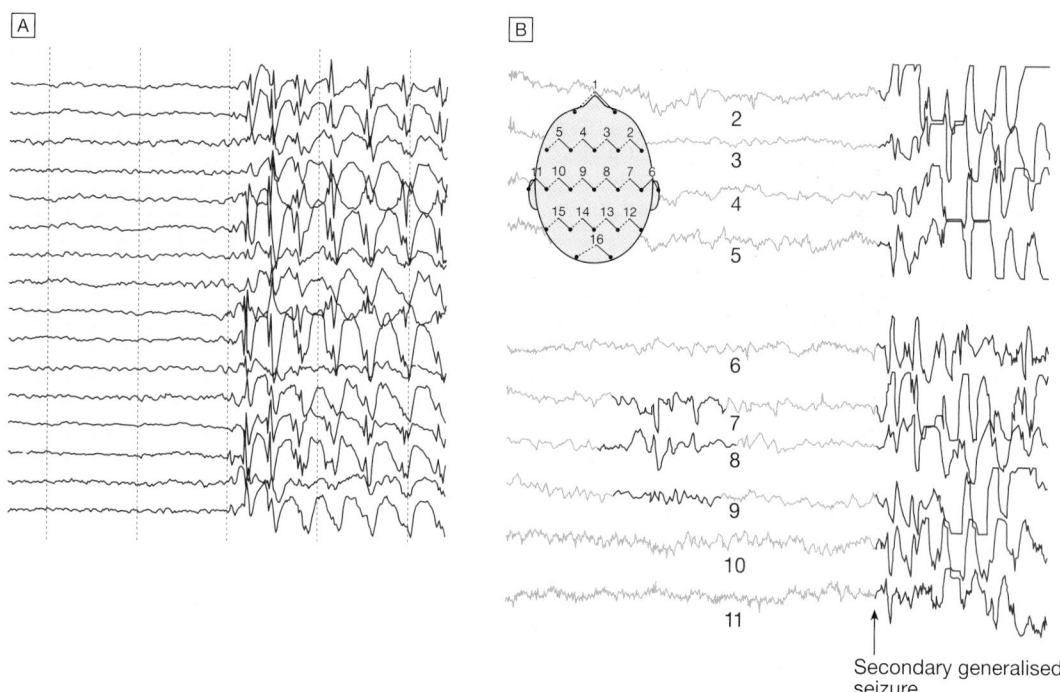

Fig. 26.10 EEGs in epilepsy. ⒶPrimary generalised epileptic discharge. ⒷFocal sharp waves over the right parietal region (between electrodes 7 and 8—shown in purple) with secondary generalised discharge.

26

The EEG is predominantly used in the diagnosis and assessment of epilepsy, to distinguish the type of epilepsy and to determine the location of an epileptic focus, particularly if surgery is contemplated. It must be stressed that only in rare circumstances will an EEG provide unequivocal evidence of epilepsy; some 50% of patients with proven epilepsy have a normal 'routine' EEG, and, conversely, the presence of features often seen in association with epilepsy does not of itself make a diagnosis (although the false-positive rate for clear-cut epileptiform features is < 1/1000). In view of this, the EEG should be used as an adjunct to clinical evaluation in the assessment of patients with suspected epilepsy. During an epileptic seizure, high-voltage disturbances of the background activity ('transients') can occur. These may be generalised, as in the 3 cycle/s 'spike and wave' of childhood absence epilepsy (petit mal), or more focal, as in partial epilepsies (see Fig. 26.10). However, it is unusual to record a seizure itself, except in the case of childhood absence epilepsy which can often be provoked by hyperventilation. Nevertheless, it is often possible to detect 'epileptiform' abnormalities in between seizures in the form of 'spikes' and 'sharp waves' that lend support to a clinical diagnosis. The likelihood of detecting these abnormalities is enhanced by hyperventilation, photic flicker, sleep and some drugs.

It is possible to enhance the information provided by EEG using a variety of techniques. For example, the usual 30-minute recording session can be lengthened to 24 hours by the use of a lightweight tape recorder. The addition of video information to the EEG allows comparison of behaviour with cerebral activity. In special circumstances, electrodes can be surgically positioned, e.g. through the foramen ovale, to record from the inferior temporal surface.

Evoked potentials

The EEG can also be used to study evoked potentials (EPs), which can be measured following visual, auditory or somatosensory stimuli if the electrodes are appropriately positioned. If a stimulus is provided—for example, to the eye—it would normally be impossible to detect the small EEG response evoked over the occipital cortex as the signal would be lost in background noise. However, when assessing EPs, EEG data from 100–1000 repeated stimuli are averaged electronically, the noise is removed and an EP is recorded whose latency (the time interval between stimulus onset and the maximum positive value of the evoked potential, P_{100}) and amplitude can be measured. In clinical practice, visual EPs are the most commonly used, but with the advent of MRI are now restricted to specialised indications, such as providing a semi-objective measure of visual function (Fig. 26.11). Abnormalities of the EP indicate damage to the relevant pathway, in the form of either a conduction delay (increased latency) or reduced amplitude, or both.

Nerve conduction studies

Nerve conduction studies (NCS) involve placing electrodes on the skin overlying peripheral nerves and recording compound action potentials (the sum of all the individual nerves' action potentials) following nerve stimulation as the impulse travels down the nerve. A normal compound action potential has an amplitude

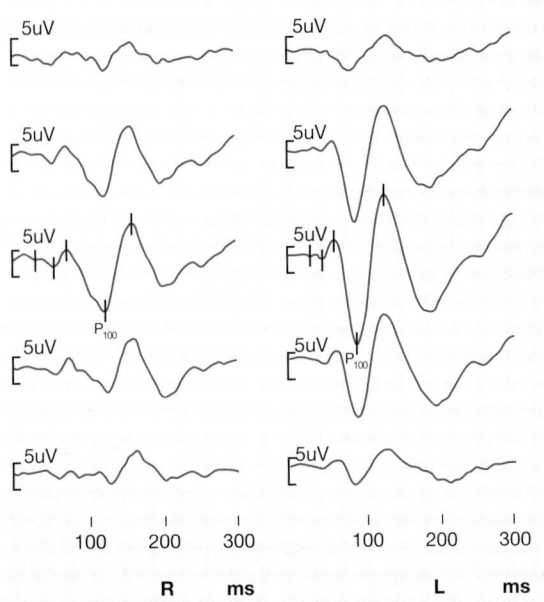

Fig. 26.11 Visual evoked responses (VER) recording showing abnormal delay on right. The latency of the P_{100} (the point of maximum positivity) on the left is 90 ms, that on the right 115 ms.

of 5–30 microvolts, depending upon the nerve; if the recorded potential is smaller than expected, this provides evidence of a reduction in the overall number of functioning axons. By measuring the response latency to stimulation of a nerve at two different points along its length, it is possible to calculate nerve conduction velocities (NCVs). This can be done for both sensory and motor nerves; typical values are 50–60 m/s. Slowing of conduction velocity is suggestive of peripheral nerve demyelination, which may be either diffuse (as in a demyelinating peripheral neuropathy) or focal (as in pressure palsies or conduction block). The principal use of NCS is to identify damage to peripheral nerves, and to determine whether the pathological process is focal or diffuse, and whether the damage is principally axonal or demyelinating. It is also possible to obtain some information about nerve roots by more sophisticated analysis of responses to impulses initially conducted antidromically (the 'wrong' way) back up to the spinal cord, and then returning orthodromically (the 'right' way) down to the stimulation point ('F waves'). Central conduction times can also be measured using electromagnetic induction of action potentials in the cortex or spinal cord by the local application of specialised coils. This is particularly useful in the investigation of disorders of the spinal cord and non-organic illness.

Electromyography

Electromyography (EMG) involves recording compound motor action potentials (CMAPs) over muscles in response to motor nerve stimulation (Fig. 26.12). These are easier to record than nerve potentials because the muscle amplifies the response, typical amplitudes being 1–20 millivolts. Fine concentric needle electrodes are inserted into muscle belly and the potentials from individual motor units recorded. It is also possible to

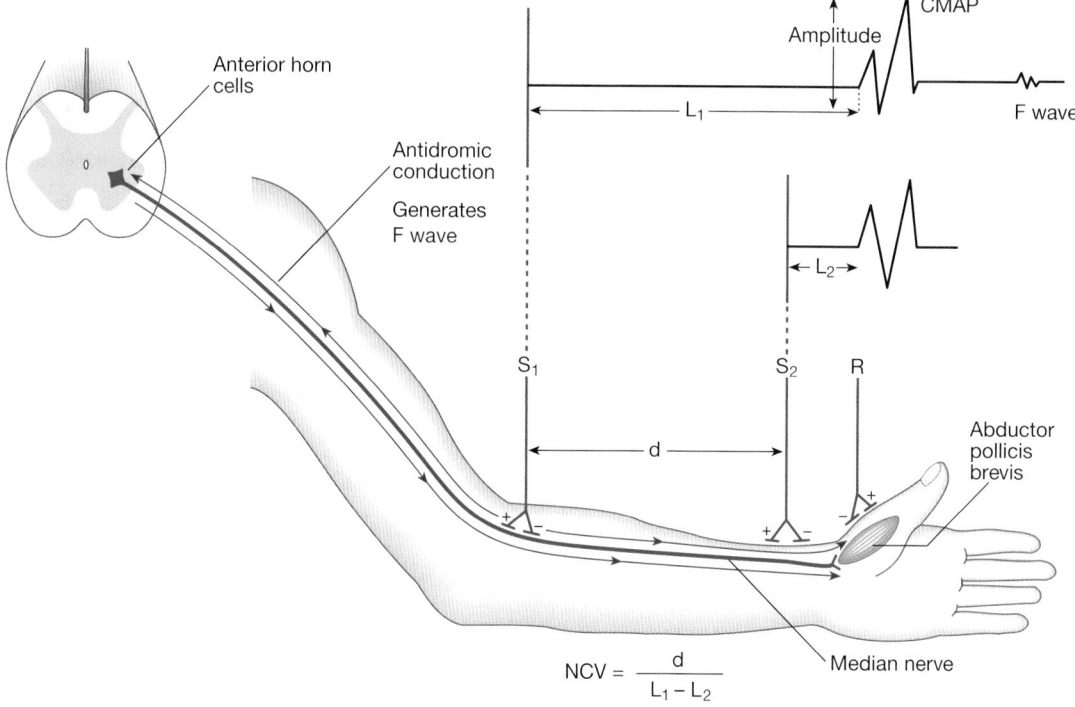

Fig. 26.12 Motor nerve conduction tests. Bipolar electrodes (R) on the muscle (abductor pollicis brevis here) record the compound motor action potential (CMAP) from stimulation at the median nerve at the elbow (S_1) and from the wrist (S_2). The CMAP amplitude is related to the number of axons, and the velocity can be determined if the distance between the two stimulating electrodes (d) is known. The latency (L) of the F wave is a measure of the conduction time in the nerve proximal to the elbow (see text). (NCV = nerve conduction velocity)

record abnormal spontaneous activity arising from muscles at rest, such as fibrillations (a sign of denervation) or myotonic discharges. Abnormalities in the shape and size of muscle potentials can help in the differential diagnosis of denervation and structural muscle diseases. Myopathies caused by metabolic abnormalities (causing electromechanical dissociation rather than loss of fibre structure) show no changes on needle EMG. Electromyography can also be used to investigate the neuromuscular junction. Repetitive stimulation of a nerve with trains of electrical impulses at 3–15/s does not normally result in a significant fall-off in the amplitude of the resulting muscle action potential. However, such a decrement is seen in myasthenia gravis (p. 1231) and provides one of the key diagnostic features. Augmentation of the response to repetitive stimulation is seen in the Lambert–Eaton myasthenic syndrome, though usually at higher stimulation frequencies.

Neuroimaging

Imaging is crucial to the identification of lesions of the nervous system in disease. Various techniques are used, including X-rays (plain X-rays, computed tomography (CT), CT angiography, myelography and angiography), magnetic resonance (MR imaging—MRI, or MR angiography—MRA), ultrasound (Doppler imaging of blood vessels) and radioisotopes (single photon emission computed tomography—SPECT, and positron emission tomography—PET). The indications, usefulness and limits of each technique are listed in Box 26.2. The choice of technique depends upon the area of the neuraxis that is being investigated.

Head and orbit

The use of plain skull X-rays is largely restricted to the diagnosis of fractures and sinus disease, and CT or MRI is needed to image pathology inside the skull. Which is used depends on what information is being sought. CT will show bone and calcium well, and will easily image collections of blood. It will also detect abnormalities of the brain and ventricles, such as atrophy, tumours, cysts, abscesses, vascular lesions and hydrocephalus. Diagnostic yield is often improved by the use of intravenous contrast and spiral CT methods. It is, however, limited in its ability to image the posterior fossa (because of the surrounding bone density), and it is poor at detecting abnormalities of white matter and at allowing detailed analysis of grey matter.

MRI is much more useful in the investigation of posterior fossa disease, as it is not affected by the surrounding bone. It is much more sensitive than CT to abnormalities of white and grey matter and is therefore useful in the investigation of inflammatory conditions such as multiple sclerosis, and in investigating epilepsy. Diffusion weighted MRI is particularly useful in diagnosing acute ischaemic stroke. MRI can also provide additional information about structural brain lesions, which may complement that available from CT. It is also useful in imaging the orbits, where special imaging sequences can be used to compensate for orbital fat and thereby allow clear views of extraocular muscles, optic nerve and other orbital structures.

Blood flow and metabolic function of the cerebral hemispheres can be assessed by using either SPECT or PET. Examples of brain imaged by the various techniques are shown in Figure 26.13.

26.2 Techniques available for imaging the nervous system

Technique	Principle	Applications	Advantages	Disadvantages	Comments
X-ray	Attenuation of X-ray beam by radio-opaque tissues and substances (bone, calcium, metal, iodinated contrast)	Plain X-rays CT, CTA Radiculography Myelography Intra-arterial angiography	Widely available Relatively cheap Relatively quick	Ionising radiation Reactions to contrast Myelography and angiography are invasive and thus carry risk	X-rays only used for showing fractures or foreign bodies. CT investigation of choice for stroke Intra-arterial angiography still 'gold standard' for vascular lesions
Magnetic resonance imaging (MRI)	Magnetic resonance of different tissues depends largely on free hydrogen/water content; signals changed by movement (e.g. flowing blood)	Structural imaging MRA Functional MRI MR spectroscopy	High-quality soft tissue imaging Good views of posterior fossa and temporal lobes No ionising radiation Non-invasive	Expensive Less widely available MRA looks at blood flow not vessel anatomy Scanners claustrophobic Pacemakers contraindicate MRI. Complications of contrast (gadolinium)	Increasing application Functional MR and spectroscopy still mainly research tools
Ultrasound	Echoes from high-frequency sound source localise structure; Doppler principle used to measure flow rate	Doppler Duplex scans	Cheap Quick Non-invasive	Operator-dependent Poor anatomical definition	Useful as screening tool to assess need for carotid endarterectomy
Radio-isotope	Radio-labelled isotopes	Isotope brain scan SPECT PET	In vivo imaging of functional anatomy (ligand binding, blood flow)	Poor spatial resolution Ionising radiation Expensive (especially PET) Not widely available	Isotope scans obsolete. SPECT and PET mainly research tools but being introduced clinically for management of epilepsy and dementia

(CT = computed tomography; MRA = magnetic resonance angiography; MRI = magnetic resonance imaging; PET = positron emission tomography; SPECT = single photon emission computed tomography)

Cervical and thoracic spine

Plain X-rays are useful in the investigation of structural damage to vertebrae, such as that resulting from trauma and from degenerative and inflammatory disease. They can also provide implicit information about intervertebral disc disease, but not detailed information about the spinal cord or nerve roots, for which myelography or MRI is needed. Use of myelography has declined with the advent of MRI, which is the imaging modality of first choice. However, myelography is still used if MRI is not available, if it is contraindicated, or if the patient cannot tolerate lying within the scanner because of claustrophobia. Myelography involves injecting radio-opaque contrast into the lumbar theca and then moving the contrast up to the cervical region by tilting the patient. The contrast outlines the nerve roots and spinal cord, thereby providing information about abnormal structure. Examples of the neck imaged by plain X-rays, myelography and MRI are shown in Figure 26.14.

Lumbo-sacral region

Plain X-rays are of value in the investigation of structural abnormalities of the lumbar spine and but are of no value in the assessment of nerve roots or the spinal canal. Contrast injection into the thecal space can be used to outline the lower nerve roots (radiculography), or it can be run up to outline the conus and spinal cord (myelography). The information obtained may be enhanced by the additional use of CT following myelography (contrast CT). Non-contrast CT of the lumbar spine can only be used to image the vertebrae and discs. As with the cervical spine, MRI provides a non-invasive way of obtaining high-resolution images of both the vertebral column and the relevant neural structures.

Blood vessels

Various techniques are available to investigate extra-ranial and intracranial blood vessels. The least invasive is ultrasound (Doppler or duplex scanning), which is

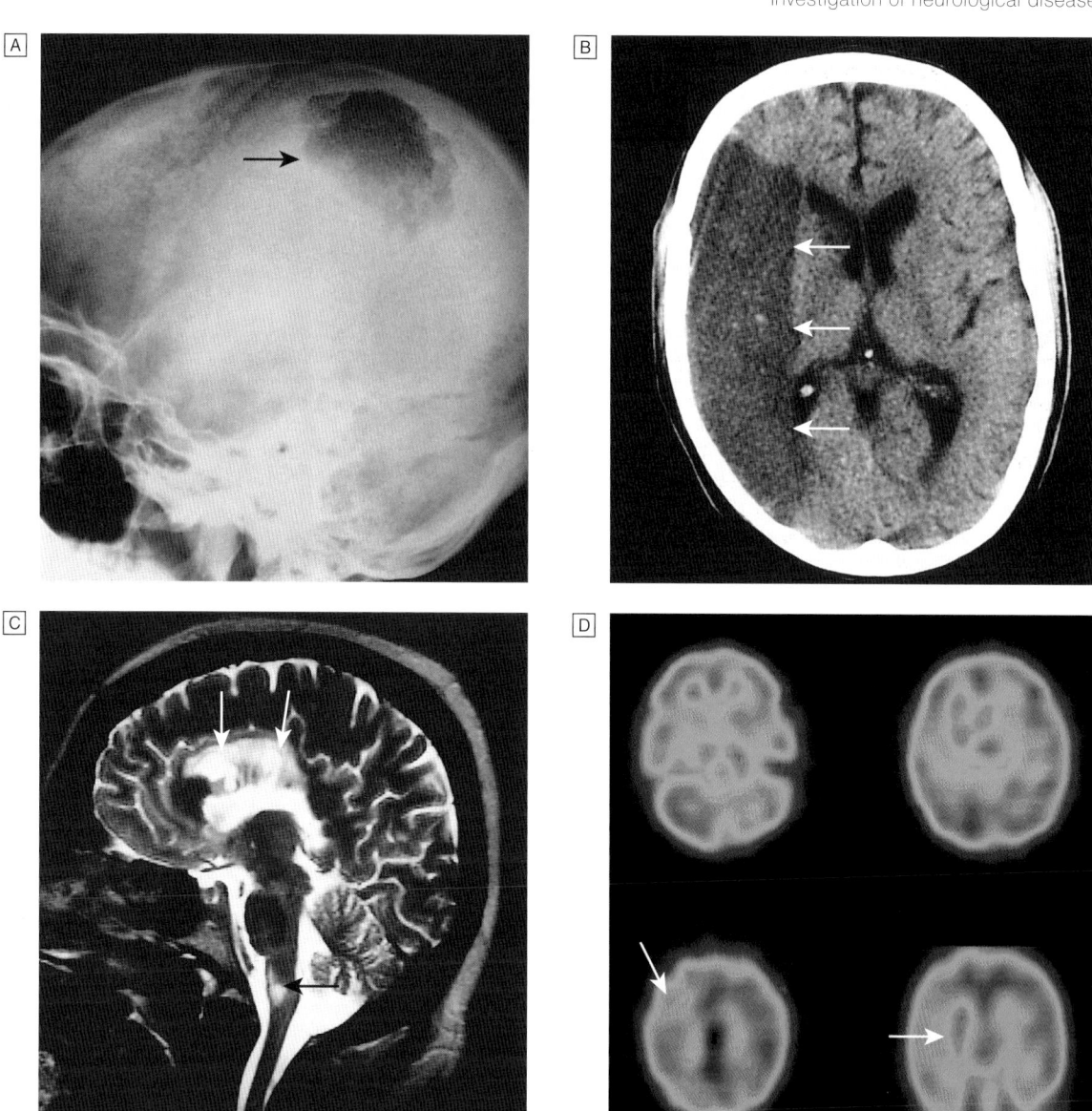

Fig. 26.13 Different techniques of imaging the head and brain. A Skull X-ray showing lytic vault lesion (eosinophilic granuloma—arrow). B CT showing complete middle cerebral artery infarct (arrows). C MRI showing widespread areas of high signal in multiple sclerosis (arrows). D SPECT after caudate infarct showing relative hypoperfusion of overlying right cerebral cortex (arrows).

used to investigate the carotid and the vertebral arteries in the neck, usually as part of the investigation of stroke. In skilled hands, reliable information can be provided about the degree of arterial stenosis, and the technique often gives useful anatomical information, such as the presence of ulcerated plaques. Information concerning the blood flow in the intracerebral vessels is also becoming increasingly possible to obtain using transcranial Doppler. While the anatomical resolution of Doppler imaging is limited, it is improving with increased experience and many centres no longer require formal angiography before performing carotid endarterectomy (p. 1189). This has the advantage of eliminating the small but significant risk of stroke or even death associated with catheter angiography.

Blood vessels can be outlined by the injection of radio-opaque contrast intravenously or intra-arterially. The X-ray images obtained can be enhanced by the use of computer-assisted digital subtraction or of spiral CT. Using the intravenous route, large amounts of contrast need to be injected and the images obtained are not generally as good as with the intra-arterial route. However, intra-arterial injections are accompanied by a higher complication rate. Intra-arterial angiography is still required to delineate lesions of the extracranial carotid artery prior to endarterectomy, and is also used to investigate abnormalities of intracerebral vessels such as arterial (berry) aneurysms or arteriovenous malformations, or to delineate the blood supply of tumours prior to surgery.

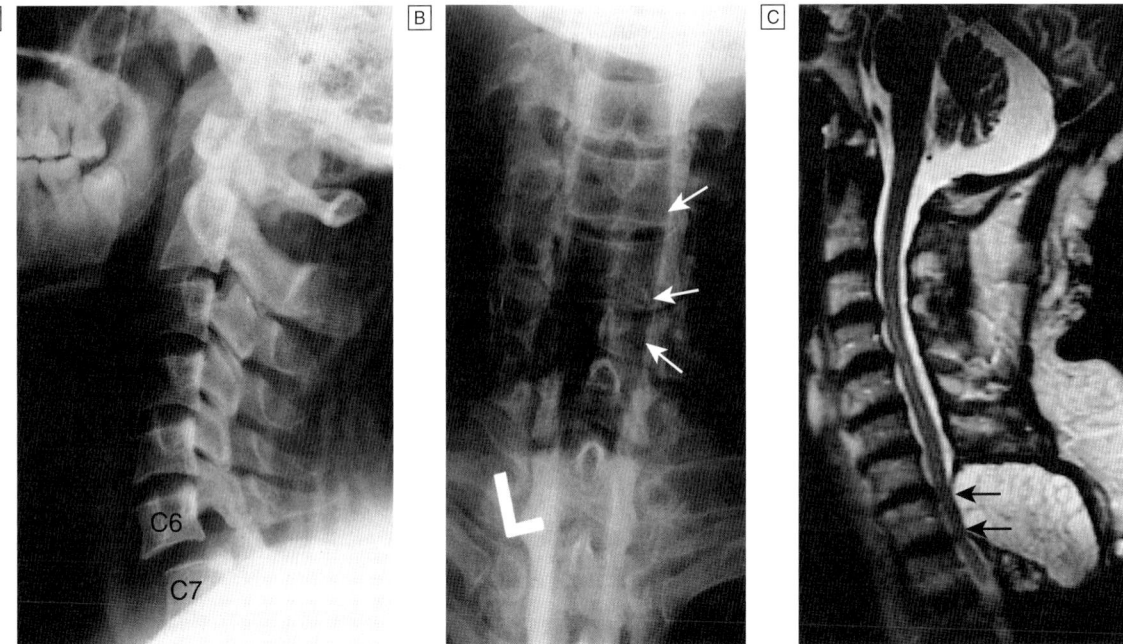

Fig. 26.14 Different techniques of imaging the cervical spine. [A] Lateral X-ray showing bilateral C6/7 facet dislocation. [B] Myelogram showing widening of cervical cord due to astrocytoma (arrows). [C] MRI showing posterior epidural compression from adenocarcinomatous metastasis to the posterior arch of T1 (arrows).

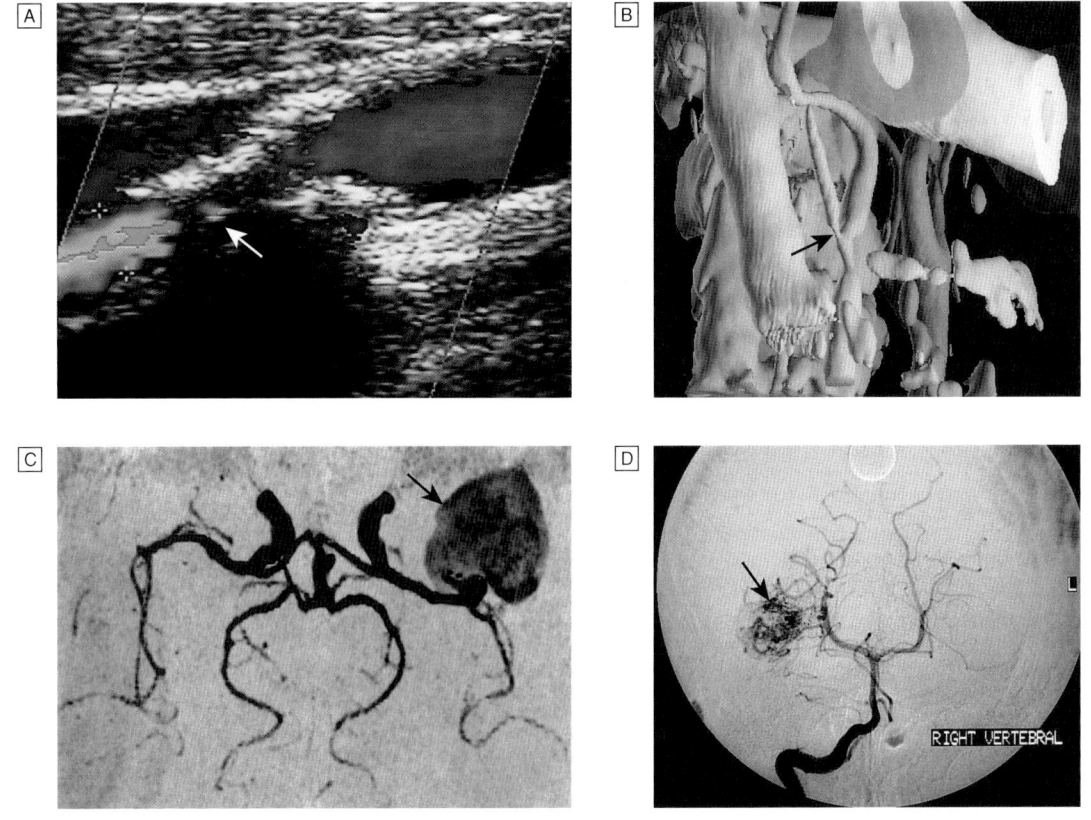

Fig. 26.15 Different techniques of imaging blood vessels. [A] Doppler scan showing 80% stenosis of internal carotid artery (arrow). [B] 3-D reconstruction of CT angiogram showing stenosis at the carotid bifurcation (arrow). [C] MR angiogram showing giant aneurysm at the middle cerebral artery bifurcation (arrow). [D] Intra-arterial angiography showing arteriovenous malformation (arrow).

Flowing blood can be detected by specialised MR sequences in MR angiography. The anatomical resolution is still not comparable to that of intra-arterial angiography, but the investigation is non-invasive and is replacing angiography in most diagnostic settings, except when MRI cannot be performed because of contraindications, such as in patients with pacemakers or in claustrophobic individuals who cannot tolerate entering the MRI scanner. Examples of these different techniques are given in Figure 26.15.

Routine blood tests

Many systemic conditions that affect the nervous system can be diagnosed with the help of blood tests: for example, confusion due to hypothyroidism, a stroke due to systemic lupus erythematosus, ataxia due to vitamin B_{12} deficiency, myelopathy due to syphilis. Acanthocytes may assist in the diagnosis of neuroacanthocytosis, creatine kinase in muscle diseases, and copper studies in Wilson's disease. Blood tests relating to general medical conditions that affect the nervous system are described in the sections dealing with individual conditions.

Immunological tests

A number of specific immunological tests are used in the diagnosis of neurological disorders. These include antibodies to acetylcholine receptors and muscle-specific tyrosine kinase (MuSK), seen in myasthenia gravis, and to voltage-gated calcium channels in Lambert–Eaton myasthenic syndrome. Antibodies to different types of ganglioside (glycoproteins expressed on nerve membranes) can be seen in various types of neuropathy, including multifocal motor neuronopathy and the Guillain–Barré syndrome (particularly the Miller–Fisher variant). Also, antineuronal antibodies provide markers of paraneoplastic cerebellar or neuropathic syndromes. Antibodies to basal ganglia neurons are found in Sydenham's chorea and encephalitis lethargica.

Genetic testing

An increasing number of inherited neurological conditions can now be diagnosed by DNA analysis (p. 56). These include diseases caused by increased numbers of trinucleotide repeats, such as Huntington's disease, myotonic dystrophy and some types of spinocerebellar ataxia. Also, defects of mitochondrial DNA can be detected in many conditions, including Leber's hereditary optic neuropathy, some syndromes causing epilepsy and stroke-like syndromes.

Lumbar puncture

Lumbar puncture is indicated in the investigation of infections (meningitis or encephalitis), subarachnoid haemorrhage, inflammatory conditions (multiple sclerosis, sarcoidosis and cerebral lupus) and some neurological malignancies (carcinomatous meningitis, lymphoma and leukaemia); it is also used to measure CSF pressure (in idiopathic intracranial hypertension). It is, of course, part of the procedure of myelography, and can be used in therapeutic procedures, either to lower CSF pressure or to administer drugs. Lumbar puncture involves inserting a needle between lumbar spinous processes (usually between L3 and L4) through the dura and into the CSF under local anaesthetic. Intracranial pressure can be measured and CSF removed for analysis. CSF is normally clear and colourless and the tests that are usually performed include a naked eye examination of the CSF, centrifugation to determine the colour of the supernatant (yellow, or xanthochromic, some hours after subarachnoid haemorrhage), biochemical analysis (glucose, total protein, and protein electrophoresis to detect oligoclonal bands), microbiological analysis (polymerase chain reaction (PCR) for herpes simplex or tuberculosis), immunology (paraneoplastic antibodies) and cytology (to detect malignant cells). Normal values and various abnormalities found in diseases are shown in Box 26.3.

26

26.3 How to interpret CSF results

	Normal	Subarachnoid haemorrhage	Acute bacterial meningitis	Viral meningitis	Tuberculous meningitis	Multiple sclerosis
Pressure	50–250 mm of water	Increased	Normal/increased	Normal	Normal/increased	Normal
Colour	Clear	Blood-stained Xanthochromic	Cloudy	Clear	Clear/cloudy	Clear
Red cell count ($\times 10^6$/L)	0–4	Raised	Normal	Normal	Normal	Normal
White cell count ($\times 10^6$/L)	0–4	Normal/slightly raised	1000–5000 polymorphs	10–2000 lymphocytes	50–5000 lymphocytes	0–50 lymphocytes
Glucose	> 60% of blood level	Normal	Decreased	Normal	Decreased	Normal
Protein	< 0.45 g/L	Increased	Increased	Normal/increased	Increased	Normal/increased
Microbiology	Sterile	Sterile	Organisms on Gram stain and/or culture	Sterile/virus detected	Ziehl–Nielson/ auramine stain or tuberculosis culture positive	Sterile
Oligoclonal bands	Negative	Negative	Can be positive	Can be positive	Can be positive	Often positive

If there is a space-occupying lesion in the head, lumbar puncture can result in a shift of intracerebral contents downwards, towards and into the spinal canal. This process is known as coning, and is potentially fatal (p. 1216). Consequently, lumbar puncture is contraindicated if there is any clinical suggestion of raised intracranial pressure (papilloedema), depressed level of consciousness, or focal neurological signs suggesting a cerebral lesion, until imaging of the head (by CT or MRI) has excluded a space-occupying lesion or hydrocephalus. Lumbar puncture is contraindicated in the presence of thrombocytopenia or disseminated intravascular coagulation, and in those on warfarin or heparin therapy, unless specific measures are taken to compensate for the clotting deficit on a temporary basis. Lumbar puncture can be safely performed in patients on low-dose aspirin. It is not safe in patients on clopidogrel or low-dose heparin due to the increased risk of epidural haematoma formation.

About 30% of lumbar punctures are followed by a headache, which is thought to be due to reduced CSF pressure. The risk of this can be reduced by using smaller needles. Other minor complications involve transient radicular pain, and pain over the lumbar region during the procedure. Infections such as meningitis are extremely rare following lumbar puncture, provided that an aseptic technique is used.

Biopsy

Nerve and muscle biopsies are occasionally required for the diagnosis of a number of neurological conditions, and it is occasionally necessary to biopsy the brain or meninges.

Nerve biopsies are sometimes necessary to investigate the cause of peripheral neuropathy. Usually, the sural nerve is biopsied at the ankle or the radial nerve at the wrist. Histological examination can help identify underlying causes such as vasculitides or infiltrative disorders like amyloid. Nerve biopsy should not be undertaken lightly since there is an appreciable morbidity; the procedure should be reserved for cases where the diagnosis is in doubt after routine investigations and where it will influence management.

Muscle biopsy is performed much more frequently and is indicated for investigation of primary muscle disease to distinguish neurogenic wasting from myositis and myopathy. These conditions can usually be distinguished by histological examination, and enzyme histochemistry can also be performed when mitochondrial diseases and storage diseases are suspected. The quadriceps muscle is most commonly biopsied but other muscles may also be sampled if they are involved clinically. Although pain and infection can follow the procedure, these are much less of a problem than after nerve biopsy.

Brain biopsy is seldom required since, in most cases, the cause of intracerebral lesions can be inferred from clinical evaluation and neuroimaging. However, there are situations in which it is important to obtain tissue for histological examination: for example, in unexplained degenerative diseases such as unusual cases of dementia and in patients with brain tumour. Most intracranial lesions can now be biopsied stereotactically through a burrhole in the skull and the complication rate of this technique is much lower than that of open craniotomy. Nevertheless, haemorrhage, infection and death still occur and brain biopsy should only be considered if a diagnosis cannot be reached in any other way.

PRESENTING PROBLEMS IN NEUROLOGICAL DISEASE

Headache and facial pain

Headache is a common presenting complaint but, unless it is accompanied by other symptoms or neurological signs, is seldom associated with significant neurological disease. Nevertheless, patients suffering from headache usually fear serious brain disease and, in order to manage them effectively, it is important to be aware of this. The likely underlying cause of headache or facial pain can usually be identified after taking a careful history and performing the appropriate general and neurological examinations (Box 26.4). Unless the history is suggestive of structural disease or another secondary cause, patients with headache who are normal on neurological examination are unlikely to have a serious disorder, however distressing their symptoms. The features of a patient's history that are helpful in making a clear diagnosis of the cause of a headache are shown in Box 26.5. In such cases, further investigations should be avoided if possible, and the patient can be reassured and provided with symptomatic treatment.

26.4 Common and important headache and facial pain syndromes

Primary headache syndromes

- Tension-type headache (persistent daily headache)
- Migraine
- Cluster headache
- Trigeminal neuralgia
- Atypical facial pain
- Benign paroxysmal headaches (see Box 26.29, p. 1170)

Secondary causes of headache

- Intracerebral bleeding (subdural haematoma, subarachnoid or intracerebral haemorrhage)
- Raised intracranial pressure (brain tumour, idiopathic intracranial hypertension)
- Infection (meningitis, encephalitis, brain abscess)
- Inflammatory disease (temporal arteritis, other vasculitis, arthritis)
- Post-herpetic neuralgia
- Referred pain from other structures (orbit, temporo-mandibular joint, neck)

26.5 How to take a history of headache

During history-taking, determine
- The overall pattern (intermittent or continuous)
- The speed of onset
- The time of day of onset of maximal pain
- The effect of posture, coughing and straining
- The location of the pain
- Any associated symptoms

Serious acute neurological disease should always be considered in patients with headaches of very sudden onset. Subarachnoid haemorrhage (p. 1190) causes a very sudden headache which may or may not be localised, although only one person in eight who has such a 'thunderclap' headache will have had a subarachnoid haemorrhage. A patient with subarachnoid haemorrhage almost invariably develops other symptoms including vomiting and neck stiffness, although the latter may take some hours to develop. The main differential diagnosis in a patient with a sudden severe headache is between subarachnoid haemorrhage (see Fig. 26.35, p. 1190) and a migraine variant. Meningitis occasionally presents apoplectically, but the headache is usually less dramatic in onset.

Headache coming on over a matter of hours is less likely to be associated with structural disease and more likely to be due to migraine, unless accompanied by other significant symptoms or signs. Patients with bacterial meningitis are usually generally ill and pyrexial, and exhibit meningism (p. 1205). Patients with viral meningitis may present with a pyrexia and quite sudden and severe headache coming on over an hour or so, but are less likely to have neck stiffness or other signs of meningism. Migraine headaches (p. 1169) may be accompanied or preceded by vomiting and focal neurological symptoms (usually in the form of zigzag 'fortification spectra' or tingling moving slowly over part of the body).

When headaches are intermittent rather than continuous over a period of days or weeks, they are most likely to be migrainous but it is worth while paying attention to the time of day they occur and to the presence or absence of precipitating factors. The headache of raised intracranial pressure is present on waking and often resolves or improves as the patient becomes upright (reducing the intracranial pressure) or takes simple analgesia (Box 26.6). It is unusual for a patient to present with such a headache alone since it is usually not sufficiently severe to cause alarm; the presentation of the causative mass lesion is more often provoked by a seizure or by focal neurological dysfunction (aphasia, hemiplegia etc.). The exceptions to this are patients with acute hydrocephalus who present with a more severe headache. As with other causes of raised intracranial pressure, this is worse when lying, bending forward or coughing, and frequently causes vomiting in the morning (especially in children). Hydrocephalus may cause no other symptoms except gait ataxia, although examination may reveal papilloedema.

Headaches that persist for weeks, are present all day and are poorly responsive to simple analgesia are very likely to be tension-type headaches, whatever their other characteristics. Headaches so well localised by the patient that a finger is used to locate the exact

26.6 Headache of raised intracranial pressure

- Worse in morning, improves through the day
- Associated with morning vomiting
- Worse bending forward
- Worse with cough and straining
- Relieved by analgesia
- Dull ache, often mild

26.7 Headaches in old age

- **Prevalence:** less common than in younger people.
- **Important causes:** giant cell arteritis, trigeminal neuralgia and post-herpetic neuralgia.
- **Less common causes:** migraine and tension headache.

spot on the skull are never associated with significant disease.

In a patient over 60 years with head pain localised to one or both temples, giant cell arteritis (p. 1115) should be considered, especially if the temporal pulses are not palpable and/or the arteries are enlarged and tender (Box 26.7).

Ocular pain

Pain in and around the eye, when not caused by ocular disease, can operationally be considered as a type of headache. This includes the dramatic pain of cluster headache (p. 1170) and rarer variants. Rarely, inflammatory or infiltrative lesions at the apex of the orbit or the cavernous sinus may cause pain in or around the eye, but tell-tale signs from involvement of the ocular motor nerves usually accompany this. Pain in the eye may accompany disorders of the carotid artery, particularly dissections, and may then be accompanied by a Horner's syndrome.

Facial pain

Pain in other parts of the face can be due to problems with the teeth or the temporo-mandibular joint. Inflamed nasal sinuses are seldom the cause of lasting facial pain in the absence of obvious nasal congestion. The very rare but serious condition of subdural empyema (p. 1212) needs to be considered if 'sinusitis' is followed by very severe unilateral facial pain and signs of cerebral irritation (seizures and/or obtundation). Destructive lesions of the trigeminal nerve causing pain are extremely rare since such lesions usually cause loss of sensation in the nerve's territory rather than pain.

Most patients with persisting pain in the face have trigeminal neuralgia, atypical facial pain or post-herpetic neuralgia. The main distinction between these is in the nature of the pain. In trigeminal neuralgia, the pain is very brief, though severe and recurrent, described as 'like lightning' and most frequently felt in the second and third divisions of the nerve. Atypical facial pain, on the other hand, is continuous and unremitting, and is centred over the maxilla, usually on the left side. It occurs most frequently in middle-aged women. Post-herpetic neuralgia is continuous and is felt as a burning pain throughout the affected territory, which is often very sensitive to light touch. The cause is usually obvious from a history of 'shingles' in the ophthalmic division of the trigeminal nerve.

Dizziness, blackouts and 'funny turns'

Episodes of lost or altered consciousness are a frequent symptom in primary care and in hospital practice (Box 26.8). A patient may complain of 'blacking out', 'going dizzy', 'having a funny turn' or other

26

- **Prevalence:** common, affecting up to 30% of people aged > 65 years.
- **Symptoms:** most frequently described as a combination of unsteadiness and lightheadedness.
- **Most common causes:** postural hypotension, cardiovascular disease, cervical spondylosis. Many patients have more than one underlying cause.
- **Arrhythmia:** can present with lightheadedness either at rest or on activity.
- **Anxiety:** frequently associated with dizziness, but rarely the only cause.
- **Falls:** multidisciplinary work required if dizziness is associated with falls.

local variants. The first task is to discover exactly what the patient means by the term used (Fig. 26.16). Some patients, for example, mean by 'blackout' that their vision darkens without alteration in consciousness (defined here as an awareness of the environment and ability to respond to it). More often 'blackout' is used to describe an episode of lost consciousness with or without falling down. The terms 'blackout' and 'funny turn' can also be used to refer to transient periods of amnesia, when the patient loses memory for a period of time. 'Dizziness' is used frequently to describe an abnormal perception of movement of the environment (vertigo), but may be used to mean a feeling of faintness, some other alteration of consciousness, or unsteadiness (p. 1171).

After a careful history from the patient, supplemented by a witness account, it should be clear whether the patient is describing an episode of loss of consciousness, altered consciousness, vertigo, transient amnesia or something else. The former two symptoms suggest a problem in mechanisms maintaining normal awareness. Vertigo is caused by an alteration in function of the peripheral vestibular organs or the central control mechanisms of balance and posture.

Loss of consciousness

Loss of consciousness, other than in sleep, suggests a global dysfunction of the brain. This most commonly occurs because of a recoverable loss of blood supply to the whole brain (syncope or faint, see below). Alternatively, loss of consciousness can occur due to

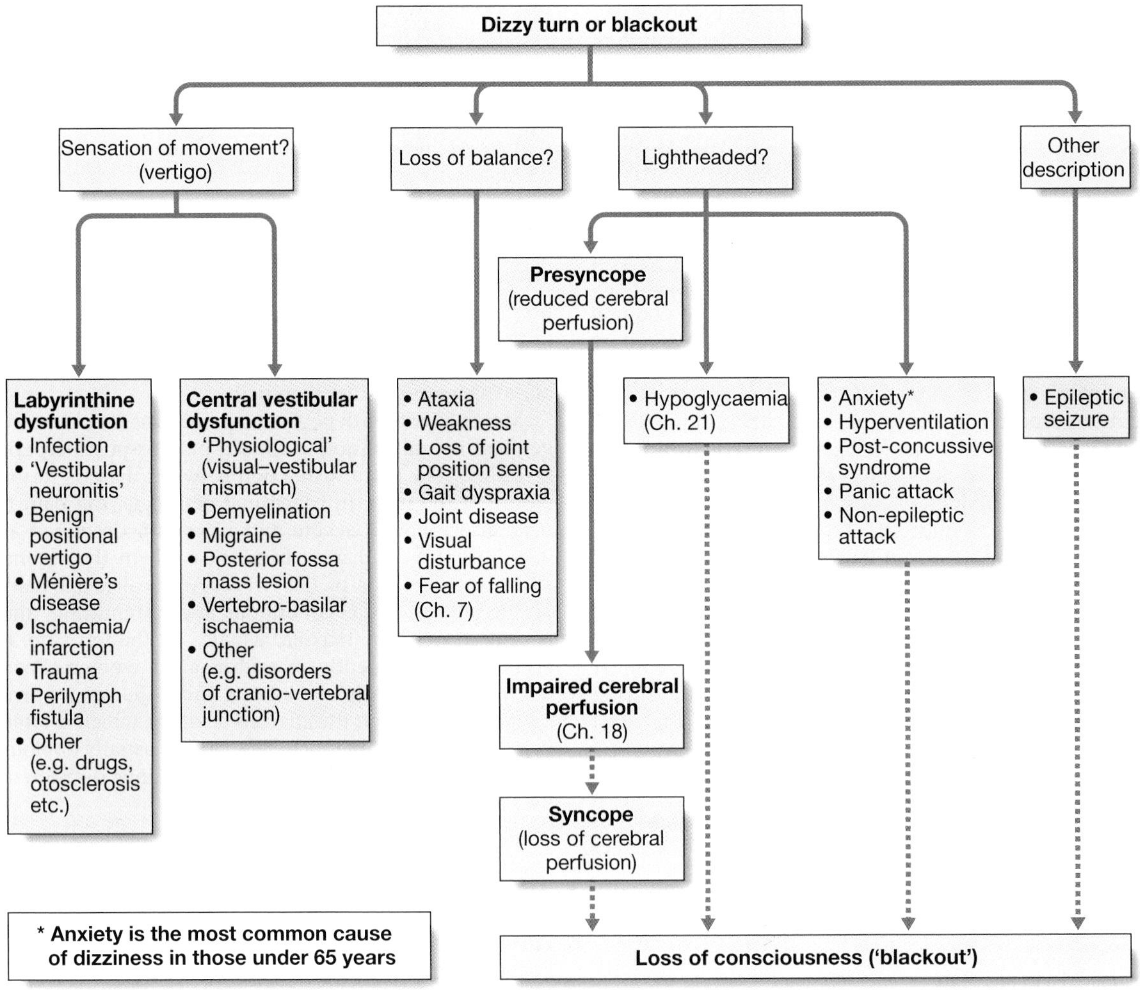

Dizzy turn or blackout

- **Sensation of movement? (vertigo)**
- **Loss of balance?**
- **Lightheaded?**
- **Other description**

Presyncope (reduced cerebral perfusion)

Labyrinthine dysfunction
- Infection
- 'Vestibular neuronitis'
- Benign positional vertigo
- Ménière's disease
- Ischaemia/infarction
- Trauma
- Perilymph fistula
- Other (e.g. drugs, otosclerosis etc.)

Central vestibular dysfunction
- 'Physiological' (visual–vestibular mismatch)
- Demyelination
- Migraine
- Posterior fossa mass lesion
- Vertebro-basilar ischaemia
- Other (e.g. disorders of cranio-vertebral junction)

- Ataxia
- Weakness
- Loss of joint position sense
- Gait dyspraxia
- Joint disease
- Visual disturbance
- Fear of falling (Ch. 7)

- Hypoglycaemia (Ch. 21)

- Anxiety*
- Hyperventilation
- Post-concussive syndrome
- Panic attack
- Non-epileptic attack

- Epileptic seizure

Impaired cerebral perfusion (Ch. 18)

Syncope (loss of cerebral perfusion)

> * Anxiety is the most common cause of dizziness in those under 65 years

Loss of consciousness ('blackout')

Fig. 26.16 A diagnostic approach to the patient with dizziness, funny turns or blackouts. (Neurological causes are shown in green.)

26.9 How to differentiate seizures from syncope

	Seizure	Syncope
Aura (e.g. olfactory)	+	−
Cyanosis	+	−
Tongue-biting	+	−
Post-ictal confusion	+	−
Post-ictal amnesia	+	−
Post-ictal headache	+	−
Rapid recovery	−	+

a sudden electrical dysfunction of the brain, as occurs during a seizure. Whilst most episodes of loss of consciousness are due to syncope or seizures, psychogenic blackouts or non-epileptic seizure can also occur and need to be considered in the differential diagnosis.

The distinction of a seizure from syncope can only be made from the patient's history, with help from a witness to the attack. No amount of investigation can replace a clear history in these circumstances. Features in the history useful in distinguishing a seizure from syncope are shown in Box 26.9.

Syncope

Typically, syncope is preceded by a brief feeling of light-headedness. There then follows a darkening of vision and there may be a ringing in the ears. Vasovagal syncope (p. 551) may be provoked by an emotional event or venepuncture, and usually occurs from the standing position. Cardiac syncope (p. 551), caused by a sudden decline in cardiac output, may be provoked by exertion in patients with severe aortic stenosis or may occur without warning in patients with cardiac arrhythmia. In vasovagal syncope, the loss of consciousness is gradual and brief, and the patient recovers quickly without confusion as long as he or she has assumed the horizontal position. It is rare for the syncope to cause injury and there is no amnesia for events that occur after regaining awareness. During a syncopal attack, incontinence of urine can occur and there is often stiffening and brief twitching of the limbs, but tongue-biting never occurs.

Seizures

The diagnosis of major seizures in which there is loss of consciousness, falling to the ground and convulsion (p. 1172) is easy but patients may also present with just a history of 'blackouts', particularly if the attacks were unwitnessed. Minor seizures, such as absences (p. 1175) or complex partial seizures (p. 1175), which cause alteration of consciousness without the patient falling to the ground, may also be described by patients as 'blackouts'.

Vertigo

Vertigo is defined as an abnormal perception of movement of the environment and occurs because of an abnormality in sensory information from the eyes, limb proprioception and the vestibular system about a person's position in space. Vertigo commonly arises from inappropriate input from the labyrinthine apparatus and is within the experience of most people, since this is the 'dizziness' which occurs after someone has spun round

vigorously and then stops. Vertigo caused by labyrinthine disorders is usually short-lived, though it may recur, whilst vertigo arising from central (brain-stem) disorders is often persistent and accompanied by other signs of brain-stem dysfunction. A careful analysis of the history will reveal the likely cause in most patients.

Sleep disturbance

Disturbances of sleep are common and in many cases are not due to neurological disease. Patients may complain of insomnia (difficulty sleeping), excessive daytime sleepiness, disturbed behaviour during night-time sleep, parasomnia (sleep walking and talking, or night terrors) or disturbing subjective experiences during sleep and/or its onset (nightmares, hypnagogic hallucinations, sleep paralysis). A careful history usually allows specific causes of sleep disturbance to be identified and these are discussed in more detail on page 1179.

Weakness

Establishing the diagnosis in a patient with weakness requires the application of basic anatomy, physiology and some pathology to the interpretation of the history and clinical findings. Points to consider are shown in Box 26.10, while physical signs and different patterns of motor loss are described in Box 26.11 and Fig. 26.17.

Weakness in only some muscles in a limb suggests a problem in the peripheral nerve(s) or motor root(s). Weakness of the whole of one limb may be due to problems in the brachial or lumbosacral plexus, or to a central lesion. Weakness in both lower limbs (paraparesis) or in all four limbs (tetraparesis) suggests either a spinal cord lesion or a diffuse peripheral nerve problem such as Guillain–Barré syndrome (p. 1129). In such cases the condition of the reflexes is the most discriminating sign. The reflexes are absent in the Guillain–Barré syndrome (or other lower motor nerve lesions) and brisk in spinal cord (upper motor neuron) lesions. The paraparesis or tetraparesis of spinal cord lesions may be associated with a specific pattern of sensory loss (p. 1156) which gives a clue to the site of the cord lesion.

Patients with a bradykinetic limb often complain of weakness. Therefore if there are no reflex, wasting or

26.10 How to assess weakness

Distribution

- A few muscles
- A limb
- Both lower limbs (paraparesis)
- Both limbs on one side (hemiparesis)

Type of weakness

- Upper motor neuron lesion
- Lower motor neuron lesion

Evolution of the weakness

- Sudden and improving
- Gradually worsening over days or weeks
- Evolving over months or years

26.11 Physical signs in different types of motor deficit

Clinical sign	Upper motor (pyramidal) lesion	Lower motor lesion	Extrapyramidal lesion	Cerebellar lesion	Functional
Power	Weak Upper limbs: extensors weaker Lower limbs: flexors weaker	Weak	No weakness	No weakness	Give-way weakness
Wasting	None	Yes, after interval	None	None	None
Fasciculation	None	Yes, after interval	None	None	None
Tone	Spastic increase (after interval)	Flaccid from onset	Rigidity (cogwheel)	Normal/reduced	Normal
Reflexes	Increased	Reduced/absent	Normal	Normal	Normal
Plantar response	Extensor	Flexor	Flexor	Flexor	Flexor
Coordination	Reduced by weakness	Reduced by weakness	Normal (but slowed)	Impaired	Normal (may be laborious)

sensory changes when a patient is complaining of weakness in a limb, extrapyramidal signs of rigidity (cogwheel or leadpipe) and bradykinesia should be sought. Patients with Parkinson's disease usually present with symptoms in one limb that may be described as weak and clumsy, especially for fine manipulations. Often the typical rest tremor is a clue to the diagnosis.

Weakness down one side of the body (hemiparesis) is almost always due to a cerebral hemisphere lesion, although it can be caused by spinal cord or brain-stem lesions. The lesion is of upper motor neuron type, and the site and often the size of the lesion can be deduced by the coexistence of other signs and symptoms, such as higher cerebral function abnormalities or sensory change. The evolution of a motor deficit over time can give a clue to the underlying pathology (Box 26.12).

Some patients may present with weakness which is not due to organic disease but which is caused by psychiatric illness such as a conversion disorder (p. 251). This type of weakness does not conform to known pathophysiological patterns and the deficit cannot be attributed to a lesion in a specific anatomical site in the nervous system. During formal testing of power, a patient's strength may appear to 'give way', yet demon-

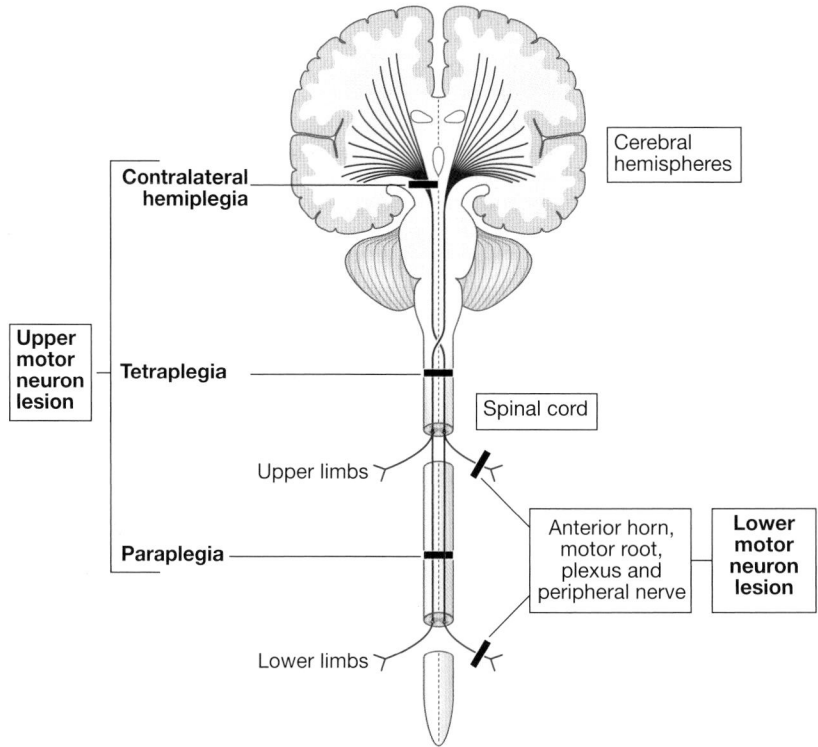

Fig. 26.17 Patterns of motor loss according to the anatomical site of the lesion.

26.12 Limb weakness: assessing the cause from typical patterns of evolution

Vascular lesions

• Sudden onset (over minutes) followed by a stable period and gradual recovery

Neoplastic lesions

• Gradual in onset and progressive over weeks or months

Inflammatory lesions

• Fairly acute in onset (over a few days), persist for a time and then improve (e.g. in multiple sclerosis)

Degenerative disorders

• Evolve over months or years (e.g. motor neuron disease or cervical spondylotic myelopathy)

strate bursts of full power at other times. Alternatively, if a 'weak' limb is held up and then suddenly allowed to drop, the limb may be momentarily held up, something which does not happen in organic weakness. Sometimes 'non-organic' weakness may occur in combination with weakness due to a neurological disorder and physical signs such as 'give-way weakness' therefore do not necessarily imply absence of pathology. Great care should therefore be exercised in making the diagnosis of functional weakness and all unusual manifestations of nervous system disease should be considered before such a diagnosis is made.

Abnormal gait

Many neurological disorders are associated with an abnormal gait and observing a patient walk can be very informative and assist in coming to a neurological diagnosis. It is also an important element of assessing disability. Various patterns of weakness, loss of coordination and proprioceptive sensory loss produce an abnormal gait. Neurogenic gait disorders need to be distinguished from those due to skeletal abnormalities, usually characterised by pain producing an antalgic gait, or limp. Gaits that do not fit either pattern may be due to psychiatric disorders and are usually incompatible with any anatomical or physiological deficit.

Pyramidal gait

Upper motor neuron lesions cause a so-called pyramidal gait in which the upper limb is held in flexion while the ankle joint in the lower limb is kept relatively extended. This causes a tendency for the toes to strike the ground while walking and in an attempt to overcome this, the leg is swung outwards at the hip (circumduction). Nevertheless, the affected foot still scuffs along the ground and the shoe on the affected side may be worn at the toes as evidence of this type of gait. In hemiplegia, the asymmetry between the affected and normal sides is obvious in walking, but in paraparesis both lower limbs swing slowly from the hips in extension and are dragged stiffly over the ground. This can often be heard as well as seen.

Foot drop

Toe strike follows heel strike in a normal gait. If there is a lower motor neuron lesion affecting the lower limb,

weakness of ankle dorsiflexion occurs, disrupting this pattern. The result is a less controlled descent of the foot which makes a slapping noise as it hits the ground. If the distal weakness is severe, the foot will have to be lifted higher at the knee to allow room for the inadequately dorsiflexed foot to swing through, resulting in a high-stepping gait.

Myopathic gait

During walking, alternating transfer of the body's weight through each leg requires careful control of hip abduction by the gluteal muscles. In proximal muscle weakness, usually caused by muscle disease, the hips are not properly fixed by these muscles and trunk movements are exaggerated, producing a rolling or waddling gait.

Ataxic gait

An ataxic gait can occur as the result of lesions in the cerebellum, vestibular apparature or peripheral nerves. Patients with lesions of the central portion of the cerebellum (the vermis) walk with a characteristic broad-based gait 'like a drunken sailor' (cerebellar function is particularly sensitive to alcohol). Patients with acute vestibular disturbances walk in a similar fashion, but the accompanying vertigo distinguishes them from those with cerebellar lesions. Less severe degrees of cerebellar ataxia can be detected by asking the patient to walk heel to toe; patients with vermis lesions are unable to do this. Defects in proprioception can also cause an ataxic gait. The impairment of joint position sense makes walking unreliable, especially in poor light. The feet tend to be placed on the ground with greater emphasis, presumably in an attempt to increase what proprioceptive input is available. This results in a 'stamping' gait which is often combined with foot drop when caused by a peripheral neuropathy, but it can also occur in disorders of the dorsal columns in the spinal cord.

Apraxic gait

In an apraxic gait, there is normal power in the legs, no cerebellar ataxia and no proprioception loss, and yet the patient still cannot formulate the motor act of walking. In this higher cerebral dysfunction, the feet appear stuck to the floor and the patient cannot walk, even though leg movement is normal on the examination couch. Gait apraxia occurs in bilateral hemisphere disease such as normal pressure hydrocephalus and diffuse frontal lobe disease.

Marche à petits pas

This gait is characterised by small, slow steps and marked instability. This looks different from the festinant gait of Parkinson's disease (see below) in that it does not have the variable pace and freezing. The usual cause is multiple small-vessel cerebrovascular disease and there are often signs of bilateral upper motor neuron disease.

Extrapyramidal gait

Patients with Parkinson's disease (p. 1199) and other extrapyramidal diseases have difficulty initiating walking and difficulty controlling the pace of their gait. Patients may get stuck whilst trying to start walking or when walking through doorways ('freezing'). Once started, they may shuffle and have problems controlling

26

the speed of their walking and sometimes have difficulty stopping. This produces the festinant gait: initial stuttering steps that quickly increase in frequency while decreasing in length.

Disorders of balance

Balance is a complicated process which involves modification of both axial and limb muscle function to compensate for the effects of gravity and alterations in body position and load (and hence centre of gravity) in order to prevent a person from falling. This process involves input from a variety of sensory modalities (visual, vestibular and proprioceptive), processing by the cerebellum and brain stem, and output via a number of descending pathways (e.g. vestibulospinal, rubrospinal and reticulospinal tracts). The process also results in a cognitive perception of vertical which is mediated through the cerebral cortex.

Disorders of balance can therefore arise from a number of different abnormalities which may affect input (loss of vision, vestibular disorders or lack of joint position sense), processing (damage to vestibular nuclei or cerebellum) or motor function (spinal cord lesions, leg weakness of any cause). The patient may complain of different symptoms depending on what is actually wrong. For example, loss of joint position sense or cerebellar function may result in a sensation of unsteadiness, while damage to the vestibular nuclei or labyrinth may result in vertigo which is an illusory sensation of movement (p. 1151). A careful history is vital. Patients may well have other associated symptoms depending on the site of damage, such as dysarthria in a cerebellar lesion. Since vision can often compensate for lack of joint position sense, patients with peripheral neuropathies or dorsal column loss will often find their problem more noticeable in the dark.

Examination of such patients may yield physical signs that depend on the site of the problem. Sensory abnormalities may be manifest as altered visual acuities or visual fields, possibly with abnormalities on fundoscopy, altered eye movements (including nystagmus), impaired vestibular function (p. 1171) or lack of joint position sense. Disturbance of cerebellar function may be manifest as nystagmus (p. 1165), dysarthria or ataxia, demonstrated as abnormalities of finger–nose testing or heel–shin testing, inability to perform alternating movements (dysdiadochokinesis) or difficulty with gait (unsteadiness or inability to perform tandem gait, p. 1153). Leg weakness, if present, will be detectable on examination of the limbs.

Abnormal movements

Abnormal movements are often caused by a disorder in the basal ganglia, in which there is disinhibition of the activity of intrinsic rhythm generators or a disorder of postural control. Some abnormal movements, like tremor, are commonplace and can be defined as a rhythmic oscillating movement of a limb or part of a limb, or of the head. Tremors can be usefully subclassified into action tremors and rest tremors. Action tremors are more common than rest tremors and the potential causes are

26.13 Causes of tremor on action

- Exaggerated physiological tremor (see Box 26.14)
- Essential tremor (may be familial)
- Parkinson's disease (rest tremor more usual)
- Wilson's disease
- Postural ('Holmes' or 'rubral') tremor
    Multiple sclerosis
    Other lesions in cerebellar outflow/red nucleus
- Intention tremor
    Cerebellar hemisphere disease

more numerous (Box 26.13). Other involuntary movements, like chorea, athetosis and dystonia, have become more common as a result of adverse effects from drugs used in the treatment of Parkinson's disease and psychiatric disease.

Rest tremor

This is pathognomonic of Parkinson's disease (p. 1199). The tremor is characteristically 'pill-rolling' and usually presents asymmetrically. However, patients with Parkinson's disease may have an abnormal action tremor as well. Tremor of the head in the upright position ('titubation') is not a rest tremor since this is a postural tremor, disappearing when the head is supported.

Physiological tremor

This is the most common type of action tremor and occurs at a frequency of 8–12 Hz. It is common in normal subjects and exaggeration occurs in anxiety and in the other situations listed in Box 26.14.

Essential tremor

Essential tremor is distinct from physiological tremor, but can resemble it superficially. It is slower and may become quite disabling. Essential tremor is often inherited and in some families is most obvious during certain specific actions such as writing or holding a glass; there is an overlap with focal dystonia (see below). Alcohol often suppresses essential tremor, sometimes to the extent that the patient becomes dependent. Centrally

26.14 Causes of exaggerated physiological tremor

Anxiety

Fatigue

Endocrine
- Thyrotoxicosis
- Cushing's disease
- Phaeochromocytoma
- Hypoglycaemia

Drugs
- β-agonists (e.g. salbutamol)
- Theophylline
- Caffeine
- Lithium
- Dopamine agonists
- Sodium valproate
- Tricyclics
- Phenothiazines
- Amphetamines

Toxins
- Mercury
- Lead
- Arsenic

Alcohol withdrawal

acting β-adrenoceptor antagonists (β-blockers) such as propranolol are often effective in treatment.

Intention tremor

This is characterised by oscillation at the end of a movement and typically occurs in cerebellar disease, due to the breakdown of control of targeted, ballistic movements. A more dramatic intention tremor occurs with lesions in the superior cerebellar peduncle (the site of the cerebellar outflow towards the red nucleus). Known variously as a 'peduncular', 'rubral' or 'Holmes' tremor, this is a violent, large-amplitude postural tremor that worsens as a target is approached. It is common in advanced multiple sclerosis and may be a source of considerable disability. Stereotactic thalamotomy can reduce the tremor, although the overall functional result is often disappointing.

Flapping tremor

Flapping tremor or asterixis is typical of metabolic disturbances (Box 26.15). It occurs as the result of intermittent failure of the parietal mechanisms required to maintain a posture. On attempts to hold the arms out with hands extended at the wrists, the posture is periodically dropped, allowing the hands to drop transiently before the posture is taken up again. Occasionally, unilateral asterixis can be seen in an acute parietal lesion, usually vascular.

26.15 Causes of asterixis

- Renal failure
- Liver failure
- Drug toxicity
- Hypercapnia
- Acute focal parietal or thalamic lesions

Chorea, athetosis and ballismus

Non-rhythmic involuntary movements may be combinations of fragments of purposeful movements and abnormal postures. All of these abnormal movements represent disorders of the balance of activity in the complex basal ganglia circuitry. Jerky, small-amplitude, purposeless involuntary movements are termed 'chorea' (the Greek for 'dance'). In the limbs they resemble fidgety movements, and in the face, grimaces; they suggest disease in the caudate nucleus (as in Huntington's disease, p. 1203) or excessive activity in the striatum due to dopaminergic drugs used to treat Parkinson's disease. There is a range of other causes (Box 26.16). More dramatic unilateral ballistic movements of the limbs (hemiballismus) can occur in vascular lesions of the subthalamic structures. Slower writhing movement of the limbs is called athetosis. This is often combined with chorea (and has a similar list of causes) and is then termed 'choreo-athetoid' movement.

Dystonia

The term 'dystonia' is used to describe sustained involuntary contraction that causes abnormal posture or movement. This may be generalised in various diseases of the basal ganglia, or may be focal or segmental as in spasmodic torticollis when the head involuntarily turns to one side. Other segmental dystonias may cause abnormal disabling postures of a limb to be taken up during certain specific actions, such as in writer's cramp or

26.16 Causes of chorea

Hereditary
- Huntington's disease
- Wilson's disease
- Neuroacanthocytosis
- Porphyria
- Paroxysmal choreoathetosis

Cerebral birth injury (including kernicterus)

Cerebral trauma

Drugs
- Levodopa
- Dopamine agonists
- Phenothiazines
- Tricyclics
- Oral contraceptive

Endocrine
- Pregnancy
- Oral contraceptive
- Thyrotoxicosis
- Hypoparathyroidism
- Hypoglycaemia

Infective/inflammatory
- Post-streptococcal (Sydenham's chorea)
- Henoch–Schönlein purpura
- Creutzfeldt–Jakob disease
- Antiphospholipid antibody syndrome
- Systemic lupus erythematosus (SLE)

Vascular
- Lacunar infarction
- Arteriovenous malformation

numerous other occupational 'cramps'. Segmental dystonias can be treated by the administration of botulinum toxin to a few of the responsible muscles, which seems to overcome the abnormal distribution of muscle activity for a period of time.

Myoclonus

Myoclonus refers to brief, isolated, random, non-purposeful jerks of muscle groups in the limbs. Myoclonic jerks occur normally at the onset of sleep (hypnic jerks). Similarly, a myoclonic jerk is a component of the normal startle response which may be exaggerated in some rare (mostly genetic) disorders. Unlike the movement disorders discussed so far, myoclonus may occur in disorders of the cerebral cortex, when groups of pyramidal cells fire spontaneously. Such myoclonus occurs in some forms of epilepsy in which the jerks are fragments of seizure activity. Alternatively, myoclonus can arise from subcortical structures or, more rarely, from diseased segments of the spinal cord. Myoclonus, especially of cortical origin, often responds to clonazepam, sodium valproate or piracetam.

Tics

Tics are repetitive semi-purposeful movements such as blinking, winking, grinning or screwing up of the eyes. They are distinguished from other involuntary movements by the ability of the patient to suppress their occurrence, at least for a short time. An isolated tic may be no more than a mild embarrassment, but may become frequent at certain times in childhood and then disappear. The uncommon syndrome of Gilles de la Tourette consists of a tendency to multiple tics and odd vocalisations, with obsessive behavioural abnormalities. The pathogenic basis is not understood, but there may be some response to major tranquillisers.

26

26

Sensory disturbance

Sensory symptoms are common but the accuracy of patients in describing sensory disturbances is very variable and so skill is often required to sift through the history in order to make anatomical and pathophysiological sense of the complaints. Although sensory symptoms are often due to neurological disease, this is not always the case; for example, tingling in the fingers of both hands and around the mouth can occur as the result of hyperventilation (p. 654) or hypocalcaemia (p. 765). Symptoms such as paraesthesia (tingling), numbness and pain may all be caused by damage to the afferent nervous pathways. When there is dysfunction of the cerebral mechanisms of somatic sensation there may be distortion of the patient's perception of the wholeness or actual presence of the relevant part of the body.

Numbness and paraesthesia

The most useful features on history are the anatomical distribution and mode of onset of the symptom. Certain patterns of onset of sensory symptoms can be recognised. For example, in a migraine attack the aura may consist of a front of tingling paraesthesia followed by numbness which takes 20–30 minutes to spread over one half of the body, often splitting the tongue. On the other hand, sensory loss due to a vascular lesion will occur more or less instantaneously and this is typically not associated with positive sensory phenomena like tingling. The rare, unpleasant paraesthesia of sensory epilepsy 'shoots' down one side of the body in seconds.

The numbness and paraesthesia of inflammatory spinal cord lesions often ascend from one or both lower limbs to a distinct level on the trunk over hours to days. Sensory symptoms of tingling and numbness can be of 'functional' or non-organic origin, as a manifestation of anxiety or as part of a conversion disorder (p. 251). The pattern of sensory symptoms in this circumstance usually does not conform to a known anatomical distribution or fit with any known pattern of sensory involvement in organic disease. As with weakness (see above), care should be taken to avoid misdiagnosing an unusual organic sensory impairment as a functional disorder.

Examination of the sensory system needs to be approached with care; it is easy to produce confusing false positive results because of the inescapably subjective nature of sensory testing. However, the distribution of sensory loss is often very useful in making a diagnosis when combined with the coexisting deficits of motor and/or cranial nerve function (Fig. 26.18).

Peripheral nerve lesions

Here the symptoms are usually of sensory loss and paraesthesia. Single nerve lesions cause disturbance in the sensory distribution of that nerve whereas in diffuse neuropathies the longest neurons are affected first, giving a characteristic 'glove and stocking' distribution. If the smaller nerve fibres are preferentially affected (e.g. in alcoholic neuropathy), temperature and pin-prick (pain) are lost, whilst vibration sense and proprioception (modalities served by the larger, well-myelinated, sensory nerves) may be spared. In contrast, vibration and proprioception are particularly affected if the

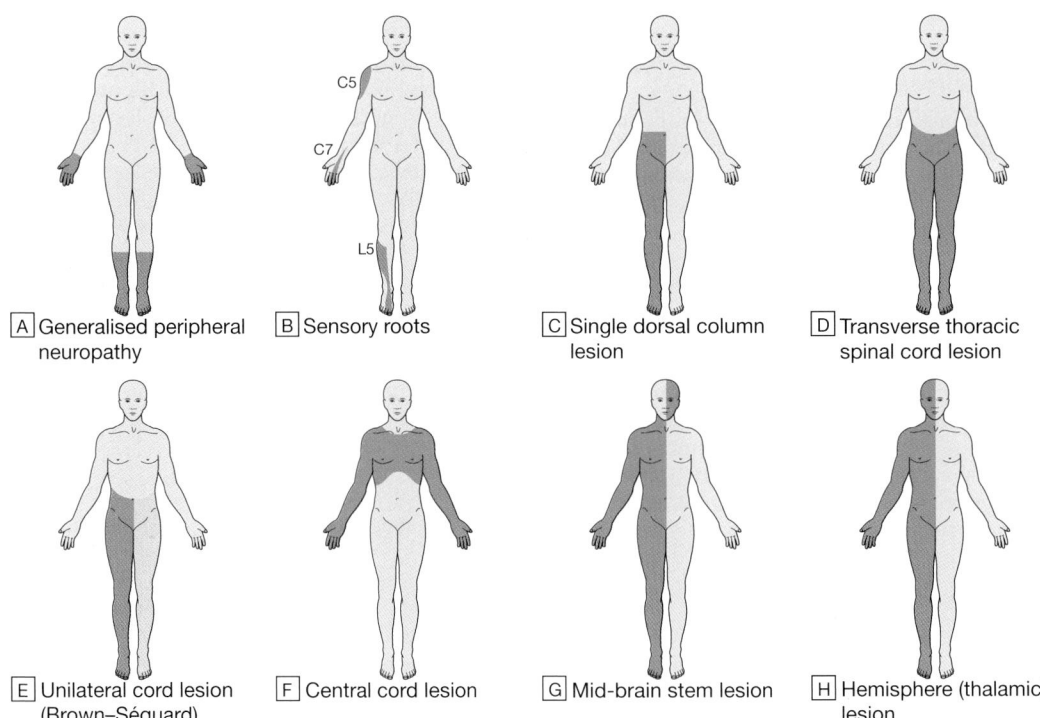

Fig. 26.18 Patterns of sensory loss. **A** Generalised peripheral neuropathy. **B** Sensory roots. **C** Single dorsal column lesion (proprioception and some touch loss). **D** Transverse thoracic spinal cord lesion. **E** Unilateral cord lesion (Brown–Séquard): ipsilateral dorsal column (and motor) deficit and contralateral spinothalamic deficit. **F** Central cord lesion: 'cape' distribution of spinothalamic loss. **G** Mid-brain stem lesion: ipsilateral facial sensory loss and contralateral loss on body below the vertex. **H** Hemisphere (thalamic) lesion: contralateral loss on one side of face and body.

neuropathy is demyelinating in character (p. 1226), producing symptoms of tightness and swelling with impairment of proprioception and vibration sensation.

Nerve root lesions

These typically present with pain as a prominent feature, either within the spine or in the limb plexuses. It is often felt in the muscles innervated by the root rather than the skin. The site of nerve root lesions may be deduced from the dermatomal pattern of sensory loss, although this is often smaller than would be expected because of the overlap of sensory 'territories'.

Spinal cord lesions

Transverse lesions of the spinal cord produce loss of all sensory modalities below that segmental level, although the level obtained clinically may differ from the level of the lesion by two or three segments. Very often there is a band of paraesthesia or hyperaesthesia at the top of the area of sensory loss. If the transverse lesion is vascular due to anterior spinal artery thrombosis, the posterior one-third of the spinal cord (the dorsal column modalities) may be spared, as this has a different blood supply.

Lesions damaging one side of the spinal cord will produce loss of spinothalamic modalities (pain and temperature) on the opposite side and of dorsal column modalities (joint position and vibration sense) on the same side of the body. This is the pattern seen in the Brown–Séquard syndrome (p. 1223).

Lesions in the centre of the spinal cord (such as syringomyelia (see Box 26.108 and Fig. 26.56 (p. 1225)) spare the dorsal columns but affect the spinothalamic fibres crossing the cord from both sides over the length of the lesion. The sensory loss is therefore dissociated (in terms of the modalities affected) and suspended (in the sense that segments above and below the lesion are spared), often with reflex loss if afferent fibres of the reflex arc within the cord are affected.

An isolated lesion of the dorsal columns is not uncommon in multiple sclerosis. This produces a characteristic unpleasant tight feeling over the limb(s) involved and, while there is no loss of pin-prick or temperature sensation, the associated loss of proprioception may severely affect the function of the limb(s).

Brain-stem lesions

Lesions in the brain stem can be associated with sensory loss, but the distribution depends on the site of the lesion. A lesion limited to the trigeminal nucleus or its sensory projections will cause sensory disturbance on that side of the face. For example, a picture resembling trigeminal neuralgia can be seen in young patients with multiple sclerosis. Because of the anatomy of the trigeminal connections, lesions in the medulla or spinal cord can give rise to 'balaclava helmet' patterns of sensory loss (p. 1140). The sensory pathways running up from the spinal cord can also be damaged in the brain stem, resulting in sensory loss of arm(s) and/or leg(s); the exact pattern depends on the site of the lesion.

Hemisphere lesions

Lesions in the hemispheres usually affect all modalities of sensation in the area(s) involved. In the thalamus, discrete lesions such as small lacunar strokes can cause isolated loss of sensation over the whole contralateral half of the body. Pure sensory loss from a lesion of the sensory cortex can occur, but the lesion has to be very small to avoid affecting the adjacent motor cortex or motor tracts deeper in the hemispheres; the resultant sensory loss is therefore usually restricted to a small area of the body such as the hand. A mixture of motor and sensory loss is much more common with cortical lesions. Substantial lesions of the parietal cortex (as in large strokes) can cause severe loss of proprioception and may even cause loss of conscious awareness of the existence of the affected limb(s). The resulting loss of function in the limb may be impossible to distinguish from paralysis.

Neuropathic pain

Neuropathic pain is caused by dysfunction of the pain perception apparatus itself, in contrast to nociceptive pain, which arises from a pathological process such as inflammation. Neuropathic pain has distinctive features and is typically described as a very unpleasant, persistent burning sensation. There is often increased sensitivity to touch, so that light brushing of the affected area causes exquisite pain (hyperpathia). Painful stimuli are felt as though they arise from a larger area than that touched and spontaneous bursts of pain may also occur. Pain may be elicited by other modalities such as loud sounds (allodynia) and this is considerably affected by emotional influences. The most common syndromes of neuropathic pain are seen where there is partial damage to a peripheral nerve ('causalgia'), to the trigeminal nerve (post-herpetic neuralgia) or to the thalamus. Treatment of these syndromes is very difficult. Drugs which modulate various parts of the nociceptive system, such as carbamazepine, tricyclics or phenothiazines, may help but usually only do so partially. Neurosurgical attempts to interrupt various pain pathways sometimes succeed but often increase the sensory deficit and may worsen the situation. Implantation of electrical stimulators has occasionally proved successful. For further information, see Chapter 12.

Coma

Persistent loss of consciousness or coma indicates disorder of the arousal mechanisms in the brain stem and diencephalon, and indicates bilateral hemisphere or brain-stem disease. There are many causes of coma (Box 26.17). The history of the mode of onset of coma and of any precipitating event is crucial to establishing the cause, and this should be obtained from family or other witnesses. As with any medical emergency, the top priority is assessment and stabilisation of the vital functions. Neurological examination may reveal important findings, such as evidence of head injury, papilloedema, meningism or an eye movement disorder. In the majority of cases, however, there are no focal neurological signs since drug overdose and metabolic disturbance are the most common causes of unexplained coma requiring hospital admission.

Assessment of conscious level is an essential component of the neurological examination of a comatose patient. This should include clear description of the patient's level of arousal and response to stimuli such as by application of the Glasgow Coma Scale (GCS) in which there is grading of coma using a numerical scale

26

26.17 Causes of coma

Metabolic disturbance

- Drug overdose
- Diabetes mellitus
  Hypoglycaemia
  Ketoacidosis
  Hyperosmolar coma
- Hyponatraemia

- Uraemia
- Hepatic failure
- Respiratory failure
- Hypothermia
- Hypothyroidism
- Thiamin deficiency

Trauma

- Cerebral contusion
- Extradural haematoma

- Subdural haematoma

Cerebrovascular disease

- Subarachnoid haemorrhage
- Brain-stem infarction/haemorrhage

- Intracerebral haemorrhage
- Cerebral venous sinus thrombosis

Infections

- Meningitis
- Encephalitis

- Cerebral abscess
- General sepsis

Others

- Epilepsy
- Brain tumour

- Functional ('pseudo-coma')

26.18 How to use the Glasgow Coma Scale

Eye-opening (E)

• Spontaneous	4
• To speech	3
• To pain	2
• Nil	1

Best motor response (M)

• Obeys	6
• Localises	5
• Withdraws	4
• Abnormal flexion	3
• Extensor response	2
• Nil	1

Verbal response (V)

• Orientated	5
• Confused conversation	4
• Inappropriate words	3
• Incomprehensible sounds	2
• Nil	1

Coma score = E + M + V

• Minimum	3
• Maximum	15

which permits serial comparison over time and may also provide prognostic information, particularly in traumatic coma (Box 26.18).

Brain death

Patents with prolonged coma as the result of severe and irreversible brain damage may nowadays survive for prolonged periods with supportive care and mechanical ventilation. In this situation diagnostic criteria for brain death have been established in order that patients

26.19 UK criteria for the diagnosis of brain death

Preconditions for considering a diagnosis of brain death

- The patient is deeply comatose
  (a) There must be no suspicion that coma is due to depressant drugs, such as narcotics, hypnotics, tranquillisers
  (b) Hypothermia has been excluded—rectal temperature must exceed 35 °C
  (c) There is no profound abnormality of serum electrolytes, acid–base balance or blood glucose concentrations, and any metabolic or endocrine cause of coma has been excluded
- The patient is maintained on a ventilator because spontaneous respiration had been inadequate or had ceased. Drugs, including neuromuscular blocking agents, must have been excluded as a cause of the respiratory failure
- The diagnosis of the disorder leading to brain death has been firmly established. There must be no doubt that the patient is suffering from irremediable structural brain damage

Tests for confirming brain death

- All brain-stem reflexes are absent
- The pupils are fixed and unreactive to light
- The corneal reflexes are absent
- The vestibulo-ocular reflexes are absent—there is no eye movement following the injection of 20 mL of ice-cold water into each external auditory meatus in turn
- There are no motor responses to adequate stimulation within the cranial nerve distribution
- There is no gag reflex and no reflex response to a suction catheter in the trachea
- No respiratory movement occurs when the patient is disconnected from the ventilator long enough to allow the carbon dioxide tension to rise above the threshold for stimulating respiration ($PaCO_2$ must reach 6.7 kPa (50 mmHg))

The diagnosis of brain death should be made by two experienced doctors, one of whom should be a consultant and the other a consultant or specialist registrar. The tests are usually repeated after an interval of 6–24 hours, depending on the clinical circumstances, before brain death is finally confirmed

without functioning brains who have no chance of recovery may be identified and have their ventilation discontinued. The diagnosis of brain death depends on meeting a set of preconditions, all of which must coexist, and then applying a series of clinical tests (Box 26.19), all of which must be fulfilled.

Acute confusional state

This is an extremely common disorder which occurs most often in the elderly. Patients demonstrate disturbance of arousal with a global impairment of mental function. This disturbance usually takes the form of drowsiness with disorientation, perceptual errors and muddled thinking. Patients typically fluctuate, and confusion is often worse at night. There may be associated emotional disturbance (anxiety, irritability or depression) or psychomotor changes (agitation, restlessness or retardation). The assessment and management of this condition is covered in more detail on page 171.

Memory loss

Loss of memory for a period of time may be due to a transient toxic confusional state, a psychological fugue state, the post-ictal period after seizure or the syndrome known as transient global amnesia. These are usually distinguished on the basis of the history. A period of amnesia often follows either a complex partial or a generalised seizure, and this may cause diagnostic confusion if the seizure was not witnessed—for example, if it occurred in sleep.

Transient global amnesia

This is a syndrome affecting predominantly middle-aged patients in which there is an abrupt, discrete loss of short-term memory function which lasts for a period of a few hours at most. During this time patients know who they are and can perform motor acts normally, but they act in a bemused way, repeatedly asking the same questions. During the attack there is retrograde amnesia for the events of the past few weeks. After 4–6 hours, memory function and behaviour return to normal but the patient has persistent, complete amnesia for the duration of the attack itself. There are none of the phenomena associated with seizures and, unlike epileptic amnesia, transient global amnesia tends not to recur. There are no associated cerebrovascular risk factors, making a vascular aetiology unlikely. Transient global amnesia is thought to be due to a benign process similar to that causing a migrainous aura, occurring in the hippocampus. The patient has no physical signs and further investigation may not be needed if epilepsy can be excluded.

Persistent amnesia

Patients with persistent memory disturbance should be assessed to exclude serious neurological disease. In general, memory problems which have been observed by relatives or colleagues are likely to be more significant than those of which only the patient is aware. Problems of concentration must be distinguished from true problems with memory, as concentration difficulties are much more likely to be due to underlying depressive or anxiety disorders.

It is important to determine for how long the problem has existed, and exactly which aspects of memory are affected. Complaints of getting lost or of forgetting to switch off burners on the kitchen stove are more likely to be significant than simply forgetting names. Disturbance of episodic memory (previously called 'short-term memory') must be distinguished from semantic memory (memory for concept-based knowledge unrelated to specific experiences). The former can be selectively impaired in Korsakoff's syndrome (often secondary to alcohol) or bilateral temporal lobe damage, but is seen in conjunction with other disturbance of cortical function in different types of dementia. Progressive deterioration over many months suggests the possibility of an underlying dementia, but it is important to take a full medical history to detect any underlying medical problem which could be responsible. A family history of a memory disorder such as dementia is clearly important.

It is important to look for features of depression (p. 233) in patients with memory loss for two reasons. First, depression can present as a 'pseudo-dementia' with concentration and memory impairment as a dominant feature, and this is often reversible with antidepressant medication. Second, many patients with dementia may develop depression in the early stages of their illness, and this is also potentially treatable.

Personality change

While this is most often due to psychiatric illness (Ch. 10), many neurological conditions present with altered personality and behaviour. This particularly applies to conditions which alter the function of the frontal lobes where control of executive function, movement and behaviour resides (see Box 26.1, p. 1136). Personality change due to a frontal lobe disorder may occur as the result of structural damage due to stroke, trauma, tumour or hydrocephalus or as the result of a metabolic disturbance.

Personality can be affected in three broad directions as a result of frontal lobe damage.

- Patients with mesial frontal lesions become increasingly withdrawn, unresponsive and mute (abulic), and this is often associated with urinary incontinence, gait apraxia and an increase in tone known as gegenhalten, in which the patient varies the resistance to movement in proportion to the force exerted by the examiner.
- Patients with lesions of the dorsolateral prefrontal cortex develop difficulties with speech and motor planning and organisation. This is known as dysexecutive syndrome.
- Those with orbitofrontal lesions of the frontal lobes become disinhibited, sometimes to the point of grandiosity, or exhibit irresponsible behaviour. Memory is substantially intact, and there may be focal physical signs such as a grasp reflex, palmomental response or pout. As the frontal lobe overlies the olfactory bulb and tracts, structural lesions such as tumours in the inferior frontal lobes may be associated with anosmia.

Personality can also be affected by damage to the temporal lobes, usually as a result of memory impairment. Disturbance to the cortical areas responsible for speech can result in speech difficulties which may be interpreted as changes in personality.

Speech and language disturbance

There are three broad categories of speech disturbance; dysphonia, which is usually caused by a local problem in the larynx; dysarthria, which can occur in association with lesions affecting the brain stem, muscle or cerebellum; and dysphasia, which is due to lesions of the cerebral cortex.

Dysphonia

Dysphonia is the term used to describe hoarse or whispered speech. This can occur because the vocal cords fail to generate sounds properly during speech, or can be due to a higher-level problem of vocal cord operation

26

(dystonia). The most common cause is laryngitis, but dysphonia can also result from a lesion of the 10th cranial nerve or a problem with the vocal cords.

Dysarthria

Dysarthria is characterised by poorly articulated or slurred speech and can occur in association with lesions of the cerebellum, brain-stem disease and lower cranial nerves, as well as in myasthenia and patients with muscle disease. Dysarthric patients have no problem with choice of words, but there is a defect in delivery of speech which can sometimes be unintelligible, depending on severity of the underlying disorder. The quality of the speech tends to differ somewhat depending on the cause, but it can be very difficult to distinguish the different types clinically (Box 26.20).

Dysphasia

Dysphasia (also termed aphasia) is a disorder of the language content of speech. It can occur with lesions over a wide area of the dominant hemisphere. The inability to produce the correct word is termed anomia. When patients with anomia are asked to name objects or parts of objects, either no word will be produced or the wrong word or a nonsense word will be produced (paraphasia). Dysphasia can be subclassified according to whether the speech output is 'fluent' or not. In fluent dysphasia, a normal or increased number of (wrong) words are produced, whereas in non-fluent dysphasia, verbal output is reduced. Patients with lesions anterior to the central (Rolandic) fissure have non-fluent aphasia whilst those with lesions posterior to the central fissure in the speech areas have a fluent aphasia (and are often mistakenly thought to be confused). If patients are tested for the comprehension of words and their ability to repeat, their aphasia can be further classified into distinct syndromes of aphasia which have localising and prognostic implications (Fig. 26.19).

If a patient is found to have difficulty with speech comprehension there is likely to be a lesion in the superior part of the posterior temporal lobe and/or the adjoining part of the parietal lobe (Wernicke's area). Patients with small lesions around the lateral (Sylvian) fissure will have difficulty with repetition, whilst those

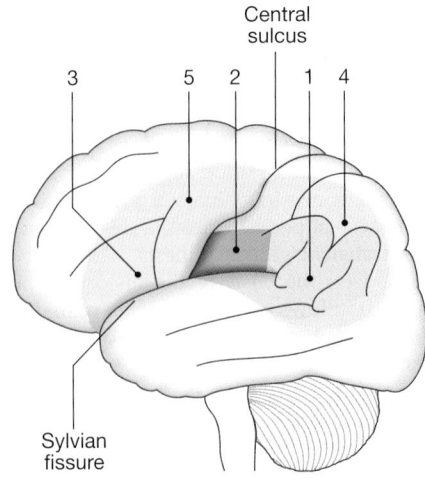

Fig. 26.19 Classification of aphasia, according to the site of the lesion and type of language deficit. All have naming difficulty (anomia). Fluent aphasias arise from lesions posterior to the central fissure; repetition is affected by lesions around the Sylvian fissure. (1) Wernicke aphasia: fluent aphasia with poor comprehension and poor repetition. (2) Conduction aphasia: fluent aphasia with good comprehension and poor repetition. (3) Broca aphasia: non-fluent aphasia with good comprehension and poor repetition. (4) Transcortical sensory aphasia: fluent aphasia with poor comprehension and good repetition. (5) Transcortical motor aphasia: non-fluent aphasia with good comprehension and good repetition. Large lesions affecting all of regions 1–5 cause global aphasia.

with lesions away from the Sylvian fissure can repeat and may do so compulsively. Patients with large lesions over much of the speech area are not testable in such a refined manner because they have no language production, and they are said to have 'global aphasia'. Patients with fluent aphasia tend not to have an associated hemiparesis since the pyramidal tract is not involved, whilst those with the more anteriorly placed lesions causing non-fluent aphasia often do have a hemiparesis.

Disorders of perception

The temporal, parietal and occipital lobes receive sensory information regarding the various different modalities

26.20 Causes of dysarthria

Type	Site	Characteristics	Associated features
Myopathic	Muscles of speech	Indistinct, poor articulation	Weakness of face, tongue and neck
Myasthenic	Motor end plate	Indistinct with fatigue and dysphonia Fluctuating severity	Ptosis, diplopia, facial and neck weakness
Bulbar	Brain stem	Indistinct, slurred, often nasal	Dysphagia, diplopia, ataxia
'Scanning'	Cerebellum	Slurring, impaired timing and cadence, 'sing-song' quality	Ataxia of limbs and gait, tremor of head/limbs Nystagmus
Spastic ('pseudo-bulbar')	Pyramidal tracts	Indistinct, breathy, mumbling	Poor rapid tongue movements, increased reflexes and jaw jerk
Parkinsonian	Basal ganglia	Indistinct, rapid, stammering, quiet	Tremor, rigidity, slow shuffling gait
Dystonic	Basal ganglia	Strained, slow, high-pitched	Dystonia, athetosis

of touch, vision, hearing and balance (see Box 26.1, p. 1136). The initial points of entry into the cortex are the respective primary cortical areas (see Fig. 26.4, p. 1137). Damage to any of these primary areas will result in reduction or loss of the ability to perceive that particular modality. This is referred to as 'negative' symptomatology. Abnormal excitation of these areas can occur in disorders such as epilepsy and migraine and result in an apparent perception which is not based in physical reality. Such 'positive' stimuli can be visual (flashing lights or formed images), somatosensory (tingling, burning or pain), auditory (noises) or vestibular (vertigo).

The parietal lobes are also involved in the higher processing and integration of the primary sensory information. This occurs in areas which may be highly specialised (e.g. the areas involved in the production and understanding of speech, p. 1159) or less specialised. Less specialised areas are referred to as 'association' cortex. Damage to the association cortex gives rise to sensory (including visual) inattention and disorders of spatial perception, and hence the disruption of spatially orientated behaviour leading to apraxia. Apraxia is the inability to perform complex, organised activity in the presence of normal basic motor, sensory and cerebellar function (after weakness, numbness and ataxia have been excluded as causes). Such complex activities include dressing, using cutlery and finding one's way around geographically. Other abnormalities which may result from damage to association cortex involve difficulty reading (dyslexia) or writing (dysgraphia), or the inability to detect that something is wrong (agnosia). The results of damage to particular lobes of the brain are given in Box 26.1 (p. 1136).

Brain-stem lesions

Lesions of the brain stem typically present with a constellation of symptoms due to cranial nerve, cerebellar and upper motor neuron dysfunction and are most commonly caused by vascular disease. This is because many different functional areas are tightly packed into the brain stem (p. 1137 and Fig. 26.5) and damage to even a small area causes major disturbance of several systems. Since the anatomy of the brain stem is very precisely organised, it is usually possible to localise the site of a lesion on the basis of careful history and examination to determine exactly which tracts/nuclei are affected. Lesions can occur singly, multiply or diffusely, but the standard neurological approach is to try to explain all of a patient's problems on the basis of a minimum number of lesions (ideally just one).

An example would be a patient presenting with sudden onset of upper motor neuron features affecting the right face, arm and leg in association with a left 3rd nerve palsy. The lesion would have to be in the left cerebral peduncle in the brain stem where the pathology is likely to have been a small stroke as the onset was sudden. This combination of signs is known as Weber's syndrome, and this is one of several well-described brain-stem syndromes which are listed in Box 26.21.

The effects of damage to the individual cranial nerves which arise in the brain stem, or to their nuclei, are discussed in the sections on eye movements (p. 1162) and on nerve and muscle, below (p. 1233). The lower cranial

26.21 Major focal brain-stem syndromes

Name of syndrome	Site of lesions	Clinical features
Weber	Anterior cerebral peduncle (mid-brain)	Ipsilateral 3rd palsy Contralateral upper motor neuron 7th palsy Contralateral hemiplegia
Claude	Cerebral peduncle involving red nucleus	Ipsilateral 3rd palsy Contralateral cerebellar signs
Parinaud	Dorsal mid-brain (tectum)	Vertical gaze palsy Convergence disorders Convergence retraction nystagmus Pupillary and lid disorders
Millard–Gubler	Ponto-medullary junction	Ipsilateral 6th palsy Ipsilateral lower motor neuron 7th palsy Contralateral hemiplegia
Wallenberg	Lateral medulla	Ipsilateral 5th, 9th, 10th, 11th palsy Ipsilateral Horner's syndrome Ipsilateral cerebellar signs Contralateral spinothalamic sensory loss Vestibular disturbance

nerves, 9, 10, 11 and 12, are frequently affected bilaterally, producing dysphagia (see below) and dysarthria (see above). The term 'bulbar palsy' is used if this results from lower motor neuron lesions, at either nuclear or fascicular level within the medulla, or from bilateral lesions of the lower cranial nerves outside the brain stem. The tongue is wasted and fasciculating and the palate moves very little. A 'pseudobulbar palsy' arises from an upper motor neuron lesion of the bulbar muscles from lesions of the corticobulbar pathways in the pyramidal tracts. Here the tongue is small and contracted, and moves

26.22 Causes of pseudobulbar and bulbar palsy

	Pseudobulbar	Bulbar
Genetic		Kennedy's disease (X-linked bulbo-spinal neuronopathy)
Vascular	Bilateral hemisphere (lacunar) infarction	Medullary infarction
Degenerative	Motor neuron disease (p. 1204)	Motor neuron disease Syringobulbia
Inflammatory/ infective	Multiple sclerosis (p. 1191) Cerebral vasculitis	Myasthenia (p. 1231) Guillain–Barré (p. 1229) Poliomyelitis (p. 1210) Lyme disease (p. 329) Vasculitis
Neoplastic	High brain-stem tumours	Brain-stem glioma Malignant meningitis

slowly; the jaw jerk is brisk. Causes of bulbar and pseudobulbar palsies are shown in Box 26.22.

Swallowing difficulty

Swallowing is a complex activity involving the coordinated action of lips, tongue, soft palate, pharynx and larynx, which are innervated by the facial nerve and cranial nerves 9, 10, 11 and 12. This mechanism is potentially vulnerable to damage in many different areas of the nervous system, resulting in dysphagia which is usually accompanied by dysarthria. Structural causes of dysphagia are considered on page 850. Acute onset of dysphagia may occur as a result of brain-stem stroke, a rapidly developing neuropathy such as the Guillain–Barré syndrome or diphtheria. The upper motor neuron innervation of the cranial nerves responsible for swallowing is bilateral, so persistent dysphagia is unusual with a unilateral upper motor lesion. However, dysphagia may occur in the early stages of such a lesion if it is very acute, such as a hemispheric stroke. Dysphagia developing subacutely may be seen in myasthenia gravis, motor neuron disease, polymyositis, basal meningitis and inflammatory brain-stem disease. More slowly developing dysphagia suggests a myopathy or possibly a brain-stem or skull-base tumour.

Visual disturbance and other ocular abnormalities

Disturbances of vision are common and often related to problems with the eye rather than disorders of the nervous system. A common reason for presentation is loss of vision, but patients may also present with positive visual symptoms, such as hallucinations. The movements of both eyes may be disturbed giving rise to double vision (diplopia) or blurred vision. Alternatively, patients may present with disordered appearance of their visual apparatus, which includes the eyelids, the globe, the eye movements, the pupils or the appearance of the optic disc on fundoscopy (e.g. papilloedema).

Visual loss

Visual loss can occur as the result of lesions anywhere from the retina to the visual cortex. Fibres from ganglion cells in the retina pass to the optic disc and then backwards through the lamina cribrosa to the optic nerve. Nasal optic nerve fibres (subserving the temporal visual field because the image on the retina is inverted) cross at the chiasm, but temporal fibres do not. Hence, all fibres in the optic tract and further posteriorly subserve both eyes' representation of contralateral visual space. From the lateral geniculate nucleus, lower fibres pass through the temporal lobes on their way to the primary visual area in the occipital cortex, while the upper fibres pass through the parietal lobe. Patterns of visual field loss are explained by this anatomy, as seen in Figure 26.20, and associated clinical manifestations are described in Box 26.23.

Transient visual loss is quite common and sudden visual loss lasting less than about 15 minutes is likely to have a vascular cause. This can affect one eye (amaurosis fugax) or one visual hemifield. Whether the field loss was monocular (carotid circulation) or a homonymous hemianopia (vertebro-basilar circulation) is crucial to further management, and this must be distinguished by careful history (e.g. did the patient try shutting each eye in turn?). Transient visual loss lasting about 20–30 minutes suggests migraine, especially if accompanied by headache and/or positive visual phenomena.

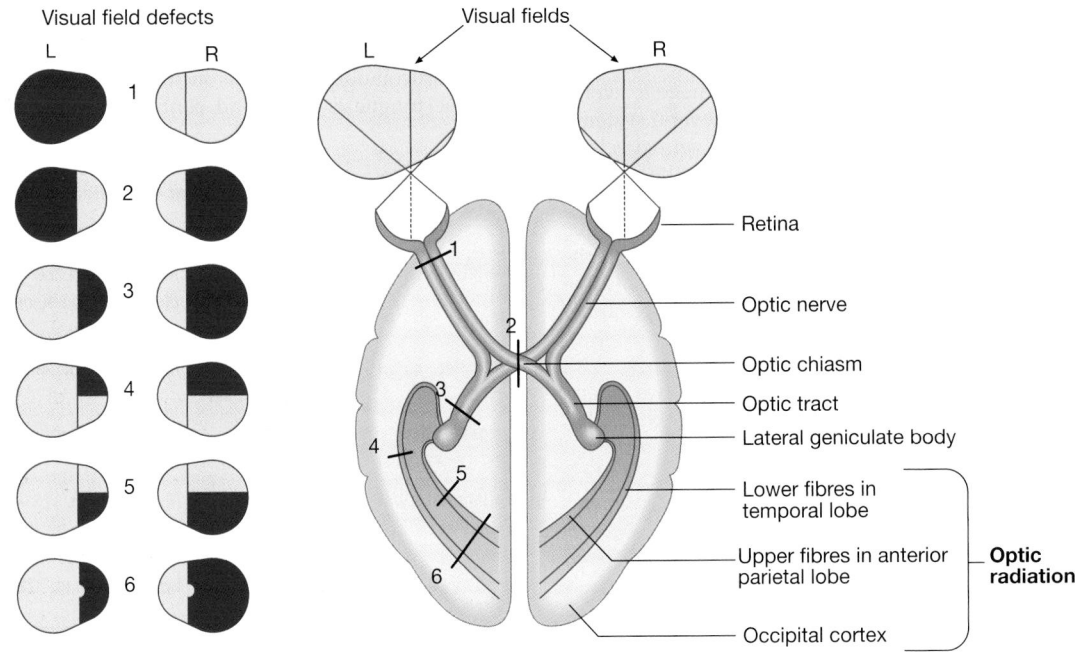

Fig. 26.20 Visual pathways and visual field defects. Schematic representation of eyes and brain in transverse section.

26.23 Clinical manifestations of visual field loss

Site	Common causes	Complaint	Visual field loss	Associated physical signs
Retina/optic disc	Vascular disease (including vasculitis) Glaucoma Inflammation	Partial/complete visual loss depending on site	Altitudinal field defect Arcuate scotoma	Reduced acuity Visual distortion (macula) Abnormal retinal appearance
Optic nerve	Optic neuritis Sarcoidosis Tumour Leber's hereditary optic neuropathy	Partial/complete loss of vision in one eye Often painful Central vision particularly affected	Central scotoma Paracentral scotoma Monocular blindness	Reduced acuity Reduced colour vision Relative afferent pupillary defect Optic atrophy (late)
Optic chiasm	Pituitary tumours Craniopharyngioma Sarcoidosis	May be none Rarely diplopia ('hemifield slide')	Bitemporal hemianopia	Pituitary function abnormalities
Optic tract	Tumour Inflammatory disease	Disturbed vision to one side of midline	Incongruous contralateral homonymous hemianopia	
Temporal lobe	Stroke Tumour Inflammatory disease	Disturbed vision to one side of midline	Contralateral homonymous upper quadrantanopia	Memory/language disorders
Parietal lobe	Stroke Tumour Inflammatory disease	Disturbed vision to one side of midline Bumping into things	Contralateral homonymous lower quadrantanopia	Contralateral sensory disturbance Asymmetry of optokinetic nystagmus
Occipital lobe	Stroke Tumour Inflammatory disease	Disturbed vision to one side of midline Difficulty reading Bumping into things	Homonymous hemianopia (may be macula-sparing)	Damage to other structures supplied by posterior cerebral circulation

Visual disturbance

The most common cause of a visual disturbance is migraine, in which patients may see silvery zigzag lines (fortification spectra) or flashing coloured lights (teichopsia) which precede the headache. Simple flashes of light (phosphenes) can also be seen as a result of damage to the retina (e.g. detachment) or damage to the primary visual cortex. Visual hallucinations may also be caused by drugs, or may be due to structural damage resulting in epilepsy or 'release phenomena', such as hallucinations which can occur in a blind visual field.

Double vision

Double vision (diplopia) arises when eye movement is impaired so that the image of an object is not projected to homologous points on the two retinae. This may result from central disorders or from disturbance of the ocular motor nerves, muscles or the neuromuscular junction. The pattern of double vision, along with any associated features, usually allows localisation of the lesion, whilst the mode of onset and subsequent behaviour (such as fatigability in myasthenia) can give a clue to the underlying cause.

Under normal circumstances, the eyes move conjugately, though horizontal vergence allows visual fusion of objects at different distances. The control of eye movements begins in the cerebral hemispheres, particularly within the frontal eye fields, and the pathway then descends to the brain stem with input from the visual cortex, superior colliculus and cerebellum. Horizontal and vertical gaze centres in the pons and midbrain, respectively, coordinate output to the ocular motor nerve nuclei (3, 4 and 6), which are connected to each other by the medial longitudinal fasciculus (MLF) (Fig. 26.21). The MLF is particularly important in coordinating horizontal movements of the eyes. The extraocular muscles are then supplied by the oculomotor (3rd), trochlear (4th) and abducens (6th) nerves.

The trochlear (4th) nerve innervates the superior oblique muscle, and the abducens (6th) nerve innervates the lateral rectus. The oculomotor (3rd) nerve innervates the remainder of the extraocular muscles along with the levator palpebrae superioris and the ciliary body (pupil constriction and accommodation). Causes of ocular motor nerve palsies are listed in Box 26.24.

Complete oculomotor (3rd) nerve lesions cause ptosis and a dilated pupil, and the eye tends to rest in a 'down and out' position due to unopposed tonic activity of the unaffected lateral rectus and superior oblique muscles. The pupil is often spared in ischaemic lesions (e.g. in diabetes), and its involvement requires that compressive lesions such as aneurysm be excluded. Trochlear (4th) nerve palsy presents with vertical diplopia (especially noticeable going downstairs), and the patient may have a head tilt to the contralateral side and double vision when looking down to the side opposite the lesion. Abducens (6th) nerve palsy causes horizontal double vision when trying to look towards the side of the lesion. In diplopia of any cause, the image projected furthest away from primary position arises from the paretic eye, and covering each eye in turn can often determine this.

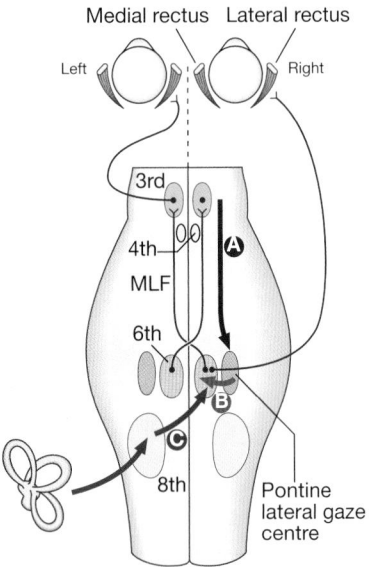

Medial rectus   Lateral rectus

Left   Right

3rd

4th

MLF

6th

8th

Pontine
lateral gaze
centre

Ⓐ

Ⓑ

Ⓒ

Fig. 26.21 Control of conjugate eye movements. Downward
projections pass from the cortex to pontine lateral gaze centre (A).
Pontine gaze centre projects to the 6th cranial nerve nucleus (B),
which innervates the ipsilateral lateral rectus and projects to the
contralateral 3rd nerve nucleus (and hence medial rectus) via the medial
longitudinal fasciculus (MLF). Tonic inputs from the vestibular apparatus
(C) project to the contralateral 6th nerve nucleus via the vestibular
nuclei.

Note that this image is not necessarily any less clear than
the image from the non-paretic eye; it is the relative position, not the clarity, of the images which is important in
determining which muscle is weak.

Myasthenia gravis (p. 1231) can cause diplopia by
affecting any or all of the extraocular muscles. It is often
associated with ptosis, and the hallmark is fatigability.
Similarly, diseases of the extraocular muscles themselves can cause diplopia. These include thyroid eye disease, myopathies and orbital myositis.

Central lesions can also give rise to diplopia. Brain-
stem lesions affecting the 3rd, 4th or 6th nerves or nuclei
will cause diplopia, as will lesions of the MLF. The
hallmark of an MLF lesion is an internuclear ophthalmoplegia (INO), most commonly seen in multiple sclerosis
(p. 1194). The lateral gaze centre in the pons sends fibres
to the ipsilateral 6th nerve nucleus. The nucleus contains
two populations of neurons. Half the cells send their
axons directly into the 6th nerve to supply the lateral
rectus, while the remaining half send their fibres into the
contralateral MLF and up to the contralateral 3rd nerve
nucleus, where they synapse with neurons destined for
the medial rectus (see Fig. 26.21). Hence, damage to the
6th nerve nucleus itself will prevent both eyes from moving ipsilaterally (gaze palsy), and a lesion of the MLF will
interfere with adduction of the ipsilateral eye (INO). In
this situation, the ipsilateral eye will either fail to adduct
past midline if the lesion is complete, or adduct very
slowly if it is partial. Nystagmus may sometimes be seen

26.24 Common causes of damage to cranial nerves 3, 4 and 6

Site	Common pathology	Nerve(s) involved	Associated features
Brain stem	Infarction Haemorrhage Demyelination Intrinsic tumour	3 (midbrain) 6 (ponto-medullary junction)	Contralateral pyramidal signs Ipsilateral lower motor neuron facial palsy Other brain-stem/cerebellar signs
Intrameningeal	Meningitis (infective/malignant)	3, 4 and/or 6	Meningism, features of primary disease course
	Raised intracranial pressure	6 3 (uncal herniation)	Papilloedema Features of space-occupying lesion
	Aneurysms	3 (posterior communicating artery) 6 (basilar artery)	Pain Features of subarachnoid haemorrhage
	Cerebello-pontine angle tumour	6	8, 7, 5 nerve lesions Ipsilateral cerebellar signs
	Trauma	3, 4 and/or 6	Other features of trauma
Cavernous sinus	Infection/thrombosis Carotid artery aneurysm Caroticocavernous fistula	3, 4 and/or 6	May be 5th nerve involvement also Pupil may be fixed, mid-position (sympathetic plexus on carotid may also be affected)
Superior orbital fissure	Tumour (e.g. sphenoid wing meningioma) Granuloma	3, 4 and/or 6	May be proptosis, chemosis
Orbit	Vascular (e.g. diabetes, vasculitis) Infections Tumour Granuloma Trauma	3, 4 and/or 6	Pain Pupil often spared in vascular 3rd nerve palsy

in the other (abducting) eye, giving rise to the archaic term 'ataxic nystagmus'.

Nystagmus

Nystagmus is the term given to describe a repetitive to-and-fro movement of the eyes. Usually the drifts are slower than the corrections giving rise to slow and fast phases. Nystagmus occurs because the control systems of the eyes are defective, causing them to drift off target; corrections then become necessary to return fixation to the object of interest, causing nystagmus. The direction of the fast phase is usually designated as the direction of the nystagmus because it is easier to see, although the abnormality is the slower drift of the eyes off target. Nystagmus may be horizontal, vertical or torsional, and is usually conjugate in that both eyes move together. Nystagmus is seen as a physiological phenomenon in response to sustained vestibular stimulation or movement of the visual world (optokinetic nystagmus). There are many different causes of pathological nystagmus, the most common being disorders of the vestibular system, the brain stem and the cerebellum.

In lesions of the vestibular system, damage to the horizontal canal or its connections on one side will allow the tonic output from the healthy, contralateral side to cause the eyes to drift towards the side of the lesion. This causes recurrent compensatory fast movements away from the side of the lesion; hence unidirectional horizontal nystagmus to the opposite side is seen. Vertical and torsional components can be seen with damage to other parts of the vestibular apparatus. The nystagmus of peripheral labyrinthine lesions disappears (fatigues) quite quickly and is always accompanied by vertigo and quite often nausea and vomiting. Central vestibular nystagmus is more persistent.

The brain stem and the cerebellum are involved in maintaining eccentric positions of gaze. Lesions will therefore allow the eyes to drift back in towards primary position. This produces nystagmus whose fast component beats in the direction of gaze (gaze-evoked nystagmus). This is the most common type of 'central' nystagmus and is most commonly bi-directional and not usually accompanied by vertigo, but there may be other signs of brain-stem dysfunction. Brain-stem disease may also cause vertical nystagmus.

Unilateral cerebellar lesions may result in gaze-evoked nystagmus when looking in the direction of the lesion, where the fast phases are directed towards the side of the lesion. Cerebellar hemisphere lesions also cause 'ocular dysmetria', an overshoot of target-directed, fast eye movements (saccades) resembling 'past-pointing' in limbs.

Nystagmus also occurs as a result of toxicity (especially drugs) and nutritional (thiamin) deficiency. The severity is variable, and it may or may not result in visual degradation, though it may be associated with a sensation of movement of the visual world (oscillopsia). Nystagmus may occur as a congenital phenomenon, in which case the nystagmus is often quasi-sinusoidal ('pendular') rather than having alternating fast and slow phases ('jerk').

Ptosis

Various disorders may cause drooping of the eyelid (ptosis) and these are listed in Box 26.25.

Abnormal pupillary responses

Abnormalities of the pupil or its response to light can develop as the result of lesions at several points between the retina and brain stem. The pupillary response to light is due to a combination of parasympathetic and sympathetic activity. Parasympathetic fibres originate in the Edinger–Westphal subnucleus of the 3rd nerve, and pass with the 3rd nerve to synapse in the ciliary ganglion before supplying the constrictor pupillae of the iris. Sympathetic fibres originate in the hypothalamus, pass down the brain stem and cervical spinal cord to emerge at T1, return up to the eye in association with the internal carotid artery and supply the dilator pupillae. Lesions in the sympathetic pathway cause Horner's syndrome (Fig. 26.22). The pupils also constrict as part of the near reflex (in association with accommodation and convergence).

Lesions of the oculomotor nerve, ciliary ganglion and sympathetic supply produce characteristic 'efferent' disorders of pupillary function. 'Afferent' defects

26

26.25 Common causes of ptosis

Mechanism	Causes	Associated clinical features
3rd nerve palsy	Isolated palsy (see Box 26.24) Central/supranuclear lesion	Ptosis is usually complete Extraocular muscle palsy (eye 'down and out') Depending on site of lesion, other cranial nerve palsies (e.g. 4, 5 and 6) or contralateral upper motor neuron signs
Sympathetic lesion (Horner's syndrome) (see Fig. 26.22)	Central (hypothalamus/brain stem) Peripheral (lung apex, carotid artery pathology) Idiopathic	Ptosis is partial Lack of sweating on affected side Depending on site of lesion, brain-stem signs, signs of apical lung/brachial plexus disease, or ipsilateral carotid artery stroke
Myopathic	Myasthenia gravis Dystrophia myotonica	Extraocular muscle palsies More widespread muscle weakness, with fatigability in myasthenia Progressive external ophthalmoplegia Other characteristic features of individual causes
Other	Pseudo-ptosis (e.g. blepharospasm) Local orbital/lid disease Age-related levator dehiscence	Eyebrows depressed rather than raised May be local orbital abnormality

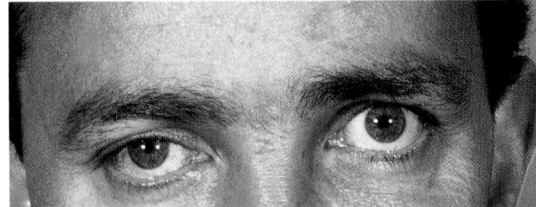

Fig. 26.22 Right-sided Horner's syndrome due to paravertebral metastasis at T1. There is ipsilateral partial ptosis and a small pupil.

occur as a result of damage to an optic nerve, impairing the direct response of a pupil to light, although leaving the consensual response from stimulation of the normal eye intact. Structural damage to the iris itself can also result in pupillary abnormalities. A summary is given in Box 26.26.

Papilloedema

There are several causes of swelling of the optic disc, but the term 'papilloedema' is reserved for swelling in association with raised intracranial pressure. In raised intracranial pressure from any cause, axoplasmic flow from retinal ganglion cells is held up at the cribriform plate. This results in swollen nerve fibres, which in turn cause capillary and venous congestion, producing papilloedema. The first sign is the cessation of normal venous pulsation seen at the disc, and the disc margins then become red (hyperaemic). The margins become indistinct and the whole disc is raised up, often with haemorrhages in the retina (Fig. 26.23).

Other causes of optic disc swelling are listed in Box 26.27. Some normal variations of disc appear-

ance can look like pathological disc swelling (pseudo-papilloedema).

Optic atrophy

Loss of nerve fibres causes the optic disc to appear pale, as the choroid becomes visible (Fig. 26.24). A pale disc (optic atrophy) follows optic nerve damage, and causes

26.27 Common causes of optic disc swelling

Raised intracranial pressure

- Cerebral mass lesion (tumour, abscess)
- Hydrocephalus, haemorrhage, haematoma
- Idiopathic intracranial hypertension

Obstruction of ocular venous drainage

- Central retinal vein occlusion
- Cavernous sinus thrombosis

Systemic disorders affecting retinal vessels

- Hypertension
- Vasculitis
- Hypercapnia

Optic nerve damage

- Demyelination (optic neuritis/papillitis)
- Leber's hereditary optic neuropathy
- Anterior ischaemic optic neuropathy
- Toxins (e.g. methanol)
- Infiltration of optic disc
- Sarcoidosis
- Glioma
- Lymphoma

26.26 Pupillary disorders

Disorder	Cause	Ophthalmological features	Associated features
3rd nerve palsy	See Box 26.24	Dilated pupil Extraocular muscle palsy (eye is typically 'down and out') Complete ptosis	Other features of 3rd nerve palsy (see Box 26.25)
Horner's syndrome (see Fig. 26.22)	Lesion to sympathetic supply	Small pupil Partial ptosis Iris heterochromia (if congenital)	Ipsilateral failure of sweating (anhidrosis)
Holmes–Adie syndrome (tonic pupil)	Lesion of ciliary ganglion (usually idiopathic)	Dilated pupil Light-near dissociation (accommodate but do not react to light) Vermiform movement of iris during contraction Disturbance of accommodation	Generalised areflexia
Argyll Robertson pupil	Dorsal mid-brain lesion (syphilis or diabetes)	Small, irregular pupils Light-near dissociation	Other features of tabes dorsalis (p. 1213)
Local pupillary damage	Trauma/inflammatory disease	Irregular pupils, often with adhesions to lens (synechiae) Variable degree of reactivity	Other features of trauma/ underlying inflammatory disease (e.g. cataract, blindness etc.)
Relative afferent pupillary defect (Marcus Gunn pupil)	Damage to optic nerve (see Box 26.23, p. 1163)	Pupils symmetrical, but degree of dilatation depends on which eye stimulated	Decreased visual acuity/colour vision Central scotoma Papilloedema/optic disc pallor

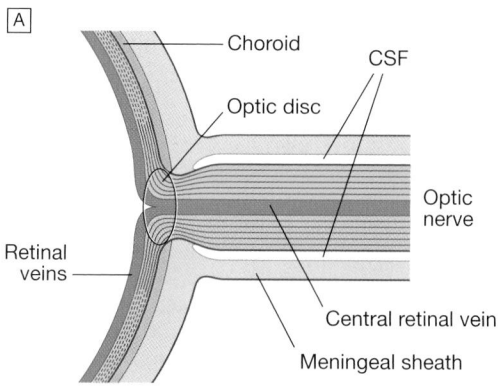

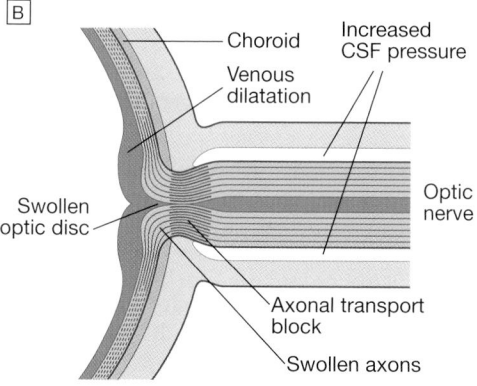

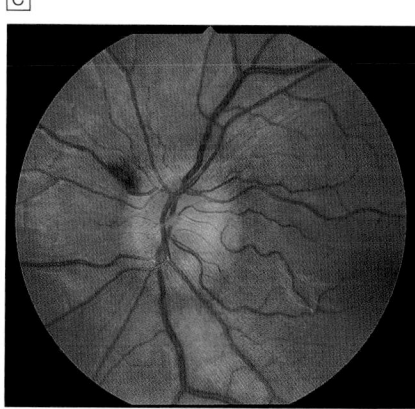

Fig. 26.23 Mechanism of optic disc oedema (papilloedema).
[A] Normal. [B] Disc oedema (e.g. due to cerebral tumour). [C] Fundus photograph of the left eye showing optic disc oedema with a small haemorrhage on the nasal side of the disc.

include previous optic neuritis or ischaemic damage, long-standing papilloedema, optic nerve compression, trauma and degenerative conditions (e.g. Friedreich's ataxia, p. 1203).

Sphincter disturbance

Incontinence and its management are discussed on pages 476 and 915. However, many different symptoms of bladder and bowel disturbance can arise as a result of nervous system dysfunction.

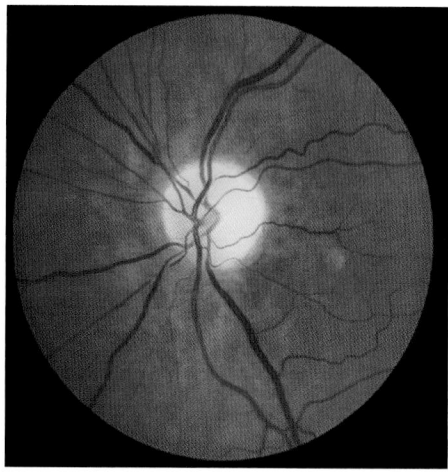

Fig. 26.24 Fundus photograph of the left eye of a patient with familial optic atrophy. Note marked pallor of optic disc.

Bladder dysfunction

The bladder is analogous to skeletal muscle in that neural control can be divided into upper and lower 'motor neuron' components. Conscious control of micturition resides within the pre-frontal cortex. Connections pass from here to the main controlling and coordinating centre in the pons, the pontine micturition centre, and from here down into the spinal cord, where they are found in the lateral columns bilaterally. The sympathetic supply to the bladder leaves from T10–L2 to synapse in the inferior hypogastric plexus, while the parasympathetic supply leaves from S2–4. In addition, a further somatic supply to the distal (voluntary) sphincter arises from S2–4, travelling via the pudendal nerves. Stimulation of sympathetic fibres causes relaxation of the detrusor muscle and contraction of the bladder neck, while stimulation of the parasympathetic fibres causes the reverse effects.

Afferent fibres from the bladder wall pass via the pelvic and hypogastric nerves. In the absence of conscious control (stroke, dementia), distension of the bladder to near-capacity evokes reflex detrusor contraction (analogous to the muscle stretch reflex). Reciprocal changes in sympathetic activation and relaxation of the distal sphincter result in coordinated bladder emptying. Normally, however, conscious control from the medial pre-frontal cortex inhibits bladder emptying until it is socially acceptable.

Damage to the 'lower motor neuron' component (the pelvic and pudendal nerves) gives rise to a flaccid bladder and sphincter with overflow incontinence, often accompanied by loss of pudendal sensation. Such damage may be due to disease of the conus medullaris or sacral nerve roots, either within the dura (as in inflammatory or carcinomatous meningitis) or as they pass through the sacrum (trauma or malignancy), or due to damage to the nerves themselves in the pelvis (infection, haematoma, trauma or malignancy).

Damage to the pons or spinal cord results in an 'upper motor neuron' pattern of bladder dysfunction due to uncontrolled overactivity of the parasympathetic supply. The bladder is small and highly sensitive to being stretched (analogous to spasticity). This results in frequency, urgency and urge incontinence.

26

Loss of the coordinating control of the pontine micturition centre will also result in the phenomenon of detrusor–sphincter dyssynergia, where detrusor contraction and sphincter relaxation are not coordinated; the spastic bladder will often try to empty against a closed sphincter. This manifests as both urgency and an inability to pass urine, which is distressing and painful, and may last some minutes before partial emptying of the bladder is achieved. There is often a post-micturition residuum of urine which is prone to infection, and the prolonged high bladder pressure may result in renal failure. More severe lesions of the spinal cord, as in spinal cord compression or trauma, can result in urinary retention; this will be painless as bladder sensation, normally carried in the lateral spinothalamic tracts, will be cut off.

Damage to the mesial frontal lobes gives rise to loss of awareness of bladder fullness and consequent incontinence. Coexisting cognitive impairment may result in inappropriate micturition. These features are seen typically in hydrocephalus, frontal tumours, dementia and bifrontal subdural haematomas.

When faced with a patient who has bladder symptoms, it is important to try to localise the lesion on the basis of history and examination, remembering that most bladder problems are not neurological unless there are overt neurological signs. Clinical features are summarised in Box 26.28.

Management of bladder disturbance involves identifying the cause and correcting it if possible. Overactive (spastic) bladders are common in neurological disease, and the unwanted detrusor activity (and hence urgency) can be lessened by anticholinergic drugs such as oxybutynin, tolterodine or imipramine. However, this will not solve the problem of detrusor-sphincter dyssynergia, and it may be necessary to teach the patient how to perform intermittent clean self-catheterisation (ISC); by emptying the bladder regularly, urinary frequency is reduced, as is the likelihood of infection. Bladder ultrasound is often helpful in this regard; a large (> 100 mL) post-micturition residual volume suggests that ISC will be necessary. Flaccid bladders are less common and unfortunately there is no effective drug treatment. These patients therefore need to perform ISC. Long-term catheterisation (urethral or suprapubic) may be necessary in either spastic or flaccid bladders, but this is avoided if at all possible as it is associated with increased infection as well as blockage.

Rectal dysfunction

The rectum has an excitatory cholinergic input from the parasympathetic sacral outflow, and inhibitory sympathetic supply similar to the bladder. Continence depends largely on skeletal muscle contraction in the puborectalis and pelvic floor muscles supplied by the pudendal nerves, as well as the internal and external anal sphincters. Damage to the autonomic components usually causes constipation but diabetic neuropathy can be associated with diarrhoea. Lesions affecting the conus medullaris, the somatic S2–4 roots and the pudendal nerves cause faecal incontinence.

Erectile failure and ejaculatory failure

These related functions are under autonomic control via the pelvic nerves (parasympathetic, S2–4) and hypogastric nerves (sympathetic, L1–2). Descending influences from the cerebrum are important for psychogenic erection, but erection can occur as a purely reflex phenomenon in response to genital stimulation. Erection is largely parasympathetic, mediated by nitric oxide, and is impaired by drugs which have anticholinergic effects and also by some antihypertensive and antidepressant agents. Sympathetic activity is important for ejaculation, and may be inhibited by α-adrenoceptor antagonists (α-blockers). For further information on erectile impotence, see page 477.

HEADACHE SYNDROMES

Headaches are often classified as primary or secondary, depending on the underlying cause (see Box 26.4, p. 1148). There are many causes of secondary headache due to structural, infective, inflammatory or vascular conditions, but these are dealt with elsewhere. The primary

---

26.28 Neurogenic bladder: clinical features and treatment

	Site of lesion	Result	Treatment
Atonic (lower motor neuron)	Lesions of sacral segments of cord (conus medullaris) Lesions of sacral roots and nerves	Loss of detrusor contraction Difficulty initiating micturition Bladder distension with overflow	Intermittent self-catheterisation In-dwelling catheterisation
Hypertonic (upper motor neuron)	Pyramidal tract lesion in spinal cord or brain stem	Urgency with urge incontinence Bladder sphincter incoordination (dyssynergia) Incomplete bladder emptying	Anticholinergics Oxybutynin (5 mg 8–12-hourly) Imipramine (25 mg 12-hourly) Tolterodine (2 mg 12-hourly) Intermittent self-catheterisation
Cortical	Post-central Pre-central Frontal	Loss of awareness of bladder fullness Difficulty initiating micturition Inappropriate micturition Loss of social control	Intermittent catheterisation

headache syndromes are discussed in the following section.

Tension-type headache

This is the most common type of headache and is experienced at some time by the majority of the population in some form.

Pathophysiology

The cause of tension headaches is incompletely understood. Emotional strain or anxiety is a common precipitant to tension-type headache and there is sometimes an associated depressive illness. Anxiety about the headache itself may lead to continuation of symptoms, and patients often become convinced of a serious underlying condition. Muscular spasms in the head and neck have been suggested to be a cause but there is little direct evidence for this.

Clinical features

The pain of tension headache is usually constant and generalised but often radiates forward from the occipital region. It is described as 'dull', 'tight' or like a 'pressure', and there may be a sensation of a band round the head or pressure at the vertex. In contrast to migraine, the pain may continue for weeks or months without interruption, although the severity may vary, and there is no associated vomiting or photophobia. The patient can usually continue normal activities, and the pain may be less noticeable when the patient is occupied. The pain is characteristically less severe in the early part of the day and becomes more troublesome as the day goes on. Local tenderness may be present over the skull vault or in the occiput but this should be distinguished from the acute pain precipitated by skin contact in trigeminal neuralgia and the exquisite tenderness of temporal arteritis. Typically, the headache does not respond well to treatment with analgesics.

Management

Careful assessment followed by discussion of likely precipitants and explanation of the fact that the symptoms are not due to any sinister underlying pathology is more likely to be beneficial than analgesics. Excessive use of analgesics, particularly of codeine, may actually worsen the headache (analgesic headache). Physiotherapy (with muscle relaxation and stress management) is usually beneficial, and low-dose amitriptyline (10 mg nocte increased gradually to 30–50 mg) sometimes helps. There is evidence that patients benefit from a perception that their problem has been taken seriously and rigorously assessed, but over-investigation can worsen a patient's anxiety.

Migraine

Migraine is a common condition which affects about 20% of females and 6% of males at some point in life. Migraine usually presents before the age of 40 and it has been estimated that 90% of migraine sufferers have their first attack by this time. Although some patients refer to any episodic paroxysmal headache as migraine, there is a characteristic presentation as discussed below.

Pathophysiology

The cause of migraine is incompletely understood but there is increasing evidence that the aura (see below) is due to dysfunction of ion channels which leads to a spreading front of cortical depolarisation (excitation) followed by hyperpolarisation (depression of activity). This process (the 'spreading depression of Leão') spreads over the cortex at a rate of about 3 mm/minute, corresponding to the spread of the symptoms of the aura. Family history is common in migraine, suggesting a genetic predisposition, and migraine-like phenomena can occur in some rare genetic disorders associated with mutations in calcium channel genes. These data are consistent with the hypothesis that the disorder may be due to abnormal function of ion channels, which in some cases is genetically determined. The great female preponderance and the tendency for some women to have migraine attacks at certain points in their menstrual cycle hint at hormonal influences. The relevance of the contraceptive pill in this context is difficult to establish, but it does appear to exacerbate migraine in many patients, and to increase the small risk of stroke in patients who suffer from migraine with aura. In some patients there are identifiable dietary precipitants such as cheese, chocolate or red wine. When psychological stress is involved, the migraine attack often occurs after the period of stress, so that some patients tend to have attacks at weekends or at the beginning of a holiday. The headache is associated with vasodilatation of extracranial vessels, but may be due to disturbed neuronal activity in the hypothalamus.

Clinical features

Migraine presents with a symptom triad of paroxysmal headache, nausea and/or vomiting, and an 'aura' of focal neurological events (usually visual). Patients with all three of these features are said to have migraine with aura ('classical' migraine). Those with paroxysmal headache (with or without vomiting) but no 'aura' are said to have migraine without aura ('common' migraine). A classical migraine attack starts with a non-specific prodrome of malaise and irritability followed by the aura of a focal neurological event, and then a severe, throbbing, hemicranial headache with photophobia and vomiting. During the headache phase, patients prefer to be in a quiet, darkened room and to sleep. The headache may persist for several days.

The aura most often takes the form of fortification spectra, which are shimmering, silvery zigzag lines which march across the visual fields over a period of about 20 minutes, sometimes leaving a trail of temporary visual field loss. In some patients there is a sensory aura which is a spreading front of tingling followed by numbness which moves, over 20–30 minutes, from one part of the body to another. If the dominant hemisphere is involved, the patient may also experience transient aphasia. Limb weakness can occur in migraine and is termed hemiplegic migraine. However, this is unusual and should be diagnosed with extreme caution. In some patients the focal events may occur by themselves ('migraine equivalent'), but in this case other structural disorders of the brain, or even focal epilepsy, need to be considered in the differential diagnosis. In a smaller number of patients, the symptoms of the aura do not resolve, leaving more permanent neurological disturbance ('complicated migraine').

26

Management

Identification and avoidance of precipitants or exacerbating factors (such as the contraceptive pill) may prevent attacks. Treatment of an acute attack consists of simple analgesia with aspirin or paracetamol, often combined with an antiemetic such as metoclopramide or domperidone. Long-term use of codeine-containing analgesic preparations should be avoided. Severe attacks can be treated with one of the 'triptans' (e.g. sumatriptan), 5-HT agonists that are potent vasoconstrictors of the extracranial arteries. These can be administered orally, sublingually, by subcutaneous injection or by nasal spray. Ergotamine preparations should be avoided since they easily lead to dependence. This is less likely to happen with the triptans, but it can occur. If attacks are frequent, they can often be prevented with propranolol (80–160 mg daily, in a sustained-release preparation), a tricyclic such as amitriptyline (10–50 mg at night), sodium valproate (300–600 mg/day) or topiramate (50–100 mg/day). Women should be warned that the small risk of ischaemic stroke attributable to taking oral contraception is increased if they have migraine with aura (see above), especially if they also smoke.

Cluster headache

Cluster headaches (also known as migrainous neuralgia) are 10–50 times less common than migraine. There is a 5:1 predominance of males and onset is usually in the third decade.

Pathophysiology

The cause is unclear. There is little evidence for a genetic predisposition, there are no provoking dietary factors and there is a male predominance. Functional imaging studies have suggested abnormal neuronal activity in the hypothalamus. Patients are usually heavy smokers with a higher than average alcohol consumption.

Clinical features

The characteristic presentation is with periodic, severe, unilateral periorbital pain accompanied by unilateral lacrimation, nasal congestion and conjunctival injection, often with the other features of Horner's syndrome. The pain, whilst being very severe, is characteristically brief (30–90 minutes). Typically, the patient develops these symptoms at a particular time of day (often in the early hours of the morning). The syndrome may occur repeatedly for a number of weeks, followed by a respite for a number of months before another cluster occurs.

Management

Acute attacks can usually be halted by subcutaneous injections of sumatriptan or by inhalation of 100% oxygen, but other migraine therapies are ineffective, probably because of the brevity of the individual attacks. Preventative therapy with the agents used for migraine is often ineffective but attacks can be prevented in some patients by verapamil (80–120 mg 8-hourly), methysergide (4–10 mg daily, for a maximum of 3 months only) or short courses of oral corticosteroids. Patients with severe and debilitating clusters can be helped with lithium therapy, although the usual precautions concerning the use of this drug should be observed (p. 243).

Other headache syndromes

There are a number of rare headache syndromes which produce pains about the eye similar to cluster headaches (Box 26.29). These include chronic and paroxysmal hemicrania, and SUNCT (short-lasting unilateral neuralgiform headaches with conjunctival injection and tearing). The recognition of these syndromes is useful

26.29 Benign paroxysmal headaches

	Character of pain	Duration	Location	Comment
Ice pick	Stabbing	Very brief (split-second)	Variable, usually temporal or parietal	Benign, more common in migraine
Ice cream	Sharp, severe	30–120 seconds	Bitemporal/occipital	Obvious trigger by cold stimuli
Exertional/coital	Bursting, thunderclap	Severe for minutes then less severe for hours	Generalised	Subarachnoid haemorrhage needs exclusion
Cough	Bursting	Seconds to minutes	Occipital or generalised	Intracranial pathology needs exclusion (especially cranio-cervical junction)
Cluster headache (migrainous neuralgia)	Severe unilateral, with ptosis, tearing, conjunctival injection, unilateral nasal congestion	30–90 minutes 1–3 times per day	Periorbital	Usually men, occurring in clusters over weeks/months
Chronic paroxysmal hemicrania	Severe unilateral with cluster headache-like autonomic features (above)	5–20 minutes, frequently through day	Periorbital/temporal	Usually women, responds to indometacin
SUNCT*	Severe, sharp, triggered by touch or neck movements	15–120 seconds, repetitive through day	Periorbital	May respond to carbamazepine

*Short-lasting, Unilateral, Neuralgiform headache with Conjunctival injection, Tearing, rhinorrhoea and forehead sweating.

since they often respond to specific treatments such as indometacin.

Trigeminal neuralgia

This is characterised by lancinating pain in the second and third divisions of the trigeminal nerve territory, usually in patients over the age of 50 years.

Pathophysiology

Trigeminal neuralgia is thought to be caused by an aberrant loop of the cerebellar arteries compressing the trigeminal nerve as it enters the brain stem. Other compressive lesions, usually benign, are occasionally found. When trigeminal neuralgia occurs in multiple sclerosis, there is a plaque of demyelination in the trigeminal root entry zone.

Clinical features

The pain is severe and very brief but repetitive, causing the patient to flinch as if with a motor tic (hence the French term for the condition, 'tic douloureux'). It may be precipitated by touching trigger zones within the trigeminal territory, by cold wind blowing on the face, or by eating. Physical signs are usually absent. Similar symptoms may occur in multiple sclerosis or, rarely, with other brain-stem lesions, in which case there may be sensory changes in the trigeminal nerve territory (and possibly other brain-stem symptoms and signs). There is a tendency for the condition to remit and relapse over many years.

Management

The pain usually responds to carbamazepine in doses of up to 1200 mg daily. It is wise to start with a low dose and increase gradually, according to effect. In patients who cannot tolerate carbamazepine, gabapentin or pregabalin may be effective. Various surgical treatments are available, the simplest of which is injection of alcohol or phenol into a peripheral branch of the nerve. Probably more effective is making a radiofrequency lesion in the nerve near the Gasserian ganglion. Care has to be taken not to cause excessive damage to sensation in the face to prevent the complication of neurogenic pain ('anaesthesia dolorosa') which is worse than the neuralgia. Alternatively, the vascular compression of the trigeminal nerve can be relieved through a posterior craniotomy, often with substantial success. This latter approach is usually favoured in younger patients in whom the other injection treatments may have to be repeated and become less effective.

Post-coital and exercise-induced headache

This usually affects men in their thirties and forties. Patients develop a sudden, severe headache at the climax of sexual intercourse. There is usually no vomiting and no neck stiffness, and it does not persist for more than 10–15 minutes, though a less severe, dull headache may persist for some hours. This type of paroxysmal headache often needs to be distinguished by CT and/or CSF examination from subarachnoid haemorrhage (see Fig. 26.35, p. 1190). A very similar headache may occur during physical exertion, especially if this is attempted with unaccustomed vigour in an unfit person. The pathogenesis is unknown. Though frightening, coital or exertional cephalgia is usually brief and may not need more than ordinary analgesia for the residual headache. The syndrome may not recur but prevention with propranolol or indometacin (75 mg daily) may be necessary.

VESTIBULAR DISORDERS

Vestibular disorders typically present with vertigo (see above) and the majority of patients with an organic cause of vertigo will have labyrinthitis, benign paroxysmal positional vertigo or Ménière's disease.

Labyrinthitis

This condition, also known as vestibular neuronitis, is the most common cause of severe vertigo, but the cause is unknown. It usually presents in the third or fourth decade as severe vertigo, with vomiting but no tinnitus or deafness. It often starts on waking, and patients are usually bedbound by the vertigo for the first few days. The vertigo usually settles over 3–4 days, though head movement may continue to provoke transient symptoms (positional vertigo) for some time and it may take a month or so before the patient feels 'back to normal'. During the acute attack, nystagmus (p. 1165) will be present but this typically disappears after a few days.

Symptomatic relief can be achieved with antihistamines such as cinnarizine, prochlorperazine, and betahistine. These agents should not be used for long-term treatment of persistent vertigo as they are ineffective and actually delay recovery in many patients. Patients with intractable symptoms may need referral to an ENT specialist for assessment, but input from an experienced vestibular physiotherapist is invaluable.

Benign paroxysmal positional vertigo

This is due to the presence of otolithic debris from the saccule or utricle affecting the free flow of endolymph in the semicircular canals (cupulolithiasis). It may follow head injury, but is more common in older patients who complain of paroxysms of vertigo occurring with certain head movements, typically looking up or turning over in bed. Each attack of vertigo lasts seconds but patients often become very distressed and reluctant to move their head, and this can produce a muscle tension-type headache. Secondary hyperventilation attacks and associated depressive features are also common. The diagnosis can be confirmed by the 'Hallpike manœuvre' to demonstrate positional nystagmus (Fig. 26.25). Although this test is often difficult to perform adequately as patients are frightened by the vertigo, it is useful since it reassures the patient that the doctor knows what is going on. Treatment comprises explanation, along with vestibular exercises designed to send the otolithic debris back from semicircular canal to saccule or utricle (such as the Epley manœuvre) and/or to re-educate the brain to cope with the inappropriate signals from the labyrinth (such as Cawthorne–Cooksey exercises). The Epley manœuvre starts with the patient sitting upright on an examination couch. They are asked to lie back with their head turned at a 45° angle to the affected side, and to hold this position for 30–60 seconds. They should then be asked to turn their head 90° to the opposite side and remain in that position for 30–60 seconds. Next, they should be asked to roll on to

26

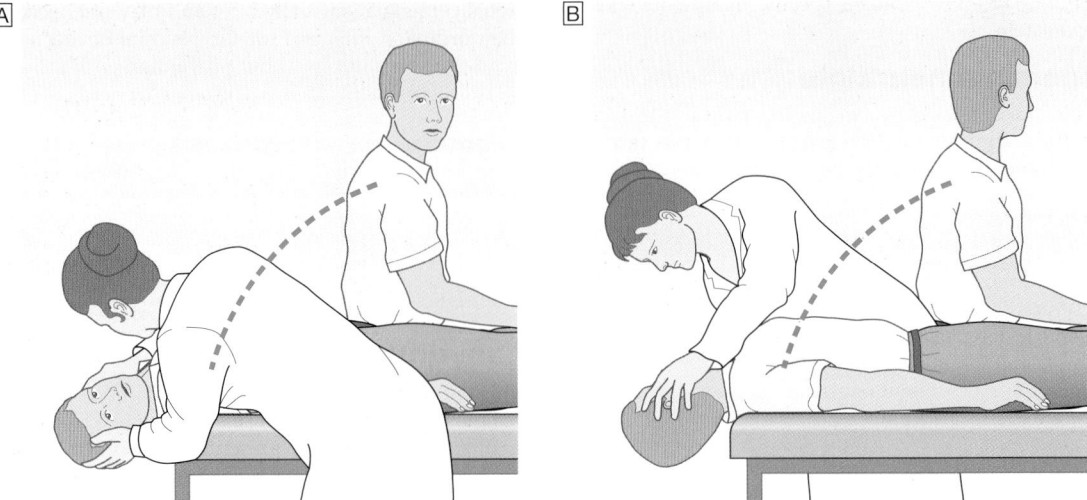

Fig. 26.25 The Hallpike manœuvre for diagnosis of benign paroxysmal positional vertigo (BPPV). Patients are asked to keep their eyes open and look at the examiner as their head is swung briskly backwards through 120° to overhang the edge of the couch. **A** Perform first with the right ear down. **B** Perform next with the left ear down. The examiner looks for nystagmus (usually accompanied by vertigo). In BPPV, the nystagmus typically occurs in A or B only and is torsional, the fast phase beating towards the lower ear. Its onset is usually delayed a few seconds, and it lasts 10–20 seconds. As the patient is returned to the upright position, transient nystagmus may occur in the opposite direction. Both nystagmus and vertigo typically decrease (fatigue) on repeat testing.

their side in the direction they are facing, so that their face is pointing towards the floor, and hold that position for 30–60 seconds before sitting up once again. Cawthorne-Cooksey exercises involve asking the patient to perform a series of eye, head and whole-body movements whilst lying down, sitting and standing. Antihistamines can be tried if the condition fails to respond to the above measures. (See page 1235 for websites.)

Ménière's disease

This is due to an abnormality of the endolymph which gives rise to paroxysms comprising a sensation of fullness in the ear followed by headache, tinnitus and profound vertigo, each attack typically lasting about 4 hours. In between attacks, patients' hearing may be distorted (typically low-tone deafness). While sensorineural hearing loss may be demonstrable, bedside examination is typically otherwise normal in between attacks, but audiometry is usually abnormal. Management is as described for labyrinthitis.

EPILEPSY

A seizure is any clinical event caused by an abnormal electrical discharge in the brain, whilst epilepsy is the tendency to have recurrent seizures. Epilepsy should be regarded as a symptom of brain disease rather than a disease itself. A single seizure is not epilepsy but an indication for investigation, and medication should generally be withheld until recurrent seizures occur. The recurrence rate after a first seizure is about 70% within the first year, and most recurrent attacks occur within a month or two of the first. Further seizures are less likely if a trigger factor is definable and avoidable (Box 26.30). In some conditions, epilepsy is the

26.30 Trigger factors for seizures

- Sleep deprivation
- Alcohol (particularly withdrawal)
- Recreational drug misuse
- Physical and mental exhaustion
- Flickering lights, including TV and computer screens (primary generalised epilepsies only)
- Intercurrent infections and metabolic disturbances
- Uncommonly: loud noises, music, reading, hot baths

26.31 Classification of epilepsy

Seizure type

• Partial (simple or complex)	• Tonic clonic
• Partial with secondary generalisation	• Tonic
	• Atonic
• Absence	• Myoclonic

Physiology (EEG)

• Focal spikes/sharp waves	• Generalised spike and wave

Anatomical site

• Cortex	• Generalised (diencephalon)
Temporal	• Multifocal
Frontal	
Parietal	
Occipital	

Pathological cause

• Genetic	• Infections
• Developmental	• Inflammation
• Tumours	• Metabolic
• Trauma	• Drugs, alcohol and toxins
• Vascular	• Degenerative

ℹ 26.32 Primary generalised epilepsies

	Incidence	Age of onset	Type of seizure	EEG features	Provoking factors	Treatment	Prognosis
Childhood absence epilepsy	6–8/100 000	4–8 yrs	Frequent brief absences	3/s spike and wave	Hyperventilation, fatigue	Ethosuximide Sodium valproate	40% develop GTCS, 80% remit in adulthood
Juvenile absence epilepsy	1–2/100 000	10–15 yrs	Less frequent absences than childhood absence	Poly-spike and wave	Hyperventilation, sleep deprivation	Sodium valproate	80% develop GTCS, 80% seizure-free in adulthood
Juvenile myoclonic epilepsy	25–50/100 000	15–20 yrs	GTCS, absences, morning myoclonus	Poly-spike and wave, photosensitivity	Sleep deprivation, alcohol withdrawal	Sodium valproate	90% remit with AEDs but relapse if AED withdrawn
GTCS on awakening	Common	10–25 yrs	GTCS, sometimes myoclonus	Spike and wave on waking and sleep onset	Sleep deprivation	Sodium valproate	65% controlled with AEDs but relapse off treatment

(GTCS = generalised tonic clonic seizure; AED = anti-epileptic drug)

only feature of underlying disease, whilst in others epilepsy is just one of the manifestations. The annual incidence of new cases of epilepsy after infancy is 20–70/100 000. The lifetime risk of having a single seizure is about 5%, whilst the prevalence of epilepsy in European countries is about 0.5%. The prevalence in developing countries is up to five times higher than in developed countries.

The classification of epilepsy is best achieved by considering the clinical events (the seizures), the abnormal electrophysiology, the anatomical site of seizure genesis and the pathological cause of the problem (Box 26.31).

Primary generalised epilepsy

The primary or idiopathic epilepsies make up some 10% of all epilepsies, including some 40% of those with tonic clonic seizures. Onset is almost always in childhood or adolescence. No structural abnormality is present and there is often a substantial genetic predisposition. Some, like childhood absence epilepsy, are relatively uncommon, whilst others, like juvenile myoclonic epilepsy, are common (5–10% of all patients with epilepsy). The more common varieties of primary generalised epilepsy are listed in Box 26.32, along with their clinical features and management.

Partial epilepsy

Partial seizures may arise from any disease of the cerebral cortex, congenital or acquired, and frequently generalise. With the exception of a few idiopathic partial epilepsies of benign outcome in childhood, the presence of partial seizures signifies the presence of focal cerebral pathology. Common causes are listed in Box 26.33.

Secondary generalised epilepsy

Generalised epilepsy may arise from spread of partial seizures due to structural disease, or may be secondary to drugs or metabolic disorders (Box 26.34). Epilepsy presenting in adult life is almost always secondary generalised, even if there is no clear history of a partial seizure before the onset of a major attack (an 'aura'). The occurrence of epilepsy in those over the age of 60 is frequently

due to cerebrovascular disease and presents specific diagnostic and management problems (Box 26.35).

Pathophysiology

Under normal circumstances, recurrent and collateral inhibitory circuits in the cerebral cortex limit synchronous discharge of neighbouring groups of neurons. The

26

🔍 26.33 Causes of partial seizures

Idiopathic

- Benign Rolandic epilepsy of childhood
- Benign occipital epilepsy of childhood

Focal structural lesions

Genetic

- Tuberous sclerosis (p. 1283)
- von Hippel–Lindau disease (p. 1219)
- Neurofibromatosis (p. 1218)
- Cerebral migration abnormalities

Infantile hemiplegia

Dysembryonic

- Cortical dysgenesis
- Sturge–Weber syndrome

Mesial temporal sclerosis (associated with febrile convulsions)

Cerebrovascular disease (p. 1180)

- Intracerebral haemorrhage
- Cerebral infarction
- Arteriovenous malformation
- Cavernous haemangioma

Tumours (primary and secondary) (p. 1216)

Trauma (including neurosurgery)

Infective (p. 1205)

- Cerebral abscess (pyogenic)
- Toxoplasmosis
- Cysticercosis
- Tuberculoma
- Subdural empyema
- Encephalitis
- Human immunodeficiency virus (HIV)

Inflammatory

- Sarcoidosis
- Vasculitis

🔍 26.34 Causes of secondary generalised epilepsy

Secondary generalisation from partial seizures
- See Box 26.33 for causes of partial seizures

Genetic
- Inborn errors of metabolism (p. 61)
- Storage diseases (p. 448)
- Phakomatoses (e.g. tuberous sclerosis, p. 1283)

Cerebral birth injury

Hydrocephalus

Cerebral anoxia

Drugs
- Antibiotics: penicillin, isoniazid, metronidazole
- Antimalarials: chloroquine, mefloquine
- Ciclosporin
- Cardiac anti-arrhythmics: lidocaine, disopyramide
- Psychotropic agents: phenothiazines, tricyclic antidepressants, lithium
- Amphetamines (withdrawal)

Alcohol (especially withdrawal)

Toxins
- Heavy metals (lead, tin)
- Organophosphates (sarin)

Metabolic disease
- Hypocalcaemia
- Hypoglycaemia
- Hyponatraemia
- Renal failure
- Hypomagnesaemia
- Liver failure

Infective
- Meningitis (p. 1205)
- Post-infectious encephalopathy

Inflammatory
- Multiple sclerosis (uncommon) (p. 1191)
- SLE (p. 1107)

Diffuse degenerative diseases
- Alzheimer's disease (uncommonly) (p. 1198)
- Creutzfeldt–Jakob disease (rarely) (p. 1214)

⏳ 26.35 Epilepsy in old age

- **Incidence and prevalence:** late-onset epilepsy is very common and the annual incidence in those over 60 years is rising.
- **Fits and faints:** the features that usually differentiate these may be less definitive than in younger patients.
- **Complex partial status epilepticus:** can present as confusion in the elderly.
- **Cerebrovascular disease** is the underlying cause of seizures in 30–50% of patients over the age of 50 years. A seizure may occur with an overt stroke or with occult vascular disease.
- **Anti-epileptic drug regimens:** keep as simple as possible and take care to avoid interactions with other drugs being prescribed.
- **Carbamazepine-induced hyponatraemia:** increases significantly with age; particularly important in patients on diuretics or those with heart failure.
- **Withdrawal of anticonvulsant therapy:** late-onset epilepsy often recurs when drug treatment is stopped, so drug withdrawal should not be attempted where it was commenced appropriately.

inhibitory transmitter gamma-aminobutyric acid (GABA) is particularly important in this role, and drugs that block GABA receptors provoke seizures. Conversely, excessive stimulation by excitatory neurotransmitters, such as acetylcholine, glutamate and aspartate, provoke seizure activity. It is likely that both reduction of inhibition and excessive excitation play a part in the genesis of most seizures. The cerebral cortex in epilepsy exhibits hypersynchronous, repetitive discharges involving large groups of neurons, intracellular recordings of which demonstrate bursts of high-frequency action potentials associated with a reduction in the transmembrane potential (paroxysmal depolarisation shift). In animal models, cells undergoing repetitive epileptic discharges undergo morphological and physiological changes which make them more likely to produce subsequent abnormal discharges ('kindling').

Seizures may be partial (focal) in which paroxysmal neuronal activity is limited to one part of the cortex, or generalised when the electrophysiological abnormality involves both hemispheres simultaneously and synchronously (Fig. 26.26). If partial seizures remain localised, the symptomatology depends on which cortical area is affected. If consciousness (the awareness of and ability to respond to the environment) is preserved, the attack is termed a 'simple partial' seizure. If consciousness is lost, this is termed a 'complex partial' seizure and this implies that the seizure activity has involved parts of the brain concerned with awareness (such as the temporal or frontal lobes). Partial seizures may spread into the

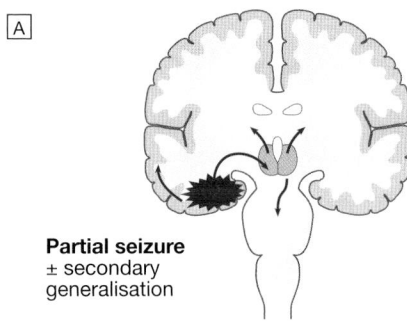

A

Partial seizure ± secondary generalisation

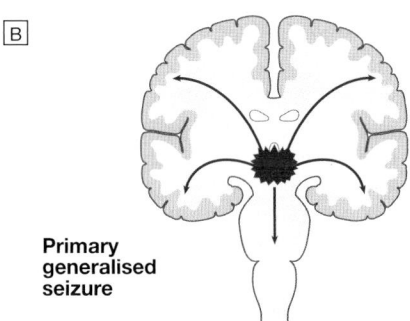

B

Primary generalised seizure

Fig. 26.26 The pathophysiological classification of seizures. [A] A partial seizure originates from a paroxysmal discharge in a focal area of the cerebral cortex (often the temporal lobe); the seizure may subsequently spread to the rest of the brain (secondary generalisation) via diencephalic activating pathways. [B] In primary generalised seizures the abnormal electrical discharges originate from the diencephalic activating system and spread simultaneously to all areas of the cortex.

diencephalon and thence throughout the rest of the cortex, leading to a 'secondarily generalised' seizure.

In 'primary generalised' seizures, the abnormal activity begins synchronously throughout the cortex without an initial partial onset. It probably originates in the central diencephalic mechanisms controlling cortical activation (see Fig. 26.26). This is recognisable on an EEG as spike and wave discharges (see Fig. 26.10, p. 1141) and quite often hyperventilation and/or photic stimulation will provoke such discharges. There are several possible manifestations of primary generalised epilepsy; some seizures may appear identical to a secondarily generalised ('tonic clonic') seizure, while in others there may be a more restricted clinical manifestation if the abnormal electrical activity fails to affect muscle tone. The latter seizures are termed 'absences'. These are typically brief and involve transient loss of consciousness but the patient remains standing or sitting. Such attacks may be difficult to distinguish clinically from complex partial seizures.

Clinical features

When taking a history from a patient with suspected seizure, it is important to clarify which type of attack is occurring, bearing in mind that there may be more than one occurring in the same patient at different times. Sometimes specific trigger factors can be identified, as discussed above (see Box 26.30, p. 1172). The type of seizure, along with further information from history and investigation, can then be used to determine the epilepsy syndrome, as discussed in the next section. Descriptions of the more common types of seizure follow.

Tonic clonic seizures

A tonic clonic seizure may be preceded by a partial seizure (the 'aura') which can take various forms, described below. However, a history of such an 'aura' is commonly not obtained, probably because the subsequent generalised seizure causes some retrograde amnesia for immediately preceding events. The patient then goes rigid and becomes unconscious, falling down heavily if standing and often sustaining injury. During this phase, respiration is arrested and central cyanosis may occur. After a few moments, the rigidity is periodically relaxed, producing clonic jerks. Some patients do not have a clonic phase and the rigidity is replaced by a flaccid state of deep coma which can persist for some minutes. The patient then gradually regains consciousness, but is in a confused and disorientated state for half an hour or more after regaining consciousness. Full memory function may not be recovered for some hours. During the attack, urinary incontinence and tongue-biting may occur. A severely bitten, bleeding tongue after an attack of loss of consciousness is pathognomonic of a generalised seizure. After a generalised seizure the patient usually feels terrible, may have a headache and will often want to sleep. Witnesses of a seizure are usually frightened by the event, often believe the person to be dying, and may not give a clear account of the episode. This in itself can be a helpful diagnostic pointer since syncope seldom produces such fear in onlookers. Patients may have no tonic or clonic phase, and may not become cyanosed or bite their tongue. However, post-ictal confusion is useful in differentiating seizures from syncope. Psychogenic non-epileptic attacks ('pseudo-seizures') may be accompanied by dramatic flailing of the limbs and arching of the back; however, these are not usually followed by the same degree of post-ictal confusion and do not usually cause cyanosis (see Box 26.9, p. 1151).

Complex partial seizures

Complex partial seizures involve episodes of altered consciousness without the patient collapsing to the ground, especially if they arise from the temporal or, less frequently, the frontal lobe. Patients stop what they are doing and stare blankly, often blinking repetitively, making smacking movements of their lips, or displaying other automatisms, such as picking at their clothes. After a few minutes, consciousness returns but the patient may be muddled and feel drowsy for a period of up to an hour. Immediately before such an attack the patient may report alteration of mood, memory or perception (such as undue familiarity—déjà vu—or unreality—jamais vu), or complex hallucinations involving sound, smell, taste, vision, emotion (fear, sexual arousal) or visceral sensations (nausea, epigastric discomfort). If these changes of memory or perception occur without subsequent alteration in awareness, the seizure is said to be a 'simple partial' seizure.

Complex partial seizures arising from the anterior parts of the frontal lobe may produce bizarre behaviour patterns including limb posturing, sleep walking, or even frenetic ill-directed motor activity with incoherent screaming. These can sometimes be very difficult to distinguish from psychogenic attacks (which are more common). However, abruptness of onset and relative brevity may help point to frontal seizures, as may a tendency to occur out of sleep.

Absence seizures

Absence seizures (petit mal) always start in childhood. The attacks can be mistaken for complex partial seizures but are shorter in duration; they occur much more frequently (20–30 times a day) and are not associated with post-ictal confusion. Absence attacks are caused by a generalised discharge that does not spread out of the hemispheres and so does not cause loss of posture.

Atonic seizures

These are seizures involving brief loss of muscle tone, usually resulting in heavy falls with or without loss of consciousness. They only occur in the context of epilepsy syndromes which involve other forms of seizure. They are not a cause of collapse in patients without epilepsy.

Partial motor seizures

Epileptic activity arising in the pre-central gyrus causes partial motor seizures affecting the contralateral face, arm, trunk or leg. Seizures are characterised by rhythmical jerking or sustained spasm of the affected parts. They may remain localised to one part, or may spread to involve the whole side. Some attacks begin in one part of the body (e.g. mouth, thumb, great toe) and spread (march) gradually to other parts of the body; this is known as a Jacksonian seizure. Attacks vary in duration from a few seconds to several hours (epilepsia partialis continua). More prolonged episodes may be followed by paresis of the involved limb lasting for several hours after the seizure ceases (Todd's palsy).

Partial sensory seizures

Seizures arising in the sensory cortex cause unpleasant tingling or 'electric' sensations in the contralateral face or limbs. A spreading pattern similar to a Jacksonian

26

seizure may occur, the abnormal sensation spreading over the body much faster (in seconds) than the march of a migrainous focal sensory attack, which spreads over 20–30 minutes (p. 1169).

Versive seizures

A frontal epileptic focus may involve the frontal eye field, causing forced deviation of the eyes and sometimes turning of the head to the opposite side. This type of attack often generalises to become a tonic clonic seizure.

Partial visual seizures

Occipital epileptic foci cause simple visual hallucinations such as balls of light or patterns of colour. Formed visual hallucinations of faces or scenes arise more anteriorly in the temporal lobes.

Investigations

After a first seizure, immediate cerebral imaging with CT or MRI is advisable, particularly in patients aged over 20 years, although the yield of structural lesions is low unless there are focal features to the seizure or there are focal signs. Other investigations for infective, toxic and metabolic causes (see Box 26.34) may be appropriate. An EEG performed immediately after a seizure may be more helpful in showing focal features than if performed after a delay.

In a situation where more than one seizure has occurred, an EEG is often useful in establishing the type of epilepsy and to guide therapy. The increasing sophistication of imaging techniques now allows the identification of the cause of epilepsy in an increasing number of patients, especially those with partial seizures. Investigations should be pursued more vigorously if the epilepsy is intractable to treatment. Investigations that may be appropriate in a patient with suspected epilepsy are shown in Box 26.36. The EEG may help to establish a diagnosis and charac-

terise the type of epilepsy. Inter-ictal records are abnormal in only about 50% of patients with definite epilepsy so the EEG cannot be reliably used to exclude the diagnosis. However, 'epileptiform changes' (sharp waves or spikes) on the EEG are fairly specific for epilepsy (falsely positive in 1/1000). The sensitivity can be increased to about 85% by prolonging recording time and including a period of natural or drug-induced sleep. Ambulatory EEG recording or video/EEG monitoring may provide helpful information when attacks are frequent.

Imaging cannot establish a diagnosis of epilepsy but it is useful in defining or excluding a structural cause. Indications for imaging are summarised in Box 26.37. Imaging is not required if a confident diagnosis of primary generalised epilepsy can be made with an EEG. CT is often sufficient to exclude a major structural cause of epilepsy. MRI of the brain may be indicated if CT shows no abnormality but a subtle structural change is still suspected, as in the case of patients with partial seizures (with or without secondary generalisation) which are resistant to therapy.

Management

It is important to explain the nature and cause of seizures to patients and their relatives, and to instruct relatives in the first aid management of major seizures (Boxes 26.38 and 26.39). Many people with epilepsy feel stigmatised by society and may become unnecessarily isolated from

26.37 Indications for brain imaging in epilepsy

- Epilepsy starting after the age of 20 years
- Seizures having focal features clinically
- EEG showing a focal seizure source
- Control of seizures difficult or deteriorating

26.36 Investigation of suspected epilepsy

Are the attacks truly epileptic?

- Ambulatory EEG
- Videotelemetry

From where is the epilepsy arising?

- Standard EEG
- Sleep EEG
- EEG with special electrodes (foramen ovale, subdural)

What is the cause of the epilepsy?

Structural lesion?
- CT
- MRI

Metabolic disorder?
- Urea and electrolytes
- Liver function tests
- Blood glucose
- Serum calcium, magnesium

Inflammatory or infective disorder?
- Full blood count, erythrocyte sedimentation rate (ESR), C-reactive protein (CRP)
- Chest X-ray
- Serology for syphilis, HIV, collagen disease
- CSF examination

26.38 How to administer first aid for seizures

- Move person away from danger (fire, water, machinery, furniture)
- After convulsions cease, turn into 'recovery' position (semi-prone)
- Ensure airway is clear, but do **NOT** insert anything in mouth (tongue-biting occurs at seizure onset and cannot be prevented by observers)
- If convulsions continue for more than 5 minutes or recur without person regaining consciousness, summon urgent medical attention
- Do not leave person alone until fully recovered (drowsiness and confusion can persist for up to 1 hour)

26.39 Immediate management of seizures

- Ensure airway is patent
- Give oxygen to offset cerebral hypoxia
- Give intravenous anticonvulsant (e.g. diazepam 10 mg) **ONLY** if convulsions are continuous or repeated (if so, manage as for status epilepticus, Box 26.45)
- Take blood for anticonvulsant levels (if known epileptic)
- Investigate cause

work and social life. It should be emphasised that any brain can develop a seizure, that epilepsy is a common disorder which affects 0.5–1% of the population, and that good control of seizures can be expected in more than 80% of patients.

Immediate care

Little can or needs to be done for a person whilst a major seizure is occurring except for first aid and common-sense manoeuvres to limit damage or secondary complications (see Box 26.38).

Lifestyle modification

As soon as possible, patients should be made aware of the riskiness of any activity where loss of awareness would be dangerous until good control of seizures has been established. Such activities include work or recreational activities involving exposure to heights, dangerous machinery, open fires or water. Only shallow baths (or showers) should be taken, preferably with someone else in the house and with the bathroom door unlocked. Cycling should be discouraged until at least 6 months' freedom from seizures has been achieved. Activities requiring prolonged proximity to water (swimming, fishing or boating) should always be in the company of someone who is aware of the risk of a seizure and who is able to rescue the patient if necessary. In the UK and many other countries, legal restrictions regarding vehicle driving apply to patients after a first unprovoked seizure and those with epilepsy, here defined as more than one seizure occurring after the age of 5 years (Box 26.40). The patient should inform the licensing authorities about the onset of seizures, and it is also wise to notify the motor insurance company. Certain occupations, such as nursery nurse or airline pilot, are not open to anyone who has ever had an epileptic seizure; further information is often available from epilepsy support organisations.

Anticonvulsant therapy

Drug treatment should be considered after more than one seizure has occurred and the patient agrees that seizure control is worthwhile. A wide range of drugs is available. The mode of action of these agents is either to increase inhibitory neurotransmission in the brain or to alter neuronal sodium channels in such a way as to prevent abnormally rapid transmission of impulses. In 80% of patients whose epilepsy is controllable, only a single drug is necessary. The combination of more than two drugs is seldom required. Dose regimens should be kept as simple as possible to promote compliance. Some guidelines are listed in Box 26.41. With the exception of absence attacks and juvenile myoclonic epilepsy, there is no hard evidence indicating that one drug is superior to another in the treatment of epilepsy. The first choice should be one of the established first-line drugs (Box 26.42), with the more recently introduced drugs as second choice. Phenytoin and carbamazepine are not ideal agents for a young woman wishing to use oral contraception, because the drugs induce liver enzymes. Phenobarbital and topiramate have similar effects. Carbamazepine, lamotrigine and sodium valproate are preferable to phenytoin as first-line drugs because of the side-effect profile of the latter and its complicated pharmacokinetics.

Monitoring therapy

With some drugs such as phenytoin and carbamazepine, occasional measurement of the blood level can be a guide to whether the patient is on an appropriate dose and is complying with the medication, but blood levels need to be interpreted carefully. The dose of anticonvulsant drug in an individual patient should primarily be governed by the efficacy of seizure control and the development of side-effects rather than blood levels alone. With sodium valproate, there is a poor relationship between blood levels and anticonvulsant efficacy, and so levels are really only useful to assess compliance. Repeated measurement of blood

26

26.40 UK driving regulations

Private use

Single seizure
- Cease driving until 1 year has passed without recurrence. Driver and Vehicle Licensing Authority (DVLA) will then restore a full licence

Epilepsy (i.e. more than one seizure over age 5 years)
- Cease driving immediately
- Licence restored when patient is free from all types of seizure for 1 year *or* seizures have occurred *exclusively* during sleep for a period of at least 3 years
- Licence will require renewal every 3 years thereafter until patient is seizure-free for 10 years

Withdrawal of anticonvulsants
- Cease driving during withdrawal period and for 6 months thereafter

Vocational drivers (heavy goods and public service vehicles)
- No licence permitted if any seizure has occured after the age of 5 years until patient is off medication and seizure-free for more than 10 years, and has no potentially epileptogenic brain lesion

---

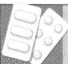

26.41 Guidelines for anticonvulsant therapy

- Start with one first-line drug (see Box 26.42)
- Start at a low dose; gradually increase dose until effective control of seizures is achieved or side-effects develop (drug levels may be helpful)
- Optimise compliance (use minimum number of doses per day)
- If first drug fails (seizures continue or side-effects develop), start second first-line drug whilst gradually withdrawing first
- If second drug fails (seizures continue or side-effects develop), start second-line drug in combination with preferred first-line drug at maximum tolerated dose (beware interactions)
- If this combination fails (seizures continue or side-effects develop), replace second-line drug with alternative second-line drug
- If this combination fails, check compliance and reconsider diagnosis (is there an occult structural or metabolic lesion or are seizures truly epileptic?)
- If this combination fails, consider alternative, non-drug treatments (e.g. epilepsy surgery, vagal nerve stimulation)
- Do not use more than two drugs in combination at any one time

26.42 Guidelines for choice of AED

Epilepsy type	First-line	Second-line	Third-line
Partial and/or secondary GTCS	Carbamazepine	Lamotrigine Sodium valproate Levetiracetam Topiramate	Tiagabine Pregabalin Gabapentin Clobazam Phenytoin Primidone Phenobarbital Oxcarbazepine Vigabatrin Acetazolamide
Primary GTCS	Sodium valproate	Lamotrigine Topiramate	Carbamazepine Phenytoin Gabapentin Pregabalin Primidone Phenobarbital Tiagabine Acetazolamide
Absence	Ethosuximide	Sodium valproate	Lamotrigine Clonazepam Acetazolamide
Myoclonic	Sodium valproate	Clonazepam	Piracetam Levetiracetam Lamotrigine Phenobarbital

N.B. Preferably one and no more than two drugs should be used at one time.

levels is not generally useful and monitoring is of most value in dealing with suspected toxicity (particularly if more than one drug is being taken), in dealing with the pharmacokinetic effects of pregnancy, or in suspected non-compliance.

Withdrawing anticonvulsant therapy

After complete control of seizures for 2–4 years, withdrawal of medication may be considered. Childhood-onset epilepsy, particularly classical absence seizures, carries the best prognosis for successful drug withdrawal. Other primary generalised epilepsies, such as juvenile myoclonic epilepsy, have a marked liability to recur after drug withdrawal. Seizures that begin in adult life, particularly those with partial features, are also likely to recur, especially if there is an identified structural lesion. Overall, the recurrence rate of seizures after drug withdrawal is about 40%. Some adult patients tend to opt for continuation of therapy because they feel that the threat of further attacks (especially the threat to driving) outweighs any drawbacks of continuing with medication. The EEG is generally a poor predictor of seizure recurrence but if the record is still very abnormal, drug withdrawal is unwise. Withdrawal should be undertaken slowly, reducing the drug dose gradually over 6–12 months. In the UK, patients must stop driving whilst withdrawing from their anti-epileptic medication and not drive for 6 months after full withdrawal of the drugs (see Box 26.40.

Contraception

Many anticonvulsant drugs, including carbamazepine, phenytoin, topiramate and barbiturates, induce hepatic enzymes and accelerate the metabolism of oestrogen, causing breakthrough bleeding and contraceptive failure. The safest policy is to use an alternative contraceptive method, but it is sometimes possible to overcome the problem by giving a higher-dose preparation of oestrogen. Lamotrigine and oxcarbazepine have little interaction, and sodium valproate has no interaction with oral contraception.

Pregnancy

Epilepsy presents specific management problems during pregnancy (Box 26.43). With the exception of gabapentin, treatment with almost all anticonvulsant drugs is associated with an increased incidence of fetal congenital abnormalities such as cleft lip, spina bifida and cardiac defects. The risk is greatest when treatment is given during the first trimester, rising from a background risk of 2–4% to about 4–8% with one anti-epileptic drug, and to about 15% with two or more drugs. Folic acid (5 mg daily) taken 2 months before conception may reduce the risk of some fetal abnormalities. Seizures often become more frequent during pregnancy, particularly during the third trimester when plasma anticonvulsant levels tend to fall. Monitoring of blood levels of anticonvulsants can be helpful with adjustment of drug doses. Occasionally, in a well-controlled patient, anticonvulsants can be withdrawn before conception, but if major seizures have occurred in the preceding year this is unwise, since uncontrolled maternal seizures represent a significant risk to the fetus.

Menstrual irregularities and polycystic ovarian disease are more common in women taking sodium valproate, and osteoporosis is more common in women taking one of the enzyme-inducing antiepileptic drugs.

Prognosis

Overall, generalised seizures are more readily controlled than partial seizures. The presence of a structural lesion makes complete control of the epilepsy less likely. The overall prognosis for epilepsy is shown in Box 26.44.

26.43 Epilepsy during pregnancy

- **Fetal malformation:** most anticonvulsants increase the risk—twofold increase in risk with one drug; fourfold increase in risk with two or more drugs. Start folic acid 5 mg daily for 2 months before conception to reduce risk.
- **Haemorrhagic disease of the newborn:** anticonvulsants increase risk. Give oral vitamin K 20 mg daily to the mother during last month. Give i.m. vitamin K 1 mg to the infant at birth.
- **Increased frequency of seizures:** monitor anticonvulsant levels and adjust the dose regimen accordingly.

26.44 Epilepsy: outcome after 20 years

- 50% are seizure-free, without drugs, for last 5 years
- 20% are seizure-free for last 5 years but continue to take medication
- 30% continue to have seizures in spite of anti-epileptic therapy

There is a 40-fold increased risk of sudden unexplained death in epilepsy (SUDEP) and patients may need to be made aware of this in order to help them rearrange their lifestyle and comply with treatment.

Status epilepticus

Status epilepticus is defined as a seizure or a series of seizures lasting 30 minutes without the patient regaining awareness between attacks. Most commonly, this refers to recurrent tonic clonic seizures (major status) and is a life-threatening medical emergency. Partial motor status is obvious clinically, but complex partial status and absence status may be difficult to diagnose because the patient may merely present in a dazed, confused state. Status is never the presenting feature of idiopathic epilepsy but may be precipitated by abrupt withdrawal of anticonvulsant drugs, the presence of a major structural lesion or acute metabolic disturbance. It tends to be more common with frontal epileptic foci. Management is summarised in Box 26.45. It should be remembered that psychogenic or non-epileptic attacks commonly masquerade as 'status epilepticus', so electrophysiological confirmation of the seizures should be obtained as early as possible.

Non-epileptic attack disorder

The episodes characterising this condition are also referred to as 'pseudoseizures' or 'psychogenic attacks'.

26.45 Management of status epilepticus

Initial

- Ensure airway is patent, give oxygen to prevent cerebral hypoxia, and secure intravenous access
- Draw blood for glucose, urea and electrolytes (including Ca and Mg), and liver function, and store a sample for future analysis (e.g. drug misuse)
- Give diazepam 10 mg i.v. (or rectally) *or* lorazepam 4 mg i.v.—repeat *once only* after 15 mins
- Transfer to intensive care area, monitoring neurological condition, blood pressure, respiration and blood gases, intubating and ventilating patient if appropriate

Ongoing

If seizures continue after 30 mins
- I.v. infusion (with cardiac monitoring) with one of:
  Phenytoin: 15 mg/kg at 50 mg/min
  Fosphenytoin: 15 mg/kg at 100 mg/min
  Phenobarbital: 10 mg/kg at 100 mg/min

If seizures still continue after 30–60 mins
- Start treatment for refractory status with intubation, ventilation, and general anaesthesia using propofol or thiopental

Once status controlled
- Commence longer-term anticonvulsant medication with one of:
  Sodium valproate 10 mg/kg i.v. over 3–5 mins, then 800–2000 mg/day
  Phenytoin: give loading dose (if not already used as above) of 15 mg/kg, infuse at < 50 mg/min, then 300 mg/day
  Carbamazepine 400 mg by nasogastric tube, then 400–1200 mg/day
- Investigate cause

Patients may present with attacks that superficially resemble epileptic seizures but which are caused by psychological phenomena and not associated with abnormal epileptic discharges in the brain. Such patients may present in apparent status epilepticus. People with epilepsy may have non-epileptic attacks as well, and this diagnosis should be considered if a patient fails to respond to anti-epileptic therapy, especially in the absence of a structural abnormality. Non-epileptic attacks may be quite difficult to distinguish from truly epileptic attacks. Clues pointing towards non-epileptic attacks include elaborate arching of the back in an attack, pelvic thrusting and/or wild flailing of limbs. Cyanosis and severe biting of the tongue are rare in non-epileptic attacks, but urinary incontinence can occur. The distinction between epileptic attacks originating in the frontal lobes and non-epileptic attacks may be especially difficult, and may require videotelemetry with prolonged EEG recordings. Non-epileptic attacks are three times more common in women than in men and have been associated with a history of sexual abuse in childhood. They are not necessarily associated with formal psychiatric illness. Treatment is often difficult and usually requires psychotherapy and/or counselling rather than drug therapy (p. 239).

DISORDERS OF SLEEP

26

Daytime somnolence

Excessive sleepiness in the day is most commonly due to inadequate night-time sleep related to fatigue and poor sleep hygiene, including the excessive use of caffeine and/or alcohol in the evening. Night-time sleep may also be disturbed by sleep apnoea (p. 722), periodic limb movements and the restless leg syndrome. Somnolence due to disturbed night-time sleep particularly occurs after meals and during dull monotonous activities, such as long car journeys. Such causes of daytime sleepiness need to be distinguished from narcolepsy.

Narcolepsy

This disorder has a prevalence of about 1 in 4000 and is associated with HLA (human leucocyte antigen) DR-1501 and DQB1-0602 in 85% of cases. This has been shown to be due to a deficiency in the hypothalamus of neurons secreting hypocretin, a neuropeptide. There is a familial tendency but a low concordance in monozygotic twins suggesting an additional pathophysiological mechanism, possibly autoimmune in nature. Recurrent bouts of irresistible sleep are experienced, during which the EEG often shows direct entry into rapid eye movement (REM) sleep. Sufferers tend to fall asleep when eating or talking, not just when understimulated. The periods of sleep are usually short and the person can be woken relatively easily. He or she usually feels refreshed after waking. In addition, patients with narcolepsy will report at least one other of the 'narcolepsy tetrad' (Box 26.46). Any of these four symptoms may occur in a given patient; most often, sleep attacks and cataplexy occur together.

Narcoleptic attacks can be treated with central nervous system (CNS) stimulants such as dexamfetamine (5–10 mg 8-hourly) or methylphenidate (10–60 mg per day) but fewer side-effects occur with modafinil

26.46 The narcolepsy tetrad
Sleep attacks
• Brief, frequent and unlike normal somnolence
Cataplexy
• Sudden loss of muscle tone set off by surprise, laughter, strong emotion etc.
Hypnagogic or hypnapompic hallucinations
• Frightening hallucinations experienced during sleep onset or waking (can occur in normal people)
Sleep paralysis
• Brief paralysis on waking (can occur in normal people)

(200–400 mg per day). Cataplexy responds to clomipramine (25–50 mg 8-hourly) or fluoxetine (20 mg per day).

Parasomnias

Automatic behaviour that is not recalled may take place during light sleep. Sleep talking and sleep walking are innocuous and common in normal children. Sleep walking is uncommon in adults and has no pathological significance. Nightmares are frightening dreams from which the sufferer wakes in a state of fear or agitation. Most normal people have experienced such phenomena and they are not of any significance in terms of organic disease.

Night terrors occur as sudden arousals from deep slow-wave sleep. They are more common in children but may affect adults. The sufferer wakes in a state of agitation, screaming and fearful. Occasionally, violent behaviour occurs. The agitation may last many minutes. Such events may be confused with nocturnal seizures, particularly those arising from the frontal lobe, or their post-ictal effects.

REM sleep behaviour disorder

In this syndrome patients and/or their bed partners notice the often violent acting out of dreams, because there is a loss of the normal muscle atonia during REM sleep. This occurs in Parkinson's disease and Lewy body dementia and can precede the recognition of these neurodegenerative disorders. Treatment is with clonazepam 0.25–2 mg at bedtime.

Restless leg syndrome

This is a common syndrome, also known as Ekbom's syndrome, affecting up to 2% of the population. Unpleasant sensations in the legs that are ameliorated by moving the legs occur when the patient is tired in the evenings and at the onset of sleep. This condition has a strong familial tendency and can present with daytime somnolence due to disturbed night-time sleep. It needs to be distinguished from the daytime sense of restlessness of the limbs known as akathisia that is a side-effect of major tranquillisers, and the related condition of periodic limb movements during sleep. Restless legs can be symptomatic of an underlying peripheral neuropathy or iron deficiency, or other general medical conditions (e.g. uraemia).

Treatment is with clonazepam (0.5–2.0 mg), small doses of levodopa (100–200 mg) or dopamine agonists (p. 1201) at night.

Periodic limb movement syndrome

In this syndrome, sleep is disturbed by repetitive jerky flexion movements of the limbs which occur in the early stages of sleep. The history of abnormal limb movements during sleep may need to be obtained from the patient's bed partner, since the patient may not be aware of the arousals that are occurring as a result of the movements, even though they may be sufficient to cause daytime somnolence. Treatment may be effected with small doses of levodopa (100–200 mg at night) or a dopamine agonist (p. 1201).

CEREBROVASCULAR DISEASE

Cerebrovascular disease is the third most common cause of death in the developed world after cancer and ischaemic heart disease, and is the most common cause of severe physical disability. Stroke is the term used to describe episodes of focal brain dysfunction due to focal ischaemia or haemorrhage. Stroke is the most frequent clinical manifestation of diseases of the cerebral blood vessels, although cerebrovascular disease may present, particularly in the elderly, as a dementia (p. 1197). Whilst subarachnoid haemorrhage (SAH) is a type of stroke based on the above definition, it will be dealt with separately in this chapter since the pathophysiology, clinical manifestations, and management are distinct from ischaemic and haemorrhagic stroke (p. 1190). Stroke is a common medical emergency with an annual incidence of between 180 and 300 per 100 000. The incidence rises steeply with age, and in many developing countries, the incidence is rising because of the adoption of less healthy lifestyles. About one-fifth of patients with an acute stroke will die within a month of the event, and at least half of those who survive will be left with physical disability.

Stroke

Acute stroke is characterised by the rapid appearance (usually over minutes) of a focal deficit of brain function, most commonly a hemiplegia with or without signs of focal higher cerebral dysfunction (such as aphasia), hemisensory loss, visual field defect or brain-stem deficit. Provided that there is a clear history of a rapid-onset focal deficit, the chance of the brain lesion being anything other than vascular is 5% or less. However, care needs to be taken to exclude other differential diagnoses if the symptoms progress over hours or days. Confusion, memory or balance disturbance are more often due to causes other than stroke. Several terms have been used to classify strokes, often based on the duration and evolution of symptoms.

• *Transient ischaemic attack (TIA)*. Describes a stroke in which symptoms resolve within 24 hours—an arbitrary cutoff which has little value in practice apart from perhaps indicating that underlying cerebral haemorrhage or extensive cerebral infarction is extremely unlikely. The term TIA traditionally also includes patients with transient monocular blindness (also known as amaurosis fugax), usually due to a vascular occlusion in the retina. Transient symptoms, such as syncope, amnesia, confusion and dizziness,

26.47 Differential diagnosis of stroke and TIA

- Primary cerebral tumours
- Metastatic cerebral tumours
- Subdural haematoma
- Peripheral nerve lesions (vascular or compressive)
- Cerebral abscess
- Todd's paresis (after epileptic seizure)
- Demyelination
- Hypoglycaemia
- Encephalitis
- Conversion disorder
- Migrainous aura (with or without headache)
- Ménière's disease or other vestibular disorder
- Focal seizures

26.48 Stroke risk factors

Fixed

- Age
- Gender (male > female, except in the very young and very old)
- Race (Afro-Caribbean > Asian > European)
- Heredity
- Previous vascular event, e.g. myocardial infarction, stroke or peripheral embolism
- High fibrinogen

Modifiable

- High blood pressure
- Heart disease (atrial fibrillation, heart failure, endocarditis)
- Diabetes mellitus
- Hyperlipidaemia
- Smoking
- Excess alcohol consumption
- Polycythaemia
- Oral contraceptives
- Social deprivation

which do not reflect focal cerebral dysfunction, are often mistakenly attributed to TIA (see Fig. 26.16, p. 1150, and Box 26.47).

- *Stroke.* This is the term reserved for those events in which symptoms last more than 24 hours. The differential diagnosis of patients with symptoms lasting a few minutes or hours is similar to those with persisting symptoms (see Box 26.47).
- *Progressing stroke (or stroke in evolution).* This describes a stroke in which the focal neurological deficit worsens after the patient first presents. Such worsening may be due to increasing volume of infarction, haemorrhagic transformation or increasing oedema.
- *Completed stroke.* This describes a stroke in which the focal deficit persists and is not progressing.

In clinical practice, it is probably most important to distinguish those patients with strokes who, when seen, have persisting focal neurological symptoms, from those whose symptoms have resolved. When assessing a patient within hours of symptom onset, it is not possible to distinguish stroke from TIA unless the symptoms have already resolved. In patients with persisting symptoms, it is necessary to confirm the diagnosis and then consider treatments to reverse the underlying pathology, prevent complications, alleviate the functional consequences of any persisting neurological impairments and reduce the risks of further stroke or other vascular events. In those patients without persisting symptoms, the emphasis should be on confirming the diagnosis and preventing further vascular events.

Pathophysiology

Of patients presenting with a stroke, 85% will have sustained a cerebral infarction due to inadequate blood flow to part of the brain and the remainder will have had an intracerebral haemorrhage. Brain imaging is required to distinguish these pathologies and to guide management. The combination of severe headache and vomiting at the onset of the focal neurological deficits increases the likelihood of a haemorrhagic stroke.

Cerebral infarction

Cerebral infarction is mostly due to thromboembolic disease secondary to atherosclerosis in the major extracranial arteries (carotid artery and aortic arch). About 20% of infarctions are due to embolism from the heart, and a further 20% are due to intrinsic disease of small perforating vessels (lenticulostriate arteries), producing so-called 'lacunar' infarctions. The risk factors for ischaemic stroke reflect the risk factors for the underlying vascular disease (Box 26.48). About 5% are due to rare causes, including vasculitis (p. 1112), endocarditis (p. 624) and cerebral venous disease (p. 1191). Cerebral infarction is a process which takes some hours to complete, even though the patient's deficit may be maximal close to the onset of the causative vascular occlusion. After the occlusion of a cerebral artery, infarction may be forestalled by the opening of anastomotic channels from other arterial territories which restore perfusion to its territory. Similarly, reduction in perfusion pressure leads to compensatory homeostatic changes to maintain tissue oxygenation (Fig. 26.27). These changes can sometimes prevent even occlusion of a carotid artery from having any clinically apparent effect.

However, if and when these homeostatic mechanisms fail, the process of ischaemia starts and ultimately leads to infarction unless vascular supply is restored. As the cerebral blood flow declines, different neuronal functions fail at various thresholds (Fig. 26.28). Once blood flow falls below the threshold for the maintenance of electrical activity, neurological deficit appears. At this level of blood flow, the neurons are still viable; if the blood flow increases again, function returns and the patient will have had a TIA. However, if the blood flow falls further, a level is reached at which the process of irreversible cell death starts. Hypoxia leads to an inadequate supply of adenosine triphosphate (ATP), which in turn leads to failure of membrane pumps, thereby allowing influx of sodium and water into the cell (cytotoxic oedema) and the release of the excitatory neurotransmitter glutamate into the extracellular fluid. Glutamate opens membrane channels, allowing the influx of calcium and more sodium into the neurons. Calcium entering the neurons activates intracellular enzymes that complete the destructive process. The release of inflammatory mediators by microglia and astrocytes produces death of all cell types in the area of maximum ischaemia. The infarction process is worsened by the anaerobic production of lactic acid (Fig. 26.29) and consequent fall in tissue pH. There have been attempts to develop neuroprotective drugs to slow down

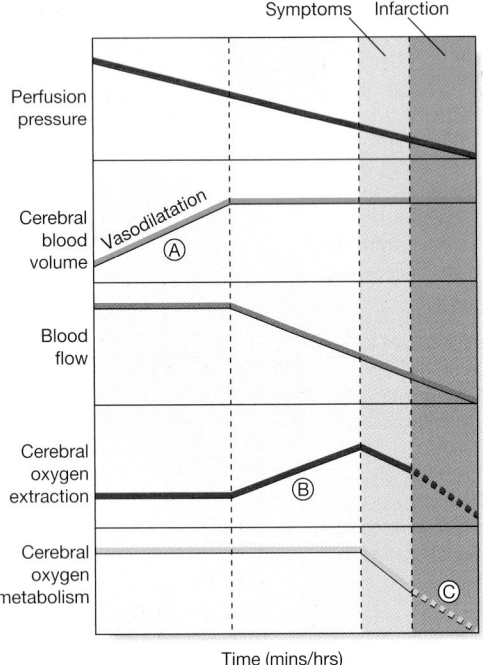

Fig. 26.27 Homeostatic responses to falling perfusion pressure in the brain following arterial occlusion. Vasodilatation initially maintains cerebral blood flow (A), but after maximal vasodilatation further falls in perfusion pressure lead to a decline in blood flow. An increase in tissue oxygen extraction, however, maintains the cerebral metabolic rate for oxygen (B). Still further falls in perfusion, and therefore blood flow, cannot be compensated; cerebral oxygen availability falls and symptoms appear, then infarction (C).

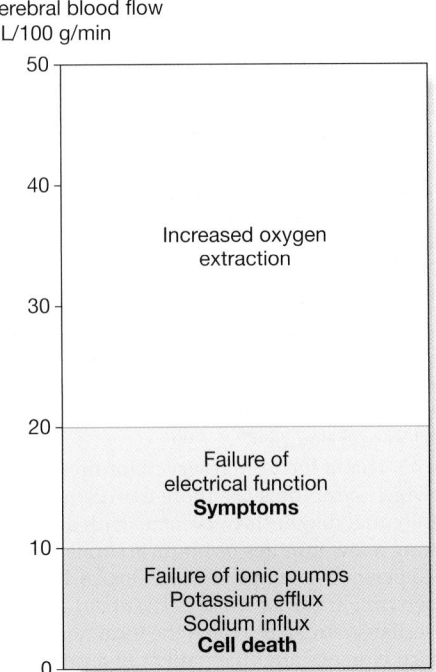

Fig. 26.28 Thresholds of cerebral ischaemia. Symptoms of cerebral ischaemia appear when the blood flow has fallen to less than half of normal and energy supply is insufficient to sustain neuronal electrical function. Full recovery can occur if this level of flow is returned to normal but not if it is sustained. Further blood flow reduction below the next threshold causes failure of cell ionic pumps and starts the ischaemic cascade, leading to cell death.

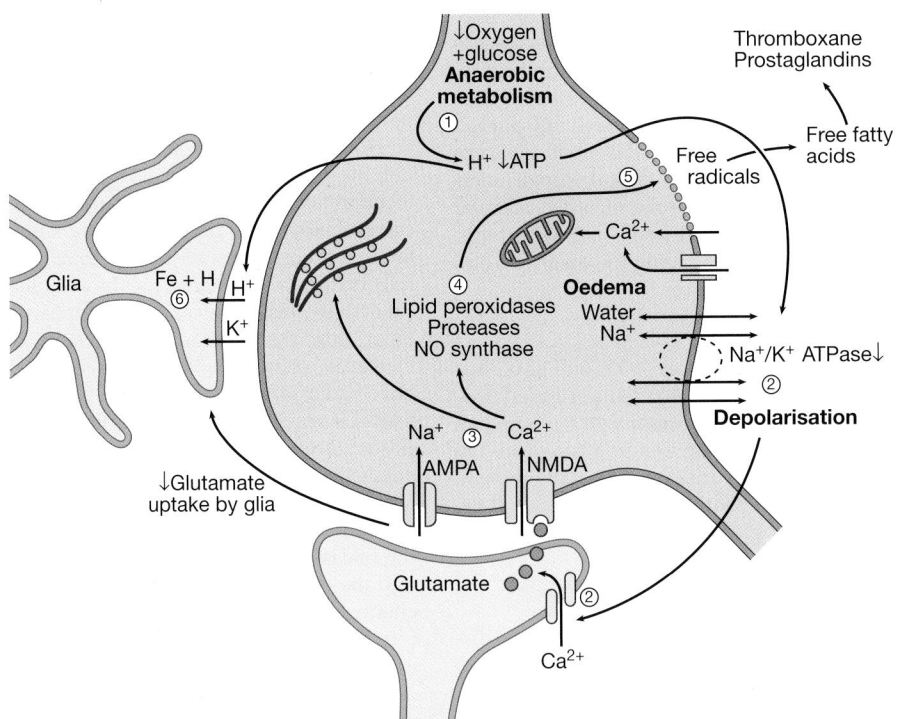

Fig. 26.29 The process of neuronal ischaemia and infarction. (1) Reduction of blood flow reduces supply of oxygen and hence ATP. H^+ is produced by anaerobic metabolism of available glucose. (2) Energy-dependent membrane ionic pumps fail, leading to cytotoxic oedema and membrane depolarisation, allowing calcium entry and releasing glutamate. (3) Calcium enters cells via glutamate-gated channels and (4) activates destructive intracellular enzymes, (5) destroying intracellular organelles and cell membrane, with release of free radicals. Free fatty acid release activates pro-coagulant pathways which exacerbate local ischaemia. (6) Glial cells take up H^+, can no longer take up extracellular glutamate and also suffer cell death, leading to liquefactive necrosis of whole arterial territory.

the processes leading to irreversible cell death but these have so far proved disappointing.

The final result of the occlusion of a cerebral blood vessel therefore depends upon the competence of the circulatory homeostatic mechanisms, the metabolic demand, and the severity and duration of the reduction in blood flow. Higher brain temperature, as might occur in fever, and higher blood sugar have both been associated with a greater volume of infarction for a given reduction in cerebral blood flow. Subsequent restoration of blood flow may cause haemorrhage into the infarcted area ('haemorrhagic transformation'). This is particularly likely to occur in patients given antithrombotic or thrombolytic drugs, and in patients with larger infarcts.

Radiologically, a cerebral infarct can be seen as a lesion which comprises a mixture of dead brain tissue that is already undergoing autolysis and tissue that is ischaemic and swollen but recoverable (the 'ischaemic penumbra'). The infarct swells with time and is at its maximal size a couple of days after stroke onset. At this stage it may be big enough to exert mass effect both clinically and radiologically; sometimes decompressive craniectomy is required at this time (see Box 26.57, p. 1188). As the weeks go by, the oedema subsides and the infarcted area is replaced by a sharply defined fluid-filled cavity.

Intracerebral haemorrhage

This usually results from rupture of a blood vessel within the brain parenchyma but may also occur in a patient with a subarachnoid haemorrhage (p. 1190) if the artery ruptures into the brain substance as well as into the subarachnoid space. Haemorrhage frequently occurs into an area of brain infarction. If the volume of haemorrhage is large, this may be difficult to distinguish from primary intracerebral haemorrhage both clinically and radiologically (see Fig. 26.31C). The risk factors and underlying causes of intracerebral haemorrhage are listed in Box 26.49. The explosive entry of blood into the brain parenchyma causes immediate cessation of function in that area as neurons are structurally disrupted and white matter fibre tracts are split apart. The haemorrhage itself may expand over the first minutes or hours, or it may be associated with a rim

of cerebral oedema, which, along with the haematoma, acts like a mass lesion to cause progression of the neurological deficit. If big enough, this can cause shift of the intracranial contents, producing transtentorial coning and sometimes rapid death (p. 1215). If the patient survives, the haematoma is gradually absorbed, leaving a haemosiderin-lined slit in the brain parenchyma (see Fig. 26.32D).

Clinical features

The clinical presentation of stroke depends upon which arterial territory is involved and the size of the lesion, both of which will have a bearing on management, such as suitability for carotid endarterectomy. The neurological deficit can be identified from the patient's history and, if the deficit is persistent, from the neurological examination. The presence of a unilateral motor deficit, a higher cerebral function deficit such as aphasia or neglect, or a visual field defect usually places the lesion in the cerebral hemisphere. Ataxia, diplopia, vertigo and/or bilateral weakness usually indicate a lesion in the brain stem or cerebellum. Different combinations of these deficits define several stroke syndromes (Fig. 26.30) which reflect the site and size of the lesion and may provide clues to underlying pathology.

Reduced conscious level usually indicates a large-volume lesion in the cerebral hemisphere but may result from a lesion in the brain stem or complications such as obstructive hydrocephalus, hypoxia or severe systemic infection.

Clinical assessment of the patient with a stroke should also include a general examination (Box 26.50) since this may provide clues to the cause of the stroke, and identify important comorbidities and complications of the stroke.

Investigations

Investigation of a patient presenting with an acute stroke aims to confirm the vascular nature of the lesion, distinguish cerebral infarction from haemorrhage and identify the underlying vascular disease and risk factors (Box 26.51).

26

26.49 Causes of intracerebral haemorrhage and associated risk factors	
Disease	**Risk factors**
Complex small vessel disease with disruption of vessel wall	Age Hypertension Low cholesterol
Amyloid angiopathy	Familial (rare) Age
Impaired blood clotting	Anticoagulant therapy Blood dyscrasia Thrombolytic therapy
Vascular anomaly	Arteriovenous malformation Cavernous haemangioma
Substance misuse	Alcohol Amphetamines Cocaine

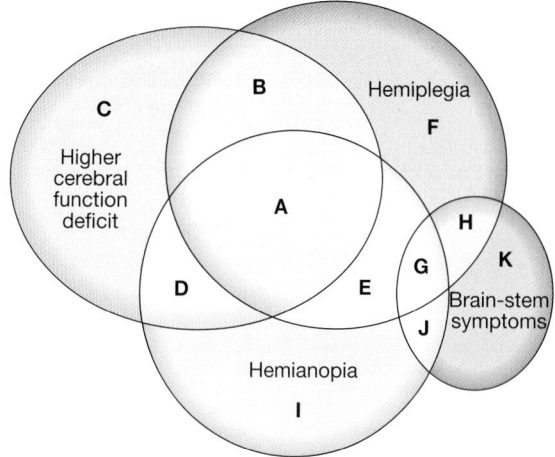

Fig. 26.30 Syndromes of acute stroke. Total anterior circulation syndrome—TACS (A). Partial anterior circulation syndromes—PACS (B, C, D and E). Pure motor stroke—lacunar syndrome (F). Posterior circulation syndromes—POCS (G, H, I, J and K).

26.50 How to examine a stroke patient

Skin

- Xanthelasma
- Rash (arteritis, splinter haemorrhages, livedo reticularis)
- Colour and temperature change (limb ischaemia/deep venous thrombosis)

Eyes

- Arcus senilis
- Diabetic changes
- Hypertensive changes
- Retinal emboli

Cardiovascular system

- Heart rhythm (atrial fibrillation)
- Blood pressure (hypertension, hypotension)
- Jugular venous pressure (heart failure, hypovolaemia)
- Murmurs (sources of embolism)
- Peripheral pulses and bruits (generalised arteriopathy)

Respiratory system

- Signs of pulmonary oedema
- Signs of respiratory infection

Abdomen

- Palpable bladder (urinary retention)

Locomotor

- Injuries sustained during collapse with stroke
- Co-morbidities which influence functional ability

26.51 Investigation of a patient with an acute stroke

Diagnostic question	Investigation
Is it a vascular lesion?	CT/MRI
Is it ischaemic or haemorrhagic?	CT/MRI
Is it a subarachnoid haemorrhage?	CT/lumbar puncture
Is there any cardiac source of embolism?	Electrocardiogram (ECG) 24-hour ECG Echocardiogram
What is the underlying vascular disease?	Duplex ultrasound of carotids Magnetic resonance angiography (MRA) CT angiography (CTA) Contrast angiography
What are the risk factors?	Full blood count Cholesterol Blood glucose
Is there an unusual cause?	ESR Serum protein electrophoresis Clotting/thrombophilia screen

Risk factor analysis

Initial investigation of all patients with stroke includes a range of simple blood tests to detect common vascular risk factors and markers of rarer causes, an electrocardiogram (ECG) and brain imaging. Where there is uncertainty about the nature of the stroke, further investigations are usually indicated. This especially

26.52 Causes and investigation of acute stroke in young patients

Cause	Investigation
Cerebral infarct	
Cardiac embolism	Echocardiography (including transoesophageal)
Premature atherosclerosis	Serum lipids
Arterial dissection	MRI Angiography
Thrombophilia	Protein C, protein S Antithrombin III Factor V Leiden, prothrombin
Homocystinuria (p. 447)	Urinary amino acids Methionine loading test
Antiphospholipid antibody syndrome (p. 1050)	Anticardiolipin antibodies/lupus anticoagulant
SLE	Antinuclear antibodies
Vasculitis	ESR CRP Antineutrophil cytoplasmic antibody (ANCA)
CADASIL (cerebral autosomal dominant arteriopathy with subcortical infarcts and leucoencephalopathy)	MRI brain Genetic analysis Skin biopsy
Mitochondrial cytopathy	Serum lactate White cell mitochondrial DNA Muscle biopsy Mitochondrial molecular genetics
Fabry's disease	Alpha-galactosidase levels in blood
Neurovascular syphilis	Syphilis serology
Primary intracerebral haemorrhage	
Arteriovenous malformation (AVM)	MRI/angiography
Drug misuse	Drug screen (amphetamine, cocaine)
Coagulopathy	Prothrombin time (PT) and activated partial thromboplastin time (APTT) Platelet count
Subarachnoid haemorrhage	
Saccular ('berry') aneurysm	MRI/angiography
AVM	MRI/angiography
Vertebral dissection	MRI/angiography

applies to younger patients who are less likely to have atherosclerotic disease (Box 26.52).

Neuroimaging

Brain imaging with either CT or MRI should be performed in all patients with acute stroke. Exceptions to this include patients in whom the results would not influence management, such as in the advanced stage of a terminal illness. CT is the most practical and widely available method of imaging the brain. It will usually exclude non-stroke lesions, including subdural haematomas and brain tumours, and will demonstrate intracerebral haemorrhage within minutes of stroke onset (Fig. 26.31). However, especially within the first few hours after symptom onset, CT changes in cerebral infarction may be completely absent or only very subtle. Changes often develop over time (Fig. 26.32), but small cerebral infarcts may never show up on CT scans. For most purposes, a CT scan performed within

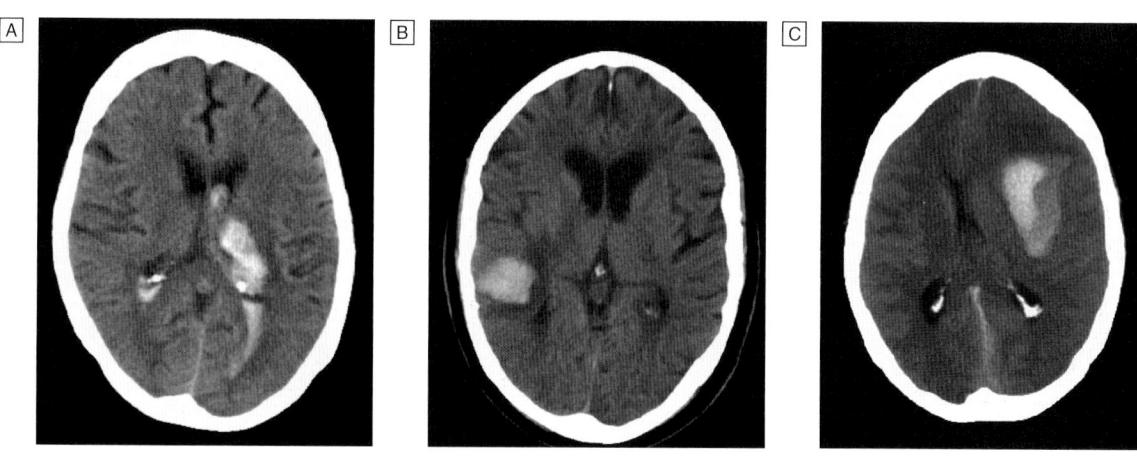

Fig. 26.31 CT scans of intracerebral haemorrhage. **A** Basal ganglia haemorrhage with intraventricular extension. **B** Small cortical haemorrhage. **C** Large haemorrhage with mass effect.

 26.53 Indications for emergency CT/MRI in acute stroke

- Patient on anticoagulants or with abnormal coagulation
- Consideration of thrombolysis or immediate anticoagulation
- Deteriorating conscious level or rapidly progressing deficits
- Suspected cerebellar haematoma, to exclude hydrocephalus

---

the first day or so is adequate for clinical care but there are certain circumstances in which an immediate CT scan is essential (Box 26.53). Even in the absence of changes suggesting infarction, abnormal perfusion of brain tissue can be imaged with CT after injection of contrast media (i.e. perfusion scanning). This can be useful in guiding immediate treatment of ischaemic stroke. MRI is not as widely available as CT, scanning times are longer, and it cannot be used in some individuals with contraindications (see Box 26.2, p. 1144). However, MRI diffusion weighted imaging (DWI) can detect ischaemia earlier than CT, and other MRI sequences can also be used to demonstrate abnormal perfusion (see Fig. 26.32). MRI is more sensitive than CT in detecting strokes affecting the brain stem and cerebellum, and, unlike CT, can reliably distinguish haemorrhagic stroke from ischaemic stroke even several weeks after the onset (see Fig. 26.32C and D). CT and MRI may reveal clues as to the nature of the arterial lesion. For example, there may be a small, deep lacunar infarct (Fig. 26.33A) indicating small-vessel disease, or a more peripheral infarct suggesting an extracranial source of embolism (see Fig. 26.33B). In a haemorrhagic lesion, the location might indicate the presence of an underlying vascular malformation, saccular aneurysm or amyloid angiopathy.

Vascular imaging

Many ischaemic strokes are caused by atherosclerotic thromboembolic disease of the major extracranial vessels. Detection of extracranial vascular disease can help establish why the patient has had an ischaemic stroke and may, in highly selected patients, lead on to specific treatments including carotid endarterectomy to reduce the risk of further stroke (p. 1189). The presence or absence of a carotid bruit is not a reliable indicator of the degree of carotid stenosis. Extracranial arterial disease can be non-invasively identified with duplex ultra-

sound, MR angiography (MRA) or CT angiography (see Fig. 26.15, p. 1146). Because of the significant risk of complications, intra-arterial contrast angiography is reserved for patients in whom non-invasive methods have provided a contradictory picture or yielded incomplete information, or in whom it is necessary to image the intracranial circulation in detail: for example, to delineate a saccular aneurysm, an arteriovenous malformation or vasculitis.

Cardiac investigations

Approximately 20% of ischaemic strokes are due to embolism from the heart. The most common causes are atrial fibrillation, prosthetic heart valves, other valvular abnormalities and recent myocardial infarction. These can often be identified by clinical examination and ECG but cardiac sources of embolism can exist without obvious clinical or ECG signs. A transthoracic or transoesophageal echocardiogram can be useful, either to confirm the presence of a clinically apparent cardiac source or to identify an unsuspected source such as endocarditis, atrial myxoma, intracardiac thrombus or patent foramen ovale. Such findings may lead on to specific treatment (Ch. 18).

Management

Management is aimed at minimising the volume of brain that is irreversibly damaged, preventing complications (Box 26.54), reducing the patient's disability and handicap through rehabilitation, and reducing the risk of recurrent episodes.

Supportive care

Early admission of patients to a specialised stroke unit facilitates coordinated care from a specialised multidisciplinary team (Ch. 7) and has been shown to reduce both mortality and residual disability amongst survivors (Box 26.55). Consideration of a patient's rehabilitation needs should commence at the same time as acute medical management. Dysphagia is common after stroke and can be detected by an early bedside test of swallowing. This allows hydration, feeding and medication to be given safely, if necessary by nasogastric tube or intravenously. In the acute phase it may be useful to refer to a checklist (Box 26.56) to ensure that all the factors

26

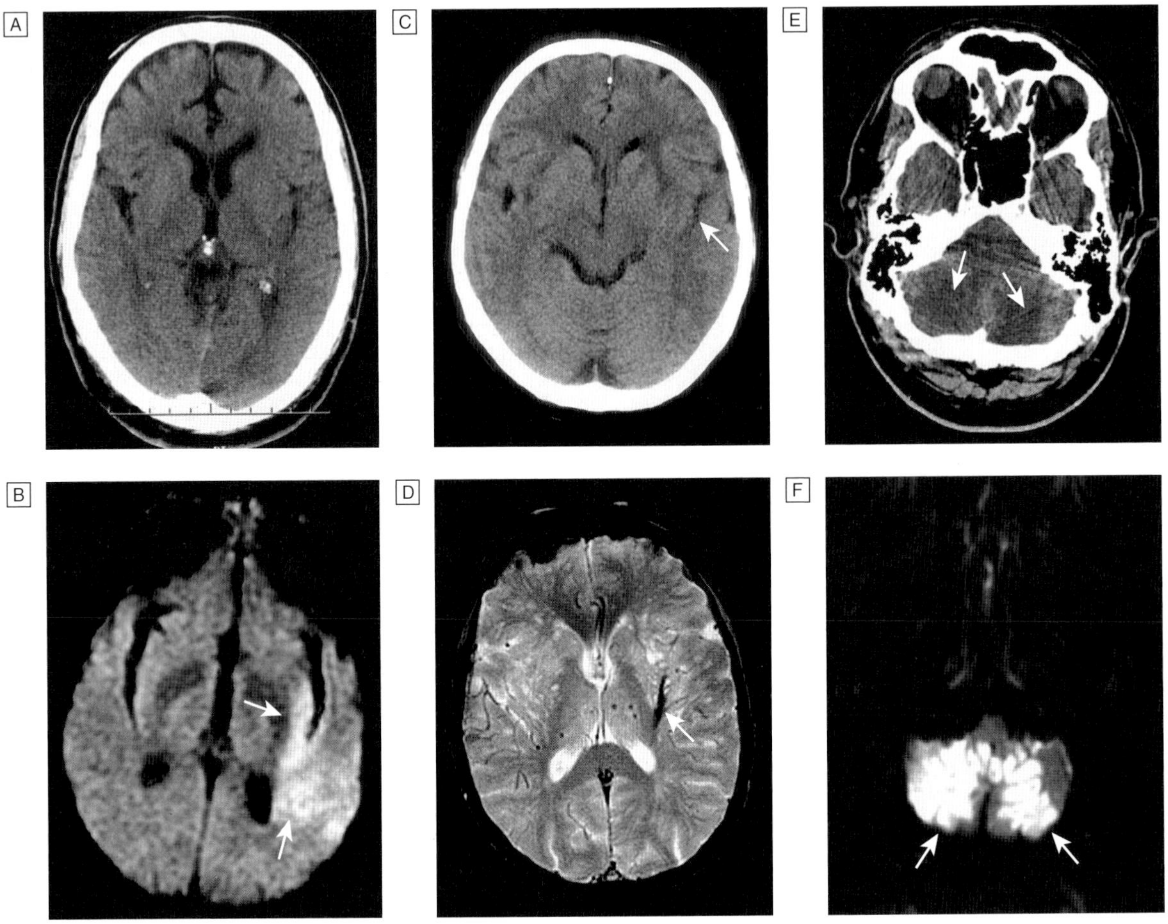

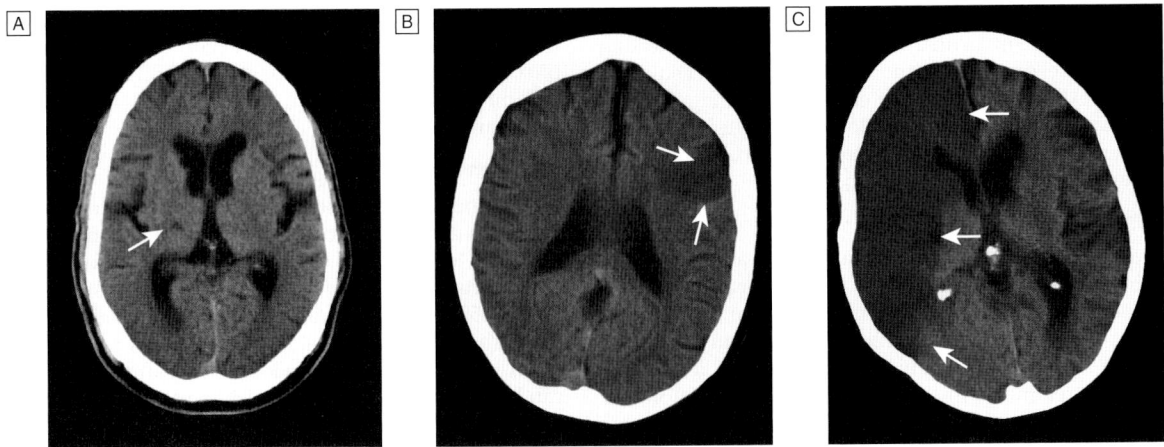

Fig. 26.32 Acute stroke seen in CT scans with corresponding MRI appearances. A CT may show no evidence of early infarction. B Corresponding image seen on MRI diffusion weighted imaging (DWI) with changes in middle cerebral artery (MCA) territory (arrows). C Late appearance of haemorrhage on CT (arrow). D Corresponding appearance on gradient echo MRI (arrow). E Subtle appearance of massive cerebellar infarction on CT (arrows). F Corresponding appearance is more obvious on DWI MRI (arrows).

which might influence the patient's outcome have been addressed.

The patient's neurological deficits may worsen during the first few hours or days after their onset. This is most common amongst those with lacunar infarc-tion but may occur in other patients, due to extension of the area of infarction, haemorrhage into it, or the development of oedema with consequent mass effect. It is important to distinguish such patients from those who are deteriorating as a result of complications such

Fig. 26.33 CT scans in ischaemic stroke. A Typical appearance of a lacunar infarct in the basal ganglia (arrow). B Small cortical infarct (arrows). C Large middle and anterior cerebral artery territory infarct with mass effect (arrows).

26.54 Complications of acute stroke

Complication	Prevention	Treatment
Chest infection	Nurse semi-erect Avoid aspiration (nil by mouth, nasogastric tube, possible gastrostomy)	Antibiotics Physiotherapy
Epileptic seizures	Maintain cerebral oxygenation Avoid metabolic disturbance	Anticonvulsants
Deep venous thrombosis/ pulmonary embolism	Maintain hydration Early mobilisation Anti-embolism stockings Heparin (for high-risk patients only)	Anticoagulation (exclude haemorrhagic stroke first)
Painful shoulder	Avoid traction injury Shoulder/arm supports Physiotherapy	Physiotherapy Local corticosteroid injections
Pressure sores	Frequent turning Monitor pressure areas Avoid urinary damage to skin	Nursing care Pressure-relieving mattress
Urinary infection	Avoid catheterisation if possible Use penile sheath	Antibiotics
Constipation	Appropriate aperients and diet	Appropriate aperients
Depression and anxiety	Maintain positive attitude and provide information	Antidepressants

---

EBM 26.55 Specialist stroke units

'Admitting 1000 patients to a stroke unit prevents about 50 patients from being dead or dependent at 6 months.'

• Langhorne P, Pollock A in conjunction with the Stroke Unit Trialists Collaboration. Age Ageing 2002; 31:365–371.

For further information: 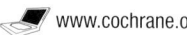 www.cochrane.org

---

26.56 Management of acute stroke

Airway
- Check that the patient can protect his/her airway and swallow without evidence of aspiration
- Perform a swallow screen and keep patient nil by mouth if swallowing unsafe

Breathing
- Check that the patient is breathing adequately; check oxygen saturation and give oxygen if saturation < 95%

Circulation
- Check peripheral perfusion, pulse and blood pressure adequate and treat with fluid replacement, anti-arrhythmics and inotropic drugs as appropriate

Hydration
- Screen for signs of dehydration and give fluids parenterally or by nasogastric tube if necessary

Nutrition
- Assess nutritional status and provide nutritional supplements if necessary
- If dysphagia persists for a day or two, start feeding via a nasogastric tube

Medication
- If the patient is dysphagic, consider alternative routes for essential medications

Blood pressure
- Unless there is heart failure or renal failure, evidence of hypertensive encephalopathy or aortic dissection, do not lower the blood pressure in the first week since cerebral perfusion may decrease. Blood pressure often returns towards the patient's normal level within the first few days

Blood glucose
- Check blood glucose and treat with insulin when levels are ≥ 11.1 mmol/L (200 mg/dL) (via infusion or glucose/potassium/insulin (GKI)). Monitor closely to avoid hypoglycaemia

Temperature
- Check for pyrexia and investigate and treat underlying cause
- Give antipyretics since raised brain temperature may increase infarct volume

Pressure areas
- Check pressure areas and introduce measures to reduce the risk of bed sores
  - Treat infection
  - Maintain nutrition
  - Provide a pressure-relieving mattress
  - Turn immobile patients regularly

Incontinence
- Check for constipation and urinary retention and treat appropriately
- Avoid urinary catheterisation unless the patient is in acute urinary retention or incontinence is threatening pressure areas

26

---

as hypoxia, sepsis, epileptic seizures or metabolic abnormalities which may be more easily reversed. Patients with cerebellar haematomas or infarcts with mass effect may develop obstructive hydrocephalus and some will benefit from insertion of a ventricular drain and/or decompressive surgery (Box 26.57). Some patients with large haematomas or infarction with massive oedema in the cerebral hemispheres may benefit from anti-oedema agents, such as mannitol or artificial ventilation, and surgical decompression to reduce intracranial pressure should be considered in appropriate patients.

Thrombolysis

Intravenous thrombolysis with recombinant tissue plasminogen activator (rt-PA) increases the risk of haemorrhagic transformation of the cerebral infarct with potentially fatal results. However, if given within 3 hours of symptom onset to highly selected patients, the haemorrhagic risk is offset by an improvement in overall outcome (Box 26.58).

Aspirin

In the absence of contraindications, aspirin (300 mg daily) should be started immediately after an ischaemic

EBM 26.57 Decompressive craniectomy after large cerebral infarction

'Early decompressive surgery in patients with large infarctions of the middle cerebral artery reduces mortality and improves functional outcome. NNT = 2 to prevent death or severe disability.'

• Vahedi K, et al. Lancet Neurol 2007; 6(3):215–222K.

EBM 26.58 Thrombolysis in acute ischaemic stroke

'rt-PA increases the risk of fatal intracranial haemorrhage, but this risk is offset by an improvement in longer-term outcome amongst survivors. The maximum benefit appears to be when thrombolysis is given within 3 hours of onset. Treating 1000 patients within 3 hours prevents about 60 patients from being dead or dependent at 3 months.'

• Wardlaw JM, et al. (Cochrane Review). Cochrane Library, issue 4, 2005. Oxford: Update Software.
• Mielke O, et al. (Cochrane Review). Cochrane Library, issue 4, 2005. Oxford: Update Software.

For further information: www.cochrane.org

stroke unless rt-PA has been given, in which case it should be withheld for at least 24 hours. Aspirin reduces the risk of early recurrence and has a small but clinically worthwhile effect on long-term outcome (Box 26.59); it may be given by rectal suppository or by nasogastric tube in dysphagic patients.

Heparin

Anticoagulation with heparin has been widely used to treat acute ischaemic stroke in the past. Whilst this does reduce the risk of early ischaemic recurrence and venous thromboembolism, these benefits are offset by a definite increase in the risk of both intracranial and extracranial haemorrhage. Furthermore, routine use of heparin does not result in better long-term outcomes, and therefore it should not be used in the routine management of acute stroke. It is unclear whether anticoagulation with heparin might provide benefit in selected patients, such as those with recent myocardial infarction, arterial dissection or progressing strokes. Intracranial haemorrhage must be excluded on brain imaging before considering anticoagulation.

Coagulation abnormalities

Coagulation abnormalities should be reversed as quickly as possible to reduce the likelihood of the haematoma enlarging. There is no evidence that clotting factors are useful in the absence of a clotting defect.

EBM 26.59 Aspirin in acute ischaemic stroke

'After an acute persistent stroke, aspirin started within 48 hours of onset improves long-term outcome. Treating 1000 patients for 2 weeks prevents 13 being dead or dependent by 6 months.'

• Gubitz G, et al. (Cochrane Review). Cochrane Library, issue 3, 2004. Oxford: Update Software.
• Chen ZM, et al. on behalf of the CAST and IST Collaborative Groups. Stroke 2000; 31:1240–1249.

For further information: www.cochrane.org

Management of risk factors

The approaches used are summarized in Fig. 26.34. The average risk of a further stroke is 5–10% within the first week of a stroke or TIA, perhaps 15% in the first year and 5% per year thereafter. The risks are not clearly different for intracerebral haemorrhage. Patients with ischaemic events should be put on long-term antiplatelet drugs (Box 26.60) and statins to lower cholesterol (Box 26.61). For patients in atrial fibrillation the risk can be reduced by about 60% by oral anticoagulation to achieve an INR of 2–3 (Box 26.62). The risk of recurrence after both ischaemic and haemorrhagic strokes can be reduced by blood pressure reduction, even for those with blood pressures in the normal range (Box 26.63).

EBM 26.60 Antiplatelet drugs in secondary prevention of ischaemic stroke

'In patients with ischaemic stroke, aspirin, clopidogrel or a combination of aspirin and dipyridamole reduces the risk of recurrent stroke, myocardial infarction and vascular deaths. Treating 1000 patients for a year prevents about 10 strokes.'

• Antithrombotic Trialists' Collaboration. BMJ 2002; 324:71–86.
• Hankey GJ, et al. Stroke 2000; 31:1779–1784.

For further information: www.cochrane.org

EBM 26.61 Statins in secondary prevention of ischaemic stroke

'In patients with ischaemic stroke, statins reduce the risk of recurrent stroke, myocardial infarction and vascular deaths. Treating 1000 patients for a year prevents about 17 strokes.'

• Heart Protection Study Collaborative Group. Lancet 2002; 360:7–22.
• Stroke Prevention by Aggressive Reduction in Cholesterol Levels (SPARCL investigators). N Engl J Med 2006; 355(6):549–559.

For further information: www.cochrane.org

EBM 26.62 Anticoagulants in secondary prevention of ischaemic stroke

'There is no net benefit to be gained in the routine use of anticoagulants after acute stroke except in the presence of atrial fibrillation, when treating 1000 patients for a year prevents about 80 strokes.'

• Hart RG, et al. Ann Intern Med 1999; 131:492–501.

For further information: www.cochrane.org

EBM 26.63 Blood pressure lowering in secondary prevention of stroke

'Lowering blood pressure even in the 'normal range' reduces the risk of recurrent stroke, myocardial infarction and vascular deaths in patients who have suffered a stroke. Treating 1000 patients for a year prevents about 22 strokes.'

• PROGRESS Collaborative Group. Lancet 2001; 358:1033–1041.

For further information: www.cochrane.org

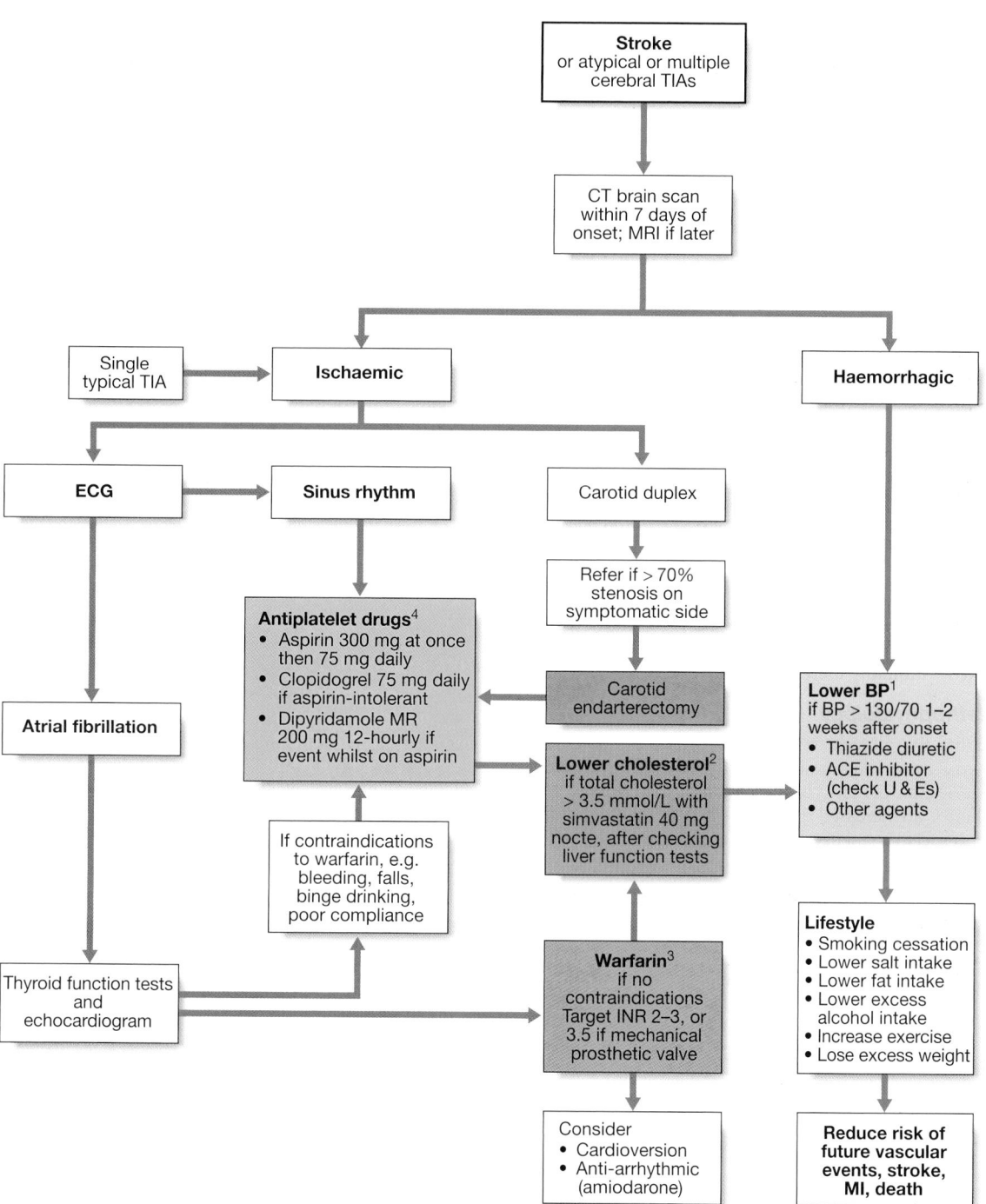

Figure 26.34 Strategies for secondary prevention of stroke. (1) Lower BP with caution in patients with postural hypotension, renal impairment or bilateral carotid stenosis. (2) Pravastatin 40 mg should be considered as an alternative to simvastatin in patients on warfarin or digoxin. (3) Warfarin and aspirin can be used in combination in patients with prosthetic heart valves. (4) The combination of aspirin and clopidogrel is only indicated in patients with unstable angina with ECG or enzyme changes.

Carotid endarterectomy and angioplasty

A small proportion of patients with a carotid territory ischaemic stroke or TIA will have a greater than 50% stenosis of the carotid artery on the side of the brain lesion. Such patients have a greater than average risk of stroke recurrence. For those without major residual disability, removal of the stenosis has been shown to reduce the overall risk of recurrence, although the operation itself carries about a 5% risk of stroke (Box 26.64). The effec-

tiveness of surgery is greatest for those with more severe stenoses (70–99%) and in those in whom surgery can be performed within the first couple of weeks after the TIA or ischaemic stroke. Carotid angioplasty and stenting are technically feasible but have not been shown to be superior to endarterectomy. Endarterectomy of asymptomatic carotid stenosis has been shown to reduce the subsequent risk of stroke, but the small absolute benefit does not justify its routine use.

26

EBM **26.64 Carotid endarterectomy in ischaemic stroke and TIA**

'Carotid endarterectomy reduces the risk of subsequent stroke in patients who have suffered a stroke in the carotid territory, when there is severe ipsilateral stenosis (70%) of the carotid artery. Operating on 1000 patients prevents about 40 strokes over the next year.

In asymptomatic carotid stenosis, endarterectomy has a smaller benefit. Operating on 1000 patients prevents about 13 strokes over the next year.'

- Rothwell PM, et al. Lancet 2003; 361:107–16.
- Executive Committee for the Asymptomatic Carotid Atherosclerosis Study. JAMA 1995; 273:1421–1428.

For further information: www.cochrane.org

Subarachnoid haemorrhage

Subarachnoid haemorrhage (SAH) is less common than other types of stroke and affects about 6/100 000 of the population. Women are affected more commonly than men and the condition usually presents before the age of 65. The immediate mortality of aneurysmal subarachnoid haemorrhage is about 30% and survivors have a recurrence, or rebleed, rate of about 40% in the first 4 weeks and 3% annually thereafter.

Pathophysiology

Eighty-five percent of SAH are caused by saccular or 'berry' aneurysms arising from the bifurcation of cerebral arteries, particularly in the region of the circle of Willis. There is an increased risk in first-degree relatives of those with saccular aneurysms, and an increased risk of SAH in patients with polycystic kidney disease and congenital connective tissue defects such as Ehlers–Danlos syndrome. In about 10% of cases, SAH are non-aneurysmal haemorrhages (so-called peri-mesencephalic haemorrhages), which have a very characteristic appearance on CT and a benign outcome in terms of mortality and recurrence. Some 5% of SAH are due to arteriovenous malformations and vertebral artery dissection.

Clinical features

Subarachnoid haemorrhage typically presents with a sudden, severe 'thunderclap' headache (often occipital) which lasts for hours or even days, often accompanied by vomiting. Physical exertion, straining and sexual excitement are common antecedents. There may be loss of consciousness at the onset, so subarachnoid haemorrhage should be considered if a patient is found comatose. About 1 patient in 8 with a sudden severe headache has SAH and, in view of this, all patients with this presentation require investigation to exclude a subarachnoid haemorrhage (Fig. 26.35).

On examination the patient is usually distressed and irritable, with photophobia. There may be neck stiffness due to subarachnoid blood but this may take some hours to develop. Focal hemisphere signs such as hemiparesis or aphasia may be present at onset if there is an associated intracerebral haematoma. A third nerve palsy may be present due to local pressure from an aneurysm of the posterior communicating artery, though this is rare. Fundoscopy may reveal a subhyaloid haemorrhage, which represents blood tracking along the subarachnoid space around the optic nerve.

Investigations

Lumbar puncture is the investigation of first choice and should be performed after 12 hours from symptom onset, if possible. The diagnosis of SAH can be made by CT, but a negative result does not exclude the diagnosis since small amounts of blood in the subarachnoid space cannot be detected by CT (see Fig. 26.35). If either of these tests is positive, cerebral angiography is required to determine the optimal approach to prevent recurrent bleeding.

Management

Insertion of platinum coils into an aneurysm (via an endovascular procedure) or surgical clipping of the

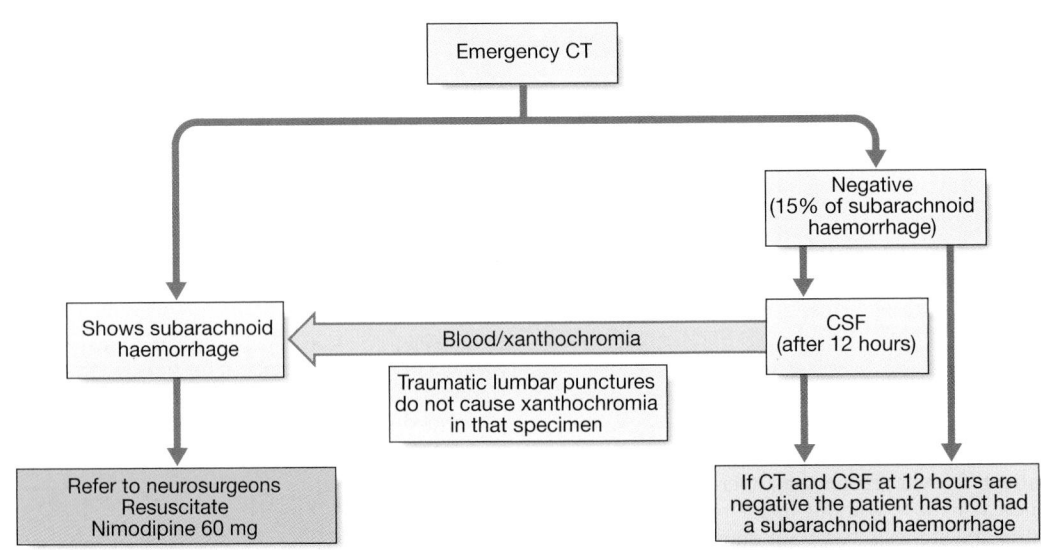

Fig. 26.35 The investigation of sudden severe headache.

aneurysm neck reduces the risk of both early and late recurrence. Coiling is associated with fewer perioperative complications and better outcomes than surgery; where feasible, it is now the procedure of first choice. Arteriovenous malformations can be managed in several different ways including surgical removal, ligation of the blood vessels that feed or drain the lesion, or injection of material to occlude the fistula or draining veins. Nimodipine (30–60 mg i.v. for 5–14 days, followed by 360 mg orally for a further 7 days) is usually given to prevent vasospasm in the acute phase. Treatment may also be required for complications of SAH, which include obstructive hydrocephalus (possibly requiring drainage via a shunt), delayed cerebral ischaemia due to vasospasm (vasodilators), hyponatraemia (water restriction) and systemic complications associated with immobility, such as chest infection and venous thrombosis.

Cerebral venous disease

Thrombosis of the cerebral veins and venous sinuses is less common than arterial thrombosis but has been recognised with increasing frequency over recent years. The causes are listed in Box 26.65.

Cerebral venous sinus occlusion causes raised intracranial pressure and patchy ischaemia, which is often haemorrhagic. The clinical features vary according to the part of the cerebral venous system involved (see below). Anticoagulation is usually beneficial, even in the presence of venous haemorrhage. In selected patients, the use of endovascular thrombolysis has been advocated. Management of underlying causes and complications, such as persistently raised intracranial pressure, is also important.

Cortical vein thrombosis

This may present with focal cortical deficits, such as aphasia and hemiparesis, and epilepsy (focal or generalised), depending on the area involved. The deficit may enlarge if spreading thrombophlebitis occurs.

Cerebral venous sinus thrombosis

The clinical features of cerebral venous sinus thrombosis depend on the sinus involved (Box 26.66). About 10% of cerebral venous sinus thrombosis is associated with infection, particularly thrombosis of the cavernous sinus. Antibiotics are obviously indicated in this situation. Otherwise, the treatment of choice is anticoagulation, as above.

26.65 Causes of cerebral venous thrombosis

Predisposing systemic causes

- Dehydration
- Pregnancy
- Behçet's disease (p. 1114)
- Thrombophilia (p. 997)
- Hypotension
- Oral contraceptive use

Local causes

- Paranasal sinusitis
- Meningitis, subdural empyema
- Penetrating head and eye wounds
- Facial skin infection
- Otitis media, mastoiditis
- Skull fracture

26.66 Clinical features of cerebral venous thrombosis

Cavernous sinus thrombosis

- Proptosis, ptosis, headache, external and internal ophthalmoplegia, papilloedema, reduced sensation in trigeminal first division
- Often bilateral, patient ill and febrile

Superior sagittal sinus thrombosis

- Headache, papilloedema, seizures
- Clinical features may resemble idiopathic intracranial hypertension (p. 1221)
- May involve veins of both hemispheres, causing advancing motor and sensory focal deficits

Transverse sinus thrombosis

- Hemiparesis, seizures, papilloedema
- May spread to jugular foramen and involve cranial nerves 9, 10, 11

Subdural haematoma

This is a collection of blood which forms between the dura and the surface of the brain, due to rupture of veins on the surface of the brain. It usually follows trauma, but may occur spontaneously, particularly in patients on anticoagulants. It is common in the elderly and in patients who misuse alcohol. There may or may not be a history of trauma. Patients present with subacute impairment of brain function, both globally (obtundation, coma) and focally (hemiparesis, seizures). Headaches may or may not be present. The diagnosis should always be considered in patients presenting with unexplained reduction of consciousness. CT is the investigation of choice, and management entails surgical drainage, usually via a burr hole.

INFLAMMATORY DISEASES

Multiple sclerosis

Multiple sclerosis (MS) is an important cause of long-term disability in adults. The prevalence is about 120 per 100 000 of the population in the UK, with an annual incidence of around 7 per 100 000. The lifetime risk of developing MS is about 1 in 400. The incidence of MS is higher in temperate climates and in Northern Europeans, and the disease is about twice as common in women as men.

Pathophysiology

There is evidence that both genetic and environmental factors play a causative role. The prevalence of MS is low in countries near the equator and increases in the temperate zones of both hemispheres. Most importantly, people retain the risk of developing the disease in the zone in which they grew up, indicating that environmental exposures during growth and development are important. The prevalence has also been found to correlate with various environmental factors, such as sunlight exposure, vitamin D and exposure to Epstein–Barr virus (EBV), although it is currently unclear exactly how all of these factors interact to cause the disease. Genetic factors are also important; the risk of familial recurrence

26

in MS is 15%, and the highest risk is in first-degree relatives (age-adjusted risk: 4–5% for siblings and 2–3% for parents or offspring). Monozygotic twins have a concordance rate of 30%. The genes that predispose to MS are incompletely defined but inheritance appears to be polygenic, with influences from the HLA region, *IL-7R* (interleukin-7 receptor), *IL-2R* (interleukin-2 receptor), *CLEC16A* (C-type lectin domain family 16 member A) and *CD226* genes. An immune mechanism is suggested by increased levels of activated T lymphocytes in the CSF and increased immunoglobulin synthesis within the CNS.

An attack of CNS inflammation in MS starts with the entry of activated T lymphocytes across the blood–brain barrier. These recognise myelin-derived antigens on the surface of the nervous system's antigen-presenting cells, the microglia, and undergo clonal proliferation. The resulting inflammatory cascade releases cytokines and initiates destruction of the oligodendrocyte–myelin unit by macrophages. Histologically, the characteristic lesion is a plaque of inflammatory demyelination occurring most commonly in the periventricular regions of the brain, the optic nerves and the subpial regions of the spinal cord (Fig. 26.36). Initially, this is a circumscribed area of disintegration of the myelin sheath, accompanied by infiltration by activated lymphocytes and macrophages, often with conspicuous perivascular inflammation. After an acute attack, gliosis follows, leaving a shrunken grey scar.

Much of the initial acute clinical deficit is caused by the effect of inflammatory cytokines upon transmission of the nervous impulse rather than structural disruption of the myelin, and this explains the rapid recovery of some deficits and probably any benefit from corticosteroids. However, the myelin loss that results from an attack reduces the efficiency of impulse propagation or causes complete conduction block, which therefore impairs the efficiency of CNS functions. Inflammatory mediators released during the acute attack (particularly nitric oxide) probably also initiate axonal damage, which is a feature of the latter stages of the disease. In established MS there is progressive axonal loss, probably due to direct damage to axonal integrity by the inflammatory mediators released in acute attacks and the subsequent loss of neurotrophic factors from oligodendrocytes. This axonal loss is the cause of the phase of the disease in which there is progressive and persistent disability (Fig. 26.37).

Clinical features

A diagnosis of MS requires the demonstration of lesions for which there is no other explanation in more than one anatomical site at more than one time (Box 26.67). Around 80% of patients have a relapsing and remitting clinical course of episodic dysfunction of the CNS with variable recovery. Of the remaining 20%, most follow a slowly progressive clinical course, with a tiny minority who have a fulminant variety leading to early death (see Fig. 26.37). The peak age of onset is in the fourth decade and onset before puberty or after the age of 60 years is rare. There are a number of clinical symptoms and syndromes suggestive of MS, some of which may occur at presentation while others may develop during the course of the illness (Box 26.68).

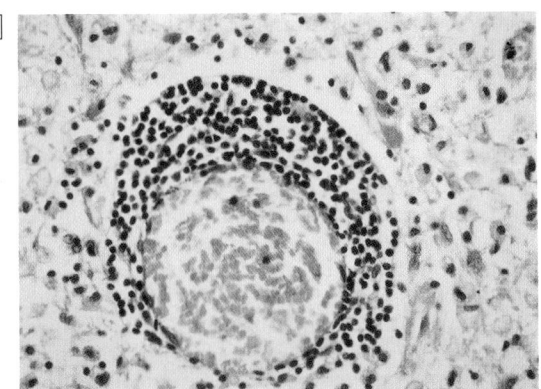

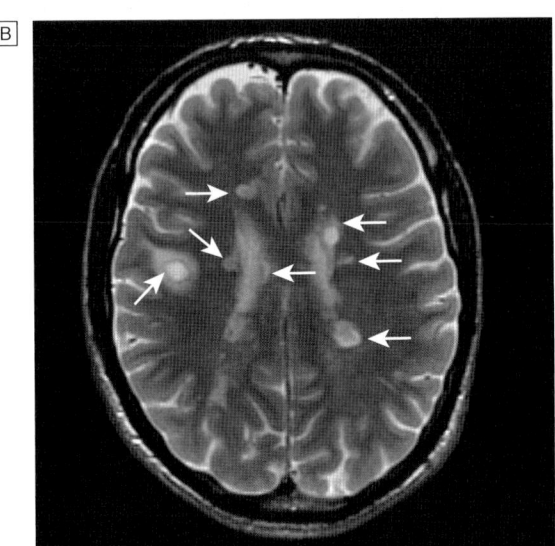

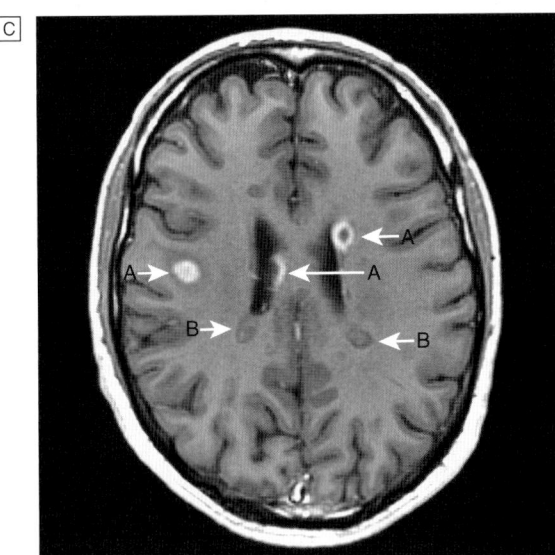

Fig. 26.36 Multiple sclerosis. **A** Photomicrograph from demyelinating plaque showing perivascular cuffing of blood vessel by lymphocytes. **B** Brain MRI in multiple sclerosis. Multiple high-signal lesions (arrows) seen particularly in the paraventricular region on T2 image. **C** In T1 image with gadolinium enhancement recent lesions (A arrows) show enhancement, suggesting active inflammation (enhancement persists for 4 weeks); older lesions (B arrows) show no enhancement but low signal, suggesting gliosis.

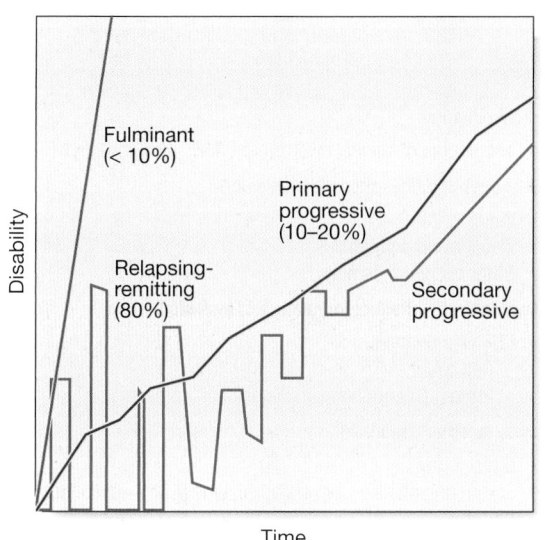

Fig. 26.37 The progression of disability in fulminant, relapsing-remitting and progressive multiple sclerosis.

Demyelinating lesions cause symptoms and signs that usually come on subacutely over days or weeks and resolve over weeks or months, although a stroke-like presentation may rarely occur. After a variable interval there may be a recurrence, often within 2 years.

Frequent relapses with incomplete recovery indicate a poor prognosis. In many patients a phase of secondary progression, caused by secondary axonal degeneration, supersedes the phase of relapse and remission. In a minority of patients, there may be an interval of years or even decades between attacks, and in some, particularly if optic neuritis is the initial manifestation, there is no recurrence. Some presentations, such as optic neuritis with purely sensory relapses, have a good prognosis.

The physical signs observed in MS depend on the anatomical site of demyelination. Combinations of spinal cord and brain-stem signs are common, possibly with evidence of previous optic neuritis in the form of an afferent pupillary deficit. Significant intellectual impairment is unusual until late in the disease, when loss of frontal functions and impairment of memory are common.

The prognosis of MS is difficult to predict with confidence, especially early in the disease. About 15% of patients have a single attack of demyelination and do not suffer further events, whilst those with relapsing and remitting MS have, on average, 1–2 events every 2 years. Approximately 5% of patients die within 5 years of onset, whilst others have a benign outcome. Overall, about one-third of patients are disabled to the point of needing help with walking after 10 years, and this rises to about 50% after 15 years.

26

26.67 The Macdonald criteria for the diagnosis of multiple sclerosis[1]

Clinical presentation[2]	Additional evidence required for diagnosis of MS
Two or more attacks separated in 'time' (at least 3 months apart) and 'space' (involving different parts of the CNS) with objective clinical evidence of two or more lesions	None
Two or more attacks separated in 'time' and 'space', but with objective clinical evidence for only one lesion	Dissemination in 'space' demonstrated by MRI (multiple lesions in several different sites) *or* Two or more MRI-detected lesions consistent with MS *and* oligoclonal bands in CSF *or* Await further clinical attack at different anatomical site
One attack with objective clinical evidence of two or more lesions in different parts of the CNS (dissemination in 'space')	Dissemination in 'time' demonstrated by serial MRI scans (looking for a new lesion developing at least 3 months after the initial presentation) *or* Await further (second) clinical attack at different anatomical site
One attack with clinical evidence of only one lesion (clinically isolated syndrome)	MRI demonstration of dissemination in 'space' and 'time' (as above) *or* Two or more MRI-detected lesions with CSF showing oligoclonal bands *and* dissemination in 'time', demonstrated by MRI *or* Await further (second) clinical attack at different anatomical site
Insidious neurological progression suggestive of MS	CSF positive for oligoclonal bands *and* Dissemination in 'space' and 'time' on MRI and/or abnormal VER[3] *or* Continued progression for a year

[1]Published by the International Panel on MS Diagnosis (Ann Neurol 2001; 50:121–127.) Starting from the clinical presentation in the left-hand column, if the evidence available fulfils the criteria in the right-hand column, the diagnosis is MS. If the criteria are not completely met, the diagnosis is 'possible MS'. If the criteria are fully explored but not met, then the patient does not have MS.
[2]Assumes other possible causes for CNS inflammation (e.g. sarcoidosis, SLE) have been excluded.
[3]VER = visual evoked response.

26.68 Clinical features of multiple sclerosis

Common presentations of multiple sclerosis

- Optic neuritis
- Relapsing and remitting sensory symptoms
- Subacute painless spinal cord lesion
- Acute brain-stem syndrome
- Subacute loss of function of upper limb (dorsal column deficit)
- 6th cranial nerve palsy

Other symptoms and syndromes suggestive of CNS demyelination

- Afferent pupillary defect and optic atrophy (previous optic neuritis)
- Lhermitte's symptom (tingling in spine or limbs on neck flexion)
- Progressive non-compressive paraparesis
- Partial Brown–Séquard syndrome (p. 1156)
- Internuclear ophthalmoplegia with ataxia (p. 1164)
- Postural ('rubral', 'Holmes') tremor (p. 1155)
- Trigeminal neuralgia (p. 1171) under the age of 50
- Recurrent facial palsy

26.69 Investigations in a patient suspected of having multiple sclerosis

Exclude other structural disease and identify plaques of demyelination

- Image area of clinical involvement (MRI, myelography)

Demonstrate other sites of involvement

- Imaging (MRI)
- Visual evoked potentials
- Other evoked potentials

Demonstrate inflammatory nature of lesion(s)

- CSF examination
    Cell count
    Protein electrophoresis (oligoclonal bands)

Exclude other conditions

- Chest X-ray
- Serum angiotensin-converting enzyme (ACE)—sarcoidosis
- Serum B_{12}
- Antinuclear antibodies—SLE
- Antiphospholipid antibodies

Investigations

There is no specific test for MS, and the results of investigation need to be considered in conjunction with the clinical picture to make a diagnosis of varying probability (see Box 26.67). The clinical diagnosis of MS should be supported by investigations to exclude other conditions, provide evidence for an inflammatory disorder and identify multiple sites of neurological involvement (Box 26.69). Following the first clinical event, investigations may help prognostically in confirming the disseminated nature of the disease. Visual evoked potentials (p. 1142) can detect clinically silent lesions in up to 70% of patients, but auditory and somatosensory evoked potentials are seldom of diagnostic value. The CSF may show a lymphocytic pleocytosis in the acute phase and oligoclonal bands of IgG in 70–90% of patients between attacks. Oligoclonal bands are not specific to MS but denote intrathecal inflammation and occur in a range of other disorders. MRI is the most sensitive technique for imaging lesions in both brain and spinal cord (Fig. 26.38) and in excluding other causes of the neurological deficit. However, the MRI appearances in MS may be confused with those of cerebrovascular disease or cerebral vasculitis. Diagnosis depends on the clinical history and examination taken in combination with the investigative findings. It is important to exclude other potentially treatable conditions such as infection, vitamin B_{12} deficiency and spinal cord compression.

Management

The management of MS involves treatment of the acute episode, prevention of future relapses, treatment of complications and management of the patient's disability.

The acute episode

In a function-threatening exacerbation of MS, pulses of high-dose methylprednisolone, either intravenously (1 g daily for 3 days) or orally (500 mg daily for 5 days), shorten the duration of the episode (Box 26.70). Pulsed

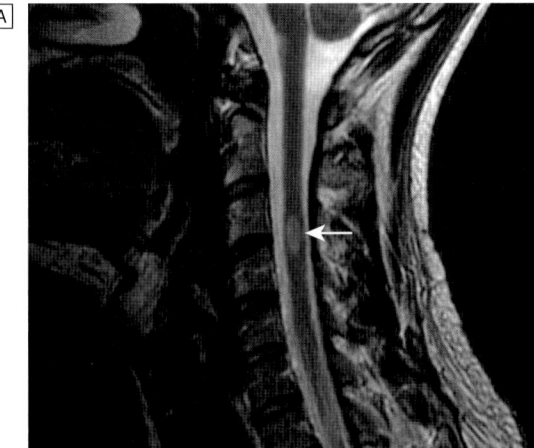

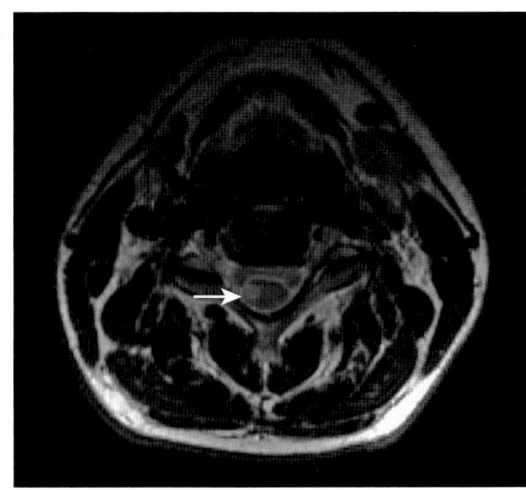

Fig. 26.38 Multiple sclerosis: demyelinating lesion in cervical spinal cord, high-signal T2 images (arrow). A Sagittal plane. B Axial plane.

EBM 26.70 **Pulsed corticosteroids in multiple sclerosis**

'In people with multiple sclerosis with acute exacerbations, corticosteroids (methylprednisolone or corticotrophin) improve symptoms compared with placebo within 5 weeks of treatment. The optimal dose, route and duration of treatment are unclear.'

• Filippini G, et al. (Cochrane Review). Cochrane Library, issue 4, 2000. Oxford: Update Software.
• Barnes D, et al. Lancet 1997; 349:902–906.

For further information: www.clinicalevidence.org

EBM 26.71 **Interferon beta in multiple sclerosis**

'In people experiencing a first demyelinating event, interferon beta decreases the risk of conversion to clinically definite multiple sclerosis over 2–3 years compared with placebo. In people with active relapsing-remitting multiple sclerosis, there is limited evidence that interferon beta reduces exacerbations and disease progression over 2 years compared with placebo.'

• PRISMS Study Group. Lancet 1998; 352:1498–1504.
• IFNB Multiple Sclerosis Study Group. Neurology 1993; 43:655–661.

For further information: www.clinicalevidence.org

steroids may also have some effect in reducing spasticity but prolonged administration of steroids does not alter the long-term outcome and should be avoided. Pulses of steroids can be given up to three times in a year but their administration should be restricted to those with significant function-threatening deficits. Prophylaxis to prevent the occurrence of steroid-induced osteoporosis (p. 1116) should be considered in patients who required multiple courses of corticosteroids.

Prevention of relapse

Immunosuppressive agents such as azathioprine appear to reduce the risk of relapses and improve long-term outcome. In relapsing and remitting MS, subcutaneous or intramuscular interferon beta reduces the number of relapses by some 30%, with a small effect on long-term disability (Boxes 26.71 and 26.72); glatiramer acetate has similar effects. Glatiramer is a polymer of four amino acids found in myelin basic protein, which is thought possibly to act as a decoy for the immune

response in patients with MS. The recently introduced agent, natalizumab, is probably somewhat more effective than both, but is usually reserved for patients with particularly aggressive disease, along with less proven therapies such as mitoxantrone and cyclophosphamide (see Box 26.72). Special diets, including a gluten-free diet or linoleic acid supplements, and hyperbaric oxygen therapy are popular with patients but are of no proven benefit.

Treatment of complications and disability

Treatment of the complications of MS is summarised in Box 26.73. It is important to provide patients with a careful explanation of the nature of the disease and its outcome. When and if disability occurs, patients and their relatives need appropriate support. Specialist nurses working in a multidisciplinary team of healthcare professionals are of great value in managing the chronic phase of the disease. Periods of physiotherapy

26

26.72 Disease-modifying treatments in MS

Treatment	Mode of action	Comment
Interferon beta	Immune modulation	In widespread use for reducing relapse rate (RCT evidence)
Glatiramer acetate	Immune modulation	Similar efficacy to interferon beta (RCT evidence)
Monoclonal antibody to alpha4-integrin (natalizumab)	Immune modulation (blocks lymphocyte entry into CNS)	Recently introduced. Possibly more effective than interferon beta and glatiramer acetate (RCT evidence)
Monoclonal antibody to CD52 (campath-1H)	Immune suppression (lymphocyte depletion)	Encouraging experimental results
Azathioprine	Immune suppression	Similar efficacy to interferon beta (RCT evidence)
Cyclophosphamide	Immune suppression (cytotoxic)	Occasionally used in aggressive disease. Not recommended for widespread use (no proven benefit in RCTs)
Mitoxantrone	Immune suppression (cytotoxic)	Early trials in aggressive disease (no proven benefit in RCTs)
Plasmapheresis	Immune modulation	Occasionally used in aggressive disease (no proven efficacy in RCTs). Probably more effective in NMO
Intravenous immunoglobulin	Immune modulation	Occasionally used in aggressive disease. Probably more effective in NMO

(NMO = neuromyelitis optica; RCT = randomised controlled clinical trial)

26.73 Treatment of complications of multiple sclerosis

Complication	Treatment
Spasticity	Physiotherapy Baclofen 15–100 mg* (oral) Dantrolene 25–100 mg* Tizanidine 18–32 mg* Intrathecal baclofen Local (i.m.) injection of botulinum toxin Chemical neuronectomy
Ataxia	Isoniazid 600–1200 mg* Clonazepam 2–8 mg*
Dysaesthesia	Carbamazepine 200–1800 mg* Gabapentin 900–2400 mg* Phenytoin 200–400 mg Amitriptyline 10–100 mg
Bladder symptoms	See Box 26.28, p. 1168
Fatigue	Amantadine 100–300 mg* Modafinil 100–400 mg* Amitriptyline 10–50 mg
Impotence	Sildenafil 50–100 mg/24 hours

*In divided doses.

and occupational therapy may improve functional capacity in those patients who become disabled, and can provide guidance in the provision of aids at home, reducing handicap. Care of the bladder is particularly important. Urgency and frequency can be treated pharmacologically (see Box 26.28, p. 1168), but this may lead to a degree of retention that promotes the development of infection. Retention can be managed initially by intermittent urinary catheterisation (by the patient, if possible), but an in-dwelling catheter may become necessary. Sexual dysfunction is a frequent source of distress. Sildenafil helps impotence in men, and skilled counselling and prosthetic aids are often useful.

Acute disseminated encephalomyelitis

This is an acute, usually monophasic, demyelinating condition in which there are areas of perivenous demyelination widely disseminated throughout the brain and spinal cord. The illness may apparently occur spontaneously but often occurs a week or so after a viral infection, especially measles and chickenpox, or following vaccination, suggesting that it is immunologically mediated.

Clinical features

Headache, vomiting, pyrexia, confusion and meningism may be presenting features, often with focal or multifocal brain and spinal cord signs. Seizures or coma may occur. A minority of patients who recover have further episodes.

Investigations

MRI shows multiple high-signal areas in a pattern similar to that of MS, although often with larger areas of abnormality. The CSF may be normal or show an increase in protein and lymphocytes (occasionally over

100×10^6 cells/L); oligoclonal bands may be found in the acute episode but do not persist upon recovery, unlike in MS. The differential diagnosis from a first severe attack of MS may be difficult.

Management

The disease may be fatal in the acute stages but is otherwise self-limiting. Treatment with high-dose intravenous methylprednisolone, using the same regimen as for a relapse of multiple sclerosis, is recommended.

Transverse myelitis

Transverse myelitis is an acute, often monophasic, inflammatory demyelinating disorder affecting the spinal cord over a variable number of segments. Patients may be of any age and present with a subacute paraparesis with a sensory level, often with severe pain in the neck or back at the onset. MRI is needed to distinguish this from a compressive lesion of the spinal cord. CSF examination shows cellular pleocytosis, often with polymorphs at the onset, and oligoclonal bands are usually absent. Treatment is with high-dose intravenous methylprednisolone. The outcome is variable; in some cases, near-complete recovery occurs despite a severe initial deficit. Some patients who present with acute transverse myelitis go on to develop MS in later years.

Neuromyelitis optica

The concurrence of transverse myelitis with bilateral optic neuritis—neuromyelitis optica (Devic's disease) — in some patients has been recognised for many years, and these clinical manifestations are more common in MS which occurs in Asia. Recent work has shown that the majority of these cases are associated with an antibody to a water channel, aquaporin 4, which is found in cells near the ventricular system of the brain. Patients typically have brain MRI scans which are either normal, or have high-signal lesions restricted to the region of the ventricular system. Spinal MRI scans show lesions which are typically longer than three spinal segments (unlike the lesions of MS which are shorter than this). Clinical deficits tend to recover less well than those of MS, and the disease may be more aggressive with more frequent relapses. Treatment with immunosuppressive agents such as steroids, azathioprine or cyclophosphamide and/or plasmapheresis seems to be more effective than in MS.

NEURODEGENERATIVE DISEASES

Many diseases cause degeneration in different parts of the nervous system without an identifiable external cause. Genetic factors are known to be involved in several cases but the cause is still unknown for the majority. Clinical features depend on which structures are affected. Degeneration of the cerebral cortex causes dementia, the most common type being Alzheimer's disease. Degeneration of the basal ganglia results in movement disorder, which may manifest as either too little or too much movement, depending on the structures involved. Examples of these conditions are Parkinson's disease and Huntington's disease. Cerebellar degeneration usually causes ataxia. Degeneration can also occur in the spinal cord or peripheral nerves, giving rise to motor, sensory or autonomic disturbance.

Dementia

Dementia is a common condition affecting up to 5% of the population over the age of 65 years; by the age of 80 the prevalence increases to 20%. Dementia therefore has major implications for health resources. It is a clinical syndrome characterised by a loss of previously acquired intellectual function in the absence of impairment of arousal. There are many underlying causes (Box 26.74) but Alzheimer's disease and diffuse vascular disease are the most common. Rarer causes of dementia should be actively sought in younger patients and those with short histories.

Pathophysiology

Dementias are often divided into 'cortical' and 'subcortical' types, depending upon their clinical features. Many of the primary degenerative diseases that cause dementia have characteristic features that may allow a specific diagnosis during life. Creutzfeldt–Jakob disease is usually relatively rapidly progressive (over months), is associated with myoclonus, and there may be characteristic abnormalities on EEG. Of the more slowly progressive dementias, fronto-temporal dementia presents with rather focal (temporal or frontal lobe) dysfunction often affecting language function early, and Lewy body demen-

tia may present with visual hallucinations. However, it is often difficult to distinguish these dementias from each other or from Alzheimer's disease during life.

Clinical features

The usual presentation is with a disturbance of personality or memory dysfunction. The first step is to exclude a focal lesion by determining that there is cognitive disturbance in more than one area. A careful history is essential and it is important to interview not just the patient but a close family member too. Simple bedside tests such as the Mini-Mental State Examination (MMSE, p. 232) are useful in assessing the cognitive deficit, but more formal help from clinical psychology may be required. General history and examination may give further clues to aetiology.

Investigations

The aim is to discover a treatable cause, if present, and to try to give an idea of prognosis using a standard set of investigations (Box 26.75). Imaging of the brain is important to exclude potentially treatable structural lesions such as hydrocephalus, cerebral tumour or chronic subdural haematoma, though often the only abnormality seen is generalised atrophy. If the initial tests fail to yield

26

26.74 Causes of dementia

Type	Common	Unusual	Rare
Vascular	Diffuse small-vessel disease	Amyloid angiopathy Multiple emboli	Cerebral vasculitis
Degenerative/inherited	Alzheimer's disease	Fronto-temporal dementia (including Pick's disease) Leucodystrophies Huntington's disease Wilson's disease Dystrophia myotonica Cortical Lewy body disease Progressive supranuclear palsy Others (e.g. cortico-basal degeneration)	Mitochondrial encephalopathies
Neoplastic (p. 1216)	Secondary deposits	Primary cerebral tumour	Paraneoplastic syndrome (limbic encephalitis)
Inflammatory	–	Multiple sclerosis	Sarcoidosis
Traumatic	Chronic subdural haematoma Post-head injury	Punch-drunk syndrome	–
Hydrocephalus (p. 1220)		Communicating/non-communicating 'normal pressure' hydrocephalus	–
Toxic/nutritional	Alcohol	Thiamin deficiency B_{12} deficiency	Anoxia/carbon monoxide poisoning Heavy metal poisoning
Infective	–	Syphilis HIV	Post-encephalitic Whipple's disease Subacute sclerosing panencephalitis
Prion diseases (p. 1214)	–	Sporadic Creutzfeldt–Jakob disease (CJD)	Variant CJD Kuru Gerstmann–Sträussler–Scheinker disease

26.75 Initial investigation of dementia

In most patients

- Imaging of head (CT and/or MRI)
- Blood tests
  - Full blood count, ESR
  - Urea and electrolytes, glucose
  - Calcium, liver function tests
  - Thyroid function tests
  - Vitamin B$_{12}$
  - Venereal Diseases Research Laboratory (VDRL) test
  - ANA, anti-dsDNA
- Chest X-ray
- EEG

In selected patients

- Lumbar puncture
- HIV serology
- Brain biopsy

an answer, more invasive investigations such as lumbar puncture or, rarely, brain biopsy may be indicated. If there is concern that the memory disturbance may be a manifestation of depressive illness, formal neuropsychological evaluation is helpful.

Management

This is directed at removing correctable causes, and providing support for patient and carers if no specific treatment exists. Anticholinesterases, such as donepezil, rivastigmine and galantamine, or NMDA (N-methyl-D-aspartate) receptor antagonists (memantine) appear to improve cognitive function to some extent in Alzheimer's disease (see Box 26.76 below).

Alzheimer's disease

Alzheimer's disease is the most common cause of dementia, which occurs mostly in patients over 45 years.

Pathophysiology

Genetic factors play an important role and about 15% of cases are familial. These fall into two main groups: early-onset disease with autosomal dominant inheritance and a later-onset group whose inheritance is polygenic. Mutations in several genes have been described which cause the disease. In addition, the inheritance of one of the alleles of apolipoprotein ε, apo ε4, is associated with an increased risk of developing the disease (2–4 times higher in heterozygotes and 6–8 times in homozygotes). However, its presence is neither necessary nor sufficient for the development of the disease, so screening for its presence is not clinically useful. Macroscopically, the brain is atrophic, particularly the cerebral cortex and hippocampus. On histological examination the disease is characterised by the presence of senile plaques and neurofibrillary tangles in the cerebral cortex. Histochemical staining demonstrates significant quantities of amyloid in the plaques (Fig. 26.39) which typically stain positive for the protein ubiquitin which is involved in targeting unwanted or damaged proteins for degradation. This has led to the suggestion that the disease may be due to defects in the ability of neuronal cells to degrade unwanted proteins. Many different neurotransmitter abnormalities have also been

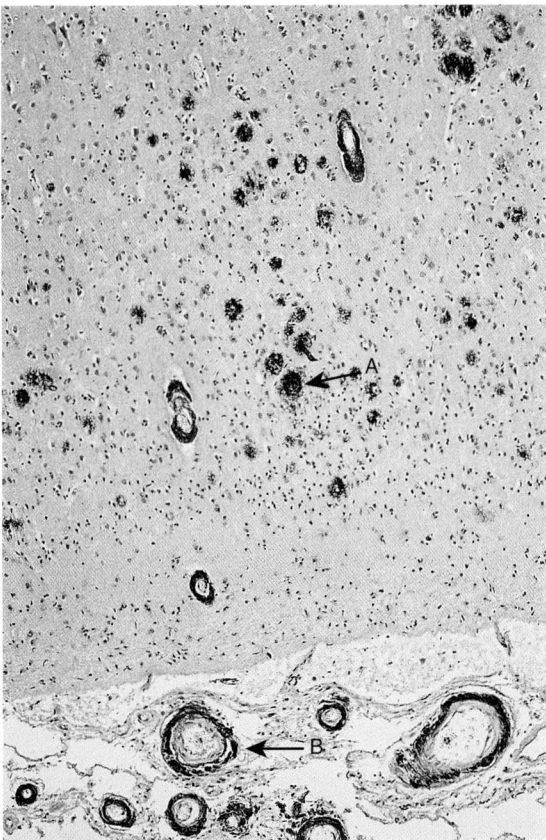

Fig. 26.39 Alzheimer's disease. Section of neocortex stained with polyclonal antibody against βA4 peptide showing amyloid deposits in plaques in brain substance (arrow A) and in blood vessel walls (arrow B).

described. In particular, there is impairment of cholinergic transmission, although abnormalities of noradrenaline, 5-HT, glutamate and substance P have also been described.

Clinical features

The key clinical feature is impairment of the ability to remember information acquired in the past. Hence, patients present with gradual impairment of memory, usually in association with disorders of other cortical functions. Short-term and long-term memory are both affected, but defects in the former are usually more obvious. Later in the course of the disease, typical features include apraxia, visuo-spatial impairment and aphasia. In the early stages of the disease patients may notice these problems, but as the disease progresses it is common for patients to deny that there is anything wrong (anosognosia). In this situation, patients are often brought to medical attention by their carers. Depression is common. Occasionally, patients become aggressive, and the clinical features are made acutely worse by coexistent intercurrent illness.

Investigations and management

Investigation is aimed at excluding other treatable causes of dementia (see Box 26.75), as histological confirmation of the diagnosis usually occurs only after death. There is no known treatment, though recently anticholinesterases such as donepezil, rivastigmine and galantamine, and

EBM 26.76 Anticholinesterases in Alzheimer's disease

'In selected patients with mild or moderate Alzheimer's disease treated for periods of up to a year, donepezil, galantamine, memantine and rivastigmine produce modest improvements in cognitive function. However, the effects on quality of life of both patient and carer are still not clear, and hence the practical importance of these drugs has not been established.'

- Areosa Sastre A, Sherriff F (Cochrane Review). Cochrane Library, issue 2, 2004. Chichester: John Wiley.
- Birks JS, Harvey R (Cochrane Review). Cochrane Library, issue 2, 2004. Chichester: John Wiley.
- Birks J, et al. (Cochrane Review). Cochrane Library, issue 2, 2004. Chichester: John Wiley.
- Olin J, Schneider L (Cochrane Review). Cochrane Library, issue 2, 2004. Chichester: John Wiley.

For further information: www.cochrane.org

the NMDA receptor antagonist, memantine, have been shown to be of some benefit (Box 26.76). Management consists largely of providing a familiar environment for the patient, and providing support for the carers. Many patients are depressed, and treatment with antidepressant medication may occasionally be helpful.

Wernicke–Korsakoff disease

This presents with an acute confusional state (Wernicke's encephalopathy) and brain-stem abnormalities such as ataxia, nystagmus and extraocular muscle weakness, particularly affecting the lateral rectus muscle. The condition is caused by deficiency of thiamin (vitamin B_1) and is often associated with alcoholism. However, other causes include generalised malnutrition, malabsorption or protracted vomiting (as in hyperemesis gravidarum). If Wernicke's encephalopathy is inadequately treated, the condition progresses to cause a dementia which is characterised by a profound disturbance of short-term memory associated with a tendency to confabulate, called Korsakoff's syndrome (p. 246). The diagnosis can be made biochemically by the finding of a reduced red cell transketolase, but this test is often difficult to obtain and so the diagnosis is usually made clinically. Because it is potentially treatable, the condition must be considered in any confused or demented patient; if there is any doubt, it is usually better to treat anyway. Treatment consists of intravenous thiamin (in the form of Pabrinex, 2 vials 8-hourly for 48 hours) initially, followed by oral (100 mg 8-hourly), in addition to treating the underlying cause.

Fronto-temporal dementia

This term encompasses a number of different syndromes, including Pick's disease and primary progressive aphasia. Patients may present with personality change due to frontal lobe involvement or with progressive aphasia. These diseases are much rarer than Alzheimer's disease, and degeneration predominantly affects the frontal and temporal lobes. Histological examination of the brain reveals argyrophilic cytoplasmic inclusion bodies of tau (τ) protein rather than the ubiquitin as in Alzheimer's disease (Fig. 26.40). Memory is relatively preserved in the early stages. There is no specific treatment.

Lewy body dementia

This is a neurodegenerative disorder clinically characterised by dementia and signs of Parkinson's disease. The cognitive state often fluctuates and there is a high incidence of visual hallucinations. Affected individuals are particularly sensitive to the side-effects of anti-parkinsonian medication and also to neuroleptic medication. The condition is associated with accumulation of abnormal protein aggregates in neurons which contain the protein alpha-synuclein in association with other proteins including ubiquitin (see Fig. 26.41). The condition is often inherited and mutations in the alpha-synuclein and beta-synuclein genes have been identified in affected patients. There is no specific treatment for this condition, although there may be clinical benefit with anticholinesterase agents such as rivastigmine.

Parkinson's disease

Parkinson's disease is a neurodegenerative condition which affects the basal ganglia and which presents with differing combinations of slowness of movement (bradykinesia), increased tone (rigidity), tremor and loss of postural reflexes. Parkinson's disease has an annual incidence of about 0.2/1000 and a prevalence of 1.5/1000 in the UK. Prevalence rates are similar throughout the

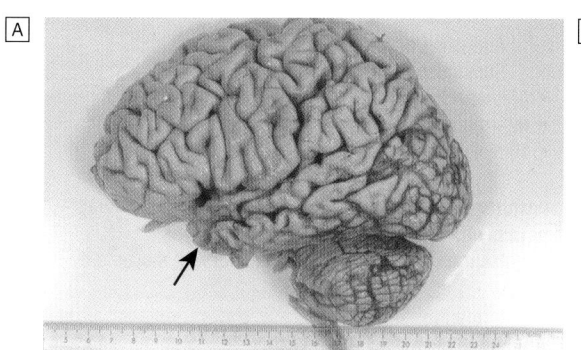
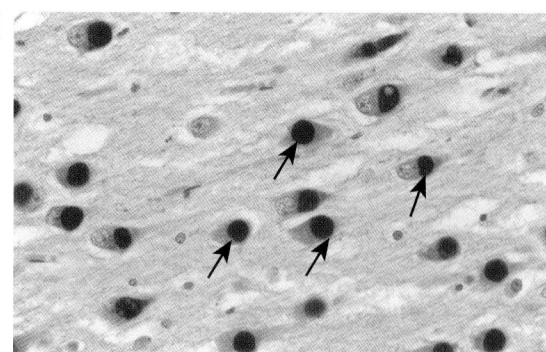

Fig. 26.40 Fronto-temporal dementia. A Lateral view of formalin-fixed brain from a patient who died of Pick's disease, showing gyral atrophy of frontal and parietal lobes and a more severe degree of atrophy affecting the anterior half of the temporal lobe (arrow). B High power (× 200) of hippocampal pyramidal layer, prepared with monoclonal anti-tau antibody. Many neuronal cell bodies contain sharply circumscribed, spherical cytoplasmic inclusion bodies (Pick bodies).

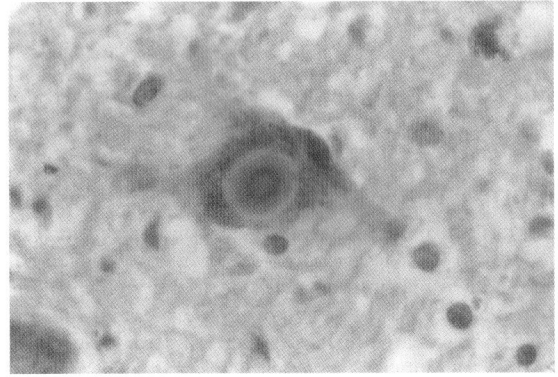

Fig. 26.41 Parkinson's disease. High power (× 400) of substantia nigra of a patient with Parkinson's disease to show classical Lewy body (haematoxylin and eosin).

world, though lower rates have been reported for China and West Africa. Whilst 10% of the patients are under 45 years at presentation, the incidence and prevalence both increase with age, the latter rising to over 1% in those over 60. Sex incidence is about equal. It is less common in cigarette smokers. The outlook for patients with Parkinson's disease is variable, and is related to age at onset. If symptoms start in middle life, the disease is usually steadily progressive and likely to shorten lifespan because of the complications of immobility and tendency to fall. Onset after 70 is unlikely to shorten life or become severe.

Pathophysiology

A small number of cases are familial in nature and mutations in several genes have now been identified as an underlying cause. However, in the majority the cause is unknown, and no strong genetic factors have been identified. The discovery that methyl-phenyl-tetrahydropyridine (MPTP) caused severe parkinsonism in young drug users suggests that the idiopathic disease might be due to an environmental toxin; many candidate toxins have been studied, but there is no strong evidence in favour of any of them. There are several features, including depletion of the pigmented dopaminergic neurons in the substantia nigra, hyaline inclusions in nigral cells (Lewy bodies—Fig. 26.41), atrophic changes in the substantia nigra and depletion of neurons in the locus coeruleus. Reduced dopaminergic output from the substantia nigra to the globus pallidus leads to reduced inhibitory effects on the subthalamic nucleus, neurons of which become more active than usual in inhibiting activation of the cortex. This in turn results in bradykinesia.

Clinical features

The classical syndrome of tremor, rigidity and bradykinesia may be absent initially, when non-specific symptoms of tiredness, aching limbs, mental slowness, depression and small handwriting (micrographia) may be noticed. The presentation is almost always unilateral, a resting tremor in an upper limb being a common presenting feature. The tremor may eventually affect the legs, mouth and tongue. It may remain the predominant symptom for some years. Bradykinesia may develop gradually. Most patients have difficulty with rapid fine

movements, and this manifests itself as slowness of gait and difficulty with tasks such as fastening buttons, shaving or writing. Rigidity, or increased muscular tone, causes stiffness and a flexed posture. Postural righting reflexes are impaired early on in the disease, but falls tend not to occur until later. As the disease advances, speech becomes softer and indistinct. There are a number of abnormalities on neurological examination, and these are listed in Box 26.77.

Although the features are initially unilateral, gradual bilateral involvement is the rule. Muscle strength and reflexes remain normal, and plantar responses are flexor. There is a paucity of facial expression (hypomimia) and the blink reflex may be exaggerated and fail to habituate (glabellar tap sign). Eye movements are normal to standard clinical testing, provided allowance is made for the normal limitation of upward gaze with age. Sensation is normal and intellectual faculties are not affected initially. As the disease progresses, about one-third of patients develop cognitive impairment.

Investigations

The diagnosis is made clinically, as there is no diagnostic test for Parkinson's disease. Sometimes it is necessary to investigate patients to exclude other causes of parkinsonism if there are any unusual features. Patients

26.77 Physical abnormalities in Parkinson's disease

General

- Expressionless face
- Greasy skin
- Soft, rapid, indistinct speech
- Flexed posture
- Impaired postural reflexes

Gait

- Slow to start walking
- Shortened stride
- Rapid, small stride length, tendency to shorten (festination)
- Reduced arm swing
- Impaired balance on turning

Tremor

Resting (4–6 Hz)
- Coarse, complex movements, usually first in fingers/thumb
  Flexion/extension of fingers
  Abduction/adduction of thumb
  Supination/pronation of forearm
- May affect arms, legs, feet, jaw, tongue
- Intermittent, present at rest and when distracted
- Diminished on action

Postural (8–10 Hz)
- Less obvious, faster, finer amplitude
- Present on action or posture, persists with movement

Rigidity

- Cogwheel type, mostly upper limbs
- Plastic (lead pipe) type, mostly legs

Bradykinesia

- Slowness in initiating or repeating movements
- Impaired fine movements, especially of fingers

presenting before the age of 50 are usually tested for Wilson's disease, and imaging (CT or MRI) of the head may be needed if there are any features suggestive of pyramidal, cerebellar or autonomic involvement, or the diagnosis is otherwise in doubt.

Management

Drug therapy

Levodopa combined with a peripheral-acting dopa-decarboxylase inhibitor provides the mainstay of treatment in Parkinson's disease but should only be started to help overcome significant disability. Other agents include anticholinergic drugs, dopamine receptor agonists, selegiline, COMT inhibitors and amantadine (Fig. 26.42).

Levodopa. Although the number of dopamine-releasing terminals in the striatum is diminished in Parkinson's disease, remaining neurons can be driven to produce more dopamine by administering its precursor, levodopa. If levodopa is administered orally, more than 90% is decarboxylated to dopamine peripherally in the gastrointestinal tract and blood vessels, and only a small proportion reaches the brain. This peripheral conversion of levodopa is responsible for the high incidence of side-effects if it is used alone. The problem is largely overcome by giving a decarboxylase inhibitor that does not cross the blood–brain barrier along with the levodopa. Two peripheral decarboxylase inhibitors, carbidopa and benserazide, are available as combination preparations with levodopa (as Sinemet and Madopar, respectively).

The initiation of levodopa therapy should be delayed until there is significant disability, since there is concern that its use makes long-term side-effects more likely. With this in mind, some authorities suggest that it is advisable to initiate treatment with a dopamine agonist (see below) or a slow-release preparation of levodopa in order to minimise or delay the onset of long-term side-effects, but evidence for this is not strong. The important point is to treat with as little medication as possible consistent with the patient being able to perform the activities of daily living. Levodopa is particularly effective at improving bradykinesia and rigidity. Tremor is also helped but rather unpredictably. The initial dose is 50 mg 8- or 12-hourly, increased if necessary. The total levodopa dose may be increased to over 1000 mg/day if necessary. Side-effects include postural hypotension, nausea and vomiting, which may be offset by the use of a peripheral dopamine antagonist such as domperidone. Other dose-related side-effects are involuntary movements, particularly orofacial dyskinesias, limb and axial dystonias, and occasionally depression, hallucinations and delusions. Unusual but important side-effects include change in personality with increased (sometimes pathological) gambling, hypersexuality and drug (levodopa)-seeking behaviour.

Late deterioration despite levodopa therapy occurs after 3–5 years in one-third to one-half of patients. Usually this manifests as fluctuation in response. The simplest form of this is end-of-dose deterioration due to progression of the disease and loss of capacity to store dopamine. More complex fluctuations present as sudden, unpredictable changes in response, in which periods of severe parkinsonism alternate with dyskinesia and agitation (the 'on-off' phenomenon). End-of-dose deterioration can often be improved by dividing the levodopa

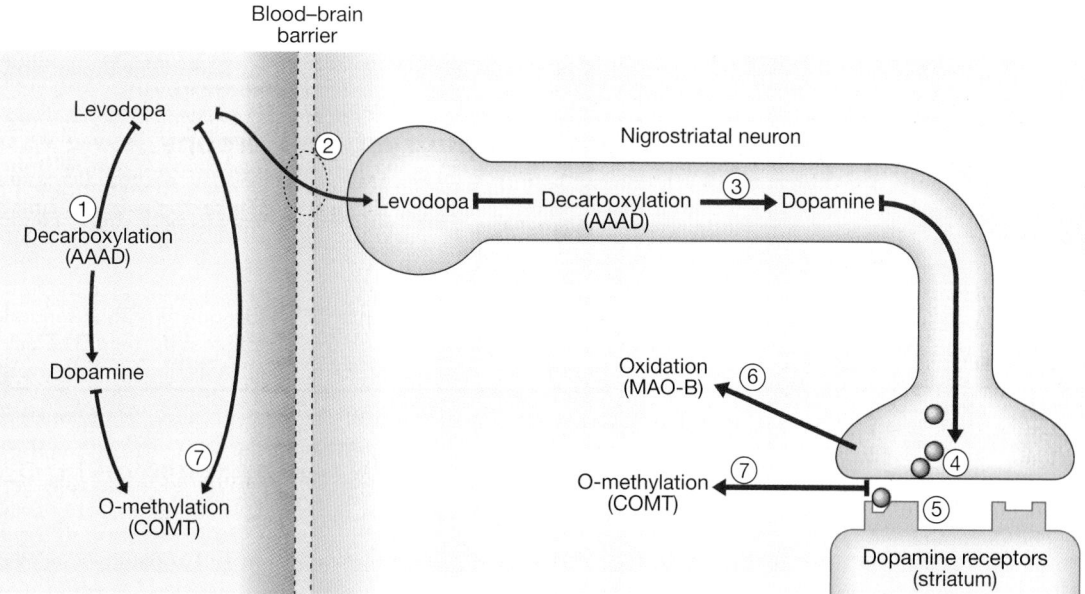

Fig. 26.42 Mechanisms of drug action in Parkinson's disease. (1) Decarboxylase inhibitors (carbidopa and benserazide) decrease side-effects by reducing peripheral conversion of levodopa to dopamine by aromatic amino acid decarboxylase (AAAD). (2) Active transport of levodopa into the brain may be inhibited by competition from dietary amino acids after a high-protein meal. (3) In the nigrostriatal neurons, levodopa is converted into dopamine. (4) Amantadine enhances the release of dopamine at the nerve terminal. (5) Dopamine agonists act directly on striatal receptors. (6) The monoamine oxidase type B (MAO-B) inhibitor selegiline increases the availability of neuronal dopamine by reducing its metabolism outside the neuron. (7) The catechol-O-methyl-transferase (COMT) inhibitor entacapone prolongs the availability of dopamine by inhibiting the metabolism of dopamine and levodopa outside the neuron.

26

into smaller but more frequent doses, or by converting to a slow-release preparation. The 'on-off' phenomenon is difficult to treat, but sometimes subcutaneous injections of apomorphine (a dopamine agonist) are helpful to 'rescue' the patient rapidly from an 'off' period.

Involuntary movements (dyskinesia) may occur as a peak-dose phenomenon, or as a biphasic phenomenon (occurring during both the build-up and wearing-off phases). Management is difficult, but involves modifying the way levodopa is administered to obtain constant levels in the brain, and the use of alternative drugs, including amantadine and dopamine agonists. Continuous infusion of apomorphine may be particularly helpful in this situation.

Anticholinergic agents. These have a useful effect on tremor and rigidity, but do not help bradykinesia. They can be prescribed early in the disease before bradykinesia is a problem, but should be avoided in elderly patients in whom they cause confusion and hallucinations. Other side-effects include dry mouth, blurred vision, difficulty with micturition and constipation. Many anticholinergics are available—for example, trihexyphenidyl (benzhexol; 1–4 mg 8-hourly) and orphenadrine (50–100 mg 8-hourly).

Dopamine receptor agonists. Several of these drugs are now available. They all have slightly different activity at the various dopamine receptors in the brain. Apomorphine given alone causes marked vomiting and has to be administered parenterally. The vomiting can be overcome by the concomitant use of domperidone, and parenteral administration achieved through continuous subcutaneous infusion from a portable pump, or by direct injection as needed. This requires considerable nursing support but, used correctly, can be very useful.

More easily administered drugs include bromocriptine, lisuride, pergolide, cabergoline, ropinirole and pramipexole, which can all be taken orally, and rotigotine which can be administered as a transdermal patch. These drugs are less powerful than levodopa in controlling features of parkinsonism, but they are much less likely to cause dose fluctuations or dyskinesia, though they will certainly exacerbate the latter once these have developed. Side-effects include nausea, vomiting, confusion and hallucinations. The dose of bromocriptine is 1 mg initially, increased to 2.5 mg 8-hourly, and thereafter up to 30 mg/day. Pergolide dose starts at 50 µg, increased to 250 µg 8-hourly, and possibly to 3000 µg/day. Dopamine agonists derived from ergot (pergolide and cabergoline) have recently been associated with the development of fibrotic reactions and thickening of heart valves. For this reason, the use of these agents is not advised.

Amantadine. This has a mild, usually short-lived effect on bradykinesia, but may be used early in the disease before more potent treatment is needed. Amantadine can be particularly useful in controlling the dyskinesias produced by dopaminergic treatment later in the disease. The dose is 100 mg 8- or 12-hourly. Side-effects include livedo reticularis, peripheral oedema, confusion and seizures.

Selegiline. Selegiline has a mild therapeutic effect in its own right. An early suggestion that it slows the progression of the disease has been discredited, as has the suggestion that it might be associated with an increased risk of sudden death. The usual dose is 5–10 mg in the morning.

COMT (catechol-O-methyl-transferase) inhibitors Entacapone (200 mg with each dose of levodopa) prolongs the effects of each dose and reduces motor fluctuations when used with levodopa. This allows the levodopa dose to be reduced and given less frequently.

Surgery

Stereotactic thalamotomy can be used to treat tremor, though this is needed relatively infrequently because of the medical treatments available. Other stereotactic lesions are currently undergoing evaluation, in particular the implantation of stimulating electrodes into the globus pallidus to help in the management of drug-induced dyskinesia. The implantation of fetal mid-brain cells into the basal ganglia to enhance dopaminergic activity remains experimental.

Physiotherapy and speech therapy

Patients at all stages of Parkinson's disease benefit from physiotherapy, which helps reduce rigidity and corrects abnormal posture. Speech therapy may help in patients where dysarthria and dysphonia interfere with communication.

Other akinetic-rigid syndromes

There are many conditions which can rarely manifest as parkinsonian syndromes, including other degenerative diseases (Huntington's disease, Wilson's disease) and infective diseases (syphilis). Drug-induced parkinsonism is much more common (particularly with neuroleptic agents and antiemetics). These conditions should always be borne in mind in the differential diagnosis. In particular there are several specific degenerative conditions that can mimic idiopathic Parkinson's disease, particularly in the early stages. These conditions are relatively uncommon, but about 10% of those thought to have idiopathic Parkinson's disease have one of these variants. The variants are notable in causing a more rapid clinical deterioration than idiopathic Parkinson's disease and in being more resistant to treatment with dopaminergic medication.

Multiple systems atrophy

Multiple systems atrophy (MSA) is a sporadic condition seen in middle-aged and elderly patients. Clinical features of parkinsonism, often without tremor, are combined with varying degrees of autonomic failure, cerebellar involvement and pyramidal tract dysfunction. The combination of parkinsonism with autonomic failure was called the Shy–Drager syndrome. The neurodegenerative process in MSA is more widespread than in idiopathic Parkinson's disease, and is associated with deposition of ubiquitin-containing inclusions in neurons. The disappointing response to levodopa and other anti-parkinsonian drugs is probably because of degeneration of post-synaptic neurons in the basal ganglia. Autonomic features include postural hypotension, sphincter disturbance and sometimes respiratory stridor; diagnosis is often assisted by performing tests of autonomic function. Management of postural hypotension includes physical measures such as sleeping with the head end of the bed elevated and wearing compression stockings, and drugs such as fludrocortisone and midodrine (p. 553). Falls are much more common than in idiopathic Parkinson's disease, and life expectancy is considerably reduced.

Progressive supranuclear palsy

This condition presents in middle-aged patients, and is due to more widespread degeneration in the brain than is seen in idiopathic Parkinson's disease. It is caused by accumulation of protein aggregates containing tau (τ) proteins rather than ubiquitin. The clinical features include parkinsonism, though with rigidity in extension rather than flexion, and tremor is usually minimal. In addition, there must be a supranuclear paralysis of eye movements, usually downgaze, for the diagnosis to be made during life. Other features include pyramidal signs and cognitive impairment.

Wilson's disease

This is an inherited disorder transmitted in an autosomal recessive manner, involving a defect of copper metabolism. It is discussed on page 960. It is a treatable cause of various movement disorders, including ataxia and akinetic rigid syndromes, and so must always be considered in the differential diagnosis of these disorders.

Huntington's disease

This is an inherited disorder with autosomal dominant transmission, affecting both males and females, which usually starts in adult life. It is due to expansion of a trinucleotide CAG repeat in the *Huntingtin* gene on chromosome 4 (p. 53). The disease frequently demonstrates the phenomenon of anticipation, in which there is a younger age at onset as the disease is inherited through generations, due to progressive expansion of the repeat. Slightly different features of the disease occur, depending on whether the abnormal gene is inherited from father or mother.

Pathophysiology

The disease is thought to be caused by accumulation of the abnormal Huntingtin protein in neurons, leading to cellular dysfunction and neuronal death.

Clinical features

Symptoms usually begin in middle adult life with the development of chorea, which gradually worsens. This is accompanied by cognitive impairment which often manifests initially as psychiatric symptoms, but later becomes frank dementia. In juvenile-onset disease, there may be parkinsonian features with rigidity (the 'Westphal variant'). Seizures may occur late in the disease.

Investigations

The diagnosis is made clinically but is supported by the finding of atrophy of the caudate nucleus on CT or MRI. Genetic testing can be used to confirm the diagnosis and provide pre-symptomatic testing for other family members after appropriate counselling (p. 60).

Management

Management is symptomatic in nature. The chorea may respond to tetrabenazine or dopamine antagonists such as sulpiride. Long-term psychological support and eventually institutional care are often needed as dementia progresses. Depressive symptoms are common, and may be helped by antidepressant medication. Genetic counselling of relatives is important.

Hereditary ataxia

This is a group of inherited disorders in which degenerative changes occur to varying extents in the cerebellum, brain stem, pyramidal tracts, spinocerebellar tracts, and optic and peripheral nerves. Onset may be in childhood or adulthood, and different disorders demonstrate recessive, sex-linked or dominant inheritance. The genetic abnormalities responsible for some types of spinocerebellar ataxia have been shown to be due to abnormal numbers of trinucleotide repeats in various genes, and these can now be detected by DNA analysis, allowing diagnostic confirmation, pre-symptomatic testing and genetic counselling. Other conditions which may manifest as progressive ataxia, including Friedreich's ataxia, are shown in Box 26.78.

26

i 26.78 Hereditary ataxias

Type	Inheritance	Onset	Clinical features
Friedreich's ataxia	Autosomal recessive	8–16 years	Ataxia, nystagmus, dysarthria, spasticity, areflexia, proprioceptive impairment, diabetes mellitus, optic atrophy, cardiac abnormalities. Usually chairbound by age 20
Ataxia telangiectasia	Autosomal recessive	Childhood	Progressive ataxia, athetosis, telangiectasia on conjunctivae, impaired DNA repair, immune deficiency, tendency to malignancies
Abetalipoproteinaemia	Autosomal recessive	Childhood	Steatorrhoea, sensorimotor neuropathy, retinitis pigmentosa, malabsorption of vitamins A, D, E, K, cardiomyopathy
Spinocerebellar ataxia (types 1–30)	Autosomal dominant	Childhood to middle age	Progressive ataxia, some types have associated retinitis pigmentosa, pyramidal tract abnormalities, peripheral neuropathy and cognitive deficit
Dentato-rubro-pallido-luysian atrophy (DRPLA)	Autosomal dominant	Childhood to middle age	Children present with myoclonic epilepsy and progressive ataxia; adults have progressive ataxia with psychiatric features, dementia and choreoathetosis
Episodic ataxias (types 1–4)	Autosomal dominant	Childhood and early adulthood	Brief episodes of ataxia, sometimes induced by stress or startle. Some develop progressive fixed ataxia

26

Motor neuron disease

This is a progressive disorder of unknown cause, in which there is degeneration of motor neurons in the spinal cord and cranial nerve nuclei, and of pyramidal neurons in the motor cortex. Between 5 and 10% of cases are familial, and in 20% of such families the disease is caused by a mutation in the superoxide dismutase (*SOD1*) gene. For the remaining 95%, possible causes include viral infection, trauma, exposure to toxins and electric shock, but no sound evidence exists to support any of these. The prevalence of the disease is about 5/100 000.

Clinical features

Patients present with a combination of lower and upper motor neuron signs without sensory involvement. The presence of brisk reflexes in wasted fasciculating limb muscles is typical. Common presenting features are listed in Boxes 26.79 and 26.80. Rarer variants present with either purely upper motor neuron features (progressive lateral sclerosis) or purely lower motor neuron features (progressive muscular atrophy). Motor neuron disease is relentlessly progressive; the mean time from diagnosis to death is 1 year, with most patients dying within 3–5 years of the onset of symptoms. Younger patients and those with early bulbar symptoms tend to show a more rapid course. Death is usually from respiratory infection and failure, and the complications of immobility. Prognosis is better for progressive lateral sclerosis and progressive muscular atrophy.

Investigations

In many patients the clinical features are highly suggestive but alternative diagnoses need to be carefully excluded. In particular, potentially treatable disorders such as diabetic amyotrophy, spinal disorders and multifocal motor neuronopathy should be excluded. Electromyography helps to confirm the presence of fasciculation and denervation, and is particularly helpful when pyramidal features predominate. Sensory nerve conduction and motor conduction studies are

26.80 Patterns of involvement in motor neuron disease

Progressive muscular atrophy

- Predominantly spinal motor neurons affected
- Weakness and wasting of distal limb muscles at first
- Fasciculation in muscles
- Tendon reflexes may be absent

Progressive bulbar palsy

- Early involvement of tongue, palate and pharyngeal muscles
- Dysarthria/dysphagia
- Wasting and fasciculation of tongue
- Pyramidal signs may also be present

Amyotrophic lateral sclerosis

- Combination of distal and proximal muscle-wasting and weakness, fasciculation
- Spasticity, exaggerated reflexes, extensor plantars
- Bulbar and pseudobulbar palsy follow eventually
- Pyramidal tract features may predominate

EBM 26.81 Riluzole and motor neuron disease

'Riluzole 100 mg per day appears to be modestly effective in prolonging survival for patients with motor neuron disease by about 2 months. However, the economics of its use have yet to be fully assessed.'

- Miller RG, et al. (Cochrane Review). Cochrane Library, issue 2, 2004. Chichester: John Wiley.

For further information: www.cochrane.org

---

normal but there may be some reduction in amplitude of action potentials due to loss of axons. Spinal imaging and brain scanning may be necessary to exclude focal spinal or cerebral disease. CSF examination is usually normal, though a slight elevation in protein concentration may be found.

Management

The glutamate antagonist, riluzole, has been shown to have a small effect in prolonging life expectancy by about 2 months (Box 26.81). Other agents such as nerve growth factor show promise. Psychological and physical support, with help from occupational and speech therapists and physiotherapists, is essential to maintain the patient's quality of life. Mechanical aids such as splints, walking aids, wheelchairs and communication devices all help to reduce handicap. Feeding by percutaneous gastrostomy may be necessary because of bulbar failure. Non-invasive ventilatory support has been shown to improve the quality of life by alleviating symptoms from weak respiratory muscles and has a small effect on prolonging life; many patients do not choose to proceed to invasive ventilation. Relief of distress in the terminal stages usually requires the use of opiates and sedative drugs (p. 280).

Spinal muscular atrophy

This is a group of genetically determined disorders affecting spinal motor and cranial motor neurons, characterised by proximal and distal wasting, fasciculation and weakness of muscles. Involvement is usually

26.79 Clinical features of motor neuron disease

Onset

- Usually after the age of 50 years
- Very uncommon before the age of 30 years
- Affects males more commonly than females

Symptoms

- Limb muscle weakness, cramps, occasionally fasciculation
- Disturbance of speech/swallowing (dysarthria/dysphagia)

Signs

- Wasting and fasciculation of muscles
- Weakness of muscles of limbs, tongue, face and palate
- Pyramidal tract involvement causing spasticity, exaggerated tendon reflexes, extensor plantar responses
- External ocular muscles and sphincters usually remain intact
- No objective sensory deficit
- No intellectual impairment in most cases

Course

- Symptoms often begin focally in one part and spread gradually but relentlessly to become widespread

26.82 Types of spinal muscular atrophy

Type	Onset	Inheritance	Features	Prognosis
Werdnig–Hoffman	Infancy	Autosomal recessive	Severe muscle-wasting/weakness	Poor
Kugelberg–Welander	Childhood, adolescence	Autosomal recessive	Proximal weakness and wasting, EMG shows denervation	Slowly progressive disability
Distal forms	Early adult life	Autosomal dominant	Distal weakness and wasting of hands and feet	Good, seldom disabling
Bulbospinal	Adult life, males only	X-linked	Facial and bulbar weakness, proximal limb weakness, gynaecomastia	Good

symmetrical but occasional localised forms occur. With the exception of the infantile form, progression is slow and the prognosis better than for motor neuron disease (Box 26.82).

INFECTIONS OF THE NERVOUS SYSTEM

The clinical features of nervous system infections depend upon the location of the infection (the meninges or the parenchyma of the brain and spinal cord), the causative organism (virus, bacterium or parasite), and whether the infection is acute or chronic. The major infections of the nervous system are listed in Box 26.83. The frequency of these varies geographically. Helminthic infections, such as cysticercosis and hydatid disease, and protozoal infections are described in Chapter 13.

26.83 Infections of the nervous system

Bacterial infections

- Meningitis
- Suppurative encephalitis
- Brain abscess
- Paravertebral (epidural) abscess
- Tuberculosis (Ch. 19)
- Neurosyphilis
- Leprosy (peripheral nerves)*
- Diphtheria (peripheral nerves)
- Tetanus (motor cells)

Viral infections

- Meningitis
- Encephalitis
- Transverse myelitis
- Progressive multifocal leucoencephalopathy
- Subacute sclerosing panencephalitis (late sequel)
- Poliomyelitis
- Rabies
- HIV infection (Ch. 14)

Prion diseases

- Creutzfeldt–Jakob disease
- Kuru

Protozoal infections

- Malaria*
- Toxoplasmosis (in immunosuppressed)*
- Trypanosomiasis*
- Amoebic abscess*

Helminthic infections

- Schistosomiasis (spinal cord)*
- Cysticercosis*
- Hydatid disease*
- Strongyloidiasis*

Fungal infections

- Candida meningitis or brain abscess
- Cryptococcal meningitis

*These infections are discussed in Chapter 13.

Meningitis

Acute infection of the meninges presents with a characteristic combination of pyrexia, headache and meningism. Meningism consists of headache, photophobia and stiffness of the neck, often accompanied by other signs of meningeal irritation including Kernig's sign (extension at the knee with the hip joint flexed causes spasm in the hamstring muscles) and Brudzinski's sign (passive flexion of the neck causes flexion of the hips and knees). Meningism is not specific to meningitis and can occur in patients with subarachnoid haemorrhage. The severity of clinical features varies somewhat according to the causative organism, as does the presence of other features such as a rash. Abnormalities in the CSF (see Box 26.3, p. 1147) are very helpful in distinguishing the cause of meningitis. Causes of meningitis are listed in Box 26.84.

26.84 Causes of meningitis

Infective

Bacteria (see Box 26.85)
- *Brucella*

Viruses
- Enteroviruses (echo, Coxsackie, polio)
- Mumps
- Influenza
- Herpes simplex
- Varicella zoster
- Epstein–Barr
- HIV
- Lymphocytic choriomeningitis
- Mollaret's meningitis (herpes simplex virus type 2)

Protozoa and parasites
- *Toxoplasma*
- *Amoeba*
- *Cysticercus*

Fungi
- *Cryptococcus neoformans*
- *Candida*
- *Histoplasma*
- *Blastomyces*
- *Coccidioides*
- *Sporothrix*

Non-infective ('sterile')

Malignant disease
- Breast cancer
- Bronchial cancer
- Leukaemia
- Lymphoma

Inflammatory disease (may be recurrent)
- Sarcoidosis
- SLE
- Behçet's disease

26

Viral meningitis

Viral infection is the most common cause of meningitis, and usually results in a benign and self-limiting illness requiring no specific therapy. It is a much less serious illness than bacterial meningitis unless there is associated encephalitis (which is rare). A number of viruses can cause meningitis (see Box 26.84), the most common being echoviruses and, where specific immunisation is not employed, the mumps virus.

Clinical features

The condition occurs mainly in children or young adults, with acute onset of headache and irritability and the rapid development of meningism. In viral meningitis, the headache is usually the most severe feature. There may be a high pyrexia, but focal neurological signs are rare.

Investigations

The diagnosis can be made by lumbar puncture. The CSF usually contains an excess of lymphocytes, but glucose and protein levels are commonly normal; the protein level may be raised. It is extremely important to verify that the patient has not received antibiotics (for whatever cause) prior to the lumbar puncture, as this picture can also be found in partially treated bacterial meningitis.

Management

There is no specific treatment and the condition is usually benign and self-limiting. The patient should be treated symptomatically in a quiet environment. Recovery usually occurs within days, although a lymphocytic pleocytosis may persist in the CSF. Meningitis may also occur as a complication of a viral infection primarily involving other organs: for example, in mumps, measles, infectious mononucleosis, herpes zoster and hepatitis. Complete recovery without specific therapy is the rule.

Bacterial meningitis

Many bacteria can cause meningitis, but different organisms tend to affect different age groups (Box 26.85). Bacterial meningitis is usually secondary to a bacteraemic illness, although infection may result from direct spread from an adjacent focus of infection in the ear, skull fracture or sinus. Bacterial meningitis has become less common but the mortality and morbidity remain significant despite the availability of an increasing range of antibiotics. An important factor in determining prognosis is early diagnosis and the prompt initiation of appropriate therapy. The meningococcus and other common causes of meningitis are normal commensals of the upper respiratory tract. New and potentially pathogenic strains are acquired by the air-borne route, but close contact is necessary. Epidemics of meningococcal meningitis occur, particularly in cramped living conditions or where the climate is hot and dry. The organism invades through the nasopharynx, producing septicaemia that is often associated with meningitis.

Pathophysiology

The meningococcus (*Neisseria meningitidis*) is now second to *Streptococcus pneumoniae* as the most common cause of bacterial meningitis in Western Europe, whilst in the USA *Haemophilus influenzae* remains common. In India, *Haemophilus influenzae* B and *Streptococcus pneumoniae* are probably the most common causes of bacterial meningitis, at least in children. *Strep. suis* is a rare zoonotic cause of meningitis associated with contact with pigs. Hearing loss is a frequent complication. The infection stimulates an immune response causing the pia–arachnoid membrane to become congested and infiltrated with inflammatory cells. A thin layer of pus forms and this may later organise to form adhesions. These may cause obstruction to the free flow of CSF leading to hydrocephalus, or they may damage the cranial nerves at the base of the brain. The CSF pressure rises rapidly, the protein content increases, and there is a cellular reaction that varies in type and severity according to the nature of the inflammation and the causative organism. An obliterative endarteritis of the leptomeningeal arteries passing through the meningeal exudate may produce secondary cerebral infarction. Pneumococcal meningitis is often associated with a very purulent CSF and a high mortality, especially in older adults.

Clinical features

Headache, drowsiness, fever and neck stiffness are the usual presenting features. In severe bacterial meningitis the patient may be comatose and later there may be focal neurological signs. Meningococcal meningitis is associated with a purpuric rash in 70% of cases. When accompanied by septicaemia, it may present very rapidly, with abrupt onset of obtundation due to cerebral oedema, probably as a result of endotoxin and/or cytokine release, and circulatory collapse. Complications of meningococcal septicaemia are listed in Box 26.86. Chronic meningococcaemia is a rare condition in which the patient can be unwell for weeks or even months with recurrent fever, sweating, joint pains and transient rash. It usually occurs in the middle-aged and elderly and those who have previously had a splenectomy. In pneumococcal and *Haemophilus* infections there may be an associated otitis media. Pneumococcal meningitis may be associated with pneumonia and occurs especially in older patients and alcoholics, as well as those without functioning spleens. *Listeria monocytogenes* has recently emerged as an increasing cause of meningitis and rhombencephalitis (brain-stem encephalitis) in the

26.85	**Bacterial causes of meningitis**	
Age of onset	**Common**	**Less common**
Neonate	Gram-negative bacilli (*Escherichia coli*, *Proteus*) Group B streptococci	*Listeria monocytogenes*
Pre-school child	*Haemophilus influenzae* *Neisseria meningitidis* *Streptococcus pneumoniae*	*Mycobacterium tuberculosis*
Older child and adult	*Neisseria meningitidis* *Streptococcus pneumoniae*	*Listeria monocytogenes* *Mycobacterium tuberculosis* *Staphylococcus aureus* (skull fracture) *Haemophilus influenzae*

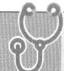

26.86 Complications of meningococcal septicaemia

- Meningitis
- Rash (morbilliform, petechial or purpuric)
- Shock
- Intravascular coagulation
- Renal failure
- Peripheral gangrene
- Arthritis (septic or reactive)
- Pericarditis (septic or reactive)

immunosuppressed, people with diabetes, alcoholics and pregnant women (p. 334). It can also cause meningitis in the neonatal period.

Investigations

Lumbar puncture is mandatory unless there are contraindications (p. 1146). Particularly if the patient is drowsy with focal neurological signs or seizures, it is wise to obtain a CT to exclude a mass lesion (such as a cerebral abscess) before lumbar puncture because of the risk of coning, but this should not delay treatment of a presumptive meningitis. If lumbar puncture is deferred or omitted, it is essential to take diagnostic specimens and to start empirical treatment (Fig. 26.43). In bacterial meningitis the CSF is cloudy (turbid) due to the presence of many neutrophils (often > 1000 × 10⁶ cells/L), the protein content is significantly elevated and the glucose reduced. Gram film and culture may allow identification of the organism. Blood cultures may be positive. Polymerase chain reaction (PCR) techniques can be used on both blood and CSF to identify bacterial DNA. These methods are useful in detecting meningococcal infection and in typing the organism.

Management

If meningococcal or other bacterial meningitis is suspected, the patient should be given parenteral benzylpenicillin immediately (intravenous is preferable to intramuscular) and prompt admission to hospital should be arranged. The only contraindication is a history of penicillin anaphylaxis. Recommended empirical therapy before the cause of meningitis is known is given in Box 26.87. Guidance as to the preferred antibiotic is given in Box 26.88 for when the organism is known after CSF examination. Adjunctive corticosteroid therapy is useful in both children (Box 26.89) and, as demonstrated more recently, adults.

In meningococcal disease, mortality is doubled if the patient presents with features of septicaemia rather than meningitis. Patients likely to require intensive care facilities and expertise include those with cardiac, respiratory or renal involvement, and those with CNS depression prejudicing the airway. Early endotracheal intubation and mechanical ventilation protect the airway and may prevent the development of the acute respiratory distress syndrome (ARDS, p. 187). Adverse prognostic features include hypotensive shock, a rapidly developing rash, a haemorrhagic diathesis, multisystem failure and an age of more than 60 years.

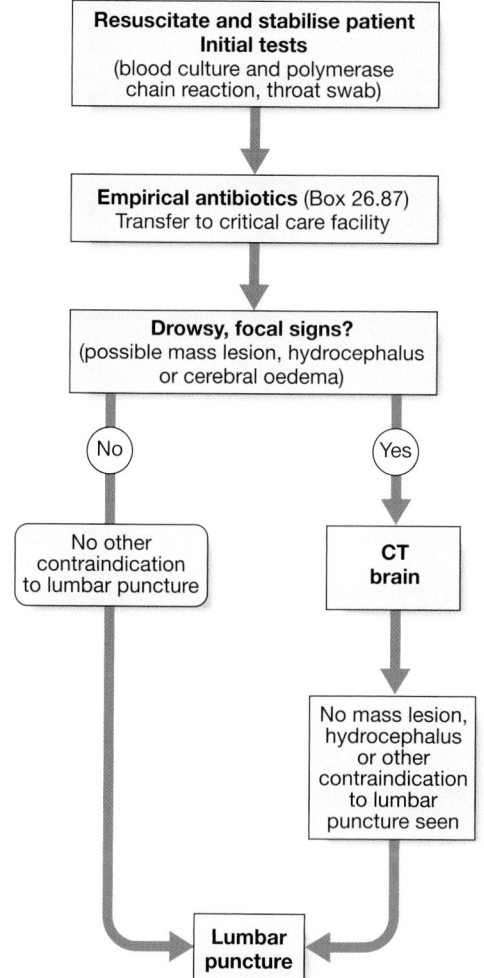

Fig. 26.43 The investigation of meningitis.

26.87 Treatment of pyogenic meningitis of unknown cause

1. Patients with a typical meningococcal rash

- Benzylpenicillin 2.4 g i.v. 6-hourly

2. Adults aged 18–50 years without a typical meningococcal rash

- Cefotaxime 2 g i.v. 6-hourly *or*
- Ceftriaxone 2 g i.v. 12-hourly

3. Patients in whom penicillin-resistant pneumococcal infection is suspected

As for (2) but add:
- Vancomycin 1 g i.v. 12-hourly *or*
- Rifampicin 600 mg i.v. 12-hourly

4. Adults aged over 50 years and those in whom *Listeria monocytogenes* infection is suspected (brain-stem signs, immunosuppression, diabetic, alcoholic)

As for (2) but add:
- Ampicillin 2 g i.v. 4-hourly *or*
- Co-trimoxazole 50 mg/kg i.v. daily in two divided doses

5. Patients with a clear history of anaphylaxis to β-lactams

- Chloramphenicol 25 mg/kg i.v. 6-hourly *plus*
- Vancomycin 1 g i.v. 12-hourly

✚ **26.88 Chemotherapy of bacterial meningitis when the cause is known**

Pathogen	Regimen of choice	Alternative agent(s)
N. meningitidis	Benzylpenicillin 2.4 g i.v. 4-hourly for 5–7 days	Cefuroxime, ampicillin Chloramphenicol*
Strep. pneumoniae (sensitive to β-lactams, minimum inhibitory concentration (MIC) < 1 mg/L)	Cefotaxime 2 g i.v. 6-hourly *or* ceftriaxone 2 g i.v. 12-hourly for 10–14 days	Chloramphenicol*
Strep. pneumoniae (resistant to β-lactams)	As for sensitive strains but add vancomycin 1 g i.v. 12-hourly *or* rifampicin 600 mg i.v. 12-hourly	Vancomycin *plus* rifampicin*
H. influenzae	Cefotaxime 2 g i.v. 6-hourly *or* ceftriaxone 2 g i.v. 12-hourly for 10–14 days	Chloramphenicol*
Listeria monocytogenes	Ampicillin 2 g i.v. 4-hourly *plus* gentamicin 5 mg/kg i.v. daily	Ampicillin 2 g i.v. 4-hourly *plus* co-trimoxazole 50 mg/kg daily in two divided doses
Strep. suis	Cefotaxime 2 g i.v. 6-hourly *or* ceftriaxone 2 g i.v. 12-hourly for 10–14 days	Chloramphenicol*

*For patients with a history of anaphylaxis to β-lactam antibiotics.

EBM **26.89 Adjunctive dexamethasone for bacterial meningitis in children**

'Adjunctive dexamethasone therapy prevents severe deafness following *H. influenzae* type B meningitis and, if commenced with or before parenteral antibiotics, in pneumococcal meningitis in childhood. Limiting dexamethasone therapy to 2 days may be optimal.'

- McIntyre PB, et al. JAMA 1997; 278:925–931.
- Coyle PK. Arch Neurol 1999; 56:796–801.

For further information: www.clinicalevidence.org

Prevention of meningococcal infection

Household and other close contacts of patients with meningococcal infections, especially children, should be given 2 days of oral rifampicin (age 3–12 months 5 mg/kg 12-hourly, > 1 year 10 mg/kg 12-hourly, adults 600 mg 12-hourly). In adults, a single dose of 500 mg of ciprofloxacin is an alternative. If not treated with ceftriaxone, the index case should be given similar treatment to clear infection from the nasopharynx before hospital discharge. Vaccines are available for the prevention of disease caused by meningococci of groups A and C, but not group B which is the most common serogroup isolated in many countries, including the UK.

Tuberculous meningitis

Tuberculous meningitis is now rare in developed countries in previously healthy individuals, but remains common in developing countries and is seen more frequently as a secondary infection in patients with AIDS.

Pathophysiology

Tuberculous meningitis occurs most commonly shortly after a primary infection in childhood or as part of miliary tuberculosis. The usual local source of infection is a caseous focus in the meninges or brain substance adjacent to the CSF pathway. The brain is covered by a greenish, gelatinous exudate, especially around the base, and numerous scattered tubercles are found on the meninges.

Clinical features

The clinical features are listed in Box 26.90. Untreated tuberculous meningitis is fatal in a few weeks but complete recovery is the rule if treatment is started before the appearance of focal signs or stupor. When treatment is started at a later stage, the recovery rate is 60% or less and the survivors show permanent neurological deficit.

Investigations

Lumbar puncture should be performed if the diagnosis is suspected. The CSF is under increased pressure. It is usually clear but, when allowed to stand, a fine clot ('spider web') may form. The fluid contains up to 500×10^6 cells/L, predominantly lymphocytes. There is a rise in protein and a marked fall in glucose. The tubercle bacillus may be detected in a smear of the centrifuged deposit from the CSF but a negative result does not exclude the diagnosis. The CSF should be cultured but, as this result will not be known for up to 6 weeks, treatment must be started without waiting for confirmation. Brain imaging may show hydrocephalus, brisk meningeal enhancement on enhanced CT and/or an intracranial tuberculoma.

Management

As soon as the diagnosis is made or strongly suspected, chemotherapy should be started using one of the regimens including pyrazinamide described on page 693. The use of corticosteroids in addition to antituberculous therapy has been controversial. Recent evidence suggests that it improves mortality but not focal neurological damage, especially if given early. Surgical ventricular drainage may be needed if obstructive hydrocephalus develops. Skilled nursing is essential during the acute phase of the illness, and measures should be put in place to maintain adequate hydration and nutrition.

26.90 Clinical features of tuberculous meningitis

Symptoms

- Headache
- Vomiting
- Low-grade fever
- Lassitude
- Depression
- Confusion
- Behaviour changes

Signs

- Meningism (may be absent)
- Oculomotor palsies
- Papilloedema
- Depression of conscious level
- Focal hemisphere signs

Other forms of meningitis

Fungal meningitis (especially cryptococcosis—p. 379) usually occurs in patients who are immunosuppressed and is a recognised complication of HIV infection (p. 400). The CSF findings are similar to those of tuberculous meningitis, but the diagnosis can be confirmed by microscopy or specific serological tests.

In some areas, meningitis may be caused by spirochaetes (leptospirosis, Lyme disease and syphilis—pp. 331, 329 and 417), rickettsiae (typhus fever—p. 345) or protozoa (amoebiasis—p. 362).

Meningitis can also be due to non-infective pathologies. This is seen in recurrent aseptic meningitis due to SLE, Behçet's disease or sarcoidosis, as well as a condition of previously unknown origin known as Mollaret's syndrome in which the recurrent meningitis is associated with epithelioid cells in the spinal fluid ('Mollaret' cells). Recent evidence suggests that this condition may be due to human herpes virus type 2, and is therefore infective after all. Meningitis can also be seen due to direct invasion of the meninges by neoplasm ('malignant meningitis'—see Box 26.84, p. 1205).

Parenchymal viral infections

Infection of the substance of the nervous system will produce symptoms of focal dysfunction (focal deficits and/or seizures) with general signs of infection depending upon the acuteness of the infection and the type of organism.

Viral encephalitis

A range of viruses can cause encephalitis but only a minority of patients have a history of recent viral infection. In Europe, the most serious cause of viral encephalitis is herpes simplex (p. 312), which probably reaches the brain via the olfactory nerves. The development of effective therapy for some forms of encephalitis has increased the importance of clinical diagnosis and virological examination of the CSF. In some parts of the world, viruses transmitted by mosquitoes and ticks (arboviruses) are an important cause of encephalitis. The epidemiology of some of these infections is changing. Japanese encephalitis (p. 323) has spread relentlessly across Asia to Australia, and there have been outbreaks of West Nile encephalitis in Romania, Israel and New York. Acute encephalitis may occur in HIV infection, occasionally at the time of infection, but more commonly as a manifestation of AIDS (p. 399).

Pathophysiology

The infection provokes an inflammatory response which causes inflammation in the cortex, white matter, basal ganglia and brain stem. The distribution of lesions varies with the type of virus. For example, in herpes simplex encephalitis, the temporal lobes are usually primarily affected, whereas cytomegalovirus can involve the areas adjacent to the ventricles (ventriculitis). Inclusion bodies may be present in the neurons and glial cells and there is an infiltration of polymorphonuclear cells in the perivascular space. There is neuronal degeneration and diffuse glial proliferation, often associated with cerebral oedema.

Clinical features

Viral encephalitis presents with acute onset of headache, fever, focal neurological signs (aphasia and/or hemiplegia) and seizures. Disturbance of consciousness ranging from drowsiness to deep coma supervenes early and may advance dramatically. Meningism occurs in many patients. Rabies presents a distinct clinical picture and is described below.

Investigations

Imaging by CT scan may show low-density lesions in the temporal lobes but MRI is more sensitive in detecting early abnormalities. Lumbar puncture should only be performed after brain imaging has excluded a mass lesion. The CSF usually contains excess lymphocytes, but polymorphonuclear cells may predominate in the early stages. Occasionally, the CSF is normal. The protein content may be elevated but the glucose is normal. The EEG is usually abnormal in the early stages, especially in herpes simplex encephalitis, with characteristic periodic slow-wave activity in the temporal lobes. Virological investigations of the CSF, including PCR for viral DNA, may reveal the causative organism but the initiation of treatment should not await this.

Management

Anticonvulsant treatment is often necessary (p. 1177) and raised intracranial pressure is treated with dexamethasone 8 mg 12-hourly. Herpes simplex encephalitis responds to aciclovir 10 mg/kg i.v. 8-hourly for 2–3 weeks. This should be given early to all patients suspected of suffering from viral encephalitis.

Even with optimum treatment, mortality is 10–30% and significant proportions of survivors have residual epilepsy or cognitive impairment. For details of post-infectious encephalomyelitis, see page 1196.

Brain-stem encephalitis

This presents with ataxia, dysarthria, diplopia or other cranial nerve palsies. The CSF is lymphocytic, with a normal glucose. The causative agent is presumed to be viral. However, *Listeria monocytogenes* may cause a similar syndrome with meningitis (and often a polymorphonuclear CSF pleocytosis) and requires specific treatment with ampicillin 500 mg 6-hourly (see Box 26.88).

Rabies

Rabies is caused by a rhabdovirus which infects the central nervous tissue and salivary glands of a wide range of mammals, and is usually conveyed by saliva through bites or licks on abrasions or on intact mucous membranes. Humans are most frequently infected from dogs. In Europe, the maintenance host is the fox. The incubation period varies in humans from a minimum of 9 days to many months but is usually between 4 and 8 weeks. Severe bites, especially if on the head or neck, are associated with shorter incubation periods. Human rabies is a rare disease, even in endemic areas. However, because it is usually fatal, major efforts are directed to limiting its spread and preventing its importation into uninfected countries such as the UK.

26

26

Clinical features

At the onset there may be fever, and paraesthesia at the site of the bite. A prodromal period of 1–10 days, during which the patient is increasingly anxious, leads to the characteristic 'hydrophobia'. Although the patient is thirsty, attempts at drinking provoke violent contractions of the diaphragm and other inspiratory muscles. Delusions and hallucinations may develop, accompanied by spitting, biting and mania, with lucid intervals in which the patient is markedly anxious. Cranial nerve lesions develop and terminal hyperpyrexia is common. Death ensues, usually within a week of the onset of symptoms.

Investigations

During life, the diagnosis is usually made on clinical grounds but rapid immunofluorescent techniques can detect antigen in corneal impression smears or skin biopsies.

Management

Established disease

Only a few patients with established rabies have survived. All received some post-exposure prophylaxis, and needed intensive care facilities to control cardiac and respiratory failure. Otherwise, only palliative treatment is possible once symptoms have appeared. The patient should be heavily sedated with diazepam 10 mg 4–6-hourly, supplemented by chlorpromazine 50–100 mg if necessary. Nutrition and fluids should be given intravenously or through a gastrostomy.

Pre-exposure prophylaxis

Pre-exposure prophylaxis is required by those who handle potentially infected animals professionally, those who work with rabies virus in laboratories and those who live at special risk in rabies-endemic areas. Protection is afforded by two intradermal injections of 0.1 mL human diploid cell strain vaccine, or two intramuscular injections of 1 mL, given 4 weeks apart, followed by yearly boosters.

Post-exposure prophylaxis

The wounds should be thoroughly cleaned, preferably with a quaternary ammonium detergent or soap; damaged tissues should be excised and the wound left unsutured. Rabies can usually be prevented if treatment is started within a day or two of biting. Delayed treatment may still be of value. For maximum protection, hyperimmune serum and vaccine are required.

The safest antirabies antiserum is human rabies immune globulin; the dose is 20 U/kg body weight. Half is infiltrated around the bite and half is given intramuscularly at a different site from the vaccine. The dose of hyperimmune animal serum is 40 U/kg; hypersensitivity reactions, including anaphylaxis, are common.

The safest vaccine, free of complications, is human diploid cell strain vaccine; 1.0 mL is given intramuscularly on days 0, 3, 7, 14, 30 and 90. In developing countries, where human rabies globulin may not be obtainable, 0.1 mL of vaccine should be given intradermally into eight sites on day 1, with single boosters on days 7 and 28. Where human products are not available and when risk of rabies is slight (licks on the skin, or minor bites of covered arms or legs), it may be justifi-

able to delay starting treatment for up to 5 days while observing the biting animal or awaiting examination of its brain, rather than use the older vaccine.

Poliomyelitis

Pathophysiology

The disease is caused by one of three polioviruses, which are a subgroup of the enteroviruses. It is much less common in developed countries following the widespread use of oral vaccines but is still a problem in the developing world, especially parts of Africa. Infection usually occurs through the nasopharynx.

The virus causes a lymphocytic meningitis and infects the grey matter of the spinal cord, brain stem and cortex. There is a particular propensity to damage anterior horn cells, especially in the lumbar segments.

Clinical features

The incubation period is 7–14 days. Figure 26.44 illustrates the various features of the infection. Many patients recover fully after the initial phase of a few days of mild fever and headache. In others, after a week of well-being, there is recurrence of pyrexia, headache and meningism. Weakness may start later in one muscle group and can progress to widespread paresis. Respiratory failure may supervene if intercostal muscles are paralysed or the medullary motor nuclei are involved. Epidemics vary widely in their incidence of non-paralytic cases and in mortality rate. Death occurs from respiratory paralysis. Muscle weakness is maximal at the end of the first week and gradual recovery may then take place for several months. Muscles showing no signs of recovery by the end of a month will probably not regain useful function. Second attacks are very rare but occasionally patients show late deterioration in muscle bulk and power many years after the initial infection.

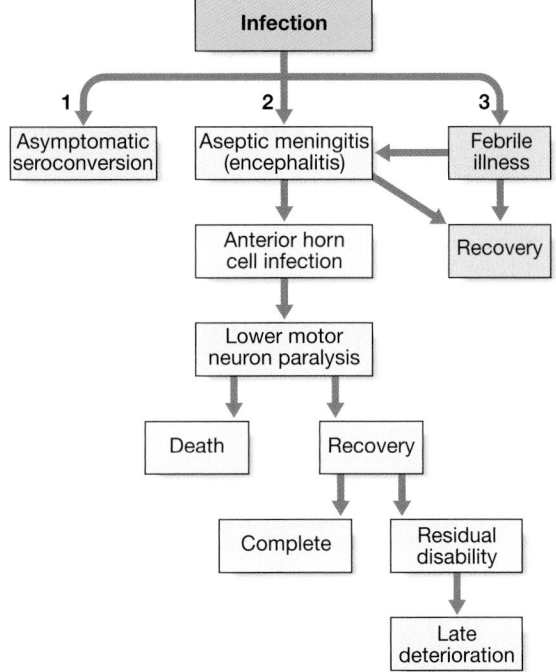

Fig. 26.44 Poliomyelitis. Possible consequences of infection.

Investigations

The CSF shows a lymphocytic pleocytosis, a rise in protein and a normal sugar content. Poliomyelitis virus may be cultured from CSF and stool.

Management

Established disease

In the early stages, bed rest is imperative because exercise appears to worsen the paralysis or precipitate it. At the onset of respiratory difficulties, a tracheostomy and ventilation are required. Subsequent treatment is by physiotherapy and orthopaedic measures.

Prophylaxis

Prevention of poliomyelitis is by immunisation with live (Sabin) vaccine. In developed countries where polio is now very rare, the live vaccine has been replaced by the killed vaccine in childhood immunisation schedules.

Herpes zoster (shingles)

Herpes zoster is the result of reactivation of the varicella zoster virus that has lain dormant in a nerve root ganglion following chickenpox earlier in life. Reactivation may be spontaneous (as usually occurs in the middle-aged or elderly) or due to immunosuppression (as in patients with diabetes, malignant disease or AIDS). Full details are given on page 314.

Subacute sclerosing panencephalitis

This is a rare, chronic, progressive and eventually fatal neurological disease caused by the measles virus, presumably as a result of an inability of the nervous system to eradicate the virus. It occurs in children and adolescents, usually many years after the primary virus infection. The onset is insidious, with intellectual deterioration, apathy and clumsiness followed by myoclonic jerks, rigidity and dementia.

The CSF may show a mild lymphocytic pleocytosis and the EEG is distinctive, with periodic bursts of triphasic waves. Although there is persistent measles-specific IgG in serum and CSF, antiviral therapy is ineffective and death ensues within years.

Progressive multifocal leucoencephalopathy

This was originally described as a rare complication of lymphoma, leukaemia or carcinomatosis. Nowadays it occurs more frequently as a feature of AIDS (p. 398). It is an infection of oligodendrocytes by human polyomavirus JC, which causes widespread demyelination of the white matter of the cerebral hemispheres. Clinical signs include dementia, hemiparesis and aphasia which progress rapidly, usually leading to death within weeks or months. Areas of low density in the white matter are seen on CT but MRI is more sensitive, showing diffuse high signal in the cerebral white matter on T2-weighted images.

Parenchymal bacterial infections

Cerebral abscess

Bacteria may enter the cerebral substance through penetrating injury, by direct spread from paranasal sinuses or the middle ear, or by haematogenous spread from septicaemia. The site of abscess formation and the likely causative organism are both related to the source of infection (Box 26.91). Initial infection leads to local suppuration followed by loculation of pus within a surrounding wall of gliosis, which in a chronic abscess may form a tough capsule. Multiple abscesses may occur, particularly with haematogenous spread.

Clinical features

A cerebral abscess may present acutely with fever, headache, meningism and drowsiness, but more commonly presents over days or weeks as a cerebral mass lesion with little or no evidence of infection. Seizures, raised intracranial pressure and focal hemisphere signs occur alone or in combination. Distinction from a cerebral tumour may be impossible on clinical grounds.

Investigations

Lumbar puncture is potentially hazardous in the presence of raised intracranial pressure, and CT should always precede it. CT reveals single or multiple

26

26.91 Aetiology and treatment of bacterial cerebral abscess			
Site of abscess	**Source of infection**	**Likely organisms**	**Recommended treatment**
Frontal lobe	Paranasal sinuses Teeth	Streptococci Anaerobes	Cefuroxime 1.5 g i.v. 8-hourly *plus* metronidazole 500 mg i.v. 8-hourly
Temporal lobe	Middle ear	Streptococci Enterobacteriaceae	Ampicillin 2–3 g i.v. 8-hourly *plus* metronidazole 500 mg i.v.
Cerebellum	Sphenoid sinus Mastoid/middle ear	*Pseudomonas* spp. Anaerobes	8-hourly *plus* either ceftazidime 2 g i.v. 8-hourly *or* gentamicin* 5 mg/kg i.v. daily
Any site	Penetrating trauma	Staphylococci	Flucloxacillin 2–3 g i.v. 6-hourly *or* cefuroxime 1.5 g i.v. 8-hourly
Multiple	Metastatic and cryptogenic	Streptococci Anaerobes	Benzylpenicillin 1.8–2.4 g i.v. 6-hourly if endocarditis or cyanotic heart disease Otherwise cefuroxime 1.5 g i.v. 8-hourly *plus* metronidazole 500 mg i.v. 8-hourly

*Monitor gentamicin levels.

1211

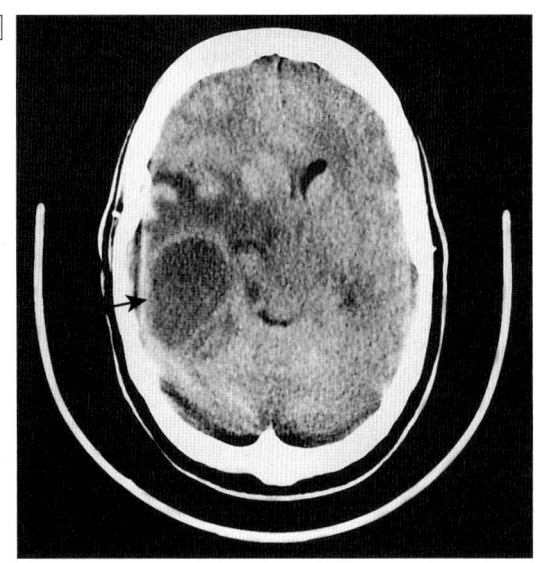
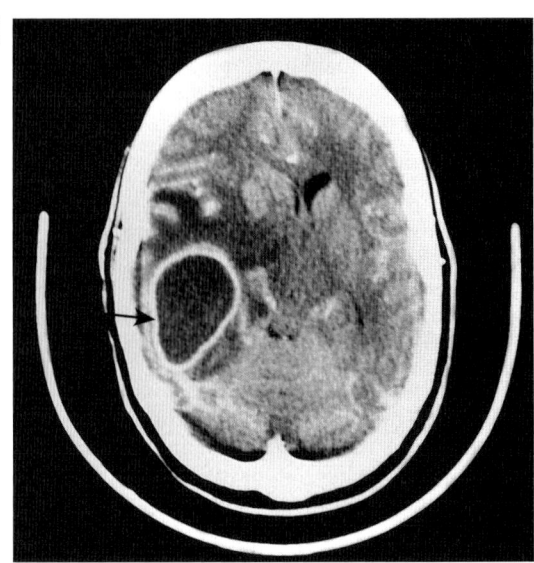

Fig. 26.45 Right temporal cerebral abscess (arrows), with surrounding oedema and midline shift to the left. $\boxed{A}$ Unenhanced CT image. $\boxed{B}$ Contrast-enhanced CT image.

low-density areas, which show ring enhancement with contrast and surrounding cerebral oedema (Fig. 26.45). There may be an elevated white blood cell count and ESR in patients with active local infection. The possibility of cerebral toxoplasmosis or tuberculous disease secondary to HIV infection should always be considered.

Management and prognosis

Antimicrobial therapy is indicated once the diagnosis is made. The likely source of infection should guide the choice of antibiotic (see Box 26.91). Surgical treatment by burr-hole aspiration or excision may be necessary, especially where the presence of a capsule may lead to a persistent focus of infection. Anticonvulsants are often necessary, as epilepsy frequently develops acutely or in the recovery phase.

The mortality rate remains at 10–20% despite an improvement in available surgical and medical treatments, and in some patients this is related to delay in diagnosis and initiation of treatment.

Subdural empyema

This is a rare complication of frontal sinusitis, osteomyelitis of the skull vault, or middle ear disease. A collection of pus in the subdural space spreads over the surface of the hemisphere, causing underlying cortical oedema or thrombophlebitis. Patients present with severe pain in the face or head and pyrexia, often with a history of preceding paranasal sinus or ear infection. The patient then becomes drowsy with seizures and focal signs such as a progressive hemiparesis.

The diagnosis rests on a strong clinical suspicion in patients with a local focus of infection. Careful assessment of a head CT (with contrast) or MRI may show a subdural collection with underlying cerebral oedema. Management requires aspiration of pus via a burr hole and appropriate parenteral antibiotics. Any local source of infection must be treated to prevent re-infection.

Spinal epidural abscess

The characteristic clinical features are pain in a root distribution and progressive transverse spinal cord syndrome with paraparesis, sensory impairment and sphincter dysfunction. Infection is usually haematogenous but a primary source of infection is easily overlooked. The resurgence of staphylococcal infection, often linked to intravenous drug misuse, has contributed to a marked rise in incidence in recent years.

Plain X-rays of the spine may show osteomyelitis but such changes are often late. MRI or myelography should precede urgent neurosurgical intervention. Decompressive laminectomy with draining of the abscess relieves the pressure on the dura. This, together with appropriate antibiotics, may prevent complete and irreversible paraplegia. Organisms may be cultured from the pus or blood.

Lyme disease

See page 329.

Neurosyphilis

Neurosyphilis may present as an acute or chronic process and may involve the meninges, blood vessels and/or parenchyma of the brain and spinal cord. In developed countries, syphilis is now most commonly seen in patients with AIDS. The clinical manifestations are diverse and, although the condition is now rare, early diagnosis and treatment remain important.

Clinical features

The clinical and pathological features of the three most common presentations are summarised in Box 26.92.

Neurological examination reveals signs appropriate to the anatomical localisation of lesions. Delusions of grandeur suggest general paresis of the insane, but more commonly there is simply progressive dementia. The pupillary abnormality described by Argyll Robertson (p. 1166) may accompany any neurosyphilitic syndrome,

26.92 Clinical and pathological features of neurosyphilis

Type	Pathology	Clinical features
Meningovascular (5 years)*	Endarteritis obliterans Meningeal exudate Granuloma (gumma)	Stroke Cranial nerve palsies Seizures/mass lesion
General paralysis of the insane (5–15 years)*	Degeneration in cerebral cortex/ cerebral atrophy Thickened meninges	Dementia Tremor Bilateral upper motor signs
Tabes dorsalis (5–20 years)*	Degeneration of sensory neurons Wasting of dorsal columns Optic atrophy	Lightning pains Sensory ataxia Visual failure Abdominal crises Incontinence Trophic changes
Any of the above		Argyll Robertson pupils (p. 1166)

*Interval from primary infection.

but most commonly tabes dorsalis; the pupils are small and irregular, and react to convergence but not directly to light.

Investigations

Routine screening for syphilis is warranted in the great majority of neurological patients. Serological tests (p. 418) are positive in the serum in most patients, but CSF examination is essential if neurological involvement is suspected. Active disease is suggested by an elevated cell count, usually lymphocytic, and the protein content may be elevated to 0.5–1.0 g/L with an increased gamma globulin fraction. Serological tests in the CSF are usually positive, but progressive disease can occur with negative CSF serology.

Management

The injection of procaine benzylpenicillin (procaine penicillin) and probenecid for 17 days is essential in the treatment of neurosyphilis of all types (p. 419). Further courses of penicillin must be given if symptoms are not relieved, if the condition continues to advance or if the CSF continues to show signs of active disease. The cell count returns to normal within 3 months of completion of treatment, but the elevated protein takes longer to subside and some serological tests may never revert to normal. Evidence of clinical progression at any time is an indication for renewed treatment.

Diseases caused by bacterial toxins

Tetanus

This disease results from infection with *Clostridium tetani*, a commensal in the gut of humans and domestic animals which is found in soil. Infection enters the body through wounds, often trivial. It is rare in the UK, occurring mostly in gardeners and farmers but with a recent increase in intravenous drug misusers. By contrast, the disease is common in many developing countries, where dust contains spores derived from animal and human excreta. If childbirth takes place in an unhygienic environment, *Tetanus neonatorum* may result from infection of the umbilical stump, or the mother may develop the disease. Tetanus is still one of the major killers of adults, children and neonates in developing countries, where the mortality rate can be nearly 100% in the newborn and around 40% in others.

In circumstances unfavourable to the growth of the organism, spores are formed and these may remain dormant for years in the soil. Spores germinate and bacilli multiply only in the anaerobic conditions which occur in areas of tissue necrosis or if the oxygen tension is low as a result of the presence of other organisms, particularly aerobic ones. The bacilli remain localised but produce an exotoxin with an affinity for motor nerve endings and motor nerve cells.

The anterior horn cells are affected after the exotoxin has passed into the blood stream and their involvement results in rigidity and convulsions. Symptoms first appear from 2 days to several weeks after injury—the shorter the incubation period, the more severe the attack and the worse the prognosis.

Clinical features

By far the most important early symptom is trismus—spasm of the masseter muscles, which causes difficulty in opening the mouth and in masticating; hence the name 'lockjaw'. Lockjaw in tetanus is painless, unlike the spasm of the masseters due to dental abscess, septic throat or other causes. Conditions that can mimic tetanus include hysteria and phenothiazine overdosage, or overdose in intravenous drug misusers.

In tetanus, the tonic rigidity spreads to involve the muscles of the face, neck and trunk. Contraction of the frontalis and the muscles at the angles of the mouth leads to the so-called 'risus sardonicus'. There is rigidity of the muscles at the neck and trunk of varying degree. The back is usually slightly arched ('opisthotonus') and there is a board-like abdominal wall.

In the more severe cases, violent spasms lasting for a few seconds to 3–4 minutes occur spontaneously, or may be induced by stimuli such as moving the patient or noise. These convulsions are painful, exhausting and of very serious significance, especially if they appear soon after the onset of symptoms. They gradually increase in frequency and severity for about 1 week and the patient may die from exhaustion, asphyxia or aspiration pneumonia. In less severe illness, convulsions may not commence for about a week after the first sign of rigidity, and in very mild infections they may never appear. Autonomic involvement may cause cardiovascular complications such as hypertension. Rarely, the only manifestation of the disease may be 'local tetanus'—stiffness or spasm of the muscles near the infected wound—and the prognosis is good if treatment is commenced at this stage.

Investigations

The diagnosis is made on clinical grounds. It is rarely possible to isolate the infecting organism from the original locus of entry.

Management

Established disease

Management of established disease should be begun as soon as possible, as shown in Box 26.93.

26

➕ 26.93 Treatment of tetanus
Neutralise absorbed toxin
• I.v. injection of 3000 U of human tetanus antitoxin
Prevent further toxin production
• Débridement of wound
• Benzylpenicillin 600 mg i.v. 6-hourly (metronidazole if allergic to penicillin)
Control spasms
• Nurse in a quiet room
• Avoid unnecessary stimuli
• I.v. diazepam—if spasms continue, paralyse patient and ventilate
General measures
• Maintain hydration and nutrition
• Treat secondary infections

🩺 26.94 The US Centers for Disease Control (CDC) definition of botulism
Three main syndromes
1. Infantile
2. Food-borne
3. Wound infection
Clinical features
• Absence of fever
• Symmetrical neurological deficits
• The patient remains responsive
• Normal or slow heart rate and normal blood pressure
• No sensory deficits with the exception of blurred vision

Prevention

Tetanus can be prevented by immunisation and prompt treatment of contaminated wounds by débridement and antibiotics. In patients with a contaminated wound the immediate danger of tetanus can be greatly reduced by the injection of 1200 mg of penicillin followed by a 7-day course of oral penicillin. For those who are allergic to penicillin, erythromycin should be used. When the risk of tetanus is judged to be present, an intramuscular injection of 250 U of human tetanus antitoxin should be given, along with toxoid which should be repeated 1 month and 6 months later. For those already immunised, only a booster dose of toxoid is required.

Botulism

Botulism is caused by the neurotoxins of *Clostridium botulinum*, which are extremely potent and cause disease after ingestion of even picogram amounts. It is classically described as the acute onset of bilateral cranial neuropathies associated with symmetric descending weakness.

Anaerobic conditions are necessary for the organism's growth. It may contaminate many foodstuffs, from canned meat and salmon to home-produced and preserved vegetables. Contaminated honey has been implicated in infant botulism, in which the organism colonises the gastrointestinal tract of infants. Wound botulism is a growing problem in injection drug-users.

The toxin causes predominantly bulbar and ocular palsies (difficulty in swallowing, blurred or double vision, ptosis), progressing to limb weakness and respiratory paralysis. Criteria for the clinical diagnosis are shown in Box 26.94.

Management includes assisted ventilation and general supportive measures until the toxin eventually dissociates from nerve endings 6–8 weeks following ingestion. A polyvalent antitoxin is available for post-exposure prophylaxis and for the treatment of suspected botulism. It specifically neutralises toxin types A, B and E and is not effective against infantile botulism.

Transmissible spongiform encephalopathies

Transmissible spongiform encephalopathies (TSEs) include a number of conditions affecting both animals and humans which are characterised by the histopathological triad of spongiform change, neuronal cell loss and gliosis in the grey matter of the brain. Associated with these changes, there is deposition of amyloid made up of an altered form of a normally occurring protein, the prion protein. These diseases can be transmitted by inoculation. The precise nature of the infective agent is not yet clear but almost certainly involves the abnormal prion protein. They may also occur spontaneously or as an inherited disorder. Diseases affecting animals include bovine and feline spongiform encephalopathies (BSE and FSE). In humans, the most common TSE is Creutzfeldt–Jakob disease (CJD). This occurs sporadically, with a world-wide incidence of approximately 1/1 000 000, but can also be transmitted by inoculation — for example, through EEG electrodes inserted into the brain, corneal grafts, neurosurgery (especially when cadaveric dura mater grafts were used) and the use of pooled cadaveric growth hormone). Some 10% of cases arise due to a mutation in the gene coding for the prion protein.

Creutzfeldt–Jakob disease

Sporadic Creutzfeldt–Jakob disease (CJD) usually occurs in middle-aged to elderly patients. Clinical features usually involve a rapidly progressive dementia, with myoclonus and a characteristic EEG pattern (repetitive slow wave complexes), although a number of other features such as visual disturbance or ataxia may also be seen. These are particularly common in CJD transmitted by inoculation. Death occurs after a mean of 4–6 months. There is no effective treatment.

Variant Creutzfeldt–Jakob disease

A variant of CJD (vCJD) has been described in a small number of patients, mostly in the UK. The causative agent appears to be identical to that causing BSE in cows, and it has been suggested that the disease appeared in humans as a result of the epidemic of BSE in the UK which started in the late 1980s. Patients affected by vCJD are typically younger than those with sporadic CJD and present with neuropsychiatric changes and sensory symptoms in the limbs, followed by ataxia, dementia and death, progressing at a slightly slower rate than patients with sporadic CJD (mean time to death is over a year). Characteristic EEG changes are not present but MRI scans of the head show characteristic high-signal changes in the pulvinar in a high proportion of cases. The brain pathology is distinct, with very florid plaques containing the prion proteins. Abnormal prion protein has been identified in tonsil specimens from sufferers of vCJD, leading to the suggestion that the disease could be transmitted by reticulo-endothelial tissue (like TSEs in animals but unlike sporadic CJD in humans). This has caused great concern in the UK, leading to precautionary measures such as leucodepletion of all blood used for transfusion, and the mandatory use of disposable surgical instruments wherever possible for tonsillectomy, appendicectomy and ophthalmological procedures. However, presumably thanks to the public health measures introduced to control BSE, the incidence of vCJD has now declined dramatically.

Other TSE syndromes

Other extremely rare inherited human TSEs include Gerstmann–Sträussler–Scheinker disease, fatal familial insomnia and kuru. Kuru occurred only in members of a cannibalistic New Guinea tribe and was probably transmitted by people eating the brains of dead tribal members. Clinical features include progressive ataxia and dementia.

INTRACRANIAL MASS LESIONS AND RAISED INTRACRANIAL PRESSURE

There are many different types of mass lesion in the head (Box 26.95). In developing countries, tuberculoma is a very common cause, but in developed countries cerebral neoplasms are the most frequent. The clinical features relate to the site of the mass, its nature and its rate of expansion. Symptoms and signs are produced by a number of mechanisms (Box 26.96).

26.95 Intracranial mass lesions	
Traumatic	
• Subdural haematoma	• Extradural haematoma
Vascular	
• Intracerebral haematoma	
Infective	
• Cerebral abscess (pyogenic, *Toxoplasma* etc.)	• Echinococcosis (as hydatid cysts, p. 375)
• Tuberculoma	• Schistosomiasis (p. 370)
• Cysticercosis (p. 373)	
Inflammatory	
• Sarcoid mass	
Neoplastic	
• Cerebral neoplasm (benign and malignant)	
Other	
• Embryonic dysplastic lesions (craniopharyngioma, hamartoma)	• Arachnoid cyst • Colloid cyst (in the ventricles)

26.96 Clinical features of intracranial mass lesions	
Local effects on adjacent brain tissue (e.g. seizures, focal signs)	
• Depends on the site of the lesion (see Box 26.1, p. 1136)	
Raised intracranial pressure	
• Headache (p. 1148)	
• Impairment of conscious level	
• Papilloedema	
• Vomiting, bradycardia, arterial hypertension	
False localising signs	
• Pupillary dilatation (ipsilateral to lesion)	
• 6th cranial nerve lesion (unilateral or bilateral)	
• Hemiparesis (ipsilateral to lesion)	
• Bilateral extensor plantar responses	

Raised intracranial pressure

Raised intracranial pressure may be caused by mass lesions (especially tumours), cerebral oedema, obstruction to CSF circulation (causing hydrocephalus) or impaired CSF absorption, as in idiopathic intracranial hypertension and cerebral venous obstruction.

Clinical features

The major features of raised intracranial pressure are listed in Box 26.96. Impairment of conscious level is related to the level of intracranial pressure. Cerebral mass lesions will tend to increase intracerebral pressure, but the amount by which the pressure is raised depends on the rate of growth of the mass. If it is slow, various compensatory mechanisms may occur, including alteration in the volume of fluid in CSF spaces and venous sinuses, thereby allowing some tumours to achieve considerable size. More rapid growth (as in highly malignant tumours or abscesses) does not allow the compensatory mechanisms to come into play, so raised intracranial pressure develops early, especially if the CSF circulation is also obstructed. Papilloedema is not always present, either because raised intracranial pressure has developed too recently, or because of anatomic anomalies of the meningeal sheath of the optic nerve. Vomiting, bradycardia and arterial hypertension develop as late features of raised intracranial pressure and usually parallel the other clinical signs; sudden vomiting may be an early feature of tumours of the cerebellum, especially in children. The rise in intracranial pressure from a mass lesion is not usually uniform within the cerebral substance and alterations in pressure relationships within the skull may lead to displacement of parts of the brain between its various compartments. Downward displacement of the temporal lobes through the tentorium due to a large hemisphere mass may cause 'temporal coning' (Fig. 26.46). This may stretch the 3rd and/or 6th cranial nerves, or cause pressure on the contralateral cerebral peduncle (causing ipsilateral upper motor neuron signs). Downward movement of the cerebellar tonsils through the foramen magnum may compress the medulla—'tonsillar coning' (Fig. 26.47). This coning may result in brain-stem haemorrhage and/or acute obstruction of the CSF pathways. As coning progresses, the patient may adopt a decerebrate posture and, unless rapidly treated, death almost invariably ensues. The process

26

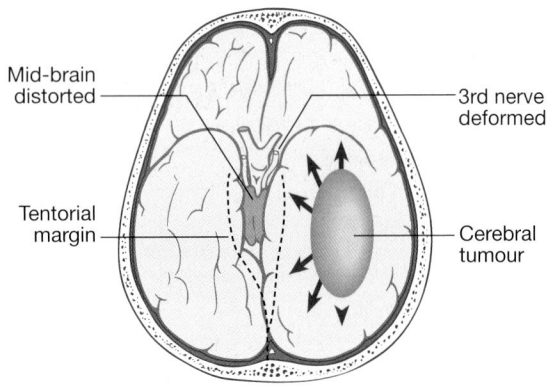

Mid-brain
distorted

3rd nerve
deformed

Tentorial
margin

Cerebral
tumour

Fig. 26.46 Cerebral tumour displacing medial temporal lobe and causing pressure on the mid-brain and 3rd cranial nerve.

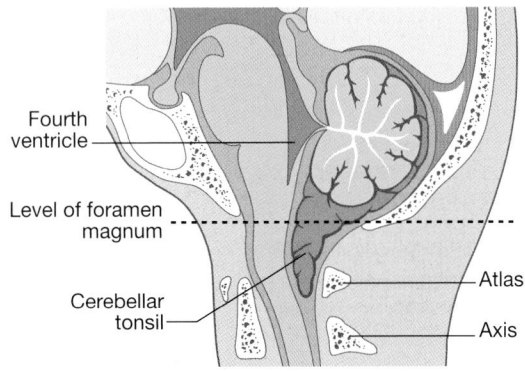

Fourth
ventricle

Level of foramen
magnum

Atlas

Cerebellar
tonsil

Axis

Fig. 26.47 Tonsillar cone. Downward displacement of the cerebellar tonsils below the level of the foramen magnum.

may be acutely accelerated if the pressure dynamics are suddenly disturbed by lumbar puncture.

Management

The management of raised intracranial pressure is largely dictated by its specific cause (see below). ICU support may be required (p. 200).

Intracranial neoplasms

In the developed world, cerebral tumours account for 2% of deaths at all ages. The majority are metastatic from malignancies outside the nervous system. Meningiomas account for about one-fifth of intracranial tumours. Benign or malignant neoplasms of CNS tissue account for the remainder.

Pathophysiology

Metastases from extracranial primary tumours are usually located in the white matter of the cerebral or cerebellar hemispheres, and common sources are bronchus, breast and gastrointestinal tract. Primary intracerebral tumours are classified by their cell of origin and degree of malignancy, and vary in incidence by age and localisation (Boxes 26.97 and 26.98). Even when malignant, they do not metastasise outside the nervous system.

26.97 Primary malignant intracranial tumours		
Histological type	**Common site**	**Age**
Glioma (astrocytoma)	Cerebral hemisphere	Adulthood
	Cerebellum	Childhood/adulthood
	Brain stem	Childhood/young adulthood
Oligodendroglioma	Cerebral hemisphere	Adulthood
Medulloblastoma	Posterior fossa	Childhood
Ependymoma	Posterior fossa	Childhood/ adolescence
Cerebral lymphoma (microglioma)	Cerebral hemisphere	Adulthood

26.98 Primary benign intracranial tumours		
Histological type	**Common site**	**Age**
Meningioma	Cortical dura	Adulthood
	Parasagittal	
	Sphenoid ridge	
	Suprasellar	
	Olfactory groove	
Neurofibroma	Acoustic neuroma	Adulthood
Craniopharyngioma	Suprasellar	Childhood/adolescence
Pituitary adenoma	Pituitary fossa	Adulthood
Colloid cyst	Third ventricle	Any age
Pineal tumours	Quadrigeminal cistern	Childhood (teratomas) Young adulthood (germ cell)

Clinical features

The presentation is quite variable. Headache is not an invariable manifestation of cerebral tumour; if present, it may have characteristics of raised intracranial pressure, or be caused by traction on the pain-sensitive intracranial structures (p. 1149). The site of the headache often does not correlate with the site of the tumour, although posterior fossa tumours often cause pain in the occiput or neck. Cerebral tumours may present with focal neurological deficits which are of slow onset and progressive. Tumours may present at an early stage in some areas, such as the brain stem where structural disturbance quickly results in a neurological deficit. In other regions, especially the frontal lobe, a tumour may be quite large before symptoms occur. The clinical features of dysfunction in the various lobes of the brain are outlined in Box 26.1 (p. 1136). Occasionally, localised oedema in the brain tissue surrounding a tumour will cause a rapid progression of symptoms. Rarely, haemorrhage into a tumour can present like an acute stroke. Tumours often present with seizures which are caused by infiltration by tumour cells of an area of cerebral cortex which excites seizure activity. The resulting seizures may be generalised or partial in nature, and the development of focal seizures in adult life should always suggest the possibility of a tumour.

Investigations

Neuroimaging by CT or MRI allows accurate localisation of the tumour and provides some guidance as to the likely histological type (Fig. 26.48). MRI is of particular value in the investigation of tumours of the posterior fossa and brain stem (Fig. 26.49), and in delineating the nature and extent of tumours prior to surgery. Distortion of intracranial structures and the size of the ventricular system can be assessed and may provide accurate evaluation of the extent of the tumour. Plain skull X-rays are rarely of diagnostic value except in pituitary tumours. Chest radiography is an important investigation and may provide evidence of a primary pulmonary tumour or other systemic malignancy.

Management

Medical

Relief of raised intracranial pressure is often required when surgery is not possible or when life is threatened before investigation has revealed the diagnosis. Dexamethasone, 8 mg 12-hourly either orally or by injection, is used to lower intracranial pressure by resolving the reactive oedema around a tumour. A striking improvement in conscious level is often produced and focal disabilities may regress. In severe and acutely raised intracranial pressure, 16–20 mg of dexamethasone may be given intravenously, or 200 mL of a 20% solution of mannitol may be infused. Prolactin- or growth hormone-secreting pituitary tumours (p. 787) may respond to treatment with the dopamine agonists bromocriptine, cabergoline or quinagolide.

Surgical

Surgery is the mainstay of treatment, although only partial excision may be possible if the tumour is inaccessible

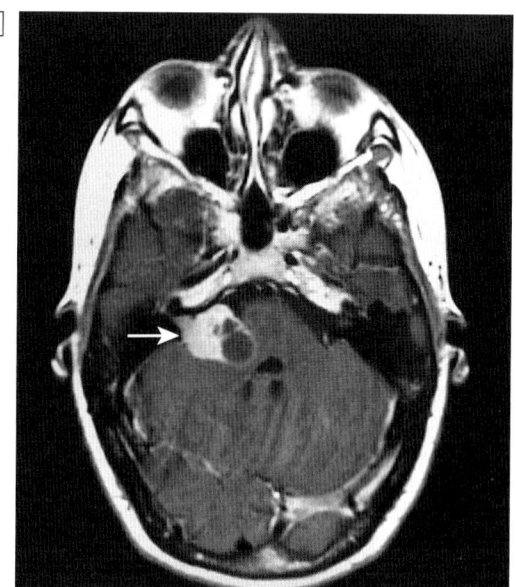

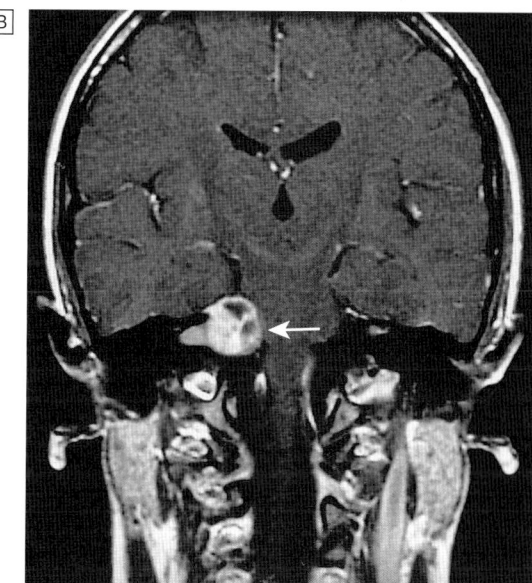

Fig. 26.49 MRI of an acoustic neuroma (arrows) in the posterior fossa compressing the brain stem. [A] Axial image. [B] Coronal image.

or if its removal is likely to cause unacceptable brain damage. Biopsy by a direct or stereotactic technique should be considered even if the tumour cannot be removed, since the histological diagnosis has important implications for management and prognosis.

Meningiomas and acoustic neuromas offer the best prospects for complete removal without unacceptable damage to surrounding structures. Meningiomas can recur, particularly those of the sphenoid ridge when partial excision is often all that is possible. Pituitary adenomas can often be removed by a trans-sphenoidal route, thereby avoiding the need for a craniotomy. Ependymomas and medulloblastomas can often be excised with minimal residual disability, but may recur with seeding of the tumour via the CSF.

Gliomas can rarely be completely excised, since infiltration often spreads beyond the radiologically

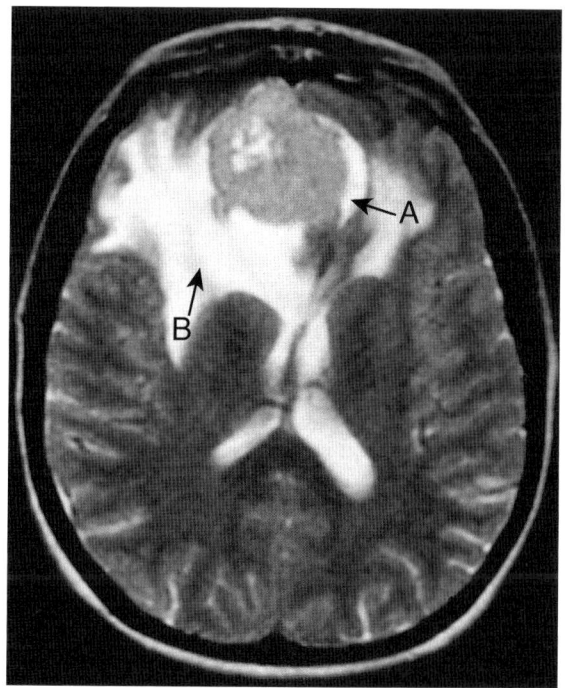

Fig. 26.48 MRI showing meningioma in frontal lobe (arrow A) with associated oedema (arrow B).

26

evident boundaries of the tumour. Recurrence is therefore common, even if the mass of the tumour is apparently removed completely. Partial excision ('debulking') may be useful in alleviating raised intracranial pressure, but survival in highly malignant gliomas is poor even if such a decompressive procedure is attempted. Prognosis is related to histological grade; patients with better grades (I–II) may survive many years, whilst only 20% of patients with grade IV gliomas (glioblastoma multiforme) survive 1 year. Oligodendrogliomas are often slow-growing and relatively benign in the early stages, but may transform to a more malignant form and behave as gliomas.

Radiotherapy and chemotherapy

Radiotherapy and chemotherapy have only a marginal effect on survival in cerebral metastases and malignant gliomas in adults, but their combination has greatly improved the prognosis in medulloblastoma in children. Radiotherapy reduces the risk of recurrence of pituitary adenoma after surgery and may also be helpful as an adjunct to operative treatment in those meningiomas whose anatomical site precludes complete excision or whose histology suggests an increased tendency to recurrence. Ependymomas, some pineal tumours and low-grade gliomas in children and young adults are often radiosensitive.

Neurofibromatosis

This disorder of autosomal dominant inheritance is caused by mutations in the *NF1* gene on chromosome 17 (type 1 neurofibromatosis, NF1) or the *NF2* gene on chromosome 22 (type 2 neurofibromatosis, NF2). Multiple fibromatous tumours develop from the neurilemmal sheaths of peripheral and cranial nerves. Most of the lesions are benign but sarcomatous change may occur. In NF1 (von Recklinghausen's disease) there are characteristic cutaneous manifestations and other extracranial manifestations (Box 26.99). Patients with NF1 are easily recognised because of the cutaneous lesions (Fig. 26.50), which increase in number throughout life. Investigation and treatment are only indicated if there are symptoms of cerebral or spinal involvement, or if malignant change is suspected. Patients with NF2 present with acoustic neuromas, often bilateral, and/or other central neoplasms, and have fewer if any cutaneous lesions. A family history of cerebral or spinal tumours should be noted with care, since relatives of patients with NF2 may require screening for acoustic neuromas.

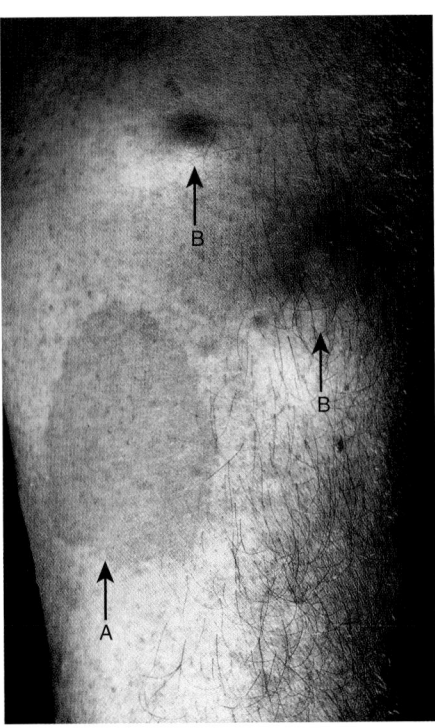

Fig. 26.50 A café au lait spot (arrow A) and subcutaneous nodules (arrows B) on the forearm of a patient with neurofibromatosis type 1.

Acoustic neuroma

This is a benign tumour of Schwann cells of the 8th cranial nerve, which may arise in isolation or as part of NF2 (see above). As an isolated finding, an acoustic neuroma occurs after the third decade and is more frequent in females. The tumour commonly arises near the nerve's entry point into the medulla or in the internal auditory meatus, usually on the vestibular division. Such lesions make up 80–90% of tumours at the cerebello-pontine angle.

Clinical features

These depend on the site of the tumour along the acoustic or vestibular nerve. Similar tumours arise rarely from the trigeminal nerve. Hearing loss is almost invariable, although it may not be the presenting feature. Sensory symptoms in the face and vertigo are also common at presentation. Distortion of the brain stem and/or cerebellar peduncle may cause ataxia and/or cerebellar signs in the limbs. Distortion of the fourth ventricle and cerebral aqueduct may cause hydrocephalus, which may be the presenting feature (see below). Facial weakness is unusual at presentation, but facial palsy may follow surgical removal of the tumour.

Investigations

MRI is the investigation of choice (see Fig. 26.49).

Management

Surgery is the treatment of choice. If the tumour can be completely removed, the prognosis is excellent. Deafness and facial weakness, if not present before surgery, often result from the operation.

26.99 Types of neurofibromatosis and their clinical features

Type 1 Peripheral form (> 70% of cases)

- Multiple cutaneous neurofibromas
- 'Soft' papillomas
- Café au lait patches
- Axillary freckling
- Iris fibromas (Lisch nodules)

- Plexiform neurofibromas
- Spinal neurofibromas
- Aqueduct stenosis
- Scoliosis
- Endocrine tumours

Type 2 Central form

- Few or no cutaneous lesions
- Cerebral and optic nerve gliomas

- Bilateral acoustic neuromas
- Meningiomas
- Spinal neurofibromas

Von Hippel–Lindau disease

This is a dominantly inherited disease caused by mutations of the *VHL* tumour suppressor gene on chromosome 3. It is characterised by the combination of retinal and intra-cranial (typically cerebellar) haemangiomas and haem-angioblastomas. There may be associated extracranial hamartomatous lesions, which may undergo malignant change. About 10% of posterior fossa tumours are cere-bellar haemangioblastomas. Von Hippel–Lindau disease needs to be considered in patients with such lesions, so that screening for other lesions and, if necessary, of family members can be instituted.

Paraneoplastic neurological disease

Neurological disease may occur with systemic malig-nant tumours in the absence of metastases. Mild degrees of myopathy and neuropathy are quite frequent with the common malignancies. Much rarer are certain dis-abling, and often fatal, paraneoplastic syndromes which often have an inflammatory basis, with associated auto-antibodies which cross-react with neural and tumour antigens (Box 26.100). In the case of the Lambert–Eaton myasthenic syndrome, the autoantibodies have a func-tional effect on neuromuscular transmission (p. 1231).

These syndromes are particularly associated with small-cell carcinoma of the lung, ovarian tumours, and lymphomas. In addition to the presence of autoantibodies in the serum and/or CSF, there is usually a lymphocytic infiltrate of the neural tissue affected.

Clinical features

These are summarised in Box 26.100. In most instances the neurological disease progresses quite rapidly over a few months. In 50% of patients with a paraneoplas-tic syndrome, the neurological disease precedes clinical presentation of the primary neoplasm. Paraneoplastic disease should be considered in the diagnosis of any unusual progressive neurological syndrome.

Investigations

The presence of characteristic autoantibodies in the context of a suspicious clinical picture may be diagnos-tic (see Box 26.100). The causative tumour may be very small and therefore CT of the chest or abdomen is often necessary to find it. The CSF often shows an increased protein and lymphocyte count with oligoclonal bands.

26

26.100 Paraneoplastic syndromes

Syndrome	Clinical features	Antibody	Associated tumours	Investigations
Retinal degeneration	Painless progressive visual loss	Antiretinal	Small-cell carcinoma of lung Melanoma	Chest X-ray, CT chest Electroretinogram
Opsoclonus-myoclonus	Arrhythmic chaotic rapid eye movements	Anti-Ri	Ovarian, lung Neuroblastoma (in children)	Chest X-ray, CT chest Pelvic ultrasound or CT
Sensory neuropathy	Limb pain, paraesthesia Distal numbness	Anti-Hu	Small-cell carcinoma of lung Hodgkin lymphoma	Chest X-ray, CT chest Nerve conduction studies
Limbic encephalitis	Memory loss, progressive dementia Seizures	Anti-Hu Anti-VGKC	Small-cell carcinoma of lung Hodgkin lymphoma	Chest X-ray, CT chest MRI (head) CSF (pleocytosis, raised protein)
Myelitis	Progressive spinal cord lesion (usually cervical cord)	Anti-Hu	Small-cell carcinoma of lung	Chest X-ray, CT chest MRI (cord, head)
Cerebellar degeneration	Progressive ataxia, nystagmus (down-beating), vertigo	Anti-Yo Anti-Hu	Small-cell carcinoma of lung Ovarian Hodgkin lymphoma	Chest X-ray, CT chest Pelvic ultrasound or CT CSF (raised protein, oligoclonal bands)
Subacute motor neuropathy	Subacute, patchy progressive, usually lower limb weakness and wasting	Anti-Hu	Hodgkin lymphoma Small-cell carcinoma of lung	Chest X-ray, CT chest Nerve conduction studies/EMG
Sensorimotor peripheral neuropathy	Mild, non-disabling peripheral limb numbness and paraesthesia	Not known	Small-cell carcinoma of lung Breast Other carcinoma	Chest X-ray, CT chest Nerve conduction studies/EMG
Lambert–Eaton myasthenic syndrome	Weakness of proximal limb muscles, fatigue with exertion after initial improvement, areflexia	Anti-VGCC	Small-cell carcinoma of lung	Chest X-ray, CT chest EMG
Dermatomyositis/polymyositis	Proximal limb weakness and pain, heliotrope skin rash, Gottron's papules on knuckles	Anti-Jo-1	Lung, breast, ovary	Chest X-ray, CT chest Creatine kinase EMG, muscle biopsy
Guillain–Barré	Ascending weakness, distal paraesthesia	Not known	Hodgkin lymphoma	Nerve conduction studies/EMG

(Anti-VGCC = antibodies to voltage-gated calcium channel; anti-VGKC = antibodies to voltage-gated potassium channels)

Management

This is directed at the primary tumour. Occasionally, successful therapy of the tumour is associated with improvement of the paraneoplastic syndrome. Some improvement may occur following administration of intravenous immunoglobulin.

Hydrocephalus

Obstructive hydrocephalus

This condition occurs as the result of an obstruction to the CSF circulation and causes dilatation of the ventricular system (Fig. 26.51). It is said to be 'communicating' if the obstruction lies outside the ventricular system (usually in the basal cisterns). Obstruction within the ventricles is most common in the narrow channels of the third ventricle and aqueduct, and may be caused by tumour or a congenital anomaly such as aqueduct stenosis (Fig. 26.52). The causes of hydrocephalus are listed in Box 26.101.

Diversion of the CSF by means of a shunt procedure between the ventricular system and the peritoneal cavity or right atrium may result in prompt relief of symptoms in obstructive or communicating hydrocephalus.

Normal pressure hydrocephalus

In this condition the dilatation of the ventricular system is caused by intermittent rises in CSF pressure, which occur particularly at night. It occurs predominantly in old age and is suggested by the combination of gait apraxia (p. 1153) and dementia, often with urinary incontinence as an early feature. This cause of dilatation of the ventricles can be very difficult to distinguish from that occurring due to cerebral atrophy, where the cortical sulci are also dilated. The result of shunting procedures for normal pressure hydrocephalus is unpredictable.

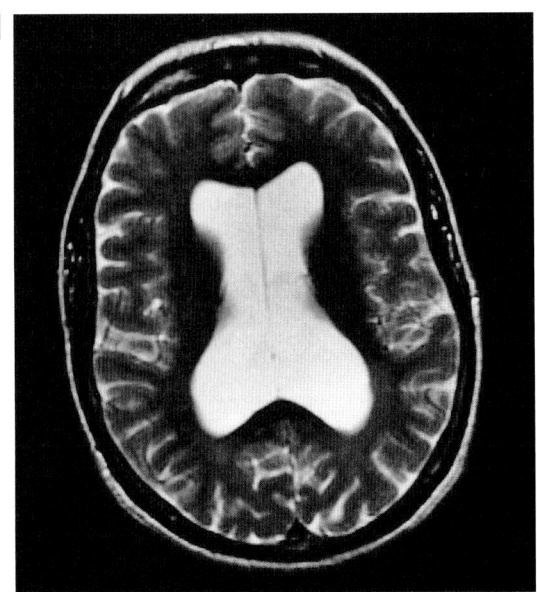

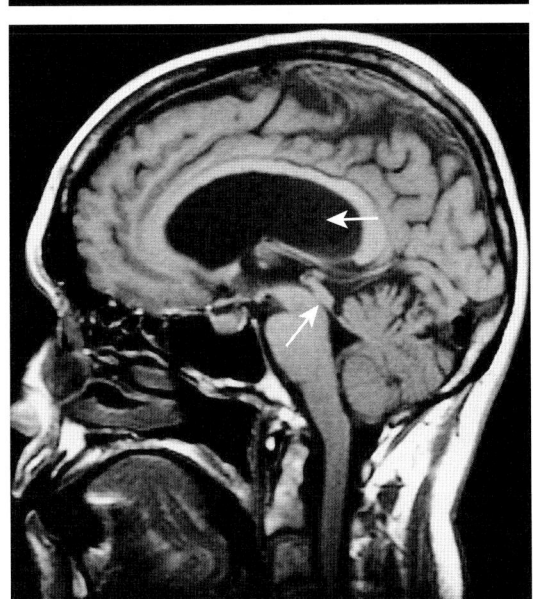

Fig. 26.52 MRI of hydrocephalus due to aqueduct stenosis.
A Axial T$_2$-weighted image (CSF appears white): note the dilated lateral ventricles. B Sagittal T$_2$-weighted image (CSF appears black): note the dilated ventricles (top arrow) and narrowed aqueduct (bottom arrow).

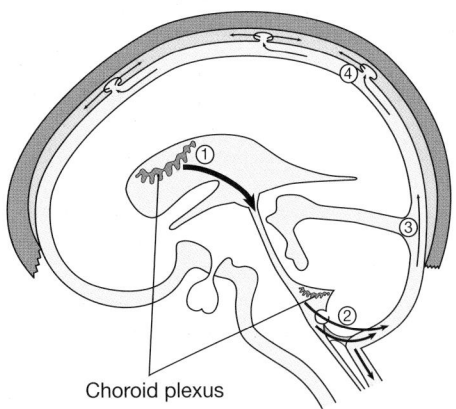

Choroid plexus

Fig. 26.51 The circulation of cerebrospinal fluid. (1) CSF is synthesised in the choroid plexus of the ventricles, and flows from the lateral and third ventricles through the aqueduct to the fourth ventricle. (2) At the foramina of Luschka and Magendie it exits the brain, flowing over the hemispheres (3) and down around the spinal cord and roots in the subarachnoid space. (4) It is then absorbed into the dural venous sinuses via the arachnoid villi.

26.101 Causes of hydrocephalus

Communicating (obstruction outside ventricular system)

- Bacterial meningitis (especially tuberculous)
- Sarcoidosis
- Subarachnoid haemorrhage
- Head injury
- Idiopathic ('normal pressure')

Non-communicating (obstruction within ventricular system)

- Tumours
- Colloid cyst
- Arnold–Chiari malformation
- Aqueduct stenosis
- Cerebellar abscess
- Cerebellar or brain-stem haematoma

Idiopathic intracranial hypertension

This condition, previously known as 'benign intracranial hypertension' and 'pseudotumour cerebri', usually occurs in obese young women. Raised intracranial pressure develops without a space-occupying lesion, ventricular dilatation or impairment of consciousness. The aetiology is uncertain but there may be a diffuse defect of CSF reabsorption by the arachnoid villi. The condition can be precipitated by drugs, including tetracycline, and vitamin A and its derivatives, the retinoids.

Clinical features

The usual presentation is with headache, sometimes accompanied by transient diplopia and visual disturbance. Clinical examination reveals papilloedema, which may be discovered incidentally at a routine visit to an optician. A palsy of the 6th cranial nerve may also be present.

Investigations

The diagnosis can be confirmed by lumbar puncture which shows raised CSF pressure, but neuroimaging must be performed before a lumbar puncture to exclude the presence of a mass lesion. Patients with idiopathic cranial hypertension have an essentially normal CT with normal-sized or small ventricles. MR angiography or cerebral venography is usually performed to exclude cerebral venous sinus thrombosis or stenosis. True papilloedema may need to be distinguished from other causes of disc swelling clinically and by fluorescein angiography which is indicated in patients where there is any doubt about the diagnosis.

Management

Any precipitating condition should be sought, relevant medication should be withdrawn and a weight-reducing diet instigated, if indicated. The carbonic anhydrase inhibitor, acetazolamide, may help to lower intracranial pressure. Repeated lumbar puncture can be considered, but is often unacceptable to the patient. Patients failing to respond, in whom chronic papilloedema threatens vision, may require optic nerve sheath fenestration or a lumbo-peritoneal shunt. In patients shown to have a fixed stenosis of the transverse venous sinus, stenting of this may be helpful.

DISORDERS OF THE SPINE AND SPINAL CORD

The spinal cord and spinal roots may be affected by intrinsic disease or by disorders of the surrounding meninges and bones. The clinical presentation of these conditions depends on the anatomical level at which the cord or roots are affected, as well as the nature of the pathological process involved. It is important to recognise when emergency surgical intervention is necessary and to plan investigations to identify such patients.

Cervical spondylosis

Cervical spondylosis is the term given to the occurrence of osteoarthritis in the cervical spine. It is characterised by degeneration of the intervertebral discs and osteophyte formation. This is extremely common and radiological changes of cervical spondylosis are very frequently found in apparently healthy individuals above the age of 50. Whilst cervical spondylosis is often asymptomatic, it may be associated with neurological dysfunction. The C5/6, C6/7 and C4/5 vertebral levels and C6, C7 and C5 roots, respectively, are most commonly affected (Fig. 26.53).

Cervical spondylotic radiculopathy

Compression of a nerve root occurs when a disc prolapses laterally, which may develop acutely, or compression may occur more gradually due to osteophytic encroachment of the intervertebral foramina.

Clinical features

The patient complains of pain in the neck that may radiate in the distribution of the affected nerve root. The neck is held rigidly and neck movements may exacerbate pain. Paraesthesia and sensory loss may be found in the affected segment and there may be lower motor neuron signs, including weakness, wasting and reflex impairment (Box 26.102).

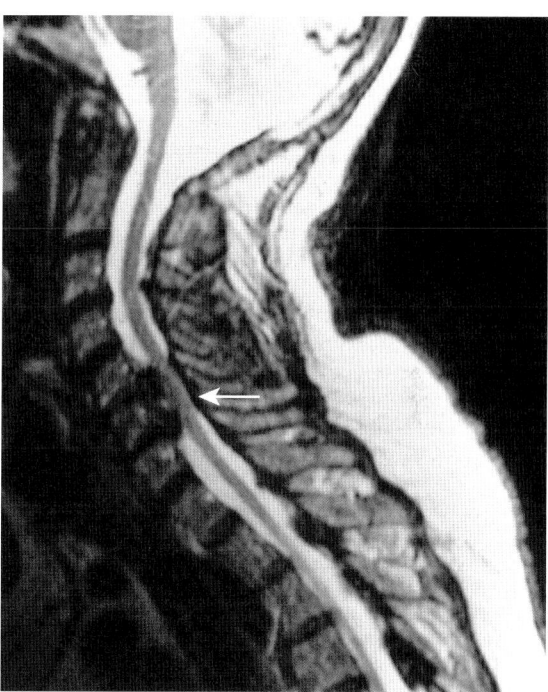

Fig. 26.53 MRI showing cervical cord compression (arrow) in cervical spondylosis.

26.102 Physical signs in cervical root compression			
Root	**Muscle weakness**	**Sensory loss**	**Reflex loss**
C5	Biceps, deltoid, spinati	Upper lateral arm	Biceps
C6	Brachioradialis	Lower lateral arm, thumb, index finger	Supinator
C7	Triceps, finger and wrist extensors	Middle finger	Triceps

26

Investigations

Plain X-rays, including lateral and oblique views, should be obtained to confirm the presence of degenerative changes and to exclude other conditions, including destructive lesions. If surgery is contemplated, MRI is required. Electrophysiological studies rarely add to the clinical examination, but may be necessary if there is doubt about the differential diagnosis between root and peripheral nerve lesions.

Management

Conservative treatment with analgesics and physiotherapy results in resolution of symptoms in the great majority of patients, but a few require surgery in the form of foraminotomy or disc excision.

Cervical spondylotic myelopathy

Dorsomedial herniation of a disc and the development of transverse bony bars or posterior osteophytes may result in pressure on the spinal cord or the anterior spinal artery which supplies the anterior two-thirds of the cord (see Fig. 26.53).

Clinical features

The onset is usually insidious and painless, but acute deterioration may occur after trauma, especially hyperextension injury. Upper motor neuron signs develop in the limbs, with spasticity of the legs usually appearing before the arms are involved. Sensory loss in the upper limbs is common, producing tingling, numbness and proprioception loss in the hands, with progressive clumsiness. Sensory manifestations in the legs are much less common. The neurological deficit usually progresses gradually and disturbance of micturition is a very late feature.

Investigations

Plain X-rays confirm the presence of degenerative changes, and MRI (see Fig. 26.53) or myelography may be indicated if surgical treatment is being considered. MRI may also show areas of high signal within the spinal cord at the level of compression. Imaging of the cervical spine should be considered if there is diagnostic doubt or if surgery is contemplated.

Management

Surgical procedures, including laminectomy and anterior discectomy, may arrest progression of disability but may not result in neurological improvement. The judgement on whether surgery should be undertaken may be difficult. Manipulation of the cervical spine is of no proven benefit and may precipitate acute neurological deterioration.

Prognosis

The prognosis of cervical myelopathy is variable. In many patients the condition stabilises or even improves without intervention, but if progressive disability does develop, surgical decompression should be considered.

Lumbar spondylosis

This is the term given to the occurrence of degenerative disc disease and osteoarthritic change in the lumbar spine. Pain in the distribution of the lumbar or sacral roots ('sciatica') is often due to disc protrusion, but can be a feature of other rare but important disorders including spinal tumour, malignant disease in the pelvis and tuberculosis of the vertebral bodies.

Lumbar disc herniation

Acute lumbar disc herniation is often precipitated by trauma, usually by lifting heavy weights while the spine is flexed. The nucleus pulposus may bulge or rupture through the annulus fibrosus, giving rise to pressure on nerve endings in the spinal ligaments, changes in the vertebral joints or pressure on nerve roots.

Pathophysiology

The altered mechanics of the lumbar spine result in loss of lumbar lordosis and there may be spasm of the paraspinal musculature. Root pressure is suggested by limitation of flexion of the hip on the affected side if the straight leg is raised (Lasègue's sign). If the third or fourth lumbar roots are involved, Lasègue's sign may be negative, but pain in the back may be induced by hyperextension of the hip (femoral nerve stretch test). The roots most frequently affected are S1, L5 and L4; the signs of root pressure at these levels are summarised in Box 26.103.

Clinical features

The onset may be sudden or gradual. Alternatively, repeated episodes of low back pain may precede sciatica by months or years. Constant aching pain is felt in the lumbar region and may radiate to the buttock, thigh, calf and foot. Pain is exacerbated by coughing or straining but may be relieved by lying flat.

Investigations

Plain X-rays of the lumbar spine are of little value in the diagnosis of lumbar disc disease, although they may show other conditions such as malignant infiltration of a vertebral body. CT, especially using spiral scanning techniques, can provide helpful images of the disc protrusion and/or narrowing of the exit foramina. MRI is the investigation of choice if available, since soft tissues are well imaged.

Management

Some 90% of patients with sciatica recover following conservative treatment with analgesia and early mobilisation; bed rest does not help recovery. The patient should be instructed in back-strengthening exercises and advised to avoid physical manoeuvres likely to strain the lumbar spine. Injections of local anaesthetic or corticosteroids may be useful adjunctive treatment

26.103 Physical signs in lumbar root compression				
Disc level	**Root**	**Sensory loss**	**Weakness**	**Reflex loss**
L3/L4	L4	Inner calf	Inversion of foot	Knee
L4/L5	L5	Outer calf and dorsum of foot	Dorsiflexion of hallux/toes	
L5/S1	S1	Sole and lateral foot	Plantar flexion	Ankle

if symptoms are due to ligamentous injury or joint dysfunction. Surgery may have to be considered if there is no response to conservative treatment or if progressive neurological deficits develop. Central disc prolapse with bilateral symptoms and signs and disturbance of sphincter function requires urgent surgical decompression.

Lumbar canal stenosis

This is due to a congenital narrowing of the lumbar spinal canal, exacerbated by the degenerative changes that commonly occur with age.

Pathophysiology

The symptoms of spinal stenosis are thought to be due to local vascular compromise secondary to the canal stenosis, rendering the nerve roots ischaemic and intolerant of the demand for increased neural activity that occurs on exercise.

Clinical features

The patients, who are usually elderly, develop exercise-induced weakness and paraesthesia in the legs ('spinal claudication'). These symptoms progress with continued exertion, often to the point that the patient can no longer walk, but are quickly relieved by a short period of rest. Physical examination at rest shows preservation of peripheral pulses with absent ankle reflexes. Weakness or sensory loss may only be apparent if the patient is examined immediately after exercise.

Investigations

The investigation of first choice is MRI, but this is not always possible because of contraindications, and if this is the case CT or myelography can be used as an alternative.

Management

Extensive lumbar laminectomy often results in complete relief of symptoms and recovery of normal exercise tolerance.

Spinal cord compression

Spinal cord compression is one of the most common neurological emergencies encountered in clinical practice and the common causes are listed in Box 26.104. A space-occupying lesion within the spinal canal may damage nerve tissue either directly by pressure or indirectly by interfering with blood supply. Oedema from venous obstruction impairs neuronal function, and ischaemia from arterial obstruction may lead to necrosis of the spinal cord. The early stages of damage are reversible but severely damaged neurons do not recover; hence the importance of early diagnosis and treatment.

Clinical features

The onset of symptoms of spinal cord compression is usually slow (over weeks), but can be acute as a result of trauma or metastases, especially if there is associated arterial occlusion. The symptoms are shown in Box 26.105.

Pain and sensory symptoms occur early, while weakness and sphincter dysfunction are usually late

manifestations. The signs vary according to the level of the cord compression and the structures involved. There may be tenderness to percussion over the spine if there is vertebral disease, and this may be associated with a local kyphosis. Involvement of the roots at the level of the compression may cause dermatomal sensory impairment and corresponding lower motor signs. Interruption of fibres in the spinal cord causes sensory loss (p. 1156) and upper motor neuron signs below the level of the lesion, and there is often disturbance of sphincter function. The distribution of these signs varies with the level of the lesion, as shown in Box 26.106.

The Brown–Séquard syndrome (see Fig. 26.18E, p. 1156) results if damage is confined to one side of the cord; the findings are explained by the anatomy of the sensory tracts (see Fig. 26.8, p. 1140). On the side of the lesion there is a band of hyperaesthesia with loss of proprioception and upper motor neuron signs below it. On the other side there is loss of spinothalamic sensation (pain and temperature). With compressive lesions there is usually a band of pain at the level of the lesion in the distribution of the nerve roots subject to compression.

26.104 Causes of spinal cord compression

Site	Frequency	Causes
Vertebral	80%	Trauma (extradural) Intervertebral disc prolapse Metastatic carcinoma (e.g. breast, prostate, bronchus) Myeloma Tuberculosis
Meninges (intradural, extramedullary)	15%	Tumours (e.g. meningioma, neurofibroma, ependymoma, metastasis, lymphoma, leukaemia) Epidural abscess
Spinal cord (intradural, intramedullary)	5%	Tumours (e.g. glioma, ependymoma, metastasis)

26.105 Symptoms of spinal cord compression

Pain
- Localised over the spine or in a root distribution, which may be aggravated by coughing, sneezing or straining

Sensory
- Paraesthesia, numbness or cold sensations, especially in the lower limbs, which spread proximally, often to a level on the trunk

Motor
- Weakness, heaviness or stiffness of the limbs, most commonly the legs

Sphincters
- Urgency or hesitancy of micturition, leading eventually to urinary retention

26

26.106 Signs of spinal cord compression

Cervical, above C5

- Upper motor neuron signs and sensory loss in all four limbs
- Diaphragm weakness (phrenic nerve)

Cervical, C5–T1

- Lower motor neuron signs and segmental sensory loss in the arms; upper motor neuron signs in the legs
- Respiratory (intercostal) muscle weakness

Thoracic cord

- Spastic paraplegia with a sensory level on the trunk

Conus medullaris

- Weakness of legs, sacral loss of sensation and extensor plantar responses

Cauda equina

- Spinal cord ends at approximately the T12/L1 spinal level and spinal lesions below this level can only cause lower motor neuron signs by affecting the cauda equina

26.107 Investigation of acute spinal cord syndrome

- Plain X-rays of spine
- Chest X-rays
- MRI of spine or myelography
- CSF
- Serum B$_{12}$

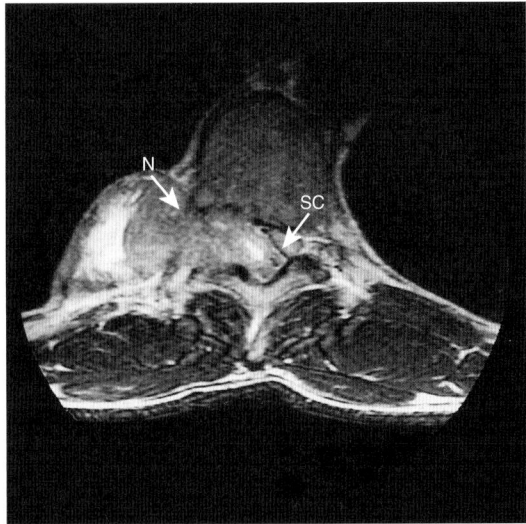

Fig. 26.54 Axial MRI of thoracic spine. A neurofibroma (N) is compressing the spinal cord (SC) and emerging in a 'dumbbell' fashion through the vertebral foramen into the paraspinal space.

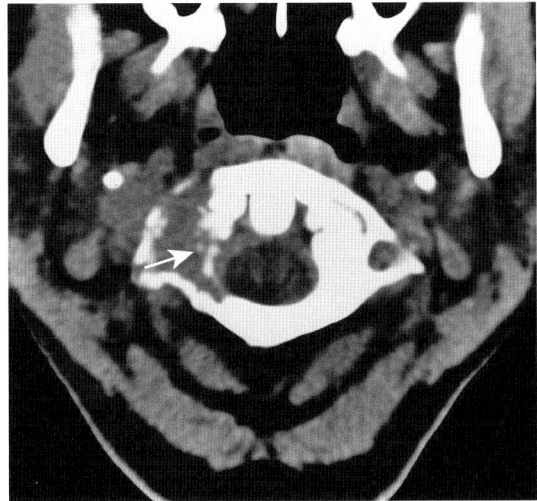

Fig. 26.55 CT myelogram of cervical spine at the level of C2 showing bony erosion of vertebra by a metastasis (arrow).

Investigations

Patients with a short history of a progressive spinal cord syndrome should be investigated urgently as listed in Box 26.107. The investigation of first choice is MRI (Fig. 26.54); but this is not always possible because of complications; in this situation, myelography can also localise the lesion and, with CT in suitable cases, can define the extent of compression and associated soft-tissue abnormality (Fig. 26.55). Plain X-rays may show bony destruction and soft-tissue abnormalities and are also an essential initial investigation. Routine investigations, including chest X-ray, may provide evidence of systemic disease. If myelography is performed, CSF should be taken for analysis; in cases of complete spinal block this shows a normal cell count with a very elevated protein causing yellow discoloration of the fluid (Froin's syndrome). Acute deterioration may develop after myelography and the neurosurgeons should be alerted before it is undertaken. In patients with secondary tumours, needle biopsy may be required to establish a tissue diagnosis, unless this has already been established.

Management

Treatment and prognosis depend on the nature of the underlying lesion. Benign tumours should be surgically excised, and a good functional recovery can be expected unless a marked neurological deficit has developed before diagnosis. Extradural compression due to malignancy is the most common cause of spinal cord compression in developed countries and has a poor prognosis, although useful function can be regained if treatment is initiated within 24 hours of the onset of severe weakness or sphincter dysfunction. Surgical decompression may be appropriate in some patients, but has a similar out- come to radiotherapy. Spinal cord compression due to tuberculosis is common in some areas of the world, and requires surgical treatment if seen early. This should be followed by appropriate anti-tuberculous chemotherapy (p. 693) for an extended period. Traumatic lesions of the vertebral column require specialised neurosurgical treatment.

Intrinsic diseases of the spinal cord

There are many disorders which interfere with spinal cord function due to non-compressive involvement of the spinal cord itself. A list of these disorders is given in Box 26.108. The symptoms and signs are generally similar to those that would occur with extrinsic compression (see Boxes 26.105 and 26.106), although a suspended sensory loss (see Fig. 26.18F, p. 1156) can only occur with intrinsic disease such as syringomyelia. Urinary symptoms

26.108 Intrinsic diseases of the spinal cord

Type of disorder	Condition	Clinical features
Congenital	Diastematomyelia (spina bifida)	Features variably present at birth and deteriorate thereafter LMN features, deformity and sensory loss of legs Impaired sphincter function Hairy patch or pit over low back Incidence reduced by increased maternal intake of folic acid during pregnancy
	Hereditary spastic paraplegia	Onset usually in adult life Autosomal dominant inheritance usual Slowly progressive UMN features affecting legs > arms Little, if any, sensory loss
Infective/ inflammatory	Transverse myelitis due to viruses (HZV), schistosomiasis, HIV, MS, sarcoidosis	Weakness and sensory loss, often with pain, developing over hours to days UMN features below lesion Impaired sphincter function
Vascular	Anterior spinal artery infarct Intervertebral disc embolus	Abrupt onset Anterior horn cell loss (LMN) at level of lesion UMN features below it Spinothalamic sensory loss below lesion but spared dorsal column sensation
	Spinal AVM/dural fistula	Onset variable (acute to slowly progressive) Variable LMN, UMN, sensory and sphincter disturbance Symptoms and signs often not well localised to site of AVM
Neoplastic	Glioma, ependymoma	Weakness and sensory loss, often with pain, developing over months to years UMN features below lesion in cord; additional LMN features in conus Impaired sphincter function
Metabolic	Vitamin B$_{12}$ deficiency (subacute combined degeneration)	Progressive spastic paraparesis with proprioception loss, absent reflexes due to peripheral neuropathy ± optic nerve and cerebral involvement (p. 113)
Degenerative	Motor neuron disease	Relentlessly progressive LMN and UMN features, associated bulbar weakness, no sensory involvement (p. 1204)
	Syringomyelia	Gradual onset over months or years, pain in cervical segments Anterior horn cell loss (LMN) at level of lesion, UMN features below it Suspended spinothalamic sensory loss at level of lesion, dorsal columns preserved. See Figures 26.18F (p. 1156) and 26.56

(AVM = arteriovenous malformation; HIV = human immunodeficiency virus; HZV = herpes zoster virus; LMN = lower motor neuron; MS = multiple sclerosis; UMN = upper motor neuron)

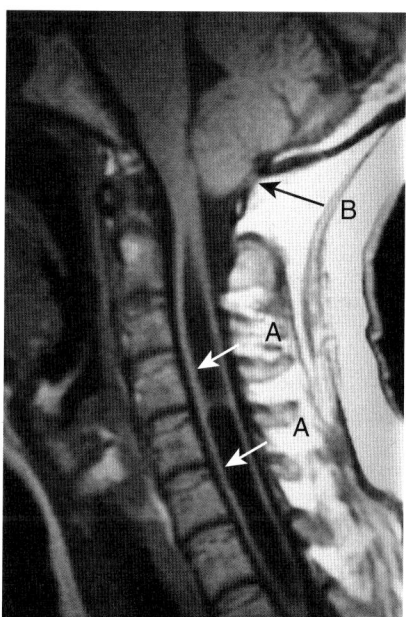

Fig. 26.56 MRI scan showing syrinx (arrows A), with herniation of cerebellar tonsils (arrow B).

usually occur earlier in the course of an intrinsic cord disorder than with compressive disorders.

Investigation of intrinsic disease starts with imaging to exclude a compressive lesion. If available, MRI provides the most information about structural lesions such as diastematomyelia, syringomyelia (Fig. 26.56), or intrinsic tumours. Non-specific signal change may be seen in the spinal cord in inflammatory (see Fig. 26.38, p. 1194) or infective conditions and others such as B$_{12}$ deficiency. Other investigations such as lumbar puncture or blood tests are required to make a specific diagnosis.

DISEASES OF PERIPHERAL NERVES

Numerous inherited and acquired pathological processes may affect peripheral nerves, targeting either the nerve roots (radiculopathy), the nerve plexuses (plexopathy) and/or the individual nerves themselves (neuropathy), as summarised in Box 26.109. Cranial nerves 3–12 share the same tissue characteristics as peripheral nerves elsewhere and are subject to the same range of diseases. Nerve fibres of different types (motor, sensory or autonomic) and of different sizes may be variably involved. Disorders may be primarily

26.109 Types and causes of peripheral neuropathy

Neurophysiology	Focal (mononeuropathy)	Multifocal (mononeuropathy multiplex)		Generalised (polyneuropathy)	
		Acute	Chronic	Acute	Chronic
Demyelinating on NCS; slowed conduction ± conduction block	Entrapment*	Diphtheria	Leprosy* Paraproteinaemia MMN HNPP	Guillain–Barré* Suramin toxicity	Hereditary* CIDP Lymphoma Osteoclastic myeloma IgM paraproteinaemia Arsenic toxicity Amiodarone toxicity Diphtheria
Axonal on NCS; reduced or absent action potentials, normal conduction velocities	Severe entrapment*	Diabetes* Vasculitis Lyme disease Cryoglobulinaemia	Diabetes* Neoplastic infiltration HIV Sarcoidosis Amyloid	Alcohol* Guillain–Barré variants Toxins Critical illness Porphyria Paraneoplastic Tick paralysis	Metabolic/endocrine diseases (including diabetes)* Alcohol* Drugs and toxins Vitamin deficiency* Hereditary* IgG paraproteinaemia Paraneoplastic Primary amyloidosis

*Common and/or important causes.
(CIDP = chronic inflammatory demyelinating peripheral neuropathy; MMN = multifocal motor neuropathy with conduction block; HNPP = hereditary neuropathy with tendency to pressure palsies; NCS = nerve conduction studies)

directed at the axon, the myelin sheath (Schwann cells) or the vasa nervorum (see Fig. 26.1, p. 1134). An acute or chronic peripheral nerve disorder may be focal (affecting a single nerve: mononeuropathy), multifocal (several nerves: mononeuropathy multiplex) or generalised (polyneuropathy).

Pathophysiology

Neuropathy can occur in association with many systemic diseases, toxins (Box 26.110) and drugs (Box 26.111) which damage function of the peripheral nerves to cause a neuropathy.

Clinical features

Motor nerve involvement produces features of a lower motor neuron lesion (p. 1152). Symptoms and signs of sensory nerve involvement depend on the type of sensory nerve involved (p. 1156). Autonomic fibre involvement may cause postural hypotension due to disruption of vasomotor control, or disturbance of sweating, cardiac rhythm, and gastrointestinal, bladder and sexual functions.

Investigations

Investigations required in a patient with peripheral neuropathy reflect this wide spectrum of causes (Box 26.112). Neurophysiological tests (p. 1142), and sometimes nerve biopsy, will help determine whether the pathology is primarily affecting the nerve axon (axonal neuropathy), the myelin sheath (demyelinating neuropathy) or the blood vessels (Box 26.109).

Entrapment neuropathy

Focal compression or entrapment is the usual cause of a mononeuropathy. However, some patients present with what initially appears to be a single nerve lesion

and then go on to develop multiple nerve lesions. This is termed mononeuritis multiplex. Symptoms and signs of entrapment neuropathy are listed in Box 26.113. In this situation pressure damages the myelin sheath, and neurophysiology studies show slowing of conduction over the relevant site. Sustained or severe pressure damages the integrity of the axons, demonstrable as loss of the sensory action potential distal to the site of compression. Certain conditions increase the propensity to develop entrapment neuropathies. These include acromegaly, hypothyroidism, pregnancy, any pre-existing mild generalised axonal neuropathy such as diabetes, and osteophytes. Patients with multiple recurrent entrapment neuropathies, especially at unusual sites, should be screened for autosomal dominant hereditary neuropathy with liability to pressure palsies (HNPP) (see Box 26.116, p. 1230). Unless axonal loss has occurred, entrapment neuropathies will recover, provided the pressure on the nerve is relieved, either by avoiding precipitating activities or limb positions, or by surgical decompression. Cranial nerves may also be the target of entrapment neuropathy. Lesions of ocular motor nerves (3rd, 4th and 6th) are reviewed on page 1163. An isolated lesion of one 8th cranial nerve usually indicates compressive pathology such as acoustic neuroma (p. 1218) in or near the cerebello-pontine angle. Isolated lesions of the 9th, 10th, 11th or 12th cranial nerves are uncommon, and anatomical considerations mean that lower cranial nerve lesions tend to occur in groups, sometimes with involvement of the ascending sympathetic innervation to the eye (Box 26.114).

Trigeminal neuropathy

Isolated trigeminal sensory neuropathy is rare. It causes unilateral facial sensory loss and is associated in some patients with scleroderma, Sjögren's syndrome or other

i **26.110 Systemic disorders and toxins associated with neuropathy**

	Metabolic/ endocrine	Toxic	Immune-mediated/ inflammatory	Infective	Neoplastic	Vitamin deficiencies
Common	Diabetes mellitus Chronic renal failure	Alcoholism Chronic liver disease Drugs	–	–	–	–
Unusual	Hypothyroidism	Lead Radiation	Systemic vasculitis SLE Rheumatoid arthritis Sjögren's disease Cryoglobulinaemia Paraproteinaemia	HIV/AIDS	Lymphoma Carcinoma (infiltration and paraneoplastic) Myeloma	Vitamin B_{12} Thiamin Pyridoxine Folic acid Vitamin E Pantothenic acid
Rare	Porphyria (p. 456) Acromegaly	Arsenic (p. 221) Mercury Thallium Organophosphates (p. 218) Acrylamide Hexacarbons (glue)	Coeliac disease Sarcoidosis Primary amyloidosis	Lyme disease	–	–

26.111 Drugs causing peripheral neuropathy

Cardiovascular agents
- Amiodarone
- Statins
- Hydralazine

Chemotherapy agents
- Cisplatin
- Thalidomide
- Paclitaxel
- Vincristine

Anti-infective agents
- Chloramphenicol
- Isoniazid
- Nitrofurantoin
- Ethambutol
- Metronidazole
- Suramin

Other
- Gold
- Disulfiram
- Pyridoxine
- Tacrolimus
- Colchicine
- Phenytoin

26.112 Investigation of peripheral neuropathy

	First-line tests	Second-line tests	Occasionally useful tests
Haematology	Full blood count ESR B_{12} and folate		
Biochemistry	Urea, electrolytes, calcium Creatinine Liver function tests Blood glucose ± tolerance test/HbA$_{1c}$ Thyroid function tests Plasma protein electrophoresis	Serum lipids, lipoproteins Cryoglobulins Toxic metal and drug screen Prostate-specific antigen Urinary porphyrins Urinary Bence Jones protein Faecal occult blood	Vitamin assays (e.g. vitamin E) Phytanic acid (Refsum's disease)
Immunology	Venereal Diseases Research Laboratory (VDRL) test Serum autoantibodies (antinuclear factor, dsDNA, rheumatoid factor, extractable nuclear antigens)	Antiganglioside antibodies Antineuronal antibodies	
Other	Nerve conduction/EMG	Genetic screening tests (hereditary neuropathies, Friedreich's ataxia) Chest X-ray/CT Mammogram Abdominal imaging	Nerve biopsy

26

26.113 **Symptoms and signs in common entrapment neuropathies**

Nerve	Symptoms	Muscle weakness/ muscle-wasting	Area of sensory loss
Median (at wrist) (carpal tunnel syndrome)	Pain and paraesthesia on palmar aspect of hands and fingers, waking the patient from sleep. Pain may extend to arm and shoulder	Abductor pollicis brevis	Lateral palm and thumb, index, middle and lateral half 4th finger
Ulnar (at elbow)	Paraesthesia on medial border of hand, wasting and weakness of hand muscles	All small hand muscles, excluding abductor pollicis brevis	Medial palm and little finger, and medial half 4th finger
Radial	Weakness of extension of wrist and fingers, often precipitated by sleeping in abnormal posture, e.g. arm over back of chair	Wrist and finger extensors, supinator	Dorsum of thumb
Common peroneal	Foot drop, trauma to head of fibula	Dorsiflexion and eversion of foot	Nil or dorsum of foot
Lateral cutaneous nerve of the thigh (meralgia paraesthetica)	Tingling and dysaesthesia on lateral border of the thigh	Nil	Lateral border of thigh

26.114 **Syndromes of lower cranial nerve lesions outside the brain stem**

Syndrome	Cranial nerves involved	Site of lesion	Cause
Vernet	9, 10 and 11	Jugular foramen (inside skull)	Metastases, neurinoma, meningioma, epidermoid, carotid body tumour
Collet–Sicard	9, 10, 11 and 12	Jugular foramen just outside skull, near foramen lacerum	Metastases, neurinoma, meningioma, epidermoid, carotid body tumour
Villaret	9, 10, 11, 12 and Horner's	Posterior retropharyngeal space, near carotid artery	Carotid dissection, metastases, neurinoma, meningioma, epidermoid, carotid body tumour
Isolated 12th	12	Skull base (hypoglossal canal)	Metastases, neurinoma, meningioma, epidermoid

connective tissue disorder. Patients with trigeminal neuralgia (p. 1171) do not have sensory loss on examination unless there have been operative procedures on the nerve. Reactivation of varicella virus in the trigeminal nerve causes herpes zoster (most frequently in the ophthalmic division) and is followed in about one-third of patients by postherpetic neuralgia (p. 314).

Facial nerve palsy

Idiopathic facial nerve palsy or Bell's palsy is a common condition affecting all ages and both sexes. The lesion is within the facial canal and may be due to reactivation of latent herpes simplex virus 1 infection. Symptoms usually develop subacutely over a few hours, with pain around the ear preceding the unilateral facial weakness. Patients often describe the face as 'numb', but there is no objective sensory loss (except possibly to taste). Hyperacusis can occur if the nerve to stapedius is involved, and there may be diminished salivation and tear secretion. Examination reveals an ipsilateral lower motor neuron facial nerve palsy. Vesicles in the ear or on the palate indicate that the facial palsy is due to herpes zoster (p. 314) rather than Bell's palsy.

Prednisolone 40–60 mg daily for a week speeds recovery if started within 72 hours. Artificial tears and ointment prevent exposure keratitis and the eye should be taped shut overnight. About 80% of patients recover spontaneously within 12 weeks. A slow or poor recovery is predicted by complete paralysis, older age and reduced facial motor action potential amplitude after the first week. Recurrences can occur but should prompt further investigation. Aberrant re-innervation may occur during recovery, producing unwanted facial movements such as eye closure when the mouth is moved, or 'crocodile tears' (tearing during salivation).

Hemifacial spasm

This usually presents after middle age with intermittent twitching around one eye, spreading ipsilaterally over months or years to affect other parts of the facial muscles. The spasms are exacerbated by talking or eating, or when the patient is under stress. The cause, as with trigeminal neuralgia, is probably an aberrant arterial loop irritating the nerve just outside the pons. The facial nerve should be imaged to exclude a structural lesion, especially in a young patient. Drug treatment is not effective but injections of botulinum toxin into affected muscles help, although these usually have to be repeated every 3 months or so. Occasionally, microvascular decompression is necessary.

Multifocal neuropathy

Multifocal neuropathy (mononeuritis multiplex) is characterised by lesions of multiple nerve roots, peripheral nerves or cranial nerves. It is due either to involvement of the vasa nervorum or to malignant infiltration of the nerves. The clinical expression of a very widespread multifocal neuropathy may become confluent so that the clinical picture eventually resembles a polyneuropathy. In this case neurophysiology may be required to identify the multifocal nature of the problem. Investigation of patients with an acute multifocal neuropathy should be urgent since vasculitis is a common cause, either as part of a systemic disease (see Box 26.110) or isolated to the nerves.

Polyneuropathy

Polyneuropathy is a generalised pathological process occurring in the longest peripheral nerves first, affecting the distal lower limbs before the upper limbs, with sensory symptoms and signs of an ascending 'glove and stocking' distribution (p. 1156). This is particularly true with axonal neuropathies where the disorder affects the metabolic processes required for axonal transport in the peripheral nerves. In inflammatory demyelinating neuropathies, the pathology may be patchier and variations from this ascending pattern occur.

Guillain–Barré syndrome

This syndrome of acute paralysis develops, in 70% of patients, 1–4 weeks after respiratory infection or diarrhoea (particularly *Campylobacter*). In Europe and North America, acute inflammatory polyneuropathy is most commonly demyelinating (acute inflammatory demyelinating neuropathy, AIDP). Axonal variants, either motor (acute motor axonal neuropathy, AMAN) or sensorimotor (acute motor and sensory axonal neuropathy, AMSAN), are more common in China and Japan. There is a predominantly cell-mediated inflammatory response directed at the myelin protein of spinal roots, peripheral and extra-axial cranial nerves, possibly triggered by molecular mimicry between epitopes found in the cell walls of some microorganisms and gangliosides in the Schwann cell and axonal membranes. The resulting release of inflammatory cytokines blocks nerve conduction and is followed by a complement-mediated destruction of the myelin sheath and the associated axon.

Clinical features

Distal paraesthesia and limb pains (often severe) precede a rapidly ascending muscle weakness, from lower to upper limbs, more marked proximally than distally. Facial and bulbar weakness commonly develops, and respiratory weakness requiring ventilatory support occurs in 20% of cases. In most patients, weakness progresses for 1–3 weeks, but rapid deterioration to respiratory failure can develop within hours. On examination there is diffuse weakness with widespread loss of reflexes. An unusual axonal variant described by Miller Fisher comprises the triad of ophthalmoplegia, ataxia and areflexia. Overall, 80% of patients recover completely within 3–6 months, 4% die, and the remainder suffer residual neurological disability which can be severe. Adverse prognostic features include older age, rapid deterioration to ventilation and evidence of axonal loss on EMG.

Investigations

The CSF protein is elevated at some stage of the illness but may be normal in the first 10 days. There is usually no rise in CSF cell number (a lymphocytosis of > 50×10^6 cells/L suggests an alternative diagnosis). Electrophysiological studies are often normal in the early stages but show typical changes after a week or

so, with conduction block and multifocal motor slowing, sometimes most evident proximally as delayed F-waves (p. 1142). Investigation to identify an underlying cause, such as cytomegalovirus, mycoplasma or *Campylobacter*, requires a chest X-ray, stool culture and appropriate immunological blood tests. Antibodies to the ganglioside GQ_{1b} are found in the Miller Fisher variant. Acute porphyria (p. 456) should be excluded by urinary porphyrin estimation, and serum lead should be measured if there are only motor signs.

Management

During the phase of deterioration, regular monitoring of respiratory function (vital capacity and arterial blood gases) is required, as respiratory failure may develop with little warning and require ventilatory support. Ventilation may be needed if the vital capacity falls below 1 L, but intubation is more often required because of bulbar incompetence leading to aspiration. General management to protect the airway and prevent pressure sores and venous thrombosis is essential. Corticosteroid therapy has been shown by RCT to be ineffective. However, plasma exchange and intravenous immunoglobulin therapy shorten the duration of ventilation and improve prognosis, provided treatment is started within 14 days of the onset of symptoms (Box 26.115).

EBM	26.115 Intravenous immunoglobulin (IVIg) and plasma exchange (PE) in Guillain–Barré syndrome

'If used within the first 2 weeks of developing the illness, IVIg and PE are equally effective in reducing the severity and duration of Guillain–Barré syndrome, but there is no advantage in combining the two treatments.'

- Plasma Exchange/Sandoglobulin Guillain–Barré Syndrome Trial Group. Lancet 1997; 349:225–230.
- Bril V. Neurology 1996; 46:100–103.

For further information: www.cochrane.org

Acute axonal polyneuropathy

There is an axonal variant of Guillain–Barré syndrome, rare in Europe and North America but more common in China and Japan. Circulating antibodies to various peripheral nerve gangliosides are often found. Other causes of acute axonal neuropathy, all rare, include drug or toxin exposure (see Box 26.110).

Chronic polyneuropathy

A chronic symmetrical polyneuropathy, evolving over months or years, is the most frequently seen form of neuropathy. In about 30% of patients no cause can be established, even after thorough investigation. These patients usually have a mild axonal neuropathy which, whilst causing unpleasant symptoms, does not lead to motor disability. Therefore, if a patient with what seems to be an idiopathic polyneuropathy progresses to significant disability, further thought needs to be given to finding a specific cause (usually inflammatory or genetic).

Chronic demyelinating polyneuropathy

This type of chronic polyneuropathy is either hereditary or immune-mediated (including those caused by abnormal paraproteins). Many inherited disorders

26

cause demyelinating peripheral neuropathies and one of the best known is Charcot–Marie–Tooth disease (CMT). Here the neuropathy produces distal wasting ('inverted champagne bottle' or 'stork' legs), often with pes cavus, and a predominantly motor clinical involvement. In 70–80% the cause is duplication of the *PMP-22* gene on chromosome 17 (autosomal dominant CMT type 1), but similar phenotypes are produced by mutations in other genes with differing modes of inheritance (Box 26.116).

Chronic inflammatory demyelinating peripheral neuropathy (CIDP) presents with a relapsing or progressive generalised neuropathy. Sensory, motor or autonomic nerves can be involved but the signs are predominantly motor; a variant causes only motor involvement (multifocal motor neuropathy, MMN). CIDP usually responds to immunosuppressive treatment, corticosteroids, methotrexate or cyclophosphamide, or to immunomodulatory treatments (plasma exchange or intravenous immunoglobulin, IVIg); MMN is best treated by IVIg.

Some 10% of patients with acquired demyelinating polyneuropathy have an abnormal serum paraprotein, sometimes associated with a lymphoproliferative malignancy.

Chronic axonal polyneuropathy

This is the most common type of chronic polyneuropathy. Where the cause can be found, it is usually a disorder affecting axonal metabolism and transport, either acquired (drugs and toxins) or genetically determined (see Box 26.109, p. 1226 and Box 26.116).

Brachial plexopathy

Trauma usually damages either the upper or the lower parts of the brachial plexus, according to the mechanics of the injury. The clinical features depend upon the anatomical site of the damage (Box 26.117). Lower parts of the brachial plexus are vulnerable to infiltration from breast or apical lung tumours (Pancoast tumour) and may be damaged by therapeutic irradiation. The lower parts of the plexus may also be compressed by anatomical anomalies at the thoracic outlet, which may be accompanied by circulatory changes in the arm due to subclavian artery compression.

An acute brachial plexopathy of probable inflammatory origin may present with 'neuralgic amyotrophy'. In

26.117 Physical signs in brachial plexus lesions

Site	Root	Affected muscles	Sensory loss
Upper plexus (Erb–Duchenne)	C5/6	Biceps, deltoid, spinati, rhomboids, brachioradialis (triceps, serratus anterior)	Patch over deltoid
Lower plexus (Déjerine–Klumpke)	C8/T1	All small hand muscles, claw hand (ulnar wrist flexors)	Ulnar border hand/forearm
Thoracic outlet syndrome	C8/T1	Small hand muscles, ulnar forearm	Ulnar border hand/forearm/ upper arm

26.116 Hereditary peripheral neuropathies

Type	Inheritance	Molecular pathology	Neurophysiology	Comments
CMT1A	Autosomal dominant	PMP-22 reduplication Chr 17p	Slowed MCV	Common
CMT1B	Autosomal dominant	PO mutation Chr 1q	Marked slowing of MCV	Common
CMTX	X-linked	Connexin-32 mutation Chr Xq	Near-normal conduction velocities	Common, females less affected
CMT2	Autosomal dominant	Not known	Axonal—normal MCV	Rare
CMT3	Dominant (usually new mutation)	PMP-22 mutation or deletion	Severely slowed MCV	Déjerine—Sottas disease, rare
CMT4	Autosomal recessive	Not known	Axonal—normal MCV	Very rare
HNPP	Autosomal dominant	PMP-22 deletion or mutation	Dysmyelination—slowed MCV	Uncommon
HSAN	Autosomal dominant (type 1) and recessive (types 2–5)	Not known	Axonal—normal MVC	Uncommon—lancinating pains, neuropathic feet, recurrent foot ulceration
Refsum's disease	Autosomal recessive	Peroxisome targeting signal 2 mutation Chr 10p	Marked slowing	Very rare, associated retinitis pigmentosa, ataxia and raised blood phytanic acid
Hereditary amyloid neuropathy	Autosomal dominant	Transthyretin mutation (in types 1 and 2) Chr 18q Other mutations (types 3 and 4)	Axonal—normal MCV	Uncommon, associated autonomic neuropathy

(Chr = chromosome; CMT = Charcot–Marie–Tooth; HNPP = hereditary neuropathy with predisposition to pressure palsies; HSAN = hereditary sensory and autonomic neuropathy; MCV = motor conduction velocity; PMP = peripheral myelin protein)

this syndrome, a period of very severe shoulder pain precedes the appearance of a patchy upper brachial plexus lesion, often affecting the long thoracic nerve which produces winging of the scapula. Recovery occurs over months and is usually complete.

Lumbosacral plexopathy

Lumbosacral plexus lesions may be caused by neoplastic infiltration or compression by retroperitoneal haematomas in patients with a coagulopathy. A small vessel vasculopathy can produce a lumbar plexopathy, especially in elderly patients when it may be the presenting feature of type 2 diabetes mellitus ('diabetic amyotrophy') or a vasculitis. This presents with painful wasting of the quadriceps with weakness of knee extension and adduction, and an absent knee reflex.

Spinal root lesions

Spinal root lesions (radiculopathy) are commonly caused by compression at or near their spinal exit foramina by prolapsed intervertebral discs or degenerative spinal disease (p. 1222). Spinal roots may also be infiltrated by spinal and paraspinal tumour masses and inflammatory or infective processes. The clinical features include muscle weakness and wasting and dermatomal sensory loss with reflex changes that reflect the pattern of roots involved. Pain in the muscles whose innervating motor roots are involved is usually a prominent feature.

DISEASES OF THE NEUROMUSCULAR JUNCTION

Myasthenia gravis

This condition is characterised by progressive fatigable weakness, particularly of the ocular, neck, facial and bulbar muscles.

Pathophysiology

The disease is most commonly caused by autoantibodies to acetylcholine receptors in the post-junctional membrane of the neuromuscular junction. These antibodies block neuromuscular transmission and initiate a complement-mediated inflammatory response which reduces the number of acetylcholine receptors and damages the end plate (Fig. 26.57). A minority of patients have other autoantibodies to epitopes on the post-junctional membrane, in particular autoantibodies to a muscle-specific kinase (MuSK), an agrin receptor which is involved in the regulation and maintenance of the acetylcholine receptors.

About 15% of patients (mainly those with late onset) have a thymoma, and the majority of the remainder have thymic follicular hyperplasia. There is an increased incidence of other autoimmune diseases, and the disease is

26

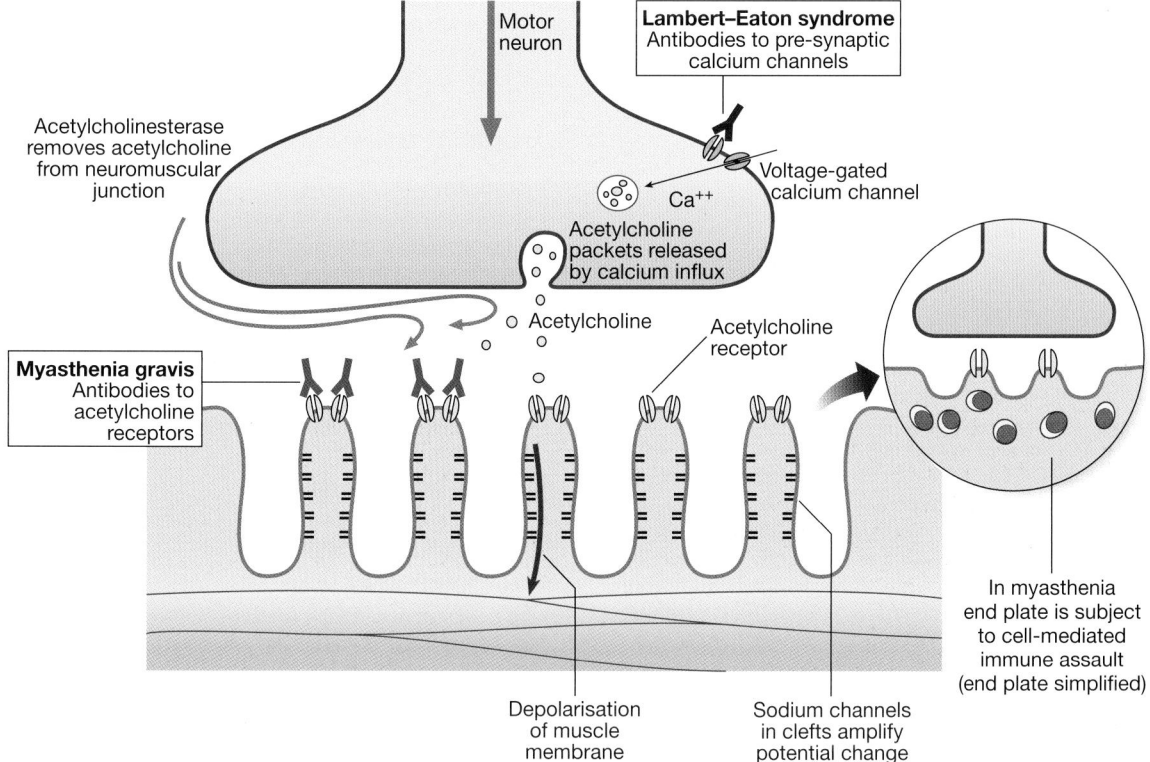

Fig. 26.57 **Myasthenia gravis and Lambert–Eaton myasthenic syndrome (LEMS).** In myasthenia there are antibodies to the acetylcholine receptors on the post-synaptic membrane which block conduction across the neuromuscular junction (NMJ). Myasthenic symptoms can be transiently improved by inhibition of acetylcholinesterase (e.g. with Tensilon—edrophonium bromide) which normally removes the acetylcholine. A cell-mediated immune response produces simplification of the post-synaptic membrane, further impairing the 'safety factor' of neuromuscular conduction. In LEMS, antibodies to the pre-synaptic voltage calcium channels impair release of acetylcholine from the motor nerve ending; calcium is required for the acetylcholine-containing vesicle to fuse with the pre-synaptic membrane for release into the NMJ.

linked with certain HLA haplotypes. Nothing is known about factors which trigger the disease itself, but penicillamine can cause an antibody-mediated myasthenic syndrome which may persist even after drug withdrawal. Some drugs, especially aminoglycosides and ciprofloxacin, may exacerbate the neuromuscular blockade and should be avoided in patients with myasthenia.

Clinical features

The disease usually presents between the ages of 15 and 50 years. Women are affected more often than men in the younger age groups while the reverse applies to older age groups. It tends to run a relapsing and remitting course, especially during the early years.

The cardinal symptom is fatigable weakness of the muscles (which is different from a sensation of muscle fatigue); movement is initially strong but rapidly weakens as muscle use continues. Worsening of symptoms towards the end of the day or following exercise is characteristic. There are no sensory signs or signs of involvement of the CNS, although weakness of the oculomotor muscles may mimic a central eye movement disorder.

The first symptoms are usually intermittent ptosis or diplopia, but weakness of chewing, swallowing, speaking or limb movement also occurs. Any limb muscle may be affected, most commonly those of the shoulder girdle; the patient is unable to undertake tasks above shoulder level such as combing the hair without frequent rests. Respiratory muscles may be involved, and respiratory failure is a not uncommon cause of death. Aspiration may occur if the cough is ineffectual. Sudden weakness from a cholinergic or myasthenic crisis (see below) may require ventilatory support. The prognosis is variable and sometimes remissions occur spontaneously. When myasthenia is confined to the eye muscles, the prognosis is excellent and disability slight. Young female patients with generalised disease have high remission rates after thymectomy, whilst older patients are less likely to have a remission despite treatment. Rapid progression of the disease more than 5 years after its onset is uncommon.

Investigations

The intravenous injection of the short-acting anticholinesterase, edrophonium bromide, is a valuable diagnostic aid (the Tensilon test); 2 mg is injected initially, with a further 8 mg given half a minute later if there are no undesirable side-effects. Improvement in muscle power occurs within 30 seconds and usually persists for 2–3 minutes. EMG with repetitive stimulation may show the characteristic decremental response (p. 1142). Anti-acetylcholine receptor antibody (AChRA) is found in over 80% of cases, though less frequently in purely ocular myasthenia (50%). Anti-MuSK antibodies are found especially in AChRA-negative patients with prominent bulbar involvement. Positive anti-skeletal muscle antibodies suggest the presence of thymoma, but all patients should have a thoracic CT to exclude this condition which may not be visible on plain X-ray examination. Screening for associated autoimmune disorders, particularly thyroid disease, is important.

Management

The principles of treatment are:

- to maximise the activity of acetylcholine at remaining receptors in the neuromuscular junctions

- to limit or abolish the immunological attack on motor end plates.

The duration of action of acetylcholine is greatly prolonged by inhibiting its hydrolysing enzyme, acetylcholinesterase. The most commonly used anticholinesterase drug is pyridostigmine, which is given orally in a dosage of 30–120 mg, usually 6-hourly. Muscarinic side-effects, including diarrhoea and colic, may be controlled by propantheline (15 mg as required). Over-dosage of anticholinesterase drugs may cause a cholinergic crisis due to depolarisation block of motor end plates, with muscle fasciculation, paralysis, pallor, sweating, excessive salivation and small pupils. This may be distinguished from severe weakness due to exacerbation of myasthenia (myasthenic crisis) by the clinical features and, if necessary, by the injection of a small dose of edrophonium.

The immunological treatment of myasthenia is outlined in Box 26.118. Thymectomy in the early stages of the disease improves overall prognosis.

Other myasthenic syndromes

There are other conditions which present with muscle weakness due to impaired transmission across the neuromuscular junction. The most common of these is the Lambert–Eaton myasthenic syndrome (LEMS), in which transmitter release is impaired, often in association with antibodies to prejunctional voltage-gated calcium channels (see Fig. 26.57). Patients may have autonomic dysfunction (and a dry mouth) in addition to muscle weakness, but the cardinal clinical sign is absence of tendon reflexes, which can return immediately after sustained contraction of the relevant muscle.

 26.118 Immunological treatment of myasthenia

Thymectomy

- Should be considered in any antibody-positive patient under 45 years with symptoms not confined to extraocular muscles, unless the disease has been established for more than 7 years

Plasma exchange

- Removing antibody from the blood may produce marked improvement but, as this is usually brief, such therapy is normally reserved for myasthenic crisis or for pre-operative preparation

Intravenous immunoglobulin

- An alternative to plasma exchange in the short-term treatment of severe myasthenia

Corticosteroid treatment

- Improvement is commonly preceded by marked exacerbation of myasthenic symptoms and treatment should be initiated in hospital
- It is usually necessary to continue treatment for months or years, often resulting in adverse effects

Other immunosuppressant treatment

- Treatment with azathioprine 2.5 mg/kg daily is of value in reducing the dosage of steroids necessary and may allow steroids to be withdrawn (Box 26.119)
- The effect of treatment on clinical disease is often delayed for several months

EBM 26.119 **Azathioprine in myasthenia gravis**

'Azathioprine as an adjunct to alternate-day prednisolone in the treatment of antibody-positive generalised myasthenia reduces the maintenance dose of prednisolone and is associated with fewer treatment failures, longer remissions and fewer side-effects. However, a small trial suggested that it is probably not useful as an initial immunosuppressive treatment on its own.'

• Palace J, et al. Neurology 1998; 50:1778–1783.
• Bromberg MB, et al. J Neurol Sci 1997; 150:59–62.

The condition is associated with underlying malignancy in a high percentage of cases, and investigation must be directed towards detecting such a cause. The condition is diagnosed electrophysiologically by the presence of post-tetanic potentiation of motor response to nerve stimulation at a frequency of 20–50/s. Treatment is with 3,4-diaminopyridine.

DISEASES OF MUSCLE

Voluntary muscle is subject to a range of hereditary and acquired disorders of either its structure or the biochemical processes whereby the chemical energy derived from cell metabolism is converted into mechanical energy. These disorders present in a limited number of ways, most commonly a symmetrical weakness of the large, power-generating proximal muscles (proximal myopathy). This weakness may be fixed or periodic. Other symptoms and signs of muscle disease include myotonia (failure of muscle relaxation) and muscle pain. Diagnosis depends upon consideration of the clinical picture along with the results of EMG studies and muscle biopsy. In some inherited muscular diseases, specific genetic abnormalities can be identified.

Muscular dystrophies

This is a group of inherited disorders characterised by progressive degeneration of groups of muscles, sometimes with involvement of the heart muscle or conducting tissue, and other parts of the nervous system (Box 26.120).

Clinical features

Onset is often in childhood, although some patients, especially those with myotonic dystrophy, may present as adults. Wasting and weakness are usually symmetrical, there is no fasciculation and no sensory loss, and tendon reflexes are preserved until a late stage, except in myotonic dystrophy where there is an associated neuropathy. Differential diagnosis is based on the age at onset, the distribution of affected muscles and the pattern of inheritance. Myotonic dystrophy may be diagnosed clinically by the distribution of muscle weakness and other features, including myotonia (see Box 26.120). Many dystrophies include cardiomyopathy (p. 635) amongst their clinical features. Patients with Duchenne

26

26.120 The muscular dystrophies

Type	Genetics	Age of onset	Muscles affected	Other features
Myotonic dystrophy (DM1)	Autosomal dominant; expanded triplet repeat chromosome 19q	Any	Face (incl. ptosis), sternomastoids, distal limb, generalised later	Myotonia, cognitive dulling, cardiac conduction abnormalities, lens opacities, frontal balding, hypogonadism
Proximal myotonic myopathy (PROMM; DM2)	Autosomal dominant; quadruplet repeat expansion in *Zn finger protein 9* gene chromosome 3q	Adult	Proximal, especially thigh, sometimes muscle hypertrophy	As for DM1 but cognition not affected Muscle pain
Duchenne	X-linked; deletions in *dystrophin* gene	First 5 years	Proximal and limb girdle	Pseudohypertrophy of calves Cardiomyopathy
Becker	X-linked; deletions in *dystrophin* gene	Late childhood/ early adult	Proximal and limb girdle	Pseudohypertrophy of calves Cardiomyopathy
Limb girdle	Autosomal dominant (type 1) Autosomal recessive (type 2) Many mutations on different chromosomes	Childhood/early adult	Limb girdle	Some have calf hypertrophy Some have cardiac conduction abnormalities
Facioscapulohumeral (FSH)	Autosomal dominant; tandem repeat deletion chromosome 4q	7–30 years	Face and upper limb girdle Distal lower limb weakness	Pain in shoulder girdle common
Oculopharyngeal	Autosomal dominant and recessive; triplet repeat expansion in *PABP2* gene chromosome 14q	30–50 years	Ptosis, external ophthalmoplegia, dysphagia, tongue weakness	Mild lower limb weakness
Emery–Dreifuss	X-linked recessive; mutations in *emerin* gene	4–5 years	Humero-peroneal, proximal limb girdle later	Contractures develop early Cardiac involvement leads to sudden death

dystrophy used to die within 10 years of diagnosis, but with improved general care they are now living into the third decade. The lifespan in limb girdle and facioscapulo-humeral dystrophies is normal. In myotonic dystrophy, there is considerable phenotypic variation and the prognosis is very variable, limited by cardiac and respiratory complications.

Investigations

The diagnosis can be confirmed by specific molecular genetic testing, supplemented with EMG and muscle biopsy if necessary. Creatine kinase is markedly elevated in Duchenne muscular dystrophy, but is normal or only moderately elevated in the other dystrophies. Screening for an associated cardiac abnormality (cardiomyopathy or dysrhythmia) is important.

Management

There is no specific therapy for these conditions, but physiotherapy and occupational therapy help patients cope with their disability. Treatment of associated cardiac failure or arrhythmia (with pacemaker insertion if necessary) may be required; similarly, management of respiratory complications (including nocturnal hypoventilation) can improve quality of life. Genetic counselling is important.

Congenital myopathy

This is rare and presents in infancy with muscular weakness and limpness. Serum muscle enzymes may be normal or slightly elevated and the EMG is usually myopathic. The syndrome may be caused by a number of specific conditions that have a variable inheritance and are defined by the type of structural abnormality present in skeletal muscle fibres. Most patients have a slowly progressive disease and there is no specific therapy.

Inherited metabolic myopathies

A large number of individually rare inherited disorders of the biochemical pathways necessary to maintain the supply of chemical energy (ATP) in muscles may present with muscle pain, weakness and fatigue. These are mostly recessively inherited deficiencies in the enzymes of the glycolytic and fatty acid metabolism pathways (Box 26.121).

Inherited disorders of the oxidative pathways of the respiratory chain in mitochondria cause a group of mitochondrial myopathies which may be associated with a range of other deficits in the nervous system, including episodic stroke-like events and myoclonic epilepsy (Box 26.122). Many of these mitochondrial myopathies (or cytopathies) are inherited via the mitochondrial

---

26.121 Inherited disorders of muscle metabolism

	Enzyme deficiency	Clinical features	Diagnosis
Carbohydrate metabolism	Myophosphorylase (McArdle's disease) Phosphofructokinase	Exercise-induced muscle cramps, myoglobinuria	CK elevated Muscle biopsy appearance Molecular genetics
	Alpha-1,4-glucosidase (acid maltase)	Proximal limb and diaphragm weakness	CK elevated Myopathic EMG Lymphocyte glycogen storage Muscle biopsy appearance Molecular genetics
Lipid metabolism	Carnitine-palmitoyl transferase (CPT) deficiency	Muscle pain on prolonged exercise, myoglobinuria	CK elevated during attacks of muscle pain, normal in between Muscle biopsy appearance

---

26.122 Mitochondrial myopathy syndromes

Syndrome	Clinical features
Myoclonic epilepsy with ragged red fibres (MERRF)	Myoclonic epilepsy, cerebellar ataxia, dementia, sensorineural deafness ± peripheral neuropathy and optic atrophy
Mitochondrial myopathy, encephalopathy, lactic acidosis and stroke-like episodes (MELAS)	Episodic encephalopathy, stroke-like episodes often preceded by migraine-like headache, nausea and vomiting
Chronic progressive external ophthalmoplegia (CPEO)	Progressive ptosis and external oculomotor palsy, proximal myopathy ± deafness, ataxia and cardiac conduction defects
Kearns–Sayre syndrome	Like CPEO but early age of onset (< 20 yrs), heart block, pigmentary retinopathy
Mitochondrial neurogastrointestinal encephalomyopathy (MNGIE)	Progressive ptosis, external oculomotor palsy, gastrointestinal dysmotility (often pseudo-obstruction), diffuse leukoencephalopathy, thin body habitus, peripheral neuropathy and myopathy

26.123 Muscle channelopathies

Channel	Muscle disease	Clinical features
Sodium	Paramyotonia congenita	Cold-evoked myotonia with episodic weakness provoked by exercise and cold
	Hyperkalaemic periodic paralysis	Brief, frequent episodes of weakness triggered by potassium ingestion
	Hypokalaemic periodic paralysis	Episodic weakness triggered by carbohydrate meal
Chloride	Myotonia congenita (Thomsen's disease)	Generalised myotonia with muscle hypertrophy
Calcium	Hypokalaemic periodic paralysis	Episodic weakness triggered by carbohydrate meal
	Malignant hyperthermia	Hyperpyrexia due to excess muscle activity, precipitated by drugs, usually anaesthetic agents

genome, down the maternal line (p. 50). There is often a characteristic 'ragged-red fibre' change on muscle biopsy.

Channelopathies

Inherited abnormalities of the sodium, calcium and chloride ion channels in striated muscle produce various syndromes of familial periodic paralysis, myotonia and malignant hyperthermia which can be recognised by their clinical characteristics, provocation by exercise or eating, and associated changes in serum potassium concentration (Box 26.123).

Acquired myopathies

Muscle weakness may be caused by a range of metabolic, endocrine, toxic or inflammatory disorders (Box 26.124). Disorders affecting the muscles' structural integrity can be distinguished by EMG from those caused by metabolic derangement. In metabolic disorders, weakness is often acute and generalised, while a proximal myopathy predominantly affecting the pelvic girdle is a feature of some endocrine disorders. This may develop without other manifestations of hormonal disturbance. A wide variety of drugs and toxins may cause myopathy and these are also listed in Box 26.124. Inflammatory myopathy (polymyositis) is described on page 1111.

Further information

Books and journal articles

Aminoff MJ, ed. Neurology and general medicine. 4th edn. Philadelphia: Churchill Livingstone; 2008.

Bradley WG, Daroff RB, Fenichel GM, Jankovic J, eds. Neurology in clinical practice. Principles of diagnosis and management. 4th edn. Philadelphia: Butterworth–Heinemann; 2004.

Mohr JP, Choi DW, Grotta JC, et al. Stroke. Pathophysiology, diagnosis, and management. 4th edn. Philadelphia: Churchill Livingstone; 2004.

Ropper AH, Samuels MA. Adams and Victor's principles of neurology. 9th edn. New York: McGraw–Hill; 2009.

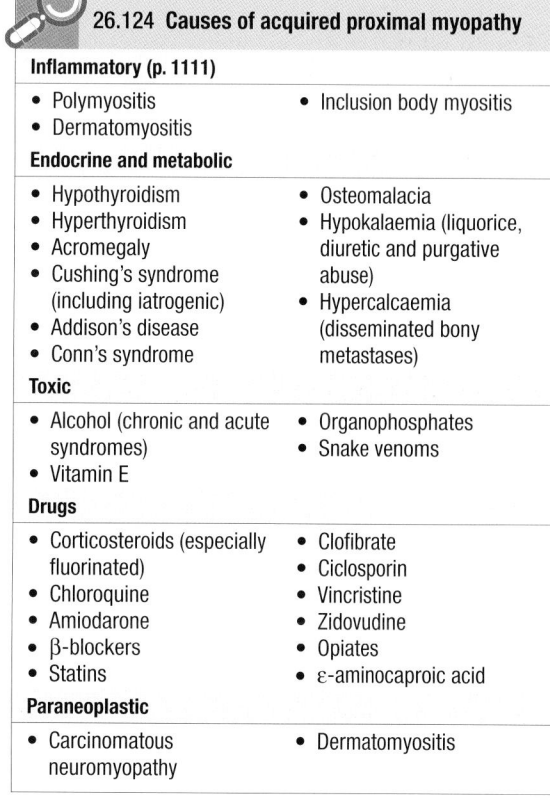

26.124 Causes of acquired proximal myopathy

Inflammatory (p. 1111)
- Polymyositis
- Dermatomyositis
- Inclusion body myositis

Endocrine and metabolic
- Hypothyroidism
- Hyperthyroidism
- Acromegaly
- Cushing's syndrome (including iatrogenic)
- Addison's disease
- Conn's syndrome
- Osteomalacia
- Hypokalaemia (liquorice, diuretic and purgative abuse)
- Hypercalcaemia (disseminated bony metastases)

Toxic
- Alcohol (chronic and acute syndromes)
- Vitamin E
- Organophosphates
- Snake venoms

Drugs
- Corticosteroids (especially fluorinated)
- Chloroquine
- Amiodarone
- β-blockers
- Statins
- Clofibrate
- Ciclosporin
- Vincristine
- Zidovudine
- Opiates
- ε-aminocaproic acid

Paraneoplastic
- Carcinomatous neuromyopathy
- Dermatomyositis

Websites

www.dizziness-and-balance.com/disorders/bppv/bppv.html and www.dizziness-and-balance.com/treatment/cawthorne.html *Diagnosing benign paroxysmal positional vertigo.*

www.ninds.nih.gov *National Institute of Neurological Disorders and Stroke.*

www.toddtroost.com/mylinks2001.html *Neuroscience links from ANA.*

www.wfneurology.org *World Federation of Neurology.*

26

O.M.V. Schofield
J.L. Rees

Skin disease

27

CLINICAL EXAMINATION IN SKIN DISEASE

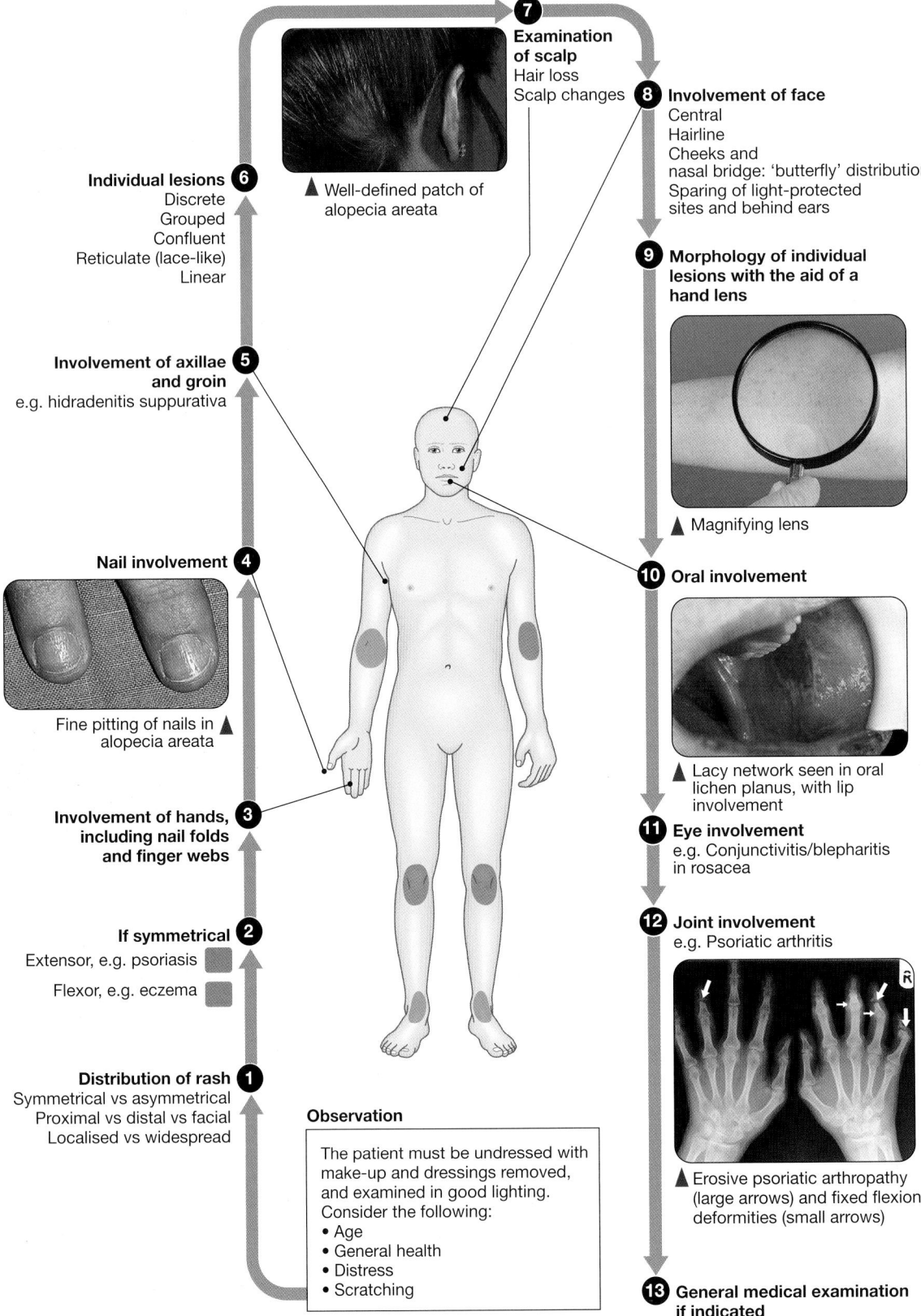

7 Examination of scalp
Hair loss
Scalp changes

▲ Well-defined patch of alopecia areata

6 Individual lesions
Discrete
Grouped
Confluent
Reticulate (lace-like)
Linear

8 Involvement of face
Central
Hairline
Cheeks and
nasal bridge: 'butterfly' distribution
Sparing of light-protected
sites and behind ears

9 Morphology of individual lesions with the aid of a hand lens

▲ Magnifying lens

5 Involvement of axillae and groin
e.g. hidradenitis suppurativa

4 Nail involvement

Fine pitting of nails in ▲ alopecia areata

10 Oral involvement

▲ Lacy network seen in oral lichen planus, with lip involvement

3 Involvement of hands, including nail folds and finger webs

11 Eye involvement
e.g. Conjunctivitis/blepharitis in rosacea

2 If symmetrical
Extensor, e.g. psoriasis
Flexor, e.g. eczema

12 Joint involvement
e.g. Psoriatic arthritis

1 Distribution of rash
Symmetrical vs asymmetrical
Proximal vs distal vs facial
Localised vs widespread

Observation

The patient must be undressed with make-up and dressings removed, and examined in good lighting. Consider the following:
• Age
• General health
• Distress
• Scratching

▲ Erosive psoriatic arthropathy (large arrows) and fixed flexion deformities (small arrows)

13 General medical examination if indicated

Terms used to describe skin lesions

Primary lesions

- **Abscess:** a localised collection of pus in a cavity, > 1 cm in diameter
- **Burrow:** a linear or curvilinear papule, caused by a burrowing scabies mite (panel A and Fig. 27.32, p. 1274)
- **Comedone:** a plug of keratin and sebum wedged in a dilated pilosebaceous orifice (panel B)
- **Macule:** a circumscribed flat area of altered colour, e.g. freckle (panel C)
- **Papilloma:** a projecting nipple-like mass, e.g. skin tag (panel D)
- **Papule:** a discrete elevation of skin that may be changed in colour (panel E). Those arising from the subcutis may be felt rather than seen. Larger lesions (> 1 cm) are referred to as nodules
- **Petechiae, purpura and ecchymosis:** petechiae are pinhead-sized flat macules of extravascular blood in the dermis. Purpura are larger and may be palpable. Ecchymosis ('bruise') is where bleeding involves deeper structures (see panel F)
- **Plaque:** a raised area of skin with a flat top, several cm in diameter, e.g. psoriasis (panel G)
- **Pustule:** a visible accumulation of pus in a blister (panel H)
- **Scale:** a flake arising from the stratum corneum, e.g. psoriasis (panel I)
- **Telangiectasia:** visible dilatation of small cutaneous blood vessels (panel J)
- **Vesicle and bulla:** a small (~ several mm) and a larger (~ several cm) fluid-filled blister respectively, e.g. pemphigoid (panel K)
- **Weal:** an evanescent discrete area of dermal oedema, usually white due to masking of local blood supply by fluid, e.g. a nettle sting (panel L)

Secondary lesions

- **Atrophy:** an area of thin, translucent skin due to loss of epidermis, dermis or subcutaneous fat, e.g. excess topical corticosteroids
- **Crust:** dried exudate of blood or serous fluid, e.g. eczema (see Fig. 27.23, p. 1269)
- **Excoriation:** a linear ulcer or erosion resulting from scratching (see Fig. 27.11, p. 1258)
- **Erosion:** an area of skin denuded by complete or partial loss of the epidermis
- **Fissure:** a slit-shaped deep ulcer, e.g. irritant dermatitis of the hands
- **Scar:** replacement of normal structures by fibrous tissue at the site of an injury
- **Sinus:** a cavity or channel that permits the escape of pus or fluid
- **Stria:** a linear, atrophic, pink, purple or white band due to connective tissue changes, e.g. Cushing's syndrome (see Fig. 20.21, p. 771)
- **Ulcer:** an area from which the epidermis and at least the upper part of the dermis have been lost (see Fig. 27.9, p. 1252)

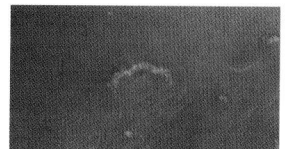

A. Burrow.

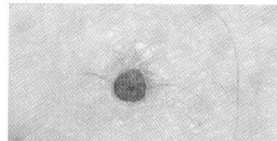

B. Comedone.

C. Macule.

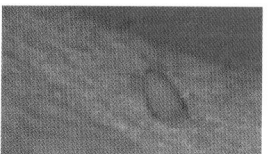

D. Papilloma.

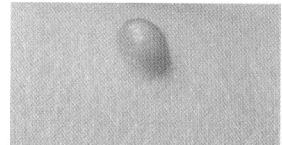

E. Papule.

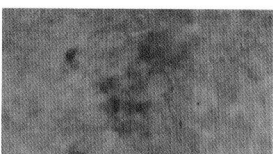

F. Petechiae and purpura.

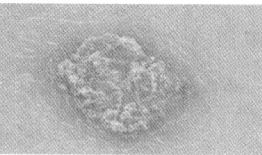

G. Plaque.

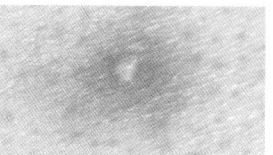

H. Pustule.

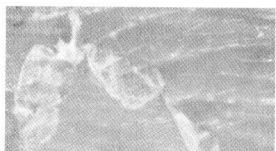

I. Scale.

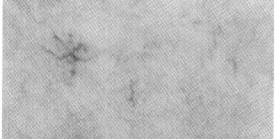

J. Telangiectasia.

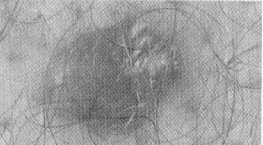

K. Vesicle.

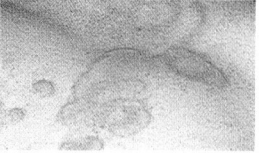

L. Weal.

Skin disease is common. European surveys suggest that approximately 1 in 7–10 consultations in primary care are for a skin problem. Skin disease appears to be becoming more common for three reasons:

- a lowered threshold for seeking medical attention
- an increase in the absolute incidence of diseases such as skin cancer and atopic dermatitis
- the availability of new and effective treatments for several skin diseases that were formerly untreatable.

Healthy and attractive skin plays a major role in most individuals' self-esteem, and is a key component of the image they present to the outside world. The appearance, texture and tactile qualities of skin play a significant role in most grooming and sexual behaviours. Patients with skin disease are often stigmatised, sometimes due to the spurious belief that their appearance is the result of a contagious disease. Population prevalence studies reveal an enormous burden of undiagnosed, untreated skin disease.

Skin complaints affect all ages, from the neonate to the elderly, and the general dermatologist sees an even distribution of patients of all ages (Fig. 27.1). This chapter concentrates on the skin conditions that are seen frequently in general practice and general medicine. Skin infections, including those related to the human immunodeficiency virus (HIV), are discussed in Chapters 13 and 14, and connective tissue diseases involving the skin in Chapter 25.

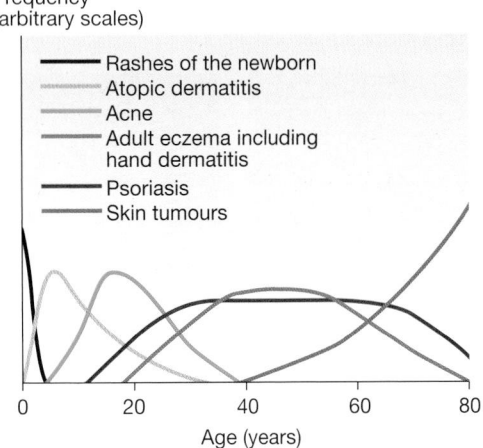

Fig. 27.1 The age distribution of some common skin conditions. Frequencies of the various rashes are not drawn to scale and are illustrative only.

FUNCTIONAL ANATOMY AND PHYSIOLOGY

The skin of an average adult covers an area of just under 2 m². The epidermis, a stratified squamous epithelium, is the outermost layer and is predominantly composed of keratinocytes. The epidermis is attached to but separated from the underlying dermis by the basement membrane. The dermis supports blood vessels and nerves, and the epidermal-derived structures such as

the appendageal structures (hair follicles, and eccrine and apocrine sweat glands). The predominant cell of the dermis is the fibroblast. Below the dermis is a layer of adipose tissue (the subcutis).

Epidermis

Keratinocytes make up approximately 90% of epidermal cells (Fig. 27.2). The proliferative compartment of the epidermis resides in the basal layer and in the layer immediately adjacent to it. The site of the keratinocyte stem cell is not known, but in hair-bearing skin is likely to be in a specialised region of the hair follicle, close to the insertion of the sebaceous gland.

Keratinocytes synthesise a range of structural proteins, such as keratins, loricrin and filaggrin (**fil**ament **agg**regating prote**in**), that play key roles in maintaining normal cutaneous physiology. There are well over 30 different types of keratin and their expression varies by site on the body, by site within the epidermis, and depending on whether the skin is healthy or diseased. Mutations of certain keratin genes result in blistering disorders such as epidermolysis bullosa simplex (p. 1249) and ichthyotic conditions (characterised by scale without dominant inflammation). As keratinocytes move out of the basal layer they differentiate, producing a variety of protein and lipid products. Keratinocytes undergo apoptosis in the granular layer before becoming the flattened anucleate cells that make up the stratum corneum. The epidermis is a site of lipid production, and the ability of the stratum corneum to act as a hydrophobic barrier is the result of its 'bricks and mortar' design; dead corneocytes with a highly cross-linked protein membrane ('bricks') lie within a metabolically active layer of lipid synthesised by the keratinocytes ('mortar'). Terminal differentiation of keratinocytes relies on the keratin filaments being aggregated. This function is in part mediated by filaggrin. It has recently been shown that mutations of the filaggrin gene are common in patients with atopic dermatitis (p. 1257) or icthyosis vulgaris.

Skin must have considerable physical resilience. Attachments between cells must be able to transmit and dissipate stress, a function performed by desmosomes. Diseases that affect desmosomes, such as pemphigus (p. 1276), result in blistering as the individual keratinocytes separate.

Three other cell types make up most of the remaining 10% of epidermal cells:

- *Langerhans cells* are dendritic, bone marrow-derived cells that circulate between the epidermis and the local lymph nodes. Their prime function is the effective presentation of foreign antigens to lymphocytes. They may also play a part in presentation of tumour antigens. Other antigen-presenting dendritic cells are also present, but in the dermis rather than the epidermis.
- *Melanocytes* are of neural crest origin and are found predominantly in the basal layer. They synthesise the pigment melanin from tyrosine, package it in melanosomes and transfer it to surrounding keratinocytes via their dendritic processes.
- *Merkel cells* are found in the basal layer and are thought to play a role in signal transduction of fine touch. Their embryological derivation is unclear.

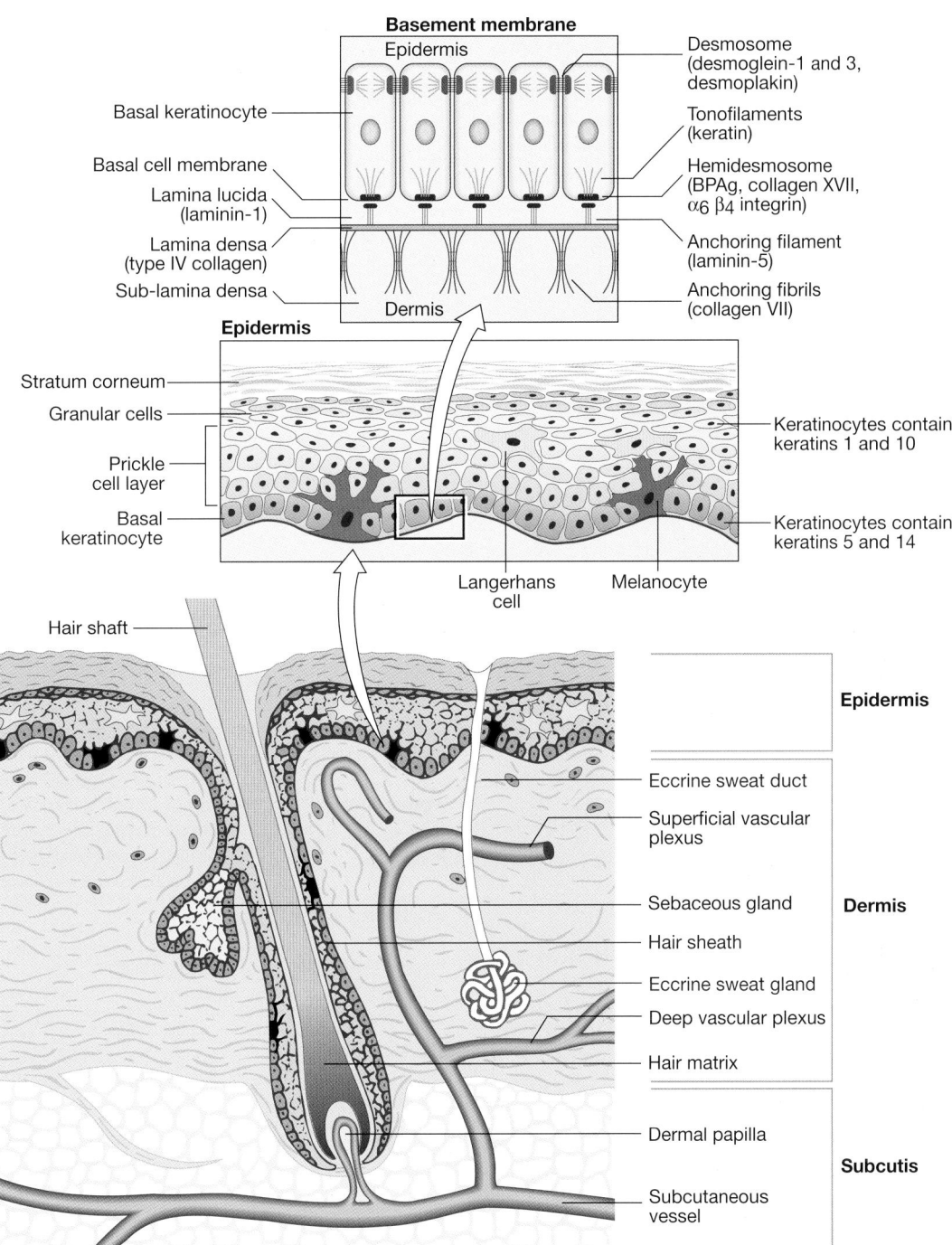

Fig. 27.2 Structure of normal skin.

Basement membrane

The basement membrane (see Fig. 27.2) acts as an anchor for the epidermis but allows movement of cells and nutrients between the dermis and epidermis. It consists of several well-defined layers. The cell membrane of the epidermal basal cell is attached to the basement membrane via hemidesmosomes. The lamina lucida is the zone immediately subjacent to the cell membrane of the basal cell, and is composed predominantly of laminin. Anchoring filaments extend through the lamina lucida to attach to the lamina densa. This electron-dense layer consists predominantly of type IV collagen; from it extend loops of type VII collagen, forming anchoring fibrils that fasten the basement membrane to the dermis.

Dermis

The dermis is vascular and supports the epidermis structurally and nutritionally. It varies in thickness from just over 1 mm on the inner forearm to 4 mm on the back. The epidermis on most sites is only 0.1–0.2 mm thick, except on the palms or soles where it can be several millimetres in thickness. The acellular part of the dermis consists

27

predominantly of fibres, including collagens I and III, elastin and reticulin, synthesised by the major cell type, fibroblasts. Support is provided by an amorphous ground substance (mostly glycosaminoglycans, hyaluronic acid and dermatan sulphate), whose production and catabolism may be influenced by hormonal changes and damage from ultraviolet (UV) radiation. Apart from fibroblasts, other cell types within the dermis include mast cells, mononuclear phagocytes, T lymphocytes, dendritic cells, nerves and vessels. Based on the pattern of collagen fibrils, the superficial part of the dermis is known as the 'papillary dermis', and the deeper and coarser part as the 'reticular dermis'.

Epidermal appendages: hair and sweat glands

Hair follicles, sweat (eccrine) and apocrine glands are epidermal structures which invaginate into the dermis. They are formed during the second trimester and number 3–5 million.

Hair follicles are found throughout the skin, with the exception of palms, soles and portions of the genitalia (glabrous skin). The highest density of hair follicles is on the scalp, which has between 500 and 1000/cm². Newborns are covered with fine 'lanugo' hairs, which are usually non-pigmented and do not have a central medulla (a central cavity). Subsequently, lanugo hair is replaced by vellus hair, which is similar but more likely to contain some pigment. By contrast, scalp hair becomes terminal hair, which is thicker with a central medulla, is usually pigmented and grows longer. At puberty, vellus hair in hormonally sensitive regions such as the axilla and the genital area becomes terminal.

Hairs in humans do not grow continuously but in a cycle with three phases:

- anagen, in which the hair grows
- catagen, a transitional phase
- telogen, a resting stage.

The individual duration of the components of the cell cycle varies by site. On the scalp, anagen will last several years, whereas catagen lasts only a few days and telogen around 3 months. The length of hair at different sites is partly a reflection of the differing lengths of anagen.

Sebaceous glands

Sebaceous glands are epidermal downgrowths, usually associated with hair follicles and comprised of modified keratinocytes. The individual cells of the sebaceous gland (sebocytes) produce a range of lipids before the cell dies, discharging its contents into the duct around the hair follicle. Sebum excretion is under hormonal control, with androgens increasing it (as do progesterones to a lesser degree) and oestrogens tending to diminish it. Sebum plays little physiological role in humans, but it is important in animals for waterproofing of hair.

Eccrine sweat glands

Eccrine sweat glands are found all over the body and their coiled ducts open directly on to the skin surface. They play a major role in thermoregulation and, unusually, are innervated by cholinergic fibres of the sympathetic rather than parasympathetic nervous system. Eccrine glands of the palms and soles are innervated differently and are activated in the 'fight or flight' response, as a small amount of sweat increases frictional forces of the palms.

Blood vessels and nerves

The abundant blood supply of the skin is arranged in superficial and deep plexuses, and is made up of arterioles, arterial and venous capillaries, and venules. The upper plexus is in the papillary dermis and communicates with the lower plexus at the junction between the dermis and the subcutis. Capillary loops arise from terminal arterioles in the horizontal papillary plexus. Blood vessels are supplied by sympathetic and parasympathetic nerves, with the relative contributions of the pathways differing by site. Sympathetic signals are important in mediating autonomic induced vasoconstriction. The blood supply of skin is far greater than that required for normal skin physiology and reflects the important role that skin plays in thermoregulation. Skin is richly innervated by nerves serving a number of different modalities, which penetrate into both the dermis and the epidermis.

Functions of the skin

These are shown in Box 27.1. Skin changes associated with ageing are shown in Box 27.2.

27.1 Functions of the skin	
Function	**Structure/cell involved**
Protection against:	
Chemicals, particles, desiccation	Stratum corneum
Ultraviolet radiation	Melanin produced by melanocytes and transferred to keratinocytes
Antigens, haptens	Langerhans cells, lymphocytes, mononuclear phagocytes, mast cells
Microbes	Stratum corneum, Langerhans cells, mononuclear phagocytes, mast cells
Maintenance of fluid balance Prevents loss of water, electrolytes and macromolecules	Stratum corneum
Shock absorber Strong, elastic and compliant covering	Dermis and subcutaneous fat
Sensation	Specialist nerve endings mediating pain leading to withdrawal, and itch leading to scratch and e.g. removal of a parasite
Vitamin D synthesis	Keratinocytes
Temperature regulation	Eccrine sweat glands and blood vessels
Protection, and fine manipulation of small objects	Nails
Hormonal Testosterone synthesis and testosterone conversion to other androgenic steroids	Hair follicles, sebaceous glands
Pheromonal (of unknown importance in humans)	Apocrine sweat glands
Psychosocial, grooming and sexual behaviour	Hair, nails, appearance and tactile quality of skin

27.2 Skin changes in old age

- **Photoageing:** most changes are a result of cumulative ultraviolet exposure rather than intrinsic ageing.
- **Typical changes:** include atrophy, laxity, wrinkling, dryness, irregular pigmentation and sparse grey hair.
- **Causes:**
  Age-related alterations in structure and function of the skin
  Cumulative effects of environmental insults, especially UV radiation
  Cutaneous consequences of disease in other organ systems.
- **Immunity:** alterations in immune surveillance and antigen presentation, and reduced cutaneous vascular supply lead to decreases in the inflammatory response, absorption and cutaneous clearance of topical medications.
- **Consequences:** the skin is less durable, slower to heal, and more susceptible to damage and disease.

27.3 Responses to Wood's light

Hypopigmentation accentuated

- Vitiligo
- Albinism
- Tuberous sclerosis

Hypopigmentation less obvious

- Post-inflammatory hypopigmentation
- Pityriasis versicolor
- Leprosy

INVESTIGATIONS AND SPECIALISED EXAMINATION

Diagnosis in dermatology relies almost entirely on clinical skills (pp. 1238–1239), and the role of investigations is limited. The relative contribution of history versus physical signs varies between particular skin disorders, but physical signs are usually the key factor in achieving the correct diagnosis. A number of visual aids are mandatory for proper clinical assessment, the simplest being a magnifying lens.

Dermatoscopy

Also known as dermoscopy or epiluminescence microscopy, this can be performed with a magnifying lens and oil applied to the skin, which reduces specular reflection and allows the observer to 'see through' the epidermis better. This is important in the assessment of pigmented lesions such as melanoma and naevi. Similar effects can be achieved by the use of illumination with polarised light and a lens, allowing non-touch imaging of the skin.

Diascopy

Distinguishing between blood and melanin, the main two pigments (or chromophores) in the skin, can be difficult. Pressing on the lesion with the corner of a glass slide will remove blood from vascular lesions, causing them to blanch. However, failure to remove blood does not reliably exclude a vascular lesion, as the vascular anatomy may sometimes be particularly convoluted. Pressing with a glass slide on some granulomatous lesions (such as cutaneous tuberculosis) gives an appearance known as 'apple jelly' nodules.

Wood's light

Exposure of skin to long wavelength ultraviolet radiation (UVA) with a Wood's light causes collagen in the dermis to fluoresce. In patients with hypopigmentation, Wood's light accentuates the difference in colour between the pigmented and non-pigmented areas because the pigment in the epidermis blocks the UVA photons before they can elicit fluorescence in the dermis. This can be helpful in mapping out the areas of depigmentation (Box 27.3). Under Wood's light, green fluorescence is seen in scalp ringworm due to *Microsporum canis* (p. 1273), a sporadic ectothrix infection, and pink fluorescence of flexural skin in seen in erythrasma (p. 1269).

Incisional biopsy and histopathology

Histopathological examination of skin biopsies is key, particularly for tumour diagnosis. The purpose of an incisional biopsy is to obtain a sample of tissue for histopathological examination rather than definitive treatment of a lesion, for which excisional biopsy is required. Skin biopsies are usually taken under local anaesthetic. It is best to select an early or typical lesion on a non-exposed site that is not affected by secondary excoriation. An ellipse biopsy, or in certain instances a punch biopsy that removes a cylindrical portion of skin, may be used. Knowing which part of a rash to biopsy, and whether an ellipse or punch biopsy will suffice, is critical to achieving a clear histological diagnosis.

Immunofluorescence

A portion of the biopsy can be frozen in liquid nitrogen for direct immunofluorescence (IF). This allows visualisation of antigens that are present in the skin using specific fluorescein-labelled antibodies. Similarly, indirect immunofluorescence can identify circulating antibodies in the serum by adding the serum to a section of normal skin or other substrate. Immunofluorescence plays a major role in the diagnosis of the autoimmune bullous disorders (p. 1275).

Microbiology
Mycology

Cutaneous scale, nail clippings and plucked hairs can be examined by light microscopy when mounted in 20% potassium hydroxide. The keratin is dissolved, allowing fungal hyphae to be identified. If the potassium hydroxide solution contains Indian ink, the typical 'spaghetti and meatballs' hyphae and spores of the yeast *Pityrosporum orbiculare* can be readily identified in pityriasis versicolor. Samples can also be sent for culture but there is a significant false negative rate for dermatophytes in some laboratories.

Bacteriology

Bacterial swabs may identify a causative infective agent. However, organisms identified from the surface of the skin may not be implicated in the underlying disease, but reflect colonisation of skin damaged by a primary

27

disease. Conversely, in diseases such as cellulitis, swabs often do not reveal the causative agent. If pustules are present, one should be punctured with a fine sterile needle and the pus exuded gently on to a swab.

Virology

A number of techniques, including immunofluorescence and polymerase chain reaction (PCR), are available to diagnose herpes simplex or herpes zoster viruses (p. 136).

Prick tests

Prick tests are a way of detecting cutaneous type I (immediate) hypersensitivity to various antigens such as pollen, house dust mite or dander. The skin is pricked with commercially available stylets through a dilution of the appropriate antigen solution. Alternatively, specific IgE levels to antigens can be measured in serum. These tests are described in detail on page 88.

Patch tests

Patch tests detect type IV (delayed or cell-mediated) hypersensitivity. A 'battery' of around 20 common antigens, including common sensitisers such as nickel, rubber and fragrance mix, are applied to the skin of the back under aluminium discs for 48 hours. The sites are examined for a positive reaction 48 hours later. An eczematous reaction in the absence of an irritant reaction suggests a type IV hypersensitivity to that particular allergen. The relevant antigens for a particular clinical case may not be in the standard battery of tests so expert advice may be needed. A negative patch test does not exclude a pathogenic role for a particular antigen, nor does a response to an antigen mean that it is necessarily causing the clinical disease.

Phototesting

Diagnostic phototesting is an essential component of the investigation of presumed photosensitive drug reactions and idiopathic photodermatoses such as solar urticaria. It involves exposing skin (often on the back) to a graded series of doses of ultraviolet radiation (UVR) of known wavelength, either on one occasion or repeatedly. In many photodermatoses, erythema will occur at a lower dose of UVR than in the normal population (e.g. drug-induced photosensitivity), or the time course of erythema may be prolonged (as in xeroderma pigmentosum). Alternatively, UVR will provoke lesions with the morphology of the underlying photodermatosis, such as may occur in lupus erythematosus or solar urticaria.

PRESENTING PROBLEMS IN SKIN DISEASE

The major presentations in dermatology are outlined below. Important points of clinical assessment are discussed, but detail about the underlying disorders is given in the disease sections later in the chapter.

New or changing skin lesion

Many patients present with a solitary skin lesion, which may or may not represent a skin cancer. The diagnostic challenge is to distinguish between benign tumours or hamartomas (e.g. angiomas, melanocytic naevi, seborrhoeic keratoses) and any of the major types of skin cancer such as melanoma, basal cell carcinoma and squamous cell carcinoma (pp. 1277–1281). It is not always possible to distinguish melanocytic lesions clinically from other highly pigmented lesions which are primarily keratinocytic (e.g. seborrhoeic keratosis, p. 1281). A particular concern is when a patient notices new changes in a lesion that has been present for some time, particularly in the case of a melanocytic naevus (mole).

Melanocytic naevus versus malignant melanoma

The following approach helps differentiate these:
- Determine the precise nature of the change. Is it the development of itch, inflammation, bleeding or ulceration, or does it relate to the colour, size, shape or surface of the lesion?
- Subtle changes should not be ignored, as many patients are good observers and 'know' their own moles well. If the change has settled, could it have been due to an insult such as nicking a facial naevus when shaving, plucking hairs from a naevus or the irritant effect of a depilatory?
- Is the patient worried about change in one or many moles? Concern relating to many moles is paradoxically reassuring, as presentation with multiple melanoma is extremely unusual; the patient may thus be needlessly anxious, or have constitutionally unusual but benign naevi.
- Does the patient have other pigmented lesions? The morphology of the other melanocytic naevi may provide useful diagnostic information about the patient's 'constitutional' mole type. Seborrhoeic warts are usually multiple. If a naevus, especially a changing one, appears significantly different in colour, shape or size from others (the 'ugly duckling' sign), it should be treated with suspicion.
- Is there a positive family history of melanoma? Fewer than 10% of melanomas occur in individuals with a strong family history, but in some families, up to 50% of individuals develop melanoma. A suspicious mole on a patient with a first-degree relative with melanoma probably warrants excision.

The ABCDE 'rule' is a guide to the characteristic features of melanoma (Box 27.4 and Fig. 27.3). Loss of normal skin markings is suggestive but not diagnostic of melanoma. Conversely, normal skin markings and fine hairs dispersed evenly over a lesion are reassuring, but do not exclude melanoma.

27.4 ABCDE features of malignant melanoma

- **A**symmetry
- **B**order irregular
- **C**olour irregular
- **D**iameter often > 0.5 cm
- **E**levation irregular

(+ Loss of skin markings)

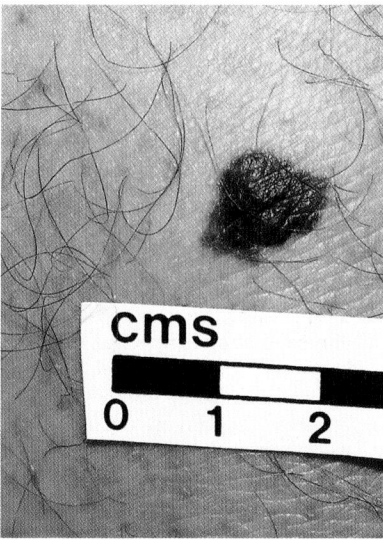

Fig. 27.3 Malignant melanoma. A changing mole which fails the ABCDE test.

Management

Any changing lesion which is suspected of being a malignant melanoma should be excised with a clear margin, without delay. Depending on the Breslow thickness of the tumour (p. 1281), further excision may be required. Some argue that, if the diagnosis is uncertain and the degree of suspicion low, the patient should be reviewed or the lesion photographed, and then re-assessed in a couple of months and rephotographed. Not all agree, given that melanomas may show only slow or intermittent progression in their early course.

Other new or changing skin lesions

These may be benign (p. 1281), pre-malignant (p. 1279) or maligant (p. 1277) and need careful assessment:

- *History*. Is the lesion of recent onset or has it been present for years? Is it growing fast or slowly? Is there any itch, pain, or bleeding and ulceration?
- *The individual*. What age is the patient (see Fig. 27.1)? Are they fair-skinned? Have they had a lot of sun exposure? Have they always been careful about photoprotection?
- *The site*. Is it in a sun-exposed or covered area? Common areas for sun-induced lesions are the scalp, face, arms and back in men, and the face, hands and lower legs in women.
- *Are there other similar lesions?* If there are many, e.g. actinic keratoses (see Fig. 27.39, p. 1279) on a balding scalp, or seborrhoeic keratoses (see Fig. 27.43, p. 1281) over a person's back, then the lesions are more likely to be benign.
- *Morphology of the lesion*. Assessment with a lens helps identify specific characteristics, e.g. the pearly thread-like border of a superfical basal cell carcinoma (p. 1277) or the poorly defined erythema and scaling of an actinic keratosis.
- *Dermatoscopy*. This is useful in lesions that are not melanocytic, and enhances typical morphological features such as keratin cysts in a seborrhoeic keratosis, or the telangiectasia of a basal cell carcinoma.

In cases of diagnostic doubt, incisional or excisional skin biospy should be performed, the latter as definitive treatement for malignant lesions.

Itch (pruritus)

Pruritus is defined as an unpleasant sensation that provokes the desire to scratch. Despite being a major symptom of skin disease, it remains poorly understood. Itch can arise from primary cutaneous disease or from systemic disease, which may cause itch via central or peripheral mechanisms. Even when the mechanism is thought to be peripheral, there may be few or no signs of primary skin disease; in a rare condition called aquagenic pruritus, water on the skin induces itch, but there are no other features.

The nerve endings that signal itch lie either within the epidermis or very close to the dermo-epidermal junction. Sensory information is transmitted via C fibres, which have slow conduction speeds, via the spinothalamic tract to the thalamus and on to a cortical representation. There seems to be an antagonistic or inhibitory relationship between pain and itch. Scratching may either cause inhibition of the itch receptors by stimulating ascending sensory pathways which inhibit itch at the spinal cord (Wall's 'gate' mechanism), or interfere with itch fibres lying superficially in skin which may be damaged directly by scratching. In the presence of a focal lesion causing itch, touch on the surrounding areas may be conducted along non-itch fibres but be centrally reinterpreted as itch (a phenomenon known as 'alloknesis', analogous to allodynia in pain).

The mechanism of itch in most systemic diseases is unknown, but in liver disease there is evidence that abnormal circulating opioids stimulate itch centrally.

Clinical assessment

Assessment of the itchy patient is difficult. Helpful pointers from the history include:

- *Time course*. This may be sudden, as in infestations and urticaria, or chronic, as in eczema.
- *Localisation*, including the site of onset. Is the itch confined to certain sites, as in localised skin disease such as lichen planus and lichen simplex, or generalised, as in eczema and scabies? The itch in diabetes is often in the genital region.
- *Exacerbating factors*. Most causes of itch are increased by heat and reduced by cooling. In cholinergic urticaria, exercise or heat dramatically induces itching (and weals on the skin surface); in aquagenic pruritus and aquagenic urticaria, water induces itch and weals respectively. In cold urticaria, cold stimuli such as ice or very cold air may induce weals and itch directly.
- *Involvement of other family members or close contacts*, as in a scabietic infestation. Insect bites usually affect only one member of the family.
- *General health* of the patient. A range of general medical conditions can precipitate itch, the symptoms of which should be sought.

It is important to determine whether there is a primary skin condition or whether the only visible clinical features are secondary to excoriation, but this may be

27

27.5 Primary skin diseases causing pruritus

Generalised pruritus

- Eczema
- Scabies
- Urticaria/dermographism
- Pruritus of old age and xeroderma

Localised pruritus

- Eczema
- Lichen planus
- Dermatitis herpetiformis
- Pediculosis

difficult. Try to classify the patient into one of the following groups:

- *Pruritus associated with skin disease* (Box 27.5). Atopic eczema and scabies infestation can be difficult to distinguish clinically, particularly in children. Secondary eczematisation occurs in scabies, giving rise to an eczematous rash all over the body. Scabietic burrows should be carefully sought, particularly in the finger and toe webs, along the borders of both the hands and the feet and at the wrists, and the mite should be extracted with a needle and examined under a microscope to make a definitive diagnosis. The genitalia and the nipples are particular sites for burrows. Even after successful treatment for scabietic infestation (p. 1274), the itch persists for several weeks or more.
- *Pruritus in pregnancy* (Box 27.6). A number of different conditions cause pruritus in pregnancy, some of which are important to fetal health.

Collaboration between a dermatologist and the obstetrician is important.

- *Pruritus associated with systemic disease* (Box 27.7). Itch is a common symptom in primary biliary sclerosis and may precede other symptoms. Classically, the itch of polycythaemia rubra vera begins soon after stepping out of the bath and lasts for 30–60 minutes. No visible skin signs are present. This can also occur in aquagenic pruritus, in which case follow-up for the development of myeloproliferative disorder is necessary. Although patients with other itchy conditions report worsening with heat or after a bath, the clinical picture is rarely as clear-cut as that seen in aquagenic pruritus or polycythaemia rubra vera. Itch is rarely associated with malignancy. The mechanisms involved are unclear but may be central, or localised secondary to tumour irritation of nerve roots. Lymphoma, particularly Hodgkin's, is important to consider, as the itch may precede other signs of the disease.

27.6 Causes of pruritus in pregnancy

Condition	Gestation and features	Treatment
Polymorphic eruption (urticarial papules) of pregnancy	3rd trimester, after delivery. Polymorphic lesions with urticaria	Chlorphenamine, emollients and topical steroids
Obstetric cholestasis	3rd trimester. Associated with abnormal liver function tests and increased risk to the fetus	Emollients. Chlorphenamine. Colestyramine. Early delivery
Pemphigoid gestationis	3rd trimester. Pruritus followed by blistering starting around the umbilicus. Diagnosed by histology and immunofluorescence	Topical or oral corticosteroids
Prurigo gestationis	2nd trimester. Excoriated papules	Emollients. Topical corticosteroids. Chlorphenamine
Pruritic folliculitis	3rd trimester. Aseptic pustules on trunk	Topical corticosteroids

27.7 Medical conditions associated with pruritus

Medical condition	Cause of pruritus	Treatment*
Liver disease	Central opioid effect. Elevation in bile salts may contribute	Naltrexone. Colestyramine. Rifampicin. Sedative antihistamines. UVB
Renal failure	Unknown; unlikely to involve histamine	Oral activated charcoal
Blood disease		
Anaemia	Iron deficiency	Iron replacement
Polycythaemia rubra vera	Unknown	
Lymphoma Leukaemia Myeloma	Unknown	
Endocrine disease		
Diabetes mellitus	May be associated with genital candidiasis	Clotrimazole
Thyrotoxicosis	Generalised due to dry skin	Emollients
Hypothyroidism	Localised; may be due to *Candida*	
Carcinoid syndrome (p. 782)	5HT-mediated	
HIV infection	Infection, infestation, e.g. *Candida*. Eosinophilic folliculitis. Unknown	Treatment of opportunistic infection. Local corticosteroids, UVB. UVB
Malignancy	Unknown	
Psychogenic	Unknown	Psychotherapy, anxiolytics, antidepressants

*In addition to specific treatment of primary condition.

In some patients, despite extensive investigations, no cause is found. Rare patients have a true delusional state in which they complain of a sensation of insects crawling across or emerging from the skin. Sometimes they produce scales or other cutaneous matter which they believe to be evidence of the insects. Psychiatric assessment is required.

Management

Treatment of itch depends on the cause and may require several trials of therapy. If there is a reversible cutaneous or systemic cause, this should be treated specifically.

A number of factors are known to exacerbate or precipitate itch. For instance, xerosis (dry skin) can be due to over-frequent bathing, soap and staying in a hot bath too long. Minimising soap and water exposure and using emollients can help. In patients with atopic dermatitis, nails need to be kept short and manicured. Although the evidence is unclear, emollients or cooling creams, such as menthol and aqueous cream, may be helpful.

If histamine is involved in pathogenesis, as in urticaria, then antihistamines are useful. The most appropriate are the non-sedative H$_1$ antagonists, e.g. fexofenadine, loratadine. If one fails, it is worth trying another. Historically, sedative antihistamines have been used in conditions such as atopic dermatitis which are not mediated via histamine; they act as sedatives which may reduce scratching, but their primary action on itch is unclear.

Phototherapy may help a wide variety of pruritic conditions but is particularly useful in atopic dermatitis and the itch secondary to renal disease. Opiate antagonists are effective in the itch of hepatic disorders. Rifampicin may also have a role in cholestatic pruritus. Capsaicin has been used in some localised causes of itch such as lichen simplex.

Although frequently the subject of ridicule, significant itch may incapacitate, embarrass, disrupt sleep and ruin patients' self-image. Its impact is easily underestimated.

Red scaly rashes (papulosquamous eruptions)

The red scaly rash is a common presenting complaint. The main causes are listed in Box 27.8 and the diagnosis is usually made on the basis of the clinical history and careful assessment of the rash. Key questions are:

- *How long has the rash been present?* Atopic eczema often starts in early childhood. Pityriasis rosea and psoriasis usually occur between the ages of 15 and 40 years. Pityriasis versicolor can persist for many years in one individual. More recent onset is seen in drug eruptions, temporally related to drug ingestion. Secondary syphilis is a transient eruption.
- *Where on the body did it start and how has it evolved?* Atopic eczema usually starts on the cheeks in infancy and spreads to involve the flexures of the limbs. Chronic plaque psoriasis tends to favour the extensor surfaces, but guttate ('raindrop') psoriasis has a rapid onset and is widespread. Facial involvement is uncommon in psoriasis. Drug eruptions evolve over a few days to 3 weeks after starting the culprit drug; they often resolve with desquamation. Fungal infections can affect any

part of the body, including the face, and continue to appear in other sites over time.
- *Is the rash itchy?* Eczema and tinea corporis are always itchy. Psoriasis and drug eruptions can be itchy but pityriasis rosea, pityriasis versicolor and syphilis are rarely so.
- *Was there a preceding illness or systemic symptoms?* Guttate psoriasis is often precipitated by a β-haemolytic streptococcal sore throat. Systemic symptoms, such as fever, malaise and joint pains, are common in drug eruptions. Although the majority of individuals are not allergic to penicillins, almost all patients with infectious mononucleosis (p. 316) treated with amoxicillin will develop

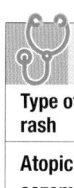

27.8 Causes and clinical features of common scaly rashes

Type of rash	Distribution	Morphology	Associated clinical signs
Atopic eczema (p. 1257)	Face/flexures	Poorly defined erythema and scaling Lichenification	Shiny nails Infra-orbital crease 'Dirty neck' (grey-brown discoloration)
Psoriasis (p. 1260)	Extensor surfaces	Well-defined plaques with a silvery scale	Nail pitting and onycholysis Scalp involvement Axillae and genital areas often affected
Pityriasis rosea (p. 1264)	'Fir tree' pattern on torso	Well-defined erythematous papules and plaques with collarette of scale	
Drug eruption (p. 1286)	Widespread	Maculopapular erythematous scaly areas which merge. Subsequent exfoliation	
Pityriasis versicolor (p. 1265)	Upper torso and upper shoulders	Hypo- and hyperpigmented scaly patches	
Lichen planus (p. 1265)	Distal limbs, especially volar aspect of wrists Lower back	Shiny, flat-topped violaceous papules with Wickham's striae	White lacy network buccal mucosa Nail changes (rare)
Tinea corporis (p. 1273)	Asymmetrical, often isolated lesions	Scaly red plaques which expand with central healing	Nail involvement (see Fig. 27.55, p. 1291)
Secondary syphilis (p. 1264)	Torso and proximal limbs Palms and soles	Red macules and papules which change to a 'gun-metal' grey	Systemic symptoms, e.g. malaise and fever

27

an erythematous maculopapular eruption. The widespread red scaly eruption of secondary syphilis follows a history of a chancre at the site of inoculation.

The extent and symmetry of the rash should be carefully examined. If symmetrical, it is likely to be due to an endogenous cause, such as eczema, psoriasis, drug eruptions, pityriasis rosea and syphilis. Exogenous eruptions, such as contact allergic dermatitis and tinea corporis, are asymmetrical, initially appearing only in the area where either the allergen or the culprit fungus has affected the skin. The morphology of the rash and the individual lesions is important, particularly whether the lesions are well or poorly defined (Box 27.8). Use of a magnifying lens may help determine this. It is not usually necessary to take a biopsy to confirm the diagnosis of red scaly eruptions, but it may help where there is doubt.

Erythroderma

Eczema, psoriasis, drug eruptions and lichen planus rarely progress to erythroderma, defined as erythema, with or without scaling, affecting almost all the body surface. In dark skin, the presence of pigmentation may mask the erythema, giving a purplish hue. Other causes include cutaneous T-cell lymphoma (Sézary's syndrome, p. 1282), the psoriasis-like condition pityriasis rubra pilaris, and rare types of ichthyosis. Erythroderma may occur at any age and is associated with severe morbidity but rarely mortality. Older people are at greatest risk. It may appear suddenly or evolve slowly.

Erythrodermic patients, especially the elderly, may be systemically unwell with shivering and hypothermia, secondary to excess and uncontrolled heat loss caused by increased blood flow to their skin. However, they may also be pyrexial, and unable to lose heat due to damage to sweat gland function and sweat duct occlusion. Tachycardia and hypotension may be present, due to volume depletion. Peripheral oedema is common in erythroderma, due to low albumin and high-output cardiac failure. Lymph nodes may be enlarged, either reactive to skin inflammation, or rarely due to lymphomatous infiltration.

Urticaria (nettle rash, hives)

Urticaria refers to an area of focal dermal oedema secondary to a transient increase in capillary permeability. On certain body sites such as the lips or hands, the oedema spreads deeper and is referred to as angioedema. By definition, the swelling lasts less than 24 hours. Acute urticaria may be associated with angioedema of the lips, face, throat and rarely wheezing, abdominal pain, headaches and even anaphylaxis (p. 89). Whilst severe angioedema can be life-threatening due to respiratory obstruction, this is extremely rare in a dermatological context.

Although the time frames are somewhat arbitrary, it is useful to ask:

- How long does the individual lesion last?
  < 24 hours (urticaria)
  > 24 hours (urticarial vasculitis)

- How long has the condition been present?
  < 6 weeks (acute urticaria)
  > 6 weeks (chronic urticaria)

Knowing the length of time that an individual weal lasts may be of some use in distinguishing urticaria from urticarial vasculitis. Urticarial vasculitis is much less common than urticaria, and many patients are unable to distinguish the development of new weals and disappearance of old ones, from individual weals which persist for more than 1 day. This may be clarified by drawing around a weal with a pen and examining the patient 24 hours later.

A directed history is the best way to elicit any causes or precipitants of urticaria (Box 27.9). Possible allergens, including drugs, should be determined. The physical urticarias can be identified by asking appropriate questions and subsequent challenge testing. A family history must be sought in cases of angioedema. Examination may reveal nothing as this is a transient eruption, or may uncover the classical weals which vary from papules to large extensive plaques (Fig. 27.4). Pathogenesis, investigations and management are described on page 1266.

27.9 Causes of urticaria

Acute and chronic urticaria

- **Autoimmune** due to production of antibodies that cross-link the IgE receptor on mast cells
- **Allergens** (in foods, inhalants and injections)
- **Drugs** (see Box 27.41, p. 1287)
- **Contact**, e.g. animal saliva, latex
- **Physical**, e.g. heat, cold, pressure, sun, water
- **Infection**, e.g. viral hepatitis, infectious mononucleosis, HIV seroconversion
- **Other conditions**, e.g. systemic lupus erythematosus (SLE), pregnancy, intestinal parasites
- **Idiopathic**

Urticarial vasculitis

- Hepatitis B
- SLE
- Idiopathic

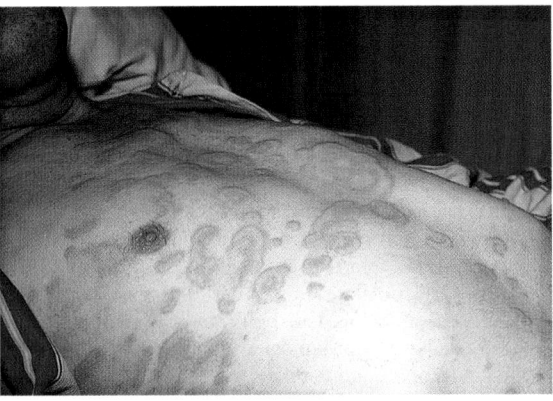

Fig. 27.4 Widespread acute urticaria. In this case urticaria was due to penicillin allergy.

Blisters

Blisters have a limited differential diagnosis (Box 27.10). Loss of adhesion within the skin leads to a potential space which, because of negative extracellular pressure, fills with fluid and forms a blister. Although an artificial distinction, the size (vesicle < 0.5 cm; bulla > 0.5 cm) can be a useful pointer in terms of diagnosis. Much of our understanding of the adhesion mechanisms within the skin has come from the study of a rare group of genetic blistering skin conditions, epidermolysis bullosa (Box 27.11), which, with other genodermatoses, present with blistering at birth.

In acquired blistering disorders, the clinical presentation depends on the site or level of blistering within the skin and this in turn is due to the underlying pathogenesis (p. 1275).

- If blisters occur high up in the epidermis, i.e. below the stratum corneum, the blister is so fragile that it ruptures easily and only an erosion is seen (e.g. pemphigus foliaceus, staphylococcal scalded skin syndrome and bullous impetigo).
- Blisters within the epidermis can be more obvious but may be erosions (e.g. eczema, particularly contact allergic eczema, pemphigus vulgaris, toxic epidermal necrolysis).
- Subepidermal blisters are more robust and can be very tense, as seen in bullous pemphigoid (Fig. 27.5), epidermolysis bullosa acquisita and porphyrias. In dermatitis herpetiformis, an autoimmune blistering disorder (p. 1276), the blisters are deep-seated but so itchy that only excoriations or erosions are seen.

A history of onset, progression, mucosal involvement, drugs and associated systemic symptoms should be taken. Clinical assessment of the distribution, extent and morphology (vesicular/bullous or mixed) of the rash should be made. The Nikolsky sign is useful; sliding pressure from a finger on normal-looking epidermis can dislodge the epidermis in conditions with intra-epidermal defects, e.g. pemphigus and toxic epidermal necrolysis.

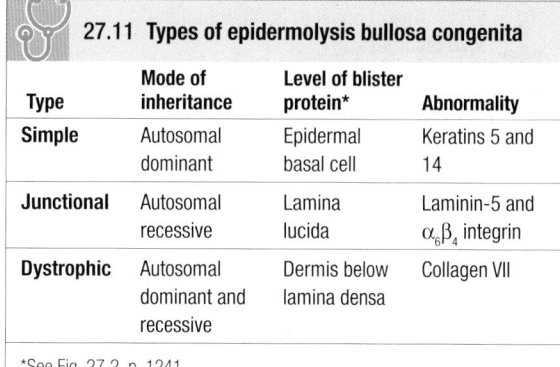

27.11 Types of epidermolysis bullosa congenita

Type	Mode of inheritance	Level of blister protein*	Abnormality
Simple	Autosomal dominant	Epidermal basal cell	Keratins 5 and 14
Junctional	Autosomal recessive	Lamina lucida	Laminin-5 and $\alpha_6\beta_4$ integrin
Dystrophic	Autosomal dominant and recessive	Dermis below lamina densa	Collagen VII

*See Fig. 27.2, p. 1241.

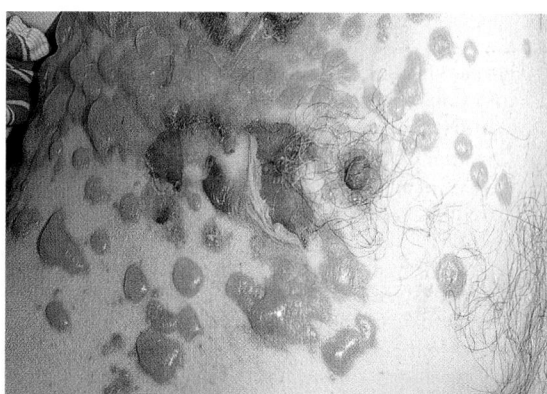

Fig. 27.5 Bullous pemphigoid. Large tense and unilocular blisters clustered in and around the axilla.

A systematic approach to diagnosis is required:
1. Exclude blistering as a *less common manifestation of a common skin problem*, e.g. severe peripheral oedema, cellulitis, allergic contact dermatitis, eczema and pompholyx.

27.10 Causes of acquired blisters

| | Localised | Generalised | |
		Mucosal involvement	No mucosal involvement
Vesicular	Herpes simplex Herpes zoster Impetigo Pompholyx	Eczema herpeticum	Eczema herpeticum Dermatitis herpetiformis Epidermolysis bullosa acquisita
Bullous	Impetigo Bullous cellulitis Bullous stasis oedema Acute eczema Insect bites Fixed drug eruptions	Pemphigus Bullous pemphigoid Bullous erythema multiforme/Stevens–Johnson syndrome Toxic epidermal necrolysis Epidermolysis bullosa acquisita	Acute eczema Erythema multiforme Bullous pemphigoid Epidermolysis bullosa acquisita Bullous lupus erythematosus Pseudoporphyria Porphyria cutanea tarda Drug eruptions, e.g. barbiturates

2. Exclude *infection,* e.g. viral infections with herpes simplex or varicella zoster or bacterial infections, e.g. staphylococcal bullous impetigo or staphylococcal scalded skin syndrome (SSSS).

3. Consider a bullous form of a *reactive skin eruption,* such as drug eruptions (particularly a fixed drug eruption, p. 1286), erythema multiforme (p. 1284) and vasculitis (p. 1112). The morphology and distribution of these eruptions are distinctive. More severe blistering, usually due to drug reactions, is seen in toxic epidermal necrolysis (TEN, p. 1275); the patient is systemically unwell, the skin is shed in large sheets and mortality is significant.

4. Consider an *immunobullous skin disorder* (p. 1275). The age of the patient can be a helpful pointer (Box 27.12).

Routine investigations include full blood count, urea and electrolytes, and also:

- swabs for virology and microbiology
- skin snip to differentiate between SSSS and TEN (p. 1270)

- skin biopsy for histology and direct immunofluorescence
- serum sample for indirect immunofluorescence if an immunobullous disorder is suspected.

Treatment is directed towards the underlying cause but significant mucosal involvement and widespread blistering need immediate topical therapy. Skin loss can be painful and fluid loss significant, so analgesia and fluid replacement are important. Blisters can be pierced to release fluid and prevent extension. Topical therapy and dressings may be very soothing (p. 1254). Patients with extensive skin loss may require treatment in an intensive care setting.

Photosensitivity

Ultraviolet radiation is the main cause of skin malignancies in most populations and is responsible for photo-ageing. Whilst UV radiation, by definition, causes a range of photodermatoses, it is also used therapeutically for some of these and for a wide range of other skin diseases, notably psoriasis and cutaneous T-cell lymphoma. It is also necessary for the production of vitamin D in keratinocytes.

UV radiation is divided by convention into three wavebands (Fig. 27.6):

- *UVC* (280–300 nm), which is effectively blocked by the earth's atmosphere
- *UVB* (300–320 nm), which forms a small component of ambient UV radiation but is much more potent biologically and accounts for most of the sunburning activity in natural sunlight
- *UVA* (320–400 nm), the dominant waveband found at the earth's surface, which is biologically less active than UVB.

Both UVB and UVA may induce rashes in sensitive individuals, and in the majority of instances both wavebands

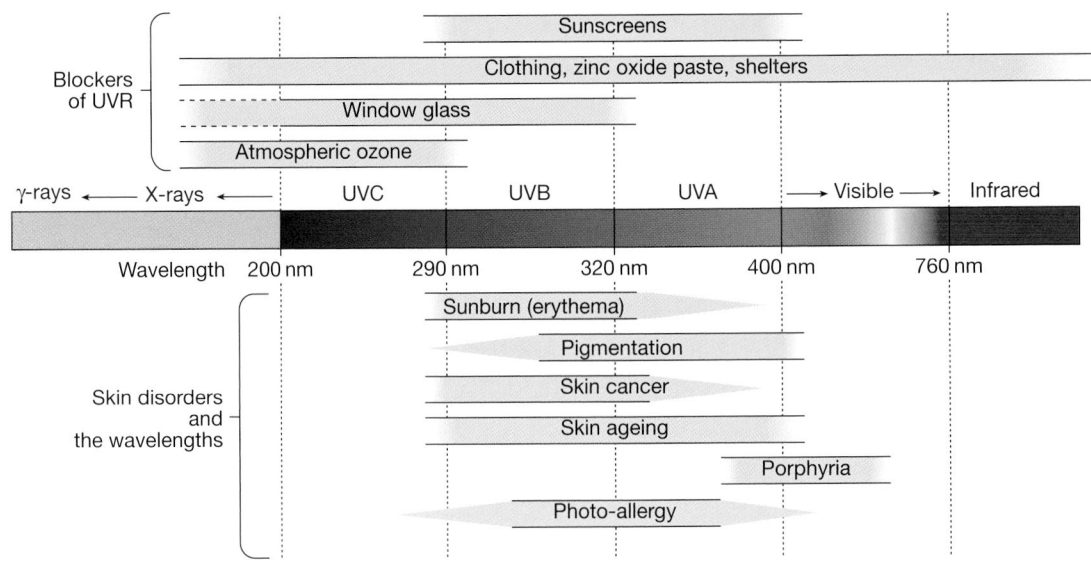

Fig. 27.6 The electromagnetic spectrum. For some conditions the action spectrum is approximate and may vary between patients (e.g. lupus erythematosus, polymorphic light eruption). The action spectrum for non-melanoma skin cancer mirrors that for erythema. The action spectrum for melanoma is not known but certainly involves UVB. (UVR = ultraviolet radiation)

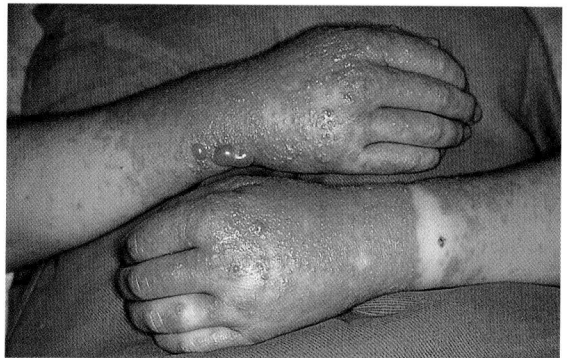

Fig. 27.7 Bullous photosensitive eruption. Note the sharp cut-off at the wrists, due to protection by the shirt sleeves, and sparing of the skin under watch and strap.

are active. In some individuals, pathological sensitivity even extends into the visible spectrum (> 400 nm).

Clinical assessment

The history may clearly indicate that the rash is temporally related to sun exposure. The sites that received the most sunshine will tend to be affected: the face, the nose and the cheeks (but excluding the eyelids, an area under the chin and an area in the shadow of the nose), and the dorsa of the forearm and the hands (Fig. 27.7). Sometimes, however, the diagnosis is not straightforward; the rash may develop on some sun-exposed sites but extend to sun-protected sites, and may not be most prevalent on the areas that have received the maximum ultraviolet exposure. Some rashes, such as solar urticaria, have a clear temporal relation with UV exposure, while others, such as lupus erythematosus, may take up to 10 days to develop following exposure. Common causes are shown in Box 27.13.

Management

If photosensitivity is suspected, an attempt should be made to provoke the rash with phototesting (p. 1244). Only longer wavelength radiation, such as UVA, will pass through normal window glass. If photosensitivity is due to UVB only, individuals will not be at risk when they are behind plain glass, which may be diagnostically useful. Management depends on the diagnosis. In some disorders, such as solar urticaria or polymorphic light eruption, carefully controlled graded exposure to UVR in a phototherapy cabinet seems to lead to a reduction in symptoms. The mechanism is unclear but may involve down-regulation of the cutaneous immune system or skin hardening (increased resistance to the harmful effects of UVR) due to tanning and epidermal thickening. Other therapeutic strategies include sun avoidance, use of sunblocks and antihistamines (useful in solar urticaria), correction of associated metabolic disorders (e.g. porphyria), or removal of an offending drug.

Sunscreens

Chemical sunscreens absorb specific wavelengths of UVR, while physical sunscreens reflect UVR and visible light. Most available products are a combination of UVA and UVB chemical sunscreens. The individual may be sensitive to visible light as well as UVR, but the agents that block visible light are obvious and have limited cosmetic acceptability.

Sunblocks are graded in terms of their sun protection factor (SPF). The SPF is the ratio of the time it takes to induce a certain degree of erythema with and without sunblock. An SPF of 10 means than 90% of the radiation is blocked, and therefore it would take an exposure 10 times as long as that without the sunblock to obtain the same degree of erythema. Thus, for a given unit of time exposure, as the SPF gets larger, the additional benefit is marginal. However, the average individual applies only about one-third of the density of sunblock per unit skin

27

27.13 The photosensitive dermatoses

Cause	Condition	Clinical features
Drugs	Phototoxic drug eruption	Common; exaggerated sunburn occurs minutes after sun exposure e.g. Phenothiazines, amiodarone, tetracyclines
	Photo-allergic drug eruption	Occurs > 24 hrs after sun exposure Dermatitis or lichen planus-like reaction, may become permanent (persistent light reactor) e.g. Thiazides, enalapril, hydroxychloroquine, quinine, phenothiazines or topical photosensitisers, e.g. fragrances
Metabolic	Porphyrias	Particularly porphyria cutanea tarda (pp. 456 and 1284)
	Pellagra	Dermatitis due to dietary lack of tryptophan (see Fig. 16.17, p. 457)
Exacerbation of pre-existing conditions	Lupus erythematosus	Page 1107
	Erythema multiforme	Page 1284
	Herpes simplex	Page 321
Idiopathic	Polymorphic light eruption	Itchy papulovesicular eruption on exposed sites within hours of UV exposure; more frequent in women
	Solar urticaria	Urticaria within minutes of sun exposure
	Chronic actinic dermatitis	Disabling, itchy dermatitis on sun-exposed sites in elderly men

used in the calculation of SPF figures, so that a sunblock with an SPF of 15 will only actually have an SPF of 5.

Leg ulcers

Ulceration of the skin is due to complete loss of the epidermis and part of the dermis. When present on the lower leg, it is usually due to vascular disease, and around 75% of cases are due in part to venous hypertension. For each cause of leg ulceration there are several different underlying pathologies that have to be considered (Box 27.14). Venous ulcers usually start in middle age. Leg ulcers are more likely to occur and persist in obese people.

Clinical assessment

The history of the onset of the leg ulceration and any underlying predisposing conditions should be sought, and the site and surrounding skin carefully assessed. Varicose veins are often present but are not inevitable. The first symptom in venous ulceration is frequently heaviness of the legs, followed by the development of oedema. Haemosiderin pigmentation and ivory-coloured scarring may then be seen, sometimes associated with venous eczema (p. 1256). This progresses to lipodermatosclerosis—firm induration due to fibrosis of the dermis and subcutis, which may produce the well-known 'inverted champagne bottle' appearance. Ulceration, often precipitated by minor trauma or infection, soon occurs. The site of ulceration on the lower leg can give a good indication of the underlying cause (Fig. 27.8). Venous ulcers are seen typically around the medial malleolus but may encircle the ankle (Fig. 27.9). Arterial and vasculitic ulcers may have a punched-out appearance. Neuropathic ulcers appear at maximum pressure points, such as the heel.

Appropriate investigations include:

- *Urinalysis* for glycosuria.
- *Full blood count* to detect anaemia and blood dyscrasias.
- *Bacterial swab* if there is a purulent discharge, rapid extension, cellulitis, lymphangitis or septicaemia.

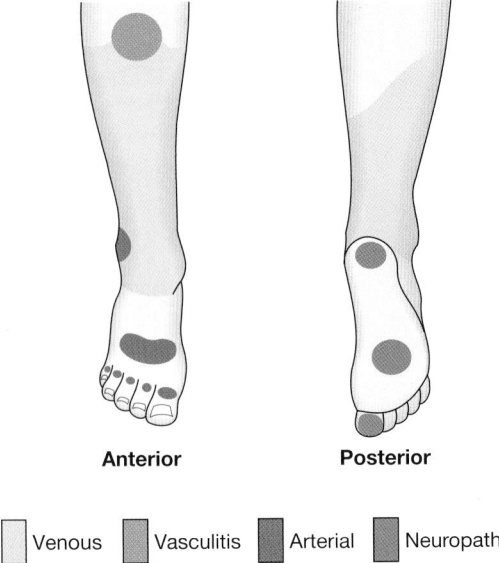

Anterior   **Posterior**

☐ Venous ☐ Vasculitis ☐ Arterial ☐ Neuropathic

Fig. 27.8 Causes of lower leg ulceration.

- *Doppler ultrasound* to assess arterial circulation. If the ratio of ankle systolic pressure to brachial systolic pressure (ABPI) is < 0.8, there is significant arterial disease. However, in some patients with diabetes, arterial calcification of the lower limb vessels produces a spuriously high result.
- *Venography*, which is occasionally useful in detecting surgically remediable venous incompetence.
- *Duplex scanning* to delineate arterial disease in those with an ABPI < 0.8.

Management depends on the cause but usually involves some form of dressing (p. 1288).

27.14 Causes of leg ulceration

Venous hypertension

Arterial disease
- Atherosclerosis
- Vasculitis
- Buerger's disease

Small-vessel disease
- Diabetes mellitus
- Vasculitis

Haematological disorders
- Sickle-cell disease
- Cryoglobulinaemia
- Spherocytosis
- Immune complex disease

Neuropathy
- Diabetes mellitus
- Leprosy
- Syphilis

Tumour
- Squamous cell carcinoma
- Basal cell carcinoma
- Malignant melanoma
- Kaposi's sarcoma

Trauma
- Injury
- Artefact

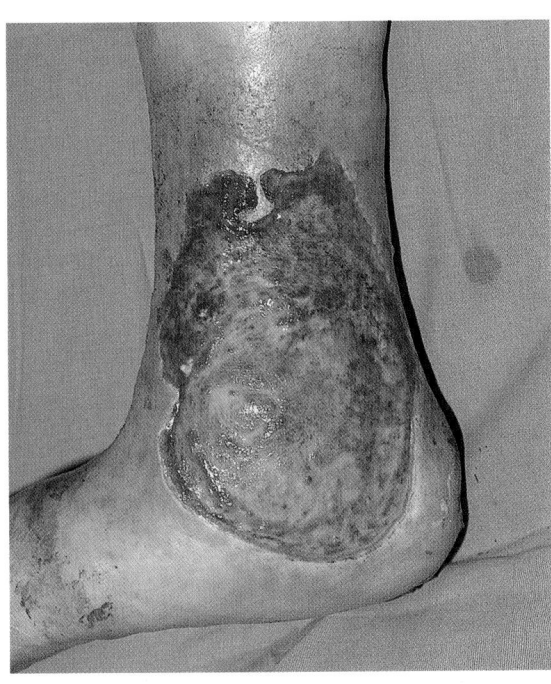

Fig. 27.9 A large venous ulcer overlying the medial malleolus.

Abnormal skin colour

Decreased pigmentation

The main disorders to consider are albinism and vitiligo. However, a number of others may produce secondary hypopigmentation:

- pityriasis alba, a type of eczema presenting as depigmented areas on the face, particularly in children, with or without scale
- pityriasis versicolor, a yeast infection characterised by hyperpigmentation early in its pathogenesis but leading to multiple areas of hypopigmentation on the trunk, particularly the back
- idiopathic guttate hypomelanosis, characterised by numerous small areas of depigmentation in areas of skin that have been exposed to the sun
- very rarely, phenylketonuria (p. 447) and hypopituitarism.

Oculocutaneous albinism

Albinism results from a range of genetic abnormalities leading to reduced melanin biosynthesis in the skin and eyes; the number of melanocytes is normal (in contrast to vitiligo). There are a number of different forms of albinism, and considerable variation even within one genetic type. Albinism is usually inherited as an autosomal recessive trait.

Type 1 albinism is due to a defect in the tyrosinase gene, whose product is rate-limiting in the production of melanin. Affected individuals have an almost complete absence of pigment in the skin and hair at birth, with resulting pale skin and white hair, and failure of melanin production in the iris and retina. Patients have photophobia, poor vision not correctable with refraction, rotatory nystagmus, and an alternating strabismus associated with abnormalities in the decussation of nerve fibres in the optic tract.

A second form of albinism is due to a defect in the *P* gene, which encodes an ion channel protein in the melanosome. Patients may have gross reduction of melanin in the skin and in the eyes, but may be more mildly affected than type 1 albinos. Establishing the subtype of albinism requires genetic analysis, as there is considerable heterogeneity in the phenotype of the various subtypes.

Oculocutaneous albinos are at grossly increased risk of sunburn and skin cancer. In equatorial regions, many die from squamous cell carcinoma or, more rarely, melanoma in early adult life. They may, however, show pigmented melanocytic naevi and may freckle in response to sun damage.

Management

Avoidance of sun exposure with protective clothing and hats is important, as is a lifestyle that avoids the mid-day sun in particular, with indoor rather than outdoor occupations. Sunblocks may be useful but can be expensive. Early diagnosis and treatment of skin tumours is essential.

Vitiligo

Vitiligo is an acquired condition in which circumscribed depigmented patches develop; it affects 1% of the population world-wide. Unlike albinism, vitiligo involves focal areas of melanocyte loss. There may be a positive family history of the disorder in those with generalised vitiligo, and this type is associated with autoimmune diseases such as diabetes, thyroid and adrenal disorders, and pernicious anaemia. Trauma and sunburn may precipitate the appearance of vitiligo. A number of hypotheses have been advanced to explain the pathogenesis, including that the melanocytes are the target of a cell-mediated autoimmune attack, but why only focal areas are affected remains unexplained.

Clinical assessment

Segmental vitiligo is restricted to one part of the body but not necessarily a dermatome. Generalised vitiligo is often symmetrical and frequently involves the hands, wrists, knees and neck, as well as the area around the body orifices. The hair of the scalp and beard may also depigment (Fig. 27.10). The patches of depigmentation are sharply defined, and in Caucasians may be surrounded by light brown 'café au lait' hyperpigmentation. Some spotty perifollicular pigment may be seen within the depigmented patches and is sometimes the first sign of repigmentation. Sensation in the depigmented patches is normal (unlike in tuberculoid leprosy, p. 341). Examination with a Wood's light enhances the contrast between the pigmented and non-pigmented skin. The course of vitiligo is unpredictable but most patches remain static or enlarge; a few repigment spontaneously.

Management

This is unsatisfactory. Protecting the patches from excessive sun exposure with clothing or sunscreen may be helpful in reducing episodes of burning and potential skin cancer. Camouflage cosmetics may also be helpful, particularly in those with dark skin, as can potent topical corticosteroids. Phototherapy with PUVA (psoralen + UVA) or more recently narrow band UVB has been used (p. 1263) but evidence is limited. PUVA therapy increases pigmentation in normal skin, so the cosmetic effect (an increase in contrast) may actually be worse than no treatment, except in very dark-skinned individuals. When repigmentation occurs, it is frequently seen as small foci of dark areas of skin surrounding hair follicles within the vitiliginous area. The absence of whiteness of the hairs in the area of vitiligo is a good prognostic feature. Transplantation, using a range of techniques including split-skin grafts and blister roof grafts, is occasionally used on to dermabraded recipient skin.

27

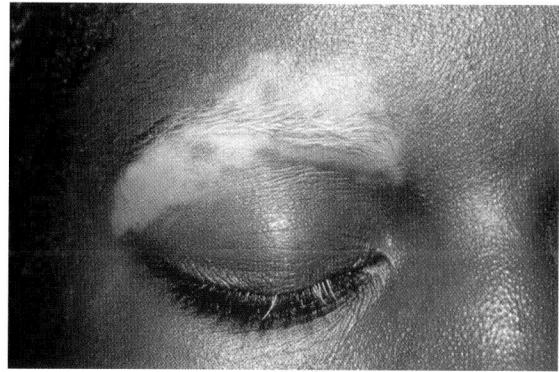

Fig. 27.10 Vitiligo. Localised patches of depigmented skin, including some white hairs.

The impact of vitiligo differs markedly between populations. In the Indian subcontinent, the effects of vitiligo are more readily discernible than in pale-skinned individuals in northern Europe. Depigmentation is also seen in leprosy, which means that individuals with vitiligo are often stigmatised. The use of more novel treatments, such as grafting, is often pursued more extensively in such populations.

Increased pigmentation

- *Diffuse hyperpigmentation.* This is mostly due to hypermelanosis but other pigments may be deposited in the skin. Orange discoloration suggests carotenaemia; bronze, haemochromatosis (p. 959); and other hues, drug eruptions.
- *Endocrine pigmentation.* This may occur in a number of conditions. Chloasma describes discrete patches of facial pigmentation which occur in pregnancy and in some women taking oral contraceptives. The basis of the focal increased sensitivity to hormonal control is unknown. Diffuse pigmentation, sometimes worse in the skin creases, may be a feature of Addison's disease (p. 774), Cushing's syndrome (p. 770), Nelson's syndrome (p. 773) and chronic renal failure. This is due to increased levels of pituitary melanotrophic peptides, including adrenocorticotrophic hormone (ACTH. p. 773).
- *Drug-induced pigmentation* (Box 27.15). This is not always due to hypermelanosis but may sometimes be due to deposition of the drug or its metabolite, either of which may be complexed with melanin.
- *Focal hypermelanosis.* This is seen in lesions such as freckles and lentigines, characterised by focal areas of increased pigmentation.

27.15 Drug-induced pigmentation	
Drug	**Appearance**
Amiodarone	Slate-grey; exposed sites
Arsenic	Diffuse bronze pigmentation with superimposed raindrop depigmentation
Bleomycin	Often flexural; brown
Busulfan	Diffuse brown
Chloroquine	Blue-grey; exposed sites
Clofazimine	Red
Mepacrine	Yellow
Minocycline	Slate-grey; scars, temples, shins and sclera
Phenothiazines	Slate-grey; exposed sites
Psoralens	Brown; exposed sites

TOPICAL TREATMENT OF SKIN DISEASE

Topical treatments are a mainstay of the management of many skin conditions. The use of the correct active ingredient (or drug) and the vehicle in which it is applied is important.

Active ingredient

Many topical formulations are available for use in skin disease. Compound formulations are becoming increasingly available. Drugs penetrate the skin according to their molecular weight and their lipid–water coefficients, water-soluble ions and polar molecules being excluded. When the stratum corneum is impaired in disease states, drug absorption increases, but as the skin heals, it diminishes accordingly. If occlusion is applied—for example, under dressings—absorption is increased. Agents may be formulated in different potencies, as with topical corticosteroids, or by different concentrations, as with anthralins, coal tar preparations and first-generation topical retinoids. Most other agents are formulated in one strength, e.g. topical antibiotics, second-generation topical retinoids and vitamin D analogues.

Vehicle (base)

Besides containing the active ingredient, the vehicle of a topical treatment has other roles. It can hydrate and cool the skin, and has antimicrobial and soothing qualities. Creams and ointments are the most common vehicles used. Gels (both non-hydrous and aqueous) and lotions (aqueous) are convenient for use in hair-bearing areas. The properties of different vehicles are listed in Box 27.16. Many active treatments are available in more than one formulation.

Topical corticosteroids

Glucocorticoids are formulated as both ointments and creams. Creams are used in acute exudative conditions, whereas ointments are better in chronic dry skin conditions. Corticosteroids come in a variety of strengths and potencies (Box 27.17), and should be prescribed according to the site of application, the age of the patient and the length of time that the corticosteroids are to be used. Mild topical corticosteroids are used on sensitive sites, such as the face or genital area, in both adults and children. Superpotent corticosteroids are used under occlusion on chronic persistent lesions such as nodular prurigo. Local side-effects of topical corticosteroids include cutaneous atrophy and telangiectasia. These are rarely seen and undertreatment is a more common problem, and can be the cause of apparent treatment failure. There are no rules about the length of time for which a topical corticosteroid may be used safely in a particular individual on any one site, but in general the least potent corticosteroid should be used for the shortest possible time. Corticosteroid-responsive dermatoses should be treated initially with a more potent topical corticosteroid, switching to a less potent one as the condition improves. Long-term treatment is often given intermittently because of tachyphylaxis.

Dressings

An appropriate covering, such as a wound dressing (e.g. Jelonet), a simple tubular bandage (e.g. Tubifast) or a medicated bandage (e.g. Steripaste or Ichthopaste), is known as a dressing. Box 27.18 shows the indications for their use. The choice of dressing should be made according to the active agent, vehicle and covering of the skin. Wet lesions should be treated

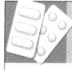

27.16 Definition of vehicles used in topical treatments

Vehicle	Definition	Use	Site	Cosmetic acceptability	Risk of contact sensitisation
Creams	Emulsions of oil and water, e.g. aqueous cream	Acute presentations Cooling, soothing and well absorbed Mild emollients	All sites, including mucous membranes and flexures, but not hair-bearing areas	Very good	May contain antimicrobials and preservatives
Ointments	Greasy preparations Insoluble in water, e.g. white soft paraffin Soluble, e.g. Macrogol	Chronic dry areas of skin Mostly occlusive and protective; help rehydrate the skin Mildly anti-inflammatory	Avoid hair-bearing areas and flexures	Moderate	Low risk
Gels	Hydrophilic and hydrophobic bases	For specific sites	Hair-bearing areas and the face	Good	Low risk
Lotions	Water-based	Cooling effect Used to clean the skin and remove exudates Often antiseptic and astringent (e.g. potassium permanganate)	Large areas of the skin and the scalp	Good, but can sting if in an alcoholic base	Rare
Pastes	Semi-stiff preparations containing finely powdered solids suspended in an ointment	Characteristically substantive and bland Used for circumscribed skin lesions, e.g. psoriasis, lichen simplex chronicus	Any area of skin Often used in medicated bandages	Moderate	Moderate

27

27.17 Strengths of topical corticosteroids*

Mild
- 0.5%, 1%, 2.5% hydrocortisone

Moderate
- Clobetasone butyrate 0.05% (Eumovate)
- Betamethasone 0.025% (Betnovate RD)

Potent
- Mometasone furoate 0.1% (Elocon)
- Betamethasone 0.1% (Betnovate)
- Betamethasone 0.1% and fusidic acid 2% (Fucibet)
- Fluticasone propionate 0.05% and 0.005% (Cutivate)

Very potent
- Clobetasol propionate 0.05% (Dermovate)

*UK trade names are given in brackets.

27.18 Indications for dressings

- Protection
- Symptomatic relief from pain or itch
- Maintenance of direct application of topical treatment
- Acceleration of healing time
- Reduction of exudates

with wet dressings; for example, acute eczema is best treated with potassium permanganate soaks, a topical corticosteroid in a cream formulation and a paste bandage to soothe and cool the skin. In acute blistering, an astringent and antiseptic, such as potassium permanganate or 2% aqueous eosin, is applied first, followed by a non-adherent dressing such as Jelonet or Allevyn; antiseptic creams (e.g. Flamazine), topical steroid creams or emollients may also be useful. Chronic dry itchy eczema is best treated with a potent topical corticosteroid in an ointment formulation and a paste bandage to ease itching and scratching. Dressings for venous leg ulcers are described on page 1288. Patients with leg ulcers have an increased risk of contact allergy to medicaments, so potential allergens, such as topical antibiotics, antiseptics and lanolin, should be avoided.

DERMATOLOGICAL SURGERY

A large number of surgical procedures can be carried out under local anaesthetic. Incisional biopsy is described on page 1243. The choice of procedure is important; for example, inappropriate excision of lesions such as seborrhoeic keratoses results in scar formation; these lesions should be treated by cryosurgery or curettage instead.

Excisional biopsy

The lesion is removed and submitted for histopathological examination. The most common indication is the clinical suspicion of malignant disease (e.g. basal cell carcinoma). Most procedures can be carried out under local anaesthetic, but in certain sites local cutaneous blocks are useful (e.g. fingers, plantar aspects of the foot and the nose). Knowledge of local anatomy is important, particularly vessels and nerves. Certain body sites are associated with particular risks:

- biopsies on the upper torso of young persons are likely to lead to keloidal scarring
- biopsies over the scapulae tend to leave unsightly scars
- biopsies on the lower legs of older people are at risk of delayed healing and ulceration.

The lesion and the line of excision should be marked out. Basal cell carcinomas should usually be excised with a 4 mm margin, whereas initial biopsies of suspicious pigmented lesions may be excised with a 2 mm margin and then further excised with 1 or 2 cm margin following histopathological confirmation of melanoma (depending on the Breslow thickness, p. 1281). It is important to excise down to the appropriate anatomical plane. Depending on body sites, a range of procedures can be used to minimise the resulting defect, including undermining, Z-plasties, flaps and grafts. On some concave sites in the elderly, healing by secondary intention can lead to surprisingly good cosmetic results.

Mohs micrographic surgery

Mohs micrographic surgery aims to ensure adequate tumour excision margins, while conserving as much tissue as possible. It is most commonly used for the management of basal cell carcinomas and, to a lesser degree, for squamous cell carcinomas. Initially, the tumour may be debulked with curettage and then an excision is performed, orientated with ink or sutures; horizontal (rather than vertical) cross-sections are cut and examined immediately using the frozen section technique. Any areas of tumour that abut onto the edge can then be orientated back onto the patient and further tissue removal in that particular direction is undertaken. This iteration is continued until the margins are clear of tumour. The procedure is time-consuming and requires particular surgical and pathological skills but is popular. It should be considered especially for morphoeic or otherwise ill-defined basal cell carcinomas, and in sites where tissue conservation is important, such as close to the eye. It is not appropriate for melanoma. Subsequently, appropriate reconstruction can be undertaken in collaboration with oculoplastic/plastic surgery.

Cryotherapy

Cryotherapy is performed as an application of liquid nitrogen either with a cotton wool bud or using a jet gun. Liquid nitrogen can be used to treat a wide range of lesions from viral warts to actinic keratoses, including invasive tumours such as basal or squamous cell carcinomas. The cosmetic effects and morbidity are variable. If neoplasia is suspected, it is wiser to carry out an incisional biopsy first. In general, superficial or 'stuck-on' lesions will require less intense therapy that will be more acceptable to the patient. Melanocytic naevi should not be treated with liquid nitrogen.

Curettage

Curettage involves scraping a small, spoon-shaped implement (curette) across the lesion, not only as a definitive treatment but also as a way of obtaining histological material. The latter, however, may be compromised because epidermal structures are over-represented and the anatomy of the lesion as it descends into the dermis is not preserved; it may therefore be difficult to determine whether a lesion with intra-epidermal dysplasia shows any evidence of invasion. Curettage is suitable for many seborrhoeic keratoses, actinic keratoses or areas of intra-epidermal carcinoma. Some superficial basal cell carcinomas can be treated with curettage but other variants, such as morphoeic forms, require excision.

Laser therapy

Laser therapy exploits the fact that certain pigments, such as melanin or blood, absorb certain wavelengths of electromagnetic radiation more readily than others. A variety of lasers have been produced which allow selective destruction of structures containing the absorbing pigment. By concentrating the light into short pulses, the damage is restricted to a particular area. Some lasers are better for dealing with primarily vascular lesions, such as port wine stains, while others are more useful for pigmented lesions or for destruction of exogenous pigments, such as tattoo pigments or drug deposits (e.g. minocycline).

By contrast with the vascular laser, the carbon dioxide laser emits infrared light which is absorbed by tissue water. When crudely used, the carbon dioxide laser is therefore similar to a diathermy but the depth of lesion can be controlled to a fraction of a millimetre, and it can therefore be useful for resurfacing and for face lifts. A general anaesthetic is required.

Photodynamic therapy

Photodynamic therapy is based on the pathological processes that underpin the photosensitivity seen in porphyria, i.e. the presence of potent endogenous photosensitisers which results in tissue damage when exposed to light. In photodynamic therapy, topical photosensitisers are applied to the tumour, which is subsequently exposed to visible light. Some tumours may selectively absorb the photosensitiser, thus enhancing the therapeutic ration. Photodynamic therapy is particularly useful for relatively flat lesions, such as some intra-epithelial carcinomas and superficial basal cell carcinomas, and may be preferable to surgery or other treatment. The treatment is time-consuming, as the sensitiser needs to be applied for several hours before exposure to the light source; as with porphyria, exposure may be painful.

Miscellaneous procedures

Keloids (scar tissue that outgrows the original scar) may require corticosteroid injections after freezing or excision. Silicone sheeting may flatten keloids, although the mechanism is obscure. Scars and wrinkles can be filled using collagen or silicone. Liposuction can be used to remove fat, and tissue folds around the eyes can be easily excised. Small acne scars can be excised and larger, more superficial lesions treated with a carbon dioxide laser. Areas of depigmentation in vitiligo or piebaldism may be treated with epidermal grafts from normal skin.

ECZEMA

The terms 'eczema' and 'dermatitis' are synonymous. They refer to distinctive reaction patterns in the skin, which can be either acute or chronic and are due to a number of causes. In the acute stage, oedema of the epidermis (spongiosis) progresses to the formation of

27.19 Classification of eczema

• Atopic	• Asteatotic
• Seborrhoeic	• Gravitational
• Discoid	• Lichen simplex
• Irritant	• Pompholyx
• Allergic	

intra-epidermal vesicles, which may enlarge and rupture. In the chronic stage there is less oedema and vesiculation, but more thickening of the epidermis (acanthosis); this is accompanied by a variable degree of vasodilatation and T-cell lymphocytic infiltration in the upper dermis.

Clinical features

There are several patterns of eczema (Box 27.19); some have identifiable environmental causes, whereas others are more complex. The clinical signs are similar in all types and vary according to the duration of the rash. The features of acute and chronic eczema are listed in Box 27.20.

Atopic eczema

Atopy is a genetic predisposition to form excessive IgE, which leads to a generalised and prolonged hypersensitivity to common environmental antigens such as pollen and house dust mite. Atopic individuals manifest one or more of a group of diseases that includes asthma, hay fever, food and other allergies, and atopic eczema. Although any of these conditions tends to be over-represented in families of those with any atopic disease, one particular disease type tends to run more strongly in a particular family. The diagnosis of atopic eczema is made using clinical criteria (Box 27.21). The prevalence of atopic eczema has increased between

27.20 The eczema reaction

Acute

• Redness and swelling, usually with ill-defined margins
• Papules, vesicles and, more rarely, large blisters
• Exudation and cracking
• Scaling

Chronic

• May show all of the above, but usually less vesicular and exudative
• Lichenification, a dry leathery thickening with increased skin markings, secondary to rubbing and scratching
• Fissures and scratch marks
• Hypo- or hyperpigmentation

27.21 Diagnostic criteria for atopic eczema

Itchy skin and at least three of the following:
• History of itch in skin creases (or cheeks if < 4 yrs)
• History of asthma/hay fever (or in a first-degree relative if < 4 yrs)
• Dry skin (xeroderma)
• Visible flexural eczema (cheeks, forehead, outer limbs if < 4 yrs)
• Onset in first 2 yrs of life

twofold and fivefold over the last 30 years, and the disease now affects 1 in 10 schoolchildren.

Aetiology

Genetic factors are important, with concordance in 86% of monozygotic but only 21% of dizygotic twins. Atopic diseases show a degree of maternal imprinting, i.e. they are inherited more often from the mother than the father. A pair of null alleles in the filaggrin gene (R501X and 2282del4), predisposing to atopic eczema and to asthma in association with eczema, have been identified. Filaggrin is an important component of the barrier of the skin (p. 1240) and these findings suggest that this structural defect is important in the development of atopic eczema. Environmental factors, such as exposure to allergens either in utero or during childhood, also have an aetiological role and 60–80% of individuals are genetically susceptible to the induction of IgE-mediated sensitisation to environmental allergens such as food and animal hair.

It is thought that the decreased barrier function of the skin may allow greater penetration of environmental allergens through the epidermis, and so cause stimulation of the immune system in susceptible individuals, precipitating an inflammatory response. In addition, IgE autoantibody production occurs in some individuals, perhaps related to scratching, but whether this is the basis of the 'atopic march' from eczema to food allergies and asthma has yet to be confirmed.

Clinical features

The cardinal feature of atopic eczema is itch, and scratching accounts for many of the signs. Widespread dryness (felt as roughness) of the skin is another feature. The distribution and character of the rash vary with age (Box 27.22; Figs 27.11 and 27.12). Complications are listed in Box 27.23.

Seborrhoeic eczema

This is characterised by a red scaly rash and classically affects the scalp (dandruff), central face, nasolabial folds, eyebrows and central chest. It is due to *Pityrosporum ovale* infection of the skin. When severe, it may resemble psoriasis. Seborrhoeic eczema is a feature of AIDS, in which case it can be very severe.

Discoid eczema

This common form of eczema is recognised from discrete coin-shaped eczematous lesions, particularly on the limbs of young and elderly men. It can occur in children with atopic eczema and may be difficult to treat.

27.22 Atopic eczema: distribution and character of rash

Infancy

• Often acute and involves the face and trunk
• Frequent sparing of the napkin area

Childhood

• Backs of the knees, fronts of the elbows, wrists and ankles (see Fig. 27.11)

Adults

• Face and trunk (see Fig. 27.12) are involved; lichenification is common

27

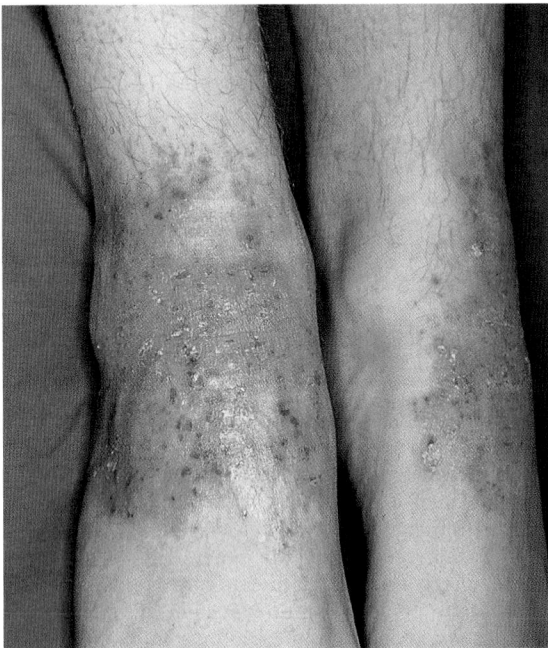

Fig. 27.11 Atopic subacute eczema on the fronts of the ankles of a teenager. These are sites of predilection, along with the cubital and popliteal fossae, in atopic eczema.

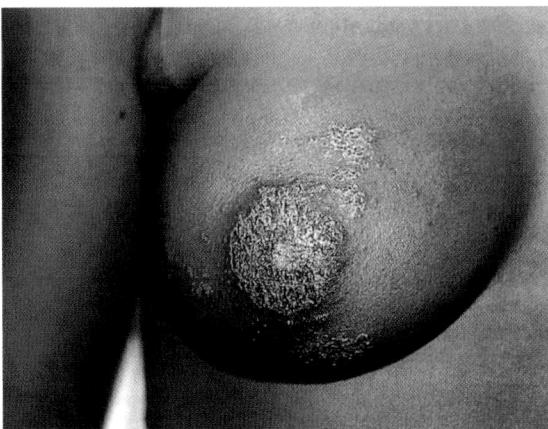

Fig. 27.12 Nipple eczema. This is frequently bilateral in atopic dermatitis.

Irritant eczema

Strong irritants elicit an acute reaction at the site of contact, whereas weak irritants most often cause chronic eczema, especially of the hands, after prolonged exposure. Detergents, alkalis, acids, solvents and abrasive dusts are common causes. There is a wide range of susceptibility to weak irritants. Irritant eczema accounts for the majority of occupational cases and work loss. The elderly, those with fair and dry skin, and those with an atopic background are especially vulnerable.

27.23 Complications of atopic eczema	

Superinfection

Bacterial
- (*Staphylococcus aureus*) most common

Viral
- Herpes simplex virus causes a widespread severe eruption—eczema herpeticum
- Papillomavirus and molluscum contagiosum may be encouraged by use of local corticosteroids

Irritant reactions
- Defective barrier function

Sleep disturbance
- Loss of schooling and behavioural difficulties

Food allergy
- Eggs, cow's milk, protein, fish, wheat and soya may cause an immediate urticarial eruption rather than exacerbation of eczema

Allergic contact eczema

This is due to a delayed hypersensitivity reaction following contact with antigens or haptens. Previous exposure to the allergen is required for sensitisation and the reaction is specific to the allergen or closely related chemicals. Common allergens are listed in Box 27.24.

The eczema reaction occurs wherever the allergen is in contact with the skin and sensitisation persists indefinitely. It is important to determine the original site of the rash before secondary spread obscures the picture, as this often provides the best clue to the allergen. There are many easily recognisable patterns, e.g. eczema of the earlobes, wrists and back due to contact with nickel in costume jewellery, watches and bra clips; or eczema of the hands and wrists due to rubber gloves. Oedema of the lax skin of the eyelids and genitalia is a frequent concomitant of allergic contact eczema (Fig. 27.13).

Asteatotic eczema

This is frequently seen in the hospitalised elderly, especially when the skin is dry; low humidity caused by central heating, over-washing and diuretics are contributory

27.24 Common allergens	
Allergen	**Present in**
Nickel	Jewellery, jean studs, bra clips
Dichromate	Cement, leather, matches
Rubber chemicals	Clothing, shoes, tyres
Colophony	Sticking plaster, collodion
Paraphenylenediamine	Hair dye, clothing
Balsam of Peru	Perfumes, citrus fruits
Neomycin, benzocaine	Topical applications
Parabens	Preservative in cosmetics and creams
Wool alcohols	Lanolin, cosmetics, creams
Epoxy resin	Resin adhesives

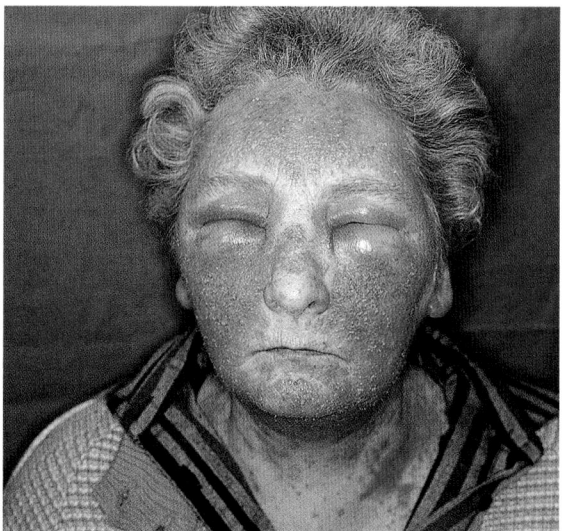

Fig. 27.13 Allergic contact eczema. This was caused by the application of an antihistamine cream. The acute eczematous reaction and bilateral periorbital oedema are typical.

factors. It occurs most often on the lower legs as a rippled or 'crazy paving' pattern of fine fissuring on an erythematous background.

Gravitational (stasis) eczema

This occurs on the lower legs and is often associated with signs of venous insufficiency: oedema, red or bluish discoloration, loss of hair, induration, haemosiderin pigmentation and ulceration.

Lichen simplex

This describes a plaque of lichenified eczema due to repeated rubbing or scratching, as a habit or in response to stress (Fig. 27.14). Common sites include the nape of the neck, the lower legs and the anogenital area.

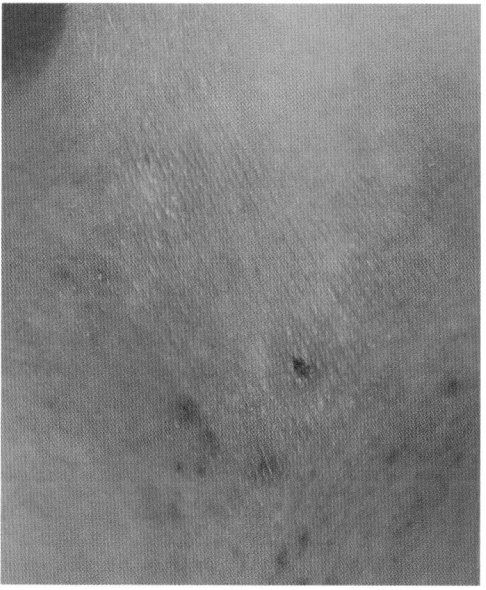

Fig. 27.14 Lichen simplex chronicus on the neck showing increased skin markings and excoriations.

Pompholyx

Recurrent vesicles and bullae occur on the palms, palmar surface of the fingers and soles, and are excruciatingly itchy. This form of eczema can occur in atopic eczema and in irritant and contact allergic dermatitis. It can be provoked by heat, stress and nickel ingestion in a nickel-sensitive patient but is often idiopathic.

Investigation of eczema

Patch tests are performed in suspected cases of contact allergic dermatitis (Box 27.25). Prick tests or IgE and specific IgE tests are occasionally performed to support the diagnosis of atopic eczema and to determine specific environmental allergens, e.g. pet dander, horse hair, house dust mite, pollens and foods. Bacterial and viral swabs for microscopy and culture are useful in suspected secondary infection. Bacteria are invariably present, but antibacterial treatment should be reserved for those cases with evidence of clinical infection. Individuals with atopic eczema have an increased susceptibility to herpes simplex virus (HSV), and are at risk of developing a widespread infection, eczema herpeticum. The presence of small punched-out lesions on a background of worsening eczema suggests the possibility of secondary HSV infection.

General management of eczema

Regular use of bland emollients (e.g. emulsifying ointment) is the mainstay of treatment in all forms of eczema. They prevent excessive water loss from an already dry skin and help to reduce the amount of local corticosteroid used. Emollients are used as a bath additive, a soap substitute and directly onto the skin.

Topical corticosteroids

Lotions and creams are preferable in acute eczema, and ointments in chronic, and are usually applied once or twice daily. Only 1% hydrocortisone should be used on the face, except under expert advice. It is seldom necessary to prescribe more than 200 g of a low-potency corticosteroid (e.g. 1% hydrocortisone), 50 g of a moderately potent corticosteroid (e.g. 0.05% clobetasone butyrate) or 30 g of a potent corticosteroid (e.g. 0.1% betamethasone valerate, 0.1% mometasone furoate) per

27

EBM 27.25 Contact dermatitis

Patch tests

'Pre-prepared patch tests are significantly more reliable than operator-prepared tests.'

'False negative results occur if a potent topical steroid is applied 2 days or less before testing.'

Management of hand dermatitis

'Second-line treatments, such as psoralen UVA (PUVA), azathioprine and ciclosporin, are useful in steroid-resistant chronic hand dermatitis.'

• Bourke J, et al. Brit J Dermatol 2001; 145(6):102–105.

For further information: www.BAD.org.uk

⏳ **27.26 Eczema in old age**

- **Loss of elasticity:** with advancing age, the skin becomes less pliable and drier. This increases the tendency to irritant dermatitis.
- **Topical corticosteroid usage:** causes more local side-effects, such as purpura or ecchymoses.
- **Prognosis:** widespread eczema is potentially life-threatening, particularly in the presence of comorbidity.

week. Very potent topical corticosteroids (e.g. 0.05% clobetasol propionate) should not be used long-term. The side-effects of strong or extensive local corticosteroid therapy are important when patients are applying these as a long-term measure, and include skin thinning (with striae, fragility and purpura), enhanced or disguised infections, and systemic absorption (causing suppression of the hypothalamic–pituitary–adrenal axis and Cushingoid features). There are no absolute guidelines for the amount of topical corticosteroid that should be used and there is marked variation in sensitivity to their harmful effects, but particular care should be taken on certain sites such as the face and flexures and in the elderly (Box 27.26). The least potent corticosteroid that is effective should be used for the shortest possible time.

Other topical immunosuppressants, including the topical calcineurin inhibitors tacrolimus (a macrolide with immunosuppressant activity) and pimecrolimus (an ascomycin with anti-inflammatory properties), are available. They are expensive but useful in the second-line treatment of facial atopic eczema and contact allergic dermatitis.

Sedative antihistamines (e.g. alimemazine tartrate) are useful if sleep is interrupted, but evidence for their use is limited.

Atopic eczema

Patient information and support are vital and are provided by the health-care system and patient support groups such as the National Eczema Society in the UK. Treatment involves the regular use of emollients and the least possible use of topical steroids. Topical steroids are needed for inflamed areas and can be used with a variety of types of dressing, such as tar and ichthammol paste bandages. Allergen avoidance may have a role in selected patients. Pimecrolimus cream and tacrolimus ointment are used as second-line treatments. Phototherapy is useful as a temporary third-line measure in adolescents and adults, but should never be used in individuals continuing to require topical calcineurin inhibitors. Rarely, systemic treatments are required, including intermittent ciclosporin A, oral steroids, azathioprine or methotrexate. Azathioprine is useful in adult chronic eczema. Baseline measurement of thiopurine methyl transferase (TPMT) levels is useful in determining azathioprine dose and avoiding toxicity.

Seborrhoeic eczema

Antipityrosporal agents, such as ketoconazole shampoo and creams, form the basis of treatment, supplemented with weak corticosteroids if needed. Treatments may need to be repeated at intervals.

Irritant eczema

This is treated by the regular use of emollients, protective clothing (e.g. gloves) and avoidance of irritants.

Contact allergic eczema

Avoidance of the culprit allergen is the most important intervention; this may entail lifestyle modifications, such as a change in occupation or hobbies. Measures used for irritant eczema are also helpful.

Gravitational eczema

Topical corticosteroids should only be applied to eczematous areas and should be avoided on ulcers. Sensitisation to topical antibiotics (neomycin) and preservatives (e.g. chlorocresol) is common. Associated peripheral oedema is treated by elevation of the leg and graded compression bandages.

PSORIASIS AND OTHER ERYTHEMATOUS SCALY ERUPTIONS

Psoriasis

Psoriasis is a non-infectious, chronic inflammatory disease of the skin, characterised by well-defined erythematous plaques with silvery scale, with a predilection for the extensor surfaces and scalp, and a chronic fluctuating course. The prevalence is approximately 2% in European populations but may be lower in African and some Asian populations, e.g. Japanese. Psoriasis may start at any age but is unusual before 5 years. There are two epidemiological patterns of psoriasis, sometimes referred to as type 1 and type 2. The first has an onset in the teenage and early adult years, often with a family history of psoriasis and an increased prevalence of the HLA group Cw6. The onset of the second is in the fifties or sixties, when a family history is less common and HLA Cw6 is not so prominent.

The clinical course of psoriasis is very variable. In general, the earlier the age of onset and the more severe the initial presentation, the more severe is the lifetime course of the disease.

Aetiology

Psoriasis is genetically complex and a large number of genes are thought to be important in its pathogenesis. There is a large familial component. Formal estimates from twin studies suggest a hereditability of around 80%, and in monozygotes perhaps one-third will be concordant for psoriasis. Empirical estimates suggest that if one parent has psoriasis, then the chance of a child being affected is in the order of 15–20%; if both parents have the disease, this figure rises to 50%. Both estimates are increased if one sibling already has the disease.

The histological changes of psoriasis are shown in Figure 27.15. There are two key pathophysiological features in psoriatic plaques:

- The keratinocytes hyperproliferate with a grossly increased mitotic index and an abnormal pattern of differentiation, leading to the retention of nuclei in the stratum corneum, not normally present as the stratum corneum cells are dead.
- There is a large inflammatory cell infiltrate.

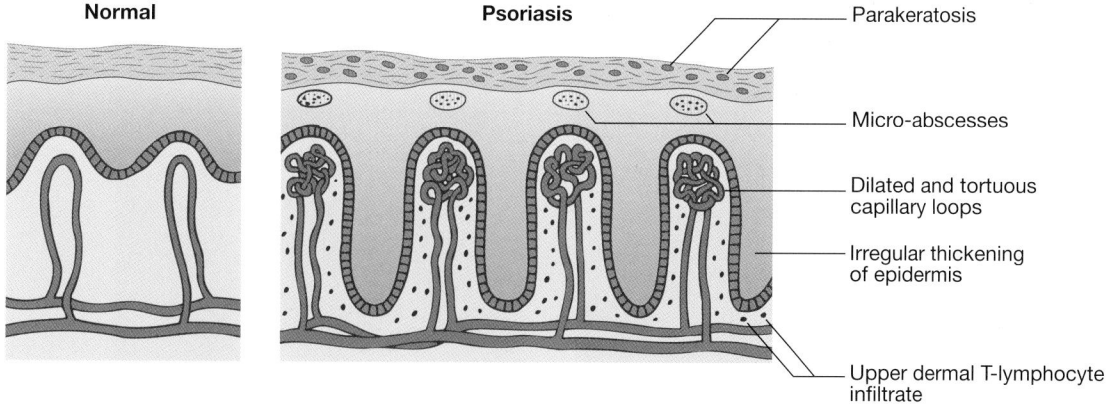

Fig. 27.15 The histology of psoriasis.

It is uncertain which of these is primary. Traditionally, psoriasis was viewed as a disorder of cell turnover, but it may be that the hyperproliferation is secondary to the inflammatory infiltrate and a consequence of inflammatory cell mediators or signalling.

Disordered cell proliferation in psoriasis is reflected by the increase in the number of mitoses visible in the psoriatic plaque. The transit time, i.e. the time it takes for keratinocytes in the basal layer to leave the epidermis, is shortened in psoriasis from perhaps 28 to 5 days, so that cells that are not fully mature or functional reach the stratum corneum prematurely. The non-plaque skin also shows an elevated rate of proliferation, but this is modest. The nails of patients with psoriasis, even when clinically unaffected, grow more quickly than those of controls.

The evidence implicating a key role for an immune pathogenesis includes the association with HLA Cw6; the success of immunosuppressive drugs, e.g. ciclosporin in treatment; the development of psoriasis in recipients of bone marrow transplants from donors with psoriasis and the precise molecular mechanisms by which the immune system causes the putative cutaneous abnormalities are unclear.

Psoriasis is characterised by variation in both temporal and spatial extent, most of which cannot be explained. At any one time, around 10% of people who have psoriasis have no lesions, and perhaps 15% report remissions of 5 years or more. Factors thought to precipitate exacerbations are listed in Box 27.27. A causal role for stress in exacerbations is not established. Certain studies suggest that alcohol consumption is greater amongst some psoriasis patients, but it is not clear whether this is a cause or result of the disease.

Clinical features

There are several different forms of psoriasis.

Stable plaque psoriasis

This is the most common. Individual lesions are well demarcated and range from a few millimetres to several centimetres in diameter (Fig. 27.16). They are red, with a dry silvery-white scale, which may only be obvious after scraping the surface. The elbows, knees and lower back are commonly involved. Other sites of predilection include:

27.27 Factors causing exacerbations of psoriasis

Trauma

- Lesions appear in areas of skin damage such as scratches or surgical wounds (Köbner phenomenon) when the condition is erupting

Infection

- β-haemolytic streptococcal throat infections often precede guttate psoriasis

Sunlight

- UVR rarely

Drugs

- Antimalarials, β-adrenoceptor antagonists (β-blockers) and lithium
- 'Rebound' after systemic corticosteroids or potent local corticosteroids are stopped

Emotion

- Anxiety

- *Scalp.* This is involved in approximately 60% of patients and it is not clear why this is so common. It typically shows well-demarcated, easily palpable areas, but on occasion a diffuse, fine scaling difficult to distinguish from classical seborrhoeic dermatitis may be present. Temporary hair loss is not uncommon and rarely permanent focal hair loss may occur.
- *Nails.* Involvement is common, with 'thimble pitting', onycholysis (separation of the nail from the nail bed, Fig. 27.17) and subungual hyperkeratosis.
- *Flexures.* Psoriasis involving the natal cleft and submammary and axillary folds is not scaly but red, shiny and symmetrical.
- *Palms.* Individual plaques may be poorly demarcated and barely erythematous, making this type of psoriasis difficult to differentiate from eczema of the palms.

Guttate psoriasis

This is most commonly seen in children and adolescents, and may follow a streptococcal sore throat. In

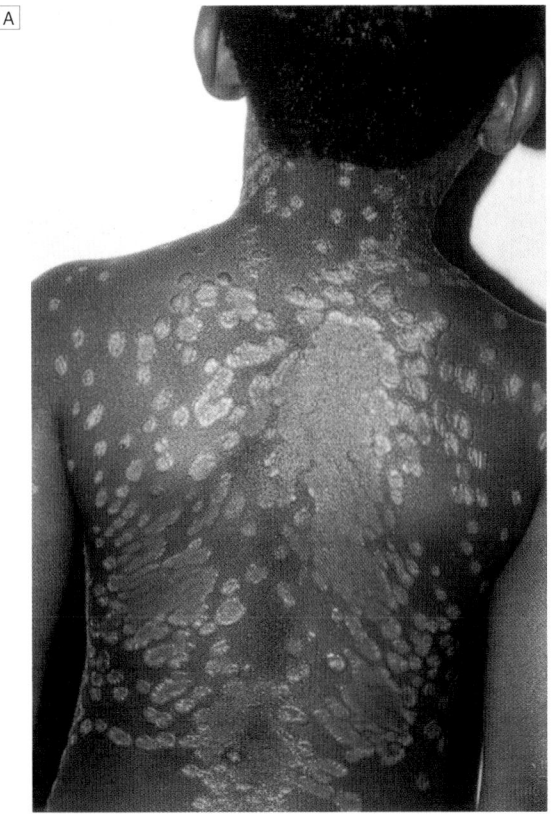

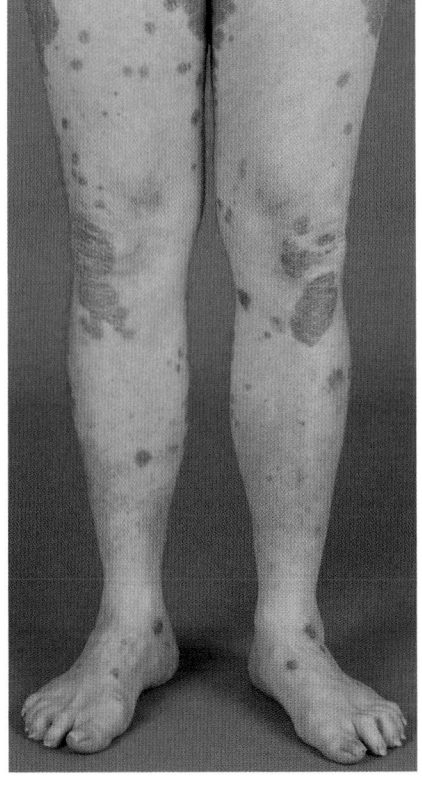

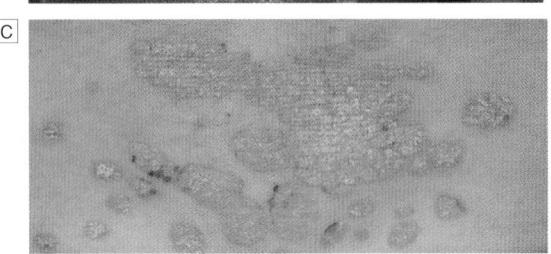

Fig. 27.16 Psoriasis. [A] Plaques of varying size in a child. [B] Plaques on the flexor surfaces of the knees. [C] Plaque detail.

many, it is the first presentation of the disease. The rash often appears rapidly. Individual lesions are droplet-shaped, seldom over 1 cm in diameter and scaly. Bouts of guttate psoriasis may clear within a few months but respond well to early treatment with phototherapy. The

majority of patients go on to develop plaque psoriasis later in life.

Erythrodermic psoriasis

The skin becomes universally red or scaly, or more rarely just red with very little scale. As in other forms of erythroderma, temperature regulation becomes compromised with a danger of either hypothermia or hyperthermia.

Pustular psoriasis

There are two varieties of pustular psoriasis. The generalised form is rare but serious. The onset is usually sudden, with large numbers of small sterile pustules erupting on a red base. The patient may rapidly become ill with a pyrexia coinciding with the appearance of new pustules, and will usually require urgent assessment and hospital admission. A localised form, which primarily affects the palms and soles, is more common. This is chronic and comprises small sterile pustules which lie on a red base, and resolve to leave brown macules or scaling. The relationship between pustular psoriasis of the palms and the soles (palmoplantar pustulosis) and psoriasis remains disputed, although they commonly coexist.

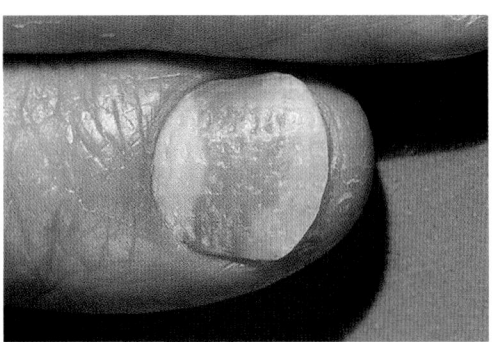

Fig. 27.17 Coarse pitting of the nail and separation of the nail from the nail bed (onycholysis). These are both classic features of psoriasis.

Arthropathy

Between 5 and 10% of individuals with psoriasis develop a chronic seronegative inflammatory arthropathy which can take on a number of patterns (p. 1095).

Investigations

Biopsy is seldom necessary and contributes little. Throat swabbing for streptococci or other evidence of recent infection may occasionally be useful in suspected guttate psoriasis. Joint symptoms, unless minor, require a formal rheumatology assessment.

General management of psoriasis

Explanation, reassurance and instruction are vital. Patients may be very distressed by their appearance and doctors should be aware of the impact that psoriasis can have. Parents may admit that they cannot take their young children swimming because of the alarm their rash causes to other swimmers. Similarly, blood on bed sheets and the ubiquitous scale on bedclothes and carpets may adversely affect personal relationships.

In the vast majority of cases, psoriasis is not life-threatening and therefore, if the treatment is worse than the disease, it should be stopped. Patients should be encouraged to share decision-making about treatment with their physician.

Treatment

Treatment can be classed in four broad categories (Box 27.28). Traditionally, therapies such as inpatient dithranol, when combined with UVR in Ingram's regimen, were capable of inducing clearance of the disease in most patients. The duration of remission varied considerably from less than 1 month to over a year. By contrast, more acceptable treatments such as calcipotriol rarely clear psoriasis, but do reduce the thickness, scaling and redness of the individual plaques to a varying degree. Depending on the extent of disease, the patient and physician need to choose an appropriate endpoint of treatment, and this may be a compromise between side-effects and practical considerations, such as time available to attend hospital.

Topical agents

A large number of topical agents are used to treat psoriasis. Emollients have a modest effect in reducing scale and diminishing itch, and many patients feel more comfortable using them.

Dithranol and tar

These were the traditional gold standard of therapy. Both are potent producers of free radicals, which are pro-inflammatory and stimulate hyperproliferation when applied to normal skin but, for reasons that remain unclear, normalise differentiation and inhibit proliferation when applied to psoriatic plaques.

Dithranol is used in two main regimens. In Ingram's regimen, the plaques are covered with low concentrations of dithranol in a zinc oxide paste following a tar bath and UVR exposure, and then covered in talcum powder and bandages, which are left in situ for 24 hours. More recently, short-contact dithranol therapy has been developed, in which higher concentrations are applied for between 15 and 30 minutes and then washed off. The main clinical limitation of dithranol is its pro-inflammatory action on normal skin, which causes 'burning' with pain and erythema that peaks 72 hours after application. Dithranol also results in brown staining of the skin and can cause a purple discoloration in individuals with light hair colour. Use of dithranol or coal tar as an inpatient treatment has drastically diminished over the last 30 years due to low patient acceptability, the increasing use of outpatient phototherapy, and the therapeutic options provided by newer immunomodulatory treatments. Attempts have been made to make dithranol and tar easier to use and more cosmetically acceptable, but efficacy is reduced.

Calcipotriol

Calcipotriol is a vitamin D agonist. It seldom clears plaques of psoriasis but reduces plaque thickness and diminishes scaling. It is applied twice or once daily and, providing no more than 100 g of ointment is used each week, does not cause hypercalcaemia or hypercalciuria. Patients like calcipotriol because it is odourless and colourless, and does not stain. Irritation, usually transient, is the main side-effect. It is a mainstay of primary care management of psoriasis and may be combined with corticosteroids.

Corticosteroids

Corticosteroids may cause local skin atrophy, and when they are stopped the psoriasis tends to return. Nevertheless, they are invaluable for many sites, particularly the flexures, and short bursts of moderately potent corticosteroids can be invaluable. Use of potent topical corticosteroids on the face or hair margins requires close medical supervision.

Ultraviolet and PUVA therapy

UV therapy

Ultraviolet radiation (UVR) is the mainstay of outpatient management of those with moderate to severe psoriasis. The main risks are burning in the short term, and increased skin cancers in the long term.

It has been known for almost a century that ultraviolet B (UVB) administered therapeutically improves psoriasis in many patients, and many sufferers notice a spontaneous improvement in summer. More recently, a particular type of UVB radiation produced by the Philips TL01 lamp (narrowband UVB), delivered 2–5

27.28 Treatment categories in psoriasis

Topical agents

- Emollients, corticosteroids, vitamin D agonists, 'weak' tar or dithranol preparations

UV therapies

- UVB or PUVA

Systemic agents

- Methotrexate, retinoids
- Immunosuppressives, e.g. ciclosporin, mycophenolate
- Newer 'biological' agents, e.g. infliximab, etanercept

Intensive inpatient or day-patient care

- Topical agents and UVR under medical supervision

times a week on an outpatient basis, has become a popular treatment. This lamp peaks at 311 nm, as shorter radiation, while inflammatory, has little therapeutic efficacy. The long-term safety of this lamp is unclear, particularly with regard to whether it is more or less carcinogenic than traditional broadband UVB sources.

PUVA therapy

Psoralens are natural photosensitisers found in a number of plants. Psoralen molecules intercalate between the two strands of DNA and, upon excitation with UVA, photons cross-link the DNA strands. It is thus a pro-drug that is distributed throughout the body after oral administration, but only activated by UVR in skin that is exposed to UVA. Alternatively, psoralens can be applied in a bath before irradiation with UVA ('bath PUVA').

PUVA treatment induces clearance to a similar degree to intensive dithranol therapy. Short-term side-effects are minimal. The therapy can be delivered between 2 and 5 times a week and clearance may be expected in more than 75% of individuals within 8 weeks. Some patients may develop nausea in response to the psoralen. Because the psoralen is present in the eye, patients must wear UVR-resistant sunglasses for 24 hours after therapy. The long-term hazards of PUVA therapy are the result of its mutagenicity; patients who have received a large amount of PUVA therapy, particularly 'maintenance therapy' (continuous PUVA lasting for 6 months to a year), are at increased risk of squamous and basal cell carcinoma. The risk of melanoma may also be increased. Because of this and the increasing availability of other modalities of treatment, the use of PUVA is decreasing in many countries.

Systemic treatment

There are now a large number of systemic agents that can be used for psoriasis. These range from the classical agents, such as methotrexate and hydroxyurea, through standard immunosuppressives such as ciclosporin and mycophenolate to the newer 'biological' therapies.

Methotrexate

Methotrexate is highly effective and is given once weekly. Its mechanism of action is primarily on the immune system (p. 1079) rather than having a direct effect on keratinocyte or epidermal hyperproliferation. The main hazards are immunosuppression and bone marrow suppression, particularly due to interactions with other commonly used drugs such as non-steroidal anti-inflammatories (NSAIDs). Long-term use is associated with hepatic fibrosis and cirrhosis. Because of this, regular monitoring of liver function tests and full blood count is required. An alternative is hydroxyurea, but this is less effective and carries an increased risk of bone marrow suppression.

Oral retinoids

Oral retinoids, such as acitretin, are effective in some patients with psoriasis, particularly pustular psoriasis of the palms and soles, but are also widely used to improve plaque psoriasis. Systemic retinoids are potent teratogens. Following use of acitretin, pregnancy is not safe for at least 2 years. Retinoids may cause raised triglycerides and rarely hepatitis, so regular monitoring of lipids and liver function tests is required.

Ciclosporin

Ciclosporin (p. 1080) is an immunosuppressive used in psoriasis and other inflammatory skin disease. Side-effects include hypertension, nephrotoxicity and immunosuppression, leading to opportunistic infection and an increased risk of skin and other cancers in the long term. Ciclosporin is highly effective in inducing and maintaining clearance of individuals with psoriasis, but continuous use is difficult to justify. It may be used over a 3–4-month period to induce clearance or prior to treatment with other systemic agents.

Biological therapies

Recently, a range of new agents, including monoclonal antibodies, fusion proteins and cytokines, have been shown to have striking activity against psoriasis and appear as effective as classical agents. The long-term role of biological therapies in psoriasis is not yet defined; they are currently extremely expensive and long-term toxicity has still to be established. Of these agents, the anti-tumour necrosis factor (TNF) therapies are the best studied. These include etanercept, which is a human recombinant TNF receptor fusion protein, while infliximab is a human-murine anti-TNF-α monoclonal antibody. Both bind TNF, preventing its action, and both seem highly effective in clearing psoriasis. They have to be given either by infusion or by subcutaneous injection, which may cause adverse reactions. Potential side-effects include reactivation of latent tuberculosis and the development of other opportunistic infections.

Pityriasis rosea

This is an acute, benign, self-limiting exanthem that particularly affects adults and occurs world-wide. It usually occurs during the spring and summer, but although this suggests an infective aetiology, no causal agent has been identified and its aetiology is unknown. It is more common in women than men (1.4:1).

Clinical features and management

Pityriasis rosea is characterised by the appearance of a 'herald patch', an oval lesion (1–2 cm) with a central pinkish (salmon-coloured) centre, a darker periphery and a characteristic collarette of scale. It is followed 1–2 weeks later by a widespread symmetrical papulosquamous eruption which is characteristically arranged in a symmetrical 'fir-tree' pattern on the torso. Individual lesions show a collarette of scale. An inverse variant is recognised with flexural involvement. Mucosal involvement is rare. There is a 3% recurrence rate. No treatment is required, although itch may be helped by emollients and mild topical steroids. Post-inflammatory hyperpigmentation can be a problem, particularly in darker skin types.

Secondary syphilis

Syphilis is caused by the spirochaete *Treponema pallidum*, which is transmitted sexually or in utero. There has been a massive increase in its incidence since 2000 due to HIV co-infection and increasing high-risk sexual behaviour. The initial site of infection is identified by a chancre occurring at the site of inoculation up to 3 months later. Between 4 and 10 weeks after inoculation, the rash of secondary syphilis develops, and 40% of untreated cases progress to tertiary syphilis. Secondary syphilis is a widespread eruption which consists of macules, papules and occasionally pustules. It affects the trunk and proximal limbs, and characteristically involves the palms, soles and face. The lesions are red, changing to a 'gun-metal' grey as they resolve. Systemic symptoms, such as malaise, fever, myalgia, arthralgia and lymphadenopathy, are usual.

Serological diagnosis and current recommendations for treatment are described on pages 418–420.

Pityriasis versicolor

Pityriasis versicolor is a benign superficial skin condition caused by sensitivity to a common skin commensal, *Malassezia furfur*, the generic term for several yeast-like fungi. It occurs with equal incidence in men and women and in different races. It is more common in warmer months and in areas with higher humidity, and tends to be more severe in the immunocompromised. It is characterised by scaly hypo- and hyperpigmented macules predominantly on the upper torso. Treatment is with selenium sulphide or ketoconazole shampoos, and topical or systemic azole antifungal agents. The change in pigmentation can persist for months after treatment.

Pityriasis lichenoides chronica

This is a rare condition that usually presents within the first three decades of life. The aetiology is unclear but the condition is part of a spectrum, all of which remit spontaneously. The more acute variety (pityriasis lichenoides et varioliformis acuta, PLEVA) presents as papules which rapidly evolve with central necrosis, each attack lasting up to 3 months. The more chronic variety presents as a persistent widespread scaly eruption. Characteristically, the lesions are papules, slightly brown in colour and covered with a mica-like scale (like a stuck-on 'cornflake'). The condition fluctuates but can persist for several months or even years. Treatment with UVB is effective at inducing temporary remissions. Topical emollients and steroids, and long-term oral erythromycin can occasionally be helpful.

Tinea corporis (p. 1273)

This fungal infection may cause a scaly rash.

Maculopapular drug eruptions

These are not common but are an important differential diagnosis in the erythematous scaly eruption (p. 1286). They often evolve with exfoliation ('peeling' of the skin) and may leave post-inflammatory hyperpigmentation.

LICHEN PLANUS AND LICHENOID ERUPTIONS

Lichen planus

Lichen planus is a rash characterised by intensely itchy polygonal papules with a violaceous hue involving the skin and, less commonly, the mucosae, hair and nails.

Aetiology and pathology

The cause is unknown but an immune pathogenesis is suspected, as there is an association with some auto-immune diseases such as myasthenia gravis (p. 1231) and with thymoma and graft-versus-host disease (GVHD) (p. 1014). There is hyperkeratosis, a prominent granular layer, basal cell degeneration and a heavy T-lymphocyte infiltration in the upper dermis. Degenerating basal cells are seen as colloid (apoptotic) bodies. The T cell–basal cell interaction leaves a 'sawtooth' dermo-epidermal junction, suggesting an immune reaction to an unknown epidermal antigen.

Clinical features

Lichen planus tends to start on the distal limbs, most commonly on the volar aspects of the wrists (Fig. 27.18) and on the lower back. Intensely itchy, flat-topped, pink-purplish papules appear and some develop a characteristic fine white network on their surface (Wickham's striae). New lesions may appear at the site of trauma (Köbner phenomenon) and the rash may spread rapidly to become generalised. Individual lesions may last for many months, and the eruption as a whole tends to last about 1 year, often leaving marked post-inflammatory pigmentation. Mucous membrane involvement, comprising an asymptomatic fine white lacy network of pinhead-sized white papules, occurs in about two-thirds of patients (see figure, p. 1238). The nails are affected in 10%, with changes ranging from longitudinal grooving to destruction of the nail fold and bed. Variants of the classic picture are rare but often diagnostically challenging, and include annular, atrophic, bullous, follicular, hypertrophic and ulcerative types.

Diagnosis

This is usually clear-cut clinically but a skin biopsy can be helpful. Other erythematous scaly conditions should be considered, including guttate psoriasis, pityriasis rosea, pityriasis lichenoides and drug eruptions.

Management

The condition is usually self-limiting, although rarely, particularly with oral lichen planus, it may persist for more than 10 years. Potent local corticosteroids may help with the intense itch but systemic corticosteroids may be indicated, and ciclosporin, retinoids or phototherapy may be required. Topical corticosteroids applied to the buccal mucosa may also be needed.

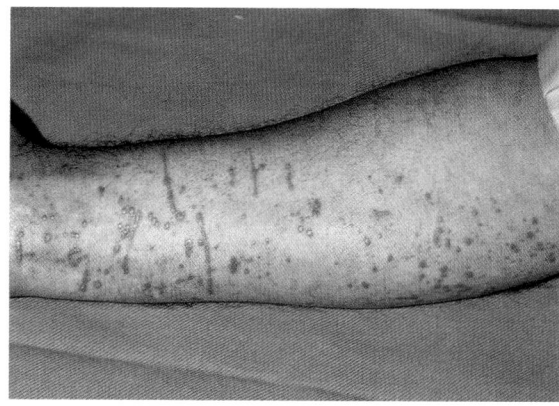

Fig. 27.18 Lichen planus. Glistening discrete papules involving the volar aspects of the forearm and wrist. Note the lesions along scratch marks (Köbner phenomenon).

Lichenoid eruptions

Rashes with clinical and histological features of lichen planus can occur in chronic active hepatitis, in hepatitis B and C infections, and with specific drugs, the most common culprits being gold, proton pump inhibitors, sulphonamides, penicillamine, antimalarials, antituberculous drugs and thiazide diuretics. They also occur in people handling colour developers.

Graft-versus-host disease (GVHD)

In the acute stage of GVHD, there is a distinctive dermatitis associated with hepatitis. After about 3 months, chronic GVHD can present with a lichenoid eruption on the palms, soles, face and upper trunk. Progressive sclerodermatous thickening of the skin can lead to contractures and limited mobility.

URTICARIA

The symptoms and signs of urticaria are due largely to mast cell degranulation with release of histamine and a variety of other vasoactive mediators (Fig. 27.19). More than histamine is clearly involved, as although potent histamine blockers frequently improve the itch of urticaria and the number of weals, they do not abolish them. Causes, clinical features and assessment are described on page 1248. There is an autoimmune pathogenesis for the most common form of disease, chronic idiopathic urticaria, which is defined by the presence of urticarial episodes for more than 6 weeks; self-reacting antibodies appear to cause cross-linking of the surface IgE receptor on mast cells with subsequent cellular degranulation.

Investigations

These should be directed at the possible underlying cause, as elicited from the clinical history. Some or all of the following may be appropriate:

- *full blood count*, including eosinophil count in case of underlying parasites
- *erythrocyte sedimentation rate* (ESR): may be elevated in cases of vasculitis
- *urea and electrolytes, thyroid and liver function tests*: may reveal an underlying systemic disorder
- *total IgE and specific IgE to possible allergens*, e.g shellfish or peanuts
- *antinuclear factor*: may be positive in chronic urticaria or urticarial vasculitis
- *CH50*: indicates the level of complement activation; C_3 and C_4 levels may reveal complement consumption
- C_1 *esterase inhibitor*: may be quantitatively reduced or more rarely functionally deficient, as in hereditary angioedema
- *skin biopsy*: helpful if urticarial vasculitis is suspected
- *appropriate challenge test*: to confirm physical urticarias.

Frequently no cause can be found for acute episodes, whereas in chronic urticaria an autoimmune pathogenesis will account for the majority of cases.

Management

Non-sedative antihistamines, such as loratadine, fexofenadine or cetirizine, are effective for perhaps one-third of patients with chronic urticaria; one-third show moderate benefit, whilst the remaining third show minimal benefit. If a patient fails to respond to one of these agents after 2 weeks of therapy, then it may be worth changing to another non-sedative antihistamine and adding in an H_2-blocker such as cimetidine or ranitidine. Other agents have been used, including mast cell stabilisers or protease and leukotriene inhibitors, but efficacy is not clear. Systemic corticosteroids are widely prescribed for urticaria, although there is little evidence of benefit. Patients with a history of life-threatening angioedema or anaphylaxis, as is seen in allergy to peanuts and wasp stings, should carry a self-administered injection kit of adren-

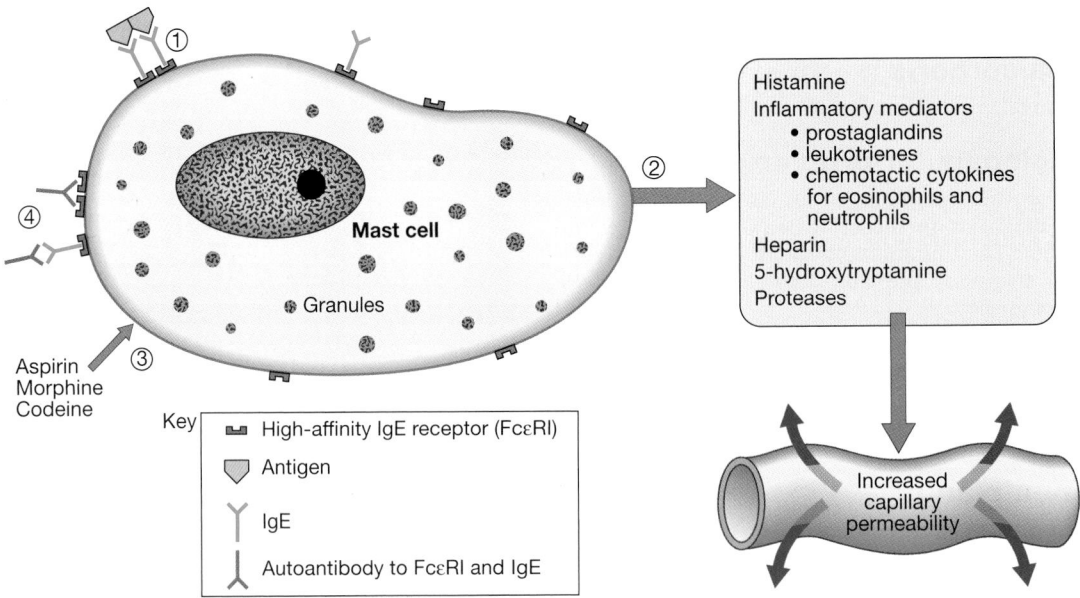

Fig. 27.19 Pathogenesis of urticaria. Mast cell degranulation occurs in a variety of ways. (1) Type I hypersensitivity causing massive degranulation and sometimes anaphylaxis. (2) Spontaneous mast cell degranulation in chronic urticaria. (3) Chemical mast cell degranulation. (4) Autoimmunity, which accounts for 30% of chronic urticaria.

aline (epinephrine). The management of anaphylactic shock and the treatment and prevention of acute attacks of hereditary angioedema are discussed on pages 89–91.

Urticaria may be precipitated by aspirin or NSAIDs. If there is a clear history of these agents precipitating attacks, they should be avoided, and even in the absence of a clear history it may be advisable to suggest alternatives such as paracetamol. Codeine and opioids can also induce urticaria.

ACNE AND ROSACEA

Acne vulgaris

Acne is almost ubiquitous in the teenage years, individual differences relating to severity and the extent of scarring. Peak severity is in the late teenage years but acne may persist into the third decade and beyond, particularly in females.

Aetiology

The pathogenic factors in acne are shown in Figure 27.20. There is a clear relation between severity of acne and sebum excretion rate, but while increased sebum excretion is necessary for the development of acne, it is not sufficient to cause it alone. The main determinants of sebum excretion are hormonal, accounting for the onset in the teenage years. Androgens are the principal sebotrophic hormones, but progestogens also increase sebum excretion, whilst oestrogens reduce it. However, the vast majority of patients with acne have a normal endocrine profile. There is some evidence for a familial component for sebum excretion, but the genetics of acne have been little studied.

In addition to the increased sebum secretion rate, *Propionibacterium acnes* colonises the pilosebaceous ducts and acts on lipids to produce pro-inflammatory factors, and the pilosebaceous unit becomes occluded.

Clinical features

Lesions are usually limited to the face, shoulders, upper chest and back, but may extend to the buttocks. Seborrhoea (greasy skin) is often obvious. Open comedones (blackheads) due to plugging by keratin and sebum of the pilosebaceous orifice, or closed comedones (whiteheads) due to accretions of sebum and keratin deeper in the pilosebaceous ducts, are usually

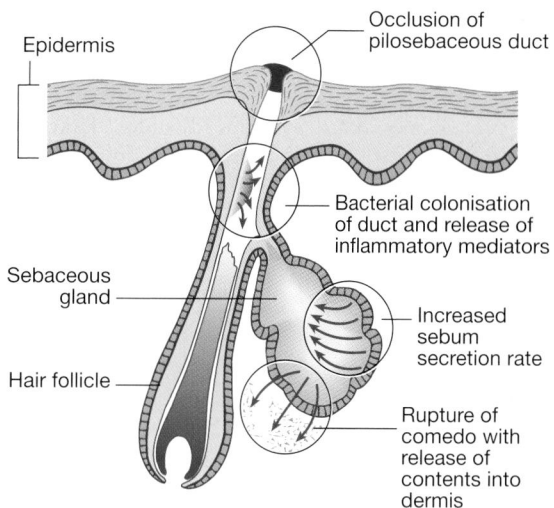

Fig. 27.20 Pathogenesis of acne.

evident. It is thought that the combination of keratin breakdown products and bacterial products gives rise to the black colour seen in blackheads. Inflammatory papules, nodules and 'cysts' occur (Fig. 27.21), with one or two types of lesion predominating. Scarring may follow.

A number of descriptive terms are applied to clinical variants of acne.

* *Conglobate acne* is characterised by comedones, nodules, abscesses and sinus tracks, often accompanied by keloidal scarring, although true cysts are rare in the acute phases and are more likely to reflect inflamed nodules. Epidermoid cysts are common later on in acne.
* *Acne fulminans* is severe acne accompanied by fever, joint pains and markers of systemic inflammation such as a raised ESR.
* *Acne excoriée* refers to the effects of scratching or picking, principally on the face of teenage girls with acne.

A mild form of acne dominated by the presence of comedones may be due to exogenous substances such as tars, chlorinated hydrocarbons or oily cosmetics. A primarily pustular rash may also be seen in those being treated with corticosteroids, lithium, oral contraceptives

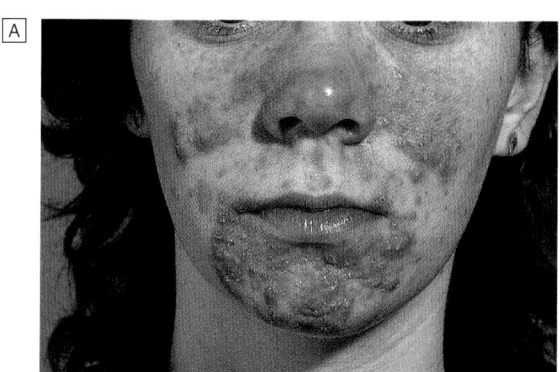
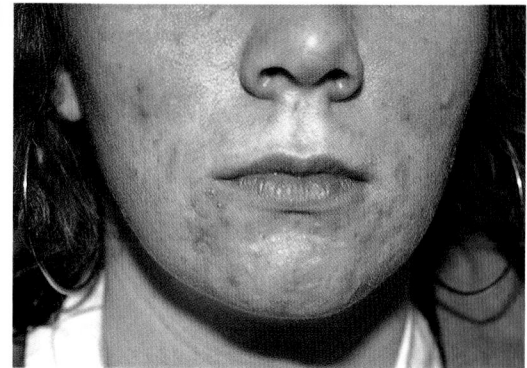

Fig. 27.21 Unpleasant cystic acne in a teenager. **A** Before treatment. **B** After prolonged systemic antibiotic treatment.

and anticonvulsants, but these forms are usually clinically distinct from the usual variety developing in adolescence.

Individuals with moderate or even severe acne very rarely have any other systemic disorder. However, those with polycystic ovary syndrome (p. 760) are more likely to have severe acne, and menstrual irregularities require investigation. If there is associated cutaneous virilism or other features of an androgen-secreting tumour, further endocrine investigation and assessment are warranted.

Investigations

Investigations are rarely required. It is important to enquire about the details of previous treatments and their duration; for example, antibiotics are commonly prescribed for too short a period of time or without the appropriate advice that most tetracyclines need to be taken separately from dairy products. It is also important to establish the patient's expectations.

Management

Mild disease

In individuals with fairly minor disease, particularly dominated by the presence of comedones, topical agents such as benzoyl peroxide or tretinoin should be used. Both may be irritant, which may be important in their therapeutic effect (sunshine or UVB may also be useful therapeutically in some instances for similar reasons). They are initially applied for short intervals of time and the strength and duration gradually increased. Although a number of other topical remedies, including washes, soaps and antiseptics, are recommended, there is little evidence of effectiveness.

Patients with anything but minor degrees of acne require antibiotic therapy, either systemic or local. Topical antibiotics (clindamycin or erythromycin) are used more widely than previously and should be considered prior to systemic antibiotics or in relatively minor disease, and in combination with other topical agents. The principal oral antibiotic is oxytetracycline, taken on an empty stomach without food, in a dose of up to 1.5 g a day if tolerated. Oxytetracycline has a good safety profile, even with long-term use. Minocycline is no longer a first-choice drug, although it may be used if other antibiotics fail, because it is associated with autoimmune hepatitis and requires frequent monitoring.

If an individual has been treated continuously for up to 3 months with little response, the regime should be changed to erythromycin (up to 1 g per day in divided doses). In women, oestrogen-containing oral contraceptives can be a useful adjunct, as they are associated with a small reduction in sebum secretion. Alternatively, oral contraception in the form of a combined oestrogen and anti-androgen (such as cyproterone acetate) may be used. If these topical and systemic agents fail to produce an adequate clinical response within 3–6 months, the patient should be referred for consideration for treatment with isotretinoin (13 cis-retinoic acid).

Moderate–severe disease

Isotretinoin has revolutionised the treatment of severe or moderate acne unresponsive to other therapy. When used at a dose of 0.5–1 mg/kg, it inhibits sebum excretion by > 90% over 4 months. Although sebum excretion gradually returns to normal over the course of the year after the drug is stopped, the clinical benefit lasts much longer. Many patients will not require any further treatment, but in a significant minority a second or third course of isotretinoin may be required. Sometimes low-dose continuous isotretinoin is used for up to 1 year, in selected patients who have previously been treated with high-dose isotretinoin.

Side-effects, especially drying of the skin and mucous membranes, are common but well tolerated and relate to the drug's effects on the function of modified sebaceous glands on the lips, and on lipid biosynthesis in the interfollicular epidermis. Rarely, abnormalities of liver function occur and limit treatment. Isotretinoin may increase serum triglycerides; levels should be checked before therapy and monitored during it. Depression and suicide have been reported, although it is difficult to disentangle the role of the drug from that of the underlying disease and age groups at risk; it is currently under investigation, but a brief psychiatric history and screening for depressive symptoms should be recorded before prescribing it. Like all systemic retinoids, isotretinoin is highly teratogenic; females must have a negative pregnancy test before treatment and must be checked regularly and following cessation of therapy.

Physical measures

Inflamed nodules can be incised and drained under local anaesthetic, and 'cysts' excised. Intralesional injections of triamcinolone acetonide (0.1–0.2 mL of a 10 mg/mL solution) hasten the resolution of stubborn inflamed nodules. Scarring following acne is uncommon if patients receive adequate care. Small deep acne scars can be excised and other forms of more extensive but shallower scars can be treated by carbon dioxide laser.

Rosacea

Rosacea is a persistent facial eruption of unknown cause. Sebum secretion is normal.

Clinical features and diagnosis

The disorder is most common in middle age. The cheeks, chin and central forehead are affected (Fig. 27.22). Intermittent blushing is followed by fixed erythema and telangiectasia. Dome-shaped papules and pustules, but no comedones, occur. Rhinophyma, with erythema, sebaceous gland hyperplasia and overgrowth of the soft tissues of the nose, is sometimes associated. Blepharitis and conjunctivitis are complications. The diagnosis is often obvious on clinical grounds but must be distinguished from acne, seborrhoeic eczema, photosensitivity and systemic lupus erythematosus (SLE).

Management

The pustular component of rosacea normally responds well to oral oxytetracycline. Once the disease is controlled (usually within a few months), the dose can be reduced but some patients may need to stay on antibiotics long-term or require repeated courses. Topical metronidazole also shows some efficacy in rosacea, but may cause irritation (Box 27.29). Unfortunately, the erythema and telangiectasia do not respond to antibiotic therapy but vascular laser therapy may be helpful, depending on the extent of the disease.

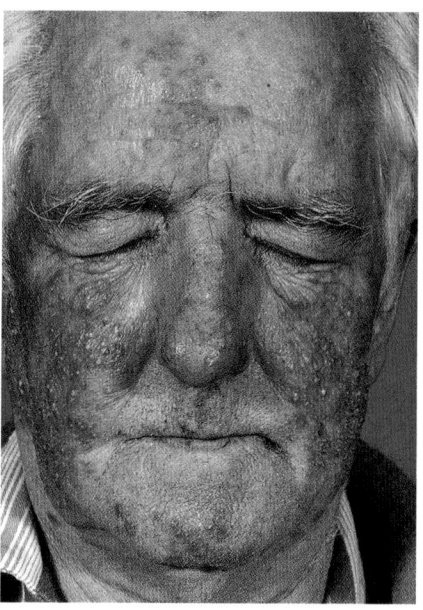

Fig. 27.22 Rosacea. The colour is distinctive and the typical papulopustular rash involves the cheeks, centre of forehead and chin.

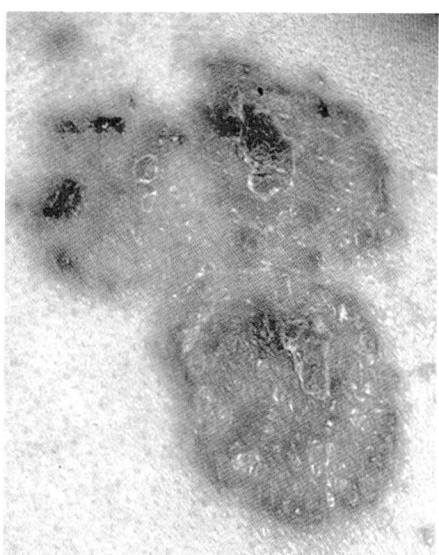

Fig. 27.23 Non-bullous impetigo.

EBM 27.29 Rosacea

'Topical metronidazole and azelaic acid are effective treatments, but the former is more cost-effective.'

• Von Zuuren EJ, et al. (Cochrane Review). Cochrane Library, issue 2, 2005.
• Thomas K, et al. J Dermatol Treat 2008; 21:1–4.

COMMON SKIN INFECTIONS AND INFESTATIONS

Bacterial infections

Impetigo

Impetigo is a common superficial purulent infection of skin caused by either *Streptococcus* or *Staphylococcus*. Two forms exist: non-bullous (Fig. 27.23) and bullous impetigo. Non-bullous impetigo can be caused by either *Staphylococcus aureus* or *Streptococcus* or a combination, and it is not completely clear which is more important. In warmer climates *Streptococcus* is more likely to be the primary organism, but in temperate climates *Staphylococcus* predominates. It affects all age groups but particularly young children, often in late summer. It is contagious and found most commonly in situations of overcrowding and communal living. Other skin diseases, such as eczema and infestations, predispose to it.

The initial lesion is a thin-walled vesicle which rapidly ruptures, with the formation of golden crust on an erythematous base. The sites usually affected are the face and the limbs. Lesions may be single but often become multiple and coalesce. A bacterial swab should be taken prior to starting treatment to determine the culprit organism.

Treatment is usually with a topical preparation such as mupirocin, which is active against both organisms, or fusidic acid. This limits the spread of infection and, together with washing with soap and water, helps the removal of the infected crusts. In severe or extensive cases, an oral antibiotic such as flucloxacillin or erythromycin is indicated. Glomerulonephritis can follow infection with a nephritogenic *Streptococcus* (p. 501). Advice should be given on measures to minimise cross-infection.

Bullous impetigo is primarily caused by *Staphylococcus* and most frequently occurs in children. Bullae (often quite large) are caused by a staphylococcal epidermolytic toxin, and develop and last for 2–3 days, initially clear and then becoming cloudy. Once the blisters have burst, crusts develop and management is the same as for the non-bullous form of the disease.

Erythrasma

Erythrasma is a mild localised infection of the skin with *Corynebacterium minutissimum*, often part of the normal skin flora. It can cause an asymptomatic or mildly itchy eruption between the toes and in the flexures. The lesions tend to be well defined and reddish-brown in colour, with some scale. *C. minutissimum* is identified by coral pink fluorescence with Wood's light. Treatment is with a topical azole cream such as miconazole or a topical antibiotic. Oral erythromycin can be used in cases that fail to respond.

Ecthyma

Ecthyma is a purulent skin infection caused by either *Staphylococcus* or *Streptococcus*, and characterised by ulceration under an exudative crust. It is associated with poor hygiene and malnutrition, and minor trauma can predispose to development of the lesions. It affects any age group and is commonly seen in drug misusers.

27

27

Folliculitis, furuncles and carbuncles

Folliculitis can be superficial, involving just the ostium of the hair follicle (folliculitis), or deep (furuncles and carbuncles).

Superficial folliculitis

This extremely common condition can be subacute or chronic. It is often infective, caused by *Staph. aureus*, but can also be caused by physical (e.g. traumatic epilation) or chemical (e.g. mineral oil) injury, in which case the folliculitis is usually sterile. Staphylococcal folliculitis is most common in children and often occurs on the scalp or limbs (Fig. 27.24). The pustules usually heal in 7–10 days but can become more chronic, and in older children and adults can progress to a deeper form of folliculitis.

Deep folliculitis (furuncles and carbuncles)

A furuncle (or boil) occurs most commonly in adolescence and early adult life. Epidemics can occur with a particular staphylococcal strain but infection is more usually sporadic. Males are more commonly affected than females. Any body site can be involved but often it is the neck, buttocks and anogenital area. Predisposing factors include tight clothing, such as neckties. The affected individual may carry the culprit strain of *Staph. aureus* in the nares or perineum. The lesions start as an inflammatory nodule, which becomes pustular and fluctuant and is often very tender. There may be associated constitutional disturbance. The lesions eventually rupture to discharge pus and, because they are deep, leave a scar. They can progress to form a carbuncle, which implies the involvement of several contiguous hair follicles (Fig. 27.25). This usually occurs in middle-aged men, and conditions such as diabetes or immunosuppressive therapy predispose to it. A carbuncle is an exquisitely tender nodule, often on the neck, shoulders or hips, and associated with severe constitutional symptoms. The nodules can be up to 10 cm in size and discharge after several days. Treatment, as for furuncles, is with

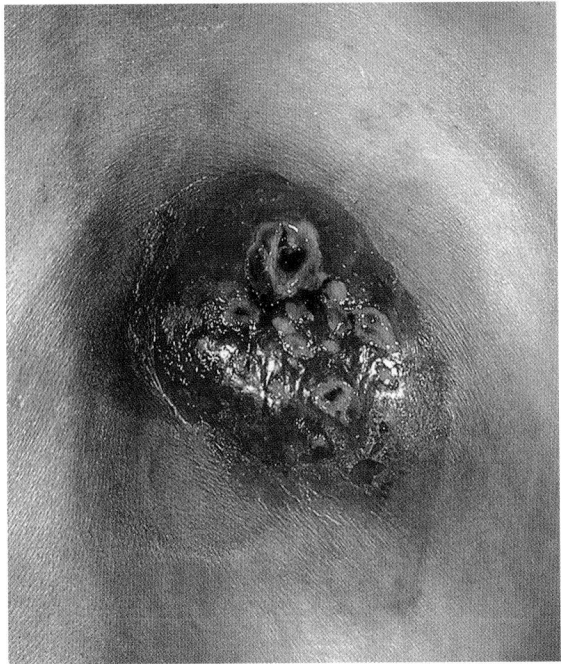

Fig. 27.25 Staphylococcal carbuncle.

an antistaphylococcal antibiotic, e.g. flucloxacillin, and occasionally incision and drainage.

Staphylococcal scalded skin syndrome (SSSS)

SSSS (Fig. 27.26) is a potentially serious exfoliating cutaneous disease that occurs predominantly in children, particularly neonates. It is caused by blood-borne exfoliative toxins from a focus of infection with *Staph. aureus*, which specifically cleave desmoglein-1 (see Fig. 27.2, p. 1241). The focus of infection may be the umbilicus or urinary tract, or it may stem from colonisation of the nasopharynx. The child presents with fever, irritability, skin tenderness and, in severe cases, erythema, starting in the groin, axilla and around the mouth. Blisters and superficial erosions develop within 24–28 hours, and can rapidly involve large areas of the skin with severe systemic upset. Bacterial swabs should be taken from obvious primary sites of infection, the nose and throat. A skin snip should be taken for rapid histological examination. This is a sample of the superficial peeling skin removed by 'snipping with scissors'. No local anaesthetic is required. It shows a split beneath the stratum corneum, and differentiates it from toxic epidermal necrolysis in which the whole epidermis is affected. Systemic antibiotics (e.g. flucloxacillin) and intensive supportive measures should be commenced at once. Bacterial swabs from nostrils, axilla and groin should be taken from the patient's relatives to exclude staphylococcal carriage.

Cellulitis and erysipelas

Cellulitis (Fig. 27.27) is inflammation, usually infective, of subcutaneous tissue. Erysipelas (Fig. 27.28) is a more superficial involvement of the subcutaneous tissue and lower dermis, but the distinction between the two

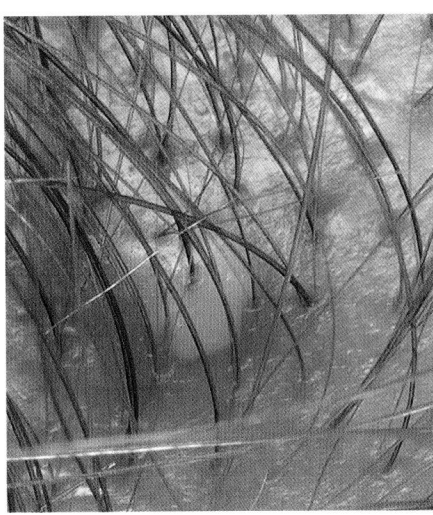

Fig. 27.24 Pustular folliculitis.

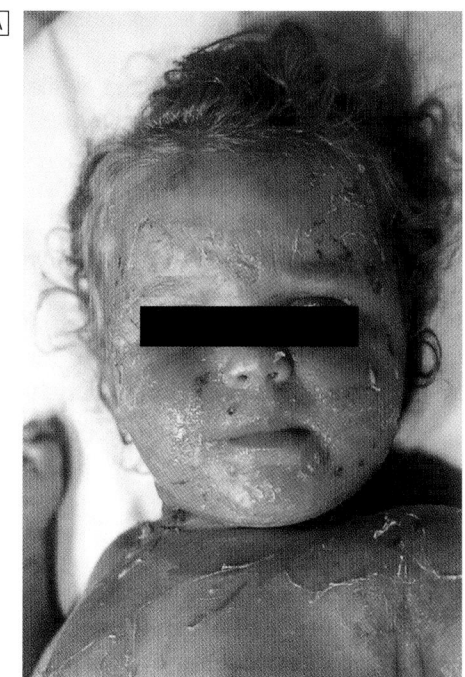

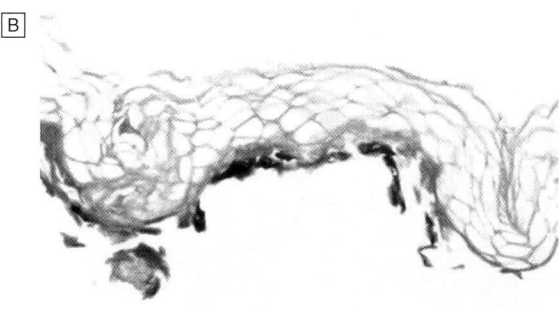

Fig. 27.26 Staphylococcal scalded skin syndrome (SSSS).
A Erythema and superficial peeling of the skin. B The condition was rapidly diagnosed by examination of a frozen section of skin snip.

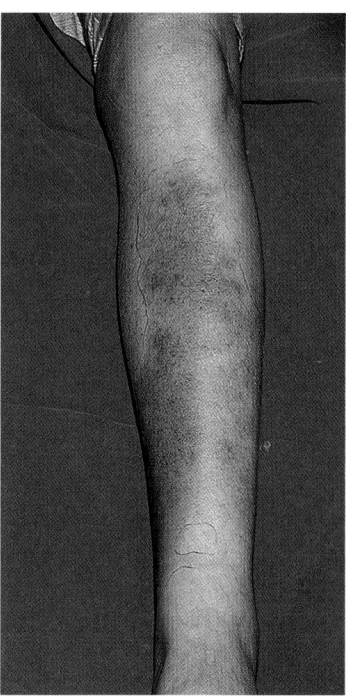

Fig. 27.27 Acute cellulitis of the leg. Note that the margin has been marked to assess progression.

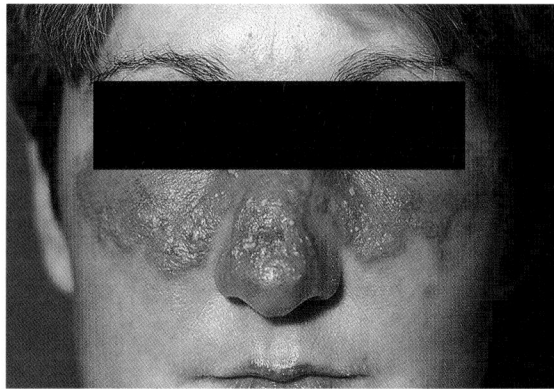

Fig. 27.28 Erysipelas. Note the blistering and crusted rash with raised erythematous edge.

conditions can be difficult. The most common organism causing both these conditions is group A *Streptococcus*. Isolating and identifying the organism is difficult but the presence of fever and a raised white cell count usually allow a firm diagnosis. There is often a predisposing portal of entry for infection, e.g. tinea pedis, or underlying predisposition to infection such as varicose leg ulcer or diabetes. Erythema, heat, swelling and pain are constant clinical features. Erysipelas has a characteristic raised erythematous edge, indicating involvement of the dermis. It usually affects the face or the legs, while cellulitis most commonly involves the legs. Blistering occurs in both conditions. Treatment is with an antistreptococcal agent such as phenoxymethylpenicillin, or in cases of penicillin sensitivity, erythromycin or ciprofloxacin. In severe cases, intravenous antibiotics are indicated.

Necrotising soft tissue infections and anthrax

Necrotising soft tissue infections are discussed on pages 300–302 and anthrax on page 341.

Viral infections

Herpes virus infections

There are eight members of the human herpesvirus group and their cutaneous manifestations are described on pages 321–322.

Papillomaviruses and viral warts

Viral warts are extremely common and are due to infection with the DNA human papillomavirus (HPV), of which there are over 90 subtypes on the basis of DNA sequence analysis. Different subtypes appear to be responsible for different clinical wart variants. Genital warts occur most commonly during the sexually active years (p. 423).

27

Transmission is by direct contact with the virus, in either living skin or fragments of shed skin, and is encouraged by trauma and moisture (e.g. in swimming pools, fishmongers etc.). Genital warts are spread by sexual activity, and show a clear relationship with cervical and intra-epithelial cancers of the genital area. HPV 16 and 18 appear to inactivate tumour suppressor gene pathways and lead to squamous cell carcinoma of the cervix or intra-epithelial carcinoma of the genital skin. Vaccinations are now available against HPV 16 and 18 (e.g. Gardasil) and are recommended for adolescent females before they become sexually active. In contrast, the relation between HPV of the skin and subsequent skin cancer is unclear. Individuals who are systemically immunosuppressed, e.g. after organ transplantation, show greatly elevated risks of skin cancer and a much higher prevalence of infection with HPV, but it is not certain that HPV is causally involved in the development of neoplasia.

Clinical features

Common warts appear initially as smooth, skin-coloured papules. As they enlarge, their surface becomes irregular and hyperkeratotic, producing the typical warty appearance. They are most common on the hands (Fig. 27.29) but may also be seen on the face, genitalia and sun-exposed surfaces of the arm and leg. Multiple warts are common. Plantar warts (verrucae) are characterised by a rough surface protruding only slightly from the skin and are surrounded by a horny collar; they may be painful and disabling. On paring, the presence of capillary loops distinguishes these plantar warts from corns.

Other varieties of wart include:
- *mosaic warts*, mosaic-like plaques of tightly packed individual warts (Fig. 27.30)
- *plane warts*, smooth, flat-top papules seen most commonly on the face and backs of hands which frequently may hyperpigment and consequently be misdiagnosed
- *facial warts*, often filiform
- *genital warts*, which may be papillomatous and protuberant.

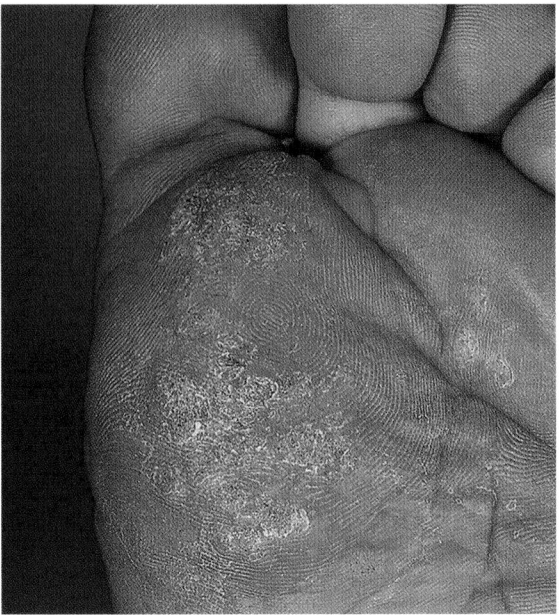

Fig. 27.30 Mosaic plantar wart. A plaque of closely grouped warts on the sole of the foot.

Management

The vast majority of viral warts will resolve spontaneously. However, this may take several years and there is often considerable pressure for treatment from the patient. The majority of treatments are based on destruction of keratinocytes, irrespective of whether they are HPV-infected or not.

Treating warts that are asymptomatic or not causing distress should be avoided. Initial treatment is with salicylic acid or salicylic and lactic acid combinations, together with frequent and regular paring of the hyperkeratotic skin. This needs to continue for several months before convincing effects will be apparent. If this fails, or as an alternative, warts can be treated by cryotherapy using liquid nitrogen. At some sites and in particular individuals, this is accompanied by significant pain, but needs to be repeated at intervals of 2–4 weeks, although the optimum strategy is not defined. Over-aggressive treatment with cryotherapy, particularly on the hands, can lead to significant complications, including tendon rupture. Warts close to or under the nails can be a particular problem. Liquid nitrogen treatment may exacerbate them due to inflammatory swelling, and skilled cutting of the nail and electrodesiccation or another destructive therapy may be necessary.

Viral warts can be a particular problem in individuals who are immunosuppressed following organ transplantation. The prevalence of warts in this group approaches 100% after 5 years and therapy appears less effective than in immunocompetent individuals. Not only are the warts particularly unsightly, but painful verrucae can also limit mobility and require intensive treatment.

Beyond the therapies described above, a number of other treatments have been claimed to be effective; these include systemic retinoids, intralesional injections of bleomycin or interferon, and the application

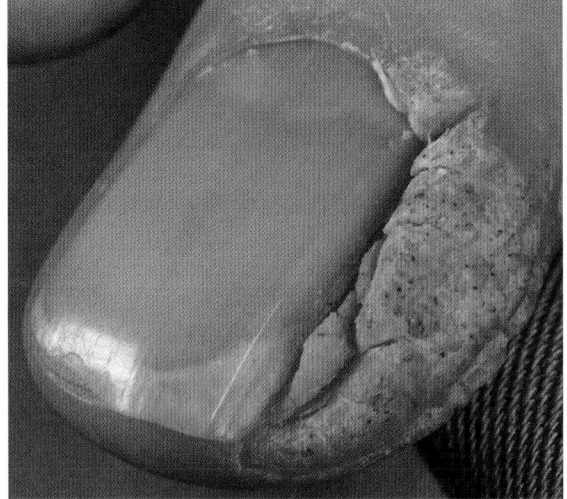

Fig. 27.29 Viral wart on finger.

of contact sensitisers such as diphencyprone or dinitrochlorobenzene to the warts. The topical immuno-modulator, imiquimod, is useful in treating stubborn anogenital warts.

Molluscum contagiosum

Molluscum contagiosum is a common cutaneous infection with a poxvirus. It can affect any age group but usually targets children over the age of 1 year. The prevalence is also high in individuals who are immuno-suppressed. The classic lesion is a dome-shaped, 'umbilicated', skin-coloured papule with a central punctum (p. 384). The lesions tend to be multiple and are often found in sites of apposition such as the side of the chest and the inner arm; they resolve spontaneously but can take several months to do so. Prior to resolution, they often become inflamed and may leave small, discrete, depressed scars. A wide range of treatments has been tried but none is very effective and they can be painful; no treatment is an acceptable option. Individual lesions can be removed by curettage under local anaesthetic but the lesions are commonly multiple. Gentle squeezing with forceps after bathing can stimulate regression. Topically applied chemicals such as salicylic acid (topical 5% acidified nitrite co-applied with 5% salicylic acid), podophyllin (topical 0.5% podophyllotoxin) and trichloroacetic acid cause marked inflammation and results vary. Cryotherapy can be tried but is not as effective as gentle squeezing. Physical occlusion with duct tape is advocated by some groups. Topical 5% imiquimod cream has recently been shown to be effective.

Orf

Orf is an occupational hazard for those who work with sheep and goats, which transmit a parapoxvirus. Inoculation of the virus, usually into the skin of a finger, causes significant inflammation and necrosis which usually resolve within 2–6 weeks. No specific treatment is available, unless there is evidence of secondary infection. Erythema multiforme (p. 1284) can be provoked by orf infection.

Erythrovirus

This is described on page 311.

Fungal infections

Dermatophytes are fungi capable of causing superficial skin infections known as ringworm or dermatophytosis. The causative fungi belong to three genera (*Microsporum*, *Trichophyton* and *Epidermophyton*). They can originate from the soil (geophilic) or animals (zoophilic), or be confined to human skin (anthropophilic).

Clinical forms of cutaneous infection include tinea corporis (involvement of the body), tinea capitis (scalp involvement, p. 1288), tinea cruris (groin involvement), tinea pedis (involvement of the feet) and onychomycosis (nail involvement, p. 1291).

Tinea corporis

The clinical features of tinea corporis are variable, so the disease should be considered in the differential diagnosis of any red scaly rash. Classically, the lesions are

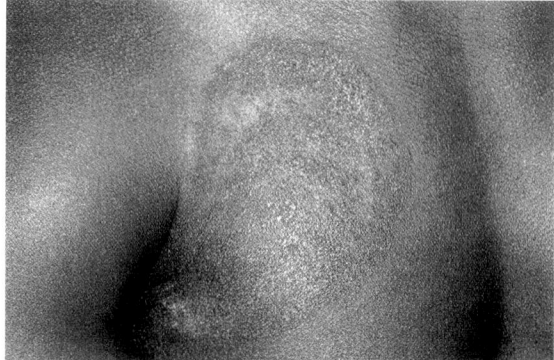

Fig. 27.31 Tinea corporis in a dark-skinned patient.

erythematous, annular and scaly, with a well-defined edge and often central clearing. They may be single or multiple, and are usually asymmetrical (Fig. 27.31). The degree of associated inflammation depends on the causative fungus and host immunity. *Microsporum canis* (from dogs) and *Trichophyton verrucosum* (from cats) are common culprits. Inadvertent topical corticosteroid application leads to disguising and worsening of the signs (tinea incognito).

Tinea cruris

This common world-wide ringworm affects the groin and is usually caused by *Trichophyton rubrum*. Itchy erythematous plaques extend from the groin flexures on to the thighs.

Tinea pedis (athlete's foot)

This is the most common form of ringworm in the UK and USA; it is usually caused by anthropophilic fungi, such as *Trichophyton rubrum*, *T. mentagrophytes* and *Epidermophyton floccosum*. Clinical features are an itchy rash between the toes, with peeling, fissuring and maceration. Involvement of one sole or palm (in the case of tinea manuum) with a fine scaling is characteristic of *T. rubrum* infection. Vesiculation or frank blistering is more commonly seen with *T. mentagrophytes*.

Diagnosis and management

In all cases of suspected dermatophyte infection, the diagnosis should be confirmed by skin scraping or nail clippings (p. 1243). Treatment can be topical with terbinafine or miconazole cream, or systemic with terbinafine, griseofulvin or itraconazole.

Scabies

Scabies is caused by the Acarus, *Sarcoptes scabiei*, with an estimated global prevalence of 300 million. The infestation causes considerable discomfort and can lead to secondary infection. Scabies spreads in households and environments where there is intimate personal contact. Diagnosis is made by identifying the scabietic burrow (p. 1246 and Fig 27.32) and by extracting the mite using a blunt needle. Inappropriate application of scabietic treatments can cause considerable irritation in other conditions. In small children the palms and soles can be involved with pustule formation (Fig. 27.33).

27

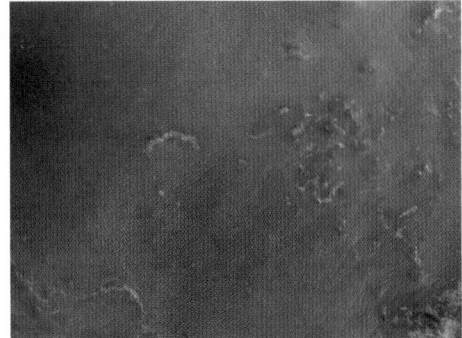

Fig. 27.32 Scabietic burrow.

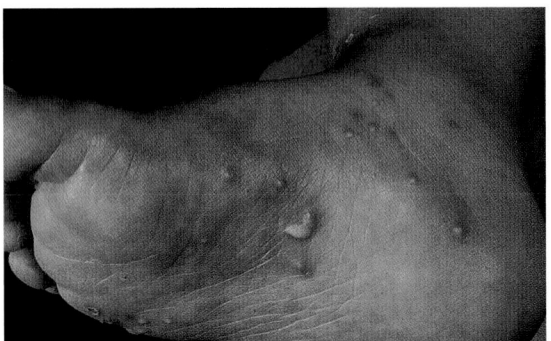

Fig. 27.33 **Scabies.** Pustules at a common site in a child. Burrows were present but cannot be seen at this distance.

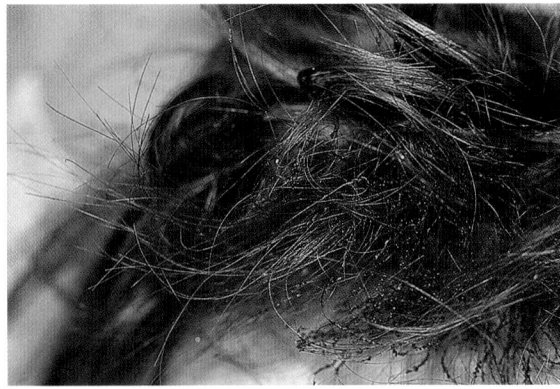

Fig. 27.34 **Head lice.** 'Nits' (empty egg cases) adhere strongly to the hair shafts.

Involvement of the genital area in boys is pathognomonic. The main symptom is itch. The clinical features include secondary eczematisation elsewhere on the body; the face and scalp are never involved, except in the case of infants. Even after successful treatment, the itch can continue and occasionally nodular lesions persist.

Topical treatment of scabies is required for the affected individual and all asymptomatic family members/physical contacts to ensure eradication. Two applications 1 week apart of an aqueous solution of either permethrin or malathion to the whole body, excluding the head, are usually successful. If there is poor compliance, immunocompromise or heavy infestations (Norwegian scabies), systemic treatment with ivermectin (200 μg/kg) as a single dose is appropriate.

Lice

Head lice

Infestation with head louse, *Pediculus humanus capitis*, is common; it is highly contagious, spread by direct head-to-head contact. Itching of the scalp leads to scratching which causes secondary infection and cervical lymphadenopathy. The diagnosis is confirmed by identifying the living louse or nymph on the scalp or on a black sheet of paper after careful fine-toothed combing of wet hair that has had conditioner applied. The empty egg cases ('nits') are easily seen along the hair shaft (Fig. 27.34) and are characteristically difficult to dislodge.

Treatment is recommended for the infected individual and any infected household/school contacts. Eradication in school populations has proved difficult because of poor compliance and resistance to certain treatments. The standard treatments are malathion, permethrin and carbaryl in a lotion or aqueous formulation, which are applied on two separate occasions at 7–10 days' interval. Many advise rotational treatments within a community to avoid resistance. Regular 'wet-combing' (physical removal of the live lice by regular combing of slippery, conditioned wet hair) seems less effective than pharmacological treatments. Involvement of the eyebrows/eyelashes is treated by topical Vaseline 12-hourly for at least a fortnight.

Body lice

These are similar to head lice but live on clothing, particularly in seams, and feed on the skin. They are found on individuals with poor hygiene and in overcrowded conditions. Itch is the principal symptom. The skin is excoriated and secondary infection is common. It is managed by dry cleaning and high-temperature washing or insecticide treatment of clothes.

Pubic (crab) lice

These are usually sexually acquired and cause pruritus. An aqueous-based treatment of either malathion or carbaryl is the treatment of choice, applied on two occasions to the whole body, as body hair can also be infested. Contacts should also be treated.

BULLOUS DISORDERS

Blistering disorders usually present acutely to the general physician and dermatologist. Better understanding of the mechanisms of adhesion within the skin (pp. 1240–1242) has revealed the pathogenesis of many blistering disorders. In pemphigus, an autoantibody acts on the adhesion protein, desmoglein-1, while in SSSS this is due to a staphylococcal protease directly cleaving desmoglein-1. Blisters can arise at any level within the skin, and the underlying defect and level of blistering accounts for the different clinical presentations (p. 1249). Primary blistering disorders are described here.

Toxic epidermal necrolysis (TEN)

TEN is a life-threatening mucocutaneous blistering eruption that is generally drug-induced, most commonly by anticonvulsants, sulphonyl drugs (e.g. sulphonamides, sulphonylureas), NSAIDs, allopurinol and antiretroviral therapy. Keratinocyte apoptosis is triggered via the Fas receptor. TEN occurs world-wide and has a high mortality rate. Clinically, 1–3 weeks after drug ingestion, the patient develops a systemic illness with pyrexia, erythema and blisters arising centrally and progressing rapidly to involve all the skin. The blisters coalesce and denude, and the underlying skin is erythematous and extremely tender (Fig. 27.35). Mucous membrane involvement is common, with erythema, oedema, blistering and haemorrhage. A standard disease severity score (Box 27.30) is used in assessing prognosis. The main differential diagnosis of this severe blistering disorder is SSSS and early diagnosis is made rapidly by skin snip (p. 1270) or skin biopsy. Initial management includes discontinuation of the possible causative agent and transfer to an intensive care or burns unit. Treatment is primarily supportive, with regular sterile dressings and care-ful monitoring for infection and of other organ systems, including for eye involvement. Studies support the use of intravenous immunoglobulins. The use of intravenous steroids is contraindicated, as they are associated with a higher mortality rate.

Immunobullous diseases

In the immunobullous disorders (Box 27.31), the diagnosis is made by taking a skin biopsy from the edge of a fresh blister. This is divided and half is immersed in 10% formalin for histology; the remainder is snap-frozen for direct immunofluorescence studies.

Bullous pemphigoid (BP)

BP is a chronic autoimmune bullous disorder that occurs world-wide and is the most common subepidermal blistering disorder in Europe. The average age of onset is 65 years and the disease affects men and women equally. Autoantibodies BP 230 and BP 180 are directed against the hemidesmosomal BP antigens, BP Ag-1 (intracellular) and BPAg-2 (transmembranous type XVII collagen), respectively. The autoantibodies bind to these, activating complement and inflammatory mediators which damage hemidesmosomes, leading to blistering. There may also be other antibodies to alternative target antigens.

Clinical features and diagnosis

Individuals present with widespread itchy, often urticated skin lesions and tense bullae (see Fig. 27.5, p. 1249). Mucosal involvement affects only 10–25%. Histology shows subepidermal blistering with an inflammatory infiltrate and a predominance of eosinophils. Direct immunofluorescence shows the presence of IgG and C3 at the basement membrane (Fig. 27.36). Differentiating this from epidermolysis bullosa acquisita (see below) requires indirect immunofluorescence studies using the patient's serum on salt split skin. In BP, the immunoreactants localise to the epidermal side (hemidesmosome) of the split skin, whereas in epidermolysis bullosa acquisita they localise to the base of the split (type VII collagen/anchoring fibrils).

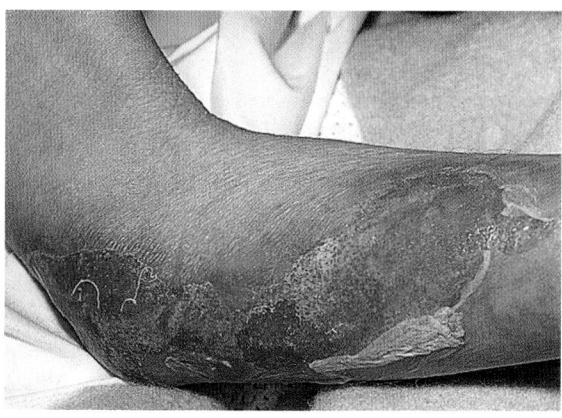

Fig. 27.35 Toxic epidermolytic necrolysis in an adult. Peeling of the skin involving the whole epidermis is usually secondary to a drug reaction.

 27.30 Disease severity score for toxic epidermal necrolysis (TEN): SCORTEN

Factor

- Age > 40 years
- Heart rate >120 beats per minute
- Cancer or haematological malignancy
- Involved body surface area > 10%
- Blood urea > 10 mmol/L (28 mg/dL)
- Serum bicarbonate < 20 mmol/L (20 mEq/L)
- Blood glucose ≥ 14 mmol/L (252 mg/dL)

Mortality rates

- 0–1 factor present = 3%
- 2 factors = 12%
- 3 factors = 35%
- 4 factors = 58%
- ≥ 5 factors = 90%

Bastuji-Garin S, et al. J Invest Dermatol 2000; 115:149–153.

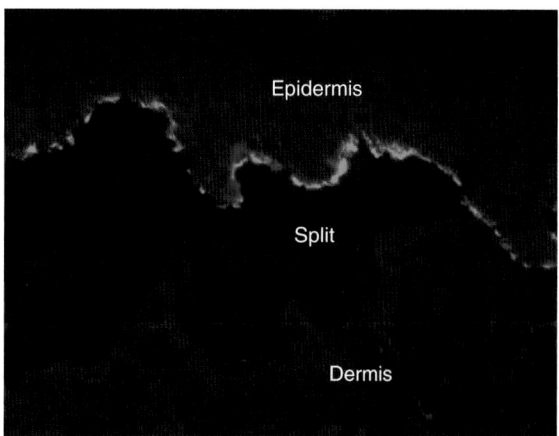

Fig. 27.36 Bullous pemphigoid. Direct immunofluorescence on salt-split skin.

27

i **27.31 Clinical and investigation findings in immunobullous disorders**

Disease	Site of blisters	Nature of blisters	Mucous membrane involvement	Antigen	Circulating antibody (indirect IF)	Fixed antibody (direct IF)
Pemphigus vulgaris	Torso, head	Flaccid and fragile, many erosions	100%	Desmoglein-1 and 3 (120 kD)	IgG	IgG, C_3 intercellular (epidermal)
Bullous pemphigoid	Trunk (especially flexures) and limbs	Tense	Occasional	BP-230 and 180	IgG (70%)	IgG, C_3 at BMZ
Dermatitis herpetiformis	Elbows, lower back, buttocks	Excoriated and often not present	No	Unknown	None	Granular IgA in papillary dermis
Linear IgA disease	Widespread	Tense, often annular configuration, 'string of beads'	Frequent	Unknown	50% have low titres of circulating antibody	Linear IgA at BMZ
Pemphigoid gestationis	Periumbilical and limbs	Tense	Rare	Collagen XVII (part of hemi-desmosome BP-180)	Circulating antibody to BPAg2 (type XVII collagen)	C_3 at BMZ
Epidermolysis bullosa acquisita	Widespread	Tense, scarring	Common (50%)	Type VII collagen	IgG (anti-type VII collagen)	IgG at BMZ
Bullous lupus erythematosus	Widespread	Tense	Rare	Type VII collagen	Anti-type VII collagen	IgG, IgA, IgM at BMZ

(BMZ = basement membrane zone; IF = immunofluorescence)

Management

BP can be managed with very potent topical steroids in frail elderly patients, but in most patients a high-dose systemic corticosteroid or azathioprine is required. With appropriate management, the disease tends to remit within about 5 years.

Pemphigus

Pemphigus is an uncommon autoimmune disorder that can present with mucosal symptoms only, usually in the mouth. It is usually due to IgG1 and IgG4 auto-antibodies, directed against desmogleins-1 and 3 and causing intra-epidermal blistering, but it can also be drug-induced (e.g. by penicillamine or captopril) and is rarely associated with an underlying malignancy ('para-neoplastic pemphigus'). In pemphigus foliaceus, a very superficial form, the autoantibodies are directed solely against desmoglein-1, therefore affecting only the most superficial epidermis.

Clinical features and diagnosis

Flaccid blisters occur on the skin, usually on the upper trunk and back. As the blisters are superficial, they are fragile and may look like erosions. The Nikolsky sign is positive. Mucosal involvement can be severe, increasing the morbidity and risk of mortality. Pemphigus can be associated with other autoimmune disorders and full assessment for these is mandatory. In the acute situation, histology from a Tzank smear (taken from the base of the blister with a scalpel) reveals acantholysis, i.e. separation of the epidermal cells. Disease activity can be monitored by measuring the level of circulating autoantibody in serum by indirect immunofluorescence. Investigations should also include full blood count, ESR, urea and electrolytes, liver function tests, chest X-ray and other imaging, particularly if paraneoplastic pemphigus is suspected.

Management

Systemic treatment with high-dose oral steroids is required, but the disease is more difficult to control than BP and life-long treatment is generally required. Azathioprine and cyclophosphamide are alternatives. Intravenous IgG may be used to gain rapid control in severe cases.

Dermatitis herpetiformis (DH)

DH is an autoimmune blistering disorder associated with coeliac disease. Up to 20% of individuals with coeliac disease have DH. The pathogenesis is unclear.

It presents as an extremely pruritic eruption, usually on the extensor surfaces of the arms, knees and buttocks, but other sites including the face are often involved. Vesicles are occasionally seen but usually it is just excoriations that are apparent, as the disorder is so itchy.

Histology reveals neutrophils and eosinophils in the dermal papillae, which form pustules and vesicles. Granular IgA is found in the papillary dermis. Up to 90% of individuals with DH have coeliac disease (p. 879) and so antiendomysial antibodies and tissue transglutaminase should be checked, and jejunal biopsy should be performed if indicated. Treatment is with a gluten-free diet and dapsone.

Linear IgA disease

This self-limiting autoimmune blistering disorder occurs in both children (chronic bullous disease of childhood) and adults. Several drugs have been implicated in its pathogenesis, notably vancomycin.

Mucosal involvement is common and regular ophthalmic assessment is important in the prevention of long-term scarring. Blisters occur on normal-looking, erythematous and urticated skin and have been described as 'clusters of jewels' (herpetiform) and 'string of beads' (annular/polycyclic). Direct immunofluorescence shows linear IgA at the basement membrane, which localises to either the roof or the floor of salt-split skin.

Treatment is with dapsone, sulphapyridine, prednisolone, colchicine or intravenous immunoglobulin. Most cases remit within a few years.

Epidermolysis bullosa acquisita

This condition is known as the great mimicker because its varied clinical presentation can simulate other autoimmune blistering diseases. It is a chronic blistering disease of the skin and mucous membranes and can be associated with inflammatory bowel disease, rheumatoid arthritis, multiple myeloma and lymphoma. It is due to an IgG autoantibody to type VII collagen and blisters often occur following trauma, with milia formation. Histologically, there is a subepidermal blister with a mixed inflammatory infiltrate in the dermis. The disease can be resistant to treatment with immunosuppressives.

Porphyria cutanea tarda and pseudoporphyria may also cause blistering (p. 1284).

SKIN TUMOURS

The diagnosis and management of skin cancer and lesions that may be confused with skin cancer form a major part of dermatological practice. A number of lesions which are not strictly tumours, but which present clinically as solitary lesions that can be confused with malignant tumours, are included in this section.

Pathogenesis of skin malignancy

In most Caucasian populations, skin cancer is the most common human malignancy. It can be categorised as melanoma and non-melanoma skin cancer (i.e. basal cell carcinomas and squamous cell carcinomas). Melanomas are less common than the non-melanoma skin cancers, but their biological behaviour is more aggressive and they have a higher case fatality rate. Non-melanoma skin cancer is much more common, but can usually be cured.

Ultraviolet radiation is the dominant cause of nearly all forms of skin cancer. The evidence for this is as follows:

- Many skin cancers, such as squamous cell carcinomas and pre-malignant conditions such as actinic keratoses, are most common on sites that receive the most exposure to UVR; for example, squamous cell carcinoma is most common on the heads of bald-headed individuals, on the tops of the ears and on the backs of the hands.
- Individuals who have pale skin, which contains less melanin, are at greatest risk of skin cancer. Melanin is a highly effective sunblock protecting normal skin from the mutagenic load of UVR.
- Skin cancer is most common in those areas which have the greatest ambient UVR (if other factors such as skin colour are kept constant). Dramatically increased tumour rates are seen in those with pale skin who have migrated from areas of relatively low to relatively high UVR exposure.
- There is a grossly elevated risk of skin cancer in patients with xeroderma pigmentosa, a rare autosomal recessive genodermatosis characterised by an inability to repair UVR-induced DNA damage. Affected individuals present in early childhood with

---

> **EBM** 27.32 **Sunscreens and skin cancer**
>
> 'In a high ambient UVR environment, sunblocks reduce the incidence of actinic keratoses, squamous cell carcinomas and melanocytic naevi in children.'
>
> • Gallagher RP, et al. JAMA 2000; 283:2955–2960.

marked photosensitivity and subsequently develop a range of skin tumours, including squamous cell carcinomas and melanomas.

Although UVR is the major environmental determinant of skin cancer, the various tumour types show different body distribution. While squamous cell carcinomas and actinic keratoses occur at the sites of highest cumulative UVR exposure, basal cell carcinomas tend to be disproportionately common on the face, perhaps reflecting their appendageal origins, and melanoma is relatively more common on areas of skin that may have received intermittent sun exposure, which has led to the suggestion that this or episodes of burning may be important for its pathogenesis.

Whereas squamous cell carcinomas seem to relate to cumulative UVR exposure, there is some evidence that continuous low-grade exposure of the skin, or the maintenance of a tan year-round, is associated with lower melanoma rates. The increase in melanoma incidence with ambient UVR exposure is not as steep as that seen for squamous cell carcinoma. However, it remains agreed that minimisation of UV exposure should reduce skin cancer, at least at the population level (Box 27.32).

Non-UVR causes of skin cancer

Patients on long-term immunosuppression following organ transplantation (especially kidney and heart) are at dramatically increased risk of non-melanoma skin cancer. Any increased risk of melanoma would appear to be marginal. Patients who have received frequent PUVA treatment for psoriasis are also at increased risk of non-melanoma skin cancer and arguably melanoma. Ionising radiation, such as that from radiotherapy, and a variety of xenobiotics including arsenic may also increase the risk of non-melanoma skin cancer.

Malignant tumours

Basal cell carcinoma (BCC)

This is the most common human cancer. Rates are five times higher than for squamous cell carcinoma in European countries. Classically, lesions are slow-growing and ulcerated, with a pearly and telangiectatic edge, and occur on the face of an elderly individual. The tumour invades locally but rarely metastasises. It is managed as though it does not metastasise, unless it is particularly large or has been present for a long time. 'Rodent ulcer' is a term commonly used for slowly expanding ulcerative basal cell carcinoma. The malignant cells resemble basal keratinocytes.

Clinical features

In the nodulo-ulcerative form, the earliest lesion is a small, glistening, skin-coloured papule, often with

27

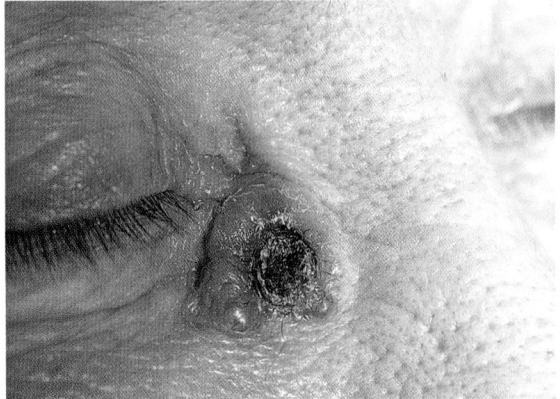

Fig. 27.37 Basal cell carcinoma. A slowly growing pearly nodule just below the inner canthus. The central crust overlies an ulcerated area.

EBM 27.33 **Management of non-melanoma skin cancer**

Basal cell carcinoma

'Surgical excision is the preferred treatment. Mohs micrographic surgery is an effective treatment for high-risk primary and recurrent BCC. Topical imiquimod appears effective in the treatment of some primary superficial BCC. Photodynamic therapy is good for primary superficial BCC. BCC in patients with Gorlin's syndrome should not be treated with radiotherapy.'

Squamous cell carcinoma

'Clinically well-defined, low-risk tumours less than 2 cm in diameter should be surgically excised with a 4 mm margin around the tumour border. Around 95% of recurrences and metastases of SCCs occur within 5 years; current guidelines suggest patients should be followed up for this period.'

• Telfer NR, et al. Br J Dermatol 2008; 159(1):35–48.
• Motley R, et al. Br J Dermatol 2002; 146(1):18–25.

For further information: www.bad.org.uk

fine telangiectatic vessels on the surface, which slowly enlarges. Central necrosis may occur, leaving an ulcer surrounded by a rolled pearly edge (Fig. 27.37). Without treatment, lesions may reach 1–2 cm in diameter over 5–10 years. Slow but relentless growth causes local tissue destruction. Sometimes the tumour becomes cystic or pigmented. The morphoeic variant is a slowly expanding, yellow or grey waxy plaque with an ill-defined edge. Fibrosis often follows ulceration and crusting, and the lesion may appear as an enlarging scar. The superficial (multifocal) variant is seen most often on the trunk; it appears as a slowly enlarging pink or brown scaly plaque with a fine 'whipcord' edge and may resemble a patch of intra-epidermal carcinoma (see below). If left, it may grow to 10 cm in diameter.

Management

The majority of BCCs are easily treated with local destruction. Metastasis is extremely rare; nevertheless, problems may arise: for example, in tumours close to the eye margins where local invasion can cause considerable management difficulty, or in tumours which track down nerves such as the infra-orbital.

Possible treatments include surgery, cryotherapy, radiotherapy, photodynamic therapy or the topical immunostimulant imiquimod. Surgery is increasingly used first choice, as it allows proper histological assessment of the tumour and examination of tumour margins (Box 27.33). Curettage and cautery also show good results for some small low-risk lesions, particularly if they are superficial and not close to the eye. Cryotherapy has a significant morbidity when used for anything other than superficial lesions. Radiotherapy is now used rarely.

The importance of control of tumour margins is widely debated. Some tumours can be misleading in terms of clinical assessment of their margins, as they are often more extensive than they first appear. Particular caution is required with morphoeic BCCs. If the primary tumour is not completely excised, it is often suggested that the lesion may just be followed up because not all tumours that appear to be incompletely excised recur. This policy makes sense in many body sites but not for high-risk tumours, such as those close to the eye, or with obviously morphoeic BCCs. Whatever modality

of treatment is used, in expert hands the cure rate should be greater than 90%. Tumour recurrences are treated using the same modalities as above.

Squamous cell carcinoma (SCC)

SCC is the second most common skin cancer after BCC and, like other forms of skin cancer, is increasing in age-specific incidence.

Aetiology

As well as the risk factors discussed above, SCC may arise in long-standing areas of inflammation such as around a chronic cutaneous ulcer, or in patients with scarring genetic syndromes of the skin such as dystrophic epidermolysis bullosa, in which up to 50% of patients may develop SCC.

Clinical features

SCC is a proliferative tumour that grows over a few months. Varying clinical presentations include keratotic nodules (Fig. 27.38), exophytic erythematous nodules, infiltrating firm tumours and ulcers with an indurated edge. Histological grade also varies from well differentiated to anaplastic. SCCs of the lip behave more

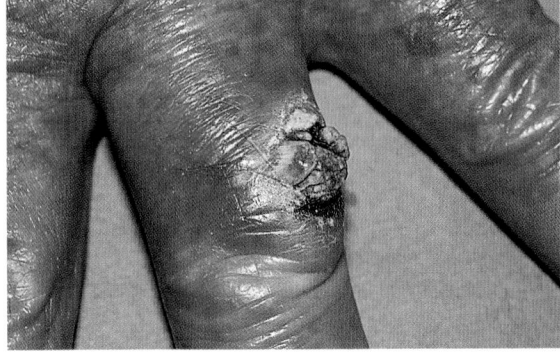

Fig. 27.38 Squamous cell carcinoma. A warty nodule with induration of the adjacent skin.

aggressively and show a greater frequency of metastasis. It is said that SCCs of the pinnae may also be more aggressive, although this may reflect inadequate primary treatment.

Management

As with BCC, a number of modalities may be used but generally excision is preferred (see Box 27.33). Some small SCCs may be treated with curettage and cautery, or with radiotherapy. Because of the definite but small risk of metastasis, assessment of margins (using standard histology) or Mohs micrographic surgery (p. 1256) is required. For straightforward SCC, excision with a 3–4 mm margin has a cure rate of 90% or more. Poorly differentiated SCC or SCC on the ears or at the site of previous burns should be treated more cautiously. Radiotherapy can be used in selected cases.

Pre-malignant tumours

Actinic keratosis

Actinic keratoses are small, scaly, red areas on sun-exposed sites that show focal areas of dysplasia on histological examination (Fig. 27.39). They are extremely common and frequently multiple; in some surveys over half the population aged over 40 have one or more lesions. The rate of progression to SCC appears low (1:1000 per year per lesion) and a large proportion of actinic keratoses may spontaneously involute. By contrast, many SCCs arise without evidence of a previous actinic keratosis. If an actinic keratosis rapidly increases in size, ulcerates, bleeds or becomes painful, then transformation to SCC should be considered.

Management

Actinic keratoses are treated effectively with liquid nitrogen. If there are a large number of lesions, then the topical cytotoxic 5-fluorouracil may be required; alternatively, topical imiquimod or photodynamic therapy

Intra-epidermal carcinoma (Bowen's disease)

Clinical features

This usually presents as a slow-growing, red, scaly area with some resemblance to a plaque of psoriasis, on the lower leg of elderly females. Histology reveals full-thickness dysplasia. Lesions may occur at other sites (Fig. 27.40) and occasionally transform into SCC, but with a higher frequency than actinic keratoses.

Investigations and management

An initial incisional biopsy may be required and treatment is by local destruction. Alternatively, the lesions may be managed with curettage and subsequent histology. Curettage, however, does not usually allow an SCC to be positively diagnosed or excluded because the tissue architecture is not preserved. Alternatives are cryotherapy, photodynamic therapy or imiquimod.

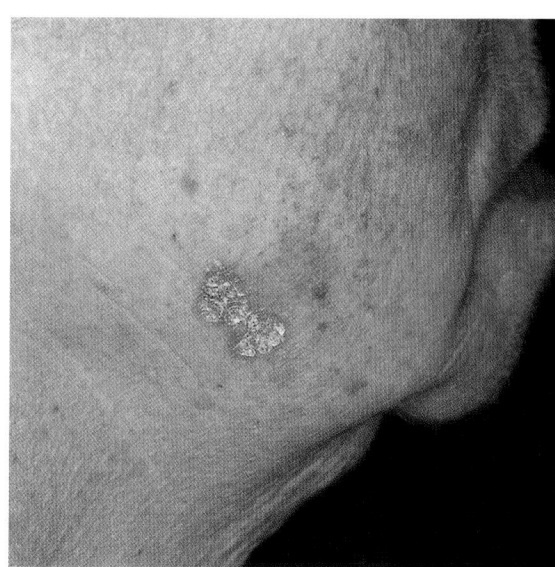

Fig. 27.40 Intra-epidermal carcinoma (right cheek). This persistent psoriasis-like plaque recurred after the original (anterior) lesion was treated by freezing.

Keratoacanthoma

This is a striking benign keratinocyte tumour, characterised by a period of rapid growth over a month or two, which develops into a tumour that may be 4 or 5 cm across or even larger. It has a volcano shape with a central keratin plug in a dome-shaped nodule (Fig. 27.41). Spontaneous resolution occurs but may take months. Clinically and histologically, the lesion resembles an SCC but has a different natural history. It is better to excise these lesions because clinically they are frequently hard to distinguish from a fast-growing SCC, and they often leave an unsightly scar which can be improved by surgical removal of the lesion. In order to make a positive diagnosis of keratoacanthoma, a large wedge biopsy or cross-sectional biopsy is required.

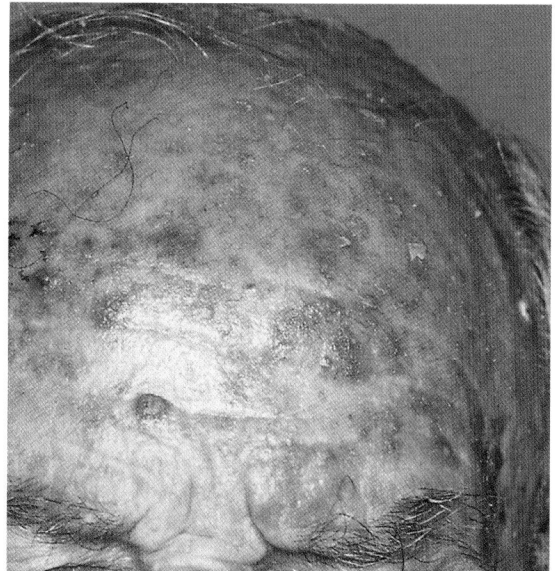

Fig. 27.39 Numerous actinic keratoses in a white patient who had lived for years in the tropics.

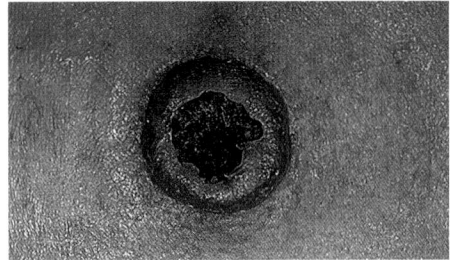

Fig. 27.41 Keratoacanthoma.

Melanoma

Malignant melanoma, like other forms of skin cancer, has increased in incidence over recent decades, even when figures are adjusted for changes in the age structure of the population. It has a case fatality rate of approximately 10–20%. Therapy for metastatic melanoma is unsatisfactory and therefore primary prevention and early detection are important. The main risk factors for melanoma are UVR exposure, pale skin, naevi number and family history. Fewer than 10% of melanomas occur in the context of a significant family history, but within this group there are rare kindreds in whom the lifetime risk of melanoma may approach 50%. Melanomas are common on the upper back in men and the lower legs in women.

Clinical features

The classification of invasive malignant melanomas is shown in Box 27.34.

Two-thirds of invasive melanomas are preceded by a superficial and radial growth phase characterised by an expanding, irregularly pigmented macule or plaque. Its margin is usually irregular with reniform projections (Fig. 27.42). Lentigo maligna (in situ changes of malignancy only) and lentigo maligna melanoma occur most often on the exposed skin of the elderly. A speckled macular lentigo maligna may have been present for many years before a nodule of invasive melanoma appears within it. The in situ phase of superficial spreading melanoma, the most common type in Caucasians, seldom lasts for longer than 2 years, usually shows much colour variation and is often palpable. Acral lentiginous melanoma occurs on the palms and soles and the absolute incidence rates are the same in all populations; by contrast, the rates at other body sites are low in African races, the Chinese and the Japanese, which suggests that this variant of melanoma is not related to UVR exposure. Nodular

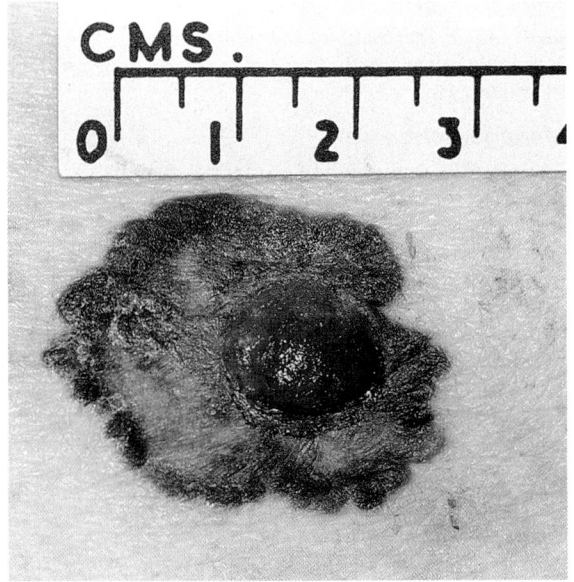

Fig. 27.42 Superficial spreading melanoma. The radial growth phase was present for about 3 years before the invasive amelanotic nodule developed within it. Note the irregular outline, asymmetrical shape and different hues, including depigmented areas signifying spontaneous regression.

melanoma develops as a pigmented nodule with no preceding in situ phase. All changing pigmented lesions deserve careful examination remembering the 'ABCDE' features of malignant melanoma (see Box 27.4 and Fig. 27.3, p. 1245). About 30–50% of melanomas appear to develop in a preceding melanocytic naevus. A change in any naevus should raise suspicion of malignant transformation.

True amelanotic melanomas occur but are rare; flecks of pigmentation can usually be seen with a lens. Subungual melanomas present as painless, expanding areas of pigmentation under a nail and usually involve the nail fold.

The clinical stages of malignant melanoma are shown in Box 27.35. The diagnosis is established by an initial excision of the lesion with a 2 mm margin wherever possible.

Management

Surgical excision is usually required, although very rarely radiotherapy may play a role. The extent of normal tissue that needs to be removed around a melanoma remains a subject of debate. Most would agree that a clear margin needs to be present so that there is little doubt that the tumour is fully excised; the deeper the tumour, the more caution is warranted (Box 27.36). The majority of tumours can be excised without the need

i 27.34 **Classification of cutaneous malignant melanoma**

Type of invasive melanoma	Presence of preceding in situ/radial growth phase
Superficial spreading	+
Lentigo maligna	+
Nodular	−
Acral lentiginous	+

i 27.35 **Clinical stages of malignant melanoma**

Stage I	Primary lesion only
Stage II	Regional nodal disease
Stage III	Distant disease (nodal or visceral)

EBM 27.36 **Margin of excision of melanoma**

'Radical surgery (4–6 cm excision margins) provides no greater benefit for local recurrence or survival than more conservative surgery (1–2 cm excision margins). Recommended excision margins for malignant melanoma depend on their Breslow thickness: melanomas < 1 mm in depth should have a 1 cm margin; melanomas > 1 mm in depth need a 2 cm margin.'

- Roberts DL, et al. on behalf of the Melanoma Study Group. Br J Dermatol 2002; 146:7–18.

For further information: www.sign.ac.uk

for grafting. The role of local lymph node dissection in the absence of evidence of tumour spread is uncertain. Recently, attempts have been made to determine whether the local nodes are 'subclinically' involved by sentinel lymph node biopsy. The draining lymph node is identified by injection of radioisotope adjacent to the primary tumour and by radioscintigraphy, and is then removed and examined for 'occult' tumour using histology with or without immunohistology or PCR amplification of melanocyte gene products. Such a biopsy provides some prognostic information, and some would argue that local lymph nodes should be removed if affected. There is, however, no evidence for better outcome in those in whom sentinel node biopsy is performed than in those in whom it is not. Palpable local nodes in stage II patients should be removed by block dissection. Chemotherapy is curative only exceptionally but may play an important palliative role in those with stage III disease or earlier. Interferon-alpha may have a role in individuals at high risk of metastasis.

Prognosis

Fewer than 10% of those with clinical stage III disease survive 2 years; those with stage I disease have a 70% chance of surviving 5 years. The thickness of the tumour can be measured microscopically by Breslow's method, which gives the distance between the granular cell layer and the deepest part of the tumour. This is a reliable predictor of prognosis for patients with stage I disease. Over 90% of those with tumours less than 1 mm thick survive 5 years, but the prognosis worsens with thicker tumours. The 5-year survival of patients with tumours greater than 3.5 mm thick is about 50%. Females generally fare better than males and tumours at certain sites (e.g. lower leg) are less aggressive.

Lesions that may be confused with skin cancers

Although the distinction between melanoma and non-melanoma skin lesions based on cell type would appear clear-cut, in practice it is not always so. For instance, melanocytic naevi which are comprised of melanocytes are frequently but not always markedly pigmented. Seborrhoeic keratosis, even in the hands of experts, can be confused with melanocytic naevi and melanoma. Therefore, in some instances, histology will be required.

Freckle (ephelis)

Freckles are focal increases in melanin in keratinocytes, but with a normal number of melanocytes. They are common in fair-skinned patients, particularly those with red hair, and there is a familial tendency. In sensitive individuals, freckles may develop at most body sites. Clinically they are flat, tanned brown lesions with irregular borders. They are common on the face and darken in response to UVR.

Lentigines

A lentigo is defined as an area of increased melanocyte proliferation along the basement membrane, but without the formation of the nests that are seen in melanocytic naevi. Confusingly, the solar lentigo is not a true lentigo but a flat form of seborrhoeic keratosis; there is increased undulation of the rete pegs and dermal papillae, associated with a normal number of melanocytes, but increased melanin in the surrounding keratinocytes. These lesions are usually seen in sun-exposed skin, become more common with age and are often referred to as 'liver' or 'age spots'. They can vary in colour from light tan to dark brown. Histopathological examination confirms plain or reticulated seborrhoeic keratoses. Their importance is as a differential diagnosis for a superficial spreading melanoma or a lentigo maligna melanoma.

Haemangiomas

Benign vascular tumours or hamartomas are not uncommon; they include Campbell de Morgan spots which present as bright pink or red smooth papules on the upper half of the body. They can sometimes be difficult to distinguish from melanocytic lesions, particularly if they are thrombosed or occur on particular sites such as the lip or the genitalia.

Seborrhoeic warts (basal cell papilloma)

Seborrhoeic warts (seborrhoeic keratoses) are common benign epidermal tumours (Fig. 27.43). Despite their name and oily appearance, they do not involve the sebaceous glands. They are usually a cosmetic issue but may mimic melanoma. As outlined above, some lesions that are commonly referred to as lentigos are flat seborrhoeic keratoses. The latter, however, may frequently become elevated and are more commonly found on the trunk and the face. Both sexes are equally affected. The lesions take on a myriad of appearances, varying in colour from

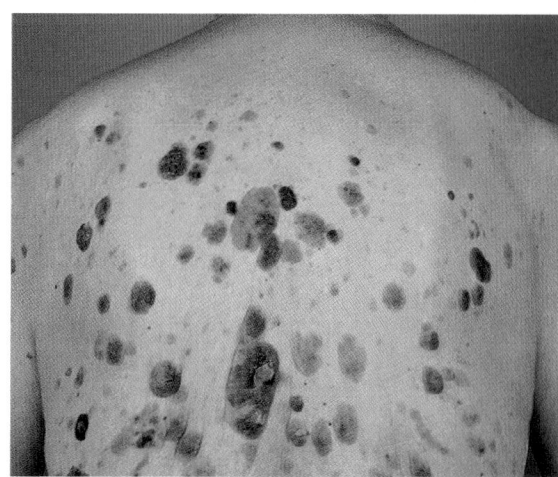

Fig. 27.43 Multiple seborrhoeic warts.

light yellow to very dark brown and almost black, and in shape from fairly flat to a protuberant and 'stuck-on' appearance. They may even be pedunculated. The surface often appears greasy and may reveal pinpoint keratin plugs, most easily seen with a lens. If there is no doubt about the diagnosis, they can be readily treated with either cryotherapy or curettage and cautery. Otherwise, an excision biopsy and histology should be performed as, if the lesion is a melanoma, prognostic information, such as the Breslow thickness, is required.

Melanocytic naevi

Melanocytic naevi (moles) are localised benign proliferations of melanocytes, which are clonal. Their cause is unknown but may relate to abnormalities of the normal migratory pattern of melanocytes during development. It is quite normal to have 20–50, but individuals with red hair have fewer. The number reflects both genetic and environmental characteristics. Individuals who have had greater sun exposure have higher numbers of moles, and monozygotic twins show a higher concordance than dizygotes. With the exception of congenital melanocytic naevi (which are present at birth or appear shortly after), most melanocytic naevi appear in childhood and early adult life, or during pregnancy or oestrogen therapy. The onset of a new mole is less common after the age of 25.

Clinical features

Acquired melanocytic naevi are classified according to the microscopic location of the clumps of melanocytes in the skin (Fig. 27.44). Junctional naevi are usually circular and macular; their colour ranges from mid- to dark brown and may vary within a single lesion. Compound and intradermal naevi are similar in appearance; both are nodules of up to 1 cm in diameter, although intradermal naevi are usually less pigmented than compound. Their surface may be smooth, cerebriform or even hyperkeratotic and papillomatous, and are often hairy.

Using a variety of criteria, some naevi have been labelled atypical or dysplastic, suggesting that the individual is at an increased risk of melanoma. Unfortunately, such terms have been poorly defined and used to describe both a clinical and a histological appearance, but these do not coincide. Some individuals have abnormal naevi in the sense that they seem to have larger numbers, or they may have naevi on the scalp and the palmar and plantar surfaces, as well as the buttocks. Some may appear pinkish and even show an inflamed halo. Such naevi are known to occur in some rare families with an inherited predisposition to melanoma. Otherwise, the significance

of such changes is unclear and criteria for management and follow-up are not agreed.

Whereas it is said that 30–50% of malignant melanomas develop from melanocytic naevi, only a minute percentage of melanocytic naevi become malignant. Malignant change is most likely in large congenital melanocytic naevi (where the risk may correlate with the size or mass of the melanocyte lesion) and possibly in those families who have been diagnosed as showing large numbers of atypical naevi with a history of melanoma. The value of self-examination has not been established in trials. A change in a mole (p. 1244) may be a harbinger of melanoma but is usually not. In the majority of Caucasian populations, any change in a mole requires careful clinical assessment, remembering that the negative specificity of clinical assessment of early melanomas is poor. Excision with histology is therefore frequently recommended.

Management

Melanocytic naevi are normal and do not require excision, except when malignancy is suspected or when they become repeatedly inflamed or traumatised. Some individuals wish to have them removed for cosmetic reasons.

Blue naevi

These are melanocytic naevi in which there is a dermal proliferation of spindled melanocytes relatively deep within the dermis. Light scattering means that the pigment appears blue rather than the usual brown. They may be difficult to distinguish from nodular melanomas.

Dermatofibromas

A dermatofibroma is a firm, often pigmented, raised lesion most common on the lower legs. Its aetiology is unclear and it is uncertain whether it represents a reactive process or a tumour. There is frequently a ring of pigment around the lesion, firmness, and dimpling when the skin is pinched, which reflects the fact that the dermatofibroma is tethered to the epidermis. These lesions are commonly confused with melanocytic naevi.

Acrochordons (skin tags)

These are harmless pedunculated lesions which are common in the skin flexures but can occur at other sites. They may be confused with melanocytic naevi but are easily excised.

Lipomas

These are benign tumours of adipocytes which have a characteristically soft consistency, and are usually easily distinguished from epidermal skin tumours because they arise more deeply within the skin. A variant, called an angiolipoma, is characteristically painful.

Cutaneous T-cell lymphoma (mycosis fungoides)

Cutaneous T-cell lymphoma develops slowly over many (sometimes 20 or 30) years from a plaque stage often resembling psoriasis, through to nodules and finally a systemic stage. B-cell lymphomas, on the other hand, usually present as nodules or plaque-like tumours. The diagnosis of cutaneous T-cell lymphoma requires a high

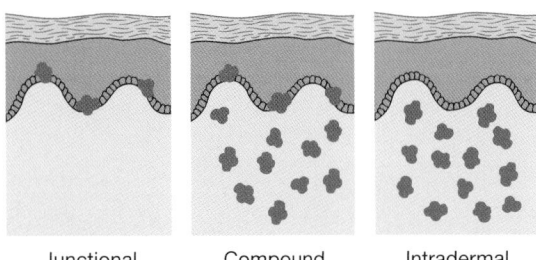

Junctional   Compound   Intradermal

Fig. 27.44 Classification of melanocytic naevi. Classification is based on microscopic location of the clumps of naevus cells.

index of suspicion, particularly in patients thought to have unusual forms of eczema or psoriasis who have failed to respond to treatment. The treatment of cutaneous T-cell lymphoma is symptomatic and there is no evidence that specific modalities of treatment alter prognosis.

In the early stages of cutaneous T-cell lymphoma, either systemic or local corticosteroids may be indicated; alternatively, PUVA or narrow band UVB phototherapy may be employed, although these are of symptomatic benefit only and are not risk-free. Once lesions have moved beyond the plaque stage, electron beam radiation or systemic anti-lymphoma regimens may be required. Management requires careful collaboration between dermatologists, pathologists and haematological oncologists.

SKIN PROBLEMS IN GENERAL MEDICINE

Many skin conditions present to a number of medical specialty clinics. These are listed in Box 27.37 and the most common of those not discussed elsewhere are described below.

Vasculitis

Vasculitis typically presents with palpable purpura (see Fig. 25.42, p. 1113). The causes include drugs, infection, connective tissue disease, malignancy and idiopathic

 27.37 Skin problems in general medicine

Primary skin problems

- Cellulitis
- Vasculitis
- Leg ulcers
- Pressure sores

Skin involvement in multisystem disease

- Genetically determined (e.g. neurofibromatosis and tuberous sclerosis complex)
- Xanthomas
- Amyloidosis
- Porphyria
- Sarcoidosis

Non-specific and variable skin reactions to systemic disease

- Urticaria
- Erythema multiforme
- Annular erythemas
- Erythema nodosum
- Pyoderma gangrenosum
- Sweet's syndrome
- Generalised pruritus

Skin conditions associated with malignancy

- Dermatomyositis
- Generalised pruritus
- Acanthosis nigricans
- Superficial thrombophlebitis

Skin problems associated with specific medical disorders

- Liver: generalised pruritus, pigmentation, spider naevi and palmar erythema
- Kidney: generalised pruritus and pigmentation
- Diabetes mellitus: necrobiosis lipoidica
- Cutaneous Crohn's disease

Skin problems secondary to treatment of systemic disease

- Drug eruptions

Miscellaneous

- Granuloma annulare
- Morphoea

conditions (e.g. Henoch–Schönlein purpura). The diagnosis is confirmed by skin biopsy, with histology and immunofluorescence examination. Investigation for systemic involvement (particularly renal) and for the precipitating cause is important.

Pressure sores

Pressure sores are caused by prolonged pressure-induced ischaemia, when the interface pressure between the patient's body and its supporting surface exceeds capillary closing pressure. Up to 5% of patients aged over 70 years in hospital develop pressure sores, but this may rise to 30% in those with a fractured neck of femur. The morbidity and mortality of those with deep ulcers are high.

Aetiology

The main risk factors for pressure sores include:
- *immobility*, e.g. coma, neurological disease with paralysis, surgery, pain, overuse of sedatives, depression
- *hypotension*, e.g. shock, dehydration
- *reduced oxygen delivery*, e.g. anaemia, fever, infection
- *peripheral vascular disease*, including diabetic microangiopathy
- *under-nutrition*, e.g. malignant cachexia, alcoholism
- *skin condition*, e.g. atrophy due to age or topical corticosteroids, dry/cracked and moist/chapped.

Clinical features

The sore starts as a localised area of erythema and progresses to a superficial blister or erosion. If the cause is not corrected, deeper damage occurs; a black eschar develops which, when removed or shed, leaves a deep and penetrating ulcer, often colonised by *Pseudomonas aeruginosa*. The skin overlying bony prominences, such as the sacrum, greater trochanter, ischial tuberosity, calcaneal tuberosity and lateral malleolus, is especially susceptible.

Management

This is not easy but the following are important:
- prevention by regular repositioning of immobile patients and use of pressure-reducing mattresses in those at high risk
- treatment of risk factors including undernutrition
- débridement of necrotic tissue either by surgery or by enzymatic necrolysis
- systemic antibiotics for spreading infection
- dressings to keep the wound wet and enhance granulation; regular cleansing with normal saline or 0.5% aqueous silver nitrate; semi-permeable dressings such as OpSite
- consideration of plastic surgical reconstruction when the ulcer is clean.

Tuberous sclerosis complex

This is an autosomal dominant condition with hamartomas affecting many systems. Two genetic loci have been identified: TSC-1 (chromosome 9) encoding hamartin and TSC-2 (chromosome 16) encoding tuberin.

The classic triad of clinical features comprises learning disability, epilepsy and skin lesions but there is a wide spectrum of clinical expression. The skin signs include small white oval (ash leaf) macules which usually present in early childhood, pink or yellowish

27

papules on the centre of the face ('adenoma sebaceum' due to angiofibromas) occurring later on in adolescence, periungual and subungual fibromas, and connective tissue naevi (cobblestone-like plaques at the base of the spine, sometimes called shagreen patches). Other features may include hyperplastic gums, retinal phakomas (fibrous overgrowth), renal, lung and heart tumours, cerebral gliomas and calcification of the basal ganglia.

Xanthomas

These deposits of fatty material in the skin, subcutaneous fat and tendons may be the first clue to primary or secondary hyperlipidaemia and are described in detail on pages 452–453.

Amyloidosis

Deposits of amyloid in the skin often appearing as waxy plaques around the eyes; they are prominent in primary systemic amyloidosis (p. 84) and in amyloid associated with multiple myeloma, but uncommon in systemic amyloidosis secondary to rheumatoid arthritis or other chronic inflammatory diseases. 'Pinch purpura' appears where the skin is traumatised due to amyloid infiltration of blood vessels and may be a striking feature. Macular amyloid is a pruritic eruption more common in darker skin types. Clinically, there is macular or patches of grey-brown discoloration, usually on the back. Treatment is difficult but potent topical steroids can be helpful.

Porphyria

The porphyrias are described in detail on page 456.

- *Porphyria cutanea tarda* is the most common porphyria. It usually starts in adulthood and can be inherited or acquired due to alcohol, iron overload, oestrogens, hepatitis C and HIV disease. The cutaneous features are increased skin fragility, blistering (Fig. 27.45), erosions and milia occurring on light-exposed areas such as the backs of the hands. Patients rarely associate their symptoms with acute light exposure. Facial hypertrichosis and hyperpigmentation may also be seen.
- *Erythropoietic protoporphyria* is rare and starts in childhood, with burning and pain on light-exposed areas due to ferrochelatase deficiency. Scars occur, particularly on the nose. Protoporphyrins are found in the red cells, plasma and stool.

- *Variegate porphyria* has cutaneous features similar to those of porphyria cutanea tarda, and systemic as those of acute intermittent porphyria.
- *Hereditary coproporphyria* is associated with photosensitivity in 30%. Systemic features are as those of acute intermittent porphyria.
- *Pseudoporphyrias* are associated with sunbed usage, NSAIDs (particularly naproxen) and renal failure, which give rise to skin lesions that mimic the photosensitive porphyrias, particularly porphyria cutanea tarda. The pathogenesis is unclear.

Sarcoidosis

Skin lesions are seen in about one-third of patients with systemic sarcoidosis (p. 708) and include erythema nodosum (see Fig. 19.54, p. 709), granulomatous deposits in long-standing scars, dusky infiltrated plaques on the nose and fingers (lupus pernio), and scattered brownish-red, violaceous or hypopigmented papules or nodules which vary in number, size and distribution.

Erythema multiforme

This is a reaction pattern of multiform erythematous lesions. The precipitating factor may not be found in some cases, but attacks are provoked by the factors listed in Box 27.38.

The multiform erythematous lesions may be urticaria-like and some have obvious 'bull's-eye' or 'target' lesions. Blisters may be seen in the centre or around the edges of the lesions (Fig. 27.46). In some cases blisters

27.38 Provoking factors in erythema multiforme
- Viral infections, e.g. herpes simplex, orf
- Bacterial infections, e.g. *Mycoplasma*
- Drugs, especially sulphonamides, penicillins and barbiturates
- Systemic malignancy
- Radiotherapy

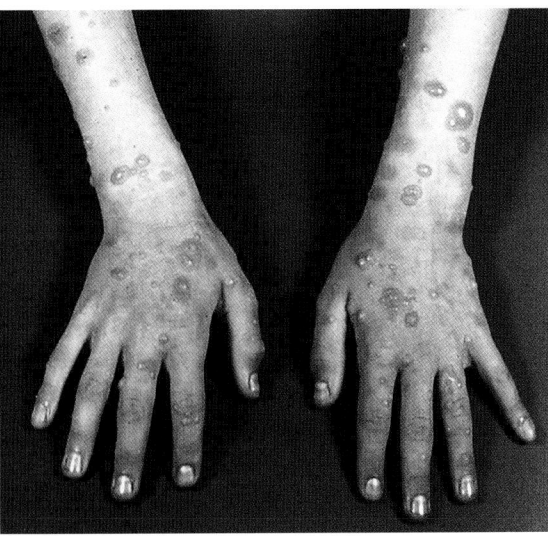

Fig. 27.46 Erythema multiforme with blistering lesions in a young woman.

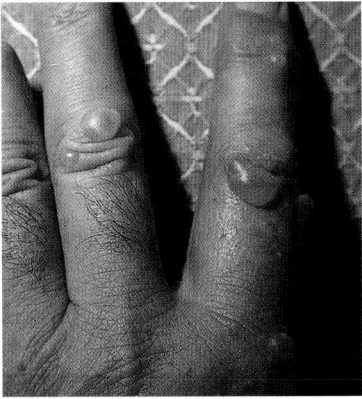

Fig. 27.45 Cutaneous hepatic porphyria. Recent skin fragility and blistering on the backs of the fingers.

dominate the picture; the Stevens–Johnson syndrome is severe bullous erythema multiforme with marked mucosal involvement including the mouth, eyes and genitals, and constitutional disturbance.

Usually no treatment is required, although symptomatic relief can be obtained with simple dressings. Stevens–Johnson syndrome can be treated with a short course of intravenous immunoglobulin. Corticosteroids are best avoided.

Erythema nodosum

This characteristic reaction pattern (see Fig. 19.54, p. 709) is due to a vasculitis in the deep dermis and subcutaneous fat. Provoking factors are listed in Box 27.39. Painful, palpable, dusky blue-red nodules are most commonly seen on the lower legs. Malaise, fever and joint pains are common. The lesions resolve slowly over a month, leaving bruise-like marks. The underlying cause should be determined and treated. Bed rest and oral NSAIDs may hasten resolution. Tapering systemic corticosteroid courses may be required in stubborn cases.

27.39 Provoking factors in erythema nodosum
Infections
• Bacteria, e.g. streptococci, mycobacteria, *Brucella*, *Mycoplasma*, *Rickettsia*, *Chlamydia*
• Viruses
• Fungi
Drugs
• e.g. Sulphonamides, oral contraceptives
Systemic disease
• e.g. Sarcoidosis, ulcerative colitis and Crohn's disease

Pyoderma gangrenosum (PG)

PG predominantly occurs in adults between the ages of 25 and 54 years. The eruption starts as an inflamed nodule or pustule which breaks down centrally and rapidly progresses to an ulcer with an indurated or undermined purplish or pustular edge (Fig. 27.47). Lesions may be single or multiple and are classified as ulcerative, pustular, bullous and vegetative. Although PG may arise in the absence of any underlying disease, it is often

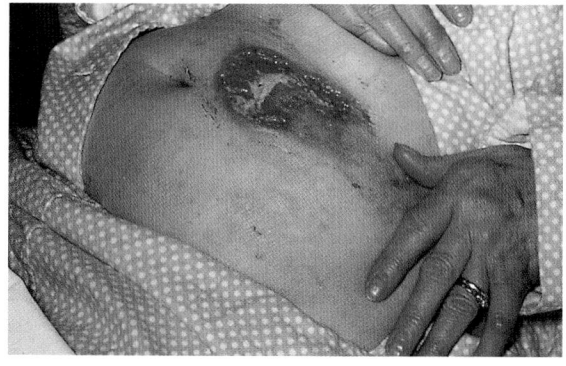

Fig. 27.47 Pyoderma gangrenosum. A large indolent ulcer in a patient with rheumatoid arthritis. Note healing in one part.

associated with a systemic disease such as inflammatory bowel disease, arthritis (both rheumatoid arthritis and seronegative arthropathies), immunodeficiency and immunosuppression including HIV disease, monoclonal gammopathies and leukaemia. Investigation for these should be performed. There are no diagnostic features on skin biopsy and the diagnosis is primarily clinical. Local management includes pain relief, prevention of secondary bacterial infection and dressings. Systemic therapy that can be tried includes oral corticosteroids in a tapering dose, dapsone, minocycline, sulfasalazine and ciclosporin. Once the patient is clear of disease, recurrences are only intermittent.

Acanthosis nigricans

This is a velvety thickening and pigmentation of the major flexures, particularly the axillae (see figure, p. 796). There are several types. The most common form is an obesity-associated weight-dependent mild acanthosis nigricans. When the patient loses weight, the cutaneous features regress. It can also be associated with various syndromes, including insulin resistance syndrome (see p. 802 and Box 21.4). Acanthosis nigricans can also be associated with malignancy, particularly gastric (60%). Pruritus is a feature of malignancy-associated acanthosis and regression occurs after the tumour is excised. Acanthosis nigricans sometimes recurs with metastatic disease.

Necrobiosis lipoidica

This condition is associated with diabetes mellitus. Less than 1% of people with diabetes have necrobiosis, but more than 85% of patients with necrobiosis will have or will develop diabetes. Typically, the lesions appear as shiny, atrophic and slightly yellow plaques on the shins (Fig. 27.48). Underlying telangiectasia are easily seen. Minor knocks may precipitate slow-healing ulcers. No treatment is very effective. Topical and intralesional corticosteroids are used, as is long-term PUVA.

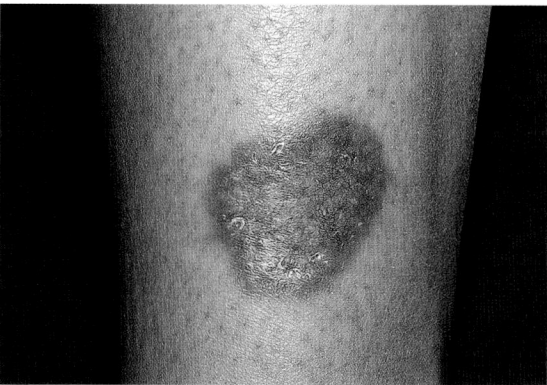

Fig. 27.48 Necrobiosis lipoidica. An atrophic yellowish plaque on the skin of a person with diabetes.

Cutaneous Crohn's disease

Skin involvement in Crohn's disease (p. 896) is rare but can be severely disabling. The skin manifestations can be categorised as specific (perianal, oral and peristomal), non-specific (erythema nodosum, neutrophilic

27

dermatoses) and secondary to nutritional deficiency. The specific changes include sinuses, fistulae, oedema, oral granulomatous disease and so-called 'metastatic' Crohn's, in which typical non-caseating granulomatous histology is found in a variety of skin eruptions. Treatment is of the underlying disease with mesalazine, steroids, immunosuppressives or anti-TNF-α therapy.

Granuloma annulare

This is a common cutaneous condition of uncertain aetiology; an association with diabetes is now thought to be spurious. Dermal nodules occur singly or in an annular configuration. They are asymptomatic but commonly occur on highly visible sites such as the hands and feet. Histologically, palisading granulomas are found in the dermis. Intralesional corticosteroids can be helpful, but the natural history is spontaneous resolution over a few months to a couple of years.

Morphoea

Morphoea is a localised form of scleroderma that can affect any site at any age. It usually presents as a thickened plaque of skin but can be more generalised or linear. There is no systemic involvement.

DRUG ERUPTIONS

Cutaneous drug reactions are common and almost any drug can cause them. They should be included in the differential diagnosis of most skin diseases. Although the mechanisms are poorly understood, drug eruptions may be classified as shown in Box 27.40.

Clinical features and investigations

Box 27.41 shows the patterns of drug eruptions that may occur. They usually start within a few days or weeks of taking the culprit drug. The possibility of a drug eruption should be considered particularly when a rash is atypical of a known skin disease (Fig. 27.49). It is essential to take a careful history of medications and preceding illnesses from at least 4 weeks prior to the onset of the rash. Further clues pointing to the diagnosis are included in Box 27.42 but no specific investigations help. While an affected individual will usually have the same reaction to the specific drug or to those chemically related on a further challenge, rechallenging with the suspected drug as a diagnostic test is unwise unless the reaction is mild and there is no suitable alternative.

Management

The first step is to withdraw the suspected drug(s), except in the case of suspected drug-induced photodermatoses, where if possible phototesting should be carried out when the patient is on the drug, and then again at a later date when the drug has been withdrawn. Drug withdrawal may not be easy, or even possible if there is no alternative available. The decision will depend on many factors, including the severity and nature of the drug reaction, its potential reversibility and the probability that the drug caused the reaction. Supportive treatment with antihistamines or a course of systemic corticosteroids may be indicated, depending on the type of skin reaction. The management of anaphylactic shock is described on page 89.

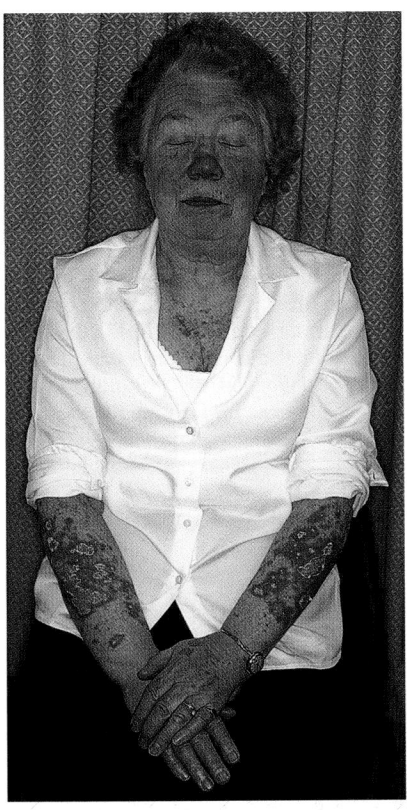

Fig. 27.49 Drug eruption. A bizarre but symmetrical erythematous scaly rash with a distribution suggesting a degree of photosensitivity. The rash persisted until the recently prescribed sulphonylurea was withdrawn.

27.40 Drug eruptions and their mechanisms	
Mechanism	**Examples**
Non-immunological (non-allergic)	
Pharmacological effect	Striae due to corticosteroids; mouth ulcers due to methotrexate
Drug overdose or failure to eliminate	Morphine rashes with liver disease/failure
Drug interaction	Bruising with warfarin and aspirin
Idiosyncratic reaction	Drug-induced variegate porphyria
Phototoxic reaction	Chlorpromazine-induced light reactions
Altered skin mycology	Tetracyclines and vaginal candidiasis
Exacerbation of pre-existing skin condition	Lithium and β-blocker worsen psoriasis
Immunological (allergic)	
Immediate hypersensitivity	Penicillin-induced urticaria
Immune complex reaction	Drug-induced vasculitis or erythema multiforme
Delayed hypersensitivity	Drug-induced exfoliative dermatitis or photoallergic reactions

27.41 Clinical patterns of drug eruptions

Reaction pattern	Clinical features	Associated drugs
Toxic erythema	Erythematous plaques Morbilliform, sometimes with urticarial or erythema multiforme-like elements	Antibiotics (especially ampicillin) Sulphonamides, thiazide diuretics, para-aminosalicylic acid (PAS)
Urticaria	Itchy weals, sometimes accompanied by angioedema	Salicylates, codeine and NSAIDs Antibiotics, dextran and ACE inhibitors
Erythema and scaling	Small, scaly, pink papules to large, scaly, red papules	Antibiotics (e.g. penicillins, sulphonamides including co-trimoxazole) Gold, penicillamine and NSAIDs, particularly ibuprofen Anticonvulsants, ACE inhibitors, barbiturates, anti-thyroid drugs and cytokine modulators, e.g. adalimumab
Allergic vasculitis	Painful, palpable purpura developing into necrotic ulcers	Sulphonamides, indometacin, phenytoin and oral contraceptives
Erythema multiforme	Target-like lesions and bullae on the extensor aspects of the limbs	Sulphonamides and barbiturates
Purpura	Widespread purpura in the absence of thrombocytopenia or a coagulation defect	Thiazides, sulphonamides, sulphonylureas, adalimumab, infliximab, barbiturates and quinine
Bullous eruptions	May be associated with erythema and purpura May occur at pressure sites in drug-induced coma	Barbiturates Penicillamine Nalidixic acid, vancomycin
Exfoliative dermatitis	Universal redness and scaling, shivering	PAS, isoniazid and gold
Acute generalised exanthematous pustulosis/toxic pustuloderma	Rapid onset of sterile, non-follicular pustules on an erythematous base	Ampicillin/amoxicillin, quinolones, sulphonamides, pristinamycin, terbinafine Diltiazem and hydroxychloroquine
Fixed drug eruptions	Round, erythematous, sometimes bullous plaques developing at same site every time drug is given. Pigmentation on resolution.	Tetracyclines, sulphonamides Quinine and barbiturates
Acneiform eruptions	Rash resembles acne	Lithium and anticonvulsants Oral contraceptive, androgenic or glucocorticoid steroids Antituberculosis drugs, biological therapy (cetuximab)
Toxic epidermal necrolysis	Rash resembles scalded skin (see Fig. 27.35, p. 1275)	Barbiturates, phenytoin, lamotrigine, fluoxetine Penicillin, co-trimoxazole, nevirapine and allopurinol
Hair loss	Diffuse	Cytotoxic agents, infliximab and acitretin Anticoagulants, antithyroid drugs and oral contraceptives
Hypertrichosis	Excessive hair growth in non-androgenic distribution	Diazoxide, minoxidil and ciclosporin
Photosensitivity	Rash limited to exposed skin	Thiazide diuretics and phenothiazines Tetracyclines, sulphonamides and nalidixic acid NSAIDs, retinoids and psoralens
Pigmentation	See Box 27.15 (p. 1254)	
Psoriasiform rash	Rash like psoriasis	Lithium, β-blockers and anti-TNF-α therapy (infliximab)

27

27.42 Diagnostic clues to drug eruptions

- Past history of reaction to suspected drug
- Introduction of suspected drug a few days before onset of rash
- Recent prescription of a drug commonly associated with rashes (e.g. penicillin, sulphonamide, thiazide, allopurinol)
- Symmetrical eruption which fits with a well-recognised pattern caused by a current drug

LEG ULCERS

Leg ulceration due to venous disease

Damage to the venous system of the leg results in oedema, haemosiderin deposition, eczema, fibrosis and ulceration.

Aetiology

In the normal leg, there is a superficial low-pressure venous system connected to the deep, high-pressure veins by perforating veins. Muscular activity, aided by valves in the veins, pumps blood from the superficial to the deep system and towards the heart. Incompetent valves in the deep and perforating veins result in retrograde flow of blood to the superficial system, causing a rise in capillary hydrostatic pressure ('venous hypertension'). Fibrinogen is forced out through the capillary walls and fibrin is deposited as a pericapillary cuff. It is thought that growth and repair factors are trapped in the macromolecular cuff so that minor trauma cannot be repaired and ulcers develop.

Incompetent veins leading to venous hypertension may be due to previous deep venous thrombosis (p. 1004), congenital or familial valve incompetence, infection or deep venous obstruction (e.g. by a pelvic tumour). If conditions are favourable, the ulcers will heal by granulation with small epithelial islands at the base and epithelial growth from the edges. Healing is often slow and may never be complete. Recurrent ulceration is common. Clinical assessment and investigations are described on page 1252.

Complications

Chronic venous ulcers are invariably colonised by bacteria. Systemic antibiotic treatment is only required if signs of infection develop. Contact dermatitis to an ointment, dressing or bandage is not uncommon. The usual culprits are preservatives, lanolin and neomycin. Lipodermatosclerosis may cause lymphoedema, leading to hyperkeratosis and the so-called 'mossy foot'. Rarely, an SCC developing in a venous ulcer (Marjolin's ulcer) is responsible for its failure to heal.

Management

- Dietary advice is required in the obese and all should be encouraged to take gentle exercise.
- Oedema is reduced by the regular use of compression bandages, elevation of the legs when sitting and the judicious use of diuretics. In the absence of compromised arterial supply (ABPI > 0.8), graduated compression bandages applied from the toes to the knees enhance venous return and have been shown to be beneficial in healing (Box 27.43). Those individuals with an ABPI < 0.8 should be assumed to have arterial disease and compression bandaging must be avoided.
- Exudate and slough should be removed with normal saline solution, 0.5% aqueous silver nitrate or 5% aqueous hydrogen peroxide. If the ulcer is very purulent, soaking the leg for 15 minutes in 1:10 000 dilution of aqueous potassium permanganate may be helpful.
- Dressings commonly used for venous ulceration include antibiotic-impregnated tulle dressings, non-adhesive absorbent dressings (alginates, charcoals, hydrogels or hydrocolloids) and dry non-adherent dressings.
- The frequency of dressing changes depends on the state of the ulcer. Very purulent and exudative ulcers may need daily dressings whilst a clean, healing ulcer may only require dressings changed every week.
- Paste bandages, impregnated with zinc oxide or ichthammol, help to keep dressings in place and provide protection.
- Surrounding venous eczema is treated by a mild or moderately potent topical corticosteroid, but it should not be applied to the ulcer itself.
- Short courses of oral antibiotic therapy are only necessary for the treatment of overt infection. An anabolic corticosteroid, stanozolol, may help lipodermatosclerosis but fluid retention and hepatotoxicity limit its use.
- Vein surgery may help some younger patients with persistent venous ulcers. Pinch grafts may hasten the healing of clean ulcers but do not influence their rate of recurrence.

Leg ulceration due to arterial disease

Deep, painful and punched-out ulcers on the lower leg, especially if they occur on the shin and foot and are preceded by a history of intermittent claudication, are likely to be due to arterial disease. Risk factors include smoking, hypertension, diabetes mellitus and hyperlipidaemia. The foot is cyanotic and cold, and the skin surrounding the ulcer is atrophic and hairless. The peripheral arterial pulses are absent or reduced. Doppler studies are required and if arterial insufficiency (ABPI < 8) is confirmed, a vascular surgical assessment should be sought (p. 599).

Leg ulceration due to vasculitis

This is described on page 1112.

Leg ulceration due to neuropathy

The most common cause of a neuropathic ulcer is diabetes. The ulcers occur over weight-bearing areas such as the heel. Microangiopathy also contributes to ulceration in diabetes (p. 833).

HAIR DISORDERS

Patients may present with too much hair (hirsutism) or too little hair (alopecia, Box 27.44). Detailed assessment allows a specific diagnosis.

Tinea capitis

Fungal scalp infection is becoming increasingly common in urban areas in the UK, where it is most frequently spread by contact between children. Clinical features are variable due to associated inflammation, with patchy hair loss and some scaling. Affected individuals should have the area scraped and affected hairs plucked for mycological microscopy and culture. Endothrix (within the hair shaft) infections, e.g. *Trichophyton tonsurans*, cause relatively uninflamed patchy baldness with breakage

---

EBM 27.43 **Compression bandaging in leg ulceration**

'Compression bandaging is effective in those individuals with an ABPI > 0.8, measured by hand-held Doppler.'

- SIGN. The care of patients with chronic leg ulcer; 2005.

For further information: www.sign.ac.uk

27.44 Classification of alopecia

Localised	Diffuse
Non-scarring	
Tinea capitis	Androgenetic alopecia
Alopecia areata	Telogen effluvium
Androgenetic alopecia	Metabolic
Traumatic (trichotillomania,	Hypothyroidism
traction, cosmetic)	Hyperthyroidism
Syphilis	Hypopituitarism
	Diabetes mellitus
	HIV disease
	Nutritional deficiency
	Liver disease
	Post-partum
	Alopecia areata
	Syphilis
Scarring	
Idiopathic	Discoid lupus erythematosus
Developmental defects	Radiotherapy
Discoid lupus erythematosus	Folliculitis decalvans
Herpes zoster	Lichen planus pilaris
Pseudopelade	
Tinea capitis/kerion	

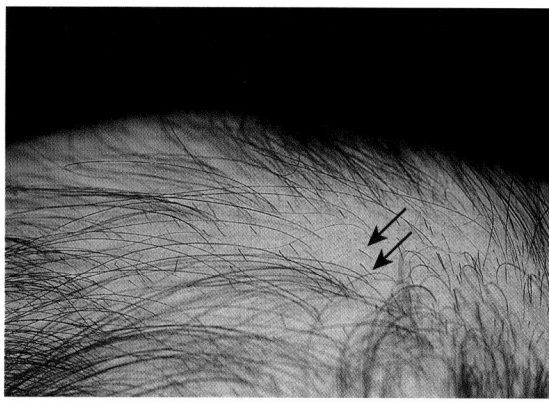

Fig. 27.50 Alopecia areata. Marked hair loss with diagnostic exclamation mark hairs (arrows).

of the hairs at the skin surface ('black dot'). There is no fluorescence under Wood's light. Ectothrix (outside the hair shaft) species of fungi, such as *Microsporum audouinii* (anthropophilic), show minimal inflammation; *Microsporum canis* (from dogs and cats) infections are more inflamed and can be identified by green fluorescence with Wood's light. Kerions are boggy, highly inflamed areas of tinea capitis and are usually caused by zoophilic (from animals, e.g. cattle ringworm) species of fungi (e.g. *Trichophyton verrucosum*). Accurate diagnosis of the culprit fungus allows treatment and control of the spread of infection.

Treatment is systemic with oral terbinafine, griseofulvin or itraconazole. Topical therapy, such as an antifungal shampoo, is recommended as an adjunct and arachis oil is used to remove crusting. Kerions sometimes require short courses of oral corticosteroids in addition to systemic antifungal therapy to reduce the inflammation.

Alopecia areata

This non-scarring condition appears as sharply defined non-inflamed bald patches, usually on the scalp. During the active stage of hair loss, pathognomonic 'exclamation mark' hairs are seen (broken-off hairs 3–4 mm long, which taper off towards the scalp, Fig. 27.50). An uncommon diffuse pattern on the scalp is recognised. The condition may affect the eyebrows, eyelashes and beard. Pitting and longitudinal wrinkling of the nail may be seen. The hair usually regrows spontaneously in small bald patches, but the outlook is less good with larger patches and when the alopecia appears early in life or is associated with atopy. Alopecia totalis describes complete loss of scalp hair, and alopecia universalis is complete loss of all hair. There is an association of alopecia areata with autoimmune disorders, atopy and Down's syndrome.

Androgenetic alopecia

Male-pattern baldness is physiological in men over 20 years old, although rarely it may be extensive and develop at an alarming pace in the late teens. It also occurs in females, most obviously after the menopause. The well-known distribution (bitemporal recession and then crown involvement) is described as 'male-pattern' but hair loss in females is often diffuse.

Investigations and management

A full blood count, ESR, urea and electrolytes, liver and thyroid function tests, an autoantibody profile and syphilis serology help determine the cause of non-scarring alopecia. Specialised tests, including the hair pluck test in which up to 50 hairs are removed with epilating forceps to determine the anagen:telogen ratio, are seldom necessary. Mycological assessment is advisable in cases of localised hair loss with scaling. In scarring alopecia, scalp biopsy, with direct immunofluorescence, may help to confirm a diagnosis of lichen planus of the scalp or discoid lupus erythematosus.

Successful treatment of alopecia is difficult, and patients require support and reassurance. Any underlying condition should be treated. Alopecia areata sometimes responds to topical or intralesional corticosteroids such as 0.3 mL triamcinolone (10 mg/mL). Some males with androgenetic alopecia may be helped by systemic finasteride or topical 2% minoxidil solution. In females, anti-androgen therapy such as cyproterone acetate is used. A wig may be appropriate for extensive alopecia. Scalp surgery and autologous hair transplants are expensive but sometimes effective in androgenetic alopecia.

Hirsutism

Hirsutism is the growth of terminal hair in a male pattern in a female, and is discussed in detail in on pages 759–760. The cause of most cases of hirsutism is unknown and, while it may occur in hyperandrogenism, Cushing's syndrome and polycystic ovary syndrome, only a small minority have a demonstrable hormonal abnormality.

27

27

NAIL DISORDERS

The condition of the nails may reflect both local and systemic disease. The nail plate arises from the nail matrix and lies on the nail bed (Fig. 27.51). The keratinous plate is produced by cells of the (dorsal) matrix and, to a much lesser extent, the (ventral) bed. Finger nails grow about 1 cm every 3 months and toe nails at about one-third of this rate.

Examination of the nail folds may reveal the inflammation and swelling of paronychia. Chronic paronychia is seen frequently in those with a poor peripheral circulation, those involved in wet work, those with diabetes mellitus, and in over-enthusiastic manicuring of cuticles. Ragged cuticles and dilated or thrombosed capillaries in the proximal nail folds are important pointers to connective tissue disease (Fig. 27.52).

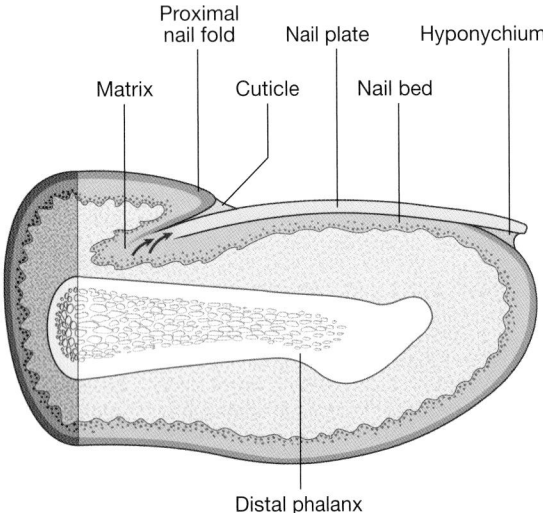

Fig. 27.51 **The nail plate and bed.** Arrows indicate the direction of nail growth.

Nail plate disorders

Longitudinal ridging and beading of the nail plate is not abnormal and increases with age. Similarly, occasional white transverse flecks (striate leuconychia) are seen frequently in normal nails and are due to airspaces within the plate and not to insufficient calcium.

Congenital disease

Pachyonychia congenita is a rare autosomal dominant condition. Most cases arise due to mutations in a particular group of keratin genes. The nails are grossly thickened, especially at the free edge, and discoloured from birth.

Trauma

- *Splinter haemorrhages* are fine linear dark brown flecks running longitudinally in the plate (see Fig. 18.93, p. 626). They are most commonly due to trauma, particularly when distal, but may be seen in nail psoriasis, and less commonly in infective endocarditis (p. 624).
- *Subungual haematomas* may appear as a crimson, purple or grey-brown discoloration of the nail plate, most frequently that of the big toe (Fig. 27.53). Sometimes but not always, there is a history of trauma. They appear suddenly and the nail folds remain uninvolved. As the nail grows out, a normally coloured band develops proximally. They may be confused with subungual melanoma and biopsy may be necessary.
- *Habit-tic dystrophy* is common, and is due to habitual picking of the proximal nail fold of the thumb. This produces a ladder pattern of transverse ridges and furrows up the centre of the nail.
- *Chronic trauma* from ill-fitting shoes and from sport may cause malalignment and thickening of the nails known as onychogryphosis, and lead to ingrowing toenails.

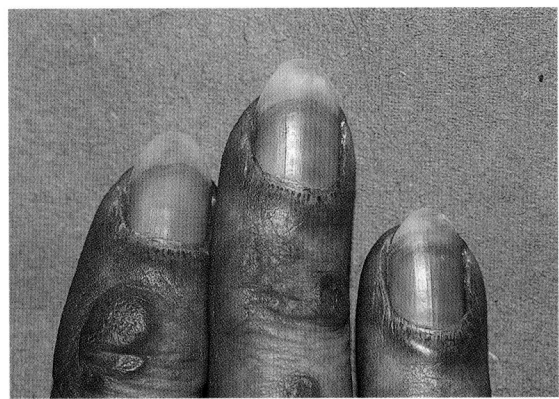

Fig. 27.52 **Dermatomyositis.** The erythema, dilated and tortuous capillaries in the proximal nail fold and the Gottron's papules on the digits are important diagnostic features (p. 1111).

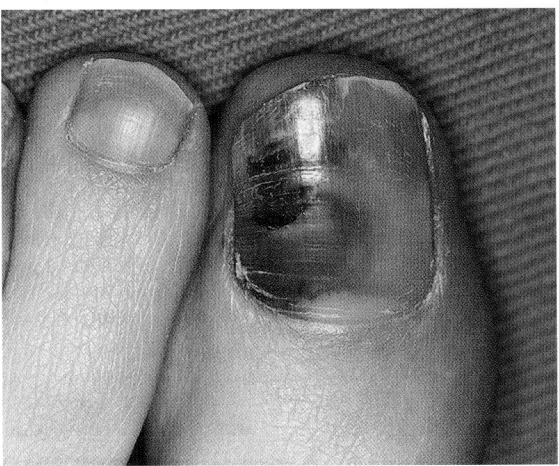

Fig. 27.53 Subungual haematoma.

The nail in systemic disease

- *Koilonychia* is a concave or spoon-shaped deformity of the plate which is a sign of iron deficiency (Fig. 27.54A). It is seen most often in countries where under-nutrition is prevalent.
- *Beau's lines* are transverse grooves which appear at the same time on all nails a few weeks after an acute illness, moving out to the free margins as the nails grow (Fig. 27.54B).
- *Digital clubbing* in its most gross form is seen as a bulbous swelling of the tip of the finger (Figs 27.54C and D) or toe. The normal angle between the proximal part of the nail and the skin is lost. Causes may be:

  respiratory—bronchogenic carcinoma, asbestosis (especially with mesothelioma), suppurative lung disease (empyema, bronchiectasis, cystic fibrosis), fibrosing alveolitis

  cardiac—cyanotic congenital heart disease, infective endocarditis

  other—inflammatory bowel disease, biliary cirrhosis, thyrotoxicosis, familial.
- *Whitening of the nails* is a rare sign of hypoalbuminaemia. 'Half and half' nails (white proximally and red-brown distally) are seen in some patients with renal failure. Rarely, drugs (e.g. antimalarials) may discolour nails.

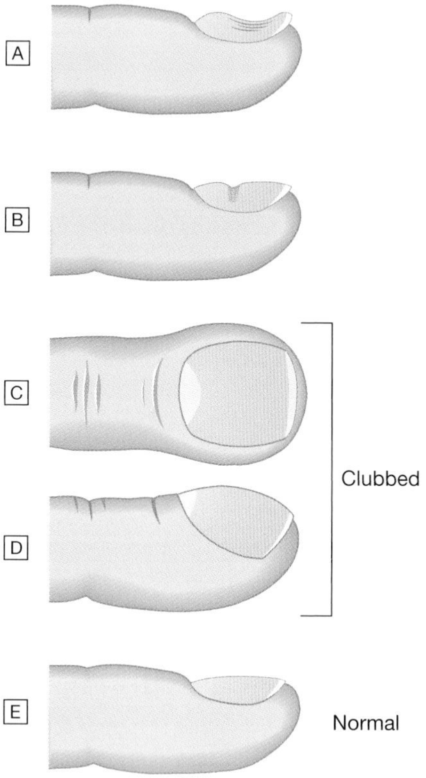

The nail in common skin diseases

- *Psoriasis* may cause coarse pitting of the nail plate, onycholysis (separation of the nail plate from the nail bed) and subungual hyperkeratosis (see Fig. 27.17, p. 1262).
- *Eczema* may feature shiny nails, which signify frequent rubbing of eczematous skin elsewhere. When eczema involves the distal phalanges, the nail may be deformed, with transverse ridging and thickening of the plate.
- *Lichen planus and severe alopecia areata* may cause trachyonychia, a fine roughness and white discoloration of the nail plate.
- *Dermatophyte infection* causes yellow-brown discoloration and crumbling of the plate which usually starts distally and spreads proximally (Fig. 27.55). Usually only a few nails (more commonly toenails than fingernails) are affected and frequently only on one foot or hand. Diagnosis relies on clippings being examined for hyphae and culture, and systemic rather than topical antifungal treatment (e.g. terbinafine) is required.

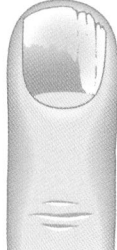

Fig. 27.55 Dermatophyte infection. This causes discoloration and crumbliness of the nail plate.

Further information

Journal articles

McMillan JR, Akiyama M, Shimizu H. Epidermal basement membrane zone components: ultrastructural distribution and molecular interactions. Journal of Dermatological Science 2003; 31:169–177.

Websites

www.bad.org.uk *Guidelines for many skin diseases.*
www.eczema.org *National Eczema Society in the UK.*
www.nice.org.uk *Guidelines for skin tumours, melanoma and atopic eczema.*
www.sign.ac.uk *No. 72: cutaneous melanoma (Feb. 2004). No. 26: care of the patient with chronic leg ulcer (July 2005).*

27

A

B

C

Clubbed

D

E

Normal

Fig. 27.54 The nail in systemic disease. A Koilonychia. B Beau's lines. C and D Digital clubbing. E Normal nail.

S.W. Walker

Laboratory reference ranges

28

NOTES ON THE INTERNATIONAL SYSTEM OF UNITS (SI UNITS)

Système International (SI) units are a specific subset of the metre–kilogram–second system of units and were agreed upon as the everyday currency for commercial and scientific work in 1960, following a series of international conferences organised by the International Bureau of Weights and Measures. SI units have been adopted widely in clinical laboratories but non-SI units are still used in many countries. For that reason, values in both units are given for common measurements throughout this textbook and commonly used non-SI units are shown in this chapter. However, the SI unit system is recommended.

Examples of basic SI units

Length	metre (m)
Mass	kilogram (kg)
Amount of substance	mole (mol)
Energy	joule (J)
Pressure	pascal (Pa)
Volume	The basic SI unit of volume is the cubic metre (1000 litres). For convenience, however, the litre (L) is used as the unit of volume in laboratory work.

Examples of decimal multiples and submultiples of SI units

Factor	Name	Prefix
10^6	mega-	M
10^3	kilo-	k
10^{-1}	deci-	d
10^{-2}	centi-	c
10^{-3}	milli-	m
10^{-6}	micro-	µ
10^{-9}	nano-	n
10^{-12}	pico-	p
10^{-15}	femto-	f

Exceptions to the use of SI units

By convention, blood pressure is excluded from the SI unit system and is measured in mmHg (millimetres of mercury) rather than pascals.

Mass concentrations (e.g. g/L, µg/L) are used in preference to molar concentrations for all protein measurements and for substances which do not have a sufficiently well-defined composition.

Some enzymes and hormones are measured by 'bioassay', in which the activity in the sample is compared with the activity (rather than the mass) of a standard sample that is provided from a central source. For these assays, results are given in standardised 'units', or 'international units', which depend upon the activity in the standard sample and may not be readily converted to mass units.

LABORATORY VALUES

Reference ranges are largely those used in the Departments of Clinical Biochemistry and Haematology, Lothian Health University Hospitals Division, Edinburgh, UK. Values are shown in both SI units and, where appropriate, non-SI units. Many reference ranges vary between laboratories, depending on the assay method used and on other factors; this is especially the case for enzyme assays. The origin of reference ranges and the interpretation of 'abnormal' results are discussed in Chapter 1. No details are given here of the collection requirements which may be critical to obtaining a meaningful result. Unless otherwise stated, reference ranges shown apply to adults; values in children may be different.

Many analytes can be measured in either serum (the supernatant of clotted blood) or plasma (the supernatant of anticoagulated blood). A specific requirement for one or the other may depend on a kit manufacturer's recommendations. In other instances, the distinction is critical (e.g. plasma is required for measurement of fibrinogen since it is largely absent from serum; serum is required for electrophoresis to detect paraproteins because fibrinogen migrates as a discrete band in the zone of interest).

28.1 Urea and electrolytes in venous blood

Analysis	Reference range	
	SI units	Non-SI units
Sodium	135–145 mmol/L	135–145 meq/L
Potassium (plasma)	3.3–4.7 mmol/L	3.3–4.7 meq/L
Potassium (serum)	3.6–5.1 mmol/L	3.6–5.1 meq/L
Chloride	95–107 mmol/L	95–107 meq/L
Urea	2.5–6.6 mmol/L	15–40 mg/dL
Creatinine	60–120 µmol/L	0.68–1.36 mg/dL

28.2 Arterial blood analysis

Analysis	Reference range	
	SI units	Non-SI units
Bicarbonate	21–29 mmol/L	21–29 meq/L
Hydrogen ion	37–45 nmol/L	pH 7.35–7.43
PaCO_2	4.5–6.0 kPa	34–45 mmHg
PaO_2	12–15 kPa	90–113 mmHg
Oxygen saturation	> 97%	

28.3 Hormones in venous blood

Hormone	Reference range	
	SI units	Non-SI units
Adrenocorticotrophic hormone (ACTH) (plasma)	1.5–11.2 pmol/L (0700–1000 hrs)	7–51 pg/mL
Aldosterone		
Supine	30–440 pmol/L	1.09–15.9 ng/dL
Erect	110–860 pmol/L	3.97–31.0 ng/dL
Cortisol	Dynamic tests are required—see Ch. 20	
Follicle-stimulating hormone (FSH)		
Male	1.0–10.0 U/L	0.2–2.2 ng/mL
Female	3.0–9.0 U/L (early follicular, luteal)	0.7–2.0 ng/mL
	< 30 U/L (mid-cycle)	< 6.7 ng/mL
	> 30 U/L (post-menopausal)	> 6.7 ng/mL
Gastrin (plasma, fasting)	< 57 pmol/L	< 120 pg/mL
Growth hormone (GH)	< 0.5 µg/L excludes acromegaly (if IGF1 in reference range) > 6 µg/L excludes GH deficiency Dynamic tests are usually required—see Ch. 20	–
Insulin	Highly variable and interpretable only in relation to plasma glucose and body habitus	–
Luteinising hormone (LH)		
Male	1.0–9.0 U/L	0.11–1.0 µg/L
Female	2.5–9.0 U/L (early follicular, luteal)	0.3–1.0 µg/L
	Up to 90 U/L (mid-cycle)	Up to 10 µg/L
	> 20 U/L (post-menopausal)	> 2.2 µg/L
17β-Oestradiol		
Male	< 160 pmol/L	< 43 pg/mL
Female	110–180 pmol/L (early follicular)	30–49 pg/mL
	550–2095 pmol/L (mid-cycle)	150–570 pg/mL
	370–770 pmol/L (luteal)	101–209 pg/mL
	< 150 pmol/L (post-menopausal)	< 41 pg/mL
Parathyroid hormone (PTH)	1.0–6.5 pmol/L	10–65 pg/mL
Progesterone		
Male	< 2.0 nmol/L	< 0.63 ng/mL
Female	< 2.0 nmol/L (follicular)	< 0.63 ng/mL
	> 15 nmol/L (mid-luteal)	> 4.7 ng/mL
	< 2.0 nmol/L (post-menopausal)	< 0.63 ng/mL
Prolactin (PRL)	60–500 mU/L	–
Renin activity		
Erect	1.0–4.2 ng/mL/hr	–
Supine	0.5–2.6 ng/mL/hr	–
Testosterone		
Male	10–30 nmol/L	2.88–8.64 ng/mL
Female	0.4–3.0 nmol/L	0.12–0.87 ng/mL
Thyroid-stimulating hormone (TSH)	0.2–4.5 mU/L	–
Thyroxine (free) (free T$_4$)	9–21 pmol/L	700–1632 pg/dL
Triiodothyronine (T$_3$)	0.9–2.4 nmol/L	59–156 ng/dL

Notes

1. A number of hormones are unstable and collection details are critical to obtaining a meaningful result. Refer to local laboratory handbook.
2. Values in the table are only a guideline; hormone levels can often only be meaningfully understood in relation to factors such as sex (e.g. testosterone), age (e.g. FSH in women), time of day (e.g. cortisol) or regulatory factors (e.g. insulin and glucose, PTH and [Ca^{2+}]).
3. Reference ranges may be critically method-dependent.

28

28 **28.4 Other common analytes in venous blood in adults**

Analyte	Reference range SI units	Non-SI units	Analyte	Reference range SI units	Non-SI units
α_1-antitrypsin	1.1–2.1 g/L	110–210 mg/dL	Ethanol	Not normally detectable	
Alanine aminotransferase (ALT)	10–50 U/L	–		Marked intoxication 65–87 mmol/L	300–400 mg/dL
Albumin	35–50 g/L	3.5–5.0 g/dL		Stupor 87–109 mmol/L	400–500 mg/dL
Alkaline phosphatase	40–125 U/L	–		Coma > 109 mmol/L	> 500 mg/dL
Amylase	< 100 U/L	–	Gamma-glutamyl transferase (GGT)	Male 10–55 U/L Female 5–35 U/L	–
Aspartate aminotransferase (AST)	10–45 U/L	–	Glucose (fasting)	3.6–5.8 mmol/L	65–104 mg/dL
Bilirubin (total)	3–16 µmol/L	0.18–0.94 mg/dL		See p. 806 for definitions of impaired glucose tolerance and diabetes mellitus, and p. 781 for definition of hypoglycaemia	
Calcium (total)	2.1–2.6 mmol/L	4.2–5.2 meq/L or 8.50–10.50 mg/dL	Glycated haemoglobin (HbA$_{1c}$)	4.0–6.0% 20–42 mmol/mol Hb	–
Carboxy-haemoglobin	0.1–3.0%	–	Immunoglobulins (Ig)		
Caeruloplasmin	0.2–0.6 g/L	20–60 mg/dL	IgA	0.8–4.5 g/L	–
Cholesterol (total)	Ideal level varies according to cardiovascular risk (see cardiovascular risk chart, p. 580) so reference ranges can be misleading. The following values were described by the European Atherosclerosis Society:		IgE	0–250 kU/L	–
			IgG	6.0–15.0 g/L	–
			IgM	0.35–2.90 g/L	–
			Lactate	0.6–2.4 mmol/L	5.40–21.6 mg/dL
	Mild increase 5.2–6.5 mmol/L	200–250 mg/dL	Lactate dehydrogenase (total)	208–460 U/L	–
	Moderate increase 6.5–7.8 mmol/L	250–300 mg/dL	Lead	< 1.0 µmol/L	< 21 µg/dL
	Severe increase > 7.8 mmol/L	> 300 mg/dL	Magnesium	0.75–1.0 mmol/L	1.5–2.0 meq/L or 1.82–2.43 mg/dL
HDL-cholesterol	Ideal level varies according to cardiovascular risk so reference ranges can be misleading. According to the National Cholesterol Education Programme Adult Treatment Panel III (ATPIII), a low HDL-cholesterol is:		Osmolality	280–296 mmol/kg	–
			Osmolarity	280–296 mosm/L	–
			Phosphate (fasting)	0.8–1.4 mmol/L	2.48–4.34 mg/dL
	< 1.0 mmol/L	< 40 mg/dL	Protein (total)	60–80 g/L	6–8 g/L
Complement			Triglycerides (fasting)	0.6–1.7 mmol/L	53–150 mg/dL
C3	0.73–1.4 g/L	–	Troponins	Values consistent with 'myocyte necrosis' or myocardial infarction are crucially dependent upon which troponin is measured (I or T) and on the method employed	
C4	0.12–0.3 g/L	–			
Total haemolytic complement	0.086–0.410 g/L	–			
Copper	13–24 µmol/L	83–153 µg/dL	Tryptase	0–135 mg/L	–
C-reactive protein	< 5 mg/L Highly sensitive CRP assays also exist which measure lower values and may be useful in estimating cardiovascular risk		Urate		
			Male	0.12–0.42 mmol/L	2.0–7.0 mg/dL
			Female	0.12–0.36 mmol/L	2.0–6.0 mg/dL
Creatine kinase (total)			Vitamin D		
Male	55–170 U/L	–	25(OH)D	25–170 nmol/L	10–68 ng/mL
Female	30–135 U/L	–	1,25(OH)$_2$D	20–120 pmol/L	7.7–46 pg/mL
Creatine kinase MB isoenzyme	< 6% of total CK	–	Zinc	11–22 µmol/L	72–144 µg/dL

28.5 Common analytes in urine

Analyte	Reference range	
	SI units	Non-SI units
Albumin	Definitions of microalbuminuria are given on page 481 Proteinuria is defined below	
Calcium (normal diet)	Up to 7.5 mmol/24 hrs	Up to 15 meq/24 hrs or 3–300 mg/24 hrs
Copper	< 0.6 µmol/24 hrs	< 38 µg/24 hrs
Cortisol Overnight (early morning sample) 24-hr collection	< 20 nmol cortisol/mmol creatinine 25–250 nmol/24 hrs	< 67 µg cortisol/g creatinine 9.1–91 µg/24 hrs
Creatinine	10–20 mmol/24 hrs	1130–2260 mg/24 hrs
5-hydroxyindole-3-acetic acid (5-HIAA)	10–42 µmol/24 hrs	1.9–8.1 mg/24 hrs
Metadrenalines Normetadrenaline Metadrenaline	0.4–3.4 µmol/24 hrs 0.3–1.7 µmol/24 hrs	73–620 µg/24 hrs 59–335 µg/24 hrs
Oxalate	0.04–0.49 mmol/24 hrs	3.6–44 mg/24 hrs
Phosphate	15–50 mmol/24 hrs	465–1548 mg/24 hrs
Potassium*	25–100 mmol/24 hrs	25–100 meq/24 hrs
Protein	< 0.3 g/L	< 0.03 g/dL
Sodium*	100–200 mmol/24 hrs	100–200 meq/24 hrs
Urate	1.2–3.0 mmol/24 hrs	202–504 mg/24 hrs
Urea	170–600 mmol/24 hrs	10.2–36.0 g/24 hrs

*The urinary output of electrolytes such as sodium and potassium is normally a reflection of dietary intake. This can vary widely. The values quoted are appropriate to a 'Western' diet.

28.6 Cerebrospinal fluid analysis

Analysis	Reference range	
	SI units	Non–SI units
Cells	< 5 × 10⁶ cells/L (all mononuclear)	< 5 cells/mm³
Glucose[1]	2.3–4.5 mmol/L	41–81 mg/dL
IgG index[2]	< 0.65	–
Total protein	140–450 mg/L	0.014–0.045 g/dL

[1]Interpret in relation to plasma glucose. Values in CSF typically approximately two-thirds plasma levels.
[2]A crude index of increase in IgG attributable to intrathecal synthesis.

28

28.7 Haematological values

Analysis	Reference range	
	SI units	**Non-SI units**
Bleeding time (Ivy)	< 8 mins	–
Blood volume		
Male	75 ± 10 mL/kg	–
Female	70 ± 10 mL/kg	–
Coagulation screen		
Prothrombin time	10.5–13.5 secs	–
Activated partial thromboplastin time	26–36 secs	–
D-dimers		
To detect disseminated intravascular coagulation	< 200 µg/L	< 200 ng/mL
To detect venous thromboembolism	< 500 µg/L	< 500 ng/mL
Erythrocyte sedimentation rate	Higher values in older patients are not necessarily abnormal	
Adult male	0–10 mm/hr	–
Adult female	3–15 mm/hr	–
Ferritin		
Male	20–300 µg/L	20–300 ng/mL
Female	14–150 µg/L	14–150 ng/mL
Fibrinogen	1.5–4.0 g/L	0.15–0.4 g/dL
Folate		
Serum	5.0–20 µg/L	5.0–20 ng/mL
Red cell	257–800 µg/L	257–800 ng/mL
Haemoglobin		
Male	130–180 g/L	13–18 g/dL
Female	115–165 g/L	11.5–16.5 g/dL
Haptoglobin	0.4–2.4 g/L	0.04–0.24 g/dL
Iron	10–32 µmol/L	56–178 µg/dL
Leucocytes (adults)	$4.0–11.0 \times 10^9$/L	$4.0–11.0 \times 10^3$/mm^3
Differential white cell count		
Neutrophil granulocytes	$2.0–7.5 \times 10^9$/L	$2.0–7.5 \times 10^3$/mm^3
Lymphocytes	$1.5–4.0 \times 10^9$/L	$1.5–4.0 \times 10^3$/mm^3
Monocytes	$0.2–0.8 \times 10^9$/L	$0.2–0.8 \times 10^3$/mm^3
Eosinophil granulocytes	$0.04–0.4 \times 10^9$/L	$0.04–0.4 \times 10^3$/mm^3
Basophil granulocytes	$0.01–0.1 \times 10^9$/L	$0.01–0.1 \times 10^3$/mm^3
Mean cell haemoglobin (MCH)	27–32 pg	–
Mean cell volume (MCV)	78–98 fl	–
Packed cell volume (PCV) or haematocrit		
Male	0.40–0.54	–
Female	0.37–0.47	–
Platelets	$150–350 \times 10^9$/L	$150–350 \times 10^3$/mm^3
Red cell count		
Male	$4.5–6.5 \times 10^{12}$/L	$4.5–6.5 \times 10^6$/mm^3
Female	$3.8–5.8 \times 10^{12}$/L	$3.8–5.8 \times 10^6$/mm^3
Red cell lifespan		
Mean	120 days	–
Half-life (^{51}Cr)	25–35 days	–
Reticulocytes (adults)	$25–85 \times 10^9$/L	$25–85 \times 10^3$/mm^3
Transferrin	2.0–4.0 g/L	0.2–0.4 g/dL
Transferrin saturation		
Male	25–56%	–
Female	14–51%	–
Vitamin B$_{12}$	251–900 ng/L	–

Picture credits

We are grateful to the following individuals and organisations for the loan of illustrations:

Page ii: Portrait of Sir Stanley Davidson, Royal College of Physicians of Edinburgh.

Chapter 5: Fig. 5.17A Institute of Ophthalmology.

Chapter 6: Fig. 6.9 Disc kindly supplied by Charlotte Symes.

Chapter 11: Fig. 11.4 Dr J Wilsdon, Freeman Hospital, Newcastle upon Tyne.

Chapter 13: Page 290 inset (splinter haemorrhages) Dr Nick Beeching, Royal Liverpool University Hospital. Page 290 inset (Roth's spots) Prof Ian Rennie, Royal Hallamshire Hospital, Sheffield. Page 291 insets (streptococcal toxic shock syndrome, meningococcal sepsis, shingles), Fig. 13.1 inset (cellulitis of the leg), Figs 13.6ABD, 13.19, 13.42B, 13.43B, 13.49 Dr Ravi Gowda, Royal Hallamshire Hospital, Sheffield. Fig. 13.1 inset (pulmonary tuberculosis) Dr Ann Chapman, Royal Hallamshire Hospital, Sheffield. Fig. 13.1 insets (empyema, pyogenic liver abscess, diverticular abscess, tuberculous osteomyelitis) Dr Robert Peck, Royal Hallamshire Hospital, Sheffield. Fig. 13.3C Dr Julia Greig, Royal Hallamshire Hospital, Sheffield. Fig. 13.6C Dr Rattanaphone Phetsouvanh, Mahosot Hospital, Vientiane, PDR Laos. Fig. 13.14 Prof Goura Kudesia, Northern General Hospital, Sheffield. Fig. 13.27 Institute of Ophthalmology, Moorfields Eye Hospital, London. Fig. 13.31 inset (malaria retinopathy) Dr Nicholas Beare, Royal Liverpool University Hospital. Fig. 13.31 insets (blood films of *P. vivax* and *P. falciparum*) Dr Kamolrat Silamut, Mahidol Oxford Research Unit, Bangkok, Thailand. Fig. 13.39 Dr S Sundar and Dr HW Murray. Fig. 13.40B Dr EE Zijlstra. Fig. 13.51 Dr Wendi Bailey, Liverpool School of Tropical Medicine, Liverpool. Fig. 13.55 insets (dimorphic fungi) Beatriz Gomez and Angela Restrepo, CIB, Medellín, Colombia.

Chapter 14: Page 384 inset (oral hairy leucoplakia) Audiovisual Dept, St Mary's Hospital, London.

Chapter 15: Figs 15.1, 15.5 Dr P Hay, St George's Hospital, London.

Chapter 17: Page 461AB Dr GM Iadorola and Dr F Quarello, G Bosco Hospital, Turin (from www.sin-italia.org/imago/sediment/sed.htm). Figs 17.1CE, 17.29ACDE Dr JG Simpson, Aberdeen Royal Infirmary. Figs 17.4AB, 17.5AB, 17.6, 17.33, 17.35, 17.38AB Dr AP Bayliss and Dr P Thorpe, Aberdeen Royal Infirmary. Fig. 17.10 Dr P Robinson, St James's University Hospital, Leeds. Fig. 17.29F–H Dr R Herriot. Fig. 17.30BC Dr J Collar, St Mary's Hospital, London.

Chapter 18: Fig. 18.82E Dr T Lawton. Fig. 18.83AB Dr B Cullen.

Chapter 19: Page 642 inset (idiopathic kyphoscoliosis) Dr I Smith, Papworth Hospital, Cambridge. Page 642 insets (serous, mucopurulent and purulent sputum) Dr J Foweraker, Papworth Hospital, Cambridge. Fig. 19.24B British Lung Foundation. Fig. 19.34 Dr William Wallace, Dept of Pathology, Royal Infirmary of Edinburgh. Fig. 19.38 Adam Hill. Fig. 19.61 Prof NJ Douglas.

Chapter 20: Figs 20.4 inset (toxic multinodular goitre), 20.23B Dr PL Padfield, Western General Hospital, Edinburgh.

Chapter 21: Page 796 inset (exudative maculopathy), page 797 (background and proliferative retinopathy) Dr AW Patrick and Dr IW Campbell. Fig. 21.4 insets (normal islet, beta-cell

destruction) Dr A Foulis, Dept of Pathology, University of Glasgow.

Chapter 22: Fig. 22.14AB Sarah Douglas.

Chapter 23: Figs 23.10, 23.42, 23.45, 23.48 Dr D Redhead, Royal Infirmary of Edinburgh.

Chapter 26: Page 1132 insets (winging of scapula, 12th nerve palsy, wasting of thenar eminence) Dr RE Cull, Western General Hospital, Edinburgh. Figs 26.13A–C, 26.14A–C, 26.15A–D Dr D Collie. Fig. 26.23C Dr B Cullen. Figs 26.31A–C, 26.32A–F, 26.33A–C Dr A Farrell and Prof J Wardlaw. Fig. 26.37 Prof DAS Compston. Figs 26.39, 26.40AB, 26.41 Dr J Xuereb.

The following figures, boxes and tables are reproduced with publishers' permission as listed:

Chapter 1: Fig. 1.4 Edwards A, Elwyn G, Mulley A. Explaining risks: turning numerical data into meaningful pictures. BMJ 2002; 324:827–830, reproduced with permission from the BMJ Publishing Group.

Chapter 2: Fig. 2.2 Brater DC, Chennavasin P, Day B, et al. Bumetanide and furosemide. Clin Pharmacol Ther 1983; 34:207–213; reproduced with permission of Mosby Inc., St Louis, Missouri; and Chennavasin P, Seiwell R, Brater DC. Pharmacokinetic-dynamic analysis of the indomethacin–furosemide interaction in man. J Pharmacol and Exp Ther 1980; 215:77–81. With permission of the American Association for Pharmacology and Experimental Therapeutics.

Chapter 4: Fig. 4.11 Helbert M. Flesh and bones of immunology. Edinburgh: Churchill Livingstone; 2006; copyright Elsevier.

Chapter 5: Fig. 5.1 Adapted by Rao M, Prasad S, Adshead F, et al. The built environment and health. Lancet 2007; 370:1112, from an original model by Whitehead M, Dahlgren G. What can be done about inequalities in health? Lancet 1991; 338:1059–1063. Fig. 5.17B WHO. Report of a joint WHO/USAID meeting, vitamin A deficiency and xerophthalmia (WHO technical report series no. 5 W); 1976. Fig. 5.18 Karthikeyan K, Thappa DM. Pellagra and skin. Int J Dermatol 2002; 41:476–481. Fig. 5.19AB Ho V, Prinsloo P, Ombiga J. Persistent anaemia due to scurvy. Journal of the New Zealand Medical Association 2007; 120(1262):62. Reproduced with permission. Box 5.3 Based on Coleman T. Smoking cessation: integrating recent advances with clinical practice. Thorax 2001; 56:579–582, with permission from the BMJ Publishing Group.

Chapter 6: Fig. 6.10 Adapted from Samaranayake L. Essential microbiology for dentistry. 3rd edn. Edinburgh: Churchill Livingstone; 2006 (Fig. 1.1); copyright Elsevier. Fig. 6.11 Based on the 'How to Handwash' URL: http://www.who.int/gpsc/5may/How_To_Handwash_Poster.pdf © World Health Organization 2009. All rights reserved.

Chapter 7: Page 164 insets (wasted hand, kyphosis) Afzal Mir M. Atlas of clinical diagnosis. 2nd edn. Edinburgh: Saunders; 2003; copyright Elsevier. Page 164 inset (senile purpura) Forbes CD, Jackson WF. Clinical medicine. 3rd edn. Edinburgh: Mosby; 2004 (p. 438, Fig. 10.101); copyright Elsevier.

Chapter 9: Page 204 inset (self-cutting) Douglas G, Nicol F, Robertson C. Macleod's clinical examination. 11th edn. Edinburgh: Churchill Livingstone; 2005 (p. 48, Fig. 2.16); copyright Elsevier. Page 204 inset (chemical burn) www.firewiki.

PICTURE CREDITS

1300

net. Page 204 inset (needle tracks) www.deep6inc.com. Page 204 inset (pinpoint pupil) http://drugrecognition.com/images. Page 204 inset (injected conjunctiva) http://knol.google.com.

Chapter 11: Fig. 11.1 Statistics from Cancer Research UK website (http://info.cancerresearchuk.org).

Chapter 12: Fig. 12.2 Adapted from McQuay H. Acute pain. In: Trames M, ed. Evidence-based resource in anaesthesia and analgesia. London: BMJ Books; 2000; reproduced with permission from the BMJ Publishing Group. Fig. 12.3 WHO. Cancer pain relief. 2nd edn. Geneva: WHO; 1996. Fig. 12.5 Reproduced from Murray SA, Kendall M, Boyd K, et al. Illness trajectories and palliative care. BMJ 2005; 330:7498; reproduced with permission from the BMJ Publishing Group.

Chapter 13: Fig. 13.12 Reproduced from Halstead SB. Dengue. Medicine 1997; 25:1 and Monath TP. Yellow fever. Medicine 1997; 25:1. By kind permission of the Medicine Publishing Company and Dr TP Monath. Fig. 13.21 Reproduced by permission of WHO. Fig. 13.25 Based on Bryceson ADM, Pfaltzgraff RE. Leprosy. 3rd edn. Edinburgh: Churchill Livingstone; 1990; copyright Elsevier. Fig. 13.33 Parry E, Godfrey R, Mabey D, Gill G. Principles of medicine in Africa. 3rd edn. Cambridge: Cambridge University Press; 2004. Fig. 13.37 Knight R. Parasitic disease in man. Edinburgh: Churchill Livingstone; 1982; copyright Elsevier. Fig. 13.40A Sundar S, Kumar K, Chakravarty J, et al. Cure of antimony-unresponsive Indian post-kala-azar dermal leishmaniasis with oral miltefosine. Trans R Soc Trop Med Hyg 2006; 100(7):698–700. Fig. 13.43A Knight R. Parasitic disease in man. Edinburgh: Churchill Livingstone; 1982; copyright Elsevier. Fig. 13.45 Gibbons LM. SEM guide to the morphology of nematode parasites of vertebrates. Farnham Royal, Slough: Commonwealth Agricultural Bureau International; 1986. Fig. 13.51 Cook GC, ed. Manson's tropical diseases. 20th edn. London: WB Saunders; 1995; copyright Elsevier. Box 13.57 WHO. Severe falciparum malaria. In: Severe and complicated malaria. 3rd edn. Trans Roy Soc Trop Med Hyg 2000; 94 (suppl. 1): S1–41.

Chapter 15: Page 410 inset (perianal warts), Figs 15.6, 15.7, 15.8 McMillan A, Scott GR. Sexually transmitted infections: a colour guide. Edinburgh: Churchill Livingstone; 2000; copyright Elsevier. Page 410 inset (coronal papillae), page 411 inset (inflammation), Figs 15.3, 15.4 McMillan A, Young H, Ogilvie MM, Scott GR. Clinical practice in sexually transmissible infections. Edinburgh: Saunders; 2002; copyright Elsevier.

Chapter 17: Fig. 17.24 Beutler JJ, Koomans HA. Malignant hypertension: still a challenge. Nephrol Dial Transplant 1977; 12:2019–2023; photograph courtesy of Prof PJ Slootweg, University Hospital, Utrecht. By permission of Oxford University Press. Fig. 17.28 Reprinted from Feehally J, Johnson R. Comprehensive clinical nephrology. London: Mosby; 2000; copyright Elsevier.

Chapter 18: Page 522 insets (splinter haemorrhage, jugular venous pulse, malar flush, tendon xanthomas), Fig. 18.12B, 18.91A–D, 18.92 inset (Doppler echo), 18.93 insets (petechial rash, nail-fold infarct) Newby D, Grubb N. Cardiology: an illustrated colour text. Edinburgh: Churchill Livingstone; 2005; copyright Elsevier. Figs 18.19, 18.69 Scottish Intercollegiate Guidelines Network (SIGN) 93; Feb 2007; pp. 42 (annex 1) and 47 (annex 4). Figs 18.34, 18.35 Resuscitation Council (UK) guidelines. Fig. 18.60 Stary HC, et al. Circulation 1995; 92:1355–1374. © 1995 American Heart Association. Fig. 18.61 Joint British Societies Cardiovascular Risk Prediction Chart, reproduced with permission from the University of Manchester. Figs 18.84, 18.85 National Institute for Clinical Excellence (NICE). CG34 Hypertension: Management of Hypertension in Adults in Primary Care. London: NICE; 2006. Available from www.nice.org.uk/CG34. Reproduced with permission. Fig. 18.86 inset (erythema marginatum) Savin JA, Hunter JAA, Hepburn NC. Skin signs in clinical medicine. London: Mosby–Wolfe; 1997;

copyright Elsevier. Fig. 18.94 Adapted from Drews U. Colour atlas of embryology. Stuttgart: Georg Thieme; 1995 (Fig. 6.9, p. 299). Box 18.63 Thygesen K, et al. Eur Heart J 2007; 28:2525–2538. Box 18.115 Moreillon P, et al. Lancet 2004; 363:139–149.

Chapter 19: Page 643 inset (right upper lobe collapse) http://3.bp.blogspot.com. Page 643 inset (right pneumothorax) http://chestatlas.com. Page 643 inset (large right pleural effusion) www.ispub.com. Fig. 19.2 www.Netter.com Illustrations 155 (bronchus, acinus) and 191 (circulation), Elsevier. Fig. 19.4 Innes JA. Davidson's Essentials of Medicine. Edinburgh: Churchill Livingstone; 2009 (Fig. 19.4, p. 791); copyright Elsevier. Fig. 19.5A–C http://radiology.rsnajnls.org. Fig. 19.7 Adapted from Flenley D. Lancet 1971; 1:1921. Fig. 19.12 WHO Global surveillance, prevention and control of chronic respiratory diseases: a comprehensive approach. Fig. 19.19 Global Initiative for Asthma, http://www.ginasthma.com. Fig. 19.26 Global Initiative for Chronic Obstructive Lung Disease, www.goldcopd.com. Fig. 19.33 Maartens G, Wilkinson RJ. Tuberculosis. Lancet 2007; 370: 2030–2043. Fig. 19.48 Johnson N McL. Respiratory medicine. Oxford: Blackwell Science; 1986. Fig. 19.54 inset (erythema nodosum) Savin JA, Hunter JAA, Hepburn NC. Skin signs in clinical medicine. London: Mosby–Wolfe; 1997; copyright Elsevier. Box 19.5 Based on Crompton GK. The respiratory system. In: Munro JF, Campbell IW. Macleod's clinical examination. 10th edn. Edinburgh: Churchill Livingstone; 2000 (p. 119); copyright Elsevier. Box. 19.13 Adapted from Radiology 2005; 237:395–400. Box 19.55 Adapted from Grange JM. In: Davies PDO, ed. Clinical tuberculosis. London: Hodder Arnold; 1998.

Chapter 21: Fig. 21.1 Wild S, Gojka R, Green A, et al. Global prevalence of diabetes. Diabetes Care 2004; 27:1047–1053; copyright © American Diabetes Association; reprinted with permission from the American Diabetes Association. Fig. 21.6B Adapted from Holman RR. Diabetes Res Clin Pract 1998; 40 (Suppl.):S21–S25. Fig. 21.8 Adapted from UK Prospective Diabetes Study Group. UKPDS 33. Lancet 1998; 352:837–853. Fig. 21.11 Nutrition Subcommittee of British Diabetic Association. Dietary recommendations for people with diabetes: an update for the 1990s. Diabet Med 1992; 9:196 (Fig. 1). Copyright John Wiley & Sons Ltd, reproduced with permission. Fig. 21.15 De Fronzo RA, Ferrannini E, Keen H, Zimmet P, eds. International textbook of diabetes mellitus. 3rd edn. Chichester: John Wiley; 2004.

Chapter 22: Fig. 22.40AB Hayes P, Simpson K. Gastroenterology and liver disease. Edinburgh: Churchill Livingstone; 1995; copyright Elsevier.

Chapter 23: Page 920 inset (spider naevi) Hayes P, Simpson K. Gastroenterology and liver disease. Edinburgh: Churchill Livingstone; 1995; copyright Elsevier. Page 920 inset (aspiration of ascitic fluid) Strachan M. Davidson's clinical cases. Edinburgh: Churchill Livingstone; 2008 (Fig. 65.1). Fig. 23.41 Shearman DC, Finlayson NDC. Diseases of the gastrointestinal tract and liver. 2nd edn. Edinburgh: Churchill Livingstone; 1989; copyright Elsevier. Box 23.30 Based on: Hayes P. Cirrhosis. In: Shearman DC, Finlayson NDC, Camilleri M, Carter D. Diseases of the gastrointestinal tract and liver. 3rd edn. Edinburgh: Churchill Livingstone; 1997 (originally from Powell LW, Mortimer R, Harris OD. Cirrhosis of the liver: a comparative study of the four major aetiological groups. Med J Aust 1971; 1:941–950).

Chapter 24: Fig. 24.24 Hoffbrand AV, Pettit JE. Essential haematology. 3rd edn. Edinburgh: Blackwell Science; 1992. Box 24.19 Wells PS. New Engl J Med 2003; 349:1227; copyright © 2003 Massachusetts Medical Society.

Chapter 27: Fig. 27.7 Munro JF, Edwards CRW, eds. Macleod's clinical examination. 9th edn. Edinburgh: Churchill Livingstone; 1995. Figs 27.10, 27.12, 27.16A, 27.31 White GM, Cox NH. Diseases of the skin. London: Mosby; 2000; copyright Elsevier. Fig. 27.26A Savin JA, Dahl M, Hunter JAA. Clinical dermatology. 3rd edn. Oxford: Blackwell; 2002.

Index

1340

1346